U0225248

Insall & Scott 膝关节外科学

上卷

第 6 版

人民卫生出版社

·北 京·

图书在版编目（CIP）数据

Insall & Scott 膝关节外科学 = Insall & Scott
Surgery of the Knee，6e：上、下卷：英文 /（美）
W. 诺尔曼·斯考特（W. Norman Scott）主编 . —北京：
人民卫生出版社，2021.10
　ISBN 978−7−117−32174−7

　Ⅰ.①I… 　Ⅱ.①W… 　Ⅲ.①膝关节 – 外科学 – 英文
Ⅳ.①R687.4

　中国版本图书馆 CIP 数据核字（2021）第 201311 号

人卫智网　www.ipmph.com	医学教育、学术、考试、健康，购书智慧智能综合服务平台	
人卫官网　www.pmph.com	人卫官方资讯发布平台	

图字：01-2021-5355 号

Insall & Scott 膝关节外科学
Insall & Scott Xiguanjie Waikexue
（上、下卷）

主　　编：W. Norman Scott
出版发行：人民卫生出版社（中继线 010-59780011）
地　　址：北京市朝阳区潘家园南里 19 号
邮　　编：100021
E - mail：pmph @ pmph.com
购书热线：010-59787592　010-59787584　010-65264830
印　　刷：廊坊一二〇六印刷厂
经　　销：新华书店
开　　本：889×1194　1/16　　总印张：147.5
总 字 数：7316 千字
版　　次：2021 年 10 月第 1 版
印　　次：2021 年 11 月第 1 次印刷
标准书号：ISBN 978-7-117-32174-7
定价（上、下卷）：1800.00 元

打击盗版举报电话：010-59787491　E-mail：WQ @ pmph.com
质量问题联系电话：010-59787234　E-mail：zhiliang @ pmph.com

Insall & Scott
SURGERY of the KNEE

VOLUME 1

Sixth Edition

EDITOR-IN-CHIEF

W. NORMAN SCOTT, MD, FACS

Clinical Professor of Orthopaedic Surgery
New York University Langone Medical Center
Hospital for Joint Diseases;
Joan C. Edwards School of Medicine
Marshall University
Founding Director
Insall Scott Kelly Institute for Orthopaedic Sports
    Medicine
New York, New York

ASSOCIATE EDITORS

DAVID R. DIDUCH, MS, MD

Alfred R. Shands Professor of Orthopaedic Surgery
Vice Chairman, Department of Orthopaedic Surgery
Head Orthopaedic Team Physician
University of Virginia
Charlottesville, Virginia

ARLEN D. HANSSEN, MD

Professor
Department of Orthopedic Surgery
Mayo Clinic
Rochester, Minnesota

RICHARD IORIO, MD

Dr. William and Susan Jaffe Professor of Orthopaedic Surgery
Chief Division of Adult Reconstructive Surgery
Department of Orthopaedic Surgery
New York University Langone Medical Center
Hospital for Joint Diseases
New York, New York

WILLIAM J. LONG, MD, FRCSC

Director,
Attending Orthopaedic Surgeon
Insall Scott Kelly Institute
St. Francis Hospital
Lenox Hill Hospital
New York, New York

ELSEVIER

Elsevier (Singapore) Pte Ltd.
3 Killiney Road,
#08-01 Winsland House I,
Singapore 239519
Tel: (65) 6349-0200; Fax: (65) 6733-1817

Notice
Practitioners and researchers must always rely on their own experience and knowledge in evaluating and using any information, methods, compounds or experiments described herein. Because of rapid advances in the medical sciences, in particular, independent verification of diagnoses and drug dosages should be made. To the fullest extent of the law, no responsibility is assumed by Elsevier, authors, editors or contributors in relation to the adaptation or for any injury and/or damage to persons or property as a matter of products liability, negligence or otherwise, or from any use or operation of any methods, products, instructions, or ideas contained in the material herein.

SECTION EDITORS

Arthur Atchabahian, MD
Professor of Clinical Anesthesiology
Department of Anesthesiology
New York University School of Medicine
New York, New York

Geoffrey S. Baer, MD, PhD
Department of Orthopedic Surgery and
    Rehabilitation
Division of Sports Medicine
University of Wisconsin—Madison
Madison, Wisconsin

Asheesh Bedi, MD
Chief, Sports Medicine and Surgery
Harold and Helen Gehring Professor
Department of Orthopaedic Surgery
University of Michigan
Ann Arbor, Michigan

Jenny T. Bencardino, MD
Attending Radiologist
Department of Radiology
New York University Hospital for Joint
    Diseases
New York, New York

Henry D. Clarke, MD
Consultant, Department of Orthopedics
Professor of Orthopedics
Mayo Clinic
Phoenix, Arizona

David R. Diduch, MD, MS
Alfred R. Shands Professor of Orthopaedic
    Surgery
Vice Chairman, Department of
    Orthopaedic Surgery
Head Orthopaedic Team Physician
University of Virginia
Charlottesville, Virginia

Andrew G. Franks, Jr., BA, MD
Clinical Professor
Internal Medicine (Rheumatology)
New York University School of Medicine
Director
Autoimmune Connective Tissue Disease
    Section
New York University School of Medicine
Attending Rheumatologist
Hospital for Joint Diseases
New York University School of Medicine
New York, New York

George J. Haidukewych, MD
Division of Orthopaedic Trauma and
    Complex Adult Reconstruction
Department of Orthopaedic Surgery
Orlando Regional Medical Center
Orlando, Florida

Arlen D. Hanssen, MD
Professor
Department of Orthopedic Surgery
Mayo Clinic
Rochester, Minnesota

Richard Iorio, MD
Dr. William and Susan Jaffe Professor of
    Orthopaedic Surgery
Chief Division of Adult Reconstructive
    Surgery
Department of Orthopaedic Surgery
New York University Langone Medical
    Center
New York, New York

Mininder S. Kocher, MD, MPH
Professor of Orthopaedic Surgery
Harvard Medical School
Associate Director
Division of Sports Medicine
Boston Children's Hospital
Boston, Massachusettes

**Richard D. Komistek, BSME, MSME,
PhD**
Fred M. Roddy Professor
Biomedical Engineering
Co-Center Director
Center for Musculoskeletal Research
University of Tennessee
Knoxville, Tennessee

William J. Long, BSc, MD, FRCSC
Director,
Attending Orthopaedic Surgeon
Insall Scott Kelly Institute,
St. Franics Hospital,
Lenox Hill Hospital,
Hospital for Joint Diseases
New York, New York

Milad Nazemzadeh, MD
Clinical Assistant
Professor of Anesthesiology
Department of Anesthesiology,
    Perioperative Care, and Pain Medicine
New York University Langone Medical
    Center
New York, New York

Mary I. O'Connor, MD
Director and Professor
Center for Musculoskeletal Care at Yale
    School of Medicine and Yale—New
    Haven Hospital
Yale School of Medicine
New Haven, Connecticut

Susan Craig Scott, MD, FACS
Clinical Assistant Professor
Department of Orthopaedic Surgery
Division of Hand Surgery
NYU Hospital for Joint Diseases
Assistant Attending
Department of Orthopedics
Department of Veterans Affairs
New York Harbor Healthcare System
New York, New York

W. Norman Scott, MD, FACS
Clinical Professor of Orthopaedic Surgery
NYU Hospital for Joint Disease Joan C.
    Edwards School of Medicine
Marshall University Founding Director
Insall Scott Kelly Institute for Orthopaedics
    and Sports Medicine
New York, New York

It's been stated that the "family" is the "smallest unit of society,"
yet it's the most complex. While the commitments can be intimidating the
rewards are awesome!

To my wife, Susan, the pillar of our family, your sacrifices have made us one!
My life has been so enriched because of you. You are where my heart resides!

To our children, Eric, Will, and Kelly, we never stop counting our blessings!
The three of you exude success because of your character, personality,
compassion, and work ethic. "To whom much has been given, much is
required." The three of you have overachieved!

To Nina, Danielle, and Erik, we love the expansion of our family. We have been
blessed by your inclusion in our family and look forward to an incredible
future.

To Ella and Layla, and your cousins to come, you bring joy to our hearts
and your successes in life will be abundant because of your parents!

Thank you ALL!

W. Norman Scott, MD

CONTRIBUTORS

Matthew P. Abdel, MD
Associate Professor of Orthopedic Surgery
and Senior Associate Consultant
Department of Orthopedic Surgery
Mayo Clinic
Rochester, Minnesota

Aryeh M. Abeles, MD
Associate Clinical Professor
Department of Rheumatology
University of Connecticut
Farmington, Connecticut

Ronald S. Adler, MD, PhD
Professor of Radiology
New York University School of Medicine;
Department of Radiology
Langone Medical Center
New York, New York

Paolo Adravanti, MD
Chief of Orthopedics
Department of Orthopedics
Clinic Città di Parma
Parma, Italy

Vinay K. Aggarwal, MD
Resident Physician
Hospital for Joint Diseases
NYU Langone Medical Center
New York, New York

Eduard Alentorn-Geli, MD, MSc, PhD, FEBOT
Duke Sports Science Institute
Department of Orthopedic Surgery
Duke University
Durham, North Carolina

Azhar A. Ali, MD
Center for Orthopaedic Biomechanics
University of Denver
Denver, Colorado

Sana Ali, MD
Resident in Diagnostic Radiology
Department of Diagnostic Imaging
Maimonides Medical Center
Brooklyn, New York

Hassan Alosh, MD

Aaron Althaus, MD
Fellow
Department of Orthopedic Surgery
Insall Scott Kelly
New York, New York

Annunziato Amendola, MD
Department of Orthopedic Surgery
Division of Sports Medicine
Duke University
Durham, North Carolina

Ned Amendola, MD

Priyadarshi Amit, MS Ortho, DNB Ortho, MRCSEd
Sicot Fellow
Department of Orthopedics and
Traumatology
Fondazione IRCCS Policlinico San Matteo
Università degli Studi di Pavia
Pavia, Italy;
Department of Orthopedics
Max Institute of Medical Sciences
New Delhi, India

Aldo Ampollini, MD
Orthopaedic Surgeon
Department of Orthopaedic Surgery
Clinic Città di Parma
Parma, Italy

Allen F. Anderson, MD
Orthopaedic Surgeon
Tennessee Orthopaedic Alliance/The
Lipscomb Clinic
Nashville, Tennessee

Christian N. Anderson, MD
Orthopaedic Surgeon
Tennessee Orthopaedic Alliance/The
Lipscomb Clinic
Nashville, Tennessee

Thomas P. Andriacchi, MD

Shawn G. Anthony, MD, MBA
Assistant Professor, Sports Medicine
Department of Orthopaedic Surgery
Icahn School of Medicine at Mount Sinai
Mount Sinai Health System
New York, New York

Jason D. Archibald, MD
New England Orthopedic Specialists
Peabody, Massachusetts

Elizabeth A. Arendt, MD
Professor and Vice Chair
Department of Orthopaedic Surgery
University of Minnesota
Minneapolis, Minnesota

Jean Noël Argenson, APHM
Institute for Locomotion
Department of Orthopaedic Surgery
Sainte-Marguerite Hospital;
Professor
Aix-Marseille University
Marseille, France

Yeseniya Aronova, MD
Resident Physician
Department of Anesthesiology,
Perioperative Care, and Pain Medicine
New York University Langone Medical
Center
New York, New York

Arthur Atchabahian, MD
Professor of Clinical Anesthesiology
Anesthesiology
New York University School of Medicine
New York, New York

Matthew S. Austin, MD
Professor
Department of Orthopaedic Surgery
Rothman Institute at Thomas Jefferson
University Hospital
Philadelphia, Pennsylvania

Christophe Aveline, MD
Department of Anesthesia and Surgical
Intensive Care
Private Hospital Sevigne
Cesson Sevigne, France

Bernard R. Bach, Jr., MD
Professor
Orthopaedic Surgery
Division of Sports Medicine
Rush University Medical Center
Chicago, Illinois

Geoffrey S. Baer, MD, PhD
Department of Orthopedic Surgery and
Rehabilitation
Division of Sports Medicine
University of Wisconsin—Madison
Madison, Wisconsin

Giovanni Balato, MD
Department of Public Health
School of Medicine
Federico II University
Naples, Italy

Andrea Baldini, MD, PhD
Institute Director
Department of Orthopaedics—Adult
    Reconstruction
IFCA Institute
Florence, Italy

Mark A. Baldwin, MD
Center for Orthopaedic Biomechanics
University of Denver
Denver, Colorado

Laura W. Bancroft, MD
Chief of MSK Radiology
Department of Radiology
Florida Hospital;
Adjunct Professor
University of Central Florida School of
    Medicine
Orlando, Florida;
Clinical Professor
Florida State University School of Medicine
Tallahassee, Florida

Sue D. Barber-Westin, BS
Director Clinical Studies
Noyes Knee Institute
Cincinnati, Ohio

William L. Bargar, BAAE, MMAE, MD
Medical Director
Joint Replacement Center
Sutter Medical Center Sacramento;
Assistant Clinical Professor
Department of Orthopaedic Surgery
UC Davis
Sacramento, California

Christopher P. Beauchamp, MD
Associate Professor
Department of Orthopaedics
Mayo Medical School
Mayo Clinic
Phoenix, Arizona

John P. Begly, MD
Resident Physician
Orthopaedics
New York University Hospital for Joint
    Diseases
New York, New York

Johan Bellemans, MD, PhD
Professor in Orthopaedics
Department of Orthopaedics and
    Traumatology
ZOL Hospitals
Genk, Belgium

Javier Beltran, MD, FACR
Chairman
Radiology
Maimonides Medical Center
Brooklyn, New York

Luis S. Beltran, MD
Assistant Professor of Radiology
Department of Radiology
New York University Langone Medical
    Center
New York, New York

Francesco Benazzo, MD
Professor of Orthopedics and Traumatology
Department of Orthopedics and
    Traumatology
Fondazione IRCCS
Policlinico San Matteo
Università degli Studi di Pavia
Pavia, Italy

Jenny T. Bencardino, MD
Attending Radiologist
Department of Radiology
New York University Hospital for Joint
    Diseases
New York, New York

Matthew Beran, MD
Attending Physician
Department of Orthopedic Surgery
Nationwide Children's Hospital;
Clinical Assistant Professor
The Ohio State University
Columbus, Ohio

Keith R. Berend, MD

Jeffrey S. Berger, MD, MS
Professor of Medicine and Surgery
Leon H. Charney Division of Cardiology
New York University School of Medicine
New York, New York

Thomas Bernasek, MD

Daniel J. Berry, MD
Past L.Z. Gund Professor and Chairman
Department of Orthopedic Surgery
Mayo Clinic
Rochester, Minnesota

Michael R. Boniello, MD, MS
Eastern Virginia Medical School
Norfolk, Virginia;
Orthopedic Surgery Resident
Cooper Bone and Joint Institute
Camden, New Jersey

Kevin F. Bonner, MD
Orthopedic Surgeon
Jordan-Young Institute
Virginia Beach, Virginia;
Assistant Professor
Department of Surgery
Eastern Virginia Medical School
Norfolk, Virginia

Joseph A. Bosco III, MD
Department of Orthopedic Surgery
New York University Langone Medical
    Center
New York, New York

Jan Boublik, MD, PhD
Department of Anesthesiology,
    Perioperative and Pain Medicine
Stanford University School of Medicine
Stanford, California

Seth Bowman, MD
Department of Orthopaedic Surgery
Medical University of South Carolina
Charleston, South Carolina

Adam C. Brekke, MD
Resident
Department of Orthopaedics and
    Rehabilitation
Vanderbilt University Medical Center
Nashville, Tennessee

Claire L. Brockett, MD
Institute of Medical and Biological
    Engineering
School of Mechanical Engineering
University of Leeds
Leeds, United Kingdom

James A. Brown, MD
Associate Professor and Division Head of
    Adult Reconstruction
Department of Orthopaedic Surgery
University of Virginia
Charlottesville, Virginia

Michael K. Brooks, MD, MPH
Clinical Assistant Professor of Radiology
    SUNY-Stony Brook
Musculoskeletal Radiology and
    InterventionWinthrop University
    Hospital
Mineola, New York

Jarett S. Burak, MD
Assistant Professor of Radiology
Hofstra-Northwell School of Medicine;
Medical Director
Northwell Health Imaging at Syosset
Northwell Health—Department of
    Radiology
Greak Neck, New York

Christopher John Burke, MBChB FRCR
Doctor/Assistant Professor
Department of Radiology
New York University;
Doctor/Assistant Professor
Department of Radiology
New York University, Langone Medical
    Center;
Doctor/Assistant Professor
Department of Radiology
New York University, Hospital for Joint
    Diseases
New York, New York

M. Tyrrell Burrus, MD
Resident Physician
Orthopaedic Surgery
University of Virginia Health System,
Charlottesville, Virginia

Charles Bush-Joseph, MD
Professor
Divsion of Sports Medicine
Department of Orthopaedic Surgery
Rush University Medical Center
Chicago, Illinois

Frank A. Buttacavoli, MD
Orthopedic Surgeon
Orthopedic Care Center
Aventura, Florida

Asokumar Buvanendran, MD, MBBS
Professor
Vice Chair Research & Director of
    Orthopedic Anesthesia
Department of Anesthesiology
Rush University Medical Center
Chicago, Illinois

Matthew G. Cable, MD
Clinical Assistant Professor
Department of Orthopaedics
Section of Musculoskeletal Oncology
Louisiana State University Health Sciences
    Center
New Orleans, Louisiana

Giuseppe Calafiore, MD
Orthopaedic Surgeon
Department of Orthopedics
Clinic Città di Parma
Parma, Italy

Tristan Camus, BSc (Hons), MD, FRCSC
Fellow
Department of Orthopaedic Surgery, Adult
    Reconstruction
New York University Langone Medical
    Center
Insall Scott Kelly
New York, New York

Jourdan M. Cancienne, MD
Resident Physician
Department of Orthopaedic Surgery
University of Virginia Health System
Charlottesville, Virginia

Thomas R. Carter, MD
The Orthopedic Clinic Association, PC
Phoenix, Arizona

Simone Cerciello, MD
Casa di Cura Villa Betania
Rome, Italy;
Marrelli Hospital
Crotone, Italy

Jorge Chahla, MD
Regenerative Sports Medicine Fellow
Center for Translational and Regenerative
    Medicine Research
Steadman Philippon Research Institute
Vail, Colorado

Eric Y. Chang, MD
Assistant Professor
Department of Radiology
VA San Diego Healthcare System;
Assistant Professor
Department of Radiology
University of California, San Diego Medical
    Center
San Diego, California

Anikar Chhabra, MD, MS
Assistant Professor
Department of Orthopedic Surgery
Mayo Clinic Arizona,
Phoenix, Arizona;
Head Team Orthopedic Surgeon
Arizona State University
Tempe, Arizona

Brian Chilelli, MD
Regional Medical Group Orthopaedics
Northwestern Medicine
Warrenville, Illinois

J.H. James Choi, MD
Duke Sports Science Institute
Department of Orthopedic Surgery
Duke University
Durham, North Carolina

Constance R. Chu, MD

Christine B. Chung, MD
Professor of Radiology
University of California School of
    Medicine;
Professor of Radiology
Veterans Affairs Medicine Center
San Diego, California

Michael P. Clare, MD
Director
Foot and Ankle Fellowship
Florida Orthopaedic Institute
Tampa, Florida

Henry D. Clarke, MD
Consultant
Department of Orthopedic Surgery
Mayo Clinic
Phoenix, Arizona;
Professor of Orthopedics
Mayo Clinic College of Medicine
Rochester, Minnesota

David E. Cohen, MD

Brian J. Cole, MD, MBA
Department of Sports Medicine
Rush University Medical Center
Chicago, Illinois

Kristopher D. Collins, MD
Fellow in Adult Reconstruction
Department of Orthopaedic Surgery
ISK Institute
New York, New York

Christopher R. Conley, MD
Consultant
Laboratory Medicine and Pathology
Mayo Clinic
Phoenix, Arizona;
Assistant Professor of Pathology
Mayo Clinic College of Medicine
Rochester, Minnesota

Raelene M. Cowie, MD
Institute of Medical and Biological
    Engineering
School of Mechanical Engineering
University of Leeds
Leeds, United Kingdom

David A. Crawford, MD

Brian M. Culp, MD
Orthopaedic Surgeon
Princeton Orthopaedic Associates
Princeton, New Jersey

John H. Currier, MS
Research Engineer
Thayer School of Engineering at
    Dartmouth College
Hanover, New Hampshire

Fred D. Cushner, MD

Brian P. Dahl, MD
Fellow
Hofmann Arthritis Institute
Salt Lake City, Utah

Diane L. Dahm, MD
Professor of Orthopedics, Mayo Clinic
    College of Medicine
Department of Orthopedic Surgery
Mayo Clinic
Rochester, Minnesota

Timothy A. Damron, MD
Vice-Chairman and David G. Murray
    Endowed Professor of Orthopedic
    Surgery
Department of Orthopedic Surgery
SUNY Upstate Medical University
Syracuse, New York

Chase S. Dean, MD
Steadman Philippon Research Institute
Vail, Colorado

Jospeh P. DeAngelia, MD, MBA
Carl J. Shapiro Department of
    Orthopaedics
Beth Israel Deaconess Medical Center
Boston, Massachusetts

David DeJour, MD
Orthopedic Surgeon
Lyon, France

Craig J. Della Valle, MD
Professor and Chief
Division of Adult Reconstruction
Department of Orthopaedic Surgery
Rush University Medical Center
Chicago, Illinois

Edward M. DelSole, MD
Resident Physician
Department of Orthopaedic Surgery
New York University Langone Medical
    Center/Hospital for Joint Diseases
New York, New York

Douglas A. Dennis, MD
Colorado Joint Replacement;
Adjunct Professor of Bioengineering
Department of Mechanical and Materials
    Engineering
University of Denver
Denver, Colorado;
Adjunct Professor
Department of Biomedical Engineering
University of Tennessee
Knoxville Tennessee;
Assistant Clinical Professor
Department of Orthopaedics
University of Colorado School of Medicine
Aurora, Colorado

Edward J. Derrick, MD

Ajit J. Deshmukh, MD
Assistant Professor
Orthopaedic Surgery
New York University Langone Medical
    Center/New York University Hospital
    for Joint Diseases;
Assistant Chief
Department of Orthopaedics
Surgery
VA New York Harbor Healthcare System
New York, New York

**Ian D. Dickey, MD, P Eng (HON)
FRCSC**
St. Luke's/Presbyterian Hospital
Denver, Colorado

Sorosch Didehvar, MD
Department of Anesthesiology
New York University Langone Medical
    Center
New York, New York

David R. Diduch, MD, MS
Alfred R. Shands Professor of Orthopaedic
    Surgery
Vice Chairman, Department of
    Orthopaedic Surgery
Head Orthopaedic Team Physician
University of Virginia
Charlottesville, Virginia

Lisa V. Doan, MD
Assistant Professor
Department of Anesthesiology,
    Perioperative Care, and Pain Medicine
New York University School of Medicine
New York, New York

Christopher A.F. Dodd, FRCS
Consultant Orthopaedic Surgeon
Nuffield Orthopaedic Centre
Oxford University Hospitals NHS Trust
Oxford, Great Britain

Shawna Dorman, MD
Assistant Professor of Anesthesiology and
    Assistant Director of Ambulatory
    Surgery
Department of Anesthesiology
New York University Langone Hospital for
    Joint Diseases
New York, New York

James C. Dreese, MD

Kostas Economopoulos, MD
The Orthopedic Clinic Association, PC
Phoenix, Arizona

Michele N. Edison, BS, MD
Department of Radiology
Florida Hospital;
Assistant Professor
University of Central Florida College of
    Medicine
Orlando, Florida

Nima Eftekhary, MD
Resident Physician
Orthopaedic Surgery
New York University Hospital for Joint
    Diseases
New York, New York

Brandon J. Erickson, MD
Orthopaedic Surgery Resident
Department of Orthopaedic Surgery
Rush University
Chicago, Illinois

Jean-Pierre Estèbe, MD, PhD
Department of Anesthesiology, Intensive
    Care, and Pain Medicine
University Hospital of Rennes
Rennes, France

Cody L. Evans, BS, MD
Resident Physician
Orthopaedic Surgery
University of Virginia
Charlottesville, Virginia

Gregory C. Fanelli, MD
Orthopaedic Surgeon
GHS Orthopaedics
Danville, Pennsylvania

Jack Farr, MD
OrthoIndy Cartilage Restoration Center
Professor of Orthopaedic Surgery
Indiana University Medical Center
Indianapolis, Indiana

Andrew Feldman, MD
Assistant Professor
Department of Orthopaedic Surgery
New York University Hospital for Joint
    Diseases
New York, New York

Jonathon T. Finoff, MD

John Fisher, MD
Institute of Medical and Biological
    Engineering
School of Mechanical Engineering
University of Leeds
Leeds, United Kingdom

Wolfgang Fitz, MD
Assistant Professor
Orthopedic Surgery
Brigham and Women's and Faulkner
    Hospital, Harvard Medical School
Boston, Massachusetts

Clare K. Fitzpatrick, MD
Center for Orthopaedic Biomechanics
University of Denver
Denver, Colorado

Vincenzo Franceschini, MD
Department of Orthopaedics and
    Traumatology
"Sapienza" University of Rome, ICOT
Latina, Italy

Corinna C. Franklin, MD
Pediatric Orthopaedic Surgeon
Shriners Hospital for Children,
Philadelphia, Pennsylvania

Andrew G. Franks, Jr., BA, MD
Clinical Professor
Department of Internal Medicine
    (Rheumatology)
New York University School of Medicine;
Director
Autoimmune Connective Tissue Disease
    Section
New York University School of Medicine;
Attending Rheumatologist
Hospital for Joint Diseases
New York University School of Medicine
New York, New York

Richard J. Friedman, MD, FRCSC
Department of Orthopaedic Surgery
Medical University of South Carolina
Charleston, South Carolina

Nicole A. Friel, MD

Mark Froimson, MD, MBA
Executive Vice President, Chief Clinical
    Officer
Trinity Health
Livonia, Michigan

**Freddie H. Fu, MD, DSc (Hon),
DPs (Hon)**
Distinguished Service Professor
University of Pittsburgh;
David Silver Professor and Chairman
Department of Orthopaedic Surgery
University of Pittsburgh School of
    Medicine;
Head Team Physician
Departmento of Athletics
University of Pittsburgh
Pittsburgh, Pennsylvania

John P. Fulkerson, MD
Orthopaedic Associates of Hartford
Hartford, Connecticut

Theodore J. Ganley, MD
Associate Professor of Orthopaedic Surgery;
    Director of Sports Medicine
Division of Orthopaedic Surgery
Children's Hospital of Philadelphia
Philadelphia, Pennsylvania

Donald S. Garbuz, MD
Professor and Head
Division of Lower Limb Reconstruction
    and Oncology
Department of Orthopaedics
University of British Columbia
Vancouver, British Columbia, Canada

Christopher Gharibo, MD
Associate Professor of Anesthesiology &
    Orthopedics
New York University School of Medicine
New York, New York

Matteo Ghiara, MD
Department of Orthopedics and
    Traumatology
Fondazione IRCCS Policlinico San Matteo
Università degli Studi di Pavia
Pavia, Italy

Thomas J. Gill, AB, MD
Director
Boston Sports Medicine and Research
    Institute
New England Baptist Hospital
Boston, Massachusetts

Megan M. Gleason, MD
Fellow
Department of Orthopedic Surgery
University of Virginia
Charlottesville, Virginia

Alyssa Reiffel Golas, MD
Resident
Hansjorg Wyss Department of Plastic
    Surgery
New York University Langone Medical
    Center
New York, New York

Gregory Golladay, MD

Andreas H. Gomoll, MD
Associate Professor of Orthopaedic Surgery
Harvard Medical School;
Orthopaedic Surgery
Brigham and Women's Hospital
Boston, Massachusetts

Felix M. Gonzalez, MD

Guillem Gonzalez-Lomas, MD
Assistant Professor
Orthopaedic Surgery
New York University Hospital for Joint
    Diseases
New York, New York

**John A. Grant, MD, PhD, FRCSC, Dip
Sport Med**
Assistant Professor
MedSport, Orthopaedic Surgery
University of Michigan
Ann Arbor, Michigan

Stephen Gregorius, MD
Department of Orthopaedics
University of Utah
Salt Lake City, Utah

Justin Greisberg, MD
Associate Professor
Department of Orthopaedic Surgery
Columbia University
New York, New York

Ulrik Grevstad, MD, PHD
Associate Professor
Anesthesia and Intensive Care
Gentofte Hospital
Copenhagen, Denmark

Trevor Grieco, BS
Graduate Research Assistant
Mechanical, Aerospace, and Biomedical
    Engineering
University of Tennessee
Knoxville, Tennessee

Justin W. Griffin, MD
Sports and Shoulder Surgery Fellow
Department of Orthopaedic Surgery
Rush University Medical Center
Chicago, Illinois

Daniel Guenther, MD

F. Winston Gwathmey, Jr., MD
Assistant Professor
Department of Orthopaedic Surgery
University of Virginia Health System
Charlottesville, Virginia

George J. Haidukewych, MD
Division of Orthopaedic Trauma and
    Complex Adult Reconstruction
Department of Orthopaedic Surgery
Orlando Regional Medical Center
Orlando, Florida

Christopher A. Hajnik, MD

Arielle J. Hall, MD
Research Intern
Sports and Shoulder Service
Hospital for Special Surgery
New York, New York

David A. Halsey, MD
Professor
University of Vermont College of Medicine
and Rehabilitation
Burlington, Vermont

William R. Hamel, PhD, MS, BS
Professor
IEEE Fellow, ASME Fellow
Department of Mechanical, Aerospace, &
Biomedical Engineering
The University of Tennessee–Knoxville
Knoxville, Tennessee

Arlen D. Hanssen, MD
Professor
Department of Orthopedic Surgery
Mayo Clinic
Rochester, Minnesota

John M. Hardcastle, MD
Crystal Run Healthcare
Middletown, New York

Christopher D. Harner, MD
Department of Orthopaedic Surgery
University of Texas
Houston, Texas

Joe Hart, PhD, ATC
Associate Professor
Department of Kinesiology
University of Virginia;
Director of Clinical Research
Department of Orthopaedic Surgery
University of Virginia
Charlottesville, Virginia

William L. Healy, MD

Emma Heath, MPhty, BAppSc
North Sydney Orthopaedic and Sports
Medicine Centre
Sydney, New South Wales, Australia

Petra Heesterbeek, PhD
Research Co-ordinator/Senior Researcher
Orthopedic Research
Sint Maartenskliniek
Nijmegen, The Netherlands

Tarek M. Hegazi, MD

Yonah Heller, MD
Orthopedic Resident
Department of Orthopedics
Northwell Health
New Hyde Park, New York

Shane Hess, MD

Benton E. Heyworth, MD
Assistant Professor of Orthopaedic Surgery
Harvard Medical School
Division of Sports Medicine
Boston Children's Hospital
Boston, Massachusetts

Betina B. Hinckel, MD
Orthopaedic Surgeon
Department Institute of Orthopedics and
Traumatology
Clinical Hospital
Medical School
University of São Paulo
São Paulo, Brazil

Richard Y. Hinton, MD, MPH
Director, Sports Medicine Fellowship
MedStar Sports Medicine
MedStar Union Memorial Hospital/
MedStar Washington Hospital Center;
Attending
Department of Orthopaedics
MedStar Union Memorial Hospital
Baltimore, Maryland

Jason P. Hochfelder, MD
Fellow
Adult Reconstruction
Insall Scott Kelly Institute
New York, New York

Aaron A. Hofmann, MD
Director
Center for Precision Joint Replacement
Salt Lake Regional Medical Center
Salt Lake City, Utah

Ginger E. Holt, MD
Department of Orthopaedics and
Rehabilitation
Vanderbilt Medical Center
Nashville, Tennessee

Mohammed M. Hoque, MD
Radiology Resident, R2
Department of Radiology
Maimonides Medical Center
Brooklyn, New York

Stephen M. Howell, MD
Professor of Biomedical Engineering
Department of Mechanical Engineering
University of California at Davis
Davis, California;
Orthopedic Surgeon
Methodist Hospital
Sacramento, California

Johnny Huard, PhD

Maury L. Hull, BS, MS, PhD
Distinguished Professor
Department of Biomedical Engineering
University of California Davis;
Distinguished Professor
Department of Mechanical Engineering
University of California Davis
Davis, California

Ian D. Hutchinson, MD
Research Fellow
Sports Medicine and Shoulder Service
Hospital for Special Surgery
New York, New York

Lorraine H. Hutzler, BA
Department of Orthopaedic Surgery
NYU Hospital for Joint Diseases
NYU Langone Medical Center
New York, New York

John N. Insall, MD[†]
Formerly Clinical Professor of Orthopedic
Surgery
Albert Einstein College of Medicine
Bronx, New York;
Director
Insall Scott Kelly Institute for Orthopedics
and Sports Medicine
Beth Israel Medical Center
New York, New York

Richard Iorio, MD
Dr. William and Susan Jaffe Professor of
Orthopaedic Surgery
Chief Division of Adult Reconstructive
Surgery
Department of Orthopaedic Surgery
New York University Langone Medical
Center
New York, New York

Sebastián Irarrázaval, MD
Department of Orthopaedic Surgery
Pontificia Universidad Católica de Chile
Santiago, Chile

[†]Deceased.

Ghislaine M. Isidore, MD
Clinical Assistant Professor of
   Anesthesiology
Anesthesiology, Perioperative Care and Pain
   Medicine
New York University Langone Medical
   Center
New York, New York

Pia Jæger, MD, PhD
Doctor
Department of Anaesthesia, Centre of Head
   and Orthopeadics
Rigshospitalet
Copenhagen, Denmark

Andre M. Jakoi, MD
Fellow
Department of Orthopaedic Surgery
University of Southern California
Los Angeles, California

James G. Jarvis, MD, FRCSC
Associate Professor of Surgery
University of Ottawa;
Division of Orthopaedic Surgery
Children's Hospital of Eastern Ontario
Ottawa, Ontario, Canada

Jason M. Jennings, MD, DPT
Colorado Joint Replacement
Porter Adventist Hospital
Denver, Colorado

Louise M. Jennings, PhD
Associate Professor of Medical Engineering
Institute of Medical and Biological
   Engineering
School of Mechanical Engineering
University of Leeds
Leeds, United Kingdom

William A. Jiranek, MD
Professor and Chief of Adult
   Reconstruction
Dept. of Orthopaedic Surgery
Virginia Commonwealth University School
   of Medicine
Richmond, Virginia

Charles E. Johnston II, MD
Assistant Chief of Staff (Emeritus)
Texas Scottish Rite Hospital for Children;
Professor
Department of Orthopedic Surgery
University of Texas Southwestern Medical
   School
Dallas, Texas

Justin B. Jones, MD
Fellow
Adult Reconstruction
Isall Scott Kelly Institute
New York, New York

V. Karthik Jonna, MD

Daniel J. Kaplan, BA
Research Fellow
Orthopaedic Surgery
New York University Langone Medical
   Center
New York, New York

Jonathan Katz, MD
Department of Orthopaedic Surgery
Medical University of South Carolina
Charleston, South Carolina

Erdan Kayupov, MSE
Research Fellow
Orthopaedic Surgery
Rush University Medical Center
Chicago, Illinois

Saurabh Khakharia, MD

Arif Khan, MD

Harpal S. Khanuja, MD
Associate Professor
Chief of Adult Reconstruction
Department of Orthopaedic Surgery
The Johns Hopkins University;
Chair
Department of Orthopaedic Surgery
Johns Hopkins Bayview Medical Center
Baltimore, Maryland

Nayoung Kim, BS
Rothman Institute
Philadelphia, Pennsylvania

Raymond H. Kim, MD
Colorado Joint Replacement;
Adjunct Associate Professor of
   Bioengineering
Department of Mechanical and Materials
   Engineering
University of Denver
Denver, Colorado;
Clinical Associate Professor
Department of Orthopedic Surgery
Joan C. Edwards School of Medicine at
   Marshall University
Huntington, West Virginia

Sung-Hwan Kim, MD
Assistant Professor
Department of Othopaedic Surgery
Arthroscopy and Joint Research Institute
Yonsei University College of Medicine;
Assistant Professor
Department of Orthopaedic Surgery
Gangnam Severance Hospital
Seoul, Republic of Korea

Sung-Jae Kim, MD, PhD
Emeritus Professor
Department of Orthopaedic Surgery
Yonsei University College of Medicine;
Director
Department of Orthopaedic Surgery
Gangdong Yonsesarang Hospital
Seoul, Republic of Korea

Yair D. Kissin, MD

Kevin Klingele, MD
Chief
Department of Orthopaedic Surgery
Nationwide Children's Hospital
Columbus, Ohio

Kevin R. Knox, MD
Indiana Hand to Shoulder Center
Indianapolis, Indiana

Mininder S. Kocher, MD, MPH
Professor of Orthopaedic Surgery
Harvard Medical School;
Associate Director
Division of Sports Medicine
Boston Children's Hospital
Boston, Massachusettes

Richard D. Komistek,
BSME, MSME, PhD
Fred M. Roddy Professor
Biomedical Engineering,
Co-Center Director
Center for Musculoskeletal Research
University of Tennessee
Knoxville, Tennessee

Dennis E. Kramer, MD
Assistant Professor of Orthopaedic Surgery
Orthopedic Center
Boston Childrens Hospital
Boston, Massachusetts

Mark J. Kransdorf, MD
Consultant
Diagnostic Radiology
Mayo Clinic,
Phoenix, Arizona;
Professor of Radiology
Mayo Clinic College of Medicine
Rochester, Minnesota

Tomas J. Kucera, MD

Christopher M. Kuenze, PhD, ATC
Assistant Professor
Department of Kinesiology
Michigan State University
East Lansing, Michigan

Vinícius Canello Kuhn, MD
Orthopedic Surgeon
Instituto de Ortopedia e Traumatologia de
    Passo Fundo
Passo Fundo, Brazil

Shinichi Kuriyama, MD
Professor and Chairman
Department of Orthopedic Surgery
Kyoto Univeristy
Kyoto, Japan

Anne Kuwabara, BA
Department of Physical Medicine and
    Rehabilitation
The Johns Hopkins University
Baltimore, Maryland

Paul F. Lachiewicz, MD
Consulting Professor
Department of Orthopaedic Surgery
Duke University,
Orthopaedic Surgeon
Veterans Administration Medical Center
Durham, North Carolina;
Orthopaedic Surgeon
Chapel Hill Orthopedics Surgery & Sports
    Medicine
Chapel Hill, North Carolina

Michael T. LaCour, BS
Graduate Research Assistant
Mechanical, Aerospace, and Biomedical
    Engineering
University of Tennessee
Knoxville, Tennessee

Claudette Lajam, MD
Assistant Professor of Orthopaedic Surgery
Department of Orthopaedics
New York University Langone Medical
    Center
New York, New York

Alfredo Lamberti, MD
Orthopaedics, Adult Reconstruction
IFCA Institute
Florence, Italy

Jason E. Lang, MD
Attending Surgeon
Blue Ridge Bone and Joint
Asheville, North Carolina

Joshua R. Langford, MD
Division of Orthopaedic Trauma and
    Complex Adult Reconstruction
Department of Orthopaedic Surgery
Orlando Regional Medical Center
Orlando, Florida

Robert F. LaPrade, MD, PhD
The Steadman Clinic;
The Steadman Philippon Research Institute
Vail, Colorado

Nicholas J. Lash, MD
Clinical Fellow
Department of Orthopaedics
University of British Columbia
Vancouver, British Columbia, Canada

Sherlin Lavianlivi, MD
MSK Fellow/Radiologist
Department of Radiology
Maimonides Medical Center
Brooklyn, New York

Gary Lawera, BS, CMPE
Chief Operating Officer
University of Toledo Physicians, LLC
Toledo, Ohio

Peter J. Laz, MD
Center for Orthopaedic Biomechanics
University of Denver
Denver, Colorado

Cheng-Ting Lee, MD
Anesthesiology Resident
Columbia University Medical Center
New York, New York

Gabriel Levi, MD

Richard G. Levine, MD

Dieter Lindskog, MD
Associate Professor
Department of Orthopaedics and
    Rehabilitation
Yale University School of Medicine
New Haven, Connecticut

Davidm R. Lionberger, MD

Frank A. Liporace, MD
Division of Orthopaedic Trauma and
    Complex Adult Reconstruction
Department of Orthopaedic Surgery
Jersey City Medical Center
Jersey City, New Jersey

Sanford M. Littwin, MD
Associate Professor of Anesthesiology,
Clinical Director Operating Rooms
UPP Department of Anesthesiology
UPMC Presbyterian and Montefiore
    Hospitals
Pittsburgh, Pennsylvania

Phillip Locker, MD

Adolph V. Lombardi, MD

William J. Long, BSc, MD, FRCSC
Director,
Attending Orthopaedic Surgeon
Insall Scott Kelly Institute,
St. Francis Hospital, Lenox Hill Hospital,
Hospital for Joint Diseases
New York, New York

Jess H. Lonner, MD
Attending Orthopaedic Surgeon
Rothman Institute;
Associate Professor
Department of Orthopaedic Surgery
Thomas Jefferson University
Philadelphia, Pennsylvania

Walter R. Lowe, MD

Sébastien Lustig, MD, PhD
Albert Trillat Center
Orthopedic Surgery
Lyon North University Hospital
Lyon, France

Thomas Luyckx, MD, PhD
Full Professor of Orthopedics and
    Traumatology
Chair, Department of Orthopedics and
    Traumatology
Ghent University
Ghent, Belgium

Dana Lycans, MD
Resident
Department of Orthopaedic Surgery
Marshall University
Huntington, West Virginia

Steven Lyons, MD
Florida Orthopedic Institute
Tampa, Florida

Samuel D. Madoff, MD
Department of Radiology
New England Baptist Hospital
Boston, Massachusetts

Robert A. Magnussen, MD, MPH
Associate Professor
Department of Orthopaedics
The Ohio State University
Columbus, Ohio

Suzanne A. Maher, PhD
Associate Scientist,
Associate Director
Department of Biomechanics,
Associate Director
Tissue Engineering Regeneration and
    Repair Program
Hospital for Special Surgery
New York, New York;
Associate Professor of Applied
    Biomechanics in Orthopaedic Surgery,
Adjunct Professor of Biomedical
    Engineering
Department of Biomedical Engineering
Weill Cornell Medical College
Cornell University
Ithica, New York

Mohamed R. Mahfouz, MS, PhD
Professor of Biomedical Engineering
Mechanical Aerospace and Biomedical
    Engineering
University of Tennessee
Knoxville, Tennessee

Amun Makani, MD
Attending Surgeon
Department of Orthopaedic Surgery
Watson Clinic
Lakeland, Florida

Eric C. Makhni, MD
Department of Sports Medicine
Henry Ford Health Center
Detroit, Michigan

Parul R. Maniar, MD
Consultant Ophthalmologist
Nook Clinic, Santacruz (W)
Mumbai, India

**Rajesh N. Maniar, MS, MCh Orth (UK),
DNB**
Head
Department of Orthopaedics & Joint
    Reconstruction
Lilavati Hospital & Research Centre;
Consultant and Joint Replacement Surgeon
Department of Orthopaedics & Joint
    Reconstruction
Breach Candy Hospital
Mumbai, India

Patrick G. Marinello, MD
Resident Orthopaedic Surgery
Cleveland Clinic Foundation
Cleveland, Ohio

Milica Markovic, MD
Assistant Professor
Department of Anesthesiology
Weill Cornell Medical College
New York Presbyterian Hospital
New York, New York

J. Bohannon Mason, MD

Bassam A. Masri, MD, FRCSC
Professor and Chairman
Department of Orthopaedics
University of British Columbia
Vancouver, British Columbia, Canada

Henry Masur, MD
Chief
Critical Care Medicine Department
Clinical Center, National Institutes of
    Health
Bethesda, Maryland

Kevin R. Math, MD
Associate Professor of Radiology
Hospital for Special Surgery
New York, New York

Kenneth B. Mathis, MD

Shuichi Matsuda, MD, PhD
Professor and Chairman
Department of Orthopedic Surgery
Kyoto University
Kyoto, Japan

Tomoyuki Matsumoto, MD, PhD
Assistant Professor
Department of Orthopaedic Surgery
Kobe University Graduate School of
    Medicine
Kobe, Japan

Chan-Nyein Maung, MD
Clinical Instructor of Anesthesiology
Department of Anesthesiology,
    Perioperative Care, and Pain Medicine
New York University Langone Medical
    Center
New York, New York

Kristen E. McClure, MD

Brian J. McGrory, MD, MS
Clinical Professor
Department of Orthopaedic Surgery
Tufts University School of Medicine
Boston, Massachusetts;
Co-Director
Maine Joint Replacement Institute
Portland, Maine

David C. McNabb, MD
Colorado Joint Replacement
Porter Adventist Hospital
Denver, Colorado

Brad Meccia, BS
University of Tennessee, Knoxville
Knoxville, Tennessee

Michael B. Mechlin, MD
Assistant Professor of Radiology
New York University School of Medicine
New York, New York

Patrick A. Meere, MD, CM
Clinical Associate Professor
Orthopaedic Surgery
New York University Langone Hospital for
    Joint Diseases
New York, New York

R. Michael Meneghini, MD
Associate Professor
Orthopaedic Surgery
Indiana University School of Medicine;
Director of Lower Extremity Adult
    Reconstruction Fellowship
Indiana University School of Medicine
Indianapolis, Indiana;
Director of Joint Replacement
IU Health Saxony Hospital
Fishers, Indiana

John J. Mercuri, MD, MA
Chief Resident
Department of Orthopaedic Surgery
Hospital for Joint Diseases
New York University Langone Medical
    Center
New York, New York

Maximilian A. Meyer, MD
Department of Sports Medicine
Rush University Medical Center
Chicago, Illinois

Cory Messerschmidt, MD
Department of Orthopaedic Surgery
Medical University of South Carolina
Charleston, South Carolina

Matthew D. Milewski, MD
Assistant Professor
Department of Orthopaedic Surgery
Connecticut Children's Medical Center—
    Elite Sports Medicine
Farmington, Connecticut

Mark D. Miller, MD
S. Ward Casscells Professor
Department of Orthopaedics
University of Virginia
Charlottesville, Virginia

Patrick J. Milord, MD, MBA
Interventional Pain Management Fellow
Department of Anesthesiology,
    Perioperative Care and Pain Medicine
New York University Langone Medical
    Center
New York, New York

Claude T. Moorman III, MD
Duke Sports Science Institute
Department of Orthopedic Surgery
Duke University
Durham, North Carolina

Vincent M. Moretti, MD
Rothman Institute
Philadelphia, Pennsylvania

William B. Morrison, MD
Professor
Department of Radiology
Thomas Jefferson University
Director
Division of Musculoskeletal and General
    Diagnostic Radiology
Thomas Jefferson University Hospital
Philadelphia, Pennsylvania

James R. Mullen, MD
Orthopedic Resident
Northwell Health
New Hyde Park, NY

Hirotsugu Muratsu, MD
Department of Orthopaedic Surgery
Steel Memorial Hirohata Hospital
Himeji, Japan

David Murray, MD
Professor of Orthopaedic Surgery
Nuffield Department of Orthopaedics
Rheumatology and Musculoskeletal
    Sciences
University of Oxford;
Consultant and Orthopaedic Surgeon
Nuffield Orthopaedic Centre
Oxford University Hospitals NHS Trust
Oxford, Great Britain

Volker Musahl, MD
Associate Professor
Department of Orthopaedic Surgery
University of Pittsburgh
Pittsburgh, Pennsylvania

Zan A. Naseer, BS
New York Medical College
New York, New York

Amit Nathani, MD, MS
Resident
Department of Orthopaedic Surgery
University of Michigan
Ann Arbor, Michigan

Milad Nazemzadeh, MD
Clinical Assistant,
Professor of Anesthesiology
Department of Anesthesiology,
    Perioperative Care, and Pain Medicine
New York University Langone Medical
    Center
New York, New York

Michael D. Neel, MD
Department of Orthopaedic Surgery
St Jude Children's Research Hospital
Memphis, West Virginia

Charles L. Nelson, MD
Chief of Adult Reconstruction
Associate Professor of Orthopaedic Surgery
University of Pennsylvania
Philadelphia, Pennsylvania

Nathan A. Netravali, MD

Michael P. Nett, MD
Orthopedic Surgeon, Coordinator of
    Quality and Clinical Arthroplasty
Department of Orthopedic Surgery
North Shore Long Island Jewish
    Orthopedic Institute @ Southside
    Hospital
Bay Shore, New York

Phillipe Neyret, MD, PhD
Head of Department
Orthopaedic Surgery and Traumatology
Hospices Civils de Lyon—Centre Albert
    Trillat
Lyon, Rhône, France

Jesse Ng, MD
Clinical Assistant Professor of
    Anesthesiology

Carl W. Nissen, MD
Physician
Elite Sports Medicine
Connecticut Children's Medical Center;
Professor
Department of Orthopaedics
University of Connecticut
Farmington, Connecticut

Philip C. Noble, BE, MES, PhD

Frank R. Noyes, MD
President and Medical Director
Noyes Knee Institute
Cincinnati, Ohio

Mary I. O'Connor, MD
Director and Professor
Center for Musculoskeletal Care at Yale
    School of Medicine and Yale—New
    Haven Hospital
Yale School of Medicine
New Haven, Connecticut

Khalid Odeh, BA

Russell M. Odono, MD
Orthopaedic Surgeon
Department of Orthopaedic Surgery
Insall Scott Kelly Institute
New York, New York

Louis Okafor, MD
Department of Orthopaedic Surgery
The Johns Hopkins University
Baltimore, Maryland

Andrew B. Old, AB, MD
Fellow
Orthopaedics and Adult Reconstruction
New York University
New York, New York

Ali Oliashirazi, MD
Chairman
Department of Orthopaedic Surgery
Marshall University
Huntington, West Virginia

Matthieu Ollivier, APHM
Institute for Locomotion
Department of Orthopaedic Surgery
Sainte-Marguerite Hospital;
Professor
Aix-Marseille University
Marseille, France

Mark W. Pagnano, MD
Chairman and Professor of Orthopedic
    Surgery
Department of Orthopedic Surgery
Mayo Clinic
Rochester, Minnesota

Christopher J. Palestro, MD
Professor
Department of Radiology
School of Medicine of Hofstra University
Hempstead, New York;
Chief of Nuclear Medicine & Molecular
    Imaging
New Hyde Park, New York

**Hemant Pandit, FRCS (Orth), D Phil
(Oxon)**
Professor
Nuffield Department of Orthopaedics,
    Rheumatology and Musculoskeletal
    Sciences
University of Oxford
Oxford, Great Britain;
Professor of Orthopaedics and Honorary
    Consultant
University of Leeds
Leeds, Great Britain

Bertrand W. Parcells, MD

Sebastien Parratte, APHM
Institute for Locomotion
Department of Orthopaedic Surgery
Sainte-Marguerite Hospital;
Professor
Aix-Marseille University
Marseille, France

Brian S. Parsley, MD

Javad Parvizi, MD, FRCS
Professor
Department of Orthopaedic Surgery
Rothman Institute of Orthopaedics at
    Thomas Jefferson University
Philadelphia, Pennsylvania

Alopi Patel, MD
Resident
Department of Anesthesiology
Mount Sinai St. Luke's—Roosevelt Hospital
    Center
New York, New York

Hersh Patel, MD

Jay Patel, MD
Hoag Orthopaedic Institute
Irvine, California;
Orthopaedic Specialty Institute
Orange, California

Henrik Bo Pedersen, MD
Director Medical Multimedia
Insall Scott Kelly Institute
New York, New York

Dawn Pedinelli, RN, MBA
Director of Research
Trinity Health
Livonia, Michigan

Vincent D. Pellegrini, Jr., MD
John A. Siegling Professor and Chair
Department of Orthopaedics
Medical University of South Carolina;
Director
Musculoskeletal Integrated Center of
    Clinical Excellence
Medical University of South Carolina;
Adjunct Professor
Department of Bioengineering
Clemson University
Charleston, South Carolina

Kevin I. Perry, MD
Mayo Clinic
Rochester, Minnesota

Catherine N. Petchprapa, MD
Assistant Professor
Department of Radiology
New York University Langone Medical
    Center—Hospital for Joint Diseases
New York, New York

Christopher L. Peters, MD
Professor, George S. Eccles Endowed Chair
Department of Orthopaedics
University of Utah
Salt Lake City, Utah

Lars Peterson, MD,PhD
Professor of Orthopaedics
Institutions for Surgical Sciences,
    Gothenburg University
Gothenburg, Vastra Gotaland, Sweden

Christopher R. Pettis, MD
Clinical Assistant Professor of Radiology
    UCF/FSU
Department of Radiology
Florida Hospital
Orlando, Florida

Michael H. Pillinger, MD
Professor of Medicine and Biochemistry
    and Molecular Pharmacology,
Director, Rheumatology Training,
Director, Masters of Science in Clinical
    Investigation Program,
New York University School of Medicine;
Section Chief
Department of Rheumatology
New York Harbor Health Care System—NY
    Campus
Department of Veterans Affairs
New York, New York

Leo A. Pinczewski, MBBS, FRACS
Associate Professor Department of
    Orthopaedics
Notre Dame University;
Consultant Orthopaedic SurgeonMater
    Hospital;
North Sydney Orthopaedic and Sports
    Medicine Centre
Sydney, New South Wales, Australia

Mark Pinto, MD, MBA
Orthopedic Surgeon
Chelsea Orthopedic Specialists
Chelsea, Michigan;
Medical Director
Perioperative Services
Trinity Health
Livonia, Michigan

William R. Post, MD
Mountaineer Orthopedic Specialists
Morgantown, West Virginia

Ian Power, MD

Jared S. Preston, MD

Peter Pyrko, MD, PhD
Assistant Professor
Department of Orthopedic Surgery
Loma Linda University
Loma Linda, California

Sridhar R. Rachala, MD
Assistant Professor of Orthopaedic Surgery
University at Buffalo
Buffalo, New York

Craig S. Radnay, MD, MPH
Director
Insall Scott Kelly Institute for Orthopaedics
    and Sports Medicine;
Clinical Assistant Professor
Department of Orthopaedic Surgery
New York University/Hospital for Joint
    Diseases
New York, New York;
Attending Physician
Department of Orthopaedic Surgery
St Francis Hospital
Roslyn, New York

Adam Rana, MD
Attending Orthopedic Surgeon
Orthopedic Surgery
Maine Medical Center
Portland, Maine

R. Lor Randall, MD
The L.B. & Olive S. Young Endowed Chair
  for Cancer Research,
Director
Sarcoma Services
Huntsman Cancer Institute, University of
  Utah;
Medical Director
Huntsman Cancer Institute Surgical
  Services,
Professor
Department of Orthopaedics
University of Utah
Salt Lake City, Utah

Amer Rasheed, MD
University of Illinois
Illinois

Parthiv A. Rathod, MD
Assistant Professor
Department of Orthopaedic Surgery
New York University Langone Medical
  Center/Hospital for Joint Diseases;
Chief of Orthopaedics
Woodhull Hospital Center
New York, New York

Robert S. Reiffel, MD
Attending Physician
Department of Surgery/Plastic Surgery
White Plains Hospital
White Plains, New York

Timothy G. Reish, MD, FACS
Associate Professor
Orthopaedic Surgery
New York University Langone Medical
  Center, Hospital For Joint Diseases;
Director
Insall Scott Kelly Institute for Orthopaedics
  and Sports Medicine
New York, New York

Daniel L. Riddle, PT, PhD, FAPTA
Otto D. Payton Professor of Physical
  Therapy
Department of Orthopaedic Surgery and
  Rheumatology
Virginia Commonwealth University
Richmond, Virginia

Samuel P. Robinson, MD
Orthopedic Surgeon
Jordan-Young Institute
Virginia Beach, Virginia

Scott A. Rodeo, MD
Professor of Orthopaedic Surgery
  (Academic Track)
Weill Medical College of Cornell University;
Co-Chief
Emeritus Sports Medicine and Shoulder
  Service
Hospital for Special Surgery;
Attending Orthopaedic Surgeon
Hospital for Special Surgery;
Head Team Physician
New York Giants Football
New York, New York

David Rodriguez-Quintana, MD

Gregory J. Roehrig, MD
Orthopaedic Institute of Central Jersey
Hackensack Meridian Health;
Director of Joint Replacement Program
Jersey Shore University Medical Center
Neptune, New Jersey

Aaron G. Rosenberg, MD
Professor of Surgery
Department of Orthopedic Surgery
Rush Unuiversity Medical College
Chicago, Illinois

Pamela B. Rosenthal, MD

Stefano M.P. Rossi, MD
Clinica Ortopedica e Traumatologica
Fondazione IRCCS
Policlinico San Matteo
Università degli Studi di Pavia
Pavia, Italy

Paul J. Rullkoetter, PhD
Professor
Department of Mechanical & Materials
  Engineering
Center for Orthopaedic Biomechanics
University of Denver
Denver, Colorado

Neda Sadeghi, BS, MD
Resident
Department of Anesthesiology
Mount Sinai St. Lukes Hospital
New York, New York

Paulo R.F. Saggin, MD
Orthopedic Surgeon
Instituto de Ortopedia e Traumatologia de
  Passo Fundo,
Passo Fundo, Brazil

Lucy Salmon, PhD
North Sydney Orthopaedic and Sports
  Medicine Centre
Sydney, New South Wales, Australia

Matthew J. Salzler, MD
Clinical Instructor
Department of Orthopaedics
Tufts Medical Center
Boston, Massachusetts

Thomas L. Sanders, MD
Orthopedic Surgery Resident
Department of Orthopedic Surgery
Mayo Clinic
Rochester, Minnesota

Sarah Sasor, MD
Indiana University Division of Plastic
  Surgery
Indiana

Adam A. Sassoon, MD
Department of Orthopaedics and Sports
  Medicine
University of Washington
Seattle, Washington

Robert C. Schenck, Jr., MD

Kurt F. Scherer, MD

**Oliver S. Schindler, BSc (Hons), PhD,
FMH, MFSEM (UK), FRCSEd, FRCSEng,
FRCS (Orth)**
Consultant Orthopaedic Surgeon
Bristol Arthritis & Sports Injury Clinic
Chesterfield Hospital
Bristol, United Kingdom;
The Manor Hospital
Oxford, United Kingdom;
Exeter Nuffield Hospital
Exeter, Devon, United Kingdom

Jason M. Schon, BS
Research Assistant
BioMedical Engineering
Steadman Philippon Research Institute
Vail, Colorado

Verena M. Schreiber, MD
Cincinnati Children's Hospital Medical
  Center
Division of Pediatric Orthopaedic Surgery
Cincinnati, Ohio

Kelly L. Scott, MD
Resident
Department of Orthopedic Surgery
Mayo Clinic
Phoenix, Arizona

Susan Craig Scott, MD
Clinical Assistant Professor
Department of Orthopaedic Surgery
Hansjorg Wyss Department of Plastic
    Surgery
New York University School of Medicine;
Surgeon
Department of Hand Surgery
NYU Hospital for Joint Diseases;
Assistant Attending
Department of Orthopedics
Bellevue Hospital Center;
Consulting Physician
Departments of Surgery and Orthopedic
    Surgery
Department of Veterans Affairs
New York Harbor Healthcare System
New York, New York

W. Norman Scott, MD, FACS
Clinical Professor of Orthopaedic Surgery
New York University Langone Medical
    Center
Hospital for Joint Diseases;
Joan C. Edwards School of Medicine
Marshall University
Founding Director
Insall Scott Kelly Institute for Orthaepedic
    Sports Medicine
New York, New York

Giles R. Scuderi, MD
Vice President
Orthopedic Service Line
Northwell Health;
Fellowship Director
Adult Knee Reconstruction
Lenox Hill Hospital
New York, New York;
Associate Clinical Professor of Orthopedic
    Surgery
Hofstra Northwell School of Medicine
Hempstead, New York

Elvire Servien, MD, PhD
Professor
Department of Orthopedic Surgery

Erik P. Severson, MD
Minnesota Center for Orthopaedics
Crosby/Aitkin, Minnesota

Nicholas A. Sgaglione, MD
Professor and Chair
Department of Orthopaedic Surgery
Northwell Health,
New Hyde Park, New York

Peter F. Sharkey, MD
Rothman Institute
Philadelphia, Pennsylvania

Adrija Sharma, PhD
Research Assistant Professor
Mechanical Aerospace and Biomedical
    Engineering
University of Tennessee
Knoxville, Tennessee

Kevin G. Shea, MD
Orthopedic Surgeon
Department of Sports Medicine
St. Luke's
Boise, Idaho;
Associate Professor
Department of Orthopaedics
University of Utah
Salt Lake City, Utah

Courtney E. Sherman, MD
Assistant Professor of Orthopedics
Department of Orthopedics
Mayo Clinic Jacksonville
Jacksonville, Florida

Jodi Sherman, MD
Assistant Professor of Anesthesiology
Yale University, School of Medicine
New Haven, Connecticut

Seth L. Sherman, MD
Attending Orthopaedic Surgeon
Department of Orthopaedic Surgery
University of Missouri
Columbia, Missouri

Michael S. Shin, MD

Rafael J. Sierra, MD
Associate Professor of Orthopedics
Department of Orthopedic Surgery
College of Medicine
Mayo Clinic
Rochester, Minnesota

Tushar Singhi, MD
Associate Professor
Department of Orthopedics
Padamshree D Y Patil Medical College
Navi Mumbai, India

David L. Skaggs, MD, MMM
Children's Orthopaedic Center
Children's Hospital Los Angeles
Los Angeles, California

Harris S. Slone, MD
Assistant Professor
Department of Orthopaedics
Medical University of South Carolina
Charleston, South Carolina

James D. Slover, MD, MS
Associate Professor
Adult Reconstruction Division
Department of Orthopaedic Surgery
Hospital for Joint Diseases
New York University Langone Medical
    Center
New York, New York

Nathaniel R. Smilowitz, MD
Professor of Medicine and Surgery
Leon H. Charney Division of Cardiology
New York University School of Medicine
New York, New York

Daniel C. Smith, MD
Adult Reconstruction Fellow
Department of Orthopaedic Surgery
New York University Langone Hospital for
    Joint Diseases
New York, New York

Gideon P. Smith, MD PhD
Director of Connective Tissue Diseases
Department of Dermatology
Mass General Hospital of Harvard University
Boston, Massachusetts

Gary E. Solomon, MD
Associate Professor
Department of Medicine
New York University Langone School of
    Medicine
New York, New York

Jeffrey T. Spang, MD
Assistant Professor
Department of Orthopaedics
University of North Carolina
Chapel Hill, North Carolina

Kurt P. Spindler, BS, MD
Vice Chairman of Research
Director Orthopaedic Clinical Outcomes
Academic Director
Cleveland Clinic Sports Health
Orthopaedic and Rheumatologic Institute
Cleveland Clinic
Cleveland, Ohio;
Adjoint Professor
Department of Orthopaedics
Vanderbilt University Medical Center
Nashville, Tennessee

Bryan D. Springer, MD
Attending Orthopaedic Surgeon
OrthoCarolina Hip and Knee Center
Charlotte, North Carolina

Ryan Stancil, MD
Department of Orthopaedics and Sports
    Medicine
University of Washington
Seattle, Washington

Samuel R.H. Steiner, MD
Department of Orthopedic Surgery and
    Rehabilitation
Division of Sports Medicine
University of Wisconsin—Madison
Madison, Wisconsin

James Bowen Stiehl, MD
Chief of Surgery
St Mary's Hospital
Centralia, Illinois

Jonathan A. Stone, MD
Resident
Department of Orthopedic Surgery
Tufts Medical Center
Boston, Massachusetts

Eric J. Strauss, MD
Assistant Professor
Department of Orthopaedic Surgery
New York University Hospital for Joint
    Diseases
New York, New York

Joseph J. Stuart, MD
Duke Sports Science Institute
Department of Orthopedic Surgery
Duke University
Durham, North Carolina

Nathan Summers, MD

Stephanie J. Swensen, MD
Resident Physician
Department of Orthopaedic Surgery
New York University Hospital for Joint
    Diseases,
New York, New York

Monica Tafur, MD
Joint Department of Medical Imaging
University Health Network
Mount Sinai Hospital and Women's College
    Hospital
Toronto, Ontario, Canada

Timothy Lang Tan, MD
Resident
Department of Orthopaedic Surgery
Rothman Institute
Philadelphia, Pennsylvania

David P. Taormina, MD
New York University Hospital for Joint
    Diseases
New York, New York

Majd Tarabichi, MD
Research Fellow
Department of Research
Rothman Institute
Philadelphia, Pennsylvania

Sam Tarabichi, MD
Director General & Consultant Orthopedic
Surgeon
Burjeel Hospital for Advanced Surgery
Dubai, United Arab Emirates

Dean C. Taylor, MD
Duke Sports Science Institute
Department of Orthopedic Surgery
Duke University
Durham, North Carolina

Kimberly Templeton, MD
Professor of Orthopaedic Surgery
Department of Orthopaedic Surgery
University of Kansas Medical Center
Kansas City, Kansas

Emmanuel Thienpont, MD, MBA
Department of Orthopaedic Surgery
University Hospital Saint Luc
Brussels, Belgium

Nicholas T. Ting, MD
Department of Orthopaedic Surgery
RUSH University Medical Center
Chicago, Illinois

Marc A. Tompkins, MD
Assistant Professor
Department of Orthopaedic Surgery
University of Minnesota
Minneapolis, Minnesota

Gehron Treme, MD
Department of Orthopaedic Surgery
University of New Mexico
Albuquerque, New Mexico

Alfred J. Tria, Jr., MD
Clinical Professor of Orthopaedic Surgery
Department of Orthopaedic Surgery
Robert Wood Johnson Medical School;
Chief of Orthopaedic Surgery
Division of Orthopaedic Surgery
St. Peters University Hospital
New Brunswick, New Jersey

Hans K. Uhthoff, MD, FRCSC
Professor Emeritus
Department of Surgery
University of Ottawa
Ottawa, Ontario, Canada

Uchenna O. Umeh, MD
Assistant Professor of Anesthesiology
Department of Anesthesiology,
    Perioperative Care and Pain Medicine
New York University Langone Medical
    Center
New York, New York

Thomas Parker Vail, MD
James L. Young Professor and Chairman
Department of Orthopaedic Surgery
University of California, San Francisco
San Francisco, California

Douglas W. Van Citters, PhD
Assistant Professor
Thayer School of Engineering at
    Dartmouth College
Hanover, New Hampshire

Geoffrey S. Van Thiel, MD, MBA
OrthoIllinois
Rockford, Illinois

Rishi Vashishta, MD
Resident
Department of Anesthesiology,
    Perioperative Care, and Pain Medicine
New York University Langone Medical
    Center
New York, New York

Haris S. Vasiliadis, MD, PhD
Orthopädie Sonnenhof
Bern, Switzerland;
Molecular Cell Biology and Regenerative
    Medicine
Sahlgrenska Academy, University of
    Gothenburg
Gothenburg, Sweden

Sebastiano Vasta, MD
Department of Orthopaedics and Trauma
    Surgery
University Campus Bio Medico of Rome
Rome, Italy

Jan Victor, MD, PhD
Full Professor of Orthopedics and
    Traumatology
Ghent University;
Chair Department of Orthopedics and
    Traumatology
University Hospital Ghent
Ghent, Belgium

Jonathan M. Vigdorchik, MD
Assistant Professor of Orthopaedic Surgery,
Co-Director of Robotics
New York University Langone Hospital for
    Joint Diseases
New York, New York

Shaleen Vira, MD
Resident Physician
Department of Orthopaedic Surgery
New York University Hospital for Joint
    Diseases
New York, New York

Pramod B. Voleti, MD
Department of Orthopaedic Surgery
Montefiore Medical Center
New York, New York

Brian E. Walczak, MD
Department of Orthopedic Surgery and
    Rehabilitation
Division of Sports Medicine
University of Wisconsin—Madison
Madison, Wisconsin

Andrew Waligora, MD

Andrew Wall, MD

Daniel M. Walz, MD
Assistant Professor
Department of Radiology
Hofstra-North Shore LIJ School of
    Medicine
Great Neck, New York

Lucian C. Warth, MD
Assistant Professor
Department of Orthopaedic Surgery;
Assistant Director of Lower Extremity
    Adult Reconstruction Fellowship
Indiana University School of Medicine
Indianapolis, Indiana

Christopher W. Wasyliw, MD

Jonathan N. Watson, MD
Department of Orthopaedic Surgery
University of Illinois at Chicago
Chicago, Illinois

Nicholas P. Webber, MD
Medical Director
Sarcoma Services and Orthopaedic
    Oncology at Aurora Cancer Care;
Chief of Orthopaedics
Aurora St. Lukes Medical Center
Aurora Healthcare
Milwaukee, Wisconsin

Jennifer Weiss, MD
Southern California Permanente Medical
    Group
Los Angeles Medical Center
Los Angeles, California

Barbara N. Weissman, MD
Vice Chair Emeritus
Professor of Radiology
Harvard Medical School;
Musculoskeletal Radiologist
Brigham and Women's Hospital
Boston, Massachusetts

Jarrett D. Williams, MD
Department of Orthopedic Surgery
New York University Langone Medical
    Center
New York, New York

Riley J. Williams III, MD
Attending Surgeon
Department of Orthopaedic Surgery
Hospital for Special Surgery;
Associate Professor
Department of Orthopaedic Surgery
Weill Medical College of Cornell University
New York, New York

Adam S. Wilson, MD
Resident
Department of Orthopaedic Surgery
University of Virginia
Charlottesville, Virginia

Robert J. Wilson II, BA, MD
Orthopaedic Surgical Resident
Vanderbilt Department of Orthopaedics
    and Rehabilitation
Vanderbilt Orthopaedic Institute
Nashville, Tennessee

Lisa Mouzi Wofford, MD
Assistant Professor
Department of Anesthesiology
Baylor College of Medicine
Houston, Texas

Paul Woods, MD, MS
Senior Vice President
Physician Networks
Trinity Health
Livonia, Michigan

Clint Wooten, MD
Orthopedic Surgeon
Mountain Orthopedic
Bountiful, Utah

Ate Wymenga, MD, PhD
Consultant Orthopedic Surgeon
Department of Orthopedic Surgery
Saint Maartenskliniek
Nijmegen, The Netherlands

John W. Xerogeanes, MD
Department of Orthopaedic Surgery
Emory University
Atlanta, Georgia

Grace Xiong, MD

Zaneb Yaseen, MD

Yi-Meng Yen, MD, PhD, MS
Assistant Professor of Orthopaedic Surgery
Harvard Medical School
Boston Children's Hosptial
Boston, Massachusetts

Richard S. Yoon, MD
Division of Orthopaedic Trauma and
    Complex Adult Reconstruction
Department of Orthopaedic Surgery
Orlando Regional Medical Center
Orlando, Florida

Adam C. Young, MD, BS
Assistant Professor
Director of Acute Pain Service
Department of Anesthesiology
Rush University Medical Center
Chicago, Illinois

Stephen Yu, MD
Adult Reconstruction Research Fellow
Department of Orthopaedic Surgery
New York University Hospital for Joint
    Diseases
New York, New York

Biagio Zampogna, MD
Department of Orthopaedics and Trauma
    Surgery
University Campus Bio Medico of Rome
Rome, Italy

Ian M. Zeller, BS, MS
Graduate Research Assistant
Department of Mechanical, Aerospace and
    Biomedical Engineering
University of Tennessee
Knoxville, Tennessee

Adam C. Zoga, MD
Associate Professor
Department of Radiology
Thomas Jefferson University;
Vice Chair for Clinical Practice
Department of Radiology
Thomas Jefferson University Hospital
Philadelphia, Pennsylvania

FOREWORD

It is fair to say that *the Insall & Scott Surgery of the Knee* series has served as the definitive chronicle to the evolution of modern reconstructive surgery of the knee. So it is with the Sixth Edition of this comprehensive textbook that we, as interested readers, are once again privileged to avail ourselves of this carefully curated knowledge from today's leaders in knee surgery. It is a vibrant time to be a knee surgeon as intellectual excitement permeates our field and opportunities to alleviate pain and improve function for our patients continue to expand.

As an orthopedic community we are indebted to the foresight of John Insall and W. Norman Scott to recognize in the early 1980s the coming sea-change in the efficacy of knee surgery and to initiate the process that captured that collective knowledge in written form. Knee surgery has progressed dramatically over the past four decades from a last-resort option reserved for the markedly disabled to a largely elective surgical option that definitively improves the quality of life for patients with a spectrum of problems involving the bone, cartilage, or ligaments of the knee. Within the field of knee replacement, Dr. Insall helped carefully push the boundaries of patient age and activity that now allow us to successfully treat a wide spectrum of patients with knee arthroplasty. Within the field of ligament reconstruction, Dr. Scott brought to light what was possible at the highest levels of sport after cruciate ligament reconstruction. Together Drs. Insall & Scott shared a vision of improving patient care and advancing the understanding of reconstructive knee surgery for which we all have reaped benefit.

The Sixth Edition continues the long and academically rich history associated with this text that began in 1984. This series was so thoughtfully conceived that every surgeon performing total knee arthroplasty today could improve their fundamental understanding of contemporary knee replacement surgery by reading Dr. Insall's chapter on surgical technique and instrumentation from the First Edition. Subsequent versions of the textbook have preserved the fundamental spirit of the original which was to be at once comprehensive yet still accessible and relevant for the practicing orthopedic surgeon. The editor of the Sixth Edition has wisely chosen from amongst today's experts in contemporary knee surgery and the individual chapters are written in keeping with that spirit of comprehensive yet accessible and relevant. With national and international experts authoring each chapter the depth and breadth of real-world experience is evident throughout each of the chapters in this text.

The Sixth Edition *of Insall & Scott Surgery of the Knee* incorporates a broad international perspective that recognizes the rich contributions that surgeons from around the globe make to the field of knee surgery. Technology has fostered broader connections amongst orthopedic surgeons in disparate parts of the world and has quickened the pace of discovery and translation of new ideas into clinical practice. The Sixth Edition incorporates such technology and includes robust, high-quality illustrations, video demonstrations, and advanced electronic media resources that aid the process of education for the interested reader. The combination of text, illustration, and video material has been carefully balanced and clearly hits the mark for educational excellence.

I invite you to enjoy this textbook as more than just a source for knowledge about knee surgery. Insall & Scott's Surgery of the Knee also captures the energy, enthusiasm, and intellectual curiosity of today's most creative, innovative, and industrious knee surgeons. I hope that excitement is evident to you as a reader and inspires you to continually improve your individual skills and to support our collective-efforts to improve knee surgery for patients in our communities, patients nationwide, and patients world-wide.

Mark W. Pagnano, MD
Professor and Chairman
Department of Orthopaedic Surgery
Mayo Clinic
Rochester, Minnesota

FOREWORD

When the late Dr. John Insall wrote the preface of the First Edition of *Insall & Scott Surgery of the Knee* in 1984, he already had a vision of a comprehensive evolutionary textbook related exclusively to knee pathology and surgery. Some 33 years later this book is now in its Sixth Edition due to the continued efforts and innovations brought by Dr. Insall's original partner and friend Dr. W. Norman Scott. This book is not only covering all aspects of knee surgery such as ligament reconstruction, meniscus disease, cartilage repair, fractures about the knee, and knee arthroplasty, but also is considering the clinical, anatomical, biomechanical, and imaging evaluation of the knee joint. This book is also considering the patient himself in terms of demographic differences, expectations of the surgery, and perioperative management such as postoperative pain control.

The computer world has overwhelmed the field of continuous medical education and the Sixth Edition of *Insall & Scott Surgery of the Knee* has beautifully taken up the challenge of providing, both for the young and committed orthopedic surgeons, an evolving video technique section to maintain the status of the book as current as possible. This Sixth Edition also expands the world-wide contributions from the United States, Europe, and Asia, focusing on all aspects of clinical examinations, MRI imaging, knee anatomy, sports medicine, and reconstructive knee surgical techniques. Dr. Insall's decision in the First Edition was to reach out of the walls of his own hospital in New York City in order to include additional expertise. This Sixth Edition of *Insall & Scott Surgery of the Knee* further expands the horizon across the oceans, East, and West, with more than 20 chapters from International contributors.

Understanding the biomechanics of the knee starts with a correct comprehension of the anatomy and Rayesh Maniar from India describes the features of the Asian knee. The field of articular cartilage repair has now reached the time of maturity, consensus, while controversies will continue to be beneficial in the pursuit of progress. Lars Peterson from Sweden provides an international overview and results with autologous chondrocyte implantation techniques. Dr. Pinczewski from Australia, a pioneer in ACL reconstruction, and Dr. Kim from Korea likewise for PCL reconstruction, demonstrate their own vast experiences. The surgical correction of bony deformity both for the patella-femoral or the tibio-femoral joint has always been a trade-mark of the Lyon school in France, and respectively, Dr. Dejour and Dr. Neyret with their co-authors detail their own specific contribution.

Considering the knee as three separate articulations has led to selective compartmental replacement, a tradition in Europe for several decades. Contributions in that field come from the United Kingdom with Chris Dodd; Italy with Paolo Adravanti and Francesco Benazzo; Belgium with Emmanuel Thienpont; and France with Jean-Noel Argenson, Matthieu Ollivier, and Sebastien Parratte. The last three decades in the field of total knee arthroplasty has been fraught with debates, controversies, and most importantly success. The Sixth Edition of *Insall & Scott Surgery of the Knee* includes PCL retaining or substituting options provided respectively by Ate Wymenga from the Netherlands and Sam Tarabichi from the Middle East. Dr. Schindler from the UK and Dr. Matsumoto from Japan reflect on the debate regarding resurfacing of the patella or not. Both inside and outside the United States we are seeing new interpretations about alignment considerations and surgical options to obtain a mobile and stable knee after the arthroplasty. Johan Bellemans and Jan Victor from Belgium discuss the issues exhaustively. Intraarticular or extraarticular deformities at the time of total knee arthroplasty are world-wide challenges and Shuichi Matsuda from Asia and Andrea Baldini for Europe accurately describe their successful approaches. These surgical techniques are also often applicable to the use of specific technologies such as computer, robotics, or custom guides, and Emmanuel Thienpont details these approaches in an expert fashion.

The Sixth Edition of *Insall & Scott Surgery of the Knee* maintains this book's reputation as "The" reference for knee surgery providing the orthopedic surgeon from the United States, Europe, Middle East, or Asia with a considerable number of principles, details, and experiences covering all aspects of knee pathology, evaluation, and surgical treatments. While the spirit of late Dr. John Insall is still evident in the Sixth Edition of *Insall and Scott Surgery of the Knee,* the considerable and unique contributions of Dr. W. Norman Scott and his section editors in the organization of this book and its video section is now even more evident with the inclusion of so many international innovators and experts throughout the world.

Jean-Noel A. Argenson, MD
Professor and Chairman
Department of Orthopedic Surgery
The Institute for Locomotion, Aix-Marseille University
Marseille, France

It would have been inconceivable 33 years ago when the First Edition of this text book was drafted that the success of knee surgery would lead to a revolutionary approach to health care economics and care delivery. The projected increase of demand for total knee replacement over the next 20 years and the current and projected cost of the procedure have caused the value based health care movement to focus on the treatment of arthritis of the knee. For the first time, *Insall & Scott Surgery of the Knee* has focused an entire section (Economics, Quality, and Payment Paradigms for Total Knee Arthroplasty) on the value based issues facing knee surgeons in the next decade.

Since the passage of the Patient Protection and Affordable Care Act (PPACA) in 2010 and Medicare Access and CHIPS Reauthorization Act (MACRA) in 2015, the Center for Medicare and Medicaid Services (CMS) has been mandated to transform from a passive consumer to an active purchaser of health care. Orthopaedic surgeons are well positioned to provide leadership and detailed analysis of the processes related to the provision of orthopaedic care. Early and active involvement by orthopaedic surgeons in the development and implementation of care improvement processes in bundled payment systems such as the BPCI, CJR and any future initiatives is critical for the efficacy and sustainability of value-based orthopaedic care pathways. Moreover, orthopaedic surgeons need to be involved in all components of health care delivery that impact the care of their patients in order to preserve access and maintain affordability. In the next 5 years, physicians will be individually held accountable for cost and quality measures affecting their patients. The Merit Based Incentive Payment System (MIPS) will change reimbursement from not just a hospital at risk, quality driven model but also to a physician at risk, quality driven model.

The Bundled Payment for Care Initiative (BPCI) was begun in 2013 by CMS. Under the voluntary BPCI program, organizations entered into payment arrangements that include financial and performance accountability for episodes of care. A successful BPCI requires that quality is maintained and that care is delivered at a lower cost. CJR is a mandatory extension of Model 2 BPCI with hospital quality and Patient Reported Outcome Measures (PROM's) reporting requirements in addition to financial performance measures. This requires physicians and hospitals to align their interests and in this context, orthopaedic surgeons must assume a leadership role in cost-containment, surgical safety, and quality assurance so that cost-effective care is provided. Because most orthopaedic surgeons practice independently and are not hospital-employed, models of physician-hospital alignment such as physician-hospital organizations or contracted gainsharing arrangements between practices and hospitals may be necessary for bundled pricing to succeed. Under BPCI, hospitals, surgeons, or third parties can share the rewards, but also assume the risk for the bundle. It is forecast that most TKA cases covered under private and public insurance will be compensated under a bundled, quality driven program within the next 5 years.

For patients, cost savings must be associated with maintenance or improvement in quality metrics. However, the manner in which quality is defined and measured and what processes and outcomes are rewarded can vary. Risk-stratified allowances for nonpreventable complications must be incorporated into bundled pricing agreements to prevent the exclusion of patients with significant comorbidities and the anticipated higher care costs. Bundled pricing depends on economies of scale for success and it may not be appropriate for smaller orthopaedic groups or hospitals, where one costly patient could impact the success of the entire program. Furthermore, significant investment in infrastructure is required to develop programs to improve the quality and coordination of care, to manage quality data, and to distribute payments. Perhaps, smaller groups of surgeons can be joined together under advanced alternative payment models in the future so that all patients can benefit from bundled, value-based care.

In the current unsustainable healthcare environment, hospitals and administrators are facing increased pressure to optimize the value equation by decreasing the risk of complications. The ethical implications of reducing provider (physician and hospital) complication rates following joint replacement is compelling. Additionally, public transparency concerning provider complication rates would help patients make more informed decisions as to where to have their TJA performed. Nevertheless, it is morally incumbent on providers and policy makers to aggressively explore options for lowering cost while maintaining access and improving quality. Patients, physicians, and health care administrators must begin to see themselves acting not just as individuals involved in the decision to undergo TKA, but rather, as part of a system that administers health care within a larger societal context. It is simply unsustainable for surgeons and hospitals to perform elective surgery in higher risk patients with modifiable risk factors without increasing efforts to reduce them. Risk modification is a component of a larger, new era of medicine in which all stakeholders ought to accept some share of responsibility to create a safer, more cost-efficient health system. As TKA surgery shows, true shared decision making which involves patients, their physicians, the hospital, and the payers in a paradigm where interventions are provided only after modifiable risk factors have been addressed, can be an effective tool for delivering high quality, ethical health care at a reasonable price with a minimum of complications. We hope the information provided within the Sixth Edition of *Insall & Scott Surgery of the Knee* will help make this transition easier for all knee surgeons and the patients they care for.

Joseph D. Zuckerman, MD
Richard Iorio, MD
Dr. William and Susan Jaffe Professor of Orthopaedic Surgery
Chief Division of Adult Reconstructive Surgery
Department of Orthopaedic Surgery
New York University Langone Medical Center
Hospital for Joint Diseases
New York, New York

PREFACE

Why write a textbook in 2017? All pertinent information is now at our fingertips, the APP should be sufficient (if it works!) right? Electronic media is all we need or is it? Search engines are often "a mile wide and an inch deep" in detailing medical specifics in general and subspecialty knowledge in particular. Just think of our patients "surfing the net" and becoming fully cognizant of all aspects of knee surgery! Thus the need for a textbook for the lifelong students of the diagnosis and treatment of knee disorders.

Obviously the successes achieved in the field of knee surgery since the 1970s are absolutely incredible. The prefaces for the last five editions of *Insall & Scott Surgery of the Knee* are included in the Sixth Edition to reflect the historical perspective and to illustrate "how far we've (patients and physicians) come." And if we are to continue succeeding we need to learn by past mistakes to minimize the future ones.

Welcome to the Sixth Edition of *Insall & Scott Surgery of the Knee* (and yes we do have a companion electronic version).

The Sixth Edition of *Insall & Scott Surgery of the Knee* has greatly expanded on the Fifth Edition. Reviewing, refreshing and updating the excellent chapters of previous authors were, of course, a must. Almost all of these lead contributors added new authors to assure the viewer would receive the most recent subject information. The Sixth Edition, unlike the Fifth, has two complete volumes, and is accompanied not only by an e-version (at expertconsult.com) but also by an enhanced video section and a glossary. There are 14 sections and more than 78 new chapters!

Dr. Henry Clarke, the section editor for Basic Science has in this section enhanced the multifaceted anatomic perspective. I believe this comprehensive (microscopic, gross, arthroscopic, and radiographic) anatomy section is the best in the knee literature.

Dr. Jenny Bencardino, an orthopedic radiologist has taken over the imaging section of *Insall & Scott Surgery of the Knee* and has added 4 new chapters with the help of 14 expert radiologists. Similarly, Rick Komistek, PhD has updated the excellent Biomechanics section (Section III) with two new chapters.

One of the two largest sections of the Sixth Edition of *Insall & Scott Surgery of the Knee* has been organized and completed by associate editor, David Diduch. David has worked with section editors Asheesh Bedi and Geoff Baer to present 53 chapters spanning the basic science, diagnoses, and treatment of cartilage, ligament, and patella femoral conditions. This is an awesome contribution to the education of the innumerable "sports medicine" students throughout the world.

Dr. Andrew Franks, a renowned Professor of Rheumatology and Dermatology has once again modernized and updated the fundamental aspects of diagnosing and treating the most common systemic arthritic conditions that orthopedists will encounter. Topics such as gout and other crystalline arthropathies, psoriatic arthritis, degenerative arthritis, and rheumatoid arthritis are discussed succinctly. Dr. Franks has also devoted a chapter to arthropathies associated with hemophilia and pigmented villondular synovitis and discussed in detail a subject pertinent to all reconstructive orthopedic surgeons, systemic allergic dermatitis in total knee arthroplasty (TKA).

One of orthopedic surgery's major advances in patient care has been the diminution of postoperative complications and more recently patients' postoperative discomfort. It is for this reason that we have devoted an entire section to anesthesia for knee surgery. Dr. Arthur Atchabahian has put this section, "Anesthesia for Knee Surgery," together by stressing different aspects: preoperative evaluation, perioperative management of inpatient and ambulatory procedures, and a section on peripheral nerve blocks. These chapters are well organized, practical, concise, and essential for successful patient care. The orthopedist needs to be cognizant of these pain modality specifics.

Wound problems are the bane of any orthopedic procedures and we are once again honored to have Drs. Susan Scott and Robert Reiffel discuss prevention and treatment of these situations, which left unrecognized or untreated will destroy any knee arthroplasty.

Under the direction of Dr. George Haidukwych, the discussions and treatments of fractures about the knee have been updated with more recent data supporting alternative treatments. This is especially helpful in the treatment of periprosthetic fractures, an increasing problem due to the abundance of replacements in more active patients.

The overlap of treating pediatric, adolescent, and adult knee conditions is often daunting for the nonpediatric orthopedist. Dr. Min Kocher and his contributors in Section XI skillfully updated the eight chapters on pediatric knee problems; these chapters now allow all orthopedists to be current and to undertake treatments or, if necessary, to refer patients appropriately.

The largest section in the book, Sections XII A and XII B, Joint Replacement and Its Alternatives and Revision Complex Knee Arthroplasty, consists of 59 chapters and to my knowledge, is the most comprehensive compendium of an exhaustive discussion on these topics in one textbook. These sections represent an international approach to knee arthroplasty and the authors are pioneers and active clinicians in this discipline. In particular, Dr. Arlen Hanssen's contributions to the world of knee arthroplasty are legendary, and this section, thankfully, has his fingerprints all over it!

The other contributors in Sections XII A and XII B, too numerous to mention in a Preface, truly comprise the majority of worldwide knee arthroplasty innovators, surgeons, academicians, and teachers to us all. This section is a "must read" for any serious student in the field of knee arthroplasty.

In addition to the obvious importance of design and surgical technique in the world of knee arthroplasty, we as surgeons have continued to strive to make our patients safe, comfortable, happy, and convinced that they experienced both an excellent and cost effective knee arthroplasty procedure.

As section editor, Dr. Rich Iorio has enhanced the Sixth Edition of *Insall & Scott Surgery of the Knee* by discussing in over 20 chapters the present day approach to perioperative and hospital management of our patients in a comprehensive cost effective paradigm. In today's complicated and controversial health care environment, these chapters represent the foundation for the future of cost effective *and* superb care for our patients.

Mary O'Connor has once again assembled an outstanding faculty to discuss "Tumors about the Knee". From evaluation to diagnosis (benign or malignant) and treatment (local, extensive, or even a situation requiring a mega prosthesis) the authors have done an excellent job in providing us with current and practical approaches to treating these tumors.

As mentioned, the Sixth Edition of *Insall & Scott Surgery of the Knee* will once again include an extensive video section. In the Fifth Edition, we had 168 videos which we have now expanded to approximately 236 technique-oriented videos. In addition to this update of pediatric, sports, and knee arthroplasty surgical techniques, we plan to remain current, to add approximately 10-12 videos of both surgical techniques and superb seminars on a monthly basis until the publication of the Seventh Edition of *Insall & Scott Surgery of the Knee*. This approach, I believe, allows the book to never be out of date.

In a similar fashion the glossary of knee prosthesis has been updated and we thank the various companies' voluntary submissions. We requested the companies' cooperation, without any compensation or advertising, and are delighted with their collective enthusiasm. We also have the ability to electronically update our glossary and have invited all companies to take advantage of this educational opportunity.

I would personally like to thank my associate editors, Drs. Diduch and Hanssen; all the section editors and all the contributors, Residents, Fellows, attendings, private practitioners, academicians, and professors. All of us students working together to advance our subspecialty are rewarded when we see our patients' happiness and gratitude.

W. Norman Scott, MD

PREFACE TO THE FIFTH EDITION

There is nothing that "succeeds like success," and for the last five decades the treatment of knee disorders has been a major success story. From the First Edition of *Surgery of the Knee* to the present Fifth Edition, inclusive of approximately 1000 National and International contributors, we have been fortunate to chronicle these tremendous advancements. Although history is often overlooked, we think it is important, so important in fact, that we have included the prefaces for the first four editions of *Surgery of the Knee* to hopefully facilitate the progressive understanding of the anatomic, physiologic, clinical, diagnostic, and therapeutic advances that allow students of the knee to "push the envelope" even further. It requires, however, an understanding of the historical failures in the scientific pursuit of helping our patients if we are to minimize the chances of repeating past mistakes and hopefully avoid future ones. The authors throughout this edition attempt to highlight these potential pitfalls.

The Fifth Edition of *Surgery of the Knee* contains one textbook, a complete e-version, an e-glossary of knee implants, and a video section that we believe is the most comprehensive sports and adult reconstruction video section in any knee textbook. The book has 14 sections, 2 more than the previous edition, and 153 chapters written by almost 200 worldwide contributors. The Fifth Edition will be enhanced by quarterly updates in a video journal format and updates to the glossary of knee replacement designs, past and present, as presented by all the manufacturers who chose to participate. Similar to the quarterly updates, the manufacturers will have the opportunity to update their prosthetic designs to keep the information timely.

In Section 1, Basic Science of Anatomy, Anatomic Aberrations, and Clinical Examination are updated and now include a more detailed video on the examination of the knee. Section 2, Imaging, has been rewritten by an orthopedic radiologist, Dan Walz, and presents the most current diagnostic criteria for knee imaging. Similarly, the Biomechanics section also has a new leader in Rick Komistek, who has assembled a stellar group of contributors.

The Sports Medicine section, almost a third of the book, has been spearheaded by David Diduch. It is a tremendous enhancement to the work of previous editors, and David's work in putting this section together has truly been Herculean! From articular cartilage biology and biomechanics, extensor mechanism issues, meniscal repair, resection, or replacement, isolated or combined cruciate and collateral ligament treatments, the information in the Fifth Edition is truly state of the art. And, of course will remain current via the aforementioned quarterly updates.

Section 7, developed by Andy Franks, pertains to the current concepts regarding the diagnosis of knee arthritis, both inflammatory and noninflammatory.

Sections 8 and 9 include updates on synovium, hemophilia, HIV, and plastic surgery as it relates to wound healing and skin coverage options about the knee.

In Section 10, George Haidukewych, once again, has done an outstanding job of organizing fractures about the knee and periprosthetic fractures, probably one of the major causes for TKR revision today.

Likewise, in Section 11, Min Kocher presents today's state of the art treatment of pediatric knee disorders, which will continue via the quarterly updates.

Section 12, Joint Replacement and Its Alternatives, includes another new feature, the International and National Roundtables Discussions. We believe that this approach really allows the reader to comprehend the international differences and similarities in understanding worldwide controversial areas. Gil Scuderi did an excellent job in organizing these discussions and the 40 other chapters encompassing the totality of the treatment of the arthritic knee. Similar to the other sections, the surgical video techniques enhance the learning experience.

Section 13 includes the extremely controversial orthopedic medical issues such as DVT prophylaxes management and comprehensive pain management protocols associated with knee surgery.

In Section 14, Mary O'Connor once again has her contributors present the latest evidence on treating tumors about the knee. The mega prosthesis chapter, of course, is often apropos to the nontumor arthritic or revision TKR and is necessary reading for the TKR revision surgeon.

A new feature on the e-version, the glossary of implants, is presented in the spirit of helping the practicing physician determine the implant that he or she is evaluating whether in a primary or revision setting. We thank the companies for their cooperation and welcome their updates since the glossary is presented as an e-version which does not require the rigors of print media.

In the last five decades, better understanding of the basic sciences has allowed the knee community to develop much more of a consensus in the treatment of the "sports knee" and the arthritic knee. From a surgical perspective, techniques are continuing to be refined but one has to question whether "better is now the enemy of good?" It is a fine line and the surgical techniques cannot be the sole indication for treatment. For instance, registries in joint replacement are often at odds with published series by experts. Is this an indication, surgical technique, or patient expectation problem? We must be able to address and solve these issues before the publication of the Sixth Edition of *Surgery of the Knee*.

In the 1980s, Dr. Insall penciled an often quoted statement that one should not perform a revision TKR, unless the etiology of the failure was thoroughly understood. If he were with us today, I am sure that he would likewise want us to ascertain the indications for procedures based on a careful analysis of resultant treatments, whether it be nonoperative or operative. Better analysis of patient demographics and expectations, design considerations, biologic advances, and evidence-based results will allow us to better develop the treatment of knee disorders as a science rather than just an art. Physicians specializing in knee disorders must understand the practical consequences of all treatments to truly give our patients the best advice.

Once again, a tremendous "thanks" to all our contributors who join me in hoping that the "knee student" truly gains from studying the text, e-version, videos, and updates in the Fifth Edition of *Surgery of the Knee!*

W. Norman Scott, MD

In 1984, John Insall almost single-handedly wrote the First Edition of *Surgery of the Knee*. There were only 24 contributors to that single volume. In 1993, the Second Edition had 40 contributors and 4 associate editors and consisted of 2 volumes. In 2001, we combined efforts (*The Knee*, Mosby, 1994) to enhance the Third Edition (159 contributors) of *Surgery of the Knee*. Thus in 17 years, 3 Editions were published, and now the Fourth Edition has published less than 5 years later. This shortened publication time reflects our interest in being current and in using the latest technology and leading experts to inform our readers. In this Fourth Edition of *Surgery of the Knee*, we have updated basic chapters and introduced new information utilizing text and visual aids (DVDs), and we are inaugurating a new feature, a companion online e-dition: www.scottkneesurgery.com. The e-dition website will include full text search, hyperlinks to PubMed, an image library, and monthly content updates, to minimize the customary complaint of the "perpetual lag" inherent with textbooks in general. Our goal is to create an interactive current environment for all students of the diagnosis and treatment of knee disorders.

The Fourth Edition of *Surgery of the Knee* has 12 sections, 112 chapters, and 191 international contributors. The DVD sections include (1) a classic video recorded in 1994 (Drs. Insall and Scott) detailing "Exposures, Approaches and Soft Tissue Balancing in Knee Arthroplasty"; (2) interactive anatomic and physical examination recordings, which enhance the material presented in Chapters 1, 2, 3, 5, 6, and 7; and (3) three commonly used minimally invasive surgical techniques for knee arthroplasty.

In Section I, Basic Science, Chapters 1 to 5, the core information presented in the Third Edition is updated. The DVD of the Anatomy Section is interactive with the imaging in Section II, so the reader can see the normal and abnormal findings side by side. Chapter 3, Clinical Examination of the Knee, now, as mentioned, has the added feature of an actual examination on the DVD to enhance the text.

Section III, Biomechanics, has been expanded under the guidance of A. Seth Greenwald, DPhil (Oxon), to include soft tissue and implant considerations that are essential to executing surgical decisions.

With the plethora of Internet information available to patients today, it behooves the knee physician to be absolutely familiar with the various nonoperative and operative alternatives for the treatment of articular cartilage and meniscal disorders (Section IV). Dr. Henry Clarke has done a magnificent job in assembling the innovators in the field. The 18 chapters in this section truly capture the basic science, including the potential of gene therapy, biomechanics, and various treatment options, presented in great detail with the most current results. The section is further highlighted by Dr. Clarke's algorithm for clinical management of articular cartilage injuries.

The advances in the treatment of knee ligament injuries since 1984 are, needless to say, overwhelming. The success achieved today in the treatment of ligament injuries would have been unimaginable 25 years ago. As Section Editor of Section V, Ligament Injuries, Dr. Fred Cushner has assembled most of the people associated with these improvements. The foundations for treatments, controversies, and specific techniques are well chronicled throughout this section. Similarly, Section VI, Patellar and Extensor Mechanism Disorders, represents an updated comprehensive review by Dr. Aglietti and surgical chapters by Drs. Fulkerson and Scuderi.

Sections VII and VIII are "must reads" for all knee clinicians. In addition to discussing the normal and abnormal synovium, we have recruited distinguished authors to discuss the application of current topics of concern to both the patient and clinician, e.g., HIV and hepatitis (Chapter 59), anesthesia for knee surgery (Chapter 60), and an understanding of reflex sympathetic dystrophy (Chapter 61). The orthopaedic knee surgeon must have an absolute awareness of the potential problems inherent in the skin about the knee. In Chapter 63, Soft-Tissue Healing, Drs. Susan Scott and Robert Reiffel give us a foundation for avoiding and treating these potential problems.

Section IX focuses on fractures about the knee and has been organized by Dr. George Haidukewych. These fracture experts have covered all the fractures that occur, including the difficult periprosthetic fractures. Treatment modalities are detailed and reflect the current options with the latest equipment.

Section X, Pediatric Knee, has been reinvigorated with the help of Carl Stanitski. We decided to present the orthopaedic pediatric approach, rather than the sole view-point of the knee physician who treats pediatric injuries. The section is well organized, comprehensive, and, I believe, an improvement over the Third Edition of *Surgery of the Knee*.

The largest section in this two-volume edition is Section XI, Joint Replacement and Its Alternatives. Dr. Gil Scuderi has organized this section of the surgical treatment of the arthritic knee, including osteotomy, unicompartment replacement, patellofemoral arthroplasty, total knee replacement, and the more challenging revision surgery. While establishing the indications and contraindications for techniques, he has been careful to include the identification and management of difficult complications, such as infection, bone defects, extensor mechanism disruption, blood management, and thrombophlebitis. The tremendous success achieved in knee arthroplasty has paralleled the improvements in surgical instrumentation. In this section, several authors have detailed the current concepts of computer and navigation surgery, a truly exciting recent development. In the aforementioned e-dition version of *Surgery of the Knee*, the first several streaming videos will focus on specific techniques. Thus, these chapters provide an excellent foundation for interpreting the subsequent e-version techniques.

Dr. Mary O'Connor has developed Section XII, Tumors about the Knee, in a concise, clinically rational framework for those physicians who do not necessarily treat many of these difficult problems. Chapters 106 to 112 are well written and are truly outstanding contributions to this text.

Surgery of the Knee is a text that includes audiovisual teaching aids and now a monthly means of communicating current information in a timely audiovisual manner. To me, it's very exciting, and I look forward to integrating the contributions of these authors into a rapidly current technology for the benefit of all our patients.

W. Norman Scott, MD

PREFACE TO THE THIRD EDITION

Twenty-five years ago, the adolescent with knee pain unresponsive to immobilization, with subsequent atrophy and increasing disability afterwards, underwent a totally unnecessary arthrotomy and meniscectomy, sometimes preceded by a very inaccurate athrography.

When symptoms persisted, the other meniscus was usually considered the source of discomfort, and the treatment was unsuccessfully repeated. Then, with the evolution of failed arthrotomies, the patella was believed to be the culprit. Unfortunately, there was no nonoperative or operative intervention that was universally successful. Surgically, distal and then proximal realignments were performed on almost all types of "chondromalacia" complaints. Anterior cruciate ligament injuries, if diagnosed, were treated in a spectrum from purposeful neglect to an assortment of combined intra- and extra-articular reconstructions. The recovery from these procedures was truly, in today's perspective, a tribute to the dedication of the patient and therapist and somewhat of a warning to avoid surgery!

Unfortunately, many of these patients' knee disorders led to posttraumatic arthritis unresponsive to most nonsteroidal anti-inflammatory medicines; thus, they were candidates for an osteotomy. Even though the osteotomy would probably not be indicated today, there were no other surgical options. Today, a better understanding of clinical diagnosis, imaging techniques, and rehabilitative modalities has eliminated many unnecessary surgeries. Arthroscopy has revolutionized the diagnosis and treatment of cartilage lesions and ligament disruptions. Total knee arthroplasty, on the other hand, has yielded unparalleled success in alleviating patients' discomfort while eliminating their disability.

This 25-year retrospective view is, I believe, somewhat predictive of how we will perceive the contribution of classic textbooks to continuing medical education. As we enter the digital century, if not millennium, it is increasingly difficult to accept the analog world's perpetual lag of inadequacy of the published word while attempting to enhance education and subsequently new breakthrough treatments for our patients. Thus, we have attempted in this two-volume comprehensive color text to "bridge the gap" between the analog and digital worlds. In combining our two previous textbooks, *Surgery of the Knee* and *The Knee,* we have solicited the contributions of national and international experts recognized worldwide by serious knee students.

This textbook consists of 95 chapters divided into 11 sections. In Basic Science (Section I) we have introduced an interactive CD-ROM combining the anatomic and imaging chapters. While we believe this approach, either by CD or through Internet access, is the future, practical considerations precluded us from presenting the entire book in this format at this time. The CD takes studying, browsing, and researching anatomy and imaging in a new direction. Thanks to Drs. Clarke and Pedersen, the CD contains an extensive collection of medical data pertaining to anatomy, anatomic aberrations, imaging, and surgical exposures. We believe this is truly a breakthrough in understanding comprehensive knee anatomy.

In Biomechanics (Section II), Dr. Michael Freeman has truly enhanced our understanding of the dynamics of knee motion in an extensive MRI-controlled model of knee motion. The remainder of this section reinforces basic principles of knee biomechanics and explains the relationship of the knee to normal and abnormal gait.

Healing articular cartilage defects has enticed orthopaedists since the beginning of our specialty. Today, the enthusiasm seems to be at fever pitch. Thus, we have included many, if not all, of the therapeutic approaches by the recognized international originators of the technique. From Europe to the United States, contributors lay the foundation for what will hopefully be therapeutic success in the year to come.

Although the more than 150 contributors to this edition are too numerous to focus on individually, there are some especially innovative chapters that deserve special attention. Chapter 41, "Revision ACL Surgery: How I Do It," allows the reader to see step-by-step the "pearls" of various experts on how they approach this difficult problem in the operating theater.

With increasing focus on recreational athletics, the problems with the pediatric knee are becoming more manifest. Thus, Chapters 64 to 68 give the reader the opportunity to learn from pediatric orthopaedists on normal growth and development, congenital deformities, physeal fractures, and dealing with ACL injuries in skeletally immature patients.

Almost a quarter of this text is devoted to knee replacement and surgical alternatives. The success of the former necessitates such an approach. Osteotomy, however, must not be forgotten; thanks to Drs. Hanssen and Poilvache, we get both the European and American perspective. The standard issues with knee replacement, designs, technique, thrombophlebitis, skin problems (Section VII), infection, and complications requiring revision surgery are extensively detailed. Just as with revision ACL surgery, there are six sections devoted to revision TKR surgery. The diversity of surgical approaches and "tips" is truly priceless.

It is a true honor to have collaborated with my mentor, partner, and, most importantly, friend in publishing this comprehensive text. Dr. Insall's published works on all aspects of knee surgery are unparalleled. For me to have continued my "residency" under his guidance for the past 2 years has been a gift beyond measure.

On behalf of all the authors, we hope that you, the reader, are stimulated by this text to learn, analyze your observations, challenge thoughtfully, and make a contribution that will ultimately help your patients!

W. Norman Scott, MD

This textbook is larger than before, a change made necessary by the many advances made in knee surgery since the First Edition was published 10 years ago. Radiology of the knee has been revolutionized by computed tomography (CT) and magnetic resonance imaging (MRI), which have added a degree of certainty to the diagnosis of meniscal and some ligament injuries. Clinical acumen and careful examination are, of course, still required, but when these state of the art investigations are available, precise diagnosis will avoid unnecessary surgery. The ligament chapters are completely new, reflecting greater understanding of the pathology of ligament injuries. The classification of these injuries was in disarray in the early 1980s without true recognition of the role of the cruciate ligaments in causing knee instability. Anteromedial and anterolateral instabilities and the tests for their diagnosis were previously discussed without mentioning the anterior cruciate ligament (ACL), and it was still widely believed that the ACL was not an important stabilizer of the knee. Lesions of the posterior cruciate ligament (PCL) were also poorly understood, and the terminology was complexed and confusing. Due to the work of the late John Marshall and his successors, ligament injuries and laxities are today logically classified. The contribution to knee stability of the ACL in particular is universally accepted. It is fitting that Russell Warren, who followed Marshall as the Director of Sports Medicine at The Hospital for Special Surgery, coauthored the chapter on acute ligament injuries.

Arthroscopy was included in the First Edition only to outline general principles. Today such limited treatment is impossible because arthroscopy has become a major part of knee surgery. Norman Scott, who has himself written a text on arthroscopy, has comprehensively described the techniques and advances in this subspecialty.

The chapters on knee arthroplasty are all new. Very little has been carried over except for historical reference. Advances in knee prostheses and especially in surgical instrumentation and technique have made the operation reliable and predictable. A preeminent bioengineer, Peter Walker, has contributed the section on knee prosthesis design. Clement Sledge and C. Lowry Bames have written on PCL retention in knee arthroplasty, and Richard Scott describes the role of unicompartmental replacement. George Galante and Aaron Rosenberg make the case for cementless fixation. However, not all of these innovations have proven successful and new problems such as polyethylene wear have recently become a major clinical issue. Osteolysis caused by polyethylene debris is an even newer complication. The extent and severity of both problems will have to wait the passage of time and further evaluation.

I may have suggested in the earlier preface that I was a "complete" knee surgeon: even if this was once true, it most certainly is not today. I do not believe that one surgeon can be equally expert in all of the conditions that affect even a single joint such as the knee: for example, since 1984 over 500 articles have been published in the three major English language journals on the subject of total knee arthroplasty alone. Therefore, to prepare this edition, I have enlisted the help of four associate editors, all of whom I have trained at some stage of their careers and who have continued to work closely with me. In addition to their editorial functions, they have also contributed material of their own. Paolo Aglietti has revised his previous chapters on fractures of the knee and in this edition provides additional chapters on chronic ligament injuries and the management of the patellofemoral joint. Norman Scott, calling upon his vast experience in athletic injuries, has contributed chapters on arthroscopy and the classification of ligament injuries. Russell Windsor has written on the management of infection, arthrodesis, and soft-tissue disorders. Michael Kelly has revised the chapters on anatomy and physical examination. Between us it is hoped that we covered the material adequately.

Mrs. Martha Moore has labored on this edition as she did on the first one, again earning my profound gratitude. I also thank Ms. Virginia Ferrante and Ms. Elizabeth Roselius for the new illustrations.

John N. Insall, MD

If the 1960s saw a revolution in hip surgery, the knee had its turn during the 1970s. Much has changed and is still changing. Arthroscopic surgery has emerged as a new discipline; knee arthroplasty has become a reliable treatment for gonarthrosis; and concepts in the treatment of ligament injuries have altered radically in the last 10 years. Also, surgeons interested in the knee have separated into three groups, their major involvement being either in arthroscopy, sports medicine, or knee replacement. As one who has dabbled in all of these areas, it is my hope that this book will have some unifying benefit.

However, there is still no unanimity of opinion about how to treat all disorders of the knee joint, and for one who has the temerity to edit a textbook on the subject, there is the certain knowledge that he cannot please everyone. On the other hand, a textbook must have cohesion so that one chapter does not contradict the next. My solution to this dilemma is to present the current opinion and practice at The Hospital for Special Surgery, and, therefore, most of the contributors are past or present members of the staff. Where there are significant areas of controversy, I have also sought other viewpoints, notably on ligament surgery, the place of cruciate ligaments in knee arthroplasty, and the fixation of prosthetic components to bone. I have also reached beyond the walls of my own hospital for additional expertise, and well-known authorities have written chapters on osteochondrosis dissecans, hemophilia, surgical pathology of arthritis, and arthroscopy.

With regard to the chapter on arthroscopy, I foresee that this chapter may be considered too short in an era when arthroscopic surgery and knee surgery are becoming synonymous in the minds of many surgeons. This decision to keep this chapter short was made deliberately for two reasons: (1) Excellent textbooks devoted specifically to the techniques of arthroscopic surgery already exist, and (2) both Doctor McGinty and I felt that, because arthroscopic surgery has not been placed in full perspective, some currently popular arthroscopic techniques may become discredited with time.

I also decided not to include specific details of AO surgical techniques in the fracture chapter as these are also very well described elsewhere.

It would not have been possible to complete this book without the invaluable assistance of my secretary, Mrs. Martha Moore, who has put in as much effort as I and must now know every word and every reference by heart. I also wish to thank Ms. Joelle Pacht for her endless retyping of the manuscript, Miss Dottie Page and the Photographic Department at The Hospital for Special Surgery for their assistance in preparing the photographic material, and Mr. William Thackeray who has done most of the book's illustrations and drawings.

John N. Insall, MD

It would be impossible to undertake a book, especially a two volume e-version with 374 contributors and approximately 237 videos, without the unbelievable help of a dedicated team.

- Dr. Henrik Bo Pedersen has been extensively involved in the Third, Fourth, Fifth and now the Sixth Editions of *Insall & Scott Surgery of the Knee*. His devotion to detail has allowed us to produce "top of the line" photographs and videos that have been a major aspect of our success.
  Thank you, Henrik.

- Likewise, Ruth Pupke has been involved since the Third Edition. Her involvement has been immeasurable. Connecting editors, authors and their staff, and the publishers is a never ending task without which it's likely these editions would never have been produced.
  Thank you, Ruth.

- For 25 years, Kathleen Lenhardt has been the "hub" of the Insall Scott Kelly (ISK) Fellowship, (now the NYU Langone/ ISK Adult Reconstruction Fellowship). She has also been the person responsible for the organization of the selection process, and coordination of both the involvement of the Insall Travelling Fellowship with the Knee Society and the host medical centers throughout the United States. Her importance to this edition of *Insall & Scott Surgery of the Knee* is especially manifest in the number of ISK Fellows and Insall Travelling Fellows who are significant contributors to the Sixth Edition.
  Thank you, Kathy.

- Dina Potaris, last but certainly not least, is the "lynchpin" who kept everything together for the Sixth Edition of *Insall & Scott Surgery of the Knee*. She was the star!
  Thanks, Dina.

W. Norman Scott, MD

CONTENTS

ONLINE CONTENTS

View Expertconsult.com for periodic updates.

Basic Science

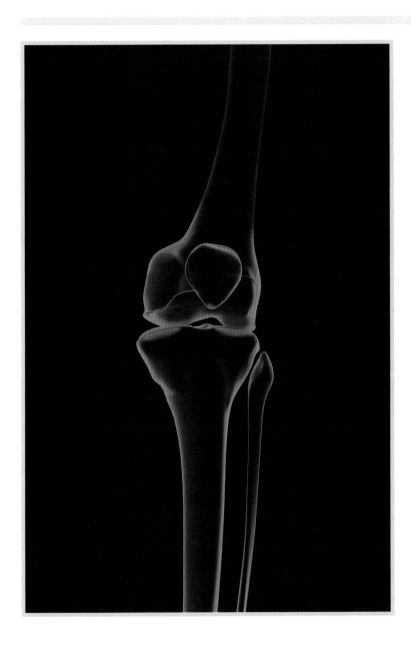

1

Anatomy*

*Henry D. Clarke, Mark J. Kransdorf, Christopher R. Conley,
Henrik Bo Pedersen, W. Norman Scott*

The anatomy of the knee can be examined on a number of levels from microscopic to gross and with a variety of techniques, including physical examination, anatomic dissection, radiographic and cross-sectional imaging, and arthroscopic examination. Any physician interested in diagnosing and treating disorders of the knee must have a detailed understanding of both normal and abnormal regional anatomy. Furthermore, the ability to interpret and correlate information obtained from different sources is highly beneficial. However, it is also paramount that the clinician gain the knowledge required to interpret the significance of an identifiable anatomic abnormality within the context of a patient's complaints. The goal of this chapter is to present a thorough review of knee anatomy to help the reader to successfully assimilate the material presented in subsequent chapters. To provide a comprehensive description of pertinent anatomic details, text, illustrations, arthroscopic photographs, radiographs, and pictures from cross-sectional imaging studies are used. In addition, in many situations the same structures are presented from different perspectives. Rather than being redundant, we hope that this approach will facilitate the development of a more complete appreciation of the anatomy of the knee. The descriptions that follow are taken in part from standard anatomic texts.[3,10,80,134]

NORMAL SKELETAL STRUCTURES

Bone Physiology

Bone is composed of mineral crystals embedded in an organic matrix. Of the dry weight of bone (~10% of the actual weight in situ), approximately 70% is mineral content and 30% is organic matter. The mineral primarily consists of calcium and phosphorus in a ratio of 2:1. The organic matter is composed of collagen, noncollagenized matrix, and proteins. Collagen is the main extracellular component of bone and is composed of fibrils. Collagen fibrils, which form a parallel, highly organized arrangement, are known as *intrinsic fibers*, whereas those that tend to anchor ligaments and tendons at attachment sites and often insert in a perpendicular manner are *extrinsic fibers*. The matrix is populated by mesenchymal cells, which differentiate into osteocytes, osteoblasts, and osteoclasts. These cells perform key functions in the turnover and remodeling of bone in

response to both physical and metabolic stimuli. Osteoblasts are cuboid in nature and have abundant cytoplasm. The main function of osteoblasts is to produce osteoid, a collagenized protein that mineralizes at the tidemark zone as hydroxyapatite crystals are incorporated (Fig. 1.1). As the matrix becomes mineralized bone, these cells become embedded and are transformed into osteocytes. The osteocyte is in contact with the osteoblast through the cannular system. Osteoclasts are multinucleated macrophage-like cells that perform bone resorption at mineralized bone surfaces (Fig. 1.2). Other associated tissues, such as periosteum (Fig. 1.3), fatty and hematopoietic marrow elements, and tendon and ligament attachments, create a complex system with mechanical, metabolic, and hematopoietic functions.

Bony Architecture

The knee joint consists of three bony structures—femur, tibia, and patella—that form three distinct and partially separated compartments: medial, lateral, and patellofemoral compartments.

Patella. The patella, the largest sesamoid bone in the body, sits in the femoral trochlea. It is an asymmetrical oval with its apex directed distally. The fibers of the quadriceps tendon envelop it anteriorly and blend with the patellar ligament distally. The articulation between the patella and the femoral trochlea forms the anterior or patellofemoral compartment (Fig. 1.4).

The posterior aspect of the patella is described as possessing seven facets. The medial and lateral facets are divided vertically into approximately equal thirds, whereas the seventh or odd facet lies along the extreme medial border of the patella. Overall, the medial facet is smaller and slightly convex; the lateral facet, which consists of approximately two-thirds of the patella, has both a sagittal convexity and a coronal concavity (Fig. 1.5). Six morphologic variants of the patella have been described (Fig. 1.6). Types I and II are stable, whereas the other variants are more likely to give rise to lateral subluxation, as a result of unbalanced forces.[12,133] The facets are covered by the thickest hyaline cartilage in the body, which may measure up to 6.5 mm in thickness.[133] The relationship between surface degeneration of this articular surface, or chondromalacia, seen arthroscopically in adolescents and young adults, and pain is unclear.

The femoral trochlea is separated from the medial and lateral femoral condyles by indistinct ridges; the lateral ridge is more prominent. The patella fits into the trochlea of the femur imperfectly, and the contact patch between the patella and the femur

*The authors thank John N. Insall for his thoughtful guidance and contributions to previous editions of this chapter and Kevin R. Math, Vincent J. Vigorita, and Fred D. Cushner for their prior work.

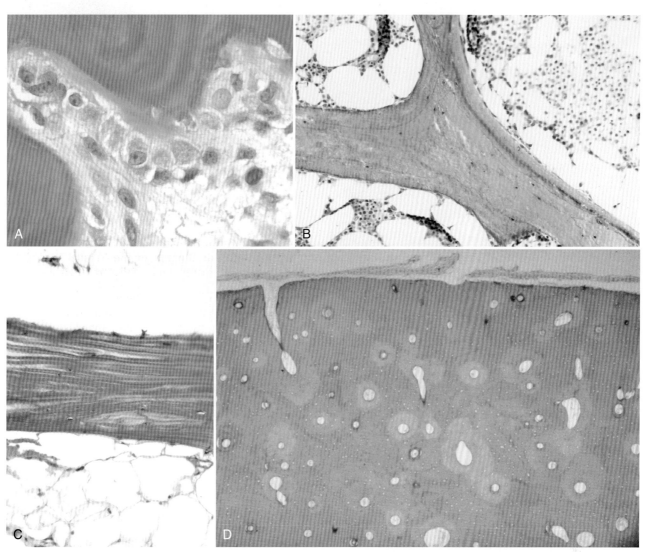

FIG 1.1 (A) Osteoblasts. Plump, cytoplasm-rich osteoblasts actively making osteoid, the type I collagen that in the normal sequence of events becomes the fibrous matrix of mineralized bone. (B) Normal cancellous (trabecular, spongy) bone bathed in normal hematopoietic marrow. Bone surfaces are smooth. Osteoid deposition (light pink surface) is interfaced with mature bone by the basophilic mineralization front. (C) Normal cancellous bone. With the use of polarized light microscopy, the organized lamellar or pleated deposition of the collagen matrix of mineralized bone is appreciated. (D) Cross-section of cortical bone showing numerous haversian systems of varying age. The cortical bone is surrounded on its surface by periosteum. The cortical bone itself is composed of haversian bone systems, which represent interwoven longitudinal, circumferential, and concentric bone-forming units (osteons) characterized by central haversian canals of various size and shape. Remodeling is ongoing throughout life; most of it occurs in an axial direction down the shaft.

varies with position as the patella sweeps across the femoral surface. The contact patch has been investigated by dye[44] and casting techniques.[2] Both methods produce very similar results and indicate that the area of contact never exceeds about one-third of the total patellar articular surface. At 10 to 20 degrees of flexion the distal pole of the patella first contacts the trochlea in a narrow band across the medial and lateral facets (Fig. 1.7).[44,61] As flexion increases, the contact area moves proximally and laterally. The most extensive contact is made at approximately 45 degrees, where the contact area is an ellipse in continuity across the central portion of the medial and lateral facets. By 90 degrees, the contact area has shifted to the upper part of the medial and

lateral patellar facets. With further flexion, the contact area separates into distinct medial and lateral patches.[2,44,61] Because the odd facet makes contact with the femur only in extreme flexion (such as in the act of squatting), this facet is habitually a noncontact zone in humans in Western cultures—which is thought to have some pathologic significance.

The main biomechanical function of the patella is to increase the moment arm of the quadriceps mechanism.[69] The load across the joint rises as flexion increases, but, because the contact area also increases, the higher force is dissipated over a larger area. However, if extension against resistance is performed, the force increases while the contact area shrinks, and

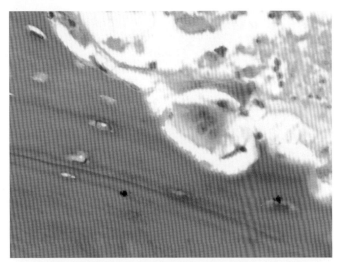

FIG 1.2 Osteoclast A multinucleated osteoclast is resorbing bone at a crenated surface, Howship lacuna.

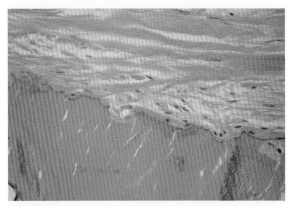

FIG 1.3 Periosteum The often inconspicuous, spindle-shaped, fibroblast-like cells of the periosteum belie their remarkable capacity to become activated as bone-forming cells.

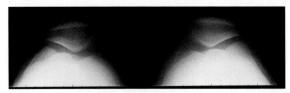

FIG 1.4 Merchant View Radiograph of a Normal Patello-femoral Joint The tibial tubercle is superimposed over the apex of the femoral trochlea.

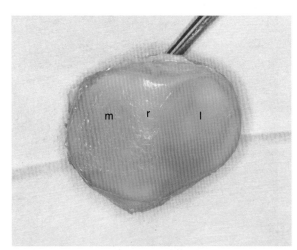

FIG 1.5 Articular Surface of the Patella The median ridge *(r)* divides the smaller medial facet *(m)* from the larger lateral facet *(l)*.

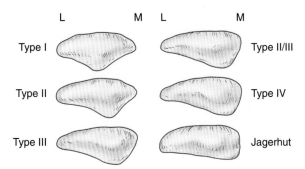

FIG 1.6 Wiberg and Baumgartl's Patella Types[12,133]

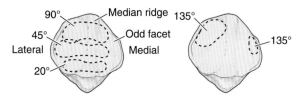

FIG 1.7 Patellofemoral Contact Areas at Different Degrees of Flexion.

this may exacerbate pain from the patellofemoral region. Straight-leg raises eliminate force transmission across the patellofemoral joint because in full extension the patella has not yet engaged the trochlea.[61]

Femur. The architecture of the distal end of the femur is complex. Furthermore, this area serves as the attachment site of numerous ligaments and tendons (Fig. 1.8). In shape and dimensions, the femoral condyles are asymmetrical; the larger medial condyle has a more symmetrical curvature. The lateral condyle viewed from the side has a sharply increasing radius of curvature posteriorly. The femoral condyles viewed from the surface, articulating with the tibia, show that the lateral condyle

is slightly shorter than the medial. The long axis of the lateral condyle is slightly longer and is placed in a more sagittal plane than the long axis of the medial condyle, which is oriented at a mean angle of approximately 22 degrees and opened posteriorly.[68] The lateral condyle is slightly wider than the medial condyle at the center of the intercondylar notch. Anteriorly, the condyles are separated by a groove known as the femoral trochlea (Fig. 1.9). The sulcus represents the deepest point in the trochlea. Relative to the midplane between the condyles, the sulcus lies slightly laterally.[33] Reproducing this anatomic relationship is important for accurate patellofemoral mechanics after total knee replacement.

The intercondylar notch separates the two condyles distally and posteriorly. The lateral wall of the notch has a flat impression, where the proximal origin of the anterior cruciate ligament (ACL) arises. On the medial wall of the notch is a larger site, where the posterior cruciate ligament (PCL) originates. The mean width of the notch is narrowest at the distal end and

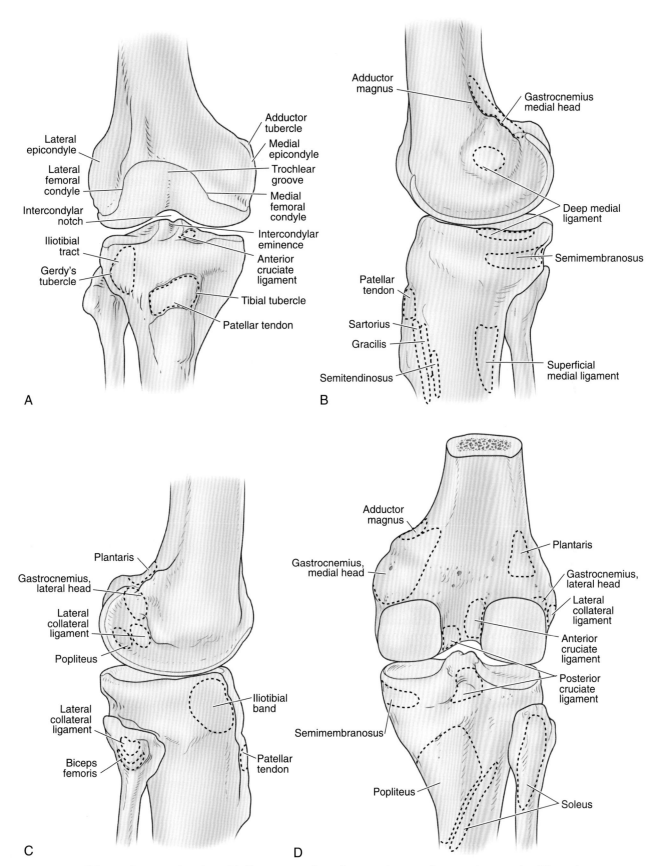

FIG 1.8 Bony landmarks with ligament and tendon attachment sites on the anterior (A), and medial (B). Medial (C) and posterior (D) aspects of the knee.

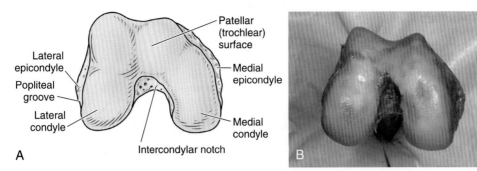

FIG 1.9 (A) Bony architecture of the distal femur. (B) Anatomic specimen of the distal femur. The femoral trochlea separates the lateral and medial femoral condyles. The deepest point lies slightly offset to the lateral side. The anterior aspect of the lateral condyle is more prominent than the medial side.

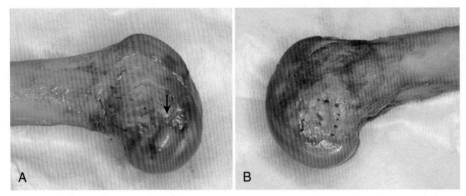

FIG 1.10 (A) Bony landmarks of the lateral aspect of the distal femur. The characteristic groove for the popliteus tendon lies just proximal to the articular surface of the lateral condyle. The prominence of the lateral epicondyle *(arrow)* is located posterior to this groove. (B) Bony landmarks of the medial aspect of the distal femur. The center of the sulcus of the C-shaped, ridgelike medial epicondyle *(both marked)* represents the center of attachment of the medial collateral ligament.

widens proximally (1.8 to 2.3 cm); in contrast, the height of the notch is greatest at the midportion (2.4 cm) and decreases proximally (1.3 cm) and distally (1.8 cm).[75] The dimensions of the notch have become an important topic because of the association between narrow notch width and increased risk for ACL tear. This risk does not seem to be related to the intrinsic characteristics of the ACL because normal-size ligaments have been identified in specimens with narrow notches.[94] Therefore the increased risk of ACL failure is probably because of impingement on the ligament.[43,77,94] Notchplasty or sculpting of the intercondylar notch to increase the dimensions has become an integral part of ACL reconstruction.

The lateral condyle has a short groove just proximal to the articular margin, in which lies the tendinous origin of the popliteus muscle. This groove separates the lateral epicondyle from the joint line. The lateral epicondyle is a small but distinct prominence to which the lateral (fibular) collateral ligament (LCL) is attached. On the medial condyle the prominent adductor tubercle is the insertion site of the adductor magnus. The medial epicondyle lies anterior and distal to the adductor tubercle and is a C-shaped ridge with a central depression or sulcus (Fig. 1.10). Rather than originating from the ridge, the medial collateral ligament (MCL) originates from the sulcus. The epicondylar axis passes through the center of the sulcus of the medial epicondyle and the prominence of the lateral epicondyle (Fig. 1.11). This line serves as an important reference line in total knee replacement.

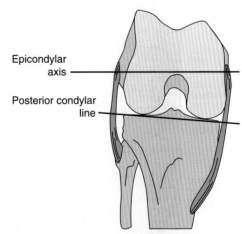

FIG 1.11 The epicondylar axis, which connects the prominence of the lateral epicondyle and the sulcus of the medial epicondyle, is externally rotated relative to the posterior condylar line.

In relation to a line tangent to the posterior femoral condyles, the epicondylar axis is externally rotated approximately 3.5 degrees in males and 1 degree in females with normal knees.[13] In patients with osteoarthritis and valgus knee alignment the transepicondylar axis has been shown to be externally rotated up to 10 degrees, relative to the posterior condylar line.[46]

In recent years, important anatomic variations in the morphology of the distal femur have been identified in males and females and in different racial groups. Measurements of the distal femur in both Asian and white populations suggest that women have narrower femurs in the medial-lateral dimension than males do, for any given anterior-posterior dimension.[14,20,22,54,84] This concept has been defined in terms of the aspect ratio of the distal femur, where the medial-lateral width is divided by the anterior-posterior dimension × 100.[20,54] In females the aspect ratio tends to be smaller than in males in both Asian and white populations.[20,54] However, this aspect ratio is also affected by race, with Japanese females displaying a greater medial-lateral width than white females, for any given anterior-posterior dimension.[124] In addition to these findings, racial differences appear to exist in the rotational anatomy of the distal femur, with more natural external rotation of the transepicondylar axis versus the posterior condylar line in Asian populations.[136] These racial differences and gender dimorphism among humans may have significant implications for both prosthesis development and surgical technique in total knee arthroplasty.[104] This information has stimulated vigorous debate regarding whether gender-specific femoral components and knee prostheses designed for different racial groups are needed.[29,45,84,92,124,126] In particular, implants with a narrower medial-lateral geometry for a given specific anterior-posterior dimension have been advocated by some for use in females.[45,54,84] A similar prosthesis has been suggested for use in Indian populations, among which greater variability in medial-lateral width for any given anterior-posterior dimension has been noted.[126] Although a gender bias has been demonstrated for some contemporary knee prostheses, it is unclear whether this bias has adversely affected the outcomes of total knee arthroplasty in females versus males.[34,54,91,92]

Tibia. In a macerated skeleton, inspection of the tibial plateau suggests that the femoral and tibial surfaces do not conform at all. The larger medial tibial plateau is almost flat and has a squared-off posterior aspect that is distinct on a lateral radiograph.[29] In distinction, the articular surface of the narrower lateral plateau borders on convexity. Both surfaces have a posterior inclination of approximately 10 degrees with respect to the shaft of the tibia. However, lack of conformity between the femoral and tibial articular surfaces is more apparent than real. In an intact knee the menisci enlarge the contact area considerably and increase the conformity of the joint surfaces. As previously noted for the femur, gender and race appear to affect the morphology of the proximal tibia.[54,76] This may again have implications for prosthesis design in total knee arthroplasty.[54,76] However, because flexibility in coverage and position of the tibial component are generally greater on the prepared surface of the tibial plateau in total knee arthroplasty, the implications of this variability have not been well researched at this time.

The median portion of the tibia between the plateaus is occupied by an eminence: the spine of the tibia. Anteriorly a depression is seen—the anterior intercondylar fossa—to which, from anterior to posterior, the anterior horn of the medial meniscus, the ACL, and the anterior horn of the lateral meniscus are attached. Behind this region are two elevations: the medial and lateral tubercles. They are divided by a gutter-like depression: the intertubercular sulcus. On an anteroposterior radiograph the medial tubercle usually projects more superiorly than the lateral tubercle; on a lateral radiograph the medial tubercle is located anterior to the lateral tubercle (Fig. 1.12). The tubercles do not function as attachment sites for the cruciate ligaments or menisci but may act as side-to-side stabilizers by projecting toward the inner sides of the femoral condyles. In concert with the menisci the tibial spine enhances the

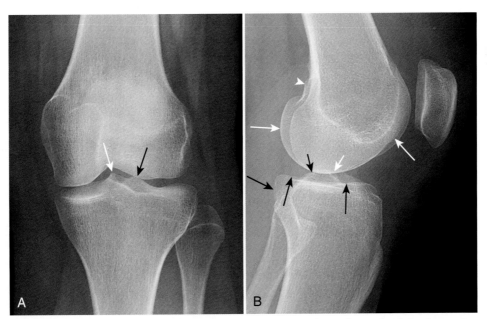

FIG 1.12 Normal Radiographic Anatomy (A) Anteroposterior radiograph of the knee shows the medial *(white arrow)* and lateral *(black arrow)* tubercles divided by a gutter-like depression. (B) Lateral radiograph showing the medial tubercle *(thin white arrow)* anterior to the lateral tubercle *(thin black arrow)*. Note the larger medial femoral condyle *(large white arrows)* with a more symmetrical radius of curvature. The inconstant adductor tubercle *(white arrowhead)* is a reliable marker for the medial femoral condyle when present. The larger medial tibial plateau is readably identified by its "squared-off" posterior margin *(large black arrows)*.

impression of cupping seen in intact specimens. In the posterior intercondylar fossa, behind the tubercles, the lateral and then the medial menisci are attached anteriorly to posteriorly. Most posteriorly the PCL inserts on the margin of the tibia between the condyles. On the anterior aspect of the tibia the tuberosity is the most prominent feature and is the attachment site of the patellar tendon. Approximately 2 to 3 cm lateral to the tibial tubercles is Gerdy's tubercle, which is the insertion site of the iliotibial band (ITB).

Tibiofibular Joint. In an embryo, both the fibula and the tibia are in contact with the femur. However, because the tibia grows at a faster rate than the fibula does, the distance from the femorotibial articulation to the fibula increases. The portion of the capsule that initially surrounds the knee is retained by the fibula and forms the superior tibiofibular joint. The articular surface of the head of the fibula is directed superiorly and slightly anteromedially to articulate with the posterolateral (PL) portion of the tibial metaphysis. The styloid process projects superiorly from the PL aspect of the fibula and is the insertion site for the LCL, biceps femoris tendon, fabellofibular ligament, and arcuate ligament.

The superior tibiofibular joint is lined with synovial membrane and possesses a capsular ligament that is strengthened by anterior and posterior ligaments. In contrast, the inferior tibiofibular joint is a syndesmosis, and the bones are joined by a strong intraosseous ligament. The intraosseous membrane originates from the intraosseous border of the fibula, and the fibers run distally and medially to attach to the intraosseous border of the tibia. A large opening that is present superiorly allows passage of the anterior tibial vessels.

The anterior aspect of the superior tibiofibular joint and the adjoining portions of the tibia and fibula give rise to the origins of the tibialis anterior, extensor digitorum longus, and peroneus longus muscles. The posterior aspect of the same region gives

rise to a portion of the soleus muscle. The anterior tibial artery, the terminal branch of the popliteal artery, enters the anterior compartment of the leg through the opening in the intraosseous membrane, two fingerbreadths below the superior tibiofibular joint. A recurrent branch contributes to anastomosis around the knee. The anterior tibial nerve and a terminal branch of the common peroneal nerve also pierce the anterior intermuscular septum between the extensor digitorum longus and the fibula and come to lie at the lateral side of the artery. The superficial peroneal nerve arises from the common peroneal nerve on the lateral side of the neck of the fibula and runs distally and forward in the substance of the peroneus longus muscle.

HYALINE AND ARTICULAR CARTILAGE

Articular cartilage is a specialized connective tissue composed of hydrated proteoglycans within a matrix of collagen fibrils. Proteoglycans are complex glycoproteins consisting of a central protein core to which glycosaminoglycan chains are attached. The structure of hyaline cartilage is not uniform, but rather can be divided into distinct zones based on the arrangement of the collagen fibrils and the distribution of chondrocytes. The density of chondrocytes is highest close to subchondral bone and decreases toward the articular surface (Fig. 1.13). Calcification occurs in a distinct basophilic zone at the deepest level of chondrocyte proliferation termed the *tidemark*. Beneath this region is a zone of calcified cartilage that anchors the cartilage to the subchondral plate. Cartilage is avascular, and chondrocytes in the superficial zones are believed to derive nutrition from synovial fluid. Deeper zones probably obtain nutrition from subchondral bone.

Examination of gross specimens or arthroscopic visualization reveals normal cartilage to consist of a white, smooth, firm material. Articular cartilage damage or degeneration, termed *chondromalacia*, can be readily identified (Fig. 1.14). These

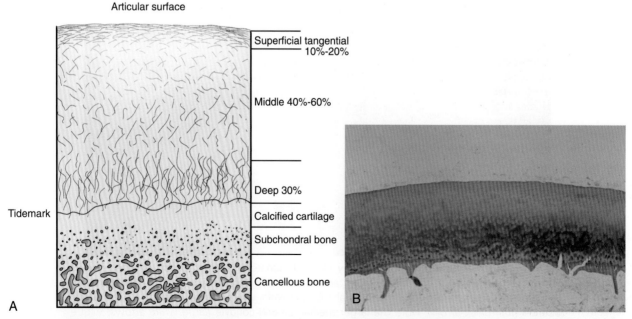

FIG 1.13 (A) Diagrammatic representation of the transition from articular cartilage to bone. (B) Normal articular (hyaline) cartilage composed of water, collagen, and proteoglycan. The sparsely cellular, smooth superficial zone becomes increasingly cellular in deeper layers. A distinct basophilic line, the mineralization front, can be seen where cartilage becomes calcified.

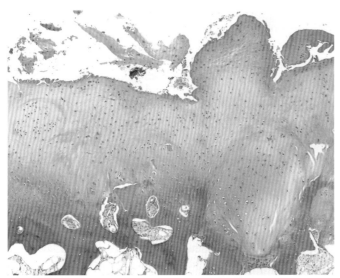

FIG 1.14 Degenerative or Chondromalacic Articular Cartilage Irregular thickness, surface fibrillation, longitudinal slits, increased chondrocyte cellularity, and altered matrix staining are evident.

characteristic changes seen during arthroscopic examination have been classified by Outerbridge[98]: grade 0 is normal, white-appearing cartilage; grade I is swelling or softening of an intact cartilage surface; grade II is represented by fissuring and fibrillation over a small area (<0.5 inch); grade III includes the same pathologic changes over a larger area (>0.5 inch); and grade IV changes represent erosion to subchondral bone and are indistinguishable from osteoarthritis. Chondral flap tears caused by delamination of the articular cartilage may also be encountered (Fig. 1.15). These changes in articular cartilage cannot be directly visualized on conventional radiographs but may be seen on magnetic resonance imaging (MRI) studies. High-grade cartilage damage (grade III or IV chondromalacia) is visible as thinning, irregularity, and fissuring of the cartilage on MRI (Fig. 1.16). However, MRI is less reliable for detecting early damage (grade I and II chondromalacia) that may appear as foci or areas of diffuse abnormal signal with a normal surface.

Damage to the articular cartilage and joint surface may result indirectly from pathologic changes in subchondral bone. Both osteonecrosis and osteochondritis dissecans (OCD) may lead to destruction of the articular surface. In the knee, OCD tends to occur on the intercondylar aspect of the medial femoral condyle in young people. These lesions may separate from the surface and form a loose body. The base of these lesions, if débrided, will reveal vascular subchondral bone (Fig. 1.17). Classic radiographic findings include a lucent osseous defect that may have a fragmented or corticated osseous density within the lucency (Fig. 1.18). On MRI studies, increased signal about the defect on T2-weighted images represents joint fluid surrounding the lesion; irregularity of the articular surface may also be noted (Fig. 1.19). Osteonecrosis results in a similar osteochondral fragment but tends to occur in elderly patients on the weight-bearing aspect of the medial femoral condyle (Fig. 1.20). In distinction to the lesions in OCD, fragments in osteonecrosis separate from a bed of avascular bone (Fig. 1.21). Again, radiographs may reveal a lucent defect at the involved site, but MRI is more reliable for evaluation of these defects (Fig. 1.22). A curvilinear area of low signal with variable bone edema is characteristic. Although the articular cartilage is initially normal,

both processes may lead to detachment of osteochondral loose bodies, fragmentation, and collapse of the articular surface with resultant degenerative changes.

MENISCI

The menisci are two crescentic fibrocartilage structures that serve to deepen the articular surfaces of the tibia for reception of the femoral condyles (Fig. 1.23). The most abundant components of the menisci include collagen (75%) and noncollagenized proteins (8% to 13%). Glycosaminoglycans and glycoproteins are also key constituents. Although four main types of collagen are present in the menisci, type I collagen is the predominant component and accounts for approximately 90% of the total collagen. Histologic examination reveals a population of fibroblasts and fibrocartilaginous cells dispersed in an organized matrix of eosinophilic collagen fibrils. The collagen bundles are arranged in a circumferential pattern that is optimal for absorption of compressive loads (Fig. 1.24). Radial fibers found at the surface and in the midsubstance parallel to the plateau may act to increase structural rigidity and help to prevent longitudinal splitting.[107] Elastin fibers, which constitute approximately 0.6% of the dry weight of the meniscus, seem to help in recoil to the original shape after deformation.[127] In degenerative menisci, metaplasia of the cell population occurs with a trend toward chondroid cell appearance (Fig. 1.25).

Each meniscus covers approximately the peripheral two-thirds of the corresponding articular surface of the tibia. The peripheral border of each meniscus is thick, convex, and attached to the capsule of the joint; the opposite border tapers to a thin, free edge. The proximal surfaces of the menisci are concave and in contact with the femoral condyles; the distal surfaces are flat and rest on the tibial plateau. On MRI studies, normal menisci are best seen on sagittal views and have low-signal characteristics with no or little internal signal. The posterior horn of the medial meniscus is larger than the anterior horn, whereas the anterior and posterior horns of the lateral menisci are typically of similar size (Fig. 1.26). Increased signal within the menisci may be noted and classified on a scale ranging from I to III. Patchy areas of increased signal that do not touch the inferior and superior borders of the menisci represent grade I changes. Grade II changes typically have a linear configuration, but again they do not touch the superior and inferior surfaces. These signal changes probably represent the normal aging process in the menisci. Increased signal with a linear appearance that contacts one of the articular surfaces of the menisci is classified as grade III change and represents a true meniscal tear (Fig. 1.27).[85,118] A variety of meniscal tears may be identified on MRI but are best delineated by arthroscopic examination (Fig. 1.28). Patterns include vertical and horizontal cleavage tears, radial tears, bucket handle tears (detachment of the body of the menisci at the periphery with intact anterior and posterior horn attachments), and complex degenerative tears (Fig. 1.29). The technique of arthroscopic repair and partial meniscectomy has superseded open meniscectomy; therefore examination of intact resected specimens is rarely possible (Fig. 1.30).

Calcification may occur within the fibrocartilage of the menisci and is referred to as *chondrocalcinosis*. This abnormality has classically been described in association with calcium pyrophosphate dihydrate deposition disease. However,

Text continued on p. 16

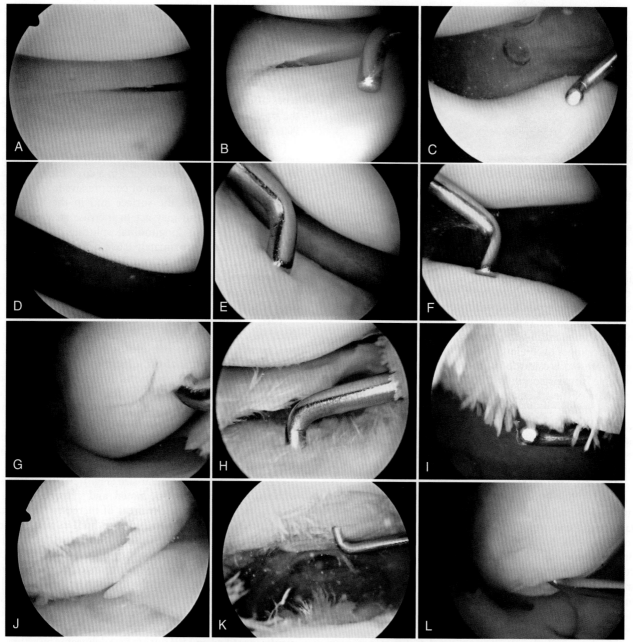

FIG 1.15 Arthroscopic Views of Articular Cartilage Normal, white, smooth articular cartilage (Outerbridge grade 0) in the medial (A), lateral (B), and patellofemoral compartments (C and D). Softening of the articular surface of the lateral tibial plateau (E) and the patellofemoral articulation (F) with indentation at the probe tip (Outerbridge grade I) is noted. (G) A small fissure and fibrillation of the medial femoral condyle (Outerbridge grade II). Extensive fibrillation of the articular cartilage involving the tibial plateau (H) and the patella (I) (Outerbridge grade III). Erosion of articular cartilage to subchondral bone involving the medial femoral condyle (J) and patella (K) (Outerbridge grade IV). Arthroscopic view of a chondral flap tear (L); the probe tip is deep to a flap of delaminated articular cartilage on the medial femoral condyle.

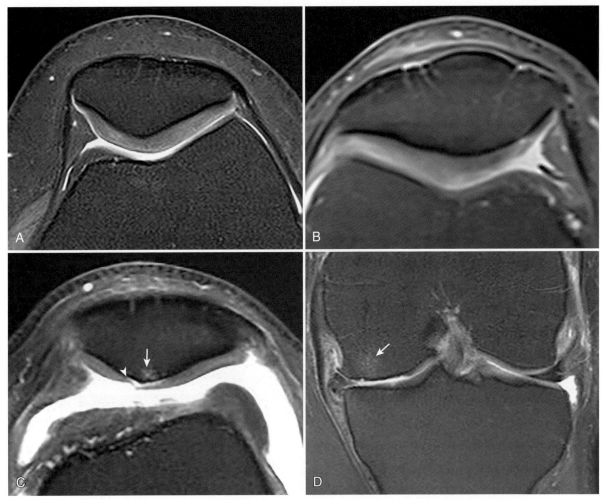

FIG 1.16 Normal and Abnormal Cartilage as Seen on Fat-Suppressed Proton Density (PD) Imaging (A) Axial image of normal patellar cartilage. (B) Axial image demonstrating grade 1 chondromalacia of the lateral patellar facet and more prominent grade 1 to 2 chondromalacia of the medial facet. (C) Axial image identifying focal grade 4 change at the patellar apex *(short arrow)* with abnormal signal in the subchondral bone. Note flap tears *(arrowhead)* of the adjacent cartilage margin. (D) Coronal image showing extensive medial compartment chondromalacia with large areas of complete cartilage loss and focal grade 4 change *(arrow)*.

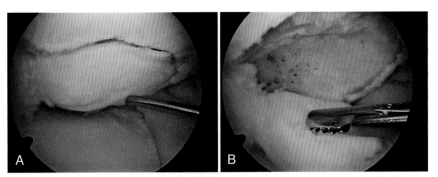

FIG 1.17 Arthroscopic View of Osteochondritis of the Femoral Condyle (A) Osteochondral fragment of the articular surface of the femoral condyle. (B) Punctate bleeding from the base of vascular subchondral bone with the osteochondral fragment mobilized.

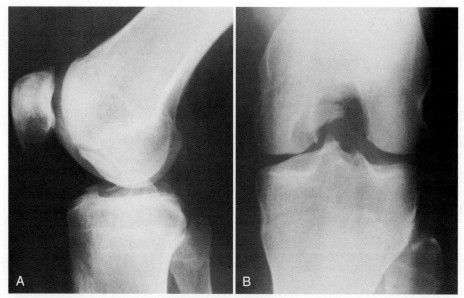

FIG 1.18 Radiographs of Osteochondritis Dissecans Lateral (A) and tunnel (B) views show an osseous density within a lucent defect on the medial femoral condyle.

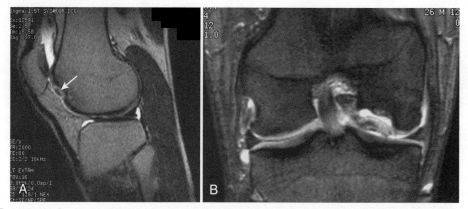

FIG 1.19 (A) Sagittal MRI demonstrating a well-demarcated osteochondral lesion *(arrow)* in the anterior aspect of the lateral femoral condyle. (B) Coronal MRI showing high-signal fluid about a loose osteochondral fragment of the medial femoral condyle. (Courtesy Martin Broker, MD.)

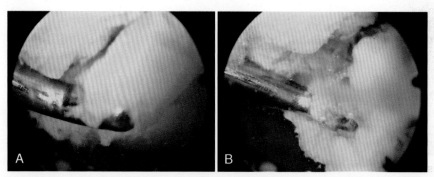

FIG 1.20 Arthroscopic Views of Osteonecrosis of the Femoral Condyle (A) Disruption of the articular surface by a detached osteochondral fragment. (B) A probe elevates the loose fragment to reveal a base of almost completely avascular, dead subchondral bone.

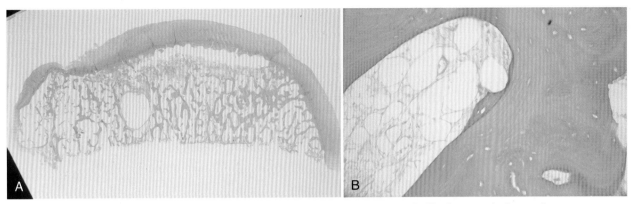

FIG 1.21 (A) Osteonecrosis. A subchondral lucent zone is surrounded by intact articular cartilage and a thin plate of subchondral bone superficially with collapsed necrotic bone and granulation tissue inferiorly. (B) Osteonecrosis (high power). Dead bone is characterized by marrow fat necrosis imparting a foggy, acellular appearance and bone devoid of osteocytes (empty lacunar spaces) and bone-lining cells.

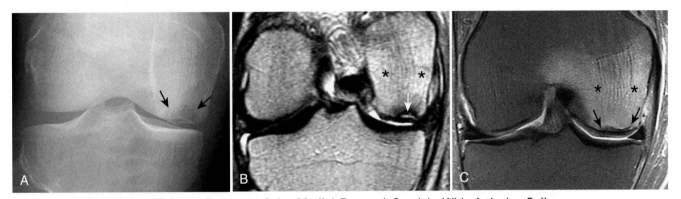

FIG 1.22 Insufficiency Fracture of the Medial Femoral Condyle With Articular Collapse (Previously Termed *Spontaneous Osteonecrosis*) (A) Anteroposterior radiograph of the knee shows collapse of the weight-bearing articular surface of the medial femoral condyle with surrounding, subtler, lucency *(arrows)*, obtained 5 months following onset of symptoms. (B) Corresponding coronal T2-weighted spin-echo (SE) magnetic resonance imaging shows the articular collapse *(white arrow)* with extensive edema-like change *(asterisks)* in the medial femoral condyle. (C) Similar lesion in a different patient with coronal fat-suppressed PD magnetic resonance image obtained prior to radiographic changes shows subtle flattening of the weight bearing surface of the medial femoral condyle with well-defined subchondral fracture line *(arrows)* and associated edema-like change *(asterisks)*.

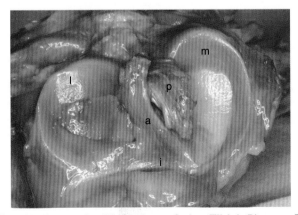

FIG 1.23 Anatomic Dissection of the Tibial Plateau The menisci act to increase the conformity of the articular surface of the tibial plateau. The medial meniscus *(m)* is C shaped, whereas the lateral meniscus *(l)* is more circular. Remnants of the ACL *(a)* and PCL *(p)* are also marked, as is the transverse intermeniscal ligament *(i)*.

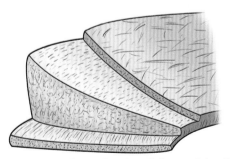

FIG 1.24 Trilaminar Cross-Sectional Area of the Meniscus

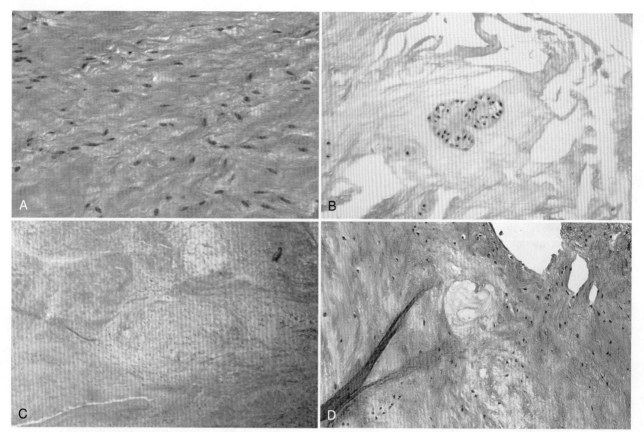

FIG 1.25 Cross-section of the medial meniscus (fibrocartilage) demonstrating the eosinophilic collagen matrix in interwoven bands, within which can be seen the nuclei of fibroblasts, here more prominent than those seen in tendons and ligaments, with occasional perinuclear spaces, often similar to immature cartilaginous cells (A). With trauma or degeneration, chondroid metaplasia (B), loss of matrix (C), and cystic changes (D) take place.

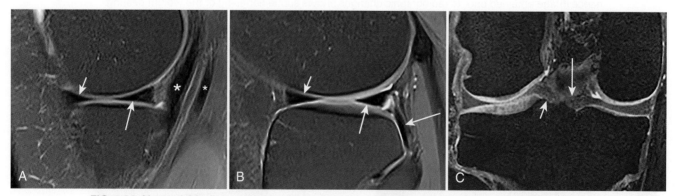

FIG 1.26 Normal Medial and Lateral Meniscus (A) Sagittal fat-suppressed PD image of the midmedial meniscus demonstrates the normal triangular shape and uniform decreased signal intensity. Note the relative increased size of the posterior horn *(long arrow)* in comparison with the anterior horn *(small arrow)*. The semimembranosus tendon *(large asterisk)* is seen as it inserts to the posterior medial tibia, with the semitendinosus tendon *(small asterisk)* just posterior to it. (B) Similar image of the midlateral meniscus. The anterior *(short arrow)* and posterior *(long arrow)* horn are generally similar in size. Note the popliteal tendon *(large arrow)* coursing posterior to the tibia. (C) Thin coronal gradient image through the posterior aspect of the joint shows the posterior lateral *(small arrow)* and medial *(large arrow)* meniscal roots.

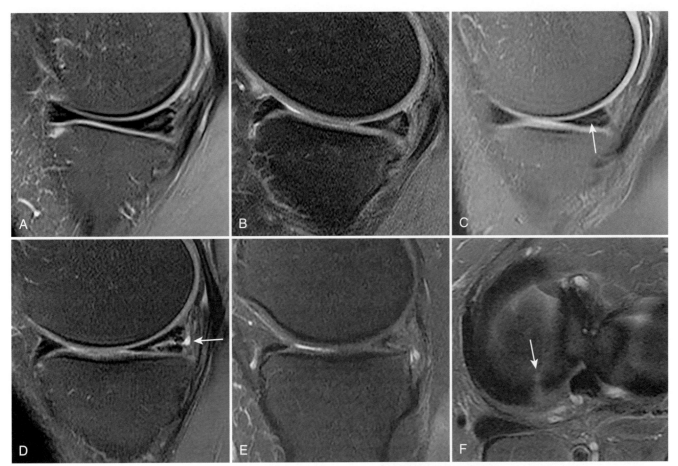

FIG 1.27 Spectrum of Meniscal Signal on Fat-Suppressed PD Magnetic Resonance Images (Demonstrated in the Posterior Horn of the Medial Meniscus) (A) Normal peripheral vascularity in a 19-year-old female. (B) Poorly defined increased signal (grade I) consistent with mucoid degenerative changes in a 45-year-old male. (C) Linear increased signal not communicating with the meniscal surface (grade II, *arrow*). (D) Linear increase signal communicating with the inferior meniscal surface (grade III) with a small associated meniscal cyst *(arrow)*. Arthroscopy confirmed an undersurface tear with a prominent horizontal component. (E and F) Complex tear of the posterior horn (E) with the axial image (F) showing the radial nature *(arrow)* to better advantage.

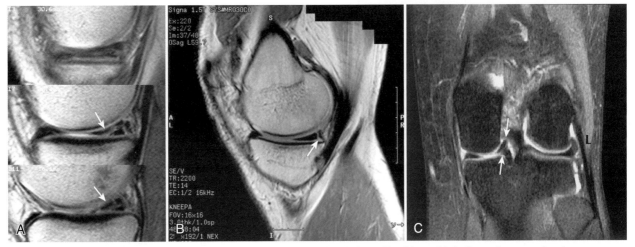

FIG 1.28 (A) Three sagittal MRI views ("meniscal windows") with multiple linear intrameniscal signals that contact the superior *(arrow, lower left image)* and inferior meniscal surfaces *(arrow, middle left image)* representing a complex degenerative tear. (B) Sagittal MRI showing a peripheral vertical cleavage tear *(arrow)* of the posterior horn of the medial meniscus. (C) Coronal MRI demonstrating a displaced bucket handle meniscal tear with the fragment displaced into the notch *(arrows)*. The LCL *(L)* is also well visualized.

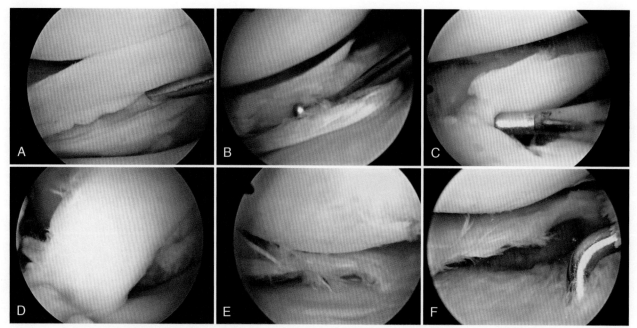

FIG 1.29 Arthroscopic Views of Meniscal Tears (A) Vertical cleavage tear with separation of the meniscus from the peripheral attachment. (B) Horizontal cleavage meniscal tear. (C) Radial tear in the midbody of the meniscus. (D) Detached meniscal bucket handle tear with a fragment displaced into the intercondylar notch. (E) Complex degenerative tear of the posterior body and horn of the medial meniscus. (F) Degenerative fraying of the meniscus without a gross tear.

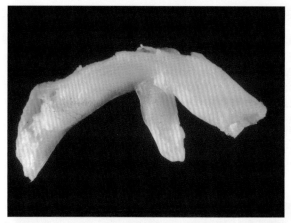

FIG 1.30 Gross Anatomic Specimen of a Torn Meniscus

chondrocalcinosis may be noted incidentally on radiographs or during arthroscopic examination (Fig. 1.31).

The menisci perform several important functions, including (1) load transmission across the joint, (2) enhancement of articular conformity, (3) distribution of synovial fluid across the articular surface, and (4) prevention of soft tissue impingement during joint motion. The medial meniscus also confers some stability to the joint in the presence of ACL insufficiency, in that the posterior horn acts as a wedge to help reduce anterior tibial translation.[83] However, the lateral meniscus does not perform a similar function.[82] The rapid progression of degenerative changes, first observed by Fairbank, that occur as a result of complete meniscectomy have been well documented.[35] These changes include (1) osteophyte formation on the femoral condyle projecting over the site of meniscectomy, (2) flattening

of the femoral condyle, and (3) narrowing of joint space in the involved compartment.

Medial Meniscus

The medial meniscus is almost semicircular in form and measures approximately 3.5 cm in length. It has a triangular cross-section and is asymmetrical, with a considerably wider posterior than anterior horn. The attachment of the posterior horn, the so-called meniscal root, is firmly attached to the posterior portion of the intercondylar fossa of the tibia, directly anterior to the PCL insertion (Fig. 1.32). The functional importance of the meniscal root has become better appreciated over the past 5 years. Tears of the meniscal root destabilize the meniscus and are associated with meniscal extrusion on MRI.[81] As a result it has been theorized that root tears appear to produce the same functional changes as total medial meniscectomy.[4,51,81,89] This is believed to be a significant risk factor in the development of early osteoarthritic changes.[4,81] In biomechanical studies, evidence to support the MRI findings has been forthcoming, with data showing increased joint contact pressures and altered knee kinematics; indeed these changes are similar to those seen after total meniscectomy that have been associated with subsequent articular cartilage damage and osteoarthritic changes.[4,89] Importantly, repair of a root tear appears to improve the function of the meniscus and may reduce the risk of early osteoarthritic changes.[4,51,89]

The anterior attachment of the meniscus is more variable; usually it is firmly attached to the anterior intercondylar fossa approximately 7 mm anterior to the anterior margin of the ACL insertion, in line with the medial tibial tubercle, but this attachment can be flimsy.[63] In addition, a fibrous band of variable thickness, the transverse intermeniscal ligament, connects the anterior horn of the medial meniscus with the lateral meniscus (Fig. 1.33). Peripherally the medial meniscus is continuously

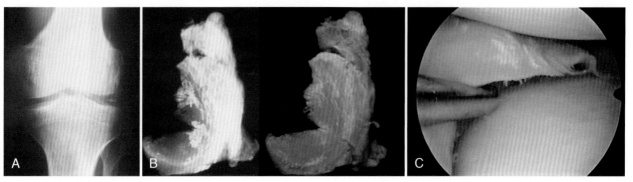

FIG 1.31 (A) Anteroposterior radiograph of a knee with calcium pyrophosphate dihydrate deposition disease. (B) Gross meniscus and specimen radiograph. (C) Arthroscopic view of chondrocalcinosis of the lateral meniscus. (From Vigorita VJ: The synovium. In Vigorita VJ, Ghelman B, editors: *Orthopaedic pathology*, Philadelphia, 1999, Lippincott Williams & Wilkins, 1999.)

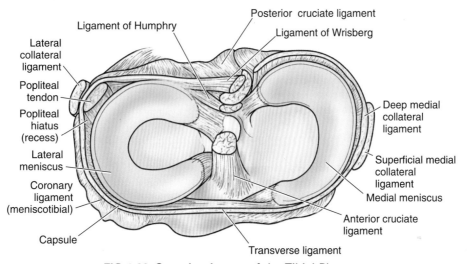

FIG 1.32 Superior Aspect of the Tibial Plateau

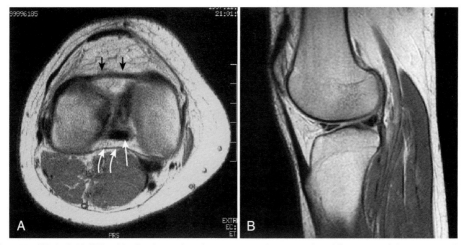

FIG 1.33 (A) Axial MRI with the low-signal transverse intermeniscal ligament *(short arrows)* connecting the anterior horns of the medial and lateral menisci. The posterior capsule *(curved arrows)* and the PCL *(long arrow)* are also identified. (B) Sagittal MRI through the lateral compartment of the knee shows the interface between the transverse intermeniscal ligament and the anterior horn of the meniscus. This may be misidentified as a meniscal tear.

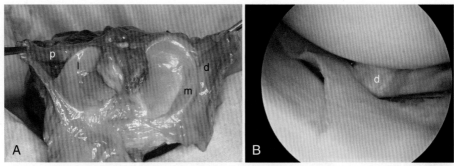

FIG 1.34 (A) Tibial plateau. The C-shaped medial meniscus has a continuous attachment to the capsule. The deep MCL (*d*, retracted in the forceps) is directly attached to the periphery of the midbody of the medial meniscus *(m)*. Laterally the popliteus tendon (*p*, retracted in the forceps) enters the joint via the popliteal hiatus. In this location the capsular attachment of the lateral meniscus *(l)* is interrupted. (B) Arthroscopic view of the deep MCL. The fibers of the deep MCL *(d)*, which represent a thickening in the medial capsule, can be seen at the tip of the probe.

attached to the capsule of the knee. The midpoint of the medial meniscus is more firmly attached to the femur via a condensation in the capsule known as the deep medial ligament (Fig. 1.34). The tibial attachment of the meniscus, sometimes known as the coronary ligament, attaches to the tibial margin a few millimeters distal to the articular surface, where it gives rise to a synovial recess. Posteromedially, according to Kaplan, the meniscus receives a portion of the insertion of the semimembranosus via the capsule.[68]

Lateral Meniscus

In contrast to the C-shaped medial meniscus, the lateral meniscus is almost circular and covers a larger portion of the articular surface (see Fig. 1.32). The anterior horn is attached to the intercondylar fossa, directly anterior to the lateral tibial tubercle and adjacent to the ACL. The posterior horn is attached to the intercondylar fossa, directly posterior to the lateral tibial tubercle and adjacent and anterior to the posterior horn of the medial meniscus.[63] Somewhat variable fibrous bands, the meniscofemoral ligaments, connect the posterior horn of the lateral meniscus to the intercondylar wall of the medial femoral condyle. These meniscofemoral ligaments, which embrace the PCL, are also known by the eponyms Humphry and Wrisberg (Fig. 1.35). The ligament of Humphry passes anterior to the PCL, whereas the ligament of Wrisberg passes posterior to the PCL (Fig. 1.36). One or the other of these meniscofemoral ligaments has been identified in 71% to 100% of cadaver knees; the ligament of Wrisberg is a more constant finding, and both ligaments together are found in only a small percentage of specimens.[107,125,128] Meniscofemoral ligaments running from the anterior horns of the medial and lateral menisci to the intercondylar notch anterior to the ACL have also been identified. Wan and Felle[128] reported a 15% incidence of both of these structures in 60 cadaver knees, and one or the other was present in 25% of specimens. In general, the ligaments of Wrisberg and Humphry were much more robust structures than either of the meniscofemoral ligaments originating from the anterior horns.

The peripheral capsular attachment of the medial meniscus is continuous, but the attachment of the lateral meniscus is interrupted by the popliteal hiatus, through which passes the popliteal tendon (Fig. 1.37). In addition, unlike the anatomy on the medial side, the lateral meniscus does not have a direct attachment to the collateral ligament. Posterolaterally at the

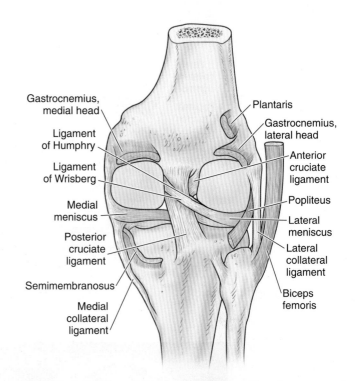

FIG 1.35 Posterior Aspect of the Knee The ligaments of Humphry and Wrisberg, which attach the posterior horn of the lateral meniscus to the medial femoral condyle, embrace the PCL. The popliteal tendon partially inserts into the PL aspect of the lateral meniscus.

popliteal hiatus the lateral meniscus is grooved by the popliteal tendon. Some fibers of the tendon insert into the periphery and superior border of the meniscus at this site.[69,70] Because the lateral meniscus is not as extensively attached to the capsule as the medial meniscus is, it is more mobile and may displace up to 1 cm. The controlled mobility of the lateral meniscus, which is guided by the popliteal tendon and meniscofemoral ligament attachments, may explain why meniscal injuries occur less frequently on the lateral side.[78,79] Although the meniscofemoral ligaments appear to perform an important function, little is known about the significance of injury to these structures.

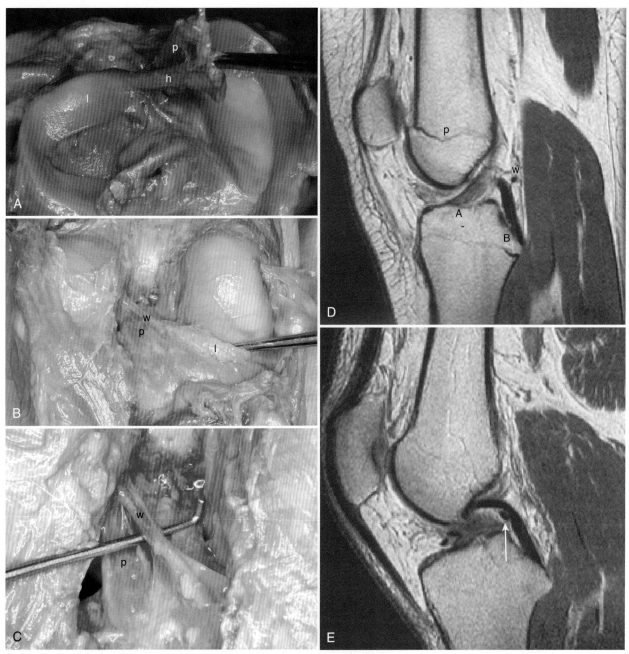

FIG 1.36 Meniscofemoral Ligaments (A) The ligament of Humphry (*h*, retracted in the forceps) arises from the posterior horn of the lateral meniscus (*l*) and passes anterior to the PCL *(p)*. (B) Posterior view of the knee with the capsule removed laterally, revealing the ligament of Wrisberg *(w)*, which originates from the lateral meniscus (*l*, tip of the forceps) and then passes posterior to the PCL *(p)*. (C) Close-up view of an anatomic dissection of the posterior aspect of the knee, with the capsule removed from the intercondylar notch. The ligament of Wrisberg *(w)* lies posterior to the PCL fibers *(p)*. (D) Sagittal MRI showing the ligament of Wrisberg *(w)* posterior to the PCL (*B*). Also identified are the ACL (*A*) and the physeal scar (*P*). (E) Sagittal MRI with the small oval ligament of Humphry identified anterior to the PCL *(arrow)*.

CAPSULE

The capsule is a fibrous membrane containing areas of thickening that may be referred to as discrete ligaments. The anterior capsule is thin, and directly anteriorly it is replaced by the patellar ligament. Proximally the capsule of the knee joint attaches to the femur approximately three to four fingerbreadths above the patella. Distally it attaches circumferentially to the tibial margin, except where the popliteal tendon enters the joint through the hiatus. Posteriorly the capsule consists of vertical fibers that arise from the condyles and walls of the intercondylar fossa of the femur. In this region the capsule is augmented by fibers of the oblique popliteal ligament, which is derived from the semimembranosus tendon. This broad, flat band is attached

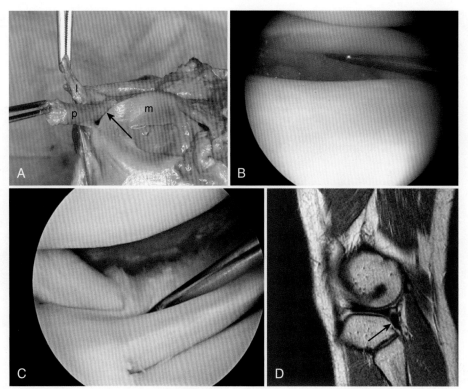

FIG 1.37 Popliteal Hiatus (A) Anatomic dissection revealing incomplete capsular attachment of the lateral meniscus *(m)*. The popliteal tendon (*p,* anterior forceps) passes deep to the LCL (*l,* posterior forceps) through the hiatus *(arrow)*. (B) Arthroscopic view of the popliteal hiatus with the lateral meniscus elevated superiorly. (C) Arthroscopic view of the popliteal tendon passing between the periphery of the lateral meniscus and the capsule. (D) Sagittal magnetic resonance image with the popliteus tendon (*arrow*) traversing the popliteal hiatus posterior to the lateral meniscus.

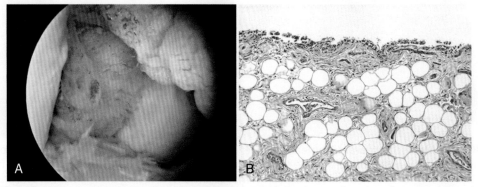

FIG 1.38 (A) Arthroscopic view of normal synovium. Normal synovium is a fine pink layer that covers the intra-articular surfaces of the knee. (B) Section of essentially normal synovium demonstrating the synovial intimal layer consisting of synoviocytes, one to two cells thick, beneath which rests the highly vascular subintimal layer, usually sparsely cellular, but containing fibroblasts, histiocytes, fat cells, and occasional mast cells.

proximally to the margin of the intercondylar fossa and posterior surface of the femur close to the articular margins of the condyles. The fascicles are separated by apertures for the passage of vessels and nerves. The oblique popliteal ligament forms part of the floor of the popliteal fossa, and the popliteal artery rests on it. At the site of the popliteal hiatus, the capsule is displaced inferiorly toward the fibula head, forming the arcuate ligament between the lateral meniscus and the fibular styloid.

SYNOVIAL CAVITY

Synovium is normally a smooth, translucent pink tissue. Histologically a thin layer of synovial cells, or synoviocytes, is found at the surface (Fig. 1.38). The synoviocytes consist of two cell populations, broadly classified into those that have macrophage-type function and those with a synthetic function. Type 1 cells contain numerous mitochondria, lysosomes,

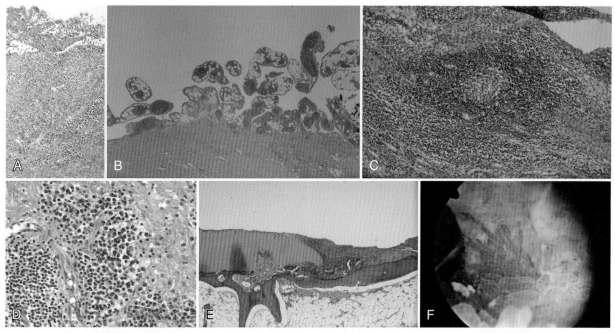

FIG 1.39 Rheumatoid Synovium In rheumatoid arthritis, the synovium becomes thickened, edematous, fibrinous, and inflamed (A). Marked lymphocytosis is seen (B, low power), along with germinal center formation (C) and plasma cell proliferation (D). The inflamed synovium or pannus (E) causes chondrolysis and invades the cartilage and bone. (F) Arthroscopic view of inflamed synovium with hypertrophic, *red villi*.

phagosomes, and surface undulations indicative of their macrophage function. Type 2 cells have rough endoplasmic reticulum and free ribosomes characteristic of secretory cells. This layer of cells, the intimal layer, lies above a fibrovascular zone, the subintimal layer, which contains arterioles, fat, and a variety of connective tissue cells, including fibroblasts and histiocytes. The fibrovascular zone gradually becomes more fibrous at capsular insertions. In specific disease processes, including rheumatoid arthritis, the synovium becomes hypertrophic and inflamed and contributes to intra-articular destruction (Fig. 1.39).

Synovium invests the interior of the knee joint and extends proximally into the suprapatellar pouch above the patella. The suprapatellar pouch is separated from the anterior surface of the femur by a layer of fat (Fig. 1.40). The uppermost limit of the pouch is attached to a small muscle, the articularis genus, which originates from the anterior surface of the femoral shaft. The articularis genus serves to prevent invagination of the suprapatellar pouch beneath the patella.

Intra-articularly the synovium invests the cruciate ligaments and the popliteal tendon. A synovial recess or sleeve extends around the popliteal tendon for a variable distance beyond the PL capsule. The synovium also lines the coronal recesses beneath the menisci and anteriorly invests the fat pad, which lies posterior to the patellar ligament and capsule. Although the synovium approximates the capsule, it is much more redundant. Synovial folds occur frequently, particularly in the suprapatellar pouch. Plicae probably represent remnants of synovial septa normally absorbed during embryonic development. The infrapatellar (ligamentum mucosum), suprapatellar, and medial patellar plicae are the three most common plicae (Fig. 1.41). Visualization of plicae on MRI studies can be difficult without an

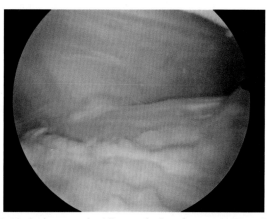

FIG 1.40 Arthroscopic View of the Suprapatellar Pouch A thin layer of translucent synovium covers the interior surfaces.

associated intra-articular effusion. In most cases sagittal and axial images provide the best detail (Fig. 1.42). Rarely, plicae, especially medial patellar plicae, can become inflamed and painful; in these circumstances, arthroscopic resection may be considered.

The posterior synovial cavity communicates with a popliteal bursa that is found between the semimembranosus tendon and the medial head of the gastrocnemius in approximately 50% of people (Fig. 1.43).[135] This bursa may be distended when dye is injected into the knee; the bursa can also become enlarged by an intra-articular effusion, resulting in a popliteal or Baker's cyst. With this exception, the synovial cavity does not normally communicate with any of the other bursae around the knee.

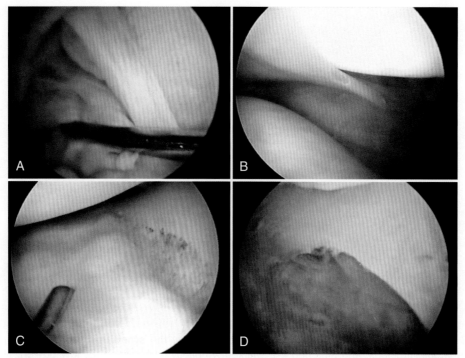

FIG 1.41 Arthroscopic Views of Intra-articular Plicae (A) The infrapatellar plica (ligamentum mucosum) passes between the intercondylar notch and the anterior fat pad. (B) A large medial patellar plica is seen interposed between the anterior surface of the medial femoral condyle and the patella. (C) Thickening along the margin of a large medial patellar plica caused by irritation and abrasion on the femoral condyle. (D) A suprapatellar plica may occlude the opening to the suprapatellar pouch. In some cases this plica may be continuous with a medial patellar plica.

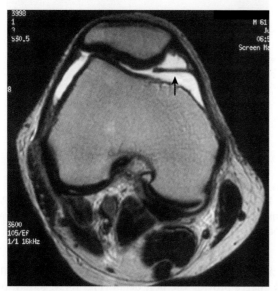

FIG 1.42 Axial magnetic resonance image with a low-signal, thick medial plica *(arrow)* that is highlighted by the large effusion.

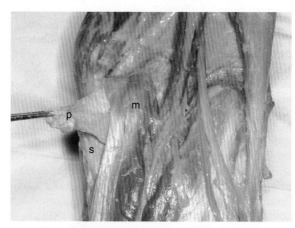

FIG 1.43 Popliteal Bursa Anatomic dissection of the popliteal fossa with a popliteal bursa *(p,* forceps) originating between the medial head of the gastrocnemius *(m)* and the semimembranosus tendon *(s).*

BURSAE

Of numerous bursae about the knee, those with the greatest clinical significance include the prepatellar, infrapatellar, and anserine bursae (Fig. 1.44). The prepatellar bursa is large and lies subcutaneously anterior to the patella. The infrapatellar bursa lies posterior to the patellar ligament and separates the ligament from the tibia and the lower portion of the fat pad. The pes anserinus bursa lies between the sartorius, gracilis, and semitendinosus tendons and the tibia; another bursa separates the superficial medial ligament from the pes tendons. These bursae may become inflamed as a result of trauma or overuse. The significance of the semimembranosus bursa has already been discussed.

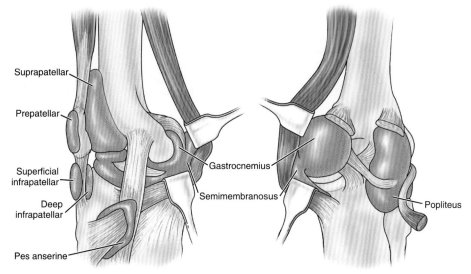

FIG 1.44 Bursae Around the Knee

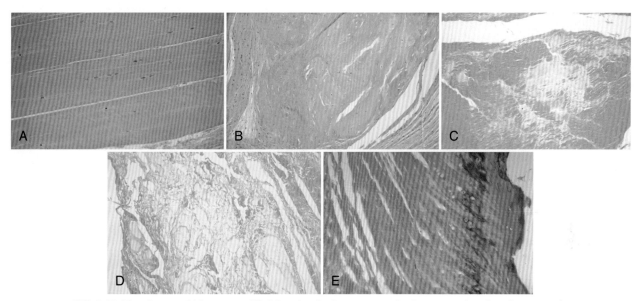

FIG 1.45 Tendon and Ligament (A) A longitudinal segment of a ligament showing the sparsely cellular, highly eosinophilic collagenized matrix. The nuclei of the fibroblasts are relatively indistinct, dark, ovoid shapes, sometimes in columns enveloped by the collagen matrix. Chondroid metaplasia (B), loss of matrix (C), and cystic changes (D) occur with injury or degeneration. (E) The fibrils of tendon and ligaments as they insert into bone provide a contiguous flow of fibrils through the calcifying zone (basophilic area) with direct continuity into the subchondral plate.

CRUCIATE LIGAMENTS

The cruciate ligaments consist of a highly organized collagen matrix, which accounts for approximately three-fourths of their dry weight. Most of the collagen is type I (90%), and the remainder is type III (10%).[32] In the ACL, collagen is organized into multiple fiber bundles 20 μm wide that are grouped into fascicles 20 to 400 μm in diameter.[26] Occasional fibroblasts and other substances, such as elastin (<5%) and proteoglycans (1%), make up the remainder of the dry weight.[32] Water constitutes 60% of the net weight under physiologic conditions. At the microscopic level, ligament and tendon insertions into bone have a characteristic structure consisting of collagen fibrils directly continuous with fibrils within the bone. A calcified front, similar to that seen between osteoid and mineralized bone, can be distinguished (Fig. 1.45).

The cruciate ligaments are named for their attachments on the tibia and are essential to function of the knee joint.[53,73,78,132] The cruciate ligaments act to stabilize the knee joint and prevent anteroposterior displacement of the tibia on the femur. The presence of numerous sensory endings also implies a proprioceptive function. These ligaments are intra-articular but, because they are covered by synovium, are considered extrasynovial. They receive their blood supply from branches of the middle genicular and both inferior genicular arteries. The anatomy of the cruciate ligaments has been studied by Girgis et al.[41] (Fig. 1.46).

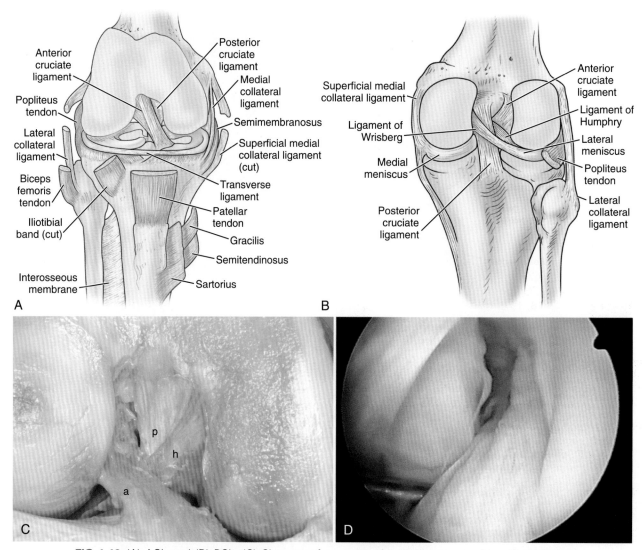

FIG 1.46 (A) ACL and (B) PCL. (C) Close-up of an anatomic specimen seen from the anterior aspect, demonstrating the relationship of the ACL *(a)*, ligament of Humphry *(h)*, and PCL *(p)* from anterior to posterior in the intercondylar notch. (D) Arthroscopic view of the contents of the intercondylar notch showing, from left to right, the ligamentum mucosum, PCL, and ACL (probe posterior to the ACL).

Anterior Cruciate Ligament

The ACL originates from the medial surface of the lateral femoral condyle posteriorly in the intercondylar notch in the form of a segment of a circle (Fig. 1.47). The anterior side of the attachment is almost straight and the posterior side convex. The ligament courses anteriorly, distally, and medially toward the tibia (Fig. 1.48). Over the length of its course the fibers of the ligament undergo slight external rotation. The average length of the ligament is 38 mm, and the average width is 11 mm.[41] Approximately 10 mm below the femoral attachment, the ligament stands out as it proceeds distally to the tibial attachment, which is a wide, depressed area anterior and lateral to the medial tibial tubercle in the intercondylar fossa (Fig. 1.49). The tibial attachment is oriented in an oblique direction and is more robust than the femoral attachment. A slip to the anterior horn of the lateral meniscus is well marked.[41]

Increasing importance has been placed on identification of discrete bundles within this ligament. Although the anatomic basis of this division has been debated for decades, with evidence to support a single anatomic structure, two discrete bundles, or even three bundles, the concept of two functional bundles is now well established.[5,41,74,97,114,137] The two bundles are defined by their respective tibial insertion with an anteromedial (AM) bundle and a PL bundle.[5,21,103,134] The AM bundle originates in the proximal part of the femoral origin and inserts in the AM portion of the tibial insertion; in distinction, the PL bundle originates distally in the femoral origin and inserts in the PL aspect of the tibial insertion.[5,21,103,137] In the coronal plane the AM bundle originates at about the 10:30 clock position, and the PL bundle originates more horizontally at the 9:30 clock position.[103,137] Increased emphasis has been placed on these anatomic details during ACL reconstruction surgery, with a trend discussed in later chapters toward more anatomic ACL reconstruction with two-tunnel, double-bundle techniques, as well as through modifications to femoral tunnel placement in single-bundle techniques.[21,50,74,114]

The ACL is the prime static stabilizer against anterior translation of the tibia on the femur and accounts for up to 86% of

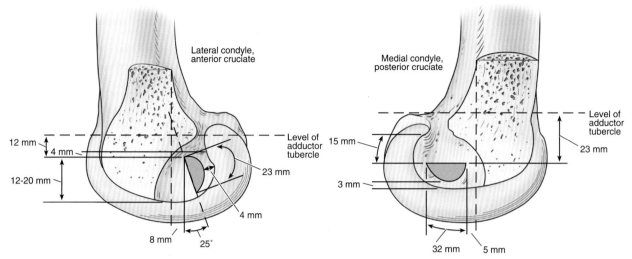

FIG 1.47 Attachments of the Anterior and Posterior Cruciate Ligaments to the Femur (From Girgis FG, Marshall JL, Al Monajem ARS: The cruciate ligaments of the knee joint. *Clin Orthop* 106:216, 1975.)

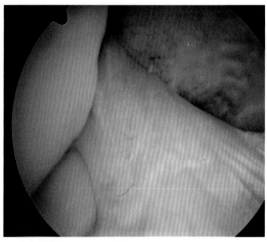

FIG 1.48 Arthroscopic View of a Normal Anterior Cruciate Ligament The fibers of the ACL fan out distally, anteriorly, and medially to insert on the tibia. The origin of the PCL can be visualized posterior to the ACL.

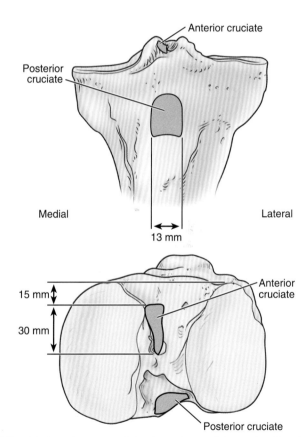

FIG 1.49 Attachments of the Anterior and Posterior Cruciate Ligaments to the Tibia (From Girgis FG, Marshall JL, Al Monajem ARS: The cruciate ligaments of the knee joint. *Clin Orthop* 106:216, 1975.)

the total force resisting anterior draw.[17,38,56,71] The bundles of the ligament are not isometric through the range of motion. Rather, at different stages of knee motion, the distinct functional bundles of the ACL have different roles in stabilizing the knee joint.[5,21,41,137] In extension the bundles are parallel, but as the knee flexes, the femoral origin of the PL bundle moves anteriorly, and the bundles cross.[5,21,38,41,132] Functionally the AM bundle tightens as the knee flexes and the PL bundle loosens; conversely, the PL bundle becomes tight as full extension is approached (Fig. 1.50).[5,21,38,41,48,132,137] Consequently, isolated rupture of the AM bundle will tend to have a greater effect on the anterior draw test (performed at 90 degrees of flexion), and failure of the PL bundle will have a greater effect on the Lachman test (performed at 30 degrees of flexion).[5,38] The PL bundle also plays an important role in resisting internal and external rotation.[5,21,137] Changes in ACL reconstruction techniques, attained through double-bundle reconstruction or by placing the femoral tunnel origin more horizontally in the

notch, have been driven by the desire to better restore the functional effects of the PL bundle in resisting rotation, as well as anterior translation.[21,50,114] The current criticism of single-bundle reconstruction methods is that when these techniques are performed through a transtibial method, the resulting femoral tunnel is placed too high in the notch; consequently, only the AM bundle is effectively reconstructed. This leads to improvement in anterior tibial translation but does not accurately restore stability through the range of motion and does not restore rotational stability.[5,50,114] In addition to the trend toward anatomic ACL reconstruction, improvements in our understanding of the anatomy and function of the ACL have stimulated the development of augmentation techniques that effectively reconstruct single functional bundles in the setting of isolated bundle tears (injuries that were previously grouped collectively under the term *partial ACL tears*).[50]

The maximum tensile strength of the ACL is approximately 1725 ± 270 N, which is less than the peak force that occurs in vigorous athletic activities.[96] Stability is enhanced by dynamic stabilizers, such as the muscles that exert a force across the knee joint. For muscles to aid in protective stabilization of the knee, effective proprioceptive feedback regarding joint position is

crucial. The ACL seems to play an important proprioceptive function because a variety of mechanoreceptors and free nerve endings have been identified.[9,32,70,111,112] In humans with ACL-deficient knees a significantly higher threshold for detecting passive motion of the involved knee has been reported.[9] Afferent and efferent signals involving the ACL are carried by branches of the posterior tibial nerve. On MRI the ACL is best visualized on sagittal images. Because of its oblique course, the ACL should be evaluated routinely on two or three sagittal sections. A normal ACL has a relatively low signal, but toward the distal insertion the ACL may appear striated (Fig. 1.51). Discontinuity in the fibers or a soft tissue mass in the notch with high signal characteristics resulting from edema and hemorrhage indicates an ACL tear. Partial ACL tears may be suggested by increased signal, thickening, or redundancy in the ligament. However, accurate diagnosis of partial injuries remains challenging (Fig. 1.52). Arthroscopic evaluation of the ACL remains the gold standard for evaluating suspected partial and complete tears (Fig. 1.53).

Posterior Cruciate Ligament

The PCL originates from the posterior part of the lateral surface of the medial femoral condyle in the intercondylar notch (see Fig. 1.47). As with the ACL the origin is in the form of a segment of a circle and is oriented horizontally. The superior boundary of the attachment is straight, and the inferior boundary is convex. The PCL has an average length of 38 mm and an average width of 13 mm.[41,125] It is narrowest in its midportion and fans out to a greater extent superiorly than it does inferiorly. The fibers are attached to the tibial insertion in a lateromedial direction, whereas in the femur they arise in an anteroposterior direction. The tibial attachment occurs in a depression posterior to the intra-articular upper surface of the tibia (see Fig. 1.49). The attachment extends up to 1 cm distally onto the adjoining posterior surface of the tibia (Fig. 1.54). Immediately proximal to the tibial attachment, the PCL sends a slip to blend with the posterior horn of the lateral meniscus.[41,125]

A normal PCL has uniformly low signal intensity on MRI studies, along with a hockey stick shape. The PCL can be well

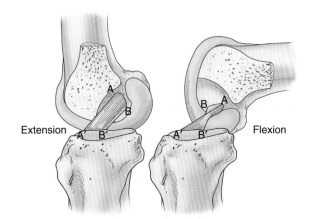

FIG 1.50 Diagram of the Anterior Cruciate Ligament in Extension and Flexion Note that in extension the PL bulk is taut, whereas in flexion the AM band is tight and the PL bulk is relatively relaxed. (From Girgis FG, Marshall JL, Al Monajem ARS: The cruciate ligaments of the knee joint. *Clin Orthop* 106:216, 1975.)

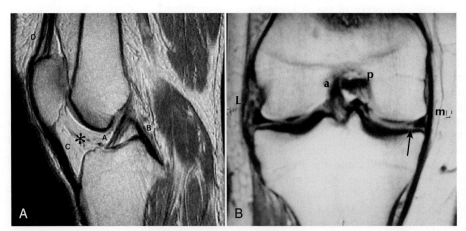

FIG 1.51 Magnetic Resonance Imaging of the Knee Sagittal view demonstrating a normal ACL (A) and PCL (B). The low-signal patellar (C) and quadriceps (D) tendons and the high-signal fat pad *(asterisk)* can be identified anteriorly. (B) Coronal view with the ACL *(a)* lateral to the PCL *(p)* in the intercondylar notch. The low-signal MCL *(m)* runs from the femur, with the superficial fibers extending distally onto the medial aspect of the tibia. The LCL *(L)* and a small tear in the medial meniscus *(arrow)* can be seen.

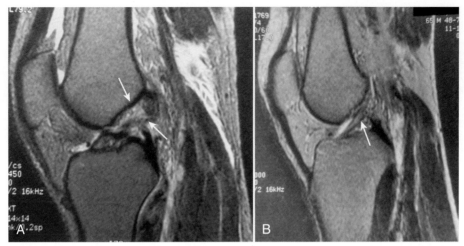

FIG 1.52 (A) Sagittal MRI of a torn ACL with disruption at the femoral origin *(arrows)* and an abnormal wavy contour. (B) Sagittal MRI showing hemorrhage about the ACL and intrasubstance signal *(arrow)* consistent with a partial ACL tear, later confirmed by arthroscopic examination.

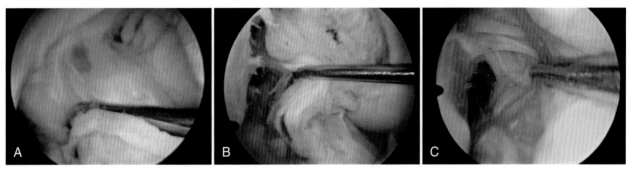

FIG 1.53 Arthroscopic Views of Anterior Cruciate Ligament Tears (A) A significant partial proximal ACL tear with a small number of intact fibers inferiorly. (B) Complete ACL tear with the remaining stump of ruptured fibers at the tibial insertion retracted medially. The bare intercondylar wall (empty wall sign) of the lateral condyle is evident. (C) Close-up view of the empty wall sign. The stump of the ACL is retracted medially to reveal that the intercondylar wall of the lateral femoral condyle is devoid of the normal ACL origin.

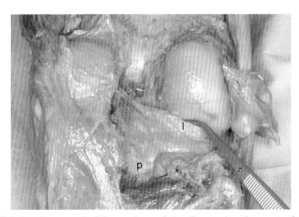

FIG 1.54 Anatomic Dissection of the Posterior Aspect of the Knee The PCL *(p)* originates on the lateral aspect of the medial femoral condyle and inserts on the posterior aspect of the tibia distal to the articular surface (*l*, probe on the superior aspect of the lateral meniscus).

visualized in both the sagittal and coronal planes (see Fig. 1.51A and B). In addition, the meniscofemoral ligaments of Humphry and Wrisberg may be identified close to the anterior and posterior aspects of the PCL. Tears of the PCL appear as bright signal intensity within the tendon substance, indicative of damage of the ligament fibers or frank discontinuity (Fig. 1.55). Chronic tears may appear as thinning or as an abnormal contour of the ligament.

The PCL is considered to be the primary stabilizer of the knee because it is located close to the central axis of rotation of the joint and is almost twice as strong as the ACL.[25,58,72,125,132] The PCL has been shown to provide approximately 95% of the total restraint to posterior translation of the tibia on the femur.[17] It is maximally taut at full flexion and becomes tighter with internal rotation (Fig. 1.56). Two inseparable components of the PCL have been identified. Anterior fibers form the bulk of the ligament and are believed to be taut in flexion and lax in extension. The opposite applies to the thinner posterior portion. The PCL appears to function in concert with the LCL and the popliteus tendon to stabilize the knee. Cutting studies have demonstrated that posterior translation in flexion significantly

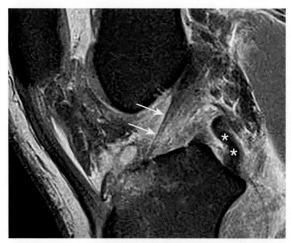

FIG 1.55 Complete Tear of the Posterior Cruciate Ligament in a 35-Year-Old Man With a History of Traumatic Knee Dislocation Sagittal fat-suppressed PD magnetic resonance image of the knee shows the torn PCL *(asterisks)* with its tibial attachment intact. The PCL was torn from its femoral attachment. At arthroscopic reconstruction the ACL *(white arrows)* was confirmed to be intact.

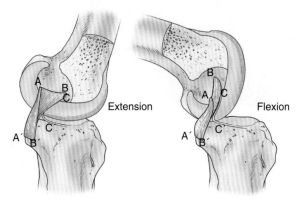

FIG 1.56 Posterior Cruciate Ligament In flexion the bulk of the ligament becomes tight, whereas in extension it is relaxed. (From Girgis FG, Marshall JL, Al Monajem ARS: The cruciate ligaments of the knee joint. *Clin Orthop* 106:216, 1975.)

increases when only the PCL is cut, but when the LCL and the popliteus are also transected, the translation is significantly greater.[42,125]

Injuries to the PCL are less common than injuries to the ACL and usually result from hyperextension or anterior blows to a flexed knee. Rarely do these injuries result in symptomatic instability, but they may be associated with chronic pain. Significant degenerative changes that involve the medial compartment in 90% of cases have been associated with chronic PCL injuries.[25]

The nature of the superior attachment of the cruciate ligaments results in twisting of the bands around their longitudinal axes on flexion. The ACL and PCL are twisted in opposite directions because they are attached to opposing surfaces. From the front, the direction of torsion will appear to be toward the center of the joint.

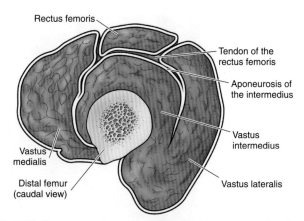

FIG 1.57 Four components of the quadriceps muscle shown through a cross-section at the junction of the middle and distal thirds of the femur. The four components then fuse to form the trilaminar tendon of the quadriceps muscle.

ANTERIOR ASPECT

The quadriceps muscle group consists of four distinct parts that share a common tendon of insertion (Fig. 1.57). The rectus femoris arises as two heads—direct and indirect—from the ilium that unite and form a muscle belly running distally in the anterior aspect of the thigh. It narrows to a tendon 5 to 8 cm proximal to the superior pole of the patella.[106] The rectus femoris accounts for approximately 15% of the cross-section of the quadriceps group. The vastus lateralis arises from a broad linear strip, beginning at the proximal end of the trochanteric line and extending halfway down the linea aspera. It also arises from the lateral intermuscular septum. A fibrous expansion from the distal margin of the vastus lateralis blends with the lateral patellar retinaculum, through which direct attachment to the tibia is attained. The vastus medialis originates from the distal part of the trochanteric line and follows the spiral line to the medial lip of the linea aspera. The most distal fibers of the muscle arise from the tendon of the adductor magnus and pass almost horizontally. This part of the muscle is sometimes described as the vastus medialis obliquus (VMO). Like the vastus lateralis the vastus medialis has a distal fibrous expansion that blends with the common tendon and inserts into the medial border of the patella. This tendinous insertion of the vastus medialis occurs at a mean of approximately 50% of the length of the patella.[55,100] However, this is variable and can occur more proximally or distally, with approximately 25% of patients on MRI noted to have an inferior insertion of the vastus medialis that occurred distal to 60% of the patellar length.[55] This insertion point has become important in the debate on the minimally invasive knee exposures, in which a central principle is to avoid violation of the quadriceps muscles and tendon. Based on anatomic observations of the vastus medialis insertion, any knee exposure that incorporates a capsular incision that extends proximal to the midportion of the patella should not be described, from a scientific perspective, as quadriceps sparing.[100] The vastus intermedius arises from the anterior and lateral aspects of the shaft of the femur; medially it partly blends with the vastus medialis. The four muscles become confluent distally and form the quadriceps tendon, which extends anteriorly about the patella and becomes the patellar tendon (ligament) (Fig. 1.58). The fibers of the rectus

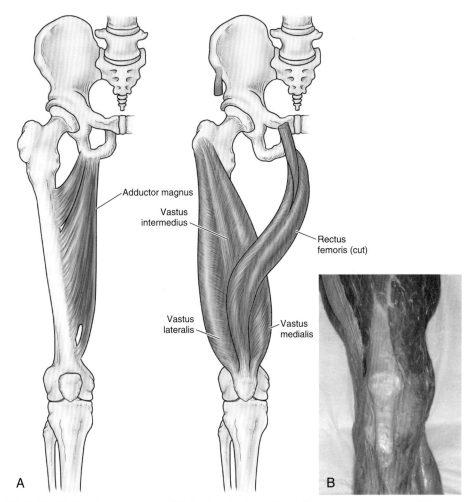

FIG 1.58 (A) Quadriceps group. (B) Anatomic dissection of the anterior aspect of the knee.

femoris and vastus intermedius insert almost perpendicularly into the superior pole of the patella, whereas the fibers of the vastus medialis and lateralis insert obliquely at mean angles of approximately 50 to 55 degrees (range, 28 to 70 degrees) and 14 degrees (range, 6 to 45 degrees), respectively.[57,100,106]

The quadriceps tendon is often depicted as a trilaminar structure; the anterior layer is formed by the rectus femoris, the intermediate layer by the vastus medialis and lateralis, and the deep layer by the tendon of the vastus intermedius.[78,106] In reality the organization is more complex and variable.[106] On MRI the multilaminar nature of the tendon may produce a striated appearance on sagittal views rather than a uniformly low signal structure (see Fig. 1.51A). Discontinuity or increased signal intensity within the tendon substance and in the surrounding tissues on T2-weighted images is suggestive of quadriceps rupture (Fig. 1.59). Distally the quadriceps tendon inserts into the patella via an expansion that passes anterior to the patella. In most cases, only fibers from the rectus femoris portion of the tendon continue in the distal expansion over the patella. However, in some cases fibers from the vastus lateralis can also directly insert distally. In addition, extensions from the medial and lateral vasti insert into the tibia via the patellar retinaculum.

The patellar tendon runs from the lower border of the patella to the tubercle of the tibia. Because the shaft of the femur has an inclination, the quadriceps muscle does not pull in a direct

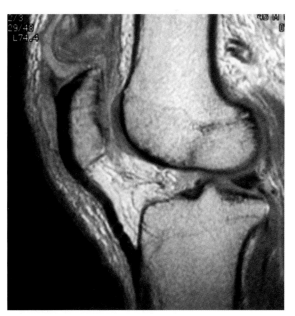

FIG 1.59 Sagittal magnetic resonance image of a complete quadriceps tendon tear with a discontinuity in the fibers at the attachment site on the superior pole of the patella.

line with the patellar tendon. The angle formed is always valgus, and the average angle is 14 degrees in males and 17 degrees in females.[1] This angle, the quadriceps (Q) angle, is accentuated by internal rotation of the femur (Fig. 1.60). The resulting tendency toward lateral patellar displacement is resisted by the lateral lip of the femoral trochlea, the horizontal fibers of the VMO, and the medial patellar retinaculum. Selective strengthening of the VMO has been proposed as treatment of patellofemoral pain and subluxation. Although the most visible function of the quadriceps group is to extend the knee (with a secondary function to flex the hip), the primary physiologic action is to decelerate flexion of the knee during the early stance phase of gait by contracting in an eccentric manner. The four segments of the quadriceps femoris are supplied by the femoral nerve.

The patellar tendon is a strong, flat ligamentous band approximately 5 cm in length. Proximally it originates from the apex and adjoining margins of the patella and the rough depression on the posterior surface. Distally the patellar tendon inserts into the tuberosity of the tibia; superficial fibers are continuous over the front of the patella with those of the tendon of the quadriceps femoris.[106] Medial and lateral portions of the quadriceps tendon pass down on either side of the patella and insert into the proximal end of the tibia on either side of the tuberosity. These expansions merge into the capsule and form the medial and lateral patellar retinacula. The patellar tendon normally has low signal intensity on MRI, but it is not uncommon for it to contain an intermediate signal at the patella or at tibial attachments. As elsewhere, focal discontinuity or high signal intensity in and about the tendon is indicative of a disruption or tear (Fig. 1.61).

The posterior surface of the patellar tendon is separated from the synovial membrane of the joint by a large infrapatellar pad of fat and from the tibia by a bursa. The fat pad fills the space between the femoral condyles and the patellar tendon and adjusts its shape as the size of this potential cavity varies with movement. The fat pad is pierced by numerous blood vessels derived from the genicular arteries. The patellar tendon forms an incomplete septum between the anterior intercondylar notch of the femur and the fat pad.

MEDIAL ASPECT

According to Warren and Marshall,[129] the supporting structures on the medial side of the knee can be divided into three layers. Layer 1 is the most superficial in that it is the first fascial plane encountered after a skin incision is made on the medial side of the knee. The plane is defined by the fascia that invests the sartorius muscle (Fig. 1.62). The sartorius inserts into this network of fascial fibers and does not have a distinct insertion distally on the tibia. Posteriorly a layer of fatty tissue lies between

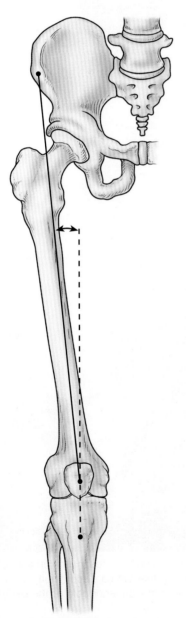

FIG 1.60 Quadriceps (Q) Angle.

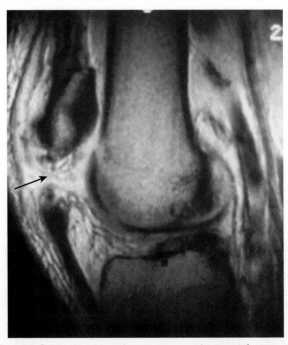

FIG 1.61 Sagittal magnetic resonance image of a patellar tendon tear at the inferior pole of the patella (arrow).

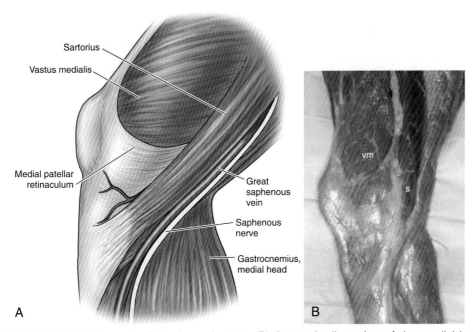

Sartorius

Vastus medialis

Medial patellar
retinaculum

Great
saphenous
vein

Saphenous
nerve

Gastrocnemius,
medial head

A

B

vm

s

FIG 1.62 (A) Medial aspect of the knee, layer 1. (B) Anatomic dissection of the medial knee. Layer 1 on the medial aspect of the knee is defined by the fascial layer, which invests the sartorius muscle *(s)*. *vm,* Vastus medialis.

layer 1 and the deeper structures. The gracilis and semitendinosus tendons lie in the plane between layers 1 and 2 (Fig. 1.63). Farther posteriorly layer 1 is a fascial sheet that overlies the two heads of the gastrocnemius and the structures of the popliteal fossa. This layer serves as a support for muscle bellies and neurovascular structures in the popliteal region. Layer 1 can always be separated from the underlying parallel and oblique portions of the superficial MCL. If a vertical incision is made posterior to the parallel fibers of the ligament, the anterior portion of layer 1 can be reflected anteriorly to expose the superficial MCL. Approximately 1 cm anterior to the superficial MCL, layer 1 blends with the anterior portion of layer 2 and the medial patellar retinaculum derived from the vastus medialis. Anteriorly and distally layer 1 joins the periosteum of the tibia.

Layer 2 is the plane of the superficial MCL. The superficial MCL, as described by Brantigan and Voshell,[16] consists of parallel and oblique portions (Fig. 1.64). Anterior or parallel fibers arise from the sulcus of the medial epicondyle of the femur and consist of heavy, vertically oriented fibers running distally to an insertion on the medial surface of the tibia. This insertion is on average 4.6 cm inferior to the tibial articular surface and is immediately posterior to the insertion of the pes anserinus. The posterior oblique fibers run from the medial epicondyle and blend with layer 3 to form the posteromedial joint capsule.

Anteriorly, according to Warren and Marshall,[129] layer 2 splits vertically. The fibers anterior to the split proceed cephalad to the vastus medialis and join the plane of layer 1 to form the parapatellar retinaculum. The fibers posterior to the split run cephalad to the femoral condyle, from which transverse fibers run forward in the plane of layer 2 to the patella and form the medial patellofemoral ligament (MPFL). This MPFL connects the patella to the medial femoral condyle and passively limits lateral patellar excursion. Indeed in biomechanical tests it has been identified as the most important soft tissue restraint during the first 20 to 30 degrees of flexion, when the patellar is

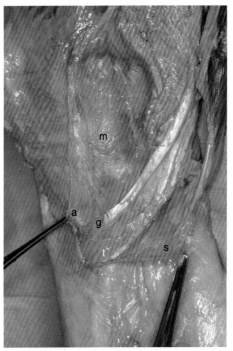

m

a

g

t

s

FIG 1.63 Anatomic Dissection of the Medial Aspect of the Knee The tendons of the gracilis *(g)* and the semitendinosus *(t)* lie between layer 1 (the fascia investing the sartorius) and layer 2 *(m,* the superficial MCL). In this specimen, layer 1 has been divided, the sartorius insertion and fascia are retracted posteriorly *(s,* inferior forceps), and the anterior fascial margin is retracted anteriorly *(a,* superior forceps).

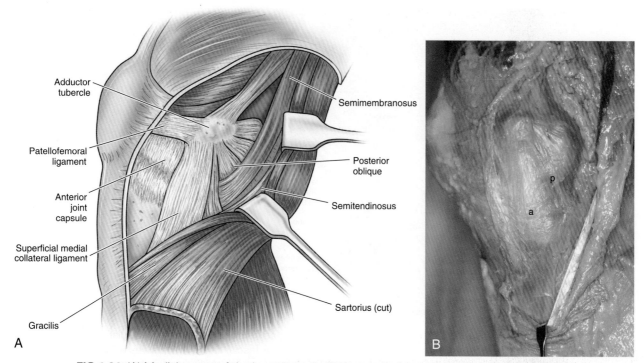

FIG 1.64 (A) Medial aspect of the knee, layer 2. (B) Anatomic dissection of the medial knee. The pes tendons are retracted distally and posteriorly to reveal the anterior parallel fibers *(a)* and the posterior oblique fibers *(p)* of the superficial MCL (layer 2).

at greatest risk of lateral dislocation, contributing between 50% and 60% of the total force.[28,31] The MPFL extends from its broad patellar attachment on the superior two-thirds of the medial patellar, with fibers also adhering to the undersurface of the vastus medialis, to a much narrower attachment on the medial femoral condyle that predisposes to injury in this location.[95,115] The precise attachment site on the medial femoral condyle is more controversial, with a number of anatomic and radiographic locations debated, including just distal to the adductor tubercle; the anterior portion of the medial epicondyle; the posterior portion of medial epicondyle; and the MCL.[95,108,115] Injuries of the MPFL and medial retinaculum that occur during lateral patellar dislocation can be visualized on routine knee MRI (Fig. 1.65). The most common locations for acute MPFL injuries include avulsions from the femoral attachment and tears of the MPFL near the femoral insertion.[95] During the past two decades, considerable knowledge has been gained about the importance of the MPFL in normal function of the patellofemoral joint. Indeed MPFL reconstruction has become the first-choice procedure for chronic lateral patellar instability.[108] However, this operation remains a challenging, with further information needed on the impact of the location of the femoral graft origin and graft tension.[108] At the inferior border of the medial patella is the medial patellomeniscal ligament, which connects the patella to the anterior horn of the medial meniscus. This structure, along with the retinacular fibers, is also an important patellar stabilizer, accounting for 10% to 20% of the total force resisting lateral dislocation.[28,31] Layer 3, the capsule of the knee joint, can be separated from layer 2 except toward the margin of the patella, where it becomes very thin (Fig. 1.66). Deep to the superficial MCL, layer 3 becomes thicker and forms a vertically oriented band of short fibers known as the deep MCL. The deep MCL extends from the femur to the midportion

of the peripheral margin of the meniscus and tibia (Fig. 1.67). Anteriorly the deep MCL is clearly separated from the superficial MCL, and a bursa is interposed, but posteriorly the layers blend because the meniscofemoral portion of the deep ligament tends to merge with the overlying superficial ligament near its cephalad attachment. However, the meniscotibial portion of the deep MCL is readily separated from the overlying superficial ligament and is referred to as the coronary ligament. Components of the MCL are well seen on MRI studies. Coronal images provide clear visualization, but axial images can provide complementary information. Normal ligament fibers have low signal intensity (see Fig. 1.51B). With partial and complete tears the fibers become less distinct, and increased signal on T2-weighted images can be identified in and adjacent to the MCL as a result of edema and bleeding (Fig. 1.68).

The posteromedial region formed by the merging of layers 2 and 3 is reinforced by five insertions of the semimembranosus tendon and tendon sheath. The semimembranosus has a direct tendinous insertion on the posteromedial corner of the tibia and a second tibial insertion deep to the superficial MCL (see Fig. 1.66). A third tract blends with the oblique fibers of the superficial MCL, and a fourth doubles back to insert proximally in the capsule over the medial meniscus. The fifth tract runs proximally and laterally across the posterior capsule and forms the oblique popliteal ligament (of Winslow) (Fig. 1.69).[129]

On the medial side the three layers are most obviously separated in the region of the superficial MCL. Anteriorly the superficial layer and a portion of the middle layer blend and merge with the overlying retinacular expansion from the quadriceps. The other cephalad portion of the middle layer, formed where it splits anterior to the superficial medial ligament, persists as a separate layer forming the patellofemoral ligament. Anteriorly the deep layer, although separate, becomes extremely thin and

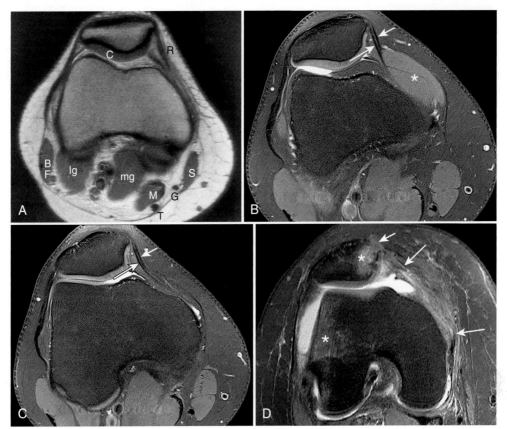

FIG 1.65 (A) High-resolution axial MRI of the knee. The popliteal vessels and the tibial nerve can be identified between the two heads of the gastrocnemius. The other following structures are marked: patella articular cartilage *(c)*, medial patellar retinaculum *(R)*, sartorius muscle *(S)*, gracilis muscle *(G)*, semimembranosus muscle *(M)*, semitendinosus tendon *(T)*, medial head of the gastrocnemius *(mg)*, lateral head of the gastrocnemius *(lg)*, and biceps femoris *(BF)*. (B and C) Normal anatomy of the medial retinaculum and MPFL on axial fat-suppressed PD MRIs. An image just distal to the superior margin of the patella (B) shows the MFPL *(short wide arrow)* as its superior margin courses obliquely from the upper pole of the patella to the adductor tubercle of the medial femoral condyle, deep to the vastus medialis muscle *(asterisk)*. The medial retinaculum *(long, thin arrow)* courses just superficial to the MPFL, although they may not be identified as distinct structures. More distally (C), below the level of the vastus medialis, they are still identified as distinct structures in this patient. (D) Axial fat-suppressed PD magnetic resonance image from a different patient immediately following first transient dislocation shows abnormal anatomy with extensive tearing of the medial retinaculum and MPFL (between *short wide arrows*). Note impaction fracture of the medial margin of the patella *(long, thin arrow)* with edema-like signal in both the medial patella and lateral femoral condyle at the site of impaction *(asterisks)*, features characteristic of transient patellar dislocation.

difficult to define. Posteriorly layer 1 becomes the deep fascia, and layers 2 and 3 blend to form the joint capsule.

The superficial MCL functions as the primary restraint against valgus stress, a restraint to external rotation of the tibia, and a weak restraint to anterior tibial translation in ACL-deficient knees.[119,130] The anterior parallel fibers of the superficial MCL are under tension from full extension to 90 degrees of flexion but become maximally taut at 45 to 90 degrees of flexion.[39,93,130] During extension the anterior fibers relax and the posterior fibers become taught.[39,93] Strain measurements in the ligament confirm that different areas of the superficial MCL experience different forces, depending on valgus load and joint position. Peak strain during valgus loading appears to occur in the fully extended position near the femoral insertion; this

finding explains the high rate of clinical injury noted to occur in this portion of the ligament.[39] Oblique fibers seem to play a minimal role in overall function of the superficial MCL. The deep MCL performs only a weak secondary role as a stabilizer against valgus stress. Understanding of the anatomy and function of the individual portions of the MCL is important during soft tissue balancing in total knee arthroplasty, as well as during evaluation of traumatic injury.

LATERAL ASPECT

Supporting structures on the lateral side of the knee have also been described by Seebacher and colleagues as consisting of three layers.[113] Layer 1 contains the superficial fascia (fascia lata), ITB, and biceps femoris, with its expansion posteriorly (Fig. 1.70). Layer 2 is formed by the quadriceps retinaculum anteriorly and is incomplete posteriorly, where it consists of two patellofemoral ligaments. Layer 3 is composed of the lateral capsule and the following structures (Fig. 1.71).[105,113] Posterior to the overlying iliotibial tract, the posterior capsule is divided into two laminae. The deep lamina is composed of the coronary ligament and the arcuate ligament and is newer phylogenetically. The superficial lamina represents the original capsule and consists of the LCL and the fabellofibular ligament. The inferior lateral geniculate artery passes between the two laminae (Fig. 1.72). The newly described anterolateral ligament (ALL) of the knee is also found in layer 3, where it represents a distinctly

thicker structure than the capsule that is found more anteriorly in the same layer (see Fig. 1.71).[24]

The ITB is a longitudinal thickening in the fascia lata that runs along the lateral side of the knee and inserts into Gerdy's tubercle on the tibia. Some of the fibers proceed across Gerdy's tubercle to the tibial tuberosity. Proximally the fascia lata is adherent to the lateral intermuscular septum, where it is attached to the femur. Posteriorly the fascia lata merges into the biceps fascia.[66] The biceps femoris muscle is formed from two heads; the long head arises in common with the semitendinosus from the ischial tuberosity, and the short head arises from the lateral lip of the linea aspera, the lateral supracondylar line, and the lateral intermuscular septum. The nerve supply of both heads is derived from the sciatic nerve, but from different branches; the long head is innervated by the tibial branch, and the short head by the common popliteal nerve. The two heads unite above the knee joint in a common tendon that folds around the LCL insertion on the fibular styloid and then divides into three layers.[88] The superficial layer spreads out and inserts as a wide expansion over the adjoining part of the proximal tibia. The middle layer is a thin, poorly defined layer that envelops the LCL and is separated from the ligament by a bursa. The deep layer bifurcates and inserts on the fibular styloid and on the tibia at Gerdy's tubercle. The biceps functions mainly as a knee flexor but additionally acts as a weaker hip extensor and external rotator of the tibia. The biceps is also believed to be an important static and dynamic stabilizer of the lateral aspect of the knee, especially as the knee flexes beyond 30 degrees.[94,122]

The lateral knee retinaculum has been described by Fulkerson and Gossling[37] (Fig. 1.73). The lateral patellar retinaculum is composed of two major components: the superficial oblique retinaculum and the deep transverse retinaculum. The superficial oblique retinaculum runs superficially from the ITB to the patella (Fig. 1.74). The deep transverse retinaculum is denser and consists of three major components. The epicondylopatellar band, also known as the transverse patellofemoral ligament, provides superolateral patellar support. The transverse retinaculum courses directly from the ITB to the

Text continued on p. 38

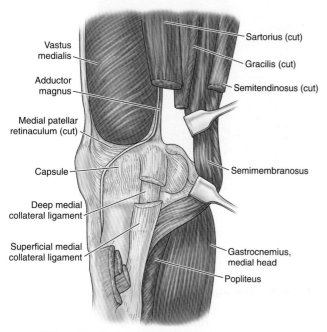

FIG 1.66 Medial Aspect of the Knee, Layer 3

Vastus medialis
Adductor magnus
Medial patellar retinaculum (cut)
Capsule
Deep medial collateral ligament
Superficial medial collateral ligament
Sartorius (cut)
Gracilis (cut)
Semitendinosus (cut)
Semimembranosus
Gastrocnemius, medial head
Popliteus

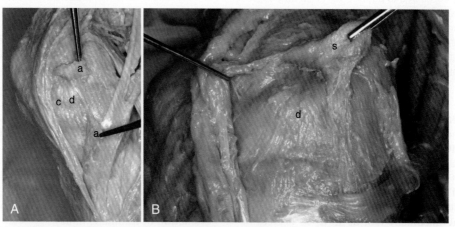

FIG 1.67 Anatomic Dissections of the Medial Aspect of the Knee (A) The anterior parallel fibers *(a)* of the superficial MCL (layer 2) have been sectioned transversely through the middle of the ligament and retracted posteriorly (both forceps) to reveal the fibers of the deep MCL *(d)* and capsule *(c,* layer 3). (B) Close-up view of fibers of the deep MCL *(d)* from the femur to the periphery of the meniscus attachment on the tibia. The superficial MCL *(s)* has been sectioned and the proximal portion retracted proximally (forceps).

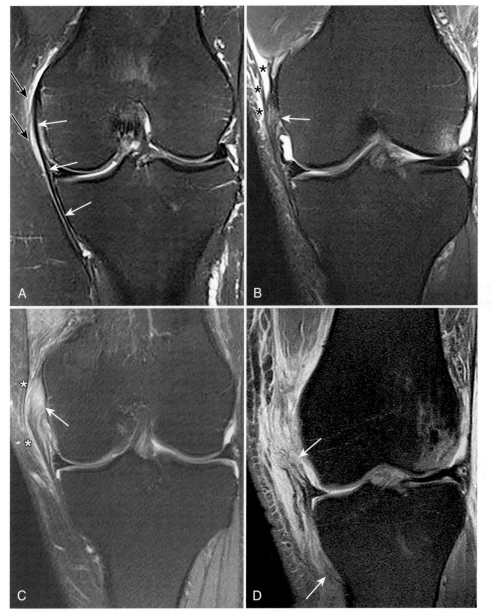

FIG 1.68 Spectrum of Medial Collateral Ligament Injuries on Coronal Fat-Suppressed PD Magnetic Resonance Images. (A) Grade I injury with an intact ligament *(white arrows)* and associated high signal and inflammatory change *(black arrows).* (B) Grade II injury to the ligament *(arrow)* with thickening and abnormal signal, as well as associated inflammatory change *(asterisks).* (C) More severe grade II injury to the ligament with more pronounced thickening, greater abnormal signal as well as disruption of fibers. Note the ligament remains taught. The decreased inflammatory change *(asterisks)* reflects the chronic nature of the injury. (D) Grade III injury with complete disruption of the ligament *(proximal arrow).* Note the extensive inflammatory change in this patient evaluated shortly after a complex knee injury. Note relative laxity of the ligament *(distal arrow),* a useful secondary sign of complete disruption.

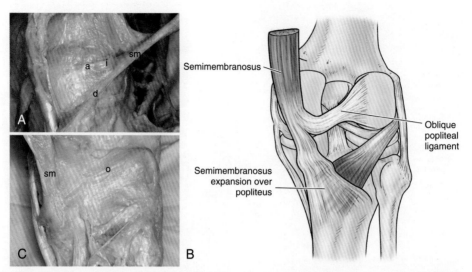

FIG 1.69 (A) Anatomic dissection of medial aspect of the knee. The superficial MCL has been sectioned and retracted to reveal the direct insertion *(i)* of the semimembranosus *(sm)* on the posteromedial tibia and the anterior extension *(a)* deep to the superficial MCL. A band of fibers *(d)* also runs distally to insert into the retracted superficial MCL. (B) Relationship of the oblique popliteal ligament *(o)* to the semimembranosus muscle. (C) Anatomic dissection of the posterior aspect of the knee, demonstrating the oblique popliteal ligament *(o)*, which passes obliquely across the posterior capsule to insert on the lateral femoral condyle.

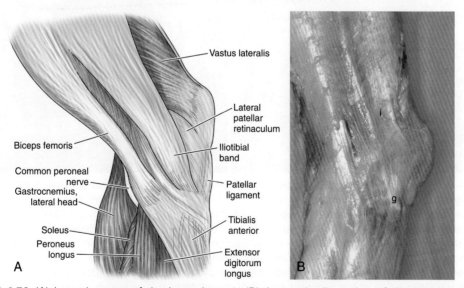

FIG 1.70 (A) Lateral aspect of the knee, layer 1. (B) Anatomic dissection of the lateral knee. Layer 1 on the lateral side of the knee with a prominent ITB *(i)* insertion on Gerdy's tubercle *(g)*.

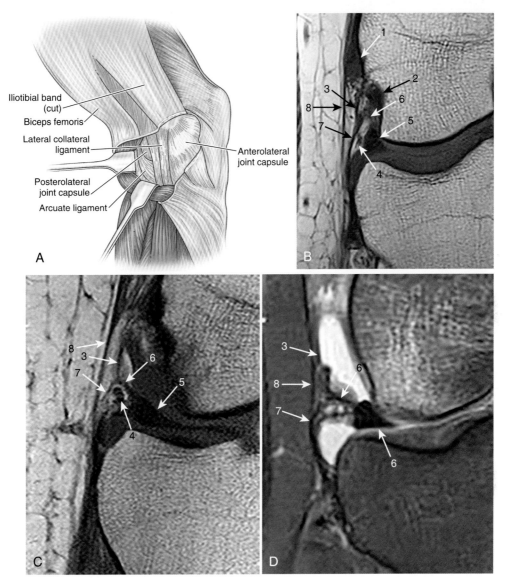

FIG 1.71 (A) Lateral aspect of the knee, layer 3. (B-D) Anatomy of the ALL on coronal T1-weighted magnetic resonance images. (B) Normal ALL. The ALL is seen with greatest clarity on coronal nonfat-suppressed images, being a fibrous structure surrounded by adipose tissue, typically 1 to 3 mm thick. The ALL is located immediately anterior to the femoral attachment of the LCL *(arrow 1)*. It extends anteroinferiorly, superficial to the popliteus tendon and popliteal groove *(arrow 2)*. It is anatomically divided into three sections: the most proximal is the femoral *(arrow 3)*, extending from the femur and bifurcating to the meniscal and tibial parts. The bifurcation is usually above and lateral to the inferior geniculate artery *(arrow 4)*, adjacent to the lateral meniscus *(arrow 5)*. The meniscal portion *(arrow 6)* is incompletely seen on this image, whereas the tibial portion is easily identified *(arrow 7)*, inserting on the tibia adjacent to the ITB *(arrow 8)*. (C and D) (same numbering as Fig. 1.71B) Coronal T1-weighted (C) magnetic resonance image in a patient being evaluated following patella dislocation shows a normal ALL. Corresponding fluid-sensitive magnetic resonance image (fat-suppressed PD image) (D) shows the ALL at the margin of the fluid-distended joint.

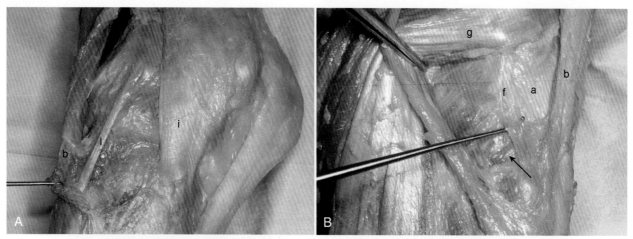

FIG 1.72 Anatomic Dissections of the Posterolateral Aspect of the Knee (A) The superficial layers along the posterior margin of the ITB *(i)* have been incised and retracted posteriorly to reveal layer 3 of the lateral aspect of the knee. The prominent LCL *(l)* inserts deep to the biceps *(b,* retracted by the probe) on the fibular head. (B) The lateral head of the gastrocnemius *(g)* has been retracted medially (forceps) to expose the fabellofibular *(f)* and arcuate ligaments *(a)*. The inferior lateral geniculate artery *(arrow)* passes between the fabellofibular ligament (superficial lamina of layer 3) and the arcuate ligament (deep lamina of layer 3) just distal to the probe placed between the two laminae *(b,* biceps femoris).

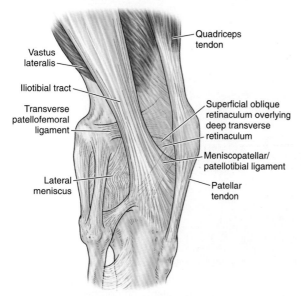

FIG 1.73 Structures of the Lateral Retinaculum.

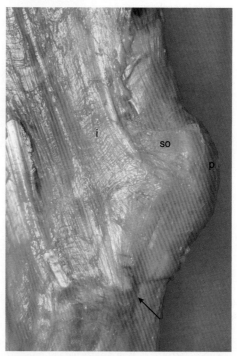

FIG 1.74 Anatomic Dissection of the Lateral Aspect of the Knee The superficial oblique *(so)* fibers of the lateral retinaculum run between the anterior margin of the ITB *(i)* and the lateral aspect of the patella *(p)* (*arrow,* Gerdy's tubercle).

midpatella and provides the primary support for the lateral patella. The patellotibial band, the third component, runs between the patella and the tibia inferiorly (Fig. 1.75). Overall the lateral retinaculum provides stronger support to the patella than is provided by its medial counterpart.

In layer 3 the lateral joint capsule is a thin, fibrous layer that is circumferentially attached to the femur and tibia at the proximal and distal margins of the knee joint. The attachment at the margin of the inferior border of the lateral meniscus, which runs to the edge of the articular margin of the tibia, has been termed the *coronary ligament.*[79,113]

The ALL of the knee, initially partially recognized in 1879 by Segond and recently more completely described by Claes et al. is a distinct ligamentous structure that is consistently found in the cadaveric specimens and is distinguishable from the anterolateral joint capsule.[24,105] The origin of the ALL is on the prominence of the lateral femoral epicondyle just anterior to and distinct from the origin of the LCL, although, while clearly separate structures, in most cases, fibers of the two structures are noted to be confluent at their origins.[24] The ALL passes

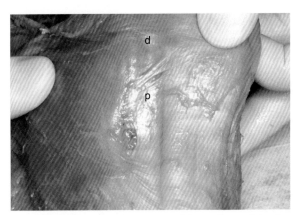

FIG 1.75 Close-Up of an Anatomic Dissection of the Lateral Retinaculum With the superficial oblique retinaculum removed, the patellotibial band *(p)* and transverse fibers *(d)* of the deep retinaculum can be identified.

obliquely to the anterolateral aspect of the proximal tibia, with attachments to the lateral meniscus and anterolateral tibia midway between Gerdy's tubercle and the tip of the fibular head.[24] Although information about the ALL is new and incomplete, this ligament appears to control internal rotation of the tibia, especially at flexion greater than 35 degrees.[24,102] The previously described lateral capsular avulsion fracture, the so-called Segond fracture, noted to be associated with ACL injury has been demonstrated to represent an avulsion, with a fleck of bone, of the insertion of the ALL from the anterolateral tibia.[23] The ALL may be difficult to completely visualize on a 1.5-T MRI, because of the oblique course and lack of familiarity with the structure. Studies have demonstrated that this normal structure is completely identified throughout its course in only 11% to 72% of cases.[52,120] Currently the best sequences for inspecting this normal structure on 1.5-T MRI appear to be in the coronal plane; however, increased magnet strength (3-T MRI) and improvements in the sequences obtained to include oblique and thinner sections will likely improve the ability to demonstrate this ligament.[52] Ultrasound may represent another useful modality for examining the integrity of the ALL.[19] Further investigation is required to better understand the importance of both isolated ALL injury and ALL injury that occurs in the presence of ACL injury. Whether ALL injuries require surgery and the optimal methods to use, if surgery is undertaken, also require further study.

The LCL originates on the lateral epicondyle of the femur, anterior to the origin of the gastrocnemius. It runs beneath the lateral retinaculum to insert into the head of the fibula, where it blends with the insertion of the biceps femoris. On MRI studies the LCL is best seen on coronal images and appears as a thin band of low signal intensity (see Fig. 1.51B). Two to three sequential images are usually required to visualize the entire structure because of the oblique course of the ligament. A tear appears as a disruption in the fibers, thickening, or increased signal on T2-weighted images in and about the ligament as a result of edema.

The fabellofibular ligament is a condensation of fibers lying between the LCL and arcuate ligaments that runs from the fabella, a sesamoid bone found in the lateral head of the gastrocnemius, to the fibular styloid.[67] The arcuate ligament has been variously described; according to Last, "In truth, there is at this part of the capsule such a complexity of fibers running

in many directions that, by artful dissection, almost any pattern desired by the dissector could be made."[79] Some fibers extend from the lateral condyle of the femur to the posterior part of the capsule. However, the strongest and most consistent fibers of the arcuate ligament form a triangular sheet that diverges upward from the fibular styloid. The lateral limb of this mass is dense and strong and is attached to the femur and the popliteal tendon. The weaker medial limb curves over the popliteal muscle and blends with the fibers of the oblique popliteal ligament. The free edge of this medial limb is crescentic, and the lateral or femoral part of the popliteus emerges beneath it to approach its tibial attachment. Three common variations in the fabellofibular and arcuate ligaments have been described. In most knees (67%) both the fabellofibular and arcuate ligaments are present, but in the case of a large fabella, the fabellofibular ligament dominates, and the arcuate ligament is absent (20%); however, in the absence of a fabella, only the arcuate ligament is present (13%).[113] Watanabe et al. further divided these categories into a total of seven types based on the presence or absence of a fibular insertion of a portion of the popliteal tendon.[131]

The popliteal muscle arises with a strong tendon approximately 2.5 cm long, from a depression at the anterior part of the groove on the lateral condyle of the femur. The tendon, which is invested in synovial membrane, passes beneath the medial limb of the arcuate ligament and forms a thin, flat, triangular muscle that inserts into the medial two-thirds of the triangular surface, proximal to the popliteal line on the posterior surface of the tibia. A direct attachment to the fibular head has been redefined.[90,131] The tendon is also attached to the arcuate ligament, and, according to Last, up to half of its fibers are attached to the lateral meniscus.[79] The synovial membrane below the meniscus herniates deep to the muscle as the popliteus bursa. The function of the popliteus is controversial, but it may act in conjunction with the meniscofemoral ligaments to control the motion of the meniscus as the knee flexes.[11,64,79,123] However, its primary role appears to be unlocking the knee to allow flexion by producing external rotation of the femur in the loaded position.[11,79,86] The nerve to the popliteus arises from the tibial nerve and runs distally across the popliteal vessels to reach the lower border of the muscle, where it enters the deep surface.

The LCL, PCL, and popliteal–arcuate complex act in concert to stabilize the PL corner of the knee, including against varus stress, external tibial rotation, and posterior translation. Damage to these structures results in posterior instability and PL rotatory instability.[8,59,60]

POSTERIOR ASPECT

The popliteal fossa is bounded laterally by the biceps femoris and medially by the semimembranosus and tendons of the pes anserine. Distally, the space is closed by the two heads of the gastrocnemius. The roof of the fossa is formed by the deep fascia; the floor consists of the popliteal surface of the femur, the posterior capsule of the knee joint, and the popliteus muscle with its fascial covering (Fig. 1.76).

The biceps femoris lies posterior to the ITB and forms the lateral wall of the popliteal fossa; it has been described previously. The semitendinosus arises from the ischial tuberosity and runs distally and medially on the surface of the semimembranosus. The semimembranosus arises from the upper and lateral impressions on the ischial tuberosity. It passes distally and

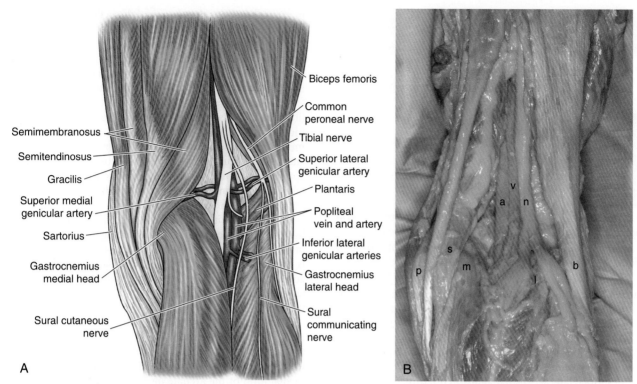

FIG 1.76 (A) Posterior aspect of the knee. The tibial nerve arises from the sciatic nerve in the thigh. The popliteal artery and vein are in close proximity. (B) Anatomic dissection of the popliteal fossa. From left to right (medial to lateral), the identified structures at the level of the joint line are the pes tendons *(p)*; semimembranosus *(s)*; medial head of the gastrocnemius *(m)*; popliteal artery *(a)*, vein *(v)*, and nerve *(n)*; lateral head of the gastrocnemius *(l)*; and biceps femoris tendon *(b)*.

medially deep to the origin of the biceps and semitendinosus (Fig. 1.77). Its tendon forms the proximal and medial boundaries of the popliteal fossa and inserts into a groove on the posteromedial aspect of the tibia. Multiple expansions reinforce the posteromedial capsule, as previously described. Directly posteriorly a robust expansion called the oblique popliteal ligament passes proximally and laterally and blends with the posterior capsule and arcuate ligament from the lateral side. The nerve supply to the hamstring muscles is derived from the tibial branch of the sciatic nerve. The gracilis muscle arises from the inferior pubic ramus and runs distally along the medial side of the thigh. In the lower third of the thigh the fibers end in a long tendon that lies medial to the tendon of the semitendinosus. It is innervated by the obturator nerve. The sartorius muscle arises from the anterior superior iliac spine and runs distally and medially across the front of the thigh, where it forms the roof of the subsartorial canal. Its nerve supply is derived from the femoral nerve. Distally the sartorius tendon is wider and less well defined than the gracilis and semitendinosus nerves. Rather than inserting directly into the tibia, the diffuse tendinous fibers blend with layer 1 of the medial aspect of the knee. Together the tendons of the sartorius, gracilis, and semitendinosus form the pes anserinus (see Fig. 1.77). The sartorius tendon expansion lies superficially and covers the insertions of the gracilis and semitendinosus. The semitendinosus inserts into the tibia just distal to the gracilis and forms a conjoint structure with a mean width of 20 mm; the proximal-most point of the insertion begins at a mean of 19 mm distal and 22.5 mm medial to

the apex of the tibial tubercle.[99] The muscles, which insert at the pes, act to flex and internally rotate the knee.

When the knee is flexed, the biceps tendon can be felt subcutaneously on the lateral side. Medially two tendons are prominent, with the gracilis lying medial to the semitendinosus.

The ischial fibers of the adductor magnus are a derivative of the hamstring group. The fibers run distally and end in a short tendon that inserts into the prominent adductor tubercle on the medial condyle of the femur. Through a gap in the insertion of this muscle, the femoral vessels enter the popliteal fossa. Similar to the hamstrings, this portion of the adductor magnus is supplied by the sciatic nerve.

The gastrocnemius muscle arises as a lateral head from the lateral aspect of the lateral femoral condyle and as a larger medial head from the popliteal surface of the femur and the medial aspect of the medial femoral condyle (Fig. 1.78). The lateral head has a largely fleshy origin, but the portion of the medial head that arises from the medial condyle adjoining the attachment of the MCL is tendinous. The two heads merge and form a common tendon with the soleus, which narrows distally and inserts into the tendo calcaneus.

The plantaris muscle has a small, fleshy belly that arises from the lateral supracondylar line of the femur deep to the lateral head of the gastrocnemius. It gives rise to a very long, narrow tendon that runs distally deep to the medial head of the gastrocnemius. The plantaris is absent in approximately 7% of individuals and is believed to represent a vestigial structure in humans.[30]

The soleus arises from multiple origins, including the upper fourth of the posterior surface of the shaft and head of the fibula, the tendinous arch crossing the posterior tibial vessels and nerve, and the soleal line of the posterior surface of the tibia. Its tendon joins the deep surface of the Achilles tendon. The gastrocnemius, plantaris, and soleus are supplied by the tibial nerve.

NERVES

Although considerable individual variation exists, predominant patterns of innervation about the knee have been identified.[40,70] Two distinct groups of afferent nerves have been differentiated. The first, a posterior group, includes the posterior articular branch of the tibial nerve and obturator nerves. The second group is anterior and includes the articular branches of the femoral, common peroneal, and saphenous nerves.

The tibial nerve (medial or internal popliteal nerve) arises from the sciatic nerve halfway down the thigh. It runs distally through the popliteal fossa, lying at first in the fat beneath the deep fascia. More distally it is found deeper in the interval between the two heads of the gastrocnemius. A cutaneous branch, the sural nerve, descends on the surface of the gastrocnemius (see Fig. 1.76). Muscular branches are given off to both heads of the gastrocnemius, plantaris, soleus, and popliteal muscles. In addition, several articular branches are present. The largest and most consistent branch, the posterior articular nerve, has a variable origin but often arises within the popliteal fossa. In other circumstances it may arise from the tibial portion of the sciatic nerve in the thigh.[40] It courses laterally and wraps

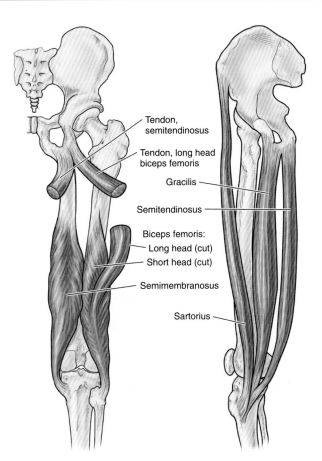

FIG 1.77 Posterior Musculature.

Labels: Tendon, semitendinosus; Tendon, long head biceps femoris; Gracilis; Semitendinosus; Biceps femoris: Long head (cut); Short head (cut); Semimembranosus; Sartorius

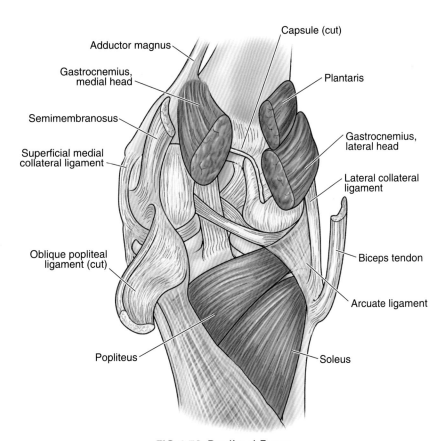

FIG 1.78 Popliteal Fossa.

Labels: Adductor magnus; Gastrocnemius, medial head; Semimembranosus; Superficial medial collateral ligament; Oblique popliteal ligament (cut); Popliteus; Capsule (cut); Plantaris; Gastrocnemius, lateral head; Lateral collateral ligament; Biceps tendon; Arcuate ligament; Soleus

around the popliteal vessels before passing deep to join the popliteal plexus. Fibers from the plexus penetrate through the oblique popliteal ligament to innervate the posterior and perimeniscal capsule and the synovial covering of the cruciates. The extent of innervation of the menisci is controversial; evidence supports penetration of both nerve fibers into the outer third of the menisci and innervation limited to the perimeniscal capsule.[3,70] The terminal branch of the posterior division of the obturator nerve, which follows the course of the femoral artery into the popliteal fossa, contributes to the popliteal plexus and thus to the innervation of the capsule and menisci.

The capsule and ligaments on the AM and anterolateral areas of the knee are innervated by the anterior afferent group, in particular, the articular branches of the nerves, which supply the quadriceps muscles. The largest branch arises from the nerve supplying the vastus medialis and supplies a portion of the AM capsule. Laterally a branch from the nerve to the vastus lateralis innervates the superolateral capsule, and anteriorly, afferent fibers from the suprapatellar pouch join nerves to the vastus intermedius. The saphenous nerve arises from the posterior division of the femoral nerve. At the lower end of the subsartorial canal, the nerve pierces the deep fascia on the medial side of the knee between the sartorius and gracilis tendons. The infrapatellar branch traverses the sartorius muscle and joins the patellar plexus; it provides innervation to the AM capsule, patellar tendon, and skin anteromedially (Fig. 1.79).[62] Distally the sartorial branch of the saphenous nerve is joined by the long saphenous vein and runs along the medial aspect of the leg (Fig. 1.80). The patellar plexus lies in front of the patella and the patellar tendon. It is formed by numerous communications between the terminal branches of the lateral, intermediate, and medial cutaneous nerves of the thigh and the infrapatellar branch of the saphenous nerve.

The common peroneal nerve (lateral or external popliteal nerve) enters the popliteal fossa on the lateral side of the tibial nerve and runs distally along the medial side of the biceps tendon (Fig. 1.81). The common peroneal nerve passes between the biceps femoris tendon and the lateral head of the gastrocnemius and runs distally posterior to the fibula head (Fig. 1.82). It next winds superficially across the lateral aspect of the neck of the fibula before piercing the peroneus longus through a fibrous tunnel and dividing into the superficial peroneal (musculocutaneous) and deep peroneal (anterior tibial) nerves. The cutaneous branches are the sural communicating nerve, which joins the sural nerve, and a small branch to the skin over the upper anterolateral aspect of the leg. Two articular branches of the common peroneal nerve are the lateral articular nerve, which arises at the level of the joint line and innervates the inferior lateral capsule and LCL, and the recurrent peroneal nerve, which ascends the anterior surface of the tibia in the peroneus longus and enters the joint anterolaterally.[70]

The individual structures involved in specific functions such as pain sensation and proprioception in the knee are controversial. Kennedy et al. indicated that deep fibrous structures, such as the ligaments and menisci, rarely contain nerve fibers, whereas both pain and specialized mechanoreceptors are found in the surrounding connective tissues of the capsule and synovium.[70] Stretching of the capsule causes pain, and effusions greater than 60 mL have been shown to cause reflex quadriceps inhibition.[70,117] Because of the numerous

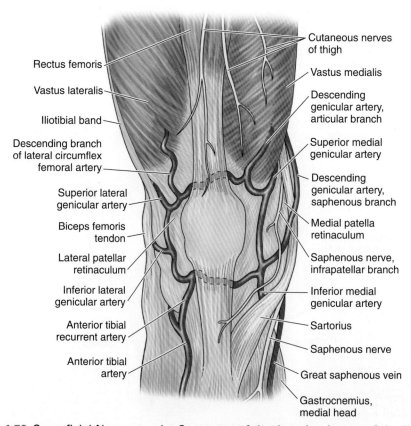

Rectus femoris

Vastus lateralis

Iliotibial band

Descending branch of lateral circumflex femoral artery

Superior lateral genicular artery

Biceps femoris tendon

Lateral patellar retinaculum

Inferior lateral genicular artery

Anterior tibial recurrent artery

Anterior tibial artery

Cutaneous nerves of thigh

Vastus medialis

Descending genicular artery, articular branch

Superior medial genicular artery

Descending genicular artery, saphenous branch

Medial patella retinaculum

Saphenous nerve, infrapatellar branch

Inferior medial genicular artery

Sartorius

Saphenous nerve

Great saphenous vein

Gastrocnemius, medial head

FIG 1.79 Superficial Neurovascular Structures of the Anterior Aspect of the Knee.

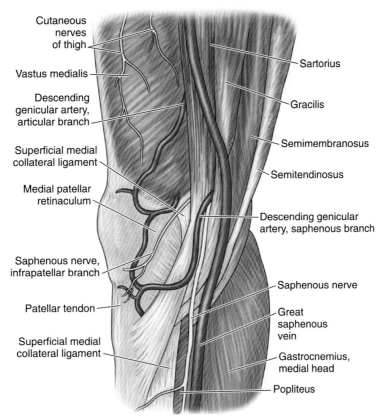

Cutaneous nerves of thigh
Vastus medialis
Descending genicular artery, articular branch
Superficial medial collateral ligament
Medial patellar retinaculum
Saphenous nerve, infrapatellar branch
Patellar tendon
Superficial medial collateral ligament

Sartorius
Gracilis
Semimembranosus
Semitendinosus
Descending genicular artery, saphenous branch
Saphenous nerve
Great saphenous vein
Gastrocnemius, medial head
Popliteus

FIG 1.80 Superficial Neurovascular Structures of the Anteromedial Aspect of the Knee.

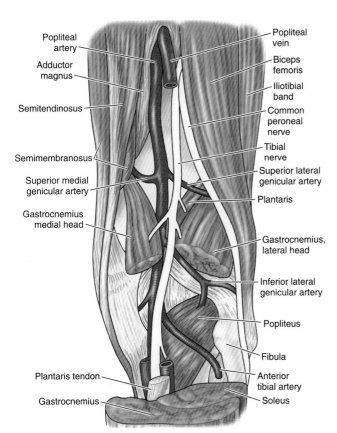

Popliteal artery
Adductor magnus
Semitendinosus
Semimembranosus
Superior medial genicular artery
Gastrocnemius medial head
Plantaris tendon
Gastrocnemius

Popliteal vein
Biceps femoris
Iliotibial band
Common peroneal nerve
Tibial nerve
Superior lateral genicular artery
Plantaris
Gastrocnemius, lateral head
Inferior lateral genicular artery
Popliteus
Fibula
Anterior tibial artery
Soleus

FIG 1.81 Neurovascular Structures of the Popliteal Fossa.

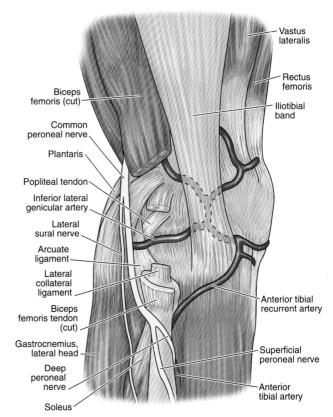

Biceps femoris (cut)
Common peroneal nerve
Plantaris
Popliteal tendon
Inferior lateral genicular artery
Lateral sural nerve
Arcuate ligament
Lateral collateral ligament
Biceps femoris tendon (cut)
Gastrocnemius, lateral head
Deep peroneal nerve
Soleus

Vastus lateralis
Rectus femoris
Iliotibial band
Anterior tibial recurrent artery
Superficial peroneal nerve
Anterior tibial artery

FIG 1.82 Superficial Neurovascular Structures of the Lateral Aspect of the Knee.

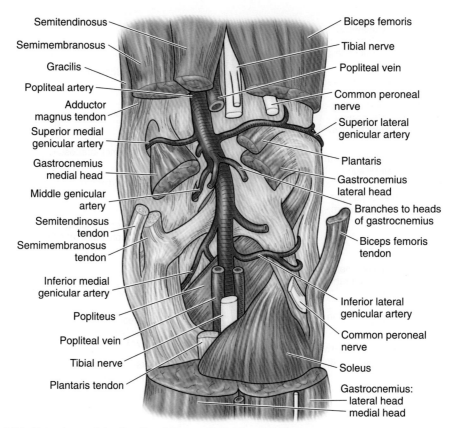

Semitendinosus
Semimembranosus
Gracilis
Popliteal artery
Adductor magnus tendon
Superior medial genicular artery
Gastrocnemius medial head
Middle genicular artery
Semitendinosus tendon
Semimembranosus tendon
Inferior medial genicular artery
Popliteus
Popliteal vein
Tibial nerve
Plantaris tendon

Biceps femoris
Tibial nerve
Popliteal vein
Common peroneal nerve
Superior lateral genicular artery
Plantaris
Gastrocnemius lateral head
Branches to heads of gastrocnemius
Biceps femoris tendon
Inferior lateral genicular artery
Common peroneal nerve
Soleus
Gastrocnemius: lateral head, medial head

FIG 1.83 Branches of the Popliteal Artery in the Popliteal Space The artery lies on the oblique posterior ligament at the level of the joint line. More proximally, it is separated from the posterior of the femur by a layer of fat. The femoral vein is interposed between the artery and the tibial nerve.

mechanoreceptors, the capsule also probably plays a significant role in proprioception.

BLOOD SUPPLY

Before passing through the adductor hiatus, the femoral artery gives off the descending genicular artery. In turn, this vessel gives off the saphenous branch, an articular branch, and the deep oblique branch. The saphenous branch travels distally with the saphenous nerve and passes the sartorius before anastomosing with the medial inferior genicular artery. The articular branch extends distally within the vastus medialis and anastomoses with the lateral superior genicular artery to contribute to the peripatellar network. The deep oblique branch courses along the medial aspect of the femur and gives off branches to the supracondylar femur, as well as collateral muscular branches. The popliteal artery exits from Hunter canal and enters the popliteal fossa at the junction of the middle and lower thirds of the femur (Fig. 1.83). Proximally it is separated from the femur by a thick pad of fat, but distally, in the region of the posterior joint line, it lies in direct contact with the oblique posterior ligament. Farther distally the artery runs superficial to the popliteus fascia and ends at the lower border of the popliteus by dividing into the anterior and posterior tibial arteries.

The popliteal artery gives off numerous muscular branches and five articular branches (Fig. 1.84). The middle genicular artery arises from the anterior aspect of the popliteal artery and

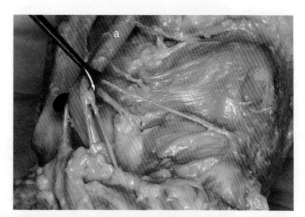

FIG 1.84 Anatomic Dissection of the Popliteal Artery The popliteal artery (a) has been elevated (probe) to reveal, from proximal to distal, the superior lateral genicular, middle genicular (passing through the posterior oblique ligament), inferior lateral and medial genicular, and two sural branches.

pierces the posterior oblique ligament to supply the posterior capsule and intracapsular structures, including the posterior horns of the menisci (Fig. 1.85).[110] Ligamentous branches of this artery traverse the synovium and form a plexus of vessels that cover both the ACL and the PCL and perforate the ligaments to anastomose with small vessels, which run parallel to the collagen fibrils.[110] The cruciates may also receive terminal

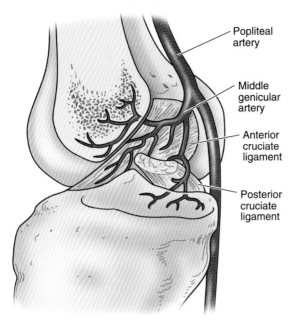

FIG 1.85 Middle genicular artery with supply to the cruciate ligaments.

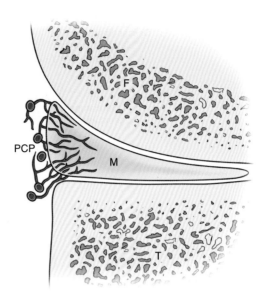

FIG 1.86 Diagrammatic representation of the peripheral blood supply to the medial meniscus *(M)*. *F,* Femur; *PCP,* perimeniscal capillary plexus; *T,* tibia.

branches from the inferior genicular arteries. The ACL receives essentially no blood supply from the ligament–bone insertion sites.[6] The medial and lateral superior genicular arteries originate from the posterior aspect of the artery and then wind around the lower end of the femur immediately proximal to the condyles. The lateral superior genicular artery passes deep to the biceps femoris tendon and then anastomoses with the descending branch of the lateral femoral circumflex artery. The medial superior genicular branch courses anteriorly deep to the semimembranosus and semitendinosus and proximal to the origin of the medial head of the gastrocnemius. Arising more distally at a level below the joint line from either side of the popliteal artery are the medial and lateral inferior genicular arteries. The inferior lateral genicular artery lies immediately adjacent to the lateral joint line. It passes deep to the LCL, proximal to the fibular head, as it traverses anterolaterally to join the anterior anastomosis. The inferior medial genicular artery passes two fingerbreadths distal to the medial joint line, deep to the MCL, and also joins the anterior anastomosis.

Branches from the inferior genicular arteries form a complex capillary network in the anterior fat pad and provide abundant supply to the fat pad, synovial cavity, and patellar tendon. Terminal branches of all four medial and lateral genicular arteries also extend into the menisci, but Arnoczky and Warren[7] have shown that the predominant vascular supply comes from the superior and inferior lateral genicular arteries. Rather than providing a uniform supply to the entire menisci, only the peripheral 30% receive these vascular branches (Fig. 1.86). Tears that occur in this peripheral vascular zone are considered to be the best candidates for repair.

The anterior anastomosis around the knee is formed by the four inferior and superior genicular arteries, branches of the descending genicular artery, the descending branch of the lateral circumflex femoral artery, and recurrent branches of the anterior tibial artery. The anastomosis thus connects the femoral artery at the origin of its profundus branch with the popliteal

and anterior tibial arteries (Fig. 1.87). Anteriorly the anastomosis forms a vascular circle around the patella, from which, according to Scapinelli, 9 to 12 nutrient arteries arise at the lower pole of the patella and run proximally on the anterior surface of the bone in a series of furrows (Fig. 1.88).[109] These vessels penetrate the anterior surface of the patella in the middle third. Additional polar vessels penetrate the patella in the apical region. The patellar retinaculum on the medial side is supplied by the anastomosis, with the main contribution coming from the descending genicular artery. The lateral retinaculum receives almost all of its supply from the lateral anastomosis formed by the superior and inferior lateral genicular arteries.[27] The arterial supply to the patellar tendon appears to be derived from two anastomotic arches that are fed by medial and lateral pedicles.[116] The descending and inferior medial genicular arteries appear to be important contributors to the medial pedicles, whereas on the lateral side, the lateral genicular arteries and recurrent tibial anterior arteries provide the greatest contributions.[116] Perforating collateral vessels from the superior (retropatellar) and inferior (supratubercular) anastomotic arches create two distinct vascular zones that anastomose in the middle third of the tendon.[116]

The skin overlying the anterior aspect of the knee receives its blood supply via three routes: direct cutaneous, musculocutaneous, and septocutaneous (intermuscular) vessels.[18,48,49] These vessels provide arterial inflow in both random perforating and axial-type distributions. Perforating vessels include terminal branches from the anterior anastomosis, as well as additional musculocutaneous terminal branches from the rectus femoris and vastus muscle group. After they have perforated through the deep fascia, these vessels run parallel to the skin surface for a considerable distance in the loose areolar layer that separates the deep fascia from subcutaneous fat. In this layer these vessels form an interconnecting fascial plexus.[48,121] Branches from this fascial plexus traverse the subcutaneous tissue and anastomose with other branches to create

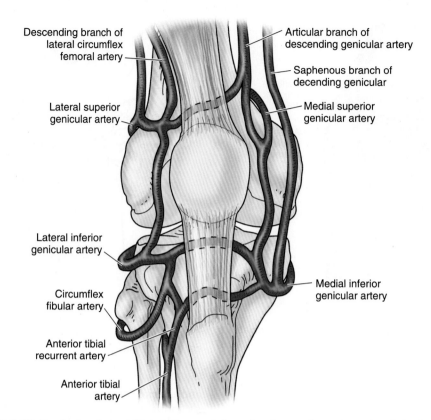

FIG 1.87 Genicular Artery Circulation and Anterior Artery Anastomosis of the Knee

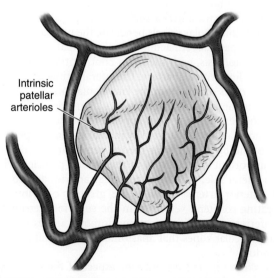

FIG 1.88 Vascular circle around the patella, which, according to Scapinelli,[109] supplies the patella via nutrient arteries that enter predominantly at the inferior pole. The genicular arteries and their branches lie in the most superficial layer of the deep fascia.

a subdermal plexus.[47,121] Because the skin relies on the distribution from the fascial plexus just superficial to the deep fascia, the true surgical plane of the anterior knee is beneath the deep fascia; consequently, undermining of the skin in a manner that creates elevated skin and subcutaneous flaps should be minimized.[47] Furthermore, although the skin receives arterial inflow

from the medial and lateral contributions to the anterior anastomosis, the principal vascular supply is provided from the medial side.[27,48] In particular the saphenous artery, which arises in a common trunk with the descending genicular vessel from the superficial femoral artery, provides a major contribution to the fascial plexus.[27,48]

Surgical exposure of the knee interrupts flow into variable portions of this network of perforating terminal branches. In a healthy individual a single midline anterior incision presents little problem for wound healing, but multiple previous incisions or ischemic disease can lead to wound complications or skin necrosis. In general, a previous transverse incision may be crossed perpendicularly. If multiple longitudinal incisions are present, the most lateral midline incision should be selected in most circumstances to avoid creating large laterally based flaps as a result of the medially biased arterial inflow.[27]

The popliteal vein enters the popliteal fossa on the lateral side of the artery; it crosses superficial to the artery and lies on the medial side in the lower part of the fossa. Throughout the popliteal fossa, it is interposed between the artery and the tibial nerve (see Fig. 1.65A).

MOTION AND FUNCTION

The knee joint is a modified hinge that possesses limited inherent stability from the bony architecture. Lack of conformity between the bony surfaces allows 6 degrees of freedom of motion about the knee, including translation in three planes (medial-lateral, anterior-posterior, proximal-distal) and rotation in three planes (flexion-extension, internal-external, and varus-valgus). Motion and stability of the joint are controlled by additional intra-articular static stabilizers, including the menisci and cruciate ligaments, as well as extra-articular static and dynamic stabilizers, such as the collateral ligaments and muscles.[56,65,87,132] In full extension, both collateral and cruciate ligaments are taut, and the anterior aspects of both menisci are snugly held between the condyles of the tibia and the femur. At the beginning of flexion the knee "unlocks" and external rotation of the femur on the tibia occurs, which, according to Last, is brought about by contraction of the popliteus muscle.[79] During the first 30 degrees of flexion, rollback of the femur on the tibia occurs and is more pronounced laterally. After 30 degrees, the femoral condyles spin at one point on the tibial condyles.[15,101] New evidence from dynamic MRI studies demonstrates that the medial condyle essentially remains static on the tibia as flexion occurs, with rollback basically limited to the lateral condyle.[36] The menisci, which are squeezed between the joint surfaces in extension, move posteriorly with the femur in flexion, the lateral more so than the medial. The articular surface of the medial femoral condyle is larger than that of the lateral femoral condyle; when the direction of motion is reversed, the lateral compartment reaches a position of full extension first before the medial compartment is fully extended. Terminal extension is achieved, and the knee is "locked" by internal rotation of the femur on the tibia—the so-called screw-home mechanism—until the medial compartment also reaches the limits of extension (Fig. 1.89).

Some portion of the superficial MCL remains taut throughout flexion, whereas the LCL is taut only in extension and relaxes as soon as the knee is flexed, thereby permitting greater excursion of the lateral tibial condyle.

The superficial MCL is the most important medial stabilizer.[130] Parallel fibers move in a posterior direction as the knee is flexed. The attachments to the femoral condyle are such that with the knee in extension, the posterior fibers are taut and the anterior fibers relax and are drawn in under the posterior part of the ligament (Fig. 1.90). With flexion of the knee, the anterior fibers move proximally and become tight and are then subjected to increasing tension as the joint is flexed (Fig. 1.91). This

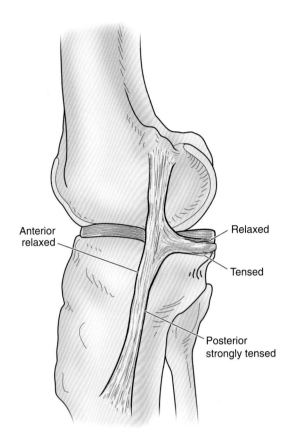

FIG 1.90 In extension the posterior margin of the MCL is tense and the anterior border relatively relaxed. Proximal anterior fibers are drawn underneath the posterior fibers.

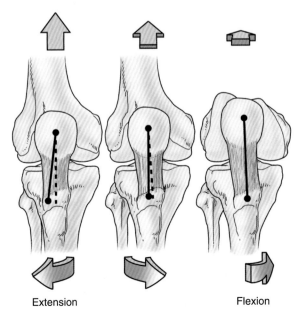

FIG 1.89 Screw-Home Mechanism At full extension the tibial tubercle lies lateral to the midpoint of the patella.

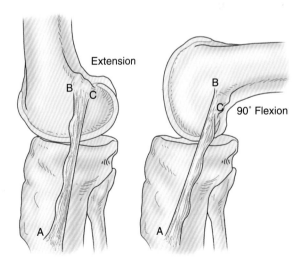

FIG 1.91 Diagram of the Superficial Medial Ligament With Flexion and Extension of the Knee Because point B moves superiorly, the anterior border is tightened in flexion. Conversely, in extension, point C moves proximally and tightens the posterior margin of the ligament. (From Warren LF, Marshall JL, Girgis FG: The prime static stabilizer of the medial side of the knee. *J Bone Joint Surg Am* 56:665, 1974.)

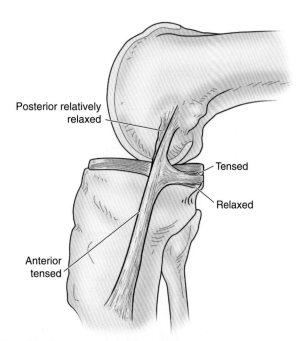

Posterior relatively relaxed

Tensed

Relaxed

Anterior tensed

FIG 1.92 The posterior oblique fibers become more tense in flexion. (From Palmer I: On the injuries to ligaments of the knee joint: a clinical study. *Acta Chir Scand* 81[Suppl 53]:3, 1938.)

action, according to Palmer, is attributable to the oval shape of the femoral origin, which changes its orientation in flexion such that the attachments of the most anterior fibers are elevated.[101] As the anterior border becomes tight, the posterior fibers slacken as the knee flexes and remain relaxed throughout flexion. The posterior oblique fibers are relaxed in extension and lie partially beneath the parallel fibers. In flexion the fibers are drawn out (Fig. 1.92); according to Palmer, because of their attachment to the capsule and the periphery of the medial meniscus, these fibers check the backward sliding of the meniscus that occurs in flexion. In the presence of intact parallel fibers, approximately 1 to 2 mm of medial opening to valgus stress is present. The joint is slightly tighter in full extension, and the greatest degree of medial opening occurs at 45 degrees.[130] Parallel fibers of the superficial MCL also control rotation; sectioning these fibers not only increases the amount of medial opening to valgus stress but also causes a significant increase in external rotation. In distinction, sectioning the capsule, the deep MCL, or the oblique fibers of the superficial MCL causes little or no increase in rotation.[130]

Lateral stability is provided by several structures.[59] In extension the fibers of the iliotibial tract are crucial, and because these fibers attach proximally to the femur and distally to the tibia, they may be regarded as a true ligament. However, Kaplan demonstrated, through electrical stimulation of the tensor fascia lata and traction on the iliotibial tract in cadavers, that contractions of the tensor fascia lata and gluteus maximus are not transmitted to the tibia; therefore the iliotibial tract does not represent a tendon.[66] As the knee flexes the iliotibial tract moves posteriorly and becomes somewhat relaxed; beyond approximately 30 degrees of flexion, the tendon of the biceps femoris may become an important lateral stabilizer.[88]

The lateral ligament is also taut in extension but is relaxed throughout flexion. The same is true of the arcuate ligament. Thus in flexion a much greater degree of rotation is possible

laterally than medially. This rotation is permitted by the attachments of the lateral meniscus and by relaxation of the supporting ligaments in flexion. A greater degree of rolling of the femur on the tibia is seen, whereas medially this motion is only slight. The attachment of the popliteal tendon to the lateral meniscus draws the meniscus posteriorly and prevents entrapment as the knee is flexed.[79]

The ACL consists of two functional bands: an AM band and a stronger, thicker PL part. In extension the ligament appears as a flat band, and the PL bulk of the ligament is taut (see Fig. 1.50). Almost immediately after flexion begins, the smaller AM band becomes tight, and the bulk of the ligament slackens. In flexion it is the AM band that provides the primary restraint against anterior displacement of the tibia.[41]

The PCL consists of two inseparable parts. An anterior portion forms the bulk of the ligament, and a smaller posterior part runs obliquely to the back of the tibia. In extension, the bulk of the ligament is relaxed, and only the posterior band is tight. In flexion the major portion of the ligament becomes tight, and the small posterior band is loose (see Fig. 1.56).[40,125]

The ACL is a check against both hyperextension and internal and external rotation. The PCL is a check against posterior instability in the flexed knee but not against hyperextension, provided that the anterior cruciate is intact.

According to Palmer, tightening of the anterior cruciate in extension fixes the lateral femoral condyle anteriorly; thus continuation of movement into hyperextension is possible only when simultaneous inward rotation of the femur occurs.[101]

Rotation occurs around an axis through the center of the medial femoral condyle, as a result of the tighter anchorage of this condyle by the superficial MCL. If this ligament is ruptured, the axis shifts laterally. According to Palmer, because of the medially shifted axis of rotation, external rotation of the tibia relaxes the ACL through forward travel of the lateral femoral condyle, at the same time stretching the PCL.[101] Internal rotation reverses this sequence, tensing the anterior cruciate, and relaxing the posterior cruciate.

A fibrous band connects the posterior cruciate with the posterior margin of the lateral meniscus (the tibiomeniscal ligament of Kaplan). This band probably restricts the forward sliding motion of the lateral meniscus in internal rotation.

Girgis et al. have shown that rotary movements of the tibia on the femur occur in all ranges of motion.[41] Their studies indicate that the anterior cruciate is a check against external rotation in flexion but does not significantly limit internal rotation. In extension the ACL is a check against external rotation and to a lesser degree against internal rotation. Thus the precise function of the cruciate ligaments with regard to rotation is a topic of some disagreement.

Action of the Muscles

The movements of the knee are flexion, extension, and rotation. Flexion is performed by the hamstrings and biceps femoris and to a lesser extent by the gastrocnemius and popliteus. Flexion is limited by the soft tissues at the back of the knee. Extension is performed by the quadriceps, and because of the shape of the articulation and the ligament attachments the femur rotates medially on the tibia in terminal extension; this is the screw-home mechanism that locks the joint. This movement is purely passive, as are other rotary movements that occur during activity, and is because of the articular geometry and static stabilizers, as previously described. The exception is lateral rotation of the femur that precedes flexion by unlocking the joint. This movement is performed by the popliteus. The sartorius, gracilis, and hamstrings are weak rotators of the knee but probably do not act as such. The sartorius, gracilis, and semitendinosus medially and the iliotibial tract laterally most often act as "guy-ropes" to stabilize the pelvis.

KEY REFERENCES

3. Agur AMR, Dalley AF: *Grant's atlas of anatomy*, ed 12, Philadelphia, 2009, Wolters Kluwer Health/Lippincott Williams & Wilkins.

10. Basmajian JV: *Grant's method of anatomy*, ed 10, Baltimore, 1980, Williams & Wilkins.

15. Brantigan OC, Voshell AF: The mechanics of the ligaments and menisci of the knee joint. *J Bone Joint Surg* 23:44, 1941.

48. Haertsch P: The blood supply to the skin of the leg: a post-mortem investigation. *Br J Plast Surg* 34:470, 1981.

63. Johnson DL, Swenson TM, Livesay MS, et al: Insertion site anatomy of the human menisci: gross, arthroscopic, and topographical anatomy as a basis for meniscal transplantation. *Arthroscopy* 11:386, 1995.

70. Kennedy JC, Alexander IJ, Hayes KC: Nerve supply of the knee and its functional importance. *Am J Sports Med* 10:329, 1982.

80. Last RJ: *Anatomy: regional and applied*, ed 6, Edinburgh, 1978, Churchill Livingstone.

93. Miyamoto RG, Bosco JA, Sherman OH: Treatment of medial collateral ligament injuries. *J Am Acad Orthop Surg* 17:152, 2009.

103. Petersen W, Zantop T: Anatomy of the anterior cruciate ligament with regard to two bundles. *Clin Orthop* 454:35, 2006.

106. Reider B, Marshall JL, Koslin B, et al: The anterior aspect of the knee joint: an anatomical study. *J Bone Joint Surg Am* 63:351, 1981.

107. Renstrom P, Johnson RJ: Anatomy and biomechanics of the menisci. *Clin Sports Med* 9:523, 1990.

109. Scapinelli R: Blood supply of the human patella: its relation to ischaemic necrosis after fracture. *J Bone Joint Surg Br* 49:563, 1967.

113. Seebacher JR, Inglis AE, Marshall JL, et al: The structure of the posterolateral aspect of the knee. *J Bone Joint Surg Am* 64:536, 1982.

129. Warren LF, Marshall JL: The supporting structures and layers on the medial side of the knee: an anatomical analysis. *J Bone Joint Surg Am* 61:56, 1979.

134. Williams PL, Warwick R: *Gray's anatomy*, ed 36, Philadelphia, 1980, WB Saunders.

The references for this chapter can also be found on www.expertconsult.com.

2

Anatomic Aberrations*

Henry D. Clarke, W. Norman Scott

Variations of normal anatomy and frankly abnormal structures are occasionally encountered by the physician. Without a fundamental understanding of the more common abnormalities, it may be difficult to identify and interpret the significance of these structures. The goal of this chapter is to provide an overview of some of the reported structural anomalies and information regarding their clinical relevance. It is not our intent to review anatomic abnormalities resulting from traumatic or degenerative causes. In addition, developmental phenomena occurring as a result of disordered maturation in the pediatric population are reviewed elsewhere.

SKELETAL ABNORMALITIES

A number of major skeletal dysplasias, including proximal femoral focal deficiencies, tibial dysplasia, fibular aplasia, amelia, and phocomelia, involve the bones of the knee joint to varying degrees but are beyond the scope of this chapter. Here we emphasize abnormalities that may represent incidental findings in some patients but can have significant clinical implications.

Femur
Trochlear Dysplasia. Trochlear dysplasia may be relatively subtle or more marked. Although trochlea dysplasia has been identified as a key factor in developing pain and patellar instability, the clinical manifestations associated with dysplasia depend not only on the extent of the dysplasia but also on other anatomic factors; patella geometry, patella alta, abnormalities in the degree of tibial tubercle lateralization determined by a tibial tubercle to trochlear groove distance exceeding 20 mm on axial computed tomography (CT), incompetence of the medial patellofemoral ligament, and abnormalities in the muscular stabilizers of the patella all likely contribute.[28,70] Symptoms may relate to chronic maltracking or frank dislocation of the patella. Pain related to the patellofemoral joint resulting from chronic patellar malalignment is typically manifested as an anterior knee ache when sitting with the knee flexed and as acute exacerbations during squatting, kneeling, and stair-climbing activities. On physical examination, crepitus from the patellofemoral joint, pain with patellar compression, and peripatellar tenderness may be noted. Specific radiologic criteria have been reported that define normal trochlear anatomy.[8,72] The sulcus

angle is defined on the Merchant view by the intersection of lines connecting the highest point of the femoral condyles to the deepest point of the femoral trochlea; the mean angle in normal knees is 130 to 137 degrees (range, 112 to 151 degrees).[1,42] Significant differences in this angle have been reported in patients with recurrent patellar dislocation and chondromalacia patellae (Fig. 2.1).[1] The lateral to medial trochlear ratio is the ratio between the segments joining the highest point of the femoral condyles to the deepest point of the trochlea. A ratio greater than 1.7 indicates trochlear dysplasia.[8] Dejour has defined four classes based on both conventional axial and lateral radiographs and axial magnetic resonance imaging (MRI) images.[72] On axial MRI, type A dysplasia is defined by a fairly shallow trochlea; type B by a flat or convex trochlea; type C by asymmetry of the trochlear facets with a hypoplastic medial condyle; and type D by asymmetry of the trochlear facets plus vertical join and cliff pattern.[72]

If nonoperative treatment, such as activity modification and physical therapy, fails to relieve symptoms, all anatomic factors that contribute to patellofemoral pain and instability must be considered and a surgical plan devised. Historically, lateral release and proximal realignment were used in patients with disabling symptoms and documented anatomic abnormalities. In carefully selected patients, 91% excellent and good results were achieved at intermediate-term follow-up by Insall et al.[56] Currently, a detailed assessment of the multiple factors that can play a role in patellar instability should be performed. Rather than a single solution, treatment is directed at correcting the major problem(s) identified in any given patient and is presented elsewhere in this textbook. In summary, surgical intervention may include a single procedure or a combination of the following: proximal soft tissue realignment, medial patellofemoral ligament repair or reconstruction, distal tibial tubercle realignment, or trochleoplasty.[14,70] For patients with severe dysplasia, especially for which other interventions have failed, trochleoplasty, or deepening and recontouring femoral trochlear groove, is becoming increasingly recognized as an important option.[14,28,70,76] Outcomes reports in which trochleoplasty were used in these difficult cases have demonstrated satisfactory results, although it is clear that patients still demonstrate limitations in their activities.[28,76]

Patella
Congenital Absence and Hypoplasia. Congenital absence of the patella and hypoplasia are extremely rare anomalies, especially as isolated findings.[11,107] An association with other abnormalities has been reported, including ischiopubic malformations,

*The authors thank John N. Insall for his thoughtful guidance and contributions to previous editions of this chapter.

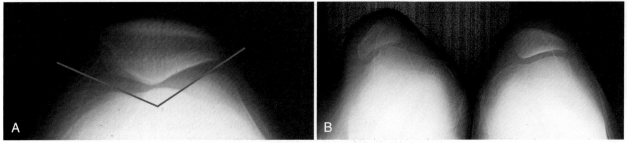

FIG 2.1 Radiographs of the Patellofemoral Joint (A) Merchant view with a normal sulcus angle of the femoral trochlea marked. (B) Bilateral Merchant view showing a severely dysplastic femoral trochlea with almost flat sulcus angles and patellar dislocation.

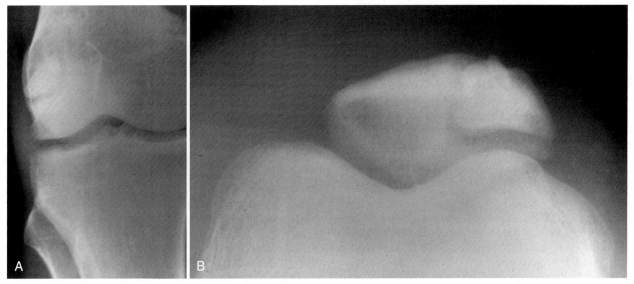

FIG 2.2 Oblique (A) and tangential axial (B) radiographs of a bipartite patella. The margins of the two fragments are relatively smooth and corticated.

and they have been described as part of the nail-patella syndrome (nail and patellar dysplasia, radial head subluxation and elbow malformation, renal abnormalities, and iliac horns).[107,110] Other patellar dysplasias include duplication in the coronal and sagittal planes; in some cases these abnormalities have been associated with multiple epiphyseal dysplasia.[43,50,91,125]

Bipartite Patella. Anomalies of patellar development are relatively common, especially failure of accessory ossification centers to fuse, which can lead to bipartite, tripartite, and multipartite patellae (Fig. 2.2). Fragmentation of the patella has been noted in approximately 2% to 5% of knees. The bipartite type accounts for most cases; approximately 50% of cases occur bilaterally.[16,108,125] The Saupe classification describes three types of patellar fragmentation based on the location of the accessory ossification center: type 1 (5%) is located at the inferior pole, type 2 (20%) at the lateral margin, and type 3, the most frequent (75%), at the superolateral pole.[16,108]

Most bipartite patellae represent incidental findings; only 13% are associated with symptoms. When pain develops, it may occur acutely after trauma or gradually.[16,20,45,108,124] In the acute setting a traumatic fracture must be ruled out. In such cases the margins of the fracture fragments usually appear more ragged on plain radiographs, whereas the accessory fragments noted in atraumatic fragmentation tend to have sclerotic smooth margins. MRI may be helpful in distinguishing

incidental fragmentation because in these cases the accessory piece demonstrates low signal intensity without surrounding marrow edema (Fig. 2.3).[108] Initial treatment may include activity modification, anti-inflammatory medication, and immobilization. In patients with persistent symptoms, successful excision of symptomatic fragments has been reported.[16,45,108,124]

LIGAMENT ABNORMALITIES

Anterior Cruciate Ligament

Congenital Absence. Congenital absence of the anterior cruciate ligament (ACL) is a rare anomaly that has been reported, in most circumstances, to occur in association with other knee abnormalities, including congenital knee dislocation, tibial dysplasia, congenital dislocation of the patella, femoral dysplasia, ring meniscus, discoid meniscus, absence of the meniscus, absence of the posterior cruciate ligament (PCL), and congenital leg length discrepancy.[3,62,82,118] An association with other musculoskeletal abnormalities not limited to the knee has also been reported, with at least one other significant anomaly noted in each patient in one series.[118] However, rare cases of isolated absence of the ACL have been reported in otherwise normal individuals.[7] On physical examination, a positive anterior draw test and a 3+ Lachman test are common findings. Complex instability may also be noted; in one study 25% of patients demonstrated medial and lateral translational instability.[118]

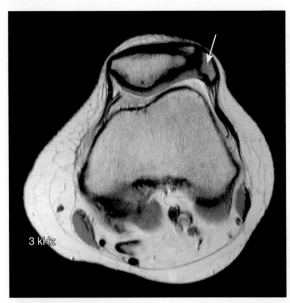

FIG 2.3 Axial magnetic resonance image demonstrating a bipartite patella with a small lateral fragment *(arrow)*. The lack of surrounding marrow edema and hemorrhage is consistent with a bipartite patella rather than an acute patellar fracture.

Therefore it is evident that this patient population is not entirely analogous to the group that experiences traumatic ACL rupture. Radiographic features that have been associated with congenital absence of the ACL include hypoplasia of the lateral aspect of the tibial spine, hypoplasia of the lateral femoral condyle, a narrow or tight A-frame intercondylar notch, and hypoplasia of the medial part of the tibial plateau.[63,118] Many patients with this anomaly are asymptomatic as children and do not complain of instability.[62] Because the long-term consequences of this type of deficiency are unknown, the need for ligament reconstruction has not been clearly defined. In several series, asymptomatic patients have been treated by observation only, with good short-term results.[7,59,118]

Other Abnormalities. An abnormal origin of the ACL has been described. Rather than the usual discrete origin, an origin extending completely between the anterior and posterior margins of the intercondylar notch was observed in a young child. Symptoms developed in this patient as a result of impingement of the abnormal ACL against the anterior portion of a discoid lateral meniscus at approximately 100 degrees of flexion.[51]

Posterior Cruciate Ligament

Abnormalities of the PCL are extremely rare. Congenital absence of the PCL has been reported in association with other congenital anomalies, including absence of the ACL, leg length discrepancies, and Larsen syndrome (multiple congenital dislocations of the elbows, knees, and hips and unusual facies).[38,59,62] The multiple anomalies present in these patients typically result in positive anterior and posterior draw tests and posterolateral rotatory instability. In one patient an anomaly of the PCL has been reported in association with congenital absence of the ACL. An anterior insertion of the PCL on the tibia was noted to compensate for the aplastic ACL.[3]

MENISCAL ABNORMALITIES

Anomalous Attachments

A variety of anomalous attachments of the medial meniscus have been described, including insertion of the anterior horn into the ACL, intercondylar notch, and infrapatellar fold and insertion of the posterior horn into the ACL.* Between 10.6% and 22.6% of all Asian patients undergoing arthroscopy were found to have anomalies of the anterior horn of the medial meniscus.[84] In a large study of 953 arthroscopies, 103 (10.8%) knees did not demonstrate the normal attachment of the anterior horn of the medial meniscus onto the tibia. Four variants of the anterior horn were observed in this study: 51 (49.5%) had only an attachment to the lateral meniscus via the transverse intermeniscal ligament, 39 (37.9%) inserted into the ACL, 11 (10.7%) inserted into the coronary ligament, and 2 (1.9%) inserted into the infrapatellar synovial fold. In these patients the abnormal anterior horn attachment rendered the anterior portion of the meniscus hypermobile, whereas the posterior body remained firmly attached. This aberration predisposed patients to symptomatic tears at the junction of the midbody and the posterior body as a result of accumulated stress.[84] Successful arthroscopic resection of symptomatic anomalous insertions has been reported.[104,109] In these cases a stable, normal-appearing anterior horn was fashioned, which relieved the preoperative knee pain. In one case symptoms appeared to be related to subluxation of the abnormal bundle under the femoral condyle with flexion.[104] Nonetheless, other authors have reported good results after observation of incidentally discovered anomalies.[12,61]

Hypoplasia and Congenital Absence

The incidence of hypoplasia and congenital absence of the medial and lateral menisci is unknown. An association with other ipsilateral knee and generalized musculoskeletal anomalies, including congenital absence of the ACL, discoid lateral meniscus, thrombocytopenia–absent radius syndrome, and anomalous insertions of the popliteus tendon, has been reported in several cases.[39,83,119,120] The association of simultaneous intra-articular anomalies in some cases is probably because of the common mesenchymal origin of several structures.[12] Condensation of the menisci occurs at approximately 7 to 8 weeks of embryologic development and occurs in concert with the intra-articular cruciate ligaments.[12,25,109]

Discoid Meniscus

The first discoid meniscus was reported by Young in 1889.[2,30,60,106] In an early report Smillie[111] described three variants: primitive, intermediate, and infantile. This classification reflected the belief that the menisci are discoid in a normal fetus and gradually assume an adult form through resorption of the central part; however, anatomic studies have suggested that this supposition is incorrect because discoid menisci do not occur during any part of routine development.[25,60,64,100] Kaplan[64] suggested that abnormal motion of the lateral menisci resulting from deficient peripheral attachments may cause a meniscus that is normal at birth to become discoid during development.[13] However, this explanation does not satisfactorily account for the

---

*References 12, 61, 66, 84, 104, and 109.

occurrence of discoid medial menisci. Rather than representing an arrest in normal development, discoid menisci are believed to be congenital anomalies.[13,30]

Medial. Discoid medial menisci are very rare phenomena. The first undisputed case was reported by Cave and Staples[22] in 1941. Its incidence in the general population is reported to be approximately 0.06% to 0.3%.[13,26,30,106] Discoid medial menisci may be asymptomatic, especially in children and adolescents. Meta-analysis has revealed that 65% of all patients with symptomatic discoid medial menisci were older than 18 years.[30] The most common symptoms associated with a discoid medial meniscus are the same as those for a medial meniscal tear and include aching medial joint line pain, intermittent swelling, locking, weakness, instability, and an inability to extend the knee fully.[13,30,60] On physical examination, a block to full extension, effusion, joint line tenderness, and a positive McMurray test may be noted.[30]

Radiographs of the involved knee are usually unremarkable; abnormalities are identified in less than 10% of patients with a discoid medial meniscus.[30] Occasionally, medial joint space widening or deepening of the medial tibial hemiplateau has been observed but may be subtle.[13,30] MRI is the best test for identifying discoid menisci. On sagittal views the menisci should be evaluated on serial images. Rather than the usual central tapering between the anterior and posterior horns as the image plane moves laterally toward the intercondylar notch, the horns remain in continuity (Fig. 2.4). Visualization of a continuous band of menisci on more than three peripheral sagittal images indicates a discoid meniscus. In addition, on coronal images, an abnormally thick meniscus, which can extend into the notch, may be visualized.[13]

Because of the rarity of this phenomenon, its treatment has not been extensively reported. Several authors have suggested that incidentally discovered intact discoid menisci may be left intact.[13,66] However, in these cases the presence of central and inferior surface cleavage tears, which may be difficult to observe, should be excluded.[26,106] In patients with intra-articular symptoms and no other abnormalities, discoid menisci should be very carefully examined for incomplete inferior or cleavage tears because they may be missed if only the superior surface is examined (Fig. 2.5).

Successful short-term results of arthroscopic débridement with partial meniscectomy and contouring of discoid medial menisci have been reported.[13,24,66] Because many symptomatic patients are initially seen as young adults, we attempt to resect the torn portion and fashion the remnant of the meniscus into as nearly normal shape as possible in the hope of minimizing the long-term degenerative changes associated with complete meniscectomy.[24,36]

Lateral. Discoid lateral menisci occur more frequently than on the medial side of the knee (Fig. 2.6). In the general population the incidence has been reported to be approximately 1.4% to 15.5%, but certain races appear to have a higher incidence.[31] Whereas a discoid lateral meniscus is thought to occur in less than 5% of white individuals, it has been identified in up to 16.6% of Asians.[21,55] Washington et al. identified three types of discoid lateral menisci based on the degree of coverage of the tibial plateau and the presence or absence of normal posterior attachments,[123] including incomplete and complete discoid menisci, which have normal posterior tibial attachments via the coronary ligament, and the Wrisberg type, which lacks the usual posterior tibial attachment, with only one attachment posteriorly via the posterior meniscofemoral ligament (ligament of

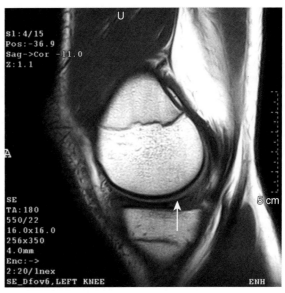

FIG 2.4 Sagittal magnetic resonance image of a discoid medial meniscus showing a blocklike appearance that was present on most sagittal cuts through the medial compartment. Intrameniscal signal was considered highly suggestive of a meniscal tear *(arrow)*.

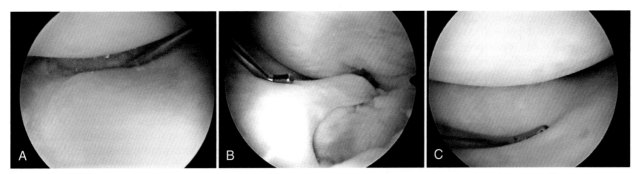

FIG 2.5 **Arthroscopic Views of the Same Patient With a Discoid Medial Meniscus** (A) The lateral margin of the discoid medial meniscus has been elevated to reveal an intact inferior surface. (B and C) The superior surface was also intact.

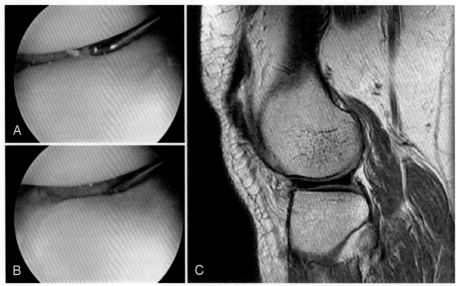

FIG 2.6 (A) Arthroscopic view of a discoid lateral meniscus with an intact superior surface. (B) Superior surface of the discoid lateral meniscus with a probe in the popliteal hiatus. (C) Sagittal magnetic resonance image of a discoid lateral meniscus with a characteristic blocklike appearance that was present on most sagittal views through the lateral compartment.

Wrisberg). Because the Wrisberg type often is not associated with a true discoid appearance, Neuschwander et al.[81] suggested that this anomaly be classified as a separate entity—the lateral meniscal variant with absence of the posterior coronary ligament. Although somewhat rare, discoid lateral menisci have been noted to occur in association with a number of other anomalies, including hypoplasia of the lateral femoral condyle, hypoplasia of the lateral tibial spine, a high fibular head, abnormal ACL attachment, and anomalous insertions of the medial meniscus.[51,66]

Patients may have symptoms related to a discoid lateral meniscus in childhood or middle age. The classic complaint of patients with a discoid meniscus is a snapping or popping knee.[2,123] However, in one large series of 62 symptomatic patients, knee pain was the most common problem (89%); other frequent complaints at initial evaluation included the classic clunk or click (58%), swelling (48%), locking (27%), and giving way (19%).[2] On physical examination the pathognomonic clunk related to abnormal motion of the meniscus as the knee is brought into full extension was elicited in 39% of patients in the same study; other frequent findings included joint line tenderness (35%), effusion (19%), and locking (11%).[2] Radiographic findings, including widening of the lateral joint line (8%), cupping of the lateral tibial plateau (5%), and sclerosis of the lateral tibial plateau (3%), were identified in a minority of patients.[2] MRI can predictably identify discoid menisci and associated meniscal tears (Fig. 2.7). Treatment of incidentally identified intact complete and incomplete discoid lateral menisci is not thought to be necessary. However, as with medial discoid menisci, tears may be difficult to see and could be missed.[47] In particular, inferior surface cleavage tears should be carefully excluded, especially in patients with intra-articular symptoms and no other identifiable lesions.

Treatment of symptomatic tears in both complete and incomplete types is somewhat controversial. Some authors reported successful results after compete sceniscectomy, and in some studies the short-term clinical results appear to surpass

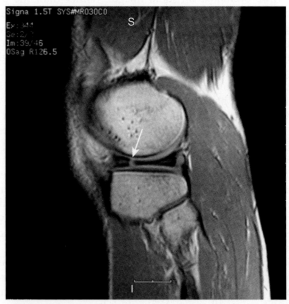

FIG 2.7 Sagittal magnetic resonance image revealing a discoid lateral meniscus with an associated radial tear *(arrow)* at the junction of the anterior horn and body.

those achieved after partial meniscectomy and saucerization.[55,123] The impact of subtotal meniscectomy for discoid lateral meniscus on the development of subsequent degenerative changes in the knee has not been unequivocally determined. Radiographic changes consistent with significant degenerative alterations in the lateral compartment after complete meniscectomy for discoid menisci in children have rarely been noted; this may reflect possible adaptive changes of the knee and mechanical alignment.[2,123] However, in one study, early degenerative changes were noted in three of eight patients at 17-year follow-up.[123] In another larger study in children, 42 knees underwent either partial meniscectomy or subtotal/total meniscectomy for treatment of a discoid lateral meniscus; significantly greater radiographic changes were noted at only 4-year follow-up in those knees treated with subtotal/total meniscectomy.[71] In another study of adult patients who were treated with subtotal meniscectomy for a torn discoid lateral meniscus, age greater than 25 years was noted to be a risk factor for the development of radiographic degenerative changes.[85] In addition to these degenerative changes noted following treatment specifically for torn discoid lateral menisci, significant long-term consequences of meniscectomy have been documented in other circumstances.[24,75] Concern regarding the potential for early degenerative disease has prompted many authors to advocate arthroscopic partial meniscectomy with salvage of the most functional remnant possible.[10,31,32,47] Excellent short-term results have been reported with this strategy.[10,31,32,90] We believe that even though the long-term outcome is not clear, the consequences associated with the development of early degenerative arthritis in this young patient population make arthroscopic partial meniscectomy and saucerization with resection to a stable, well-contoured remnant the preferred treatment of symptomatic tears of complete- and incomplete-type discoid menisci.

Treatment of a Wrisberg-type discoid meniscus, which is inherently unstable because of lack of posterior tibial attachments, has traditionally involved complete meniscectomy. However, successful reattachment by suturing the posterior horn to the capsule has been reported, and in a small series of six patients treated in this manner, no clinical re-tears were noted at a mean of 32 months.[81,99] If the long-term results are also successful, this treatment is again theoretically more appealing than complete meniscectomy when the long-term incidence of degenerative changes is not clear.

Other Structural Meniscal Anomalies

Extremely rare structural abnormalities have been reported, including ring-shaped lateral menisci and accessory lateral menisci that appear as a double-layered meniscus.[4,34,67,82,116] When symptoms were believed to be related to these abnormalities, arthroscopic resection of the abnormal portion of the meniscus has proved successful.

Meniscofemoral Ligaments

The anterior and posterior meniscofemoral ligaments (of Humphry and Wrisberg, respectively) run between the posterior horn of the lateral meniscus and the intercondylar notch (Fig. 2.8). They embrace the PCL and are named for their location relative to the ligament. The presence of the anterior meniscofemoral ligament (of Humphry) is less consistent, with an incidence of 33% to 83% in anatomic studies; the posterior meniscofemoral ligament (of Wrisberg) is a more constant structure and is noted in 90% to 93% of the same specimens.[94,122]

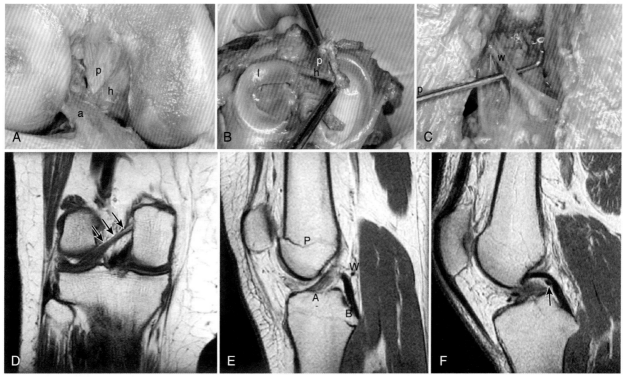

FIG 2.8 Meniscofemoral Ligaments (A) Anterior view of the intercondylar notch with the ligament of Humphry (h) passing obliquely between the ACL (a) and the PCL (p). (B) The ligament of Humphry (h, inferior forceps) originates from the lateral meniscus (l) and embraces the anterior aspect of the PCL (p). (C) Posterior view of the intercondylar notch with the ligament of Wrisberg (w) directly posterior to the PCL (p, probe deep to the ligament of Wrisberg). (D) Coronal MRI of the meniscofemoral ligaments (arrows) from the lateral meniscus to the intercondylar wall of the medial femoral condyle. (E) Sagittal MRI showing the ligament of Wrisberg (w) posterior to the PCL (B). Also identified are the ACL (A) and a physeal scar (P). (F) Sagittal MRI with the small oval ligament of Humphry identified anterior to the PCL (arrow).

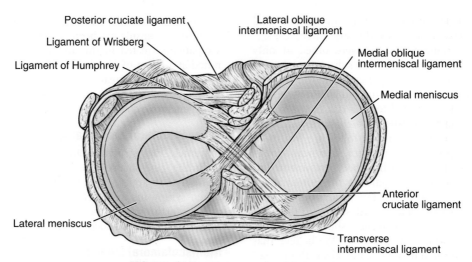

FIG 2.9 Oblique intermeniscal ligaments.

Overall, 100% of the specimens had at least one of these ligaments. In other studies one or the other of these meniscofemoral ligaments was identified in 71% to 94% of specimens.[48,97,121] In general, the ligament of Wrisberg is more robust than the ligament of Humphry.

The presence of meniscofemoral ligaments running between the anterior horns of the medial and lateral menisci and the intercondylar notch has also been observed. In Wan and Felle's study[122] an anterior medial meniscofemoral ligament running between the anterior horn of the medial meniscus and the intercondylar notch, just anterior to the ACL, was observed in 15% of specimens. A similar number of specimens (15%) demonstrated an anterolateral meniscofemoral ligament running between the anterior horn of the lateral meniscus and the intercondylar notch. At least one of these ligaments was present in 25% of specimens; however, both were present in only 5% of knees.[122] The anteromedial meniscofemoral ligament was never more than half the thickness of the ACL, whereas the anterolateral ligament was never more than a third the size of the ACL. In all cases the ligaments of Humphry and Wrisberg were more robust than the anteromedial and anterolateral meniscofemoral ligaments.[122]

Oblique Intermeniscal Ligaments

Oblique intermeniscal (meniscomeniscal) ligaments have been identified in 1% to 4% of specimens.[29,128] These ligaments derive their name from their anterior meniscal point of origin. The medial oblique intermeniscal ligament arises from the central part of the anterior horn of the medial meniscus and passes obliquely posteriorly to the posterior horn of the lateral meniscus. The lateral intermeniscal ligament runs between the anterior horn of the lateral meniscus and the posterior horn of the medial meniscus, passing between the cruciates (Fig. 2.9).[29] The functional significance of these ligaments has not been clearly defined.

MUSCLE ABNORMALITIES

Anomalous Attachments

A number of variations in the muscle attachments about the popliteal fossa have been described and are clinically significant in circumstances associated with popliteal artery compression, as described subsequently. The most commonly reported anomalies include lateral and more proximal origins of the medial head of the gastrocnemius.

Anomalous attachments of the pes muscles and hamstrings have also been observed. In one case report an abnormal attachment of the biceps femoris was noted to be the cause of painful snapping; the biceps inserted entirely on the proximal end of the tibia rather than onto the normal insertion site on the fibula.[49] During extension, subluxation of the tendon over the fibular head was noted. Transposition of the biceps insertion successfully relieved the pain and snapping.

Variations in the pes tendon insertions are common; half the specimens in one cadaver study demonstrated one of seven variations ranging from fascial loops connecting the sartorius tendon with the medial collateral ligament to separate tendon slips from each of the three tendons inserting separately into the tibia.[57] These anatomic variations can be clinically important when tendon autografts are harvested for reconstructive procedures on the knee ligaments.

Accessory or Hypertrophic Muscles

Anomalous muscles in the popliteal fossa and the posterior aspect of the knee are rare. In a report of 300 anatomic dissections over a 15-year period, the authors observed only a single anomalous muscle.[112]

The popliteus muscle normally flattens and forms a tendon before passing deep to the fibular collateral ligament. In a small number of specimens (approximately 14%) a more robust muscle with an abnormally short tendon that intruded into the joint was observed.[19] In theory, the extra bulk of this anomalous structure may impinge posteriorly and require recession during total knee replacement.

A third head of the gastrocnemius originating from the posterior and inferior aspects of the femur and joining the medial or lateral head has been noted in 2% to 5% of individuals and appears to be more common in the Japanese population.[58] Another reported anomaly is an accessory or hypertrophied semimembranosus that lies more laterally in the fossa than normal and rests superficial to the neurovascular bundle.[15,114] A hypertrophied plantaris muscle with a large and more distal origin from the medial aspect of the lateral head of the gastrocnemius has been observed. This anomalous muscle runs distally and medially and passes under the neurovascular bundle.[15] All these anomalies may lead to symptomatic compression of the popliteal vessels. However, the true incidence of these variations is unknown because many are asymptomatic.

Hypoplasia

Hypoplasia of the vastus medialis muscle may contribute to patellofemoral pathomechanics. The vastus medialis is the last muscle of the quadriceps group to form, and in some individuals this muscle develops poorly, with resultant lateral and superior displacement of the patella. This hereditary or congenital anomaly has been identified to some degree in up to 40% of individuals but is frequently asymptomatic.[41] However, in some individuals, such hypoplasia may contribute to abnormal patellar tracking and may result in subluxation, dislocation, or patellofemoral pain syndromes. Clinical findings may include observation of a poorly developed vastus medialis relative to the vastus lateralis, lateral hypermobility of the patella, pain with patellar compression, and peripatellar tenderness. Physical therapy with selective strengthening of the vastus medialis may be successful in patients with patellofemoral pain. However, as noted previously in the section on trochlear dysplasia, in cases of recurrent patellar subluxation or dislocation, identification of all anatomic abnormalities that can affect patellar stability is required followed by appropriate surgical intervention, which may include distal bony realignment of the tibial tubercle, repair or reconstruction of the medial patellofemoral ligament, proximal soft tissue realignment, and trochleoplasty.

ARTERIAL ANOMALIES

Persistent Sciatic Artery

The sciatic artery represents persistence of the embryonic axial artery that is the predominant vascular supply to the lower limb bud during early development (Fig. 2.10). The incidence of this structural anomaly has been reported to be approximately 0.01% to 0.05%.[17] In the early embryo the axial artery is a continuation of the internal iliac artery. During normal development, it involutes by the 22-mm embryo stage, and the femoral artery provides the major vascular supply to the lower extremity. The only normal remnants of the axial artery are the proximal portions of the anterior and superior gluteal vessels and the popliteal and peroneal vessels. When normal development fails and a persistent sciatic artery occurs, it may be complete or incomplete. In patients with a complete persistent sciatic artery it is the predominant arterial supply to the limb. However, in incomplete cases the sciatic artery is hypoplastic and the femoral artery predominates. In some patients a persistent sciatic vein may accompany the arterial abnormality.

A persistent sciatic artery follows a characteristic course in which it initially passes through the greater sciatic foramen below the piriform. Next it passes inferior to the gluteus maximus muscle and posterior to the greater trochanter; it then runs distally along the posterior margin of the adductor magnus muscle to the popliteal fossa.[17,74] On physical examination the presence of a persistent sciatic artery may be suspected if a pulsatile mass is found in the buttock. In addition, the presence of palpable popliteal and pedal pulses without a femoral pulse may be noted. However, in most cases the femoral artery is developed enough proximally to produce a normal pulse. Sciatic arteries have a high incidence of aneurysm formation (up to 44%), which may require revascularization procedures.[17]

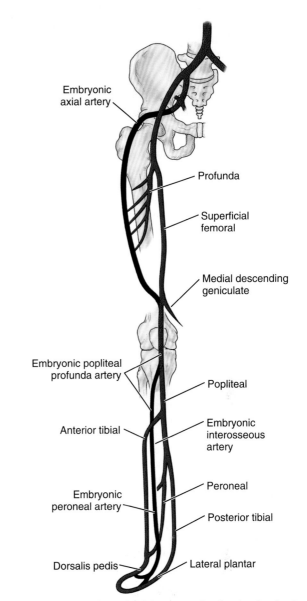

FIG 2.10 Embryonic and adult artery distribution in the lower extremity. The *black* portions regress during normal development, whereas the *red* portions form part of the adult vascular supply. (Redrawn from Mandell VS, Jaques PF, Delany DJ, et al: Persistent sciatic artery: clinical, embryologic, and angiographic features. *AJR Am J Roentgenol* 144:245, 1985.)

Visualization of this anomalous vessel along its entire course can be difficult, and the condition may be misinterpreted on routine angiograms as atherosclerotic occlusion of the superficial femoral vessel. If this anomaly is suspected, selective internal iliac artery injection or additional delayed-timing injections can assist in correct angiographic identification.[74]

Persistent Deep Popliteal Artery

During embryonic development the deep popliteal artery represents the distal continuation of the sciatic artery. The deep popliteal artery, which passes between the popliteal muscle and posterior aspects of the tibia, is normally replaced at the 18-mm crown-rump embryonic stage by the superficial popliteal artery, which runs posterior to the popliteus.[101] Persistence of the earlier embryonic artery has been reported to be a rare cause of popliteal artery entrapment syndrome, which is discussed in greater detail next.[9,101]

Popliteal Artery Entrapment Syndrome

Compression of the popliteal artery may be caused by a number of anomalous structures in the popliteal fossa, including deviation of the artery anterior and medial to the origin of the medial head of the gastrocnemius, passage of the artery through the medial head of the gastrocnemius, a high origin of the medial head of the gastrocnemius, a fibrous band running from the medial head of the gastrocnemius to the lateral condyle, hypertrophy of the plantaris muscle, an accessory head of the gastrocnemius, and hypertrophy or an accessory portion of the semimembranosus (Fig. 2.11).[9,15,46,58,101] The incidence of this syndrome was noted to be 0.165% in one large series of 20,000 patients, and it appears to be more frequent in young adult males.[15,46,101] Most cases are thought to be because of abnormalities in embryonic muscle development, but as previously noted, rare cases may result from persistence of embryonic arterial structures.[9,101]

Patients most frequently complain of activity-related claudication (54%) but can have acute signs of ischemia (5%) when arterial thrombosis occurs.[9,101] Other symptoms may include swelling, limping, or muscle cramps. On physical examination, absence of a pedal pulse or diminishment with dynamic maneuvers, including active plantar flexion and passive dorsiflexion of the foot with the knee in active extension, may be noted. Lower extremity edema or severe varicosities may be observed if compression of the popliteal vein also occurs. Diagnostic tests, such as arteriograms, ultrasonograms, and MRI, can be helpful in evaluating young people with complaints of claudication. An arteriogram may show local compression or medial deviation of the popliteal artery in patients with an abnormal origin or path of the medial head of the gastrocnemius. In patients with an acute onset, complete obstruction caused by thrombosis may be observed.[46,101] Dynamic maneuvers performed during arteriography or duplex ultrasonography may also demonstrate active compression. MRI can be quite helpful in identifying anomalous structures that compress the artery and has become the gold standard for evaluating the anatomy of the popliteal fossa (Fig. 2.12).[37,101]

In patients with documented symptomatic compression, simple release of anomalous bands or resection or transposition of abnormal or accessory muscles may be performed. However, in those with chronic scarring of the artery or acute thrombosis, revascularization procedures may be required.[9,15,101]

NERVE ABNORMALITIES

Sensory Distribution Variations

Sensation to the anterior and medial aspect of the knee is supplied by the infrapatellar branch of the saphenous nerve. In most patients, the infrapatellar branch originates after the saphenous nerve emerges through the deep fascia between the sartorius and the gracilis in the distal part of the thigh. It then traverses through the sartorius muscle and joins the patellar plexus, curving distal and medial to the patella.[54] Anterior and medial surgical approaches to the knee place these branches at risk and have been associated with neuroma formation postoperatively if transected.[23] Frequent variations in anatomy,

including more proximal origins of the saphenous nerve and infrapatellar branches, which result in a more anterior course of the infrapatellar branch, make it difficult to avoid the cutaneous nerves reliably, and we do not routinely attempt to preserve them. Multiple patterns of the cutaneous innervation to the lateral aspect of the knee have been described.[52]

CYSTS

Ganglion Cysts

Ganglion or synovial cysts have been reported to originate from numerous structures in and around the knee joint, including the ACL, PCL, popliteal tendon, and menisci. In most cases these cysts are believed to be related to cystic degeneration of the structure or herniation of synovial fluid and cells through a defect into surrounding tissue; however, in some cases they may represent congenital anomalies.[†] Symptoms related to these cysts may include palpable masses, recurrent effusions, aching pain, and locking or catching. Successful open excision and arthroscopic débridement of these cysts have been reported in a limited number of cases.[63,73,87,98,105] However, if the underlying disease is not addressed, the risk of recurrence is a concern.

Meniscal Cysts

Meniscal cysts represent a subgroup of ganglion cysts that occur in association with meniscal tears. Originally the cause of these lesions was controversial; possibilities included myxoid generation, trauma, and synovial rests. However, a link with meniscal tears has now been documented.[87,102] Cysts involve the lateral more often than the medial aspect of the knee. The most common site of occurrence is along the lateral joint line anterior to the lateral collateral ligament. Patients may note a palpable mass that disappears in flexion (Pisani sign), aching knee pain, or an effusion.[102]

MRI is the test of choice for both evaluating a suspected cyst and detecting associated meniscal tears (Fig. 2.13). Lateral cysts commonly occur at the junction of the anterior and middle thirds of the body, whereas medial cysts are located most frequently in the posterior horn.[102,117] A horizontal cleavage or transverse tear is typically identified at this site in each case.[44,87,102]

Nonoperative treatment, including aspiration and injection of cortisone into the cyst, has been used successfully, but an approximately 25% short-term recurrence rate has been reported.[78] We do not favor this approach because of the association with intra-articular disease. Surgical intervention previously consisted of open cyst excision, complete meniscectomy, or both.[67,69] However, arthroscopic partial meniscectomy of the involved torn meniscus with intra-articular cyst drainage has become the accepted initial intervention.[44,87,88,102] If intraoperative attempts at cyst decompression by the application of external pressure are unsuccessful, an 18-gauge needle can be percutaneously passed through the cyst and accompanying meniscal defect to facilitate intra-articular decompression of the loculated fluid.[88] Alternatively, an arthroscopic punch or shaver may be passed through the meniscal defect into the cyst.[44,87] With these techniques, good and excellent clinical results have been reported in approximately 90% of patients, with no recurrences observed in several series.[‡]

---

†References 63, 73, 87, 102, 105, and 113.
‡References 80, 81, 87, 88, 95, and 102.

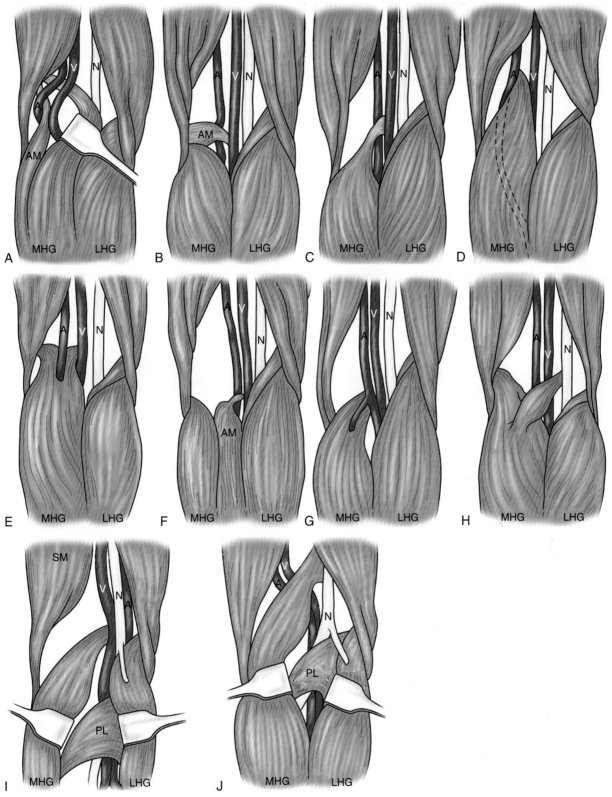

FIG 2.11 (A through J) Diagrammatic representations of abnormal muscle anatomy encountered during surgical release of symptomatic popliteal artery entrapment. Popliteal artery entrapment may be because of the presence of a variety of anomalous muscle bodies and tendons, deviation of normal muscle attachments (particularly the medial gastrocnemius), and abnormal muscle hypertrophy. *A* and *V*, Popliteal artery and vein; *AM*, anomalous muscle; *MHG* and *LHG*, medial and lateral heads of the gastrocnemius; *N*, tibial nerve; *PL*, abnormal plantaris; *SM*, hypertrophied semimembranosus. (Redrawn from Bouhoutsos J, Daskalakis E: Muscular abnormalities affecting the popliteal vessels. *Br J Surg* 68:501, 1981.)

Popliteal Cysts

The posterior synovial cavity communicates with a popliteal bursa that is found between the semimembranosus tendon and the medial head of the gastrocnemius in about 50% of people (Fig. 2.14).[126] This bursa may be distended when dye is injected into the knee; the bursa can also become enlarged by an intra-articular effusion, resulting in a popliteal or Baker cyst.[5] After being trapped in the bursa, fluid is unable to return to the joint because of a functional one-way valve. In two large series of patients who underwent MRI of the knee, a 5%

to 19% incidence of popliteal cysts was identified.[27,40,77] A higher incidence in older patients was noted.[77] In adult patients, popliteal cysts commonly occur in association with intra-articular abnormalities, including meniscal tears, ACL tears, and degenerative or inflammatory arthritis, which can all result in increased joint fluid.[27,40,77,115] Fielding et al.[40] reported an 82% incidence of posterior horn medial meniscus tears in patients with documented popliteal cysts. Histologic examination has revealed that popliteal cysts are generally lined with flattened mesothelium-like cells surrounded by fibroblasts and lymphocysts and contain a viscous, fibrin-rich fluid.[27] Burleson et al.[18] identified three types of popliteal cysts. Type 1 cysts have a thin, 1- to 2-mm fibrous wall with flat endothelial-like cells; type 2 cysts have thicker walls that are poorly defined and lined with cuboid-type cells; and type 3 cysts have walls up to 8 mm thickness with greater numbers of lymphocytes, plasma cells, and

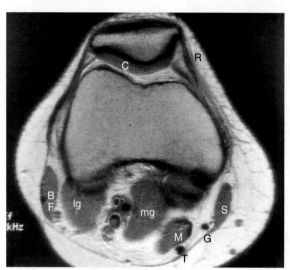

FIG 2.12 Axial Magnetic Resonance Image of the Knee The contents of the popliteal fossa and the location of the neurovascular structures between the two heads of the gastrocnemius can be readily identified. *BF*, Biceps femoris; *c*, patella cartilage; *G*, gracilis; *M*, semimembranosus muscle; *mg* and *lg*, medial and lateral gastrocnemius, respectively; *R*, medial retinaculum; *S*, sartorius muscle; *T*, semitendinosus tendon.

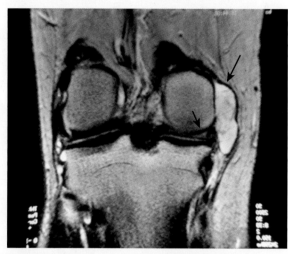

FIG 2.13 Coronal magnetic resonance image of a medial meniscal cyst *(thick arrow)* with high-signal fluid contents in association with a meniscal tear *(thin arrow)*.

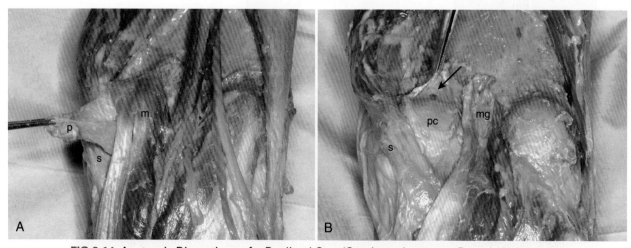

FIG 2.14 Anatomic Dissections of a Popliteal Cyst (Semimembranosus Bursa) (A) An evacuated popliteal cyst (*p*, forceps) originates between the semimembranosus (*s*) and the medial head of the gastrocnemius (*m*). (B) The wall of the cyst has been removed and the medial head of the gastrocnemius (*mg*) has been detached from its origin on the posterior aspect of the medial femoral condyle and transposed medially to reveal the posterior capsule (*pc*). A small hole in the capsule (*arrow*, inferior to the tip of the forceps) in the base of the cyst communicates with the intra-articular cavity (*s*, semimembranosus).

histiocytes. A small number of cysts could not be adequately classified and were termed *transitional types.*[18]

In pediatric patients, asymptomatic swelling in the popliteal fossa is the most common manifestation, but in adult patients, vague posterior aches or symptoms related to the intra-articular disease are commonly present. A pseudothrombophlebitis syndrome with severe calf swelling and pain related to rupture of a cyst has been described.[27,65] On examination the cyst can often be palpated in the medial aspect of the popliteal fossa as a firm mass that is best appreciated with the knee in extension.

Plain radiographs are rarely helpful for diagnosis, except to identify associated arthritic changes. Both MRI and ultrasonography can be used to distinguish between cystic and solid masses in the popliteal fossa.[27,86] However, MRI is also excellent at demonstrating associated meniscal tears and other intra-articular disease. Because of the fluid content, popliteal cysts appear bright on T2-weighted images and have low signal intensity on T1-weighted images (Fig. 2.15). The best visualization of these cysts appears to be obtained with axial fat-suppressed fast T2-weighted images.[77]

In the pediatric population, popliteal cysts rarely require operative intervention; in most patients treated by observation, the cysts spontaneously resolve within 1 to 2 years.[33] In symptomatic adults, treatment can include nonsteroidal anti-inflammatory medications, compression, and physical therapy. However, if symptoms persist or are disabling, arthroscopic examination and débridement of the associated intra-articular disease should be considered. We do not favor aspiration or injection of corticosteroids into the cysts because these solutions are rarely definitive. Open excision is rarely required, but if attempted after failure of arthroscopic management, complete excision of the cyst and stalk with simple closure of the capsular defect may be considered.[53] Transposition of a portion of the medial gastrocnemius tendon over the capsular repair has been reported to decrease the rate of cyst recurrence.[27,95]

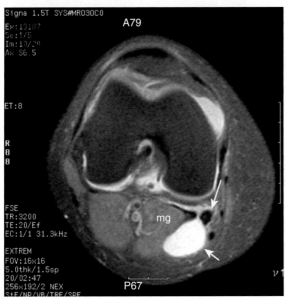

FIG 2.15 Axial magnetic resonance image of a popliteal cyst with the high signal of a fluid-filled cyst *(thin arrow)* dissecting into the popliteal fossa from its origin between the semimembranosus *(thick arrow)* and the medial head of the gastrocnemius *(mg).*

PLICAE

During fetal development the knee is separated into three compartments by synovial membranes. At approximately 4 to 5 months of embryonic development, these partitions resorb to form a single cavity; incomplete or partial resorption results in incomplete synovial folds or plicae.[35,127] Three plicae are most commonly described: suprapatellar, infrapatellar, and medial patellar. Histologic examination reveals a bland fibrous membrane (Fig. 2.16). Visualization of these plicae on MRI is difficult without an associated intra-articular effusion, but it is possible, particularly on sagittal and axial views. Rarely these plicae become inflamed and fibrotic and may become symptomatic. Arthroscopic resection has proved successful in relieving symptoms in carefully selected patients.[35,68,79,89,96]

Medial Patellar Plica

A medial patellar plica has its origin on the medial wall of the knee joint and runs obliquely distally toward and inserts into the synovium, covering the medial infrapatellar fat pad. It may occur in association with or in continuity with a suprapatellar plica. A medial patellar plica has been noted in 5% to 55% of all individuals but becomes symptomatic in only a small number of patients.[6,68,79,89,103] A fenestrated plica is less common but is more likely to be symptomatic.[6]

A previously asymptomatic plica may become symptomatic after a knee injury. It is postulated that effusion and synovitis related to the original injury may cause the plica to become edematous, which in turn produces a fibrotic reaction leading to tightening, bowstringing, and impingement of the plica against the medial femoral condyle or the medial patellar facet. This irritation leads to further thickening and contraction of the fibrous band.[79,89] Patients complain of dull, aching medial knee pain that may be exacerbated by activity or prolonged sitting. Patients may also have mechanical symptoms, such as crepitus and catching or pseudolocking. In one study the most frequent symptoms were pain (92%), snapping (80%), swelling (67%), and pseudolocking (35%).[79] Physical examination consistently reveals tenderness over the medial condyle, and a

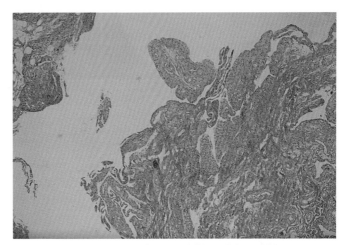

FIG 2.16 Histology of a Synovial Plica A bland fibrous membrane is lined with rather indistinct synovial-like lining cells. (From Vigorita VJ: The synovium. In Vigorita VJ, Ghelman B, editors: *Orthopaedic pathology,* Philadelphia, 1999, Lippincott Williams & Wilkins.)

painful band may be palpated approximately one fingerbreadth away from the medial border of the patella.[89] A snap or catching may also be elicited.[79]

Koshino and Okamoto[68] described two provocation tests that they found helpful in diagnosing symptomatic plicae. The first, the rotation valgus test, involves flexing the knee and applying a valgus force with internal and then external rotation of the tibia while simultaneously attempting to displace the patella medially. The second, the holding test, involves attempting to flex the knee against active resistance. If either test elicits pain, with or without a click, it is positive.

MRI is the most appropriate imaging modality and has been reported to be reliable for detection of medial patellar plicae, with a sensitivity of 93% and a specificity of 81%.[80] These plicae have low signal intensity on both T1- and T2-weighted images, which is believed to be because of recurrent synovitis and fibrosis of the plica (Fig. 2.17).[80]

Arthroscopic examination may reveal a thickened plica that impinges on the femur or patella. Sakakibara and Watanabe[103] described a classification of medial patellar plicae based on the arthroscopic appearance. Type A is a cordlike elevation in the medial wall; type B has a shelflike appearance, but it does not arthroscopically cover the anterior surface of the medial condyle; type C has a large shelflike appearance that covers the anterior surface of the medial femoral condyle; and type D is a special variation in which double insertions in the medial wall are seen.[103] Chondromalacia or groove formation may be noted at the site of impingement on the medial femoral condyle or the medial patellar facet (Fig. 2.18).[89]

Nonoperative treatment includes a reduction in activity, administration of nonsteroidal anti-inflammatory medications, and physical therapy. These modalities are all aimed at reducing the inflammation and breaking the cycle of irritation and edema within the plica. If nonoperative measures are ineffective, arthroscopic examination and plica excision may be considered. Arthroscopic débridement of symptomatic medial patellar plicae has been moderately successful in carefully selected patients, with 66% to 90% experiencing complete pain relief; however, cautions against overdiagnosis and resection of incidental plicae have been put forth.[6,68,79,89]

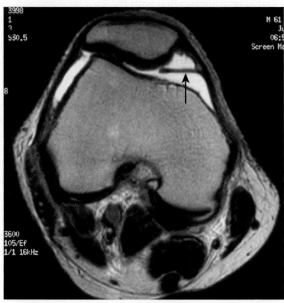

FIG 2.17 Axial magnetic resonance image with a low-signal, thick medial patellar plica *(arrow)* that is highlighted by the large effusion.

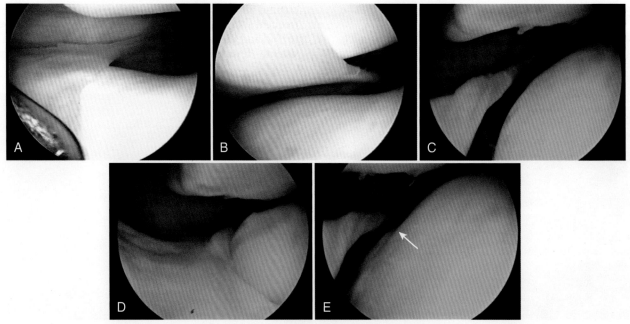

FIG 2.18 Arthroscopic Views of Medial Patellar Plicae (A and B) Superior and inferior surfaces of a large medial patellar plica that is impinging between the patella and the medial femoral condyle. (C) Thickened edge of a fibrotic medial plica. (D) Impingement by a thickened plica on the medial femoral condyle. (E) Erosion in the medial femoral condyle articular cartilage as a result of chronic impingement *(arrow)*.

Suprapatellar Plica

A suprapatellar plica is a crescent-shaped septum that may be found between the suprapatellar pouch and the knee joint. It is attached to the medial and lateral walls of the knee joint, as well as the undersurface of the quadriceps tendon (Fig. 2.19). In a large cadaver study the presence of a persistent plica was observed in 17% of specimens. In 95 of these specimens the plica was complete and divided the suprapatellar pouch into two parts, and in 8% the plica was incomplete.[127] A large suprapatellar plica may shield loose bodies and, if in continuity with a medial patellar plica, can contribute to symptomatic impingement against the femoral condyle or patella.[35,89] Symptoms may also occur in patients with division of the pouch by a complete plica.[35]

Patients have symptoms similar to those associated with patellofemoral pain syndrome; pain is aggravated by stair climbing and knee flexion. Swelling in the suprapatellar region may be noted after activity. When the pouch is completely isolated from the knee joint, it has been postulated that distention of the bursae related to activity with occasional dissection between the planes of the quadriceps mechanism leads to pain.[35,92,93] In other cases pain is probably related to impingement and entrapment of the plica. Again, MRI is the best imaging modality for identifying these plicae (Fig. 2.20). Successful arthroscopic resection of a symptomatic suprapatellar plica has been reported, although the number of cases is small.[35,79]

Infrapatellar Plica

An infrapatellar plica, commonly known as the ligamentum mucosum, traverses from the intercondylar notch to the infrapatellar fat pad. It widens from its origin in the notch and fans out as it inserts distally in the fat pad. It is the most common plica and is not considered pathologic.[79] Rarely this plica is very large and thickened; in such cases it is referred to as a persistent vertical septum (Fig. 2.21).[96] The only clinical significance of this plica relates to problems caused by the membrane during arthroscopy or arthrography. During arthroscopic examination, a large infrapatellar plica or a persistent vertical septum can be an obstacle to easy passage of the arthroscope and instruments.[79,96] Resection of these membranes when encountered facilitates easy maneuvering inside the anterior knee joint.

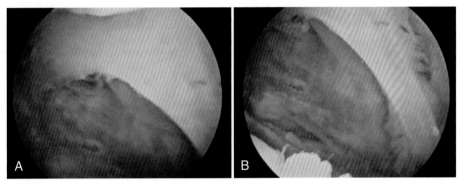

FIG 2.19 Arthroscopic Views of a Suprapatellar Plica (A) Incomplete crescent-shaped suprapatellar plica with an opening to the suprapatellar pouch. (B) Extension of the same suprapatellar plica distally and posteriorly along the intra-articular surface of the medial capsule.

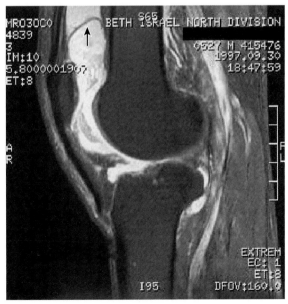

FIG 2.20 Sagittal magnetic resonance image with a curvilinear suprapatellar plica *(arrow)* outlined by an intra-articular effusion.

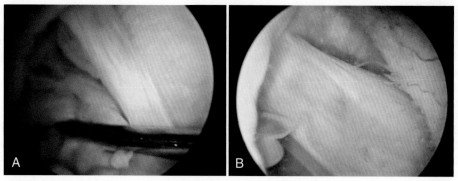

FIG 2.21 (A) Arthroscopic view of an infrapatellar plica (ligamentum mucosum) seen anterior to the anterior cruciate ligament (ACL) (probe tip posterior to the ACL). (B) Arthroscopic view of a persistent vertical septum with almost complete division of the medial and lateral compartments anterior.

SUMMARY

A large number of anatomic variations have been reported and in many cases represent incidental findings. However, in certain circumstances, such as trauma or degeneration, these structures may become symptomatic. To interpret the significance of these findings and render suitable treatment, the first step is correct identification.

KEY REFERENCES

8. Beaconsfield T, Pintore E, Maffulli N, et al: Radiological measurements in patellofemoral disorders: a review. *Clin Orthop* 308:18, 1994.
9. Becquemin J-P, Melliere D, Lamour A, et al: The popliteal entrapment syndrome. *Anat Clin* 6:203, 1984.
14. Bollier M, Fulkerson JP: The role of trochlear dysplasia in patellofemoral instability. *J Am Acad Orthop Surg* 19:8, 2011.
27. Curl WW: Popliteal cysts: historical background and current knowledge. *J Am Acad Orthop Surg* 4:129, 1996.
31. Dickhaut SC, DeLee JC: The discoid lateral-meniscus syndrome. *J Bone Joint Surg Am* 64:1068, 1982.
38. Ferrone JD, Jr: Congenital deformities about the knee. *Orthop Clin North Am* 7:323, 1976.

59. Johansson E, Aparisi T: Congenital absence of the cruciate ligaments: a case report and review of the literature. *Clin Orthop* 162:108, 1982.
71. Lee DH, Kim TH, Kim JM, et al: Results of subtotal/total or partial meniscectomy for discoid lateral meniscus in children. *Arthroscopy* 25:496, 2009.
94. Poynton AR, Javadpour SM, Finegan PJ, et al: The meniscofemoral ligaments of the knee. *J Bone Joint Surg Br* 79:327, 1997.
96. Reider B, Marshall JL, Warren RF: Brief note: persistent vertical septum in the human knee joint. *J Bone Joint Surg Am* 63:1185, 1981.
97. Renstrom P, Johnson RJ: Anatomy and biomechanics of the menisci. *Clin Sports Med* 9:523, 1990.
101. Rosset E, Hartung O, Brunet C, et al: Popliteal artery entrapment syndrome: anatomic and embryologic bases, diagnostic and therapeutic considerations following a series of 15 cases with a review of the literature. *Surg Radiol Anat* 17:161, 1995.
121. Van Dommelen BA, Fowler PJ: Anatomy of the posterior cruciate ligament: a review. *Am J Sports Med* 17:24, 1989.
126. Wilson PD, Eyre-Brook AL, Francis JD: A clinical and anatomical study of the semimembranosus bursa in relation to popliteal cyst. *J Bone Joint Surg* 20:963, 1938.
128. Zivanovic S: Menisco-meniscal ligaments of the human knee joint. *Anat Anz* 135(Suppl):35, 1974.

The references for this chapter can also be found on www.expertconsult.com.

3

Clinical Examination of the Knee

Justin B. Jones, Aaron Althaus, Jason P. Hochfelder, Timothy G. Reish, William J. Long, Michael P. Nett, Henrik Bo Pedersen, Gregory J. Roehrig, Alfred J. Tria, Jr., W. Norman Scott

HISTORY

Despite improvements in advanced imaging techniques, clinical examination of the knee remains an essential step in evaluating the knee patient. Evaluation of every patient should begin with a complete history of the symptoms and a full description of the mechanism of injury. Often, the history will direct the examiner to the area of knee involvement. This will sharpen the physical examination, result in a more accurate diagnosis, and allow the clinician to be more proficient.

OBSERVATION AND INSPECTION

The examination should begin with observation of the patient's gait, which provides critical information. The examiner should note the patient's ability to ambulate, the use of gait aids, the speed of ambulation, and the amount of discomfort present with attempted ambulation. Evaluation of the gait pattern and the stance position of the lower limb is performed while the patient ambulates. A shortened stance phase of gait (antalgic gait) will confirm the side of involvement. A short leg gait requires confirmation of limb length. This may be accompanied by a significant varus or valgus deformity at the knee or may represent an extra-articular deformity requiring further evaluation. Varus or valgus alignment should be noted, as well as any medial or lateral thrust in the stance phase of gait (Fig. 3.1). The clinical alignment of the lower part of the leg (anatomic axis) measures the femorotibial angle (Fig. 3.2) and is different from the mechanical axis of the limb (Fig. 3.3), as measured from the femoral head through the knee to the center of the ankle on a standing roentgenogram. With a goniometer applied to the anterior aspect of the thigh and the lower part of the leg and centered on the patella, the examiner can report the clinical varus or valgus alignment. This measurement should be used along with the roentgenographic measurements.

Patellar alignment must also be observed. It is influenced by femoral neck anteversion, tibial torsion, the anatomy of the individual patellar facets, and the depth and angle of the femoral sulcus (Fig. 3.4). The Q angle is drawn from the middle of the tibial tubercle to the middle of the patella and then to the anterior superior iliac spine of the pelvis. The normal angle is 10 to 20 degrees.

Clinical effusion may be apparent visually. Active range of motion should be recorded, along with any limitations to full extension or flexion. Active range of motion will be further evaluated with palpation and should be compared with passive range of motion of the knee (Fig. 3.5). It is customary that full extension should be considered 0 degrees, and flexion is recorded as an increasing number or as the distance of the heel of the foot from the buttocks. An inability to fully extend may represent lag, a locked knee, or a flexion contracture. An inability to fully flex may be because of an effusion, pain, or extension contracture.

Quadriceps atrophy is sometimes visually apparent and can help confirm the involved side. The gross appearance of quadriceps atrophy should lead to further investigation with circumferential measurement during the palpation phase of the physical examination.

PALPATION

All bony landmarks should be palpated and identified. The Q angle, Gerdy's tubercle, the fibular head, the epicondyles of the femur, the patellar margins, and the tibiofemoral joint lines can be readily palpated in most patients.

Effusions can be graded in size by compressing the suprapatellar pouch and then noting any fluid (grade 1), slight lift-off of the patella (grade 2), a ballotable patella (grade 3), or a tense effusion with no ability to compress the patella against the femoral sulcus (grade 4) (Fig. 3.6).

If muscle atrophy was noted on observation, thigh circumference should now be measured. The circumference of the thigh should be measured at a set distance (10 cm) above the patella with the knee in full extension and then compared with the opposite side. The calf should be measured at its greatest circumference in the lower part of the leg.

Crepitation in and of itself may or may not represent evidence of a disorder. The location should be recorded for future reference. It may involve the medial or lateral patellofemoral articulation, the medial tibiofemoral articulation, or the lateral tibiofemoral articulation.

THE PATELLOFEMORAL JOINT

Examination of the patellofemoral joint includes both static and dynamic evaluation. Visual inspection should be performed to note any evidence of quadriceps atrophy or vastus medialis obliquus hypoplasia. Prepatellar swelling or erythema may be present, suggesting prepatellar bursitis. The Q angle should be measured with the patient supine and the hip and knee in full extension. If the knee is allowed to flex slightly, the Q angle will decrease with internal rotation of the tibia on the femur

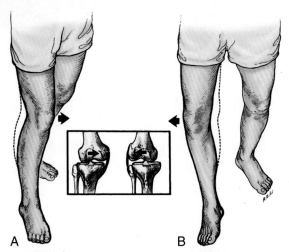

FIG 3.1 (A) Medial thrust of the femur indicates shift of the femur medially on the tibia through the stance phase of gait in the coronal plane. (B) Lateral thrust indicates lateral shift of the femur in the coronal plane. (From Tria AJ Jr, Klein KS: *An illustrated guide to the knee*, New York, 1992, Churchill Livingstone.)

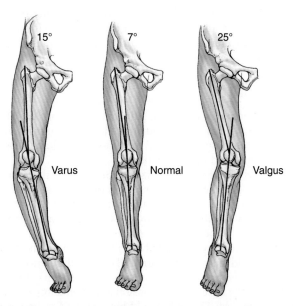

FIG 3.2 The anatomic axis is measured by drawing lines parallel to the long axis of the femur and the tibia and measuring the intercepting angle. (From Tria AJ Jr, Klein KS: *An illustrated guide to the knee*, New York, 1992, Churchill Livingstone.)

(Fig. 3.7). The average male Q angle is 14 ± 3 degrees, and the average female Q angle is 17 ± 3 degrees.[1] A Q angle greater than 20 degrees must be noted as excessive. Tracking of the patella from full extension into flexion should be recorded visually. In full extension, the patella begins with contact of the median ridge and the lateral facet with the lateral side of the sulcus. The patella moves more centrally and the facets increase their contact with the femoral condyles as flexion increases (Fig. 3.8). Excessive lateralization of the patella with full extension will result in a pathologic J sign. This may be seen in patients with recurrent lateral subluxations or excessive ligamentous laxity, or following a traumatic lateral patellar dislocation.

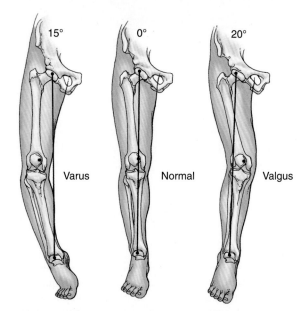

FIG 3.3 The mechanical axis of the leg is measured in the standing position with an imaginary "plumb line" dropped from the femoral head to the ground. This angular measurement gives the best functional evaluation of lower extremity alignment. (From Tria AJ Jr, Klein KS: *An illustrated guide to the knee*, New York, 1992, Churchill Livingstone.)

Because the patellar facets do not begin to contact the femoral sulcus until the knee is flexed 30 degrees, the medial and lateral patellofemoral articulation should be palpated at this degree of flexion. This can be accomplished by allowing the leg to bend slightly over the edge of the table or by placing a small pillow below the knee. Direct patellar compression is performed and may elicit pain over the medial or lateral facet, depending on the location of the pathology (Fig. 3.9). Direct compression can be performed at progressively increasing degrees of flexion to further isolate the location of a chondral lesion. The patellar grind test consists of quadriceps contraction while direct compression is placed on the patella. When performed in full extension, entrapped synovium can cause pain even with a normal patellofemoral joint, which is especially true in patients with patella alta. This is an unreliable test and is not recommended. The examiner should complete the static aspect of the examination by evaluating for the presence of tenderness over the medial and lateral facets of the patella, the medial and lateral retinacula, the insertion of the quadriceps tendon, and the insertion of the patellar tendon.

Dynamic evaluation should include observation of patellar tracking with active knee flexion and extension. This is performed with the patient seated on the edge of the examination table with knees bent over the side (Fig. 3.10). The patella can be seen engaging the trochlea at 10 to 30 degrees of flexion.[10] Any excessive lateral displacement with full extension or any maltracking should be noted. After patellar tracking is assessed, the examiner should place one hand over the anterior aspect of the patella and provide resistance to knee extension with the opposite hand. Knee extension against resistance will elicit any patellofemoral crepitus or pain from chondral pathology. The half-squat test is a different technique to load the patellofemoral joint in a similar manner. With this test, the patient is asked to

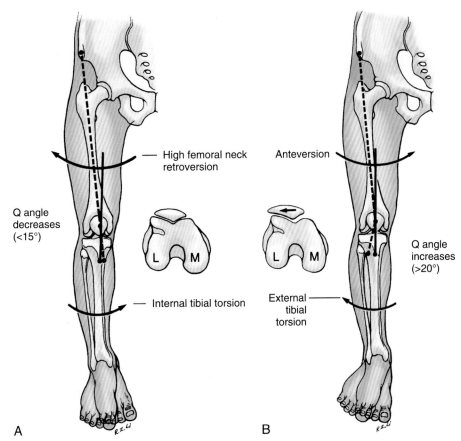

FIG 3.4 High femoral neck retroversion rotates the distal end of the femur externally. In combination with internal tibial torsion, the Q angle is decreased. Patellar tracking is improved, and patellofemoral sulcus alignment is normal. High femoral neck anteversion rotates the distal end of the femur internally. In combination with external tibial torsion, the Q angle is increased. Patellar tracking is compromised, and the patella tends to track laterally. (From Tria AJ Jr, Klein KS: *An illustrated guide to the knee,* New York, 1992, Churchill Livingstone.)

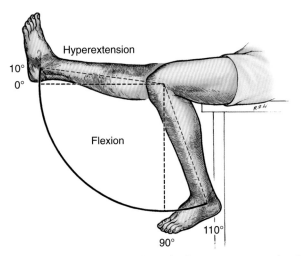

FIG 3.5 Full extension of the knee is the zero or neutral point. (From Tria AJ Jr, Klein KS: *An illustrated guide to the knee,* New York, 1992, Churchill Livingstone.)

hold the position of a half-squat and report the presence of anterior knee pain.

Patellar tilt, mobility, and the presence of patellar apprehension are then evaluated. The patient is placed in a supine position. In full extension, neutral or slight lateral tilt of the patella is normal. The inability to tilt the patella past neutral indicates an excessively tight lateral retinaculum (Fig. 3.11). With the knee flexed 20 to 30 degrees, patellar mobility is assessed. Both medial and lateral translation should be noted. Translation should not exceed two quadrants in either direction.[16] If less than one quadrant of medial translation is present, this suggests an excessively tight lateral retinaculum. Patellar apprehension should also be assessed with the knee flexed 20 to 30 degrees (Fig. 3.12).[7] Medial apprehension may be seen but is much less frequent and often iatrogenic in nature following an excessive lateral release. Lateral apprehension is more common and may suggest recurrent subluxations, traumatic lateral patellar dislocation, or excessive ligamentous laxity.

Examination of the patellofemoral joint is not complete until the hip is examined. Passive and active range of motion of the hip should be recorded. Excessive internal rotation of the hip secondary to increased femoral anteversion will result in an increased Q angle and may be part of a "miserable malalignment" type syndrome.[15] Hip rotation and femoral anteversion

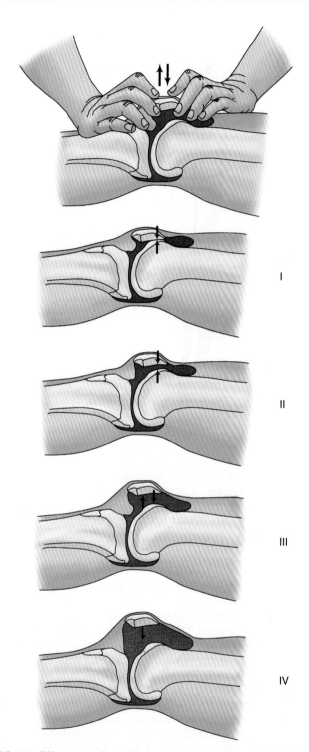

FIG 3.6 Effusions of the knee are graded from 1 to 4. (From Tria AJ Jr, Klein KS: *An illustrated guide to the knee,* New York, 1992, Churchill Livingstone.)

should be assessed with the patient in a prone position (Fig. 3.13). Internal rotation that exceeds external rotation by greater than 30 degrees is considered pathologic and should be noted.[4] Limited range of motion or pain with hip range of motion may signify hip pathology as a source of referred pain. This suggests that further evaluation of the hip should be performed before an accurate diagnosis can be made.

TABLE 3.1 Meniscal Tests	
Palpation	**Rotation**
Bragard	Apley
McMurray	Apley grind
Steinmann second	Bohler
	Duck walking
	Helfet
	Merke
	Payr
	Steinmann first

THE TIBIOFEMORAL JOINT

Examination of the tibiofemoral joint should note the presence of any cystic mass (ganglion) along the joint line, localized tenderness, crepitation, snapping, or clicking. Meniscal tears occur as a result of injury to or degeneration of fibrocartilage. Physical examination of a knee with a torn meniscus reveals joint line tenderness with a palpable click or snap and occasionally the presence of an effusion. Range of motion may be limited secondary to a displaced meniscal tear. A block to full extension may be indicative of a locked knee with a large displaced tear.

Tests for meniscal tears are divided into two groups: those that evaluate the presence of tenderness or clicks with palpation, and those that depend on symptoms of joint line pain with rotation (Table 3.1).[2]

The primary palpation tests are the Bragard, McMurray, and Steinmann second tests. The Bragard test describes that external tibial rotation and knee extension increases tenderness along the medial joint line in the presence of a medial meniscus tear. This maneuver brings the medial meniscus more anterior and closer to the examining finger, therefore eliciting more pain. Internal rotation and flexion cause less tenderness by moving the meniscus farther from the area of palpation. In the presence of a lateral meniscus tear, internal rotation of the tibia and extension will increase tenderness along the lateral joint line, while flexion and external rotation will reduce tenderness. If an articular surface irregularity of the femur or the tibia leads to tenderness, no difference between the two positions will be noted.

The McMurray test elicits a palpable click on the joint line.[21] Medially, it is demonstrated by external tibial rotation and passive motion from flexion to extension. Laterally, it is demonstrated with the tibia in internal rotation and passive motion from flexion to extension. A posterior tear may result in occurrence of a click within the initial few degrees from full flexion. If a click is palpated later as the knee is brought into greater extension, the tear is believed to be more anterior.

The Steinmann second test demonstrates joint line tenderness that moves posteriorly with knee flexion and anteriorly with knee extension. This finding is consistent with a meniscal tear that moves with range of motion of the knee. On the other hand, with a fixed joint line disorder, tenderness should remain stationary throughout the range of motion (Fig. 3.14).

The remaining tests for meniscal pathology depend on pain with rotation. The Apley grind forces the tibiofemoral surfaces together to elicit pain. A positive finding is believed to confirm a meniscal tear. On the other hand, the Apley test is performed with the knee surfaces distracted. If the Apley test (distraction) elicits less discomfort than the Apley grind (compression), the finding of a meniscal tear is favored over a fixed joint line

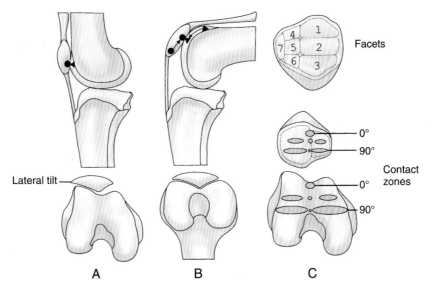

FIG 3.7 As flexion increases, the patella moves more medially, and the contact zones shift proximally and to the medial and lateral facets. (From Tria AJ Jr, Klein KS: *An illustrated guide to the knee,* New York, 1992, Churchill Livingstone.)

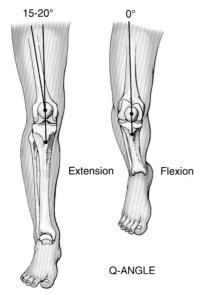

FIG 3.8 Flexion of the knee decreases the Q angle as the result of internal tibial rotation. (From Tria AJ Jr, Klein KS: *An illustrated guide to the knee,* New York, 1992, Churchill Livingstone.)

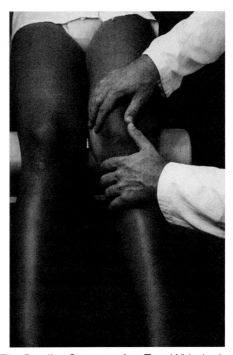

FIG 3.9 The Patellar Compression Test With the knee flexed slightly to engage the patella in the femoral trochlea, direct compression is applied to the patella.

disorder. If the distraction test and compression are equally painful, an articular surface disorder is favored (such as an irregular surface secondary to osteoarthritic erosion).

If a medial meniscus tear is expected, the Bohler test can be performed by applying a varus stress to the knee. With a medial tear, a varus stress will result in increased pain caused by compression. A lateral meniscus tear can be similarly diagnosed with a valgus stress causing compression. Duck walking increases the compressive force on the posterior horns of the menisci, thus causing pain in the presence of a posterior meniscus tear.

The Helfet test is appropriate only when the knee is locked. Because a mechanical block to normal motion is present, the tibial tubercle cannot rotate externally with extension, and the Q angle cannot increase to normal with extension of the knee. Failure of the knee to externally rotate normally with extension is a positive test result.

In the Steinmann first test, the patient is seated and the knee is flexed to 90 degrees. To assess for a possible medial meniscus tear, the tibia is suddenly externally rotated by grasping the foot. A positive result produces pain along the medial joint line. Sudden internal tibial rotation is used in a similar manner to confirm a lateral meniscus tear and will result in lateral joint line pain (Fig. 3.15).

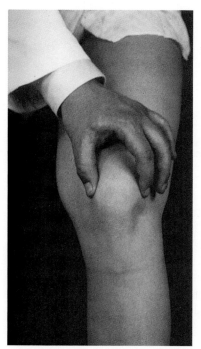

FIG 3.10 Clinical evaluation of patellar tracking is performed with the patient seated with the knee flexed to 90 degrees. During active knee extension, the examiner can detect the presence of maltracking, excessive lateral tilt, or lateral subluxation of the patella.

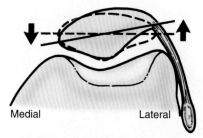

Medial   Lateral

FIG 3.11 The Passive Patellar Tilt Test In full extension, the transverse axis of a normal patella will tilt beyond the horizontal. The inability to perform this maneuver may indicate an excessively tight lateral retinaculum.

The Merke test is similar to the first Steinmann test and is performed with the patient bearing weight on the affected extremity. Internal rotation of the body over the affected limb produces external rotation of the tibia and medial joint line pain when the medial meniscus is torn. The opposite occurs with external rotation of the body over the limb when the lateral meniscus is torn.

The Payr test is performed with the patient in the "Turkish sitting position." A downward force is then applied to the knee. This results in a varus stress on the knee. A torn medial meniscus results in medial pain from increased compression. This test can be performed only for medial joint line pathology.

LIGAMENTOUS EXAMINATION

The ligamentous examination is performed to evaluate the status of the collateral ligaments, the cruciate ligaments, and the

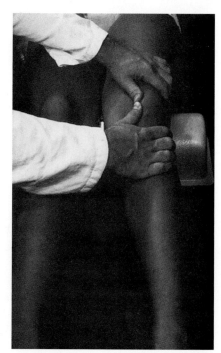

FIG 3.12 The Apprehension Test With the knee flexed 20 to 30 degrees, the examiner translates the patella laterally. With a positive test, the patient experiences apprehension, contracts the quadriceps, and attempts to push the examiner's hand from the knee.

posteromedial and posterolateral capsular structures.[12,13,20] During stress testing, the examiner should record the degree of opening and the quality of the endpoint. It can be graded from I to III or by the number of millimeters that the joint opens, as determined by the examiner.[5] Grade I corresponds to a stress examination that allows minimal to no opening, but causes pain indicating partial injury to the involved structure. Grade II corresponds to a physical examination that shows some opening of the joint but with a distinct endpoint. Grade III shows gross joint instability with no distinct endpoint to the stress evaluation.

The valgus stress test evaluates the medial collateral ligament (MCL) and the posteromedial capsule. A valgus stress applied in full extension is used to assess the MCL and the associated posteromedial capsule. In 30 degrees of flexion, the same valgus stress isolates the MCL by relaxing the capsule (Fig. 3.16). In a similar fashion, the varus stress test is performed in 30 degrees of flexion and full extension to evaluate the lateral collateral ligament and the posterolateral capsule, respectively (Fig. 3.17).

There are many ways to examine the anterior cruciate, but there are two that are most often used clinically. The test that is most often used during the ligamentous exam is the Lachman test (Fig. 3.18). The Lachman test is performed in 30 degrees of flexion with the examiner producing an anteriorly directed force on the tibia to determine the grade of laxity and quality of endpoint. Another common test is the anterior drawer (Fig. 3.19), which is performed with the knee flexed to 90 degrees and the examiner again producing an anterior directed force. The Lachman is thought to be more sensitive for the posterolateral bundle of the anterior cruciate, and the anterior drawer test more sensitive for the anteromedial bundle.

Other commonly used ACL tests in the clinical setting include the flexion rotation drawer test. It builds on the Lachman

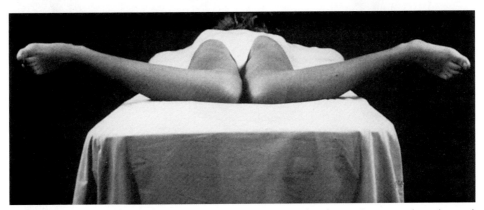

FIG 3.13 **Hip Rotation and Femoral Version** With excessive femoral anteversion, the patient will display a marked increase in hip internal rotation. This may contribute to recurrent patellar dislocations, maltracking, or lateral subluxation.

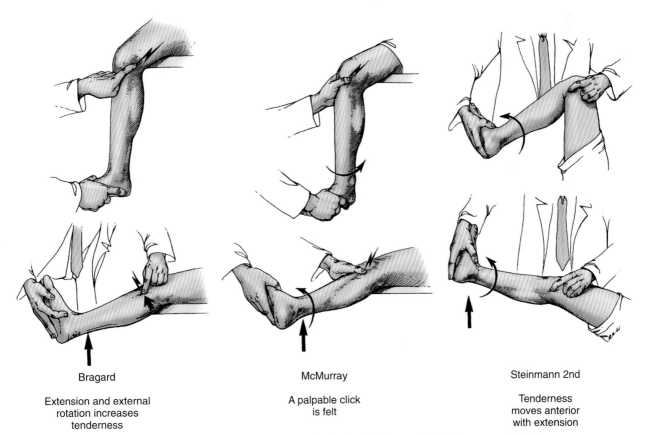

Bragard	McMurray	Steinmann 2nd
Extension and external rotation increases tenderness	A palpable click is felt	Tenderness moves anterior with extension

FIG 3.14 Meniscal tests requiring palpation include the Bragard, McMurray, and Steinmann second tests. (From Tria AJ Jr, Klein KS: *An illustrated guide to the knee*, New York, 1992, Churchill Livingstone.)

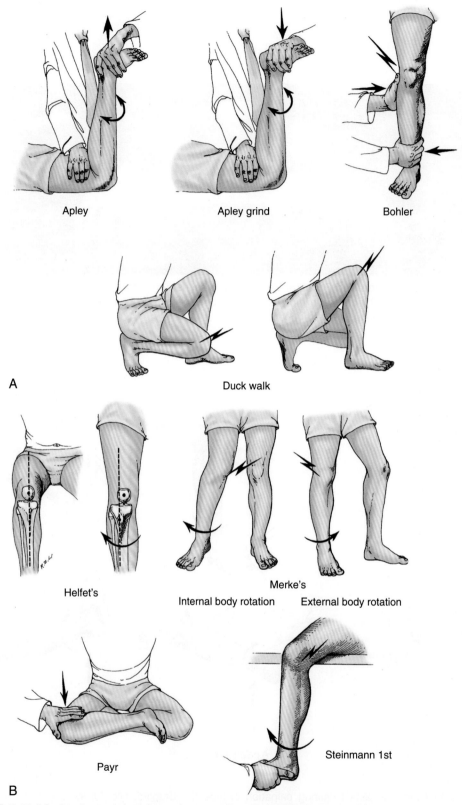

Apley   Apley grind   Bohler

A   Duck walk

Helfet's   Merke's

Internal body rotation   External body rotation

Payr   Steinmann 1st

B

FIG 3.15 Meniscal tests that depend on rotation of the knee. (From Tria AJ Jr, Klein KS: *An illustrated guide to the knee,* New York, 1992, Churchill Livingstone.)

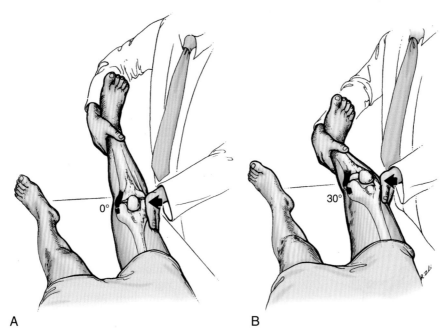

A B

FIG 3.16 Valgus stress in extension tests the MCL and the posteromedial capsule. Stress in 30 degrees of flexion tests only the MCL. (From Tria AJ Jr, Klein KS: *An illustrated guide to the knee,* New York, 1992, Churchill Livingstone.)

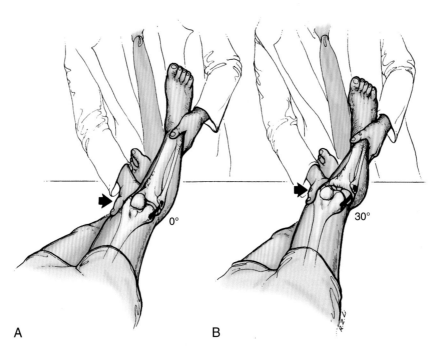

A B

FIG 3.17 Varus stress in extension tests the lateral collateral ligament and the posterolateral capsule. Stress in 30 degrees of flexion tests only the lateral collateral ligament. (From Tria AJ Jr, Klein KS: *An illustrated guide to the knee,* New York, 1992, Churchill Livingstone.)

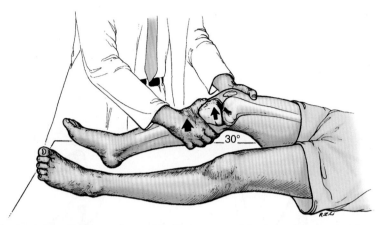

FIG 3.18 The Lachman test is performed in 30 degrees of flexion with anterior force exerted on the proximal end of the tibia. (From Tria AJ Jr, Klein KS: *An illustrated guide to the knee,* New York, 1992, Churchill Livingstone.)

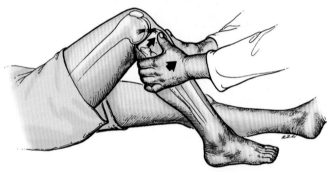

FIG 3.19 The anterior drawer test is performed with the knee flexed to 90 degrees and anterior force applied to the proximal end of the tibia. (From Tria AJ Jr, Klein KS: *An illustrated guide to the knee,* 1992, New York, Churchill Livingstone.)

test and notes tibial motion and femoral rotation from 15 to 30 degrees of flexion (Fig. 3.20).[22] Anterior force is applied to the tibia, starting at 15 degrees of flexion. This maneuver leads to anterior subluxation, much as in the Lachman test. With further knee flexion, the tibia reduces beneath the femur with a noticeable "clunk" and internal rotation of the femur. In the quadriceps active test for the ACL, the knee is held at 30 degrees of flexion and the patient is asked to extend the knee; an anterior cruciate deficient knee will pull the tibia slightly forward before the lower part of the leg begins to extend (Fig. 3.21).[6]

The pivot-shift, jerk, and Losee tests emphasize anterolateral motion of the tibia relative to the femur. Although the Lachman and anterior drawer tests can be performed with the patient in the clinical setting, the anterolateral tests produce more discomfort and are difficult to perform without sedation on a patient with an acute knee injury. In a knee with chronic instability, the anterolateral tests are easier to perform in the clinical setting.

The pivot-shift test is probably the most often used of the anterolateral provocative tests, and it begins with the knee in full extension.[8,9,11] Valgus stress is applied along with internal tibial rotation and forward pressure on the fibular head. As flexion is commenced, the lateral aspect of the tibia again comes forward and then reduces on further flexion with a palpable clunk (Fig. 3.22).

The jerk test is initiated in flexion with associated internal tibial rotation, forward pressure on the fibular head, and valgus stress (Fig. 3.23). This combination subluxates the lateral tibial condyle anteriorly. As the knee is brought into extension, the tibia reduces with a palpable clunk that is sometimes visible, indicating an insufficient anterior cruciate.

The Losee test is similar to the jerk test.[17-19] It also begins with the knee in flexion and valgus stress. The tibia, however, is initially held in external rotation. As the knee is gradually extended, the tibia is rotated internally, and the clunk of the reduction is again felt as in the jerk test. The test attempts to accentuate the subluxation with external tibial rotation (Fig. 3.24).

The posterior cruciate ligament is commonly evaluated with two tests. The posterior Lachman test is performed in 30 degrees of flexion with a posteriorly directed force on the tibia (Fig. 3.25). In the posterior drawer test (Fig. 3.26), the knee is positioned in 90 degrees of flexion, and posterior force is then applied. Grading of posterior cruciate ligament (PCL) laxity with the posterior drawer test is based on the position of the anterior tibia relative to the distal aspect of the femoral condyles. Grade I produces increased posterior tibial translation but remains anterior to the femoral condyles, grade II produces more posterior translation with the anterior tibia flush with the femoral condyles, and grade III produces posterior tibial translation past the level of the femoral condyles and often indicates multiligamentous or severe capsular injury.

A knee with chronic posterior cruciate ligament laxity will often have a posterior sag. If the patient attempts to contract the quadriceps muscle with the knee in 90 degrees of flexion, the tibia will come forward before the lower part of the leg begins to extend (quadriceps active test for the posterior cruciate ligament) (see Fig. 3.21).

The posteromedial capsule is evaluated with the Slocum test (anterior drawer test at 90 degrees of flexion with external rotation of the lower part of the leg).[3,23] When the tibia is rotated externally, the posteromedial capsule should tighten and allow less anterior excursion than with the drawer test in neutral rotation. When the posteromedial capsule is torn, the Slocum test demonstrates an increase in anterior motion of the tibia versus the drawer test in neutral, and the tibia tends to "roll out" (Fig. 3.27).

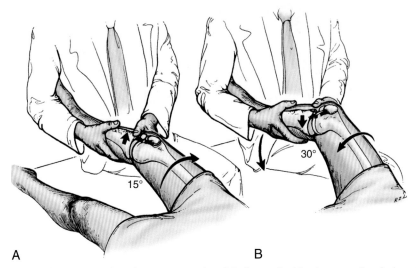

FIG 3.20 In the flexion rotation drawer test, the tibia is cradled in the examiner's hands, while the knee is flexed to demonstrate tibial reduction and internal femoral rotation. (From Tria AJ Jr, Klein KS: *An illustrated guide to the knee,* New York, 1992, Churchill Livingstone.)

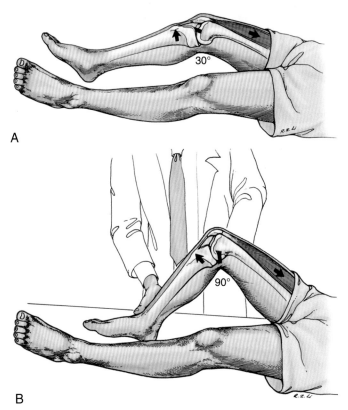

FIG 3.21 Quadriceps active test for the anterior cruciate ligament in 30 degrees of flexion (A) and for the posterior cruciate ligament in 90 degrees of flexion (B). (From Scott WN, editor: *The knee,* St Louis, 1994, CV Mosby.)

The posterolateral capsule is tested with the anterior drawer test at 90 degrees of flexion and internal tibial rotation of 15 degrees. If the posterolateral capsule is torn, the drawer test with internal rotation will show an increase in anterior motion versus the drawer test in neutral, and the tibia will tend to "roll in" (Fig. 3.28). The dial test can assess both the posterolateral structures and the posterior cruciate ligament. The patient is placed in the prone position. External rotation of the tibia is recorded at 30 and 90 degrees and is compared with the uninjured side. Increased external rotation with asymmetry at 90 degrees is indicative of an injury to the PCL. Increased external rotation with asymmetry at 30 degrees is indicative of an injury to the posterolateral structures. The hyperextension recurvatum sign correlates with injury to the posterolateral capsule. If the leg is held in full extension, the knee hyperextends and the tibia rotates externally because of the absence of the posterolateral capsule and its supporting structures (Fig. 3.29). The reverse pivot-shift test is performed with the tibia rotated externally and the knee flexed. When the knee flexes 20 to 30 degrees, tibial external rotation is seen with posterior subluxation of the lateral tibia. As the knee is extended, the tibia reduces with a palpable clunk, indicative of a deficient posterolateral capsule (Fig. 3.30).[14]

Along with a detailed history of the mechanism of injury, the physical examination is vital for the diagnosis and management of an injured knee. One must challenge the common practice of relying on an MRI as the sole diagnostic tool, as the physical exam provides important details of the patient's condition that may be overlooked by excessive use of diagnostic studies. Advanced imaging is a tremendous asset in the diagnosis and management of knee injuries and should be used as confirmation of clinical suspicion following a well-performed physical examination. It is important to use all of the information obtained from the clinical evaluation to maximize diagnostic accuracy, which will lead to the appropriate treatment plan and improved patient outcomes.

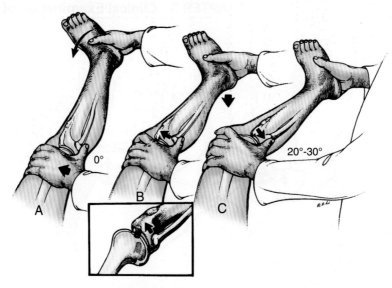

FIG 3.22 The pivot-shift test begins with the knee in full extension, and internal rotation and valgus stress are applied to demonstrate anterolateral subluxation. (From Tria AJ Jr, Klein KS: *An illustrated guide to the knee,* New York, 1992, Churchill Livingstone.)

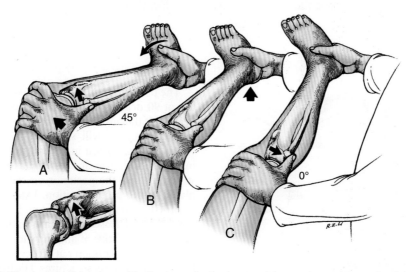

FIG 3.23 The jerk test begins with the knee in flexion, and internal rotation and valgus stress are applied to demonstrate anterolateral subluxation of the tibia. (From Tria AJ Jr, Klein KS: *An illustrated guide to the knee,* New York, 1992, Churchill Livingstone.)

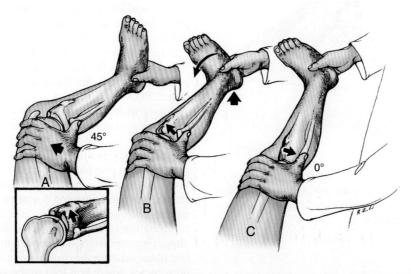

FIG 3.24 The Losee test begins with the knee in flexion, but the foot is externally rotated. Valgus stress is applied, and the tibia is internally rotated as the knee is extended. (From Tria AJ Jr, Klein KS: *An illustrated guide to the knee,* New York, 1992, Churchill Livingstone.)

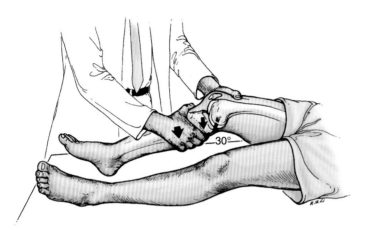

FIG 3.25 The "posterior" Lachman test applies posterior force to the proximal end of the tibia with the knee flexed 30 degrees. (From Tria AJ Jr, Klein KS: *An illustrated guide to the knee,* New York, 1992, Churchill Livingstone.)

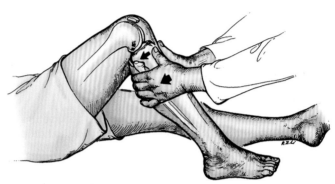

FIG 3.26 The posterior drawer test is performed in 90 degrees of flexion with posterior force on the proximal end of the tibia. (From Tria AJ Jr, Klein KS: *An illustrated guide to the knee,* New York, 1992, Churchill Livingstone.)

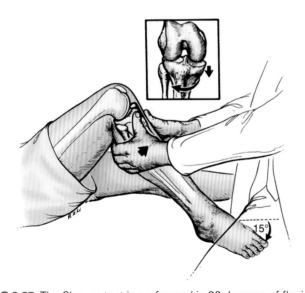

FIG 3.27 The Slocum test is performed in 90 degrees of flexion with the foot externally rotated and anterior proximal tibial force applied to test the posteromedial capsule. (From Tria AJ Jr, Klein KS: *An illustrated guide to the knee,* New York, 1992, Churchill Livingstone.)

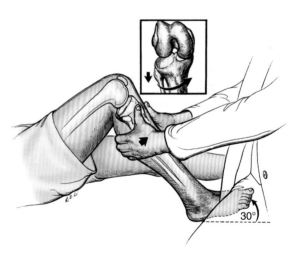

FIG 3.28 The posterolateral capsule is tested with the knee flexed to 90 degrees and anterior proximal tibial force applied with the tibia rotated internally. (From Tria AJ Jr, Klein KS: *An illustrated guide to the knee,* New York, 1992, Churchill Livingstone.)

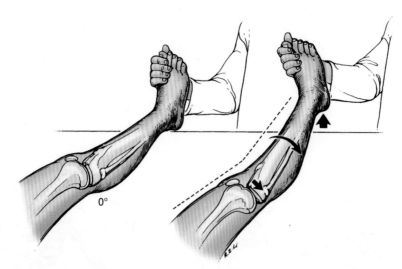

FIG 3.29 The hyperextension recurvatum test demonstrates increased extension of the knee along with external tibial rotation and drop-back. (From Tria AJ Jr, Klein KS: *An illustrated guide to the knee,* New York, 1992, Churchill Livingstone.)

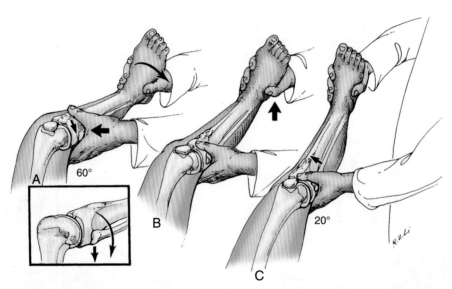

FIG 3.30 The reverse pivot-shift test begins with the knee flexed, and the tibia is externally rotated. The knee is then extended to demonstrate posterolateral capsular laxity. (From Tria AJ Jr, Klein KS: *An illustrated guide to the knee,* New York, 1992, Churchill Livingstone.)

KEY REFERENCES

1. Aglietti P, Insall JN, Cerulli G: Patellar pain and incongruence. I: measurements of incongruence. *Clin Orthop* 176:217, 1983.
2. Apley AC: The diagnosis of meniscal injuries. *J Bone Joint Surg Am* 29:78, 1947.
6. Daniel DM, Stone ML, Barnett P, et al: Use of the quadriceps active test to diagnose posterior cruciate ligament disruption and measure posterior laxity of the knee. *J Bone Joint Surg Am* 70:386, 1988.
7. Fairbank HA: Internal derangement of the knee in children. *Proc R Soc Lond* 3:11, 1937.
8. Feagin JA, Cooke TD: Prone examination for anterior cruciate ligament insufficiency. *J Bone Joint Surg Br* 71:863, 1989.
9. Fetto JF, Marshall JL: Injury to the anterior cruciate ligament producing the pivot-shift sign. *J Bone Joint Surg Am* 61:710, 1979.
12. Hughston JC, Andrews JR, Cross MJ, et al: Classification of knee ligament instabilities. Part I. The medial compartment and cruciate ligaments. *J Bone Joint Surg Am* 58:159, 1976.

13. Hughston JC, Andrews JR, Cross MJ, et al: Classification of knee ligament instabilities. Part II. The lateral compartment. *J Bone Joint Surg Am* 58:173, 1976.
18. Losee RE: Diagnosis of chronic injury to the anterior cruciate ligament. *Orthop Clin North Am* 16:83, 1985.
21. McMurray TP: The semilunar cartilages. *Br J Surg* 29:407, 1942.
22. Noyes FR, Butler D, Grood E, et al: Clinical paradoxes of anterior cruciate instability and a new test to detect its instability. *Orthop Trans* 2:36, 1978.
23. Slocum DB, Larson RL: Rotatory instability of the knee: its pathogenesis and a clinical test to demonstrate its presence. *J Bone Joint Surg Am* 50:211, 1968.

The references for this chapter can also be found on www.expertconsult.com.

4

Gene Therapy for the Treatment of Knee Disorders*

Johnny Huard, Walter R. Lowe, Freddie H. Fu

INTRODUCTION

The treatment of knee disorders has improved over the years as a consequence of new minimally invasive operative techniques, novel instruments, modern rehabilitation, medications, and increasing knowledge about the biomechanics of the knee joint. For the treatment of knee instability, sports medicine specialists focus on systematically addressing each injury, preventing degenerative osteoarthritis (OA), and allowing patients to return to their normal activities. Repair and/or reconstruction of ligamentous injuries using current techniques have been shown to restore near-normal knee stability with respect to anteroposterior translation, rotational motion (pivoting), and varus/valgus motion. In addition to addressing all other concomitant injuries (including meniscus tears and focal chondral defects), current techniques have also been shown to help to prevent premature joint degeneration—a process that dramatically reduces the long-term quality of life.[24,36,70,82]

Despite the recent advances in technical proficiency for the treatment of knee disorders, there still exist numerous opportunities to improve the care of these patients, many of which revolve around enhancing the biologic healing capacity of the injured tissues. Ligament, tendon, meniscus, and articular cartilage are tissues with inherently deficient blood supply, low cellular density, and low cellular turnover, properties that render these tissues, especially those that are exposed to synovial fluid, incapable of spontaneous healing after injury. As a result, these tissues heal very slowly, if at all, and the repaired tissue is known to be biomechanically inferior to that of native tissue.

Various cytokines and growth factors have been identified as being capable of modifying the healing processes of many musculoskeletal tissue types.[99] Growth factors are small peptides that can be synthesized both by resident cells at the site of injury (eg, fibroblasts, endothelial cells, mesenchymal stem cells [MSCs]) and by infiltrating reparatory or inflammatory cells (eg, platelets, macrophages, monocytes). These peptides are capable of stimulating cell proliferation, migration, and differentiation, as well as the synthesis of extracellular matrix components, in different tissues.[87] The genes encoding many of these growth factors have been determined and, using recombinant DNA technology, these proteins can be produced in large quantities to facilitate clinical application.[83]

Although the direct injection of these human recombinant proteins has some beneficial effects on the healing process,[22] their relatively short biologic half-life often necessitates very high doses and repeated injections. Another major limitation of using these human recombinant growth proteins to promote healing lies in their delivery to the injury site.[22] Various strategies, including the use of polymers, pumps, and heparin, have been investigated to maintain the bioactivities of these proteins for prolonged periods of time. Although these approaches have proved capable of improving the local persistence of growth factor proteins, the results remain limited. Among the different methods developed for the delivery of therapeutic proteins, gene therapy remains a promising approach, although there still exist a number of challenges that must be overcome before these techniques can be widely introduced into clinical practice.[69]

OVERVIEW OF GENE THERAPY

Definition

Gene therapy is a technique that relies on the delivery of cellular genetic information to cells to alter the expression of one or more genes to exert a desired effect. Gene therapy involves identifying a gene of interest, determining the method of transfer (in vivo vs. ex vivo), identifying a target cell (potentially stem cells), finding a method to control expression, and, finally, addressing safety and ethical issues involved in manipulating genetic material. Gene therapy was originally developed to allow researchers to manipulate germline cells for the treatment of heritable genetic disorders, but this method was greatly limited by insufficient technologies and considerable ethical concerns. However, with recent technologic advancements, the genetic manipulation of somatic cells has been heavily investigated for the regeneration of many tissue types.[69] Gene therapy may become a valuable tool in musculoskeletal medicine for the targeted delivery of growth factors and cytokines, along with other genes that are known to enhance tissue regeneration. As a result, host cells near the site of injury will be able to express proteins that are capable of improving the healing process.

Vectors

For therapeutic genes to be expressed, the transferred DNA must enter the nuclei of host cells where it either integrates into their chromosomes or remains separated from the host DNA in the form of an episome. Following the transcription of the modified DNA sequence, the resulting mRNA is transported outside the nucleus and serves as a matrix for the production of proteins (eg, growth factors, cytokines) in the ribosomes (Fig. 4.1). Treated host cells can consequently express the desired

*The authors are grateful for the editorial assistance of Ryan J. Warth, MD (Department of Orthopaedic Surgery, University of Texas Health Science Center at Houston), Jorge Chahla, MD (Steadman Philippon Research Institute, Vail, CO), and Lavanya Rajagopalan, PhD.

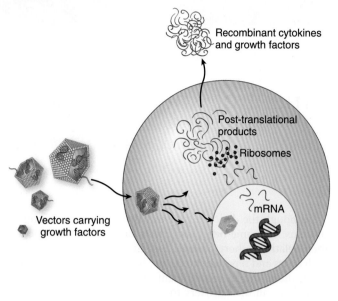

FIG 4.1 Gene transfer using a viral vector (ie, transduction).

Method of Gene Delivery	Vectors	Specifications
Nonviral	Liposomes	Low efficiency of gene delivery
		Low immunogenicity
	DNA gene gun	Easy to produce
	DNA-protein complex	Infects mitotic/postmitotic cells
		Low cytotoxicity
	Naked DNA	Immune rejection problems
		Low cytotoxicity/ immunogenicity
Viral	Adenovirus	Infects mitotically active cells only
		Low gene insert capacity
	Retrovirus	Low cytotoxicity/ immunogenicity
		High persistence of gene transfer
		Low gene insertion capacity
	Adeno-associated virus	High gene insertion capacity
		Limited size for gene of interest
		Requires helper virus for proliferation
	HSV	Infects mitotic/postmitotic cells
		Immune rejection problems
	Lentivirus	Transduces only dividing cells
		Potential for insertional mutagenesis

TABLE 4.1 **Common Vectors Used for Gene Delivery Into Cells**

HSV, Herpes simplex virus.

growth factors and cytokines and become a reservoir of secreting molecules capable of improving the healing process.

Viral and nonviral vectors can be used for the delivery of genetic material into cells (Table 4.1). Nonviral gene transfer (termed "transfection") is usually easier and induces significantly less cellular toxicity and immunogenicity than does viral gene transfer (termed "transduction"); however, the overall use of nonviral gene transfection has become less common because of its limited efficiency and low gene transfer rates. Different approaches are being investigated to improve the efficiency of nonviral gene transfer (eg, the use of electroporation,[9,10] liposomes,[54,57] DNA-polycation complexes,[25,98] the so-called gene gun[48]) but with limited success.

Viral transduction is currently the most efficient and most reliable method currently available for the transfer of exogenous genetic material, although unfavorable risk to benefit ratios do remain as a result of safety concerns.[22,86] Viral vectors have a native ability to enter target cells and express their own genetic material within the transduced cells of host tissues. Therefore, before viral transduction for gene therapy can be performed, all genes encoding pathogenic viral proteins must be deleted and replaced by the genes of interest in order to prevent the expression of harmful genes.

Common viral vectors used to transfer genetic material include herpes simplex virus (HSV), adenovirus (AdV), and adeno-associated virus (AAV), whose transferred nucleic acid sequences exist as separate episomes within the transduced cell nuclei. Lentiviral and retroviral vectors are also commonly used; their genetic materials integrate into the host genome, thereby allowing for long-term, stable expression of the inserted genes. Each of the viral vectors has a unique set of advantages and disadvantages that render them useful in certain situations but less useful in others (see Table 4.1). Although viral vectors display high efficiency of gene transfer to many cell types, their cytotoxicity (ie, HSV), immunogenicity (ie, AdV), and inability to transduce postmitotic cells (ie, retrovirus) limit their general applicability for gene therapy purposes. Consequently, new viral vectors with reduced cytotoxicity and immunogenicity are

currently being developed.[83] In general, for most musculoskeletal conditions, AdV, AAV, and lentiviral vectors are most frequently used in preclinical and laboratory studies.

Strategies

Gene transfer to the knee and the musculoskeletal system can be achieved using various gene delivery strategies, which can be classified into two delivery types: direct and systemic. Systemic delivery of a viral vector consists of injecting the vector into the bloodstream, resulting in the dissemination of the vector to the target tissues. This approach offers a major advantage when the target tissue is difficult to reach by direct injection. Moreover, systemic delivery often effects better distribution of the vector within the targeted tissues because direct injection of the vector often results in localized expression at the injection site. The major disadvantages of this technology are the high amount of vector required and the lack of specificity of expression, because much of the vector is disseminated into the lungs and the liver (major blood filter). Furthermore, the lack of blood supply in certain tissues, such as articular cartilage, portions of the menisci, and intervertebral disks, makes this approach inappropriate for some knee injuries and disorders.

Two main strategies for direct gene therapy to the musculoskeletal system have been extensively investigated. These strategies involve either (1) the direct injection of the vector carrying

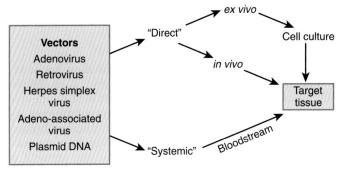

FIG 4.2 Strategies for gene delivery into the knee joint.

the desired genes into the host tissue (in vivo) or (2) the harvesting of somatic cells or stem cells from the injured tissue, genetic modification of these cells in vitro, and their reinjection into the tissue (ex vivo) (Fig. 4.2). Although the direct in vivo method is less technically demanding, ex vivo gene delivery offers an additional layer of safety because the process of genetic manipulation takes place under highly controlled conditions. Furthermore, the ex vivo approach also ensures the delivery of genetically modified host cells, thus reducing the problems associated with low rates of in vivo gene transfer. In addition, numerous tests, such as tumorigenicity and toxicity assays, can be performed on genetically modified cells, making this approach safer than direct gene transfer technology. Approaches based on tissue engineering, which aim at using cells from different tissues to deliver genes (MSCs, muscle-derived cells, dermal fibroblasts), may bring additional advantages to the healing process in various tissues of the musculoskeletal system because the injected stem cells can also participate in the healing process. Selecting the appropriate procedure depends on various factors, such as the division rate of the target cells, pathophysiology of the disorder, availability of cells from the injured tissues, vascularity of the tissues, and type of vector used.

Limitations

One of the primary concerns surrounding the use of gene therapy in any tissue is safety. Although gene therapy may represent a last resort for the treatment of malignancies and severe genetic disorders (eg, Duchenne muscular dystrophy, Gaucher's disease, cystic fibrosis), the risks for adverse side effects and the potential consequences of gene therapy are currently unacceptable in elective orthopedics. Viral vectors integrated into the cell genome pose the danger of insertional mutagenesis and oncogenesis.[14] Although abnormal regulation of cell growth (because of expression of antiapoptotic genes) and toxicity (because of overexpression of the inserted gene) are theoretically conceivable, no cases have ever been reported with regard to these adverse events. Vectors that do not integrate into the native DNA avoid these risks, but their efficacy remains greatly limited by the lack of persistent expression of the desired genes in the target tissues. Loss of expression of the transferred gene over a few weeks is a frequent occurrence and is a phenomenon that is not completely understood, especially with regard to adenoviral vectors. However, temporary and self-limiting expression of the desired gene could be useful for the treatment of acute musculoskeletal injuries for which the duration of treatment is much shorter than for longer-term conditions.

GENE THERAPY FOR THE TREATMENT OF KNEE DISORDERS

Osteoarthritis

OA has many different etiologies (eg, inflammatory, noninflammatory, infectious, hemorrhagic, and autoimmune) and is a common source of knee pain. Early intervention, before the onset of cartilage degeneration and alteration of condylar morphology, appears to be the most important strategy for the treatment of OA. This strategy requires early identification of the disease, which in turn necessitates comprehensive understanding of its pathogenesis, advanced imaging techniques, and meaningful biochemical markers.[30,81] Despite significant advances, our knowledge of the early stages of the disease is limited; studies to test biomarkers of early disease require long-term follow-up to determine disease progression and are still under way.

Using both ex vivo and in vivo methods, direct (ie, local) genetic manipulation has been successfully performed in a number of animal studies.* One promising therapeutic approach in gene therapy is the transfer of the interleukin-1 receptor antagonist protein (IRAP) into the inflamed knee joint.[7,39,80] Interleukin-1 (IL-1) is a cytokine that is highly expressed during both acute and chronic inflammatory conditions, particularly in rheumatoid arthritis and OA.[21] IL-1 is the leading proinflammatory cytokine and is responsible for inducing protease synthesis, which leads to catabolic changes within articular cartilage. Following the ex vivo transfer of the IRAP gene into extracted synovial cells using a retroviral vector, significantly increased expression of IRAP was observed, along with other antiinflammatory effects, in rabbit knee joints.[7] Among the other antiinflammatory cytokines, IL-10 has garnered increased attention over the past few decades because of its antiinflammatory properties and independent effects on T-cell reactivity.[21] It has been shown that injecting the genes for both IRAP and IL-10 together resulted in greater inhibition of cartilage breakdown, suggesting that simultaneous gene delivery may be necessary to treat OA by targeting the activities of multiple inflammatory effectors.[105] Interestingly, antiinflammatory effects were often achieved not only in the injected knees but also in the contralateral knees and in distal joints, suggesting that local gene delivery can be distributed into the systemic circulation. Similar systemic therapeutic effects of adenoviral vectors carrying IL-10 have been demonstrated in mice with collagen-induced arthritis.[2] Numerous additional studies have been performed to identify therapeutic targets for gene delivery; however, many of the current obstacles revolve around the lack of an animal model that reproduces the pathophysiologic process of primary OA (both inflammatory and non-inflammatory) that occurs in human knees.

Focal Chondral Defects

Damage to articular cartilage in the knee joint leads to premature secondary OA because of abnormal joint forces and may ultimately lead to diminished quality of life and enormous long-term health care costs.[24,36,70,82] When left untreated, focal chondral defects may potentiate cartilage degeneration, particularly along the edges of the defects.[42] Unfortunately, cartilage

---

*References 7, 17, 21, 23, 29, 39, 41, 76, 80, and 84.

has very limited healing capacity,[40] and defects isolated to the cartilage rarely exhibit adequate tissue repair, perhaps because of the lack of vascularity, cellularity, and lymphatic drainage of the tissue.[40,90] To initiate a healing response in cartilage, the injury must penetrate the calcified cartilage layer and disrupt local capillaries to allow blood and nutrients from the underlying subchondral bone to migrate into the defect, eventually producing a fibrocartilaginous scar.[26,90] This concept is the basic premise behind the development of a microfracture procedure that was introduced several decades ago for the treatment of full-thickness focal chondral defects.[94] However, the resulting regenerated tissue is predominantly composed of fibrocartilaginous scar tissue rich in type I collagen, which has inferior structural and biomechanical properties compared with native hyaline cartilage[42] (which is composed of type II collagen, aggrecan, and proteoglycans).[90]

The most common operative techniques for the treatment of chondral defects include arthroscopic débridement of unstable chondral flaps, microfracture, autologous chondrocyte transfer (with or without matrix scaffold augmentation), osteochondral autografts or allografts, or new scaffold materials.[78] Despite some promising clinical results,[68] more efficient strategies should be developed to optimize clinical outcomes and minimize surgical risks.

Gene therapy for articular cartilage regeneration has focused on upregulating growth factors that enhance the proliferation, differentiation (chondrogenesis), and matrix production of host cells and/or donor stem cells. Some of these growth factors include bone morphogenetic proteins (BMPs), basic fibroblast growth factor (bFGF), transforming growth factor beta (TGF-β), endothelial growth factor (EGF), insulin-like growth factor 1 (IGF-1), and cartilage-derived morphogenetic protein (COMP). Each of these growth factors has been shown to positively influence the activity of chondrocytes in vitro and their survival and regenerative capacities in vivo.[4,16,20,40,88]

In one study, TGF-β1 and proteoglycan synthesis levels increased after in vivo adenoviral transduction of chondrocytes in rabbit intervertebral disks.[74] It has also been shown that the ex vivo transduction of periosteal cells to express BMP-7 can also influence the healing potential of articular cartilage following in vivo transplantation[62]; the roles of BMPs in cartilage regeneration are still unclear because of the conflicting results reported by others.[†] Numerous techniques for gene therapy are currently being investigated for the treatment of cartilage defects; however, these techniques have not been introduced into clinical medicine for a number of reasons, many of which are related to ethical and safety concerns along with the inefficiencies involved with gene delivery.[46,96]

It should also be recognized that proangiogenic growth factors, such as vascular endothelial growth factor (VEGF), appear to be detrimental to cartilage regeneration. For example, Kubo et al.[52] compared cartilage regeneration within osteochondral defects after treating the defects with muscle-derived stem cells (MDSCs) transduced to express BMP-4, and either VEGF or a VEGF inhibitor (ie, sFlt-1). The authors reported improved healing when BMP-4 was expressed in combination with sFlt-1, when compared with the combination of BMP-4 and VEGF. Similar findings were reported by Matsumoto et al.[63] who observed that blocking angiogenesis with ex vivo gene

transfer also improved articular cartilage repair in a rat model of OA.

Ligamentous Injuries

The anterior cruciate ligament (ACL) is the most frequently injured intra-articular knee ligament, with more than 200,000 ACL injuries occurring each year in the United States. In contrast to the other primary stabilizing ligaments of the knee, the ACL has a very low capacity for spontaneous healing because of its relatively tenuous blood supply, the lack of close interposition between its torn ligament stumps, and the presence of matrix metalloproteinases (MMPs) and plasminogen activators (eg, urokinase) within the synovial fluid.[35] Because the ACL cannot heal spontaneously, surgical reconstruction using autograft or allograft tissue is required to restore normal knee kinematics and to prevent degenerative OA.[77,92] ACL reconstruction techniques have inherent disadvantages, including donor site morbidity following autograft harvest and infection (either from the surgical procedure itself or transmission through the implanted allograft).[1,58] The most common sources of autograft tissue for ACL reconstruction include bone-patellar tendon-bone (BPTB) autografts and hamstring tendon autografts.[92] Techniques for ACL reconstruction have dramatically improved in recent years, and we are nearing the point at which further technical modifications are not likely to significantly reduce the complications or failure rates associated with the procedure. Because we are near the plateau of technical optimization, it is important that we turn towards biologic approaches (such as gene therapy) to enhance tendon-bone integration and intra-articular remodeling (ie, "ligamentization"). Because the process of ligamentization involves active endogenous decellularization,[85] the graft progressively weakens for up to 6 months after implantation before cellular repopulation and remodeling can begin. It is for this reason that rehabilitation after ACL reconstruction must remain slow, despite the significant advances that have been made in surgical techniques.

Several studies have demonstrated the positive effects of growth factors on the metabolism of ACL fibroblasts (eg, platelet-derived growth factor AB [PDGF-AB], IGF-1, EGF, bFGF, TGF-β).[19,61,87,93] These data suggest that strategic modifications of growth factor concentrations may improve tendon-bone healing and remodeling of implanted graft tissues; these modifications can be achieved by new techniques in gene therapy.[65] Initial feasibility studies have shown that virally transduced cells can survive and express reporter genes within ligamentous tissues in vivo.[28,38,72,73] Although no transfer of a therapeutic gene has been achieved in the ACL in vivo, positive effects of therapeutic genes on both primary ligament healing and graft integration have been shown by upregulating the expression of various growth factors, especially PDGF-B and TGF-β1.

Tendon-Bone Integration

Because the use of BPTB grafts rely primarily upon bony union to achieve early graft fixation within the bone tunnels (ie, within 6 weeks), the use of soft tissue grafts is viewed as a less favorable alternative because of the prolonged time required to achieve bony ingrowth (ie, 12 weeks post graft). Although the overall time for rehabilitation is similar for both BPTB grafts and soft tissue grafts, the use of BPTB grafts allows for earlier initiation of physical therapy because of the shorter time required for bony union to occur. Some studies have shown that local

---

†References 37, 43, 51, 53, 89, and 95.

delivery of BMP-2 and several other growth factors to the tendon-bone interface may accelerate the process of bony integration of soft tissue grafts.[27]

To test the efficacy of gene therapy with BMP-2 on tendon-bone healing following ACL reconstruction with soft tissue grafts,[56] Martinek et al.[59] used AdV-BMP-2 ex vivo gene therapy to treat tendon grafts that were used for ACL reconstruction in rabbits. Histologic analysis of the AdV-BMP-2–treated autografts showed improved tendon-bone integration and statistically significant improvements in stiffness and ultimate load-to-failure. In addition, all pretreated grafts failed within the graft substance rather than at the tendon-bone interface, whereas untreated grafts failed at the tendon-bone interface.

Intra-Articular Graft Remodeling

With respect to ligamentization, Li et al.[55] used an ex vivo approach to genetically modify the expression of PDGF-β in MSCs to accelerate the revascularization and ligamentization of Achilles tendon allografts following ACL reconstruction in a rabbit model. Their results demonstrated increased type III collagen deposition at 3 weeks, increased cellularity at 3 weeks, and increased expression of PDGF-β for more than 12 weeks after implantation. However, despite these potentially favorable results, there was no evidence to support the notion that PDGF-β would accelerate graft revascularization or improve graft strength. Other studies have suggested that the amplification of VEGF expression may represent a viable strategy to accelerate angiogenesis in ACL grafts.[45] However, the initial enthusiasm for this strategy has since waned because of recent biomechanical data suggesting that exogenous VEGF temporarily decreases the stiffness of implanted ACL grafts.[104]

There has been significant interest in enhancing the expression of TGF-β1 in ACL fibroblasts to accelerate ligamentization. It has been shown that the in vivo application of TGF-β1 significantly enhanced the healing of partial ACL tears and also the ligamentization of tendon grafts.[49,50,103] Furthermore, TGF-β1 was also found to enhance the synthesis of perpendicular collagen fiber to promote bony ingrowth at the tendon-bone interface.[102]

It has been recently reported that the walls of blood vessels contain perivascular and endothelial cell markers believed to be at the origin of a multitude of stem cell lines.[12,97,106] These cells appear to be very early progenitor cells and have high regenerative potential in various tissues throughout the musculoskeletal system.[13,97,106] Taken together, these results suggest that the blood vessel walls contain stem cells that are likely the origin of various adult MSC populations, supporting the theory that most adult stem cells originate from well-vascularized tissues, whereas very few stem cells are found in poorly vascularized tissues. Indeed, it has been demonstrated that the medial collateral ligament (MCL), which is highly vascularized, heals more effectively than the less vascularized ACL. More importantly, a reduction of angiogenesis within the MCL has been shown to reduce the healing potential of the MCL, similar to that which occurs in the native ACL.[75] Subsequently, blood vessel–derived stem cells have been shown to exist within the ACL (ie, ACL-derived stem cells), and more importantly these cells can potentially be used to improve the outcome of ACL reconstruction via intra-articular injection.[64,66] ACL-derived stem cells can also be delivered using a cell sheet, which functions to immobilize cells in the immediate vicinity of the tendon graft, thus potentially improving the beneficial effects that ACL-derived stem cells impart to tendon grafts following ACL reconstruction. Improvements in clinical outcomes after ACL reconstruction using stem cell implantation technologies have been primarily attributed to the enhancement of angiogenesis and osteogenesis.[66,67] This new technology may be used in the context of gene therapy to further accelerate the process of tendon-bone healing and graft maturation following ACL reconstruction.

Meniscus Lesions

Meniscal tears can occur under a variety of circumstances, including both primary and secondary acute injuries, along with chronic injuries. Without treatment, OA develops in most patients in 5 to 10 years.[44] Treatment after meniscal depletion is limited. There exist many surgical techniques for meniscus repair that have excellent success rates[18]; however, tears that involve the relatively avascular inner two-thirds of the meniscus cannot heal effectively even after repair.[5] Exposure of tear edges to the synovial fluid also contributes to the inability of the inner two-thirds of the meniscus to heal spontaneously. As a result, these tears are often subjected to partial meniscectomy in an effort to create stable tear margins, which is thought to prevent point contact and the subsequent degeneration of load bearing surfaces.[11] Experimental studies have shown that the healing process in the avascular zone of the meniscus might be promoted by certain chemotactic or mitogenic stimuli delivered by autogenous fibrin clot, synovial tissue, or growth factors (TGF-α, TGF-β, bFGF, EGF, PDGF-AB, HGF).[‡] The future roles of gene therapy for meniscal healing may involve (1) direct in vivo viral transduction of meniscal fibroblasts surrounding the tear margins or (2) targeted delivery of transduced autologous cells expressing growth factors that favor meniscal healing ex vivo followed by cell reimplantation into the meniscus tear.

The first experiment using in vivo gene therapy for meniscal healing was performed in rabbits by transducing meniscal fibroblasts to express TGF-β1 using ex vivo techniques.[32] Based on the work of Arnoczky et al.[6] that used autologous fibrin clots as scaffolds for meniscal healing, Goto et al.[31] further tested the feasibility of gene therapy as a means of achieving prolonged growth factor release for meniscus repair using both retroviral and AdV vectors in both ex vivo and in vivo approaches. The ex vivo approach, in which scaffolds seeded with transduced cells were implanted into meniscal defects, demonstrated localized expression within the scaffold at the site of the defect for more than 6 weeks after implantation in a canine model. In a more recent study involving human tissues, Cucchiarini et al.[15] tested the ability of virally transduced human meniscal fibrochondrocytes to overexpress TGF-β within both human meniscus explants and within experimental human meniscal defects. They reported that overexpression of TGF-β1, effected using a convenient injection technique, is capable of improving the healing capacity of meniscal defects.

After a complete loss of the meniscus because of an extended injury or to repeated resections, most patients experience rapid impairment of knee function. For these patients, meniscus scaffold implantation[100] or meniscal allograft transplantation[71] can be performed. Clinical studies on this issue have become more common, but many of these studies cite high postoperative failure rates up to 2 years.[71,100] Experimental studies show

---

‡References 6, 8, 32, 34, 91, 93, and 101.

the occurrence of slow immune rejection problems in transplanted meniscal allografts.[33,71] Gene therapy has been explored as a method to accelerate healing and remodeling processes after meniscal allograft transplantation[32,60]; however, much work needs to be done to render these strategies compatible with the rigorous sterilization procedures that are required to prevent disease transmission and allograft rejection.

It is known that surgical repair of tears within the vascular regions of the meniscus heal more effectively than those in the avascular regions; therefore it is possible that vascularized regions may possess a richer supply of vascular-derived stem cells than seen in avascular regions.[79] Immunohistochemical and flow cytometric analyses have demonstrated that higher numbers of endothelial and perivascular cells exist in the peripheral regions of the meniscus than in the inner regions. Vascular-derived cells isolated from the peripheral regions of both fetal and adult menisci demonstrated multilineage differentiation capacities and were more potent than cells isolated from the inner regions. Following transplantation into the knee joints of athymic rats, these endothelial and perivascular cells were recruited to the sites of meniscal tears and contributed to the regeneration of meniscus tissue. These results suggest that the vascularized regions of the meniscus contain more stem cells compared with avascular regions and that these meniscus-derived stem cells may be used in the context of gene therapy and tissue engineering to improve meniscal regeneration.

CLINICAL APPLICATION

At this point, AAV has emerged as the virus of choice for the treatment of intra-articular knee disorders. AAV, particularly serotypes 2 and 5, has been shown to be safe for intra-articular injection with reasonable transduction efficiency, which can be improved by using an additional self-complementary viral vector.[3,47] In addition, cytokines and growth factors are typically small and will fit within the size constraints of this viral vector. Inducible promoters may allow expression of the transgenes only when disease flares occur and therefore may reduce the incidence of isolated inflammatory episodes, especially in cases of rheumatoid arthritis. With these new technologic advances, the possibility of using intra-articular gene therapy to deliver therapeutic growth factors and cytokines for the treatment of knee disorders has become safer and more effective.

FUTURE DIRECTIONS

Gene therapy applications must be refined to overcome many obstacles before achieving the status of current established therapeutic techniques. Successful delivery of therapeutic genes to the human joint has been documented, and many animal studies have indicated a benefit to the delivery of different genes to tissues throughout the musculoskeletal system. One of the main obstacles impeding the application of gene therapy into clinical medicine has to do with the availability of appropriate vectors to carry and deliver the required genes; however, great progress is being made in the development of new vectors. We

believe that the combination of gene therapy techniques, tissue engineering principles, and the use of postnatal stem cells, including bone marrow-derived stem cells, adipose-derived stem cells, MDSCs, endothelial cells, and perivascular cells, could result in the establishment of new and effective therapies to enhance the healing of tissues with inherently low regenerative capacities (eg, articular cartilage); however, numerous basic science and preclinical studies need to be performed before these techniques can be performed with the level of efficiency and safety required for clinical application. Because stem cells generally enhance the process of tissue healing via paracrine signaling and chemotaxis of host cells, a major focus of current research involves identifying these autocrine and paracrine mediators, identifying the origins of the host cells that participate in tissue healing, and developing methods to promote intercellular cross-talk between donor and host cells.

SELECTED REFERENCES

12. Crisan M, Deasy B, Gavina M, et al: Purification and long-term culture of multipotent progenitor cells affiliated with the walls of human blood vessels: myoendothelial cells and pericytes. *Methods Cell Biol* 86:295–309, 2008.

13. Crisan M, Yap S, Casteilla L, et al: A perivascular origin for mesenchymal stem cells in multiple human organs. *Cell Stem Cell* 3(3):301–313, 2008.

52. Kubo S, Cooper GM, Matsumoto T, et al: Blocking vascular endothelial growth factor with soluble Flt-1 improves the chondrogenic potential of mouse skeletal muscle-derived stem cells. *Arthritis Rheum* 60(1):155–165, 2009.

53. Kuroda R, Usas A, Kubo S, et al: Cartilage repair using bone morphogenetic protein 4 and muscle-derived stem cells. *Arthritis Rheum* 54(2):433–442, 2006.

59. Martinek V, Latterman C, Usas A, et al: Enhancement of tendon-bone integration of anterior cruciate ligament grafts with bone morphogenetic protein-2 gene transfer: a histological and biomechanical study. *J Bone Joint Surg Am* 84-A(7):1123–1131, 2002.

63. Matsumoto T, Cooper GM, Gharaibeh B, et al: Cartilage repair in a rat model of osteoarthritis through intraarticular transplantation of muscle-derived stem cells expressing bone morphogenetic protein 4 and soluble Flt-1. *Arthritis Rheum* 60(5):1390–1405, 2009.

64. Matsumoto T, Ingham SM, Mifune Y, et al: Isolation and characterization of human anterior cruciate ligament-derived vascular stem cells. *Stem Cells Dev* 21(6):859–872, 2012.

66. Mifune Y, Matsumoto T, Ota S, et al: Therapeutic potential of anterior cruciate ligament-derived stem cells for anterior cruciate ligament reconstruction. *Cell Transplant* 21(8):1651–1665, 2012.

67. Mifune Y, Matsumoto T, Takayama K, et al: Tendon graft revitalization using adult anterior cruciate ligament (ACL)-derived CD34+ cell sheets for ACL reconstruction. *Biomaterials* 34(22):5476–5487, 2013.

75. Nishimori M, Matsumoto T, Ota S, et al: Role of angiogenesis after muscle derived stem cell transplantation in injured medial collateral ligament. *J Orthop Res* 30(4):627–633, 2012.

106. Zheng B, Cao B, Crisan M, et al: Prospective identification of myogenic endothelial cells in human skeletal muscle. *Nat Biotechnol* 25(9):1025–1034, 2007.

The references for this chapter can also be found on www.expertconsult.com.

Imaging of the Knee

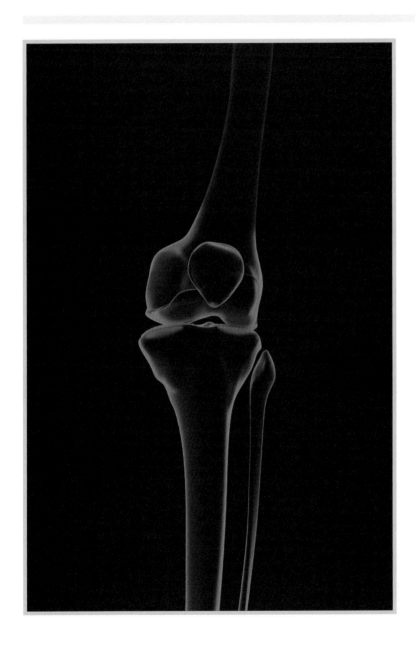

5

Knee Imaging Techniques and Normal Anatomy

Samuel D. Madoff, Jarett S. Burak, Kevin R. Math, Daniel M. Walz

RADIOGRAPHY

Applications

Radiographs are the workhorse of knee imaging. Almost any symptom or sign may be initially evaluated with an x-ray. Radiographs provide useful information across the entire spectrum of knee pathology, including congenital deformities, arthritis, trauma, oncology, sports injuries, metabolic disease, and arthroplasty evaluation.[41]

Technique

A brief orientation to x-ray technology enhances an understanding of knee imaging. An x-ray tube converts electricity into a beam of high-energy photons. The x-ray beam is aimed through the knee. A cassette containing x-ray film is positioned opposite the x-ray beam on the other side of the patient. Photons that pass through the patient strike the film, exposing it. Tissue density is the primary determinant of whether a photon successfully reaches the film. A dense tissue, such as bone, absorbs or deflects most photons. Thus few photons reach the film. Areas of unexposed film appear white, representing dense tissue. Less dense materials, such as the lung or fat, do not obstruct as many passing photons. Here the exposed film appears darker. Simplistically a radiograph is a shadow formed by high-energy light outlining the patient's anatomy.

Traditionally an exposed film was developed and hung for interpretation. Over the past 20 years, new cassette designs have replaced film with an imaging plate, creating computed radiography (CR). After exposure, the imaging plate is run through a CR reader, and the captured image is digitized. The imaging plate is subsequently reset and can be reused thousands of times. Digital radiography (DR) represents the next evolution of filmless image capture. DR dispenses with the cassette entirely and uses a flat panel detector. The detail and overall image quality of DR are superior to CR.

A remaining niche for true film radiography is the standing, frontal, long-standing view radiograph of the lower extremity. This may be requested for precise knee anatomic and mechanical axis measurements.

After an image has been acquired by a CR or DR reader, it is transmitted to the picture archiving and communication system (PACS) for interpretation. The advantages of PACS are manifold, including image manipulation (windowing, zooming, etc.), transmission (electronic), and storage (online, easily accessible). The time-honored file room has given way to a well-ventilated closet housing several hard-working computers.

Radiographic Views

Standard radiographic examination of the knee consists of three views: anteroposterior (AP), lateral, and axial (sunrise or Merchant). Tunnel, posteroanterior (PA) flexion weight-bearing (Rosenberg view), and oblique views may be performed for particular indications. In the setting of knee instability and ligamentous injury, stress radiographs may be performed. If a bilateral examination has been requested, each knee should be imaged separately.

Anteroposterior Radiograph. The AP view is obtained with the knee extended, the cassette posterior to the knee, and the central x-ray beam perpendicular to the cassette. A standing (weight-bearing) AP radiograph more accurately assesses the joint space than one obtained with the patient supine.[1,2,36,43] For this reason and to allow the estimation of valgus or varus angulation, weight-bearing images are preferable whenever possible (Fig. 5.1). Normal structures evaluated on every AP radiograph of the knee are the patella, medial and lateral femoral condyles, medial and lateral joint compartments, tibial spines, medial and lateral tibial plateaus, and fibula. The AP view also provides a gross assessment of femoral tibial alignment (Fig. 5.2A). The lateral compartment is normally slightly wider than the medial.

Lateral Radiograph. The lateral view is obtained with the knee flexed 30 degrees and the patient lying on the affected limb. The cassette is positioned under the lateral side of the knee, and the x-ray beam is directed perpendicular to the cassette. This view depicts the quadriceps tendon, patella, patellar tendons, suprapatellar bursa, distal femur, proximal tibia, and proximal fibula (see Fig. 5.2B).

The medial femoral condyle is slightly larger than the lateral condyle. The lateral femoral condyle can be identified by the presence of the lateral femoral sulcus at the anterior aspect of its weight-bearing portion.[39] Blumensaat line represents the roof of the intercondylar notch. The closed physeal scar is also evident on the lateral view, and the patella should fall between the closed scar and Blumensaat line.

The tibial plateaus slope downward as they progress posteriorly, which can aid in fracture identification. The plateaus may be differentiated by several clues. The higher of the two tibial spines belongs to the medial plateau. At its posterior extent, the medial tibial plateau projects most dorsally and is squared. In contrast, the posterior aspect of the lateral tibial plateau slopes smoothly downward with a rounded contour.

The quadriceps and patellar tendons are well evaluated on a lateral view. The distal quadriceps tendon attaches to the superior pole of the patella. The patellar tendon extends from the inferior pole of the patella to the tibial tubercle. Both structures are well demarcated by a posterior fat plane. They should be straight and of uniform thickness.

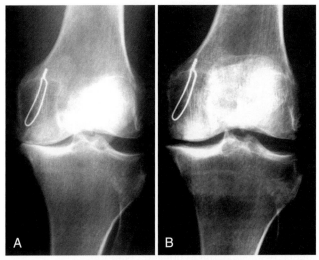

FIG 5.1 Anteroposterior Supine Versus Weight-Bearing Views Severe medial joint space narrowing is more apparent on the weight-bearing view (A) compared with the supine view (B).

In the setting of a joint effusion and suspected occult intra-articular fracture, a cross-table lateral view is useful for evaluating for lipohemarthrosis. The view is obtained with the patient supine and the knee slightly elevated. The cassette is placed adjacent to the medial knee. This positioning, in contrast to the standard lateral view, is better tolerated by a traumatized patient. The presence of a fat fluid level indicates an intra-articular fracture (most commonly, the tibial plateau) and prompts further evaluation with computed tomography (CT) or magnetic resonance imaging (MRI) (Fig. 5.3A to C).

The suprapatellar bursa is the proximal extension of the joint space. It may be identified on the standard lateral view as a slender, 1- to 2-mm, vertically oriented structure contained within the lucent area of fat formed by the anterior margin of the distal femur and the posterior margin of the quadriceps tendon.

Superoinferior positioning of the patella may be evaluated using the Insall-Salvati ratio. This is the ratio of the greatest length of the patella divided by the length of the patellar tendon. This ratio averages 1.17 and normally falls between 0.8 and 1.2 (see Fig. 5.2B). A long patellar tendon generates a ratio greater than 1.3, indicating a high patella (patella alta). Conversely, a short tendon accompanies a low patella and a ratio less than 0.8, termed patella baja.

Axial View. The axial view of choice is the Merchant view.[16,40,42] The patient is placed in the supine position on the radiography table; the knees are flexed 45 degrees (using a fixed or adjustable platform), and the cassette is placed on the proximal part of the

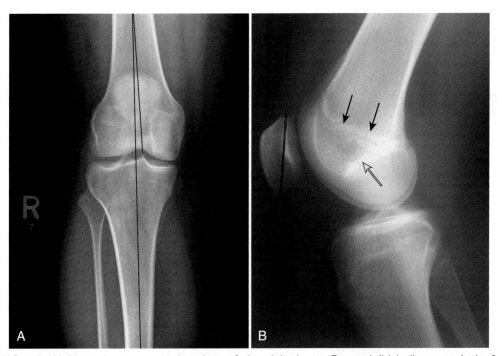

FIG 5.2 (A) Normal anteroposterior view of the right knee. Femoral-tibial alignment is in 6 degrees of valgus angulation. The lateral compartment is normally slightly wider than the medial compartment. (B) Lateral view of the knee. Blumensaat line *(open arrow)* represents the roof of the intercondylar notch. The physeal scar is indicated by the *solid arrows.* The patella is commonly located between these two lines, with the lower pole approximately at the level of Blumensaat line. The Insall-Salvati ratio is a more accurate method of assessing patellar height: the length of the patellar tendon *(dotted line)* divided by the greatest diagonal length of the patella *(solid line)* should be approximately 1 (0.8 to 1.2).

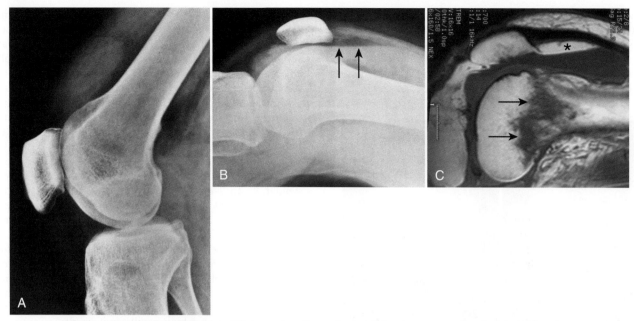

FIG 5.3 Knee Joint Effusion (A) Lateral radiograph demonstrates an oval soft tissue density representing a joint effusion within the suprapatellar pouch posterior to the quadriceps tendon. (B) Cross-table lateral view shows a fat-fluid level *(arrows)* indicative of an intra-articular fracture with lipohemarthrosis. (C) A sagittal T1-weighted magnetic resonance image obtained with the patient supine demonstrates high-signal fat *(asterisk)* floating on top of intra-articular hemorrhage. An acute supracondylar fracture is also noted *(arrows)*. (From Torg JS, Pavlov H, Morris VB: Salter-Harris type III fracture of the medial femoral condyle occurring in the adolescent athlete. *J Bone Joint Surg Am* 63:586, 1981.)

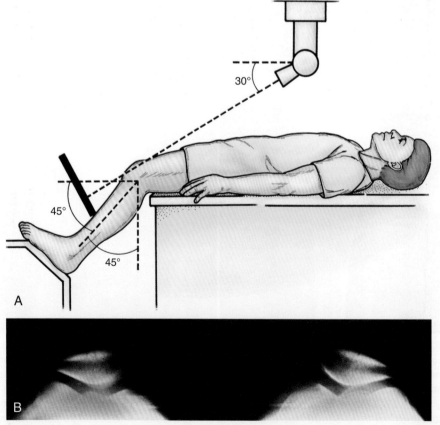

FIG 5.4 Merchant View (A) Technique. (B) Normal merchant view. Patellofemoral alignment is normal bilaterally, and the osseous structures and articular cortices are normal.

shins. Both knees are exposed simultaneously, with the x-ray beam directed toward the feet, inclined 30 degrees from the horizontal (Fig. 5.4A). This view provides an excellent assessment of patellofemoral alignment and is ideal for assessing the osseous patellofemoral articular surfaces (see Fig. 5.4B). In contrast, a skyline (or sunrise) view is obtained with the patient prone and the knee in maximum flexion. This view demonstrates the posterior surface of the patella and the anterior surface of the femur, but the imaged femoral surface is not at the patellofemoral joint. Furthermore, accurate assessment of patellofemoral alignment is limited when the knee is flexed excessively.[7,16] Some patients have difficulty tolerating this position.

Supplemental Views

The tunnel view is a frontal view obtained with the knee flexed 60 degrees. It can be obtained AP with the patient in the supine position, or PA with the patient prone or kneeling on the cassette. The x-ray beam is directed perpendicular to the tibia. This view demonstrates the posterior aspect of the intercondylar notch, the inner posterior aspects of the medial and lateral femoral condyles, and the tibial spines and plateaus (Fig. 5.5A). It is ideal for evaluating patients with suspected osteochondritis dissecans, which tends to occur more posteriorly in the intercondylar notch (see Fig. 5.5B to D).

The flexed, PA weight-bearing (Rosenberg) view is a modified tunnel view. It is obtained with the patient standing and the knee flexed 45 degrees. The patellae should touch the film cassette. The x-ray beam is centered at the level of the inferior pole of the patella and is directed 10 degrees caudad. It captures the joint space at the posterior aspect of the femorotibial joint. This view is valuable for evaluating arthritis. It detects joint space narrowing because of cartilage loss that often goes unappreciated or underestimated on a conventional AP weight-bearing view (Fig. 5.6A and B).[8,9,30,52,54] Comparisons of intraoperative and radiographic findings demonstrate that the flexed PA weight-bearing view has greater accuracy, sensitivity,

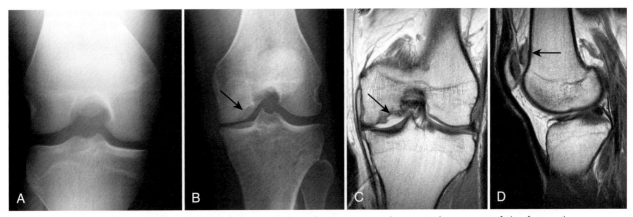

FIG 5.5 Tunnel View (A) Normal tunnel view demonstrates the posterior aspect of the femoral condyles, tibial spines, articular surfaces of the tibial plateau, and intercondylar notch. (B) Tunnel view from a different patient, demonstrating an ovoid area of lucency at the inner margin of the medial femoral condyle *(arrow)* suspicious for osteochondritis dessicans. (C) Coronal and (D) sagittal proton density MRI confirms the large osteochondral defect *(arrow)* with a completely displaced osteochondral fragment located in the suprapatellar joint recess *(arrow)*. (Case provided courtesy of the MRI Department, Hospital for Special Surgery, New York, New York.)

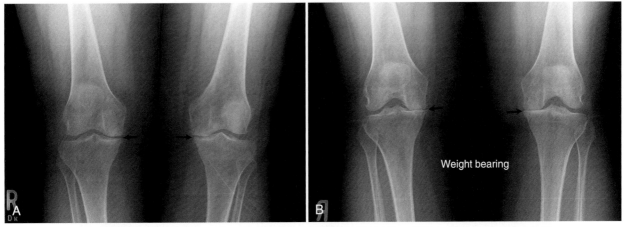

FIG 5.6 The Flexed Weight-Bearing posteroanterior (PA) View (A) Routine standing AP film demonstrates moderate bilateral medial compartment joint space narrowing with proliferative changes *(arrows)*. (B) PA flexion view demonstrates the findings to be more severe with marked narrowing of bilateral medial joint compartments, complete loss of the joint space, and bone-on-bone apposition *(arrows)*.

and specificity than the conventional extension weight-bearing radiograph.[54]

Oblique radiographs complement a routine examination. Occult fractures and tibiofibular arthritis may be more easily detected with oblique views than with routine AP radiographs. Bilateral oblique views are obtained at 45 degrees of internal and external rotation, with the patient supine, the affected knee extended, and the cassette behind the knee. The x-ray beam should be directed 5 degrees cephalad. Views should demonstrate the patella, femoral condyles, tibial plateaus, and fibula. In external rotation the tibia and fibula are superimposed on each other. With internal rotation there is less superimposition between the tibia and fibula (Fig. 5.7A and B).

Various stress views have been described for evaluation of instability and include *valgus and varus stress* radiographs for evaluation of the collateral ligaments and *anterior drawer stress* radiographs for evaluation of the anterior cruciate ligament (ACL). These require use of a mechanical stress device or lead gloves worn by the x-ray technologist and manually stress the knee joint. In current clinical practice these views are seldom ordered because MRI is considered the gold standard for evaluation of internal derangement and stress views often need to be performed with local anesthesia for pain control.

Special Considerations and Anatomic Variants

Two sesamoid bones commonly identified on knee radiographs are the fabella and the cyamella. The fabella is located within the lateral head of the gastrocnemius. It overlies the lateral femoral condyle on the frontal view and sits posterior to the distal femur on the lateral view. The cyamella lies within the popliteus tendon. On a frontal radiograph it may be found at the insertion of the popliteus in the notch of the lateral femoral condyle (Fig. 5.8A to C).

Normal variants also occur in the patella, which can have two or more osseous centers, referred to as a bipartite or multipartite patella (Fig. 5.9A and B). A bipartite patella is the more common variant, seen in 1% of the population. It is bilateral 50% of the time.[40] The smaller pieces of the patella are located superolaterally and should fit neatly together like pieces of a jigsaw puzzle. The width of a bipartite patella is usually greater than that of the contralateral patella when assessed on a tangential axial view. MRI depicts intact cartilage overlying a bipartite patella, whereas a fracture displays disrupted osteochondral integrity. These features help to dismiss the suspicion of a fracture.[40] Rarely (<2% of the time), a bipartite patella can be symptomatic. MRI of the knee may demonstrate bone marrow edema on one or both sides of the synchondrosis.

A dorsal defect of the patella is another anatomic variant, usually detected incidentally. It appears as a lucent area of the superolateral patella (Fig. 5.10).[21,31] Pathologically the lesion is composed of fibrous tissue and spicules of bone. This uncommon entity is seen in children and typically fills in with normal or sclerotic bone in adulthood.

Patellofemoral Alignment. Merchant views can evaluate patellofemoral malalignment, which can be quantified with the sulcus and congruence angles. The sulcus angle is formed by drawing lines outward from the deepest portion of the

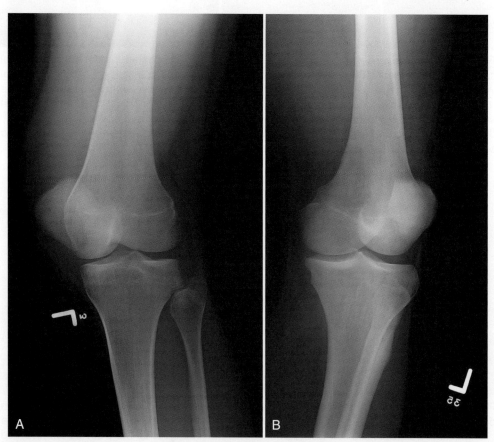

FIG 5.7 Internal (A) and external (B) rotational views of the knee in different patients. In external rotation the tibia and fibula are superimposed on each other; with internal rotation there should be less superimposition. A suprapatellar joint effusion is seen on the internally rotated view.

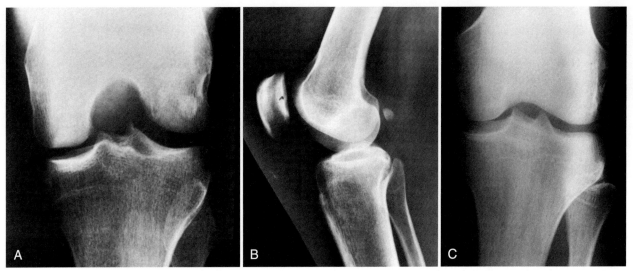

FIG 5.8 Fabella and Cyamella The fabella is a circular osseous density, a sesamoid, in the lateral head of the gastrocnemius muscle. (A) On the AP view it is superimposed on the lateral femoral condyle. (B) On the lateral view the fabella is posterior to the femoral condyles. (C) A cyamella is a sesamoid bone in the popliteus tendon. On the AP view the cyamella is seen within the notch at the lateral aspect of the lateral femoral condyle.

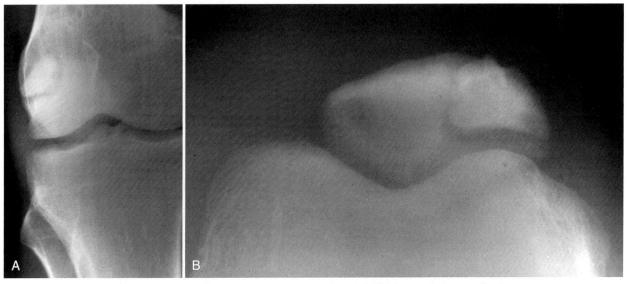

FIG 5.9 Bipartite Patella Oblique (A) and tangential axial (B) views of the patella demonstrate a crescentic radiolucency traversing the superolateral aspect of the patella. This lucency forms the interface between the two osseous centers of the bipartite patella. The superolateral location is typical of this entity.

trochlear sulcus to the tops of the femoral condyles. The angle normally measures 138 degrees (±6 degrees).[23] A shallow sulcus greater than 144 degrees is associated with recurrent patellar dislocation.

The congruence angle provides an index of subluxation. To measure it, the sulcus angle is bisected to create a reference line. An additional line is then drawn from the deepest portion of the trochlear sulcus to the patellar apex. The angle formed between this line and the reference line is the congruence angle. If the patellar apex falls lateral to the reference line, then the value of the congruence angle is positive. If the apex falls medial to the reference line, then the value of the congruence angle is negative. The normal congruence angle is 6 degrees (±11 degrees) (Fig. 5.11).[23,42]

Patellar tilt is another measure of patellofemoral alignment. It is measured by the angle formed between a horizontal line and a line drawn between the medial and lateral corners of the patella. In a study performed by Grelsamer and colleagues the mean tilt angle of a group of patients with signs and symptoms suggesting patellofemoral malalignment was 12 degrees (±6 degrees); in a similar group of control subjects it was 2 degrees (±2 degrees). Tilting of 5 degrees was taken to be the limit of normal. It is noteworthy that in the Grelsamer study, the knee was held in 30 degrees of flexion, rather than 45 degrees of flexion in the normal Merchant view.[24] Other imaging techniques (CT scans performed at various degrees of flexion) are sometimes necessary to detect patients with subtle or transient lateral patellar subluxation (Fig. 5.12A and B).

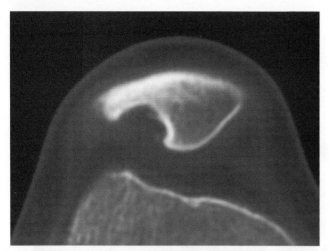

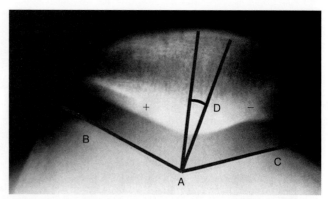

FIG 5.11 Merchant View; Measurement of the Sulcus and Congruence Angles The sulcus angle *(BAC)* is bisected by the reference line. A second line *(AD)* is then drawn from the sulcus to the patellar ridge. If the patellar apex is lateral to the reference line, the value of the angle is positive; if it is medial, the value of the angle is negative.

FIG 5.10 Dorsal Defect of the Patella Axial computed tomography image demonstrates a large lucent dorsal defect involving the majority of the lateral facet of the patella. The patient had a smaller, similar lesion in the contralateral patella. This finding is bilateral in approximately one-third of individuals.

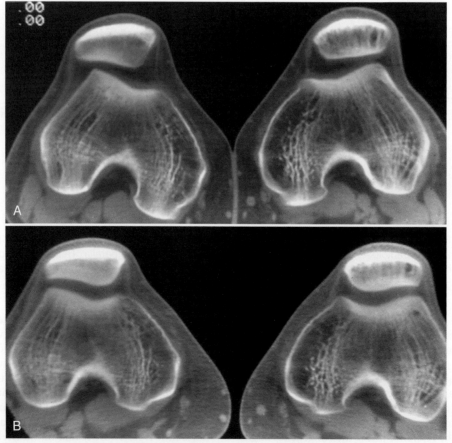

FIG 5.12 CT Assessment of Patellar Tracking Axial CT images obtained at 30 degrees (A) and 45 degrees (B) of flexion demonstrate transient bilateral lateral patellar subluxation. The patellar subluxation present at 30 degrees reduces at 45 degrees of flexion, thus explaining the normal Merchant view in this symptomatic patient.

Short- Versus Long-Standing Views. Short-standing frontal views (weight-bearing AP or Rosenberg) are typically sufficient for measuring the anatomic axis of the knee joint. The normal anatomic axis is 6 to 7 degrees of valgus angulation. If the exact quantitative measurement of the mechanical axis is required, then a long-standing frontal view of the lower extremity may be performed. The mechanical axis (weight-bearing axis) of the lower extremity is defined by a line drawn from the center of the femoral head to the center of the tibial plafond. In the normal setting this line should pass through the inner aspect of the medial compartment of the knee joint. If genu valgus is excessive, then the mechanical axis will shift laterally. A medially shifted mechanical axis indicates genu varus. Knowledge of the mechanical axis and how it relates to the anatomic axis is important in evaluating patients who are about to undergo or have undergone total knee arthroplasty and/or revision arthroplasty. It is also helpful in evaluating patients with posttraumatic deformities, malalignment, or limb length discrepancies.

Obtaining long-standing radiographs requires a long cassette. If a long cassette is not available, a CT scanogram can be obtained. CT scanning to obtain the mechanical axis is not advocated by the authors because it is not weight bearing, does not provide functional information, and may fail to take account of ligamentous laxity. In addition, CT scanograms entail higher radiation dosage exposure compared with conventional radiographs (Fig. 5.13).

Arthrography

Radiographic arthrography entails intra-articular injection of x-ray dye, typically an iodine-based product. Arthrography has many uses, including confirming placement before joint aspiration. Commonly, after radiographs or real-time ultrasound confirm dye placement within the joint space, a CT or MRI is performed to better evaluate meniscal or articular cartilage pathology and or component loosening (Fig. 5.14).

Safety

Radiography necessitates exposing the patient to ionizing radiation. The associated risk is low, particularly in the extremities. Special consideration should be given to children and young adults to minimize their exposure.

COMPUTED TOMOGRAPHY

Applications

CT provides detailed information about osseous structures and generally functions as a problem-solving modality once the limits of radiography have been reached. Specialized knee applications include evaluation of complex trauma, such as tibial plateau fractures, fracture healing, and joint loose bodies. CT is used with increasing frequency for preoperative joint replacement planning, arthroplasty complications, and revision arthroplasty preparation.[10,34,38,51] Extensor mechanism and patellofemoral joint evaluation in the setting of knee pain has also been reported.[25,32,33,37]

CT arthrography may be requested to evaluate menisci and/or articular cartilage when a patient is unable to undergo an MRI. This situation is commonly encountered in patients with claustrophobia or MRI-contraindicated metallic devices, such as pacemakers.[46,65]

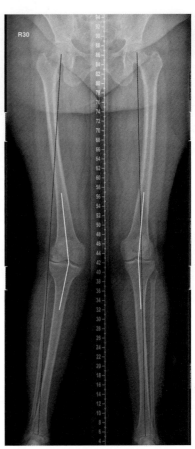

FIG 5.13 Long-Standing Views of Bilateral Lower Extremities Mechanical axis *(long black lines)*, anatomic axis *(shorter white lines)*. On the left the anatomic axis is normal (6 degrees of valgus), and the mechanical axis (the line drawn from the center of the femoral head to the center of the tibial plafond) passes through the inner aspect of the medial compartment of the femorotibial joint. On the right, genu valgus angulation is excessive, and the mechanical axis is shifted laterally. Ruler included for limb length validation.

Technique

CT scanning is a radical extension of radiography. A radiograph is obtained in a single projection, but a tomogram is the fusion of multiple projections to form an image. The notion is similar to looking at an object, say a car, only from the front versus walking around the car to appreciate it from multiple perspectives. The computed element of CT involves having a computer generate an image as the x-ray beam strikes multiple detectors from multiple locations.

Similar to radiographs, CT scanners measure a single parameter, tissue density. Hounsfield units (HU) are the standard for measuring density. Water is zero HU. Less dense materials, such as fat (−120 HU) and air (−1000 HU), appear darker. Denser materials, such as muscle (40 HU) and bone (400 HU), appear brighter. Thus a CT image can be thought of as a density map plotted along a gray scale. Contrast is provided by the different densities of adjacent tissues.

CT technology has evolved quickly over the past several decades. Early on, a scanner moved stepwise through the anatomy of interest, acquiring a single slice at a time. Studies required several minutes to complete. Nowadays, scanners

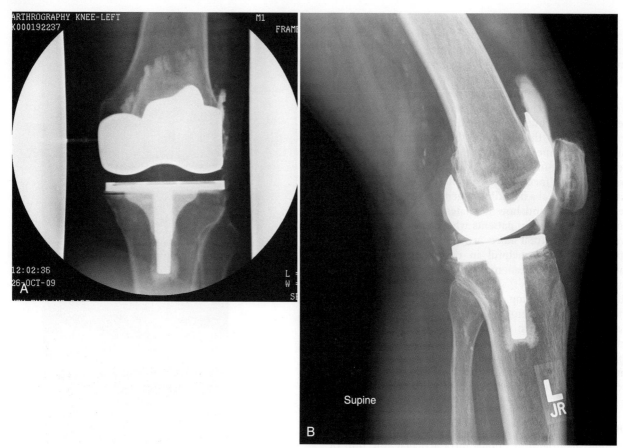

FIG 5.14 Normal Knee Arthrogram in a Patient With a Total Knee Arthroplasty AP (A) and lateral views (B) of the knee after intra-articular injection of radiopaque contrast material. Needle noted on the AP view.

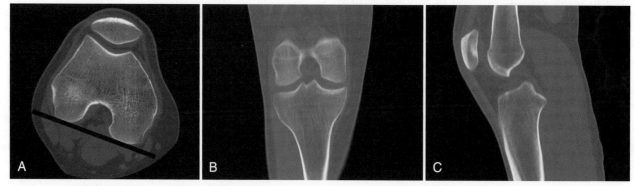

FIG 5.15 Normal axial (A), coronal (B), and sagittal (C) CT images of the knee. A line drawn along the posterior aspect of the femoral condyles (A) on axial images demonstrates the correct plane selection for coronal reconstruction.

move helically, acquiring multiple slices in fractions of a second. Entire examinations are routinely finished in a few seconds.

In addition, modern technology allows the acquisition of isotropic voxels. Voxels are the three-dimensional (3D) analogues of pixels. They are the building blocks of an image. Each voxel represents a discrete density (HU) at a discrete location. A voxel is isotropic if it is equal in each of its three dimensions (ie, cubic). This permits multiplanar reformatting. Thus data acquired in a standard axial fashion with isotropic voxels can be reworked into sagittal and coronal planes or any other plane

desired. One pass of the scanner allows you to look at the knee from any perspective you want!

Practically, the knee is imaged axially with thin sections (1.25 or 0.625 mm). The coronal reformats are prescribed via a line connecting the posterior aspects of the femoral condyles. The sagittal plane is generated along a line perpendicular to the coronal plane (Fig. 5.15A to C).

Slice thickness is user dependent. Thicker slices, such as 2.5 or 5 mm, reduce the number of overall images, making the dataset more manageable. It is easier and more efficient to scroll through 50 images rather than 200. In contrast, thin slices may provide finer detail that is effectively averaged out on thicker reformats. A balance is usually sought in slice thickness to provide a digestible number of images with adequate diagnostic information. Datasets are malleable, and additional reformats may be requested as necessary.

Several techniques are available for reducing metal-related artifact. First off, patient positioning is important. When possible, the goal is to position the patient so the beam penetrates the smallest cross-sectional area of metal. The high density of metal is challenging for a CT scanner because it prohibits the passage of photons. This may be partially overcome by increasing the peak kilovoltage (kVp) and milliampere seconds (mAs). kVp is the maximum voltage applied across an x-ray tube. A higher voltage results in higher-energy photons, which possess greater penetrating power. mAs is the quantity of photons produced by the x-ray tube. Raising the mAs means that more photons are available to penetrate the metal and contribute to the image. The pitch may be decreased, typically to less than one, to increase the overlap of slices (think of a tight spiral). This effectively increases the number of image-generating photons. The trade-off in increasing each of these parameters is increased radiation exposure to the patient. During postprocessing, choosing thicker sections reduces image noise, combating metal-related artifact. In addition, because bone algorithms worsen artifact, using a standard reconstruction filter is preferable (Fig. 5.16).

Image Interpretation

A knee CT scan is read in any of three standard imaging planes: axial, sagittal, or coronal. An advantage of a PACS environment is that images can be instantaneously adjusted to focus on a specific range of densities to best show the tissue(s) of interest. A center density is identified, termed the *level*. The second setting, the *window*, is the range of densities around the level. For example, to evaluate fine bony detail, a level of 500 HU and a window of 2000 HU might be elected. In contrast, to assess soft tissue structures, such as the menisci or cruciate ligaments, a level of 40 HU and a window of 400 may be chosen. These different bone and soft tissue settings are often programmed

into the PACS and can be quickly selected at the touch of a button (Fig. 5.17A to C).

In addition, 3D volume and surface-rendered reconstructions can be created at an independent workstation. These are useful in the setting of complex osseous trauma, as well as in obtaining a more global view of implanted hardware (Fig. 5.18A and B).

Computed Tomography Arthrography

CT arthrography is a two-step process. First, under fluoroscopic or ultrasound guidance, at least 15 mL of iodinated contrast is instilled into the knee joint. To provide double contrast, some physicians choose to instill several milliliters of air as well. The amount of air and contrast varies significantly among radiologists, but the point is to coat the joint surfaces with contrast so as to make abnormal extension of contrast into tears visible. The patient then is transported to the CT suite and scanned.

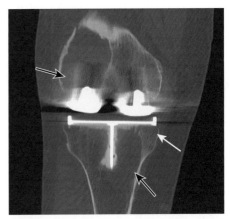

FIG 5.16 Coronal reconstructed CT image of the knee, using metal artifact reduction techniques, clearly demonstrates large areas of osteolysis *(black arrows)* surrounding both the femoral and tibial components of a total knee arthroplasty, including a region immediately subjacent to the tibial plate *(white arrow).*

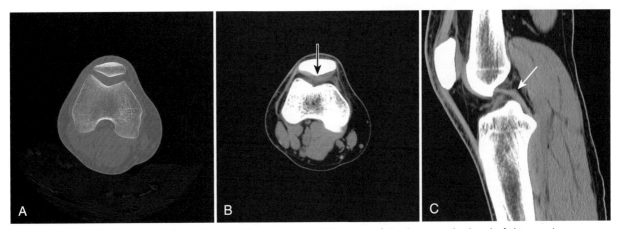

FIG 5.17 **Bone and Soft Tissue Windows** Axial CT image of the knee at the level of the patellofemoral joint, using a bone reconstruction filter (A) is useful for demonstrating fine osseous detail. An image obtained at the same level using a soft tissue window (B) can evaluate soft tissue structures, such as patellar cartilage *(arrow)*. Sagittal image of the knee using a soft tissue window (C) demonstrates ligamentous structures such as the PCL *(arrow)*.

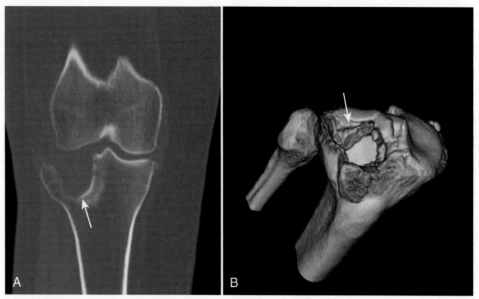

FIG 5.18 Three-Dimensional Reconstruction A coronal reformatted image of the knee (A) demonstrating a markedly depressed fracture of the lateral tibial plateau *(white arrow)*. Postprocessed 3D volume rendered reconstruction with the soft tissues and femur cut away (B) shows the depressed fracture from a cranial oblique vantage point *(white arrow)* and may be useful for preoperative planning.

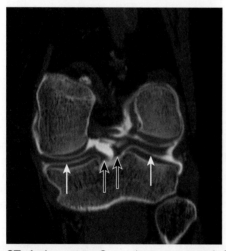

FIG 5.19 CT Arthrogram Coronal reconstructed CT arthrographic image of the knee demonstrates normal appearing medial and lateral menisci *(white arrows)*, including normal posterior root attachments *(black arrows)*. No imbibition of contrast material into the menisci occurs to indicate a meniscal tear.

Contrast fills cartilage defects and meniscal tears. Loose bodies are outlined by contrast, appearing as filling defects (Fig. 5.19).

Artifacts and Special Considerations

Currently CT artifacts are notably few in orthopedic applications. Modern scanners have almost eliminated several traditionally nagging artifacts. Motion artifact from patient movement renders an image blurry with indistinct margins. This now is rarely an issue because scanning a knee takes only a few seconds (or less). Partial volume effects occur when the scanner has difficulty processing adjacent tissues of markedly different density (eg, bone and fat). The scanner resolves this discrepancy by generating an average density that represents neither tissue. Sharp edges become blurred. The ability to obtain thin slices (ie, <1 mm) has greatly diminished partial volume effects.

Beam hardening occurs when the x-ray beam encounters a dense material, such as contrast or metal. The outcome is one of two distortions: cupping or streaks/dark bands. Cupping, as the name implies, is the appearance of a curved contour to an object when none actually exists. Streak artifact manifests as dark bands that radiate from a dense material, obscuring nearby anatomy. In the past this artifact rendered the evaluation of metallic implants challenging. Current sophisticated software and filtration algorithms are able to minimize these artifacts (see Fig. 5.16).

It is important to keep in mind that the cost of reducing an artifact may be increased radiation to the patient. Although it is less of an issue when imaging an extremity of an adult patient, radiation exposure remains an issue at the forefront of protocol planning and patient safety, especially in the pediatric population.

Safety

Similar to radiography, CT uses ionizing radiation to generate an image. The difference lies in the amount of exposure. The effective dose of a CT scan is an order of magnitude greater than that of a radiograph. By virtue of comparison, a chest x-ray results in a 10-millirem effective dose, whereas a chest CT requires 600 millirem. When a CT scan is performed, determining and considering the radiation exposure are warranted, particularly in younger patients.

MAGNETIC RESONANCE IMAGING

Applications

MRI is an extremely powerful tool that has supplanted other imaging modalities as the most versatile and effective technique for evaluating patients with internal derangement and cartilage disorders.[4,6,47] MRI is also invaluable for evaluating other pathologic processes, such as tumor, infection, metabolic bone disease, and suspected knee arthroplasty complications. When used appropriately, after careful physical examination, MRI can be a useful tool in the surgical decision-making process and for preoperative planning.[3,45,64] Many orthopedic hardware manufacturers (Zimmer-Biomet, Conformis) now use MRI to create patient-specific instruments by using custom implant protocols.

Technique

The MRI scanner is a large, powerful magnet. A 1.5-T machine is 30,000 times stronger than the earth's magnetic field. This mighty device exposes a patient to strong magnetic forces and measures the resulting tiny, very fast movements of atoms.

Clinical imaging centers upon hydrogen atoms (protons), which are ubiquitous throughout the body. Inherent qualities of each tissue dictate how its protons will respond in the MRI environment. In contrast to a CT scanner that measures density, the MRI scanner is capable of measuring multiple tissue properties, such as T1, T2, and proton density (PD). MRI scanners are calibrated to measure a specific property by prescribing values for several variables—altogether termed a *sequence*. Two of these variables are time to echo (TE) and time to repetition (TR). In general, a T2-weighted sequence necessitates a long TR on the order of several thousand milliseconds and a TE near a hundred milliseconds. A T1-weighted sequence uses a relatively short TR (hundreds of milliseconds) and a short TE (<50 ms). Sequences vary considerably across manufacturers and field strengths.

Bearing this in mind, different tissues in the body behave in a reproducible manner on specific pulse sequences, and knowledge of these characteristics is helpful for detection of pathologic processes. For example, adipose tissue and acute hemorrhage are hyperintense (bright) on T1-weighted sequences; hematopoietic bone marrow is lower in signal intensity on T1- and T2-weighted images than fatty marrow because of its lower fat content (Fig. 5.20A and B). Water is bright on T2-weighted images and dark on T1-weighted images. Because pathologic processes (tumor, infection, contusion, and ligament and tendon injury) are typically associated with increased water content, abnormalities usually appear hyperintense to adjacent tissues on fluid-sensitive sequences and lower in signal intensity on T1-weighted images. Increased signal intensity or bone marrow edema pattern becomes more conspicuous when fat suppression is applied. Fat suppression can be accomplished by preferentially saturating the fat protons (chemical saturation) or by a technique known as short tau inversion recovery (STIR) imaging. The former technique is more commonly used in the knee. Fat suppression serves to make the presence and extent of pathologic processes more conspicuous on T2-weighted and PD sequences.

As the scanner executes the sequence, protons in a patient's tissues generate signal. A receiver coil, a device analogous to a highly engineered antenna, then collects signal and transmits it back to the scanner, which then produces an image. The coil is an important determinant of image quality. The more signal that is accurately captured, the better is the image. Optimal coils are designed for a specific body part. For example, a wrist coil is used for the wrist and a knee coil is used for the knee. Using

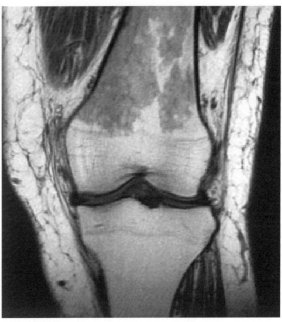

FIG 5.20 MRI of Marrow Signal A coronal T1-weighted image shows bright marrow signal in the tibia and at the distal end of the femur, which represents fatty marrow. The dark signal in the metaphysis and distal shaft of the femur represents hematopoietic marrow hyperplasia. Note that the red marrow almost never crosses the growth plate scar.

a coil not designed for the body part of interest may result in images of lower quality.

Advances in MRI and decreases in cost have further placed it at the forefront in evaluation of the knee. Among these advances includes 3.0-T strength magnet systems, improved cartilage imaging, 3D imaging, and multichannel (8 or 16) dedicated knee receiver coils.

In addition, metal reduction techniques now allow for comprehensive evaluation of suspected arthroplasty complications.[18] In the past, metallic implants in MRI would cause substantial image artifacts, including signal loss, failure of fat suppression, geometric and magnetic field distortion, and bright pile-up artifacts, which greatly limited diagnostic usefulness.[26] Optimized conventional and advanced (designer) pulse sequences can now result in significant and substantial metallic artifact reduction and improved evaluation of bone-implant interfaces and periprosthetic soft tissues.[18]

So-called MARS or metallic artifact reducing sequence improve visualization by varying sequence parameters. Typically used techniques include imaging at 1.5 T instead of 3.0 T, STIR (or Dixon technique) for fat suppression (spectral fat suppression performs better in a homogeneous field) instead of chemical fat saturation, use of fast spin echo (FSE) instead of gradient echo, maintaining good signal-to-noise ratio (SNR), increased bandwidth during slice selection and readout, view-angle-tilting (VAT), use of intermediate echo times, using a high number of excitations, and using a large matrix in the frequency direction (eg, 512).[18,26]

More advanced implant- and vendor-specific protocols are now commercially available and include multiacquisition variable-resonance image combination (MAVRIC), which is a specialized sequence designed to minimize metallic artifact around metallic prostheses.[27] Another technique used for addressing through-plane metal artifacts is Slice Encoding for Metal Artifact Correction (SEMAC), in which an additional slice-encoding gradient is added to a standard FSE sequence.[58] The combination of the MAVRIC and SEMAC technique is known as MAVRIC-SL.[12]

Although these improvements have helped to create fast and sophisticated imaging protocols, one must remember that tremendous variation and quality are seen among clinically available MRI systems. The spectrum of clinically available systems ranges in strength from open 0.2 T without dedicated coils to 3.0-T magnets with 16 channel receiver coils. The deficiencies of these lower field strength systems are exposed most conspicuously when subtle meniscal and hyaline cartilage injuries are imaged.

Plane and Protocol Selection. MRI of the knee is performed in axial, sagittal, and coronal planes. The axial plane is a true anatomic transverse plane through the knee. The coronal plane is typically prescribed from the axial plane based on a line drawn along the posterior aspect of the femoral condyles (Fig. 5.21). The sagittal plane is then chosen perpendicular to the coronal plane. Most knee structures may be evaluated in three planes, although each plane has particular advantages. For example, axial images best display the patellar cartilage and subchondral bone. In contrast, the trochlear sulcus cartilage is seen to best advantage in the sagittal plane. The sagittal and coronal planes best demonstrate meniscal and femorotibial cartilage anatomy and pathology. Although the sagittal plane is most often used for preliminary evaluation of the ACL and posterior cruciate ligament (PCL), it is essential to use the coronal and axial planes to follow the entire course of each ligament to the level of the osseous attachments.

Wide variation in protocol planning and sequence selection has been noted. PD sequences with or without fat suppression are commonly used to evaluate ligaments, tendons, and articular cartilage. Fat-suppressed PD or T2-weighted sequences are useful for imaging osseous contusion and/or the bone marrow edema pattern, as well as muscle, tendon, and ligament tears and strains. T1-weighted images (with and without fat suppression and both before and after intravenous gadolinium contrast administration) are often obtained to evaluate the marrow cavity in cases of suspected tumor or osteomyelitis. Fat-saturated, T1-weighted imaging is used when MR arthrography

is performed after intra-articular administration of dilute gadolinium.

Three-dimensional volumetric acquisitions are also readily available and have been used in various musculoskeletal applications for years.[59] Until fairly recently these consisted primarily of gradient-recalled echo (GRE) sequences, allowing for very thin slices which afforded for high "through-plane" resolution. Although more commonly used in the hand and wrist (to evaluate thin structures, such as the triangular fibrocartilage complex (TFCC) and intercarpal ligaments), GRE sequences in the knee were primarily used for cartilage imaging and had more limited utility for evaluating knee ligaments, the menisci, and for bone marrow signal abnormalities.[59] Many vendors now offer 3D pulse sequences with FSE technique for clinical use. For example, widely available sequences include SPACE (sampling perfection with application of optimized contrasts using different flip angle evolution) and CUBE (3-dimentional fast spin echo imaging sequence with variable tilt angle). The advantage of a SPACE 3D sequence over GRE sequences is that they can mimic the imaging properties and appearance of more conventional two-dimensional (2D) FSE PD and T2-weighted acquisition and therefore potentially allow a more comprehensive evaluation of the knee joint.[59] Another advantage using 3D SPACE is that the entire isotropic, volumetric dataset is acquired during a single pulse sequence, and then that data can be reformatted into any additional plane required. This is analogous to axial CT acquisitions that can also be reformatted into additional planes and has the potential to reduce overall scan time. A typical 3D SPACE sequence of the knee takes approximately 5 minutes to complete. Up until now 3D SPACE sequences have been shown to be comparable to conventional 2D FSE pulse sequences for evaluation of knee ligaments but have shown to be slightly inferior to conventional 2D FSE pulse sequences for evaluation of the menisci.[59]

Three example protocols are presented here. The first two protocols are based on the use of a 3.0-T MRI (Siemens Verio) with a 15-channel dedicated knee coil (Table 5.1). MRI using a metal reduction (MARS) protocol is based on a 1.5-T MRI (Siemens Aera) and also using a 15-channel dedicated knee coil (see Table 5.1).

Normal Anatomy

Ligaments. The ACL functions primarily to restrain anterior tibial translation. It courses from the inner or medial aspect of the lateral femoral condyle, traveling inferiorly and obliquely, parallel to Blumensaat line, to insert on the anteromedial tibia adjacent to the medial tibial spine. The ligament is composed of anteromedial and posterolateral bundles. In the sagittal plane the ACL is typically visualized over several images because of its oblique course. The ACL is also well evaluated on standard images obtained in the coronal and axial planes. Dedicated imaging can be performed in an oblique sagittal plane to produce images within the same plane as the ligament. However, this is not believed to be necessary because of the accuracy of imaging ACL injuries using standard imaging planes.[35] The normal appearance of the ACL is that of a low-signal band on all imaging sequences with an intrasubstance linear intermediate to bright signal from normal interposed fat and synovium (Fig. 5.22A to C).

The PCL limits posterior tibial translation and is larger and stronger than the ACL. The PCL originates at the inner aspect of the medial femoral condyle and inserts on the posterior tibia.

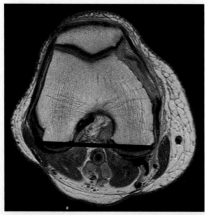

FIG 5.21 Axial PD FSE image of the knee with a black line connecting the posterior aspects of the femoral condyles. This line is the correct plane choice for coronal imaging.

TABLE 5.1 Knee Magnetic Resonance Imaging Protocols

3.0 T SIEMENS MAGNATOM VERIO — ROUTINE KNEE

Sequences	TR	TE	Turbo Factor	Matrix	ST (mm)	Gap (mm)	Flip Angle	Average/Nex	FOV
Axi PD FS	4000	33	7	307 × 384	3	0.7	150	2	150
COR PD	4000	28	12	358 × 512	3.5	0	150	2	160
Cor T2 FS	5000	72	16	307 × 384	3.5	0	150	2	160
Sag PD	4000	28	13	448 × 336	3.5	0	150	2	160
SAG PD FS	4000	28	11	448 × 313	3.5	0	150	2	160
Sag PD Space	1500	36	67	224 × 256	0.6	0	160	1	150

3.0 T SIEMENS MAGNATOM VERIO — TUMOR OR INFECTION KNEE

Sequences	TR	TE	Turbo Factor	Matrix	ST (mm)	Gap (mm)	Flip Angle	Average/Nex	FOV
Ax T1	900	12	3	240 × 384	3	0.7	140	2	160
AX T2 FS	4000	76	13	240 × 384	3	0.7	140	2	160
Sag T1	900	12	3	240 × 384	3	0.7	140	2	160
Sag T2 FS	4000	76	13	240 × 384	3	0.7	140	2	160
Cor T1	900	12	3	240 × 384	3	0.7	140	2	160
Cor T2 FS	4000	76	13	240 × 384	3	0.7	140	2	160
Ax T1 FS PRE	950	12	3	256 × 320	3	0.7	140	2	160
Contrast	—	—	—		—	—	—	—	—
Ax T1 FS C+	950	12	3	256 × 320	3	0.7	140	2	160
Sag T1 FS C+	950	12	3	256 × 320	3	0.7	140	2	160
Cor T1 FS C+	950	12	3	256 × 320	3	0.7	140	2	160

1.5 T SIEMENS MAGNATOM AERO — METAL REDUCTION PROTOCOL/KNEE

Sequence	TR	TE	Turbo Factor	Matrix	ST (mm)	Gap (mm)	Flip Angle	Average/Nex	TI	FOV	BW
Cor Stir	4510	30	17	240 × 320	3	0.8	150	3	150	190	504
Cor PD	2500	33	17	346 × 384	3	0.8	150	3		190	501
Axi Stir	5100	34	17	204 × 256	3.5	0.9	150	4	150	180	501
Axi PD	2560	22	17	224 × 320	3.5	0.9	150	4		180	504
Sag Stir	3940	30	17	240 × 320	3	0.6	150	3	150	190	504
Sag PD	2500	25	17	288 × 384	3	0.6	150	3	—	190	449

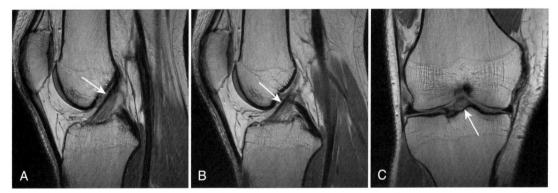

FIG 5.22 Consecutive sagittal PD FSE images of the knee (A and B) demonstrate a normal appearing ACL *(arrow)*. Coronal PD FSE image (C) shows a normal tibial insertion of the ACL *(arrow)*. Intermediate to bright signal is seen interposed between the ligament fibers, consistent with fat and synovium.

The cross-sectional area of the PCL is largest at its femoral origin and decreases toward the tibial insertion. The PCL tibial attachment extends over the dorsal rim of the posterior tibial shelf.[53] Similar to the ACL the PCL can be divided into two functional units: anterolateral and posteromedial bundles. The normal MRI appearance of the PCL is that of a low-signal band on all imaging sequences; it is typically visualized on one or two consecutive images on sagittal pulse sequences. The PCL is taut in flexion and tends to become more lax with extension—the typical position in which the knee is placed during MRI. It should have a gently curved configuration when viewed in the sagittal plane (Fig. 5.23).[53]

The medial collateral ligament (MCL) provides support to the medial aspect of the knee. Its primary functions are to stabilize the femorotibial joint when valgus stresses are applied and to stabilize against lateral subluxation or dislocation of the patella. Although the MCL has been described as a simple band-like structure, it is rather a ligamentous complex composed of

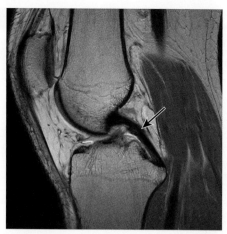

FIG 5.23 Sagittal PD FSE image of the knee demonstrates a normal appearing PCL *(arrow)*.

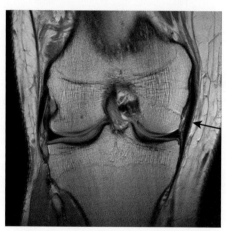

FIG 5.24 Coronal PD FSE image of the knee demonstrates a normal appearing MCL *(arrow)*.

three layers. It blends imperceptibly with the surrounding joint capsule and other medial supporting structures.[5] The MCL consists of deep and superficial components. The superficial fibers of the MCL reside in layer 2 of the medial supporting structures and take their origin at the medial femoral condyle (layer 1 primarily consists of crural fascia).[61] Superficial MCL fibers run slightly anteromedially to insert on the tibia, approximately 5 cm from the joint line, just posterior to the pes anserinus tendons.[62] The deep fibers or capsular layer includes the meniscofemoral and meniscotibial (coronary) ligaments. The deep and superficial fibers are separated by the medial collateral bursa, which in the normal setting should be collapsed and imperceptible on MRI. The MCL should appear with uniformly low signal on all pulse sequences. It is best appreciated on coronal and axial sequences (Fig. 5.24). MCL injuries range from sprains, in which the ligament will be normal in appearance with surrounding fluid signal, to partial- and full-thickness tears with disruption of the superficial and/or deep fibers.

The lateral collateral ligament (LCL) functions to resist varus stress and provide posterolateral stability. This complex is composed of three layers. The superficial layer (layer 1) includes the iliotibial band anteriorly and the superficial portion of the biceps femoris posterolaterally.[61] The iliotibial band inserts at the far anterior aspect of the lateral tibia at Gerdy's tubercle. The biceps femoris inserts on the fibular styloid. The middle layer (layer 2) includes the lateral retinaculum anteriorly and two discrete areas of ligamentous thickening that originate from the lateral patella.[61] The deep layer (layer 3) forms a portion of the lateral joint capsule. It is composed of the LCL proper (fibulocollateral ligament), the arcuate complex, and several posterolateral corner structures.[61] The fibulocollateral ligament originates from the lateral femoral condyle and courses posterolaterally to insert upon the fibular head, combining with the deep fibers of the biceps femoris tendon to form the conjoined tendon.[61] The contents of the posterolateral corner include the popliteus tendon, the LCL proper, the lateral head of the gastrocnemius muscle, and the arcuate, popliteofibular, and fabellofibular ligaments.

The components of the LCL complex and the posterolateral corner are normally of homogeneously low signal. Coronal images display them optimally (Fig. 5.25A to G), although axial images are also illustrative. Tears of any portion of the LCL complex manifest themselves as signal hyperintensity and discontinuity of ligament/tendon fibers. Tears of the LCL proper are closely associated with posterolateral corner injuries, which can lead to posterolateral instability.[5]

Menisci. The menisci are wedge-shaped, semilunar fibrocartilaginous structures that lie between the femoral condyles and the tibia. The primary function of the menisci is to increase surface area and distribute the load evenly across the femoral condyles. The menisci also act as shock absorbers and play a role in chondrocyte nutrition and joint lubrication. In the ACL-deficient knee the menisci act as AP stabilizers. The absence of a normal meniscus can lead to irreversible and accelerated degenerative changes.[19]

Each meniscus is arbitrarily divided into anterior horn, body, and posterior horn. The periphery of each meniscus is thick, and the inner aspect is thin. Thus the menisci appear triangular in cross-section, except at the body, where the menisci maintain a "bow-tie" appearance on sagittal images. The central edge of the meniscus is termed the free edge or apex. It should appear as a sharp point. The superior surfaces of the menisci are concave and serve to deepen the contact area with the femoral condyles; the inferior aspects are flat and rest on the tibial plateau. The menisci are almost entirely avascular structures. The posterior and peripheral aspects of the menisci have a vascular supply and therefore are termed the *red zone*. It has been proposed that tears in this region have a greater tendency to heal.[28,44,63]

The menisci cover 50% of the medial and 70% of the lateral surface of the tibial plateau.[19] The medial meniscus is C-shaped, and the posterior horn is approximately 2 times larger than the anterior horn (Fig. 5.26). The medial meniscus is attached to the joint capsule throughout its course peripherally, limiting its mobility and making it more prone to injury than the lateral meniscus. The anterior horn has a root attachment centrally, just anterior to the ACL attachment on the tibia. The posterior horn attachment is to the posterior aspect of the tibia within the intercondylar fossa.

The lateral meniscus is semicircular, and its two horns are symmetrical. The lateral meniscus is more mobile than the medial meniscus. It attaches only to the anterior and far posterior aspects of the joint capsule. Its capsular attachment is interrupted at the body and much of the posterior horn to

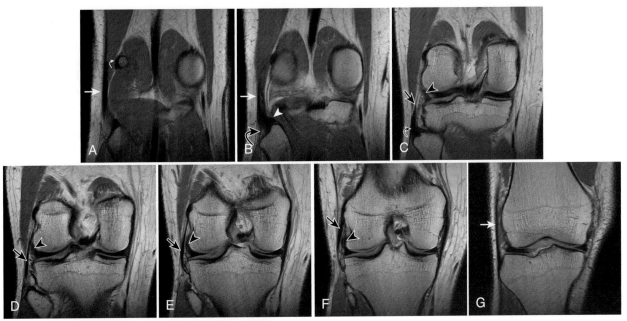

FIG 5.25 The lateral collateral ligament complex and selected structures of the posterolateral corner. Multiple coronal PD images starting at the far posterior aspect of the knee and progressing anteriorly (A to G) demonstrate the normal-appearing fabella and fabellofibular ligament *(curved white arrow)*, biceps femoris tendon *(straight white arrow)*, conjoined tendon inserting on the fibula *(curved black arrow)*, popliteofibular ligament *(white arrowhead)*, fibulocollateral ligament *(straight black arrow)*, popliteus tendon *(black arrowhead)*, and iliotibial band *(wide white arrow on image G)*. Images A through F are consecutive, and image G is located more anteriorly.

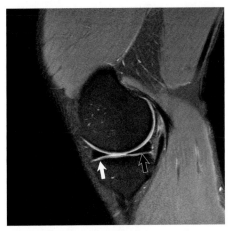

FIG 5.26 Normal Medial Meniscus Sagittal fat-suppressed PD image demonstrates both the anterior and posterior horns to be normal in signal (diffusely low) and morphology (appear as triangles with a sharp free edge), with the posterior horn *(black arrow)* approximately 50% larger than the anterior horn *(white arrow)*.

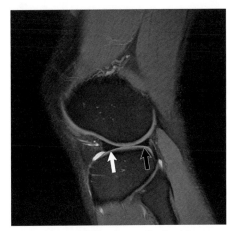

FIG 5.27 Normal Lateral Meniscus Sagittal fat-suppressed PD image demonstrates both the anterior and posterior horns to be normal in signal (diffusely low) and morphology (appear as triangles with a sharp free edge), with the posterior horn *(black arrow)* approximately the same size as the anterior horn *(white arrow)*.

accommodate the popliteus tendon coursing through the popliteal hiatus (Fig. 5.27). Small fascicles attach the popliteus to the lateral meniscus, allowing the meniscus to be pulled posteriorly during knee flexion (Fig. 5.28).

The meniscofemoral ligaments of Humphrey and Wrisberg extend from the posterior horn of the lateral meniscus to the inner aspect of the medial femoral condyle. They cross anterior and posterior to the PCL, respectively (Fig. 5.29A and B).

Meniscofemoral ligaments are inconsistently and variably present (ie, patients may have one, both, or neither and may be considered normal).

The menisci are homogeneous, low-signal structures that should be evaluated on both sagittal and coronal images. On sagittal images, normal menisci should appear as black signal triangles with sharp central edges. The body segment, the portion between the anterior and posterior horns, appears as a low-signal, bow tie–shaped structure at the peripheral aspect of the sagittal images. Coronal images through the menisci allow evaluation of the root attachments and cross-sectional evaluation of the meniscal bodies.

Tears of the menisci manifest as linear bright signal abnormalities on fluid-sensitive sequences that reach an articular surface, or as alterations in normal meniscal morphology.[14,50,60]

Meniscal variants include the discoid meniscus and the transverse meniscal ligament (TML). A discoid meniscus, instead of having a semicircular or C shape, is shaped like a disk. Discoid menisci are much more common on the lateral side and have a reported incidence of 0.4% to 16.6%. Three types of discoid menisci have been described: complete, incomplete, and Wrisberg variants. Visualization of a continuous band of meniscus on more than three contiguous peripheral sagittal images (5 mm or less in thickness) indicates a discoid meniscus (Fig. 5.30).[56] A meniscal body on coronal images greater than 15 mm wide or extending into the intercondylar notch also suggests the diagnosis. Discoid menisci have an increased incidence of tears and degeneration.[19]

The transverse or anterior intermeniscal ligament connects the anterior horns of the medial and lateral meniscus. It is present in 44% to 58% of patients.[19] On sagittal images the interface of this structure with the anterior horn of the lateral meniscus often simulates a tear (Fig. 5.31).[15,29] Following this "pseudotear" on sequential images helps to identify this normal structure.

Tendons. The extensor mechanism of the knee consists of the quadriceps and patellar tendons. The quadriceps is composed of the rectus femoris tendon anteriorly, the vastus medialis and

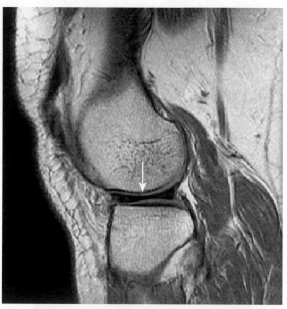

FIG 5.30 Discoid Lateral Meniscus Sagittal PD image demonstrates a blocklike continuous band of meniscus *(white arrow)*; the lateral meniscus had this configuration on almost all sagittal images. A normal meniscus has this appearance only on the more peripheral images and assumes the appearance of two separate triangles (anterior and posterior horns) centrally in the region of the intercondylar notch.

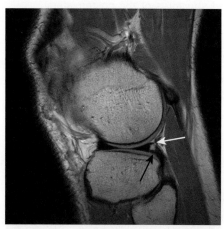

FIG 5.28 Sagittal PD FSE image of the knee demonstrates a normal-appearing posterior horn of the lateral meniscus with intact superior *(white arrow)* and inferior *(black arrow)* fascicular attachments *(arrows)* to the popliteus tendon.

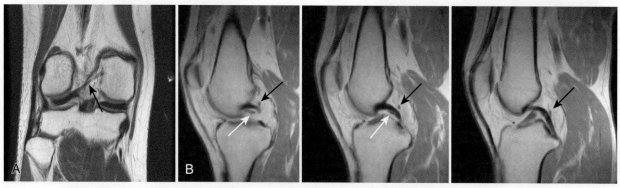

FIG 5.29 Meniscofemoral Ligaments Coronal PD image of the knee (A) demonstrates the normal course of the meniscofemoral ligament *(arrow)* extending from the posterior horn of the lateral meniscus to the inner aspect of the posterior medial femoral condyle. Three consecutive sagittal PD images of the knee (B) in a different patient, with the meniscofemoral ligaments of Humphrey *(white arrow)* and Wrisberg *(black arrow)* noted anteriorly and posteriorly to the PCL, respectively.

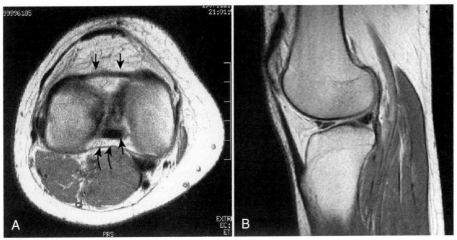

FIG 5.31 Transverse Meniscal Ligament (A) Axial PD image shows the low-signal TML *(short arrows)* connecting the anterior horns of the lateral and medial menisci. Also seen on this image are the posterior cruciate ligament *(long arrow)* and the posterior joint capsule *(curved arrows)*. (B) Sagittal PD image through the lateral meniscus shows a linear interface between the anterior margin of the anterior horn of the lateral meniscus and the TML. The TML can be mistaken for a portion of the lateral meniscus; the interface can therefore simulate a tear.

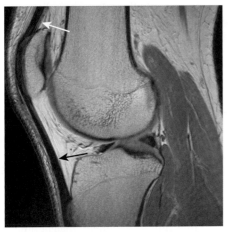

FIG 5.32 Extensor Mechanism Sagittal PD FSE image of the knee demonstrates normal homogeneously low signal patellar *(white arrow)* and quadriceps *(black arrow)* tendons.

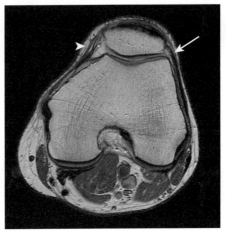

FIG 5.33 Axial PD FSE image of the knee demonstrates intact medial *(white arrowhead)* and lateral *(white arrow)* patellar retinaculi.

lateralis tendons centrally, and the vastus intermedius posteriorly. The normal quadriceps tendon is low signal on all pulse sequences, with internal striations of brighter signal representing the divisions of the previously described tendons. The quadriceps inserts on the superior pole of the patella. The patellar tendon is composed primarily of fibers from the rectus femoris, which continue below the patella to insert on the tibial tubercle. Its normal appearance is homogeneously low signal. The extensor mechanism is best visualized in the sagittal plane (Fig. 5.32). The axial plane provides ideal visualization of the medial and lateral retinaculi, which originate from the patella to insert on the medial and lateral femoral condyles, respectively (Fig. 5.33).

The semimembranosus and pes anserinus tendons course along the posteromedial aspect of the knee. They are low-signal structures. The semimembranosus has multiple slips that insert on both the medial tibia and the joint capsule. The pes anserinus is made up of three tendons: gracilis, sartorius, and semitendinosus. The three tendons insert on the medial aspect of the tibia anterior to the MCL insertion. They are well demonstrated on axial images (Fig. 5.34).

The popliteus tendon originates at the lateral aspect of the lateral femoral condyle and courses posteroinferiorly to join the muscle belly, which inserts on the proximal posteromedial aspect of the tibia. Superior and inferior popliteomeniscal fascicles serve as attachments between the lateral meniscus, popliteus tendon, and capsule to form the roof and floor of the popliteal hiatus. At least one fascicle is visualized in 97% of patients with an intact lateral meniscus. The fascicles control the motion of the lateral meniscus in flexion and extension and appear as thin low signal structures that extend from the posterolateral aspect of the lateral meniscus to the joint capsule (see Fig. 5.28). Disruption of one or more of the fascicles allows increased motion of the meniscus and can result in pain and/or locking.[19]

Cartilage. Various techniques are used to evaluate cartilage within the knee joint. Fat-suppressed, PD-weighted images provide increased conspicuity of lesions, given their high resolution and clear differentiation between fluid and cartilage. Properly obtained non–fat-suppressed FSE PD images can also provide exquisite cartilage detail. Some authors believe this sequence is inferior to fat-suppressed sequences in evaluating for commonly associated subchondral bone abnormalities.[62] Other advanced but less frequently clinically used techniques include T2 mapping, T1RHO, and delayed gadolinium-enhanced MRI of cartilage. T1 fat-saturation sequences can also be used after placement of intra-articular gadolinium to provide images analogous to nonarthrographic fat-saturation PD FSE. Although the optimal pulse sequence is controversial, the Articular Cartilage Imaging Committee, a subcommittee of the International Cartilage Repair Society, recommends using FSE imaging with PD-weighted imaging with or without fat saturation, T2-weighted imaging with or without fat saturation, or

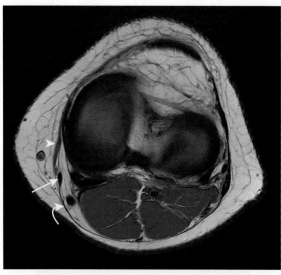

FIG 5.34 The Pes Anserinus Axial PD image demonstrates the normal-appearing, low-signal sartorius *(white arrowhead)*, gracilis *(straight white arrow)*, and semitendinosus *(curved white arrow)* tendons coursing anteriorly and inferiorly along the medial aspect of the knee at the level of the knee joint toward their insertion on the anteromedial aspect of the tibia.

T1-weighted gradient echo imaging for the evaluation of both native and repaired cartilage.[55]

The articular cartilage of the femorotibial joint covers the entirety of the femoral condyles and the tibial plateau. The femoral cartilage anterior to the anterior horns is termed the *trochlear cartilage*. This cartilage articulates with the patella. Posteriorly on the femoral condyles is cartilage that is not in contact with the tibia during routine MRI. During flexion, this surface contacts the tibial surface. It is important not to overlook cartilaginous defects in this region. The cartilage of the patellofemoral joint is evaluated in both the axial and sagittal planes. Patellar cartilage represents the thickest cartilage in the body. Axial PD FSE sequences, either with or without fat saturation, display it nicely. The patellar cartilage comprises medial and lateral facets, as well as a median ridge (patellar apex). The medial facet sometimes contains an extra flat surface termed the odd facet. The trochlear cartilage is better evaluated in the sagittal plane, because of its obliquity within the axial plane (Fig. 5.35A to D).

On non–fat-suppressed FSE images performed with an intermediate TE, the zonal architecture of the articular cartilage will be apparent. The deep zone will appear hypointense because of the closely aligned collagen fibers of the radial zone, which are highly ordered and markedly restrict water mobility. Water is less restricted in the middle and superficial zones, which have more randomly ordered collagen fibers. Thus these areas have a higher signal compared with the deep zone and subchondral bone. This subtly increasing signal is referred to as gray-scale stratification.[55] The most superficial layer of cartilage, the so-called lamina splendins, is extremely thin and is not visible at clinically relevant field strengths.

Arthroplasty. When proper image acquisition technique is used, MRI allows for detailed evaluation of the prosthesis-bone interface, as well as the surrounding soft tissues, synovium, and capsular supporting structures. Common arthroplasty complications including, polyethylene wear-induced synovitis, periprosthetic osteolysis, and implant loosening are all well evaluated (Figs. 5.36 to 5.38). Additional complications, such as arthrofibrosis, infection, component malalignment, extensor mechanism injuries, and periprosthetic fractures are also readily assessed.[18]

Safety. When used appropriately, MRI is an extremely safe imaging modality. An MRI examination causes no pain, and the

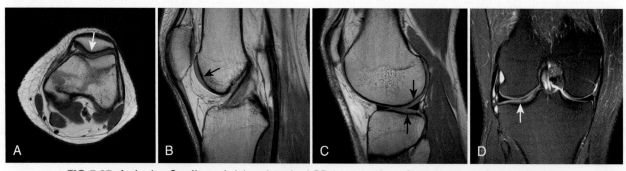

FIG 5.35 Articular Cartilage Axial and sagittal PD images (A to C) and coronal fat-suppressed PD image (D) demonstrating normal patellar (A), trochlear (B), and femorotibial articular cartilage (C and D). Note the higher signal in the middle and superficial zones compared with the deep zone and subchondral bone. This is normal and is referred to as gray scale stratification.

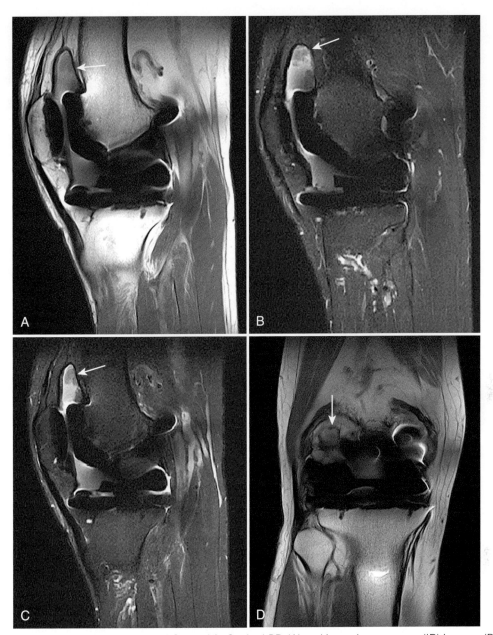

FIG 5.36 Polyethylene-Induced Synovitis Sagittal PD (A) and inversion recovery (IR) images (B and C) using a metal reduction protocol demonstrate a moderate-sized knee effusion with confluent and nodular synovial debris in the suprapatellar pouch *(white arrow)* in this patient who is status post total knee arthroplasty. The findings are more conspicuous on the IR sequence because of fat suppression technique *(white arrow)*. A coronal PD image (D) in the same patient shows a small area of osteolysis along the superior as aspect of the femoral component in the laterally femoral condyle *(white arrow)*.

magnetic fields produce no known tissue damage of any kind. The MR scanner may make loud tapping or knocking noises during the procedure. However, using earplugs usually alleviates problems associated with these noises. In addition, some patients who are claustrophobic may not tolerate being in the bore of the magnet long enough to complete an MRI examination, or may require anti-anxiolytic medication prior to imaging.

However, an MRI scanner is an extremely powerful magnet, and therefore great care is taken to be certain ferromagnetic metallic objects are not brought into the MR system area. In addition, it is vital that patients remove any metallic belongings in advance of an MRI exam, including hearing aids, watches, jewelry, and items of clothing that have metallic threads or fasteners. Makeup, nail polish, or other cosmetics that may contain metallic particles also should be removed. Some patients that have implanted metallic devices, such as spinal cord stimulators, cardiac pacemakers, or ferromagnetic aneurysm clips, are not able to undergo MRI exams because the powerful magnet filed may cause these devices to malfunction and much more importantly may cause severe injury to the patient.[66]

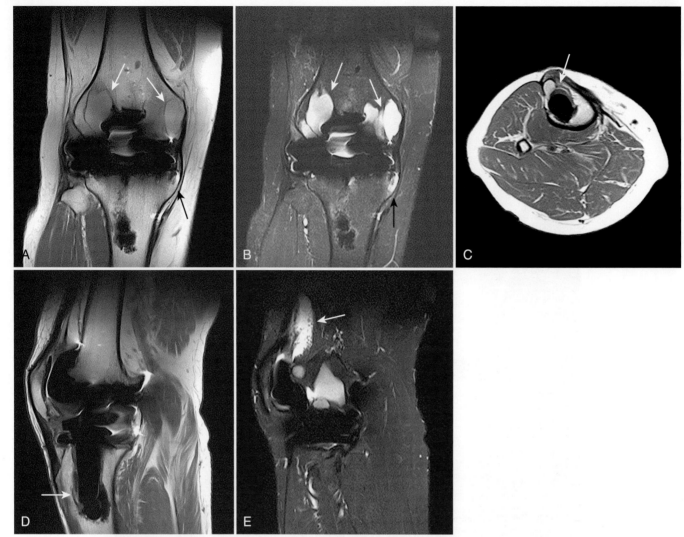

FIG 5.37 Femoral and Tibial Osteolysis With Component Loosening Coronal PD (A) and inversion recovery (IR) images (B) using a metal reduction protocol demonstrate large area of osteolysis surrounding the femoral component *(white arrow)* and small area of osteolysis in the medial tibial plateau *(black arrow)* in this patient who is status post total knee arthroplasty. Axial and sagittal PD sequences (images C and D) in the same patient show near circumferential intermediate-to-high signal surrounding the keel of the tibial component also consistent with osteolysis *(white arrow)*. The tibial component was noted be loose during revision arthroplasty. Inversion recovery (IR) sagittal image (E) showing particulate and nodular synovial debris in the suprapatellar pouch consistent with polyethylene-induced synovitis *(white arrow)*.

ULTRASOUND

Applications

Ultrasound of the knee excels in evaluation of the popliteal fossa. Vascular structures, such as popliteal artery aneurysms, can be fully depicted, and their flow characteristics analyzed. Popliteal cysts can also be imaged, often with the goal of ultrasound-guided aspiration (Fig. 5.39). Another application of ultrasound is evaluation of the extensor mechanism. A range of maladies, such as patellar tendon tears and prepatellar bursitis, may be identified. Ultrasound also may be used to evaluate patients with meniscal and parameniscal symptoms. The availability of high-frequency, high-resolution linear transducers permits diagnosis and treatment of symptomatic parameniscal cysts.[11,13,49]

Technique

Ultrasound, as the name implies, aims high-frequency sound waves through tissue to form an image. The transducer acts as both the emitter and receiver of the signal. The image represents a map of how much sound is reflected to the transducer from each location in an imaging plane (ie, depth). Bright (echogenic) objects, such as calcifications, strongly reflect the ultrasound beam. Substances such as water allow the sound waves to pass through easily and reflect little signal. As a result simple fluid appears dark (hypoechoic). The contrast in the images represents how much (or little) of the sound wave is reflected back to the transducer by any two adjacent tissues. The ultrasound machine uses high-level math and the speed of sound to map the signals it receives, thereby forming a 2D image.

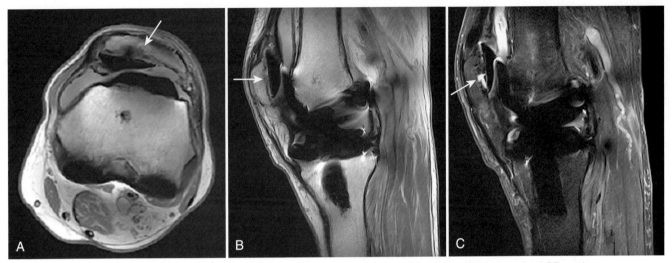

FIG 5.38 Loose Patellar Component With Migration Axial PD image (A) and sagittal PD and inversion recover (IR) images (B and C) demonstrate a 2- to 3-mm rim of osteolysis undermining the patellar backing in the patient who is status post total knee arthroplasty *(white arrow)*. The component has migrated superiorly and medially which is indicative of loosening.

Image Interpretation

Ultrasound is heavily operator dependent. Therefore views are labeled according to their location and plane of imaging to orient those interpreting the images. Ultrasound affords great freedom in scanning. A handheld probe is used to investigate a structure in real time at virtually any angle, allowing appreciation of its relationship to other nearby anatomy. Cine clips are short movies saved during an examination that allow valuable segments of the real-time examination to be reviewed on the PACS.

Artifacts and Special Considerations

Ultrasound artifacts may be broadly separated into technical and tissue factors. If recognized, technical artifacts may be addressed while scanning (and hopefully eliminated). As for artifacts intrinsic to the tissue, strong reflectors, such as bone, calcium, and metal, distort the sound wave, thereby altering its return course to the transducer. This results in a variety of appearances, such as reverberation artifact. Interfaces between two very different tissues also disrupt ultrasound transmission. This may create a mirror image artifact.

Safety

Concerns regarding ultrasound safety are minimal, particularly in the extremities. It is notable that high-intensity exposure may cause tissue heating, but this is rarely, if ever, a factor when imaging the knee.

NUCLEAR MEDICINE

Applications

Nuclear medicine has myriad applications. Examinations of the knee are requested for occult fractures, stress injuries, infection, arthroplasty complications, arthritis, metabolic bone disease, and tumor workup. Bone scanning is also frequently used to image the entire skeleton to determine the presence and distribution of osseous metastatic disease.

Nuclear medicine scans of the knee are complementary to anatomic studies, such as radiographs, CT scans, or MRI. It is useful to have correlative examinations available while interpreting a bone scan because this helps to localize abnormal radiotracer activity. Bone scans may also elucidate pathology not visible on other modalities, such as osteomyelitis and occult fracture.

Technique

In contrast to anatomic imaging, nuclear medicine stands out in its ability to capture and characterize physiologic processes, such as increased blood flow, abnormal lung ventilation, or altered renal function. Rather than pass an x-ray beam through a patient, nuclear scintigraphy relies on injecting a radiopharmaceutical and measuring the resulting gamma ray emissions coming from within the patient. A radiopharmaceutical is a combination of a tracer and a radioisotope. A tracer is a substance whose uptake, distribution, and metabolism are predictable. For example, a phosphate analogue, such as diphosphonate (MDP), is preferentially taken up by bone. A tracer may consist of the patient's own cells. For example, labeled white blood cells (WBCs) may be used to seek out inflammation or infection.

Radioisotopes are usually byproducts of nuclear power plants. These radioactive molecules emit gamma rays as they decay, providing measurable emissions to create an image. Examples include technetium-99m (Tc-99m) and indium-111 (In-111). Each radioisotope is characterized by a distinctive half-life and gamma ray energy (measured in kiloelectron volt). Half-life is important because it guides imaging time and helps to determine radiation exposure to the patient. A short half-life, 6 hours in cases of Tc-99m, necessitates imaging within a few hours. The later imaging is attempted, the fewer gamma rays will be available for detection. Conversely, a longer half-life, such as 2.8 days for In-111, allows imaging over several days. Radiation exposure is directly related to half-life (physical *and* biologic). A relatively short half-life means that the radioisotope exposes the patient to less radiation. In general, if the half-life is longer, radiation exposure is higher.

Images are acquired with cameras sensitive to the gamma rays emitted by the radioisotopes. This is known as scintigraphy. In brief, a gamma camera performs three complementary functions. It converts a gamma ray into light, assigns a location to this emission, and counts the number of emissions from a particular location over time. As the number of counts increases for a given position, the image reflects more activity at this location. The number of counts a gamma camera receives is related to the amount of pharmaceutical administered and the length of time the patient spends under the camera. It may take 30 minutes or longer to acquire sufficient counts to generate a diagnostic image. The anatomy of interest should be as close to the camera as possible to get the maximum counts within the shortest time. If pathology of the patella is suspected, the camera should be positioned anterior to the knee. If a popliteal process is being investigated, the camera is positioned posterior to the knee. Some gamma cameras simultaneously obtain images in anterior and posterior projections.

Most nuclear medicine images are planar (ie, 2D) frontal or oblique projections. The spatial resolution of nuclear medicine images is inherently restricted by a number of factors beyond discussion in this review. Small or closely positioned structures may not be readily identified or delineated.

Single-photon emission CT is a technique used to acquire a dataset in multiple planes, similar to a CT scan. A special camera that rotates around the patient is required. Additional imaging time is necessary, as compared with standard, static planar images. Once complete, the area of interest can be manipulated on the viewing station so that abnormalities can be more precisely localized. This is particularly helpful around hardware and in the spine.

Multiple examinations may be performed to further heighten diagnostic specificity. For example, a Tc-99m sulfur colloid (SC) performed in tandem with an In-111 WBC scan increases the specificity of the WBC scan when evaluating a joint prosthesis for infection.

Technetium 99m-Methylene Diphosphonate Scan.

The Tc-99m-MDP (Tc-MDP) bone scan is the most commonly performed nuclear medicine examination for orthopedic purposes. Imaging may be performed in one or three phases. For a single-phase scan, delayed planar images are acquired 2 or 3 hours after administration of the radiotracer. This type of examination is commonly requested for metastatic disease, primary bone tumors, and metabolic disease. A three-phase scan involves acquiring images immediately and within several minutes of radioisotope dispensation. These first two phases, blood flow and blood pool, respectively, yield information about perfusion to bones and joints, as well as periosseous and periarticular soft tissues. Standard delayed whole body and spot images are obtained 2 or 3 hours later, similar to the single-phase examination, and reflect bone metabolic activity. The three-phase examination is helpful when osteomyelitis, septic arthritis, aseptic synovitis, or fractures are diagnostic considerations.

Timed images, such as the blood flow and blood pool phases, rely upon the appearance (or cessation) of activity within an appropriate time window. A normal blood flow phase reveals expected arterial activity without focal activity in the bone. A normal blood pool phase has no increased bone or soft tissue activity. A normal delayed phase reveals symmetrical osseous distribution of radioisotope.

The mechanism of action of Tc-MDP is chemisorption. Tc-MDP is taken up by cortical bone and is bound to the hydroxyapatite crystal. The degree of delayed skeletal uptake is largely determined by ongoing bone formation and blood flow.[22] Areas of abnormally increased bone turnover (whether secondary to fracture, infection, inflammation, arthritis, metabolic bone disease or neoplasm, etc.) will have increased uptake relative to the remainder of the surrounding skeleton.

In all phases of imaging, it is critical to compare for symmetry. This includes comparing the right and left knees, as well as analogous structures within a single knee, such as the medial and lateral femoral condyles. Skeletally immature patients have normally increased activity at the physes (Fig. 5.40A and B). Notably, implants appear as photopenic defects.

Labeled White Blood Cell Scan.

Labeled WBC scans augment the workup of suspected infection, whether it be osteomyelitis, septic arthritis, or soft tissue abscess. The specificity and sensitivity of this examination are superior to gallium-67 citrate. WBCs are isolated from a sample of the patient's blood, labeled in vitro with In-111 (or Tc-99m), and reinjected into the patient. Images may be obtained 3 or 4 hours later. Some departments image at 24 hours. A normal scan demonstrates no focal area of increased uptake. Abnormal radioisotope deposition indicates inflammation or infection with sensitivity and specificity approaching 90%. Most labeled cells are neutrophils and therefore have a strong predilection for sites of bacterial infection.

In the presence of infection, blood work for C-reactive protein and erythrocyte sedimentation rate is often elevated. For the exclusion of septic arthritis, knee aspiration is preferred because it has the highest specificity and sensitivity. Aspirate is sent for cell count with differential, Gram stain, and culture and sensitivity. In equivocal cases, nuclear medicine scanning can be useful.

Labeled leukocyte imaging is the radionuclide procedure of choice for diagnosing so-called complicating osteomyelitis. It often must be performed in conjunction with bone marrow (Tc-SC) scanning to maximize specificity and accuracy.[48] Normal labeled leukocyte scans have a high negative predictive value for infection.

Although the sensitivity and negative predictive value of indium-WBC scans are very high, approaching 95% and 100%, respectively, a positive indium scan, in and of itself, is of limited value.[41] This dilemma is addressed by performing the labeled WBC scan in conjunction with a Tc-99m SC scan.

Technetium-99m Sulfur Colloid Scan.

A Tc-99m SC scan is used as a problem-solving tool. It complements the In-111 WBC scan, increasing specificity and accuracy for diagnosing infection after total knee arthroplasty.[48] Imaging occurs within a few hours of injection. Tc-99m SC localizes to the reticuloendothelial system: bone marrow, liver, and spleen.

The rationale behind Tc-99m SC examination is that accumulation of In-111 WBCs may occur in infection or hyperplastic marrow. Hyperplastic marrow is a relatively common finding after arthroplasty implantation. Tc-99m SC differentiates these two entities because it will localize to reactive marrow but not to a site of infection. Thus, if results are congruous on both In-111 WBC and Tc-99m SC scans, infection is unlikely (Fig. 5.41A and B). On the contrary, increased activity on the In-111 WBC scan, as compared with Tc-99m SC images, indicates a high likelihood of infection (>90%).[41]

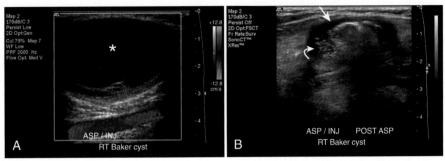

FIG 5.39 Ultrasound images performed before (A) and after (B) ultrasound-guided aspiration and injection of a Baker cyst *(asterisk)*. Postprocedure image (B) demonstrates the collapsed cyst *(straight arrow)* with small dependent echogenic foci *(curved arrow)* reflecting injected steroid and anesthetic.

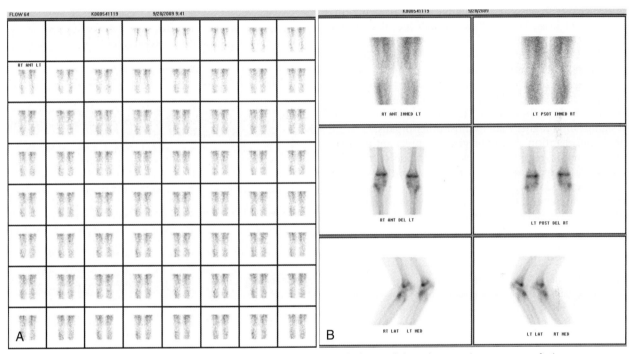

FIG 5.40 Normal triple-phase technetium-99m methylene diphosphonate bone scan of the knees, demonstrating normal blood flow (A), normal blood pool (top two images of B), and delayed skeletal uptake of radiotracer (bottom four images of B). Symmetrical areas of increased uptake in the physeal regions bilaterally reflect ossification at the growth plates in this skeletally immature patient.

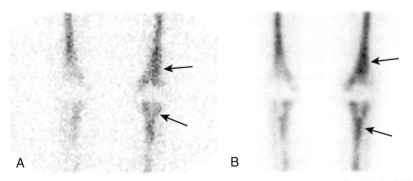

FIG 5.41 A 71-year-old male with bilateral total knee arthroplasties, left side in 2000 and right side in 2002, with pain on the left side. Apparent asymmetrical and increased uptake on the indium-111–labeled white blood cell scan in the distal left femur and proximal tibia (A) *(arrows)* is related to marrow expansion and *not* infection, as demonstrated by matching (congruent) areas of uptake on the technetium (Tc)-sulfur colloid scan (B) *(arrows)*.

Gallium-67 Citrate Scan. Gallium-67 citrate scans have largely been replaced by labeled leukocyte scans and are less commonly performed. Images are acquired 48 and 72 hours after injection. This radioisotope acts as both a calcium and iron analogue, resulting in its incorporation into bone and bone marrow. It localizes to sites of infection or inflammation, in part because it binds the iron-carrying proteins transferrin and lactoferrin. Gallium was traditionally used in the evaluation of infection, particularly chronic osteomyelitis and septic arthritis. In the setting of a normal WBC count, labeled leukocyte scans are preferred because they have higher sensitivity and specificity. In the immunocompromised patient (WBC < 2000) or for spinal infection, gallium scanning may be favored.[48]

Safety

Nuclear medicine uses ionizing radiation. The patient is exposed from the time the radiotracer is administered until it has decayed sufficiently to become a negligible source of radiation, at least four half-lives. For Tc-99m the half-life of 6 hours renders radiation exposure negligible after 24 hours for a standard 20 mCi dose. In-111 has a longer half-life of 2.8 days, resulting in greater radiation exposure.

Specific organs may receive disproportionate radiation exposure. For example, Tc-MDP is primarily eliminated via the kidneys and collects in the bladder. Therefore bladder exposure may be significantly higher than in most other organs.

Careful consideration should be given to pregnant women and children before requesting nuclear medicine scans. The dose to the fetus may be particularly high if the radiopharmaceutical is excreted via the genitourinary tract, given the bladder's proximity to the uterus. Consultation with a radiologist or nuclear medicine physician is recommended.

KEY REFERENCES

5. Beall D, Googe J, Moss J, et al: Magnetic resonance imaging of the collateral ligaments and the anatomic quadrants of the knee. *Radiol Clin North Am* 45:983–1002, 2007.

13. De Maeseneer M, Vanderdood K, Marcelis S, et al: Sonography of the medial and lateral tendons and ligaments of the knee: the use of bony landmarks as an easy method for identification. *AJR Am J Roentgenol* 178:1437–1444, 2002.

14. DeSmet AA, Norris MA, Yandow DR, et al: MR diagnosis of meniscal tears of the knee: importance of high signal in the meniscus that extends to the surface. *AJR Am J Roentgenol* 161:101, 1993.

18. Fritz J, Lurie B, Potter HG: MR imaging of knee arthroplasty implants. *Radiographics* 35(5):1483–1501, 2015.

19. Fox M: MR imaging of the meniscus: review, current trends, and clinical implications. *Radiol Clin North Am* 45:1033–1053, 2007.

23. Greenspan A: *Orthopedic imaging, a practical approach*, ed 4, Philadelphia, 2004, Lippincott Williams & Wilkins.

26. Hargreaves BA, Worters PW, Pauly KB, et al: Metal-induced artifacts in MRI. *AJR Am J Roentgenol* 197(3):547–555, 2011.

39. Manester BJ, Roberts CC, Andrews CL, et al: *Diagnostic and surgical imaging anatomy: musculoskeletal*, ed 1, Philadelphia, 2006, Lippincott Williams & Wilkins.

41. Math KR, Zaidi SF, Petchprapa C, et al: Imaging of total knee arthroplasty. *Semin Musculoskelet Radiol* 10:47–63, 2006.

42. Merchant AC, Mercer RL, Jacobsoen RH, et al: Roentgengraphic analysis of patellofemoral congruence. *J Bone Joint Surg Am* 56:1391, 1974.

48. Palestro CJ, Love C: Radionuclide imaging of musculoskeletal infection, conventional agents. *Semin Musculoskelet Radiol* 11:336–339, 2007.

49. Parker L, Nazarian NL, Carino JA, et al: AIUM practice guidelines: musculoskeletal ultrasound. <http://www.aium.org/publications/guidelines/musculoskeletal.pdf>, 2007.

53. Roberts CC, Towers JD, Spangehl MJ, et al: Advanced MR imaging of the cruciate ligaments. *Radiol Clin North Am* 45:1003–1016, 2007.

54. Rosenberg TD, Paulos LE, Parker RD, et al: The forty-five degree posterior anterior flexion weightbearing radiograph of the knee. *J Bone Joint Surg Am* 70:1479, 1988.

55. Shindle MK, Foo LF, Kelly BT, et al: Magnetic resonance imaging of cartilage in the athlete: current techniques and spectrum of disease. *J Bone Joint Surg Am* 88(Suppl 4):27–46, 2006.

62. Stoller DW, Li AE, Anderson LJ, et al: The knee. In Stoller DW, editor: *Magnetic resonance imaging in orthopedics and sports medicine*, ed 3, Philadelphia, 2007, Lippincott Williams & Wilkins.

The references for this chapter can also be found on www.expertconsult.com.

6

Fractures

Michael B. Mechlin

DIAGNOSIS AND IMAGING PROTOCOLS

Radiography

Trauma to the knee is a relatively common injury, accounting for a significant number of visits to emergency rooms, urgicenters, and orthopedic offices. However, not all of these knee injuries will present as fractures. When evaluating trauma to the knee and potential fractures about the knee, conventional radiographs have been, and should continue to be, the first approach. Rules have been devised to select the patients for whom radiographs should be obtained.[56,57] The Ottawa decision rule for radiography in acute knee trauma includes any of the following indications: patient 55 years or older, tenderness at the head of the fibula, isolated tenderness of the patella, inability to flex 90 degrees, or inability to bear weight immediately following injury and in the emergency department. The presence of one or more of these findings has identified those patients who are more than likely to have a fracture and has reduced the number of radiographic examinations.[57]

The standard radiographic examination for knee trauma should include at least four projections: anteroposterior (AP), lateral, and 45-degree internal and external rotation oblique projections, with the following caveat that if patella trauma is suspected, then an axial or tangential view of the patella should be performed. In addition, a tunnel frontal projection (or notch view) may be of benefit if trauma to the intercondylar notch or posterior aspect of the knee is suspected. The AP view generally will allow for adequate evaluation of the distal femur (including the medial and lateral femoral condyles) and the proximal tibia (including the medial and lateral tibial plateaux and tibial spines, as well as the proximal fibula, although the head of the fibula may be overlapped by the lateral margin of the tibia on the AP view). In addition, the tibial plateaux slope posteriorly and are not visualized tangentially on this projection. The oblique views may be helpful if there are obliquely oriented fractures involving the tibial plateaux or femoral condyles or an avulsion fracture of the fibula head and may be the only views to demonstrate those fractures. A tunnel view obtained in the posteroanterior projection with the knee flexed may be useful to evaluate the posterior femoral condyles and posterior tibial plateaux; because it provides a clear look into the intercondylar notch, it may provide the best way to see fractures of the intercondylar eminences and tibial spines and to evaluate for ossific bodies and fracture fragments within the knee joint. The patella is not optimally evaluated on any of the above projections because it is superimposed upon the distal femur, but a lateral view as part of the standard radiographic series will generally be able to assess the patella/femoral relationship to evaluate for fractures of the patella (Fig. 6.1). The lateral view also has the benefit of providing assessment for a knee joint effusion (which cannot be reliably seen on any of the other views). If the lateral view is performed in the erect position or if a cross-table lateral view is performed with the patient supine, it can also demonstrate a fat-fluid level, indicating a lipohemarthrosis (Fig. 6.2), which is highly suggestive of an intra-articular fracture in which blood and marrow fat escape into the joint space.[7] If patella trauma is suspected, in addition to the lateral view, an axial or tangential view of the patella will often be necessary and to assess for any patellar dislocation and to diagnose longitudinal fractures of the patella in the sagittal plane that will be missed on the conventional lateral view (Fig. 6.3).

Computed Tomography

Computed tomography (CT) is typically acquired in the axial plane, preferably with thin axial slices and processed with a bone algorithm to provide maximum spatial resolution. Reconstructed images are then obtained in the coronal and sagittal planes and are an important adjunct in the evaluation of knee fractures. Three-dimensional (3D) reconstructions can be created, providing the orthopedic surgeon with a global view of complex fractures, and is frequently used in preoperative planning. One advantage is the ability to perform the examination through splints and casts, which often limit the radiographic examination for detection of the subtle minimally displaced or nondisplaced fractures (Fig. 6.4). Thus CT has a role in the evaluation of knee trauma for those patients in whom a fracture is suspected based on clinical findings or on the basis of a cross-table lateral radiograph demonstrating a lipohemarthrosis and in which no fracture is demonstrated on the initial set of radiographs. In addition, CT will better visualize the degree of comminution of an already detected fracture. With the use of coronal and sagittal reconstructions, CT can give a more accurate delineation of the degree of depression of the articular surfaces, especially important in the evaluation of tibial plateau fractures (Fig. 6.5).[32] CT may help in evaluating for subtle articular surface injuries, such as osteochondral injuries, which may not be apparent on the plain film radiographs.

Magnetic Resonance Imaging

Magnetic resonance imaging (MRI), as is well established, is the imaging modality of choice to evaluate for soft tissue injuries about the knee, including cruciate and collateral ligament injuries, meniscal injuries, and quadriceps and other muscle and tendon injuries. However, MRI also has a role in the diagnosis of knee fractures. Because of its ability to detect bone marrow edema, it can easily diagnose areas of bone contusion or bone

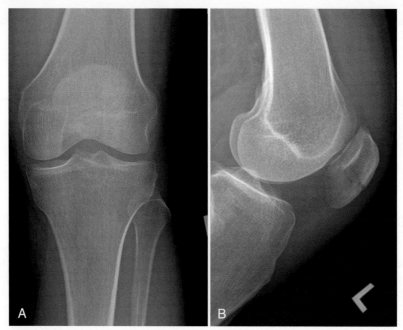

FIG 6.1 Patellar Fracture AP radiograph (A) does not demonstrate the patella fracture, but the lateral radiograph (B) clearly shows a nondisplaced transverse patella fracture.

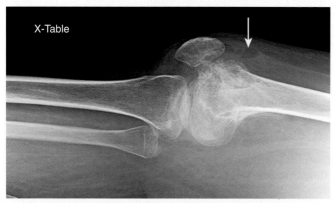

FIG 6.2 Lipohemarthrosis Cross-table lateral radiograph demonstrates fat-fluid levels in a patient with a supracondylar femoral fracture, indicating the presence of a lipohemarthrosis *(white arrow)*.

bruise due to direct trauma. Within the bone marrow edema pattern, MRI can find occult fractures that are nondisplaced or that were missed or not identified on the initial radiographic or CT examinations (Fig. 6.6).[7,10] In addition, because of its ability to see the ligaments, MRI can often demonstrate or better define ligamentous avulsion fractures. MRI also is vastly superior to radiographs to evaluate osteochondral fractures of the joint surface and is the modality of choice to diagnose early stress or insufficiency fractures, which often are not apparent on radiographs, CT, or even bone scintigraphy.[18]

Angiography

In the cases in which there is high-energy trauma causing dislocations of the knee or in those patients with supracondylar fractures or markedly displaced tibial fractures, angiographic evaluation of the status of the popliteal artery is often required,

prior to surgical fixation.[54] The popliteal artery may be injured by displaced or angulated fracture fragments. If there is a pulseless, cold extremity distal to the knee fracture site or if there is suspicion for decreased pulse and coolness of the lower extremity, the status of the arterial system should be assessed. In the presence of an arterial injury the artery must be repaired as soon as possible, and if there is definitive clinical evidence of an arterial injury, repair should not be delayed for the performance of an arteriographic examination in the radiology department, but rather the examination can be performed by percutaneous femoral artery injection in the operating room at the time of the reduction of the fracture or dislocation. If it is a nonemergent situation and there is only possible arterial injury, the popliteal artery can be evaluated by conventional radiographic angiography. More recently, both CT angiography and MR angiography may play a role in evaluating the arterial system in nonemergent situations.[42,58]

DISTAL FEMORAL FRACTURES

Incidence and Etiology

The incidence of distal femoral fractures has a bimodal distribution—young adults with high-energy injuries and elderly patients with lower-energy injuries. Distal femoral fractures occur less commonly than fractures of the proximal femur, accounting for approximately 6% of all femoral fractures.[13,33] The supracondylar fracture in young adults typically results from a large external force, such as that from a motor vehicle collision, a fall from a height with axial loading, or other heavy industrial accidents.[33] The amount of energy required to cause a distal femoral or supracondylar fracture in young patients with no existing bone pathology is usually significant. Thus there is often fracture comminution and displacement (Fig. 6.7), and the fracture is often seen in conjunction with other associated fractures and ligamentous injuries.[8] Intra-articular extension into the knee joint is common from these injuries,

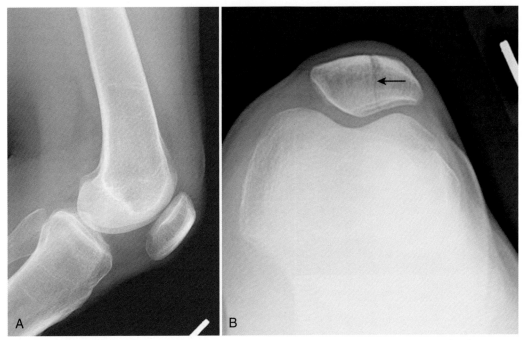

FIG 6.3 Sagittally Oriented Longitudinal Patella Fracture Lateral radiograph (A) does not demonstrate a fracture, but the sagitally oriented nondisplaced fracture *(black arrow)* is seen on the sunrise view (B).

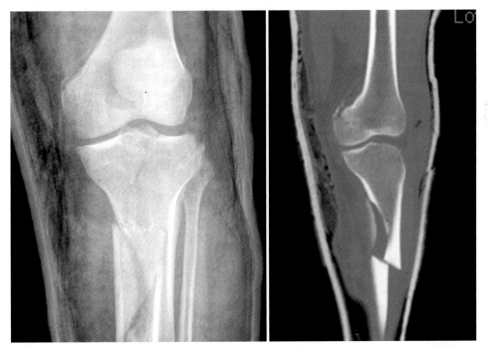

FIG 6.4 (A) AP radiograph performed through a splint demonstrates the comminuted proximal tibial fracture, but the reconstructed coronal CT image (B) better demonstrates the additional medial femoral condyle fracture.

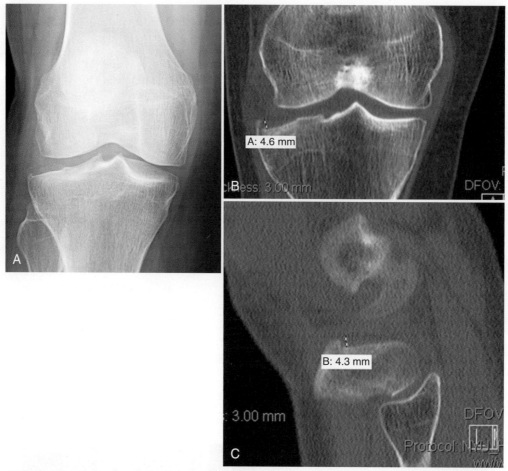

FIG 6.5 AP radiograph (A) visualizes some depression of the lateral tibial plateau, but the CT reconstructed in the coronal (B) and sagittal (C) planes better demonstrates the amount of depression.

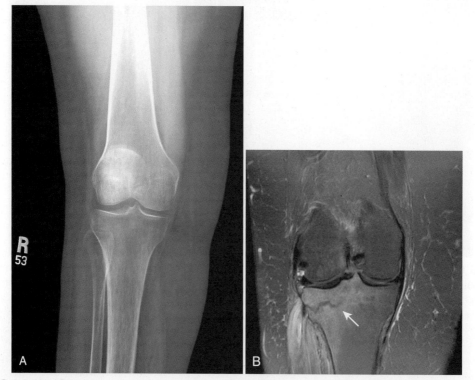

FIG 6.6 (A) AP radiograph of the knee does not demonstrate any tibial fracture, but (B) coronal fat-suppressed T2-weighted image of the knee performed 1 week later demonstrates linear low-signal *(white arrow)* with surrounding marrow edema consistent with an occult fracture.

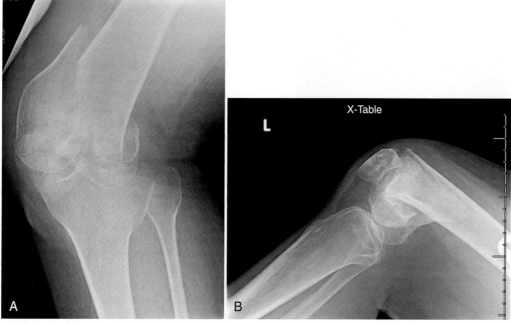

FIG 6.7 Supracondylar Fracture AP (A) and cross-table lateral (B) radiographs demonstrate a displaced and posteriorly angulated supracondylar fracture.

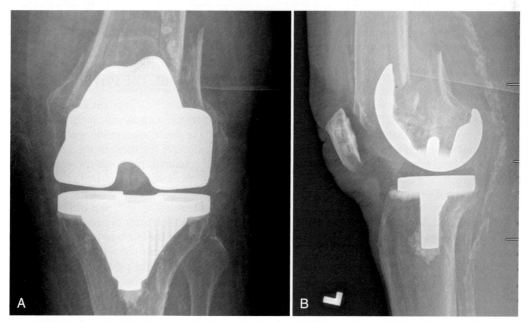

FIG 6.8 Periprosthetic Fracture Radiographs in the AP (A) and lateral (B) projections demonstrate the fracture at the superior aspect of the femoral component of a total knee arthroplasty.

and this is important to know in planning the therapeutic approach. In elderly patients, lower-energy injuries, such as that sustained with low-level falls, or twisting injuries can cause these fractures because of underlying osteopenia or osteoporosis or in those patients with prosthetic devices or other metallic implants because of stress shielding in the transition area between the prosthesis and native bone. Examples include the area just proximal to a total knee arthroplasty (Fig. 6.8) or the area distal to a long femoral nail or long stem hip prosthesis (Fig. 6.9). Bedridden and wheelchair-bound patients generally

have decreased bone density in the femoral bones due to the lack of activity and stress placed on these bones (Wolff's law) and thus are at increased risk for a distal femoral fracture through falls from a bed or wheelchair during transfer.

Classification

Numerous classification schemes have been proposed in the past to categorize distal femoral fractures. One commonly used system is one developed by the Orthopedic Trauma Association[40]: type A, extra-articular; type B, unicondylar; and type C,

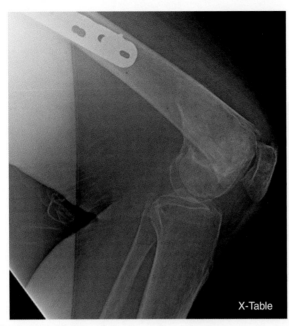

X-Table

FIG 6.9 Lateral view of the knee demonstrates a supracondylar fracture of the femur distal to a femoral plate.

bicondylar, which is further subdivided by the degree of comminution (Fig. 6.10). The type C or bicondylar fractures can be T or Y shaped with the vertically oriented component extending down into the intercondylar notch. In this type the condyles may become widely separated.

Although most of the distal femoral fractures will fall into the previously mentioned grouping, there are other types of fracture of the distal femur that are not as easily categorized by the previously mentioned scheme. These include the osteochondral (or chondral) impaction fracture of the articular surface of the distal femoral condyle (Fig. 6.11), usually resulting from a shearing force or axial impaction. This may result in a cartilaginous fragment originating from the articular surface, with varying degrees of attached subchondral bone. The resultant fragment may remain in situ or may become displaced, if unstable, and may be a loose body in the joint. The appearance may be similar to the lesion of osteochondritis dissecans (OCD), which has an unclear etiology but may result from repetitive trauma and which classically involves the medial femoral condyle but also can be seen in the lateral femoral condyle.[7] In addition, subchondral insufficiency fracture (previously known as spontaneous osteonecrosis of the knee [SONK]) with a predilection for the weight-bearing surface of the medial femoral condyle can occur. This is often seen in osteoporotic individuals with minimal trauma or in those who have altered mechanics related to meniscal tears (Fig. 6.12).[20]

Imaging Diagnosis

As with any fracture, orthogonal AP and lateral radiographs of the knee are the barest minimum that needs to be done if there is suspicion for a supracondylar fracture. However, it is advisable to obtain both femur and knee radiographs to fully evaluate the fracture and to determine the proximal extent of the fracture, as well as to assess for segmental fracture patterns and exclude additional fractures.[13] In addition, oblique views of the knee are often necessary to visualize nondisplaced or minimally displaced supracondylar or condylar fractures and should be

part of the routine radiographic series in the setting of trauma. The lateral view is most helpful in identifying coronal condylar intra-articular fractures (Hoffa fractures), which must not be missed because the presence of such coronal splits influences the selection of fixation devices.[4,25]

CT with axial scans and sagittal and coronal reconstructions is indicated as an additional study for all comminuted fractures to better localize the fracture fragments. In addition, CT should be performed if there is concern that all fracture lines, including intra-articular extension, cannot be adequately visualized on the provided radiographs. This would include the previously mentioned Hoffa fractures, many of which are not seen with radiographs alone. Osteochondral impaction fractures can be seen on plain film radiographs, especially if the fragment is displaced but may be better visualized and detailed with CT or MRI.

To diagnose a chondral fracture if it involves only the articular cartilage without the subjacent bone, MRI would be necessary. In addition, MRI would provide a more thorough evaluation of OCD lesions, in that it can more accurately detect the depth of the lesion and the involvement of the subchondral bone,[38] and there are guidelines on MRI to determine whether the OCD lesion is stable or not.[14,43] In addition, MRI would be the modality of choice to make the diagnosis of a subchondral insufficiency fracture in the femoral condyle articular surface. Many other traumatic conditions about the distal femur, such as bone bruises or contusions and nondisplaced fractures confined to the intramedullary bone, would not be detected on radiographs and would require MRI to make the diagnosis (Fig. 6.13).

FRACTURES OF THE PHYSIS

Although children can sustain displaced fractures of the supracondylar femur with significant trauma, the physis or growth plate is the most susceptible portion of the bone in these patients. Physeal fractures in the knee may occur at the distal femoral, proximal tibial, or proximal fibula growth plates. However, those that occur in the distal femur are the most common and are the most significant because of the potential for growth disturbance[30,47] and will be discussed here. The prognosis for such fractures depends on such factors as the age of the patient and the fracture type and location.

The Salter-Harris classification system[47] is used to describe fractures involving the physis everywhere in the childhood skeleton. Five types of Salter-Harris fractures are described. Type I fractures are those that occur through the plane of the growth plate, with separation of the epiphysis from the metaphysis, without a fracture fragment, whereas type II and III fractures extend through the physeal plate for a variable distance and then exit through the metaphysis (type II) or epiphysis (type III). Thus these type III fractures are usually intra-articular fractures. All three of these types usually result from shearing or avulsive forces and carry more favorable prognoses than type IV or V. Salter-Harris type IV is an intra-articular fracture that extends from the joint through the epiphysis, across the thickness of the growth plate, and into portion of the metaphysis (Fig. 6.14). Type V fractures usually result from a severe crush injury to the physis, which may separate, and has the worst prognosis but is uncommon.

The diagnosis of physeal injury (especially types II to V) can usually be made from radiographs. However, type I fractures, although often evident on radiographs if there is severe

Types:

A. Extra-articular

Groups:

Femur, distal, extra-articular

A1. Simple   A2. Metaphyseal wedge   A3. Metaphyseal complex

B. Partial articular

Femur, distal, partial articular

B1. Lateral condyle, sagittal   B2. Medial condyle, sagittal   B3. Frontal

C. Complete articular

Femur, distal, complete articular

C1. Articular simple, metaphyseal simple   C2. Articular simple, metaphyseal multifragmentary   C3. Multifragmentary articular fracture

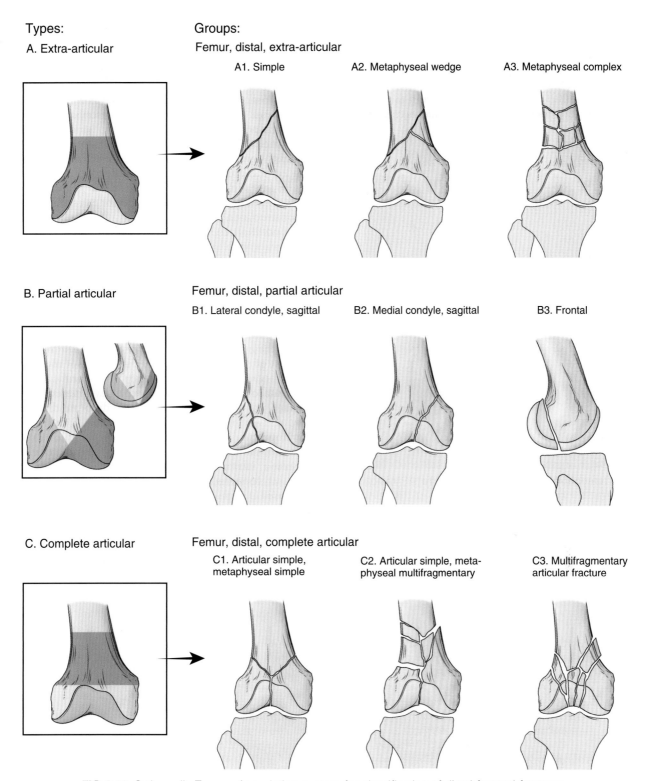

FIG 6.10 Orthopedic Trauma Association system for classification of distal femoral fractures.

widening of the physis, may be missed if there is only subtle widening of the physis. In those cases a comparison AP view of the contralateral knee may be of benefit to assess for any asymmetry. In addition, MRI has been used to detect subtle physeal injury, which is not as radiographically evident[23,30,38] because bone marrow edema may be evident on both sides of the physis (Fig. 6.15). However, one potential pitfall is what has been termed the focal periphyseal edema (FOPE) zone, a focal bone marrow edema pattern seen on MRI centered about the closing physis in adolescents, often associated with pain.[63] FOPE lesions are usually central in location, and because the physis are in the process of closing, the physes are usually narrowed in these patients, thus allowing for differentiating these lesions from Salter-Harris I fractures in most patients.

FRACTURES AND DISLOCATIONS OF THE PATELLA

Incidence and Etiology

The patella is prone to injury due to its superficial location, making it susceptible to a direct blow, and because the patella is subjected to significant contractive forces from the extensor mechanism, with falls and motor vehicle accidents constituting

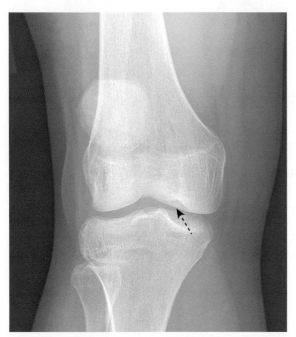

FIG 6.11 Osteochondral Impaction Fracture AP radiograph demonstrates an osteochondral impaction of the articular surface of the medial femoral condyle *(black interrupted arrow).*

the most common causes.[9] Direct trauma can result in a comminuted fracture, whereas excessive quadriceps contraction, such as that due to severe squatting, in otherwise native, nonoperative knees causes a distracted transverse fracture.[50] Patellar fractures have also been seen in chronic conditions where there is focal loss of bone due to erosions, such as that seen with gout.[2] Fractures of the patella have also been described in patients who are status post total knee arthroplasty[12,50,51] and status post anterior cruciate ligament (ACL) reconstruction, especially in those patients in which a portion of the patella and the infrapatellar tendon was used as graft for a bone-tendon-bone ACL reconstruction.[55] However, it is still rare following ACL reconstruction, with an incidence of 0.2% in one large series of ACL reconstructions.[31]

In addition, the fact that the patella maintains a small area of contact with the femur, especially with higher degrees of flexion, makes the patellofemoral relationship unstable. Throughout flexion the area of patella-femoral contact changes. Patella dislocation can result when there is internal rotation of the femur on a fixed, externally rotated tibia, such as what occurs when there is a sudden change in direction while running with the foot planted and the knee in a flexed valgus position.[48] When the quadriceps contracts, the patella then migrates laterally out of the trochlear groove. Dislocation of the patella may occur because of a traumatic tear in the medial patellar retinaculum or may be secondary to a developmental anatomic variant that would predispose one to dislocate the patella following even minor or incidental trauma. Examples of such developmental anomalies include abnormality of the position and shape of the patella, such as a high riding patella or patella dysplasia (flattened articular surface), abnormality of the femoral condyles, such as a shallow trochlear groove, an increased Q angle (the angle between vertical axis of the femoral shaft and that of the patella which is normally around 15%),

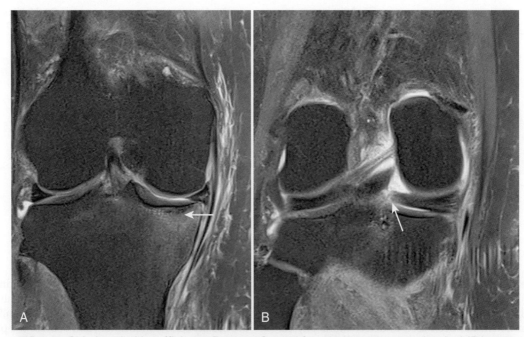

FIG 6.12 Subchondral Insufficiency Fracture Coronal fat-suppressed proton density MR image (A) demonstrates a subchondral insufficiency fracture *(white arrow)* in a patient with a posterior meniscal root tear *(white arrow)* seen on another coronal MR image more posteriorly (B).

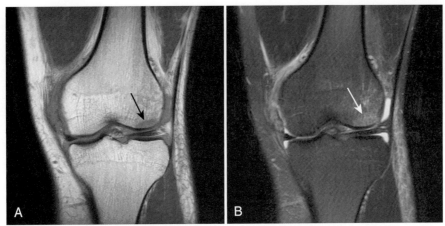

FIG 6.13 Bone Contusion on Magnetic Resonance Imaging Coronal T1-weighted (A) and coronal fat-suppressed T2-weighted (B) images demonstrate a focal area of low-signal intensity within the bone marrow in the subarticular region of the lateral femoral condyle on T1-weighted imaging *(black arrow)* with a corresponding region of increased signal intensity involving the same region on T2-weighted imaging *(white arrow)*.

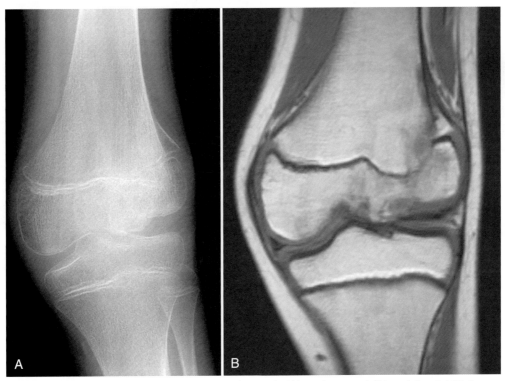

FIG 6.14 Salter-Harris IV Fracture AP radiograph (A) and coronal T1-weighted MR image (B) demonstrate the Harris IV fracture extending from the articular surface of the lateral femoral condyle cephalad through the epiphysis and growth plate and into the metaphysis with proximal displacement of the fracture fragment.

and a dysplastic distal one-third of the vastus medialis obliquus muscle.[16] These anomalies would make one susceptible to recurrent dislocations. Indeed, recurrent dislocation of the patella following relatively minor trauma or twisting injury in which the femur is internally rotated on a fixed, externally rotated tibia is considered to be more common than acute traumatic dislocation from direct blow to the side of the knee. Patella dislocation much more often occurs laterally, rather than medially, because of the normal valgus alignment of the knee,

as well as the relative weakness of the vastus medialis and the medial patellar retinaculum compared with the lateral stabilizers.[17,48] These patella dislocations may be transient and often are reduced spontaneously with the patella in appropriate position in the trochlea groove on subsequent imaging studies. The only imaging clue to the diagnosis of a lateral patellar dislocation may be a small bone fracture fragment at the medial aspect of the patella on the axial radiograph, although rarely seen (Fig. 6.16), or the typical bone marrow contusion pattern in the

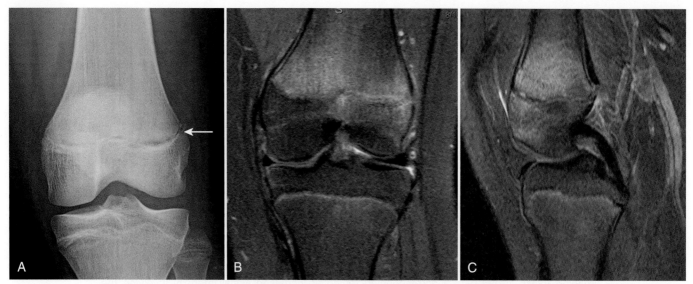

FIG 6.15 Salter-Harris I Fracture AP radiograph (A) demonstrates equivocal widening of the lateral aspect the distal femoral physis with possible a tiny fracture fragment laterally *(white arrow)*. Coronal fat-suppressed proton density (B) and sagittal fat suppressed proton density (C) MR images confirm the presence of a Salter-Harris I fracture with edema on both sides of the physis.

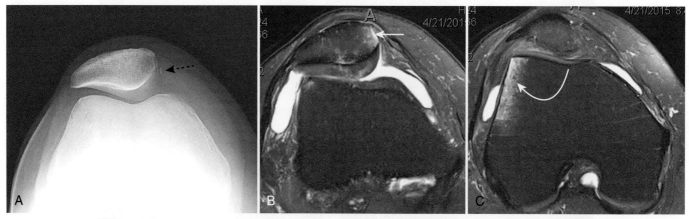

FIG 6.16 Transient Lateral Patellar Dislocation and Relocation Sunrise view of the patella (A) demonstrates a small fleck of bone at the medial aspect of the patella *(black interrupted arrow)*. Fat-suppressed T2 axial image (B) demonstrates corresponding bone marrow edema in the medial patella *(white arrow)*, whereas another fat-suppressed T2-weighted image more inferiorly (C) demonstrates bone marrow edema in the lateral femoral condyle anteriorly *(white curved arrow)*, the typical bone marrow contusion pattern from transient lateral patellar dislocation.

medial patella and anterolateral femoral condyle, as seen on the subsequent MRI (to be discussed later). Medial dislocations of the patella are extremely rare but have been reported in patients who have had recurrent lateral patellar subluxation treated by lateral retinacular release.[35]

Fracture Classification

In the past, classification systems involved describing fracture patterns according to mechanism of injury.[9] Contemporary schemes, such as the Orthopedic Trauma Association classification system (Fig. 6.17), involve classifying the fracture of the patella according to the degree of displacement, the location of the fracture on the patella, the geometric pattern of fracture lines (transverse, vertical, marginal or apical, comminuted or

stellate, osteochondral, or sleeve avulsion), and whether the fracture is extra-articular (type A), partial articular (type B), and complete articular with a disrupted extensor mechanism (type C).[40] In skeletally immature patients a special category of patellar sleeve avulsions occur when a distal pole fragment with a large surface of the articular surface is avulsed.[16] However, no specific classification system based on the proposed mechanism of injury, fracture pattern, or degree of displacement has proved effective in determining long-term results.

Nondisplaced Fractures. These fractures can be transverse, stellate, osteochondral, or vertical, although stellate and transverse fractures can also be displaced. In all these nondisplaced fractures the patellar retinacular structures are not torn, the

Types:

A. Patella extra-articular

Groups:

Patella, extra-articular

A1. Patella, extra-articular, avulsion   A2. Patella, extra-articular isolated body

B. Partial articular, vertical

Patella, partial articular, vertical

B1. Patella, partial articular, vertical, lateral   B2. Patella, partial articular, vertical, medial

C. Complete articular, non-vertical

Patella, complete articular, non-vertical

C1. Patella, articular, transverse   C2. Patella, articular, transverse plus second fragment   C3. Patella, articular, comminuted

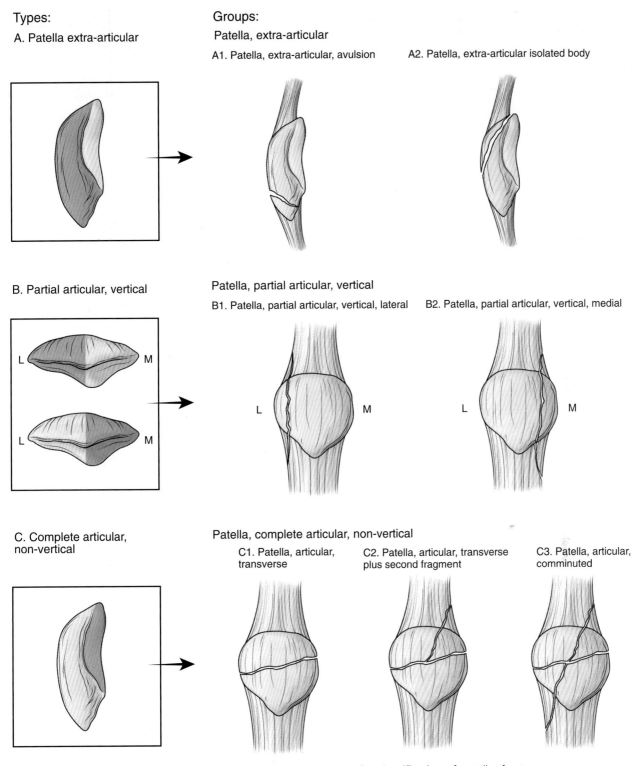

FIG 6.17 Orthopedic Trauma Association system for classification of patellar fractures.

extensor mechanism remains competent, and reduction is achieved nonoperatively.

Nondisplaced transverse fractures often result from indirect longitudinal forces that fracture the patella but are insufficient to tear the patellar retinacular structures. A majority of these fractures occur in the middle-to-lower third of the patella (Fig. 6.18).[6,9]

Stellate fractures typically occur when there is a direct blow to the patella while the knee is in a partially flexed position. Articular surface injury can occur in these fractures because of that mechanism of injury, producing osteochondral lesions.

Osteochondral fractures are often seen in association with stellate fractures or can be seen in isolation after a patellar dislocation. With a patellar dislocation or relocation a

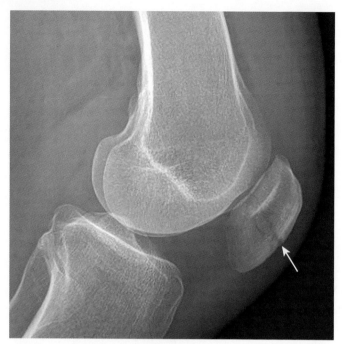

FIG 6.18 Lateral radiograph demonstrating a transverse nondisplaced fracture of the patella involving the mid-to-lower pole (*white arrow*).

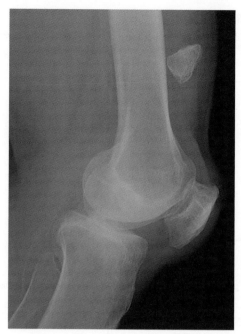

FIG 6.19 Lateral radiograph demonstrates a quadriceps avulsion fracture of the superior aspect of the patella with resultant inferior displacement of the remainder of the patella (patella baja).

characteristic pattern of osteochondral fracture fragments from the lateral femoral condyle and/or medial patellar facet often results.[48]

Vertical or longitudinal fractures can result when a hyper-flexed knee is subjected to direct compression or can be the result of a lateral avulsion fracture. In these fractures the fracture line is most commonly seen between the lateral and middle third of the patella, involving the lateral patella facet. These vertical fractures are not as uncommon as was previously thought.[6,9]

Displaced Fractures. Transverse, stellate, or polar fractures can be displaced. Transverse fractures are the most common, making up approximately 50% of all displaced patella fractures.[9] The stellate fractures that are displaced typically are markedly comminuted and result from a high-energy direct blow to the patella. Polar fractures can also be displaced. Fractures of the superior pole of the patella usually result from quadriceps avulsion fractures with resultant patella baja (Fig. 6.19), whereas fractures of the inferior pole of the patella are usually bone avulsions of the patellar tendon, resulting in patella alta (Fig. 6.20). In these inferior pole patella fractures, knee extension is often lost, with retinacular disruption almost always occurring.[6] A type of inferior pole avulsion fracture is the patellar sleeve avulsion, as seen in children, in which there is a cartilaginous avulsion from the lower pole of the patella, and often a small osseous fragment can also be avulsed following vigorous contraction of the quadriceps in a flexed knee.[16] In addition, in adolescents one can see Sinding-Larsen-Johansson disease, a chronic condition in which the lower pole of the patella becomes separated and may be fragmented and the infrapatellar tendon may exhibit calcification and ossification (Fig. 6.21).

One potential pitfall in evaluating for a displaced patella fracture is the bipartite or multipartite patella, which is a normal anatomic variant that can be misdiagnosed as a displaced patella

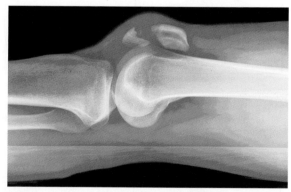

FIG 6.20 Lateral radiograph of the knee demonstrates a patellar tendon avulsion fracture of the inferior pole of the patella with high riding of the remainder of the patella (patella alta).

fracture. The bipartite patella is the result of incomplete fusion of the accessory patella ossification center and typically occurs in the superolateral aspect of the patella with a well-corticated fragment. Bipartite patella is thought to have an incidence of approximately 8% and is often bilateral.[6] Unilateral bipartite patellae are rare and may actually be the result of an old marginal patellar fracture.[15] The bilaterality may help in differentiating a bipartite patella from a fracture if it is seen in both knees, if contralateral knee radiographs are also performed (Fig. 6.22). In addition, the ossification center of a bipartite patella does not fit perfectly into the defect in the patella to form a normal patella if the apparent fragments are put together, as a fracture usually does. In addition, the bipartite ossification center has well-corticated margins, as does the opposing surface of the main body of the patella, another way to differentiate a bipartite patella from an acute fracture.

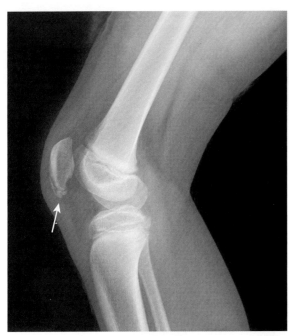

FIG 6.21 Sinding-Larsen-Johansson Disease Lateral radiograph of the knee demonstrates fragmentation and ossification of the patellar tendon insertion on the patella *(white arrow)*.

Imaging Diagnosis

Radiography. Plain film radiographs are usually adequate to make the diagnosis of a patella fracture, assuming that the radiographic examination consists of standard AP, lateral, and oblique radiographs of the knee, and an additional tangential or axial view of the patellofemoral joint. AP and oblique views will be most helpful in diagnosing a bipartite patella in the superolateral quadrant of the patella and can diagnose comminuted or stellate patellar fractures, especially if slightly overpenetrated.

The lateral view is most helpful in determining if there is any articular step off and in determining the degree of displacement, especially with transverse fractures. Superior or inferior pole avulsion fractures are best demonstrated on the lateral view. The lateral view is the only view that will reliably diagnose a knee joint effusion, a finding that should be seen with intraarticular patellar fractures. If the lateral view is performed in the cross-table lateral projection, a lipohemarthrosis may be seen, clueing one into the diagnosis of an intra-articular fracture. Ideally the lateral view should be obtained in some degree of flexion (approximately 30 degrees), which will allow calculation of the Insall-Salvati ratio (length of the patellar tendon relative to the length of the patella). A ratio of 0.8 to 1.2 is considered normal, whereas a ratio of greater than 1.2 indicates patella alta and less than 0.8 indicates patella baja.[27,29] Because patellar shape is known to be variable, which may influence classification of patella height, and because of relative elevation of the patella with full extension and relative descent of the patella with knee flexion, the Insall-Salvati ratio may not be accurate in some cases, and some modifications have been advocated.[22,29] In addition, sagittal MR images can be used to assess for patella alta and baja.[52]

Although a lateral view may be all that is necessary to diagnose a transverse patella fracture, a tangential view may be necessary to visualize a nondisplaced or minimally displaced longitudinal fracture (Fig. 6.23) that would be in the sagittal plane of the patella on the lateral view and may be obscured by the overlapping femur on the AP view. A tangential view may also help in either evaluating for marginal fractures or diagnosing a bipartite patella. The axial or tangential view may also be the only radiographic projection that would suggest either a recent patellar subluxation or dislocation with the patella not completely centered within the trochlear groove or the demonstration of a small fracture fragment at the medial aspect of the patella. This fracture occurs when the medial aspect of the patella impacts against the anterolateral femoral condyle during relocation. The tangential view that is most commonly used is the sunrise view, in which the patient is prone with the knee flexed 115 degrees with the x-ray beam directed toward the patella with approximately 15 degrees of cephalad angulation. However, because of extreme flexion required for this view, the patella may be positioned deeply within the trochlear groove, limiting evaluation of the patellofemoral articular surfaces. To better visualize the patellofemoral joint itself, an axial Merchant view may be performed. The Merchant view is a tangential view that is taken with the patient in a supine position with positioning of the knee at 45 degrees of flexion at the edge of the table with the central beam directed caudally through the patella at a 30-degree angle from horizontal.[34] This view will better demonstrate any osteochondral fractures of the patella because the Merchant view better demonstrates the articular facets of the patella. The Merchant view will also better demonstrate any patellar subluxation because the sunrise view requires a greater degree of flexion, which decreases the amount of patellar subluxation.

Computed Tomography. Although CT is rarely necessary to diagnose patellar fractures, which are usually evident radiographically, CT may be of benefit in the detection of nondisplaced patellar fractures that are not seen radiographically but which are suspected clinically, especially in light of the presence of a lipohemarthrosis. This is especially helpful in the evaluation of fractures that are best seen in the axial plane, such as those that are longitudinal in nature, which may be not evident radiographically except on an axial view. CT also has a role in evaluation of comminuted fractures, in assessing the number and displacement of multiple fracture fragments. CT also may be used in suspected cases of nonunion and malunion to further define the degree or lack of healing. CT has also been used historically to diagnose stress fractures of the patella in the elderly with osteoporosis, although MRI has for the most part supplanted CT in that regard.

Magnetic Resonance Imaging. MRI, because of its high contrast resolution and ability to detect bone marrow edema in the patella, has the capacity to detect patellar fractures that were not evident on other studies but were suspected clinically, such as posttraumatic fractures or stress fractures that are nondisplaced. This can be seen on MRI performed for other reasons, such as that to detect internal derangement. One caveat to remember when assessing the patella for bone marrow edema is that the patella is a superficial structure and if there is inhomogeneous fat suppression on conventional fat-saturated T2 images, one might see spurious increased T2 signal in the patella, which would be artifactual. MRI would be of value in evaluating for osteochondral fractures of the patella because of its inherent ability to detect bone marrow edema and cartilage

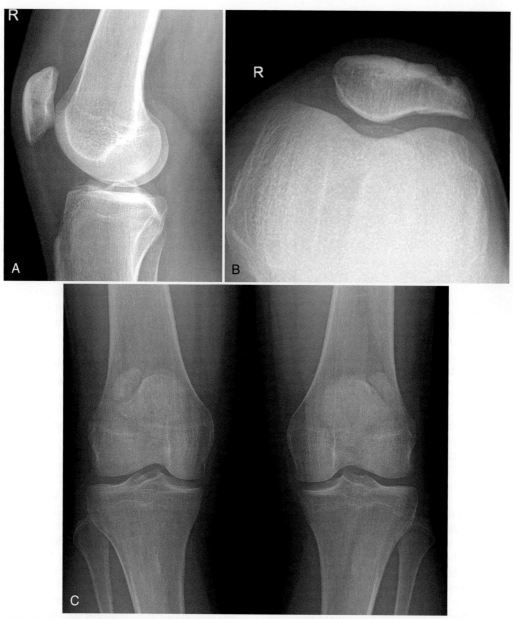

FIG 6.22 Bipartite Patella Lateral (A) and sunrise (B) radiographs of the right knee demonstrate some irregularity of the superior and lateral aspects of the right patella respectively suspicious for a bipartite patella or an old fracture. AP view of both knees (C) confirms the presence of bilateral bipartite patellae.

defects, which may not be radiographically evident. This is especially indicated in the adolescent, in whom determination of patellar sleeve avulsion fracture with a large amount of cartilage detached would be important to differentiate from Sinding-Larsen-Johansson.[16,21] MRI can also be used in those patients with patella baja or patella alta to detect patella avulsion fractures related to extensor mechanism injuries because of its ability to diagnose tears of the quadriceps or infrapatellar tendon respectively. In addition, MRI is the modality of choice in the evaluation of suspected patella dislocation because of the typical bone marrow edema pattern that is seen in the lateral femoral condyle anteriorly and in the medial aspect of the patella, which may or may not be associated with a fracture fragment along the medial patella.[48] MRI also has the advantage

in these cases because of its ability to detect the tear of the medial patellar retinaculum, which is demonstrated in these patients with lateral patellar dislocation. These findings will be seen even after relocation of a previously dislocated patella, a not uncommon scenario, because approximately 50% to 75% of patella dislocations will have self-relocated at the time of initial presentation.[16]

FEMOROTIBIAL KNEE DISLOCATIONS

Knee dislocation at the femorotibial joint is a rare but potentially catastrophic injury. It usually occurs secondary to high-energy trauma, such as motor vehicle collisions, falls from heights, or high-energy athletic injuries.[19,42]

Dislocations may be categorized as anterior, posterior, medial, lateral, or rotatory, depending on the direction of the tibial dislocation relative to the femur.[45] There can also be associated fractures of the distal femur and proximal tibia. Anterior dislocation can occur after a severe hyperextension injury and is the most common, whereas posterior dislocation usually results from a direct blow to the anterior tibia, such as a fall on a flexed knee or a dashboard-type injury, and is the second most common. Medial, lateral, and rotatory are associated with varus, valgus, or rotatory stresses, respectively. Occasionally, spontaneous reduction after the dislocation occurs, limiting the

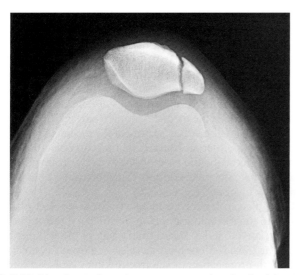

FIG 6.23 Merchant view demonstrates a longitudinal fracture of the patella along the lateral patella facet.

usefulness of the directional classification scheme. Thus a classification system based on the extent and pattern of associated ligamentous injuries has been developed.[24,45]

As can be anticipated, ligament and soft tissue damage with this type of dislocation is usually very severe and can involve the menisci, tendons, and neurovascular bundle.[37,45] Injury to both cruciate ligaments, especially the ACL, is almost universal, especially with the anterior or posterior dislocations, whereas injuries to the collateral ligaments, menisci, and tendinous attachments commonly occur. Of significance and particular importance is that the popliteal artery and common peroneal nerve[41,45] can also be injured in a significant proportion of these dislocations.

Although radiographs would be diagnostic in the setting of femorotibial dislocation and would be done as the first imaging procedure, other studies will be necessary if that is indeed diagnosed or if the knee dislocation has been reduced spontaneously or by manipulation. Radiographs can also be helpful to assess for any associated fractures (Fig. 6.24). MRI would be crucial to evaluate the ligamentous structures that are invariably injured, as well as to evaluate for any meniscal tear or tendon disruption. MRI can be of benefit in evaluating the peroneal nerve.

Angiography may also be warranted to exclude popliteal artery injury.[54] Asymmetrical distal pulses with question of a diminution of the pulse in the affected extremity, coolness of that extremity, or an ankle brachial index (ABI) below 0.9 on a pulse volume recording (PVR) study would be an indication for angiographic examination.[45,54] Angiography may be helpful in localizing the injured area, which is often at the site of a displaced fracture fragment. In these cases CT angiography may be of benefit because the CT can show the displaced fracture fragments and the angiographic portion of the exam with

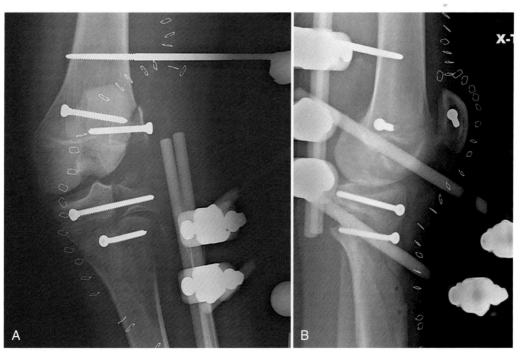

FIG 6.24 Posterior Knee Dislocation Status Reduction AP (A) and lateral (B) radiographs demonstrate multiple fixated fractures in a patient who had a posterior dislocation reduced and externally fixated.

reconstructions can show the effect of the fracture on the adjacent vessels (Fig. 6.25).[42,44]

MR angiography has recently been advocated as a technique to be used in the evaluation of these dislocations instead of conventional angiography because it can be performed at the same time as the MRI is being done to evaluate the supporting soft tissue structures.[58] However, any of these tests should not delay vascular exploration at the time of surgery if the leg is obviously ischemic, such as a cold, pulseless extremity. In those cases, angiography should be performed in the operating room while external fixation of the fracture is performed, to expedite the care of the patient if significant arterial injury is suspected.

TIBIAL PLATEAU AND PROXIMAL TIBIA AND FIBULA FRACTURES AND DISLOCATIONS

Incidence and Etiology

Fractures of the tibial plateau represent only 1% to 2% of all fractures, but account for approximately 8% of the fractures occurring in older adults, indicating that there is a higher risk in advancing age, due to osteoporosis.[46] These fractures are by definition intra-articular because they involve the articular surface of the proximal tibia. However, in addition to involving the articular surface, these fractures can also involve the epiphysis, metaphysis, and even the diaphysis in severe injuries. There can be associated or isolated injuries of the tibial spines and proximal fibula.

The mechanism of injury for tibial plateau fractures is generally one with axial loading, with concomitant varus or valgus stress. This can be seen with high-energy injuries, such as motor vehicle accidents, or with low-energy trauma, such as that due to a fall from a standing height. The more an axial load predominates, the more likely a patient is to sustain a bicondylar injury. These tend to be seen in the high-energy injuries in younger patients due to the severe axial loading in combination with shearing injuries. The greater the amount of energy directed to the proximal tibia, as seen with axial loading, the more comminution and displacement of the fracture fragments.[3] Isolated valgus or varus loading tends to cause isolated lateral or medial fractures, respectively, with the simple depression-type injuries often the result of lower-energy injuries in older patients with osteoporosis. Younger patients with stronger bones tend to have split fractures with little depression, whereas older osteoporotic patients generally have more depression than splitting. Because of the normal slight valgus alignment of the knee and because it is more common for trauma to be on the lateral rather medial side, the proximal tibia is more likely to be subjected to a valgus load. Thus the lateral plateau is more commonly involved in these types of fractures, in 55% to 70% of cases, with medial plateau or bicondylar involvement occurring in 10% to 30% of cases.[46] Varus injuries can lead to medial tibial plateau fractures, although this mechanism is less common but can be seen with the knee flexion, varus, and internal rotation of the medial femoral condyle. This can result in a posteromedial shearing fracture of the medial tibial plateau, manifesting as either an isolated split fracture or a bicondylar fracture pattern.[5] In the case of stress fractures involving the proximal tibia, the medial aspect of the proximal tibia is more commonly involved (Fig. 6.26).[10]

Tibial plateau fractures can also occur as a result of direct trauma to the metaphyseal region in which a direct force, such as that related to a dashboard injury, fall, or other direct blow, causes the tibial shaft to become separated from the tibial condyles, with propagation of the fracture lines cephalad into the tibial plateaux. These fractures can have severe associated injuries, such as open fractures, soft tissue ligament or meniscal injury, vascular injury, or compartment syndrome.[1,53,62]

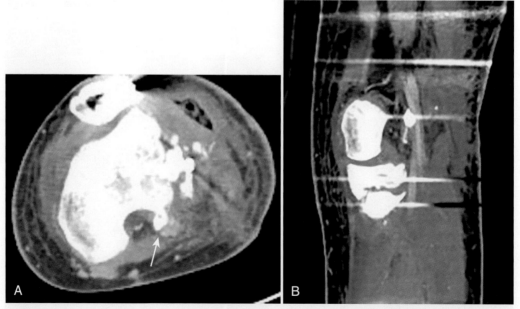

FIG 6.25 Axial CT image (A) and reconstructed coronal CT image (B) in the same patient as in Fig. 6.24 who had a prior knee dislocation reduced and externally fixed. Note the comminuted fracture of the distal femur with one fracture fragment in the vicinity of the popliteal artery *(white arrow)* but with patency of the popliteal artery demonstrated on the coronal CT reconstructed image.

Other types of fractures can also occur about the proximal tibia and fibula and generally are of the avulsive type. Avulsion of the anterior tibial tuberosity from infrapatellar injury with resultant patella alta, avulsion of the fibula styloid/head from lateral collateral ligamentous injury or lateral corner injury, and avulsion of the anterior tibial spine or intercondylar eminence at the ACL insertion (Fig. 6.27) are all examples of ligamentous avulsion fractures. Avulsion of the fibular styloid process has been termed the *arcuate sign* and can occur after a force is directed against the anterior tibia with the knee in extension and has been associated with posterolateral knee instability.[26,60]

Avulsion of the anterior tibial intercondylar eminence at the ACL insertion in adults can be seen after a hyperextension injury, rather than the more common scenario of disruption of the ACL itself. However, this fracture is more common in children and young adolescents[21] because the chondroepiphyseal insertion site is weaker than the ACL itself and occurs following forced flexion of the knee with internal rotation of the tibia, such as that which might occur after a fall from a bicycle. Avulsions of the anterior tibial intercondylar eminence are often isolated injuries in children, but if seen in adults with severe hyperextension injuries, they are usually associated with other injuries, such as PCL and MCL tears.[7,21,59] Avulsion fracture of the posterior surface of the tibial plateau related to posterior cruciate ligament insertion (Fig. 6.28) is rare but can be seen after severe hyperextension or dashboard-type injury and is unlikely to be isolated, usually associated with more severe ligamentous injuries.[21] In addition, posteromedial tibial plateau avulsion at the semimembranosus tendon insertion,[11] as well as the Segond fracture related to lateral capsular ligament avulsion of the lateral tibial condyle posterior to Gerdy's tubercle,[21] would also be included in this category. The Segond fracture (Fig. 6.29) is a thin longitudinal linear avulsion fracture of the lateral tibia just posterior to the insertion of the iliotibial band on Gerdy's tubercle. These latter two avulsion fractures are particularly of importance, due to their high association with ACL tears. In all these types of avulsion fractures, treating the avulsion fracture itself may not be as important as the treating the underlying associated or causative ligamentous injury.

Tibiofibular joint and proximal fibula injuries can also occur following knee injury. Dislocations and subluxations about the proximal tibiofibular joint are uncommon, manifesting with either anterolateral, posteromedial, or superior displacement of the head of the fibula, with anterolateral dislocation being the most common but still rare.[19,39] These can occur after a fall on a flexed knee with the foot inverted and plantar flexed.[19] This can be seen in various sports activities that require twisting motions of the flexed knee, such as in wresting, parachute jumping, gymnastics, skiing, and football.[28] These are often missed at initial

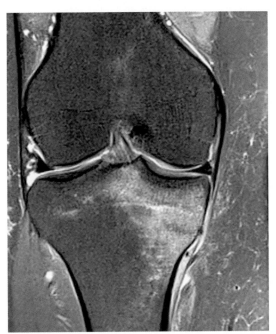

FIG 6.26 Medial Tibial Stress Fracture Coronal fat-suppressed T2-weighted MR image demonstrates medial proximal tibial stress fracture line with surrounding bone marrow edema.

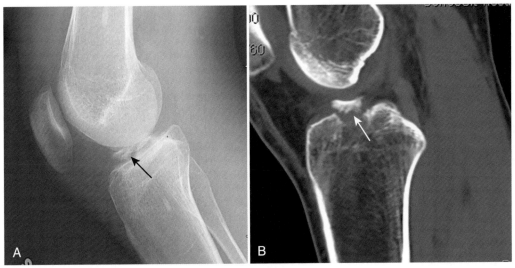

FIG 6.27 Anterior Cruciate Ligament Avulsion Lateral radiograph of the knee (A) demonstrates an avulsed osseous fragment arising from the tibial attachment site of the ACL at the intercondylar eminence *(black arrow)*. The reconstructed sagittal CT image (B) confirms the presence of the osseous fragment which is attached to the ACL *(white arrow)*.

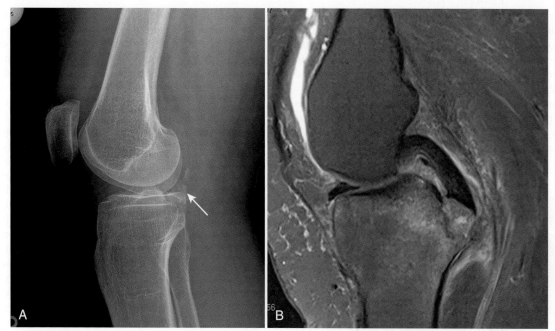

FIG 6.28 Posterior Cruciate Ligament Avulsion Lateral radiograph of the knee (A) demonstrates a bony fragment *(white arrow)* along the posterior tibial plateau. Sagittal T2-weighted fat-suppressed MR image (B) confirms that the osseous fragment is an avulsion fracture related to the PCL insertion, with the PCL itself intact.

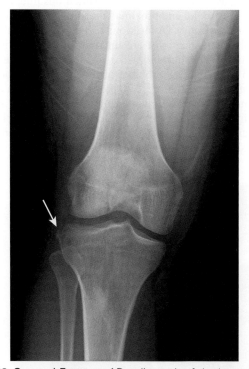

FIG 6.29 Segond Fracture AP radiograph of the knee demonstrates a small avulsion fracture from the lateral aspect of the proximal tibia *(white arrow)*.

presentation and require a high degree of clinical suspicion, and close inspection of the lateral radiograph needs to be made to assess the congruity of the proximal tibiofibular joint.[10]

Although direct impaction can result in an isolated fracture of the head of the fibula, fibula head and neck injuries are

usually associated with more significant knee ligamentous disruptions or fractures of the tibial plateau and rarely occur in isolation. Thus whenever a fracture of the proximal fibula is identified, one must search for other commonly associated injuries. Fracture of the fibula head can be seen following a valgus force, which also results in lateral tibial plateau fracture and medial collateral ligament injury, and a varus force can also cause an avulsion fracture of the proximal fibula or styloid process with other associated ligamentous injuries. Fractures located more distally in the neck of the fibula can also be the result of a Maisonneuve injury, an external rotational injury of the ankle in which the force is transmitted cephalad through the tibiofibular interosseous membrane and spirals upward, causing a spiral/oblique fracture of the proximal fibula. In that case there may be an associated fracture of the medial malleolus about the ankle, a distal tibial fracture, and/or a distal tibiofibular syndesmotic injury.

Fracture Classification

Because of the complex and varied appearance of the fractures about the tibial plateau, classification schemes have been developed to attempt to better categorize these fractures to guide the treatment plan for better patient outcomes and to lower the risk of complications. Anatomic classifications, such as the AO (Arbeitsgemeinschaft für Osteosynthesefragen) or the Orthopedic Trauma Association classification,[40] for articular fractures are well suited for tibial plateau fractures (Fig. 6.30) and have been used in the past because they are well accepted, especially for research purposes and trauma databases. It has several advantages, in that it identifies articular and nonarticular fractures, can subclassify these fractures based on the degree of comminution, and provides a way to separate proximal tibial fractures from tibial shaft fractures. It had been considered somewhat cumbersome but has been recently updated and

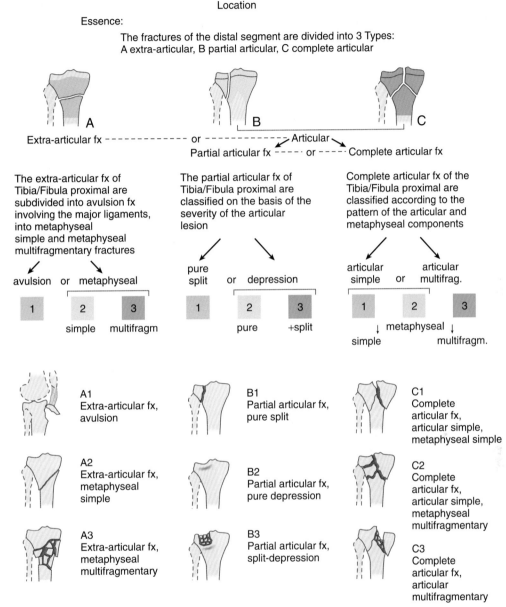

Location

Essence:

The fractures of the distal segment are divided into 3 Types:
A extra-articular, B partial articular, C complete articular

A

B

C

Extra-articular fx ----------- or ------------ Articular
Partial articular fx ---- or ---- Complete articular fx

The extra-articular fx of Tibia/Fibula proximal are subdivided into avulsion fx involving the major ligaments, into metaphyseal simple and metaphyseal multifragmentary fractures

avulsion or metaphyseal

| 1 | 2 | 3 |

simple multifragm

The partial articular fx of Tibia/Fibula proximal are classified on the basis of the severity of the articular lesion

pure split or depression

| 1 | 2 | 3 |

pure +split

Complete articular fx of the Tibia/Fibula proximal are classified according to the pattern of the articular and metaphyseal components

articular simple or articular multifrag.

| 1 | 2 | 3 |

↓ metaphyseal ↓
simple multifragm.

A1
Extra-articular fx, avulsion

A2
Extra-articular fx, metaphyseal simple

A3
Extra-articular fx, metaphyseal multifragmentary

B1
Partial articular fx, pure split

B2
Partial articular fx, pure depression

B3
Partial articular fx, split-depression

C1
Complete articular fx, articular simple, metaphyseal simple

C2
Complete articular fx, articular simple, metaphyseal multifragmentary

C3
Complete articular fx, articular multifragmentary

FIG 6.30 AO-ASIF classification of tibial plateau fractures. (From Muller ME, Nazarian S, Koch P, Schatzker J: The comprehensive classification of fractures of long bones, Bern, Switzerland, 1995, ME Muller Foundation)

republished[40] and is increasingly being used again as a well-accepted way to categorize proximal tibial fractures in the international orthopedic community.[61]

The Schatzker classification system (Fig. 6.31) continues to be the most clinically used classification system.[32,37,49] In the Schatzker classification system a type I injury is a pure split fracture of the lateral tibial plateau without any articular depression (Fig. 6.32), the type of fracture often seen in young patients with strong bones, as discussed previously. These split fractures can be associated with a peripheral tear of the lateral meniscus

if there is significant displacement.[37] Type II fractures (Fig. 6.33) are combined split depression fractures, often caused by axial loading combined with a lateral bending force. Type III fractures are pure depression fractures of the lateral tibial plateau and are often seen in older osteoporotic patients following lower-energy trauma. The type III fracture is the most common fracture pattern.[49] Type IV fractures are fractures isolated to the medial tibial plateau (Fig. 6.34); because the medial tibial plateau is intrinsically stronger than the lateral plateau, these fractures generally are secondary to higher-energy injuries and

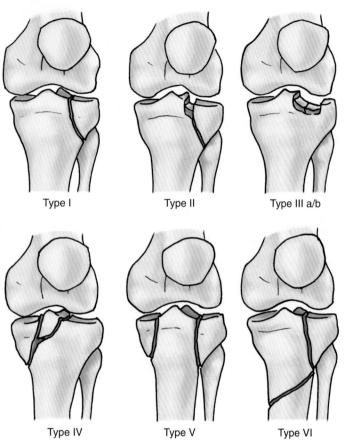

Type I   Type II   Type III a/b

Type IV   Type V   Type VI

FIG 6.31 Schatzker classification of tibial plateau fractures *I,* Lateral plateau fracture without depression. *II,* Lateral plateau fracture with depressed fragment. *III,* Compression fracture of lateral (a) or central (b) plateau. *IV,* Medial tibial plateau. *V,* Bicondylar fracture. *VI,* Diaphyseal dissociation with variable condylar component.

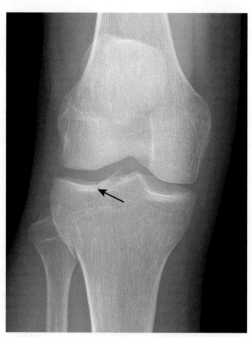

FIG 6.32 Schatzker I Tibial Plateau Fracture AP radiograph demonstrates a split fracture of the lateral tibial plateau *(black arrow)* without significant depression.

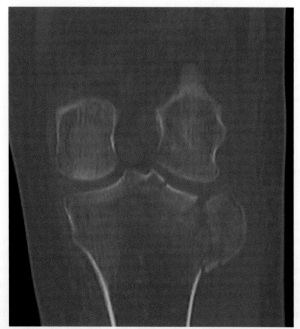

FIG 6.33 Schatzker II Tibial Plateau Fracture CT coronal reconstructed image demonstrates a combined split and depression fracture of the lateral tibial plateau.

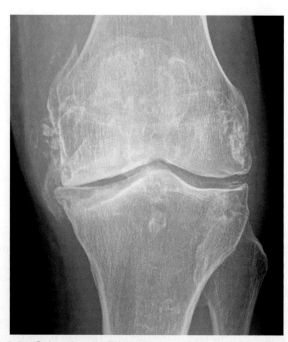

FIG 6.34 Schatzker IV Tibial Plateau Fracture AP radiograph demonstrates a depression fracture of the medial tibial plateau from an impaction injury with an accompanying comminuted fracture of the medial femoral condyle.

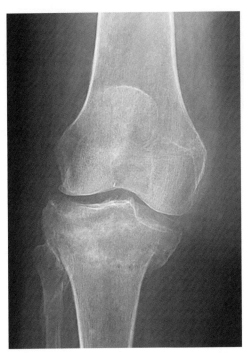

FIG 6.35 Schatzker VI Tibial Plateau Fracture AP radiograph demonstrates fractures of the lateral and medial tibial plateaux with extension inferiorly into the metadiaphyseal region. Note also the minimally displaced proximal fibula fracture.

often have significant soft tissue damage. Type V fractures involve both the medial and lateral tibial plateaux (bicondylar) and are often secondary to a pure axial load while the knee is in full extension. An example of this might happen in a motor vehicle accident when a driver suddenly brakes right before a front-end collision. Type VI fractures also involve both the medial and lateral tibial plateaux but with extension into the metadiaphyseal region with diaphyseal discontinuity and are caused by the highest-energy injuries (Fig. 6.35).

Although there are these two well-accepted and commonly used classification systems for tibial plateau fractures, radiologists and surgeons still often classify them by description. If descriptive terminology is used, then the location of the fracture must be described (medial or lateral tibial plateau or both), as well as the type of fracture (split, split depression, pure focal depression, or bicondylar). In addition, whether the fracture is comminuted, displaced, or angulated and whether there is subluxation or dislocation are standard descriptions. In addition, the amount of articular surface depression measured in millimeters can quantify the severity of the fracture and can be used as a guide for surgical management.

Many of these tibial plateau fractures are often associated with significant soft tissue injuries that can be as important, if not more important, for the surgeon to address than the underlying fracture.[32]

Imaging Diagnosis

In the case of diagnosing fractures of the proximal tibia and fibula, oblique radiographs are extremely helpful, in addition to AP and lateral views, to diagnose minimally displaced fractures of the tibial plateau and fibula head and neck. Because the fracture of the tibial plateau may be obliquely oriented and nondisplaced or minimally displaced, oblique views are often necessary to diagnose the fracture because it may not be obvious on AP and lateral radiographs. Tunnel views may help to diagnose posterior tibial plateau fractures, and tibial plateau views obtained in the AP projection with the knee in 10 to 15 degrees of flexion or with the x-ray tube angled 10 to 15 degrees inferiorly may help to define the fracture and degree of depression of the articular surface.[10]

CT with sagittal and coronal reconstructions, as well as 3D reconstructions, can be a valuable tool in the evaluation of suspected tibial plateau fractures as an adjunct to plain film radiographs because of its ability to detect occult tibial plateau fractures that are not seen on plain film radiographs. CT can also be obtained through casts and splints, which in some cases may obscure the fracture on conventional radiographs. CT also has a role in defining the complex nature of these intra-articular fractures and can help in surgical planning due to its ability to accurately detect the degree of the depression of the tibial plateau in the reconstructed sagittal and coronal planes and to more accurately define the fracture planes and localize the fracture fragments.

MRI is superior to CT in detection of occult fractures and in determining damage to the supporting ligaments and menisci about the knee, which are often injured in these type of fractures.[36] Thus MRI should be used in those cases where the clinical exam or the fracture patterns that are seen would make one suspect that there is associated soft tissue menisci or ligament injury that would impact surgical management. Examples of indications for MRI would include those cases in which there is depression of the tibial plateau where meniscal or collateral ligament injury would be suspected, those cases in which radiographs detect linear avulsion fractures where ligamentous injury is suspected, or in those cases of fibula head and neck injury in which ligament injury would be important to rule out. The benefit of MRI in these cases lies largely in the detection of significant meniscal or ligament injuries in patients who might otherwise be treated nonoperatively. In addition, MRI has value in assessing for occult fractures about the knee due to its ability to detect bone marrow edema. This would be helpful to assess for subtle tibial plateau fractures (Fig. 6.36), in addition to osteochondral or insufficiency fractures, which would otherwise not be detected by radiographs alone. Suspected stress fractures would also fall into this group because neither radiographs nor CT can reliably detect these early in the acute setting. MRI also has a role in the evaluation of peroneal nerve injuries that can be seen after displaced comminuted tibial plateau fractures, and especially after proximal fibula fractures and proximal tibiofibular joint injuries. The peroneal nerve is susceptible in these type of injuries because of its location as it courses over the head and around the neck of the fibula.[41] In addition, because compartment syndrome may be a complication of severe acute trauma in those cases in which there is direct trauma to the tibial metaphysis, forcing it to separate from the tibial condyles, as in Schatzker type VI fractures, MRI of the calf may be helpful in those cases in which that diagnosis of compartment syndrome is in doubt.[62] However, serial intracompartmental pressure measurements remain the procedure of choice to evaluate in the acute setting in which physical exam findings, such as pain with passive stretching and tense compartments, would raise the likelihood for compartment syndrome.

Angiography may be also be indicated in select cases when the vascularity of the traumatized lower extremity is in question, because of the potential for arterial injury from complex

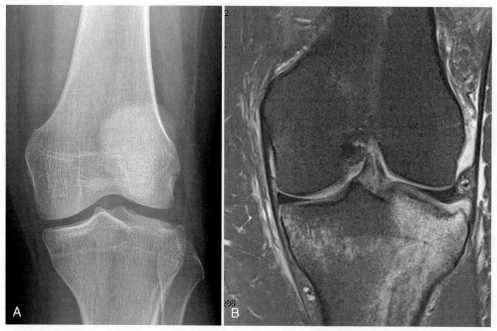

FIG 6.36 Schatzker III Lateral Tibial Plateau Fracture AP radiograph (A) demonstrates a suggestion of the depressed lateral tibial plateau fracture, but the coronal T2-weighted fat-suppressed MR image (B) confirms the diagnosis as it shows the depressed tibial plateau with marked reactive bone marrow edema.

markedly displaced proximal tibial fractures, as was discussed in the section on femorotibial dislocations, because of the proximity of the popliteal artery and trifurcation.

KEY REFERENCES

7. Berquist TH: Osseous and myotendinous injuries about the knee. *Radiol Clin North Am* 45:955–968, 2007.
10. Capps GW, Hayes CW: Easily missed injuries around the knee. *Radiographics* 14:1191–1210, 1994.
16. Dupuis CS, Westra SJ, Makris J, et al: Injuries and conditions of the extensor mechanism of the pediatric knee. *Radiographics* 29(3):887–896, 2009.
19. Gimber LH, Scalcione LR, Rowan A, et al: Multiligamentous injuries and knee dislocations. *Skeletal Radiol* 2015. [Epub ahead of print].
21. Gottsegen CJ, Eyer BA, White EA, et al: Avulsion fractures of the knee: imaging findings and clinical significance. *Radiographics* 28:1755–1770, 2008.
24. Heinrichs A: A review of knee dislocations. *J Athl Train* 39:365–369, 2004.

32. Markhardt BK, Gross JM, Monu JUV: Schatzker classification of tibial plateau fractures: use of CT and MR imaging improves assessment. *Radiographics* 29:585–597, 2009.
37. Newton EJ, Love J: Emergency department management of selected orthopedic injuries. *Emerg Med Clin N Am* 25:763–793, 2007.
40. Orthopaedic Trauma Association Classification, Database, and Outcomes Committee: Fracture and dislocation classification compendium–2007. *J Orthop Trauma* 21:S1–S160, 2007.
45. Robertson A, Nutton RW, Keating JF: Dislocation of the knee. *J Bone Joint Surg Br* 88:706–711, 2006.
47. Salter RB, Harris R: Injuries involving the epiphyseal plate. *J Bone Joint Surg* 45:587–622, 1963.
48. Sanders TG, Medynski MA, Feller JF, et al: Bone contusion patterns of the knee at MR imaging. *Radiographics* 20:S135–S151, 2000.
49. Schatzker J, McBroom R, Bruce D: The tibial plateau fracture. The Toronto experience, 1968–1975. *Clin Orthop Relat Res* 138:94–104, 1979.
60. Vinson EN, Major NM, Helms CA: The posterolateral corner of the knee. *Am J Roentgenol* 190:449–458, 2008.

The references for this chapter can also be found on www.expertconsult.com.

7

Imaging of the Meniscus

Monica Tafur, Jenny T. Bencardino

INTRODUCTION

Meniscal tears are among the most common knee injuries. Abnormal biomechanics after a meniscal injury expose the underlying articular cartilage to increased axial and sheer stress, leading to articular cartilage lesions and early osteoarthritis (OA).[1,47,83] The choice of treatment and ultimate prognosis associated with meniscal tears are influenced by such factors as tear orientation, extent, and location.[21] In the United States arthroscopic partial meniscectomy is one of the most commonly performed orthopedic operations, with approximately 1 million patients undergoing surgery each year.[67]

Magnetic resonance imaging (MRI) has been considered the imaging modality of choice in diagnosing meniscal pathology since its first introduction into the clinical practice. MRI accuracy in detecting and characterizing meniscal tears has been extensively reported, with high reported sensitivities and specificities in several studies.[11,44,83,98,99]

Accurate and prompt diagnosis of meniscal injury is critical to initiate proper treatment and reduce morbidity. Knowledge of the detailed anatomy of the menisci and closely related structures, meniscal pathology, and postoperative changes is critical for an adequate interpretation of knee magnetic resonance (MR) examinations.

NORMAL ANATOMY

The menisci are fibrocartilaginous structures located between the tibial plateau and femoral condyles. Distributing load, delivering congruency, enhancing stability, and contributing to lubrication and nutrition are major functions of normal menisci. Once these functions are impaired, the risk of degenerative changes and morbidity increases.[47,58,68]

The shape of the meniscus can be described as an elongated semilunar or C-shape triangle with a concave superior surface and a flat inferior surface. The meniscus is generally divided into thirds: anterior horn, body, and posterior horn (Figs. 7.1 and 7.2).[33] Each meniscus attaches to the flat surface of the tibial plateau via the anterior and posterior root ligaments and accommodates the convex surface of the femoral condyles.[98]

The anterior and posterior meniscal root ligaments are the strongest of the structures that attach the meniscus to the tibial plateau (Fig. 7.3). Some similarities between meniscal roots and other ligamentous structures have been demonstrated on scanning electron microscopy and histology studies of meniscal attachments, leading to the term *meniscal root ligaments*.[26,117] Other insertions of the medial and lateral menisci are the meniscotibial ligaments, which attach the meniscal body to the tibia, and a loose attachment of the meniscal body to the capsule.[22,92,117,120]

Medial Meniscus

The medial meniscus has an open, C-shape configuration and is longer in its anteroposterior dimensions compared with the lateral meniscus in the axial plane. In cross-section the medial meniscus has a nonuniform, wedge-shape morphology with the posterior horn twice as large as the anterior horn.[75,76] Although larger, the medial meniscus covers a smaller percentage of the articular surface of the tibia (50% to 60% compared with 70% for the lateral meniscus).[26,98,110]

Medial meniscus root ligaments are located more superficially compared with lateral meniscus root ligaments because of the more open C-shape of the medial meniscus. Four insertion patterns of the anterior root ligament of the medial meniscus have been described: type I insertion, which is the most frequent, is located in the flat intercondylar region of the tibial plateau; type II insertion is more medial, close to articular tibial surface; type III insertion is more anterior, on the downward slope from the medial tibial plateau; type IV insertion shows no bony attachment.[13,110] The attachment site of the posterior horn of the medial meniscus is located posterior to the medial tibial eminence and anteromedial to the posterior cruciate ligament (PCL) insertion (see Fig. 7.3).[13,60,110]

The medial meniscus is entirely attached to the joint capsule, with the exception of a small area at the medial collateral ligament (MCL). The medial meniscus serves as origin of the meniscocapsular ligaments, meniscofemoral ligament, and meniscotibial or coronary ligament, which are structures that belong to the deep portion of the MCL. The meniscofemoral ligament originates from the outer superior margin of the meniscus to blend either with the superficial portion of the MCL or the femoral condyle 1 to 2 cm above the level of the joint space. The meniscotibial or coronary ligament is shorter compared with the meniscofemoral ligament and originates from the outer inferior margin of the meniscus to attach to the tibia, distal to the joint space. Fibrofatty tissue and the MCL bursa separate the medial meniscus and deep portion of the MCL from the superficial or main portion of the MCL (Fig. 7.4).[37,76] The meniscocapsular ligaments are not the only medial supporting structures closely related to the medial meniscus. The posterior portion of the MCL designated as the posterior oblique ligament fuses with the deep portion of the MCL and attaches closely to the posteromedial meniscus. Along the posterior aspect of the knee, the posterior oblique ligament envelops the posteromedial aspect of the medial femoral condyle where it takes the name of oblique popliteal ligament.[37]

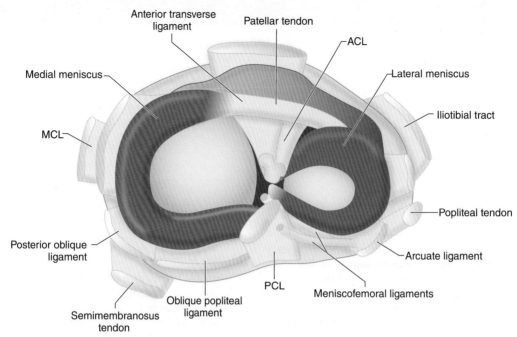

FIG 7.1 Normal Anatomy of the Knee The C-shaped morphology of the menisci is demonstrated. The medial meniscus is larger than the lateral meniscus, particularly in its anteroposterior dimension. The closely related structures that can mimic meniscal tears are depicted in the drawing. The relationship of the meniscofemoral ligaments with the ligament of Humphry anterior to the PCL and the ligament of Wrisberg posterior to the PCL is observed. *ACL,* Anterior cruciate ligament; *PCL,* posterior cruciate ligament.

Lateral Meniscus

The lateral meniscus appears more rounded with a closed C-shape configuration in the axial plane. In cross-section the lateral meniscus has a uniform, wedge-shape morphology minimally and gradually enlarging from anterior to posterior.[33,76]

The root ligament of the anterior horn of the lateral meniscus inserts immediately lateral to the origin of the anterior cruciate ligament (ACL). The posterior attachment of the lateral meniscus is located posteromedial to the lateral tibial eminence, anterior to the PCL insertion, and anterolateral to the medial meniscus posterior attachment (see Fig. 7.3).[60]

The lateral meniscus is attached to the joint capsule only in the anterior and far posterior portions. A deep lamina of the capsule, part of the deep layer of the lateral supporting structures of the knee, travels deep to the lateral collateral ligament (LCL) and gives rise to the coronary ligament.[52] In the lateral portion of the knee, the popliteal hiatus interrupts the meniscal capsular attachment at the body and portion of the posterior horn. The proximal intra-articular insertion of the popliteus tendon is situated within a shallow concavity in the lateral aspect of the femur, designated the popliteal sulcus. The tendon then takes a posteroinferior oblique course to the posterolateral corner of the knee. As it passes the posterior horn of the lateral meniscus, the popliteus tendon becomes extra-articular (Fig. 7.5).[76,87]

Related Structures

Knowledge of closely related structures to the meniscus is critical because they may simulate pathology and can also be injured. Some of these structures include the meniscofemoral ligaments, meniscomeniscal ligaments, ligamentum mucosum

or infrapatellar plica, popliteomeniscal fascicles, and patellomeniscal ligament.

The meniscofemoral ligaments of Humphry and Wrisberg originate from the posterior horn of the lateral meniscus and insert onto the lateral aspect of the posterior medial femoral condyle, with the ligament of Humphry coursing anterior to the genu of the PCL and the ligament of Wrisberg coursing behind the genu of the PCL (Figs. 7.6 and 7.7). The incidence of the meniscofemoral ligaments ranges from 50% to 76% in the literature. The ligament of Wrisberg is more frequently found than the ligament of Humphry, with a reported incidence of 90% and 17%, respectively, in a series of cadaveric specimens by Cho et al.[28] Meniscofemoral ligament proximal insertion may vary, attaching only at the femoral condyle or attaching at the femoral condyle while some fibers blend with the PCL. In the latter type a hump in the PCL can be observed on sagittal MR images. The Wrisberg ligament is thicker than the Humphry ligament and is usually depicted with clarity on sagittal and coronal sections, whereas the Humphry ligament is better visualized on sagittal sections (see Figs. 7.6 and 7.7).[18] In general, the attachment of the meniscofemoral ligaments to the posterior horn of the lateral meniscus should not extend greater than 14 mm beyond the lateral border of the PCL, otherwise a meniscal tear should be suspected.[28,84]

Literature describes four types of meniscomeniscal ligaments: the anterior transverse meniscal ligament, posterior transverse meniscal ligament, and medial and lateral oblique meniscomeniscal ligaments.[25] The anterior transverse (geniculate) ligament of the knee is a structure frequently identified posterior to Hoffa fat pad, connecting the anterior convex margin of the lateral meniscus to the anterior horn of the

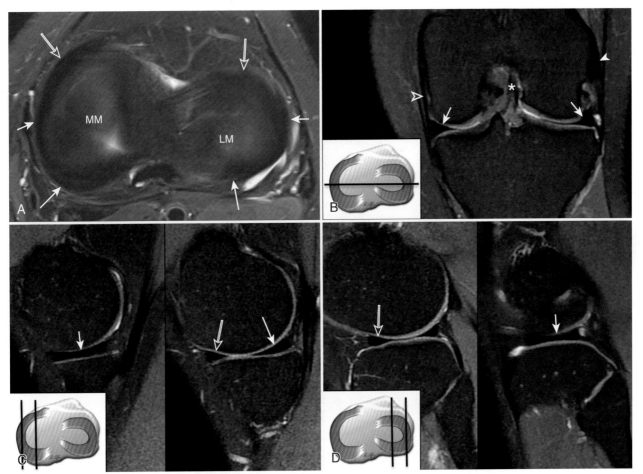

FIG 7.2 Axial (A), coronal (B), and sagittal (C and D) proton density (PD) fat-saturated (FS) MR images show the normal MR anatomy of the lateral and medial meniscus. Normal semilunar morphology of the menisci is observed on the axial MR image (A). The medial meniscus (MM) has a more open C-shape configuration than the lateral meniscus (LM). Each meniscus is divided in three portions: anterior horn *(open arrows)*, body *(thick arrows)*, and posterior horn *(thin arrows)*. The body of the medial and lateral meniscus *(thick arrows)* appears as a wedged, hypointense structure on coronal MR images (B), whereas the anterior *(open arrows)* and posterior *(thin arrows)* horns of the medial (C) and lateral (D) meniscus have a wedged configuration on sagittal MR images. The body of the menisci take on a more bow tie configuration when imaged parallel to its longitudinal axis *(thick arrows* in C and D). *Open arrowhead* indicates the medial collateral ligament; *white arrowhead* indicates lateral collateral ligament.

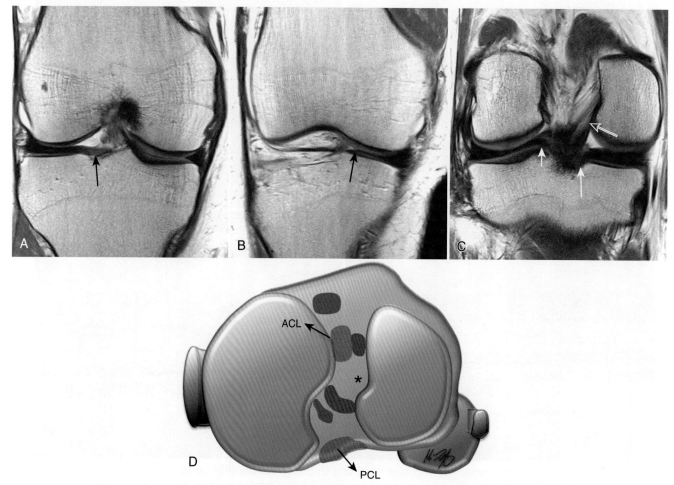

FIG 7.3 Normal Anatomy of the Root Ligaments (A-C) Coronal T1-weighted MR images demonstrating the anterior root ligament of the lateral meniscus (*arrow* in A), the anterior horn of the medial meniscus (*arrow* in B), and the posterior root ligaments of the posterior horn of the lateral meniscus *(thick arrow)* and the medial meniscus *(thin arrow)*. The anterior root ligament of the medial meniscus (*arrow* in B) inserts closer to the articular surface compared with the lateral meniscus (*arrow* in A). The close relation of the posterior root ligaments (*white arrows* in C) with the posterior cruciate ligament (PCL) *(open arrow)* is demonstrated. (D) Illustration of the root ligaments insertion sites. Insertions of the lateral meniscus are depicted in red and medial meniscal insertions in purple. *Asterisk* indicates lateral tibial tubercle.

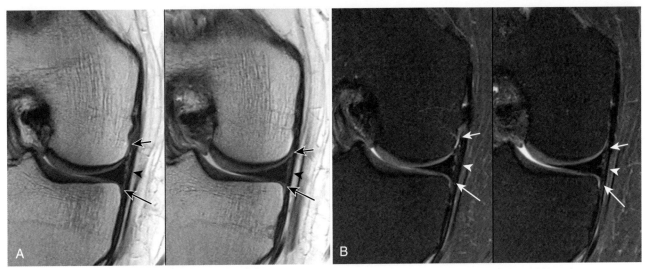

FIG 7.4 Normal Anatomy of the Medial Supporting Structures Coronal T1-weighted (A) and PD FS (B) MR images through the body of the medial meniscus demonstrating the deep portion of the medial collateral ligament (MCL) formed by the meniscocapsular ligaments: the meniscofemoral ligament *(thick arrows)* and the meniscotibial or coronary ligament *(thin arrows)*. Fibrofatty tissue and the MCL bursa separate the medial meniscus and the meniscocapsular ligaments from the main portion of the MCL *(arrowheads)*.

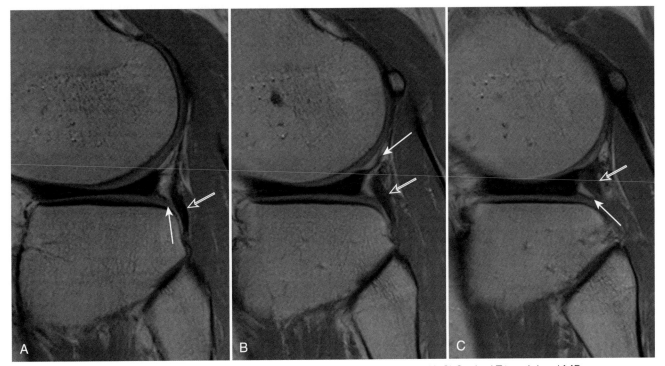

FIG 7.5 Normal Anatomy of the Lateral Supporting Structures (A-C) Sagittal T1-weighted MR images through the lateral meniscus show the three popliteomeniscal fascicles. (A) The posteroinferior popliteomeniscal fascicle *(arrow in A)* is the most central of the fascicles and is located medial to the popliteal hiatus. (B) The posterosuperior popliteomeniscal fascicle *(arrow in B)* forms the roof of the popliteal hiatus. (C) The anteroinferior popliteomeniscal fascicle *(arrow in C)* is the most lateral of the fascicles and forms the floor of the popliteal hiatus. The popliteal tendon *(open arrows)* is seen within the popliteal hiatus adjacent to the posterior horn of the lateral meniscus.

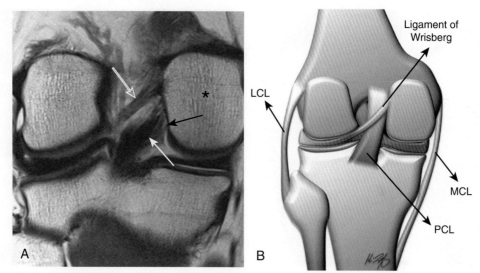

FIG 7.6 Normal Anatomy of the Meniscofemoral Ligaments (A) Coronal T1-weighted MR image through the posterior root ligaments showing the meniscofemoral ligaments of Wrisberg *(open arrows)* and Humphrey *(white arrows)* and their close relationship with the PCL *(black arrow).* The meniscofemoral ligament of Wrisberg inserts superior to the PCL and the ligament of Humphry in the medial femoral condyle *(asterisk).* (D) Drawing showing the meniscofemoral ligament of Wrisberg and its relationship with the PCL. *LCL,* Lateral collateral ligament; *MCL,* medial collateral ligament; *PCL,* posterior cruciate ligament.

medial meniscus (Fig. 7.8). This ligament is present in 50% to 90% of gross specimens and has an important function in restricting anteroposterior excursion of the anterior horn of the medial meniscus during the early phase of knee flexion.[34] The anterior transverse ligament of the knee is closely related to the ligamentum mucosum or infrapatellar plica, a structure that extends from Hoffa fat pad to the apex of the intercondylar notch of the femur (Fig. 7.9). In some cases the ligamentum mucosum may have an attachment to the inferior pole of the patella. A synovial cleft may be found beneath the ligamentum mucosum in the posteroinferior portion of Hoffa fat pad in 11% to 14% of individuals.[3] The posterior transverse meniscal ligament has a reported prevalence of 1% to 4% and connects the posterior horns of the medial and lateral menisci.[103] The medial and lateral oblique meniscomeniscal ligaments are intrameniscal ligaments that run obliquely from the anterior horn of one of the meniscus to the posterior horn of the opposite meniscus. Their combined prevalence in the literature ranges from 1% to 4%. Each oblique meniscomeniscal ligament receives its name from its anterior meniscal origin and passes between the anterior and PCLs as it traverses the intercondylar notch.[103] In addition to the classical four intermeniscal ligament variants, two new structures have been reported: unilateral medial and lateral intermeniscal ligaments.[25]

The popliteomeniscal fascicles attach the popliteus tendon to the lateral meniscus and are considered important meniscal stabilizers (see Fig. 7.5). Two fascicles have been commonly recognized: anteroinferior and posterosuperior fascicles. The anteroinferior popliteomeniscal fascicle extends from the lateral edge of the body of the meniscus to the inferior portion of popliteal paratenon and forms the floor of the popliteal hiatus. The lateral portion of the fascicle fuses with the popliteofibular ligament to form a conjoined attachment at the fibular styloid process. The posterosuperior popliteomeniscal fascicle extends from the body and portion of

the posterior horn of the lateral meniscus to the superior portion of the popliteal paratenon and the capsule and forms the roof of the popliteal hiatus. This fascicle has a posterior course and attaches to the posterior capsule.[76,87] Some authors have described a third popliteomeniscal fascicle, known as the posteroinferior popliteomeniscal fascicle. The posteroinferior popliteomeniscal fascicle is located medial to the popliteal hiatus extending from the inferior margin of the posterior horn of the lateral meniscus near the posterior meniscofemoral ligament of Wrisberg to the medial aponeurosis of the popliteus muscle.[87]

The patellomeniscal ligament, part of the middle layer of the lateral supporting structures of the knee, travels from the patella to the lateral meniscus deep to the iliotibial tract.[52]

Meniscal Tissue Composition

The meniscal blood supply is derived from the medial and lateral geniculate arteries. In adults the peripheral 20% to 30% of the meniscus is vascularized (red zone), whereas the inner two-thirds are relative avascular (white zone). A mixed-vascularity pink zone is described at the red-white junction. The extent of meniscal vascularization is similar in both lateral and medial menisci and appears to be more pronounced at the anterior and posterior horn than in the body. The vascular and avascular zones can be differentiated histologically but not with direct inspection.[11,55]

Meniscal tissue is mainly composed of water (72% water), with the remaining composed of organic matter, mostly extracellular matrix and cells. A collagen network is the main component of the organic matter (75%), and different collagen types exist in varying quantities in each region of the meniscus. Collagen type I predominates in the red zone of the meniscus, and collagen types I and II are present in the white zone of the meniscus.[47,120] Collagen fibers are arranged in three distinct layers in the meniscus cross section: (1) superficial network, a

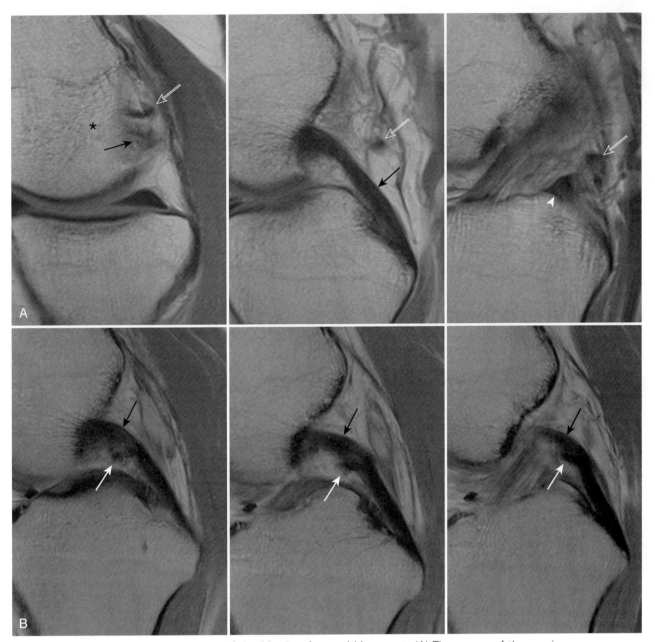

FIG 7.7 Normal Anatomy of the Meniscofemoral Ligaments (A) The course of the menisco-femoral ligament of Wrisberg is demonstrated on consecutive sagittal T1-weighted MR images where the ligament extends from the medial femoral condyle *(asterisk)* to the posterior horn of the lateral meniscus *(arrowhead)*. The ligament of Wrisberg courses behind the posterior cruciate ligament (PCL) *(black arrow)*. (B) The course of the meniscofemoral ligament of Humphrey is shown on consecutive sagittal T1-weighted MR images where the ligament is seen anterior to the genu of the PCL *(black arrows)*. Blending of the ligament of Humphrey with the PCL is seen in the sagittal image to the right where a hump in the PCL is formed.

meshwork of thin fibers at tibial and femoral meniscus surfaces; (2) lamellar layer, beneath the superficial network; and (3) central main layer, which has the circular bundles of collagen fibers oriented parallel to the longitudinal axis of the meniscus and the radial fibers, traveling perpendicular to the long axis of the meniscus (Fig. 7.10A).[2,89] Although the principal orientation of the collagen fibers is circumferential, the radial fibers appear on both femoral and tibial meniscal surfaces and within the substance of the menisci. The longitudinally oriented fibers predominate at the meniscal periphery and that could explain why longitudinal tears occur more frequently at the periphery of the meniscus. The "middle perforating" or "tie" fibers are condensed, radially oriented fibers located in the substance of meniscal tissue, which could explain the frequent location of radial tears in this location. Knowledge of the collagen architecture of the meniscus is important to understand the different types of meniscal tears and the appropriate use of meniscal repair techniques.[2]

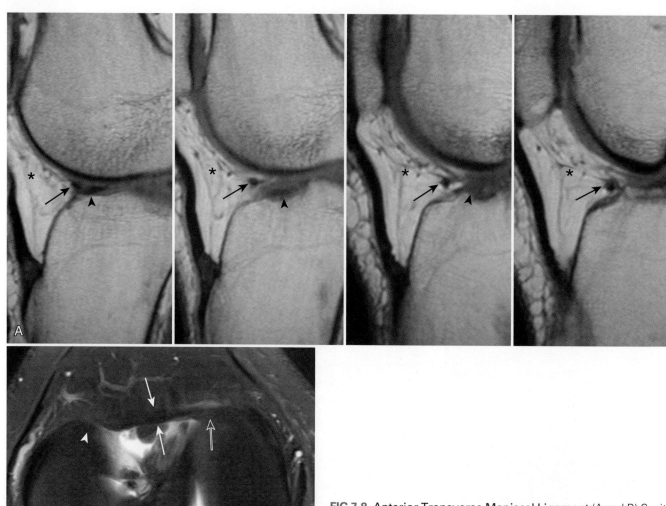

FIG 7.8 Anterior Transverse Meniscal Ligament (A and B) Sagittal T1-weighted (A) and axial PD FS (B) MR images showing the anterior transverse meniscal ligament extending from the anterior horn of the lateral meniscus *(arrowheads)* to the anterior horn of the medial meniscus *(open arrow)*. The ligament is clearly depicted on consecutive sagittal T1-weighted MR images coursing posterior to the hyperintense Hoffa fat pad *(asterisk)*.

In histologic studies the root ligaments demonstrate the typical structure of an enthesis at the attachment to the tibia, transitioning from the meniscal substance to uncalcified fibrocartilage, calcified cartilage, and ultimately bone.[120] The midsubstance of the root ligaments has a microstructure very similar to that of other ligaments. It is composed of parallel collagen bundles and a connective tissue sheath embracing them.[117] Attachment of the anterior and posterior horns of the menisci via root ligaments have been characterized in cadavers and by MRI because proper selection of the anchoring sites at surgery is critical to restore normal meniscal function.[60]

BIOMECHANICAL PROPERTIES OF THE MENISCUS

The menisci perform several important functions in the knee joint: (1) increase stabilization of the knee by deepening the contact between femoral condyles and tibial plateau; (2) distribute axial loads and absorb shock by distributing hoop forces evenly across the articulating surfaces; (3) assist in joint lubrication and facilitate nutrient distribution; and (4) aid in proprioception because of the nerve fibers located in the anterior and posterior thirds.[11,81]

During knee flexion, the medial meniscus moves an average of 2 to 5 mm, whereas the lateral meniscus is more mobile, with an anteroposterior displacement of approximately 9 to 11 mm along the tibial articular surface. The lateral meniscus moves as a single unit, whereas the medial meniscus anterior horn is more mobile than its posterior horn. The posteromedial portion of the medial meniscus is the least mobile region of the meniscus because of the constraint of the adjacent posterior oblique ligament. Changes in meniscal morphology during flexion and extension allow meniscal surface to maintain contact with the femur and tibia throughout movement.[47]

The arrangement of meniscal collagen fibers is ideal for transferring a vertical compressive load into circumferential "hoop" stresses. Collagen fibers are oriented circumferentially in the deeper layers of the meniscus, parallel to the peripheral border. These fibers blend the ligamentous connections of the

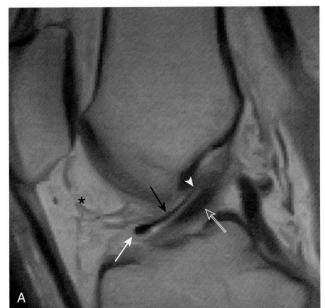

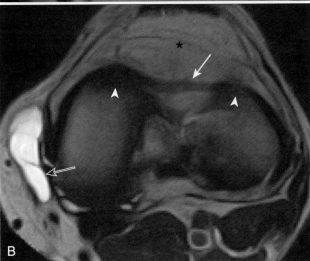

FIG 7.9 Ligamentum Mucosum or Infrapatellar Plica (A) Sagittal T2-weighted MR image demonstrating the ligamentum mucosum or infrapatellar plica extending from the anterior transverse meniscal ligament *(white arrows)* located posterior to Hoffa fat pad *(asterisks)* to the intercondylar notch of the femur *(arrowhead in A)*. This structure locates anterior to the PCL *(open arrow in A)* as it traverses the intercondylar notch. (B) Axial T2-weighted MR image through the menisci of the same subject shows the anterior transverse meniscal ligament *(white arrow)* coursing between the anterior horns of the menisci *(arrowheads in B)*. A medial parameniscal cyst is also noted *(open arrow in B)*.

meniscal horns to the tibial articular surface.[47] Hoop stresses are generated as axial forces and converted to tensile stresses along the circumferential collagen fibers of the meniscus (see Fig. 7.10B). The wedge shape of the meniscus gives it a tendency to extrude from between the femoral and tibial condyles and firm attachments via root ligaments prevent the meniscus from extruding peripherally during load bearing. Studies have demonstrated that 70% of the load in the lateral compartment and 50% of the load in the medial compartment is transmitted

through the menisci.[1,47,77] The thinner radial tie fibers are interposed perpendicular to the circumferential fibers and act to tie bundles together, preventing the circumferential fibers to split apart when hoop stress is applied to the meniscus.[55,83]

Radial tears extending to the periphery disrupt the collagen fibers and may reduce meniscal hoop strength, severely impairing meniscal function (see Fig. 7.10C).[12] In contrast, only compressive loads are observed across longitudinal tears with maximum loads at full knee extension or at 90-degree knee flexion.[94]

Injuries that involve root ligaments severely affect meniscal biomechanics and kinematics, leading to accelerated degenerative changes within the knee joint. Injuries to the posterior meniscus root ligaments, including root avulsion, full-length tears, and radial tears of the posterior horn adjacent to the root, have been associated with significant meniscal extrusion. Meniscal extrusion may impair hoop stress force transmission, increasing peak tibiofemoral contact pressures similar to that of meniscectomy.[15,64,77]

In 1948 Fairbank described an increased incidence and predictable degenerative changes of the articular surfaces in completely meniscectomized knees.[46] After Fairbank's report, numerous studies have confirmed these findings. After total meniscectomy the contact areas decrease by 50% to 75% and the contact pressure increases two to three times.[1,49] The increased load may contribute to cartilage injury and degeneration. Misalignment, concurrent articular pathology, and ligament instability have been associated with an accelerated development of OA in meniscectomized knees.[1,72] A higher prevalence of late OA has been found in partially meniscectomized knees compared with normal knees, with radiographic signs of OA four to seven times more frequent in the partially meniscectomized knees. Individuals with partial meniscectomy have better functional outcome than those with total meniscectomy. The amount of meniscal tissue excised has been shown to be inversely related to the proper function of the meniscus. Specifically those individuals with large resection of the posterior horn will have the worst functionality.[1] Demonstration of biomechanical alterations and higher risk of OA after partial or total meniscectomy has led to surgical techniques in which the goal is to maintain the tissue intact whenever possible.[75]

IMAGING OF THE MENISCUS

MRI has evolved into the preferred noninvasive imaging modality for evaluating internal knee derangement since its first use in the clinical setting. During the past two decades MRI has been the modality of choice in the imaging diagnosis of meniscal tears. MRI has demonstrated high sensitivity and specificity for detection of meniscal tears, with arthroscopy as the reference standard.[44,83,99]

Normal Magnetic Resonance Appearance of the Meniscus

Menisci are hypointense on T1- and T2-weighted MR images, with intermediate to long time to echo (TE) because of their fibrocartilaginous composition. The MR properties of meniscal tissue relate to the extremely rapid T2 relaxation resulting from the high intrameniscal content of collagen and other short T2 components.[88,95] Higher signal intensity may be demonstrated in the peripheral third of the meniscus in young individuals, representing normal vascularity or tie fibers.[11]

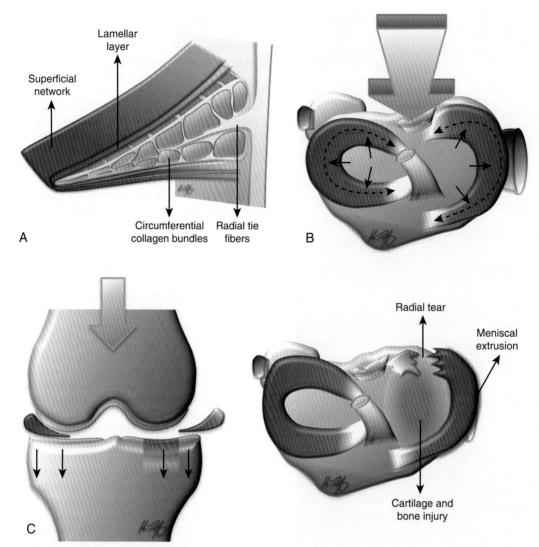

FIG 7.10 (A) Illustration of the collagen fiber arrangement in the meniscus in three distinct layers: (1) superficial network, (2) lamellar layer, and (3) central main layer. The last layer is constituted by the circumferential and the radial or tie fibers. (B) Representation of the normal biomechanics of the meniscus. Hoop stresses *(black arrows)* are generated as axial forces *(blue arrow)* are converted to tensile stresses *(dashed arrows)* along the circumferential fibers of the meniscus. (C) Radial tears extending to the periphery disrupt the circumferential collagen fibers and reduce meniscal hoop strength. Axial forces *(blue arrow)* result in meniscal extrusion with increased peak tibiofemoral contact pressures leading to cartilage and bone injury *(red and yellow areas)*.

The MR appearance of the meniscus depends on the orientation of the imaging plane with respect to the axis of the meniscus (see Fig. 7.2). On axial MR images menisci have a semilunar or C-shape configuration, and the differences between lateral meniscus with a closed C-shape and medial meniscus with a more open C-shape can be demonstrated. When imaged perpendicular to the meniscal longitudinal axis, menisci have a triangular or wedge appearance. Therefore the anterior and posterior horns are seen as triangular or wedged structures on sagittal MR images, whereas the meniscal body is seen as a triangular or wedged shape on coronal MR images. The apex of the triangle points to the intercondylar notch, the base is oriented peripherally, the superior surface of the triangle is slightly concave and accommodates the femoral condyle, and the inferior surface is flat and lies on the tibial plateau. Menisci take on a more slab or bow tie configuration when the imaging plane is oriented parallel to the long axis of the meniscus (ie, anterior and posterior horns on coronal MR images and meniscal body on coronal MR images).[98,33] Differences in size between the anterior and posterior horns of the meniscus can be appreciated on sagittal sections in which anterior and posterior horns of the lateral meniscus are similar, whereas the posterior horn of the medial meniscus can be twice as large as the anterior horn.[76,99]

Magnetic Resonance Imaging Sequences

Several sequences have been advocated for imaging of meniscal tears. MR images with short TEs and high-resolution MR images are required to improve detection of meniscal tears.

Although protocols may vary, most meniscal tears are best demonstrated on the sagittal plane. It has been shown that up to 97% of medial and 96% of lateral meniscal tears can be identified on sagittal MR images.[38] Proton density (PD) sequences which use long time to repetition (TR) and short TEs are optimal in the detection of the increased signal intensity seen in meniscal tears. Most recent articles support the use of either conventional spin echo (SE) PD sequences or fast spin echo (FSE) PD sequences to detect meniscal tears.[19,45] Rubin et al. found similar sensitivities and specificities when comparing FSE and SE PD sequences with arthroscopy as the reference standard.[100] The major advantage of FSE is faster imaging times with decreasing motion artifacts but with an increase in image blurring. The use of lower echo train lengths (four or less), high-performance extremity gradient coils, and longer bandwidths (in the 30s or higher) allows a decrease in image blurring.[99]

Spatial resolution can be improved by maximizing the matrix size while maintaining a small field of view (FOV) and thin section thickness. These parameters will result in a decrease in the signal-to-noise ratio (SNR), which can be partially compensated for by increasing the number of excitations (NEX of 2) and using dedicated high-performance extremity gradient coils. Typical parameters for meniscal imaging include an FOV of 16 cm or less, a matrix size of at least 192 (phase-encoding direction) × 256 (frequency-encoding direction), and slice thickness of 3 to 4 mm.[83,99]

Three tesla (3 T) MRI allows for a higher SNR compared with 1.5-T imaging. This can be used to improve imaging acquisition speed or resolution. However, there is increased sensitivity to magnetic susceptibility artifacts and chemical shift artifacts compared with 1.5 T.[73] Despite the advantages in SNR, speed, and resolution with the 3-T MRI, studies have found comparable accuracies between 1.5- and 3-T imaging.[53,115]

EVALUATION OF MENISCAL TEARS

Meniscal tears are among the most common knee injuries. The prevalence of meniscal tears increase with age, and meniscal tears are often associated with and contribute to degenerative joint disease. Tears are more common in the posterior horn of the menisci, especially in the medial meniscus, because of its decreased mobility compared with the lateral meniscus.[83]

Meniscal tears can be traumatic or degenerative. Traumatic tears result when an excessive force is applied to a normal meniscus during trauma, exceeding the capacity of the meniscal tissue to deform. Radial and vertical tears are most frequently created with this mechanism of injury, although horizontal or oblique tears may also occur. Degenerative tears on the other side occur from normal forces acting on degenerated tissue and are mostly horizontal cleavage tears.[93]

MRI has proved to be highly accurate in detection of meniscal injuries, with excellent arthroscopic correlation. A meta-analysis of published articles between 1991 and 2000 reported a pooled sensitivity and specificity of 93% and 88%, respectively, for medial meniscal tears and 79% and 96%, respectively, for lateral meniscal tears. Several factors, such as sample size, technical parameters, and accuracy of arthroscopic findings, the current reference standard, accounted for differences in accuracy.[99] Reported sensitivity and specificity of conventional SE and FSE MRI at 1.5 T for diagnosing meniscal tears compared with arthroscopy ranges from 86% to 97% and 84% to 94%, respectively, for medial meniscus and from 70% to 92% and 89% to 98%, respectively, for lateral meniscus.[44]

The diagnosis of meniscal tears has been based on two main criteria: linear intrameniscal signal intensity extending into the superior and/or inferior surfaces and morphologic alterations of the meniscus in the absence of prior surgery.[34,81] To assist with correct classification of a tear, meniscal signal has been categorized into different grades: grade 0 consists of a normal, uniform, low-signal intensity; grade 1 consists of an intrameniscal globular or ovoid high signal that is not communicating with an articular surface; grade 2 consists of an intrameniscal linear or wedge-shape signal that is not communicating with an articular surface; grade 3a is an intrameniscal signal that equivocally contacts the articular surface; and grade 3b is an intrameniscal signal that clearly contacts the articular surface. Only grade 3 signal represents a tear. Grade 1 or 2 signal does not indicate a tear and is associated with normal vascularity in children and tissue degeneration in adults.[32,48] There is a high probability for a meniscus to be torn when abnormalities in signal intensity or morphology are seen in two or more MR images and considerably less likely to be torn when abnormalities are seen in only one MR image. De Smet et al. have presented these findings as the "two-slice-touch" rule and have found an increase in positive predictive values (PPVs) compared with the standard diagnostic criteria using one or more MR images. In their study the PPV increased from 91% to 94% for medial meniscal tears and from 83% to 96% for lateral meniscal tears.[44]

Despite the high accuracy of MRI for diagnosing tears, false-positive diagnoses still occur and are more common in the medial meniscus than in the lateral meniscus. False-positive diagnoses are frequently associated with longitudinal, root ligament and radial tears compared with bucket-handle, complex, flap, and horizontal tears, with complex tears having the lowest frequency of false-positive diagnosis. Of all the meniscal tear types, longitudinal tears have the lowest reported PPV, especially those located at the meniscocapsular junction.[43] Spontaneous meniscal healing may contribute to a false-positive diagnosis, particularly in those cases in which arthroscopy is performed 6 weeks after the MR examination.[43,63] The sensitivity of MRI for diagnosing meniscal tears has been consistently lower for lateral meniscal tears compared with medial meniscal tears and may vary with tear location, extension, and type. It has been shown that tears that involve one-third or less of the meniscus, tears located at the posterior horn, or longitudinal type tears are the most frequently missed meniscal tears in the lateral meniscus.[42]

Meniscal Tear Classification

The choice of treatment and ultimate prognosis associated with meniscal tears are influenced by such factors as tear orientation, extent, and location. The location of the tear is critical because tears located in the red zone (vascular portion) are far more likely to heal than tears located in the white zone (avascular portion) of the meniscus. Tears located in the red zone of the meniscus may be treated with meniscus-preserving techniques such as suture repair, whereas tears in the white zone typically are treated by means of débridement.[55]

No classification system has been widely accepted. There are several types of meniscal tears described in the literature, based on tear morphology, including basic and displaced types of meniscal tears. Basic meniscal tears include longitudinal, radial, and complex types. Longitudinal tears can be further divided into longitudinal horizontal and longitudinal vertical tears.

Displaced types include bucket handle, displaced flap, and free fragment tears. The more recently described root ligament tears are also included in this section.[38,83,93]

Longitudinal Horizontal Tears

Longitudinal horizontal tears are common, with a reported prevalence of 32%.[38] These tears run parallel to the tibial plateau, involve either one of the articular surfaces or the free edge of the meniscus, and extend toward the periphery, thus dividing the meniscus into superior or inferior portions. These tears have also been designated as horizontal, fish-mouth, or cleavage tears. Longitudinal horizontal tears usually involve the posterior horn of the menisci, with variable anterior extension separating rather than violating the circumferential collagen fibers.[93] Horizontal tears occur most commonly in individuals older than 40 years without a specific history of trauma,

probably secondary to tissue degeneration. On MRI this type of tear is demonstrated as a horizontal hyperintense line extending from the center to the periphery of the meniscus on sagittal and coronal planes (Fig. 7.11).[38,83]

Early reports suggested that the diagnosis of degenerative meniscal tears on MRI was more difficult compared with traumatic tears because of the progression from meniscal degeneration to meniscal tear. A significantly high rate of false-negative findings was reported when interpreting grade 2 signal meniscal lesions.[118] However, subsequent studies have shown that patients with intrameniscal hyperintensity do not have an increased likelihood of developing a meniscal tear compared with patients with homogeneous low signal intensity meniscus on MRI.[38]

Parameniscal cysts have been associated with horizontal meniscal tears and have been described involving almost twice as often the medial compartment than the lateral

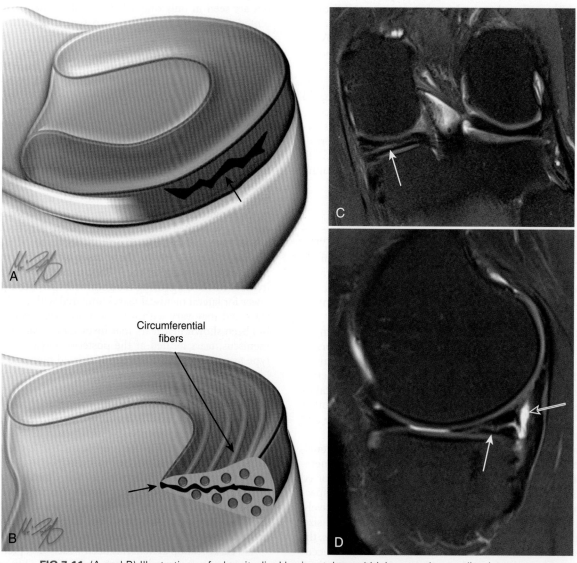

FIG 7.11 (A and B) Illustrations of a longitudinal horizontal tear *(thick arrows)* extending between the circumferential collagen bundles. Coronal (C) and sagittal (D) PD FS MR images show a longitudinal horizontal tear *(white arrows)* of the posterior horn of the medial meniscus extending from the free edge to the periphery of the meniscus. A fluid-filled parameniscal cyst *(open arrow)* is seen communicating with the tear.

compartment.[24] Those parameniscal cysts adjacent to the anterior horn of the lateral meniscus are the only parameniscal cysts not associated with an underlying meniscal tear.[41] Several theories for cyst formation have been proposed, with the dominant theory suggesting that synovial fluid is forced out through the underlying tears accumulating at the meniscocapsular to form a cyst. Medial cysts are often located adjacent to the posterior horn and lateral cysts are often located adjacent to the body or the anterior horn of the lateral meniscus

(Fig. 7.12). Large cysts tend to form in the medial side near the MCL, penetrate the capsule, and expand more that lateral cysts, which are more likely to be contained within the joint capsule. Large parameniscal cysts formed posterior to the MCL can be confused with popliteal cysts and when extending into the region of the PCL may mimic a ganglion cyst. Demonstration of communication of the parameniscal cyst with the adjacent horizontal tear is useful to avoid misinterpretations.[23] Treatment often involves débridement of the meniscal leaf and

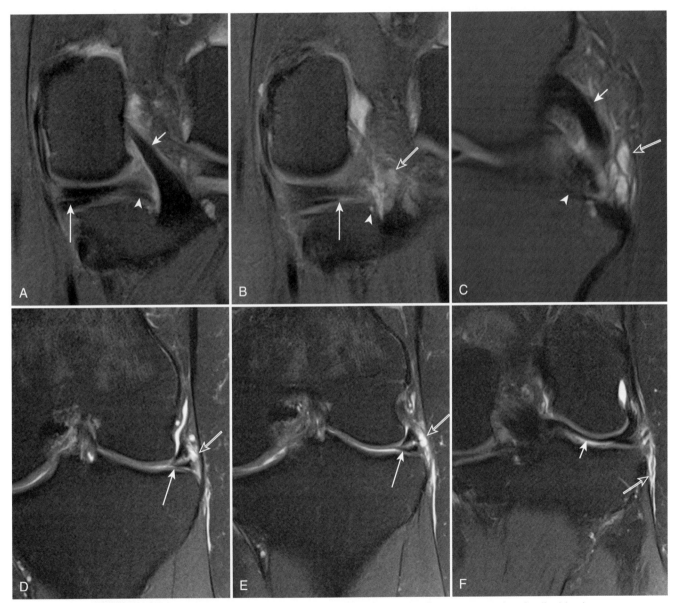

FIG 7.12 Coronal (A and B) and sagittal (C) PD FS MR images demonstrate a longitudinal horizontal tear of the posterior horn of the medial meniscus contacting the inferior articular surface *(thin arrows)*. An adjacent multilobulated, septated parameniscal cyst *(open arrows)* is seen extending into the intercondylar notch close to the PCL *(thick arrows)*. A thickened and hyperintense posterior root ligament of the medial meniscus with bone cystic changes is noted *(arrowheads)*. (D-F) Coronal PD FS MR images show a hyperintense longitudinal horizontal tear of the body of the lateral meniscus extending from the free edge to the periphery *(thin arrows)*. The tear involves the inferior articular surface of the posterior horn, which appears thinned *(thick arrow)*. A parameniscal cyst adjacent to the body of the lateral meniscus with inferior extension is demonstrated *(open arrows)*.

decompression of the associated parameniscal cyst or particle meniscectomy with open cystectomy to avoid recurrence of the parameniscal cyst.[83]

Longitudinal Vertical Tears

Longitudinal vertical tears are oriented along the longitudinal or anteroposterior axis of the meniscus, perpendicular to the tibial plateau, dividing the meniscus into a central and a peripheral portion.[83,93] Pure longitudinal vertical tears do not involve the free edge of the meniscus. This type of tear has been referred to as longitudinal vertical tear as the tear extends in the anteroposterior and the superoinferior dimensions between the circumferential collagen bundles of the meniscus. Some longitudinal vertical tears may have a slightly oblique course violating some of the collagen bundles. Longitudinal vertical tears are more common in the medial meniscus than in the lateral, often involving the peripheral third and less frequently the central third of the meniscus. Longitudinal vertical tears almost always involve the posterior horn of the menisci. On MRI images, longitudinal vertical tears are seen as a hyperintense vertical line contacting the superior, the inferior, or both surfaces of the meniscus (Figs. 7.13 and 7.14).[38,83,93]

There is a close relationship between ACL tears and peripheral longitudinal vertical tears, particularly those tears located in the periphery of the posterior horn of the menisci. Specifically, 90% of medial meniscus and 83% of lateral meniscus peripheral longitudinal tears have an associated ACL tear. It has been shown that meniscal tears associated with ACL injuries are more difficult to detect on MRI because of their location and configuration with lower sensitivities compared with meniscal

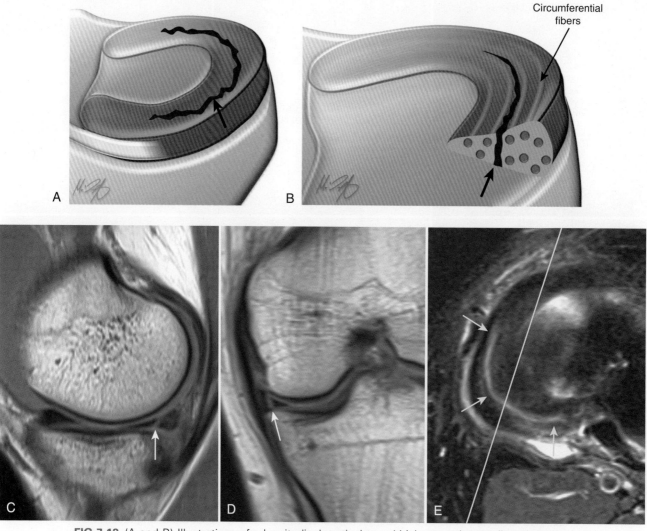

FIG 7.13 (A and B) Illustrations of a longitudinal vertical tear *(thick arrows)* extending along the longitudinal axis of the meniscus between the circumferential collagen bundles. The tear contacts both articular surfaces. Sagittal (C) and coronal (D) T1-weighted MR images demonstrate a longitudinal vertical tear involving the posterior horn *(thin arrow* in D) and the body *(thin arrow* in E) of the medial meniscus. The tear extends from the superior to the inferior articular surfaces of the meniscus. (E) Axial T2-weighted MR image through the medial meniscus in the same subject shows the longitudinal vertical tear in its anteroposterior dimension extending from the body to the posterior root ligament of the meniscus *(yellow arrows)*. The *yellow line* represents the sagittal plane used in C.

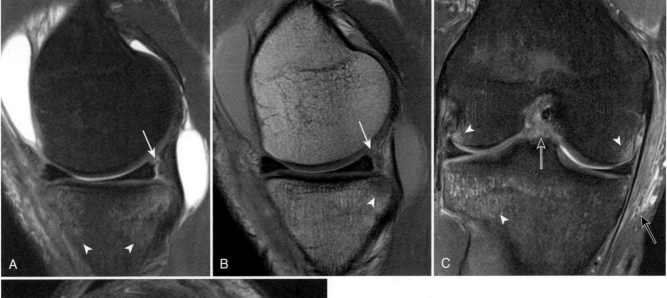

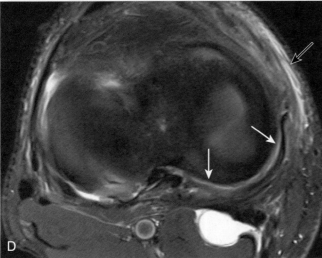

FIG 7.14 Sagittal PD FS (A), PD non–fat-saturated (NFS) (B), coronal PD FS (C), and axial PD FS MR images showing a longitudinal vertical tear at the meniscocapsular junction. A peripheral longitudinal vertical tear located at the meniscocapsular junction of the medial meniscus is seen on the sagittal MR images (A and B). The tear extends from the superior to the inferior articular surfaces *(thin arrows)*, appears hyperintense on the PD FS MR images (A) and can be easily missed on the NFS PD MR images (B). The anteroposterior dimension of the tear is well demonstrated on the axial MR image where it involves the posterior horn of the meniscus *(thin arrows)*. Bone contusions in the tibial plateau and femoral condyles *(arrowheads)*, soft tissue edema adjacent to the MCL *(thick arrow)*, irregularity and increased signal intensity of the proximal ACL *(open arrow)* are also demonstrated.

tears in the absence of ACL injury (88% vs. 97% for medial meniscal tears and 69% vs. 94% for medial meniscal tears).[40] Longitudinal vertical peripheral tears of the posterior horn of the lateral meniscus were the most commonly missed tears that could be seen in retrospect in a study by De Smet et al. Probable causes include the smaller size of tears in this region, oblique visualization of the posterior horn because of the sloping upward course at its attachment and the small radius of the curvature of the lateral meniscus, the more complex anatomy of the posterior horn and related structures, magic angle phenomenon, and arterial pulsation artifact.[42]

Tears at the junction of the posterior horn of the lateral meniscus, referred to as the *Wrisberg rip*, are seen frequently in association with ACL tears. This particular tear type occurs as a result of traction from the ligament of Wrisberg upon the posterior horn of the lateral meniscus in cases of ACL injury where there is anterior translation of the tibia.[9] In general, if the meniscofemoral ligament is identified on four or more consecutive sagittal MR images lateral to the PCL (with a 3-mm slice thickness and a 0.5-mm slice gap) or if it extends beyond than 14 mm lateral to the lateral edge of the PCL, a peripheral longitudinal tear of the posterior horn of the lateral

meniscus should be suspected, especially in the setting of an ACL tear.[84,98]

A disrupted or absent superior popliteomeniscal fascicle on sagittal MR images has been considered an indirect sign to diagnose lateral meniscal tears with a moderately high PPV (79%).[20] Abnormal superior popliteomeniscal fascicle and pericapsular edemas are two indirect signs that have been found to be significantly associated with ACL tears.[20]

Because longitudinal meniscal tears occur most often in the peripheral third of the meniscus, which is the vascularized (red zone) of the meniscus, these tears may heal spontaneously or may be amenable to repair.[11]

Radial Tears

Radial tears have a reported prevalence of 15% in a series of 196 consecutive knee arthroscopy patients.[54] Radial tears run perpendicular to the tibial plateau and to the longitudinal axis of the meniscus and violate the circumferential collagen bundles as they extend from the free edge toward the periphery of the meniscus. This type of meniscal tear may be complete, reaching the periphery of the meniscus, or incomplete, involving the inner portion of the meniscus and preserving its outer portion.

When the radial tear is long, it transects many collagen fibers and severely disrupts the meniscal hoop strength, resulting in a dramatic loss of function and meniscal extrusion. In these cases the meniscus opens up at the site of the tear, and a fluid-filled gap may be found.[93]

Radial tears have been reported to be difficult to visualize on MR images, and these tears account for a large percentage of meniscal tears missed by MRI.[73] These tears occur more frequently at the center of the posterior horn of the medial meniscus or at the junction of the anterior horn and body of the lateral meniscus.[38,54] The appearance of radial tears on MRI is variable and depends on the location of the tear and the imaging plane used (Fig. 7.15). When radial tears involve the body of the meniscus, the free edge appears truncated on coronal MR images, and the bow tie seen on the sagittal MR images displays a blunted configuration of one or its both halves. The ghost meniscus sign refers to an absent or minimal meniscal tissue seen when a gap develops at the tear site and the imaging plane is oriented along the axis of the tear. Conversely, a tear involving the posterior horn would appear as truncated or ghost meniscus on sagittal MR images and as a cleft on coronal MR images. Radial tears may be oriented obliquely rather that perpendicular to the longitudinal axis of the meniscus. In these cases the "marching cleft" sign is present and appears as a cleft moving

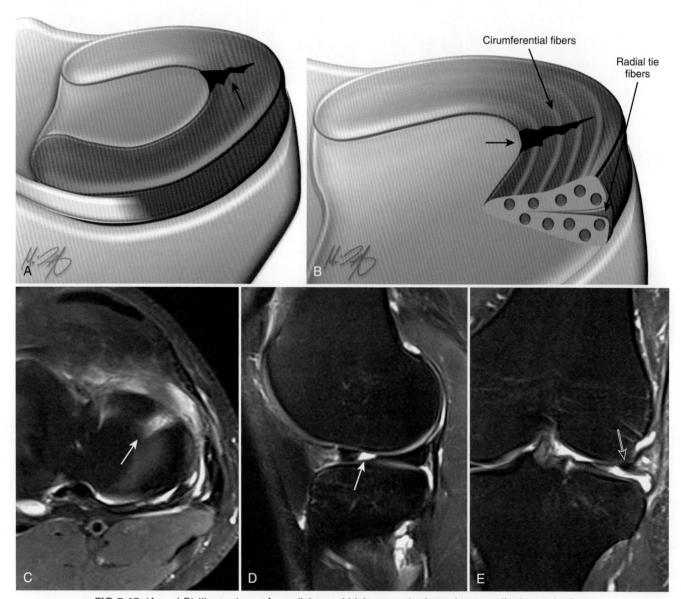

FIG 7.15 (A and B) Illustrations of a radial tear *(thick arrows)* oriented perpendicular to the longitudinal axis of the meniscus involving the free edge. The tear violates the circumferential collagen bundles impairing the ability of the meniscus to resist hoop stress. Axial (C), sagittal (D), and coronal (E) PD FS MR images show a radial tear *(thin arrows)* located at the junction of the anterior horn and body of the lateral meniscus. The tear extends from the free edge to the periphery of the meniscus with a fluid-filled gap and therefore is an unstable tear. The free edge of the anterior horn of the meniscus appears truncated on the sagittal MR image (D). The meniscal body appears small *(open white arrow)* on the coronal image (E).

away from the free edge of the meniscus on consecutive MR images. The cleft sign is not specific for radial tears and can be observed also in longitudinal vertical tears. The location of the cleft determines which type of tear is present because the cleft in radial tears is located in the inner portion of the meniscus and the cleft in longitudinal vertical tears locates in the outer portion of the meniscus.[38,54,83] When using the four signs (ie, the truncated meniscus, cleft, marching cleft, and ghost meniscus signs), identification improved from 37% to 89% of the cases in a study by Harper et al.[54]

A sharp tear involving the free edge of the meniscus is usually associated with a radial tear, and an irregular tear involving the free edge of the meniscus is usually associated with a horizontal or cleavage tear.[93] Because radial tears can lie between image slices in one plane, they may only be visible on one orthogonal image and are an exception to the two-slice-touch rule.[33]

Free edge radial tears are frequently treated with débridement. Repair of radial tears is infrequently attempted because these tears occur commonly in the avascular (white zone) of the meniscus and have a low likelihood of healing.[54]

Complex Tears

Complex tears include a combination of radial, longitudinal horizontal, and/or longitudinal vertical tears.[83] On MRI there is considerable distortion of the meniscal architecture and multiple lines of high signal intensity to the meniscal surface indicating that multiples flaps will be found at arthroscopy (Fig. 7.16).[6,38] Because of the extent of these tears, the collagen fibers are typically injured, severely disrupting the ability of the meniscus to bear weight and to resist hoop strain.[33,98]

Displaced Meniscal Tears

Displaced meniscal tears are common, representing most symptomatic meniscal lesions with joint pain and locking. Identification of displaced fragments is crucial because they may be missed at arthroscopy if their location is difficult to visualize and the residual meniscal surface appears healthy. Various classification systems have been proposed in the literature but displaced meniscal tears can be divided into three basic types: bucket handle, flap tear, and free fragment tears.[78]

Bucket Handle Tears

Bucket handle tears are the most frequent type of displaced meniscal tears. These tears represent longitudinal vertical or oblique tears with an attached fragment displaced away from the meniscus. Bucket handle tears occur seven times more frequently in the medial meniscus and usually involve the entire meniscus. Isolated involvement of the anterior horn, posterior horn, or body can occur. The displaced fragment is usually located in the intercondylar notch, the anterior compartment, or both.[4,10]

Several MR signs of bucket handle tears have been described on MRI, including the double PCL, fragment-in-notch, double anterior horn, flipped meniscus, and absent bow tie signs (Fig. 7.17). The double PCL sign refers to a band of low signal intensity seen anterior and parallel to the PCL on sagittal MR images.

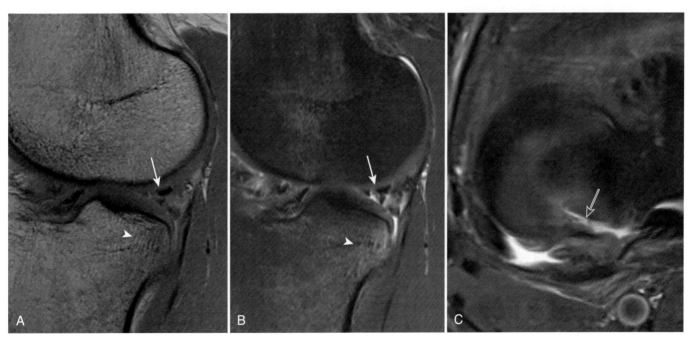

FIG 7.16 Sagittal PD non–fat-saturated (NFS) (A), PD FS (B), and axial PD FS (C) showing a complex meniscal tear involving the posterior horn of the lateral meniscus. Meniscal morphology is completely distorted with a multidirectional hyperintense tear extending from the superior to the inferior articular surfaces of the meniscus *(thin arrows)*. On the axial MR image an oblique radial component of the tear is demonstrated involving the posterior horn and posterior root ligament of the meniscus *(open arrow)*. The severe distortion and the presence of fluid within the tear are findings indicative of lesion instability. Bone contusion in the posterior region of the lateral tibial plateau is noted on sagittal MR images *(arrowheads)*.

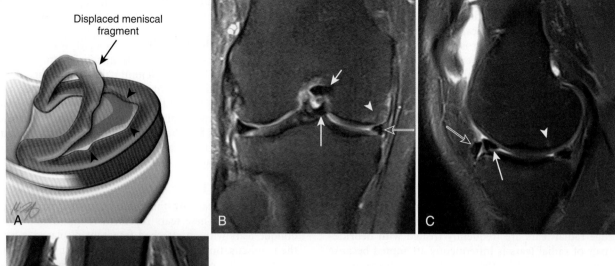

Displaced meniscal fragment

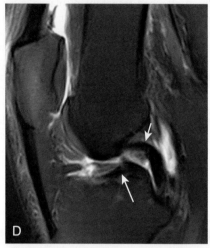

FIG 7.17 (A) Illustration of a bucket handle tear showing the centrally displaced meniscal fragment. This type of tear results from a longitudinal vertical tear *(arrowheads)* when the central portion of the meniscus displaces. Coronal (B) and sagittal (C and D) MR images showing a bucket handle tear of the medial meniscus. The body of the meniscus appears small *(open arrow)* on the coronal MR image (B). A hypointense structure is seen in the intercondylar notch representing the displaced meniscal fragment *(thin arrows)*. The double anterior horn sign is observed in C where hypointense meniscal tissue *(thin arrow)* is seen posterior to the anterior horn of the meniscus *(open arrow)*. The double PCL sign is demonstrated in D where the displaced meniscal fragment *(thin arrows)* is seen as a band of low signal intensity anterior to the PCL *(thick arrows)*. Bone edema-like signal intensity *(arrowheads)* in the medial femoral condyle is also noted.

The double PCL sign is observed mostly in medial bucket handle tears. The fragment-in-notch sign refers to a meniscal fragment within the intercondylar notch and is seen as a band-like area of low signal intensity within the notch appearing on a different slice than the PCL. The fragment-in-notch sign is usually associated with lateral bucket-handle tears. The fragment of a bucket handle tear can also be displaced into the anterior compartment, where it can be located either superior or posterior to the ipsilateral anterior horn. The double anterior horn sign refers to a well-defined meniscus shape, which constitutes the displaced fragment, seen immediately posterior to the anterior horn of the meniscus on sagittal MR images. The flipped meniscus sign is observed when the fragment displaces superior to the anterior horn, and it is seen as an abnormally tall anterior horn (<6 mm) on sagittal MR images. The double anterior horn and flipped meniscus signs can be observed with either lateral or medial bucket handle tears and can be seen in association with double PCL and fragment-in-notch signs.[101,121] The absent bow tie sign refers to the absence of the normal bow tie appearance of the meniscal body in two consecutive sagittal MR images. On coronal MR images the body of the meniscus with a bucket handle tear may appear truncated, deformed, or small.[56] The "disproportional posterior horn sign" is seen when the meniscal fragment of a bucket handle tear is displaced posterocentrally. On sagittal MR images the disproportional posterior horn sign is seen as a larger meniscal posterior horn in the central section than in the peripheral sections (Fig. 7.18).[27]

Bucket handle tears are treated with arthroscopic repair of the displaced fragment or arthroscopic resection when the tear is irreparable. Although repair is attempted whenever possible, bucket handle tears in the avascular zone, tears already accompanied by degenerative changes, the inability to obtain anatomic reduction of the displaced fragment, and deformation of a torn fragment may be indications for partial meniscectomy.[4]

Displaced Flap Tears

Displaced flap tears are those tears in which the tear extends in more than one plane creating separate flaps of meniscus. Although less frequent than bucket handle tears, flap tears are not rare, accounting for 19% of symptomatic meniscal injuries in one series.[101] When a piece of torn meniscus is displaced or can be displaced by a probe during arthroscopy, that piece is termed a "flap." Displaced flap tears are associated most commonly with longitudinal horizontal tears, and these tears will always have a superior flap and an inferior flap. A radial tear located perpendicular to the longitudinal axis of the meniscus will not have a flap, but an oblique radial tear can result in a free edge flap. Oblique radial tears with displaced flaps are also called "parrot beak" tears, as the curved beak flap resembles de beak of a parrot. The term parrot beak has been used mostly in arthroscopy.[38] On MRI, thin-section or well-placed axial MR images confirm that the tear is not a simple radial tears but rather an oblique radial tear (Fig. 7.19). Adjacent normal structures can simulate a displaced flap tear, such as the transverse

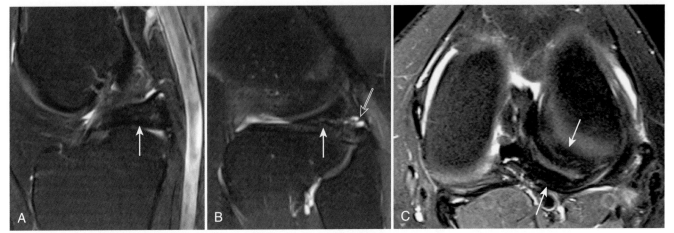

FIG 7.18 Sagittal PD FS (A and B) and axial PD FS (C) MR images showing a posteriorly flipped lateral meniscus. The disproportional posterior horn sign is seen on sagittal MR images where the posterior horn appears enlarged more medially (*thin arrow* in A) as compared with the lateral portion of the meniscus (*thin arrow* in B). A hyperintense longitudinal horizontal tear is seen in the lateral portion of the posterior horn of the lateral meniscus (*thin arrow* in B) communicating with a small parameniscal lobulated cyst *(open arrow)*. The posterocentrally displaced meniscal fragment *(thick arrows)* is well demonstrated on the axial MR image (C).

meniscal ligament, meniscofemoral ligaments, and popliteus tendon.[33]

Several studies have found that displaced flap tears are more common in the medial meniscus, with frequencies ranging from 82% to 87%, than in the lateral meniscus. Displaced flaps tears involving the medial meniscus are located most commonly at the body (71%) and at the posterior horn (26%) and those tears involving the lateral meniscus occur most commonly at the posterior horn (62%). Displaced flap tears at the body of medial meniscus may be superiorly or inferiorly displaced (Fig. 7.20). When located at the posterior horns the meniscal flap often displaces into the intercondylar notch. Inferiorly displaced flap tears are an important finding on MRI because these fragments are typically invisible at arthroscopy. Superiorly displaced tears located anteriorly in the superior recess, are difficult to visualize on coronal MR images and should not be confused with the patellofemoral ligament.[67,78]

The size of the displaced flap has been positively correlated with the degree of cartilage loss and joint pain. Displaced flap tears are treated with meniscal débridement, with average removal of 49% of the meniscus.[67]

Root Ligament Tears

Interest in meniscal root ligaments has increased because injuries at or near the root ligament insertion have been reported to significantly alter tibiofemoral contact biomechanics, leading to accelerated progression of OA. Complete tearing of a meniscal root ligament results in a complete loss of hoop stress, which is almost functionally identical to that of total meniscectomy.[30]

Meniscal root ligament tears have been reported to occur in both acute and chronic settings. The posterior horns of medial and lateral menisci transmit more load than the anterior horns, especially at 90 degrees of flexion. The posterior root ligament of the medial meniscus has the least mobility of all the meniscal root attachments, with the highest reported incidence (10% to 21%) of tears compared with the other root ligaments.[15] Several

reports have suggested that tears of the root ligament of the posterior medial meniscus are relatively common, particularly in the middle-aged and older adult population.[30] Ligament root tears of the posterior root ligament of the lateral meniscus are more frequent in the presence of an ACL tear.[39]

In the absence of highly sensitive and specific history and physical examination findings, MRI has become increasingly used to diagnose meniscal root tears, with variable reported sensitivity and specificity.[15,39] The standard MR criteria of meniscal distortion and high signal intensity extending to the surface can be used to diagnose meniscal root ligament tears.[39] Using standard MR criteria, MR has shown sensitivities of 86% to 94% and specificities of 89% to 100% for diagnosing tears of the posterior root ligaments, using knee arthroscopy as the reference standard. To accurately diagnose a tear of the posterior root ligament of the lateral meniscus, the root ligament needs to be assessed on both the coronal and sagittal MR images.[39,70]

Meniscal root ligament lesions are usually radial type tears, although other patterns may exist and several classification systems have been proposed. These systems classify root ligament lesions into distinct types based on several characteristics, such as tear width, longitudinal extension, location within the root ligament, and communication to adjacent meniscal tears. In addition to the radial tear of the root ligament, these classifications include longitudinal and oblique tear patterns.[30,69]

Radial tears of root ligaments have been described on MRI as a radial tear within 1 cm from tibial attachment of the meniscal root ligament. Several MRI signs have been used to diagnose radial tears of meniscal root ligament: a linear high signal intensity perpendicular to the longitudinal axis of the meniscus in the axial plane, a fluid cleft in the coronal plane, a vertical linear defect on the meniscal root ligament (the truncation sign), and a diffuse area of increased signal intensity in the root ligament (the ghost meniscus sign) in the sagittal plane (Fig. 7.21).[29] Tears of the posterior root ligament of the lateral meniscus may exhibit more irregular morphologic distortion and abnormal signal than the typical cleft and ghost meniscus signs.[33]

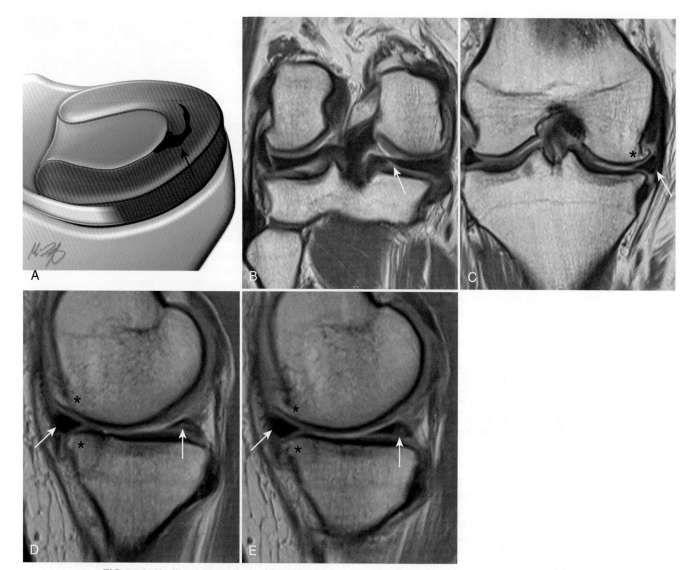

FIG 7.19 (A) Illustration of an oblique radial tear *(arrow)*. The tear contacts the free edge of the meniscus and results is a free edge flap. Coronal (B and C) and sagittal PD non–fat-saturated (NFS) (D and E) MR images showing an oblique radial tear with a flap or parrot beak tear. The tear is seen as an increased signal intensity cleft at the posterior horn of the medial meniscus, which contacts the inferior articular surface *(thin arrows)*. A small displaced flap at the tear site is observed in B. Anteromedial meniscal extrusion and osteoarthritic changes with osteophyte formation and cartilage thinning in the medial compartment of the knee *(asterisks)* are also observed.

Associated findings include concurrent meniscal tears, meniscal extrusion, insertional osseous changes at the root ligament insertion, regional synovitis, and osteoarthritic changes.[30]

Treatment of root ligament tears of menisci has evolved from partial meniscectomy into a variety of repair strategies to restore meniscal function both biomechanically and clinically.[15]

Unstable Meniscal Tears

Stability of a meniscal tear is an important criterion in deciding the appropriate treatment and is best determined by direct visualization and palpation at arthroscopy. Unstable tears are those lesions in which the meniscus or a fragment of it can be inappropriately displaced by a probe into the femorotibial joint. Although it is widely accepted as an accurate technique for

diagnosing meniscal tears, its use to predict the reparability of meniscal tears is less established.[14] Vande Berg et al. described four MR signs of meniscal instability. When using these four criteria, high specificities (94% to 100%) and PPVs (92% to 100%) and low sensitivities (18% to 54%) and negative predictive values (39% to 52%) were found.[116] The first sign corresponds to a displaced meniscal fragment on MRI, which is considered a direct evidence of an unstable meniscal lesion. Displaced meniscal lesions have been described previously in this section and include bucket handle tears, inferiorly or superiorly displaced horizontal tears, displaced radial oblique or parrot beak tears, and free meniscal fragments.[67,78,121] The second sign of meniscal instability is a tear that is visible on more than 3-mm thick coronal and two 4-mm thick sagittal

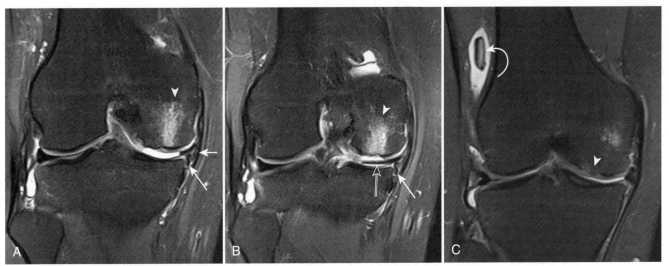

FIG 7.20 Coronal PD FS MR images (A-C) demonstrate a longitudinal horizontal tear involving the posterior horn *(open arrow)* and body *(thick arrow)* of the medial meniscus. The tear extends from the periphery to the free edge of the meniscus. A hypointense thin flap *(thin arrows)* is displaced into the meniscotibial or coronary recess. Extensive bone marrow edema and full-thickness chondral loss at the medial femoral condyle are observed *(arrowheads)*. An intra-articular body is seen in the lateral recess *(curved arrow)*.

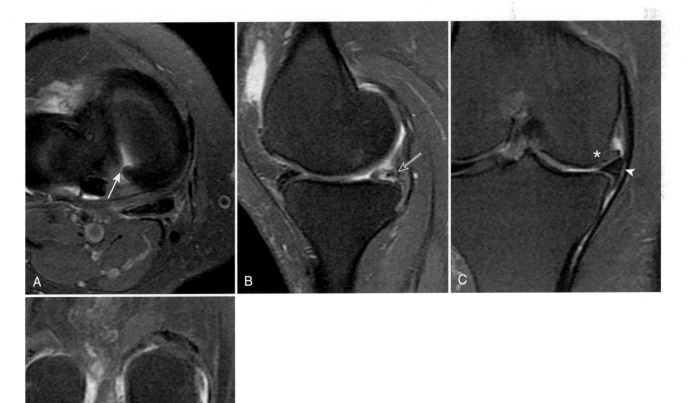

FIG 7.21 Axial (A), sagittal (B) and coronal (C and D) PD FS MR images showing a root ligament tear. A radial tear with a fluid-filled gap *(thin arrows)* is demonstrated in the posterior root ligament of the medial meniscus. The tear is oriented perpendicular to the longitudinal axis of the meniscus in the axial plane (A). The cleft sign is observed in D *(thin arrow)* contacting both articular surfaces. The ghost meniscus sign is observed on the sagittal MR image (B) where some fragments of the posterior root ligament are visualized *(open arrow)*. Extrusion of the meniscal body *(arrowhead)* and degenerative changes at the medial compartment with osteophyte formation *(asterisk)* are observed in C.

images, which approximately corresponds to a 10-mm long tear. It has been accepted in the orthopedic literature that a tear must be long enough (longer than 10 mm) to cause instability of the torn portion.[14] Third, having more than one orientation plane or more than one tear pattern has also been considered a sign of meniscal tear instability. Vande Berg et al. recognized lesion instability if more than one plane or lesion pattern, including contour irregularity, peripheral meniscus separation, and meniscal tear, was found in the same meniscal area.[116] The fourth MR sign is represented by fluid-like signal intensity in the meniscus on T2-weighted images. Accumulation of fluid within a tear occurs when the torn edges are moderately separated, thus allowing joint fluid to enter into the tear.[116]

Displacement of the meniscus rather than a fragment has also been considered a sign of meniscal instability in arthroscopy. Severe meniscal degeneration, complex tears patterns, large radial tears with gaps, and tears involving meniscal root ligaments have been associated with meniscal extrusions of more than 3 mm on midcoronal images.[15]

ANATOMIC VARIANTS AND PITFALLS

The literature describes numerous potential pitfalls and sources of error in evaluation of the meniscus for potential tears. Causes of such misinterpretations include anatomic variants, closely related structures, and technique-related artifacts.[81]

Anatomic Variants in Meniscal Morphology

Discoid meniscus represents a frequent morphological variation defined as an enlarged meniscus with further central extension onto the tibial articular surface. The two major criteria to diagnose a discoid meniscus on MRI are a mediolateral width of the meniscus at the center of the body greater than 15 mm or more than two meniscal body segments on consecutive 5-mm-thickness sagittal MR images, in which the meniscus takes on a bow tie appearance. It has been described in 1.5% to 15.5% lateral menisci and in 0.1% to 0.3% medial menisci.[97,108]

Watanabe and Takeda described three subgroups of discoid menisci: (1) complete discoid, (2) incomplete discoid, and (3) Wrisberg variant. The complete discoid meniscus has a thicker inner margin and wider meniscal surface covering almost the entire surface of the tibial plateau compared with the incomplete discoid meniscus (Fig. 7.22).[83,111] The incomplete discoid type is difficult to diagnose because meniscal width changes with age. Arthroscopically an incomplete discoid meniscus covers between 70% and 80% of the tibial plateau. Studies have evaluated the usefulness of the meniscal to tibial transverse diameters ratio showing higher values in incomplete discoid menisci compared with normal menisci.[85] Of meniscal variations the incomplete discoid type is the most frequent (17% to 31%) and the complete discoid type is second (31.8%).[102]

The Wrisberg variant is a less frequently found variation, with arthroscopically proven prevalence of 0.2%. In the Wrisberg variant the meniscus lacks the normal posterior coronary ligament and capsular attachments, and the posterior horn of the lateral meniscus is mobile. The meniscus can occasionally subluxate, producing such symptoms as knee pain, snapping, or locking.[109] Other rare morphological variations of menisci are the ring-shaped and double-layered types. The ring-shaped meniscus has been described in the lateral meniscus and differential diagnoses include a displaced bucket handle tear or a

complete discoid meniscus with a central perforation. Similar to the discoid meniscus, the ring-shaped meniscus displays the "central bow tie sign," which is the bow tie appearance extending more than two consecutive sagittal MR images.[66] The extremely rare double-layered meniscus has been described in the lateral meniscus and is an accessory meniscal tissue seen as a triangular hypointense structure adjacent to the normally located meniscal tissue on T1- and T2-weighted MR images.[50]

Meniscal Flounce

Meniscal flounce is a rippled appearance of the free inner edge of the medial meniscus, which can be observed in 0.2% to 0.3% of asymptomatic knees. This meniscal fold, first described in arthroscopy, is thought to be a transient physiologic distortion and has been related with knee valgus, flexion or rotation, and redundancy of medial meniscal tissue.[86] On MRI the meniscal flounce has been associated with active knee positioning in the surface coil with changes in meniscal flounce at varying knee positions. On coronal MR images, meniscal flounce may simulate a truncated meniscus and mimic a radial tear.[83,65] Occasionally, meniscal tears can produce a flouncelike morphology, but other abnormal findings indicating a meniscal tear help to differentiate them from the normal anatomic variation. Excessive folding or waviness along the free edge of the meniscus usually differentiates a tear from the single symmetric fold typical of a meniscal flounce.[124]

Anatomic Variants in Meniscal Insertions

The anterior horn of the medial meniscus has common patterns of attachment as described earlier. Anomalous insertions of the anterior horn of the medial meniscus into the intercondylar notch are rare. The anterior meniscofemoral ligament is an infrequently demonstrated structure that travels from the medial meniscus running parallel to the ACL and attaching into the intercondylar notch anterior to the ACL insertion. The anterior meniscofemoral ligament is a separate structure from the ligamentum mucosum.[5] The anterior horn of the medial meniscus root ligament has been also found to attach to the ACL and the anterior transverse ligament lacking a normal tibial attachment. Discoid menisci have a greater incidence of anomalous ACL insertion, with a reported incidence rate of 5.5%, but this anatomic variation has been also described in normally shaped menisci.[91]

The anterior horn of the lateral meniscus root ligament has been localized to the last few millimeters of meniscal tissue, stretching and angling down to the tibial plateau attachment in the intercondylar notch.[68] A speckled or comblike pattern of increased signal intensity of the root ligament has been considered a normal variant. This frequent appearance has been associated with the insertion of some ACL fibers into the meniscus and should not be confused with a tear.[105] The shared embryological origin between the ACL and menisci may explain the intimate anatomic relationship of these structures.[8,16,105] Isolated tears of the anterior horn of the lateral meniscus are rare and account for approximately 16% of lateral meniscus tears.[81] Signal alterations in the anterior horn of the medial or lateral meniscus commonly do not represent clinically significant lesions with high percentage of false-positive results when comparing MRI and arthroscopic findings. Isolated abnormalities in the anterior horns should be interpreted with caution and should be correlated with physical examination.[106] A rare case of anomalous primary insertion of the ACL into the lateral

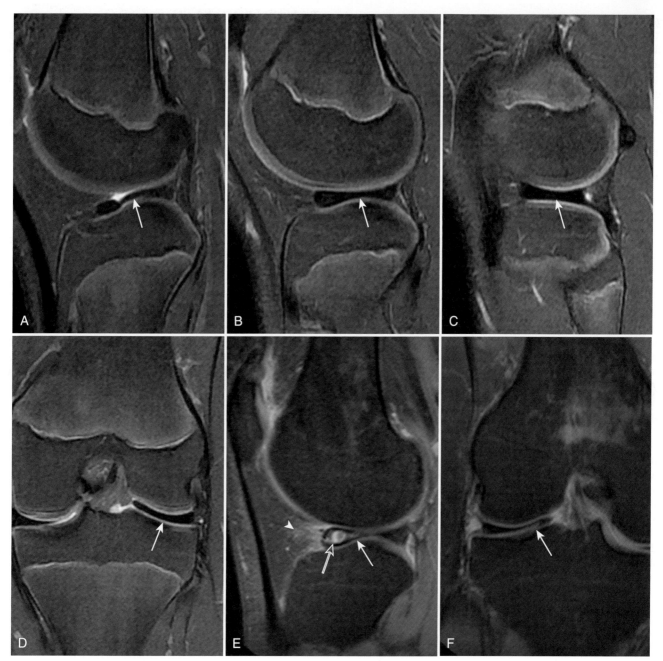

FIG 7.22 (A-D) Sagittal (A-C) and coronal (D) PD FS MR images of a 13-year-old female showing a complete discoid lateral meniscus. The meniscal body extends to the medial aspect of the articular surface covering the lateral tibial plateau *(thin arrows)*. The abnormal meniscal morphology with an enlarged and thickened body *(thin arrow)* is well appreciated on the coronal MR image. Sagittal (E) and coronal (F) PD FS MR images demonstrate a discoid meniscus tear. A longitudinal horizontal tear contacting the inferior articular surface is observed in the anterior horn of the lateral meniscus *(thin arrows)*. There is a fluid-filled intrameniscal cyst in the anterior horn of the meniscus *(open arrow)* and edema in adjacent Hoffa fat pad *(arrowhead)*. The complete discoid morphology of the lateral meniscus is confirmed on the midcoronal MR image (F).

meniscus has been reported in a teenager who presented with an ACL avulsion.[112]

A meniscoligamentous band between the posterior horn of the lateral meniscus root ligament and the ACL has also been described in few cadaveric studies. This band is a small expansion of a fibrous-like structure with variations in thickness that provides the lateral meniscus more stability while conserving its mobility.[125]

Meniscal Variations in Children

High signal intensity on MRI that is not associated with a tear likely represents normal vascularity in children and myxoid degeneration in adults. The meniscus is fully vascularized at birth, but the area of vascularity recedes toward the periphery with age, until it reaches the adult pattern at approximately 10 years of age. Prevalence of abnormal signal intensity unrelated to a tear on MRI is significantly higher in children than in adults. High signal intensity has been shown to decrease with age, with a prevalence of 60% in children younger than 13 years and 30 in individuals older than 14 years.[48] The higher vascularity in the young meniscus provides better healing of meniscal tears compared with the adult meniscus.[107]

Pitfalls Caused by Closely Related Structures

Normal anatomic structures closely related to the meniscus with similar signal intensity can easily mimic a tear. The junction of the anterior transverse ligament with the anterior horn of the medial and lateral menisci can be misinterpreted as an oblique tear if consecutive sagittal images are not carefully followed and if axial images are not used for confirmation.[81]

The close relationship of the oblique meniscomeniscal ligament with the lateral meniscus may be confused for a displaced meniscal fragment, simulating a flap tear or bucket handle tear. This potential misdiagnosis may be avoided by following the ligament on consecutive MR images, thus confirming its extension between the anterior horn of one of the meniscus to the posterior horn of the opposite meniscus.[81,103]

A significant association between apparent far lateral meniscal attachment of the meniscofemoral ligament and tear of the posterior horn of the lateral meniscus has been demonstrated. A pseudotear is seen as a high signal intensity band located between the meniscofemoral ligaments and the posterior horn of the lateral meniscus and has been found to have a high prevalence in MRI and cadaveric studies (63%). The orientation of pseudotears in this location is typically from an anterosuperior to a posteroinferior direction. Slice thickness may be associated with this pitfall because pseudotears can represent volume-average artifacts of the meniscofemoral-meniscus junction.[35,114]

The popliteus tendon and its hiatus are structures closely related to the posterolateral region of the lateral meniscus. Signal intensity from any of these structures could be mistaken for a meniscal tear on both sagittal and coronal sections. On the most superficial sagittal section, the popliteus tendon is seen above the lateral meniscus moving behind the meniscus on the next medial sagittal section. The tendon locates then inferior to the meniscus on the two next medial sagittal sections. A true peripheral lateral meniscal tear usually presents with a different obliquity than that described for the popliteus tendon sheath. Any separate structure above the lateral meniscus seen on sagittal sections, excepting the most superficial section, should be considered suspicious of a tear in the posterior horn of the lateral meniscus.[76,79,87]

Small recesses may be present at the meniscocapsular junction of the posterior horn of the medial meniscus, simulating meniscocapsular separation. Normal recesses should not compromise the entire meniscocapsular junction length.[81] In contrast, true meniscocapsular separations extend from the superior surface of the meniscocapsular junction to its inferior surface (see Fig. 7.14). Other signs indicative of a meniscocapsular separation include meniscal displacement relative to the tibia, concurrent meniscal corner tear, perimeniscal fluid, extension of contrast material along the outer aspect of the meniscus, irregular meniscal margin, and meniscocapsular extension of a meniscal tear.[36]

Technique-Related Artifacts

In addition to normal structures closely related to the menisci that may mimic meniscal tears, some technique-related artifacts can either mimic a tear or obscure true meniscal tears.

Truncation artifact can appear especially in images acquired in 128×256 matrices as lines through the menisci, which can be confused with meniscal tears. These artifacts result from the use of Fourier transform methods to construct MR images of high-contrast boundaries, such as the articular cartilage and the meniscus in the knee. Typically the lines are oriented horizontally within the meniscus, approximately two pixels away from the cartilage. The truncation artifact can be a source of error for those unaware.[113]

Horizontal lines of hyperintensity could be produced artifactually in the superficial sections through the meniscus because of partial volume averaging. Partial volume averaging of the normal concavity at the outer edge of the meniscus can mimic a horizontal tear on sagittal MR images. This potential pitfall can be avoided by examining the coronal images, which fail to show a horizontal tear of the body of the meniscus.[79]

Meniscal fibrocartilage normally exhibits a uniformly low signal intensity on all pulse sequences (TEs > 20 ms). However, increased signal intensity is frequently seen at the junction of the posterior horn with the root ligament junction secondary to the "magic-angle" effect. This phenomenon refers to spuriously increased signal intensity that occurs when collagen fibers are oriented at 55 degrees relative to the external magnetic field (B_0) because of changes in dipole-dipole interactions. The posterior horn and root ligament of the medial meniscus travel at approximately 55 degrees from B_0 to attach at the tibia, rendering this particular region susceptible to the magic-angle effect.[51,88]

Increased signal intensity can be seen in the absence of meniscal tears because of tissue degeneration or in the context of trauma, because of meniscal contusion.[81] Increased signal intensity can also be observed in normal menisci acutely following exercise or in children representing normal vascularity. Because of the multiple causes of nonspecific high signal intensity within the meniscal tissue, this finding has to be interpreted with caution.[11,31,81]

RELATED MENISCAL PATHOLOGY

Meniscal pathology other than meniscal tears includes meniscal extrusion, meniscal degeneration, meniscal contusion, chondrocalcinosis, and meniscal ossicles.

Meniscal extrusion defined as partial or total displacement of the meniscus from the tibial articular cartilage has been highly correlated with root ligament tears, particularly at the medial side.[30] Meniscal extrusion results after extensive injury of the circumferential collagen fibers, leaving the meniscus unable to resist hoop strain. Tear patterns associated with meniscal extrusion have been already described under the unstable meniscal tears section because meniscal extrusion has been considered a sign of meniscal instability. A significant association between meniscal extrusions of more than 3 mm and articular cartilage degeneration has also been found.[15] A retrospective review of 300 knee MRIs with arthroscopy correlation found that meniscal extrusion of more than 3 mm on MRI had a sensibility of 92% and a specificity of 93% for medial meniscus posterior root ligament tears.[17]

Meniscal degeneration results in an abnormal high signal intensity within the substance of the meniscus that does not reach the articular surface. Histologically, the increased signal intensity corresponds to areas of mucoid degeneration and eosinophilic degeneration within the meniscus.[11]

Meniscal contusions represent a transient injury to the meniscus without a definite tear. Cothran et al. have defined meniscal contusion as amorphous signal intensity in the meniscus, abutting an articular surface without a linear component, suggesting a meniscal tear. Usually a bone contusion adjacent to the abnormal meniscus is demonstrated. Meniscal contusion may be a source of false-positive interpretations in the preoperative evaluation of the posttraumatic knee.[31]

Chondrocalcinosis refers to calcifications in the menisci or articular cartilage because of deposition of calcium pyrophosphate dehydrate crystals, dicalcium phosphate dehydrate, calcium hydroxyapatite crystals, or a combination of these. These deposits are seen as punctate or linear calcifications on knee radiographs. On MRI, chondrocalcinosis results in increased signal intensity on T1- and T2-weighted MR images that can simulate or mask a meniscal tear, thus decreasing the sensitivity and specificity of MRI.[61]

The presence of a meniscal ossicle is an uncommon finding with ossification within the substance of the meniscus. The prevalence of meniscal ossicles in the knee has been reported as 0.15% in the literature. There are three theories proposed about the origin of the meniscal ossicle. One theory proposes a congenital origin and suggests that the meniscal ossicle is a congenital vestigial structure similar to those seen in certain animal species. The second theory affirms that meniscal ossicles result from mucoid degeneration and interval mineralization within the meniscus. The third and most popular theory affirms that meniscal ossicles have a posttraumatic origin and result from either heterotopic ossification within the meniscus or an avulsion injury of the root ligament attachment of the meniscus off the tibial spine.[80] On MRI a meniscal ossicle is seen as a rounded structure with a characteristic isointensity to adjacent normal bone marrow and a hypointense cortical rim within the substance of the meniscus.[96]

POSTOPERATIVE MENISCUS

In general, there are three general surgical strategies (known as the 3 Rs) to approach meniscal tears: resection, repair, and replacement or reconstruction. Each of the three techniques results in a different MRI appearance of the postoperative meniscus.[21]

The conventional diagnostic criteria used to diagnose meniscal tears cannot be applied to the postoperative meniscus for the following reasons: (1) when a partial meniscectomy is performed, hyperintense intrasubstance signal intensity may extend to the remodeled articular surface, thus simulating a tear; and (2) a healing tears may be seen as hyperintense signal intensity because of granulation tissue.[104]

MR arthrography has shown improved accuracy for detecting residual or recurrent meniscal tears following meniscectomy or meniscal repair. Several studies have found an increase in overall accuracy from 38% to 82% using conventional MRI to 88% to 92% using MR arthrography.[7,104]

Despite the advantages of MR arthrography, conventional MRI is often performed first because of several reasons. MR arthrography is an invasive technique usually associated with discomfort and potential risk of infection and allergic reaction to contrast material. Some tears do not fill with

contrast material, and areas of intermediate signal intensity may be difficult to interpret if a precontrast MRI is also performed. Parameniscal cysts, which are specific findings of a meniscal tear, usually do not fill with contrast material on arthrographic examinations.[21]

MR criteria commonly used to diagnose recurrent meniscal tears include: fluid entering the meniscal substance, separation or displacement of the meniscus, a grossly irregular meniscal contour, or a combination of these findings (Figs. 7.23 and 7.24).[57,62,104]

Resection

Indications for partial meniscectomy include a meniscal tear not amenable to repair, symptoms refractory to conservative treatment that affect daily living, mechanical symptoms (locking, catching, and giving way), and coexisting degenerative changes. Irreparable tears usually include horizontal, oblique flap, or parrot beak or complex tears involving the inner two-thirds or the avascular zone of the meniscus. Tears that are stable (<1 cm in length) or MRI-detected horizontal tears in the posterior horn do not need meniscectomy. MRI-detected horizontal tears with cartilage loss need to be assessed with special caution because cartilage injuries can progress rapidly after a particle meniscectomy.[21,59]

In partial meniscectomy, damaged or loose tissue is removed arthroscopically with a probe until firm tissue is reached. The remaining meniscus is tapered and contoured to prevent further tearing that can be caused by drastic changes in the shape of the meniscus. It is recommended to preserve as much meniscus as possible, including those portions where damage is uncertain, and the meniscocapsular junction. Rarely a complete meniscectomy is performed.[59]

MR appearance depends on the extent of partial meniscectomy with volume loss and blunting of the inner edge of the meniscus on sagittal MR images (Fig. 7.25).[71] Diagnostic accuracy of MR arthrography improves when there was high-grade partial meniscectomy (more than 25% of the meniscus resected).[7] Radial tears are more frequent in meniscal remnants (32% vs. 14%), probably because of an alteration in knee biomechanics after partial meniscectomy. Redistribution of stress to the meniscus may make them more prone to injury.[74]

Repair

The ideal indication for meniscal repair is an acute, 1- to 2-cm, longitudinal peripheral tear that can be repaired in conjunction with ACL reconstruction in young patients. Other authors include tears extending into the avascular zone in patients less than 20 years of age, whereas several authors recommend meniscal repair to be performed whenever possible regardless of age. The reparability of meniscal tears depends on several factors, such as vascularity, type of tear, chronicity, and size.[123]

Arthroscopic repair can be divided into four categories: inside-out techniques, outside-in techniques, all-inside techniques, and a combination of techniques. The inside-out technique with vertical mattress sutures is the gold standard with which other repair techniques are compared. The inside-out technique can be performed using double-armed needles with an absorbable or nonabsorbable suture passing through single-lumen, zone-specific repair cannulas. Suturing is performed by passing a long needle with a suture attached through the cannula and then through the meniscus to exit superficially. The outside-in technique was introduced to decrease the risk of

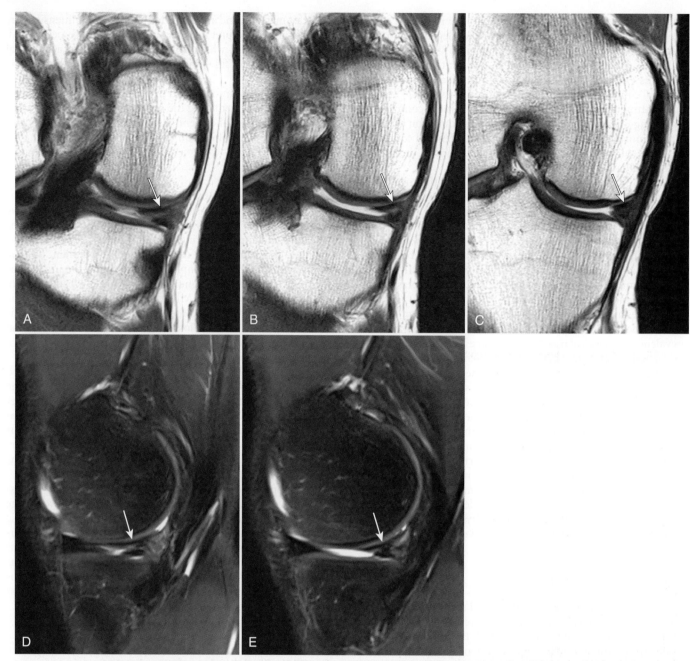

FIG 7.23 Postoperative Meniscus With Remnant Tear Coronal T2-weighted (A-C) and sagittal PD FS (D-E) MR images show a complex tear of the body and posterior horn of the medial meniscus *(arrows)* with multiple displaced flaps, severe distortion of meniscal morphology, and fluid within the tear indicating meniscal instability. A small body is seen on the midcoronal MR image secondary to postoperative changes.

injury of the peroneal nerve during lateral meniscal repair. The outside-in technique can be used for most of the meniscal tear patterns and locations, especially those tears located in the anterior horn. The all-inside repair technique can be used for repairing posterior horn tears. This technique is usually performed using suture hooks and more recently self-adjusting suture devices. Advantages of the all-inside technique include ease of use, avoidance of unnecessary incisions, shorter operating time, and less risk to neurovascular structures. Disadvantages include meniscal or chondral damage from manipulation of the devices, implants migration, foreign body reactions, and higher cost.[21,123]

On conventional MRI, signal alterations at the site of meniscal repair reaching the articular meniscal surface and displaying a signal as high as that of joint fluid are considered meniscal remnant tears. In contrast, low-to-intermediate signal intensity within the meniscus is considered as scar tissue formation secondary to a healed suture repair.[57,104] Useful signs suggesting a remnant tear are frank fluid within the line extending to the meniscal surface, a displaced meniscal fragment, or a definite change in configuration compared with the previous tear.[11] Follow-up studies have demonstrated a poor correlation between signal intensity grading on conventional MRI and

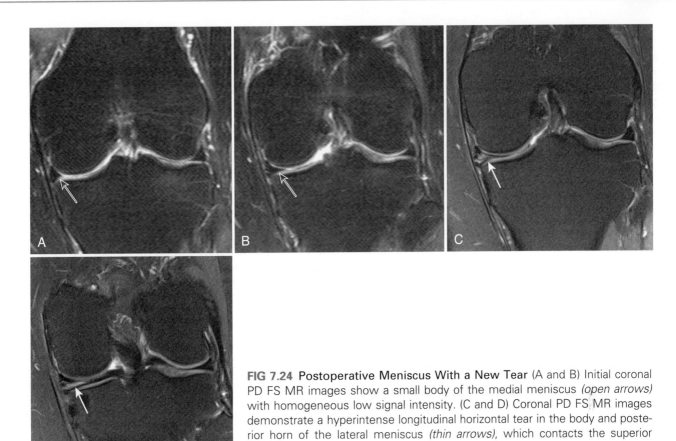

FIG 7.24 Postoperative Meniscus With a New Tear (A and B) Initial coronal PD FS MR images show a small body of the medial meniscus *(open arrows)* with homogeneous low signal intensity. (C and D) Coronal PD FS MR images demonstrate a hyperintense longitudinal horizontal tear in the body and posterior horn of the lateral meniscus *(thin arrows)*, which contacts the superior articular surface. The tear was not visualized on the initial MR images and therefore constitutes a new tear.

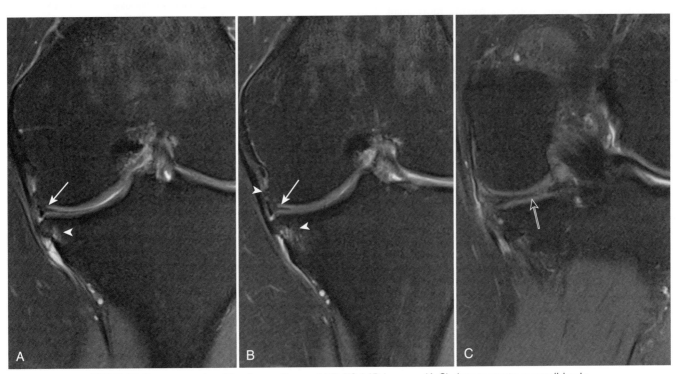

FIG 7.25 Postoperative Meniscus Coronal PD FS MR images (A-C) demonstrate a small body *(thin arrows)* and a thinned posterior horn *(open arrow)* of the medial meniscus secondary to partial medial meniscectomy. Degenerative changes in the medial compartment of the knee secondary to altered biomechanics are observed with osteophyte formation and adjacent bone marrow edema-like signal intensity *(arrowheads)*.

clinical outcomes probably secondary to a functional scar tissue. MRI following meniscal repair does not permit distinction between successful and ineffective meniscal healing, and signal abnormalities can last more than 10 years after surgery.[57,90]

MR arthrography has proved to be useful in the evaluation of repaired menisci with a sensitivity of 80%, specificity of 100%, and overall accuracy of 84%.[62] On MR arthrography, a remnant tear at the surgical site is diagnosed by visualizing extension of contrast into the substance of the meniscus.[11]

Replacement

Two meniscal replacement techniques have been developed: meniscus allograft transplantation and synthetic meniscus implantation. Synthetic meniscus implantation techniques can be used after extensive partial meniscectomies, provided that the peripheral rim is still intact, the defect is greater than two-thirds of the meniscal width and less than 5 cm, and the anterior and posterior root ligaments are intact. Upon resection of damaged tissue the resulting space is filled with a custom-sized, synthetic, porous material, which serves as a scaffold to regenerate meniscus-like tissue. After total or subtotal meniscectomies, in which the peripheral rim is not intact anymore, the load-bearing capacity of a total meniscal substitute should exceed that of partial substitutes. Total synthetic meniscus implantation is still under investigation.[119]

For several decades, symptomatic total meniscectomy patients with minor cartilage damage have been treated by implantation of meniscal allograft. Meniscal allografts are harvested from human donors and then transplanted most commonly with attached bone as anchors, using bone plugs.[21] This procedure is usually performed to relieve joint line pain after a total or subtotal meniscectomy. Diffuse Outerbridge grade III-IV degeneration, joint space narrowing more than 2 to 3 mm, and a higher than II grade degeneration according to the Fairbank classification are contraindication for meniscal allograft transplantation.[82]

Common findings observed on MRI include changes in morphology and signal intensity of the transplanted allograft over the first postoperative year, which include increased signal intensity and decreased width and increased thickness of the body. The incidence of complications has been reported to be approximately 21%. Progressive cartilage loss, allograft extrusion, allograft shrinkage, arthrofibrosis, and synovitis are relatively common postoperative complications.[82,122]

In this chapter we have reviewed the basic anatomy and histologic composition of the knee menisci. A detailed description of the closely related structures, anatomical variations of the menisci, and potential pitfalls, which may help to avoid MRI misinterpretations, has been presented. Common classification of meniscal tears based on tears patterns and postoperative changes of the meniscus were discussed and correlated with illustrations and MR images.

KEY REFERENCES

10. Aydingoz U, Firat AK, Atay OA, et al: MR imaging of meniscal bucket-handle tears: a review of signs and their relation to arthroscopic classification. *Eur Radiol* 13(3):618–625, 2003.

11. Barber BR, McNally EG: Meniscal injuries and imaging the postoperative meniscus. *Radiol Clin North Am* 51(3):371–391, 2013.

21. Boutin RD, Fritz RC, Marder RA: Magnetic resonance imaging of the postoperative meniscus: resection, repair, and replacement. *Magn Reson Imaging Clin N Am* 22(4):517–555, 2014.

24. Campbell SE, Sanders TG, Morrison WB: MR imaging of meniscal cysts: incidence, location, and clinical significance. *AJR Am J Roentgenol* 177(2):409–413, 2001.

42. De Smet AA, Mukherjee R: Clinical, MRI, and arthroscopic findings associated with failure to diagnose a lateral meniscal tear on knee MRI. *AJR Am J Roentgenol* 190(1):22–26, 2008.

43. De Smet AA, Nathan DH, Graf BK, et al: Clinical and MRI findings associated with false-positive knee MR diagnoses of medial meniscal tears. *AJR Am J Roentgenol* 191(1):93–99, 2008.

44. De Smet AA, Tuite MJ: Use of the "two-slice-touch" rule for the MRI diagnosis of meniscal tears. *AJR Am J Roentgenol* 187(4):911–914, 2006.

46. Fairbank TJ: Knee joint changes after meniscectomy. *J Bone Joint Surg Br* 30B(4):664–670, 1948.

63. Kijowski R, Rosas HG, Lee KS, et al: MRI characteristics of healed and unhealed peripheral vertical meniscal tears. *AJR Am J Roentgenol* 202(3):585–592, 2014.

69. LaPrade CM, James EW, Cram TR, et al: Meniscal root tears: a classification system based on tear morphology. *Am J Sports Med* 43(2):363–369, 2015.

78. McKnight A, Southgate J, Price A, et al: Meniscal tears with displaced fragments: common patterns on magnetic resonance imaging. *Skeletal Radiol* 39(3):279–283, 2010.

81. Mohankumar R, White LM, Naraghi A: Pitfalls and pearls in MRI of the knee. *AJR Am J Roentgenol* 203(3):516–530, 2014.

83. Nguyen JC, De Smet AA, Graf BK, et al: MR Imaging-based diagnosis and classification of meniscal tears. *Radiographics* 34(4):981–999, 2014.

87. Peduto AJ, Nguyen A, Trudell DJ, et al: Popliteomeniscal fascicles: anatomic considerations using MR arthrography in cadavers. *AJR Am J Roentgenol* 190(2):442–448, 2008.

99. Rosas HG, De Smet AA: Magnetic resonance imaging of the meniscus. *Top Magn Reson Imaging* 20(3):151–173, 2009.

The references for this chapter can also be found on www.expertconsult.com.

8

Cruciate Ligaments

Felix M. Gonzalez, Adam C. Zoga

Noncontrast magnetic resonance imaging (MRI) is standard of care imaging in the posttraumatic knee with clinical findings suggestive of ligamentous injury. MRI readily delineates injuries of the cruciate ligaments and offers a distinct advantage in preventing unnecessary arthroscopy by assessing the severity of the anterior cruciate ligament/posterior cruciate ligament (ACL/PCL) tear and other coexisting injuries. In addition, MRI is ideally suited for the evaluation of pain or instability in the postoperative patient by allowing assessment of graft integrity, graft ganglia formation, or hardware failure. MRI findings of partial and complete, and acute and chronic ligament tears throughout the knee are well described. With this in mind, MRI review should be systematic, with every effort made to identify the injury mechanism, and thus should focus on osseous, ligamentous, and cartilaginous structures at risk for acute trauma, while identifying chronic and degenerative lesions that might not be related to the recent injury.

ANTERIOR CRUCIATE LIGAMENT

Normal Anterior Cruciate Ligament Anatomy

The ACL arises proximally from the intercondylar notch of the lateral femoral condyle and inserts distally on the anteromedial (AM) tibial plateau in the anterior intercondylar region, which follows an oblique course with a mean sagittal angle of 54 to 55.5 degrees (angle measured between the ACL and the tibial plateau).[10,20] The ligament is intra-articular but extrasynovial surrounded by a synovial layer separating it from the joint space, which contains a periligamentous arterial plexus that supplies the ACL with its own blood supply. The hemarthrosis that occurs with an acute ACL disruption is secondary to the disruption of this periligamentous plexus. Its fibers are distributed into two bundles with nomenclature according to their tibial insertions, known as the anteromedial bundle (AMB), which attaches proximally at the lateral femoral condyle more superomedially, and the posterolateral bundles (PLBs), which attaches the lateral femoral condyle more laterally and distally. It measures approximately 38 mm in length and 11 mm in width.[14] The AMB is longer and measures approximately 34 to 39.8 mm in length and 4.3 to 5.7 mm in width,[6] whereas the PLB is shorter and measures 18 to 23 mm in length and 4.6 to 6 mm in width.[6]

Biomechanics of the Anterior Cruciate Ligament

There is a reciprocal tension pattern shared between the AM and posteromedial ACL bundles. In flexion the AM band becomes taut while the posterolateral band is lax; however, during extension the opposite occurs when the posterolateral band becomes taut and the AM band is lax. This process maintains the ACL under tension throughout the different phases of normal biomechanics by activating the different ligamentous bundles, allowing for knee stability; especially during flexion, the stronger AM band provides the necessary stability.

There is a natural tendency of anterior tibial translation, which is prevented by both bundles of the ACL based on the position of the knee. In flexion, the main stability against anterior tibial translation is provided by the AM band. The anterior drawer tests for deficiency of this bundle, which is performed at 90 degrees of flexion—the knee position that places most tension on the AM bundle. Conversely, with the knee in extension, the PLB becomes "activated," preventing anterior tibial translation; thus posterolateral band deficiencies are more commonly identified by the Lachman test and the pivot shift exam. Furthermore, the PLB plays a pivotal role in maintaining rotational stability during terminal extension of the knee, allowing tibial external rotation relative to the femur and aiding to "lock" the knee in extension.[9]

ANTERIOR CRUCIATE LIGAMENT MECHANISM OF INJURY

The most important sign of an ACL tear is disruption or discontinuity of the fibers. ACL tears can be classified as partial or complete. Partial tears represent less than a third of the cases and can be further described as minor tears involving just a few fibers, a low-grade partial-thickness tear (involving less than 50% of the ligament thickness), or a high-grade tear (involving more than 51% of the ligament thickness but not the entire width). An attempt should be made to describe the degree of involvement based on ligamentous thickness affected. A partial tear can involve both or only a single bundle to varying degrees. Sometimes ACL insufficiency can be caused by plastic deformity without fiber discontinuity.[22] Visualization of distal partial tears near the tibial insertion may be somewhat challenging, but presence of diffuse, high signal intensity with nonvisualization of the normal, linear, high signal intensity of the distal stripes qualifies as a partial distal tear of one or both bundles depending on the anatomic distribution of signal alteration.

An acute, complete ACL tear presents as ligament discontinuity with abnormal high signal intensity and complete ligamentous disruption (direct signs of ACL tear). The tear can occur proximally, at its midsubstance, or distally and may present with a mechanical block caused by the stump with resultant surrounding inflammation and fibrosis. Complete disruption most often occurs in the middle of the ACL and often leads to an abnormal slope or posterior bowing of the distal fibers. Secondary signs may be seen in the majority of complete ACL tears and include lateral tibiofemoral compartment contusions like the ones present in "pivot-shift" injuries involving the terminal sulcus of the lateral femoral condyle and the posterior aspect of the lateral tibial plateau, less than 45-degree angles between the lateral tibial plateau and a buckled course of the PCL with indentation of the distal part of the PCL and anterior displacement of the tibia.[22] These indirect signs lack sensitivity, and the absence of these signs does not exclude presence of an ACL tear.[10]

The main mechanism of injury of the ACL includes internal rotation of the femur relative to a fixed tibia with the foot planted beyond the stretching ligamentous capability in a sudden deceleration and rotation maneuver common in contact sports, such as football, or while skiing. Partial ACL tears most commonly involve the AM band of the ACL. Injury mechanisms as a whole are the same for partial tear and complete tear. The most common contact-related injury is the "clipping" type injury sustained in football. Pivot shift is a low-energy noncontact injury common in such sports as basketball, football, or rugby that can occur with the knee in flexion while the foot is fixated, by applying a valgus (lateral) force to the knee, causing internal rotation of the tibia or external rotation of the femur, which can produce an O'Donoghue unhappy triad comprised of an ACL tear, a medial collateral ligament (MCL) tear/sprain, and a medial meniscal tear. The pivot-shift mechanism of injury is one of the most common mechanisms resulting in tear of the ACL. This type of injury occurs during rapid deceleration combined with simultaneous sudden change of direction. After the ACL tears, it allows the tibia to translate anteriorly relative to the femur, resulting in impaction of the tibia against the femur, giving rise to the reciprocal bone bruise pattern in the lateral femoral condyle and posterolateral tibial plateau, known as the "pivot-shift" marrow edema pattern.

Hyperextension injuries can occur during jumping or high kick maneuvers with or without a varus force can result in ACL disruption and frequently occur without associated collateral ligament or meniscal injury.[51] This kissing contusion pattern associated with this type of injury results from impaction of the anterior tibia against the anterior femur. The third mechanism is external rotation of the tibia relative to the femur with a varus (medial) stress leading to impaction/bone bruise in the medial knee compartment and distraction laterally resulting in avulsion of the lateral tibial rim (Segond fracture) and injury/tear of the lateral collateral ligament (LCL).

BONE MARROW CONTUSION PATTERNS

Careful observation and assessment of osseous contusions about the knee should serve as a guide for interrogation regarding suspect soft tissue structures likely to be injured based on specific mechanisms. Osseous contusion patterns often elucidate the mechanism of injury and guide the evaluation for subsequent pathology. Five dominant osseous contusion patterns described by Sanders and associates play a key role in diagnostic MRI interpretation of knee ligament trauma.[36] These include pivot-shift injury, dashboard injury, hyperextension injury, clip injury, and lateral patellar dislocation. MRI evaluation for osseous contusion is facilitated by the use of T2 fat-saturated sequences. Contusions appear as subcortical or subchondral regions of increased T2 signal and decreased T1

signal, often with a flame-shaped configuration, without a discrete fracture line.

Following a pivot-shift injury, osseous contusions most commonly involve the posterolateral tibial plateau and the lateral femoral condyle (Fig. 8.1). The presence of this contusion pattern indicates acute or chronic ACL disruption because it is failure of this ligament that leads to tibial subluxation and impaction. Other associated pathology includes posterolateral corner injury and subsequent instability. Osseous contusion of the medial tibial plateau has also been described with a pivot-shift mechanism of injury, present in approximately 20% of cases and associated with posteromedial peripheral tears of the medial meniscus.

The dashboard injury is related to a direct blow to the knee, often during an automobile accident. This mechanism manifests as contusions involving the anterior tibia and posterior subchondral patella. Concomitant soft tissue injury with a dashboard contusion pattern often includes PCL and posterior capsule disruption. Hyperextension injury results in impaction of the anterior tibia and anterior femoral condyle and subsequent osseous contusions (Fig. 8.2). Associated ligamentous pathology with this mechanism can include ACL or PCL injury.

A clip injury is related to valgus stress to the knee and results in a dominant contusion within the lateral femoral condyle from direct impaction, along with a smaller focus of bone marrow edema within the medial femoral condyle related to avulsive force at the origin of the MCL. Injury to the MCL is common with this mechanism, ranging from low-grade sprains to frank disruption. In addition, ACL injury and medial meniscal injury have been described with clip injuries. Osseous contusions following lateral patellar dislocation involve the lateral, nonarticular portion of the lateral femoral condyle, as well as the medial patellar facet (Fig. 8.3). Associated soft tissue injuries include medial patellar retinaculum and medial patellofemoral ligament (MPFL) sprain or disruption. Cartilaginous injury has

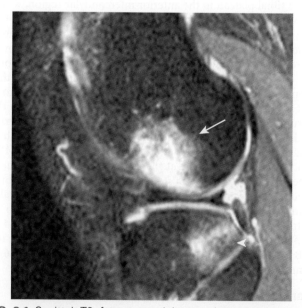

FIG 8.1 Sagittal T2 fat-saturated image demonstrates bone marrow edema, with the lateral femoral condyle *(arrow)* and the posterolateral tibia *(arrowhead)* representing osseous contusions secondary to a pivot-shift injury during a fall while skiing.

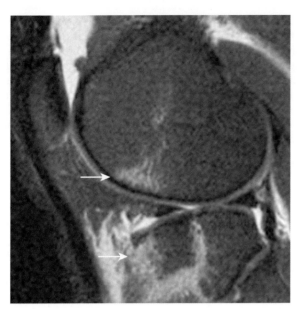

FIG 8.2 Sagittal T2 fat-saturated image shows bone marrow edema in the anterior tibia and femoral condyle compatible with osseous contusions *(arrows)* related to hyperextension injury in a 20-year-old soccer player.

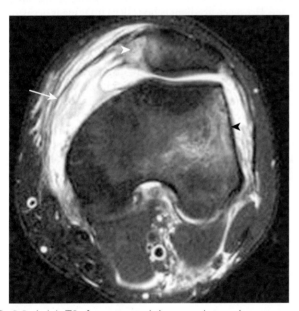

FIG 8.3 Axial T2 fat-saturated image shows bone marrow edema in the medial patella and lateral femoral condyle *(arrowheads)* representing osseous contusions secondary to prior lateral patellar dislocation in a 15-year-old field hockey player. Edema surrounds the medial patellar retinaculum *(arrow)*.

also been reported with transient lateral patellar dislocations, with delamination of cartilage at the medial patellar facet or at the anterolateral margin of the lateral femoral condyle, sometimes leading to intra-articular cartilaginous bodies.

NORMAL MAGNETIC RESONANCE APPEARANCE OF THE ANTERIOR CRUCIATE LIGAMENT

On MRI, the ACL is low in signal relative to muscle on all sequences and parallels the intercondylar roof on sagittal images

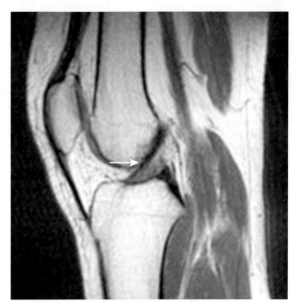

FIG 8.4 Sagittal proton density image showing a normal anterior cruciate ligament *(arrow)*.

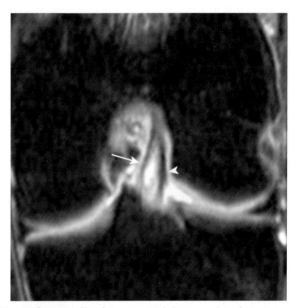

FIG 8.5 Coronal T2 fat-saturated image showing a normal anterior cruciate ligament with intact anteromedial *(arrow)* and posterolateral *(arrowhead)* bundles.

(Blumensaat line). Proximally the ACL usually displays a homogeneous low signal intensity, whereas distally the ligament demonstrates a striated appearance with fat and synovium interspersed between the AMB and PLB.[46] Familiarization with this appearance is key to avoid misinterpreting the distal ligament appearance for a tear (Fig. 8.4). With the knee in full extension, the ACL should parallel the roof of the intercondylar notch (Blumensaat line). All three planes should be used for the most accurate assessment of the ACL. The sagittal sequence (see Fig. 8.4) is most useful and can be performed in an oblique sagittal plane parallel to the orientation of the ACL as prescribed from an axial localizer image with 3- to 4-mm image thickness to decrease volume averaging. The axial and coronal images (Fig. 8.5) are useful in evaluating the ligamentous attachments and confirming abnormalities seen on the sagittal sequence. Axial images are particularly helpful for assessing the integrity of individual ACL bundles in the setting of sprain or partial tear.

RADIOGRAPHY

The use of radiographs in the assessment of acute ACL injuries is limited to osseous abnormalities. There are several indirect findings that could indicate an underlying ACL injury, such as avulsion fractures of the ACL at the tibial insertion or femoral origin. Avulsion fractures of the intercondylar eminence more commonly occur in children than adult patients and usually come about because of extreme hypertension. There are three types of tibial avulsion fractures: type I describes a minimally distracted fracture; type II encompasses a partially displaced fracture fragment; and a type III is commonly associated with complete separation.[28]

Other radiographic signs that correlate highly with disruption of the ACL include the deep lateral femoral sulcus sign, best seen on lateral radiographs of the knee, which is defined as deepening (more than 2 mm) and cortical irregularity of the lateral femoral sulcus (Fig. 8.6). An avulsion fracture at the lateral aspect of the lateral tibial rim (Segond fracture; Fig. 8.7) can be associated in 75% to 100% of the time with ACL injury and occurs in approximately 9% to 12% of all ACL tears.[16,44] It is characteristically secondary to an avulsion fracture of the iliotibial band (ITB), although the term has also been applied when there is avulsion of the anterior oblique band (AOB) of the LCL.[4] Lastly, other less specific radiographic signs include a large joint effusion following an acute injury and cortical irregularity or fracture of the posterior aspect of the lateral tibial plateau.

COMPUTED TOMOGRAPHY

The use of computed tomography (CT) in the assessment of ACL injury is limited as well. The gold standard imaging modality currently used in the setting of an ACL injury is MRI because it can diagnose or exclude a tear in patients with equivocal physical examination findings. An area in which CT imaging excels is in allowing more accurate characterization of comminuted fractures and in CT arthrography with sensitivities and specificities of 90% and 96% for the detection of ACL injury, respectively, at initial interpretation.[49] These results are compatible to those previously published with MRI.[15,29,35,50]

ANTERIOR CRUCIATE LIGAMENT MAGNETIC RESONANCE IMAGING

The ideal MR sequences for visualization of the ACL are two-dimensional (2D) fast spin echo (FSE) sequences either with or without fat suppression. The standard protocol typically includes a short echo time (TE) sequence (proton density [PD]) in the sagittal and coronal imaging planes. These images are best suited for detecting meniscal pathology. A preferred standard knee protocol comprises the following three sequences: (1) T2-weighted fat-suppressed sequence performed in the axial, sagittal, and coronal imaging plane; (2) FSE sagittal PD-weighted sequence; and (3) spin echo (SE) coronal T1-weighted with fat-suppression sequence. PD- or T2-weighted images with fat saturation are best suited for the evaluation of the articular cartilage. However, gradient echo (GRE) imaging is occasionally also used for this purpose.

MRI plays an important role in the assessment of suspected ACL injury. The majority of ACL tears are complete (approximately 80%) and most commonly occur at the midsubstance or middle third and less frequently occur proximally (near the femoral attachment in 7% of the time) or distally (near the tibial attachment with a frequency of almost 3%). The remainder 20% presents as incomplete tear demonstrating various degrees of involvement.[22]

Both primary and secondary signs of ACL rupture have been seen on MRI. Primary signs of rupture include a discontinuous

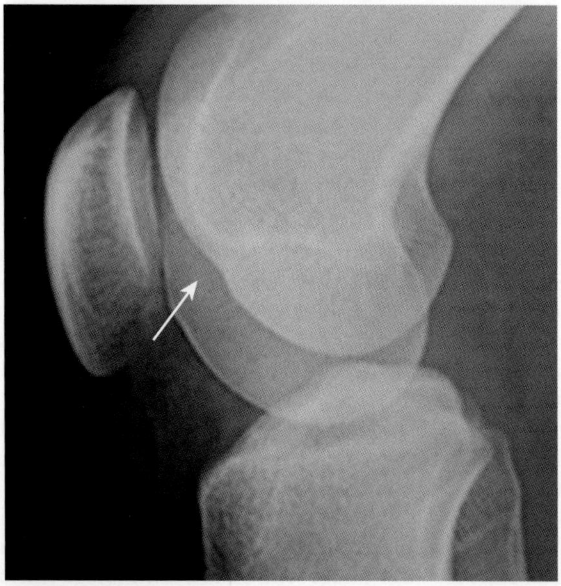

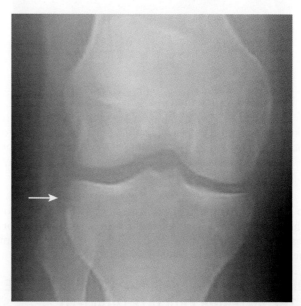

FIG 8.6 Radiographic lateral view of a knee demonstrating a deep sulcus sign at the lateral femoral condyle *(arrow).*

FIG 8.7 Anteroposterior radiograph of the right knee shows a small avulsion fracture *(arrow)* of the lateral aspect of the proximal tibia, consistent with a Segond fracture.

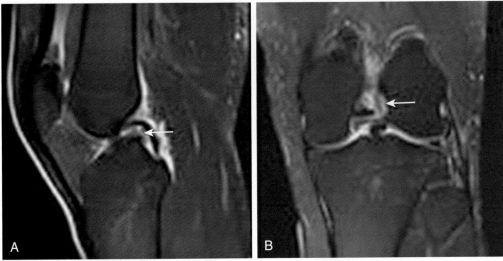

FIG 8.8 Sagittal (A) and coronal (B) T2 fat-saturated images show a complete anterior cruciate ligament tear. On the sagittal image (A), the fibers are horizontally oriented *(arrow)*. On the coronal image (B), hematoma replaces the expected location of the ligament *(arrow)*. Sagittal proton density image showing a normal anterior cruciate ligament *(arrow)*.

ligament or an abnormal course of the ligament, no longer paralleling Blumensaat line.[46] With a discontinuous ligament, the fibers may appear wavy or horizontal in orientation (Fig. 8.8A). Often the ligament is replaced with amorphous increased signal related to edema and hemorrhage when tears are subacute; fibers appear as if they have been cut with scissors in more acute injuries (see Fig. 8.8B). Secondary signs of ACL tear include buckling of the PCL, anterior translation of the tibia, uncovering of the posterior horn of the lateral meniscus, and characteristic osseous contusion patterns. Buckling of the PCL, uncovering of the posterior horn of the lateral meniscus, and anterior translation of the tibia are all related to anterior subluxation of the tibia relative to the femur secondary to ACL incompetence. Anterior translation of the tibia, referred to as the MRI equivalent of an anterior drawer sign, is assessed using the sagittal imaging plane (Fig. 8.9). The distance between the posterior tibia and the femoral condyle is measured using lines parallel to the long axis of the image. With this method, Vahey et al. demonstrated high specificity (93%) and positive predictive value (95%) of subluxation of 5 mm or more for ACL disruption. A 7-mm or greater subluxation had 100% specificity and positive predictive value.[48] The characteristic osseous contusion pattern for ACL disruption involves the posterolateral tibial plateau and the lateral femoral condyle. Contusion may also be seen at the posteromedial tibial plateau. Complete rupture of the ACL is often accompanied by joint effusion and hemarthrosis. A fluid-fluid level representing layering blood products may be identified in the suprapatellar recess as related to patient positioning during the examination. In skeletally immature patients, ACL injury commonly manifests as an avulsion fracture at its insertion onto the tibia. MRI will demonstrate an intact ligament with an associated displaced osseous fragment at the medial tibial spine or the intercondylar tibial eminence (Fig. 8.10). Subchondral bone marrow edema may be seen within the proximal tibial epiphysis related to the fracture. With this injury, the immature epiphyseal bone is weaker than the mature ligament. Identification of the avulsed tibial fragment on radiography or MRI is essential because treatment

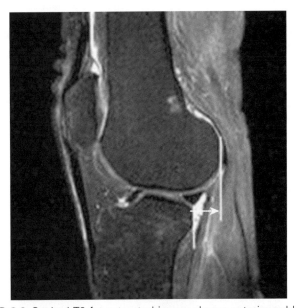

FIG 8.9 Sagittal T2 fat-saturated image shows anterior subluxation of the tibia with respect to the femur and demonstrates the measurement used to assess anterior drawer.

options differ considerably from those used with a traditional ACL rupture.

Partial tears of the ACL are more difficult to detect with MRI and are defined as abnormal intrasubstance signal within an otherwise intact ligament or as discontinuity of some of the ligamentous fibers not involving the full width (Fig. 8.11). Commonly, the most proximal portion of the anterolateral bundle of the ACL is disrupted with an intact posteromedial bundle. Although this type of injury can be confidently called a partial ACL tear on MRI, ligamentous integrity is not easily established without a dedicated and properly performed physical examination. MRI is not a sensitive tool for determining the

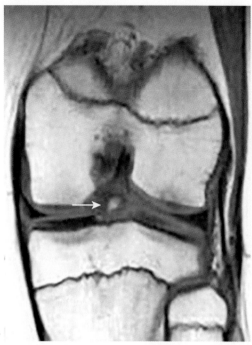

FIG 8.10 Coronal T1 image shows an avulsion fracture *(arrow)* of the intercondylar tibial eminence at the anterior cruciate ligament insertion in a skeletally immature 12-year-old football player.

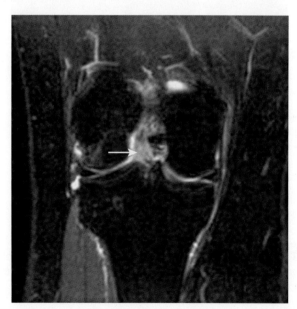

FIG 8.11 Coronal T2 fat-saturated image shows abnormal intrasubstance signal within intact anterior cruciate ligament fibers *(arrow)* compatible with partial tear in a 35-year-old snowboarder.

integrity of a partially torn ACL, although secondary signs such as pivot-shift osseous contusions or an MRI anterior drawer can be helpful in suggesting ligamentous incompetence. In general, abnormal T2 hyperintense signal about or within a partially or completely intact ACL with a recent trauma history should be described as a partial tear of the ACL or low-grade ACL injury by MRI. This should be followed by a thorough description of the findings, the presence or lack of pivot-shift contusions, and other findings that might suggest ligament incompetence.

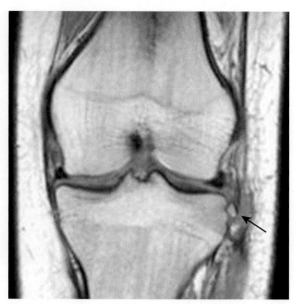

FIG 8.12 Coronal T1 image shows an avulsion fracture at the proximal tibia *(arrow)*, a Segond fracture, at the site of lateral capsular ligament insertion.

ACL tears are often accompanied by other injuries of the ipsilateral knee. MCL sprain and meniscal tear are the most commonly associated injuries, with a particular prevalence of peripheral vertical tears in the posterior horn of either meniscus. Peripheral meniscus tears just above points of osseous contusion on the posterolateral or posteromedial tibial plateau are also commonly seen. Injuries to the posterolateral corner have also been described in association with ACL disruption. The Segond fracture, an avulsion fracture from the lateral tibia at the lateral capsular ligament insertion, is an indicator of ACL disruption that can be seen on MRI, as well as on plain radiographs (Fig. 8.12).

Nonvisualization of the ACL is the most common MRI presentation of a chronic tear. On axial images, fluid in the lateral intercondylar notch, where the normal ACL is found, described as the empty notch sign, can be seen in chronic ACL tears (Fig. 8.13). The ligament may be attenuated or residual fibers may have a horizontal orientation. The chronically torn ACL may scar and adhere to the PCL and clinically may present with an endpoint on anterior drawer examination.[46] Pivot-shift contusions suggest ACL incompetence but not necessarily an acute tear. A patient with a chronic and long-standing ACL tear can acutely pivot shift, leading to new contusions and a hemarthrosis, as well as injury to other ligamentous and cartilaginous structures. Therefore pivot-shift contusions and no visible ACL fibers at MRI should be interpreted as an age-indeterminate ACL tear, with a recent pivot-shift injury. In contrast, mucoid degeneration of the ACL manifests as increased T2 signal, enlargement, and ill definition of an otherwise intact ligament. This pattern of ACL abnormality at MRI should not show a pivot-shift contusion pattern and does not suggest the presence of acute ACL trauma but more likely chronic and repetitive abnormal ACL biomechanics related to meniscal tear or osteoarthritis. Mucoid degeneration of the ACL or PCL can be associated with osseous cystic formation at the cruciate attachments, distal more common than proximal. These intraosseous cruciate cysts are likely a variant of cruciate ganglion cysts, which show homogeneous increased T2 signal similar to that of fluid, insinuating between intact ligament bundles. They are loculated cysts often with lobulation and generally extending along the length of the ligament (Fig. 8.14).[33]

ANTERIOR CRUCIATE LIGAMENT RECONSTRUCTION

The most common type of ACL reconstruction is a single-bundle ACL reconstruction aimed at reconstructing the anatomy of

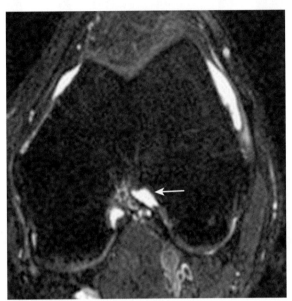

FIG 8.13 Axial T2 fat-saturated image shows absence of fibers at the lateral intercondylar notch *(arrow)* representing a chronic anterior cruciate ligament tear after a basketball injury.

the AMB of the ACL.[45] Nonetheless, up to 25% of patients after single-bundle reconstruction report persistent pain and instability, and for this reason double-bundle reconstructions focused at reconstituting the anatomic courses of the AMB and PLB, have been promoted.[45]

ACL graft material may include autografts (graft taken from the same patient) or allografts (grafts harvested from cadavers), with the most commonly used choices for autograft being the bone-patellar tendon-bone (BPTB) and hamstring tendons. The BPTB graft (Fig. 8.15) is harvested from the central third of the patellar tendon and contains a bone plug collected from the patellar attachment on one end of the graft and from the tibial attachment on the other end of the graft. The bone plugs facilitate fixation of the graft in the femoral and tibial tunnels. BPTB graft reconstructions have the advantage of stable fixation and improved strength but may be associated with postoperative anterior knee pain and an increased incidence of arthrofibrosis.[25] On the other hand, the hamstring graft comprises the gracilis and semitendinosus tendons typically harvested from the ipsilateral knee, sutured together side by side and then folded on themselves until a 4-strand graft construct is produced. The hamstring graft requires fixation by interference screws, surgical staples, cross-pins, or EndoButtons.

Autografts are still considered the most reliable type of ACL reconstruction, with BPTB and hamstring grafts used with approximately equal frequency. The BPTB graft is perhaps more frequently used in competitive athletes who are planning on returning to full strength as quickly as possible because it provides stronger fixation early on the path of recovery; however, increased harvest site morbidity (anterior knee pain and patellar tendinopathy) and complications associated with the extensor mechanism can lengthen the rehabilitation process. As a comparison, the strength of a hamstring graft can be

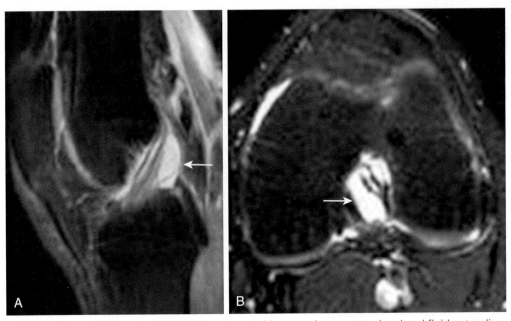

FIG 8.14 Sagittal (A) and axial (B) T2 fat-saturated images demonstrate loculated fluid extending along the length of the anterior cruciate ligament *(arrows)* representing an anterior cruciate ligament ganglion. Axial T2 fat-saturated image demonstrates a Baker cyst between the semimembranosus *(arrow)* and the medial head of the gastrocnemius *(arrowhead)* tendon. Axial T2 fat-saturated image demonstrates a ruptured Baker cyst with fluid dissecting along the subcutaneous tissues *(arrow)*.

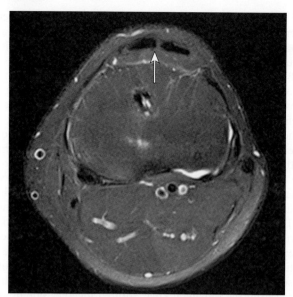

FIG 8.15 Axial T2 fat-saturated image demonstrates postsurgical changes of bone-patellar tendon-bone graft harvesting *(arrow)*.

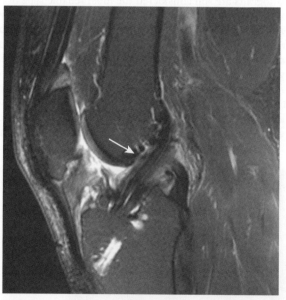

FIG 8.16 Sagittal T2 fat-saturated image demonstrates postsurgical changes of an intact anterior cruciate ligament reconstruction *(arrow)*.

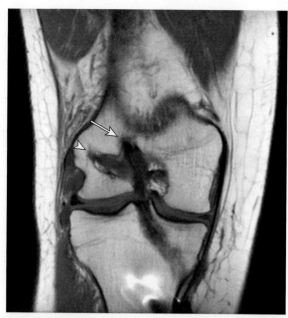

FIG 8.17 Coronal T1 image demonstrates a double-bundle anterior cruciate ligament reconstruction of the right knee. The anteromedial bundle tunnel is seen at the 1 to 2 o'clock position *(arrow)*, and the posterolateral bundle tunnel is seen at 2 to 3 o'clock position *(arrowhead)*.

slightly lower during the first year after surgery compared with a BPTB graft because of the lack of firm bone plug fixation. There is also lower morbidity associated with the hamstring graft harvest as well. Because of increased incidence of synthetic graft complications and foreign body reactions, synthetic graft materials are not commonly used nowadays.

NORMAL ANTERIOR CRUCIATE LIGAMENT GRAFT IMAGING

The type of ACL graft used and the time interval after surgery determines the MRI appearance of the graft. Immediately after surgery, the normal ACL graft displays a homogeneous low signal intensity and is of uniform caliber (Fig. 8.16).[18] The patellar tendon graft being a solid single structure initially demonstrates a homogeneous low signal intensity on all pulse sequences, whereas with a hamstring graft, the individual graft construct strands may be visualized as linear striations, representing the separate bundles of the graft.

During the initial 3 months, the grafts are avascular and demonstrate signal intensity similar to the native harvest site. Between 3 and 8 months postoperatively, the graft undergoes a process of remodeling and revascularization as a synovial-vascular lining develops with small vessels penetrating the graft.[2] During this period, the graft may demonstrate intermediate or increased MR signal intensity on T1- and T2-weighted images. By 12 months, ACL grafts usually undergo a process known as "ligamentization," in which the grafts exhibit a signal intensity similar to the native harvest site. Small foci of intermediate-to-high signal intensity may be seen in normal grafts beyond 18 months postoperatively.

One- to 2-mm longitudinal defect is classically seen at the central third of the patellar tendon graft harvest sites, which heals with granulation tissue by 2 years postoperatively. Low signal intensity with persistent thickening of the patellar tendon can be seen as a normal postoperative finding.[47] Similarly, postsurgical changes with scar tissue formation may be seen at the site of the hamstring graft harvest region.

Femoral and tibial tunnel positioning is essential in ACL reconstruction by allowing stability and avoiding graft impingement. On sagittal MR images, the region of the roof of the intercondylar notch and the posterior femoral cortex corresponds to the optimal opening of the femoral tunnel. On coronal images, the femoral tunnel opening should be situated at the 10 to 11 o'clock position in the right knee (Fig. 8.17) or 1 to 2 o'clock position in the left knee. In the cases of double-bundle ACL grafts, the femoral tunnel for the AMB is preferably selected to be at the 10 to 11 o'clock (right knee) or 1 to 2 o'clock (left knee). In the right knee the PLB should be located at 9 to 10 o'clock (see Fig. 8.17), whereas in the left knee the PLB should be situated at 2 to 3 o'clock of the intercondylar notch.[5] In the sagittal plane the tibial tunnel should be located with the anterior aspect of the ACL graft parallel and posterior to the roof of the intercondylar notch (Blumensaat line).[17]

In the coronal plane the graft should be positioned with an angle measuring between 60 and 65 degrees with respect to the joint line, with the lateral margin of the tibial tunnel in line with the lateral tibial spine. In double-bundle reconstruction the epicenter of the AM tibial tunnel should be positioned at the junction of the anterior and middle thirds of the tibia, with the epicenter of the PLB posterior to the midpoint of the tibia (Fig. 8.18).[17]

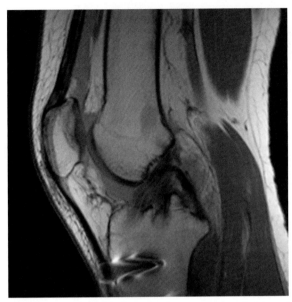

FIG 8.18 On sagittal T1 image, the anteromedial bundle is noted anteriorly with tibial attachment at the junction of anterior to middle third of the tibia. The posterolateral bundle is seen more posteriorly with tibial attachment just posterior to the midpoint of the tibia.

MAGNETIC RESONANCE IMAGING OF COMPLICATIONS OF ANTERIOR CRUCIATE LIGAMENT RECONSTRUCTION

Patients who present with complications in the setting of ACL reconstructions usually complain of pain or symptoms of recurring instability secondary to graft disruption or graft laxity, which on MRI may appear with graft discontinuity or buckling with posterior bowing. The primary imaging signs of graft tears include graft discontinuity, signal intensity alteration within the graft, a change in the caliber of the graft and posteroinferior bowing of the graft. The sensitivity and specificity of MRI for the detection of complete and partial-thickness ACL graft tears have been reported to be 36% and 80%, respectively.[17] A sensitivity of 100% and specificity of 89% to 100% can be achieved with MR arthrography.[26] A graft injury on the sagittal and coronal imaging planes has the highest specificity for full-thickness tears. A graft with no change in caliber has 100% specificity and positive predictive value in excluding a full-thickness tear. A change in signal intensity has limited reliability in helping to detect graft tears and may be seen in intact and stable grafts.[37] Posteroinferior bowing of a graft may be appreciated in the setting of graft tearing resulting in laxity and graft stretching. The detection of partial-thickness graft tears by MRI is poor, with the most useful imaging property being a change in caliber with associated altered signal intensity.[17]

GRAFT IMPINGEMENT

Development of graft impingement is primarily related to improper positioning of the tibial tunnel, which may lead to loss of normal knee joint extension predisposing to graft tearing. With graft impingement related to an abnormally anteriorly placed tibial tunnel, the graft will show increased signal in the distal two-thirds, with visible deflection or angulation at the intercondylar roof on sagittal sequences acquired in near full knee extension (Fig. 8.19).[46,51]

After notchplasty, a subsequent osteophyte in the region of the roof of the intercondylar notch can also result in graft

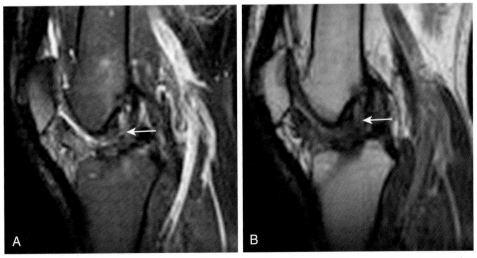

FIG 8.19 Sagittal T2 fat-saturated (A) and sagittal proton density (B) images demonstrate abnormal signal within the anterior cruciate ligament (ACL) graft *(arrows)* related to impingement by osseous proliferation at the distal femur in an NFL player 11 months after ACL reconstruction.

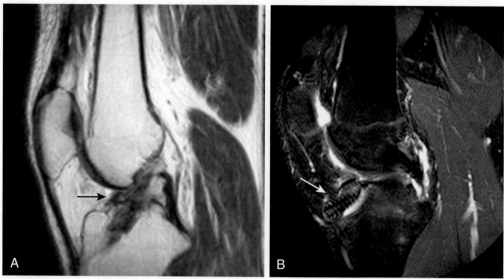

FIG 8.20 (A) Sagittal proton density image shows a hypointense nodular mass of fibrous tissue *(arrow)* anterior to the anterior cruciate graft compatible with arthrofibrosis in a patient with limited knee extension. (B) Sagittal T2 fat-saturated shows post–anterior cruciate ligament reconstruction with lysis of the tibial tunnel and migration of the interference screw into Hoffa fat *(arrow)*.

impingement. If the anterior wall of the tibial tunnel is placed too far anteriorly (anterior to the Blumensaat line), the graft can impact the roof of the intercondylar notch during knee extension, predisposing to roof impingement. In addition, if the ACL graft is positioned too vertically, graft roof impingement can be seen during extreme knee flexion. MRI findings of graft impingement include increased signal intensity within the distal two-third of the graft (the intercondylar portion), roof osteophytes abutting the graft at the site of caliber change, and abnormal contact between the graft and roof of the interchondylar notch, resulting in posterior bowing of the graft. The normal ACL graft should parallel but should never contact the roof of the intercondylar notch. Positioning of the tibia tunnel either too far anterior or too far posterior can cause impingement of the graft.

ARTHROFIBROSIS

A nodular mass of fibrous tissue anterior to the graft at the joint line and proximal to the tibial tunnel with intermediate-to-low signal on T1- and T2-weighted images is typical for postoperative arthrofibrosis (Fig. 8.20A).[3,34] It can also manifest as a fibrotic process that surrounds the graft. On MRI, a somewhat speculated, ill-defined region of intermediate low T1 signal and T2 signal intensity is seen centered within the Hoffa fat pad along the trajectory taken to access the anterior joint. Both focal and diffuse forms of arthrofibrosis can result in pain, locking, catching, or decreased range of motion. It occurs with a frequency of 1% to 10% after ACL reconstructions and may lead to restricted knee extension similar to that seen with graft impingement.[34] In more severe cases of arthrofibrosis, repeat arthroscopic surgery to release the scar tissue can be performed. In less severe cases, aggressive physical therapy is recommended initially as an attempt to break up the scar tissue.

OTHER ANTERIOR CRUCIATE LIGAMENT GRAFT COMPLICATIONS (GANGLION CYST FORMATION AND TUNNEL WIDENING)

Tunnel enlargement or lysis has been reported after ACL reconstruction surgery, which can contribute to knee laxity. The etiology of tunnel lysis is thought to be multifactorial but results in poor fixation of the graft fibers within the osseous tunnel. This phenomenon may be clinically relevant in revision surgery because the enlarged tunnels may complicate graft placement and fixation. Tunnel lysis (see Fig. 8.20B) characteristically occurs within the initial 3 months after ACL reconstruction. A small amount of fluid signal intensity within a hamstring ACL graft can be seen during the first 12 to 18 months. Fluid accumulation without tunnel expansion can occur within the osseous tunnel and fibers of the hamstring graft at the time of surgery and then gradually disappears over the subsequent 12 to 18 months. An expanded tunnel can complicate graft revision, which must be performed in two stages in this setting: bone grafting of the enlarged tunnel must be performed first, and then a delayed graft revision after the tunnel enlargement has been corrected with new bone and granulation tissue can be carried out.

HARDWARE FAILURE

Loss of graft fixation and knee instability can result from early postoperative hardware complications, such as fracture, malpositioning, and displacement. In the event of a fractured or dislodged ACL graft construct, mechanical joint symptoms can arise from displaced intra-articular bodies. Patients with intra-articular bodies can present with locking, catching, or restricted range of motion. Loose bodies may originate from articular cartilage damage that occurred during the initial injury or may

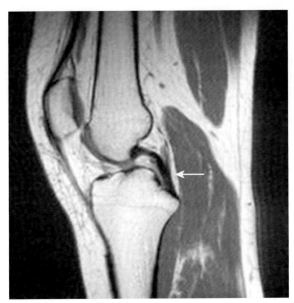

FIG 8.21 Sagittal proton density image demonstrating a normal posterior cruciate ligament *(arrow).*

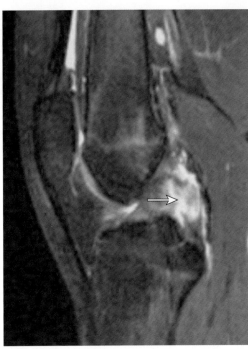

FIG 8.22 Sagittal T2 fat-saturated image shows disruption of the posterior cruciate ligament *(arrow)* compatible with complete tear after a motor vehicle accident and dashboard injury.

result from hardware failure or dislodgement after ACL graft placement.

POSTERIOR CRUCIATE LIGAMENT

Normal Posterior Cruciate Ligament Anatomy and Biomechanics

The PCL is the main restraint to posterior tibial translation, especially translation during knee flexion. It consists of two bundles, which are functionally assisted by the meniscofemoral ligaments: the anterolateral bundle and the posteromedial bundle. The anterolateral bundle is taut in knee flexion, and the posteromedial bundle is taut during knee extension. These bundles insert approximately 1 cm inferior to the articular surface of the proximal tibial posteriorly.

Normal Posterior Cruciate Ligament Magnetic Resonance Imaging

The normal appearance of the PCL on MR images is a well-defined continuous band of low signal intensity in all pulse sequences. The PCL is best evaluated on T2-weighted sagittal images of the knee, where it generally exhibits homogeneously low signal with a slightly curved morphology (Fig. 8.21). Although the coronal and axial images may add additional information, they are not completely necessary to make the diagnosis of a PCL injury. Axial images are suited for the examination of the vertical component and the coronal images for visualization of the horizontal component. The PCL is usually visualized on one or two consecutive sagittal images. It demonstrates a curved appearance with horizontal, genu, and vertical components from proximal to distal. Magic angle phenomenon may be seen at the genu on short TE pulse sequences.

The meniscofemoral component of the PCL is best visualized on sagittal or coronal images and can be seen as a small bandlike extending either anterior (Humphrey) or posterior (Wrisberg) to the PCL and spanning from the posterior horn of the lateral meniscus to attach on the inner aspect of the medial femoral condyle.

Magnetic Resonance Imaging of Posterior Cruciate Ligament Injury

PCL injury is less frequently encountered on MRI than ACL lesions, commensurate with published ligament injury rates.[46] MRI signs of complete tear of the PCL include nonvisualization of the ligament with or without hematoma in its expected location or focal, discrete disruption (Fig. 8.22).[25] Partial or intrasubstance PCL tearing, defined as abnormal MRI signal within the ligament, or fiber discontinuity, is more frequently encountered. Partial tears of the PCL more commonly involve its anterolateral bundle on MRI, and there is often focal ill definition and enlargement of the ligament at its middle third.[32] There is no pathognomonic osseous contusion pattern to confirm a PCL tear, but high-grade PCL injuries can be seen with both dashboard and hyperextension contusion patterns. Osseous avulsion injury is uncommon but most frequent at the tibial attachment, with irregularity of the tibial cortex and an osseous fragment attached to the free end of the otherwise intact ligament (Fig. 8.23).[43] Subchondral bone marrow edema and hemorrhage may be present between the fragment and the tibia.[46] A grading system has been described for PCL evaluation on MRI: grade 0 is normal, grade 1 is abnormal intrasubstance signal (intrasubstance tear), grade 2 injury is partial interruption of the anterior or posterior border (partial tear), and grade 3 injury is complete disruption, but correlating MRI findings with physical examination and surgery using this system can be difficult, and a descriptive MRI report may be of greater use to treating orthopedists. Osseous avulsion at the AM aspect of the medial tibial plateau has been termed a reverse Segond fracture or an AM impingement fracture. This injury represents an avulsion of the deep portion of the MCL and is an insensitive but highly specific finding for PCL tear. Indeed, if an osseous fragment is identified on radiographs in this location and there is a history of trauma, knee MRI is indicated to assess the PCL.[8]

PCL injuries are an isolated finding on MRI in only approximately 25% of PCL sprains or tears. Concomitant injuries include meniscal tears, medial slightly more common than lateral, and ligamentous injury, most commonly involving the ACL. Posterolateral corner injury and avulsion fractures of the fibular head are also associated with PCL disruption. This

fracture has been described as the arcuate sign, related to avulsion at the insertion of the arcuate complex, consisting of the fabellofibular, popliteal-fibular, and arcuate ligaments. In one small series, all patients with an avulsion at the fibular head had concomitant PCL injury.[19] In contrast to the torn ACL, at imaging follow-up, the PCL can have a normal appearance, even with complete disruption on initial MRI. Therefore MRI appearances of a PCL tear do not correlate as well with long-term PCL dysfunction as those indicating ACL tear do with ACL dysfunction. Chronic tears may also present with abnormal morphology, such as a hyperbuckled or U-shaped appearance,[1] or they may have intermediate intrasubstance signal.[46]

PCL injuries sustained during motor vehicle accidents represent approximately 45% of all PCL injuries.[38] Dashboard injury is a type of mechanism of injury sustained during high-energy impacts with an anterior blow to the proximal tibia, forcing the tibia posteriorly relative to the femur, resulting in PCL and concomitant ligamentous and posterior capsular injuries.

In the athletic population, PCL injuries are seen with a frequency of approximately 40%.[38] In these cases a fall on a flexed knee and hyperextension injuries are common injury mechanisms. Hyperextension injuries can selectively injure the anterolateral bundle without damaging the posteromedial bundle,[38] with more severe injuries additionally causing ACL and posterolateral corner or posteromedial corner injuries.

The function of the meniscofemoral ligaments is somewhat controversial. They are often identified by MRI, best in the sagittal plane, with the meniscofemoral ligament of Humphrey anterior to the PCL and the ligament of Wrisberg posterior to the PCL (Fig. 8.24). Some authors propose a mechanical role of the mensicofemoral ligaments in supplementing the PCL.[11] At imaging, the meniscofemoral ligament can mimic a tear of the posterior horn of the lateral meniscus. Following the ligament medially on subsequent sagittal images to its femoral attachment aids in interpretation. A prominent meniscofemoral ligament of Humphrey on sagittal T2-weighted images with surrounding soft tissue edema should tip the interpreter off to the possibility of a primary PCL sprain.

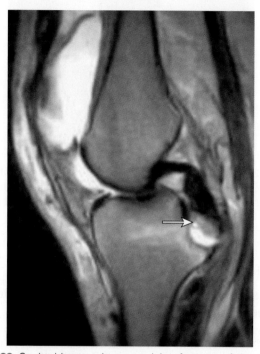

FIG 8.23 Sagittal image shows avulsion fracture of the tibia at the posterior cruciate ligament insertion *(arrow)* in a football player with knee hyperextension.

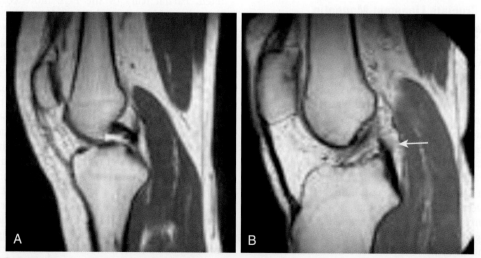

FIG 8.24 Sagittal proton density images show the meniscofemoral ligaments of Humphrey *(arrow* in A) and Wrisberg *(arrow* in B), anterior and posterior to the posterior cruciate ligament, respectively.

The posterior drawer test helps to assess the integrity of the PCL clinically by evaluating the degree of posterior translation of the tibia relative to the femur during 90-degree knee flexion. Hence tears are demarcated on the basis of functional integrity of the ligament rather than the presence or absence of complete disruption. During arthroscopy, laxity to probing is diagnostic of a tear.

Posterior Cruciate Ligament Reconstruction

The PCL is injured at a frequency far less than the ACL, accounting for up to 23% of all knee ligament injuries in the general population. Most PCL injuries are commonly seen as a result of motor vehicle accidents and sports-related injuries. As a result, PCL reconstruction is typically uncommon and performed following multiligamentous injuries, which emphasizes the importance of a thorough search for other associated ligamentous injuries of internal derangement in the setting of an obvious PCL injury. The appropriate surgical treatment of PCL injuries is controversial with isolated injuries been treated nonoperatively.[40] However, studies have demonstrated a PCL-deficient knee will likely progress to premature osteoarthritis if left untreated in physically active patients, such as high-performance athletes, or in patients with multiple concurrent ligamentous injuries because of altered biomechanics.[13,24] The BPTB graft and hamstring graft are the two most common graft materials used to reconstruct the PCL. Traditionally the objective of arthroscopic transtibial techniques has been to reconstruct the stronger anterolateral bundle of the native PCL using a single-bundle surgical technique; however, the results of this technique have been disappointing.[12,13] Tibial graft fixation may be accomplished by using either a tibial tunnel or a tibial inlay procedure with a BPTB graft. Late graft failure is more commonly seen with tibial tunnel fixation because as the graft exits the tibial tunnel it must make an acute turn around the proximal posterior tibia (at the opening of the tunnel), resulting in a "killer turn," which causes stress leading to abrasive wear of the graft at the edge of the tibial tunnel (Fig. 8.25). On the other hand, tibial inlay fixation consists of PCL graft bone plug fixation to the posterior cortex of the proximal tibia, avoiding the killer turn, and is performed by a combined arthroscopic and open technique through a posterior incision in the region of the popliteal fossa.

OTHER LIGAMENTOUS KNEE STRUCTURES

Medial Collateral Ligament

The MCL is injured with valgus stress to a flexed knee (Fig. 8.26). On MRI, it is evaluated primarily on the coronal fat-saturated T2 or short tau inversion recovery (STIR) sequences. Axial fat-saturated fluid-sensitive sequences supplement and confirm those findings on the coronal sequence. Injury to the MCL, as with other ligaments, is graded 1 to 3 by MRI. Findings of a grade 1 injury include an intact ligament, normal in signal, with surrounding edema and/or hemorrhage (Fig. 8.27). Edema surrounding the MCL should be evaluated in context with the overall knee pathology. Mimickers of grade 1 MCL injury include a ruptured Baker cyst, medial compartment pathology (such as osteoarthritis or meniscal tear), and lateral patellar dislocation. All of these injuries can present with edema insinuating around the MCL. A grade 2 injury, or partial rupture, manifests as abnormal signal within the ligament itself and/or fluid surrounding the ligament in the MCL bursa (Fig. 8.28).[39]

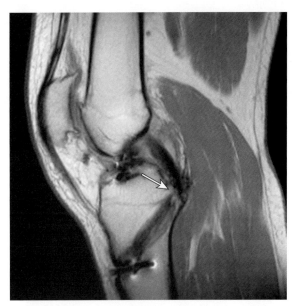

FIG 8.25 Sagittal proton density image shows a posterior cruciate ligament reconstruction using a tibial tunnel fixation technique demonstrating an intact graft with the typical angulation or "killer turn" of the graft at the opening of the tibial tunnel *(arrow)*, which may predispose to graft attrition and tear.

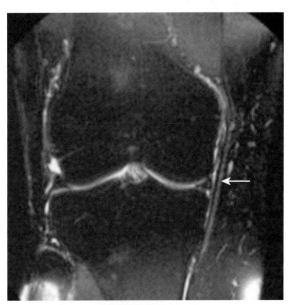

FIG 8.26 Coronal T2 fat-saturated image shows a normal medial collateral ligament *(arrow)*.

A grade 3 injury, or complete rupture, is characterized by frank disruption and discontinuity of the ligament (Figs. 8.29 and 8.30). Osseous contusions of the medial femoral condyle or lateral tibial plateau may accompany grade 2 or 3 sprains. Injury to the MCL should prompt close evaluation of the other structures of the knee because it is associated with tears of the ACL and medial meniscus.[39] Osseous avulsion is most common at the femoral attachment, with the osseous fragment best appreciated on T1 non–fat-saturated images.[32]

Because MCL injuries often present clinically with medial joint line tenderness, the medial meniscus and meniscocapsular

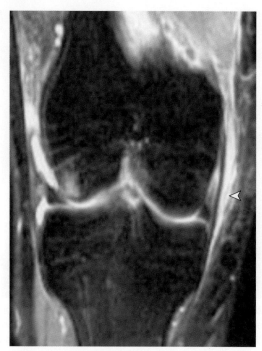

FIG 8.27 Coronal T2 fat-saturated image demonstrates edema signal *(arrowhead)* surrounding an intact medial collateral ligament representing a grade 1 sprain.

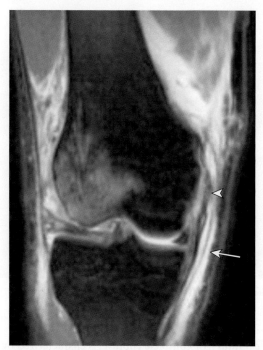

FIG 8.28 Coronal T2 fat-saturated image shows abnormal intrasubstance signal *(arrowhead)* and edema surrounding *(arrow)* the medial collateral ligament compatible with a grade 2 sprain in a soccer player.

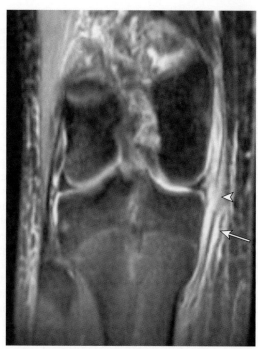

FIG 8.29 Coronal T2 fat-saturated image shows complete disruption of the midsubstance of the medial collateral ligament *(arrowhead)* and surrounding edema *(arrow)* representing a grade 3 sprain (full-thickness tear) sustained in a football injury with a blow to the lateral knee.

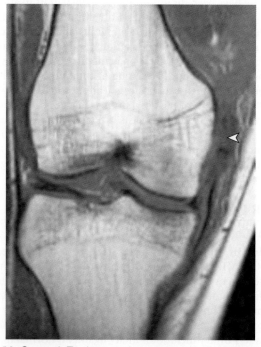

FIG 8.30 Coronal T1 image demonstrates disruption of the proximal medial collateral ligament *(arrowhead)* representing a grade 3 sprain in a skier after a valgus injury.

attachments should be carefully interrogated on MRI in the setting of a valgus trauma or MCL sprain. In addition, especially with contact sports injuries, the lateral knee structures should be evaluated thoroughly for osseous and soft tissue contusions and for fibular head fractures that may be occult to radiographs.

A peroneal neuropathy paired with an MCL sprain is a common scenario identified on MRI because the common peroneal nerve can be contused or impinged at the site of lateral impaction that led to the valgus stress. Chronic injury to the MCL may result in ligamentous thickening or the radiographic finding of calcification or ossification along the medial knee, also known as a Pellegrini-Steida lesion. On MRI, the chronically sprained MCL is often hypointense on all sequences and larger and more irregular than the normal MCL.

Lateral Collateral Ligament and Posterolateral Corner

Injury to the static and dynamic stabilizers of the posterolateral corner of the knee, including the fibular collateral ligament (FCL), popliteus and biceps femoris muscles and tendons, popliteal-fibular ligament, arcuate ligament, and fabellofibular ligaments, can be evaluated with MRI. Coronal and axial T2 fat-saturated sequences are most frequently used in examination of the posterolateral corner. Isolated injury is uncommon and therefore it should prompt close inspection of the other structures of the knee. Cruciate ligament pathology is often encountered with posterolateral corner injury, as well as MCL, meniscal, and peroneal nerve pathology. Posterolateral corner injury and instability can be somewhat occult clinically, especially in the setting of a recent pivot-shift mechanism, so interrogation of these structures at MRI is essential. In one series by Miller et al., 3 of 30 posterolateral corner injuries were detected by physical examination. Posterolateral instability has been cited as a cause of ACL graft failure and persistent instability following PCL repair. Therefore preoperative assessment of these structures can be of clinical import for surgical planning.

FCL (LCL proper) injury is less common than MCL injury (Fig. 8.31). In a prospective study by LaPrade et al.,[21] MRI detected FCL injury with 94% sensitivity and 100% specificity. Most commonly, FCL injury manifests as complete midsubstance disruption with surrounding soft tissue edema. Injury to the LCL complex can be graded on MRI, with a similar system used for other ligamentous structures about the knee. Edema surrounding an intact ligament is defined as a grade 1 sprain. Intrasubstance ligamentous signal, possibly with ligamentous thickening or thinning and surrounding edema, is considered a grade 2 sprain. Frank disruption and discontinuous fibers represent a grade 3 injury (Fig. 8.32). Osseous avulsion fractures at the ligamentous attachments, most commonly involving the fibular head, can also be seen at MRI (Fig. 8.33), although radiographs are more sensitive for small avulsed bony fragments. Biceps femoris tendon injury is usually related to chronic repetitive trauma. On MRI, the tendon will appear thickened just proximal to its insertion and may demonstrate abnormal signal. Acute injury may manifest as abnormal intrasubstance signal with surrounding edema or an avulsion fracture at its insertion with the FCL on the fibular head.

With its oblique course, the popliteus muscle and tendon are best evaluated with both sagittal and coronal MRI sequences (Fig. 8.34). They are most commonly injured at the musculotendinous junction (Fig. 8.35).[32] Increased T2 signal extends along the distal muscle fibers to the tendon, giving a feathery or herringbone appearance. Injury to the popliteus tendon manifests as increased intrasubstance signal or complete disruption. Subjacent bone marrow edema within the lateral femoral condyle has also been described (Fig. 8.36). A strain at the proximal myotendinous junction of the popliteus, a dynamic posterolateral stabilizer, should raise concern for traumatic injury to the static posterolateral corner stabilizers. Indeed, in the setting of a traumatic knee injury and subsequent MRI, the popliteus can be considered the "window to the posterolateral corner." Smaller static posterolateral stabilizers include the arcuate ligament, the popliteal-fibular ligament, and the fabellofibular ligament. These are variable in size and, in the case of the fabellofibular ligament, may or may not be present in the normal knee. The arcuate ligament is a multidirectional condensation of ligamentous and capsular fibers, often out of plane and difficult to identify on standard MRI sequences. Therefore nonvisualization of these structures in isolation cannot be

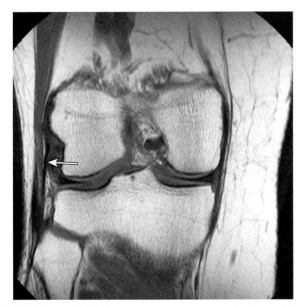

FIG 8.31 Coronal T1 image shows a normal fibular collateral ligament *(arrow)* extending from the femoral condyle to the fibula.

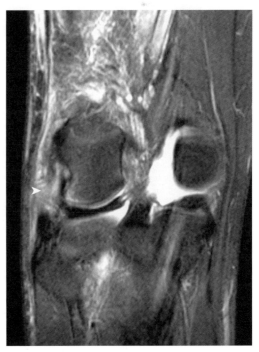

FIG 8.32 Coronal T2 fat-saturated image shows disruption of the fibular collateral ligament *(arrowhead)* representing a grade 3 sprain after a basketball injury.

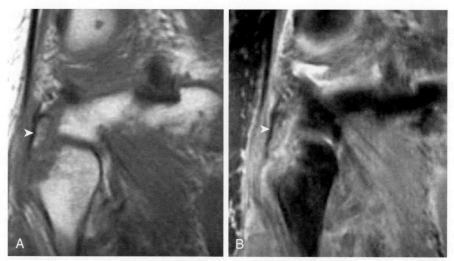

FIG 8.33 Coronal T1 (A) and coronal T2 fat-saturated (B) images show an avulsion fracture of the proximal fibula at the insertion of the fibular collateral ligament *(arrowhead)*.

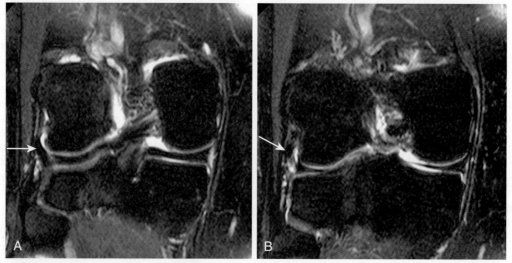

FIG 8.34 Consecutive coronal T2 fat-saturated images (A and B) demonstrate a normal popliteus tendon *(arrows)*.

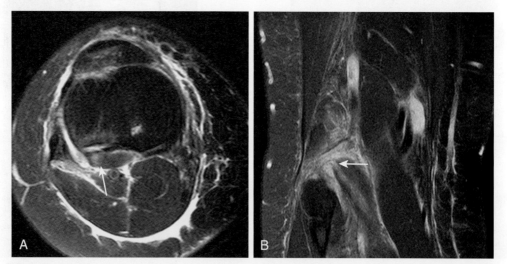

FIG 8.35 Axial (A) and coronal (B) T2 fat-saturated images demonstrate increased signal at the musculotendinous portion of the popliteus muscle indicative of a strain *(arrows)* without injury to the posterolateral corner stabilizers in a football player.

interpreted as disruption. Yu et al.[52] proposed using an oblique coronal plane, paralleling the course of the popliteus tendon for better visualization of these structures; however, this has not become a part of the routine evaluation of the knee at most institutions. Injury to the popliteal-fibular ligament was detected at MRI with a reported sensitivity of 69% and specificity of 68% in one series.[21] However, a systematic approach using standard T2-weighted fat-suppressed coronal imaging should increase this sensitivity. If a traumatic strain is evident at the proximal myotendinous junction of the popliteus, as well as edema about the posterolateral soft tissues, an irregular or ill-defined and injured popliteal-fibular ligament can often be identified as a dark structure bridging the popliteus to the fibula amidst the bright edema. With this constellation of findings, especially in the presence of pivot-shift contusions, concern for posterolateral corner stabilizer injury should be reported (Fig. 8.37).[52]

Posteromedial Corner

Components of the posteromedial corner of the knee include the posterior oblique ligament, semimembranosus expansions, meniscotibial ligaments, oblique popliteal ligament, and posterior horn of the medial meniscus. Although physical examination is the most reliable diagnostic tool for posteromedial corner injuries,[41] MRI can aid in evaluation. The intimate relationship of the meniscus, posterior oblique ligament, and capsule is demonstrated on MRI. Injury can manifest as increased signal within the semimembranosus tendon on a fluid-sensitive fat-saturated sequence or as meniscocapsular disruption. Evaluation of the posteromedial corner is best on sagittal and coronal imaging sequences. On MRI, posteromedial corner injuries are frequently associated with peripheral (red zone) meniscus tears. Occasionally patients with focal medial joint line tenderness without evidence of internal derangement will have abnormal signal within the distal semimembranosus insertion, representing an underlying tendinopathy.

Extensor Mechanism

The extensor mechanism is composed of the quadriceps muscle and tendon, the patella and patellar tendon, and the retinacula. Injuries to the extensor mechanism can be characterized by MRI. The quadriceps tendon routinely exhibits a trilaminar appearance on MRI, where it converges on the superior pole of the patella (Fig. 8.38). The most anterior component consists of fibers of the rectus femoris, middle component fibers from the vastus medialis and vastus lateralis, and posterior component fibers from the vastus intermedius. Quadriceps tendon tears most often occur in the occasional athlete or weekend warrior and have been associated with systemic conditions,

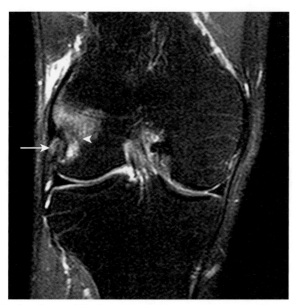

FIG 8.36 Coronal T2 fat-saturated image shows popliteus tendinopathy *(arrow)* and subjacent bone marrow edema within the lateral femoral condyle *(arrowhead)*.

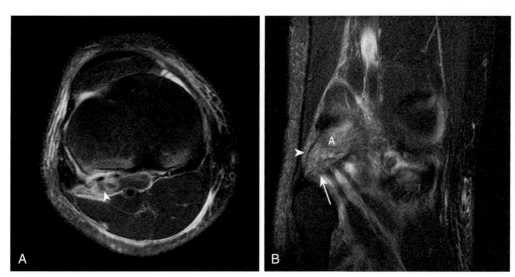

FIG 8.37 Axial (A) and coronal (B) T2 fat-saturated images show a severe posterolateral corner injury following a skiing accident. Along with a complete anterior cruciate ligament tear (not shown), images reveal a strain of the popliteus muscle, sprain of the fabellofibular ligament *(arrowhead* in B), soft tissue edema *(arrow* in B), and a sprain of the popliteofibular ligament *(arrow* in A). Arcuate fibers are denoted by *A* in part B.

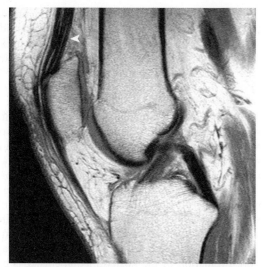

FIG 8.38 Sagittal proton density image demonstrates a normal quadriceps tendon with a trilaminar appearance *(arrowhead)*.

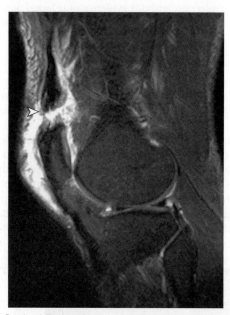

FIG 8.39 Sagittal T2 fat-saturated image shows a complete tear of the quadriceps tendon with fluid signal at the site of disruption *(arrowhead)* in a middle-aged recreational basketball player.

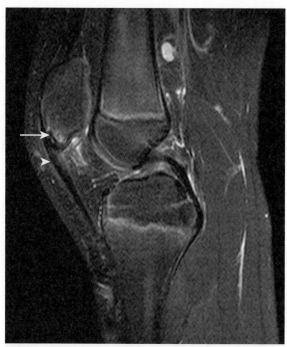

FIG 8.40 Sagittal T2 fat-saturated image shows abnormal signal within the proximal patellar tendon *(arrowhead)* and bone marrow edema within the inferior patella *(arrow)* in this skeletally immature patient (note femoral and tibial physes). Findings represent patellar tendinitis or jumper's knee.

such as chronic renal failure, rheumatoid arthritis, diabetes, and long-term steroid therapy.[32] The quadriceps tendon can be evaluated on MRI on the sagittal fluid-sensitive sequences. Partial tears appear as abnormal increased signal within the tendon, with intact fibers coursing around or through the tear.[42] With a complete tear, T2 or fluid-sensitive signal is increased at the site of the tear, and no intact fibers can be identified (Fig. 8.39). The proximal tendon edge may be wavy or balled up, owing to quadriceps muscular contraction. The patella may be tilted anteriorly and displaced inferiorly.[42] An assessment of the cranial-caudal gap or retraction should be made on sagittal MRI in the setting of quadriceps rupture.

Patellar tendon injury is more commonly attributed to overuse and repetitive microtrauma. Patellar tendinitis, or jumper's knee, is seen in adolescent and young adult basketball players, volleyball players, and other athletes as the result of repetitive quadriceps muscle contraction. Although this condition may be asymptomatic, patients can present with focal infrapatellar pain. Therefore it is important to identify early signs of patellar tendon disease with imaging. On MRI, the proximal patellar tendon will appear thick with foci of increased T2 signal (Fig. 8.40).[32] Chronic patellar tendon degeneration, a disease of adulthood, can be seen anywhere along the length of the tendon. Imaging reveals areas of intermediate T1 and T2 foci within the tendon, with or without tendon thickening (Fig. 8.41). Foci of increased fluid-sensitive signal may be related to mucinous degeneration and interstitial cyst formation. Using the quadriceps tendon as a reference is often helpful because a patellar tendon that is equal in thickness to the quadriceps tendon is abnormal.[42] Rupture of the patellar tendon may be related to chronic degeneration, most commonly at the proximal aspect, or to acute forced flexion against a contracted quadriceps muscle, most commonly at its midportion.[32] The patellar tendon will be discontinuous on sagittal imaging sequences, with superior displacement of the patella (Fig. 8.42). Acute and chronic avulsion injuries of the patellar tendon affect adolescents and include patellar sleeve avulsion, Osgood-Schlatter disease, and Sinding-Larsen-Johansson syndrome. Patellar sleeve avulsion occurs secondary to an acute forceful contraction of the quadriceps muscle and results in a tear of the proximal patellar tendon with an avulsed osteochondral fragment from the patella. On MRI, the fracture line through the patella will be seen on fluid-sensitive sequences with the retracted patellar tendon and its bony fragment distally (Fig. 8.43). Osgood-Schlatter disease and Sinding-Larsen-Johansson syndrome are similar in pathology and mechanism, affecting the distal and proximal patellar tendon, respectively. Both are related to chronic microavulsion of the patellar tendon. In Osgood-Schlatter disease, MRI will demonstrate enlargement of the tendon with foci of ossification (Fig. 8.44). Although there is normal variant anatomy of the tibial eminence ossification centers, the presence of surrounding edema and fluid in the deep infrapatellar bursa supports a diagnosis of Osgood-Schlatter disease. Sinding-Larsen-Johansson syndrome has similar MRI characteristics at the proximal patellar tendon with tendon thickening, abnormal intrasubstance signal, and areas of ossification.[42]

Lateral patellar dislocation is often transient, and patients as well as clinicians may not realize that it has occurred. MRI plays an important role with this lesion, as it has been reported that between 45% and 73% of lateral patellar dislocations are clinically unsuspected. Characteristic MRI findings in lateral patellar dislocation include joint effusion and hemarthrosis, medial retinacular injury, and osteochondral injury to the anterolateral lateral femoral condyle and medial patella. Osseous contusions secondary to patellar dislocation and subsequent relocation will be seen as foci of increased signal at the nonarticular, subcortical lateral femoral condyle, and at the medial patellar

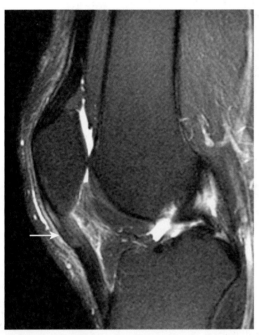

FIG 8.41 Sagittal T2 fat-saturated image demonstrates thickening and abnormal signal within the proximal patellar tendon (*arrow*), suggesting a chronic patellar tendinosis.

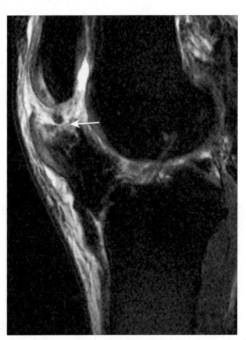

FIG 8.42 Sagittal T2 fat-saturated image shows a complete tear of the patellar tendon with fluid signal at the site of the tear and retraction of tendon fibers (*arrow*) in a middle-aged soccer player.

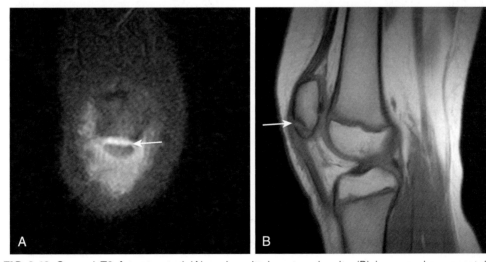

FIG 8.43 Coronal T2 fat-saturated (A) and sagittal proton density (B) images show a patellar sleeve avulsion in a 15-year-old basketball player with abnormal signal in the patellar tendon and a transverse fracture through the inferior patella (*arrow* in A) with mild inferior displacement of the osteochondral fragment (*arrow* in B).

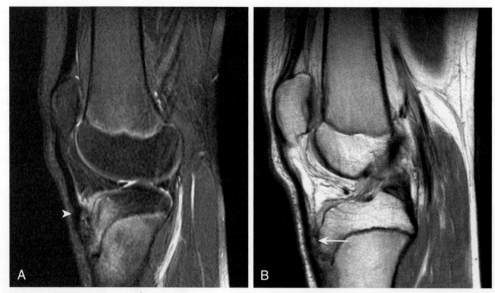

FIG 8.44 Sagittal T2 fat-saturated (A) and sagittal proton density (B) images demonstrate bone marrow edema at the tibial tuberosity and abnormal signal within the distal patellar tendon (*arrowhead* in A). Osseous fragmentation is evident at the tibial tuberosity (*arrow* in B). Findings represent Osgood-Schlatter disease.

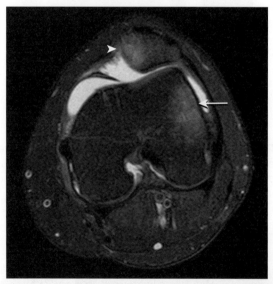

FIG 8.45 Axial T2 fat-saturated image shows bone marrow edema and osseous contusions within the medial patella (*arrowhead*) and lateral femoral condyle (*arrow*) compatible with recent transient lateral patellar dislocation in this 16-year-old lacrosse player.

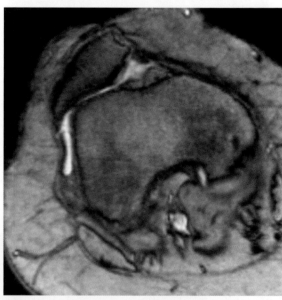

FIG 8.46 Axial gradient echo image shows lateral patellar tilt in a female with a long-standing lateral patellofemoral tracking syndrome.

facet on bone marrow edema–sensitive images (Fig. 8.45). The medial retinaculum is invariably injured and may be thickened or disrupted. However, injury to the MPFL may hold greater clinical importance and should be recognized at MRI. With disruption of the MPFL, fluid signal dissects under the distal, oblique fibers of the vastus medialis, which has been disrupted from its adductor tubercle attachment. Often, a torn MPFL can be identified as a wavy hypointense structure amid this soft tissue edema.[7] Injury can also be seen within the infrapatellar fat pad, manifested by increased fluid-sensitive signal, or even shear injury, as fluid-filled clefts within the fat pad.[32] Patellar

malalignment and abnormal tracking are related to incongruence between the patella and femur that results in patellofemoral joint instability. The patellofemoral compartment is best evaluated in the axial plane. Excessive lateral pressure syndrome manifests on MRI with lateral patellar tilt (Fig. 8.46), cartilage abnormality along the lateral patellar facet, and/or edema within the lateral patella (Fig. 8.47).[32] Dynamic assessment of patellar tracking with varying degrees of flexion and quadriceps contraction have been described with MRI using GRE sequences. The Insall-Salvati ratio has also been used with MRI. The longest patellar measurement and the length of the patellar

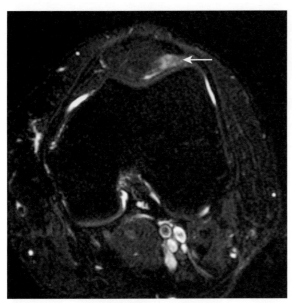

FIG 8.47 Axial T2 fat-saturated image shows edema within the lateral patella *(arrow)* and within the lateral aspect of Hoffa fat typical for abnormal patellofemoral tracking.

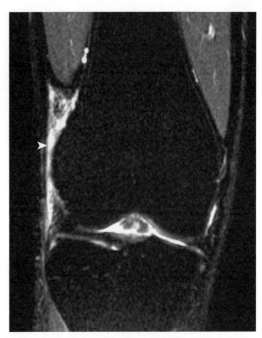

FIG 8.48 Sagittal T2 fat-saturated image demonstrates extensive soft tissue edema deep to the ITB *(arrowhead)* compatible with ITB friction syndrome in a 33-year-old distance runner.

tendon at its mid portion are used. If the ratio of patellar tendon length to patellar length is 1.3 or greater, then patella alta is present. Patella infera or patella baja occurs with a ratio of 0.8 or less.

Iliotibial Band

The ITB is an aponeurosis formed from the more proximal tensor fascia lata, gluteus maximus muscle, and gluteus medius muscle. It inserts onto the lateral femoral condyle and more distally onto the anterolateral tibia at Gerdy's tubercle. ITB friction syndrome is a condition most often seen in runners and cyclists and is related to repetitive flexion and extension, causing compression of vascularized and innervated fat between the ITB and the lateral femoral condyle.[32] Fluid-sensitive fat-saturated coronal and axial images are most sensitive, demonstrating increased signal or soft tissue edema deep to the ITB adjacent to the lateral femoral condyle (Fig. 8.48). Increased signal may extend into and even superficial to the ITB, and focal fluid collections have been described.[30,31] The ITB itself may be normal in signal and morphology or mildly enlarged with this overuse syndrome, and reciprocal bone marrow edema is occasionally present in the nonarticular lateral femoral condyle (Fig. 8.49).

Multiligament Knee Injuries

Although this term is more prevalent in the orthopedics and sports medicine literature than in radiology journals, it is important for imagers to accept and even expect associated soft tissue injuries in the knee, once an injury mechanism or ligamentous lesion has been identified. Injuries previously labeled as knee dislocations are now often more appropriately categorized under the term multiligament knee injury, indicating that at least two of the knee-stabilizing structures discussed in this chapter have been injured during a traumatic episode. Rather than review each MRI with a checklist, investigating each tendon and ligament individually, a more effective mechanism for interpretation of the traumatized knee is to identify the

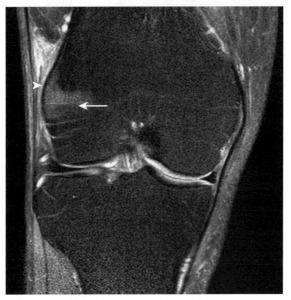

FIG 8.49 Sagittal T2 fat-saturated image demonstrates a more advanced case of iliotibial band friction syndrome with edema deep to the iliotibial band *(arrowhead)* and bone marrow edema within the lateral femoral condyle *(arrow)*.

mechanism and primary ligamentous injury, and then interrogate the other structures likely to be secondarily involved. Often, imaging findings can raise concern for a ligament sprain or tendon strain, but the actual integrity and stability of the secondarily injured structure must be confirmed at physical examination or sometimes at surgery. Common multiligament knee injury patterns include ACL tear with posterolateral corner injury with or without an MCL sprain, PCL tear and FCL sprain with or without posterolateral corner injury, and

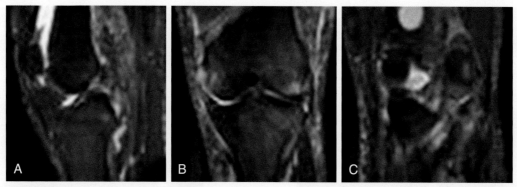

FIG 8.50 Sagittal (A) and coronal (B and C) T2 fat-saturated image shows tears of the anterior cruciate, posterior cruciate, and medial collateral ligaments with associated posterolateral corner injury (C).

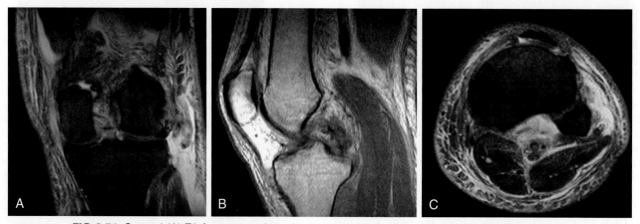

FIG 8.51 Coronal (A) T2 fat-saturated, sagittal proton density (B), and axial T2 fat-saturated (C) images show tears of the anterior cruciate, posterior cruciate, and lateral collateral ligaments.

tears of both cruciate ligaments with FCL and posterolateral corner injury—a pattern more appropriately labeled as a knee dislocation (Figs. 8.50 and 8.51).[23,27]

Often articular cartilage defects, lesions, and meniscal tears in specific locations are associated with ligament injuries and mechanisms; these associations should drive the imager to take a second look at structures in jeopardy. A transient lateral patellar dislocation is associated not only with MPFL injury, but also with a shear-type, delaminating articular cartilage lesion at the anterolateral margin of the lateral femoral condyle. In this regard, effective MRI interpretations often log specific lesions under an umbrella mechanism, such as "constellation of MRI findings," consistent with a recent pivot-shift injury at the right knee, including an acute, midsubstance, complete tear of the ACL, a grade 2 sprain of the popliteal-fibular ligament, a vertical tear at the posteromedial periphery of the medial meniscus, and a 4 × 3 mm focal grade 4 articular cartilage lesion at the terminal sulcus of the lateral femoral condyle.

CONCLUSION

The posttraumatic knee MRI review should be injury mechanism based, including a second look or careful evaluation of soft tissue and osseous structures likely to be injured based on the biomechanics of the injury. Recognition of reproducible injury patterns will lead to a thorough and useful imaging interpretation that can effectively guide therapeutic options.

Grading cruciate injuries as complete versus partial (high grade vs. low grade) is essential in clinical management, for which MRI is the imaging modality of choice. MRI offers a high sensitivity and specificity for the recognition of complete tears and a limited accuracy in the setting of chronic and partial tears. MRI readily delineates injuries of the cruciate ligaments and offers a distinct advantage in preventing unnecessary arthroscopy by assessing the severity of the ACL/PCL tear and other coexisting injuries.

KEY REFERENCES

7. Elias DA, White LM: Imaging of patellofemoral disorders. *Clin Radiol* 59:543–557, 2004.
19. Huang GS, Yu JS, Munshi M, et al: Avulsion fracture of the head of the fibula (the "arcuate" sign): MR imaging findings predictive of injuries to the posterolateral ligaments and posterior cruciate ligament. *AJR Am J Roentgenol* 180:381–387, 2003.
21. LaPrade RF, Gilbert TJ, Bollom TS, et al: The magnetic resonance imaging appearance of individual structures of the posterolateral knee: a prospective study of normal knees and knees with surgically verified grade III injuries. *Am J Sports Med* 28:191–199, 2000.
36. Sanders TG, Medynski MA, Feller JF, et al: Bone contusion patterns of the knee at MR imaging: footprint of the mechanism of injury. *Radiographics* 20:S135–S151, 2000.
41. Sims WF, Jacobson KE: The posteromedial corner of the knee. *Am J Sports Med* 32:337, 2004.

The references for this chapter can also be found on www.expertconsult.com.

9

Imaging of Synovium and Cartilage of the Knee

Tarek M. Hegazi, Kristen E. McClure, William B. Morrison

SYNOVIUM

INTRODUCTION

It is important for the surgeon to understand the principles for imaging the synovial compartments and articular cartilage of the knee. This chapter summarizes the anatomy, normal variations, pathologic conditions, and the strengths and weaknesses of the available imaging modalities.

SYNOVIAL ANATOMY

The synovium surrounding a joint has an outer fibrous capsule and an inner thinner synovial membrane. The inner vascular synovial membrane lines the nonarticular portions of the synovial joint and the intra-articular ligaments and tendons. It secretes synovial fluid, which nourishes and helps lubricate the joint, and maintains joint integrity by assisting with removal of debris. Within the knee joint anteriorly, the synovial lining extends superior to the patella and deep to the quadriceps femoris to form the suprapatellar recess. Below the patella, the infrapatellar fat (Hoffa's fat pad) displaces the synovium posteriorly away from the patellar tendon toward the intercondylar notch. The synovium then extends posteriorly within the intercondylar notch covering the cruciate ligaments, which divides the knee into medial and lateral compartments with an interposed extrasynovial space containing the cruciate ligaments.[16] A posterior recess at midline is identified posterior to the posterior cruciate ligament and is an extension from the medial tibiofemoral compartment. Other posterior recesses are seen between the posterior aspect of the femoral condyles and the deep surface of the lateral and medial heads of the gastrocnemius. Posterolaterally, the synovial membrane extends around the popliteus tendon at the popliteal hiatus, and extends inferiorly forming the popliteus bursa. The recesses are important when magnetic resonance imaging (MRI) is reviewed concerning important findings, such as intra-articular bodies and synovial disease, often present in these locations.

The normal synovium is barely perceptible on MRI and hence its visualization suggests the presence of synovial pathology. MRI and power Doppler ultrasound are the most sensitive imaging modalities to demonstrate abnormal synovium, but findings are usually nonspecific. Proliferative synovium exudes fluid and hence effusions are the most common and most sensitive finding of joint pathology. Synovial thickening and proliferation can be seen as *complex* or *dirty* fluid on T2-weighted images with careful windowing applied. Synovitis can be a diffuse or localized process. MRI with administration of intravenous gadolinium contrast shows the extent of synovitis more accurately because it provides strong, rapid enhancement; contrast can differentiate proliferative synovium from joint effusion. Power Doppler ultrasound can also demonstrate synovial inflammation quite effectively.

THE SYNOVIAL PLICAE

A plica is a fold of vascularized synovial tissue that is a remnant of cavitation junction formation during embryologic development. The most commonly seen plicae are the infrapatellar plica, the suprapatellar plica, and the medial patellar plica. They are usually asymptomatic and normally found in the knee, but any chronic inflammation may cause these plica to be symptomatic, with the medial patellar plica being the most common.[12] At MRI, the plica appear as low-signal-intensity bands within the high-signal-intensity joint fluid on T2-weighted images (Fig. 9.1). There are no size or morphologic criteria on MRI to determine whether a plica is clinically significant, although a symptomatic plica usually appears thickened with associated synovitis.

The suprapatellar plica divides the suprapatellar recess from the knee joint cavity. It courses obliquely downward from the anterior femoral metaphysis to the posterior aspect of the quadriceps tendon and inserts proximal to the superior pole of the patella. On MRI, it appears as a band-like low-signal-intensity structure posterior to the patella and is best seen on sagittal images.

The infrapatellar plica (ligamentum mucosum) is the most common plica in the knee. It has a dumbbell or fan-shaped appearance, originates from the intercondylar notch, and extends horizontally through the infrapatellar fat pad. On MRI, it is identified as a low-signal-intensity linear structure anterior and parallel to the anterior cruciate ligament (ACL) on sagittal images.

The medial patellar plica (plica alaris or patellar meniscus) is the most important clinically. It arises from the medial wall of the joint and courses obliquely, to insert on the infrapatellar fat pad. Sakakibara[24] classified medial patellar plicae into four types on the basis of size: Type A is a cord-like elevation in the synovial wall, Type B has a shelf-like appearance that does not cover the anterior surface of the medial femoral condyle, Type C is large with a shelf-like appearance covering the anterior surface of the medial femoral condyle, and Type D is a plica with central fenestration. Types A and B are usually asymptomatic and an incidental finding in many patients, while types C and D can impinge between the medial femoral condyle and the patella, be symptomatic, and even occasionally cause

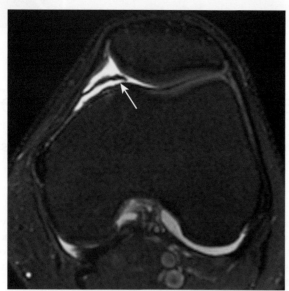

FIG 9.1 Medial Patellar Plica Axial T2-weighted fat-suppressed image shows a linear low-signal band *(arrow)* within the high-signal-intensity joint fluid without significant thickening or fibrosis. This was asymptomatic and an incidental finding in this patient.

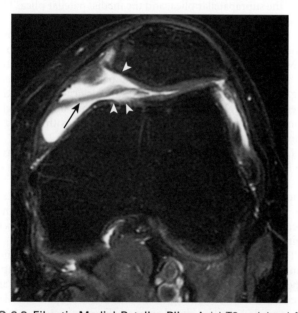

FIG 9.2 Fibrotic Medial Patellar Plica Axial T2-weighted fat-suppressed image shows a thick and irregular medial patellar plica *(arrow)* extending into the trochlear notch and interposed between the medial trochlea and patella. Note the cartilage loss *(arrowheads)* at the medial patellar facet and medial femoral trochlea.

cartilage loss at the femoral condyle and patella. Plica syndrome is defined as painful impairment of knee function, with a thickened fibrotic plica. It can be secondary to trauma, chronic repetitive activity, or other inflammatory process, and when the plica becomes thick and fibrotic, it causes friction over the medial femoral condyle and patella during knee flexion and extension (Fig. 9.2). On MRI, the plica will appear thickened and irregular associated with a joint effusion.[6]

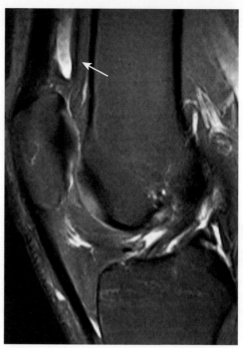

FIG 9.3 Obstructing Suprapatellar Plica Sagittal T2-weighted fat-suppressed image shows abnormal fluid in the suprapatellar recess *(arrow)* with mass effect, and not communicating with the remainder of the knee joint, suggestive of failure of regression of the suprapatellar plica and subsequent isolation of the compartment.

BURSAE

Bursae are synovial-lined structures containing synovial fluid that function to facilitate movement and reduce friction where tendons and muscles pass over bony prominences. They are typically not visible on imaging because they contain limited fluid, however with inflammation, they become visible on MRI as fluid collections with low signal on T1-weighted images and high signal on T2-weighted images. They may or may not be communicating with the synovial membrane of the knee joint itself. Anteriorly, the suprapatellar recess is located between the quadriceps and femur in midline. It normally communicates with the knee joint, but failure of regression of the suprapatellar plica leads to obstruction of the recess.[11] It may be found incidentally, or present as a mass above the knee joint when large (Fig. 9.3). The prepatellar bursa is located anteriorly between the patella and the overlying subcutaneous soft tissues. Bursitis in that location is commonly caused by chronic repeated trauma such as kneeling (housemaid's knee). MRI shows a fluid signal intensity lesion in the subcutaneous soft tissues anterior to the patella. The superficial infrapatellar bursa is located between the tibial tubercle and the overlying skin and a bursitis is usually caused from chronic overuse. On MRI, it will appear as a focal localized fluid collection anterior to the patellar tendon. The deep infrapatellar bursa lies posterior to the distal patellar tendon and anterior tibia, and bursitis usually results from extensor mechanism overuse. On the medial aspect of the knee, the pes anserine bursa separates the pes anserine tendons (sartorius, gracilis, and semitendinosus tendons) from the adjacent medial tibial condyle. On MRI, it will appear as a high-signal-intensity fluid collection on T2-weighted images along the pes anserine tendons in the posteromedial aspect of the knee that does not communicate with the knee joint. The medial collateral ligament bursa is located between the superficial and deep layers of the medial collateral ligament at the level of the joint line. On the lateral aspect of the knee, the iliotibial band bursa is located between the distal portion of the iliotibial band near its insertion on Gerdy's tubercle and the adjacent tibial surface. On MRI, iliotibial band bursitis appears as a localized fluid collection between the distal iliotibial band insertion and the lateral aspect of the tibia.

JOINT EFFUSION

Knee effusions are common and occur in a variety of settings (eg, trauma, degenerative, infection, or inflammatory conditions). On radiographs, knee effusions are only reliably seen on a lateral projection. A few signs have been described as sensitive for joint effusion including a rounded soft tissue density in the suprapatellar recess and loss of the normal posterior fat plane of the quadriceps tendon. A fat pad separation sign has been described that reflects the base of the suprapatellar bursa, which is located between the periarticular fat pads; a measurement greater than 10 mm is described as being diagnostic for an effusion.[9] MRI is extremely sensitive to the presence of fluid. Although there is no consensus on when to call a joint effusion pathologic versus normal physiologic fluid, an anteroposterior measurement of 10 mm or less in the lateral aspect of the suprapatellar pouch is considered a reasonable threshold for distinguishing physiologic from pathologic fluid.[14]

HEMARTHROSIS

Hemarthrosis is most commonly seen after trauma, but is also observed in various arthropathies, bleeding disorders such as hemophilia, and tumor-like conditions such as synovial hemangioma and pigmented villonodular synovitis (PVNS). Layering will be seen in the acute setting with the serum above and cells below. The presence of a fat-fluid level indicates a lipohemarthrosis, which is considered a strong indicator for an intra-articular fracture.[15] In the subacute phase, the effusion will be of relatively high signal on both the T1- and T2-weighted images. In the chronic phase, the synovium will show low signal on both T1- and T2-weighted images because of hemosiderin deposition and can show a blooming artifact (expansive black signal) on the gradient recalled echo (GRE) sequences.

SYNOVIAL PATHOLOGY

Inflammatory Arthropathies

Inflammatory arthropathy is a generic term representing synovial disease and includes septic arthritis, rheumatoid arthritis, psoriatic arthritis, reactive arthritis, and crystalline arthropathies such as gout. There is too much overlap of the imaging findings to discriminate septic arthritis from other inflammatory arthropathies. The clinical features of the disease, the number of affected joints, and the distribution of disease is crucial in arriving at the correct diagnosis.[5] In the early phases of an inflammatory arthropathy, radiographs are usually normal or show nonspecific joint effusion; however, a joint effusion is not a must and the diagnosis of an inflammatory arthropathy should not be ruled out on the basis of a lack of effusion; joint aspiration still remains the primary means of excluding infection. MRI is more sensitive than radiographs for demonstration of early disease and allows better evaluation of the joint and surrounding soft tissues. MRI will usually show the extent of the synovitis and erosions, which start marginally with progression to diffuse cartilage loss and associated bone marrow edema (Fig. 9.4). Surrounding soft tissue edema maybe seen as well.

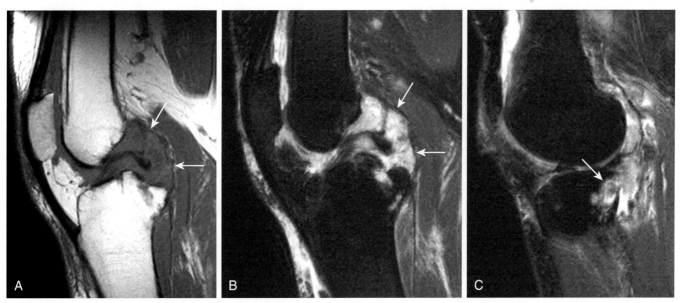

FIG 9.4 Rheumatoid Arthritis Sagittal T1-weighted image (A) shows intermediate mass-like synovial proliferation in the posterior aspect of the knee *(arrows)* with mass effect on the posterior capsule. Sagittal T2-weighted fat-suppressed image (B) shows the mass-like synovial proliferation to be of high signal intensity with a more complex or "dirty" appearance *(arrows)*. Sagittal T2-weighted fat-suppressed image (C) shows marginal erosion in the posterior aspect of the lateral tibia *(arrow)* typical of rheumatoid arthritis.

The presence of *rice bodies*, which represent sloughed necrotic debris in the joint, may suggest rheumatoid arthritis. They appear as small rod-shaped bodies measuring a few millimeters in size, and are of intermediate signal on T1- and T2-weighted images.[5]

Primary Synovial Chondromatosis

Primary synovial chondromatosis is a benign proliferative disorder characterized by synovial metaplasia of unknown cause. It is a monoarticular disorder affecting large joints, with the knee being most common. It is typically a self-limited process that tends to recur locally. Cartilaginous nodules can become calcified or ossified, in which case, the term *synovial osteochondromatosis* is used.[20] Radiographs show numerous bodies of similar small size distributed evenly throughout the joint, disproportionate to the degree of osteoarthritis (Fig. 9.5). The joint spaces are usually maintained and periarticular osteopenia is usually absent. Chronic erosions, which can be seen in other smaller joints, are less common in the knee because of its capacious volume. Computed tomography (CT) is usually not necessary to make the diagnosis because approximately 70% to 95% of bodies calcify and can be seen on radiographs; however, some bodies can be so small and faintly calcified that they may be missed on radiographs, making CT the ideal imaging modality for identifying and characterizing calcifications when radiographs are normal or equivocal.[20] On MRI, the imaging findings are variable depending on the extent of ossification. When nonmineralized, the synovium shows intermediate to high signal intensity on T2-weighted images, although a slightly lower signal than joint fluid. When calcified or ossified, bodies show low-signal intensity on all sequences (Fig. 9.6).[21]

Pigmented Villonodular Synovitis

PVNS is a benign, mono-articular synovial proliferative disorder with the knee the most commonly affected joint, representing approximately 60% to 80% of cases.[19] It is characterized by hyperplasia of the synovial lining with infiltration by multinucleate giant cells and hemosiderin-laden macrophages. PVNS is usually a diffuse process but it can have a focal, localized form[29]; a nonpigmented form is also rarely observed. Diffuse PVNS presents with a joint effusion and hemarthrosis and usually has a frond-like appearance with hemosiderin deposition usually more abundant than in the localized form. Radiographs may appear normal with bone density and the joint space usually preserved. Sometimes periarticular swelling or joint effusion representing hemarthrosis may be seen.[2] Erosions are uncommon at the knee joint as compared to other smaller-capacity joints such as the hip and ankle. MRI is the preferred imaging modality because it provides specific imaging features to distinguish PNVS from other synovial processes. MRI reveals diffuse or localized intra-articular soft tissue masses. In the diffuse form, the entire synovium may be involved, whereas the focal form usually shows a well-defined solitary nodule or mass. Lesions are usually intermediate on T1-weighted images but relatively low on T2-weighted and gradient echo sequences because of hemosiderin deposition (Fig. 9.7).[2] The synovium is significantly enhanced after intravenous gadolinium contrast administration. Rust-colored hemosideric synovium has been described as a "shaggy red bread" on visual inspection.

Lipoma Arborescens

Lipoma arborescens is a benign process with villous synovial proliferation; the subsynovial fat undergoes hyperplasia

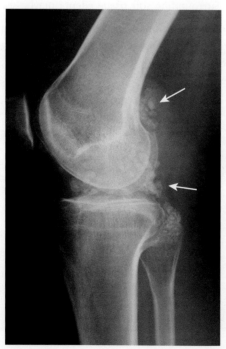

FIG 9.5 Synovial Osteochondromatosis on Radiograph Lateral view shows classic imaging findings of multiple small round bodies *(arrows)*, all of similar size, extending into the posterior joint space out of proportion to the degree of osteoarthritis.

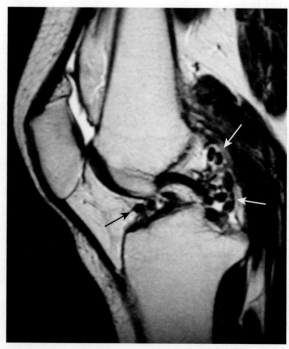

FIG 9.6 Synovial Osteochondromatosis on Magnetic Resonance Imaging Sagittal T2-weighted image shows a joint effusion with multiple round low-signal-intensity filling defects of similar size, consistent with ossified bodies *(arrows)*.

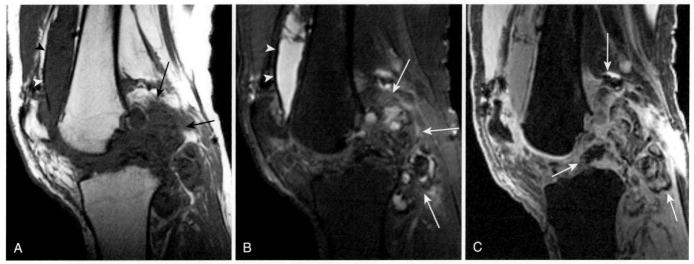

FIG 9.7 Pigmented Villonodular Synovitis Sagittal T1-weighted image (A) and sagittal T2-weighted fat-suppressed image (B) show a large suprapatellar effusion *(arrowheads)* and low-signal-intensity nodularity along with thickened synovium within the posterior knee joint *(arrows)* and erosion into the posterior aspect of the medial femoral condyle. The sagittal T2* gradient recalled echo (GRE) image (C) shows the nodules *(arrows)* as larger and lower in signal intensity than on the T2-weighted images (referred to as a "blooming" artifact) because of hemosiderin, which confirms the diagnosis.

resulting in predominantly fatty tissue signal on MRI.[10] It is a nonspecific finding but likely results from reactive synovial inflammation from chronic inflammatory conditions rather than a primary neoplastic process. It is usually associated with joint effusions and underlying degenerative arthritis and appears to represent a "burned out" process of subclinical inflammation leaving behind subsynovial fat proliferation.[28] Radiographs are usually of limited value but may demonstrate nonspecific fullness and soft tissue density in the suprapatellar recess. CT will demonstrate characteristic fat density villous fronds interspersed between thickened synovium and a joint effusion. MRI is considered the imaging modality of choice and the findings are usually diagnostic with villous lipomatous proliferation showing signal intensity similar to that of fat on all sequences (Fig. 9.8).[25]

Synovial Hemangioma

Synovial hemangioma is a rare benign vascular malformation usually affecting children and young adults. The knee is the most common joint affected, with the suprapatellar recess the most common location in the knee.[17] Radiographs are usually normal but can show a soft tissue mass, sometimes with phleboliths observed. MRI findings are usually characteristic with a lobulated intra-articular mass that has intermediate to low signal on T1-weighted images and high signal intensity on T2-weighted images related to slow blood flow in vascular spaces (Fig. 9.9).[8] Linear low-signal-intensity septations can be seen within the lesion representing fibrous septae or flow voids.[8]

Synovial Cyst

A synovial cyst is defined as a juxta-articular fluid collection that is lined with synovial cells and represents a focal extension of joint fluid communicating with the joint. The most common synovial cyst in the knee is in the gastrocnemius-semimembranosus bursa located posterior to the medial

femoral condyle, and is also called a *popliteal cyst* or *Baker cyst* (Fig. 9.10). They usually form as a result of chronic effusion secondary to any degenerative, traumatic, or inflammatory process, and can appear simple or multiloculated and may contain debris or bodies. MR imaging of a simple cyst is low signal on T1-weighted images and fluid signal on T2-weighted images.[18] When a cyst ruptures, it results in edema in the surrounding fascial planes with fluid tracking along the medial gastrocnemius muscle. Other complications include infection, hemorrhage, or compression of the neurovascular bundle, which can be identified on MRI. Other less common synovial cysts in the knee include cysts in the proximal tibiofibular joint, which can cause pain and foot drop secondary to impingement on the common peroneal nerve.

Ganglion Cysts

Ganglion cysts are lobulated outpouchings of the joint capsule containing clear viscous fluid surrounded by connective tissue but lacking a synovial lining. There is no consensus on the pathogenesis of ganglion cysts around the knee, but they have been classified as myxoid lesions and are believed to result from degeneration of the connective tissue from repeated trauma or capsular pressure from chronic or repeated joint effusion.[4] Ganglion cysts are generally classified as juxta-articular, intra-articular, and intra-osseous. Most are asymptomatic and discovered incidentally; however, they can compress adjacent structures or extend to the subcutaneous tissues and be perceived as a mass. In fact, ganglion cysts are so much more common than soft tissue tumors that a palpated mass at the knee is best evaluated by a noncontrast MRI that evaluates for communication with the joint and associated effusion and internal derangement rather than a tumor. Intra-articular ganglion cysts are most commonly seen in association with cruciate ligament mucoid degeneration; if large, these can cause a mass effect within the joint resulting in pain and limited range

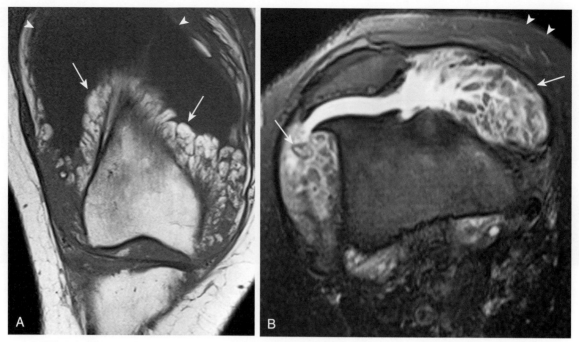

FIG 9.8 Lipoma Arborescens Coronal T1-weighted image (A) shows a grossly distended knee joint. This distension is because of frond-like fatty proliferation of the synovium *(arrows)* and a joint effusion *(arrowheads)*. The axial T2-weighted fat-suppressed image (B) in the same patient shows the frond-like synovial masses *(arrows)* have low signal, following the signal of subcutaneous fat *(arrowheads)*, confirming fat composition.

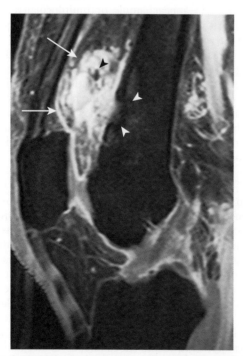

FIG 9.9 Synovial Hemangioma Sagittal T1-weighted fat-suppressed post-gadolinium contrast image shows a well-defined lobulated intra-articular mass *(arrows)* in the suprapatellar recess with avid enhancement and multiple low-signal fibrous septa. Note the oval low-signal foci within the lesion *(black arrowhead)*, most likely representing a phlebolith. There is minimal erosion into the anterior aspect of the femur *(white arrowheads)*.

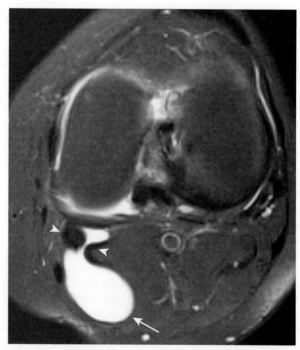

FIG 9.10 Popliteal (Baker) Cyst Axial T2-weighted fat-suppressed image shows a well-defined fluid signal lesion *(arrow)* in the posterior knee with a "dumbbell" shape located between the semimembranosus and medial gastrocnemius tendons *(arrowheads)*.

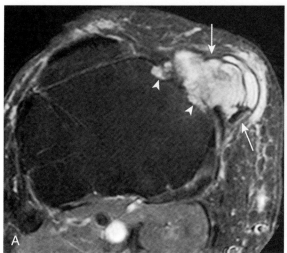
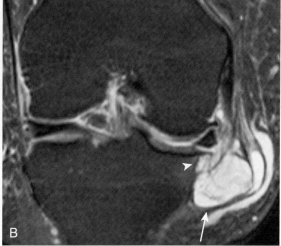

FIG 9.11 Ganglion Cyst Axial T2-weighted fat-suppressed image (A) and coronal T2-weighted fat-suppressed image (B) show a multilobulated fluid signal cystic mass *(arrows)* at the medial joint line with multiple septations and debris. Also note mild scalloping of the medial tibial plateau *(arrowheads)* consistent with intraosseous extension.

of motion. Intra-osseous ganglion cysts are most commonly seen at the tibial plateau associated with the ACL or posterior cruciate ligament (PCL) insertion. Intra-articular or juxta-articular ganglion cysts can also extend into the adjacent bone. On MRI, ganglion cysts are lobulated and show fluid signal occasionally with debris present within (Fig. 9.11).[13]

CARTILAGE

CARTILAGE AND OSTEOCHONDRAL INJURIES

Hyaline cartilage covers the articular surface of the knee joint and is composed of chondrocytes surrounded by a medium of collagen, proteoglycans, and electrolytes. Hyaline cartilage aids in resistance against compressive and shearing forces, predominantly by dissipating the forces to the menisci and subchondral bone.[22] Because of the prevalence of degenerative osteoarthritis, imaging of hyaline cartilage has become an important focus of diagnostic radiology research.

MAGNETIC RESONANCE IMAGING OF HYALINE CARTILAGE

To adequately image hyaline cartilage in the knee, adequate difference in signal intensity (contrast) must be evident among the joint fluid, hyaline cartilage, and the subchondral bone. Additionally, spatial resolution must be optimized, allowing for differentiation among cartilage thinning, fissuring, and partial-thickness and full-thickness defects.

No universal dedicated MRI sequence has been dedicated for hyaline cartilage imaging. Proton density and T2-weighted fast spin echo sequences with fat suppression provide sufficient contrast between the higher signal joint fluid and intermediate signal cartilage to detect chondral abnormalities. Both proton density and T2-weighted fast spin echo sequences produce high signal-to-noise ratio images with relatively short acquisition times. Short T1 inversion recovery (STIR) images may also provide sufficient contrast resolution to evaluate for chondral

abnormalities, but intrinsically have a lower signal-to-noise ratio and spatial resolution. Two- or three- dimensional (2D or 3D) gradient imaging sequences can improve resolution and can more accurately evaluate the superficial surface of the cartilage; however, these sequences generally require a longer acquisition time, are limited for use in evaluation of the deeper cartilage layers, and are more susceptible to imaging artifacts.[26] MRI diagnostic capabilities in low-grade cartilage lesions are limited by contrast and spatial resolution, partial volume averaging, and artifact.

Normal articular cartilage has a homogeneous or laminar appearance with a smooth surface contour. Articular cartilage has intermediate signal on both T1- and T2-weighted images (Fig. 9.12). Fat-suppression techniques can be used on any sequence and have the advantage of increasing the apparent signal of the hyaline cartilage relative to other tissues (ie, cartilage appears bright on fat-suppressed images, regardless of the sequence used).

Chondral abnormalities are diagnosed on MRI by recognizing a contour defect within the cartilage, focal thinning compared to the thickness of the adjacent cartilage, and/or signal alteration within the cartilage (Fig. 9.13 to 9.17). A secondary sign of a cartilage defect includes underlying bone marrow edema, as manifested by increased signal in the subchondral bone on fat-suppressed proton density and T2-weighted images. Subchondral bone marrow edema is a nonspecific finding that may be seen with acute injury (bone contusion or bruise, fracture), a mechanical disturbance such as stress response or overlying meniscal tear, and many other conditions including metabolic and neoplastic lesions. However, a flame-shaped or rounded focus of marrow edema in the subchondral bone should initiate a search for an overlying hyaline cartilage abnormality.

Cartilage damage can be related to acute trauma, prolonged and repetitive stress, and degeneration. Numerous classifications have been proposed to grade cartilage lesions based largely on arthroscopic findings, and less so on MRI findings. These classification systems describe articular cartilage damage

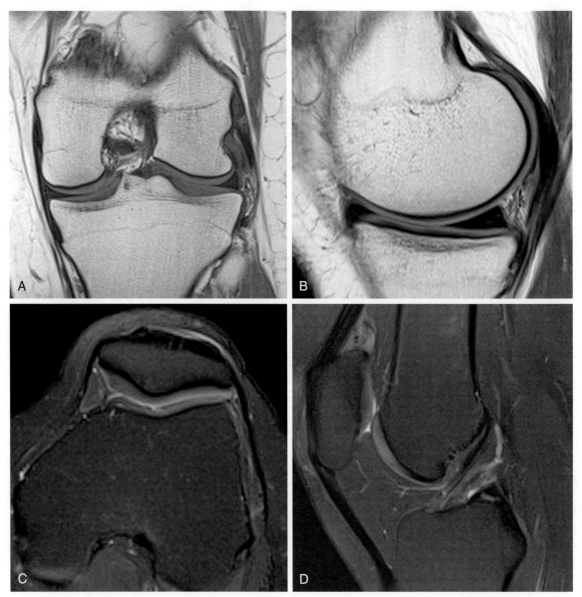

FIG 9.12 Normal Articular Cartilage Normal cartilage is demonstrated on coronal T1 (A), sagittal proton density (B), axial T2-weighted fat-suppressed (C), and sagittal T2-weighted fat-suppressed (D) images. Articular cartilage has intermediate signal on T1- and T2-weighted images; on most sequences, fat suppression results in higher relative cartilage signal. Achieving high resolution and a pronounced difference in brightness of cartilage and joint fluid is essential for imaging cartilage abnormalities. Note the poor contrast between cartilage and joint fluid on the T1-weighted image (A).

ranging from swelling and signal heterogeneity to fissuring, ulceration, partial-thickness defects, and full-thickness defects with exposure of the subchondral bone.

The Outerbridge scale classifies cartilage abnormalities based on arthroscopic findings. Grade I includes softening or swelling of the articular cartilage. Grade II is described as cartilage fragmentation and fissuring less than 1.5 cm in diameter. Grade III includes cartilage fragmentation and fissuring greater than 1.5 cm in diameter, and Grade IV involves cartilage erosion to bone.[23] The International Cartilage Repair Society has adopted a classification system described by Yulish & Associates. Grade 0 represents normal cartilage, Grade 1 describes increased T2 signal within the cartilage, Grade 2 refers to a partial-thickness

defect that is less than 50% of the normal cartilage thickness, Grade 3 represents a partial-thickness defect greater than 50% of the normal cartilage thickness, and Grade 4 describes a full-thickness defect.[22] In the Noyes system, Grade 1 depicts an intact cartilage surface, Grade 2A reflects cartilage damage with less than 50% cartilage thickness involved, Grade 2B cartilage defects involve greater than half of the cartilage thickness, and Grade 3 represents full-thickness cartilage defects with exposed subchondral bone (3A cortical surface is intact, 3B cortical has surface cavitation) (Table 9.1).

Aside from grading cartilage loss, assessing the location, size, and morphology of the cartilage defect is also important. Chondral injuries in weight-bearing areas have a worse

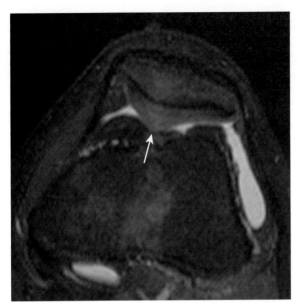

FIG 9.13 Low-Grade Chondromalacia Axial T2-weighted fat-suppressed image shows swollen, T2 hyperintense cartilage *(arrow)* along the median ridge of the patella.

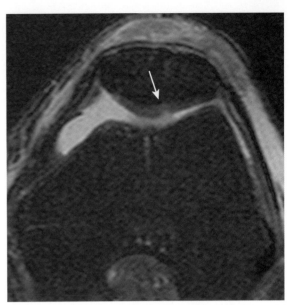

FIG 9.14 Partial-Thickness Cartilage Defect Axial T2-weighted fat-suppressed image demonstrates diffuse patellar cartilage thinning with focal partial-thickness cartilage loss at the lateral facet *(arrow)*, accounting for less than 50% of the normal cartilage thickness.

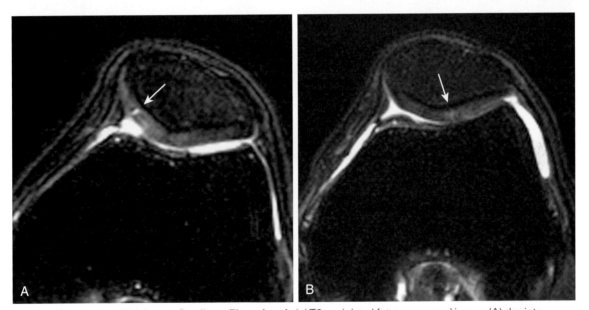

FIG 9.15 Full-Thickness Cartilage Fissuring Axial T2-weighted fat-suppressed image (A) depicts a small fissure at the medial patellar facet *(arrow)*. Axial T2-weighted fat-suppressed image of a different patient (B) shows a more broad area of cartilage surface irregularity at the lateral facet with a full-thickness fissure *(arrow)*.

prognosis and different treatment implications than those in non–weight-bearing areas. Traumatic chondral injuries are usually focal and may have acute margins with adjacent shoulders. They may be partial thickness or full thickness and can shear off from the cortex, resulting in an intra-articular body.[27]

In osteoarthritis, the cartilage thins particularly along weight-bearing aspects and degenerates with fraying, fissuring, ulceration, and sometimes delaminating defects. Accompanying osteophyte formation, subchondral cystic change, bone marrow edema, and sclerosis may occur. Several studies have demonstrated that meniscal root tears, large radial meniscal tears, and severe meniscal degeneration are strongly associated with major meniscal extrusion and may precede or even accelerate the development of osteoarthritis with cartilage loss.[27]

Inflammatory arthritides result in diffuse, uniform cartilage thinning throughout the joint, with uniform joint space narrowing. Focal cartilage defects are not typical. However, in areas

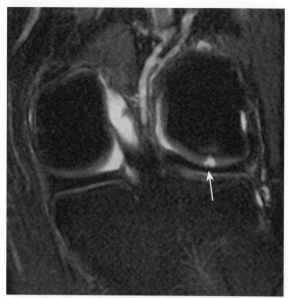

FIG 9.16 Focal Full-Thickness Defect Coronal T2-weighted fat-suppressed image shows a focal full-thickness cartilage defect *(arrow)* along the lateral femoral condyle. Reactive underlying subchondral bone marrow edema is evident.

TABLE 9.1	Chondral Injury Classifications		
Outerbridge	**ICRS**	**Noyes**	
Grade I: Softening and swelling of cartilage	Grade 0: Normal cartilage	Grade 1: Intact cartilage surface	
Grade II: Cartilage fragmentation and fissuring <1.5 cm diameter	Grade 1: Increased T2 signal in the cartilage	Grade 2A: Cartilage surface damaged with <50% thickness involved	
Grade III: Fragmentation and fissuring >1.5 cm diameter	Grade 2: Partial-thickness defect <50% of normal cartilage thickness	Grade 2B: Cartilage defects involve >50% cartilage thickness	
Grade IV: Cartilage erosion to bone	Grade 3: Partial-thickness defect >50% of normal cartilage thickness	Grade 3: Bone exposed (3A cortical surface intact, 3B cortical surface cavitation)	
	Grade 4: Full-thickness defect		

ICRS, International Cartilage Repair Society.

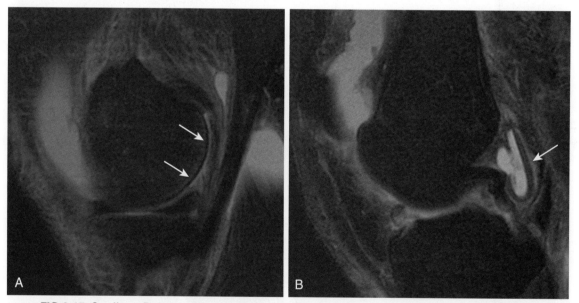

FIG 9.17 Cartilage Delamination (A) Sagittal T2-weighted fat-suppressed images demonstrate a broad area of full-thickness cartilage loss from the posterior aspect of the medial femoral condyle *(arrows)*. (B) The cartilage has delaminated from the femoral condyle and is seen displaced into the posterior joint space *(arrow)*.

of inflammatory pannus, focal cartilage and bony erosions may be found. Significant osteophyte formation should not occur.[27]

OSTEOCHONDRAL LESIONS

The term *osteochondral lesion* is used to describe a spectrum of disease from traumatic osteochondral injury to chronic osteochondritis dissecans (OCD). Lesions may arise from forces applied to the chondral surface in a single traumatic event, or over time as the result of repeated minor injury. Damage to the

underlying subchondral bone ensues. The bone may become necrotic and collapse. If the cartilage surface is damaged, fluid can extend from the joint into the bone and the fragment can separate, eventually detaching and forming a loose body. Alternatively, especially if the overlying cartilage remains intact, the underlying bone can heal. Overlying cartilage can itself delaminate and become displaced as an intra-articular body, or it may degenerate and become thinned and fissured. Osteochondral lesions are most commonly encountered in the talus, femoral condyles, and elbow.

TRAUMATIC OSTEOCHONDRAL LESIONS

A traumatic osteochondral lesion occurs when shearing, compressive, or rotational forces are transmitted between two articular surfaces, resulting in a chondral or subchondral fracture (Fig. 9.18). A cartilage flap or an osteochondral fragment may form, depending on the depth of the fracture line. This injury is typically associated with tenderness, a joint effusion, and sometimes even hemarthrosis. Elevated intra-articular pressure is thought to force synovial fluid into the cartilage flap or beneath the osteochondral fragment, resulting in resorption of the subchondral bone and cystic change. Sometimes the cartilage flap or osteochondral fragment dissociates from the underlying bone, resulting in an intra-articular body.[22]

OSTEOCHONDRITIS DISSECANS

OCD is a somewhat outdated term, although still in common use; a better term is *osteochondral lesion*. Nevertheless, the term *OCD* typically refers to an osteochondral lesion that is often discovered incidentally and is presumed to represent a chronic injury. The classic OCD is most commonly seen in young patients between 10 and 20 years of age. The idiopathic variety of OCD often occurs in the lateral aspect of the medial femoral condyle, along the non–weight-bearing aspect near the intercondylar notch, possibly related to microtrauma between the tibial spine and the medial femoral condyle during internal rotation of the tibia. Repetitive microinjuries are thought to disrupt blood supply to the subchondral bone, sometimes resulting in osteonecrosis, and progressing to an osteochondral lesion. The natural progression of stable OCD (ie, with intact overlying cartilage) is spontaneous healing. However, if the lesion is painful and unstable, surgery is usually indicated.

MRI should be performed to accurately characterize OCD, to evaluate size and location, and to determine the stability of the lesion (Fig. 9.19). The osteonecrotic fragment has low-signal intensity on T1- and T2-weighted images. Measurement is generally performed using T1-weighted images. Surrounding bone marrow edema is variable and may represent healing response or irritation from lesion instability, so this finding is

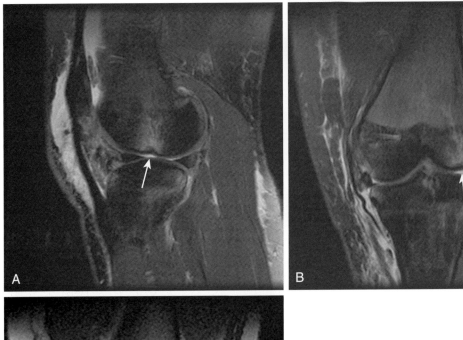

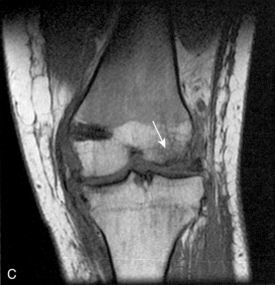

FIG 9.18 Osteochondral Impaction Injury Sagittal T2-weighted fat-suppressed (A), coronal T2-weighted fat-suppressed (B), and coronal T1-weighted (C) images show an osteochondral impaction injury along the lateral femoral condyle *(arrows)* consistent with a pivot shift injury mechanism.

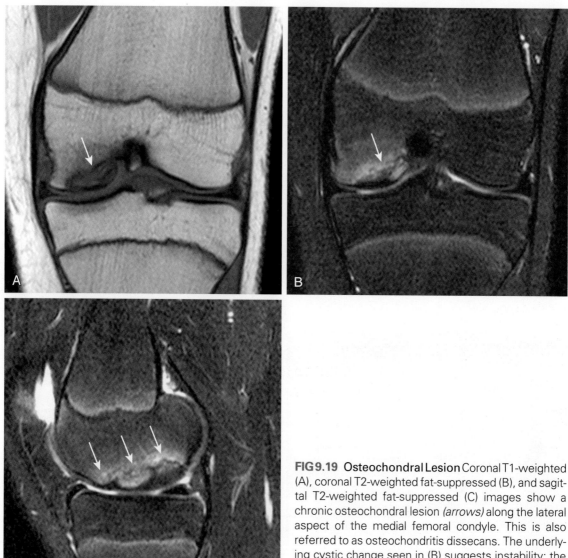

FIG 9.19 Osteochondral Lesion Coronal T1-weighted (A), coronal T2-weighted fat-suppressed (B), and sagittal T2-weighted fat-suppressed (C) images show a chronic osteochondral lesion *(arrows)* along the lateral aspect of the medial femoral condyle. This is also referred to as osteochondritis dissecans. The underlying cystic change seen in (B) suggests instability; the black signal in (A) in the subchondral bone suggests underlying necrosis.

nonspecific; however, it is often the case that the more bone marrow edema is present the more painful the lesion is. An unstable lesion is identified by one or more of the following findings on T2-weighted fat-suppressed images or STIR images: (1) linear high signal intensity surrounding the osteochondral fragment, (2) cystic change interposed between the osteochondral fragment and normal bone, or (3) overlying cartilage defect or fissuring.[1] Intra-articular gadolinium may dissect beneath the osteochondral fragment, also indicating lesion instability.

OCD was initially graded by Berndt and Harty into four stages, with the first two stages indicating lesion stability, and the last two stages signifying instability. Stage 1 demonstrates no discontinuity between the osteochondral lesion and surrounding bone, stage 2 describes a partially detached but stable osteochondral lesion, stage 3 refers to a completely detached osteochondral lesion that is not dislocated, and stage 4 represents a completely detached and displaced osteochondral

fragment. The Anderson MRI classification of OCD is more widely used; it was initially created to describe osteochondral lesions of the talus (OLT), but can also be applied to the knee and other areas. Stage I refers to the presence of bone marrow edema, stage IIa describes underlying subchondral cystic change, stage IIb refers to a partially detached osteochondral lesion with bone marrow edema, stage III lesions have fluid undermining a nondisplaced and completely detached osteochondral lesion, and stage IV describes a completely detached and displaced osteochondral fragment (Fig. 9.20). One criticism of this classification is that bone marrow edema may be present at any stage and appears to be a nonspecific finding.[3]

A healed osteochondral lesion will not demonstrate fluid bright signal between the osteochondral fragment and the host bone. Normal bone marrow fat signal will return to the osteochondral fragment once it heals. The overlying articular cartilage may be intact, without contour irregularities or may exhibit degeneration, thinning, or fraying.

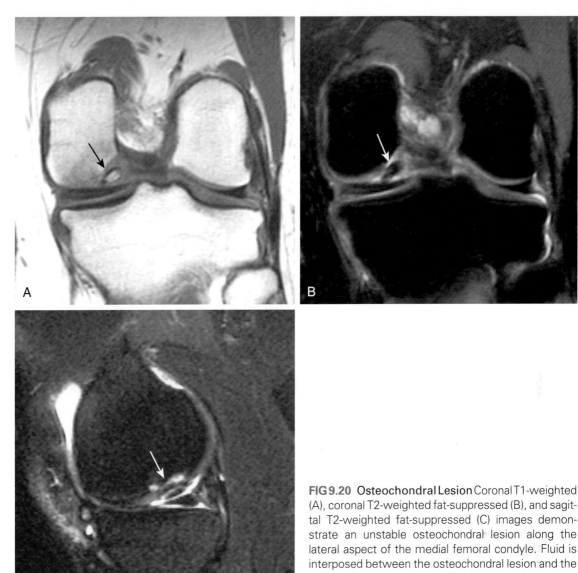

FIG 9.20 Osteochondral Lesion Coronal T1-weighted (A), coronal T2-weighted fat-suppressed (B), and sagittal T2-weighted fat-suppressed (C) images demonstrate an unstable osteochondral lesion along the lateral aspect of the medial femoral condyle. Fluid is interposed between the osteochondral lesion and the normal femoral condyle. The fragment is partially detached. This corresponds to Anderson stage IV.

RECENT ADVANCES IN MAGNETIC RESONANCE IMAGING OF CARTILAGE

Current MR imaging of articular cartilage uses 2D multislice acquisitions with small gaps between slices. Three-dimensional imaging, typically spoiled GRE with fat suppression, allows for volumetric image acquisition, producing high contrast between signal of cartilage and adjacent joint fluid. Three-dimensional spoiled gradient recalled (SPGR) sequence is the standard for evaluating cartilage volume and thickness, but is limited in evaluating internal cartilage abnormalities (eg, degeneration, delamination) and other joint pathology.

Driven equilibrium Fourier transform (DEFT) imaging uses a 90-degree pulse to return magnetization to the *z*-axis, and increases signal from tissues with long T1 relaxation time. This results in high-signal synovial fluid and improved contrast between cartilage and fluid at a short time to repetition (TR). The contrast between cartilage and synovial fluid with DEFT imaging is superior to that with SPGR, proton density fast spin echo, and T2-weighted fast spin echo images.[7]

Balanced steady-state free precession (SSFP) is also known as true FISP (true fast imaging with steady-state precession, Siemens Healthcare, Malvern, Pennsylvania), FIESTA (fast imaging employing steady-state acquisition, GE Healthcare, Buckinghamshire, UK), or BFFE (balanced fast-field echo imaging, Philips Healthcare, Andover, Massachusetts), depending on the MRI scanner manufacturer. Images are 3D volumetric acquisitions, synovial fluid is hyperintense, and the tissue contrast is sufficient for evaluation of cartilage and for imaging internal derangement.[7]

T2 relaxation time mapping is based on the knowledge that T1 and T2 relaxation times are constant for a given tissue at specific MRI field strengths. Alteration of relaxation time within a given tissue may be related to pathology or introduction of a contrast agent. T2 relaxation time mapping detects the water content within cartilage, with altered water content correlating to cartilage damage. A color or gray-scale map depicting the T2 relaxation time is created, illustrating areas of cartilage damage.[7]

Delayed gadolinium-enhanced MRI of cartilage (dGEMRIC) refers to the use of gadolinium-based contrast in the evaluation of cartilage damage. Gadolinium contrast carries a negative ionic charge, which facilitates its diffusion into cartilage and concentration in areas of depleted glycosaminoglycan (GAG), which is also negatively charged. A T1 map is created, demonstrating GAG content. Areas of decreased GAG correspond to damaged cartilage.[7]

KEY REFERENCES

1. DeSmet AA, Fisher DR, Graf BK, et al: Osteochondritis dissecans of the knee: value of mr imaging in determining lesion stability and the presence of articular cartilage defects. *AJR Am J Roentgenol* 155:549–553, 1990.

4. Fenn S, Datir A, Saifuddin A: Synovial recesses of the knee: MR imaging review of anatomical and pathological features. *Skeletal Radiol* 38:317–328, 2009.

5. Flemming DJ, Hash TW, II, Bernard SA, et al: MR imaging assessment of arthritis of the knee. *Magn Reson Imaging Clin N Am* 22:703–724, 2014.

6. Garcia-Valtuille R, Abascal F, Cerezal L, et al: Anatomy and MR imaging appearances of synovial plicae of the knee. *Radiographics* 22:775–784, 2002.

7. Gold GE, Chen CA, Koo S, et al: Recent advances in MRI of articular cartilage. *AJR Am J Roentgenol* 193:628–638, 2009.

11. Janzen DL, Peterfy CG, Forbes JR, et al: Cystic lesions around the knee joint: MR imaging findings. *AJR Am J Roentgenol* 163:155–161, 1994.

16. Lee SH, Petersilge CA, Trudell DJ, et al: Extrasynovial spaces of the cruciate ligaments: anatomy, MR imaging, and diagnostic implications. *AJR Am J Roentgenol* 166:1433–1437, 1996.

18. McCarthy CL, McNally EG: The MRI appearances of cystic lesions around the knee. *Skelet Radiol* 33:187–209, 2004.

19. Murphey MD, Rhee JH, Lewis RB, et al: Pigmented villonodular synovitis: radiologic-pathologic correlation. *Radiographics* 28:1493–1518, 2008.

20. Murphey MD, Vidal JA, Fanburg-Smith JC, et al: Imaging of synovial chondromatosis with radiologic-pathologic correlation. *Radiographics* 27:1465–1488, 2007.

21. Narvaez JA, Narvaez J, Ortega R, et al: Hypointense synovial lesions on T2-weighted images: differential diagnosis with pathologic correlation. *AJR Am J Roentgenol* 181:761–769, 2003.

22. Pope TL, Bloem HL, Beltran J, et al: *Imaging of the musculoskeletal system*, ed 1, Philadelphia, PA, 2008, Saunders Elsevier, pp 567–596, 665–689.

26. Sonin AH, Pensy RA, Mulligan ME, et al: Grading articular cartilage of the knee using fast spin-echo proton density weighted MR imaging without fat suppression. *AJR Am J Roentgenol* 179:1159–1166, 2002.

27. Verstraete KL, Almqvist F, Verdonk P, et al: Magnetic resonance imaging of cartilage and cartilage repair. *Clin Radiol* 59:674–689, 2004.

28. Vilanova JC, Barcelo J, Villalon M, et al: MR imaging of lipoma arborescens and the associated lesions. *Skeletal Radiol* 32:504–509, 2003.

The references for this chapter can also be found on www.expertconsult.com.

10

Lateral Supporting Structures: Posterolateral Corner Structures and Iliotibial Band

Eric Y. Chang, Christine B. Chung

INTRODUCTION

The lateral supporting structures, including the posterolateral corner and iliotibial band, are important for knee stability and injuries to these structures are more common than historically recognized. Using magnetic resonance imaging (MRI) exams in patients presenting with acute knee trauma, authors have recently found that injuries to the posterolateral corner structures occur in up to 21% of cases[40] and injuries to the iliotibial band occur in up to 58% of cases.[38] This is in contrast to previously reported figures as low as 6% for injury to the posterolateral corner structures[42] and as low as 0% for iliotibial band injury in the setting of posterolateral corner injury.[59] The true prevalence likely lies somewhere in between, but in general these injuries are underdiagnosed.

Isolated injuries to the posterolateral corner are rare, typically occurring after an impact is directed at the anteromedial knee during extension,[8] although posterolateral twisting[12] or a varus force in flexion[9] can also be mechanisms. Rather, the overwhelming majority of posterolateral corner and iliotibial band injuries involve concurrent injuries to other ligaments, most commonly the anterior cruciate ligament.[34,38] Cruciate ligament injuries may dominate the clinical picture and, when deficiency of the lateral supporting structures is overlooked or mistreated, persistent knee instability can lead to cruciate ligament graft failure and poor patient outcomes.[45] The appropriate diagnosis and treatment of injuries to the lateral supporting structures has historically been challenging, because of a combination of poorly understood anatomy, limitations in noninvasive diagnostic techniques, and nonanatomic reconstructive procedures.[29]

In more recent years, improvements to our understanding of anatomy and the use of biomechanically validated anatomic reconstructive techniques have led to improved patient outcomes.[29,33] Furthermore, advances in imaging techniques have increased diagnostic accuracy.[35,36] Although ultrasound can also be used,[11] MRI has been and remains the standard imaging modality for comprehensive evaluation of the lateral supporting structures. This chapter reviews the MRI examination of the anatomy and diagnosis of abnormalities to the lateral supporting structures, focusing on acute injuries to these structures.

GENERAL ANATOMIC CONSIDERATIONS

Traditionally, a layered approach has been used to describe the soft tissue supporting structures about the knee, including those of the posterolateral corner.[50] While this approach has historic significance and can be helpful during hands-on cadaveric dissections, the most common method of learning and understanding the anatomy of the lateral and posterolateral knee is to name individual anatomic structures.

The major source of confusion regarding the lateral knee structures is nomenclature, and the naming of individual structures differs among authors. LaPrade reviewed over 250 years of literature and systematically outlined the historical confusion regarding the posterolateral corner structures.[26] After highlighting the controversy around the term *arcuate ligament*, it was recommended that this term be dropped. In short, previous authors who did not recognize the *popliteofibular ligament* usually called it the *arcuate ligament*, including Seebacher et al.,[50] whose article is one of the most highly cited of all time with regard to detailing the posterolateral corner structures. A subsequent publication from authors from the same institution later recognized the *popliteofibular ligament* and redefined the *arcuate ligament*,[39] but we now know that their description represents the *capsular arm* of the short head of the biceps femoris.[26] Others have referred to the *fabellofibular ligament* as the *arcuate ligament*.[26] LaPrade defines the *arcuate ligament* as being comprised having two limbs: a medial limb, composed of the oblique popliteal ligament, and a lateral limb, composed of the many structures that course from the posteromedial aspect of the fibular styloid to the posterolateral capsule, including the *popliteofibular ligament*, *fabellofibular ligament*, and capsular arm of the short head of the biceps femoris.[25,57] Recently other authors have used the same term to describe the functional unit composed of the *popliteofibular ligament*, *fabellofibular ligament*, *popliteomeniscal fascicles*, *anterolateral ligament*, and capsular arm of the short head of the biceps femoris.[58] It is generally agreed that the arcuate ligament is not a single, distinct ligament but rather several structures that form an arched appearance.[25,57] Therefore a strong argument can be made to describe the important individual components rather than continue using the confusing term *arcuate ligament*, which has nearly as many definitions than there are structures in the posterolateral corner.

Rediscovery, renaming, and clarification of ligamentous structures persists to this day, most recently with the highly publicized *anterolateral ligament*.[7,22,47] The need for standardization of terminology is imperative for communication. Unfortunately, despite the long history of conflicting nomenclature and numerous calls for standardization,[25] no universally accepted set of terms has emerged. This chapter uses the terminology proposed by LaPrade,[25] which is based on consistent anatomic attachments and relationships, to readily identified anatomic structures, such as the inferior lateral genicular artery and popliteus.

GENERAL IMAGING CONSIDERATIONS

It is emphasized that the need for surgery is determined based on a clinical exam. However, imaging assessment can play an important role in acute and chronic injuries. In the acutely injured knee, a complete physical examination may be difficult and MRI is particularly helpful. Similar to a complete physical exam, complete imaging assessment of the injured knee involves evaluation of the lateral supporting structures. If edema or any post-traumatic abnormality is detected in the posterolateral corner, careful analysis of all supporting structures is necessary because of the high frequency of associated injuries.

Visualization of the posterolateral corner structures can be dependent on the MRI protocol. Conventional MRI protocols are based on two-dimensional (2D) sequences, typically in the axial, coronal, and sagittal oblique (prescribed parallel to the lateral border of the lateral femoral condyle or anterior cruciate ligament) imaging planes.[44] Conventional sequences provide high in-plane resolution but typically use relatively thick 4-mm slices, which may suboptimally evaluate many of the posterolateral knee structures.[24] Even with highly optimized sequences using 2-mm slice thickness,[28] the through-plane resolution is at least 4 to 6 times the in-plane resolution. This is well suited for structures that are large or course within or orthogonal to the imaging plane. However, structures that are small or have an oblique course relative to the plane of imaging tend to be less consistently identified on standard 2D imaging, such as the fabellofibular ligament.

The 2D coronal oblique imaging plane has been reported to improve visualization of the fabellofibular and popliteofibular ligaments[62]; however, it is clear that three-dimensional (3D) sequences will ultimately provide the best assessment. Rajeswaran et al. used a 0.8-mm isotropic 3D water excitation double-echo steady-state (WE-DESS) sequence acquired in 2 minutes on a 1.5T system and reported visualization of the popliteofibular ligament in 91% of cases compared with 71% using the 2D coronal-oblique plane. Imaging technology continues to improve, most recently with 3D variable flip angle fast-spin echo (FSE) sequences such as SPACE (Siemens, Erlangen, Germany), CUBE (GE Medical Systems, Milwaukee, WI), and VISTA (Philips, Eindhoven, Netherlands), which can provide improved contrast compared with gradient echo–based 3D sequences. Many centers have incorporated 3D-FSE sequences into their routine protocols using isotropic voxel sizes less than 0.6 mm. However, studies comparing the different 3D sequences and use of different imaging parameters for the assessment of the lateral supporting structures have not yet been performed to our knowledge. As part of the 3T knee protocol at our institution, we use a non–fat-suppressed, intermediate-weighted 3D-FSE sequence and routinely, but not invariably, visualize most of the structures described in this chapter using standard or reconstructed oblique planes (Fig. 10.1).

For accurate identification of the posterolateral corner structures, a thorough understanding of the osseous and soft tissue anatomy is imperative. Familiarity with the typical cross-sectional appearance of osseous contours and the soft tissue attachment sites aids in the recognition of structures on individual images. The styloid process projects upward from the posterior portion of the fibular head at approximately the middle third and is a particularly important landmark (Fig. 10.2). For instance, the expected attachment of the popliteofibular ligament is at, and just medial to, the superior tip of the styloid process.

Although signal abnormality is a hallmark of pathology, not all increases in signal are pathologic or indicative of a tear. Choi et al. found that intrasubstance signal alteration and thickening is frequently present in the fibular collateral ligament and popliteus tendon in patients with minor internal derangements in otherwise stable knees.[4] However, structural discontinuity is indicative of a tear. Although failure of ligaments and tendons can occur at any location, including within their substance, at the enthesis (soft tissue–bone attachment), or at bone in the form of an osseous avulsion, there are more typical patterns of failure for each of the lateral supporting structures. The location of failure is important because it has implications for treatment, particularly for surgical candidates. For instance, midsubstance injuries are not typically amenable to primary repair, but osseous avulsions are. Soft tissue avulsions of the structures that attach to the proximal fibula or tibia may be repaired back to their attachment sites, but femoral soft tissue avulsions tend to be constructed.[27,43] In the following section, anatomic considerations and imaging features of individual components of the lateral supporting structures are further discussed.

Fibular Collateral Ligament

The fibular collateral ligament (FCL), also known as the *lateral collateral ligament*, is one of the most important lateral supporting structures for preventing varus instability. The FCL originates from the femur proximal and posterior to the lateral epicondyle, extends posteroinferiorly, and attaches to the lateral aspect of the fibular head, mostly in a small bony depression (see Figs. 10.1 and 10.2).[32,52]

Using conventional 2D MRI, the FCL is best evaluated in axial and coronal imaging planes.[28] Because of its oblique course, it is not typically visualized in a single imaging plane, and when it can easily be seen on a single coronal image, this may be because of anterior tibial translation.[20] As mentioned previously, thickening and increased intrasubstance signal of the proximal portion of the FCL can be a frequent finding in patients with minor internal derangements but otherwise stable knees.[4]

The FCL most typically fails at its midsubstance, but other failure sites can occur.[14,39,43,48] When an osseous avulsion is present that involves the FCL, portions of the biceps femoris may also be attached to the displaced fragment.[21] In these cases the osseous fragment involving the fibular head is larger than those involve only the styloid process and may be more proximally retracted because of muscle contraction. Osseous avulsions of the fibular head involving the FCL have been termed the *arcuate sign* by some authors.[21] However, other authors have used the same term to refer to styloid process fractures involving the popliteofibular and fabellofibular ligaments.[18] Use of the term *arcuate sign* is therefore ambiguous, reinforcing the concept that the term *arcuate* should be dropped in favor of less confusing and more accurate descriptions.

Popliteus Musculotendinous Complex

In addition to the FCL, the components of the popliteus musculotendinous complex are the most important structures for

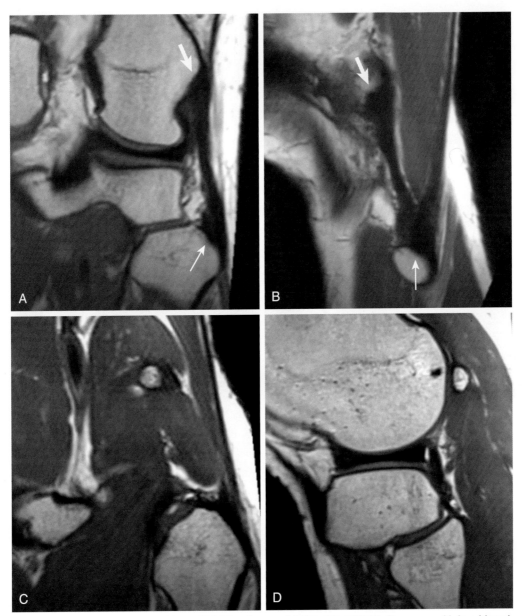

FIG 10.1 Left Knee of a 35-Year-Old Man Imaged With 3D SPACE Sequence Using Voxel Dimensions of 0.47 × 0.47 × 0.58 mm³ (A and B) The fibular collateral ligament is well visualized on reconstructed oblique coronal and sagittal images, coursing from the femoral attachment *(thick arrows)* to a small bony depression at the lateral aspect of the fibular head *(thin arrows)*. (C and D) Although the patient has a large ossified fabella and the capsular arm of the short head of the biceps tendon could be identified (not shown), a discrete fabellofibular ligament was not seen on imaging.

posterolateral knee stability.[25] The popliteus muscle is extra-articular and arises from the popliteal fossa at the posteromedial aspect of the tibia. The myotendinous junction begins at the lateral one-third of the popliteal fossa and the tendon becomes intra-articular as it courses anterolaterally around the posterior aspect of the lateral femoral condyle.[32] The tendon attaches to the femur at the proximal half and anterior fifth of the popliteal sulcus, in a location anterior and inferior to the FCL.[32]

Because of its helicoid course, the popliteus musculotendinous complex should be evaluated using all three imaging planes through its entire course. The popliteus tendon near the

femoral insertion is typically evaluated with axial and coronal images.[19,28] Similar to the FCL, thickening and increased intra-substance signal of the proximal portion of the popliteus tendon can frequently be seen in stable knees and should not be over-interpreted (Fig. 10.3).[4] There are multiple causes of increased intratendinous signal intensity, including artifacts such as the magic angle effect, which is most evident as the long axis of anisotropic collagenous structures approaches 55 degrees relative to the main magnetic field[23] or volume averaging with adjacent fluid or synovial tissue. Other causes include the variable presence of intratendinous fibrocartilage as it wraps around the femur, or tendon degeneration.[1] Normal anatomy such as

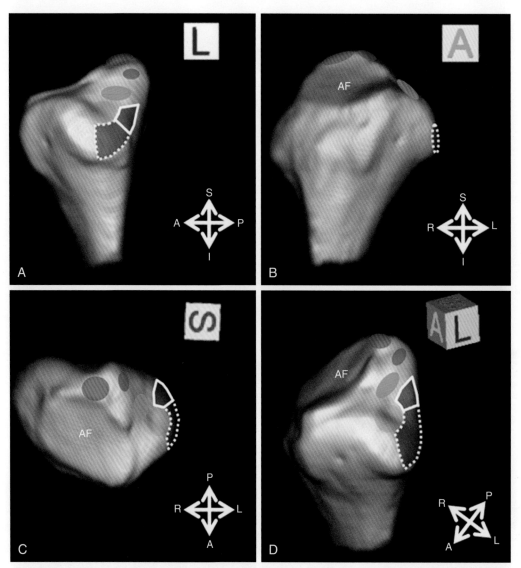

FIG 10.2 Approximate footprint locations on the left proximal fibula of a 35-year-old man, viewed from the left lateral (A), anterior (B), superior (C), and anterior-superior-lateral (D) projections. The articular facet (AF) projects upward, forward and medially. The fibular collateral ligament *(green oval)* inserts in a small bony depression of the fibular head. The popliteofibular ligament *(red oval)* inserts at the medial aspect and tip of the fibular styloid. The long head of the biceps femoris tendon has direct *(white outline)* and anterior *(dashed outline)* arms that insert at the posterolateral edge of the fibular head. The short head of the biceps femoris *(pink oval)* has a direct arm that inserts onto the fibular head lateral to the styloid. The fabellofibular ligament *(blue oval)*, which is the distal edge of the capsular arm of the short head of the biceps, inserts just lateral to the tip of the fibular styloid. 3D orientation cubes and orientation axes are present on the right side of each image, indicating left (L), right (R), anterior (A), posterior (P), and superior (S) sides.

the subpopliteal recess,[13] which is an inferior extension of the joint cavity beneath the popliteal hiatus, and the appearance of multiple popliteal intramuscular tendon slips should not be misinterpreted as pathologic. Tears of the popliteus tend to involve the muscle belly and musculotendinous junction, although osseous or tendinous avulsions from the femur can occur (Fig. 10.4).[19]

Popliteofibular Ligament

The popliteofibular ligament (PFL) originates from the myotendinous junction of the popliteus and attaches to the fibular styloid at the tip and along the medial aspect, coursing at an angle of approximately 53 degrees (range 50 to 68 degrees) relative to the main magnetic field.[32] The PFL has two divisions (anterior and posterior), but the posterior division is more functionally important because it is more than twice as wide.[32] The average combined width of the PFL measures 9.6 mm at the myotendinous origin and 8.4 mm at the fibular styloid.[32] The PFL is the only distinct ligamentous structure that courses deep to the inferior lateral genicular artery, which is an important landmark when comparing anatomic studies using different terminology.[25,26]

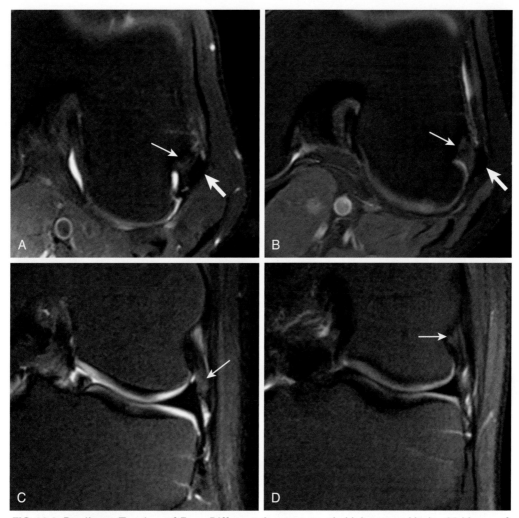

FIG 10.3 Popliteus Tendon of Four Different Asymptomatic Volunteers Under 30 Years of Age Without History of Knee Injuries (A and B) Axial fluid-sensitive images show the tendon insertion at the popliteal sulcus *(thin arrows)*. Note the tendon is higher in signal intensity than the adjacent fibular collateral ligament *(thick arrows)*. (C and D) Coronal fluid-sensitive images show focal regions of high signal intensity inside the tendons *(thin arrows)*.

Using conventional 2D images, the PFL can be evaluated in all three imaging planes. It is typically visualized in the sagittal oblique imaging plane because it extends from the popliteus toward the fibular styloid.[19,40,46] Less frequently a single coronal image can show the PFL, and when more prominent, it may be followed along its course on axial images. Because of obliquity, it is not surprising that a coronal oblique imaging plane can be used to improve visualization,[62] and with 3D-FSE sequences, this ligament can routinely be visualized in a single reformatted plane (Fig. 10.5).

Tears of the popliteofibular ligament most commonly occur through the midsubstance (Fig. 10.6).[39] When an osseous avulsion is present that involves the popliteofibular ligament, portions of the fabellofibular ligament may also be attached to the small bone fragment because of their close attachments to the styloid process. Huang et al. reported on 13 cases of styloid process avulsions and noted that the bony fragment measured 8 to 10 mm in length, 2 to 5 mm in width, with mean displacement of 5 mm (Fig. 10.7).[18] All of their cases had injuries to the posterior cruciate ligament and no case had a tear of the anterior cruciate ligament. As described previously, although the term *arcuate sign* has been used to describe these styloid process avulsion fractures, the same term has been used to describe larger fractures of the fibular head. Therefore the term should be dropped and less confusing and more accurate descriptions should be used instead.

Popliteomeniscal Fascicles

The popliteomeniscal fascicles attach the posterior horn of the lateral meniscus to the popliteus. There are three popliteomeniscal fascicles including the anteroinferior, posterosuperior, and posteroinferior fascicles.[57] In most cases the anteroinferior popliteomeniscal fascicle forms a conjoined fibular attachment with the popliteofibular ligament.[57] The posteroinferior popliteomeniscal fascicle courses in a posteromedial direction from the posterior horn of the lateral meniscus and attaches to the posterior joint capsule. This portion of the joint capsule connects the popliteus, lateral meniscus, and posterior cruciate ligament and has been referred to as the *proximal popliteal capsular expansion*[25] or the *medial aponeurotic expansion* of the

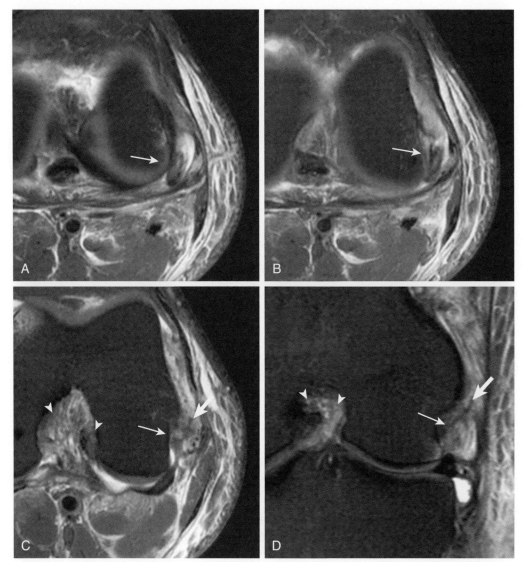

FIG 10.4 Left Knee of a 25-Year-Old Man With Multiligamentous Injury After a Motorcycle Accident (A to C) Axial fluid-sensitive images show an avulsion of the popliteus tendon from the femur *(thin arrows)* and rupture of the fibular collateral ligament *(thick arrow)*. Bi-cruciate ligament injury is evident within the intercondylar notch *(arrowheads)*. (D) Coronal fluid-sensitive image confirms the tendon avulsion from the popliteal sulcus *(thin arrow)* and fibular collateral ligament tear *(thick arrow)*.

popliteus.[46,57] The popliteomeniscal fascicles can be well visualized on conventional 2D sagittal oblique images (Fig. 10.8).[46] However, in healthy knees, it is estimated that a discrete low-signal-intensity band is absent in the expected region of the anteroinferior and posterosuperior popliteomeniscal fascicles in up to 30% and 50% of cases, respectively.[49] Peduto et al. found that the posteroinferior popliteomeniscal fascicle could not be identified in 60% of their cadavers.[57] Tears of the popliteomeniscal fascicles can lead to hypermobile meniscus syndrome, where the posterior horn of the lateral meniscus becomes entrapped during knee flexion; these tears can be repaired (Fig. 10.9).[27,31]

Anterolateral Ligament

Much has been learned about the anterolateral ligament in recent years. The anterolateral ligament is a true ligament that appears as a thickening of the lateral joint capsule.[7,15] It comes under tension during internal rotation at 30 degrees of knee flexion.[22] The femoral origin of the anterolateral ligament is posterior and proximal to the FCL attachment, although this has been debated in the literature.[22] A source of confusion in previous studies may be the misinterpretation of the fine fascial expansion that extends anteriorly and distally from the anterolateral ligament over the fibular collateral ligament attachment and lateral epicondyle.[22] As the ligament courses anterolateral from its origin, there are thick attachments to the body of the lateral meniscus. These can be divided into meniscofemoral and meniscotibial portions of the anterolateral ligament.[7] At the level of the body of the lateral meniscus, the anterolateral ligament courses superficial to the inferior lateral genicular vessels. The tibial attachment is approximately midway between the center of Gerdy's tubercle and the anterior margin of the fibular head.[22]

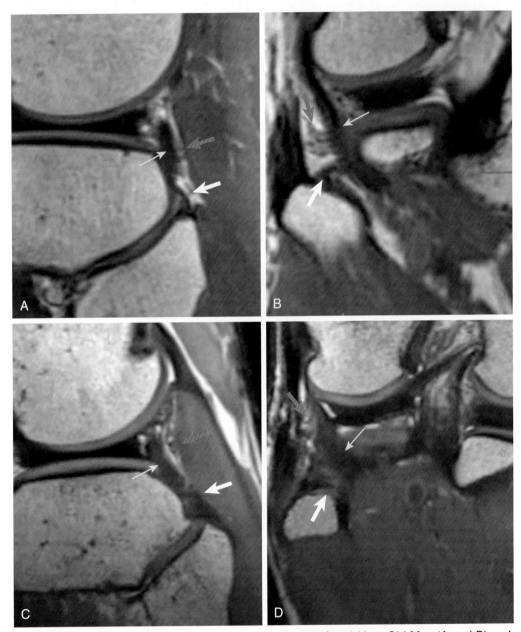

FIG 10.5 **Popliteofibular Ligaments in the Right Knees of a 43-Year-Old Man (A and B) and a 31-Year-Old Man (C and D) on 3D SPACE Images** (A and B) Sagittal and reformatted coronal oblique planes demonstrate a lax but normal popliteofibular ligament *(white arrows)*. (C and D) Sagittal and reformatted coronal oblique planes show a markedly thick, but intact popliteofibular ligament that is increased in signal intensity, consistent with degeneration. On all images, the popliteus tendon *(yellow arrows)* and the inferior lateral genicular vessels *(orange arrows)* are marked.

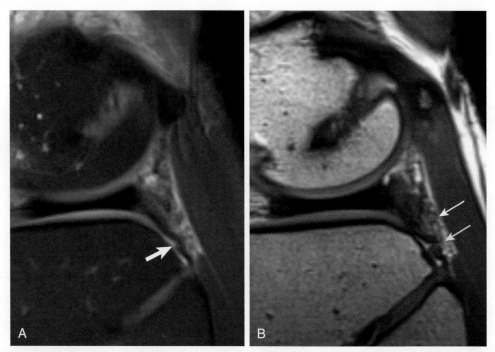

FIG 10.6 **A 43-Year-Old Man With a Tear of the Popliteofibular Ligament** (A) Conventional sagittal fluid-sensitive image shows the popliteofibular ligament *(thick white arrow)*, which appears irregular but intact. (B) Sagittal isotropic 3D SPACE images show a complete tear of the popliteofibular ligament *(yellow arrow)*. Inferior lateral genicular vessels *(thin white arrows)* are well seen on SPACE images but are poorly delineated on conventional image.

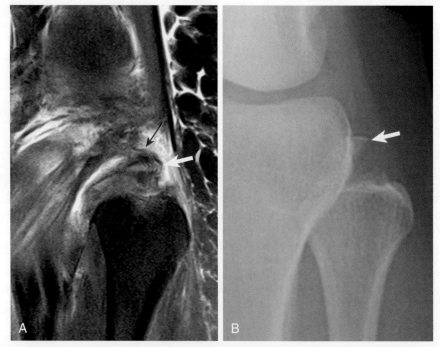

FIG 10.7 **A 54-Year-Old Woman With Bony Fibular Styloid Avulsion** (A) Coronal fluid-sensitive image shows a 4 × 8 mm² osseous avulsion *(white arrow)* at the fibular attachment of the popliteofibular ligament *(red arrow)* with 5 mm of retraction. (B) Radiograph confirms the small bony avulsion from the fibular styloid.

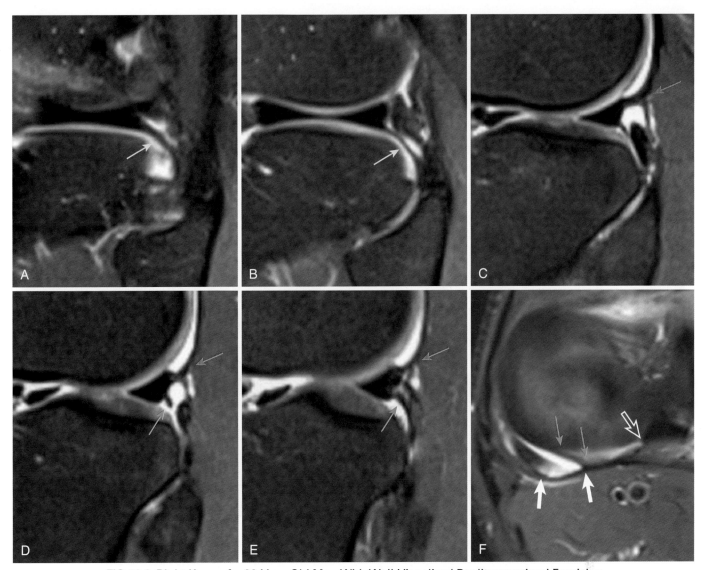

FIG 10.8 Right Knee of a 32-Year-Old Man With Well-Visualized Popliteomeniscal Fascicles
(A to E) Sagittal oblique fluid-sensitive images from lateral (A) to medial (E) show the anteroinferior *(yellow arrows)*, posterosuperior *(orange arrows)*, and posteroinferior *(blue arrows)* popliteomeniscal fascicles. (F) Axial fluid-sensitive image shows the posteroinferior popliteomeniscal fascicle *(blue arrows)* as it attaches to the medial aponeurotic expansion of the popliteus *(thick white arrows)*. The inferomedial extension of the medial aponeurosis attaches to the posterior cruciate ligament *(open arrow)*.

Using conventional 2D images, the anterolateral ligament can typically be visualized on coronal and axial images.[28] Reported visualization of the anterolateral ligament on MRI varies greatly, ranging from 51% to 100%.[16,28,47,53] Coronal images may show the entire course of the anterolateral ligament or may visualize only a portion of it because of its oblique course. When the anterolateral ligament appears discontinuous on coronal images, cross-referencing to the axial images and attention to the osseous landmarks is important to avoid misinterpreting an out-of-plane ligament as a tear (Fig. 10.10A). With oblique reformatted images obtained from a 3D dataset, the entire course of the anterolateral ligament can typically be readily visualized on a single image (see Fig. 10.10B).

Tears of the anterolateral ligament can occur within the midsubstance, as soft tissue avulsions from either femoral (see Fig. 10.10D and E) or tibial attachments, or at the tibia in the form of a bone avulsion.[5,9,22] Anterolateral ligament tears are strongly associated with anterior cruciate ligament tears.[5] Osseous avulsions of the anterolateral ligament are known as *Segond fractures.* Some authors believe these fractures are purely because of the anterolateral ligament,[6,22] while others have found that both the anterolateral ligament and posterior fibers of the iliotibial band insert onto this fragment.[3,10]

Biceps Femoris Complex

The biceps femoris is composed of long and short heads that form a common biceps tendon before dividing into numerous distinct components. The long head originates together with the semitendinosus muscle from the ischial tuberosity and the distal myotendinous junction is approximately 5 cm above the knee joint line.[60] Approximately 1 cm proximal to the fibula, the tendon divides into direct and anterior arms.[25] The direct

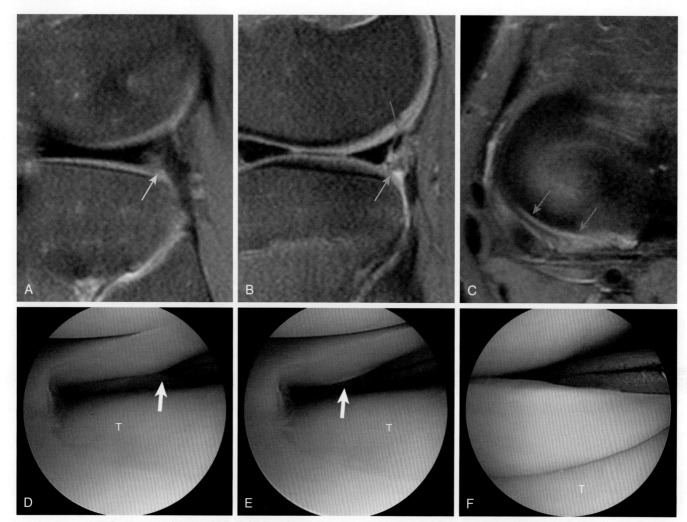

FIG 10.9 A 14-Year-Old Girl After Right Knee Injury (A and B) Sagittal fluid-sensitive images show a tear of the anteroinferior *(yellow arrow)*, posterosuperior *(orange arrow)* and posteroinferior *(blue arrow)* popliteomeniscal fascicles. (C) Axial fluid-sensitive image shows the course of the posterosuperior popliteomeniscal fascicle tear *(orange arrows)*. (D to F) Arthroscopic images with scope in the anterolateral portal shows the probe tip extending through the torn popliteomeniscal fascicles *(white arrows)*. The posterior horn of the lateral meniscus was easily translated beyond the midpoint of the tibial articular surface (T), which is diagnostic of a hypermobile lateral meniscus.

arm inserts on the posterolateral edge of the fibular head and the anterior arm inserts at the lateral edge of the fibular head, lateral to the fibular collateral ligament.[56] A small synovial-lined bursa is consistently located between the anterior arm and fibular collateral ligament.[30] In addition to the two main tendinous components of the long head of the biceps femoris, three fascial components are present, including the *lateral aponeurosis, reflected arm,* and *anterior aponeurosis.*[56] The lateral aponeurosis arises from the anterior edge of the anterior arm and courses to the posterolateral aspect of the FCL (Fig. 10.11C to F, dashed yellow arrows). The reflected arm originates just proximal to the fibular head and courses anterior to insert onto the iliotibial band (see Fig. 10.11E, dashed red arrow). The anterior aponeurosis is visible after the anterior arm crosses the FCL and continues over the anterior compartment of the leg (see Fig. 10.11G and H, dashed blue arrows).

The short head originates medial to the linea aspera of the distal femur and the distal myotendinous junction is located at

approximately the knee joint line.[60] The short head has a *proximal muscular attachment* to the anteromedial aspect of the long head tendon (see Fig. 10.11A, green arrow), but the first main attachment that courses toward the posterolateral structures is the *capsular arm* (see Fig. 10.11A to D, red arrows). The capsular arm is a main component of the biceps femoris complex and has a broad attachment onto several structures, including the posterolateral joint capsule, fabella or fabella analogue, and lateral gastrocnemius.[25] The distal edge of the capsular arm is the *fabellofibular ligament,* which attaches just lateral to the tip of the fibular styloid.[25,57] Distal to the capsular arm is a fascial confluence that connects the short head of the biceps femoris to the iliotibial tract, termed the *biceps-capsulo-osseous iliotibial tract confluens* (see Fig. 10.11E to G, white arrows).[56] Similar to the long head, the short head also has a *lateral aponeurosis,* which courses anteriorly and attaches to the posteromedial aspect of the FCL (see Fig. 10.11C and D, yellow arrows). Just above the fibula, the short head divides into a direct arm, which

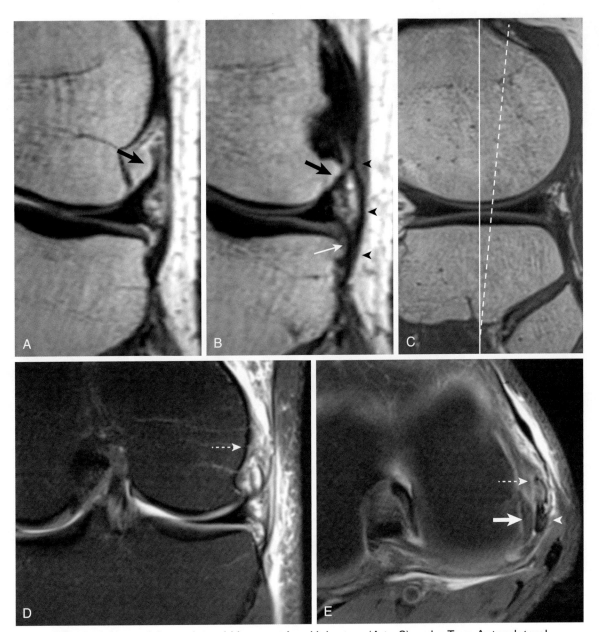

FIG 10.10 Normal Anterolateral Ligament in a Volunteer (A to C) and a Torn Anterolateral Ligament in a 43-Year-Old (D and E) (A) Coronal 3D SPACE image shows apparent discontinuity of the meniscofemoral portion because of oblique course relative to imaging plane *(thick black arrow)*. (B) Coronal oblique reformatted image shows the entire course of the intact anterolateral ligament *(black arrowheads)*, including the meniscofemoral *(thick black arrow)* and meniscotibial portions *(white arrow)*. (C) Sagittal image shows the coronal *(solid line)* and coronal oblique *(dashed line)* planes used for A and B, respectively. (D) Coronal fluid-sensitive image shows a complete tear of proximal anterolateral ligament *(dashed arrow)*. (E) Axial fluid-sensitive image confirms the complete tear *(dashed arrow)* and shows a partial tear of the more posterior fibular collateral ligament *(white arrowhead)*. The popliteus tendon was intact *(thick white arrow)*.

inserts on the fibular head lateral to the styloid,[56] and an anterior arm, which inserts onto the tibia, posteroinferior to the anterolateral ligament.[22]

On MRI, the main tendinous arms (direct and anterior) of the long and short heads of the biceps femoris complex are usually visualized, although the smaller components may not be routinely seen.[28] However, when carefully evaluated, many of the previously described anatomic structures are typically visible, particularly when abnormal, either in the setting of chronic repetitive stress, where the components maybe thickened (see Fig. 10.11), or after acute injury where edema may improve contrast (Fig. 10.12). The fabellofibular ligament, although reported to always be present on anatomic dissections,[25] may be difficult to identify with MRI studies using 2D sequences with visibility ranging from 0% to 48%.[2] An important landmark for identification of the fabellofibular ligament

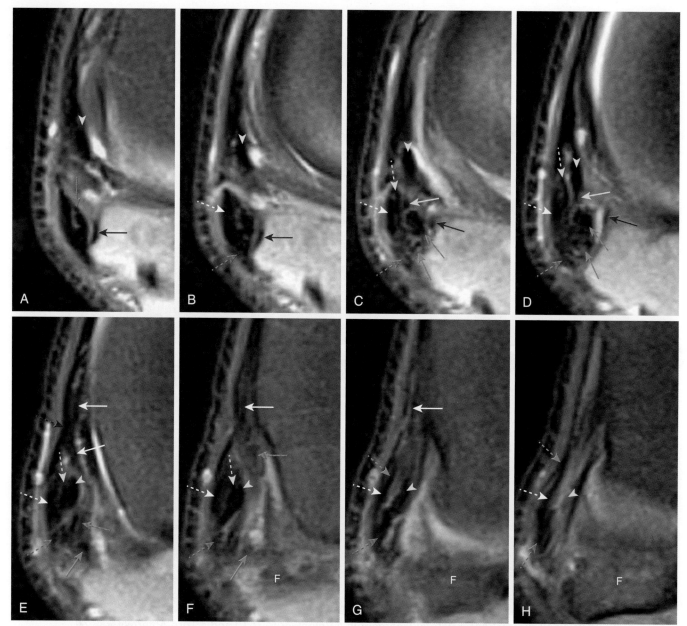

FIG 10.11 Right knee of a 31-year-old man obtained as a comparison after acute injury to his left knee, showing prominent distal biceps femoris components because of chronic stress since there was no history of discrete traumatic injury to this knee. (A to H) Axial fluid-sensitive images from superior to inferior, beginning at the first slice where the common biceps tendon divides. The fibular collateral ligament, which is increased in signal at its fibular insertion, is marked on all images with a yellow arrowhead, whereas all components of the long head are in dashed arrows and the short head in solid arrows. The long head has two main tendinous components, the anterior *(dashed white arrows)* and the direct *(dashed orange arrows)* arms. The long head has a *lateral aponeurosis (dashed yellow arrows)* that arises from the anterior edge of the anterior arm and courses to the posterolateral aspect of the fibular collateral ligament, a *reflected arm (dashed red arrow)* that courses anterior and inserts onto the posterior aspect of iliotibial band, and an *anterior aponeurosis (dashed blue arrows)* that continues over the anterior leg. The short head has a *proximal muscular attachment* to the long head *(green arrow)*, a *capsular arm (red arrows)* that attaches to the posterolateral joint capsule, a *biceps-capsulo-osseous iliotibial tract confluence (white arrows)* that courses medial to the superficial layer of the iliotibial band and attaches onto tibia, and a *lateral aponeurosis (yellow arrows)* that attaches to the posteromedial aspect of the FCL. The tendinous direct *(blue arrows)* and anterior *(pink arrows)* arms of the short head attach to the fibula and tibia, respectively, and are increased in signal and irregular in this patient, consistent with degeneration.

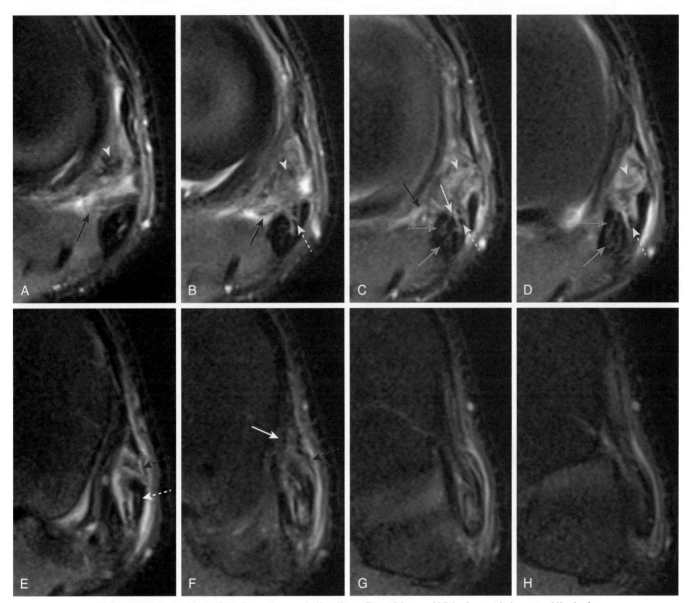

FIG 10.12 A 31-Year-Old Experienced Jiu-Jitsu Practitioner With Acute Injury to His Left Knee (Same Patient as in Fig. 10.10) (A to H) Axial fluid-sensitive images from superior to inferior. There is a complete tear of the fibular collateral ligament *(yellow arrowheads)* along with the *lateral aponeurosis* of the long *(dashed yellow arrows)* and short heads *(yellow arrows)* of the biceps femoris. The short head has low-grade tearing of the direct *(blue arrows)* and anterior *(pink arrows)* arms and tearing of the *capsular arm (red arrows)*. The *reflected arm (dashed red arrow)* of the long head is torn. The *biceps-capsulo-osseous iliotibial tract confluence (white arrow)* of the short head is thick, but intact.

is the inferior lateral genicular artery, which is situated superficial to the popliteofibular ligament but deep to the fabellofibular ligament.[25] Multiple authors have reported that the size and thickness of the fabellofibular ligament is related to the presence of an ossified fabella.[25] The presence of an ossified fabella may be related to ethnicity; for instance, cadaveric studies in a Brazilian sample[51] showed 3% with ossified fabellae whereas a Chinese sample[63] showed ossified fabellae in 55% of cases. In cases without an ossified fabella, a cartilaginous fabella is reported to be present instead.[25] The fabellofibular ligament may be seen on coronal or coronal-oblique images; however, the variable imaging prevalence of this ligament, even with isotropic 3D sequences (see Fig. 10.1), makes it particularly difficult to confidently diagnose pathology unless torn edges are visualized that are superficial to the inferior lateral genicular artery (Fig. 10.13).

The most common site of injury of the distal biceps femoris complex is debated, with some showing the most common sites involving the capsular arm (see Fig. 10.11A to C) and biceps-capsulo-osseous iliotibial tract confluens of the short head,[56] the myotendinous junction,[37] or at the fibular enthesis as a soft tissue avulsion.[48] As mentioned previously, osseous avulsions may occur in conjunction with the fibular collateral ligament because of their close attachments. These avulsions of the fibular head may be proximally retracted because of muscle contraction (Fig. 10.14).

Iliotibial Band

The iliotibial band, or iliotibial tract, is a thickening of the deep fascia of the thigh, which is also known as the *fascia lata*. At the hip and pelvis, the iliotibial band consists of three layers (superficial, intermediate, and deep) that merge with the gluteal aponeurotic fascia and course distally along the entire lateral thigh.[17] Although the iliotibial band is often viewed as a band of fascial tissue that passes over the lateral epicondyle and attaches to Gerdy's tubercle, it is a much more complex structure with a wide periarticular insertion and interconnections to the femur, patella, and tibia.[61]

At the knee, the iliotibial band is composed of *superficial*, *deep*, and *capsulo-osseous layers*.[57,61] The main component is the superficial layer, which covers a large portion of the lateral aspect of the knee, and primarily attaches to Gerdy's tubercle (Fig. 10.15A). There is an anterior expansion of the superficial layer that courses over the anterior aspect of the patella, known as the *iliopatellar band* (also known as *arciform fibers* or the *superior oblique retinaculum*) (see Fig. 10.15B).[41] Although the iliopatellar band is functionally intimate with the iliotibial tract and plays an important role in patellofemoral tracking, some have described it as anatomically separate,[57,61] whereas others have described it as a fourth component of the iliotibial band itself.[25] The deep layer begins 5 to 6 cm proximal to the lateral epicondyle and broadly originates from the lateral intermuscular septum and lateral epicondyle (Fig. 10.16A to C).[54,57,61] The deep and superficial layers fuse distal to the lateral epicondyle of the femur.[61] The capsulo-osseous layer begins deep to the other layers as the investing fascia of the lateral gastrocnemius, short head of the biceps femoris, and plantaris, and merges with the deep layer and posterior portion of the superficial layer to insert onto the tibia just posterior and proximal to Gerdy's tubercle.[54,57,61] Derivatives from the iliotibial band, including the iliopatellar band, are important contributors to the lateral retinaculum.[41]

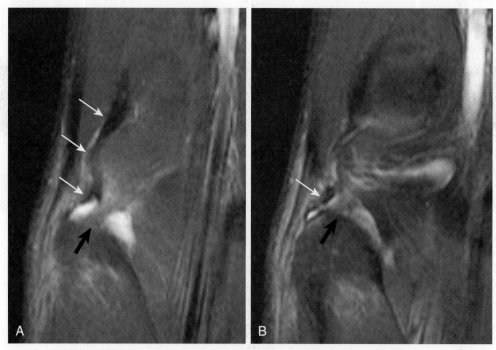

FIG 10.13 Right Knee of a 22-Year-Old Man After Soccer Injury (A and B) Coronal fluid-sensitive images show a distal soft tissue avulsion of the fabellofibular ligament *(white arrows)* with 6 mm of retraction, resulting in a wavy appearance to the ligament. The more medial popliteofibular ligament *(thick black arrows)* is increased in signal intensity, but intact, consistent with a low-grade sprain. The inferior lateral genicular vessels coursed between these two structures on other imaging planes (not shown).

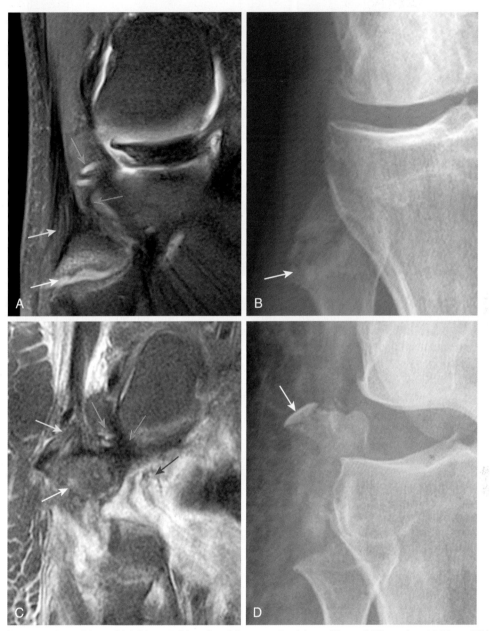

FIG 10.14 A 63-Year-Old Man 3 Months After an Accident (A and B) and a 46-Year-Old Woman 4 Days After Injury (C and D) (A) Coronal fluid-sensitive image shows a fibular head avulsion fracture *(white arrows)* with edema at the edges and fluid between fracture fragments. (B) Frontal radiograph shows the large avulsion fracture without evidence of osseous union *(white arrow)*. (C) Coronal fluid-sensitive image shows a displaced and rotated fibular head avulsion fracture *(white arrows)*. The popliteus is completely torn at the myotendinous junction *(red arrows)*. (D) Frontal radiograph shows the comminuted fracture *(white arrow)*, which is retracted to the level of the widened lateral joint space. In both patients, the distal biceps tendon *(yellow arrows)* and popliteofibular ligaments *(orange arrows)* attach to the fracture fragments. The inferior lateral genicular vessels *(blue arrows)* are located superficial to the popliteofibular ligaments.

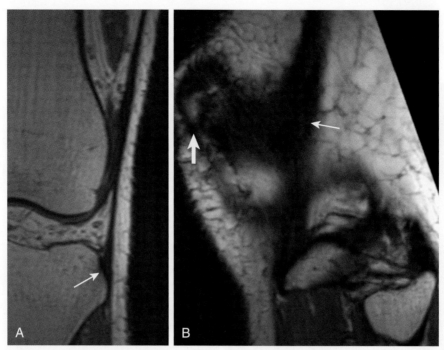

FIG 10.15 A 43-Year-Old Man With Normal Left Iliotibial Tract Imaged Using 3D SPACE Sequence (A) Coronal reformatted image shows the superficial layer of the iliotibial band as it inserts onto Gerdy's tubercle *(thin arrow)*. (B) Double-oblique reformatted image obtained parallel to the lateral retinaculum at the level of the patella shows the iliopatellar band as it courses from the iliotibial tract *(thin arrow)* toward the patella *(thick arrow)*.

Traumatic iliotibial band injuries have not been widely addressed. Mansour et al. evaluated 200 knee MRI exams in patients with acute trauma and found the iliotibial band injured in 58%, most typically characterized by edema at the superficial and deep sides of an intact iliotibial band.[38] Terry and Jones estimated that 50% of iliotibial band injuries occur in the deep layer (found in the area of the lateral intermuscular septum) (see Fig. 10.16D to G), 25% occur at the midportion of the iliotibial band at the biceps capsulo-osseous confluence, and 25% at the tibial attachment of the capsulo-osseous iliotibial tract, either with or without a bone fragment (Fig. 10.17).[55] Osseous avulsions can also occur from Gerdy's tubercle (see Fig. 10.17). In patients with grade 3 posterolateral knee injuries who went to surgery, LaPrade found that tears to the deep layer occurred in 71% (5 of 7 cases) whereas injuries to the superficial layer occurred 14% (1 of 7 cases).[28]

CONCLUSION

In summary, although there is no widely accepted nomenclature of the lateral supporting structures at this time, the terminology proposed by LaPrade and used in this chapter is based on consistent anatomic attachments and relationships to readily identified structures. Standardization of terminology is necessary to improve communication, and the terms *arcuate ligament* and *arcuate sign* should not be used because they are ambiguous and confusing. Although the need for surgery is based on clinical exam, MRI can play an important role in acute and chronic injuries. With optimized imaging protocols and a thorough understanding of anatomy, the lateral supporting structures of the knee can be assessed with exquisite detail and pathology can be readily diagnosed.

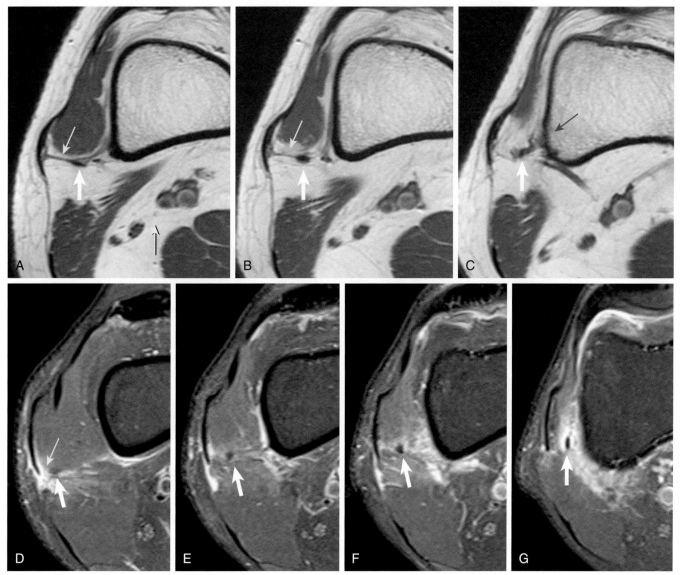

FIG 10.16 Right Iliotibial Bands in an Asymptomatic 23-Year-Old Woman (A to C) and a 40-Year-Old Man After Varus Flexion Injury While Wakeboarding (D to G) (A to C) Axial T1-weighted images show the deep layer of the iliotibial band originating from the lateral intermuscular septum *(thick white arrow)*, which attaches to the lateral supracondylar line of the femur *(red arrow)*. (D to G) Axial fluid-sensitive images show a tear of the deep fascia of the thigh and deep layer of the iliotibial band *(yellow arrow)*. Edema surrounds the lateral intermuscular septum as it courses toward the femur *(thick white arrows)*.

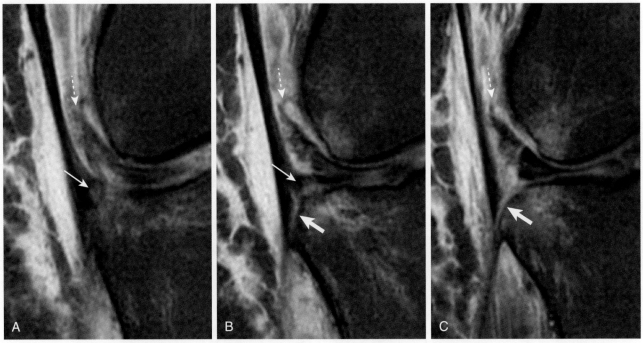

FIG 10.17 Right Knee of a 37-Year-Old Woman Who Was Hit by a Car (A to C) Coronal fluid-sensitive images show an avulsion fracture of Gerdy's tubercle from the superficial layer of the iliotibial band *(white arrows)*. There is also high-grade tearing and stripping of the iliotibial band posterior to Gerdy's tubercle, where all three contributing layers insert *(thick arrows)*. The anterolateral joint capsule and meniscofemoral portions of the anterolateral ligament are also completely torn *(dashed arrows)* with extravasation of joint fluid into the soft tissues.

KEY REFERENCES

6. Claes S, Luyckx T, Vereecke E, et al: The Segond fracture: a bony injury of the anterolateral ligament of the knee. *Arthroscopy* 30:1475–1482, 2014.

7. Claes S, Vereecke E, Maes M, et al: Anatomy of the anterolateral ligament of the knee. *J Anat* 223:321–328, 2013.

8. Covey DC: Injuries of the posterolateral corner of the knee. *J Bone Joint Surg Am* 83-A:106–118, 2001.

24. Clinical examination of posterolateral knee injuries. In LaPrade RF, editor: *Posterolateral knee injuries: anatomy, evaluation, and treatment*, New York, NY, 2006, Thieme, p xv. 238 pp.

25. Comprehensive anatomy of the structures of the posterolateral knee. In LaPrade RF, editor: *Posterolateral knee injuries: anatomy, evaluation, and treatment*, New York, NY, 2006, Thieme, p xv. 238 pp.

26. History of the nomenclature and study of the anatomy of the posterolateral knee. In LaPrade RF, editor: *Posterolateral knee injuries: anatomy, evaluation, treatment*, New York, NY, 2006, Thieme, p xv. 238 pp.

27. Treatment of posterolateral knee injuries. In LaPrade RF, editor: *Posterolateral knee injuries anatomy, evaluation, and treatment*, New York, NY, 2006, Thieme, p xv. 238 pp.

28. LaPrade RF, Gilbert TJ, Bollom TS, et al: The magnetic resonance imaging appearance of individual structures of the posterolateral knee.

A prospective study of normal knees and knees with surgically verified grade III injuries. *Am J Sports Med* 28:191–199, 2000.

32. LaPrade RF, Ly TV, Wentorf FA, et al: The posterolateral attachments of the knee: a qualitative and quantitative morphologic analysis of the fibular collateral ligament, popliteus tendon, popliteofibular ligament, and lateral gastrocnemius tendon. *Am J Sports Med* 31:854–860, 2003.

33. LaPrade RF, Moulton SG, Nitri M, et al: Clinically relevant anatomy and what anatomic reconstruction means. *Knee Surg Sports Traumatol Arthrosc* 23(10):2950–2959, 2015.

39. Maynard MJ, Deng X, Wickiewicz TL, et al: The popliteofibular ligament. Rediscovery of a key element in posterolateral stability. *Am J Sports Med* 24:311–316, 1996.

46. Peduto AJ, Nguyen A, Trudell DJ, et al: Popliteomeniscal fascicles: anatomic considerations using MR arthrography in cadavers. *AJR Am J Roentgenol* 190:442–448, 2008.

52. Song YB, Watanabe K, Hogan E, et al: The fibular collateral ligament of the knee: a detailed review. *Clin Anat* 27:789–797, 2014.

54. Terry GC, Hughston JC, Norwood LA: The anatomy of the iliopatellar band and iliotibial tract. *Am J Sports Med* 14:39–45, 1986.

57. Terry GC, LaPrade RF: The posterolateral aspect of the knee. Anatomy and surgical approach. *Am J Sports Med* 24:732–739, 1996.

The references for this chapter can also be found on www.expertconsult.com.

11

Medial Supporting Structures: Medial Collateral Ligament and Posteromedial Corner

Sherlin Lavianlivi, Sana Ali, Mohammed M. Hoque, Luis S. Beltran, Javier Beltran

INTRODUCTION

The posteromedial corner of the knee (PMC) is a significant anatomic structure that is as important as the posterolateral corner in multiligamentous injuries. Even though it is easily seen on modern high-field magnetic resonance (MR) imaging systems, it is often unnoticed and there is a lack of knowledge of its complex anatomy and function. Appropriate understanding of its structures, including knowledge about its normal appearance on MR imaging and specific biomechanical function can help in easy recognition of PMC injuries.

The posteromedial corner of the knee is between the posterior margin of the longitudinal fibers of the superficial medial collateral ligament (MCL) and the medial border of the posterior cruciate ligament (PCL). Some variations exist due to certain investigators including the posterior oblique ligament (POL) as a part of the MCL, and others referring to the posteromedial joint capsule as all structures posterior to the superficial MCL. Even though there is some controversy regarding the structures in this area, five major components have been consistently described in the literature.

The PMC plays a significant role in stabilizing the medial corner of the knee and preventing excessive anterior translation and external rotation of the medial tibial plateau with respect to the femur. Injuries to the PMC and therefore disruptions of its supporting structures can cause anteromedial rotational instability (AMRI).

Posteromedial corner injuries also usually occur simultaneously with injuries to other important knee-stabilizing structures such as the anterior cruciate ligament (ACL) and the PCL. Overlooked PMC injuries may be a cause of failure of surgical management, such as ACL and PCL graft failures and increased stress and tension on reconstructed knee ligaments. Having good knowledge and understanding of the anatomic structures of the PMC and their static and dynamic roles in supporting the knee can help detect various forms of injuries. Consequently, the ability to recognize PMC injuries is highly invaluable in determining proper diagnosis, which may alter or even require further surgical management. This chapter reviews the anatomy of the PMC, its function in supporting the medial knee, and common PMC injuries including the associated clinical symptoms and available treatment options.

ANATOMY OF THE POSTEROMEDIAL CORNER

The medial-side supporting structures of the knee can be divided into three layers: Layer I, crural fascia including the pes anserine tendons; Layer II, superficial MCL and the oblique popliteal ligament (OPL); and Layer III, the joint capsule, semimembranosus, and the deep medial collateral ligament (Figs. 11.1 and 11.2).[32] Structures between the posterior margin of the superficial MCL and the medial margin of the PCL combine to form the PMC.

The PMC is a complex anatomic region containing several structures important for the stability and proper biomechanical functioning of the knee. It is difficult to delineate the separate structures of the PMC owing in large part to anatomic variability and relatively thin capsular components. There are five main components of the PMC: the semimembranosus tendon complex, the OPL, the POL, the posteromedial joint capsule, and the posterior horn of the medial meniscus (Figs. 11.3 to 11.9).[10,20]

Semimembranosus Tendon Complex

The semimembranosus tendon is the most important dynamic stabilizer of the PMC. It originates at the posterolateral aspect of the ischial tuberosity. Distally, it divides into five anatomically distinct tendinous branches, each inserting into the posteromedial region of the knee: (1) the direct arm (principal attachment), (2) the capsular arm, (3) the extension to the OPL (OPL insertion), (4) the anterior arm (tibial or reflected arm, pars reflexa), and the (5) inferior (popliteal) arm[2,12,29] (see Figs. 11.3 to 11.9). The insertion sites include the infraglenoid tubercle of the posteromedial tibial plateau, the posterior capsule, the posterior horn of the medial meniscus, and a portion of the capsule deep to the MCL. Axial MR images may often demonstrate a small amount of fat accumulation between the different arms of the semimembranosus tendons at the level of the joint line, which is considered a normal variant. Axial sections obtained at the level of the upper portion of the femoral condyles may demonstrate the semimembranosus tendon before it branches into the five different arms as a "C"-shaped structure or as a "3"-shaped structure adjacent to the distal semimembranosus muscle.

The direct arm has an anterior course deep to the anterior arm and inserts at the tubercle on the posteromedial tibial condyle, also known as the *tuberculum tendinis*.[18] Immediately prior to its tibial insertion, it attaches to the posterior aspect of the coronary ligament of the posterior horn of the medial meniscus. The insertion site of the direct arm is best visualized on both sagittal and axial images. The anterior and direct arms together may form a low-signal-intensity band along the posteromedial aspect of the tibia, distal to the articular margin and inseparable from each other (see Figs. 11.3 to 11.9).

Text continued on p. 221

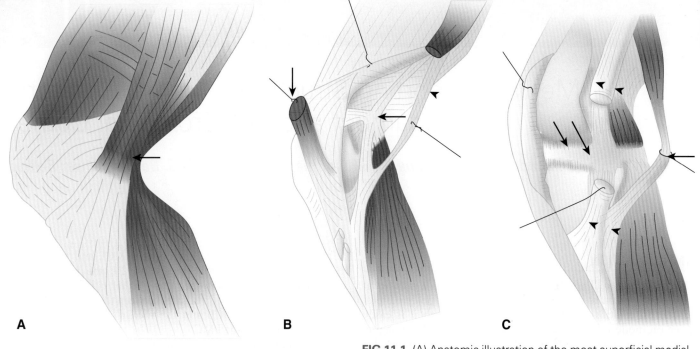

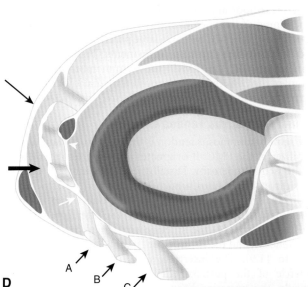

FIG 11.1 (A) Anatomic illustration of the most superficial medial structure of the knee. This illustration highlights layer I, which is the deep crural fascia. Arrow points to the sartorius muscle. (B) Anatomic illustration of the medial corner structures depicting layer II, which includes the superficial MCL *(long arrow)*. Arrowhead depicts the semimembranosus tendon. Short arrow depicts the sartorius muscle, which is cut and retracted. (C) Sagittal anatomic illustration of layer III, which includes the joint capsule, semimembranosus, and the deep medial collateral ligament (MCL, *long arrow*). Superficial MCL *(arrowheads)* is cut and retracted in this illustration. Short arrow depicts the semimembranosus tendon. (D) Axial anatomic illustration of the layers of the PMC of the knee. Layer I is the crural fascia *(thin arrow)* and also includes the pes anserinus [(A) sartorius tendon, (B) gracilis tendon, and (C) semitendinosus tendon]. Layer II *(long arrow)* is the superficial MCL. Layer III *(white arrowhead)* includes the joint capsule, semimembranosus, and the deep MCL. Also illustrated is the POL *(white arrow)*.

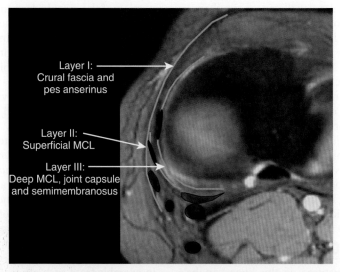

FIG 11.2 Three Layers of the Medial Corner Structures Axial short tau inversion recovery (STIR) MR image demonstrating the three layers of the medial corner of the knee. *MCL,* Medial collateral ligament.

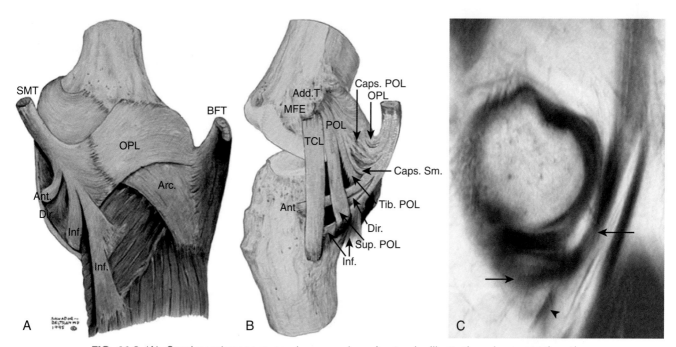

FIG 11.3 (A) Semimembranosus tendon complex: Anatomic illustration demonstrating the various arms/divisions of the complex and their relationships to each other, the oblique popliteal ligament (OPL), the arcuate ligament, and the biceps femoris tendon (BFT). This illustration highlights the semimembranosus tendon (SMT) located in the posterior medial aspect of the knee and its five divisions: [1] anterior arm *(Ant)*, [2] direct arm *(Dir)*, [3] inferior arm *(Inf)*, [4] OPL, and [5] capsular arm. The capsular arm is located deeper and not depicted in this image. Note the relationship between the OPL and the arcuate ligament *(Arc)*. The biceps femoris tendon (BFT) is seen in the posterolateral aspect of the knee. *BFT,* Biceps femoris tendon; *OPL,* oblique popliteal ligament; *SMT,* semimembranosus tendon. (Beltran J, Matityahu A, Hwang K, et al: The distal semimembranosus complex: normal MR anatomy, variants, biomechanics and pathology. *Skelet Radiol.* 32:435–445, 2003.) (B) Semimembranosus tendon complex: Anatomic illustration demonstrating the various arms/divisions of the complex and their relationships to each other, the oblique popliteal ligament (OPL), the arcuate ligament, and the tibial collateral ligament (TCL). This medial view of the knee demonstrates the anterior arm *(Ant)* as it curves anteriorly, inserting in the medial aspect of the proximal tibia, deep to the tibial collateral ligament (TCL). Note the inferior arm *(Inf)* with its popliteal extension. The capsular arm of the semimembranosus *(Caps. Sm.)* intertwines with the capsular bundle of the posterior oblique ligament *(Caps. POL)*. The superior bundle of the POL *(Sup. POL)* covers the anterior, direct, and inferior arms of the semimembranosus. The tibial bundle of the POL *(Tib. POL)* is located more posteriorly and deeper. The TCL and the POL originate in the adductor tubercle *(Add. T)* in the medial aspect of the distal femoral epicondyle (MFE). *MFE,* Medial aspect of the distal femoral epicondyle; *OPL,* oblique popliteal ligament; *POL,* popliteal oblique ligament; *TCL,* tibial collateral ligament. (Beltran J, Matityahu A, Hwang K, et al. The distal semimembranosus complex: normal MR anatomy, variants, biomechanics and pathology. *Skelet Radiol* 32:435–445, 2003.) (C) Semimembranosus tendon complex: Anterior and inferior divisions/arms and their relationships to each other. Sagittal proton density MR image demonstrates the semimembranosus tendon *(long arrow)*, the anterior arm *(short arrow)*, and the inferior arm *(arrow head)*. (Beltran J, Matityahu A, Hwang K, et al. The distal semimembranosus complex: normal MR anatomy, variants, biomechanics and pathology. *Skelet Radiol* 32:435–445, 2003.)

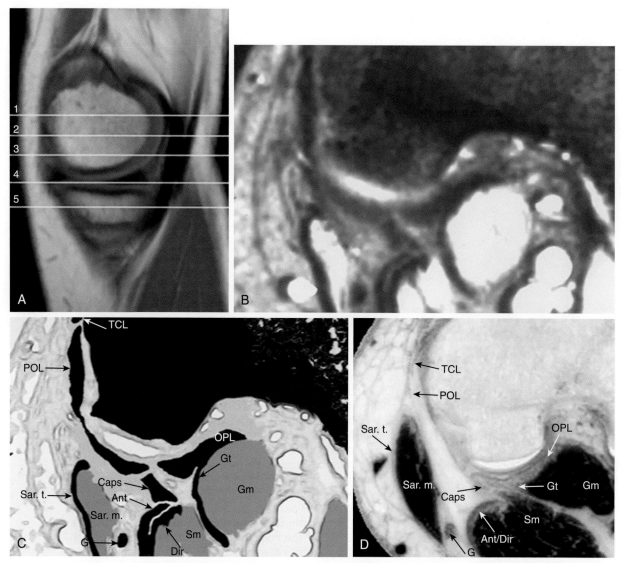

FIG 11.4 Semimembranosus Tendon Complex and Its Divisions/Arms and Their Relationships to Their Surrounding Structures at Various Levels Through the Knee: Level 1—The Most Upper Level: Upper Portion of the Femoral Condyles A sagittal proton density image though the distal semimembranosus tendon. (A) The numbered white horizontal lines correspond to the selected axial planes shown in subsequent Figs. 11.5 to 11.8. Anatomic components of the semimembranosus complex are labeled only in the schematic representations of the axial images depicted separately in Figs. 11.5 to 11.8. This series of axial MR images demonstrate the normal anatomy of this area. The cadaveric sections are depicted for correlation. (B) Axial gradient echo MR image, (C) schematic depiction of the same image, and (D) cadaveric section through level 1 located at the upper portion of the femoral condyles. At this level the capsular arm, anterior arm, direct arm, and OPL are already identified as separate structures in this normal volunteer. Note the gastrocnemius muscle *(Gm)* and tendon *(Gt)*, the semimembranosus muscle *(Sm)*, the gracilis tendon (G), and the sartorius muscle *(Sar. m.)* and tendon *(Sar. t.)*. The OPL is already seen at this level due to its upward direction. *Ant,* Anterior arm; *Caps,* capsular arm; *Dir,* direct arm; *G,* gracilis tendon; *Gm,* gastrocnemius muscle; *Gt,* gastrocnemius tendon; *OPL,* oblique popliteal ligament; *Sm,* semimembranosus muscle; *Sar. m.,* sartorius muscle; *Sar. t.,* sartorius tendon. (Beltran J, Matityahu A, Hwang K, et al: The distal semimembranosus complex: normal MR anatomy, variants, biomechanics and pathology. *Skelet Radiol* 32:435–445, 2003.)

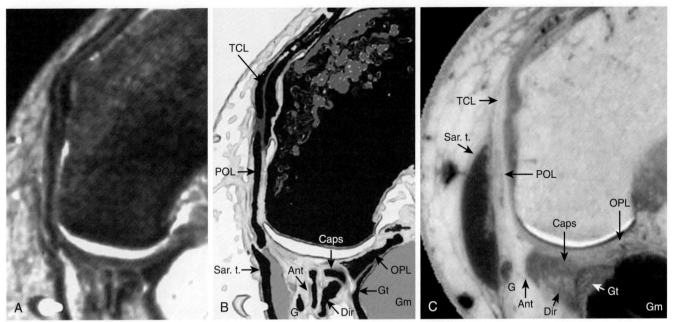

FIG 11.5 Semimembranosus Tendon Complex and Its Divisions/Arms and Their Relationships to Their Surrounding Structures at Various Levels Through the Knee: Level 2—Mid-Portion of the Femoral Condyles (A) Axial gradient echo image, (B) schematic depiction of the same image, and (C) cadaveric section through level 2 (Fig. 11.4A) located at the mid-portion of the femoral condyles. Abbreviations are as in Fig. 11.4. (Beltran J, Matityahu A, Hwang K, et al: The distal semimembranosus complex: normal MR anatomy, variants, biomechanics and pathology. *Skelet Radiol* 32:435–445, 2003.)

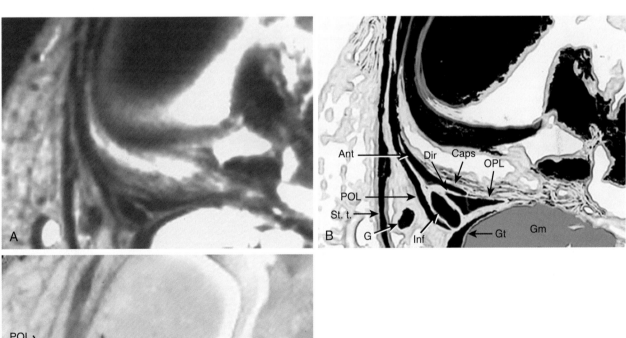

FIG 11.6 Semimembranosus Tendon Complex and Its Divisions/Arms and Their Relationships to Their Surrounding Structures at Various Levels Through the Knee: Level 3—Lower Portion of the Femoral Condyles (A) Axial gradient echo image, (B) schematic depiction of the same image, and (C) cadaveric section through level 3 (Fig. 11.4A) located at the lower portion of the femoral condyles. Note the posterior oblique ligament covering the different tendinous arms of the semimembranosus. Abbreviations are as in Fig. 11.4. (Beltran J, Matityahu A, Hwang K, et al: The distal semimembranosus complex: normal MR anatomy, variants, biomechanics and pathology. *Skelet Radiol* 32:435–445, 2003.)

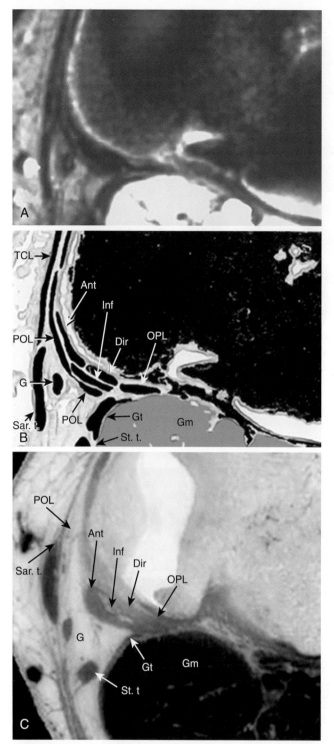

FIG 11.7 Semimembranosus Tendon Complex and Its Divisions/Arms and Their Relationships to Their Surrounding Structures at Various Levels Through the Knee: Level 4—Just Below the Joint Line (A) Axial gradient echo image, (B) schematic depiction of the same image, and (C) cadaveric section through level 4 (Fig. 11.4A) located just below the joint line. Note the semimembranosus tendon *(St. t.)*. Abbreviations are as in Fig. 11.4. (Beltran J, Matityahu A, Hwang K, et al: The distal semimembranosus complex: normal MR anatomy, variants, biomechanics and pathology. *Skelet Radiol* 32:435–445, 2003.)

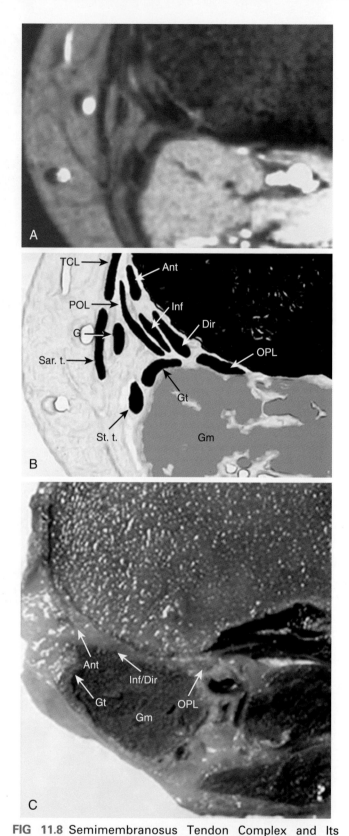

FIG 11.8 Semimembranosus Tendon Complex and Its Divisions/Arms and Their Relationships to Their Surrounding Structures at Various Levels Through the Knee: Level 5—Proximal Tibia (A) Axial gradient echo image, (B) schematic depiction of the same image, and (C) cadaveric section through level 5 (Fig. 11.4A) located at the proximal tibia. Note that the skin, subcutaneous fat, TCL, part of the posterior oblique ligament, sartorius tendon, and gracilis tendon have been resected in the cadaveric section (C). Abbreviations are as in Fig. 11.4. (Beltran J, Matityahu A, Hwang K, et al: The distal semimembranosus complex: normal MR anatomy, variants, biomechanics and pathology. *Skelet Radiol* 32:435–445, 2003.)

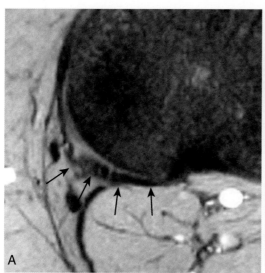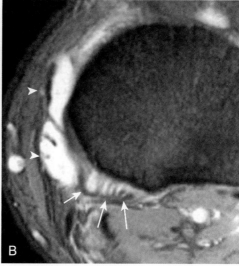

FIG 11.9 Semimembranosus Complex With and Without Presence of a Joint Effusion (A) Axial proton density MR image of the semimembranosus complex without a joint effusion. (B) Axial STIR MR image with a joint effusion. The image shown in A illustrates a more frequent depiction of the semimembranosus complex. The direct, capsular, and anterior arms form a low-signal-intensity band in the medial posterior aspect of the tibia *(arrows)*. The different arms separated by fat planes are frequently not seen as separate structures. A joint effusion (B) separates the fibers of the capsular arm, direct arm, and capsular bundle of the posterior oblique ligament *(arrows)*. Note also the presence of a semimembranosus bursitis *(arrow heads)*. (Beltran J, Matityahu A, Hwang K, et al: The distal semimembranosus complex: normal MR anatomy, variants, biomechanics and pathology. *Skelet Radiol* 32:435–445, 2003.)

The capsular arm of the semimembranosus tendon is best visualized on axial images. This arm is seen as a deep-lying, flat, striated structure arising from the posterior medial aspect of the tibial plateau, which then combines with the posteromedial capsule to join the capsular portions of both the OPL and POL. This arm is better appreciated as a separate structure when the joint is distended by fluid, although this is not very common. Hence, the capsular arm is seen as a flat striated structure located in the posterior medial aspect of the tibial plateau, inseparable from the adjacent direct and anterior arms arm while continuous to the OPL (see Figs. 11.3 to 11.9).

The anterior or tibial arm, also known as the *reflected arm*, extends anteriorly, passing under the POL, and inserts on the medial aspect of the proximal tibia under the tibial collateral ligament. Most commonly, this arm is seen on medial peripheral sagittal images as a low-signal-intensity structure curving anteriorly and taking an almost horizontal course.[12,18] When the knee is fully extended, there is angulation of the anterior arm, resulting in a focal area of high signal intensity within the tendon with a echo time (TE) of 20 ms consistent with a magic angle artifact (Fig. 11.10). On sequential coronal images, the horizontal portion of the anterior arm is seen as a round or oval hypointense or as a thin structure adjacent to the medial aspect of the tibia, under the tibial collateral ligament and POL (Fig. 11.11). The thickness of the anterior arm varies significantly between normal individuals. On sequential axial images, the anterior arm is demonstrated as a hypointense structure adjacent to the posterior medial aspect of the tibia, extending anteriorly in consecutive sections (see Figs. 11.4 to 11.9).

The inferior or popliteal arm extends more distally than the anterior and the direct arms. It passes under the distal tibial

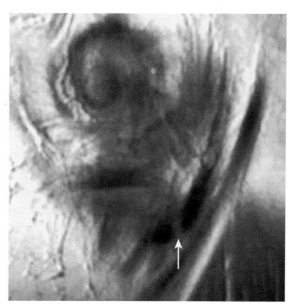

FIG 11.10 Semimembranosus Tendon Complex and the Magic Angle Artifact of the Anterior Division Sagittal proton density MR image demonstrates the anterior arm. Note a focal area of increased signal intensity *(arrow)* representing a magic angle artifact. (Beltran J, Matityahu A, Hwang K, et al. The distal semimembranosus complex: normal MR anatomy, variants, biomechanics and pathology. *Skelet Radiol* 32:435–445, 2003.)

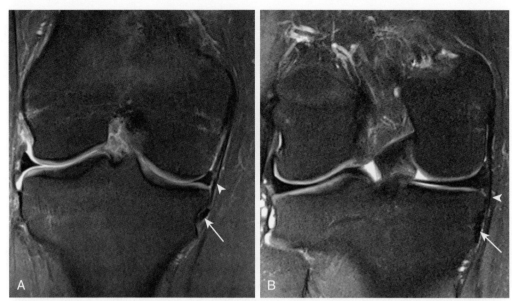

FIG 11.11 Semimembranosus tendon complex Anterior division/arm: Coronal fat-saturated proton density MR images demonstrating the anterior arm (A) as a round or oval, thick low-signal-intensity tendon *(arrow)* or (B) as a thin tendon *(arrow)*. Note the POL *(arrowheads* in A and B) covering the anterior arm. (Beltran J, Matityahu A, Hwang K, et al: The distal semimembranosus complex: normal MR anatomy, variants, biomechanics and pathology. *Skelet Radiol* 32:435–445, 2003.)

segments of the POL and the tibial collateral ligament, inserting just above the tibial attachment of the tibial collateral ligament. On sequential axial MR images, the inferior arm is seen as a low-signal-intensity structure extending inferiorly and anteriorly from the posterior margin of the joint line, deep to the MCL. The anterior arm is sometimes further divided into medial and lateral divisions, with the attachment to the medial tibia forming the medial division and the lateral division extending over the popliteal fascia (see Figs. 11.3 to 11.9).*

Posterior Oblique Ligament (Ligament of Winslow)

The POL or ligament of Winslow originates in the adductor tubercle of the femur. Its anterior margin combines with the posterior margin of the superficial MCL and its posterior margin joins the joint capsule, which is part of layer III.[5,12,18,30] The POL has three bundles of attachment that are inseparable: (1) the superficial arm, or fascial tissue of the pes anserinus, (2) the tibial arm, or the posterior medial aspect of the tibia and the posterior horn of the medial meniscus, and (3) the capsular arm, which merges with the capsular arm of the semimembranosus tendon (SMT) and OPL (see Fig. 11.3). The tibial arm is considered the thickest and most important of these arms. This arm extends posteriorly and obliquely and inserts into the posteromedial aspect of the medial meniscus and the adjacent posteromedial aspect of the tibia, migrates deep to the anterior arm of the semimembranosus tendon, and finally merges with the main part of the tendon (see Fig. 11.3). The tibial arm is seen best on the sequential coronal and axial images, running immediately posterior to the superficial MCL as it joins with the capsule while inserting into the medial meniscus and the adjacent tibia.[5,12] The capsular arm of the POL lies superior to the joint line of the knee. This arm is continuous with the posterior joint capsule and combines with the capsular arm of the semimembranosus tendon to form the proximal aspect of the OPL (see Fig. 11.3). Using the axial images, the capsular arm is commonly seen at the level of the femoral condyle, while on coronal images it presents as a thin hypointense band that extends posteriorly from the superficial MCL to combine with the medial aspect of the posterior capsular structures. Finally, the superficial arm inserts into the sheath and tibial insertion points of the semimembranosus tendon, combines with the posterior margin of the superficial MCL, and passes superficially to the anterior arm of the semimembranosus tendon[12,18,29,30] (see Fig. 11.3). The superficial arm is best visualized on coronal images as a thin hypointense band superficial to the direct insertion of the semimembranosus tendon and extends from its origin to insert into the medial aspect of the tibial plateau.

Oblique Popliteal Ligament

The OPL is a thin, broad, lateral extension of the semimembranosus tendon. It both covers and blends with the posterior medial capsule to extend beyond the midline of the joint and unites with the arcuate ligament from the posterolateral aspect of the knee. The OPL originates from both the capsular arm of the POL and the lateral expansion of the semimembranosus. It transcends laterally to insert into the osseous or cartilaginous fabella, the meniscofemoral portion of the posterolateral joint capsule, and the plantaris muscle (see Fig. 11.3). The fibrous attachment of the OPL attaches to the lateral aspect of the PCL facet.[18] Coronal and sagittal images may demonstrate this thin structure as a low-signal-intensity line indistinguishable in most cases from the posterior capsule but in continuity with the main tendon of the semimembranosus (Figs. 11.12 and 11.13).[7]

---

*References 5, 14, 15, 18, 26, and 31.

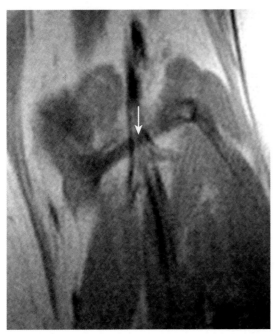

FIG 11.12 Oblique Popliteal Ligament Coronal T1 MR image demonstrating the OPL *(arrow)* as a broad, flat, low-signal-intensity band extending from the lateral femoral condyle to the medial condyle of the tibia.

Posteromedial Joint Capsule and Posterior Horn of the Medial Meniscus

The knee joint capsule forms part of layer III of the medial corner of the knee. Along with its meniscotibial and meniscofemoral components, it forms the deep MCL along the medial aspect of the knee. Then the knee joint capsule extends posteriorly and is reinforced externally by the POL, which is a part of layer II and together forms the posteromedial joint capsule. Further distally, the posteromedial joint capsule runs deep to the medial head of the gastrocnemius extending laterally to form the posterior joint capsule. The posterior joint capsules together with the posteromedial side of the knee are strengthened by both the POL and expansions from the semimembranosus. The meniscotibial ligament fastens the medial meniscus to the tibia while the meniscus attaches to the capsule posteromedially.

FUNCTION AND BIOMECHANICS OF THE POSTEROMEDIAL CORNER

The meniscal, myotendinous, and ligamentous components of the posteromedial corner of the knee provide both dynamic and static support and also restrict anteromedial rotation of the knee.[29] The myotendinous structures and their respective aponeuroses provide dynamic support of the PMC. Static support

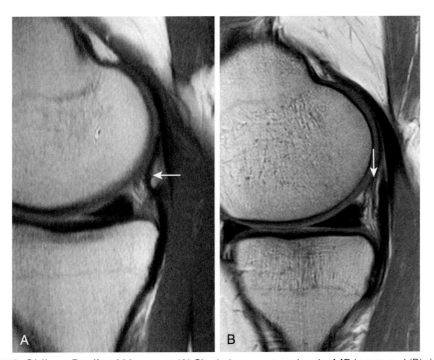

FIG 11.13 Oblique Popliteal Ligament (A) Single-layer proton density MR image and (B) double-layer proton density MR image demonstrating the OPL/posterior capsular line *(white arrows)* seen in the sagittal plane in two different patients. When present, these structures can easily be identified by their S-shaped configuration. (Beltran J, Matityahu A, Hwang K, et al: The distal semimembranosus complex: normal MR anatomy, variants, biomechanics and pathology. *Skelet Radiol* 32:435–445, 2003.)

is provided by the joint capsule and regional ligaments.[12,18] Several muscles and ancillary structures provide active support relative to knee position. The semimembranosus muscle supports the superficial MCL and POL during active flexion, the pes anserinus muscles and tendons actively support the knee when flexed, and the vastus medialis muscle in knee extension.[11,12] The posterior horn of the medial meniscus delivers passive support and rotational support is provided by the deep meniscotibial connections.

The POL is naturally relaxed with knee flexion and taut in extension. In full knee extension, the tibia externally rotates, tightening the PMC and its components to create a pouch around the medial femoral condyle. In initial knee flexion with internal rotation of the tibia, the semimembranosus is contracted, tightening the posteromedial capsule. However, with growing flexion, the posteromedial capsule subsequently relaxes and envelops itself.[11,12,28,30]

The main dynamic stabilizer of the PMC of the knee is the semimembranosus, which also has protective effects on the posterior horn of the medial meniscus preventing injury during full knee flexion. The semimembranosus flexes and internally rotates the tibia during contraction. When the knee is extended, it actively prevents valgus motion and in flexion it prevents external rotation. It also places traction on the posterior horn of the medial meniscus and the semimembranosus tendon protects it from compression between the femur and tibia.[7] The semimembranosus is positioned parallel to the femur and its protective effect is greatest at 90 degrees of knee flexion. This decreases as the knee slowly extends. The semimembranosus also further stabilizes the OPL and posterior joint capsule in the PMC. It adds to the stability of the posterolateral corner by working synergistically with the popliteus and works alongside the biceps femoris muscle to dynamically stabilize the knee in internal and external rotation.[6,11,12,13,29]

The medial meniscus and meniscotibial ligament synergistically play a role in the brake stop mechanism of support of the knee. In situations where the meniscus is securely on its tibial platform and the meniscotibial ligament is undamaged, the posterior horn of the medial meniscus provides a brake stop function preventing posterior translation of the tibia. In meniscotibial ligament insufficiency, the posteromedial meniscus becomes unstable on its tibial platform, and ultimately the brake stop mechanism is lost. This subsequently causes the meniscus and femoral condyle to move together and slide over the tibial articular surface. There are then no stabilizing functions and there is increased risk of injury and stress to the meniscus and the tibial articular surface. This PMC injury causes lack of support of the knee, absence of the brake stop mechanism, and decreased dynamic function of the medial meniscus.[11,12,19,24,29]

The POL has many functional roles including restricting internal and external rotation, valgus stress, and anterior and posterior tibial translation. It has been shown that after sectioning of the MCL, there were significant increases in load to the POL with both external and valgus rotation. The POL is also an essential stabilizer against internal rotation at all knee flexion angles. The oblique popliteal ligament constrains knee hyperextension and plays a key role in preventing genu recurvatum.[8,23,25,33]

The primary restraint to valgus stress at all angles of flexion is the superficial MCL, with the deep MCL providing secondary static stabilization. The PMC additionally delivers one-third of the support to stabilize the knee and restrict valgus stress when in knee extension. In the setting of an isolated MCL injury, the POL provides secondary stabilization for both rotation and valgus stress.[†]

The PMC plays a crucial role in the secondary stabilization of pure anterior tibial translation. This is seen in many athletes with ACL ruptures who still function at a high level despite their injuries. Patients who undergo ACL reconstruction with overlooked preexisting PMC injuries have an increased risk of ACL graft failure.[12,27,29] The POL also delivers secondary stabilization in posterior tibial translation, mainly in knee extension. Its supporting role increases with tibial internal rotation. Similar to the PMC, which helps prevent excessive anterior tibial translation in ACL-deficient knees, the POL is important in supporting against posterior tibial translation in PCL-deficient knees.[9,25,27,30]

POSTEROMEDIAL COMPARTMENT INJURIES

As discussed earlier in the chapter, the posteromedial compartment is composed of many structures, which, when injured, can lead to anteromedial rotational instability. Anteromedial rotational instability can put undue stress on other supporting structures of the knee, compromising their integrity, especially after repair. Anteromedial rotational instability is defined as external rotation with anterior subluxation of the medial tibial plateau relative to the distal femur.[7] This instability can be better understood if we consider the dynamics of an MCL injury. When the MCL is injured, it allows for excess opening of the medial compartment of the knee via additional abduction of the lower leg. In anteromedial rotational instability, there is simultaneous anteromedial rotational subluxation of the medial tibial condyle about the axis of the PCL, in addition to the excess opening of the medial compartment of the knee. This rotational subluxation can potentiate stress on the ACL and PCL, possibly delaying healing after a repair. This is especially important considering that in the majority of patients with symptomatic ACL or MCL injuries, one or more components of the posteromedial corner of the knee are also usually injured.[30]

Semimembranosus Injury

The main stabilizing muscle of the PMC is the semimembranosus muscle. It is commonly affected in posteromedial knee injuries and frequently associated with injuries of the ACL, MCL, and medial meniscus. Semimembranosus injuries can lead to avulsion fractures at the insertion site along the posteromedial tibia, tears of the tendon, or chronic injury tendinosis. Avulsion fractures can occur when there is forced abduction at the knee and external rotation of the tibia on an internally rotated, flexed knee. Avulsion fractures usually occur where the direct arm of the tendon attaches to the tibia and usually present with a bone bruise and a low-signal fracture line on MRI (Figs. 11.14 to 11.18). The insertional tendon is stronger than the insertional site at the bone, so tendon tears are less common than avulsion fractures.[3] Complete tears are visualized as a discontinuous tendon with intervening hemorrhage (see Fig. 11.16). Partial tears and strains are visualized as increased signal within the tendon with associated edema (see Fig. 11.17).

[†]References 4, 6, 8, 9, 11, 27, 30, and 33.

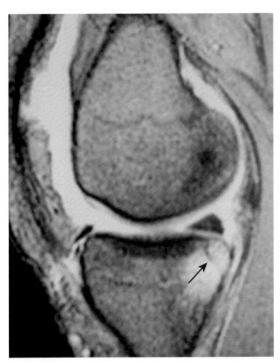

FIG 11.14 Semimembranosus Avulsion Injuries Sagittal T2 MR image through the knee demonstrating partial avulsion fractures of the posterior medial aspect of the tibia at the insertion of the semimembranosus tendon. Note the fracture line *(black arrow)* with surrounding bone marrow edematous changes. (Beltran J, Matityahu A, Hwang K, et al: The distal semimembranosus complex: normal MR anatomy, variants, biomechanics and pathology. *Skelet Radiol* 32:435–445, 2003.)

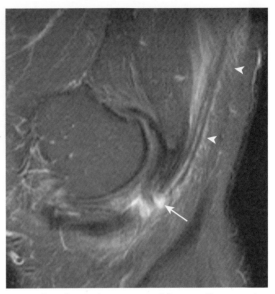

FIG 11.15 Semimembranosus Myotendinous Junction Injury Sagittal STIR MR image demonstrating a focus of hyperintense signal intensity at the semimembranosus myotendinous junction consistent with a partial tear *(arrow)*. Arrowheads depict the semimembranosus tendon.

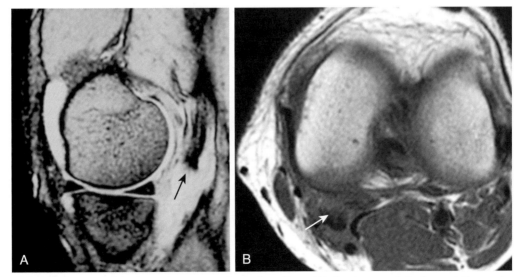

FIG 11.16 Acute Semimembranosus Complete Tear (A) Acute complete tear of the main semimembranosus tendon with tendon retraction *(black arrow)* seen on sagittal gradient recalled echo (GRE) MR image and (B) axial T1-weighted images *(white arrow)*. (Beltran J, Matityahu A, Hwang K, et al: The distal semimembranosus complex: normal MR anatomy, variants, biomechanics and pathology. *Skelet Radiol* 32:435–445, 2003.)

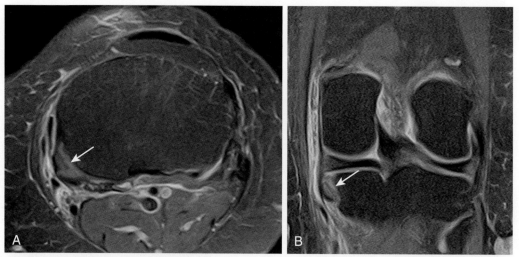

FIG 11.17 Partial Tear of the Semimembranosus Tendon Axial and coronal STIR MR images demonstrating a linear hypointense signal intensity within the distal semimembranosus tendon with adjacent hyperintense signal intensity consistent with a partial longitudinal tear of the distal semimembranosus tendon *(arrows)* with surrounding hyperintense signal intensity representing edematous changes.

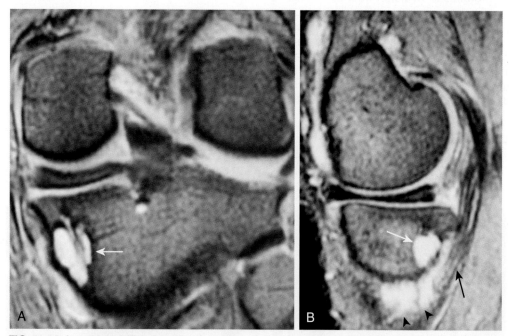

FIG 11.18 Insertional Tendinosis of the Distal Semimembranosus Tendon (A) Coronal and (B) sagittal GRE MR images demonstrate a partial longitudinal tear of the tendon *(black arrow* in B) and bone cyst formation at the level of the tibial insertion *(white arrow* in A and B). Note the presence of fluid distending the semimembranosus bursa (double arrowheads in B). (Beltran J, Matityahu A, Hwang K, et al: The distal semimembranosus complex: normal MR anatomy, variants, biomechanics and pathology. *Skelet Radiol* 32:435–445, 2003.)

Increased signal intensity within the tendon can also be seen with tendinosis, but accumulation of fat, which is a normal variant, can cause increased signal as well. In tendinosis, there is increased signal in the distal semimembranosus tendon insertion and irregularity and cystic changes at the level of the posterior medial tibia (see Fig. 11.18).

Posterior Oblique Ligament and Oblique Popliteal Ligament Injuries

In a study looking at surgically repaired knees with medial-sided injuries and symptomatic AMRI, 99% of cases had an associated POL injury.[28] POL injuries can be classified the same

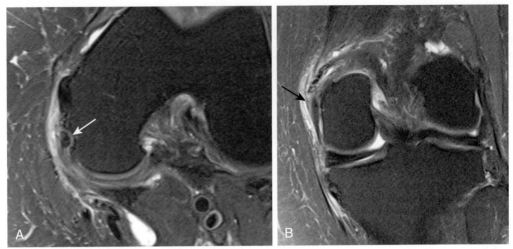

FIG 11.19 Posterior Oblique Ligament Partial Tear (A) Axial and (B) coronal STIR MR images demonstrating hyperintense signal intensity (*white arrow* in A and *black arrow* in B) partially involving the POL consistent with an incomplete tear. (Beltran J, Matityahu A, Hwang K, et al: The distal semimembranosus complex: normal MR anatomy, variants, biomechanics and pathology. *Skelet Radiol* 32:435–445, 2003.)

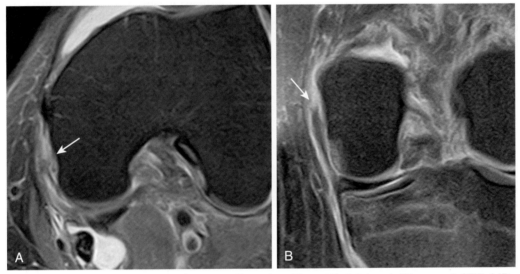

FIG 11.20 Posterior Oblique Ligament Complete Tear (A) Axial and (B) coronal STIR MR images demonstrating hyperintense signal intensity *(arrows)* in the region of the expected POL consistent with a complete tear.

way as MCL tears.[12] A sprain is a grade I injury and is characterized by a normal-sized ligament with no discontinuity and no associated edema. A grade II injury is a partial-thickness injury, with partial discontinuity of the ligament with thickening, edema, and surrounding hemorrhage (Fig. 11.19). A grade III injury is a complete tear, with complete ligament discontinuity, edema, and hemorrhage (Fig. 11.20). Injuries to the oblique popliteal ligament are difficult to visualize explicitly and are usually implied when the posterior joint capsule is injured; these injuries are seen as increased signal intensity and surrounding edema (see Fig. 11.19).

Medial Meniscus and Stop Brake Injury

The posterior aspect of the medial meniscus plays an important role in the stability of the knee during weight bearing. The posterior third of the medial meniscus prevents posterior translation of the medial femoral condyle on the tibia when the tibia bears the weight of the medial femoral condyle. Damage to the medial meniscus or the meniscotibial ligament allows for uninhibited posterior translation of the femoral condyle relative to the tibia. Unsurprisingly, this could lead to injury of other components of the knee or delayed healing of already injured components. On imaging, meniscotibial ligament injuries are seen as disruption, thickening, or increased signal of the ligamentous fibers with associated edema. Edema and increased signal intensity that are superficial to the posteromedial capsule can also be seen in more benign cases, such as a ruptured popliteal cyst, so imaging findings must be paired with clinical history to ensure that a wrong diagnosis is not made.[12]

Anterior Cruciate Ligament Injuries and the Posteromedial Corner

It is important to understand the relationship between injuries of the PMC and the ACL. A majority of patients with medial-sided knee injuries concurrently have associated ACL injuries.[22] There are subsets of patients with ACL injuries that are able to perform at a high level physically. It is thought that in these patients, an uninjured PMC compensates for an injured ACL. In patients with injuries to both the ACL and the PMC of the knee, healing of the ACL may be significantly delayed due to the lack of compensatory action from the PMC. Accurately identifying patients with PMC injuries can allow surgeons to better predict outcomes in repair surgeries.

CLINICAL MANIFESTATIONS OF POSTEROMEDIAL CORNER INJURIES

Injuries to the PMC usually do not present with specific symptoms that would point a clinician to this specific part of the knee. The symptoms usually suggest injuries to parts of the knee to which attention is more classically paid, such as the ACL, MCL, PCL, and menisci. Most injuries are sports related, but non–sports-related traumatic events are also culprits.[16] Patients who present with medial knee pain are usually examined for injuries to the ACL, MCL, and PCL by performing the anterior and posterior drawer test, and the abduction stress test. In the abduction stress test, the medial joint space is assessed with the knee in zero flexion and with the knee flexed at 30 degrees. Normally, there should not be any medial joint space opening at zero flexion. If there is, the PMC is injured. Furthermore, PMC injuries allow for increased joint space laxity at 30 degrees of flexion and anterior rotary subluxation of the medial tibial plateau. AMRI is defined as a positive anterior drawer test with the tibia in external rotation. Simultaneous injury of the PCL and the posteromedial corner is demonstrated with a positive posterior drawer test with the tibia in internal rotation.[17] In addition to physical exam findings, performing an MRI is important for complete anatomic evaluation, especially in settings where pain can mask physical exam findings.

Although x-rays can be and usually are obtained in the acute setting, the findings are usually nonspecific. Additionally, radiographs with valgus and posterior stress may be obtained to assess medial-sided and combined PCL and capsular-collateral ligament injury. Computed tomography (CT) may be helpful to evaluate acute osseous abnormalities including fractures. MR imaging may play an important role in identifying concealed PMC injuries, especially in situations where clinical examination is limited, as well as presurgical planning.

TREATMENT OF POSTEROMEDIAL CORNER INJURIES

As mentioned earlier, PMC injuries most commonly occur in association with other injuries and require surgical treatment. When they occur alone, conservative management is the treatment of choice.[12,29,30] Surgical treatment is the optimal management for symptomatic functional AMRI, whether in isolation or occurring in association with other injuries, such as ACL, PCL, and PMC injuries.[1,29]

For multiligamentous injuries (ACL, PCL, and MCL), the surgeon's opinion determines whether to treat medial-side injuries conservatively or surgically.[16,30] Different techniques such as plication, advancement, augmentation, and reconstruction with autografts and allografts are commonly used to repair and reconstruct the POL along with reconstruction of the MCL.

It is imperative to surgically correct simultaneous PMC injuries when aiming for optimal ACL reconstruction outcomes. Isolated PCL injuries that are not surgically treated will derange the dynamics of the medial compartment, leading to osteoarthritis of the medial compartment. This is further exacerbated when PCL and PMC injuries occur simultaneously, leading to increased posterior translation of the tibia. Hence, early repair of PMC injuries along with appropriate cruciate ligament reconstruction can effectively restore knee stability for patients with PMC injuries associated with cruciate ligament ruptures. Complications resulting from cruciate and PMC surgeries are infrequent and include knee stiffness and saphenous nerve injury, among others.[30]

CONCLUSION

The PMC of the knee is often overlooked and neglected. This should not be the case, as PMC injuries are a significant source of morbidity in patients with knee injuries. Appropriate understanding of its anatomy, including knowledge about normal appearance on MR imaging and specific biomechanical function, can help in better recognizing PMC injuries. Detailed attention to this area can help avoid serious morbidity in patients with acute knee injuries, especially in the setting of multiligamentous injuries.

KEY REFERENCES

1. Bauer KL, Stannard JP: Surgical approach to the posteromedial corner: indications, technique, outcomes. *Curr Rev Musculoskelet Med* 6:124–131, 2013.
2. Benninger B, Delamarter T: Distal semimembranosus muscle-tendon-unit review: morphology, accurate terminology, and clinical relevance. *Folia Morphol* 72:1–9, 2013.
4. Cohen M, Astur DC, Branco RC, et al: An anatomical three-dimensional study of the posteromedial corner of the knee. *Knee Surg Sports Traumatol Arthrosc* 19:1614–1619, 2011.
7. Geiger D, Chang EY, Pathria MN, et al: Posterolateral and posteromedial corner injuries of the knee. *Magn Reson Imaging Clin N Am* 22:581–599, 2014.
12. House CV, Connell DA, Saifuddin A: Posteromedial corner injuries of the knee. *Clin Radiol* 62:539–546, 2007.
20. Loredo R, Hodler J, Pedowitz R, et al: Posteromedial corner of the knee: MR imaging with gross anatomic correlation. *Skeletal Radiol* 28:305–311, 1999.
21. Lundquist RB, Matcuk GR, Jr, Schein AJ, et al: Posteromedial corner of the knee: the neglected corner. *Radiographics* 35:1123–1137, 2015.
27. Robinson JR, Sanchez-Ballester J, Bull AM, et al: The posteromedial corner revisited. An anatomical description of the passive restraining structures of the medial aspect of the human knee. *J Bone Joint Surg Br* 86:674–681, 2004.
28. Sims WF, Jacobson KE: The posteromedial corner of the knee: medial-sided injury patterns revisited. *Am J Sports Med* 32:337–345, 2004.
29. Tibor LM, Marchant MH, Jr, Taylor DC, et al: Management of medial-sided knee injuries, part 2: posteromedial corner. *Am J Sports Med* 39:1332–1340, 2011.

The references for this chapter can also be found on www.expertconsult.com.

12

Imaging of the Extensor Mechanism

Catherine N. Petchprapa

IMAGING OF THE EXTENSOR MECHANISM

The extensor mechanism of the knee plays an important role in normal lower extremity function. It is a complex of interconnected structures in the anterior knee that includes the quadriceps muscle group, quadriceps tendon, patella, patellar tendon, tibial tubercle, retinaculum, and adjacent soft tissues.[4] Functionally, the extensor mechanism allows for knee extension when the leg is elevated, and acts as a stabilizer and decelerator when standing.[22] In addition, the structures of the extensor mechanism play a vital role in patellofemoral stability.[4]

Magnetic resonance imaging (MRI) is ideal for the evaluation of the bony and soft structures that comprise the extensor mechanism and is the focus of this chapter. MRI provides a comprehensive, multiplanar examination of the knee and allows for detailed evaluation of the bone and bone marrow, articular cartilage, and surrounding soft tissue structures. MRI identifies clinically suspected and unsuspected pathology and helps stratify patients for treatment.

The extensor mechanism is well evaluated on routine MRI of the knee. Imaging with closed 3 Tesla and newer 1.5 Tesla MR scanners is preferred over older MR scanners or open MR systems, as they provide higher resolution examinations and shorter scan times. Use of a dedicated knee coil is essential to maximize signal to noise (SNR), which is needed for high-resolution images. The knee is imaged in three planes: sagittal, coronal, and axial. Specific imaging sequence protocols may vary slightly between imaging centers. The proton density weighted sequence is the workhorse sequence for musculoskeletal imaging and the mainstay of knee imaging protocols; it provides high resolution, high SNR images with excellent soft tissue contrast, in addition to being particularly sensitive to abnormalities of the cartilage. Adding fat suppression to imaging sequences increases the conspicuity of fluid, which is often seen in pathologic conditions; the resulting sequences are commonly known as fluid-sensitive sequences. An inversion recovery sequences such as short tau inversion-recovery (STIR) is also sensitive to fluid; it has the added advantage of being less affected by the presence of metal and can be used when relatively small amounts of metal are present. When the extensor mechanism is evaluated in the presence of significant metal, such as an arthroplasty, specialized metal artifact reduction techniques are extremely effective at mitigating the strong, metal-induced local susceptibility artifacts. Intravenous or intra-articular gadolinium is not necessary for routine imaging; it may be helpful in specific conditions such as in the evaluation of soft tissue masses, inflammatory arthritis, and the postoperative knee. A routine, high-resolution MR examination of the knee can be completed in less than 15 minutes in a 3 T MR scanner and less than 20 minutes in a 1.5-T MR scanner when dedicated, multichannel knee coil and parallel imaging techniques are used.

Disorders of the extensor mechanism commonly manifest as anterior knee pain and may be the result of degeneration, acute, or chronic injury. In this chapter, we review the MRI findings seen in the range of disorders associated with the extensor mechanism, which include lateral patellar dislocation; quadriceps and patellar tendon pathology; abnormalities of the prepatellar quadriceps continuation; abnormalities of bursae, fat pads, and plicae; and bipartite patellae.

PATELLAR DISLOCATION

Acute Injury

Traumatic lateral patellar dislocation (LPD) most commonly occurs as a result of a noncontact injury where internal femoral rotation occurs on a fixed tibia when the knee is partially flexed; direct injury to the medial knee is a less common mechanism of injury. The resultant lateralizing force on the patella places tension on the medial patellar retinacular complex and causes it to tear partially or completely. As the patella translates over the lateral femoral condyle, shear forces can result in a chondral or osteochondral injury of the median ridge of the patella and lateral femoral trochlea. Once completely dislocated from the trochlear groove, the lower aspect of the patella impacts on the lateral femoral condyle, and upon relocation, a contusion, chondral, or osteochondral injury of the inferior medial patellar facet may result.[68]

Traumatic LPD may be clinically unsuspected in up to 73% of cases,[44] as spontaneous relocation is common and physical examination of the painful, swollen knee can be a challenge.

Initial plain radiographs are nonspecific and most often show joint effusion, soft tissue swelling, and lateral patellar subluxation. Occasionally, a displaced osteochondral fragment may be seen; termed the "sliver sign," the finding of a displaced osteochondral fragment in the setting of joint effusion correlates with recent LPD.[31] An avulsion fracture or ossification adjacent to the medial patella on tangential patellar views also correlates with a history of previous subluxation or dislocation (Fig. 12.1).[35]

On MRI, the patella may be laterally tilted or laterally subluxed, and there is often a joint effusion or hemarthrosis (Figs. 12.2 and 12.3).[24] MRI also depicts the extent and location of characteristic bone and soft tissue injuries, which include bone contusion; chondral/osteochondral injury; injury of the medial patellar retinacular complex, including the medial patellofemoral ligament; and injury of the vastus medialis obliquus muscle.

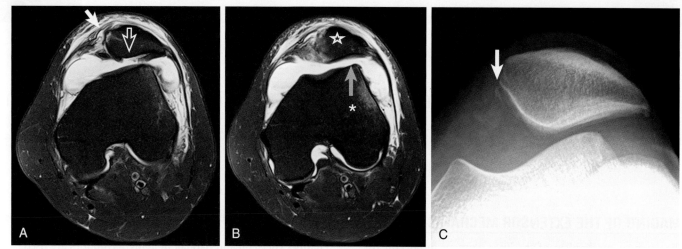

FIG 12.1 Transient Patellar Dislocation Axial fat suppressed T2 weighted images obtained at the level of the upper (A) and mid trochlea (B) and tangential view of the patella (C). The medial retinaculum is torn at its patellar origin (*white arrow*, A) and there are impaction injuries of the inferomedial patella *(star, B)* and nonarticular lateral femoral condyle (*asterisk*, B). There is an osteochondral injury of the median ridge patellar articular cartilage with cartilage delamination (*open white arrow*, A) and chondral defect along the far lateral trochlea (*gray arrow*, B). The patella is laterally subluxed, and there is an avulsion fracture of the medial patella on the plain radiograph (*long white arrow*, C).

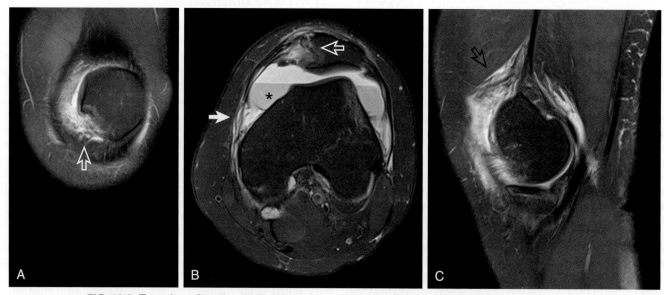

FIG 12.2 Transient Patellar Dislocation Coronal fat suppressed proton density (A), axial fat suppressed T2 (B), and sagittal fat suppressed proton density (C) weighted MR images. There is a concave inferomedial patellar osteochondral impaction fracture (*open white arrows*, A and B), rupture of the medial retinaculum at its femoral origin (*white arrow*, B), hemarthrosis (*asterisk*, B) and injury to vastus medialis obliquus muscle with muscle stripped and elevated (*open black arrow*, C).

Bone Contusion. The characteristic anterolateral, nonarticular femoral condylar and medial patellar bone contusions[24] related to translational injury are manifest by increased marrow signal on fluid sensitive sequences or decreased marrow signal on T1 weighted sequences (see Fig. 12.1). These may be associated with depression of the overlying cortical or subchondral bone.

Medial Patellar Retinacular Complex, Medial Patellofemoral Ligament and Vastus Medialis Obliquus Muscle Injury. At shallow flexion angles, the patella is reliant on soft tissue stabilizers for stability. The medial patellar retinaculum, specifically the medial patellofemoral ligament and vastus medialis obliquus (VMO) muscle, contribute important static and dynamic soft tissue stability to the patella.

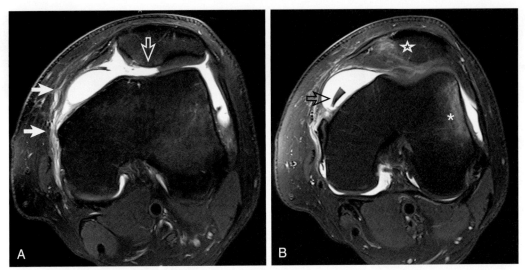

FIG 12.3 Transient Patellar Dislocation Axial fat suppressed T2 MR image obtained at the time of injury (A) shows femoral side medial patellofemoral ligament rupture *(arrow)* and hemarthrosis *(black asterisk)*. Axial fat suppressed T2 MR image after medial patellofemoral ligament repair (B) shows intact ligament *(open arrow)* and bone anchor *(white asterisk)*.

The medial patellar retinaculum is a complex of structures that includes the patellotibial, patellomeniscal, and medial patellofemoral ligaments. It receives a fibrous expansion from vastus medialis.[4] The medial patellofemoral ligament (MPFL) is considered most important in providing restraint to lateral patellar displacement[3] and is injured in 97% of acute patellar dislocations.[4]

The MPFL is located within the second anatomic layer of the three-layered fascial structure of the medial knee. It is widest at its broad origin from the upper two-thirds of the patella.[94] Although there is variation as to the site of the femoral insertion of the MPFL in anatomic studies in the literature,* more recent studies have shown it to insert on the femur posterior to the medial epicondyle and distal to the adductor tubercle.[8,20] Furthermore, Baldwin's cadaveric study[8] revealed both a bony and soft tissue origin of the MPFL: distal transverse fibers from a bony groove between the adductor tubercle and medial epicondyle, and proximal oblique fibers from the edge of the medial collateral ligament. Both fiber groups joined the VMO tendon and formed a conjoint structure that inserted along the upper two-thirds medial border of the patella.

On MRI, the MPFL is best seen on axial images. It is a well-defined low signal intensity band that arises from the upper patella[46] and courses over the femoral origin of the medial collateral ligament to its insertion; it may be inseparable from the VMO muscle along part of its course.[20] Complete tears are manifest by full thickness discontinuity of the ligament and local soft tissue edema seen as increased or fluid signal on MRI.[19] Partial tears are manifest by partial thickness ligament disruption or irregularity of the ligament in association with soft tissue edema (Fig. 12.4).[19] The MPFL can be injured at its patellar origin (see Fig. 12.1),[41,44] at or near its femoral insertion (see Figs. 12.2 and 12.3),[6,57,58] at its midsubstance,[6] or in more than one location.[6,24]

MR is reported to be 85% sensitive and 80% accurate in detecting MPFL injury and has been found to be better than arthroscopy[7] at detecting injuries at its femoral insertion.

MPFL injury is often associated with stripping and elevation of vastus medialis obliquus muscle from its adductor tubercle attachment.[24] Edema and hemorrhage along the inferior border of the VMO are best appreciated on sagittal images (see Fig. 12.2).

Chondral/Osteochondral Injury. Patellar, trochlear, and lateral femoral condylar chondral/osteochondral injuries are reported to occur in up to 95% following LPD.[60,87] These are often radiographically occult. MR has been shown to be highly sensitive and specific for the detection of high-grade cartilage lesions in the setting of LPD.[87]

There are two sites of patellar cartilage injury: at the median ridge related to dislocation, and at the inferomedial patellar facet related to patellar relocation.[68] Injuries to the median ridge patellar articular cartilage are related to shear and can result in a partial or full thickness injury (see Figs. 12.1 and 12.5). Injuries at the inferomedial patella are related to impaction and can result in a concave osteochondral injury (see Figs. 12.1, 12.2, 12.4, and 12.5); this finding was shown to be 44% sensitive and 100% specific for LPD.[24]

Femoral cartilage injuries are less common than patellar cartilage injuries[60,73,87] and occur in two distinct and separate regions. Those that occur along the lateral femoral trochlea are thought to be secondary to shear injury. These full or partial thickness articular cartilage defects of the femoral trochlea are best appreciated on axial images (see Fig. 12.1). Osteochondral injuries can also occur along the central surface of the midlateral femoral condyle.[68] These injuries of weight-bearing femoral condylar articular cartilage are likely the result of pivot-shift mechanism of injury and are best seen on coronal and sagittal images (see Fig. 12.4). In Zlatkin's study, 50% of patients had osteochondral injuries of the lateral femoral condyle, 30% had osteochondral injuries of the femoral trochlea, and 20% had both.[68]

*References 3, 14, 18, 25, 59, and 84.

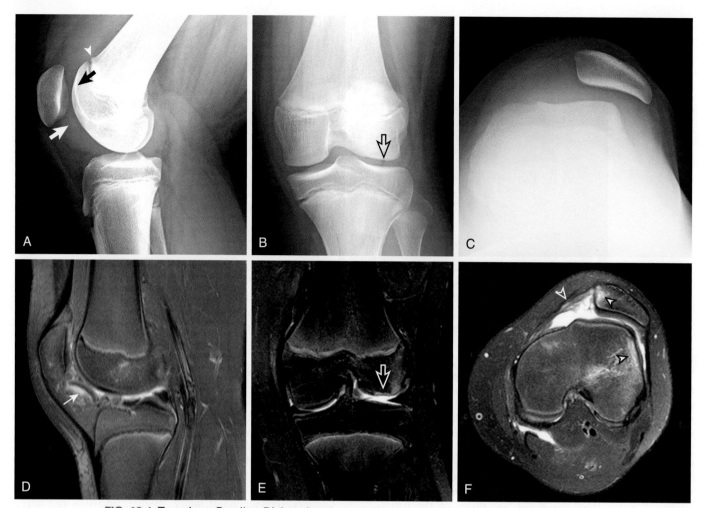

FIG 12.4 Transient Patellar Dislocation Lateral (A), frontal (B), and tangential patellar (C) radiographs, and sagittal fat suppressed proton density (D), coronal fat suppressed proton density (E), and fat suppressed T2 (F) MRI of the knee in an 11-year-old who presented after sports injury. Radiographs show osteochondral fragment in the anterior joint (*white arrow*, A), loss of lateral femoral cortical outline (*open black arrow*, B), and lateral patellar subluxation (C). "Crossing sign" (*black arrow*, A) and small supratrochlear spur (*white arrowhead*, A) indicate TD, and there is patella alta. MRI obtained 1 week later confirms the displaced osteochondral fragment (*white arrow*, D), lateral femoral condylar donor site (*open white arrow*, E), medial patellar osteochondral injury and lateral femoral condylar bone contusion (*open black arrowheads*, F), and partial mid-substance tear of the stretched medial retinaculum (*open white arrowhead*, F). The lateral trochlear facet is convex and the medial facet hypoplastic (F).

RISK FACTORS FOR LATERAL PATELLAR DISLOCATION

Patellar dislocation commonly occurs in anatomically pre-disposed knees.[10] Increased risk of LPD has been associated with patella alta, trochlear dysplasia (TD), abnormal patellar morphology, lateral patellar displacement, increased Q angle with lateralized tibial tuberosity, genu valgum, vastus medialis muscle hypoplasia, ligament hyperlaxity, external tibial torsion, subtalar joint pronation, and increased femoral anteversion.[78] Individuals who suffer from recurrent dislocation have been shown to have more than one anatomic risk factor.[77] Patella alta, TD, and increased tibial tubercle-trochlear groove (TT-TG) distance can be evaluated on a routine MR examination of the knee.

Patella Alta

In extension and early flexion, before patellar-trochlear engage-ment, the patella is dependent on soft tissues for its stability and therefore more vulnerable to displacement. Because a knee with high riding patella must be in deeper flexion before the trochlea can provide constraint, those with patella alta are at higher risk for patellar dislocation.[49] The radiographic method of Insall-Salvati is commonly used for patellar height assessment and has been validated for MR[55,74] for its accuracy and reproducibility. Using this method, patella alta is diagnosed with a threshold of greater than 1.3.[55]

Trochlear Dysplasia

The trochlea provides the major restraint to lateral patellar displacement once the knee is flexed beyond 30 degrees.[48] A

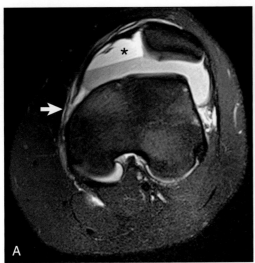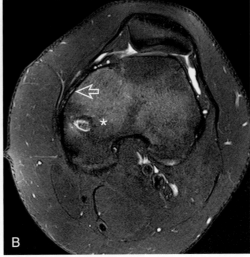

FIG 12.5 Transient Patellar Dislocation Axial fat suppressed T2 weighted images obtained at the level of the upper (A) and mid trochlea (B). The medial retinaculum is torn at its femoral insertion and at its midsubstance (*white arrow*, A), and there are impaction injuries of the infero-medial patella (*star*, B) and nonarticular lateral femoral condyle (*asterisk*, B). There is an osteo-chondral injury of the median ridge patellar articular cartilage (*open white arrow*, B) with displaced osteochondral fragment (*open black arrow*, B).

dysplastic trochlea is shallow, short, and geometrically abnormal and thus morphologically less able to resist lateral patellar displacement.[10,94] TD is a risk factor for LPD; it is seen in 96% of individuals with patellar instability[17] and in up to 85% in those with recurrent instability.[17] It is also associated with abnormalities of patellar tracking, increased contact pressures, and patellofemoral osteoarthritis.[37,85]

Assessment of trochlear morphology is classically made on properly positioned lateral radiographs on which the femoral condyles superimpose. Imaging findings include the crossing sign, double contour sign, and supratrochlear spur, which is discussed in greater detail elsewhere in this text (Fig. 12.6). However, as little as 5 degrees rotation can result in false positive and false negative diagnosis of TD.[45] Axial views taken in 30 degrees flexion can also underdiagnose TD, because dysplastic morphology is more common in the proximal aspect of the trochlea.[80]

Cross sectional imaging (MR, CT) can be used to evaluate trochlear morphology and is less affected by differences in patient positioning. Pfirrmann et al.[65] studied TD on MRI and established several quantitative and qualitative criteria for TD. Trochlear groove depth less than 3 mm, 3 cm above the joint was 100% sensitive and 96% specific. Ventral trochlear prominence greater than 8 mm, measured on the sagittal image at the deepest point in the groove, was 75% sensitive and 83% specific. Trochlear facet asymmetry with the medial facet much smaller than the lateral facet was seen in dysplastic trochlea; when measured 3 cm above the joint, a medial to lateral facet length ratio greater than 0.4 was 100% sensitive and 96% specific. Lateral patellar position greater than 6 mm with respect to the lateral femoral condyle was found to be 75% sensitive and 83% specific.[65] Carrillon et al. also found flattening of the lateral trochlear angle, measured by the lateral trochlear inclination angle at the most proximal aspect of the trochlea, to be 93% sensitive and 87% specific for identifying TD when a threshold value of 11 degrees or less was used.[13]

Tibial Tubercle-Trochlear Groove Distance

First described by Goutallier et al.[29] on plain radiographs and later modified for CT by Dejour et al.,[17] the TT-TG distance is a measure of the degree of tibial tubercle lateralization and an indirect assessment of the inferolateral force vector on the patella. The TT-TG distance reflects the linear distance between the center of the tibial tubercle and the deepest point of the bony trochlear groove with the knee extended and can be measured on axial CT or MR images.[72] Increased TT-TG distance, which indicates greater lateralization of the tibial tubercle, is associated with increased risk of LPD. It has been shown that patients with recurrent LPD have TT-TG distances that measure greater than 20 mm.[17]

QUADRICEPS AND PATELLAR TENDINOPATHY AND TENDON TEAR

The quadriceps muscle group is made up of the rectus femoris muscle and three vastus muscles, whose tendons converge to form the quadriceps tendon. The quadriceps tendon, primarily central rectus femoris fibers, continues over the surface of the patella to become the patellar tendon.[4] The patella, a sesamoid bone embedded in the quadriceps tendon, links the quadriceps and patellar tendons and assists the quadriceps muscle group by directing its forces and increasing its mechanical advantage.[26] Together, the quadriceps and patellar tendons and the patellar retinacular complex form a strong connective tissue network that allows the quadriceps muscle group to function as a knee extensor.[92]

The quadriceps tendon anatomy is reflected in its MRI appearance. On sagittal MR images, the stratified tendon arrangement results in a multilaminar structure, with low signal tendons separated by interspersed high signal fat on short TE sequences (proton density, T1) without fat suppression. The deepest layer is formed by the vastus intermedius tendon. The middle layer is formed by the vastus lateralis and vastus medius

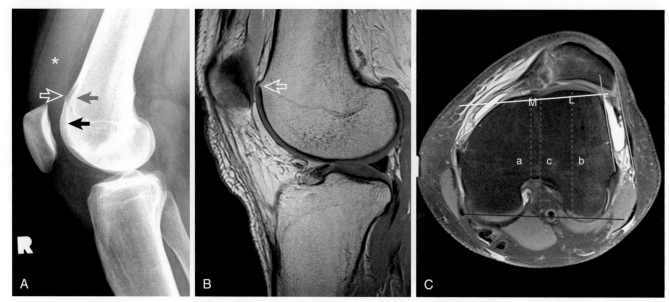

FIG 12.6 Transient Patellar Dislocation-Trochlear Dysplasia 27-year-old woman who presented after patellar dislocation. Lateral radiograph (A) shows crossing sign *(black arrow)*, double contour sign *(gray arrow)*, and supratrochlear spur *(open white arrow)*. There is a joint effusion *(asterisk)*. Sagittal proton density MR image (B) shows supratrochlear spur *(open white arrow)*. Axial fat suppressed proton density weighted MR image 3 cm above the joint (C) shows convex lateral trochlea. Trochlear groove is shallow; its depth is calculated as the average of the maximum AP measurement of the medial *(a)* and lateral *(b)* femoral condyle minus the distance between the deepest point of the trochlear groove and a line connecting the posterior outlines of the femoral condyles ([a + b]/2 − c). The lateral trochlear inclination angle, formed by a line connecting the posterior outlines of the femoral condyles and one along the lateral trochlea, is diminished. The patella is lateralized; the lateral most point of the patella is more than 6 mm lateral to a line paralleling the lateral surface of the femoral condyle. There is significant facet asymmetry; the medial facet *(M)* is much shorter than the lateral *(L)*.

tendons, which may appear as a single layer or two separate layers. The rectus femoris tendon forms the most superficial layer; its fibers continue over the patella to form the patellar tendon. The deep surface of the tendon is lined with synovium.[76]

The patellar tendon fans out to insert on the anterior tibia and tibial tubercle.[56] The patellar tendon is generally homogeneously low signal on MRI, regardless of pulse sequence. Subtle intermediate intratendinous signal may be seen along its deep surface at its origin and insertion in asymptomatic individuals.[16]

Tendinopathy

Patellar tendinopathy is a potentially disabling overuse injury of the extensor mechanism. It is a common injury in athletes who participate in sports with high demands on the leg extensors.[50]

In the setting of tendinopathy, increased tendon signal may be accompanied by an increase in tendon size and reactive changes in the adjacent bone and surrounding soft tissues. This is most common in the medial, deep tendon fibers at their patellar insertion,[93] where tensile stress is greatest.[54] Distal tendon pathology has been observed in volleyball players but is much less common.[70] Deep surface tendon tears are depicted by intratendinous fluid signal and tendon fiber discontinuity (Fig. 12.7).[2]

Clinically significant quadriceps tendinopathy is less common than patellar tendinopathy, although it has been reported in

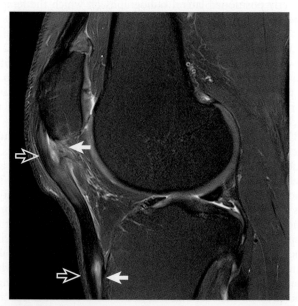

FIG 12.7 Patellar Tendinopathy Sagittal fat suppressed proton density MR image. Diffuse thickening and increased signal in the proximal and distal patellar tendons compatible with proximal and distal insertional tendinopathy *(open white arrows)*. There is superimposed partial tear of the deep tendon at its origin and focal intrasubstance tendon tear of the distal tendon near its insertion *(white arrows)*.

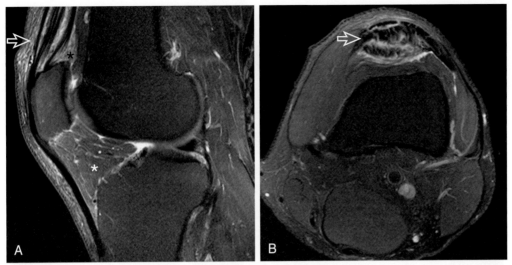

FIG 12.8 Quadriceps Tendinopathy Sagittal fat suppressed proton density (A) and axial fat suppressed T2 MR images. The quadriceps tendon is thickened and increased in signal as a result of tendinopathy (*open arrow*, A and B). There is reactive edema in the quadriceps fat pad (*black asterisk*, A). The signal in the infrapatellar fat pad, in comparison, is normal (*white asterisk*, A).

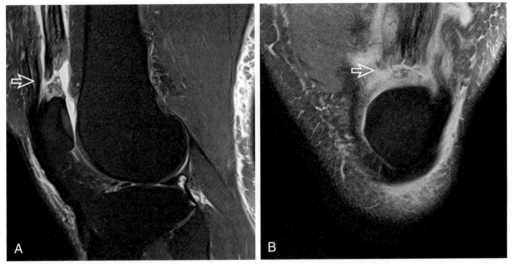

FIG 12.9 Quadriceps Tendon Rupture Sagittal (A) and coronal (B) fat suppressed proton density MR images show complete distal quadriceps tendon rupture (*open arrows*, A and B).

elite volleyball players.[64] MRI findings include increased tendon signal and size.[91] There may also be reactive edema in the quadriceps fat pad (Fig. 12.8).

Tendon Tear

In general, normal tendons do not rupture under stress,[39] although in some rare instances healthy tendons can rupture as a result of acute tendon overload. More commonly, chronic overuse or intrinsic tendon degeneration results in tendinopathy, which weakens the tendon and makes it more vulnerable to rupture.

Quadriceps tendon rupture tends to occur in individuals over the age of 40 and in tendons compromised by systemic disease, chronic use of certain medications, or underlying tendon degeneration. History and clinical exam findings are often dramatic and diagnostic of quadriceps tendon ruptures;

however, in the acute setting, clinical diagnosis can be missed in up to 50% of cases.[69] Active knee extension may be preserved when the quadriceps tendon is only partially torn or the integrity of the retinaculae are preserved.[8] Joint effusion, suprapatellar masses, osseous avulsion, and patella baja on plain radiographs may infer injury if present.[38] Tendon pathology can be readily assessed on MRI or ultrasound, but MR is more specific for distinguishing between complete and partial tears.[63,81] MR can confirm the diagnosis, delineate the extent of injury, and quantify the amount of tendon retraction.

Partial quadriceps tendon tears are manifest by disruption of any of the tendon layers; full thickness tears involve all tendon layers.[92] Complete quadriceps tendon tears most commonly occur at the patellar insertion and may involve the full width (Figs. 12.9 and 12.10) or partial width (Fig. 12.11) of the tendon.[56] There is often a fluid filled gap or hemorrhage

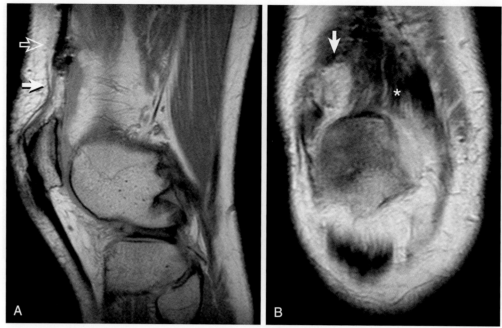

FIG 12.10 Quadriceps Tendon Repair, Two Patients Sagittal fat suppressed proton density MR image in one patient (A) shows a tract (*open arrow*, A) through the upper portion of the patella and susceptibility artifact in the distal quadriceps tendon related to previous quadriceps tendon repair. The tendon is intact although the tendon no longer has a multilaminar appearance. Sagittal fat suppressed proton density MR image in another patient (B) shows full thickness tear of the tendon (*arrow*, B) in a patient who had previous quadriceps tendon repair indicated by susceptibility artifact in the torn and retracted tendon and in the patella (*asterisk*, B).

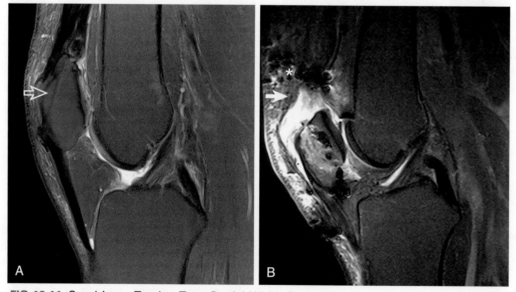

FIG 12.11 Quadriceps Tendon Tear, Partial Width Sagittal (A) and coronal (B) proton density MR images shows full thickness tear of the lateral portion of the quadriceps tendon (*arrows*, A and B). The medial tendon is intact (*asterisk*, B). Susceptibility artifact is seen in the distal tendon related to previous tendon repair (*open arrow*, A).

at the site of rupture, which is best seen on sagittal and axial images. The torn tendon can be proximally retracted. The patella may be displaced distally, and the patellar tendon can appear redundant or lax.

Patellar tendon rupture is less common[56]; those affected are younger than 40 years and have a history of chronic tendinopathy.[75] The tendon most commonly ruptures at its patellar origin (Fig. 12.12).[39]

MRI can be used to evaluate the status of the repaired tendon. The repaired quadriceps tendon may no longer have the normal laminar appearance after repair as a result of scar remodeling (see Fig. 12.10). The diagnosis of a re-tear is made

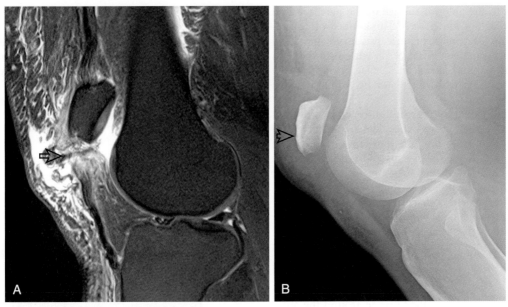

FIG 12.12 Patellar Tendon Rupture Sagittal fat suppressed proton density MR image (A) and lateral knee radiograph (B) shows complete rupture of the patellar tendon at its patellar origin (*open black arrow*, A). The patella is proximally retracted (*arrow*, B).

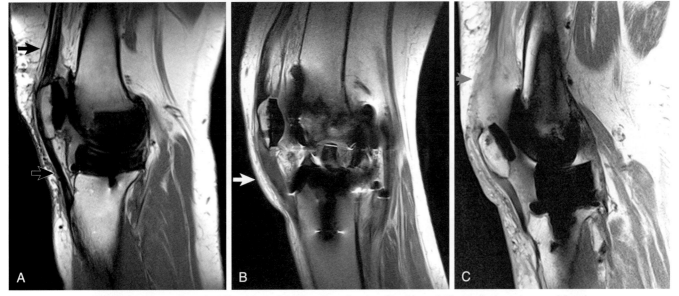

FIG 12.13 Imaging the Extensor Mechanism in the Setting of Knee Arthroplasty—Metal Artifact Reduction Techniques in Three Patients Sagittal proton density WARP view angle tilting (VAT) MR image (A) shows normal appearance of the quadriceps and patellar tendons *(black arrows)*. Sagittal slice-encoding metal artifact correction (SEMAC) MR image (B) in another patient shows diffuse thickening and increased signal in the patellar tendon in the setting of diffuse patellar tendinopathy *(white arrow)*. Sagittal proton density WARP VAT MR image (C) in a third patient with complete rupture of the quadriceps tendon *(gray arrow)*.

when fluid filled tendon gaps are identified (see Figs. 12.10 and 12.11).

Quadriceps or patellar tendon rupture is a rare but devastating complication of total knee arthroplasty.[21] It affects the quadriceps tendon in 0.1% to 1.1% of cases[5,21] and the patellar tendon in 0.17% to 1.4% of cases.[51,66] Tendon ruptures are well seen on MRI, particularly if metal artifact reduction techniques are used (Fig. 12.13).

PREPATELLAR QUADRICEPS CONTINUATION

In their anatomic studies, Dye et al.[23] revealed three separate layers of tissue anterior to the patella: a superficial fascial layer, an intermediate aponeurotic layer, and a deep layer composed of those rectus femoris tendon fibers that continue distally to form the patellar tendon. Anatomic bursae were found in between each layer except deep to the rectus femoris layer,[23] which is attached to the anterior surface of the patella via an irregular fibrocartilaginous interface.[89] This aponeurotic structure was termed the "prepatellar quadriceps continuation" in a cadaveric study by Wangwinyuvirat et al., who also observed merging of the medial and lateral retinaculae, formed by the aponeurosis of vastus medialis and lateralis, with this deep central aponeurotic band.[89]

Normally, the individual layers are not discernible as distinct structures on sagittal MRI; instead a low signal intensity band can be appreciated coursing over the anterior surface of the patella, continuous with the quadriceps and patellar tendons and not discernible as a separate structure from the patellar cortex on MR.[89] When the prepatellar bursa is fluid distended, two or three laminae may be seen, corresponding to the superficial fascial and intermediate aponeurotic layers.[1]

Disruption of the prepatellar quadriceps continuation can occur without injury to the quadriceps and patellar tendons (Fig. 12.14).[52,89]

Bursae

There are three commonly identified bursae around the anterior knee: the deep and superficial infrapatellar bursae and the superficial prepatellar bursa. Bursae are present at sites of mechanical friction, providing cushion and facilitating gliding.

The superficial prepatellar bursa is located in the soft tissues anterior to the patella (Fig. 12.15) and may have a multilaminar appearance resulting from variably present prepatellar fascial layers.[23]

The deep infrapatellar bursa is located deep to the tibial insertion of the patellar tendon. It can be compartmentalized by the presence of an apron-like projection of the infrapatellar fat pad[47] giving it a V shaped appearance on sagittal MR images when fluid filled (Fig. 12.16). Deep infrapatellar bursitis can develop as a result of overuse injury of the extensor mechanism, particularly of runners and jumpers. The bursa can also be affected by infection, gout, and ankylosing spondylitis.[86]

The superficial infrapatellar bursa is located in the soft tissues superficial to the distal patellar tendon (Fig 12.17).

It may become distended as a result of chronic mechanical friction.

On MRI, bursitis is diagnosed when fluid distends these anatomic bursae. Inflammation and hemorrhage can result in a more heterogeneous appearance, and inflammatory changes in the surrounding soft tissues may be present.[79] A small amount of fluid in the deep infrapatellar bursa is commonly seen on MRI in asymptomatic individuals (see Fig. 12.17).[83]

Fat Pad Impingement

There are three intracapsular, extrasynovial fat pads around the knee[76]: the suprapatellar or quadriceps fat pad, the prefemoral or supratrochlear fat pad, and the infrapatellar or Hoffa's fat pad. The roles the fat pads play in normal knee function are

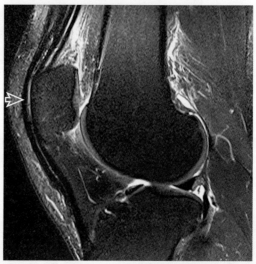

FIG 12.14 Old Prepatellar Quadriceps Continuation Injury Sagittal fat suppressed proton density MR image. The superficial fibers of the quadriceps tendon are anteriorly displaced from the patellar cortex *(open arrow)*.

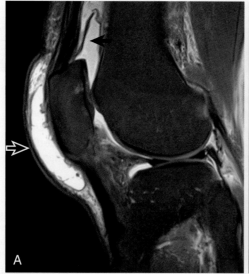
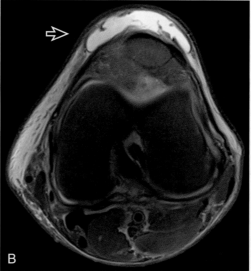

FIG 12.15 Prepatellar Bursitis Sagittal fat suppressed proton density (A) and axial fat suppressed T2 MR image. There is a well-defined fluid collection anterior to the patella *(open arrow, A and B)*. A superior plica is noted incidentally *(black arrow, A)*.

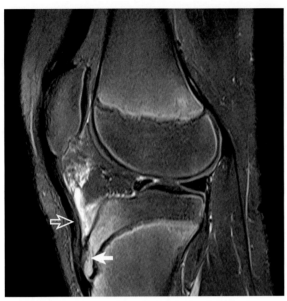

FIG 12.16 Deep Infrapatellar Bursitis Sagittal fat suppressed proton density MR image. There is a V shaped collection deep to the patellar tendon near its tibial insertion *(open arrow)*. Edema in the tibial tubercle *(white arrow)* is also present in this patient with Osgood Schlatter's disease.

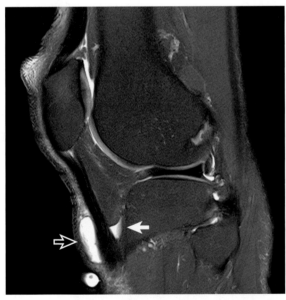

FIG 12.17 Superficial Infrapatellar Bursitis Sagittal fat suppressed proton density MR image. There is a well-defined fluid collection anterior to the patellar tendon near its tibial insertion *(open arrow)*. Small amount of fluid is present in the deep infrapatellar bursa *(white arrow)*.

debated; they may enhance gliding, provide a protective cushion, and facilitate distribution of synovial fluid in the joint.[67]

The infrapatellar fat pad (IPF) has been most vigorously studied. It is richly innervated by type IV free nerve endings, which transmit information on pain and inflammation, and nerve fibers positive for substance P, a neuropeptide that plays a role in the transmission of pain.[9,94] A preliminary

immunohistochemical study showed increased concentration of substance P positive nerves in the infrapatellar fat pad in patients with anterior knee pain; this supports a role of the IPF in anterior knee pain.[90] There is also early evidence to support its role in the development of osteoarthritis.[33]

Infrapatellar Fat Pad

The IFP, also known as Hoffa's fat pad, fills the space between the patella and patellar tendon, and the tibia and the femoral condyles. It projects into the intercondylar notch via two synovial folds that fuse to form the infrapatellar plica,[67] which secures it to the femur. It is also attached to the inferior patella, the patellar tendon and anterior joint capsule, and the anterior horns of the menisci and proximal tibia.[27] The IFP has been shown to have a consistent shape, composed of a thick central body and thinner medial and lateral extensions[27] that overlie the anterior aspect of the distal femur.[67]

The infrapatellar fat pad is easily evaluated on axial and sagittal MR images as a homogenous structure with signal characteristic typical of fat (see Fig. 12.8). On sagittal images, the central body may be interrupted by two synovial-lined clefts (the vertical and horizontal clefts), which are most conspicuous in the presence of a joint effusion or pathology. The vertical cleft is located within the superior aspect of the fat pad and the horizontal cleft more posterior and inferior.[27,67] The superolateral extension of the IFP can be evaluated on axial and sagittal images.

The IFP may be affected by intrinsic disease (Hoffa's disease, localized nodular synovitis, postsurgical fibrosis) and extrinsic disease (articular, synovial, and extracapsular).[34]

Hoffa's disease is the result of chronic fat pad impingement, whereby a potentially self-perpetuating pathologic process results in chronic inflammation of the IFP. Whether incited by acute or repetitive trauma, the resulting hemorrhage and inflammation can lead to fat pad enlargement, which makes it more prone to repeated impingement between the femur and tibia.[30,32]

Fluid-sensitive MR sequences reveal increased signals in the fat pad resulting from edema and hemorrhage in the acute stage (Fig. 12.18).[34] The enlarged fat pad may cause the patellar tendon to bow from its mass effect. Later, fibrosis, hemosiderin deposition, and rarely calcification can develop; this is manifest as a decreased signal on T1 and fluid sensitive sequences.[34]

Abnormalities of the superolateral extension of the IPF have recently been studied with regard to patellar maltracking and anterior knee pain. Patella alta, increased TT-TG distance, lateral patellar tilt, and lateral patellar displacement have all been seen on MR examinations in patients with edema in superolateral Hoffa's fat.[12,36,53] These findings, however, may not always be symptomatic.[30] Edema of the superolateral extension of the IPF, often between the lateral retinaculum and lateral femoral condyle, can be appreciated on fluid sensitive axial and sagittal images (Fig 12.19).

Quadriceps Fat Pad

Triangular in sagittal cross section, the quadriceps fat pad (QFP) fills the gap between the deep surface of the quadriceps tendon and the superior aspect of the patella. It articulates with the prefemoral fat when the knee is extended and the trochlear cartilage when the knee is flexed, and it provides a gliding surface for the deep portion of the distal quadriceps tendon.[76]

Increased signal in the QFP may be seen in the setting of underlying quadriceps tendon pathology (see Fig. 12.8). As an isolated finding, however, QFP edema and mass effect (based on increased T2 signal and convex margin of the joint facing surface) may or may not be symptomatic.[82,88]

Prefemoral Fat Pad

The literature is limited to a case report of symptomatic prefemoral fat pad abnormalities. Kim et al. reported a case of a 27-year-old woman with years of continuous knee pain, worsening with knee flexion and associated with intermittent mechanical symptoms, who had mass-like fatty tissue in the prefemoral fat on MRI and at arthroscopy.[43] Edema in the prefemoral fat can be seen on fluid sensitive axial and sagittal images (see Fig. 12.18).

PLICA

Synovial plicae are believed to represent incompletely resorbed embryonic synovial membranes. These can be seen on MRI as thin, linear low signal structures in characteristic locations[28]: the suprapatellar joint (superior plica), medial and lateral joint (medial and lateral plica), and anteroinferior joint (inferior plica). Normally thin and pliable, plica can become thick and inflexible as a result of acute or repetitive injury, or synovitis.[71] These pathologic plica appear thickened on MRI and may be seen with synovitis and wear of femoral or patellar cartilage.[28]

The superior plica extends from the anterior femoral metaphyseal synovium to the posterior surface of the quadriceps tendon above the patella.[28] It may be variably fenestrated or completely separate the suprapatellar recess from the remainder of the joint. Complete plica may be associated with recurrent effusions; fenestrated plica may act like valves to allow fluid to accumulate in the suprapatellar region of the joint above the plica.[15,71] The superior patellar plica is best seen on sagittal MR images as a low signal linear tissue in the suprapatellar joint (see Fig. 12.15).[28]

The inferior plica (ligamentum mucosum) arises from the intercondylar notch of the femur anterior to the anterior cruciate ligament (ACL) and traverses through the infrapatellar fat, where it may terminate or continue on to insert on inferior patella.[15] It forms the roof of the horizontal cleft. The inferior plica varies in thickness; when seen, the intercondylar component appears as a linear low signal intensity structure paralleling the distal ACL on sagittal MR images and is more conspicuous when outlined by fluid. The portion of the plica that traverses Hoffa's fat is rarely

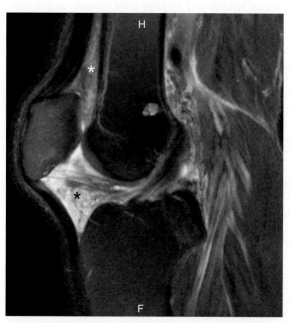

FIG 12.18 Hoffa's Disease Sagittal fat suppressed proton density MR image. Diffuse edema and enlargement of Hoffa's fat pad (*black asterisk*). There is also edema in the prefemoral (*white asterisk*) and quadriceps fat pads in this patient.

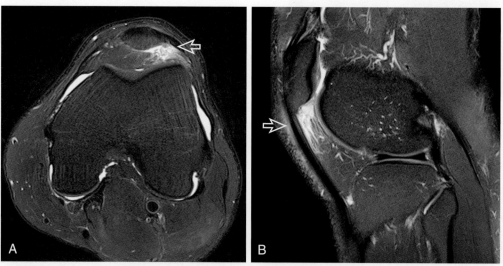

FIG 12.19 Superolateral Hoffa's Fat Pad Impingement Axial fat suppressed T2 (A) and sagittal fat suppressed proton density (B) MR image. There is localized edema in superolateral Hoffa's fat (*open arrow*, A and B). There is patella alta.

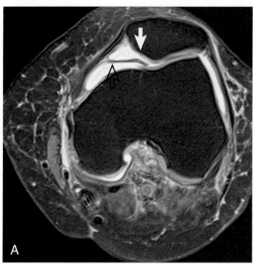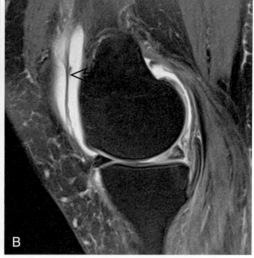

FIG 12.20 Medial Patellar Plica Axial fat suppressed T2 (A) and sagittal fat suppressed proton density (B) MR images. The medial patellar plica is thickened and interposed between the medial patella and trochlea *(open arrow)*. There is a partial thickness cartilage loss of the subjacent medial patellar facet *(white arrow)*.

visualized. Pathologic inferior plica have rarely been implicated in anterior knee pain; this is limited to case reports in the literature.[11]

The medial plica is a sheet-like structure oriented in the coronal plane that arises from the medial knee synovium and inserts on the synovial lining of the infrapatellar fat pad.[28] Of the knee synovial plica, the medial plica is most commonly symptomatic. A large, shelf-like medial plica may interpose itself between the femoral condyle and patella and impinge on the medial patellar or medial femoral cartilage (Fig. 12.20).[28] The medial plica can be seen on sagittal and axial images; the associated articular cartilage injuries are best depicted on axial images (Fig. 12.21).

The lateral plica is not common. An arthroscopic study by Kim et al. found the incidence of lateral plica to be 1.3% in their study group (as opposed to the 87%, 72%, and 86% incidence of superior, medial, and inferior plica, respectively).[42] It is not known to be a common cause of symptoms.

BIPARTITE PATELLA

The patella is formed via fusion of primary and secondary ossification centers. When accessory ossification centers fail to fuse in adolescence, bipartite or multipartite patellae result. Failure of fusion commonly occurs in the superolateral quadrant (at the insertion of vastus lateralis, type III); it is more common in men and frequently bilateral.[40] Unfused ossification centers may also occur at the inferior pole (type 1) and lateral margin (type 2) of the patella. The bipartite patella is considered a normal variant that occurs in 1% to 2% of the population[61] and is identified incidentally on MRI. Edema in the bipartite fragment and on either side of the synchondrosis or pseudoarthrosis on fluid sensitive sequences, however, may correlate with anterior knee pain (Fig. 12.22)[40] and be the result of motion or stress at the synchondrosis.[61] The presence of a sclerotic margin and rounded contour and presentation with

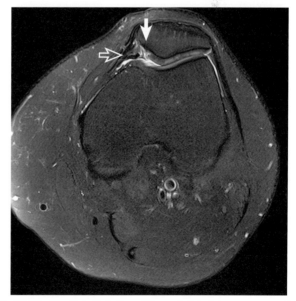

FIG 12.21 Medial Patellar Plica Axial fat suppressed T2 weighted MR image. The medial patellar plica is thickened and interposed between the medial patella and trochlea *(open arrow)*. There is a full thickness cartilage defect of the subjacent medial patellar facet *(white arrow)*.

dull ache after trauma can help differentiate between a bipartite patella and acute fracture.[62]

CONCLUSION

Disorders of the extensor mechanism are responsible for a wide range of pathologic conditions. MRI is a relatively fast, noninvasive method for the evaluation of the knee and is well suited for the assessment of the extensor mechanism.

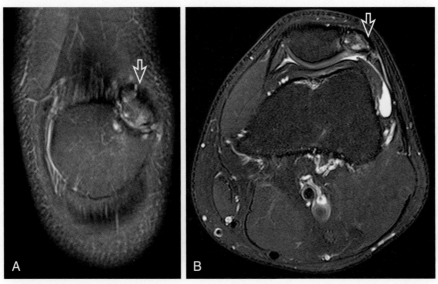

FIG 12.22 Type III Bipartite Patella Coronal fat suppressed proton density (A) and axial fat suppressed T2 (B) MR image. There is an unfused superolateral accessory ossification center (*open arrow*, A and B). Edema in the os and in the adjacent patella and at the synchondrosis has been shown to be associated with symptoms.

KEY REFERENCES

4. Andrikoula S, Tokis A, Vasiliadis HS, et al: The extensor mechanism of the knee joint: an anatomical study. *Knee Surg Sports Traumatol Arthrosc* 14(3):214–220, 2006.

10. Bollier M, Fulkerson JP: The role of trochlear dysplasia in patellofemoral instability. *J Am Acad Orthop Surg* 19(1):8–16, 2011.

19. Diederichs G, Issever AS, Scheffler S: MR imaging of patellar instability: injury patterns and assessment of risk factors. *Radiographics* 30(4):961–981, 2010.

24. Elias DA, White LM, Fithian DC: Acute lateral patellar dislocation at MR imaging: injury patterns of medial patellar soft-tissue restraints and osteochondral injuries of the inferomedial patella. *Radiology* 225(3):736–743, 2002.

28. García-Valtuille R, Abascal F, Cerezal L, et al: Anatomy and MR imaging appearances of synovial plicae of the knee. *Radiographics* 22(4):775–784, 2002.

30. Grando H, Chang EY, Chen KC, et al: MR imaging of extrasynovial inflammation and impingement about the knee. *Magn Reson Imaging Clin N Am* 22(4):725–741, 2014.

40. Kavanagh EC, Zoga A, Omar I, et al: MRI findings in bipartite patella. *Skeletal Radiol* 36(3):209–214, 2007.

64. Pfirrmann CWA, Jost B, Pirkl C, et al: Quadriceps tendinosis and patellar tendinosis in professional beach volleyball players: sonographic findings in correlation with clinical symptoms. *Eur Radiol* 18(8):1703–1709, 2008.

65. Pfirrmann CWA, Zanetti M, Romero J, et al: Femoral trochlear dysplasia: MR findings. *Radiology* 216(3):858–864, 2000.

68. Sanders TG, Paruchuri NB, Zlatkin MB: MRI of osteochondral defects of the lateral femoral condyle: incidence and pattern of injury after transient lateral dislocation of the patella. *AJR Am J Roentgenol* 187(5):1332–1337, 2006.

89. Wangwinyuvirat M, Dirim B, Pastore D, et al: Prepatellar quadriceps continuation: MRI of cadavers with gross anatomic and histologic correlation. *AJR Am J Roentgenol* 192(3):W111–W116, 2009.

94. Zaffagnini S, Dejour D, Arendt EA, editors: *Patellofemoral pain, instability, and arthritis: clinical presentation, imaging, and treatment*, Heidelberg, New York, NY, 2010, Springer, p 331.

The references for this chapter can also be found on www.expertconsult.com.

13

Imaging of Total Knee Arthroplasty

Michael K. Brooks, Christopher J. Palestro, Barbara N. Weissman

Total knee arthroplasty (TKA) results in improvement in overall quality of life in more than 90% of patients.[117] This remarkable success and factors such as an aging population have led to a dramatic increase in the number of procedures performed and to a corresponding increase in the number of imaging studies obtained for assessment. In addition to radiography, computed tomography (CT), magnetic resonance imaging (MRI), ultrasonography (US), arthrography, and a number of nuclear medicine studies are now available for evaluation of knee arthroplasty. It is the responsibility of both imagers and clinicians to provide the most efficacious and cost-effective examinations in a particular clinical situation. This chapter reviews some available imaging techniques, expected findings in uncomplicated and complicated cases, and the efficacy of various techniques in assessing complications.

IMAGING

Radiographs

Preoperative Radiographs. Preoperative radiographs often include supine anteroposterior (AP) and lateral and tangential patellar views of the affected knee, as well as standing AP and flexed posteroanterior (PA) views of both knees and an AP standing radiograph of both legs.[104] At the Brigham and Women's Hospital, lateral radiographs are usually obtained cross-table lateral with the knee in maximal extension. When digital radiographs are used, a standard-sized reference object is placed alongside the knee to allow assessment of magnification.

The standing view of both legs allows the mechanical axis (a line drawn from the center of the femoral head to the center of the talus) and anatomical axis (a line drawn along the length of the intramedullary canal of either the femur or the tibia) to be defined.[30] Normally, the mechanical axis passes through the center of the knee or just medial to it, and the angle between the anatomic axis of the femur and the mechanical axis measures 5 to 8 degrees.[30,107] Standing radiographs of the legs are used to plan the femoral resection, so as to re-create normal mechanical alignment. McGrory et al., however, found that this examination did not significantly aid in obtaining a neutral mechanical axis as compared with performing a standard femoral cut of 5 degrees.[104] Huang et al. found measurement of the mechanical axis to have a variability of 1 to 3 degrees.[72]

Postoperative Radiographs. Imaging performed immediately after surgery may not be ideal because the radiographs are obtained supine and may not reflect the correct alignment as determined on subsequent standing radiographs.[133] Typically at the Brigham and Women's Hospital, radiographs are instead performed at the first postoperative visit. At that time, both supine radiographs (AP, lateral, and tangential patellar views) and standing radiographs[144] are obtained.

Normal Postoperative Radiographic Appearances

Alignment. Because coronal malalignment can lead to decreased implant survival[29] and accelerated wear, careful analysis of component position and leg alignment is warranted. Radiographs are an effective means of evaluating component position in sagittal and coronal planes.

Anteroposterior and lateral knee radiographs. Component position on AP and lateral knee radiographs can be assessed as in Fig. 13.1. The tibial resection is generally perpendicular to the anatomic axis of the tibia.[11] Femoral resection is more complex because of the desire to remove the femur perpendicular to its mechanical axis. Approximately 5 to 8 degrees of valgus is present between the femoral condyles and the anatomic axis of the femur.[107] The posterior/inferior tilt of the tibial component can be assessed on the lateral radiograph. Various axis reference lines have been used for this assessment. Increased down sloping of the tibial component (with posterior cruciate ligament [PCL] retaining components) can increase maximum flexion, but excessive tibial downslope can lead to anterior tibial subluxation, posterior polyethylene (PE) wear, and lack of extension.[16]

Standing radiographs

Axial alignment. Angulation of the knee in the coronal plane can be measured on standing radiographs of the legs. Conventional radiographs or digital radiographs can be used for this assessment.[149]

The mechanical axis. A line drawn from the center of the femoral head to the center of the talus (Maquet's line) should intersect the center of the knee (Fig. 13.2).[78,107] The femoral and tibial components should be perpendicular to this line,[107] and the joint space should be parallel to the ground.[169] Deviations from this alignment should be minimal (within 3 degrees of the normal mechanical axis).[180] Because higher loosening rates have been described in this situation, some authors consider axial malalignment as mechanical alignment outside the range of 1 degree varus to 2 degrees valgus.[18] However, the significance of deviations from this line on implant survival has been questioned.[129]

The joint line. In 1986, Figgie et al. noted that restoration of the tibial patellofemoral relationships had an impact on function in patients receiving posterior stabilized condylar knee prostheses.[46] Change of 8 mm or less in the height of the joint line (JL) (measured as the perpendicular distance from the weight-bearing surface of the tibial plateau to the tibial tubercle) resulted in better functional knee scores, improved range of

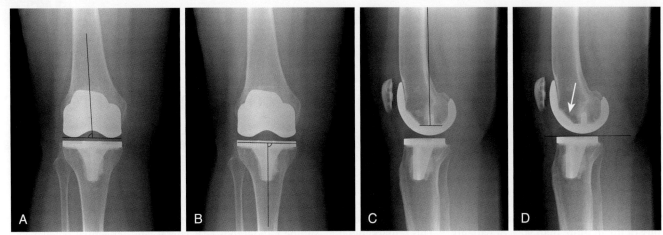

FIG 13.1 Normal Component Positioning on Standing Knee Radiographs (A) AP view of the knee demonstrates the method of measuring femoral component alignment. (B) The tibial tray should be 90 degrees to the long axis of the tibial shaft. (C) Lateral radiographs show the femoral component parallel to the femoral shaft. (D) The tibial tray is at approximately 90 degrees to the tibial shaft. Osteopenia *(arrow)* is seen about the femoral component, consistent with stress shielding.

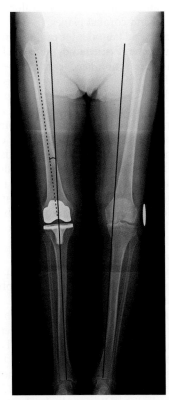

FIG 13.2 The Mechanical Axis Ideally, the mechanical axis (drawn from the center of the femoral head to the center of the tibial plafond in this case) falls through the center of the knee. Standing AP radiograph of both legs shows that the mechanical axis on the right *(solid line)* falls through the center of the knee arthroplasty, whereas the anatomic femoral axis *(dashed line)* is 6 degrees valgus to the mechanical axis. On the left, the mechanical axis passes through the medial tibial plateau indicating varus alignment, in this case because of osteoarthritis with medial joint space narrowing.

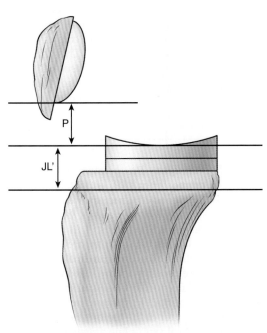

FIG 13.3 Assessing Joint Line and Patellar Height Diagram of a method for measuring JL and patellar height. *JL,* Joint line; *P,* patellar. (From Figgie HE, Goldberg VM, Heiple KG, et al: The influence of tibial-patellofemoral location on function of the knee in patients with the posterior stabilized condylar knee prosthesis. *J Bone Joint Surg Am* 68:1035–1040, 1986.)

motion, and absence of patellofemoral pain or mechanical symptoms (Fig. 13.3).

Hofmann et al. used measurements from the adductor tubercle to the JL of the distal femur (in comparison with the normal side or the preoperative radiograph) to assess "proximalization" or "distalization" of the JL (Fig. 13.4).[68] Restoration of the JL to within 4 mm of the preoperative or contralateral side is said to help avoid problems such as patella baja, patella alta, extensor mechanism maltracking, lack of motion, and midflexion instability.[68]

Radiolucent lines. Development of thin radiolucent lines at the bone/cement or bone/prosthesis interface of less than 2 mm within the first 6 months in a cemented implant or during the first 1 to 2 years in noncemented implants without evidence of progression is considered normal (Fig. 13.5). Evaluation of low contact stress TKA with meniscal bearings showed that 99% of radiolucent lines were nonprogressive, but even progressive radiolucent lines did not appear to affect fixation.[2]

Lucent lines are described by their location (prosthesis-bone, prosthesis-cement, bone-cement), whether they are stable or progressive, and by whether they involve all or part of the interface surface and by their width. They are usually demarcated by an adjacent thin sclerotic line, allowing them to be distinguished from the more poorly defined lucency of osteopenia. A standardized system for monitoring lucent lines developed by The Knee Society delineates specific areas to be assessed (see Fig. 13.5).[41] This method is complex, and a simplified system has been proposed.[9,106]

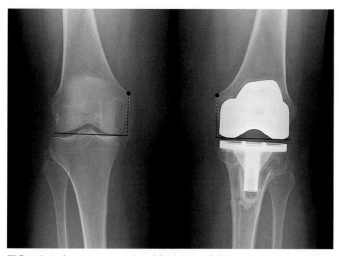

FIG 13.4 Anteroposterior Method of Measuring the Joint Line According to Hofmann and Associates The distance from the adductor tubercle to the JL on the operated side is compared with that on the nonoperated side (38.3 mm vs. 40.1 mm on the operated side).

FIG 13.5 (A) Coronal and (B) sagittal radiographic schematic of keeled and two-peg implants with zones for documentation of radiolucent lines and osteolysis. (C) Sagittal plane radiographic schematic of femoral implant with zones denoted for radiolucent lines and osteolysis. (D) Patellofemoral view radiographic schematic of multi- or single-peg patella implant with zones denoted for documentation radiolucent lines and osteolysis. Radiolucent lines should be denoted and documented as "partial" or "complete" and osteolysis documented in millimeters. (E) Less than 2 mm lucent line is present under the medial and lateral tibial baseplate with an adjacent thin sclerotic line *(arrow).* Such lucencies are seen in asymptomatic patients. (A-D from Meneghini RM, Mont MA, Backstein DB, et al: Development of a modern knee society radiographic evaluation system and methodology for total knee arthroplasty. *J Arthroplasty* 30:2311–2314, 2015.)

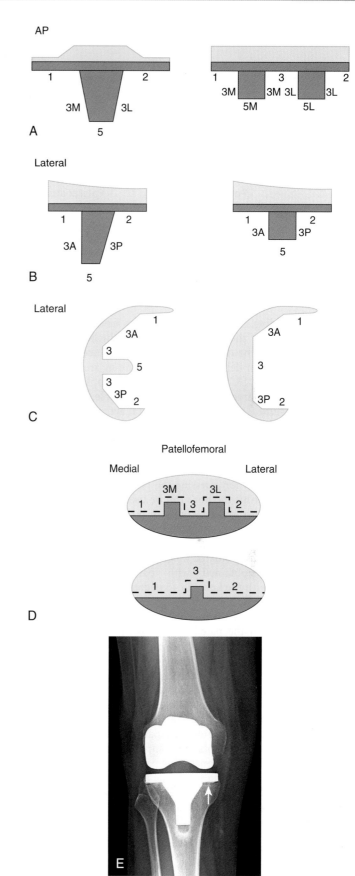

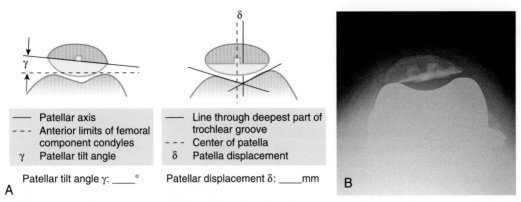

FIG 13.6 Patellar Displacement and Patellar Tilt (A) Methods of assessing patellar tilt and patellar displacement. (B) Tangential patellar view demonstrates patellar tilt with articulation between the medial patella and the femoral component. (From Meneghini RM, Mont MA, Backstein DB, et al: Development of a modern knee society radiographic evaluation system and methodology for total knee arthroplasty. *J Arthroplasty* 30:2311–2314, 2015.)

Stress shielding. Areas of decreased stress around femoral or tibial components show a diffuse decrease in bone density. These usually can be distinguished from radiolucent lines by absence of the thin delimiting sclerotic line in areas of stress shielding (see Fig. 13.1). Stress shielding develops within the first 2 years after surgery and then remains stable.[112]

Patellofemoral joint. The patellofemoral articulation can be an important cause of postoperative knee pain and prosthetic failure.[179] However, the relationship between patellar abnormalities on radiographs and knee symptoms is imperfect.[10]

Imaging techniques. Both lateral and tangential patellar views are important for assessing the patellar component and alignment. Numerous methods can be used for obtaining tangential patellar views in preoperative or postoperative individuals. Radiographic positioning alterations such as degree of flexion and weight bearing may significantly alter imaging findings.[179] Baldini et al. evaluated weight-bearing tangential patellar radiographs obtained with patients standing and semi-squatting with the knees in 45 degrees of flexion.[10] A correlation was made between anterior knee symptoms and signs and imaging findings.[10] Persistence of patellar tilt of greater than 5 degrees on the patellar dome on the weight-bearing study correlated positively with anterior knee pain.[10] None of the measurements made on non-weight-bearing radiographs correlated with pain and clinical scores.[10]

Radiographic evaluation of the patellofemoral joint includes assessment of patellar tilt, patellar dislocation or subluxation (Fig. 13.6), asymmetry in patellar component positioning,[10] "overstuffing," patellar height,[14] and patellar fracture.[46,52] Often postoperative measurements are compared with preoperative ones. CT is helpful in demonstrating patellar fracture, and MRI can be used for delineating soft tissue abnormalities.

Patellar height. Figgie et al. proposed measuring patellar height as the perpendicular distance from the inferior pole of the patellar implant to the JL of the prosthesis (see Fig. 13.3). Measurements of between 10 and 30 mm were associated with the best clinical results.[46]

Several additional measurements have been modified to evaluate patellar position after TKA, which include the Insall Salvati method,[33] the plateau-patellar angle,[141] the modified Blackburne-Peel index,[22,31] the Caton-Dechamps method,[25] and patella height.[135,142]

Patellar tilt. Patellar tilt is measured as the angle formed between a line drawn along the anterior femoral condyles and a line along the prosthesis/bone interface.[90]

Patellar tilt is not uncommon (see Fig. 13.6). For example, Bindelglass et al. found patellar tilt in 31.2% of 234 primary total knee prostheses.[21] Patellar tilting in relation to the femoral component changes the contact area and permits the thinner peripheral portion of the patellar component to be subject to maximum forces.[90] PE deformation, particle shedding, and early failure may occur. Laughlin et al. found that patellar tilt may change during the course of postoperative follow-up examinations.[90]

Asymmetry of patellar component placement. Asymmetrical resection greater than 4 mm in the mediolateral dimension or asymmetry of component position in the superior/inferior position as demonstrated on lateral views has been shown to correlate with anterior knee pain.[10] Lateral placement may cause retinacular tightness that may be avoided by medial positioning of the patellar component.[107]

Overstuffing. The postoperatively resurfaced patella should have a thickness equal to or thinner than that of the native patella.[90] A too large femoral component may produce stress on the lateral retinaculum, resulting in lateral patellar subluxation.[107] Patellar thickness greater than 26 to 28 mm is considered abnormal.[150]

Computed Tomography

Scout View. A relatively low-dose scout view obtained supine has been shown to allow accurate determination of the mechanical and anatomic axes of the femur for surgical planning.[169]

One potential limitation of this technique is the absence of weight bearing during the examination. Chauhan et al. described CT assessment of component position with relation to the mechanical axis as determined by CT scanning from the acetabular roof to the talar dome.[20,27,92]

Improvement in CT techniques has made this modality useful in evaluating complications of TKA.[80,132,146,163] Multidetector helical CT with a higher applied kilovolt peak (140 kVp) improves x-ray penetration and produces superior image quality.[96,136,139] Use of soft tissue reconstruction filters in the setting of metallic prostheses and of wide window settings (width, 3000 to 4000 Hounsfield units [HU]; level, 800 HU) allows for evaluation of bone near a prosthesis and is useful in the detection of focal areas of osteolysis.[24,159,181] Reformatted images may be helpful in minimizing artifact and demonstrating granuloma extent. Three-dimensional volume-rendered images minimize artifacts usually seen on conventional multiplanar reformatted images.[42]

Rotational Alignment of Components. Malrotation of patellar components has been associated with postoperative pain, stiffness, and patellofemoral complications.[15,89,116] Valkering et al. performed a literature review and found medium and large positive correlations between tibial and femoral component rotational alignment and better functional outcome. Revision of malrotated TKA was successful in all six cases.[170] However, a cutoff point for revision of malrotated TKA components has not yet been identified.

Several methods have been used to align the femoral component at surgery, such as the Whiteside line (the AP axis of the distal femur),[182] the posterior femoral condylar axis, and the transepicondylar axis. The surgical transepicondylar axis connects the point of the lateral epicondyle to the medial sulcus of the medial epicondyle.[20] The femoral component should be parallel to this line or slightly externally rotated. Errors in femoral component rotation are common and may lead to patellofemoral complications and anterior knee pain.[161] Berger et al. found that patellofemoral complications were associated with combined (tibial and femoral) internal rotation, and the greater the rotational abnormality, the worse the symptoms.[18]

Unfortunately, the assessment of component malrotation on imaging is not clear-cut.[3] CT scanning can be used to measure the rotation of tibial and femoral components, but the methodology is controversial and often complicated, particularly on the tibial side.[3] Thus, tibial component rotation has been determined with reference to the middle or medial third of the tibial tubercle,[15,143] the posterior tibial axis,[76] the trans-tibial axis,[38] the anterior border of the tibial plateau,[148] the tibial spines,[33] or the anatomic tibial axis.[32]

Berger et al. used the transepicondylar axis as a reference to evaluate femoral component rotation and the tibial tubercle as the reference to assess tibial component rotation on CT scans[18] (Fig. 13.7). They noted that normal rotation of the femoral condyles is 0.3 ± 1.2 degrees of internal rotation for females and 3.5 ± 1.2 degrees of internal rotation for males in comparison with the surgical epicondylar axis. On the tibial side, the native tibial articular surface (and the correctly positioned tibial component) is in 18 degrees ± 2.6 degrees of internal rotation relative to the tibial tubercle.[18] The AP tibial component axis is drawn perpendicular to the posterior edge of the tibial component.[20] When the femoral component is parallel to the transepicondylar axis and the tibial component is aligned in 18 degrees of internal rotation in relation to the tibial tubercle, normal patellar tracking results.[20] The degree of excessive combined internal rotation of the components was shown to be directly proportional to the severity of patellofemoral complications.[20]

This method has been difficult to use because the sulcus in the medial epicondyle is frequently difficult to identify. When the prominences of both epicondyles (instead of the medial sulcus) are used, the clinical transepicondylar axis produces a baseline that is more anteriorly and externally rotated (by about 6 degrees).[107] The angle between the epicondylar prominences and the posterior condyles is termed the twist angle.[4,168]

Roper et al. describe a method of using a single high definition 3D CT slice to assess tibial component rotation.[143] With this technique, the rotational axis of the tibial tray is measured relative to the junction of the medial and middle thirds of the tibial tubercle (see Fig. 13.7). Mismatch between femoral and tibial component rotation may also be problematic.[168]

Magnetic Resonance Imaging

Despite the presence of metal components, MRI has become a valuable noninvasive method for investigating complications of arthroplasty, including periprosthetic osteolysis and wear-induced synovitis (Fig. 13.8)[86,137,177,178] MRI-compatible metallic prostheses significantly degrade MR imaging for a variety of reasons. Common MRI artifacts resulting from metallic implants include signal loss from dephasing, failure of fat suppression, geometric distortion, in-plane distortion (pile-up and signal loss), and through-slice distortion. A number of techniques have been used to reduce artifacts from metal, including increasing the bandwidth, which diminishes the frequency shift caused by metallic components; increasing the signal-to-noise ratio by increasing the number of acquisitions; and using fast spin-echo techniques with longer echo-train lengths.[59,96,174] Although these modifications have been effective in reducing metal-artifact interference, susceptibility artifacts persist, limiting assessment of hardware and periprosthetic bone and soft tissues.

More recent novel pulse sequences such as multiacquisition variable-resonance image combination (MAVRIC) and slice encoding for metal artifact correction (SEMAC) have successfully reduced susceptibility artifacts, allowing bone and soft tissues around implants to be better examined, improving bone-metal interface and synovial evaluation.[157] MAVRIC technique involves combining multiple individual image datasets acquired at frequency bands incrementally offset from the dominant proton frequency.[83,84] In comparison with standard metal-artifact reduction fast spin-echo imaging, visualization of periprosthetic osteolysis was significantly better using MAVRIC techniques.[61,83,85] Additionally, SEMAC, which includes view-angle tilting, has also shown improvement in artifact reduction and detection of periprosthetic osteolysis compared to conventional protocols for improving imaging of knee hardware.[58,95,164] However, although the use of multispectral imaging methods (ie, MAVRIC or SEMAC) reduces arthroplasty-related artifacts, improves visualization of anatomic structures, and increases detection of periprosthetic osteolysis, these benefits come at the cost of increased scanning time.

Ultrasound

Ultrasound may be useful in evaluating the soft tissues around knee prostheses. Joint effusions, fluid collections, abscesses, vessels, and tendons may be assessed. The PE thickness has been investigated using ultrasound, but otherwise the prosthesis and the adjacent bone cannot be studied with this modality.[158,185]

COMPLICATIONS

Sharkey et al. reviewed the causes of revision total knee arthroplasties from 2003 to 2012 and compared the causes of revision in 2002 to those in 2012.[45,153,154] In the more recent series,[154] the most common failure mechanisms were loosening (39.9%), infection (27.4%), instability (7.5%), periprosthetic fracture (4.7%), and arthrofibrosis (4.5%). Infection was the most common failure mechanism for early revision (<2 years

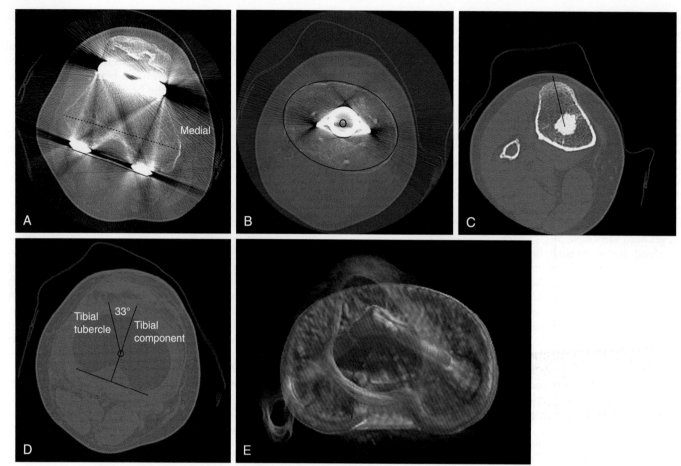

FIG 13.7 Analysis of Component Rotation on Computed Tomography According to Berger and Associates (A) Femoral component rotation. The CT slice that passes through the femoral epicondyles is used to assess femoral component rotation. The transepicondylar axis is constructed by connecting the prominence of the lateral epicondyle with the trough in the medial epicondyle *(dashed line)*. The posterior condylar line is drawn along the posterior aspects of the medial and lateral posterior condylar surfaces *(solid line)*. Ideally, the femoral component is parallel to this line or in external rotation. The angle between these lines is measured. If the angle opens medially, the component is internally rotated. Because women normally have a posterior condylar angle of 3.1 (±1.2) degrees of internal rotation, this angle may be subtracted from any measured internal rotation to determine the degree of "excessive internal rotation." (B) Tibial component rotation. Axial CT image obtained below the tibial baseplate. This image allows the center of the tibia to be located, establishing a reference point. (C) The center reference point in (B) is transposed onto the image showing the most prominent portion of the tibial tubercle, and the axis is drawn between these two points. (D) On the image through the articular PE, a line is drawn along the posterior surface of the PE liner, and a perpendicular line is drawn to that. The tibial tubercle axis from (C) is superimposed on the image, and the angle is measured. A total of 18 degrees is subtracted from the measured internal rotation to determine the excessive internal rotation. (This case demonstrates excessive internal rotation of 15 degrees.) (E) A reformatted 3D image through the proximal tibia shows the relationship between the tibial component and the tibial tubercle. Measurements can be made according to the methods proposed by Roper et al. (E, from Roper GE, Bloemke AD, Roberts CC, et al: Analysis of tibial component rotation following total knee arthroplasty using 3D high definition computer tomography. *J Arthroplasty* 28[8 suppl]:106–111, 2013.)

from primary), and aseptic loosening was the most common reason for late revision. PE wear was no longer the major cause of failure. Compared to their previous report, the percentage of revisions performed for PE wear, instability, arthrofibrosis, malalignment, and extensor mechanism deficiency has decreased.

Disorders of the Patella and Extensor Mechanism

A retrospective review of 1272 consecutive total or partial knee arthroplasties by Melloni et al. disclosed patellar complications in 3.6%.[105] Complications included instability/dislocation, fracture, osteonecrosis, infection, erosion, impingement, patellar or quadriceps tear, and loosening of the patellar component

(Fig. 13.9). The most common complication is patellar instability related to maltracking, often resulting from internal rotation of the tibial or femoral component.[105] Many patellar complications can be detected on radiography, but any underlying rotatory malalignment of components is best assessed on CT.

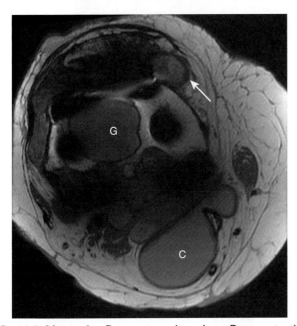

FIG 13.8 Magnetic Resonance Imaging Demonstrating Bone and Soft Tissue Changes in Granulomatous Disease Axial fast spin-echo image shows intermediate signal intensity synovitis *(arrow)*, as well as an intermediate signal region (granuloma *[G]*) adjacent to the fixation plug. A popliteal cyst *(C)* is also noted.

Patellar Fracture. Patellar fragmentation and sclerosis have been attributed by Melloni et al. to osteonecrosis (see Fig. 13.9). Patellar fractures may be difficult to identify on radiographs and may be asymptomatic.[105,150] Over-resection of the patella may predispose to fracture.[107]

Patellar Impingement. Articulation (impingement) between the unresurfaced patellar bone and the femoral component may occur. When this is extensive and associated with sclerosis of the patella on a weight-bearing tangential patellar view, a positive correlation with pain has been found.[10] However, although contact of the lateral patellar bone on the femoral component and patellar tilt have been seen in patients with impingement, they are also seen in control patients.[119]

Patellar Clunk. Pain and catching on extension may occur after TKA, and this is termed the patellar clunk syndrome. This occurs because of overgrowth of fibrous tissue at the superior pole of the patella.[51] Patella baja, a proximally positioned patellar component, and patellar subluxation or dislocation can be seen via radiography.[62] The abnormal soft tissue may be detected as a well-marginated mass of intermediate-to-low signal intensity on intermediate-weighted MR images.[51] Ultrasound can also demonstrate the size of the nodule and its position on flexion and extension.[120] Quadriceps or patellar tendon disruption may be confirmed on ultrasound examination.[105]

Polyethylene Liner Wear

Multiple factors influence tibial component PE liner wear,[99] including the weight and activity level of the patient, PE thickness, alignment, relationship between the PE component and the metal surface of the femoral and tibial components, and physical properties of the PE.[50,53,64,107] Wear leading to revision

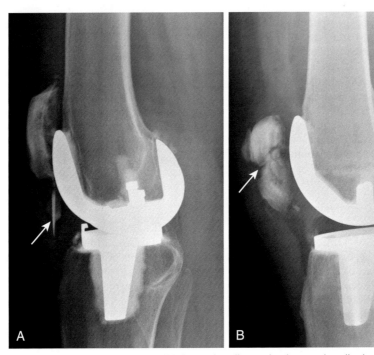

FIG 13.9 Patellar Complications (A) Lateral radiograph shows the displaced PE component *(arrow)* to lie caudal to the patella. (B) Lateral radiograph in another patient shows a patellar fracture *(arrow)*. Increased density of the fragments suggests osteonecrosis.

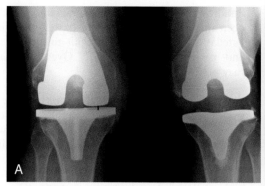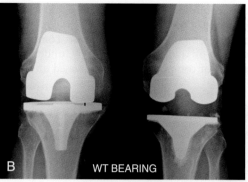

FIG 13.10 Polyethylene Wear (A) Standing flexed PA view of both knees and (B) a similar view 3 years later show that the distance between the medial femoral condyle (*vertical line* in A and B) and the tibial baseplate has decreased, indicating wear of the PE liner. Ideally, positioning should be identical to make this assessment. A mobile bearing left total knee prosthesis is shown in the opposite knee.

surgery has decreased in modern total knee arthroplasties.[154] The thickness of the PE liner depends on the tensile forces needed to balance the knee ligaments, but it should measure at least 8 mm initially.[53,64]

In TKA, PE wear may be evaluated on standing AP and lateral views, with the x-ray beam parallel to the tibial baseplate (Fig. 13.10). The distance from the femoral condyles to the tibial baseplate can then be measured. Large amounts of PE wear will be detected as moderate to severe narrowing of the distance between the femoral component and the metal backing (baseplate); early or mild joint space narrowing may be more subtle and may be appreciated only if comparison is made between serial examinations.[107] Eventually, wear may progress to allow metal-to-metal contact, erosion of the tibial metal backing, and metal synovitis (Fig. 13.11). Development of a popliteal cyst in patients with a TKA may be an indirect sign of prosthetic wear or loosening.[111,118] Fluoroscopy permits the operator to align radiographs perpendicular to the joint surface to compensate for any tilt of the tibial component. Measurement of the tibial liner thickness can then be obtained, and corrections can be made for magnification by comparison to an object of known dimension.[63,69] Ultrasound has also been used but is largely a research device for determining wear.[158,185] Cadaver study showed ultrasound measurements to be accurate to 0.5 mm with a 95% confidence interval. In vivo assessment[14] has shown a high correlation between the longitudinal measurement of the PE liner and the thickness of the radiolucent PE as measured on conventional radiographs.

Loosening, Particle Disease, and Osteolysis

Particle shedding, especially that caused by PE wear, is the primary reason for long-term failure of TKA.[17,44,113,114,154] The natural response to particulate debris begins with the release of inflammatory cytokines, which stimulate osteoclasts and inhibit osteoblasts. The biologic cascade of PE wear–related osteolysis is dependent on several factors, including the number of wear particles, the size and surface morphology of the wear particles, and the rate at which particles accumulate in periprosthetic tissues.[48,70] Particles migrate along the "effective joint space"[151] and produce changes in the joint, along the bone cement or prosthesis bone interfaces, and sometimes in adjacent soft tissues and lymph nodes. PE wear–induced synovitis can be

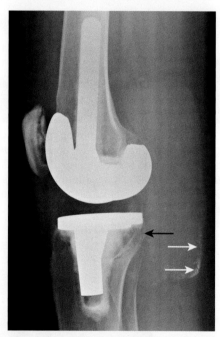

FIG 13.11 Metal Synovitis Lateral radiograph following revision of a TKA demonstrates a dense line outlining a distended popliteal cyst (metal line sign, *white arrows*), which is diagnostic of metal synovitis. Osteolysis is also seen at the posterior tibial baseplate *(black arrow)*, along with loosening of the patellar component.

seen on MRI as synovial thickening with dense synovial proliferation and debris of low-to-intermediate signal intensity with variable amounts of interspersed fluid and joint distention.[51]

Loosening. Loosening may result from mechanical stresses, osteolysis secondary to particle debris, and/or poor bone stock.[112] The tibial component loosens more frequently than the femoral component. Radiographic indicators that are suggestive of loosening include the development of focal radiolucencies greater than 2 mm, interval increases in the width of an existing radiolucency, cement fracture, changes in component position,[107] and any lucency at the metal cement or metal bone

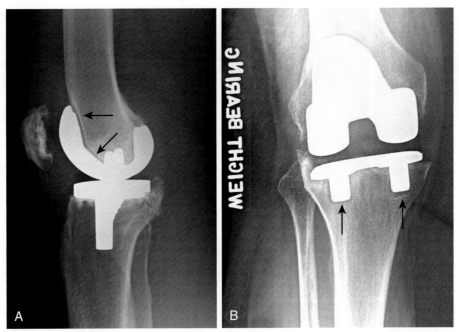

FIG 13.12 Loosening (A) Lateral radiograph shows radiolucent lines *(arrows)* along the femoral component (zones 1 and 3A). This component was proven to be loose at the time of revision surgery. (B) Weight-bearing view in another patient demonstrates radiolucent lines greater than 2 mm along the tibial baseplate *(arrows)* and subsidence of the tibial component, indicating loosening.

interface.[112] Radiolucent zones in both noncemented and cemented implants are often bordered by a thin layer of lamellar bone, which is produced by remodeling (Fig. 13.12). Wide lucent lines around the stem are more likely to be indicators of loosening than peripheral lucent zones. Detection of radiolucent lines requires that they be seen in tangent, and this is facilitated by fluoroscopy or by special views (such as an oblique posterior condylar view).[43,102,108,109,114] The tibial component tends to shift into a varus position with subsidence into the medial plateau and collapse of the cancellous bone,[97,102] whereas a loose femoral component tends to shift into flexion (see Fig. 13.12).

Disappearance of the bordering line of sclerosis may suggest infection. However, in most cases, loosening resulting from infection and loosening resulting from mechanical factors or histiocytic response cannot be distinguished on radiographs.[107]

In 23 surgically proven cases, Marx et al.[101] found the sensitivity of radiographs for tibial component loosening to be 83%, and for femoral component loosening, this was 77%. Specificity was 72% for the tibial component and 90% for the femoral component.

On MRI, as summarized by Sneag et al., a fibrous membrane is assumed when a smooth intermediate to high-signal region, less than 2 mm in thickness and bordered by a hypointense line, is present at the interface of the host bone and the cement or implant.[157] A layer greater than 2 mm between the bone and implant or bone and cement interface that may have irregular borders suggests bone resorption or osteolysis.[157]

Granulomas. Focal areas of bone destruction resulting from particle disease produce well-defined areas of osteolysis (granulomas) (Fig. 13.13). Typically these are located adjacent to the components, although extension of the process may occur and large soft tissue masses may result. Osteolysis can occur at the interfaces of a loose component. With well-fixed components, osteolysis occurs in the posterior aspects of the femoral condyles and condylar attachments of collateral ligaments, near the edges of the tibial baseplate, along the stem or screw holes, and along the patellar component interface or margins.[107]

Most patients with evidence of loosening present with pain; however, patients with focal osteolysis may be asymptomatic. Radiographs can underestimate the extent of bone involvement.[42,128,159] CT examination can be helpful, as it can demonstrate synovitis, detect more granulomas than are visible on the radiograph, and allow assessment of component rotation on the same study (see Fig. 13.13).

Because of its direct multiplanar capabilities and superior soft tissue contrast (and with the added benefit of the absence of ionizing radiation), tailored MRI can evaluate both periprosthetic osteolysis[137,177] (granulomas) and synovitis (that may precede bone loss) (see Fig. 13.13).[96,137] The osteolytic lesions are typically geographic, intermediate in signal intensity, but may appear high signal on inversion recovery images, and replace the normal periprosthetic trabecular bone and high-signal-intensity marrow fat.[51] MRI may demonstrate radiographically occult osteolytic lesions and may offer more accurate assessment of the extent and localization of osteolysis prior to revision surgery. MRI may be more sensitive for detecting osteolysis around the curved flanges of the femoral component as compared to CT.[157] MRI with metal suppression may be indicated in specific cases in which osteolysis is suspected clinically but is not visible radiographically, as well as in cases in which the extent or volume of osteolysis needs to be determined preoperatively.[50,96,157,174]

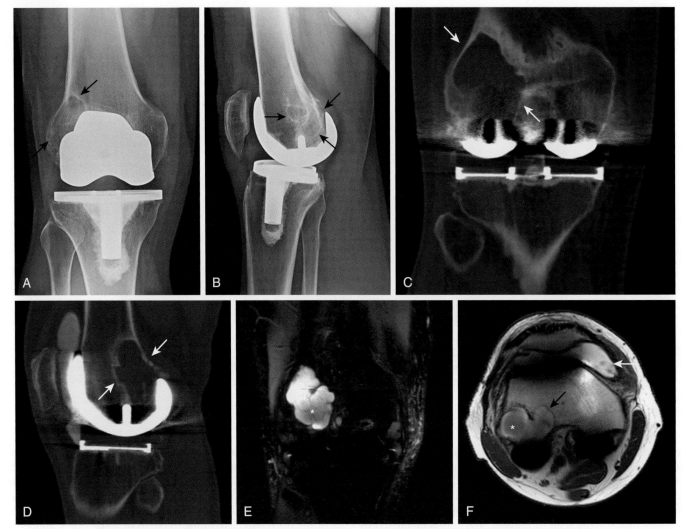

FIG 13.13 Granulomatous Disease This 47-year-old man presented with a painful right total knee replacement, as well as a deep venous thrombosis (DVT) and effusion 5 years after initial surgery. Pathologic examination revealed synovium with mononuclear histiocytic proliferation and foreign body giant cell reaction. (A) AP and (B) lateral radiographs demonstrate an eccentric lytic lesion with thin sclerotic margins in the lateral femoral condyle (*arrows* in A and B). (C) Coronal and (D) sagittal images from a CT arthrogram clearly demonstrate the large lytic lesion *(arrows)* with sclerotic margins in the posterolateral femoral condyle with disruption of the cortex posteriorly. (E) Coronal short tau inversion recovery (STIR) and (F) axial T1-weighted postcontrast images demonstrate the multilobulated lesion (*) in the posterior aspect of the lateral femoral condyle with a hypointense rim and peripheral enhancement consistent with a large granuloma. Joint distention *(arrow)* is present.

Metal Synovitis

Metal-induced chronic synovitis is the result of metal wear debris caused by abrasion of metal components that occurs after failure of the interposed PE-bearing surface.[28] A radiodense line outlining a distended knee capsule or an articular surface on radiographs, also known as the metal-line sign, is diagnostic of metal synovitis (see Fig. 13.11).[179] Erosion of the tibial metal backing may reveal the site of wear. On MRI, thickened synovium in cases of metal synovitis shows low signal intensity on all pulse sequences.

Periprosthetic and Component Fractures

The overall incidence of periprosthetic fracture is very low, with supracondylar femoral fractures reportedly in the range between 0.3% and 2.5%.[60] Risk factors for postoperative supracondylar fracture include osteopenia, femoral notching, and poor flexion,[167] as well as focal osteolysis and component loosening.[107] A decrease in the torsional strength of the femur has been reported when a 3-mm notch is present in the anterior femoral cortex,[155] with others reporting that almost 50% of periprosthetic femur fractures have associated anterior femoral

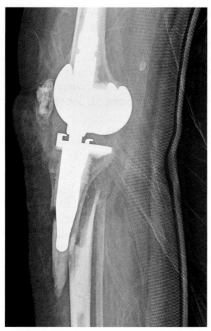

FIG 13.14 Periprosthetic Fracture Constrained TKA with a periprosthetic fracture at the distal tibial stem.

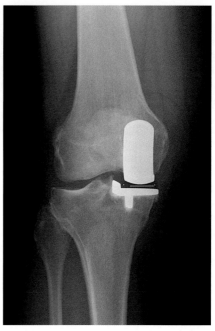

FIG 13.15 Normal Unicompartmental Arthroplasty of the Medial Compartment (Oxford Bearing) The metallic markers in the bearing allow assessment of its position.

notching.[1] The significance of femoral notching is controversial, however. Periprosthetic fractures of the proximal tibia have been reported less often than supracondylar and patellar fractures (Fig. 13.14). Fractures may also occur following medial or lateral[23,87,173,184] unicompartmental knee arthroplasty (UKA).

The Unified Classification System (UCS) provides a standardized classification system of periprosthetic fractures. It has been shown to have substantial inter-observer and almost perfect intra-observer reliability.[37,172]

Fracture of the femoral or tibial component is uncommon, with a rate of 0.2%.[71] Malalignment, uneven cement fixation, severe PE wear, and under sizing of the tibial tray have been described as causes of tibial component failure.[6,67,100] Femoral component fracture is a result of metal defects or cracks.[165,182] The PE stabilizing post in posterior stabilized total knee replacement may also fracture, resulting clinically in an extension clunk.[103]

Unicompartmental Complications

Use of the UKA has grown in acceptance and has seen resurgence over the past several years, primarily because of the introduction of minimally invasive techniques (Fig. 13.15). The aim of UKA is to resurface the medial or lateral tibiofemoral compartment in patients with uncontrolled symptoms as a result of arthritis predominantly confined to a single compartment. Unicondylar implants with a freely mobile meniscal bearing are available, distributing forces over a larger surface area, theoretically decreasing contact stresses and PE wear. An intact anterior cruciate ligament is required to maintain near-normal joint kinematics and mechanics.[36,40] Although some studies have shown comparable survival rates for total and unicompartmental knee arthroplasties, especially with conservative indications,* a direct comparative study of UKA and

TKA revealed a lower 5-year survivorship for UKA (85%) versus TKA (98%).[7] A 12-year survivorship of 80.6% has been demonstrated in patients younger than 50 years old who underwent UKA, with most revisions as a result of PE wear.[127]

Complications of UKA include infection, PE wear, osteolysis, subsidence and loosening, development of degenerative arthritis in another compartment, and stress fractures below the tibial component.[20,23,77,107] Radiolucent lines are commonly observed under the tibial component of Oxford unicompartmental knee implants, especially medially, and although the cause remains unknown, they are not thought to lead to loosening.[57,140] PE wear and axial malalignment can be evaluated on standing AP radiographs,[82] and radiographs in flexion and extension have been described for evaluation of femoral component loosening.[110]

Infection

Infection complicates 0.8% to 1.9% of knee arthroplasties.[35] Predisposing causes are categorized as those related to the patient (such as prior revision arthroplasty, prior infection of a prosthesis in the same joint, rheumatoid arthritis, and diabetes) and those related to the surgery and the postoperative period (such as simultaneous bilateral arthroplasty, long operating time, allogenic blood transfusion, wound complications, and urinary tract infection).[35]

Infection is often not obvious prior to revision surgery. Low-grade or chronic infections are particularly difficult to identify. More than half of cases are a result of staphylococci. Organisms may be introduced at the time of surgery (usually skin bacteria) or through hematogenous spread or direct contamination from compromised adjacent tissues.[35] Microorganisms adhere to the prosthesis, residing in a biofilm that limits the effects of antimicrobial agents.[35] The primary symptom of infection is pain—typically night pain or pain at rest.[91] If other signs of

---

*References 8, 19, 49, 115, 138, and 166.

infection (erythema, sinus tract) are not present, differentiation from other causes of pain, particularly aseptic loosening, can be problematic. The American Academy of Orthopaedic Surgeons (AAOS) proposes that testing strategies be planned according to the probability of infection.[130] According to the AAOS Guideline, high probability of infection is suspected in a patient with one or more symptoms *and* with one or more risk factors (eg, prior knee infection, superficial surgical site infection, operative time >2.5 hours, and immunosuppression) *or* a physical finding *or* early implant loosening/osteolysis as detected by radiographs.[130] More recently, the Parvizi workgroup of the musculoskeletal infection society proposed a standardized definition for periprosthetic infection, to increase confidence in the diagnosis of prosthetic infection.[131]

Nonimaging techniques such as C-reactive protein (CRP) may be helpful. DelPozo and Patel noted that CRP levels return to normal within 2 months, and a normal CRP level generally excludes infection.[35] A CRP of 13.5 mg per liter or more per liter is 73% to 91% sensitive and 81% to 86% specific for the diagnosis of infected TKA in the absence of other inflammatory conditions.[35] The AAOS recommends joint aspiration of patients being assessed for periprosthetic infection who have an abnormal erythrocyte sedimentation rate and/or CRP.[130]

Joint aspiration is the most valuable test for infection.[35] A cell count of greater than 1.7×10^3 per cubic millimeter or greater than 65% neutrophils is consistent with knee joint infection.[35] Barrack et al. noted that, in contrast to aspiration of total hip replacement, where false-positive results are more common, aspirations of knee joints are more likely falsely negative.[12] This was thought to result most often from antibiotic treatment.[12] At least 2 weeks off antibiotics is recommended before the aspiration is performed (with careful clinical monitoring for sepsis), but as long as 1 month may be necessary for cultures of aspirated fluid to become positive. In questionable cases, aspiration should be repeated.

Radiographs. Generally, radiographs are insensitive for diagnosing prosthetic infection (Fig. 13.16). Radiographs may not be helpful because loosening, periostitis, focal osteolysis, and radiolucent lines have been seen in infected and uninfected knees. Also, infection may be present with a "normal" radiographic appearance.

Increasing soft tissue swelling with blurring of fat lines and joint effusion, periosteal reaction, and loosening (especially with loss of the thin sclerotic demarcation lines) should suggest infection. Arthrography may show sinus tracts.

Computed Tomography and Magnetic Resonance Imaging. In the absence of a prosthesis, CT and MRI are well-recognized tools for evaluating infection. CT has less soft tissue contrast and suffers image degradation by metallic components. In spite of these limitations, considerable information can be gleaned with the use of these modalities (see Fig. 13.16). MRI can be used to evaluate soft tissues for edema, fistulas, sinus tracts, abscesses, and fluid collections. Abscess cavities can often be differentiated from bland postoperative fluid collections, as abscesses have thick, irregular, diffusely enhancing walls, and fluid collections are bounded by thin, minimally enhancing walls. MRI findings of lamellated synovitis with hyperintense signal (see Fig. 13.16F), extracapsular soft-tissue edema, extracapsular collections, and reactive lymphadenopathy make periprosthetic joint infection likely.[51]

The MRI finding of hyperintense lamellated synovitis by itself appears to be a sensitive (0.86 to 0.92) and specific (0.85 to 0.87) feature of periprosthetic knee infection when experienced individuals interpret the examination.[134] The synovium in these cases is described as thickened and composed of multiple layers with hyperintense signal compared to skeletal muscle on intermediate–echo time fast SE images.

RADIONUCLIDE IMAGING

Bone Scintigraphy

Bone scintigraphy is the most commonly performed radionuclide imaging procedure for the painful joint arthroplasty. Performed with ^{99m}Tc labeled diphosphonates, the test is highly effective for detecting complications of lower extremity prosthetic joint surgery. Although sensitive for identifying the failed joint replacement, bone scintigraphy cannot determine the cause of the failure. Evaluation of knee replacements is especially problematic because, even in the absence of complications, increased periprosthetic activity can persist for some time after implantation.[122] Rosenthall et al.[145] observed persistent periprosthetic activity around more than 60% of the femoral components and almost 90% of the tibial components of asymptomatic knee replacements more than 1 year after their implantation. Hofmann et al.[68] studied asymptomatic knee replacements with serial bone scans over a 2-year period and found that although periprosthetic activity usually decreased over time, there was considerable patient-to-patient variation. They concluded that a single study cannot reliably detect prosthetic failure and that sequential scans are needed (Fig. 13.17).

Smith et al.[156] reviewed the results of bone scintigraphy performed on 75 patients with painful knee arthroplasties. They reported that a negative study makes loosening or infection unlikely, but that periprosthetic uptake patterns in abnormal studies could not reliably differentiate between infection and aseptic loosening. Palestro et al.[126] also observed that bone scintigraphy is not specific for infection (Fig. 13.18).

Performing the bone scan as a three-phase study does not improve the accuracy of the test (Fig. 13.19). Palestro et al.[126] reported that the three-phase bone scan was neither sensitive (67%) nor specific (76%) for prosthetic knee infection.

Bone scintigraphy, with an overall accuracy of about 50% to 70%, is most useful as a screening test. A normal study makes it unlikely that the patient's symptoms are related to the prosthesis. An abnormal study requires further investigation.[93]

Sequential Bone/Gallium Imaging

In an effort to enhance the specificity of the bone scan, various radiopharmaceuticals have been investigated. One of the earliest agents studied was gallium-67 citrate (gallium) imaging. Factors that account for gallium uptake in infection include increased blood flow and vascular membrane permeability at inflammatory sites, lactoferrin binding, siderophore and bacterial gallium uptake, and direct transport by leukocytes. Imaging is typically performed 2 to 3 days after injection.[124]

Unfortunately, gallium accumulates not only in infection, but in various tumors at sites of new bone formation (such as fractures), and in aseptic inflammation (Fig. 13.20). The accuracy of sequential bone/gallium imaging for diagnosing lower extremity periprosthetic joint infection ranges between 65% and 80%, which is only slightly better than that of bone

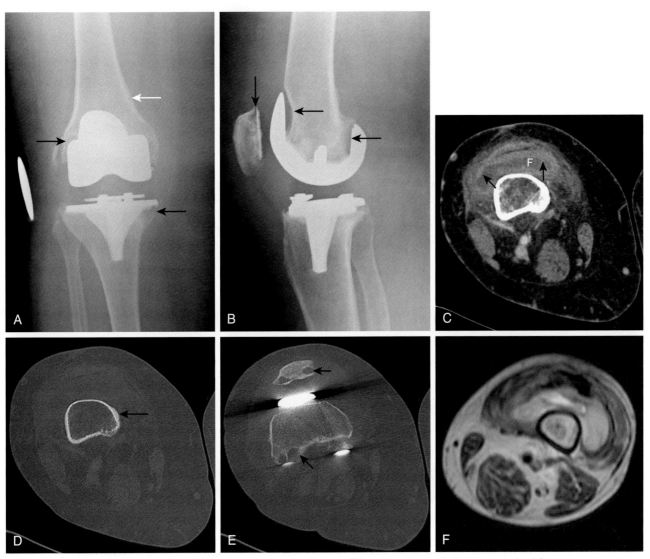

FIG 13.16 Infected total knee arthroplasties in two different patients. A-E were acquired from a 55-year-old woman presenting with a history of a painful right total knee replacement years following arthroplasty. C-reactive protein (CRP) (33.1) and sedimentation rate (67 mm per hour) were both elevated. Aspiration reveled a white count of 28,000 mm³ with 86% polymorphonuclear leukocytes. The *Abiotrophia* species was cultured. (A) Anteroposterior and (B) lateral radiographs show extensive soft tissue swelling, bone resorption along the femoral and patellar interfaces *(black arrows)*, and periosteal reaction *(white arrow* in A). A magnification marker of known size is placed alongside the knee. (C) Axial computed tomography (CT) image with soft tissue algorithm shows marked thickening of the suprapatellar recess *(arrows)*, which is distended with low attenuation fluid (F). (D) Axial CT images using a bone algorithm at the same level image C demonstrates periosteal reaction *(arrow)*. E, Axial CT image at the level of the patella confirms bone loss adjacent to the femoral and patellar components *(arrows)*. These lytic areas are not specific and may be seen with granulomatous disease. Pathologic examination showed fibrin and granulation tissue with acute inflammation. (F) Axial proton density image acquired in another patient demonstrates thickened lamellated synovium, which is hyperintense compared to adjacent skeletal muscle. Subsequent cultures revealed the presence of *Staphylococcus aureus* infection.

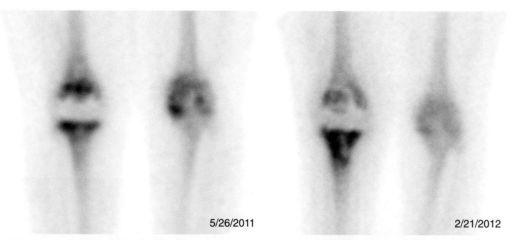

5/26/2011   2/21/2012

FIG 13.17 Aseptically Loosened Right Knee Arthroplasty Bone scan performed about 6 months after implantation *(left)*, shows mildly increased radiopharmaceutical accumulation around the femoral and tibial components. On the repeat study, performed 9 months later (15 months after implantation), there is intensely increased radiopharmaceutical accumulation around the tibial component, whereas activity around the femoral component has resolved. An aseptically loosened tibial component was revised.

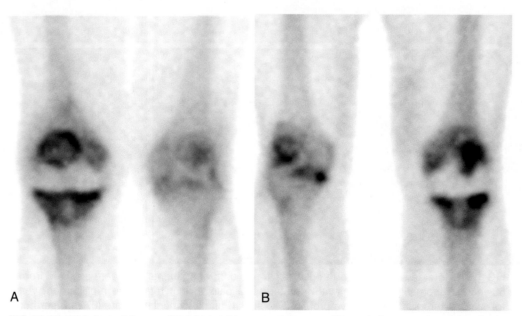

A   B

FIG 13.18 (A) Infected 1-year-old right total knee replacement. There is increased periprosthetic activity, especially around the tibial component, on the bone scan. (B) Aseptically loosened 2-year-old left total knee replacement. The increased periprosthetic activity around this knee prosthesis is virtually indistinguishable from that in (A).

scintigraphy alone. This test has largely been abandoned and replaced by labeled leukocyte (WBC) imaging.[124]

Labeled Leukocyte Imaging

The accumulation of labeled white cells at a focus of infection depends on chemotaxis, the quantity and types of white cells labeled, and the predominant cellular response in a particular situation. Neutrophils usually comprise most leukocytes labeled and consequently sensitivity of WBC imaging is highest for neutrophil-mediated inflammatory processes. When indium-111 is the radiolabel, images are acquired 18 to 30 hours after reinfusion of the labeled cells. When technetium-99m is the radiolabel, imaging is typically performed 4 to 6 and 18 to 30 hours after reinfusion.[124]

Neutrophils invariably are present around the infected prosthesis, and it might be assumed that WBC imaging would accurately diagnose prosthetic joint infection. Although WBC imaging has become the radionuclide test of choice for diagnosing prosthetic infection, its value was, for a considerable amount of time, the subject of controversy. Early results were inconsistent, with some investigators reporting that the test was sensitive but not specific and others reporting that the test was specific but

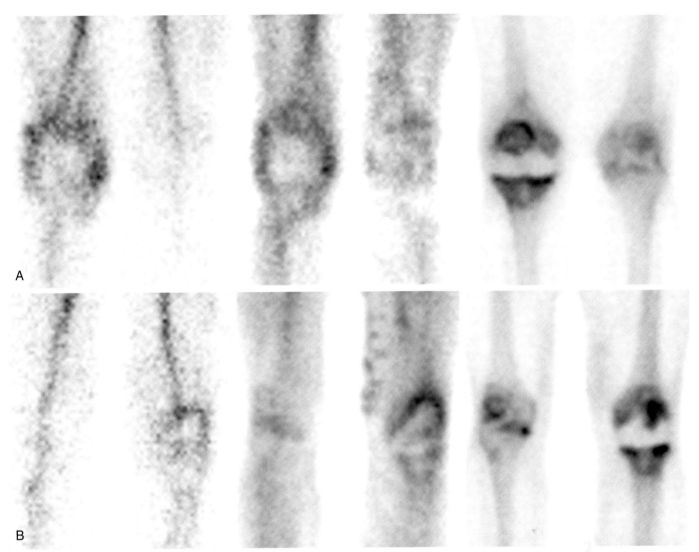

FIG 13.19 (A) Infected 1-year-old right total knee replacement (same patient illustrated in Fig. 13.18A). There is hyperperfusion and hyperemia around the right knee on the flow *(left)* and blood pool *(center)* images, with increased periprosthetic activity on the delayed image *(right)* of the three-phase bone scan. (B) Aseptically loosened 2-year-old left total knee replacement (same patient illustrated in Fig. 13.18B.). There is hyperperfusion and hyperemia around the left knee on the flow *(left)* and blood pool *(center)* phases, with increased periprosthetic activity on the delayed image *(right)* of the three-phase bone scan. Although bone scintigraphy is sensitive, it is not specific, even when performed as a three-phase study and cannot be used to differentiate aseptic loosening from infection.

not sensitive. Low sensitivity was attributed to the chronicity of the infection, whereas poor specificity was ascribed to nonspecific inflammation. Although chronicity and nonspecific inflammation may help explain inconsistent results, a more fundamental problem with this test is related to the interpretation of the images themselves. The standard practice for interpreting WBC images is to compare activity in the region of interest with activity in some normal reference point. Thus WBC studies are interpreted as positive for osteomyelitis when uptake in the region of interest exceeds uptake in the predetermined reference point, or when activity outside the normal distribution of the radiopharmaceutical is observed. Unfortunately, both the intensity of uptake in prosthetic knee infection and the normal distribution of labeled WBCs are variable (Fig. 13.21).[93,124]

Efforts to improve the accuracy of WBC imaging for diagnosing prosthetic joint infection, and musculoskeletal infection in general, have focused on the use of two combined modalities: WBC/bone and WBC/marrow imaging. Wukich et al.[183] reported that the specificity improved from 45% for WBC alone to 85% for WBC/bone imaging. Palestro et al.[126] investigated 25 painful knee replacements and reported that the sensitivity (67%) and specificity (78%) of WBC/bone imaging were not better than those of WBC imaging alone (89% sensitivity and 75% specificity).

An alternative to WBC/bone imaging is the combination of WBC and ^{99m}Tc sulfur colloid bone marrow (marrow) imaging. The principal of combined WBC/marrow imaging is based on the fact that WBC and marrow images both reflect

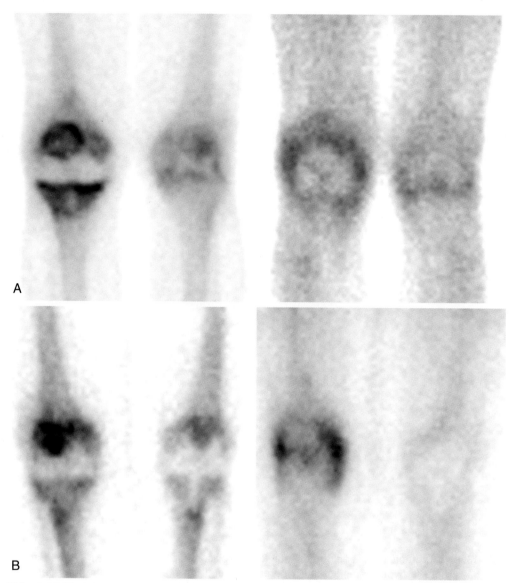

FIG 13.20 (A) Infected 1-year-old right total knee replacement (same patient illustrated in Fig. 13.18A). The abnormal activity on the bone scan *(left)* primarily is located around the tibial component, whereas the abnormal activity on the gallium scan *(right)* primarily is located around the femoral component. When the distribution of the two radiopharmaceuticals is spatially incongruent, as in this case, the combined study is positive for infection. (B) Aseptically loosened 2-year-old right total knee replacement. The abnormal activity on the bone scan *(left)* primarily is located around the femoral component, whereas the abnormal activity on the gallium scan *(right)* primarily is located along the lateral and medial margins of the knee joint itself. In this case the combined study is false positive for infection.

radiopharmaceutical accumulation in the reticuloendothelial cells, or fixed macrophages, of the marrow. The distribution of marrow activity is similar, or spatially congruent, on WBC and marrow images in normal individuals and in those with underlying marrow abnormalities. The exception is osteomyelitis, including prosthetic joint infection, which stimulates uptake of leukocytes but suppresses uptake of sulfur colloid, resulting in spatially incongruent images (Fig. 13.22).[125]

Over the years, the results of WBC/marrow imaging for diagnosing prosthetic knee infection have been remarkably consistent, with reported accuracies ranging from 83% to 100%.[122] Joseph et al.[79] reported that among the 22 knee prostheses in their investigation, 6 of which were infected, the test was 83% sensitive and 94% specific. Palestro et al.[126] reported that WBC/marrow imaging was 89% sensitive and 100% specific for diagnosing prosthetic knee infection and was superior to bone (including three-phase) scintigraphy alone, WBC alone, and WBC/bone. Love et al.[94] reported that in 19 patients with surgically, histopathologically, and microbiologically confirmed diagnoses, the test was 100% accurate for diagnosing prosthetic knee infection. El Espera et al.[39] compared WBC/bone to WBC/marrow imaging for diagnosing hip and knee prosthetic joint infection and reported that there were far fewer equivocal results and much better inter-observer agreement for WBC/

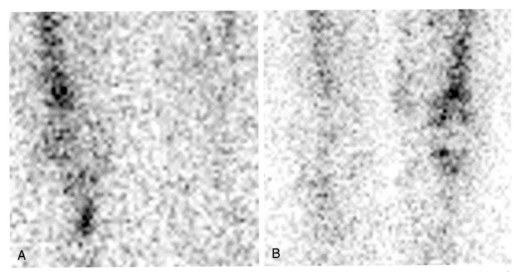

FIG 13.21 (A) Infected 1-year-old right total knee replacement. There is intense accumulation of labeled leukocytes in the distal right femur and proximal right tibia. (B) Aseptically loosened 2-year-old left total knee replacement. There is intense accumulation of labeled leukocytes in the distal left femur and proximal left tibia, similar to that in (A).

marrow than for WBC/bone imaging. Basu et al.[13] performed WBC/marrow imaging on 29 knee arthroplasties and reported that although the test was 88% specific, it was only 33% sensitive for infection. It should be noted, however, that only 3 of the 29 prostheses in this investigation were infected.

In spite of its usefulness, there are disadvantages to WBC/marrow imaging. The in vitro labeling procedure is technically demanding, not routinely available, and involves direct contact with blood products. Labeling a sufficient quantity of leukocytes to produce a diagnostically useful study may not be possible in immunocompromised individuals. Image quality, especially when using indium-111 as the radiolabel, is not ideal. The need to perform an additional study such as marrow imaging is another drawback. Radiolabeled antigranulocyte antibodies and antibody fragments and ^{18}F-fluorodeoxyglucose (FDG) have been explored as alternatives to in vitro WBC imaging.[122]

Antigranulocyte Antibodies

Besilesomab is a murine monoclonal G1 immunoglobulin that binds to normal cross-reactive antigen-95 on leukocytes.[124] Klett et al.[81] reported that by analyzing changes in periprosthetic uptake over time, ^{99m}Tc-besilesomab was 100% sensitive and 80% specific for prosthetic knee infection. Besilesomab unfortunately incites a human antimurine antibody (HAMA) response in up to 30% of patients to whom it is administered. Consequently, patients should be prescreened for HAMA, injected with no more than 250 µg antibody, and should avoid repeat administration.[124]

Antibody fragments are an attractive alternative to whole antibodies because they do not induce a HAMA response. Sulesomab is a fragment antigen binding (Fab') portion of a murine monoclonal G1 immunoglobulin that binds to nonspecific cross-reactive antigen-90 on leukocytes. Early investigations suggest that sulesomab binds to circulating neutrophils that migrate to foci of infection and to leukocytes already present at the site of infection. More recent data, however, suggest that accumulation in infection is nonspecific.[124]

von Rothenburg et al.[176] reported that ^{99m}Tc-sulesomab was 100% accurate for prosthetic knee infection. Iyengar and Vinjamuri[74] reported that the test was 100% sensitive but only 50% specific for prosthetic knee infection. Pakos et al.,[121] in an investigation that included 12 hip and 7 knee arthroplasties, reported an overall sensitivity and specificity of 75% and 86%, respectively. Vicente et al.,[175] in an investigation of 80 lower extremity joint arthroplasties, including 45 knee prostheses, reported that ^{99m}Tc-sulesomab was 80% sensitive and 89% specific for infection. Rubello et al.[147] studied 90 knee arthroplasties and reported that using dual time point imaging, at 4 and 24 hours, ^{99m}Tc-sulesomab sensitivity and specificity was 93% and 100%, respectively. Gratz et al.[54] reported sensitivity and specificity of 91% and 76%, respectively, for knee replacement infection. Sousa et al.[160] in a study of 27 hip and knee prostheses reported that the specificity of ^{99m}Tc-sulesomab increased from 20% to 100% when complementary bone marrow imaging was performed.

Although the use of antigranulocyte antibodies/antibody fragments eliminates some of the problems associated with in vitro WBCs, these agents have their own limitations. In an additional study, either bone or marrow imaging probably still needs to be performed. Furthermore, the use of whole antibodies raises concerns about immunogenicity. The use of these agents, none of which are available in the United States, typically is limited to those circumstances in which in vitro WBC imaging is not available.

Single Photon Emission Computed Tomography/ Computed Tomography

Because radiopharmaceuticals reflect primarily function, the anatomic detail necessary to differentiate physiologic from pathologic processes is often lacking. The development of hardware-based fusion imaging systems (ie, SPECT/CT and positron emission tomography [PET]/CT), where functional and morphologic studies are acquired on the same device without moving the subject, has resulted in significant improvements in both diagnostic confidence and test accuracy.

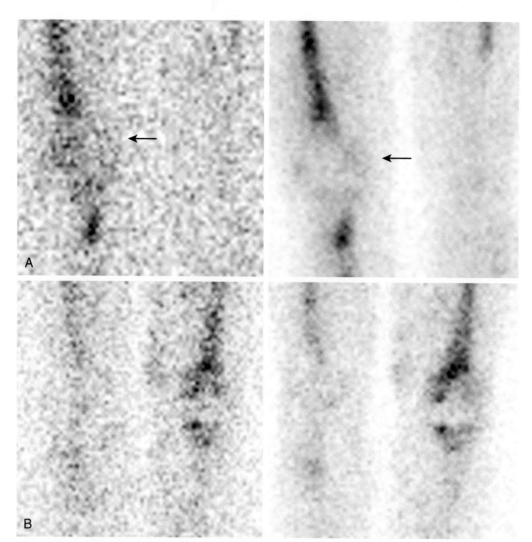

FIG 13.22 (A) Infected 1-year-old right total knee replacement (same patient illustrated in Fig. 13.21A). The distribution of activity on the labeled leukocyte *(left)* and bone marrow *(right)* images is the same except in the knee joint region *(arrows)*, where there is accumulation of labeled leukocytes, but not sulfur colloid. The images are incongruent, and the combined study is positive for infection. The areas of most intense activity on the labeled leukocyte image correspond to areas of activity on the bone marrow image and reflect marrow activity, not infection. The abnormal labeled leukocyte activity, which is in the joint region, is much less intense. (B) Aseptically loosened 2-year-old left total knee replacement (same patient illustrated in Fig. 13.21B). The distribution of activity on the labeled leukocyte *(left)* and bone marrow *(right)* images is virtually identical, and the combined study is negative for infection. Neither intensity nor distribution of labeled leukocyte activity around a joint prosthesis is a reliable criterion for diagnosing infection.

Filippi and Schillaci[47] compared ^{99m}Tc-WBC imaging with SPECT and SPECT/CT in 13 patients with hip and knee prostheses. Accuracy improved from 64% for scintigraphy with SPECT to 100% for SPECT/CT. The authors noted that SPECT/CT is valuable because it precisely localizes foci of WBC accumulation and facilitates the differentiation of soft tissue from bone infection.

Al-Nabhani et al.[5] performed ^{99m}Tc-bone SPECT/CT on 69 patients with a painful knee arthroplasty. They found that the test contributed useful information in more than 80% of the cases, helping confirm mechanical loosening and excluding other causes of pain such as infection.

Graute et al.[55] reported on 31 patients with suspected lower extremity prosthetic joint infection, including 27 with knee arthroplasties, who underwent imaging with ^{99m}Tc-besilesomab. Nine of the 31 prostheses were infected. Sensitivity, specificity, and accuracy for planar imaging were 66%, 60%, and 61%, respectively. By adding SPECT/CT, sensitivity, specificity, and accuracy increased to 89%, 73%, and 77%, respectively.

The potential impact of SPECT/CT on the diagnosis of prosthetic joint infection is significant. The examination could provide information, not only about the presence but also the extent of infection (Fig. 13.23). Joint aspiration and culture could be performed at the same time. In patients without

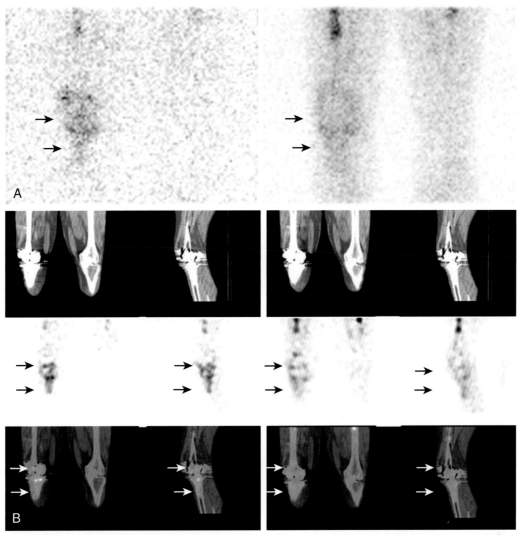

FIG 13.23 (A) Infected right total knee prosthesis (planar images). The distribution of activity in the right knee *(arrows)* on the labeled leukocyte *(left)* and bone marrow *(right)* images is spatially incongruent, and the combined study is positive for infection. (B) Infected right total knee prosthesis (dual isotope SPECT/CT). Although the planar images in (A) were sufficient to make the diagnosis of infection, the distribution of activity on the coronal and sagittal images from the labeled leukocyte *(left)* and bone marrow *(right)* SPECT/CT not only makes the diagnosis of infection but also demonstrates that the infection involves both the tibial and femoral components of the prosthesis, without evidence of extension into the adjacent soft tissues. Such information can be useful for operative planning.

infection, the test could provide information about other causes of prosthetic failure.[65,66] Patients could potentially be spared the need to undergo multiple imaging tests at different times and possibly different locations, and a diagnosis could be made in a more expeditious, cost-effective manner.

[18]F-Fluorodeoxyglucose Positron Emission Tomography

^{18}F-FDG PET has generated considerable interest as an alternative to WBC/marrow imaging for diagnosing prosthetic joint infection. FDG is transported into cells via glucose transporters but, unlike glucose, is not metabolized and remains trapped within the cell. Increased FDG uptake in inflammation presumably is due, at least in part, to increased expression of glucose transporters in inflammatory cells and increased affinity of these glucose transporters for deoxyglucose.[123]

FDG-PET (and PET/CT) has several potential advantages over conventional nuclear medicine tests. Degenerative bone changes usually show only faintly increased FDG uptake compared to infection. Normal bone marrow has only a low glucose metabolism under physiologic conditions, which could facilitate the differentiation of inflammatory cellular infiltrates from hematopoietic marrow and obviate the need for bone marrow imaging. The small FDG molecule enters poorly perfused areas quickly, and the procedure is completed within 2 hours after radiopharmaceutical injection. Images have higher spatial resolution than those obtained with single photon emitting radiopharmaceuticals. Semi-quantitative analysis by means of standardized uptake values (SUV), which is readily available with PET but less feasible with conventional nuclear techniques, potentially could be useful for differentiating infectious from non-infectious conditions and for monitoring response to therapy.[123]

The results of FDG-PET for diagnosing prosthetic knee infection have been variable. Zhuang et al.[186] evaluated FDG-PET in knee replacements and reported a sensitivity, specificity, and accuracy of 92%, 72%, and 78%, respectively, for diagnosing infection. Manthey et al.[98] studied 14 painful knee prostheses and reported that FDG-PET correctly identified the one infected device and was true negative in the 13 uninfected devices (100% accuracy). Basu et al.[13] investigated 87 knee replacements and reported that FDG-PET was 95% sensitive and 88% specific for infection. Gravius et al.[56] studied 20 patients with painful knee prostheses, 9 of which were infected. The sensitivity and specificity of FDG-PET for infection were 89% and 82%, respectively.

Van Acker et al.[171] evaluated FDG-PET in 21 patients with suspected prosthetic knee infection and reported that the test was 100% sensitive but only 73% specific for infection. When FDG-PET was interpreted together with bone scintigraphy, specificity improved to 80%. Chacko et al.[26] reviewed the results of FDG-PET scans performed on 36 knee prostheses. The sensitivity, specificity, and accuracy of FDG-PET for diagnosing prosthetic knee infection were 92%, 75%, and 81%, respectively. Delank et al.[34] reviewed FDG-PET imaging of 27 lower extremity joint replacements, including five knee arthroplasties, and reported that although a negative test excluded infection with a high degree of certainty, a positive test could not reliably differentiate between infection and aseptic inflammation. Stumpe et al.[162] studied FDG uptake in 28 patients with a painful TKA. Eighteen patients were studied with PET/CT and 10 with PET alone. Increased FDG uptake in the synovial membrane was present in 27 arthroplasties, including all three infected devices and 24/25 uninfected devices. These authors concluded that periprosthetic FDG accumulation cannot automatically be equated with infection. Love et al.[94] compared coincidence detection FDG-PET to WBC/marrow imaging for diagnosing prosthetic knee infection in 19 patients and reported an accuracy of 58% for FDG-PET, compared to an accuracy of 100% for WBC/marrow imaging. In a meta-analysis, the sensitivity and specificity of FDG-PET for diagnosing lower extremity prosthetic joint infection was 82% and 87%, respectively. Specificity was significantly lower for prosthetic knee infection (75%) than for prosthetic hip infection (90%).[88]

The ability to detect inflammatory conditions with FDG depends on glucose use by leukocytes during their metabolic burst. Aseptic loosening and prosthetic joint infection both can be accompanied by an often intense inflammatory response in which leukocytes participate, and thus the inability of FDG to accurately differentiate between these two conditions is expected. The variability in published results for FDG imaging likely is related to the prevalence of loosening and infection in the various populations studied, important information that frequently is not provided.

At the present time, the role, if any, of FDG-PET in the evaluation of knee arthroplasties remains to be determined.

SUMMARY

Currently the principal role of nuclear medicine in the evaluation of painful knee replacement is to diagnose infection. Nonspecific indicators of inflammation, such as gallium and FDG, are of limited value because of the frequency with which

inflammation accompanies aseptic loosening. Bone scintigraphy is useful for screening purposes, but combined WBC/marrow scintigraphy is the radionuclide procedure of choice for diagnosing infection. Initial data suggest that SPECT/CT, in addition to providing information about the presence and extent of infection, may be able to provide additional information about other conditions that cause joint replacements to fail.

KEY REFERENCES

20. Berger RE, Rubash HE: Rotational instability and malrotation after total knee arthroplasty. *Orthop Clin North Am* 32:639–647, 2001.

35. DelPozo J, Patel R: Infection associated with prosthetic joints. *N Engl J Med* 361:787–793, 2009.

42. Fayad LM, Patra A, Fishman EK: Value of 3D CT in defining skeletal complications of orthopedic hardware in the postoperative patient. *AJR Am J Roentgenol* 193:1155–1163, 2009.

46. Figgie HE, Goldberg VM, Heiple KG, et al: The influence of tibial-patellofemoral location on function of the knee in patients with the posterior stabilized condylar knee prosthesis. *J Bone Joint Surg Am* 68:1035–1040, 1986.

50. Frick MA, Collins MS, Adkins MC: Postoperative imaging of the knee. *Radiol Clin North Am* 44:367–389, 2006.

51. Fritz J, Lurie B, Potter HG: MR imaging of knee arthroplasty implants. *Radiographics* 35:1483–1501, 2015.

86. Koff MF, Shah P, Potter HG: Clinical implementation of MRI of joint arthroplasty. *AJR Am J Roentgenol* 203:154–161, 2014.

93. Love C, Marwin SE, Palestro CJ: Nuclear medicine and the infected joint replacement. *Semin Nucl Med* 39:66–78, 2009.

96. Malchau H, Potter HG: Implant wear symposium clinical work: how are wear-related problems diagnosed and what forms of surveillance are necessary? *J Am Acad Orthop Surg* 16(Suppl 1):S14–S19, 2008.

105. Melloni P, Valls R, Veintemillas M: Imaging patellar complications after knee arthroplasty. *Eur J Radiol* 65:478–482, 2008.

106. Meneghini RM, Mont MA, Backstein DB, et al: Development of a modern knee society radiographic evaluation system and methodology for total knee arthroplasty. *J Arthroplasty* 30:2311–2314, 2015. <http://dx.doi.org/10.1016/j.arth.2015.05.049>.

107. Miller TT: Imaging of knee arthroplasty. *Eur J Radiol* 54:164–177, 2005.

112. Mulcahy H, Chew FS: Current concepts in knee replacement: complications. *AJR Am J Roentgenol* 202(1):W76–W86, 2014.

113. Naudie DD, Ammeen DJ, Engh GA, et al: Wear and osteolysis around total knee arthroplasty. *J Am Acad Orthop Surg* 15:53–64, 2007.

122. Palestro CJ: Nuclear medicine and the failed joint replacement: past, present, and future. *World J Radiol* 6:446–458, 2014.

123. Palestro CJ: FDG-PET in musculoskeletal infections. *Semin Nucl Med* 43:367–376, 2014.

124. Palestro CJ: Radionuclide imaging of osteomyelitis. *Semin Nucl Med* 45:32–46, 2015.

126. Palestro CJ, Swyer AJ, Kim CK, et al: Infected knee prosthesis: diagnosis with In-111 leukocyte, Tc-99m sulfur colloid, and Tc-99m MDP imaging. *Radiology* 179:645–648, 1991.

131. Parvizi J, Zmistowski B, Barbara EF: New definition for periprosthetic joint infection. From the workgroup of the musculoskeletal infection society. *Clin Orthop* 469:2992–2994, 2011.

154. Sharkey PF, Lichstein PM, Shen C, et al: Why are total knee arthroplasties failing today—has anything changed after 10 years? *J Arthroplasty* 29(9):1774–1778, 2014.

157. Sneag D, Bogner EA, Potter HG: Magnetic resonance imaging evaluation of the painful total knee arthroplasty. *Semin Musculoskelet Radiol* 19(1):40–48, 2015.

159. Sofka CM, Potter HG, Adler RS, et al: Musculoskeletal imaging update: current applications of advanced imaging techniques to evaluate the early and long-term complications of patients with orthopedic implants. *HSS J* 2:73–77, 2006.

174. Vessely MB, Frick MA, Oakes D, et al: Magnetic resonance imaging with metal suppression for evaluation of periprosthetic osteolysis after total knee arthroplasty. *J Arthroplasty* 21:826–831, 2006.

179. Weissman BN, Scott RD, Brick GW, et al: Radiographic detection of metal-induced synovitis as a complication of arthroplasty of the knee. *J Bone Joint Surg Am* 73:1002–1007, 1991.

The references for this chapter can also be found on www.expertconsult.com.

14

Tumors in the Knee

Edward J. Derrick, Michele N. Edison, Kurt F. Scherer,
Christopher W. Wasyliw, Christopher R. Pettis, Laura W. Bancroft

INTRODUCTION

Tumors involving the knee can be subdivided into osseous and soft tissue neoplasms, with either benign or malignant histology. This chapter describes the patient demographics and multimodality imaging characteristics of the most common tumors about the knee, organized by the classification set forth by the World Health Organization.[37] The imaging features of these tumors are described based upon their characteristics exhibited on radiographs, computed tomography (CT), magnetic resonance imaging (MRI), sonography, and nuclear scintigraphy and F18-fluorodeoxyglucose positron emission tomography (FDG-PET).

BENIGN PRIMARY OSSEOUS TUMORS OF THE KNEE

Cartilaginous Tumors

Osteochondroma. An osteochondroma, also commonly referred to as an exostosis, is the most common primary bone tumor, accounting for approximately 25% to 50% of benign bone tumors and 10% to 15% of all bone neoplasms.[81] Most cases present prior to 20 years of age and there is a 1.5 to 3.5:1 male-to-female predominance.[81] Approximately 40% of osteochondromas occur around the knee. It is thought that trauma or congenital perichondral deficiency results in abnormal foci of metaplastic cartilage spontaneously giving rise to these benign entities[63]; however, some studies have demonstrated associated mutations of the exostosin-1 (EXT1) gene with solitary osteochondroma.[43] There is also evidence associating hematopoietic stem cell transplant[13] and radiation[102] as other risk factors. Most cases are asymptomatic and are discovered incidentally.[81] Although unusual, fracture through a pedunculated osteochondroma can compress the adjacent neurovascular structures and become symptomatic.[33,81] Malignant transformation is exceedingly rare in solitary lesions; however, approximately 18% of cases are associated with multiple hereditary exostoses and an increased risk of malignant transformation of 3% to 25%.[33,88]

An osteochondroma is a masslike structure with cortical and medullary continuity with the underlying bone.[33,81] These lesions are often found in the metaphysis or metadiaphysis of long bones, can be sessile or pedunculated, and often protrude away from the adjacent joint (Fig. 14.1). CT is very effective in demonstrating cortical and medullary continuity of the lesion with the parent bone, but assessment of the cartilage cap is variable. The cartilaginous cap typically has attenuation similar to adjacent soft tissue on CT, and is better visualized when the cap is mineralized.[33,81] Sonography can provide accurate measurement of the cartilaginous cap with accuracy similar to MRI. The cartilage cap is normally hypoechoic relative to the adjacent tissues, but echogenic foci with posterior shadowing will be evident if cartilaginous calcifications develop.[81]

MRI can add significant value in the assessment of a symptomatic or worrisome osteochondroma. The cartilage cap thickness can be assessed on MRI, as it is almost isointense to normal hyaline cartilage on all sequences and possesses a surrounding perichondrium that is typically a thin hypointense rim (Fig. 14.2).[33,81] Cap thickness greater than 2 cm has been associated with significantly increased risk of malignant transformation to sarcoma.[33,81] MRI is also excellent in assessing neurovascular complications of a symptomatic osteochondroma around the knee.[33] The common peroneal nerve is the most commonly affected nerve in the presence of lateral lesions, and MRI may identify complications such as fatty muscular atrophy of the short head of the biceps femoris and the anterior and lateral compartments of the calf. Pseudoaneurysm formation can also occur due to chronic friction of an artery against the osteochondroma, with the popliteal artery most commonly affected.[33,69,113] Symptomatic bursitis may also form adjacent to pedunculated lesions.

Enchondroma. Enchondromas (also referred to simply as chondroma) are benign neoplasms composed of lobules of hyaline cartilage. The peak age of presentation ranges between the third and fourth decade of life.[33] One study found an incidental prevalence of approximately 3%,[108] although the true prevalence is unknown, given that most patients are asymptomatic. The most commonly involved osseous structures are the bones around the knee, most often the distal femur.[33,108] Most enchondromas are centrally located and involve the metaphysis of long bones; however, cortical-based lesions are not uncommon. It is believed that enchondromas arise from the displacement of cartilaginous cells from the physis into the metaphysis during embryonic development. However, a recent retrospective analysis of 240 MRI exams of the knee failed to identify such displacement of cartilage into the metaphysis.[32] Other evidence suggests that mutations in isocitrate dehydrogenase 1 and 2 (IDH1 and IDH2) may be associated with approximately half of all low-grade cartilaginous tumors.[2] Although most enchondromas are solitary benign lesions with a low risk of malignant degeneration, patients with multiple enchondromas

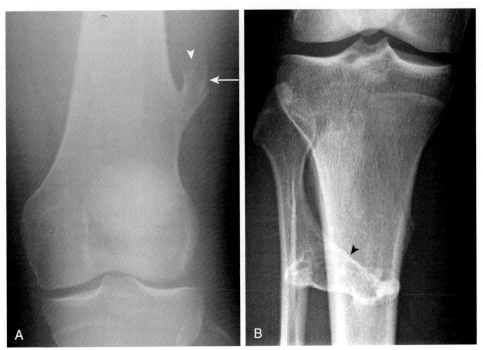

FIG 14.1 Osteochondroma (A) Anteroposterior radiograph of the knee in a 17-year-old boy demonstrates a pedunculated osteochondroma originating from the distal lateral femoral meta-diaphysis *(arrow)*. The cartilage cap is facing away from the knee joint *(arrowhead)*. Medullary and cortical continuity with the underlying normal bone is pathognomonic for this entity. (B) Pedunculated osteochondroma *(arrowhead)* of the right proximal fibula in a different patient who exhibited symptoms in the peroneal nerve distribution.

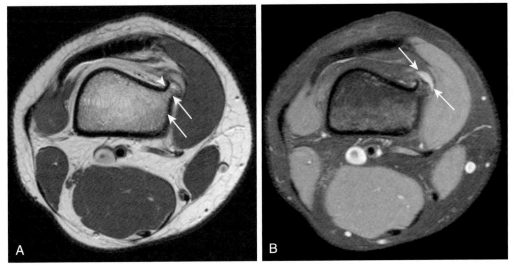

FIG 14.2 Thirteen-Year-Old Girl With Osteochondroma (A) Axial T1-weighted image through the distal femoral osteochondroma demonstrates cortical *(arrowhead)* and medullary *(arrows)* continuity with the underlying bone. (B) Axial T2-weighted image shows the normal, thin hyper-intense cartilage cap *(arrows)* and corticomedullary continuity.

have a significantly higher risk of malignant transformation. Ollier disease is manifested by multiple enchondromas, with a risk of malignant transformation as high as 50%; the risk of malignant transformation is higher than 50% in patients with Maffucci's syndrome, which is characterized by multiple enchondromas and soft tissue hemangiomata.[88,90]

An enchondroma is evident on radiographs as a central geographic lytic lesion with variable mineralization and ill-defined or lobulated margins (Fig. 14.3).[63] Lesions often measure less than 6 cm in greatest dimension and mineralization can be seen in 95% of cases.[33] Lesions may be difficult to detect if the margins have a wide zone of transition or there is an absence of matrix mineralization. Subtle endosteal scalloping, cortical thinning, and expansile remodeling of bone may occur.[33] CT is superior to radiography in the detection of subtle findings such as occult matrix mineralization and endosteal

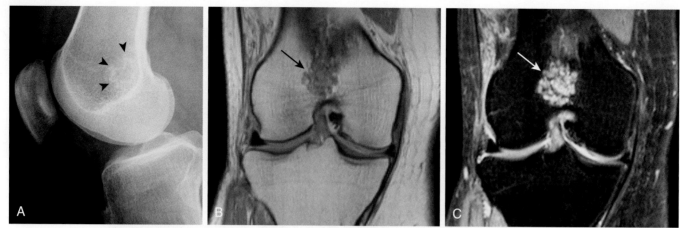

FIG 14.3 Distal Femoral Enchondroma in a 52-Year-Old Woman (A) Lateral radiograph of the knee shows the classic arcs-and-rings *(arrowheads)* pattern of mineralization in the distal femoral enchondroma. (B) Coronal T1-weighted image of the knee. There is a distinctly lobular, heterogeneous, hypointense lesion in the femoral metaphysis *(arrow)*. (C) Corresponding T2-weighted image once again demonstrates a lobular, heterogeneously hyperintense lesion with internal low-signal intensity representing chondroid calcification *(arrow)*.

scalloping. Endosteal scalloping with an enchondroma typically involves approximately 10% of the cortical thickness and extends for only a portion of the lesion.[86]

MRI demonstrates a distinctive lobular conglomeration of tiny, clustered T2-hyperintense foci, reflective of the high ratio of water to mucopolysaccharide composition in the hyaline cartilage (see Fig. 14.3). On T1-weighted images, the enchondroma is isointense to skeletal muscle and intermixed with a high signal representing medullary fat (see Fig. 14.3).[63] Murphey et al. have shown that MRI can help differentiate an enchondroma from a central chondrosarcoma in up to 90% of cases, based upon features such as depth and extent of endosteal scalloping.[86] However, a more recent study demonstrated significant variability among radiologists' ability to differentiate enchondromas from low-grade chondrosarcomas, and the addition of MRI only slightly improved the accuracy of tumor grading.[100] Skeletal scintigraphy demonstrates mild to moderate increased uptake relative to the iliac crest,[33,36] and some authors have reported increased activity on FDG-PET imaging.[30]

Periosteal Chondroma. Periosteal chondromas are rare extracortical cartilaginous tumors that arise deep to the periosteum. The peak age of presentation is between the third and fourth decades.[33] Periosteal chondromas most commonly involve the metaphysis of long bones, with the femur and tibia being the second most involved structures after the humerus.[96,112]

These lesions typically demonstrate cortical scalloping, variable sclerosis, and a thin periosteal shell with or without central chondroid mineralization on radiographs and CT (Fig 14.4). Periosteal chondromas are typically 2 to 2.5 cm in size; lesions greater than 3 to 5 cm are suspicious for periosteal chondrosarcoma. On MRI, these lesions demonstrate signal intensity isointense to hyaline cartilage on all sequences, and a thin hypointense rim on gradient echo sequences; peripheral and septal enhancement patterns can be seen with the administration of contrast.[33,96,112]

Chondroblastoma. Chondroblastomas are rare benign tumors accounting for less than 2% of all primary bone tumors and approximately 5% of all benign bone tumors.[26] Approximately

50% of chondroblastomas are located within the proximal tibia or distal femur; the majority involve the epiphysis or apophysis and commonly extend into the metadiaphysis.[33] The mean age at presentation is approximately 20 years of age with a 2 to 3:1 male prevalence.[26,33] Presenting symptoms most often include pain, local tenderness, and stiffness.

Chondroblastomas typically present radiographically as 1- to 4-cm lytic lesions with a thin, sclerotic margin. A lobular contour and matrix mineralization are present in 30% of cases.[33] Lesions are classically located in the epiphysis of long bones adjacent to the growth plate, and approximately half of cases extend into the metaphysis (Fig. 14.5).[26,33] A solid periosteal reaction is present in up to 60% of cases.[33] Nuclear scintigraphy can demonstrate increased uptake on vascular and delayed phases.[33]

On MRI, the chondroblastoma typically demonstrates an intermediate T1-weighted signal and ranges from a hypointense to hyperintense T2-weighted signal with a lobular, thin hypointense margin (see Fig. 14.5). Prominent perilesional bone marrow edema is often present (see Fig. 14.5) along with periostitis, soft tissue edema, reactive joint effusion, and synovitis. Contrast-enhanced sequences demonstrate peripheral or septal enhancement.[26,33,59] Secondary aneurysmal bone cyst (ABC) formation can occur in 15% of cases, with fluid-fluid levels identified on fluid sensitive sequences.[59]

Fibro-Osseous Tumors
Nonossifying Fibroma and Fibrous Cortical Defect. Nonossifying fibroma (NOF) and fibrous cortical defect are also known as *metaphyseal fibrous defect and fibroxanthoma*. Lesions are histopathologically identical, benign, self-limited defects that commonly occur in adolescents and children. Benign fibrous histiocytoma is also histopathologically indistinguishable from NOF and fibrous cortical defects and it is often a term used for cases with atypical radiologic appearance or clinical presentation.[63] The peak age at diagnosis is within the second decade of life, and there is a 2:1 male predominance.[11] These lesions are relatively common and may be present up to 36% of children.[63] A large percentage of cases present around the knee, most commonly in the distal femoral metaphysis. Physical exam is often

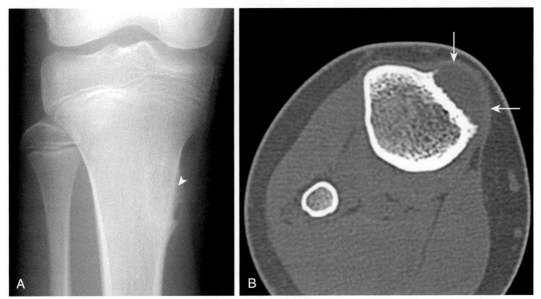

FIG 14.4 Periosteal Chondroma of the Proximal Tibia (A) AP radiograph of the knee shows an ovoid focus of peripheral hyperostosis in the proximal medial tibial metadiaphysis. (B) Axial computed tomography shows a hypodense surface lesion *(arrows)* in the proximal tibia with adjacent cortical scalloping and periosteal reaction in this biopsy-proven periosteal chondroma. *AP,* Anteroposterior.

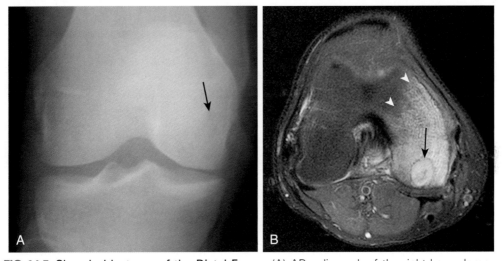

FIG 14.5 Chondroblastoma of the Distal Femur (A) AP radiograph of the right knee demonstrates a subtle lucency *(arrow)* in the medial femoral condyle. (B) Axial T2-weighted image demonstrates a predominantly hyperintense lesion *(arrow)* with a thin hypointense margin, internal intermediate signal, and intense perilesional bone marrow edema *(arrowheads)*. *AP,* Anteroposterior.

unremarkable; however, there may be occasional tenderness or pathologic fracture.[11] These lesions can grow but eventually ossify starting from the diaphyseal side toward the epiphysis.[63] Multifocal lesions may be present in 8% of patients and often should not give rise to concern in most cases. However, multiple fibroxanthomas are also a component of Jaffe-Campanacci syndrome, in addition to café au lait macules, decreased mentation, and hypogonadism or cryptorchidism.[11,12]

Radiography, in conjunction with clinical history and physical exam, is often sufficient to make the diagnosis of fibroxanthoma. Classic radiographic appearance of fibrous cortical defect is a cortically based lytic lesion with a thin sclerotic rim. These lesions typically have an oval shape and parallel the long axis of the bone. NOF is a term typically used to describe larger defects that extend into the medullary cavity (Fig. 14.6).[12,63]

CT can occasionally better characterize indeterminate lesions, but is more commonly used for preoperative planning for large lesions located in weight-bearing regions that are at risk for pathologic fracture.[12] On MRI, fibroxanthomas are most frequently located in the metaphysis, are eccentrically located, and have well-defined scalloped margins (Fig. 14.7). T2-weighted signal characteristics are variable, with areas of hyperintense, intermediate, and low-signal intensity due to the fibrous matrix and mineralization (see Fig. 14.7). Occasionally, areas of fat-isointense signal or secondary ABC formation may

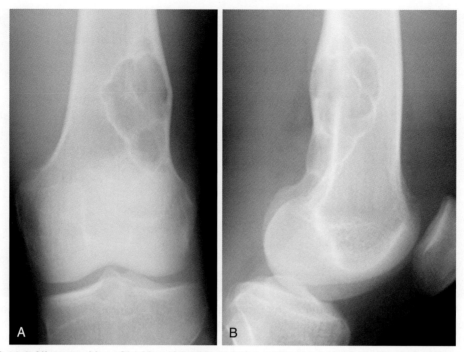

FIG 14.6 **Nineteen-Year-Old Man With Nonossifying Fibroma** AP (A) and lateral radiographs (B) show a lytic lesion in the posterolateral femoral metadiaphysis with a thin, sharp sclerotic margin characteristic for NOF. Note that the long axis of the lesion parallels the long axis of the bone. *AP,* Anteroposterior; *NOF,* nonossifying fibroma.

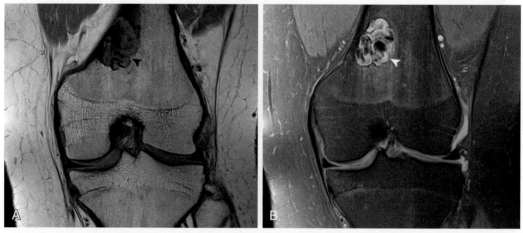

FIG 14.7 **Nonossifying Fibroma in the Left Distal Femur** (A) Coronal T1-weighted image demonstrates an eccentric, T1-hypointense medial distal femoral metaphyseal lesion with scalloped margins *(arrowhead).* (B) Corresponding T2-weighted sequence demonstrates a heterogeneous signal within the lesion *(arrowhead).*

be present. Contrast-enhanced images most often demonstrate heterogeneous, intense enhancement.[63] Nuclear scintigraphy can help differentiate the activity within the lesion as uptake varies through the evolution of these lesions, but it is not routinely performed as part of the diagnostic workup. Intense uptake indicates an active lesion or possible associated fracture. Intermediate uptake is present during the healing process as the lesion ossifies, but healed lesions should demonstrate no increased radiotracer uptake.[11]

Cortical Desmoid. The cortical desmoid is a benign, self-limited lesion considered to be a variant of NOF.[41,58] The peak age at time of diagnosis is in the second decade of life with a 3:1

male predominance.[61] It is believed that cortical desmoids arise from repeated traction on the insertion of the adductor magnus aponeurosis or the origin of the medial head of the gastrocnemius on the posterior femoral metaphysis.[41,61] Most cases are asymptomatic, although mild associated pain and localized swelling may occur.[41]

The cortical desmoid is best viewed on external rotation radiographs of the femur, and typically presents as a small radiolucent, saucer-shaped lesion or region of focal cortical roughening (Fig. 14.8). The typical location for cortical desmoids is within the posteromedial femoral metaphysis.[41] These findings, in conjunction with a physical exam and clinical history, are often sufficient for diagnosis. CT may be useful to better visualize the lesion in cases where radiographs are inconclusive, and may demonstrate a concave or convex lesion in the axial plane (see Fig. 14.8).[41]

MRI can also help in indefinite atypical cases and often demonstrates low to intermediate signal intensity on T1-weighted and intermediate to high intensity on T2-weighted sequences, often with surrounding hypointensity representing a sclerotic rim (see Fig. 14.8). On contrasted sequences, these lesions demonstrate intense enhancement. MRI can also help delineate the relationship of the cortical desmoid to the insertion of tendons.[41,61] Nuclear scintigraphy demonstrates findings similar to NOF in cortical desmoid and uptake is contingent upon the activity of the lesion. Single-photon emission computed tomography (SPECT) has been reported to have greater accuracy in the detection of small lesions, even in cases where bone scans are negative.[58,61]

Osteoid Osteoma. Osteoid osteomas are the third most common benign bone tumor, comprising 10% to 12% of all benign and 2% to 3% of all primary bone neoplasms.[56,92] It is characterized by a central nidus composed of an osteoid matrix and osteoblasts surrounded by sclerosis. Approximately 85% of osteoid osteomas occur between the ages of 5 and 24 years, with a 1.6:1 to 4:1 male predominance, and most cases occur in Caucasian populations.[14,56,103] Approximately 50% of these tumors occur in the femur and tibia.[92,103] The classic clinical presentation is pain that worsens at night and is alleviated with nonsteroidal anti-inflammatory drugs (NSAIDs). The pain is often described as deep, achy, intense, and intermittent and may last weeks to months before the diagnosis is made.[14,56] The pathogenesis of these lesions is poorly understood, but there is evidence that local increased levels of prostaglandins, prostacyclin, and cyclooxygenase-2 play a role in the localized inflammation and vasodilation.[3,56,80]

The radiographic appearance of the osteoid osteoma is contingent upon the location of the lesion. Three predominant patterns have been described in the literature—cortical, medullary, and subperiosteal. *Cortical lesions* are the most common, representing about 75% of all osteoid osteomas. These are characterized by cortical lucent lesions less than 2 cm with or without calcification within the central nidus. Sclerosis surrounding the nidus may be sufficiently thick to opacify the central lucency (Fig. 14.9).[56,68,103] *Medullary lesions* account for approximately 20% of all osteoid osteomas and typically form some eccentric sclerosis on the adjacent cortex. *Subperiosteal lesions* account for less than 5% of all osteoid osteomas and form soft tissue masses adjacent to the bone with typically no sclerosis of the adjacent osseous structures. *Intra-articular* osteoid osteomas can occur, but are uncommon in the knee.[68]

CT is the modality of choice in the diagnosis of osteoid osteoma with numerous studies showing the superiority of CT to MRI.[56,103] The nidus of the osteoid osteoma is of low attenuation (isodense to soft tissue) and surrounded by sclerosis. Focal calcifications can be present within the nidus and may be punctate, amorphous, or ringlike (Fig. 14.10).[14,56,68] The "vascular groove" sign has been found to be a relatively sensitive and specific CT sign for osteoid osteoma, with the identification of linear vascular channels surrounding the tumor.[14,75,103]

The appearance of an osteoid osteoma on MRI is variable. In general, these lesions have a low to intermediate signal on T1-weighted and an intermediate to increased signal on T2-weighted images (see Fig. 14.9). Associated bone marrow and soft tissue edema is not an uncommon finding and can mimic a malignant process (see Fig. 14.9). Enhancement is also variable, but the central nidus and surrounding edema typically enhance.[14,103]

Nuclear scintigraphy is almost 100% sensitive in the detection of osteoid osteoma.[14,56,103] These neoplasms exhibit increased uptake on all three phases[14,103] and classically demonstrate a double-density sign. This is characterized by highly intense central uptake, relating to the highly osteoblastic nidus, surrounded by a zone of less-intense uptake, which corresponds to the bone's response to the tumor.[14,56,103] Pinhole magnification has been shown as superior to planar imaging in demonstrating the double-density sign.[56] Sonography has limited usefulness in the evaluation of osteoid osteomas, but it has been used in the assessment of the vascular supply to these tumors. The feeding artery may be identified with color Doppler;

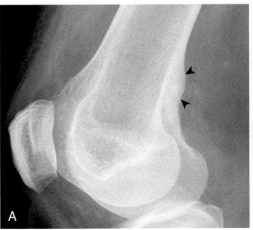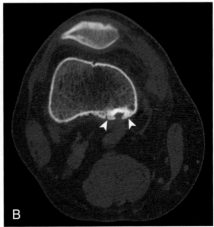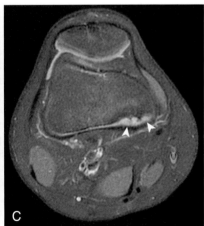

FIG 14.8 Cortical Desmoid of the Right Knee (A) Lateral radiograph of the right knee shows focal hyperostosis of the posterior metaphysis *(arrowheads)*. (B) Axial CT better defines the cortical hyperostosis in the posteromedial femur *(arrowheads)*. (C) Axial proton density image shows the cortically based intermediate intensity lesion with a thin, hypointense rim *(arrowheads)* at the tendinous origin of the medial head of the gastrocnemius muscle. Imaging features are classic for desmoid and the patient was clinically followed. *CT,* Computed tomography.

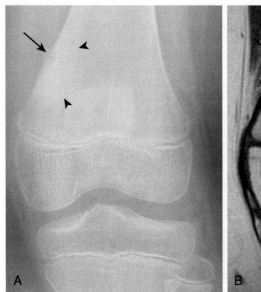 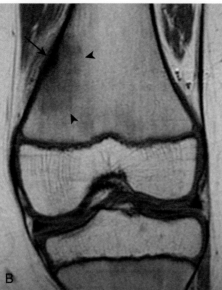 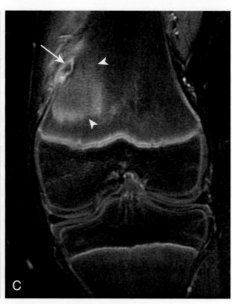

FIG 14.9 Ten-Year-Old Boy With Osteoid Osteoma of the Left Knee (A) AP radiograph of the left knee shows a cortically based lucency *(arrow)* in the medial femoral metaphysis with subtle surrounding sclerosis *(arrowheads)*. (B and C) Coronal T1 (B) and T2-weighted fat-suppressed (C) images show the cortically based lesion in the medial femoral metaphysis *(arrows)* with surrounding low T1 and high T2 signals, signifying perilesional bone marrow edema *(arrowheads)*. Surgical en bloc incision was chosen, with complete excision of the osteoid osteoma. *AP,* Anteroposterior.

however, the use of ultrasound has largely been replaced by other modalities.[14,34]

The predominant differential consideration when diagnosing osteoid osteoma is osteoblastoma. These two entities bear multiple similarities and are sometimes considered to be within the same pathologic spectrum.[56] Osteoblastomas are traditionally expansile lesions larger than 2 cm that may grow over time, whereas osteoid osteomas are nonprogressive. Osteoblastomas can also present with pain but do not usually respond to NSAIDs.[14,56,103]

Giant Cell Tumor of Bone. The giant cell tumor (GCT) of bone is generally a benign entity histologically characterized by multinucleated giant cells superimposed on a background of mononuclear stromal cells. GCTs account for approximately 20% of all benign bone tumors and 5% of all primary bone neoplasms.[19] Lesion prevalence peaks in the third decade[19] and there is a slight 1.2 : 1 female predominance.[94,104] Approximately 50% to 65% of cases occur around the knee.[19,84] Patients often present with pain. Pain can be associated with activity or can occur at rest, and is due to mechanical failure from bone destruction, which may predispose to pathologic fracture, and expansion of the periosteum. The exam may reveal direct tenderness to palpation, swelling, joint effusion, and gait abnormalities.[94,104]

Radiographs demonstrate an eccentric lytic lesion involving the subchondral bone with well-defined, nonsclerotic margins (Fig. 14.11). Ninety percent of cases are metaphyseoepiphyseal in location.[94] Locally aggressive features include cortical destruction and expansile remodeling, wide zone of transition, and extra-osseous soft tissue extension.[19] Periosteal reaction is not a common finding with these tumors.[84] Initial radiographs often show these classic findings and biopsy is performed to confirm the diagnosis.[94] Malignant transformation is exceedingly rare, with a prevalence of approximately 1% of all GCTs.[19]

Malignant GCTs of bone may also exhibit cortical permeation and soft tissue extension, preventing reliable radiologic differentiation between benign and malignant lesions.[84]

CT allows for better visualization of pathologic fractures, cortical destruction/thinning, expansile remodeling, and periosteal reaction (see Fig. 14.11). GCT soft tissue density is measured on CT, and soft tissue extension is seen in up to 44% of cross-sectional studies.[84] MRI shows the classic eccentric, metaphyseoepiphyseal location of the GCT, low to intermediate T1-weighted and increased T2-weighted signal intensity, areas of blooming on gradient echo imaging, and enhancement (Fig. 14.12).[19] There may also be fluid-fluid levels from secondary ABC development present in approximately 14% of cases.[84] Nuclear scintigraphy typically demonstrates peripheral, increased uptake with central photopenia ("donut sign").[19,84] However, this is not a specific finding and can be seen in ABCs and telangiectatic osteosarcomas. There is frequently increased uptake in the adjacent joint due to increased blood flow and local demineralization secondary to disuse, and uptake does not suggest tumor extension into the joint.[84]

GCTs of the bone have been reported to metastasize to the lungs in 1% to 6% of cases.[19] These lesions are thought to arise through hematogenous seeding of the GCT. Pulmonary metastases have imaging characteristics similar to the primary bone tumors, have benign histology, and may not require treatment.[19,94]

MALIGNANT PRIMARY OSSEOUS TUMORS OF THE KNEE

Myeloma

The myeloma is the most common primary bone tumor and predominantly affects patients in the seventh decade of life.[45]

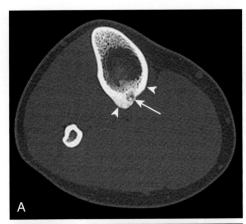

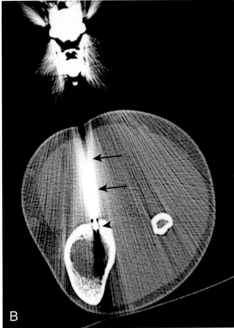

FIG 14.10 Fourteen-Year-Old Girl With Osteoid Osteoma
(A) Axial CT shows a cortically based lucency *(arrowhead)* in the posterior, proximal tibial cortex with the central mineralized nidus and surrounding sclerosis *(arrowheads)* in this girl with a 4-month history of progressive pain relieved by nonsteroidal anti-inflammatory medication. Lesion was classic for osteoid osteoma and the patient elected radiofrequency ablation. (B) Axial CT image obtained during percutaneous biopsy and radiofrequency ablation shows needle placement *(arrows)* within the nidus *(arrowhead). CT,* Computed tomography.

Myelomas are characterized by anomalous proliferation of plasma cells that produce monoclonal immunoglobulins. These cells can infiltrate bone marrow and replace the normal marrow environment, resulting in abnormal hematopoiesis. The classic findings of myeloma consist of hypercalcemia, renal insufficiency, anemia, and lytic bone lesions; pathologic fractures also occur and the myeloma entity carries significant risk of morbidity and mortality.[27,45]

Initial evaluation of a myeloma often involves a full skeletal survey, including views of the skull, spine, ribs, femurs, and knees. The long bones are affected in approximately 25% of patients.[27,28,45] Radiographic findings may include cortical thinning with or without discrete lytic lesions (Fig. 14.13) caused

by abnormal bone marrow proliferation with resultant destruction of bone. Approximately 80% of patients have detectable abnormalities on skeletal survey, however radiographs have significant diagnostic limitations.[27,45] Lesions may not be apparent until there is 30% to 50% loss of the normal bone density, and there is a false-negative rate of 30% to 70%.[28,29,44,45]

Multidetector CT allows for increased sensitivity in the detection of lytic lesions when compared to radiography and can further delineate areas at risk for pathologic fracture.[40,44,45,65] In conjunction with MRI, CT improves staging over any independent modality.[44,45] One of the primary drawbacks to whole-body CT is radiation dose; however, low-dose CT protocols have been developed for use in the screening of myeloma.[50] Whole-body MRI examination is being used more extensively in the imaging workup of myeloma, and has been shown to be effective in detection of lesions in the axial and appendicular skeleton.[9,45] Bone marrow involvement can be identified by detection of a hypointense signal relative to the normal fatty marrow on T1-weighted images and hyperintensity on T2-weighted images (see Fig. 14.13). Untreated lesions also exhibit diffuse contrast enhancement. However, these findings are nonspecific and can be seen with lymphoma, leukemia, and metastatic disease.[44] The number and pattern of lesions has been correlated with treatment outcomes.[45] There are four predominant patterns seen in MRI with myelomas:
1. Normal marrow pattern
2. Micronodular, also referred to as a variegated or salt-and-pepper pattern
3. Focal pattern
4. Diffuse pattern

Normal and micronodular patterns have been associated with stage I disease, whereas focal and diffuse patterns are more frequently associated with stage II or III disease.[44] Currently there are no universally accepted scanning recommendations with multiple whole-body MRI protocols using many different scanning sequences in the literature.[44] At some institutions, whole-body coronal and sagittal T1 and short tau inversion recovery (STIR) images are used as the standard protocol. Newer emerging MR techniques are being researched including dynamic contrast-enhanced (DCE) MRI and diffusion-weighted imaging[30] but they are not currently used in widespread clinical practice.*

FDG-PET/CT is a useful tool for the staging and prognosis of myeloma. The CT component allows for detection of osseous lesions, as described previously, and PET aids in the delineation of medullary lesions without associated bony changes and extra-osseous involvement.[27] Active lesions are characterized by increased FDG uptake. Patients with more than three focal lesions generally have a worse survival rate when compared to patients with three or fewer lesions. Lesions smaller than 10 mm may be difficult to detect and yield a false-negative result when using a standardized uptake value (SUV) threshold of 2.5.[15,44] Corticosteroid treatment may also result in false-negative results if not stopped at least 5 days prior to the examination.[44] FDG-PET/CT may also be useful in post-treatment monitoring, with decreased uptake after successful treatment. Furthermore, it is noteworthy that patients with *monoclonal gammopathy of undetermined significance* (MGUS) do not have increased uptake as seen in patients with myeloma, allowing for distinction between the two entities on PET.[44,45]

*References 27, 45-48, 67, and 89.

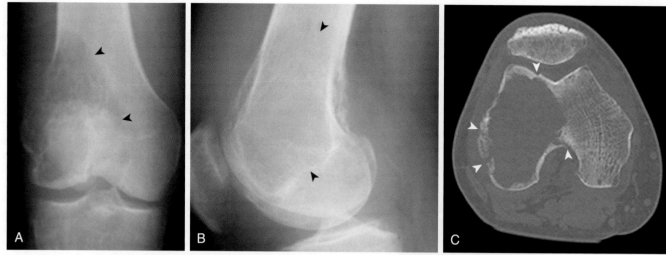

FIG 14.11 Forty-Three-Year-Old Man With Giant Cell Tumor of the Right Knee (A) AP and (B) lateral radiographs show an eccentric, lytic lesion in the distal femur with the epicenter in the metaphysis and extension into the articular end of the bone. (C) Axial CT shows the large, eccentric lytic lesion with expansile remodeling and better defines the multifocal areas of cortical destruction *(arrowheads)*. *AP*, Anteroposterior; *GCT*, giant cell tumor; *CT*, computed tomography.

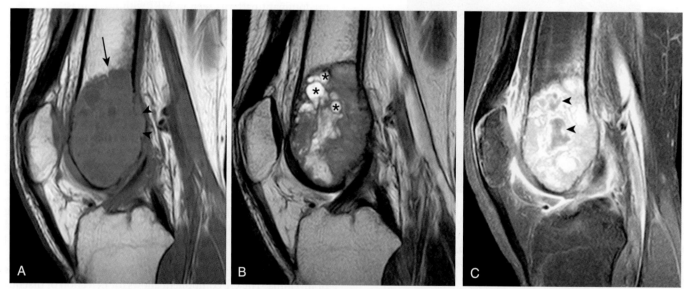

FIG 14.12 Twenty-Year-Old Man With Giant Cell Tumor and Secondary Aneurysmal Bone Cyst Formation (A) Sagittal T1-weighted image shows a marrow-replacing lesion *(arrow)* in the distal femur extending to the articular surface, with expansile remodeling of the posterior cortex *(arrowheads)*. (B) T2-weighted image shows a heterogeneous signal within the tumor, with hyperintense cystic foci *(asterisks)* corresponding to secondary ABC formation. (C) T1-weighted enhanced fat-suppressed image shows marked, diffuse enhancement with areas of nonenhancement *(arrowheads)*. *ABC,* Aneurysmal bone cyst.

Osteosarcoma

The osteosarcoma is a malignant, osteoid-forming bone tumor that is the second most common primary bone tumor, and the most common primary bone tumor in children. Osteosarcomas are most commonly located within the central medullary canal of long bones, but can also occur within the cortex, periosteum, and soft tissues.[38] There are multiple syndromes and genetic mutations that can predispose to the development of osteosarcoma including Li-Fraumeni syndrome; Rothmund-Thomson

syndrome; p53, retinoblastoma susceptibility (Rb) and murine double minute 2 (MDM2) mutations; and heterozygosity in chromosomes 3q, 13q, and 18q.[38,114] All the osteosarcoma subtypes are listed in Table 14.1,[38] but only the more common subtypes will be discussed.[38]

Central Type

Conventional osteosarcoma. The conventional osteosarcoma is a high-grade osteosarcoma and is the most common central subtype, accounting for approximately 75% of all cases.[38] It

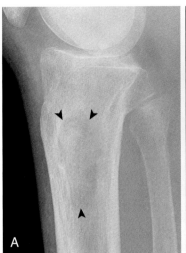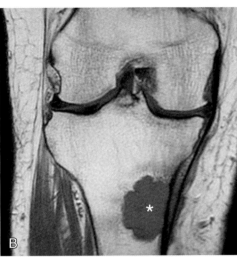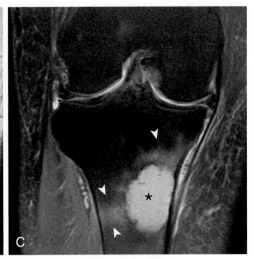

FIG 14.13 Seventy-Four-Year-Old Woman With Myeloma of the Proximal Tibia (A) Lateral radiograph demonstrates a lytic lesion in the tibial metadiaphysis *(arrowheads)* with a narrow zone of transition and non-sclerotic margins. (B and C) Coronal T1- (B) and T2-weighted fat-suppressed (C) images from prior MRI show a lobulated, well-defined, homogeneous marrow-replacing lesion *(asterisks)* with perilesional edema *(arrowheads)*. *MRI,* Magnetic resonance imaging.

TABLE 14.1 Subtypes of Osteosarcoma
1. Central type
a. Conventional
b. Epithelioid
c. Giant cell–rich
d. Osteoblastoma-like
e. Small cell
f. Telangiectatic
g. Low-grade central
2. Multifocal
3. Gnathic
4. Surface osteosarcoma
a. Parosteal
b. Periosteal
c. High-grade surface
d. Intracortical
5. Secondary

From Fox MG, Trotta BM: Osteosarcoma: review of the various types with emphasis on recent advancements in imaging. *Semin Musculoskelet Radiol* 17:123–136, 2013.

typically presents in the second to third decades with a male-to-female predisposition of approximately 2:1.[91,114] Typical presenting symptoms include swelling and pain that persists at night. Osteosarcomas most commonly involve the metaphysis of long bones, but can uncommonly present in isolated epiphyseal and diaphyseal locations.[38,101,110] There are three classic radiographic patterns depending on the osteoblastic, chondroblastic, and fibroblastic composition of the tumor.

Most osteosarcoma cases exhibit mixed osteolysis and osteosclerosis on radiographs, with cloudlike or flocculent sclerosis intermixed with permeative lucent areas. If the tumor is predominantly composed of mineralized osteoid, there is predominating osteosclerosis. If a lesion is predominantly composed of fibrous tissue or unmineralized cartilage, there is predominating osteolysis (Fig. 14.14).[101] Aggressive periosteal reaction has been associated with osteosarcomas; the most classic pattern is the "sunburst" pattern, which is almost pathognomonic for osteosarcoma (see Fig. 14.14). Codman's triangle, multilaminated, and "hair-on-end" periosteal reactions have also been described with the osteosarcoma.[38,101,111]

CT is useful in assessing tumor mineralization in cases where it may be subtle or absent on radiographs. Approximately 90% of cases that present with an associated soft tissue mass can be detected by CT examination.[101] Furthermore, high-resolution CT of the chest is useful in evaluating patients with osteosarcoma, since pulmonary metastases account for approximately 80% of all metastases.[38] About 20% of pediatric populations will have detectable metastases at presentation.[114]

MRI has limited usefulness in characterization of the osteosarcoma, but it is the modality of choice for local staging and preoperative planning.[38,101] Osteosarcomas are hypointense or isointense on T1-weighted sequences, and heterogeneously hyperintense on T2-weighted and STIR sequences. Foci of mineralization demonstrate hypointensity on all sequences (see Fig. 14.14).[101,114] Using T1 and STIR sequences on unenhanced MRI is useful for determining epiphyseal spread of the tumor.[49] Intra-articular extension is more difficult to gauge with disruption of the synovial membranes or articular cartilage being the most sensitive finding. Absence of joint effusion is also suggestive of articular sparing.[16] However, specificity is low for most of these findings, making MRI far more useful in the exclusion of intra-articular extension.[16,38] MRI is also useful in preoperative planning by delineating the soft tissue component of the tumor and invasion of adjacent neurovascular structures.[97]

Nuclear scintigraphy is sometimes performed at the time of diagnosis using thallium-201 or technetium-99m methoxyisobutylisonitrile (^{99m}Tc-MIBI) to detect metastases (see Fig. 14.14). There is some preliminary evidence showing that the washout rate of ^{99m}Tc-MIBI correlates to expression of multidrug resistance–associated protein (MRP), which may impact chemotherapeutic response.[18]

Telangiectatic osteosarcoma. Telangiectatic osteosarcomas account for up to 12.5% of all osteosarcomas[101] and have a male-to-female predominance of about 2:1. Patients typically

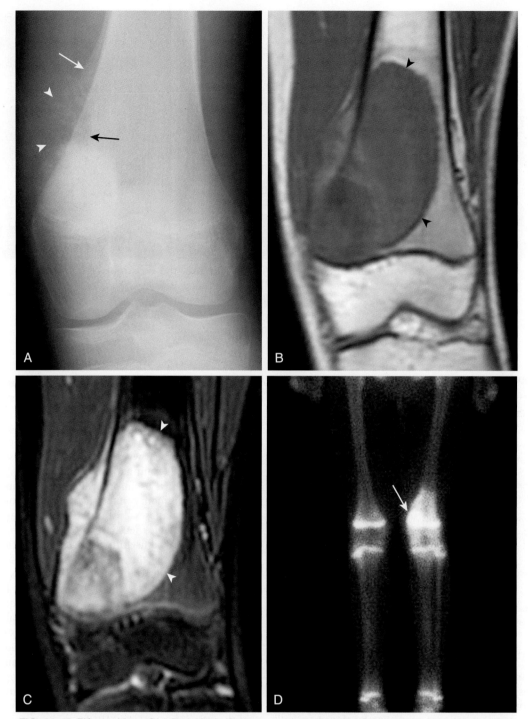

FIG 14.14 Fifteen-Year-Old Boy With Osteosarcoma of the Left Knee (A) AP radiograph of the left knee shows a lucent lesion *(arrow)* in the medial femoral metadiaphysis, with sunburst pattern *(arrowheads)* and Codman's triangle *(white arrow)* periosteal reaction. (B and C) Coronal (B) T1-weighted and (C) T2-weighted images through the left knee demonstrate a lesion *(arrowheads)* with hypointense T1-weighted signal and a heterogeneously high signal on T2. (D) Nuclear scintigraphy shows corresponding increased activity within the left distal femoral osteosarcoma *(arrow)* and no "skip lesions" within the remaining lower extremities. *AP,* Anteroposterior.

present in the second or third decades.[38,101] Pathologic fracture and metastases are present in 40% to 60% and 20% of patients, respectively. These tumors are characterized by numerous dilated blood-filled cavities with peripheral sarcomatous cells in the tumoral margin and septa.[38,87]

Telangiectatic osteosarcomas are predominantly lytic tumors with a wide zone of transition on radiographs. Expansile remodeling, cortical destruction, lack of significant sclerosis, and periosteal reaction are common findings.[38] Cross-sectional imaging demonstrates fluid-fluid levels caused by blood-filled

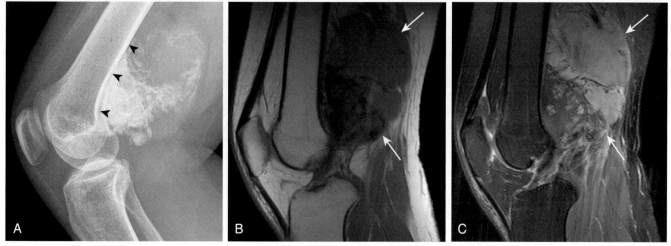

FIG 14.15 Forty-Year-Old Woman With Parosteal Osteosarcoma in Posterior Distal Femur
(A) Lateral radiograph shows a large, mineralized surface mass in the posterior femoral metadi-aphysis with a lucent line *(arrowheads)* between the mass and underlying cortex. (B and C) Sagittal (B) T1-weighted and (C) T2-weighted images through the knee. The mass is primarily hypointense on T1 *(arrows)* and slightly hyperintense to skeletal muscle of T2-weighted image. The underlying bone marrow is not involved by the mass.

cysts within the tumor, and can mimic ABC. On postcontrast images, telangiectatic osteosarcomas will typically have thick, nodular, enhancing peripheral tissue, whereas ABCs will have smooth, thin, peripheral rims less than 3 mm thick. CT can further help differentiate the two entities by detecting osteoid mineralization in the telangiectatic osteosarcoma. Furthermore, cortical destruction associated with a soft tissue mass should favor against the diagnosis of an ABC.[87,101] Nuclear scintigraphy can demonstrate a lesion with central photopenia in the con-figuration of a "donut."[38]

Surface Type

Parosteal osteosarcoma. Parosteal osteosarcomas account for 65% to 75% of all surface osseous lesions and approximately 5% of all osteosarcomas. Parosteal osteosarcomas typically present in the third to fourth decades of life with a slight 1.3:1 female predominance.[31,38,101] Patients often present with a pain-less mass, and approximately 70% arise from the posterior distal femur.[31,38]

On radiography, these lesions appear as sessile masses with dense, lobulated central sclerosis (Fig. 14.15). There is charac-teristically a lucent line between the periosteum and the cortex, representing unmineralized, thickened periosteum (see Fig. 14.15).[31,38,101,105] Invasion into the underlying medulla and adjacent soft tissues is not uncommon.[38,101] Dedifferentiation occurs in up to 27% of parosteal osteosarcomas, with medullary invasion being twice as common in these cases.[6] Areas of dedif-ferentiation are typically more lytic radiographically, unminer-alized on CT, and are more T2-hyperintense and enhancing on MRI (see Fig. 14.15). These suspicious regions should be tar-geted on image-guided biopsy to maximize detection of dedif-ferentiated tumors.[31]

Chondrosarcoma

Chondrosarcoma is a malignant cartilage-forming bone tumor. It is the third most common overall primary bone tumor after myeloma and osteosarcoma. These tumors are commonly characterized on radiographs by the chondroid "ring-and-arc"

TABLE 14.2 Subtypes of Chondrosarcoma

1. Primary
   a. Conventional
   b. Clear cell
   c. Juxtacortical
   d. Myxoid
   e. Mesenchymal
   f. Extraskeletal
   g. Dedifferentiated
2. Secondary

From Murphey MD, Walker EA, Wilson AJ, et al: From the archives of the AFIP: imaging of primary chondrosarcoma: radiologic-pathologic correlation. *Radiographics* 23:1245–1278, 2003.

pattern with aggressive features.[86] All the types of chondrosar-coma are listed in Table 14.2, however addressing each in detail is outside the scope of this chapter. Only the more common types will be discussed.

Conventional Intramedullary Chondrosarcoma. Conventional intramedullary chondrosarcomas, commonly referred to as conventional chondrosarcomas, are the most common type of primary chondrosarcoma. Conventional chondrosarcomas often present in patients between 30 and 40 years of age with a 2:1 male predominance. Symptoms are typically nonspecific and most commonly consist of pain with or without an associ-ated mass.

On radiographs, conventional chondrosarcomas present as lytic lesions with admixed sclerosis from chondroid mineraliza-tion seen in approximately 75% of cases (Fig. 14.16). The classic pattern of mineralization has been described as a "ring-and-arc" appearance; however, chondrosarcomas may form a denser, flocculent pattern of mineralization. More aggressive lesions are typically lucent and may exhibit a permeative lytic pattern. Lobulated endosteal scalloping with eventual cortical penetra-tion and soft tissue mass are present in approximately 50% of chondrosarcomas on long bone radiographs.[86,90] Pathologic fracture is also present on initial presentation in about 5% to

15% of patients.[86] CT imaging can also further characterize the chondrosarcoma and help differentiate this entity from the benign enchondroma. Ninety percent of chondrosarcomas will demonstrate endosteal scalloping greater than two-thirds of the cortical thickness and extend along the length of the lesion; conversely, enchondromas may result in mild endosteal scalloping along only a portion of the lesion in 10% of cases. Extra-osseous soft tissue extension also excludes the diagnosis of enchondroma.[36,86] Nuclear scintigraphy commonly demonstrates heterogeneously increased activity in most cases.[36,86]

MRI can also help define the extent of bone marrow involvement and soft tissue extension from the chondrosarcoma (see Fig. 14.16). Although rests of normal fatty marrow may be preserved within a chondrosarcoma, this is much more commonly present with an enchondroma. The typical lobular configuration of cartilaginous neoplasms can be appreciated at the tumor margin. Chondrosarcomas exhibit a heterogeneous high signal on T2-weighted sequences, and the mineralized matrix will be hypointense on all sequences (see Fig. 14.16). Extra-osseous soft tissue extension exhibits similar MR characteristics to the intraosseous counterpart, usually with a mild peripheral and septal enhancement pattern.

Dedifferentiated Chondrosarcoma.

Dedifferentiated chondrosarcomas account for up to 10% of all chondrosarcomas, with evidence suggesting a rate of dedifferentiation as high as 20% in all conventional chondrosarcomas. Typically these occur in older patients between the ages of 50 and 70 years of age with no gender predilection. Presenting symptoms are similar to those seen in patients with conventional chondrosarcomas—pain, pathologic fracture, and soft tissue mass.[86]

Imaging findings are largely contingent upon the proportion of high-grade involvement, and a lesion with a minimal high-grade component may be indistinguishable on imaging from a low-grade lesion. High-grade, dedifferentiated foci within a chondrosarcoma are characterized by lysis and decreased mineralization on radiographs and CT. Low-grade components demonstrate low CT attenuation, whereas high-grade foci are isodense to skeletal muscle on CT.[74,86] Furthermore, high-grade dedifferentiated foci display variable T2-weighted intensity (but are typically hypointense to the low-grade elements) and display avid diffuse enhancement.[74,86]

Secondary Chondrosarcoma.

Although the focus of this chapter is on primary tumors of the knee, it is also worthwhile to mention that up to 12% of chondrosarcomas develop secondary to pre-existing conditions including osteochondromas, enchondromatosis, fibrous dysplasia, Paget disease, or prior radiation. Osteochondromatosis, enchondromatosis, and Maffucci's syndrome all carry a significant risk of malignant degeneration estimated to be 5% to 25%, 25% to 50%, and 50% to 100%, respectively.[88,90]

Osseous Lymphoma

Osseous lymphomas account for approximately 7% of all bone malignancy.[72] Primary bone lymphomas are rare; however, secondary involvement of osseous structures is not uncommon, especially in pediatric populations. Primary lymphomas of the bone (also called *reticulum cell sarcomas*) are rare malignancies accounting for less than 5% of all primary bone tumors.[64] It is typically defined as a lymphoma within a single osseous site with or without regional nodal metastasis and no distant metastasis within 6 months of diagnosis. Most commonly, these tumors are non-Hodgkin lymphomas (NHLs) of the diffuse large cell lymphoma type.[72] In one study reviewing 237 cases, the mean age of patients was 42 years with a 1.8:1 male predominance.[79] Patients most often present with pain, B symptoms, swelling or mass, and pathologic fractures.[25] Some of the more common sites of involvement include osseous structures adjacent to the knee joint.[79] The disseminated lymphoma with osseous involvement, or secondary lymphoma of the bone, is significantly more common than the primary

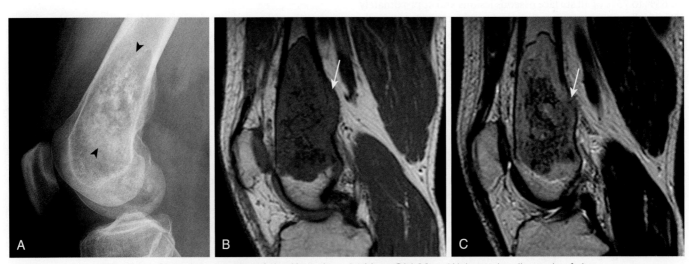

FIG 14.16 Chondrosarcoma of the Knee in a 34-Year-Old Man (A) Lateral radiograph of the knee demonstrates a large, lytic lesion *(arrowheads)* in the distal femoral shaft and metaphysis with internal chondroid mineralization. (B and C) Sagittal (B) T1 and (C) T2-weighted images through the knee better delineate the large, heterogeneous marrow-replacing lesion with hypointense foci corresponding to mineralization and posterior cortical expansile remodeling *(arrows)*. Patient underwent resection of the chondrosarcoma and reconstruction with custom total knee replacement.

bone lymphoma and occurs in both Hodgkin's and NHL. There is a tendency of these lesions to preferentially spread to the axial skeleton, but metastases can occur along any osseous structure.

Lymphomas may be radiographically occult or present as a moth-eaten or permeative lytic lesion. Periosteal reaction is occasionally present (lamellated, "onion-skin," or discontinuous patterns) and is indicative of a poor prognosis. More advanced lesions may demonstrate local invasion into the adjacent soft tissues and/or cortical destruction with an associated fracture. Less commonly, lymphomas can be of mixed density or purely sclerotic (Fig. 14.17). Sclerosis is more frequently associated with treated lesions or Hodgkin's lymphoma, although most Hodgkin's lymphoma lesions remain purely lytic.[64,72] Bony sequestra are also sometimes present.[57] CT findings are similar to those found on radiographs, but CT is more sensitive in detecting cortical or trabecular abnormalities, periosteal reaction, extra-osseous soft tissue extension, and adenopathy than radiography.[54,72] The relative absence of cortical destruction in the presence of a tumor favors the diagnosis of lymphoma over other osseous malignancies (see Fig. 14.17). Extra-osseous seeding without cortical destruction suggests that the tumor spreads via osseous vascular channels.

MRI can provide additional information regarding the extent of bone marrow and soft tissue involvement, and detect multifocal lesions. Bone marrow replacement typically exhibits diminished T1-weighted and elevated T2-weighted signal intensity (see Fig. 14.17).[64,72] T1-weighted sequences are preferred in assessing the extent of tumor burden since the elevated T2-signal can be confounded with adjacent edema. Any extra-osseous soft tissue component is typically isointense to the intraosseous tumor and will diffusely and homogeneously

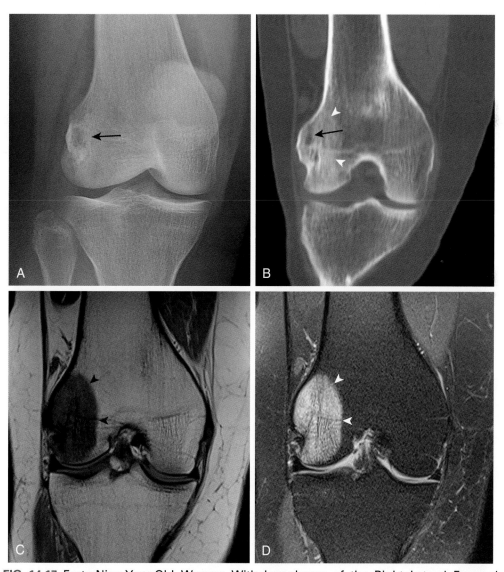

FIG 14.17 Forty-Nine-Year-Old Woman With Lymphoma of the Right Lateral Femoral Condyle Internal oblique radiograph (A) and coronal 2D reformatted image (B) of the right knee demonstrate a lytic lesion in the lateral femoral condyle *(arrow)* with some adjacent sclerosis *(arrowheads)*. Coronal T1-weighted (C) and T2-weighted (D) images show a marrow-replacing lesion *(arrowheads)* with preservation of the underlying trabecular, which is much more conspicuous compared to the radiographs.

enhance.[54] Scintigraphy is useful in detecting multifocal lesions. FDG-PET and PET/CT show intense increased uptake within involved areas and has been reported to be superior to CT/MRI in monitoring therapeutic response.[20] FDG-PET has also been shown to be more effective in determining bone marrow involvement than biopsy alone and could prove useful as an adjunct exam.[22]

BENIGN PRIMARY SOFT TISSUE TUMORS OF THE KNEE

Adipocytic Soft Tissue Tumors

Lipoma. The lipoma is the most prevalent benign soft tissue tumor.[8] However, it is not possible to estimate the incidence of lipomatous tumors since the diagnosis is commonly made clinically and tumors are often untreated.[7] Approximately 50% of all benign mesenchymal tumors are found to be lipoma at surgical excison.[7] Clinically, lipomas present as a slow-growing soft tissue mass that is usually painless and asymptomatic.[7,8,53] However, large lipomas can cause local mass effect and pain due to local nerve compression.[7,37] Lipoma has a slight female predominance and classically presents in the fifth to seventh decades.[7,8,37,53]

On gross examination, the lipoma is an encapsulated, soft, greasy, yellow mass usually without calcifications.[37,53] Lipomas are composed almost entirely of differentiated and mature adipocytes and are histologically indistinguishable from mature fat.[7,37] Lipomas are generally subcutaneous and do not involve the joint; however, intra-articular lipomas most commonly involve the knee.[53] Intra-articular lipomas can develop regions of ossification or calcification.[70] Cytogenetically, there are three major aberrations associated with the formation of benign lipomatous tumors—mutation of 12q13-15 (65%), loss of a portion of chromosome 13q (10%), or mutation of 6p21-31 (5%).[37]

Lipomas are often not visible on radiographs, but larger lesions can be detected as lucent soft tissue masses of fat density.[7] The lipoma has an almost identical appearance to subcutaneous fat on cross-sectional imaging, and imaging of lipomas is diagnostic in 70% to 90% of cases (Fig. 14.18).[7,37,53] When encapsulated, the capsule has an attenuation similar to that of skeletal muscle on CT and will be hypointense on all MRI sequences.[7] Furthermore, unencapsulated subcutaneous lipomas may be overlooked or imperceptible on imaging.[7]

Lipoma Arborescens. Lipoma arborescens is a benign proliferation of the synovial membrane forming villous, frondlike projections filled with mature adipocytes.[7,53,106] It can be thought of as a lipomatous distention of hypertrophic synovial villi, is most commonly unilateral, and seen within the suprapatellar pouch if involving the knee.[7,10,106,107] Lipoma arborescens of the knee presents clinically with slow-onset edema that can be associated with transient joint effusions.[7,10,37] It occurs most commonly in patients in their fifth to seventh decades and has a slight male predominance.[7,106] The underlying cause of lipoma arborescens is unknown, but it is thought to be associated with a preceding traumatic or inflammatory condition.[53,106]

The imaging characteristics of lipoma arborescens are usually diagnostic. However, lipoma arborescens must be differentiated from a true synovial lipoma, which is a very rare and benign adipocytic neoplasm.[107] On radiographs, lipoma arborescens often shows nonspecific fullness of the knee.[7] Sonography may show an echogenic, frondlike mass and effusion involving the suprapatellar bursa.[7] On MRI, lipoma arborescens demonstrates a villous fatty mass that is isointense to subcutaneous fat on all sequences, is most common in the suprapatellar bursa, and is often associated with a joint effusion (Fig. 14.19).[7,10,53,106]

Lipoblastoma. The lipoblastoma is a slow-growing, benign soft tissue tumor that is most commonly seen in very young children, usually less than 1 year of age.[8,35] Lipoblastomas should be considered in the differential diagnosis for any fatty mass in a child less than 3 years of age.[7,8,35]

Lipoblastomas are composed of lipoblasts and fetal adipocytic-like tissue.[8,35] There is a strong male predominance with a 3:1 male-to-female ratio.[7,8,35] Tumors most commonly occur in the trunk and extremities, and patients typically present with a nontender mass.[7,37]

There are two general subtypes of lipoblastoma—circumscribed and diffuse.[35] The *circumscribed* subtype has

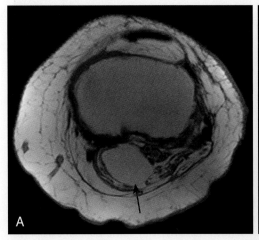
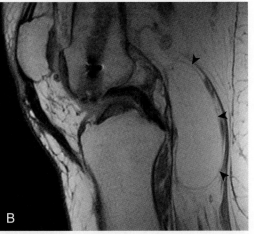

FIG 14.18 Popliteal Fossa Lipoma in a 77-Year-Old Woman Axial (A) and sagittal (B) T1-weighted images of the knee show a well-circumscribed mass *(arrow)* in the popliteal fossa that is isointense to subcutaneous fat and has a thin, low-signal margin *(arrowheads).*

septa between fat lobules and rarely recurs after resection.[35] The *diffuse* form (commonly called *lipoblastomatosis*) is an infiltrative tumor seen throughout the deep soft tissues, often in the retroperitoneum.[35] On gross examination, lipoblastoma is a soft, lobular yellow to tan mass, usually measuring 2 to 5 cm in diameter.[37] Histologically, lipoblastomas are composed of mature adipocytes, fetal adipocytes, and myxoid matrix.[7] Most cases of lipoblastoma demonstrate an aberration of chromosome 8q11-13.[37]

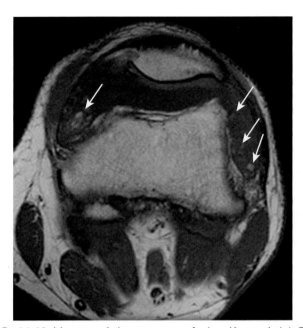

FIG 14.19 Lipoma Arborescens of the Knee Axial T1-weighted image demonstrates frondlike, villous outpouchings of hyperintense synovial fatty tissue, pathognomonic of lipoma arborescens.

On imaging, lipoblastoma is a well-circumscribed, lobulated mass with some fatty composition.[35] The imaging appearance is dependent on the histology of the tumor,[35] specifically the ratio of adipose tissue to lipoblasts and myxoid tissue.[7,35] On CT and MRI, the adipocytic portions of the tumor follow the imaging features of subcutaneous fat, while the nonadipocytic tissues have a nondescript appearance.[7] The imaging appearance of the liposarcoma is similar to that of a lipoblastoma because they both can have thin septa, can demonstrate slight hypointensity compared with subcutaneous fat on T1-weighted images, can undergo cystic transformation, and can have variable enhancement (Fig. 14.20).[8,35] However, knowledge of the patient's age is crucial, as the liposarcoma is extremely rare in very young children.[35]

Fibroblastic Soft Tissue Tumors

Desmoid-Type Fibromatosis. Fibromatosis includes desmoid tumors (most common), fibromatosis coli, congenital fibromatosis, and congenital fibrosarcoma.[78] Desmoid tumors (also known as *desmoid-type fibromatosis or aggressive fibromatosis*) are rare, benign, but locally aggressive mesenchymal tumors composed of large bundles of fibroblasts and myofibroblasts that produce intracellular collagen.[71,78] Desmoid tumors most commonly present as a painless mass in the trunk or extremity of a patient in the third to fourth decade, with a slight female predominance.[37,71] Desmoid tumors tend to be larger than 5 cm in diameter, involve deep tissue structures, exhibit rapid growth, and are associated with a high local recurrence rate after surgical excision.[71] On gross examination, a desmoid tumor is often a firm, shiny, white tumor with internal trabeculations and a gritty cut surface.[37] Histologically, a desmoid tumor has a very benign appearance with little, if any, evidence of mitosis.[71] Desmoid tumorigenesis is thought to be linked to the adenomatous polyposis coli (APC) gene on chromosome 5q22, which is also linked to familial adenomyomatous polyposis and Gardner's syndrome.[71]

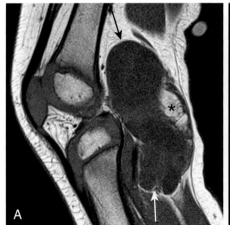
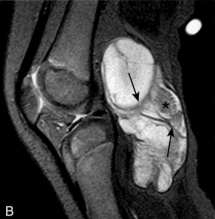
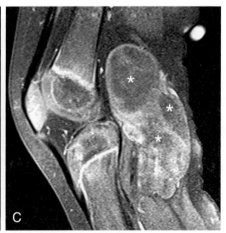

FIG 14.20 Lipoblastoma in the Popliteal Fossa (A) Sagittal T1-weighted image of a lipoblastoma in the popliteal fossa of the knee demonstrates a circumscribed, hetero-homogeneous mass *(arrows)* with nodular focus *(asterisk)* that is isointense to fat. (B) Sagittal T2-weighted fat-suppressed image shows a drop in signal within the fatty nodule *(asterisk)* and multiple cystic components separated by thin, hypointense internal septations *(arrows)*. (C) Sagittal enhanced image shows heterogeneous enhancement with lack of enhancement of the cystic regions *(asterisks)*.

While histologic tissue analysis is required for diagnosis of a desmoid tumor, imaging can aid in diagnosis.[71] A desmoid tumor is usually radiographically occult, but if seen, is a nondescript soft tissue mass.[71] On CT evaluation, a desmoid tumor is an ovoid or irregular mass that is isodense to hypodense to skeletal muscle.[71] Desmoid tumors present as relatively homogeneous, infiltrative, deep soft tissue masses on T1-weighted MRI, and are isointense to hyperintense to skeletal muscle.[8,71,78] On T2-weighed images, the desmoid is usually heterogeneous and hyperintense compared to muscle.[8,71,78] Desmoids will display intermediate to strong gadolinium enhancement in the noncollagenous portions of the tumor, and the degree of contrast enhancement is directly correlated with tumor cellularity (Fig. 14.21).[8,71,78] Desmoids have bands of low signal seen on all MR sequences, corresponding to the more fibrous component of the mass.[71] Although the desmoid tumor and soft tissue sarcoma may be confused sometimes, sarcomas tend to displace (as opposed to invade) adjacent structures. Desmoid tumors are infiltrative and violate fascial planes, but osseous invasion is rare.[71] Furthermore, soft tissue sarcomas often outgrow their blood supply leading to central necrosis, whereas desmoid tumors do not.[71]

Nerve Sheath Tumors of the Soft Tissues

Schwannoma. The schwannoma (also known as *neurilemmoma*) is a benign neoplasm composed of dedifferentiated Schwann cells of the peripheral nerves.[37,52] Schwannomas represent approximately 5% of all benign soft tissue tumors.[73] Clinically, schwannomas present as slow-growing painless mass in patients in their second to fifth decades.[52,73,77] Tumors are most commonly seen in the head and neck, but are not uncommon in the extremities.[52] In the extremities, schwannomas are most commonly seen in the cutaneous and subcutaneous tissues along the flexor surface of a joint.[37] Schwannomas are equally prevalent in males and females.[77]

The schwannoma is usually solitary and sporadic with an unknown cause.[37,73,77] However, multiple schwannomas are associated with neurofibromatosis type 2 (NF2).[37] On gross examination, the schwannoma is a white-gray, globular, fibrous tumor with interspersed bright yellow foci and an epineurium capsule.[52,77] Conventional schwannomas are entirely composed of Schwann cells, whereas the schwannomas seen in NF are composed of Schwann cells, mast cells, lymphocytes, and fibroblasts.[77] Histologically, the schwannoma is composed of regions of densely packed spindle cells (Antoni A areas) and regions of less dense myxoid tissue with poorly organized cells (Antoni B areas).[77] The most common genetic aberration associated with schwannoma formation is the loss of at least some portion of chromosome 22.[37]

Sonographic evaluation of a schwannoma will reveal a hypoechoic nodule with entering and exiting nerve fascicles.[52] On CT, a schwannoma is a circumscribed mass that is hypodense to isodense to skeletal muscle, and will demonstrate homogeneous contrast enhancement when small.[77] The enhancement pattern becomes more heterogeneous in larger tumors.[77] MR evaluation of the schwannoma can be diagnostic, evidenced by a circumscribed nodule with low T1 signal intensity and high T2 signal intensity, and entering and exiting nerve fascicles.[52] Schwannomas may demonstrate the "target sign" or the "split fat sign," as described in neurofibroma (Fig. 14.22).[73] However, one differentiating feature is that schwannomas tend to lie peripheral to the nerve, while neurofibromas lie more centrally relative to the nerve.[73] In addition, changes associated with cystic degeneration are much more common with schwannomas.[73]

Neurofibroma. Neurofibromas are benign, well-circumscribed nerve sheath tumors arising from nonmyelinating Schwann cells and are of neuroectodermal origin.[60,95] Neurofibromas are composed of Schwann cells, perineural-like cells, fibroblasts, mast cells, and neuronal axons.[37] It is the most common peripheral nerve sheath tumor and most commonly occurs within cutaneous tissues.[37] Neurofibromas represent approximately 5% of benign tumors of the soft tissues and most commonly arise in patients in the third to fourth decades.[66,73] Neurofibromas usually present as slow-growing, painless masses.[37,73,95] However, when tumors involve the deeper soft tissues, neurologic symptoms are not uncommon.[73]

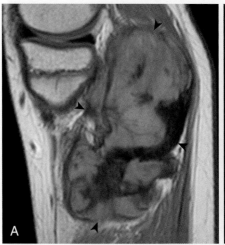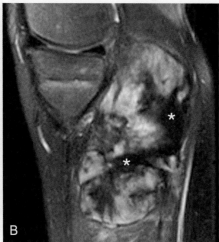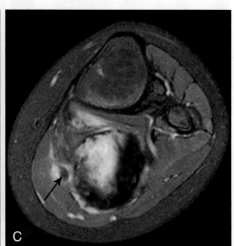

FIG 14.21 Desmoid Tumor of the Knee (A) Sagittal T1-weighted image of a desmoid tumor in the popliteal fossa shows a heterogeneous mass *(arrowheads)* with signal predominantly isointense to skeletal muscle. Sagittal (B) and axial (C) T2-weighted fat-suppressed images show low-signal intensity within the fibrous portions of the tumor *(asterisks)* and mass effect upon the posterior tibial artery *(arrow)*.

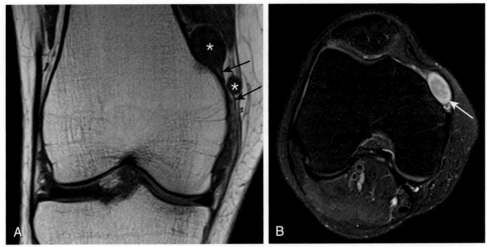

FIG 14.22 Schwannoma in a 22-Year-Old Man With Complaint of Mass (A) Coronal T1-weighted image shows two well-circumscribed nodules *(asterisks)* in the superior anteromedial knee with exiting nerves *(arrows)* surrounded by fat. (B) Axial T2-weighted image shows the "target sign," with a hyperintense rim *(arrow)* surrounding the hypointense central component. The resection specimen proved to be a schwannoma.

The neurofibroma is most commonly solitary and sporadic; however, patients with neurofibromatosis type 1 (NF1) generally have numerous neurofibromas.[37,60] Neurofibromas demonstrate one of three general growth patterns—localized, diffuse, or plexiform.[60] Regardless of the growth pattern, neurofibromas are deeply intertwined with the adjacent peripheral nerve and cannot be separated at surgical resection.[66,73] In addition, patients with NF1 tend to have larger tumors that are at increased risk of malignant degeneration.[73] Genetically, a neurofibroma is a monoclonal tumor whose tumorigenesis is due to loss of both copies of the NF1 gene on 17q, and tumors can be hereditary or sporadic in nature.[37]

The classic imaging appearance of the neurofibroma is a well-circumscribed, unencapsulated soft tissue nodule arising from a small peripheral nerve.[60] Sonographic evaluation of the neurofibroma shows a circumscribed, hypoechoic nodule.[73] CT of the neurofibroma demonstrates a fusiform, circumscribed nodule that is hypodense to skeletal muscle and shows contrast enhancement.[73] On MRI, localized neurofibromas are well-circumscribed, low-signal soft tissue nodules that are isointense to skeletal muscle on T1-weighted images and heterogeneously high in signal on T2-weighted images.[66,73] On MRI, a neurofibroma may demonstrate the classic "target sign," as previously described, and variable enhancement.[66,73] When the neurofibroma is of the plexiform subtype, it classically demonstrates an infiltrating, heterogeneous mass comprised of multiple tumor nodules, with an MRI appearance corresponding to the gross pathologic appearance of a "bag of worms" (Fig. 14.23).[66]

Vascular Soft Tissue Tumors

Synovial Hemangioma. The synovial hemangioma is a rare, benign neoplasm of vascular origin that occurs at the synovial lined surfaces of the intra-articular space or bursae, most commonly involving the knee.[23,37,42,51,99] According to one source, 97% of these tumors involve the knee.[76] Synovial hemangiomas most commonly present in children and adolescents, and demonstrate a preponderance in girls.[37,42,51,76,99] Clinically, the synovial hemangioma is often asymptomatic, but can be painful due to local destruction and hemarthrosis.[99] Approximately one-third of patients with a synovial hemangioma have pain at presentation and patients often present with swelling and effusion.[37] Up to 40% of patients with a synovial hemangioma will also have a cutaneous hemangioma.[51] Synovial hemangiomas are composed of adipose tissue, fibrous tissue, vascular channels, and muscular components and may contain thrombus within the vascular components.[42] Phleboliths can be seen in up to 30% of hemangiomas and are more commonly seen with the cavernous subtype.[99] Grossly, these tumors are soft, brown, noncircumscribed, lobulated masses; they are brown on gross examination due to hemosiderin deposition.[42] When intra-articular, synovial hemangiomas tend to be more circumscribed and often attached to the synovium by a small soft tissue pedicle.[42]

The imaging characteristics of the synovial hemangioma are relatively nonspecific.[42,51] In most cases, synovial hemangiomas are not seen on radiographs unless bone erosion or phleboliths are present.[42,51] However, when the tumor is large, a soft tissue mass may be appreciated on radiographs.[51] On CT, synovial hemangiomas are lobulated, heterogeneous soft tissue masses with overall attenuation similar to that of skeletal muscle, areas of high attenuation due to calcified phleboliths, and low attenuation foci.[23,42]

MRI is the diagnostic tool of choice.[76] On MR imaging, the hemangioma is evident as an intra-articular or juxta-articular lobulated, noncircumscribed mass.[23,42] Hemangiomas may contain internal septations and have a more circumscribed appearance on fluid-sensitive sequences (Fig. 14.24).[23,42] Hemangiomas demonstrate a low to intermediate signal on T1-weighted images and an intermediate to high heterogeneous signal on T2-weighted images.[23,99] Synovial hemangiomas are typically isointense to skeletal muscle on T1-weighed images and hyperintense to fat on T2-weighted images.[42] The heterogeneity on fluid-sensitive sequences can be attributed to the hyperintense blood in slow-flowing vascular channels, flow voids within higher-velocity channels, low signal due to calcified phleboliths, and intermediate signal within the intervening fatty and fibrous septations.[99,106] Gadolinium enhancement of the synovial hemangioma is generally homogenous, especially in comparison to extra-articular hemangioma.[99]

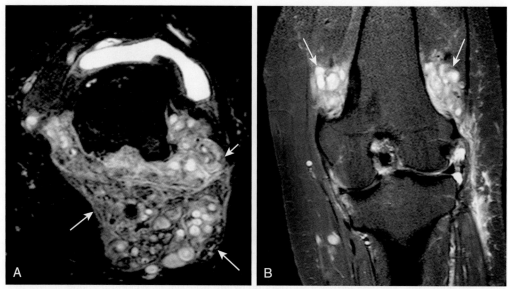

FIG 14.23 Plexiform Neurofibroma of the Knee in a Patient With Neurofibromatosis Axial (A) and coronal (B) T2-weighted fat-suppressed images through a large, biopsy-proven plexiform neurofibroma show an infiltrating, heterogeneous mass *(arrows)* comprised of multiple tumor nodules. The MRI appearance corresponds to the gross pathologic appearance of a "bag of worms." *MRI,* Magnetic resonance imaging.

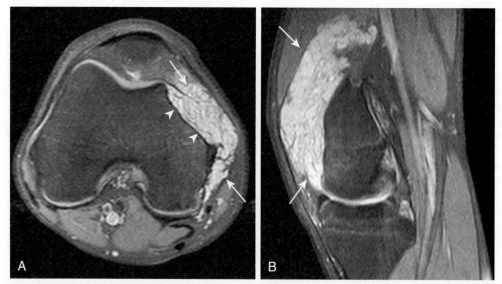

FIG 14.24 Synovial Hemangioma in an 18-Year-Old Man Presenting With Medial Knee Pain and Swelling Axial (A) and sagittal (B) T2-weighted images through the medial knee synovial hemangioma demonstrate a circumscribed mass *(arrows)* comprised of multiple serpentine, high-signal vascular channels with intervening septations. Notice the remodeling of the antero-medial femoral condyle *(arrowheads)* due to chronic pressure changes.

Chondroid Soft Tissue Tumors

Synovial Chondromatosis. Synovial chondromatosis (also known as *synovial osteochondromatosis*) is a benign proliferation of hyaline cartilage nodules in the synovial tissue of a joint, tendon sheath (tenosynovial osteochondromatosis), or bursa.[85,109] It is most commonly seen intra-articularly and approximately two-thirds of cases involve the knee.[37,109] In contrast, tendon sheath and bursal synovial involvement most commonly involve the hands and feet.[109] Synovial chondromatosis is twice as common

in men as women, and most commonly presents in the third to fifth decades.[37,85] Grossly, synovial chondromatosis presents as a multitude of light gray nodules attached to the synovial membrane.[37] Scientists have yet to discover an exact genetic mutation linked to the cause of synovial chondromatosis; however, higher expression of the hedgehog target genes *PTCH1* and *GLI1* has been reported.[37]

Primary synovial chondromatosis will radiographically demonstrate osteochondral bodies in 60% to 100% of cases, and an absence of underlying degenerative change.[85] Erosive changes of the adjacent bones are unusual in the large capacity knee joint, but may be seen in 20% to 50% of smaller capacity joints.[85] CT can better quantify the load of osteochondral bodies and is felt by some to be the imaging modality of choice for the detection of synovial chondromatosis.[85] Synovial chondromatosis can have a variable appearance on MRI, depending on the presence or absence of mineralization within the intra-articular bodies (Fig. 14.25).[85,109] Purely cartilaginous nodules will closely follow the signal characteristics of hyaline cartilage on all sequences, osteochondral bodies will demonstrate internal marrow signal, and densely calcified nodules will be hypointense and may be more conspicuous on gradient echo sequences due to magnetic susceptibility artifact.[85]

BENIGN FIBROHISTIOCYTIC SOFT TISSUE TUMORS OF THE KNEE

Localized Giant Cell Tumor

The localized type of tenosynovial GCT (also known as *nodular synovitis or GCT of the tendon sheath*) is a benign, nodular mass usually seen in the fingers and toes, but can also involve the knee.[4,109] Giant cell tumors of the tendon sheath (GCTTS) are fibrohistiocytic tumors of the tendon sheath, and nodular synovitis is the synovial-based, focal form of PVNS.[109] Clinically, nodular tenosynovitis presents as a painless mass in a patient in the fourth to sixth decades, with a slight female preponderance.[1] On gross examination, nodular synovitis is usually a small, circumscribed, light gray nodular or lobulated mass.[37] The most commonly associated genetic aberration is that of a translocation on chromosome 1.[37]

Radiography and CT are of little usefulness in the diagnosis of nodular synovitis.[1] Sonography may demonstrate a fixed, hypoechoic soft tissue nodule. Nodular tenosynovitis presents as a circumscribed, lobular soft tissue nodule with low-signal intensity on most MR sequences and exhibits avid enhancement.[4,39,109] Nodular synovitis can demonstrate a blooming artifact on gradient echo sequences due to hemosiderin deposition, similar to PVNS (Fig. 14.26).[39,109]

TUMORS OF THE SOFT TISSUES, UNCLASSIFIED

Myxoma

Juxta-articular myxomas are rare, benign tumors most commonly seen in the subcutaneous tissues adjacent to large joints.[24,37] They are composed of fibroblast-like cells that overproduce mucopolysaccharides.[83] Approximately 88% of juxta-articular myxomas occur around the knee.[37] Clinically, myxomas often present as a painful enlarging mass in a patient in the third to fifth decades.[24] Myxomas are more common in males than females, and are generally about 2 to 7 cm in size.[24] When juxta-articular, myxoma can be located within or adjacent to the joint capsule.[24] On gross examination, the tumors are shiny and gelatinous with ganglion-like cystic areas.[37] Histologically, myxomas are composed of primitive fibroblasts in a hypovascular myxoid matrix.[24] However, pathologic diagnosis is sometimes incorrect and the tumor is thought to be malignant in approximately 25% of cases.[24]

The myxoma is a nonspecific, hypoechoic solid mass on sonography.[83] On CT, it appears as a hypodense mass due to the high water content in the mucinous matrix throughout the tumor.[83] On MR, they have a low signal on T1 and a higher signal on T2-weighted imaging.[24,83] A thin rim of high signal surrounding the myxoma is common on T1-weighted imaging, and is thought to represent fatty tissue surrounding the tumor.[83] Often, intramuscular myxomas will demonstrate a very high T2-weighed signal, cystic components, and mild to moderate contrast enhancement due to their hypocellularity (Fig. 14.27).[24,83] It is difficult to differentiate myxoma and low-grade myxomatous sarcoma by imaging alone.[24]

MALIGNANT SOFT TISSUE TUMORS OF THE KNEE

Liposarcoma

Liposarcomas are the second most common soft tissue sarcoma.[93,98] Approximately 80% of liposarcomas are located in the lower extremities, and they are most commonly seen at the knee, elbow, or retroperitoneum.[62,98] Liposarcomas become increasingly common with patient age, usually present between

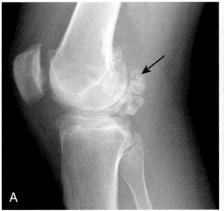
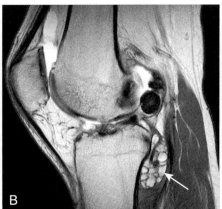
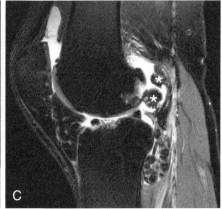

FIG 14.25 Synovial Chondromatosis of the Knee (A) Lateral radiograph shows multiple osteochondral bodies *(arrow)* in the posterior recess of the knee. (B) Sagittal proton density image shows several additional hyperintense nodules *(arrow)* distending the popliteal tendon sheath. (C) Sagittal T2-weighted image better delineates the osteochondral bodies *(asterisks on larger nodules)* outlined by joint fluid.

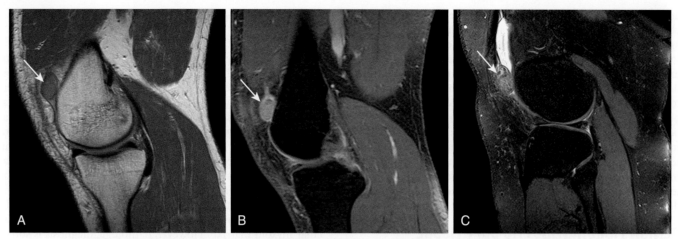

FIG 14.26 Nodular Synovitis in a 35-Year-Old Woman (A) Sagittal T1-weighted image demonstrates a soft tissue nodule *(arrow)* in the lateral suprapatellar pouch that is almost isointense to skeletal muscle. (B) Sagittal T2-weighted image shows the nodule *(arrow)* to be hyperintense to skeletal muscle. (C) Sagittal gradient echo image shows areas of "blooming" artifact in the nodule *(arrow)*, signifying hemosiderin deposition. The nodule was resected arthroscopically and proved to be nodular synovitis.

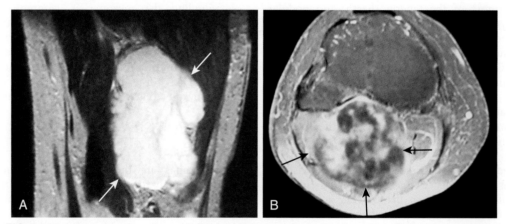

FIG 14.27 Intramuscular, Juxta-Articular Myxoma in a 79-Year-Old Woman (A) Coronal T2-weighted image shows a large, circumscribed, hyperintense mass in the popliteal fossa. (B) Axial T1-weighted enhanced fat-suppressed image shows heterogeneous enhancement of the mass *(arrows)*. The resection specimen demonstrated myxoma.

the fifth and seventh decades, and are more common in males than females.[62,98] Liposarcomas most commonly present as an enlarging painless soft tissue mass.[53,62,93,98] Liposarcomas will metastasize in about 50% of cases, most commonly to the lung.[93] Local recurrence after surgical excision is common.[93] The 5-year survival rate is 29% to 63%, depending on the source.[98]

There are four different subtypes of liposarcomas—well-differentiated, dedifferentiated, myxoid, and pleomorphic.[98] The well-differentiated liposarcoma is the most common subtype, accounting for approximately 50% of all liposarcomas, and has no metastatic potential.[93] On gross examination, a well-differentiated liposarcoma is almost identical to a lipoma.[93] The dedifferentiated liposarcoma subtype is most commonly seen in the retroperitoneum.[93] This subtype is felt to represent a well-differentiated liposarcoma that has undergone malignant degeneration and contains a histologically separate sarcoma such as a malignant fibrous histiocytoma or fibrosarcoma.[93] The myxoid-type liposarcoma is a low to mid-grade tumor.[93] For the

myxoid subtype, more aggressive tumors have greater cellularity, whereas tumors with more myxoid components are lower in tumor grade.[93] When myxoid liposarcomas metastasize, they tend to spread to extrapulmonary locations.[93] The pleomorphic variety is the least common subtype of liposarcoma, has the highest grade, and is most commonly seen in the extremities.[93]

Genetically, the liposarcoma subtypes stem from different points of mutagenesis. Well-differentiated liposarcomas (also known as *atypical lipomatous tumors*) demonstrate a supernumerary ring and giant marker chromosomes.[37] This aberration is also commonly seen in dedifferentiated liposarcoma.[37] This chromosomal formation leads to overexpression of the MDM2 gene on chromosome 12q15.[37] Myxoid liposarcoma is associated with a translocation of t(12;16)(q13;p11).[37] Pleomorphic liposarcomas demonstrate genetic anomalies that are most similar to those seen in other pleomorphic sarcomas.[37]

The liposarcoma is often not visualized radiographically, but may appear as a nondescript soft tissue mass with or without calcifications.[93] On CT and MRI, the liposarcoma is a fatty mass with a variable amount of soft tissue nodularity and/or thickened septations, and avid enhancement of the nonadipose tissue, with a variable T2 signal on MRI (Fig. 14.28).[93] Well-differentiated liposarcomas generally contain at least 75% adipose tissue, whereas the other subtypes may be composed of less than 25% adipose.[93] The myxoid subtype may show cystic, T2-hyperintense components.[93] It can be difficult to differentiate a liposarcoma from a lipoma based on imaging alone.[62] According to Kransdorf et al., a fatty mass is much more likely to be a well-differentiated liposarcoma versus a lipoma when the lesion is larger than 10 cm, there are thick internal septa greater than 2 mm in diameter, if globular or nodular nonadipose tissue is identified, and if the lesion is composed of more than 25% nonadipose tissue.[62] Calcification is also more commonly seen in malignant lipomatous tumors.[62]

Synovial Sarcoma

Synovial sarcomas are aggressive and locally destructive tumors that arise from mesenchymal cells of the tendon, tendon sheath, or bursa surrounding a joint.[5,39] Despite its name, the synovial sarcoma does not arise from synovial tissue.[5,39] The most common location is in the extra-articular tissues surrounding the knee joint and approximately 70% occur in the lower extremities.[5,17,39] Synovial sarcomas account for approximately 5% of all primary soft tissue sarcomas and are the most common soft tissue malignancy involving the knee in children and young adults.[17,39] Synovial sarcomas most commonly present as a painful mass in young adults and demonstrates a male predominance.[37,39] On gross examination, the synovial sarcoma is a circumscribed mass with variable appearance, depending on its composition.[37] Formation of a synovial sarcoma is associated with an (X:18) chromosomal translocation leading to formation of the SS18-SSX fusion gene, making polymerase chain reaction (PCR) a useful diagnostic tool.[21,37,82]

Diagnosis of a synovial sarcoma can be challenging because of its slow growth pattern and often small size at diagnosis.[82] Imaging characteristics of the synovial sarcoma may be nonspecific if lesions are smaller than 5 cm.[39] Synovial sarcomas typically present as a soft tissue mass near, but not within, the knee joint on radiographs.[82] Synovial sarcomas display calcifications in approximately 30% of cases, and approximately 50% of cases will have normal radiographs.[82] Lesions demonstrating calcifications are thought to be associated with a better prognosis.[17,55] If a soft tissue tumor demonstrates calcifications in a child, synovial sarcoma should be high in the differential diagnosis, since other calcifying lesions are exceedingly rare in children.[21] At times, synovial sarcomas may erode the adjacent bone.[82] On CT, synovial sarcomas present as a heterogeneous, nodular, lobulated mass isodense to skeletal muscle with heterogeneous enhancement.[82] There are often regions of lower attenuation that represent foci of cystic necrosis and hemorrhage.[82] When present, calcifications within a synovial sarcoma are best characterized on CT and can even be seen in some metastatic lesions.[82]

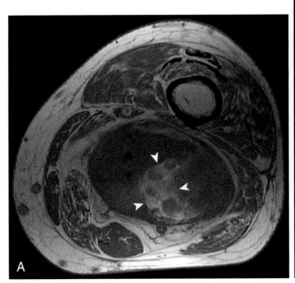
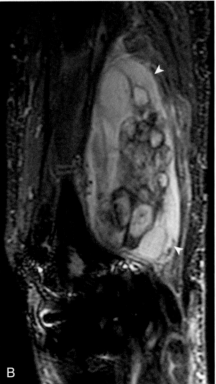

FIG 14.28 Well-Differentiated Liposarcoma in a 91-Year-Old Woman Presenting With Large, Painless Mass (A) Axial T1-weighted image through the biopsy-proven well-differentiated liposarcoma shows a large, well-circumscribed heterogeneous mass with central areas isointense to fat *(arrowheads)*. (B) Sagittal T2-weighted fat-suppressed image through the heterogeneous mass *(arrowheads)* shows a predominantly cystic mass with central areas of low-signal fat.

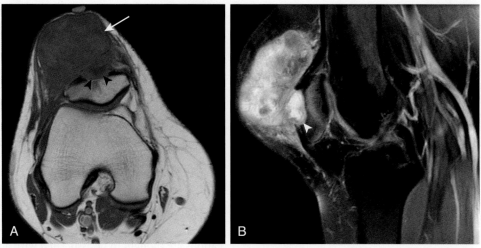

FIG 14.29 Prepatellar Synovial Sarcoma in a 38-Year-Old Woman (A) Axial T1-weighted image shows a large, lobulated prepatellar mass *(arrow)* that is isointense to skeletal muscle and invades the anterior patella *(arrowheads)*. (B) Sagittal T2-weighted image better delineates the patellar invasion *(arrowhead)* by the heterogeneous mass. The resected mass proved to be synovial sarcoma.

On MRI, a synovial sarcoma is a multiloculated cystic and lobulated mass with heterogeneous peripheral nodular or septal enhancement.[17] Synovial sarcoma is typically heterogeneous, isointense to muscle on T1-weighted images, hyperintense to fat on fluid-sensitive sequences (Fig. 14.29), and may have cystic or multilobular regions.[5] Synovial sarcomas may show the triple signal intensity sign (hypointense, isointense, and hyperintense regions all within the same lesion) on T2-weighted images, a "bowl-of-fruit" appearance, fluid-fluid levels, lobular morphology, and internal septations.[17,39] The "bowl-of-fruit" sign refers to hemorrhage, fluid, septations, and intervening cystic areas of necrosis within the tumor.[17,82]

The prognosis of patients with synovial sarcoma is variable. Patients younger than 25 years old with masses smaller than 5 cm, having the SYT-SSX2 mutation but lacking poorly differentiated cells on histologic analysis have a relatively good prognosis.[17] The converse portends a poor diagnosis. The 5-year survival rate varies between 20% and 63%.[85] Approximately 41% of patients demonstrate metastatic disease and about the same number have local recurrence postsurgical resection.[85]

CONCLUSION

Osseous and soft tissue tumors of the knee include a variety of benign and malignant lesions, as outlined by the World Health Organization. A thorough knowledge of patient age, clinical history, and musculoskeletal tumor imaging characteristics may empower the radiologist to markedly limit the differential diagnosis prior to biopsy or allow a specific diagnosis to be made in some cases. Radiographs and/or CT are helpful in identifying mineralized chondroid or osteoid tumor matrix in tumors such as enchondroma, chondrosarcoma, osteoid osteoma, and osteosarcoma. Furthermore, MRI can identify adipose, fibrous, or adjacent neural tissue within certain soft tissue tumors such as lipoma, liposarcoma, desmoid, and peripheral nerve sheath tumors. MRI is also useful in detecting the paramagnetic effect of hemosiderin deposition in GCTs, nodular synovitis, and PVNS around the knee.

KEY REFERENCES

19. Chakarun CJ, Forrester DM, Gottsegen CJ, et al: Giant cell tumor of bone: review, mimics, and new developments in treatment. *Radiographics* 33:197–211, 2013.
33. Douis H, Saifuddin A: The imaging of cartilaginous bone tumours. I. Benign lesions. *Skeletal Radiol* 41:1195–1212, 2012.
36. Flemming DJ, Murphey MD: Enchondroma and chondrosarcoma. *Semin Musculoskelet Radiol* 4:59–71, 2000.
56. Iyer RS, Chapman T, Chew FS: Pediatric bone imaging: diagnostic imaging of osteoid osteoma. *AJR Am J Roentgenol* 198:1039–1052, 2012.

The references for this chapter can also be found on www.expertconsult.com.

15

Ultrasound-Guided Procedures

Christopher John Burke, Ronald S. Adler

INTRODUCTION

The use of ultrasound guidance for knee procedures has become increasingly popular in recent years due to recognized increased accuracy compared with those performed blind, as well as an expansion in the range of both intra-articular and extra-articular knee therapies.* Indeed, in addition to aiding knee joint injections and aspirations, ultrasound guidance is widely considered the gold standard for localization in a range of procedures, including proximal tibifibular joint, patellar tendon, iliotibial band (ITB), popliteus tendon, pes anserinus bursa, Baker cyst, ganglia, and parameniscal cyst therapies, as well as biopsies.

This chapter will address the use of ultrasound in therapeutic and diagnostic procedures of the knee. The authors' technique for various procedures will also be described within the relevant sections.

INTRA-ARTICULAR PROCEDURES

Intra-articular procedures mainly include tibiofemoral joint aspiration and injection. Aspiration may be performed for therapeutic reasons (eg, to relieve the discomfort of a large effusion) or diagnostic reasons (eg, to sample fluid for potential infective, crystalline, or inflammatory etiologies). Injections may be performed for therapeutic intentions, such as with corticosteroid[3,5,23,31,46] or viscosupplementation[6,37,39,45,54] or for diagnostic purposes with arthrographic contrast.[1,7] More recently there has been interest in the intra-articular injection of platelet-rich plasma (PRP) and mesenchymal stem cells.

Misplaced intra-articular injection (eg, during corticosteroid or hyaluronic acid injection) may produce reduced therapeutic effect if injected into periarticular tissue and even lead to increased post procedure pain. Inaccurate steroid injections can result in local fat atrophy and depigmentation, hematomas, steroid articular cartilage atrophy, or crystal synovitis. Misguided arthrographic contrast injection may result in a nondiagnostic study. There is also an increased susceptibility to tendon rupture by inadvertent intratendinous injection.[30,41,52]

Numerous studies have demonstrated improved accuracy of intra-articular injections, with up to 96% accuracy with ultrasound guidance, increased responder rate to treatment, decreased pain scores, and even a reduction in overall cost per year, with ultrasound guidance.† Other studies have demonstrated the increased accuracy of ultrasound-guided extra-articular injections (eg, as much as 100% compared with 50% without guidance for the pes anserine bursa).[17]

Multiple techniques for ultrasound-guided intra-articular injection of the knee joint have been described in the literature, with the lateral patellar and suprapatellar approaches being the most commonly used,‡ although a medial patellar approach was also described with the knee fully extended.[25] The patient is usually placed in the supine position with a pillow or support under the knee so the joint is flexed to approximately 30 degrees. A high-frequency linear probe is used to scan the suprapatellar and lateral pouches for an effusion. If localized, this hypoechoic fluid collection becomes the target for the aspiration and injection (Fig. 15.1). A subclinical effusion can usually be visualized under the quadriceps tendon proximal to the patella; therefore it is important not to overly compress with the transducer. Likewise, the trochlear cartilage can be targeted with a nondistended suprapatellar pouch. A needle pathway is predetermined; this area is then marked and prepped in a sterile fashion, lidocaine is administered subcutaneously, and subsequently a needle is then advanced into the joint recess or effusion. A test dose containing a small amount of local anesthetic can be used to confirm intra-articular needle tip placement. There should be minimal resistance encountered during injection, and hypoechoic fluid should be seen filling the suprapatellar and lateral pouches.

CORTICOSTEROID INJECTIONS

Intra-articular injection of steroid is a well-established and common treatment for osteoarthritis of the knee.[23] Improvement in symptoms of osteoarthritis of the knee after intra-articular corticosteroid injection varies in the literature, with effects generally lasting up to 16 to 24 weeks.[3,46] Ultrasound also allows assessment response to intra-articular therapy in osteoarthritis of the knee.

VISCOSUPPLEMENTATION

In 1997 exogenous high-molecular-weight hyaluronan viscosupplementation was approved to treat knee osteoarthritis in the United States by the US Food and Drug Administration (FDA). Viscosupplementation with intra-articular hyaluronic acid is an alternative to the treatment of symptomatic knee osteoarthritis in patients who have failed to respond adequately to conservative therapy[45,54] and is frequently used due to ease of use and good tolerance. This has demonstrated moderate but significant efficacy (20%) versus placebo in terms of pain and

---

*References 4, 8, 13, 25, 26, 30, 44, and 49.
†References 4, 8, 13, 25, 26, 30, 44, and 49.

‡References 4, 8, 13, 26, 30, 44, and 49.

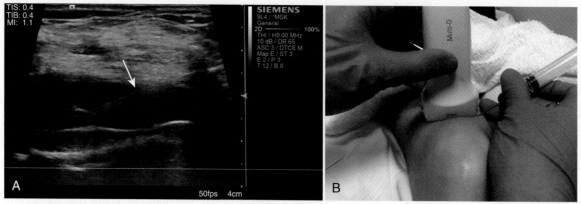

FIG 15.1 Knee Joint Effusion (A) Transverse ultrasound image at the level of the suprapatellar pouch shows aspiration of a hypoechoic knee joint effusion with the needle coming in-plane from the right *(white arrow).* (B) Example of joint effusion aspiration using a lateral suprapatellar approach demonstrating probe and needle orientation.

function, with a high rate of responders (60% to 70%) in knee osteoarthritis.[45] It may allow reduced administration of analgesics, with an improved risk to benefit ratio, and may delay joint replacement. A multitude of linear or reticulated hyaluronic acid derivatives are now commercially available, with varied characteristics and levels of evidence (eg, Gel-One Cross-linked Hyaluronate [Zimmer], Synvisc-One Hylan G-F 20 [Sanofi Biosurgery], Hyalgan [Fidia Pharma], Supartz [Bioventus], Orthovisc [DePuy], and Euflexxa [Ferring Pharmaceuticals]). Clinical efficacy shows onset 1 to 4 weeks later than with corticosteroids but is often maintained for 6 or even 12 months. The efficacy of viscosupplementation and optimal response profile is a matter of ongoing debate after discordant findings in some meta-analyses, and cartilage protection remains to be proven. The optimal indication seems to be moderate tibiofemoral osteoarthritis without swelling.[6,37]

CONTRAST

Intra-articular injection of contrast agents may be used before computed tomography (CT) and magnetic resonance (MR) arthrography. The sensitivity in detecting recurrent or residual meniscal tears after surgery has been shown to be improved when intra-articular contrast material was used, compared with conventional magnetic resonance imaging (MRI).[1,7] There has also been interest in the use of CT arthrography in the evaluation of the postoperative meniscus, as well as for assessment of cartilage and osteochondral allograft transplants.[10,55]

Platelet-Rich Plasma

Most of the studies to date assessing the efficacy of PRP intra-articular injection treatment for patients with knee osteoarthritis have suffered small sample size with inconclusive data, and there have been limited randomized controlled trials. Although the findings indicate that PRP might have better outcomes in patients with lower degree of degeneration and in younger patients, current studies remain inconclusive regarding the efficacy of intra-articular PRP treatment.[36]

Autologous Bone Marrow-Derived Mesenchymal Stem Cells

There has been interest in the efficacy of intra-articular injection of autologous mesenchymal stem cells isolated from

bone marrow and adipose tissue to promote cartilage regeneration in knee osteoarthritis[29,58] and meniscal regeneration,[43] although as yet efficacy remains to be established.

Proximal Tibiofibular Joint

Pathology involving the proximal tibiofibular joint is often overlooked as a potential cause of knee pain. Symptoms are often nonspecific, with patients presenting with anterolateral knee pain, and may be mistaken for lateral collateral ligament injury or ITB friction syndrome.[18] The proximal tibiofibular joint is also a common site for ganglion cyst formation, which can be treated with aspiration and injection (Fig. 15.2). Proximal tibiofibular joint injection can be performed with a high degree of accuracy[50] and intra-articular corticosteroid injection has demonstrated therapeutic benefits.

The technique for accessing the proximal tibiofibular joint, involves placing the patient in a lateral decubitus position with the lateral aspect of the affected knee towards the ceiling. Flexion of the knee to approximately 30 degrees widens the joint space, and the transducer is positioned in a transverse oblique orientation then rotated for optimal imaging. The joint space may be identified between the hyperechoic cortical margins of the tibia and fibula deep to the anterior proximal tibiofibular ligament which overlies the joint space.[41,50,52] The needle may be inserted out of plane perpendicular to the long axis of the transducer (short axis) or in-plane targeting the joint space (long axis).

Extra-Articular Procedures

Numerous procedures involving tendons, such as percutaneous tenotomy, PRP, prolotherapy, and peritendintous steroid injections, are commonly practiced. Therapeutic procedures involving ganglions, bursa, cysts, and nerves around the knee are also well established.

TENDON PROCEDURES

Ultrasound guidance has been increasingly used in the treatment of tendinopathies around the knee. There has been particular interest with respect to the patella tendon; however, ultrasound-guided treatments of the popliteus, ITB, and pes anserinus tendons have been also described.

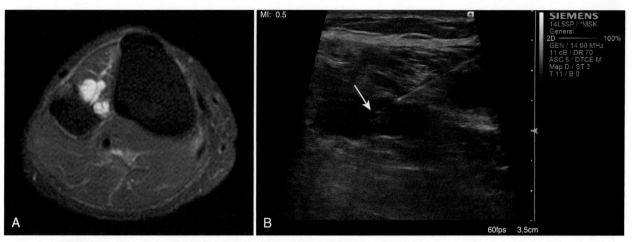

FIG 15.2 Proximal Tibiofibular Ganglion (A) Axial Short Tau Inversion Recovery (STIR) MR image demonstrating lobular hyperintense ganglion cyst arising from the proximal tibiofibular joint. (B) Ultrasound image in the same patient demonstrating guided aspiration with needle tip *(white arrow)* positioned within the cyst.

PATELLA TENDON

Patellar tendinopathy, often referred to as "jumper's knee," is well known to be refractory to conservative treatment and may represent a therapeutic challenge.[2,12,21,24,33] Tendinopathy can result in disordered regrowth of the underlying collagen matrix of the tendon, leading to regions of weakening, which often appear hypoechoic on ultrasound with loss of the normal fibrillary tendon echotexture. Multiple cycles of injury and repair can lead to chronic tendinopathy with an angiofibroblastic response seen as increased vascularity on Doppler imaging.[21,33] Multiple therapies for patella tendinopathy have been described,[2] with needle fenestration,[24] high-volume injections,[12] hyperosmolar dextrose,[47] polidocanol,[22,57] PRP,[48,56] autologous blood,[27] and ultrasound-guided high-intensity focused ultrasound ablation[42] all demonstrating reported improved outcomes.

Ultrasound-guided needle fenestration of the patellar tendon for tendinopathy is a well-established procedure. In a retrospective follow-up study by Housner et al. of 47 patellar tendons in 32 patients with recalcitrant patellar tendinopathy and diagnosis made via history, physical examination, and sonographic examination, in which ultrasound-guided needle fenestration was performed after failure of conservative management, 72% of patients reported excellent or good results when questioned regarding return to activity and 81% of patients reported excellent or good satisfaction scores, with an average time to follow-up of 45 months.[24]

In addition to percutaneous needle tenotomy of the patellar tendon, there are several studies reporting the effectiveness and safety of PRP injections.[48,56] Vetrano et al. compared PRP injections versus focused shock waves in the treatment of jumper's knee in athletes who had failed conservative management, demonstrating significantly improved outcomes with therapeutic PRP injections at 6- and 12-month follow-up.[56]

There has been recent interest in the use of high-intensity focused ultrasound ablation for the treatment of diseased tendons.[42] One commercially available device is the Tenex Health TX System, which is a surgical instrument designed to perform a percutaneous tenotomy. Using ultrasound in the same manner as for standard tenotomy for visualization, the TX MicroTip uses ultrasonic energy to cut and remove damaged tendon tissue.

Although the use of corticosteroid injections is widely practiced, in a systematic review by Coombes et al., the effects of corticosteroid injections were noted to provide only short-term benefit in studies pertaining to patella tendinopathy,[11] and concern has been raised with regard to increased risk of tendon rupture.

For procedures involving the patellar tendon, the patient is usually positioned supine with the knee flexed to approximately 30 degrees with a support placed underneath (Fig. 15.3). The probe is typically placed longitudinally, with the patella visualized proximally and Hoffa fat pad lying immediately deep to the tendon. The entire tendon should be scanned in short and long axis from the inferior patellar pole to the tibial tuberosity insertion. The probe is normally positioned in the longitudinal plane, although it may be positioned transversely. Regions of tendinopathy are targeted for fenestration or PRP injection (Fig. 15.3). After the needle is inserted, by retracting and altering direction, the amount of diseased tendon covered may increase without having to reinsert the needle through the skin. Barbotage may also be performed for any calcific deposits within the tendon.[27]

POPLITEUS TENDON

The popliteus muscle tendon complex arises primarily from the lateral femoral condyle and proximal fibula and inserts onto the posteromedial surface of the proximal tibia, acting to maintain dorsolateral knee stability and control tibial rotation. Pain arising from the popliteus muscle tendon complex may be difficult to localize on clinical examination. Popliteus tendinopathy may occur due to injury or chronic overuse especially in athletes and osteophyte impingement.[19] Ultrasound-guided popliteal tendon sheath injections can play a substantial role in providing both diagnostic and therapeutic information for pain arising from the popliteus tendon. The patient is usually positioned in the lateral decubitus position with the knee flexed approximately 30 degrees and the leg slightly internally rotated. The probe should be positioned with the lateral femoral

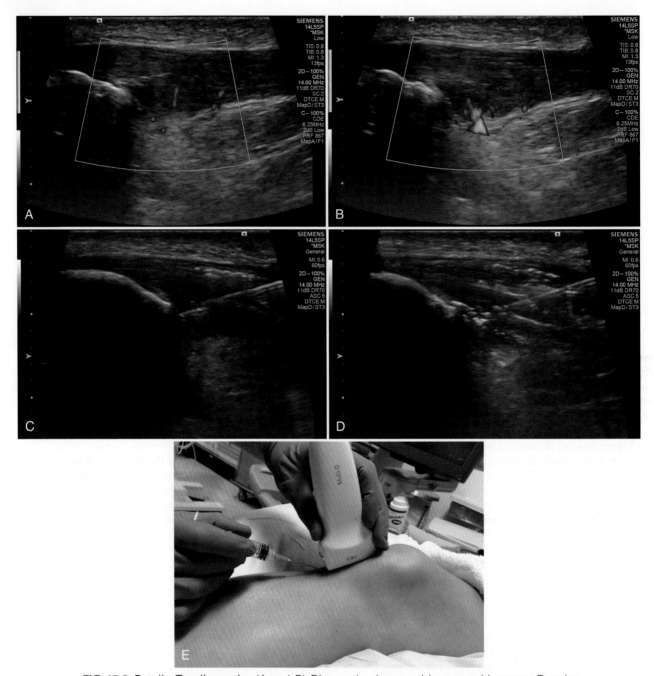

FIG 15.3 Patella Tendinopathy (A and B) Diagnostic ultrasound images with power Doppler demonstrating the appearance of patella tendinosis with regions of intrasubstance hypoechogenicity and associated neovascularization. (C and D) Ultrasound images demonstrating guided percutaneous needle tenotomy and PRP injection. (E) Example of probe orientation and needle positioning for the approach to patellar tenotomy.

epicondyle identified as a cephalad landmark and the fibula as the caudal landmark, between which the popliteus tendon is seen transversely within the groove. It is important to identify and avoid the more posterior common peroneal nerve. The needle is then passed in-plane, aiming at the superior margin of the popliteus tendon within the tendon sheath.[41,51,52]

Iliotibial Band

ITB friction syndrome is a common cause of lateral knee pain. Formed proximally by the convergence of the tensor fascia lata, gluteus maximus, and medius at the level of the trochanteric bursa, the ITB then travels distally along the lateral femur and inserts distally with two main insertions onto the lateral femoral condyle and Gerdy's tubercle. ITB friction syndrome is thought to be caused by repetitive friction of the iliotibial tract across the lateral femoral condyle, leading to chronic inflammation of the ITB bursa. Patients commonly present with pain and tenderness over the lateral femoral epicondyle at and above the lateral joint line. Corticosteroid injections have shown to provide improved pain relief compared with lidocaine alone.[20]

The ITB is a superficial structure; therefore there is a risk of local fat atrophy and depigmentation with corticosteroid injection or superficial hematoma with tenotomy or PRP. Care should be taken to avoid directly injecting the tendon because this may increase susceptibility to rupture.

BURSAE, CYSTS, AND GANGLIONS

Pes Anserinus Bursa

The pes anserinus consists of the conjoined tendon tibial insertion of the sartorius, gracilis, and semitendinosus. Pes anserine bursitis is a common source of medial-sided knee pain, often associated with knee osteoarthritis or repetitive trauma. Patients often demonstrate tenderness to palpation over the tibial insertion. The pes anserinus bursa may be poorly conspicuous on ultrasound, even when the patient is symptomatic, although is frequently thickened and edematous (Fig. 15.4). Finnoff et al. demonstrated that injection of the pes anserine bursa may be performed under ultrasound guidance with an accuracy of 100% compared with 50% without guidance,[17] and therapeutic injection has established efficacy.[59]

The patient is usually positioned with the knee in slight flexion and leg externally rotated. The probe is placed in a transverse orientation over the posterior medial knee identifying sartorius, gracilis, and semitendinosus tendons, which can be seen in cross-section and traced distally to their insertion. The pes anserine bursa and three ovoid tendons superficially should be identified. After this, the overlying skin should be marked over the middle of the pes anserinus, where it crosses the anterior margin of the medial collateral ligament. The needle is typically inserted in-plane on the proximal or distal side of the transducer, targeting the bursa between the medial collateral ligament and the pes anserinus (see Fig. 15.4).

Baker Cysts

Baker's cysts are a type of popliteal cyst resulting from the egress of fluid through a normal communication, the semimembranosus -gastrocnemius bursa interposed between the semimembranosus and medial gastrocnemius tendons, or may be caused by herniation or synovial membrane through the joint capsule.

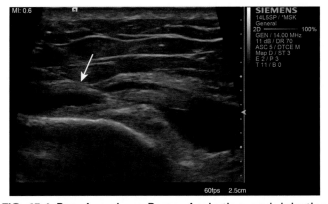

FIG 15.4 Pes Anserinus Bursa Aspiration and Injection *Gray-scale sonographic image of the medial right knee demonstrates the needle (white arrow) placed within the pes anserine bursa, which contains a small volume of fluid and synovial thickening.*

Primary Bakers cysts, common in children, infrequently communicate with the knee joint and intra-articular pathology is rare. The majority of Baker cysts are secondary to intra-articular pathology, predominantly osteoarthritis, and communicate with the knee joint acting as a mechanism for joint fluid decompression.[28]

Patients typically complain of posterior knee swelling and discomfort, although rupture can cause significant pain and calf swelling; this may be difficult to differentiate from deep vein thrombosis, although ultrasound allows accurate differentiation. Once ruptured, aspiration of a Baker cyst may become significantly more challenging due to the presence of daughter cysts and possible associated organizing hematoma. In addition, the nature of the fluid can be quite variable, from relatively nonviscous to almost gelatinous.

Baker cysts can be classified as simple and complex via ultrasonography prior to the treatment. Aspiration using ultrasound guidance is important because of the adjacent neurovascular structures and the possible complex nature of the cysts, to ensure maximal volume is aspirated. Cyst aspiration with ultrasound-guided corticosteroid injection generally yields clinical improvement and cyst volume reduction in all subgroups of patients with Baker cyst secondary to knee osteoarthritis.[9,34] Koroglu et al. reported a significant clinical improvement after percutaneous aspiration in 32 patients with knee osteoarthritis. The volume reduction of Baker cyst after the treatment significantly correlated with the clinical improvement. Following percutaneous treatment, six Baker cysts relapsed at ultrasonography, which were all of the complex type.[34] From a symptomatic perspective, it has been suggested that although cyst aspiration with corticosteroid injection provides pain relief and cyst volume reduction in patients with Baker cyst and concomitant knee osteoarthritis, results are similar to those obtained with intra-articular knee corticosteroid injection.[15]

For Baker's cyst aspiration the patient is usually positioned prone with legs extended (Fig. 15.5). The transducer is positioned over the medial gastrocnemius, identifying the semimembranosus and medial gastrocnemius tendons between which simple Baker cysts typically appear as a lobular, well-defined, thin-walled, anechoic structure as opposed to more complex cysts that may contain internal septations, synovial hypertrophy, and occasionally, osteochondral bodies. Scan transversely and longitudinally over the cyst; identify the popliteal artery, vein, and tibial nerve. Doppler can be used to avoid the popliteal artery and vein and can exclude a popliteal artery aneurysm or venous ectasia. Mark a suitable entry position, and prepare the overlying skin in a sterile fashion. Infiltrate local anesthesia to the skin and soft tissues, then insert the needle either in or out of plane under direct dynamic guidance (Fig. 15.5).

Parameniscal Cysts and Ganglions

Parameniscal cysts are usually associated with horizontal cleavage tears; however, isolated cysts without meniscal pathology may occur, which may present with signs and symptoms consistent with typical meniscal pathology. MR frequently initially confirms the presence of a suspected meniscal cyst and identifies any concurrent meniscal tear. Ultrasound-guided percutaneous aspiration of meniscal cysts is a safe and effective procedure,[40] particularly appropriate for patients unsuitable for surgical débridement or as an interim therapy (Fig. 15.6).

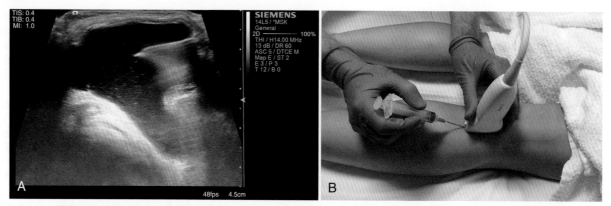

FIG 15.5 Baker (Popliteal) Cyst (A) Ultrasound image demonstrating aspiration of a large, simple hypoechoic Bakeric Baker. Note the posterior reverberation artifact from the needle that enters from the right. (B) Example of longitudinal approach to Baker cyst aspiration with the patient positioned prone.

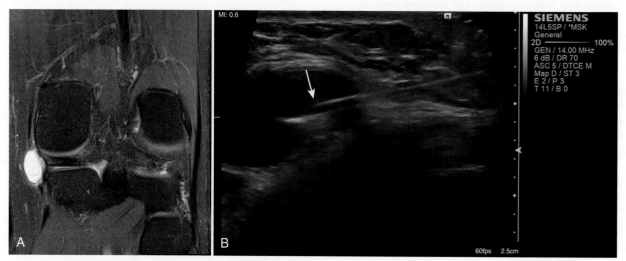

FIG 15.6 Parameniscal Cyst (A) Coronal fat-suppressed proton density magnetic resonance image demonstrates a parameniscal cyst abutting the medial meniscus. (B) Ultrasound image of the medial knee demonstrating guided aspiration with needle tip *(white arrow)* positioned within the parameniscal cyst.

Ultrasound-guided aspiration of symptomatic ganglion cysts about the knee is a valuable and routinely performed therapeutic procedure. Intra- and extra-articular ganglions, complex ganglions with both superficial and deep components, may arise around the knee, which are amenable to percutaneous aspiration and therapeutic injection (Fig. 15.7). Furthermore, ganglion cysts of the posterior[14] and anterior[35] cruciate ligaments (Fig. 15.8), tendons (including popliteus),[32] and rarely intraneural ganglion cysts may arise,[38] usually in relation to the common peroneal nerve, which is also accessible using ultrasound guidance. Percutaneous aspiration and injection with corticosteroid often provide therapeutic benefit.

Intraneural ganglion cysts are rare, benign, mucinous lesions that occur within neural sheaths and are thought to involve cystic fluid exiting from nearby synovial joints. They often present as tender masses causing paresthesias in the distribution of the involved nerve, muscle weakness or cramping, or localized or referred pain. Due to the risks of nerve and vessel damage associated with surgical resection, ultrasound-guided aspiration and injection of corticosteroid is a useful and minimally invasive alternative to surgery for managing intraneural ganglion cysts,[38] which were also reported in the pediatric population.[53]

BIOPSY

Benign and malignant soft tissue masses around the knee are frequently amenable to ultrasound-guided biopsy. The principles are the same as with biopsies elsewhere with core needle and fine needle aspiration techniques usually used for soft tissue mass lesions (Figs. 15.9 and 15.10). Some osseous and paraosseous lesions may also be amenable to ultrasound-guided biopsy, although the approach should be carefully planned if there is a possibility of seeding malignant cells and contamination of a compartment outside of a planned surgical field. Ultrasound-guided synovial biopsy has also been proposed as a reliable method for the histopathologic assessment of knee joint synovium.[16]

SUMMARY

The role of ultrasound guidance in knee procedures has expanded significantly, with an increasing range of treatments available. Improved accuracy and safety have been established with ultrasound, which is widely regarded as the standard of care for guiding knee procedures.

Text continued on p. 296

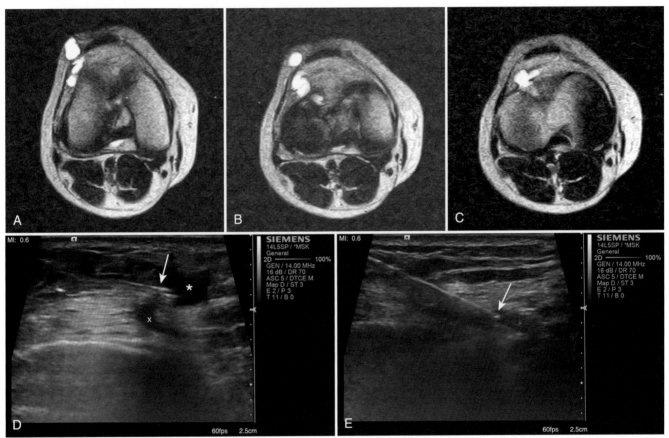

FIG 15.7 Complex Ganglion Cyst With Both Extra- and Intra-articular Components (A-C) Sequential axial T2-weighted magnetic resonance images demonstrate a lobular hyperintense mass with superficial and deep extension. (D and E) Ultrasound images demonstrating aspiration and injection of the ganglion cyst. (D) First the needle *(white arrow)* has been placed within superficial component *(asterisk)* for aspiration. (E) The tip of the needle *(white arrow)* has subsequently been repositioned within neck of the deeper component *(x)*.

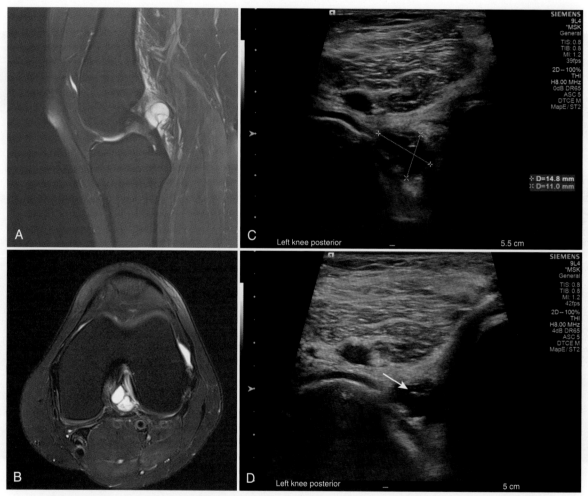

FIG 15.8 Anterior Cruciate Ligament Ganglion Cyst (A) Sagittal fat-suppressed proton density and (B) axial T2 fat-suppressed images demonstrating lobular hyperintense structure posteriorly abutting the anterior cruciate ligament (ACL) consistent with a ganglion cyst. (C) Ultrasound image of the posterior knee demonstrates the hypoechoic ACL ganglion cyst. (D) Guided aspiration with the needle tip *(white arrow)* positioned within the ganglion cyst.

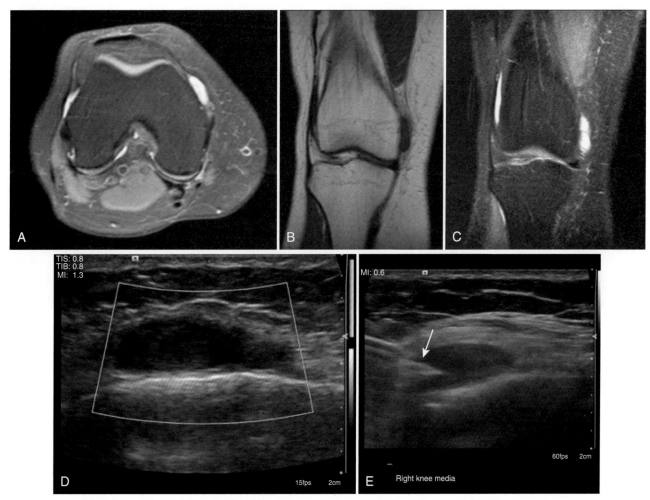

FIG 15.9 Nerve Sheath Tumor (A) Axial T2, (B) coronal proton density, and (C) coronal proton density fat-suppressed images demonstrating an ovoid lesion with internal T2 high signal initially thought to be a ganglion cyst, abutting the medial femoral condyle. (D) Ultrasound demonstrates a hypoechoic soft tissue mass. (E) Subsequent ultrasound-guided core biopsy *(white needle)* confirmed the mass to be a nerve sheath tumor.

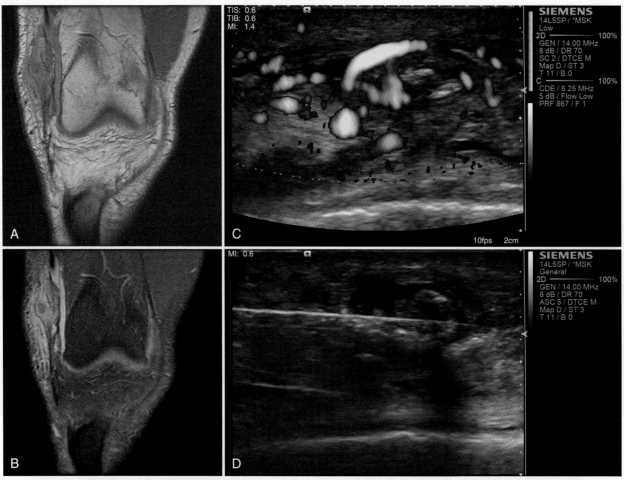

FIG 15.10 Myositis Ossificans (A) Coronal proton density and (B) coronal proton density fat-suppressed images demonstrating nodular thickening in the region of the ITB with surrounding soft tissue edema. (C) Ultrasound image with Power Doppler demonstrates marked associated vascularity. (D) Ultrasound demonstrating guided core biopsy of the lesion, which yielded tissue compatible with myositis ossificans on histopathology.

KEY REFERENCES

4. Balint PV, Kane D, Hunter J, et al: Ultrasound guided versus conventional joint and soft tissue fluid aspiration in rheumatology practice: a pilot study. *J Rheumatol* 29:2209, 2002.

6. Bellamy N, Campbell J, Robinson V, et al: Viscosupplementation for the treatment of osteoarthritis of the knee. *Cochrane Database Syst Rev* 19:2, 2006.

7. Boutin RD, Fritz RC, Marder RA: Magnetic resonance imaging of the postoperative meniscus: resection, repair, and replacement. *Magn Reson Imaging Clin N Am* 22:517–555, 2014.

9. Chen CK, Lew HL, Liao RIH: Ultrasound-guided diagnosis and aspiration of Baker's cyst. *Am J Phys Med Rehabil* 91(11):1002, 2012.

17. Finnoff JT, Nutz DJ, Henning PT: Accuracy of ultrasound-guided versus unguided pes anserinus bursa injections. *PM R* 2:732, 2010.

24. Housner JA, Jacobson JA, Morag Y, et al: Should ultrasound-guided needle fenestration be considered as a treatment option for recalcitrant patellar tendinopathy? A retrospective study of 47 cases. *Clin J Sport Med* 20:488–490, 2010.

26. Jackson DW, Evans NA, Thomas BM: Accuracy of needle placement into the intra-articular space of the knee. *J Bone Joint Surg Am* 84-A: 1522–1527, 2002.

37. Legre-Boyer V: Viscosupplementation: techniques, indications, results. *Orthop Traumatol Surg Res* 101:S101–S108, 2015.

40. Macmahon PJ, Brennan DD, Duke D, et al: Ultrasound-guided percutaneous drainage of meniscal cysts: preliminary clinical experience. *Clin Radiol* 62:683–687, 2007.

41. McNally E: Musculoskeletal interventional ultrasound. In McNally E, editor: *Practical musculoskeletal ultrasound*, ed 1, New York, 2005, Elsevier, p 30000Y.

45. Petrella RJ, Petrella M: A prospective, randomized, double-blind, placebo controlled study to evaluate the efficacy of intraarticular hyaluronic acid for osteoarthritis of the knee. *J Rheumatol* 33:951–956, 2006.

46. Raynauld JP, Buckland-Wright C, Ward R, et al: Safety and efficacy of long-term intraarticular steroid injections in osteoarthritis of the knee: a randomized, double-blind, placebo-controlled trial. *Arthritis Rheum* 48:370–377, 2003.

49. Sibbitt WL, Jr, Band PA, Kettwich LG, et al: A randomized controlled trial evaluating the cost-effectiveness of sonographic guidance for intra-articular injection of the osteoarthritis knee. *J Clin Rheumatol* 17:409–415, 2011.

52. Spinner D, Danesh H, Waheed S: Knee. In Spinner D, Kirschner JS, Herrera JE, editors: *Atlas of ultrasound guided musculoskeletal injections*, New York, 2013, Springer, pp 57–68.

56. Vetrano M, Castorina A, Vulpiani MC, et al: Platelet-rich plasma versus focused shock waves in the treatment of jumper's knee in athletes. *Am J Sports Med* 41:795–803, 2013.

The references for this chapter can also be found on www.expertconsult.com.

Biomechanics

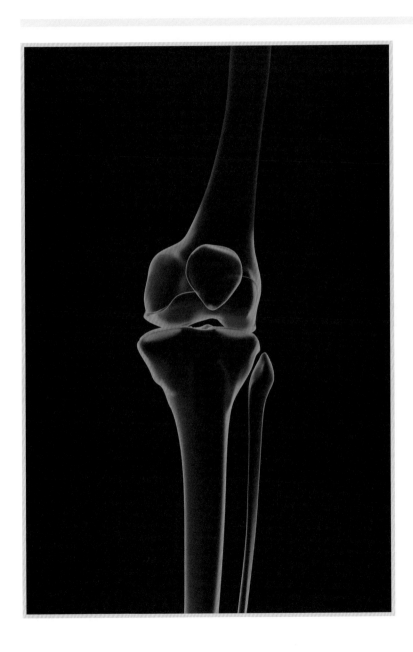

16

Three-Dimensional Morphology of the Knee

Mohamed R. Mahfouz

INTRODUCTION

Of primary interest to the author of this chapter is the analysis of the intrinsic shape differences of the knee joint between different ethnic populations for development of implantable orthopedic devices. The research presented is thus threefold: by developing a novel automatic feature-detection algorithm, a set of automated measurements can be defined based on highly morphometric variant regions, which then allows for a statistical framework when analyzing different populations' knee joint differences.

Ethnic differences in lower limb morphology have received attention in orthopedic literature, which focuses on the differences between Asian and Western populations because this variation is of great import in implant design. For example, femurs from Chinese people are more anteriorly bowed and externally rotated, with smaller intermedullary canals and smaller distal condyles than femurs from white individuals.[5,11,30,31] Similarly, femurs from white people are larger than that of the Japanese in terms of length and distal condyle dimensions.[28] The medical literature has also established ethnic differences in proximal femur bone mineral density (BMD) and hip axis length between black and white Americans.[21,27] The combined effects of higher BMD, shorter hip axis length, and shorter intertrochanteric width may explain the lower prevalence of osteoporotic fractures in black women compared with their white counterparts.[21,27] Similarly, elderly Asian and black men were found to have thicker cortices and higher BMD than white and Hispanic men, which may contribute to greater bone strength in these ethnic groups. In general, black populations have thicker bone cortices, narrower endosteal diameters, and greater BMD than do white populations.[22] However, interestingly, these traits are most pronounced when comparing African black with American black populations.[22,27]

The following analysis will consider landmarks and shape variation in the lower limb of modern black and white Americans. This chapter has been updated since initial publication to include discussion material relating morphology to kinematics and soft tissues. For a more recent treatment of ethnic differences, including larger populations and Asian subsets, the author recommends the manuscript by Mahfouz et al.[18] Three-dimensional (3D) statistical bone atlases will be used to facilitate rapid and accurate data collection in the form of automated measurements, including some measurements tested in the studies previously mentioned, as well as measurements used in biomedical studies and some newly devised measurements. The shape analysis will be conducted with a statistical treatment combining principal components analysis (PCA) and multiple discriminant analysis (MDA)[6]; analysis of landmarks and clinically relevant axes will be performed using t-tests, power tests, and linear discriminant analysis as in the study by Mahfouz et al.[18] The results of these analyses will add to the existing knowledge of morphologic variation in the knee joint and provide useful information that can be extracted for prosthesis design, preoperative planning, and intraoperative navigation.

MATERIALS AND METHODS

The foundation of the current approach derives from the use of computed tomography (CT) scans for data collection combined with the computational power and precision offered by statistical bone atlases. As such, data acquisition and analysis requires a number of distinct steps. The data acquisition and segmentation steps are described in the "Data Acquisition" section. The "Atlas Creation and Validation" section details the creation of statistical bone atlases for black and white Americans. The analysis of global morphologic differences between both ethnic groups is explained in the "Morphologic Shape Analysis" section. The "Automated Measurements" section describes the complete automated quantitative analysis of each femur and tibia, which consists of detecting bony landmarks, measuring linear features, and calculating relevant axes and angles (eg, transepicondylar axis [TEA], anatomic axis). Automation of these measurements is possible because of the vast of information contained in the ethnic-specific statistical atlases.

Data Acquisition

A dataset of 223 male individuals (183 white Americans and 40 black Americans) was scanned using CT. Only normal femurs and tibia were included in this study; femurs or tibia with severe osteophytes and other abnormalities were specifically excluded. Only one femur and tibia was chosen from each individual, with no preference taken to either right or left side.

The bones were CT scanned using 0.625 mm × 0.625 mm × 0.625 mm cubic voxels. The result is high resolution, 3D radiographs in the form of Digital Imaging and Communications in Medicine (DICOM) image slices. This stacked image data were then segmented, and surface models were generated. This process has been found to be reliable with negligible inter- and intra-observer error.[15] These models were then added to the ethnicity-specific statistical bone atlases.

Atlas Creation and Validation

Briefly, a bone atlas is an average mold, or template mesh, that captures the primary shape variation of a bone and allows for the comparison of global shape differences between groups or populations. Bone atlases were developed initially for automatic medical image segmentation[3,4,10,19]; however, it can be used as a way to digitally recreate a bone and conduct statistical shape analyses.[2,7,14,15,17,19] In addition, they have proven useful in biologic anthropology as a means of studying sexual dimorphism and for reconstructing hominid fossils and making shape comparisons among fossil species.[2,14,16,17,20]

For the ethnicity difference analysis in this study, a previously developed technique for creating a statistical representation of bone shape was used in a novel manner.[14,15,17] Two separate statistical atlases of femurs were compiled with one atlas containing only femurs of white Americans and the other only femurs of black Americans. Similarly, two separate atlases were created for the tibia and divided in the same manner (ie, tibiae of white and black Americans). The processes of creating these statistical atlases and adding bones to the atlases are outlined below.

First, all of the bone models in the dataset were compared, and a bone model with average shape characteristics was selected to act as a template mesh. The points in the template mesh are then matched to corresponding points in all of the other training models. This ensures that all of the bones have the same number of vertices and the same triangular connectivity.[15] Next, a series of registration and warping techniques was used to select corresponding points on all the other bone models in the training set. This process of picking point correspondences on new models to be added to the atlas is "nontrivial."[17] The matching algorithm described here uses several well-known techniques of computer vision, as well as a novel contribution for final surface alignment.

During the first step in the matching algorithm, the centroids of the template mesh and the new mesh were aligned, and the template mesh was prescaled to match the bounding box dimensions of the new mesh. Second, a rigid alignment of the template mesh to the new mesh was performed using a standard vertex-to-vertex iterative closest point (ICP) algorithm. Third, after rigid alignment we performed a general affine transformation without iteration. This method was applied to align the template mesh to the new mesh using 12 degrees of freedom (rotations, translations, scaling, and shear). After the affine transformation step, the template and new model have reached the limits of linear transformation, but local portions of the models still remain significantly distant. Because the goal of final surface-to-surface matching is to create new points on the surface of the new model that will have similar local spatial characteristics as the template model, a novel nonlinear iterative warping approach was developed to reduce misalignment.[17]

To achieve point correspondence (Fig. 16.1), an iterative algorithm is used in which the closest vertex-to-vertex correspondences are found from the template to the new model as before, but now we also find the correspondences from the new model to the template model. Using both of these point correspondences, points on the template mesh are moved toward locations on the new mesh, using a nonsymmetrical weighting of the vectors of correspondence. Next, a subroutine consisting of an iterative smoothing algorithm is applied to the now-deformed template mesh. This smoothing algorithm seeks to

Principle of Bone Atlas

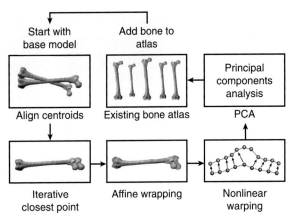

FIG 16.1 Flow chart outlining the process of the atlas creation.

average the size of adjacent triangles on the template mesh, thereby eliminating discontinuities. At the beginning of the warping algorithm, the smoothing algorithm uses the actual areas of the surrounding triangles to dictate the smoothing vector applied to each point, which aids in effectively removing outlying points with large triangles. Consequently, at the beginning of the process the template mesh makes large steps, and larger smoothing is required. However, toward the end of the process the smoothing vector is normalized by the total area of the surrounding triangles, which allows for greater expansion of the template mesh into areas of high curvature. After this procedure has been completed on all the femurs and tibiae in their respective atlases, the atlases are ready for morphologic shape analyses and automated metric comparisons.

Morphologic Shape Analysis

An innovative statistical treatment was used to analyze global shape differences between the two groups. This method uses the power of PCA both as a means of variable reduction and as a global shape descriptor. This method is designed to find points of high discrimination between and within different gender and (or) different ethnic groups when normalized against the first principal component (PC), which is considered primarily scale. This procedure highlights areas on models that would be highly discriminating without the use of any other information. The landmarks identified by this algorithm provide adequate discrimination without the use of any other landmarks between ethnic groups. We used this feature finder algorithm to examine femursl and tibial shape differences independent of the size differences between white and black Americans.

Automated Measurements

A wide array of comparisons was made using specific measurements at defined landmarks on the ethnicity-specific statistical atlases. These landmarks were chosen based on surgical importance, clinical relevance, and historical measurements. Because the atlas consists of homologous points on each femur (or tibia) model, they provide ample information for automating this process. In addition, each bone model in the atlas is aligned to the same coordinate frame. A total of 99 femur and 23 tibia measurements, angles, and indices were calculated, although only a select subset of these variables is defined here. Furthermore, for purposes of conciseness, only the most significant

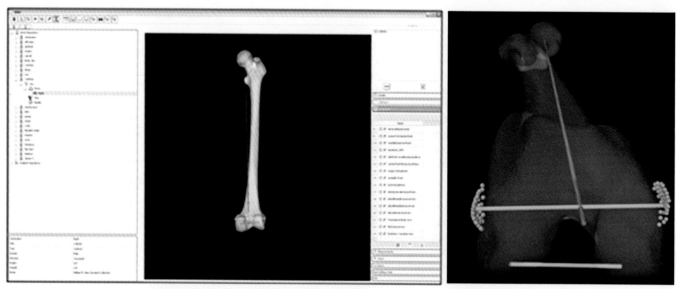

FIG 16.2 Automatic calculated landmarks using IDAS software.

measurements are discussed in the "Results" section. Unless otherwise specified, the measurements outlined below represent 3D Euclidean distances between pairs of landmarks, and angles are measured as 3D rotations between vectors. In some cases these measurements were projected onto a plane for comparison with previous work in the field. A subset of these measurements is shown in Fig. 2.4. The landmarks that define the measurement endpoints are first computed and then defined relative to surgical and anatomic axes.

Distal Femur Measurements. The following axes, landmarks, and measurements were calculated on the distal femur (see Fig. 2.3):

- *TEA:* This measurement is known in the anthropological literature as *biepicondylar breadth.* To compute the clinical TEA, rough sets of vertices were manually defined on an average femur on the most lateral prominence of the lateral epicondyle and the most medial prominence of the medial epicodyle.[1] This step was performed only once because vertices in the atlas femurs are homologous. Using these rough sets of points, a search region of 10-mm radius was defined from the centroid of the rough sets of vertices on both the lateral and medial sides. Defining the vector from each of these centroids then gives a rough direction for the TEA. A pair of points was selected by maximizing the distance in this rough direction; these selected points form the endpoints of the TEA measurement (Fig. 16.2).
- *Distal anatomic axis (DAA):* The DAA was defined by locating the shaft centroids at the distal one-third and distal one-fifth of the overall femur length.
- *Central anteroposterior axis (CAP):* Using the DAA and the TEA, a mutually perpendicular axis was defined with termini at the posterior aspect of the intercondylar notch and the most anterior portion of the intercondylar groove. The length of this axis is recorded as CAP (Fig. 16.3). This axis is similar to "height of intercondylar notch."[15]
- *Femoral saddle point:* A landmark located at the most distal extension of the intercondylar groove.
- *Knee center (K):* Using the two bndpoints of the CAP measurement and the femoral saddle point, a plane is defined

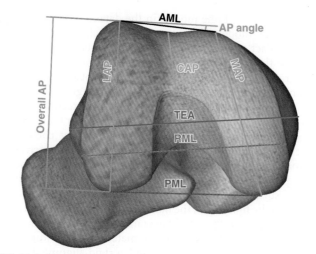

FIG 16.3 The axes, landmarks, and measurements on the distal femur.

that bisects the femur into medial and lateral sides. The intersection of this plane with the TEA is the K, which forms the distal endpoint of the mechanical axis (MA) of the femur. The proximal endpoint of the MA is the center of the femoral head (see proximal femur measurements later).
- *Anteroposterior (AP) direction:* Using the MA and TEA, a mutually perpendicular vector with its origin at the K is used to define the AP direction, resulting in a direction similar to Whiteside line.[17]
- *Anterior mediolateral width (AML) and posterior mediolateral width (PML):* The AP direction was used to locate four landmarks: the most anterior and posterior points on the medial and lateral condyles of the distal femur. Connecting the two most anterior points gives a measurement of AML along the trochlear line,[17] whereas connecting the two most posterior points gives a measure of PML measured along the posterior condylar axis (PCA)[17] (see Fig. 16.2).
- *AP length of medial and lateral condyles (MAP and LAP):* Connecting the pairs of lateral and medial vertices defined above, respectively, gives the LAP and MAP (see Fig. 16.3).

- *Posterior plane:* A unique plane containing the endpoints of the PML measurement, which is also parallel to the MA, was used to define the posterior plane.
- *Overall AP length:* The minimum distance between the prominences of the lateral anterior condyle and the posterior plane (see Fig. 16.3).
- *AP angle:* The angle of the AML vector relative to the posterior plane (see Fig. 16.3).
- *Distal mediolateral length (DML):* The most distal aspects of the medial and lateral condyles were recorded using MA as a reference direction. The distance between these two landmarks was denoted as DML.
- *Posterior angle (PA):* The angle between the vector connecting the DML length and mean axis of the femur (Fig. 16.4).
- *Condylar twist angle (CTA):* The angle between the TEA and PCA.
- *Patellar groove height (GH):* Calculated between the posterior aspect of the intercondylar notch and the midpoint between the two DML axis points (see Fig. 16.4).
- *Femoral shaft curvature (SC):* The radius of curvature of the femoral mean axis.

Distal Femur Curvature Mapping

To calculate medial profile a plane defined by the medial anterior point (most anterior point in medial condyle), the medial distal point (most distal point on medial condyle) and medial posterior point (most posterior point in medial condyle) are intersected with the distal femurs; this results in contour that corresponds to the most protruding points on medial condyle surface. The same method is used to calculate the lateral profile, as shown in Fig. 16.5.

For the sulcus profile calculation a set of contours is extracted by intersecting the distal femur with a series of planes rotating around the TEA with a 10-degree increment. The lowest points on these contours are then used to define the sulcus points, as shown in Fig. 16.5. Curvature of the medial, lateral, and sulcus profiles are then calculated by finding best number of circles passing that accurately approximate the curve, as shown in Fig. 16.6. To capture the curvature of the condylar surface the curves produced earlier by intersecting the femur with the planes around TEA are trimmed around the medial, lateral, and sulcus profiles, the circle of curvature of each of these trimmed contours are then calculated, as shown in Fig. 16.6.

Tibia Measurements. The following landmarks and measurements were identified automatically (Figs. 16.7 and 16.8):

- *Intercondylar eminence points:* The two highest projecting points on the medial and lateral intercondylar eminences.
- *Eminence midpoint:* The midpoint between the lateral and medial intercondylar eminence points.
- *Tibial tuberosity:* The most anteriorly protruding point on the tibial tuberosity.
- *Mediolateral (ML):* Maximum width of the tibia plateau in the ML direction.

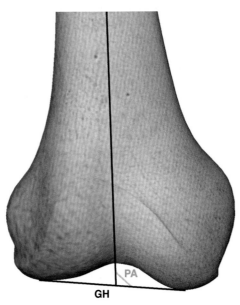

FIG 16.4 The axes, landmarks, and measurements on the distal femur.

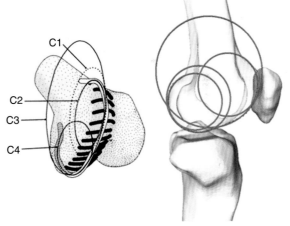

FIG 16.6 Distal femurs curvature and profile mapping using IDAS software.

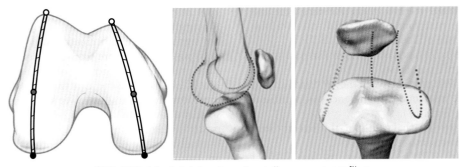

FIG 16.5 Medial, lateral, and patellar groove profiles.

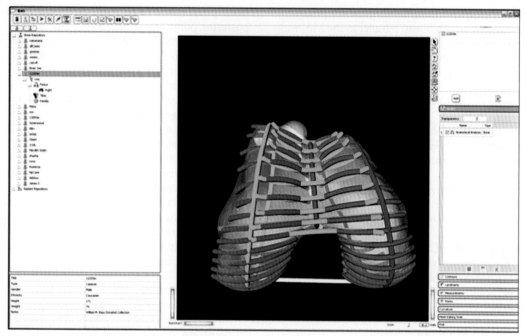

FIG 16.7 The axes, landmarks, and measurements on the proximal tibia.

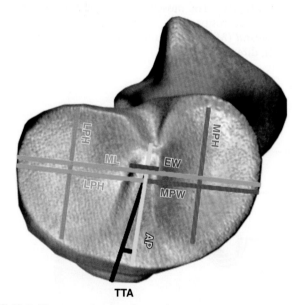

FIG 16.8 The axes, landmarks, and measurements on the proximal tibia.

- *AP:* Length of the tibial plateau in the AP direction and passing through the midpoint of the tibial intercondylar eminence (ie, eminence midpoint) (see Fig. 16.7).
- *Eminence width (EW):* Distance between medial and lateral intercondylar eminence points (see Fig. 16.7).
- *Tibial twist angle (TTA):* Angle between the AP direction and a line connecting the intercondylar eminence midpoint and tibial tuberosity (see Fig. 16.7).
- *Lateral plateau height (LPH):* Length of the lateral tibial plateau in the AP direction (see Fig. 16.7).
- *Lateral plateau width (LPW):* Length of the lateral tibial plateau in the ML direction (see Fig. 16.7).

- *Medial plateau height (MPH):* Length of the medial tibial plateau in the AP direction (see Fig. 16.7).
- *Medial plateau width (MPW):* Length of the medial tibial plateau in the ML direction (see Fig. 16.7).
- *Eminence ML ratio (EMLR):* Ratio of MPW (ie, MPW) over ML.
- *Maximum length:* Length of the tibia from the medial malleolus to the intercondylar eminence.

RESULTS

Femur

The results from the feature finder shape analysis tool highlight shape differences in the femoral shaft, lateral condyle, and greater trochanter, but in this analysis we are concentrating on the distal femur. Fig. 16.9 shows the variation captured in the 2nd to 10th PCs. The blue-colored areas denote areas with low magnitudes of difference, and the red-colored areas designate areas of greater morphologic difference between the two ethnic groups. These differences were highlighted in the t-tests and power test based on the automated measurements as well. Table 16.1 presents the results from the t-tests and power tests for the automated measurements; several of these measurements correlate with some of the shape differences highlighted in Fig. 16.9. In black American males the lateral condyle has a higher AP height ($p < 0.01$), whereas the medial condyle height was not significant, thereby creating a more trapezoid-shaped knee as opposed to the more square-shaped knee in white American males, resulting in larger AP condyle angles in black Americans. Metric comparisons indicate that black Americans have significantly longer femurs, narrower knees in the ML dimension (ie, smaller TEA width), and longer lateral condyles in the anteroposterior dimension.

Analyzing the curvature of both lateral and medial profiles we found that they can be accurately approximated by four distinct radii of curvature (C1-4, as shown in Fig. 16.10). These

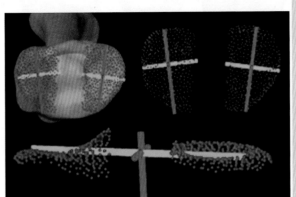
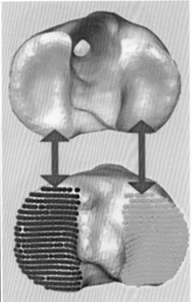

FIG 16.9 Feature finder results highlighting areas of maximum and minimum differences between black and white populations in both femur and tibia.

TABLE 16.1 Important Femur Measurements—Means, Standard Deviations, *t*-Tests, and Power Test Results

	White Mean	SD	Black Mean	SD	*t*-Test *p*-Value	Power Test
TEA	8.60	0.38	8.44	0.48	0.10	197
AML	3.61	0.4	3.65	0.54	0.71	3905
PML	5.35	0.4	3.65	0.54	0.71	3905
MAP	6.60	0.45	6.69	0.29	0.32	446
LAP	6.77	0.47	7.05	0.34	0.01	55
DML	5.50	0.47	5.58	0.54	0.48	1073
PA	98.48	3.85	98.30	2.16	0.82	7937
GH	0.78	0.26	0.81	0.18	0.59	1597
SC	115.41	16.00	128.38	23.75	0.01	62

N = 212.

TABLE 16.2 Important Tibia Measurements—Means, Standard Deviations, *t*-Tests, and Power Test Results

	White Mean	SD	Black Mean	SD	*t*-Test *p*-Value	Power Test
ML	7.81	0.37	7.88	0.40	0.41	759
AP	5.73	0.32	5.73	0.34	0.96	266,814
EW	1.32	0.58	1.44	0.79	0.40	758
TTA	82.96	34.05	79.29	33.89	0.63	2,223
LPH	4.85	0.38	5.03	0.39	0.05	127
LPW	3.26	0.37	3.22	0.38	0.64	2,425
MPH	5.13	0.33	5.15	0.43	0.75	5,382
	3.08	0.27	3.14	0.32	0.34	592

N = 110.

four radii were found to be consistent between both ethnicities (black and white Americans); however, the values of these radii were different in each ethnicity, as shown in Fig. 16.11. Difference in curvature of medial and lateral profile were noticed, mainly the flatness of the lateral profile compared with medial profile, as shown in Fig. 16.12.

Tibia (Fig. 16.13)

The feature finder results for the tibia indicate that ethnic shape differences have higher significance around tibial tuberosity area as compared with the medial and lateral plateau areas. Fig. 16.9 shows the color map reflecting the magnitudes of difference between the two ethnic groups. In addition to minor differences in the proximal anterior tibia, the only area that registered significant was the tip of the medial malleolus. The results from the *t*-tests and power test also underscore these findings. The most significant variables are those related to scale, including maximum length, measures of shaft robusticity, and several measurements of the tibial plateau. In short, tibiae

of black Americans are longer with a more robust shaft and slightly larger tibial plateau. Table 16.2 shows the automated measurements for the tibia with LPH as the most significant measurement ($p < 0.05$), which correlates to the significant difference in the lateral femoral condyle height.

DISCUSSION

Presented are novel methods to ascertain ethnic differences on the distal femur and proximal tibia on a global scale, to discover regions that were likely to offer discriminating information, and to measure relevant surgical and anatomic features to aid implanted prosthesis design. Different studies have tried to identify ethnic differences of the femur and tibia. Measurement techniques that lack accuracy or precision have been used for many years to find femoral and tibiae measurements with the largest significance. Unfortunately, these methods lack the ability to find features of smaller consequence. From the onset, the manual segmentation of the worst-case data has shown to

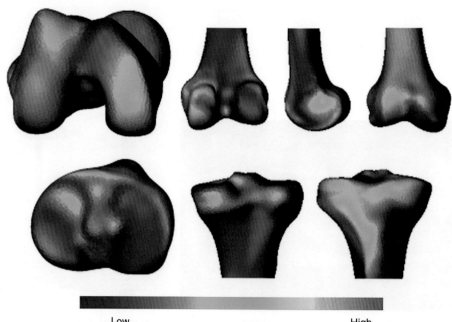

Low variation   High variation

FIG 16.10 Lateral profile radii of curvature.

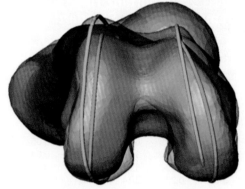

FIG 16.11 Medial and lateral profile for black *(gray)* and white *(red)* populations, normalized to same femur height.

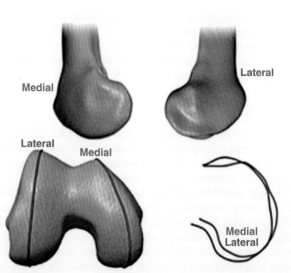

FIG 16.12 Difference in curvature between medial and lateral profile.

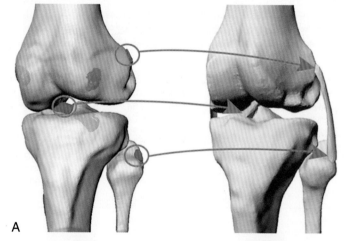

A

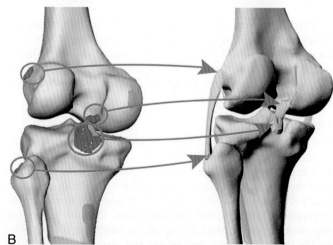

B

FIG 16.13 Ligament attachment locations extracted from segmented models. Here ligaments are segmented from magnetic resonance imaging *(right)* and mapped to the statistical atlas *(left)*.

provide surface accuracies of less than a quarter of a millimeter. Consequently, many of the automatic measurements had reliability coefficients greater than 0.97, indicating that, although the measured variable might not be significant between the genders, it would not likely lead to a statistical type II error.

The ordered series of methods that were used first showed the largest global differences, which subsequently allowed identification of isolate regions likely to be highly different using the feature finder method, and finally allowed for the coding of algorithms to locate and measure surgically relevant anatomic features with a high degree of accuracy and repeatability. In all of these comparison methods, bones with different scales were considered to have the possibility of shape changes dependent on size. In this way, correlations between measured variables and size were removed to expose demonstrable shape differences inherent to the ethnicities.

The present analysis confirms that black American males have longer, straighter femurs with narrower knees than do white American males. In addition, this study reveals differences in the dimensions and orientation of the lateral condyle that result in overall shape differences in the distal femur: black Americans have a trapezoid-shaped knee, and white Americans have a more square-shaped knee. Not unexpected, the differences in the distal femur are echoed in the adjacent tibia, whereby black Americans have a longer lateral tibial condyle. The mean ML length of the tibial plateau is slightly longer in black than in white populations, but this difference did not register as significant with the existing sample size. However, black Americans do have significantly longer and more robust tibiae. As presented in the study by Mahfouz et al.,[18] which included an Asian population in addition to white and black populations, ratios, such as the ML/AP, AML/PML, and MAP/LAP, may provide more insight than individual measurements into shape differences and more value as input to component design. These ratios led Mahfouz et al.[18] to propose a classification system identifying six distinct types of femurs (Fig. 16.14). Given these differences, clinical studies should make efforts to incorporate representative population statistics, a factor often overlooked in study design.[24]

At the time of initial publication, the author was primarily interested in morphologic features to be used as input to implant design methods. As the analysis methods presented in this work have become increasingly popular, interest has shifted towards coupling morphologic measurements with joint kinematics. When considering the cause and effect relationship between morphometric features and kinematics, the complex structures of the knee must be included—meaning exploration of the interplay between ligaments, hyaline cartilage, morphologic axes, and kinematics. Given the challenges of extracting all of this information for a single individual—much less an entire population—creative strategies are required to fuse multiple data sources. The statistical atlas provides one such tool through point correspondence.

For example, consider the following two additional axes: (1) the cylindrical axis, defined as "a line equidistant from contact points on the medial and lateral condylar surfaces from 10 to 120 degrees of flexion"[9] and (2) the spherical axis, defined as the line passing through the centers of spheres fit to the medial and lateral posterior condyles.[26] Clearly both are directly related to posterior condylar curvature, which is known to vary between populations.[18] The motivation for both of these axes is driven by kinematics; each is claimed to better represent the true axis of tibia rotation about the femur. Figs. 16.15 and 16.16 provide an example of how kinematics and morphology may relate.

As seen in this chapter, anatomic variation is present both within a population and between different populations. Although both modes of variation are important to capture in

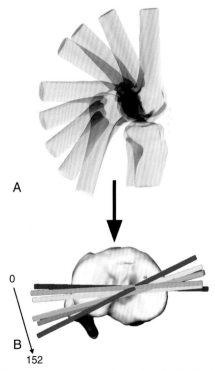

A

B

0

152

FIG 16.15 Instantaneous axes of rotation *(helical axis)* extracted from digital x-ray fluoroscopy video. (A) Models were superimposed on the fluoroscopy images at approximately 20-degree intervals starting at extension.[13] (B) The instantaneous axis of rotation was calculated between successive poses. This axis represents the true axis of rotation of the femur about the tibia. There has been significant effort to relate this true axis of rotation to anatomic axes.

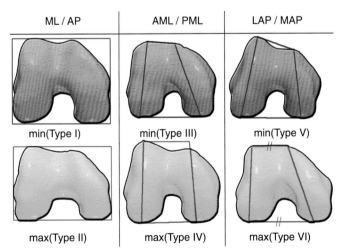

ML / AP	AML / PML	LAP / MAP
min(Type I)	min(Type III)	min(Type V)
max(Type II)	max(Type IV)	max(Type VI)

FIG 16.14 Classification system for femurs based on ratios of measured axes. Six distinct classes of femurs were identified through rigorous analysis.[18]

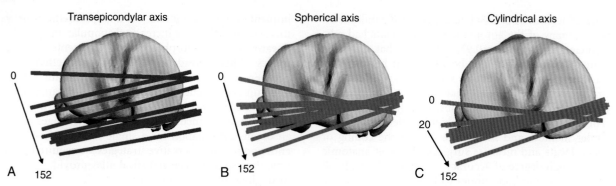

Transepicondylar axis   Spherical axis   Cylindrical axis

A   152   B   152   C   152

FIG 16.16 Three femoral axes mapped during deep knee bend (as in Fig. 16.1). Comparison with Fig. 16.15 suggests the (A) transepicondylar axis may not be as closely related to kinematics as (B) the spherical or (C) the cylindrical axes. In other words, the axes in (B) and (C) suggest direct linkage between femoral anatomy and joint motion.

design, there are also implications for joint alignment and function. For example, an AP direction for the tibia is often defined along the vector connecting the tibia tuberosity and posterior cruciate ligament insertion for the purposes of setting rotation of the tibial implant during knee surgery. As reported in the "Tibia" section the tuberosity landmark is subject to large variation. Therefore the tuberosity may not be a reliable landmark when setting implant component alignment, a suggestion reinforced by Siston et al.[23] in a study reporting 27-degree standard deviation in setting alignment using the tuberosity-PCL axis.

Understanding differences in morphology is a key step in implant design, but in a complex joint like the knee, the interplay of morphology, tissues, and kinematics requires further investigation.

ACKNOWLEDGMENTS

The author thanks Drs. Michael Johnson and Gary To for their efforts in preparing this work.

The references for this chapter can also be found on www.expertconsult.com.

17

Fluoroscopic Analysis of Total Knee Replacement

Michael T. LaCour, Richard D. Komistek

ANALYSIS METHODS

The ongoing goal of improving the outcomes of total knee arthroplasty (TKA) yields the continuing need for accurate in vivo kinematic analyses. Popular kinematic study techniques include in vivo fluoroscopic analyses, in vitro analyses using cadavers,[12] noninvasive analyses using motion tracking surface markers,[10,29] more invasive in vivo analyses using roentgen stereophotogrammetric analysis (RSA),[2,8] and quasidynamic magnetic resonance imaging (MRI) testing.[19]

Unfortunately, the mechanical actuators used to simulate muscles in cadaveric studies do not replicate in vivo motion, and hence this technique does not allow for in vivo accuracy. Video analysis using markers attached to the skin, similar to what is found in gait laboratory systems, is a popular form of kinematic analysis because it is noninvasive, effective in determining in-plane rotations, and can determine kinematics of the whole body. However, soft tissue artifact (the movement of skin markers relative to the bone) induces significant out-of-plane rotational and translational errors,[1,16] and these out-of-plane transformations are measurements that must be precise when evaluating knee kinematics for orthopedics. Although the RSA techniques are generally highly accurate and precise,[2,8] they are also highly invasive and therefore uncommon for in vivo human analyses. These tests are also conducted under quasistatic conditions, which does not allow for dynamic analysis of the knee joint. Finally, MRI testing is conducted under static, non–weight-bearing conditions, which also does not represent what is happening during daily dynamic activity.

Hence using fluoroscopy as a means of analyzing both normal and implanted joints is becoming an increasingly popular method to evaluate in vivo kinematics.*

KINEMATIC STUDIES USING FLUOROSCOPY

Data Collection

Fluoroscopy can be used to analyze a variety of activities, both weight bearing and non–weight bearing, including deep knee bend, gait, chair rise, step up, step down, ramps, and leg swings. Fluoroscopy, an imaging technique that uses traditional x-rays to create a video, allows for two-dimensional (2D) visualization of the joint throughout the entire activity. During a fluoroscopic study, the subject is asked to perform an activity while the subject's joint is under fluoroscopic surveillance (Fig. 17.1). Throughout data collection, it is advantageous to keep the knee

in the center of the video, and this is generally easier if the knee is kept as close to the image intensifier as possible. Although the optimal plane to use for analysis is activity-specific, depending on the nature of the data that is desired, fluoroscopic studies of the knee are generally conducted in the sagittal plane.

Video Processing

After patients have performed the required activities while under fluoroscopic surveillance, the videos, recorded at frame rates of 30 or 60 Hz, are stored digitally, and specific frames of interest are captured from the video and exported into the preprocessing software. Depending on the type of fluoroscopy unit used, the images may experience distortion. The extent of image distortion depends on the medium that is used to detect the x-rays. For example, analog image intensifiers generally experience much less distortion than digital flat panel detectors.

Distortion effects, such as pin cushion and spiral distortion, must be corrected to ensure that the image registration techniques are accurate. This can be performed using fiducial control markers. These control markers, generally a grid of metallic beads in precise, systematic, and known spacing, are used to transform each pixel of the fluoroscopic image until the modified image correctly matches the true, undistorted grid. After the images have been properly processed, they can be exported to a model-fitting software program for three-dimensional (3D)-to-2D registration.[26,27]

Image Registration

To find the orientation of an implanted TKA component from an x-ray image, the fluoroscopic space is virtually modeled within a computer graphical user interface (GUI). This GUI allows the user to virtually view the fluoroscopic space between the x-ray source and the image intensifier. A virtual camera represents the x-ray source, and the processed image represents the image intensifier. 3D computer-aided design (CAD) models of the TKA components are virtually placed in the space between the camera and the image (Fig. 17.2), which allows the user to superimpose (overlay) the CAD model silhouettes on top of the implant component silhouettes from the x-ray image. The nature of x-ray images is such that objects closer to the radiation source appear larger than those more distant from the source, which allows for measurements of out-of-plane translations and orientations because the portion farther away from the radiation source will appear smaller in the silhouette than the portion nearer the source. By matching a 3D CAD model of the implant component to each fluoroscopic frame of interest from the video, 3D in vivo kinematics can be extracted from a 2D image (Fig. 17.3).

---

*See references 4-7, 9, 13-15, 20-23, 25-28, 30-33.

The current state of the art matches the CAD models to the fluoroscopic silhouettes using either a manual or an iterative, computer-automated, model-fitting technique.[26,27] The automated technique is generally faster and removes the inherent human error by using a computerized algorithm to match models with implant silhouettes. The algorithm uses an

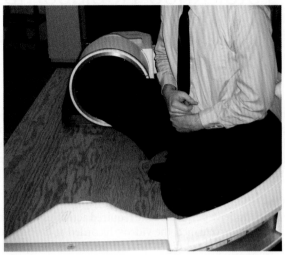

FIG 17.1 A subject performing a deep knee bend to maximum weight-bearing flexion while the knee is under fluoroscopic surveillance.

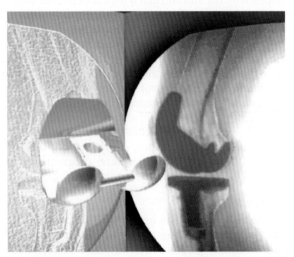

FIG 17.2 Virtual recreation of fluoroscopic space showing an implant CAD model and corresponding shadow overlaid atop the 2D fluoroscopy image.

optimization method known as simulated annealing, an energy minimization routine, to maximize the correlation value. Thus the computer quickly and accurately determines the correct positions and orientations of the TKA implants.

An unbiased error analysis comparison was initially conducted on multiple operators each using three methods: an early matching technique known as template matching, a manual matching technique, and the current automated matching technique. The analysis determined that the automated model-fitting process outperformed both the manual and template-matching methods.[26,27] In general, the errors associated with this model-fitting technique are less than 0.5 mm for in-plane translations and 0.5 degrees for rotations.[26] Out-of-plane errors are normally higher. The use of fluoroscopy units with higher frame rates and greater image resolutions will increase the accuracy of the fluoroscopic analyses.

Tracking Polyethylene Bearings

Monitoring the rotations of TKA bearing inserts can provide valuable insight into the kinematic performance of the implants as a whole, especially with rotating platform TKAs.[23,28] Unfortunately, tracking polyethylene bearings can be difficult because polyethylene is invisible in x-ray and fluoroscopic images. To account for this, specially designed polyethylene bearings must be used. These bearings contain four precisely located, metallic reference beads that are visible in fluoroscopic images. CAD models with four virtual beads placed in the exact same locations can then be used to register the polyethylene insert to the image (Fig. 17.4). A minimum of three beads must be visible in the fluoroscopy image to successfully determine the insert transformations, and more beads would further increase the registration accuracy.

Other Fluoroscopic Analysis Techniques

The fluoroscopic analyses discussed so far have been single-plane fluoroscopic analyses, thus using only one x-ray source and one image intensifier. As an alternative, biplanar fluoroscopic setups can be used. In this scenario, two offset fluoroscopy units are used to analyze the knee (Fig. 17.5). By incorporating a second fluoroscopy unit, the out-of-plane errors associated with single-plane fluoroscopy are eliminated. The errors associated with biplanar fluoroscopy have been reported to be as low as 0.36 mm for translations and 0.42 degrees for rotations,[18] similar to the in-plane errors associated with single-plane fluoroscopy. However, despite the potential for improved accuracy, the use of biplanar fluoroscopy can also limit the activities that can be analyzed because of space constraints.

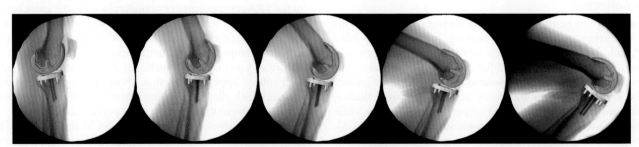

FIG 17.3 Fluoroscopic images of a patient with PCRF TKA performing a deep knee bend maneuver and corresponding 3D CAD model registered to the 2D fluoroscopy images at 30-degree increments.

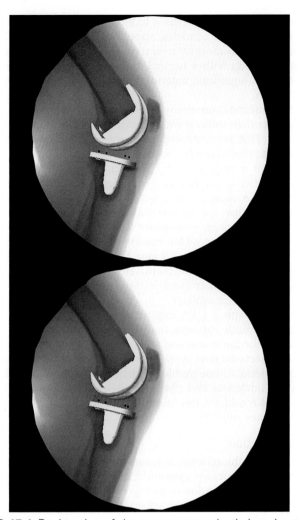

FIG 17.4 Registration of the transparent polyethylene bearing to the fluoroscopic image using four metallic beads as reference.

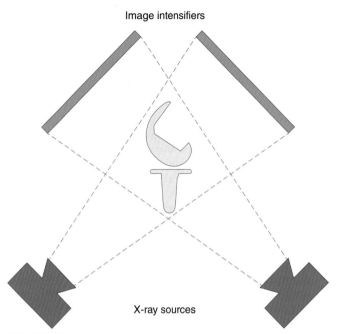

FIG 17.5 Biplanar fluoroscopic setup showing two x-ray sources and two image intensifiers, set at offset angles, being used to analyze a TKA.

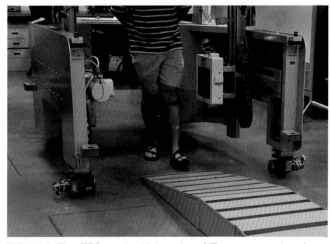

FIG 17.6 The TFS at the University of Tennessee, showing a patient completing a gait activity and about to begin a ramp activity.

A more recent advancement in fluoroscopic studies is the implementation of tracking fluoroscope system (TFS) units that are capable of following a patient around a room, keeping the knee (or any joint of interest) in the center of the fluoroscopy video at all times. These TFS units, such as the one from the Center for Musculoskeletal Research and the University of Tennessee, shown in Fig 17.6, allow for fluoroscopic evaluations of more complex activities, such as ramp activities, several stair steps in succession, and multiple gait cycles.[17] This is accomplished by (1) ensuring that the unit as a whole follows the patient's motion around a room and (2) ensuring that the x-ray source and flat panel detector move together with the motion of the patient's knee. Although fluoroscopic studies with TFS units are relatively new, it is hypothesized that these TFS studies will allow patients to conduct activities in a much more natural, unconstrained manner versus traditional C-arm fluoroscopy units, thereby yielding results that more accurately represent a patient's daily activities.[17]

With both biplanar and mobile fluoroscopy, the aforementioned model-fitting approach can still be used to extract 3D kinematics from the 2D fluoroscopy video.

Radiation Concerns

One of the primary concerns with fluoroscopy is the exposure of patients to potentially harmful x-rays. To address these radiation concerns, it is important for fluoroscopic investigators to seek to minimize patient radiation time and exposure. To minimize time, the individuals conducting the studies should set maximum exposure time limits, and they should ensure that the patient knows exactly what activities he or she is supposed to perform and how to perform them so that the patient does not receive unnecessary radiation. It can be beneficial to have the patient rehearse the activity first, before exposing them to radiation. Fortunately with the development of TFS units that accurately track the patient's joint, the patient can perform the entire set of activities in one trial with minimal practice, thereby reducing exposure time significantly. Patients may also desire to wear lead shielding over their hips, chest, and/or thyroid, which would further help to prevent unnecessary exposure. With proper practice and a concern for patient safety, radiation exposure can be easily minimized.

SAMPLE RESULTS

The model-fitting approach discussed earlier has been used to determine the kinematics of more than 3000 knees, including fixed posterior cruciate-retaining (PCRF), mobile-bearing posterior cruciate-retaining (PCRM), fixed posterior cruciate-substituting (PSF), mobile-bearing posterior cruciate-sacrificing (PCSM), mobile-bearing posterior cruciate-substituting (PSM), fixed anterior cruciate-retaining (ACRF), bicruciate-stabilizing fixed-bearing (BCSF) TKA, and both medial unicondylar knee arthroplasty (MED UKA) and lateral unicondylar knee arthroplasty (LAT UKA).

Recent developments in TKA research have led to the development of patient-specific conforming implants, which can be analyzed in the same manner. These fluoroscopy techniques have also been used to analyze normal and anterior cruciate ligament-deficient (ACLD) nonimplanted knees by creating 3D models of the bones using computed tomography (CT) scans and overlaying the bone models accordingly.[26,27]

Parameters of interest for fluoroscopy studies commonly include anteroposterior (AP) femorotibial translation, axial rotation, range of motion, incidence of femoral condylar lift-off, and cam-post engagement. Included in the following sections are sample results from a study of 1630 knees during a weight-bearing deep knee bend activity, analyzing AP translation and axial rotation, as well as references to multiple studies analyzing condylar liftoff.

Anteroposterior Translation

In Table 17.1 the AP data for the 1630 analyzed knees are shown. Subjects with a normal knee generally experienced posterior motion of both condyles throughout flexion, with the lateral condyle's motion generally being greater than that of the medial condyle (−16.4 vs. −8.9 mm). Subjects with an ACLD knee experienced similar patterns of motion (−13.3 and −5.9 mm for lateral and medial condyles, respectively), but logically these knees sat slightly more anterior throughout flexion than normal knees. Subjects with a normal knee rarely (2% of the time) experienced significant anterior slide of the knee with increasing flexion.

The kinematic variability between subjects with a TKA was far greater than subjects with normal knees. For example, four of seven TKA types showed, on average, paradoxical anterior slide of the medial condyle with increasing flexion. Similarly the amount of average posterior rollback of the lateral condyle ranged between 1.3 and 21.9 mm, depending on TKA type. Certain TKA designs (such as the BCSF TKA) are far more constrained than others; therefore ensuring that certain kinematic patterns occur throughout flexion. On average, subjects with a TKA experienced less motion of both condyles throughout flexion (−5.8 and −1.9 mm for the lateral and medial condyle, respectively), and there were far more cases of anterior slide (14%) of either condyle throughout flexion compared with normal knee subjects.

Subjects with a UKA experienced slightly more posterior motion of both condyles than the average TKAs (−6.3 and −4.4 mm for the lateral and medial condyle, respectively), but these subjects did not experience as much motion as the normal knee subjects. Although a lower frequency of anterior slide of either condyle was also observed when comparing UKA subjects to TKA subjects, this frequency was once again greater than normal knee subjects.

Axial Rotation

In Table 17.2 the axial rotation data for the 1630 analyzed knees is shown. The average amount of axial rotation in the normal knee from full extension to 90 degrees of knee flexion was 17.8 degrees. The average maximum amounts of normal and reverse rotation of any normal knee at any flexion increment were 31.6 and −7.3 degrees. Subjects with an ACLD knee experienced less axial rotation than subjects with a normal knee (9.8 vs. 17.8 mm, respectively).

Similar to the AP translation results the TKA subjects once again experienced large variations in the data, depending on the

---

TABLE 17.1 Summary of Anteroposterior Translation for 1630 Implanted and Nonimplanted Knees During Deep Knee Bend

Knee Type	POSTERIOR ROLLBACK (0-90 DEGREES)[a]		AVERAGE (±SD) MOVEMENT (0-90 DEGREES)[b]		ANTERIOR SLIDE >3.0 mm
	Lateral (%)	Medial (%)	Lateral (mm)	Medial (mm)	Any Condyle (0-90 Degrees) (%)[c]
Normal	100	98	−16.4 ± 6.8	−8.9 ± 6.0	2
ACLD	100	100	−13.3 ± 8.3	−5.9 ± 1.9	0
PCRF TKA	68	34	−2.4 ± 4.2	0.6 ± 3.7	24
PSF TKA	71	61	−8.5 ± 8.4	−4.0 ± 5.4	4
ACRF TKA	91	83	−10.4 ± 5.0	−5.6 ± 5.1	6
PCRM TKA	68	46	−1.3 ± 3.5	0.4 ± 3.8	25
PCSM TKA	85	37	−2.1 ± 2.7	0.4 ± 2.6	18
PSM TKA	59	26	−2.7 ± 4.2	0.6 ± 3.7	16
BCSF TKA	100	100	−21.9 ± 6.6	−12.5 ± 3.1	0
All TKAs	70	46	−5.8 ± 5.9	−1.9 ± 4.0	14
MED UKA	—	63	—	−4.4 ± 4.8	5
LAT UKA	100	—	−6.3 ± 7.6	—	0

ACLD, Anterior cruciate ligament-deficient; *PCRF TKA*, fixed posterior cruciate-retaining total knee arthroplasty (TKA); *PSF*, fixed posterior cruciate-substituting; *ACRF*, fixed anterior cruciate-retaining; *PCRM*, mobile-bearing posterior cruciate-retaining; *PCSM*, mobile-bearing posterior cruciate-sacrificing; *PSM*, mobile-bearing posterior cruciate-substituting; *BCSF*, bicruciate-stabilizing fixed-bearing; *MED UKA*, medial unicondylar knee arthroplasty; *LAT UKA*, lateral unicondylar knee arthroplasty.
[a]Knees exhibiting posterior motion from 0 to 90 degrees of flexion.
[b]Average ± standard deviation (SD) movement from 0 to 90 degrees of flexion.
[c]Anterior slide greater than 3.0 mm on any condyle from 0 to 90 degrees of flexion.

Knee Type	Average Rotation (0-90) (Degrees)[a]	Maximum Normal Rotation, Any Increment (Degrees)[b]	Maximum Reverse Rotation, Any Increment (Degrees)[c]
Normal	17.8	31.6	−7.3
ACLD	9.8	21.2	−9.8
PCRF	3.9	21.3	−19.0
PSF	5.0	19.1	−18.1
ACRF	5.6	20.9	−14.1
PCRM	3.9	15.6	−11.4
PCSM	3.3	11.4	−5.9
PSM	4.4	27.1	−14.9
BCSF	10.7	22.5	−4.2
All TKAs	**4.8**	**27.1**	**−19.0**
MED UKA	4.3	17.1	−15.3
LAT UKA	−0.7	13.3	−16.1

TABLE 17.2 Summary of Axial Rotation for 1630 Implanted and Nonimplanted Knees During Deep Knee Bend

ACLD, Anterior cruciate ligament-deficient; *PCRF TKA,* fixed posterior cruciate-retaining total knee arthroplasty (TKA); *PSF,* fixed posterior cruciate-substituting; *ACRF,* fixed anterior cruciate-retaining; *PCRM,* mobile-bearing posterior cruciate-retaining; *PCSM,* mobile-bearing posterior cruciate-sacrificing; *PSM,* mobile-bearing posterior cruciate-substituting; *BCSF,* bicruciate-stabilizing fixed-bearing; *MED UKA,* medial unicondylar knee arthroplasty; *LAT UKA,* lateral unicondylar knee arthroplasty.
[a]Average axial rotation from 0 to 90 degrees of flexion.
[b]Maximum normal rotation at any increment.
[c]Maximum reverse rotation at any increment.

TKA type. For example, subjects with a BCSF TKA experienced an average of 10.7 degrees of axial rotation, whereas subjects with a PCSM TKA experienced only 3.3 degrees of axial rotation. As a whole, the TKA subjects experienced less axial rotation than normal knee subjects (4.8 vs. 17.8 mm, respectively), and there were also greater magnitudes of reverse axial rotation among TKA patients compared with normal patients. Arbitrary of TKA type, the average maximum amount of normal axial rotation is 27.1 degrees, which is below that for normal knees, and the average maximum amount of reverse rotation is −19.0 degrees, which is well above that for normal knees.

The UKA subjects were also largely varied, with the lateral UKA patients averaging reverse axial rotation throughout flexion (−0.7 degrees) and the medial UKA patients averaging only 4.3 degrees of axial rotation.

Condylar Lift-Off

Femoral condylar liftoff in TKA is a concern because, when only one condyle is in contact with the bearing, the contact stresses between the femur and bearing are essentially doubled, thus resulting in large increases in wear on the bearing. Studies have shown that lift-off can occur in multiple types of TKA, on either condyle. These studies have also shown that lift-off can be dependent on surgical technique and is highly influenced by surgical errors, with liftoff frequencies of up to almost 70%.[11,24] Fortunately, with improvements in fluoroscopic analysis methods, surgical methods, and ligament balancing techniques, the frequency and magnitudes of femoral condylar lift-off have been reduced compared with older studies.[3,11,23,31-33] A study by Anderle et al.[3] in 2011 showed that lift-off can happen in patients of all body types, regardless of body mass index (BMI). Of the 284 subjects analyzed in this study, 12.3% of the subjects experienced lift-off. A study by LaCour et al.[23] in 2014 analyzed eight patients with posterior-stabilized rotating platform TKAs

and showed that, at 10 years postoperatively, not a single patient experienced condylar lift-off.

SUMMARY

Because of the highly accurate and minimally invasive nature of fluoroscopy, in vivo fluoroscopic analysis of the knee has become one of the most widely used kinematic analysis techniques in orthopedics today. With the continuing advancements in the technology, such as TFSs, the techniques will continue to improve and result in more accurate and detailed kinematic analyses. To date, fluoroscopy has been used to determine the in vivo kinematics of both normal and implanted knees, as well as other joints (including ankles, hip, and shoulders). This information has been used to help both surgeons and implant companies to develop and improve surgical techniques, surgical instrumentation, and component design, ultimately resulting in improved postoperative outcomes and greater patient satisfaction.

KEY REFERENCES

2. Allen MJ, Hartmann SM, Xacks JM, et al: Technical feasibility and precision of radiostereometric analysis as an outcome measure in canine cemented total hip replacement. *J Orthop Sci* 9:66–75, 2004.
3. Anderle MA, Zingde SM, Komistek RD, et al: Body mass index comparison of knee kinematics for obese, overweight and normal weight TKA subjects. *J Bone Joint Surg Br* 93-B(Suppl IV):S447–S448, 2011.
8. Benoit DL, Ramsey DK, Lamontagne M, et al: Effect of skin movement artifact on knee kinematics during gait and cutting motions measured in vivo. *Gait Posture* 24:152–164, 2006.
11. Daines BK, Dennis DA: Gap Balancing vs. measured resection technique in total knee arthroplasty. *Clin Orthop Surg* 6:1–8, 2014.
13. Dennis DA, Komistek RD, Mahfouz MR, et al: A multicenter analysis of axial femorotibial rotation after total knee arthroplasty. *Clin Orthop Relat Res* 428:180–189, 2004.
14. Dennis DA, Komistek RD, Scuderi GR, et al: Factors affecting flexion after total knee arthroplasty. *Clin Orthop Relat Res* 464:53–60, 2007.
17. Hamel W: Robotic in vivo fluoroscopic arthroplasty evaluations with normal patient movements. *Bone Joint J* 95-B(Suppl 15):S70, 2013.
22. Komistek RD, Kane TR, Mahfouz MR, et al: Knee mechanics: a review of past and present techniques to determine in vivo loads. *J Biomech* 38:215–228, 2005.
23. LaCour MT, Sharma A, Carr CB, et al: Confirmation of long-term in vivo bearing mobility in eight rotating-platform TKAs. *Clin Orthop Relat Res* 472:2766–2773, 2014.
26. Mahfouz MR, Hoff WA, Komistek RD, et al: A robust method for registration of three-dimensional knee implant models to two-dimensional fluoroscopy images. *IEEE Trans Med Imaging* 22:1561–1574, 2003.
27. Mahfouz MR, Hoff WA, Komistek RD, et al: Effect of segmentation errors on 3D-to-2D registration of implant models in x-rays images. *J Biomech* 38:229–239, 2005.
28. Ranawat CS, Komistek RD, Rodriguez JA, et al: In vivo kinematics for fixed and mobile-bearing posterior stabilized knee prostheses. *Clin Orthop Relat Res* 418:184–190, 2004.
31. Victor J, Mueller JKP, Komistek RD, et al: In vivo kinematics after a cruciate substituting total knee TKA. *Clin Orthop Relat Res* 468:807–814, 2010.
32. Wasielewski RC, Galat DD, Komistek RD: An intraoperative pressuremeasuring device used in total knee arthroplasties and its kinematics correlations. *Clin Orthop Relat Res* 427:171–178, 2004.
33. Wasielewski RC, Galat DD, Komistek RD: Correlation of compartment data from an intraoperataive sensing device with postoperative fluoroscopic kinematic results in TKA patients. *J Biomech* 38:333–339, 2005.

The references for this chapter can also be found on www.expertconsult.com.

18

In Vivo Kinematics of the Patellofemoral Joint

Trevor Grieco

The patellofemoral joint is an integral aspect of the knee that enhances flexion and extension. Any disturbance in the joint, such as injury, muscle weakness, and congenital or developmental abnormalities, can greatly affect the overall functionality of the joint and inherently decrease the effectiveness of one's ability to flex and extend the lower leg. Patellofemoral disorders are often difficult to diagnose and may be related to kinematics, kinetics, or soft tissue deficiency. Given its anatomy as a sesamoid bone attached at its superior pole to the quadriceps tendon and at its inferior pole to the patellar ligament, the patella can experience and withstand remarkably high contact and joint reaction forces. These high forces coupled with small overall contact areas result in high stresses and pressures in the joint. One can imagine that such an environment can lead to complications. Patellofemoral pain (PFP) is one of the most common knee problems, and because of vague patient explanations and the large quantity of variables associated with the patellofemoral joint, it is often unclear what the cause of pain is. Beyond common PFP the mechanical nature of this joint lends itself to difficult surgical decisions regarding joint replacement and resurfacing techniques in the case of debilitating arthritis in the knee. Establishing a thorough understanding of the kinematics associated with healthy, pain-ridden, and implanted patellae will shed light on these decisions and provide one with the means to more adequately administer clinical treatment.

PATELLA SIGNIFICANCE AND FUNCTION

The importance of the patella was documented as early as 1789, when John Sheldon explained "muscles extend the leg by pulling up the *Patella*, which plays in the groove between the two condyles of the *Os Femoris*, as a rope in a pulley, and therefore these muscles… act with great mechanical advantage; they not only extend the leg, but assist, likewise in keeping the thigh-bone fixed upon the *Tibia* in the erect posture; in balancing the body; and in straightening the knee-joint."[30] In 1937 the importance of the patella was challenged when Brooke concluded "the patella serves no important function in man" and that the performance of the knee could be improved via patellectomy.[5] Although this was accepted by some at the time, research has proven the removal of the patella impairs the extensor mechanism by decreasing the moment arm. After patellectomy the extensor mechanism moment arm decreases by 14% (Fig. 18.1), and Kaufer demonstrated that the extensor mechanism's power is reduced by at least 15%.[12] Such a reduction in kinetic efficiency may explain why patellectomy patients experience

difficulty extending the knee fully. Therefore preservation of the patella is now recommended whenever possible.[6,18]

Understanding the kinematics of the patella and the factors that drive these can advance biomechanical modeling, joint implant design, and clinical treatment of joint pathology.[27] The motion of the patella is primarily described with respect to its corresponding articulating body, the femur. The articulating portion of the native patella is completely covered by the thickest articular cartilage in the human body (4 to 6 mm at its central portion).[15,26] This cartilage is aneural, which allows the joint to bear high compressive loads, up to 12.9 times body weight ($\times$BW).[26] The elastic nature of the articular cartilage allows the resulting high stresses to be distributed within the cartilage and thus protects the richly innervated subchondral bone by ensuring the pain threshold is not exceeded.[15,26] The cartilage properties coupled with the synovial fluid lubrication of the knee capsule allow the patella to transmit high forces in an essentially frictionless manner.[15] As a sesamoid bone encapsulated within the extensor mechanism, the patella is free to rotate and translate in three dimensions, providing six degrees of freedom. Thus as it travels through the femoral trochlea, it rotates and translates as needed to optimize the effect of the quadriceps and to guide the extensor mechanism, thus preventing dislocation of the extensor apparatus.[26] In addition, the patella acts as an anterior constraint for the femur, effectively preventing subluxation with respect to the tibia.[26]

ANATOMY AND DESIGN FACTORS

Native Patellofemoral Joint

To investigate the kinematics further, it is important to define the anatomy and physiology associated with the joint. Various shapes on the native femur may be associated with patellofemoral kinematics. These include the lateral trochlear inclination (LTI), the sulcus angle, articular cartilage depth (ACD), the sulcus groove length, the trochlear bump, trochlear groove width, and trochlear depth.[10] Aside from the osseous features and constraints, the patella kinematics are dictated by the quadriceps tendon, the medial and lateral retinaculum, and the patellar ligament. Because the quadriceps tendon and patellar ligament effectively connect at the patella, it is sensible to define the relationship between the two anatomic structures in the form of a physical variable. This variable is referred to as the Q angle, which is specifically the angle between the quadriceps' line of pull and the patellar tendon (Fig. 18.2).[10,26] Because anatomically the quadriceps line of action is superolateral, the quadriceps creates a line of pull with an outward directed

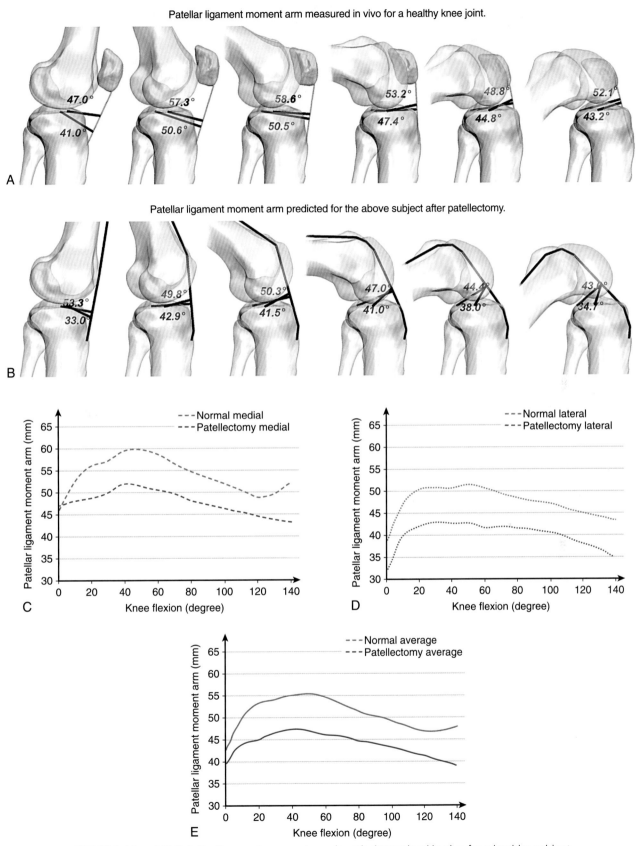

FIG 18.1 (A and B) Patellar ligament moment arm length determined in vivo for a healthy subject and the effects of patellectomy on the moment arm length simulated for the same subject. The reference points at the medial (C) and lateral (D) tibiofemoral contact points were used to determine the average moment arm lengths (E).

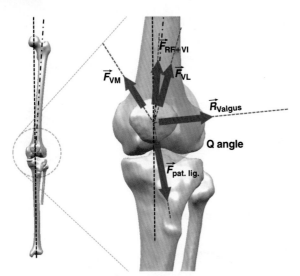

FIG 18.2 Schematic representation of the directions of the muscles of the quadriceps group and Q angle.

horizontal component when contracted (see Fig. 18.2).[15,26] Anatomic factors, including a more anterior projection of the lateral condyle compared with the medial condyle (quantified by the LTI) and more distally reaching fibers of the vastus medialis compared with those of the vastus lateralis, offset the lateral pull of the quadriceps.[29]

Patellofemoral Joint in Total Knee Arthroplasty

Intraoperative Considerations. Malpositioning of total knee arthroplasty (TKA) components is a frequent cause of patellar maltracking, which is traditionally remedied via a lateral retinacular release. Specifically internal rotation of the femur, internal rotation of the tibia, overstuffing (increasing overall thickness of the composite patella) of the patella, and lateralization of the patellar component on the native patella can promote maltracking, which most commonly manifests itself in the form of lateral patellar subluxation. Some have shown that patellar maltracking can occur regardless of component position. Patient variability demands decisions be made based on intraoperative evaluation.[4]

Modifying the joint line during TKA may also affect patellar kinematics because normal knee kinematics require a correct interrelationship between the bony anatomy and the surrounding soft tissue.[2] Elevation of the joint line in revision TKA often occurs because of distal femoral bone loss, undersizing the femoral component, and overstuffing the tibiofemoral gap. Pseudo-patella baja (because of joint line elevation as opposed to a change in the length of the patellar tendon) can lead to patellotibial impingement in deep flexion, a decreased moment arm, a decreased range of motion, increased midflexion instability, and anterior knee pain.[1,14] It has also been reported that increasing the joint line elevation will cause tibiofemoral and patellofemoral contact forces to increase considerably.[14] Overloading of the patellofemoral joint can increase the risk of patellar degeneration and can increase the risk of failure for implanted components.[14] Because of such factors, restoration of the joint line is recommended whenever possible.

Femoral Trochlea Geometry.
Design features of the femoral component that can affect patella kinematics include the pitch, depth, orientation, curvature, and symmetry of the trochlear groove. Specifically, multiple studies have shown that a shallow and symmetrical trochlea groove with abrupt changes in its sagittal radius can lead to abnormal patellar kinematics and increase the risk of maltracking.[24] Therefore femoral trochlear geometry has evolved from a fairly symmetrical design with an almost vertical path to one which exhibits a more prominent lateral inclination and a groove which is aligned proximal-lateral to distal-medial.[32] The orientation of this groove is unlike that of the native knee. The increased lateral inclination is designed to "catch" the laterally tracking patella, thus increasing medial-lateral stability.[32]

Patella Resurfacing. There are currently three basic strategies among clinicians regarding the use of patellar components. These include (1) always resurface, (2) selectively resurface, and (3) never resurface the patella. Arguments for and against patella resurfacing are numerous and detailed, and the subject has become synonymous to topics of religion or politics. Therefore this chapter will simply highlight the kinematic effects of resurfacing techniques as discussed in a comprehensive review of the literature.[24] Supporters of nonresurfacing claim this technique maintains more physiologic patellofemoral kinematics compared with the resurfaced patella, and that it avoids intraoperative errors associated with patellar resurfacing that may lead to maltracking. It is important to note that ideal tracking and performance of the nonresurfaced patella depends on the shape and design of the femoral trochlear, and because most current femoral components are designed to articulate with a corresponding implant geometry, they are ill suited to accommodate the native patella. Therefore it is critical that "patella-friendly" femoral designs are selected in nonresurfacing cases to avoid maltracking and tilt, as well as potential impingement of the retropatellar ridge apex with the intercondylar notch of the femoral component. In a case of significant patellar tilt, displacement of the patella into the notch becomes possible.

Patella implant designs span a spectrum from the symmetrical dome shape to the asymmetrical anatomic based design. All other designs are a hybrid of these. Among these hybrids are the modified dome shape that exhibits a concave surface near the circumference for increased conformity, and the medialized dome shape that exhibits a larger lateral facet to promote more normal-like contact mechanics and patellar tilt patterns. The dome-shape components are more forgiving during implantation because they are less sensitive to rotary alignment and minor malpositioning by lessening edge loading.[25] Anatomic components provide more conforming articulation that ideally increases contact area and decreases subluxation; however, these are more sensitive to malpositioning and require a higher level of precision during implantation.[25] At this point there still remains a lack of consensus as to which implant design is superior.

Mobile Bearing Total Knee Arthroplasties. Another TKA characteristic that has been reported to effect patellofemoral kinematics is the mobile bearing design.[21,23,25] Rees et al. demonstrated that the patella tendon angle to knee flexion angle for a mobile bearing prosthesis exhibited linear behavior similar to the normal knee.[21] The ability of the mobile-bearing insert to self-align with the femoral component may promote centralization of the extensor mechanism, thus preventing the incidence of excessive lateralization of the patella.[34] Such self-correcting

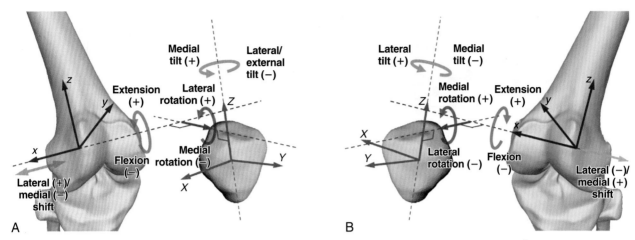

FIG 18.3 Application of the joint coordinate system proposed by Grood and Suntay[9] for the patellofemoral joint of the right (A) and left (B) knees.

features allow for the accommodation of small mismatches in the rotational position of the tibial and femoral components that can happen in fixed-bearing designs. The inability of a fixed-bearing design to correct for said mismatches can result in lateralization of the tibial tubercle, an increase in the Q angle, and an increased lateral force vector on the patella.[34] The absence of this increased lateral force vector in mobile bearing designs may reduce patellar tilt and thus enhance patellar contact mechanics. Yang et al. discussed a strict criteria based on patellar tilt and bicondylar contact of the medial and lateral patella facets through 90 degrees of flexion for determining the need for a retinacular release during TKA. Following this procedure they showed that the need for retinacular release was significantly reduced in mobile bearing designs when compared to fixed bearing designs,[34] thus suggesting that the mobile bearing design features may reduce the occurrence of excessive lateral tilt and effectively improve the contact mechanics of the implanted patella as seen intraoperatively.

PATELLOFEMORAL KINEMATICS, TRACKING, AND CONTACT

Standard Coordinate System

To study and discuss patellofemoral kinematics, it is necessary to define the six degrees of freedom in unambiguous terms. As previously stated, because the patella articulates only with the femur, its motion is described relative to the femur. The patella translates in three directions (anterior-posterior, medial-lateral, and proximal-distal) and rotates in three planes (coronal, sagittal, and transverse). Various coordinate systems have been used in the literature which leads to significant discrepancies in data. Therefore in 2002 the Standardization and Terminology Committee of the International Society of Biomechanics (ISB) recommended using the principles and joint coordinate system defined by Grood and Suntay in 1983[9] as the standard for reporting human joint kinematics. In this three-dimensional, right-handed coordinate system the body fixed coordinate systems of each body and the shared perpendicular between them (also known as the floating axis) are used to describe the rotations and translations. More specifically with respect to the patella, we can say that patella flexion/extension is defined

about the medial-lateral axis of the femur, which passes through the femoral epicondyles, medial/lateral tilt is defined about the proximal-distal axis of the patella, and medial/lateral rotation is defined about the anterior-posterior floating axis. This standard allows rotations to remain consistent with clinical terminologies throughout the range of motion and ensures that the rotations are sequentially independent. This standard is used to describe patellofemoral kinematics throughout this chapter and is illustrated in Fig. 18.3.

Patellar Shift

In the native knee at full extension the patella is positioned above the trochlear groove, because of the superior pull of the tightened quadriceps.[15] In this position the patella may not be in contact with the femur and thus is most susceptible to lateral subluxation or dislocation because of the large Q angle and lack of condylar constraint.[15] The lateral shift at or near full extension during weight-bearing conditions has been shown using real time magnetic resonance imaging (MRI) techniques to be significantly less than that exhibited in non–weight-bearing conditions.[7] This is attributed to the differences in hip alignment, quadriceps activation, and the quadriceps force associated with open-chain isometric contraction (eg, supine leg extension) and closed-chain isometric contractions (eg, squatting).[7] Lateral shift can be even more pronounced in cases of patella alta and can occur not only at full extension but also in the early phases of flexion because the patella has not yet passed into the trochlear groove and remains somewhat unconstrained.[10,29]

Numerous studies have investigated the medial-lateral shift of the native patella using in vitro, in vivo, and intraoperative techniques, with varying results (Fig. 18.4A).* Almost all the studies demonstrate lateral positioning of the patella at full extension. With the exception of the PFP symptomatic case,[33] all of the in vivo data revealed that the patella shifts medially after full extension through about 30 degrees of knee flexion. This is because with increasing knee flexion the tibia rotates internally, thus reducing the Q angle, and the patella moves distally and slightly medially, centralizing itself within the trochlea. The quadriceps are now contracting to help to balance

*See references 1, 8, 13, 17, 20, 27–29, 32, 33.

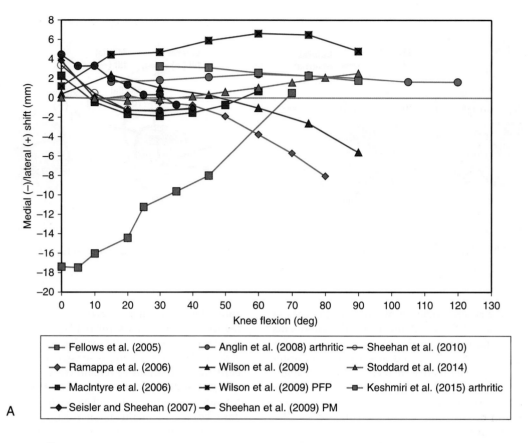

A

Legend for A:
- Fellows et al. (2005)
- Anglin et al. (2008) arthritic
- Sheehan et al. (2010)
- Ramappa et al. (2006)
- Wilson et al. (2009)
- Stoddard et al. (2014)
- MacIntyre et al. (2006)
- Wilson et al. (2009) PFP
- Keshmiri et al. (2015) arthritic
- Seisler and Sheehan (2007)
- Sheehan et al. (2009) PM

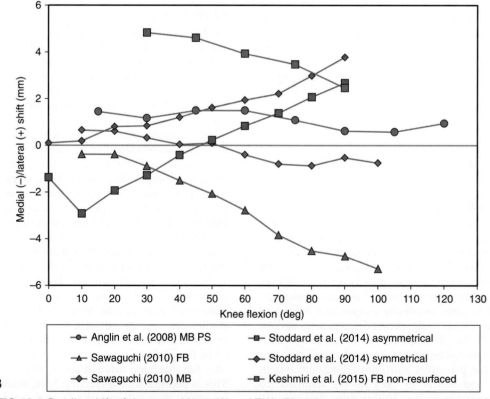

B

Legend for B:
- Anglin et al. (2008) MB PS
- Stoddard et al. (2014) asymmetrical
- Sawaguchi (2010) FB
- Stoddard et al. (2014) symmetrical
- Sawaguchi (2010) MB
- Keshmiri et al. (2015) FB non-resurfaced

FIG 18.4 Patellar shift of the natural knee (A) and TKA (B) reported in the literature measured in vitro *(green)*, in vivo *(red)*, and intraoperatively *(blue)*.

the knee and the extensor mechanism effectively pulls the patella against the femur, successfully establishing contact within the confines of the trochlea. Through the remaining range of motion the patella is effectively guided by the trochlea, thus limiting its overall medial-lateral translation. Wilson et al. and Ramappa et al. showed that the healthy patella continues to shift medially through deeper flexion,[20,33] whereas others have demonstrated that as it moves through the trochlear, the healthy patella has a tendency to move laterally.

PFP syndrome is one of the most common problems in the knee.[10] Although the mechanism of PFP syndrome is considered multifactorial, one of the most commonly accepted causes is lateral malalignment or maltracking.[31] Subjects with PFP have been shown to exhibit lateral hypermobility, and positive J sign.[29] The J sign is a simple observation made as the knee approaches full extension during a non–weight-bearing leg extension. In the case of PFP it has been shown that the patella will suddenly shift laterally and thus exhibits a reverse J-shape track within the trochlear from flexion to extension.[29] Investigations of subjects with PFP have shown that the patella is consistently shifted more laterally compared with healthy subjects.[17,22,28,33]

Overall the intraoperative studies (shown in blue in Fig. 18.4B) show that the TKA patella has a tendency to shift medially with increasing flexion.[1,13,23] Direct comparisons of preoperative with postoperative data revealed at most a difference of 1.6 mm in medial-lateral position from its original position.[1,13] A direct comparison of fixed-bearing vs mobile-bearing TKAs revealed that the fixed-bearing design exhibits larger magnitudes of shift,[23] which may be because of the self-aligning ability of the mobile bearing design previously discussed. Assessment of all the intraoperative data presented in Fig. 18.4B supports this. One in vitro investigation of two different TKA designs showed a consistent lateral shift throughout flexion.[32] The medial-lateral translation of both TKA (asymmetrical and symmetrical trochlear designs) was within 2.5 mm of the natural knee. In line with that which was previously stated, the patella in the asymmetrical trochlea was displaced medially, whereas the patella in the symmetrical trochlea was displaced laterally compared with the position of the intact joint. The differences in the shift patterns throughout knee flexion between the intraoperative and in vitro studies may be attributed to the muscle loading and the state of the tissue, as well as the relatively small sample size associated with the in vitro study.

Patellar Flexion

Patellar flexion increases with increasing knee flexion. This has been consistently shown in both the native knee and in TKA with in vitro, in vivo, and intraoperative techniques.[†] In the native knee the patella flexes at a lower rate than the femur relative to the tibia in a linear fashion (Fig. 18.5A). The regression line fitted to the data in Fig. 18.5A yields the following equation ($r^2 = 0.97$):

$$\text{Patellar Flexion} = -0.68 \times (\text{Tibiofemoral Flexion}) + 1.83 \quad \textbf{(18.1)}$$

The flexion of the patella after TKA also increases with knee flexion (see Fig. 18.5B). It behaves very similarly to the normal knee and can also be described by a linear function. The regression line fitted to the data in Fig. 18.5B yields the following equation ($r^2 = 0.99$):

$$\text{TKA Patellar Flexion} = -0.67 \times (\text{Tibiofemoral Flexion}) - 8.47$$

$$\textbf{(18.2)}$$

Patellar Rotation

Positive patellar rotation is defined as a lateral rotation such that the superior pole (base) of the patella moves laterally and the distal pole (apex) of the patella moves medially. In vitro, in vivo, and intraoperative studies of the normal tracking native patellae show that the patella exhibits a fairly neutral orientation at full extension (Fig. 18.6A).[‡] With increasing flexion the patella exhibits a positive lateral rotation of its base. This makes sense in view of the coupling effect between motion of the tibial tuberosity and the apex of the patella. As the tuberosity moves medially with increasing knee flexion, it is natural for the base of the patella to follow suit. This motion combined with the lateral pull of the quadriceps will result in a lateral rotation of the patella. Using in vivo MRI techniques both Wilson et al. and Sheehan et al. demonstrated that PFP patients and patients diagnosed with patellar maltracking exhibited negative patellar rotation such that the patellar base moved medially with increasing knee flexion.[28,33]

The TKA patella has also been shown to rotate laterally with increasing knee flexion using intraoperative and in vitro techniques (see Fig. 18.6B).[1,13,19,32] Although the overall pattern of patellar rotation throughout flexion in the TKA is similar to that of the native patella, Anglin et al. showed with computer-aided surgery (CAS) techniques that the postoperative implanted patella within a mobile-bearing TKA design, rotated up to 4.6 degrees less than the preoperative patella.[1] In a separate intraoperative study, Keshmiri et al. found no significant change in the postoperative rotation of the nonresurfaced patella implanted within a fixed-bearing TKA system when compared with its preoperative rotation using computer navigation.[13] An in vitro investigation of differences in trochlear geometry showed that the patella implanted in an asymmetrical trochlea was more medially rotated at full extension and throughout flexion compared with the native patella and the implanted patella articulating within a symmetrical trochlear design.[32] Merican et al. also found that the implanted patella was more medially rotated than the natural patella throughout flexion.[19]

Patellar Tilt

The measurement of patellar tilt in the literature varies considerably. Evaluation of in vivo, in vitro, and intraoperative patellar tilt studies since 2004 shows that during the early phase of knee flexion (0 to 30 degrees) the natural patella tilts medially from its initial orientation (Fig. 18.7A).[§] After 30 degrees the native patella has a tendency to tilt laterally through 90 degrees. The overall magnitudes of tilt vary greatly. Stoddard et al., Wilson et al., and Ramappa et al. showed very little patellar tilt (lesser than 5 degrees in magnitude) throughout knee flexion in their studies.[32,20,33] In contrast Fellows et al., Seisler and Sheehan, and Sheehan et al. all showed greater than 10 degrees of medial tilt

---

[†]See references 1, 8, 11, 16, 17, 27, 28, 29, 32, 33.

[‡]See references 1, 8, 13, 17, 19, 20, 27-29, 32, 33.
[§]See references 1, 8, 13, 17, 19, 20, 27-29, 32, 33.

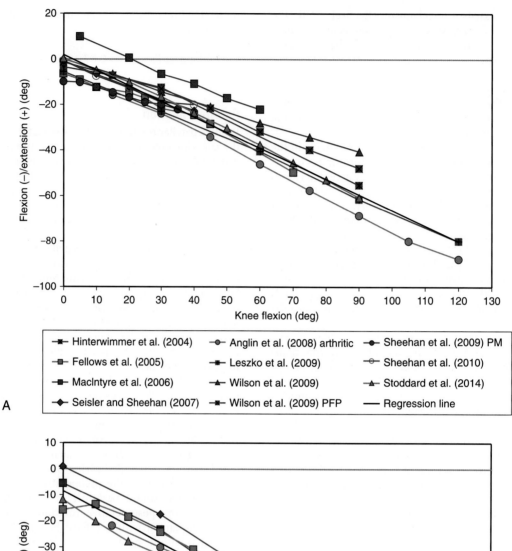

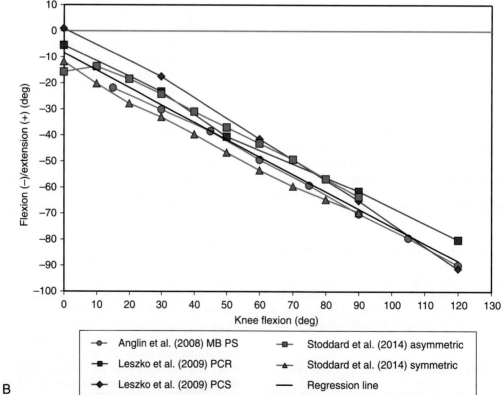

FIG 18.5 Patellar flexion of the natural knee (A) and TKA (B) reported in the literature measured in vitro *(green)*, in vivo *(red)*, and intraoperatively *(blue)*.

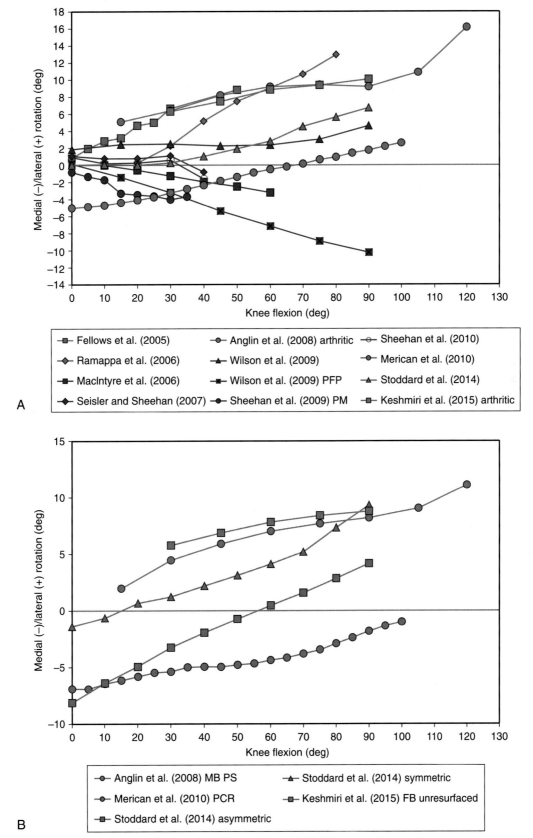

FIG 18.6 Patellar rotation of the natural knee (A) and TKA (B) reported in the literature measured in vitro *(green)*, in vivo *(red)*, and intraoperatively *(blue)*.

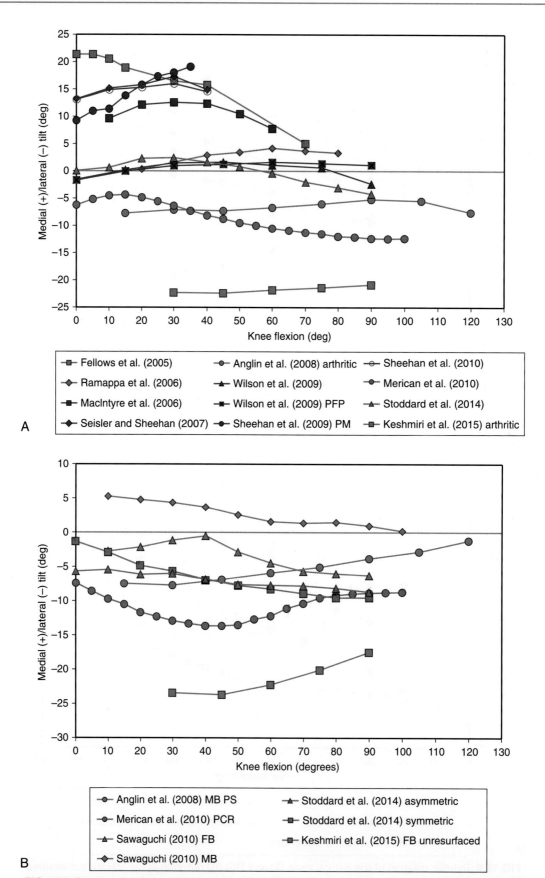

FIG 18.7 Patellar tilt of the natural knee (A) and TKA (B) reported in the literature measured in vitro *(green)*, in vivo *(red)*, and intraoperatively *(blue)*.

at full extension.[27,29,8] Interestingly, both intraoperative-based investigations showed lateral patellar tilt throughout all flexion angles with relatively small changes in tilt orientation. It is also worth pointing out that the maltracking group studied by Sheehan et al. exhibited consistent increasing degrees of medial patellar tilt through 35 degrees of knee flexion.[28]

Review of in vitro and intraoperative TKA patellar tilt data from the literature since 2004 reveals that the TKA patella has a tendency to be laterally titled throughout flexion (see Fig. 18.7B).[1,13,19,23,32] A comparison of preoperative and postoperative TKA by Anglin et al. shows no difference in patellar tilt until late flexion, at which point it appears lateral patellar tilt is reduced as a result of the surgery and mobile-bearing prosthesis.[1] Interestingly Anglin et al. did show that the female patella was significantly more laterally tilted both preoperatively and postoperatively compared with the male patella.[1] In a separate intraoperative study, Sawaguchi et al. effectively showed that the mobile-bearing design may reduce lateral patellar tilt compared with the fixed-bearing design throughout knee flexion.[23] In an in vitro study conducted by Merican et al. the implanted patella exhibited an almost opposite tilt pattern compared with its normal state, such that it first tilted laterally through 30 degrees of knee flexion followed by medial tilt through maximum flexion.[19] Looking at the data presented by Stoddard et al., it can be seen that there is little difference in the patellar tilt pattern because of trochlear design geometry.[32] As expected this study demonstrated that the asymmetrical geometry prevents excessive lateral tilt at full extension compared with the symmetrical geometry.

Patellofemoral Contact

In the healthy knee joint at full extension the patella is positioned superior to the trochlea and is not always in contact with the femoral bone (the green color in Fig. 18.8A and B represents the lower probability of contact occurrence at full extension).[15] It has been observed that the apex of the patella comes in contact with the femur between 10 and 20 degrees of knee flexion[26] and that it settles within the trochlea beyond 30 degrees of knee flexion.[15,26] The location of contact moves distally on the femur and proximally on the patella and contact across the center of the patella occurs between 30 and 60 degrees of knee flexion. After 90 degrees of knee flexion the patella continues to articulate along the femoral condyles, upon which bifurcation of the contact area occurs. Between 20 and 60 degrees of knee flexion the contact area increases linearly from approximately 150 mm^2 up to 480 mm^2 on average.[26] The contact area remains fairly constant up to 90 degrees, and then it decreases linearly to approximately 360 mm^2 at 120 degrees of knee flexion.[26] In an in vivo, weight-bearing MRI investigation, the patella contact area in female and male patients reached over 500 mm^2 and 600 mm^2, respectively.[3]

The contact area in TKA is at best 40% of that exhibited in the normal patella. This is primarily because of the difference in the elasticity of polyethylene used in the TKA patellar components versus that of cartilage in normal knees. Because cartilage is an order of magnitude softer than polyethylene, it more effectively deforms under load, subsequently leading to increased contact area.[25] The implanted patellar component deforms much less and therefore has limited ability to change its surface contact area through variations in patellofemoral load.[25] For TKA knees, the patella (assembled with the patellar button) has been found to always be in contact with the femoral component.[15] Similar to the intact patella, contact on the implanted patella moves proximally as the knee is flexed (see Fig. 18.8D). Contact area on dome-shaped patella components range from 13 mm^2 to 164 mm^2, and the contact area has been reported to reach up to 270 mm^2 in more conforming designs.[25] In contrast to the implanted patella component, the

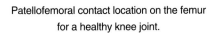

Patellofemoral contact location on the femur for a healthy knee joint.

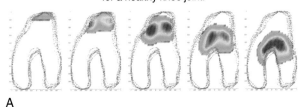

A

Patellofemoral contact location on the patella for a healthy knee joint.

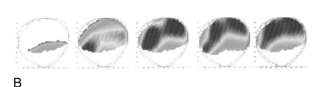

B

Patellofemoral contact location on the femoral component of TKA.

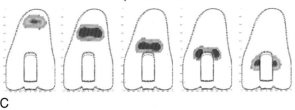

C

Patellofemoral contact location on the patellar component of TKA.

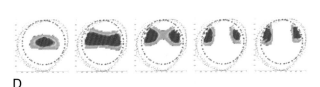

D

FIG 18.8 Normalized distance maps showing most frequent locations of patellofemoral contact for healthy (A and B) and TKA (C and D) knees at full extension and at 30, 60, 90, and 120 degrees. *Red* represents the most probable area of the contact location. *TKA*, Total knee arthroplasty.

nonresurfaced patella has been reported to maintain up to 79% of its original contact area.[24] Because of the differences in modulus of elasticity between the femoral component and the native patella, the articular surface of the patella will adapt to its articulating geometry through biologic remodeling, also described as stress contouring.[24] This natural occurrence combined with the superior deforming capabilities of native cartilage contribute to the increased contact areas of the non-resurfaced patella when compared with those of implanted patella components.

CHAPTER HIGHLIGHTS

- The patella is a critical component of the extensor mechanism. A patellectomy can reduce the length of the moment arm by 14%, and this reduction has been shown to reduce the extensor mechanism's power by at least 15%.
- Patella kinematics are constrained by osseous features that define the shape of the trochlea and are dictated by the surrounding soft tissues, including the quadriceps tendon, the medial and lateral retinaculum, and the patellar tendon. The Q angle is the angle between the quadriceps line of pull and the patellar tendon.
- Malpositioning of TKA components is a frequent cause of patellar maltracking, which is traditionally remedied via a lateral retinacular release.
- Design features of the femoral component that can affect patella kinematics include the pitch, depth, orientation, curvature, and symmetry of the trochlear groove.
- Resurfacing the patella remains a highly debated topic. Patella resurface designs span a spectrum from dome shaped to anatomic shape, and there remains a lack of consensus as to which design is superior.
- The ability of a mobile-bearing insert to self-align with the femoral component may promote centralization of the extensor mechanism, thus preventing the incidence of excessive lateralization of the patella.
- Lateral maltracking is one of the most commonly accepted causes of PFP.
- The patella flexes at approximately 68% the rate of tibiofemoral flexion.
- With increasing knee flexion the patella exhibits a positive lateral rotation of its base.
- The measurement of patellar tilt in the literature varies considerably.
- The contact area of a resurfaced patella is at best 40% of its native joint contact.

KEY REFERENCES

1. Anglin C, Ho KC, Briard JL, et al: In vivo patellar kinematics during total knee arthroplasty. *Comput Aided Surg* 13:377–391, 2008.
10. Harbaugh CM, Wilson NA, Sheehan FT: Correlating femoral shape with patellar kinematics in patients with patellofemoral pain. *J Orthop Res* 28:865–872, 2010.
13. Keshmiri A, Maderbacher G, Baier C, et al: The influence of component alignment on patellar kinematics in total knee arthroplasty: an in vivo study using a navigation system. *Acta Orthop* 86:1–7, 2015.
16. Leszko F, Sharma A, Komistek RD, et al: Comparison of in vivo patellofemoral kinematics for subjects having high-flexion total knee arthroplasty implant with patients having normal knees. *J Arthroplasty* 25:398–404, 2010.
17. MacIntyre N, Hill N, Fellows R, et al: Patellofemoral joint kinematics in individuals with and without patellofemoral pain syndrome. *J Bone Joint Surg Am* 88:2596–2605, 2006.
19. Merican AM, Ghosh KM, Iranpour F, et al: The effect of femoral component rotation on the kinematics of the tibiofemoral and patellofemoral joints after total knee arthroplasty. *Knee Surg Sports Traumatol Arthrosc* 19:1479–1487, 2011.
20. Ramappa AJ, Apreleva M, Harrold FR, et al: The effects of medialization and anteromedialization of the tibial tubercle on patellofemoral mechanics and kinematics. *Am J Sports Med* 34:749–756, 2006.
23. Sawaguchi N, Majima T, Ishigaki T, et al: Mobile-bearing total knee arthroplasty improves patellar tracking and patellofemoral contact stress: in vivo measurements in the same patients. *J Arthroplasty* 25:920–925, 2010.
24. Schindler OS: The controversy of patellar resurfacing in total knee arthroplasty: Ibisne in medio tutissimus? *Knee Surg Sports Traumatol Arthrosc* 20:1227–1244, 2012.
25. Schindler OS, Scott WN: Basic kinematics and biomechanics of the patellofemoral joint. Part 1: the native patella. *Acta Orthop Belg* 77:421–431, 2011.
26. Schindler OS: Basic kinematics and biomechanics of the patellofemoral joint. Part 2: The patella in total knee arthroplasty. *Acta Orthop Belg* 78:11–29, 2012.
27. Seisler AR, Sheehan FT: Normative three-dimensional patellofemoral and tibiofemoral kinematics: a dynamic, in vivo study. *IEEE Trans Biomed Eng* 54:1333–1341, 2007.
29. Sheehan FT, Derasari A, Fine KM, et al: Q-angle and J-sign: indicative of maltracking subgroups in patellofemoral pain. *Clin Orthop* 468:266–275, 2010.
32. Stoddard JE, Deehan DJ, Bull AMJ, et al: No difference in patellar tracking between symmetrical and asymmetrical femoral component designs in TKA. *Knee Surg Sports Traumatol Arthrosc* 22:534–542, 2014.
33. Wilson NA, Press JM, Koh JL, et al: In vivo noninvasive evaluation of abnormal patellar tracking during squatting in patients with patellofemoral pain. *J Bone Joint Surg Am* 91:558–566, 2009.

The references for this chapter can also be found on www.expertconsult.com.

19

Forward Solution Modeling: An In Vivo Theoretical Simulator of the Knee

Brad Meccia

WHAT IS MATHEMATICAL MODELING?

Mathematical modeling pertains to any simulation of a physical system using a computer. In practice, mathematical modeling is an extremely diverse field, which can be applied to any system, ranging from modeling weather patterns to analyzing artificial knees. In this chapter, mathematical modeling focuses on physics simulations of the human knee. Therefore total knee arthroplasty (TKA) mathematical models are used to analyze muscle forces, soft tissue forces, joint reaction forces, implant geometry, and in vivo kinematics to simulate a TKA patient that exists entirely on the computer (in silico). By modifying any one of these parameters, the results of the other parameters can be derived and reviewed.

Therefore mathematical modeling can be used as a powerful design tool to assess or design both existing and future TKA implants. By evaluating various implant designs and analyzing the resulting mechanics, improved designs can be created. Furthermore, those designs can be evaluated with varying soft tissue constraints to determine under which conditions they perform best.

WHY MATHEMATICAL MODELING?

The modern knee implant has a sophisticated design, which in general tries to restore the native kinematics and kinetics. Although current designs experience some success, new generations of TKA are constantly being developed. To develop more successful knee implants, it is necessary to first understand the forces that will be induced at the implant-bearing surfaces. Then the interplay between those forces and the geometry can be considered. These two factors play a major role in the determination of in vivo kinematics and the soft tissue forces.

There are two main ways of determining the loading in a post-TKA knee: telemetry and mathematical modeling. Telemetry produces the most accurate measurements of forces incurred by the TKA, which are directly measured in vivo using sensors placed within the implant. However, developing and manufacturing these implants is prohibitively expensive, so studies typically use small samples sizes of one to three subjects.

In addition to directly measuring the forces through telemetry, these bearing surface and soft tissue forces can also be calculated using mathematical models. Mathematical modeling of the knee incorporates that evaluation of all soft tissue constraints, interactive and independent motions, and muscle forces that are used to drive these motions, leading to the generation of equations of motion to solve for the desired results.

After a mathematical model has been developed and validated, it possesses many benefits that go beyond what telemetry can offer. For example, after a mathematical model has been created, conducting the theoretical analysis is extremely inexpensive. Furthermore, the model can be used to evaluate any number of patients, efficiently, after their input parameters are known. The model also allows for patient modifications to be made, in relatively short time periods that could not be accomplished using any other method. For example, the medial collateral ligament or lateral collateral ligament could be damaged or removed in a mathematical model, which could not be simulated using a living subject. These soft tissue modifications could be simulated using a cadaver, but then the test does not replicate in vivo conditions, leading to concerns that evaluation is being conducted in an altered environment not representing actual muscle forces found during in vivo conditions.

As a design tool, mathematical modeling offers unparalleled flexibility, leading to very powerful parametric analyses. The model can be used to run iterative simulations with only small design changes between each simulation, leading to a pathway design process that documents all changes that were evaluated. Alternatively, one could attempt to manufacture and test many implants modifications, but again this would be very expensive and not simulate the in vivo environment. Mathematical modeling can also provide detailed information about the internal stress on an implant, which can be very difficult to measure. This information can help to eliminate any potential stress shielding or stress concentrators on the implant or bone. Overall, mathematical modeling allows for the opportunity to conduct very efficient experiments that otherwise would be very expensive and impossible to perform in a nontheoretical environment.

BASIC CONCEPTS OF KNEE MODELING

All mathematical modeling of the dynamics of rigid body systems are derived using the principles of Newton's second law.

$$Force = Mass \times Acceleration$$

When modeling the knee, three rigid bodies—the femur, tibia, and patella—are the objects that can accelerate and decelerate within the system. The acceleration of the femur, tibia, and patella represent the right side of the above equation (mass $[M]$ × acceleration $[A]$). Muscles, ligaments, tendons, and joint interactions are the forces within the system that generate or constrain this acceleration. Mathematical modeling is the process of accurately describing all of the forces and bodies within a system.

After the system is accurately modeled, the equations of motion are determined. Equations of motion are a series of differential equations that are more complicated than the simple force $(F) = M \times A$ because they incorporate rotations as well as translations. For example, one acceleration equation within the human body leg system could amount to five pages in length, which is very complicated. Each rigid body can be defined by six equations of motion because it can move in six different ways: three translations and three rotations. By applying known forces and simultaneously solving all of the equations, the resulting accelerations of the rigid body can be computed. When deriving a mathematical model, the reverse approach could be taken in which the accelerations of the bodies are known using an experimental measuring technique, leading to a solution that solves for the muscle and bearing surface forces. Typically these kinematic parameters that induce accelerations are computed using either motion capture systems or fluoroscopic techniques.

Optimization Versus Reduction Techniques

Optimization techniques involve modeling a large number of muscles that affect knee motion using more unknowns than derived equations of motion. As a result there are many potential solutions. For example, the equation $\{X + Y = 0\}$ has an infinite number of solutions because there are two unknowns and only one equation. Optimization methods find the solution that minimizes some other variables, such as peak muscle recruitment. Optimization always results in one mathematically accurate solution out of an infinite number of possible mathematically accurate solutions, but this optimization criteria chooses which solution is most feasible, often leading to a mathematically correct solution but not a physiologically correct one.[3] Indeed most early efforts involving optimization overpredicted joint reaction forces when compared with telemetry.[6,7]

Although use of optimization techniques allows a model to incorporate more unknowns than can be solved for, reduction techniques reduce the number of unknowns so the model has only one possible solution for each unknown variable. This has been successfully accomplished by modeling only the primary muscles that drive the system motion, while assuming the other muscles do not make a significant contribution to the overall motion of the system. For example, a two-dimensional (2D) model of sitting knee extension might model only the quadriceps because it is the primary driver of motion (Fig. 19.1). Such a model would have six degrees of freedom: two translations of each body and one rotation of each body. Of these six degrees of freedom, three could be used to solve for the forces and torques exerted by the table on the femur, two more degrees of freedom would be used to solve for the anterior-posterior and superior-inferior joint reaction forces at the knee. The final degree of freedom would allow for the quadriceps muscle force to be calculated. In practice, three-dimensional (3D) models incorporating the reduction technique are much more complicated than the one just described,

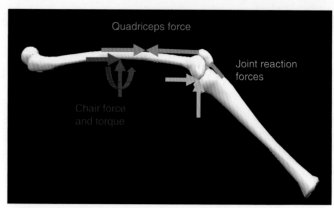

FIG 19.1 A reduced 2D model of knee extension has six degrees of freedom. This allows for the solution of two reaction forces and one reaction torque on the femur, two joint interaction forces, and one muscle force. The patella acts to redirect the quadriceps force but is not included as a separate body.

but this simple model provides a basis for understanding this methodology.

Forward Modeling Versus Inverse Modeling

Another difference in mathematical modeling is forward solution modeling versus inverse solution modeling. With each equation that comes from an equation of motion, it is possible to solve for either a movement (translation or rotation) or a force or torque acting on the body. In inverse models, the accelerations of the bodies are known and the forces and torques are solved. In forward models, forces and torques are known and the motions are then solved.

In practice, inverse models derive a solution for forces within the system, using known motion profiles and input parameters. The patterns of motion are most commonly found using either motion analysis systems or fluoroscopic methodologies. These known patterns of motion are then used as input within either a reduction or an optimization model to determine joint and muscle forces. These types of models are very useful for determining the forces within the systems, particularly the bearing surface forces between implant components.

With forward modeling, muscle forces are used as inputs that drive the motions within the system. These muscle forces commonly, at least initially, are derived using an inverse model. Then the muscle forces are applied to the forward model, and motions are the motions calculated and often compared to known motion patterns for specific patients as a validation. It may seem a bit counterintuitive to compute muscle forces from known motions, then use those muscle forces to recompute motions, but there are valid reasons to do this. For example, in a forward solution knee model including all of the ligamentous structures, it would be possible to see the resulting effect on the motion patterns if ligaments were removed or damaged. This can provide useful information about how ligaments stabilize the system, leading to various motion patterns. Furthermore, these muscle force profiles could be applied to a mathematical model in which different knee implants were virtually implanted in the same theoretical subject. In this way, the resulting motions of different knee implants could be computed. In addition, the known force profiles could then be modified, leading to a different theoretical patient.

Rigid Body Models Versus Finite Element Analysis

In reality, all materials deform under a load. However, the deformation process is very complicated and therefore often ignored when deformations are small. Models that make this assumption are known as rigid body models. When attempting to look at multiple joints involving numerous bones, these models can be ideal because they are much more computationally efficient. However, because these models assume bodies do not deform, they cannot be used to analyze the stress and strain inside of bodies. This means they are useful for determining motions and joint forces but cannot be used to look for stress concentrators in an implant design or for stress shielding inside a bone.

Models that choose to focus on the deformable nature of bodies are typically finite element analysis (FEA) models. These models assume each body can deform and contain the properties of all materials in the model. These models can generate accurate information pertaining to stress and strain within materials. However, they can require a considerable amount of time for setup and execution. For this reason they are normally used in a narrow scope and contain a limited number of bodies. For more information on FEA, see Chapter 22.

Kane's Dynamics and Autolev

Kane's dynamics is a computationally efficient method of generating simpler equations of motion than other available methods.[2] Originally designed to help the National Aeronautics and Space Administration (NASA) analyze spacecraft motion, Kane's dynamics is also applicable for any complex physical system of rigid bodies whose motion needs to be analyzed. This method uses the concept of generalize coordinates, partial velocities, and partial angular velocities to formulate the simpler equations of motions.[1] Instead of solving the $F = M \times A$ equation, Kane's dynamics uses generalized coordinated, partial velocities, and partial angular velocities to formulate a different equation:

$$F_r + F_r^* = 0$$

In this equation F_r represents the generalized active forces on the system which are any external forces, such as gravity, whereas F_r^* represents generalized inertial forces. Generalized inertial forces are internal forces that do no net work, such as joint reaction forces.

Autolev is a powerful software for creating custom rigid body models of physical systems. Its use is not exclusive to biomechanics, and it is also frequently used in aerospace engineering. The power of Autolev comes from its use of Kane's dynamics. This allows models created in Autolev to have many degrees of freedom while being fully inverse or fully forward.

Two notable models have been constructed in Autolev. The first model is an inverse kinematics approach based on discrete element analysis.[8] The model first calculates the contact forces based on a rigid body model. Then these known forces are used to drive a discrete spring network. A discrete spring network represents a body as a highly connected network of springs. The properties of springs are chosen so that the spring network possesses the actual properties of the material being modeled. This allows for the accurate computation of deformation much like an FEA model. However, it is orders of magnitude faster at solving the equations. To validate this model, a single subject was compared to telemetry for four activities: deep knee bend,

chair rise, step down, and step up.[4] For deep knee bend, telemetry found a maximum force of 3.71 × body weight (BW), whereas the model found a max of 3.76 × BW with an Root-mean-square (RMS) error of 0.07 × BW (Fig. 19.2). During chair rise, telemetry computed a maximum force of 2.17 × BW, whereas the model predicted a maximum force of 2.21 × BW with an RMS error of 0.1 × BW (Fig. 19.3). During step down, telemetry computed a maximum force of 3.05 × BW, whereas the model predicted a maximum force of 2.92 × BW (Fig. 19.4). This is an RMS error of 0.06 × BW. Finally, telemetry calculated a maximum force of 3.76 × BW during step up (Fig. 19.5). The model predicted a maximum force of 3.91 × BW and had an RMS error of 0.03 × BW.

A separate error analysis of the model also found very similar contact areas and contact pressures when compared with FEA with maximum differences of less than 10% and less than 15%, respectively.[8] However, the discrete spring network solved in under 4 minutes, whereas the FEA analysis took an average of 3.2 hours. Therefore, this model provides a validated method of computing knee forces efficiently while also providing deformation data that a rigid body model cannot.

The second model was a forward model designed to predict native and implanted knee kinematics based on the geometric constraints of the articulating tibiofemoral and patellofemoral joints.[5] This model functions based on an idealized knee flexion for an activity. This activity can be either leg extension or

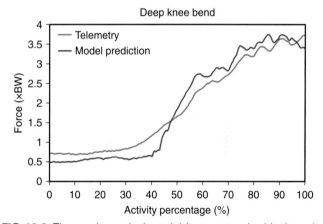

FIG 19.2 The mathematical model is compared with the telemetric results for deep knee bend.

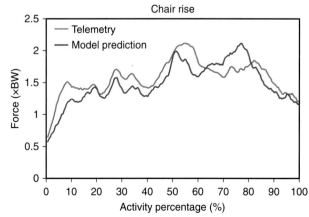

FIG 19.3 The mathematical model is compared with the telemetric results for chair rise.

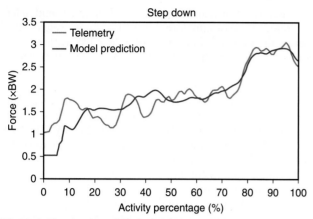

FIG 19.4 The mathematical model is compared with the telemetric results for step down.

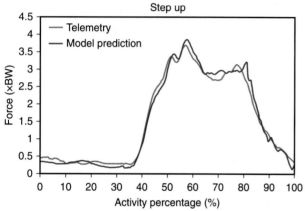

FIG 19.5 The mathematical model is compared with the telemetric results for step up.

weight-bearing deep knee bend. During the simulated activities, the quadriceps forces are adjusted based on the error between the actual knee flexion and the idealized knee flexion, and the knee mechanics are computed based on the equations of motion and the ligament forces are calculated as nonlinear springs. Constraints are based on the patellofemoral contact point on the patella and the tibiofemoral contact point on the femur remaining in contact with the surfaces of the polyethylene and trochlear groove, respectively. The deep knee bend model was validated against telemetry and found peak forces of 3.96 × BW, whereas the instrumented TKA predicted 3.84 × BW. This model is valuable in that it establishes the framework for a geometrically constrained forward solution model of the in vivo knee. These are the requirements for creating a theoretical knee simulator to help in the development of novel TKA designs.

CREATING A THEORETICAL SIMULATOR OF THE KNEE

One of the greatest challenges with mathematical modeling is to accurately predict kinematics of a novel knee implant. If this can be done, a very powerful tool will be given to design engineers who can predict results without the necessity of actually fabricating implants. This will allow many different iterations of designs before the first fabrication is required. A model that

does this would have to fulfill many requirements, which include the following:

1. Must be a forward solution model in nature.
2. Use a controller to determine muscle forces.
3. Constrain the activity fully based on geometry.
4. Analyze multiple implant designs and features.
5. Accurately represents soft tissues.

The first requirement stems from the nature of the model's use as a design tool. When evaluating a novel implant, the motions of the components are not necessarily known (because this is what the design engineers want to compare and improve); thus the only applicable model for this situation is a forward model.

For the second requirement, muscle forces must be predicted in each simulation. If the same force profile were always used, some implants may perform nonideally as a result of inaccurate force profiles and not as a result of a poor design. Because this is a forward model, the equations of motion are being used to predict the translations and rotations. Therefore the muscle forces must be predicted by a controller. The controller adjusts the theoretical muscles forces to try to match the predicted motion to known kinematics, often determined using fluoroscopy.

Next the geometry must be the only driving factor of implant interactions to ensure model predictions are truly based on the implant design and not on model assumptions. For example, abduction/adduction and axial rotation should not be a function of knee flexion as it is in some models. This principle is closely related to the mathematical model being a forward solution system.

In addition, a model should be able to analyze multiple implant types, such as posterior cruciate-retaining (PCR), posterior-stabilized (PS) mobile bearing, and fixed bearing, to allow for an accurate comparison between multiple types. Therefore the boundary conditions must be changed based on the implant type. In addition to these types, a model should be flexible enough to accommodate new designs that have not been thought of yet or are less common, such as a bistabilized TKA or a bicruciate-retaining TKA.

Finally the model must accurately represent the soft tissues present at a joint because soft tissues and implant geometry together drive a simulated activity. In addition, accurate soft tissue representations allow for the TKA to be analyzed under various conditions representing different ligament balancing techniques during surgery.

To this end, the Autolev model designed by Mueller fulfills all of these criteria.[5] However, there is still increased room for improvement. First, the Mueller model makes some simplifying assumptions about geometry. For example, the polyethylene plateaus are represented with only sagittal curvature. Second, the tibiofemoral contact point is assumed to always be the lowest point on the femur in the tibial reference frame (Fig. 19.6). This is true only if the femur rests at the dwell point and becomes increasingly inaccurate as the femur translates away from it. The model has since been improved, and further work is still going on to refine the model.

Part of the ongoing work with this model has focused on analyzing what happens with poorly balanced ligaments. For example, the translations of the medial and lateral condyles of the femoral component on the polyethylene were analyzed for both a PCR TKA with a properly balanced posterior cruciate ligament (PCL) and with an insufficient PCL. The insufficient

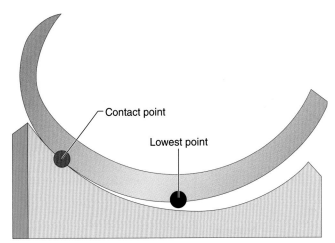

FIG 19.6 Assuming the low point that is in contact is not accurate. As the tibia slides away from the dwell point, contact moves up the curved surface of the polyethylene.

PCL was modeled as applying no force on the femur or tibia. The model computes that the medial condyle will slide an additional 1.5 mm more anterior during a deep knee bend activity and the lateral condyle will slide an additional 1.7 mm more anterior (Fig. 19.7).

In addition, a PS TKA was analyzed when both mechanically aligned and anatomically aligned. For the particular subject analyzed, the anatomically aligned implant had much more normal-like predicted axial rotations. The anatomically aligned implant had 8.9 degrees of axial rotation at full flexion, whereas the mechanically aligned implant had only 2.7 degrees of axial rotation (Fig. 19.8). However, the mechanically aligned implant had much lower predicted maximum tibiofemoral forces of $4.2 \times BW$ versus $5.3 \times BW$ for the anatomically aligned implant (Fig. 19.9).

Another improvement that is not a basic requirement but would improve the performance of the knee model as a theoretical simulator is the parametrization of the articulating geometries in the model. In essence, if the geometry of the implants is defined mathematically instead of simply as a 3D surface, it becomes possible to develop algorithms to incrementally adjust the parameters until an optimal solution is found. One method of doing this is describing the articulating surfaces as polynomials (Fig. 19.10). This allows for the curvature of the surface to be adjusted by changing the coefficients in the polynomial. A model with these features would provide a method of quickly evaluating and optimizing implant designs.

CHAPTER HIGHLIGHTS

- Mathematical modeling of the knee involves representing on a computer the knee joint and all muscles and ligaments that affect it.
- Optimization versus reduction
  - Optimization models represent more muscles than can be solved within the system. Therefore there are an infinite number of feasible mathematical solutions, and a solution is chosen that minimizes a second criteria, such as muscle activations.
  - Reduction methods consider only the major muscles driving an activity so that the system has only one solution. The complexity of the model is "reduced" to make it solvable.

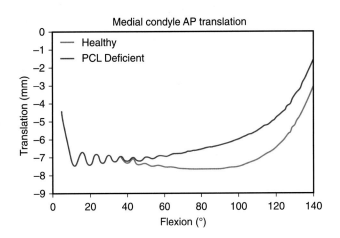

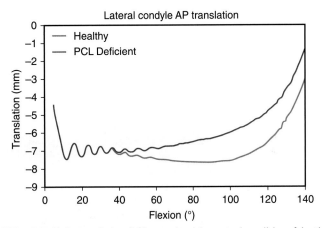

FIG 19.7 Failure of the PCL resulted in anterior slide of both the medial and lateral condyles.

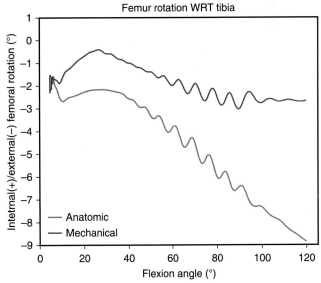

FIG 19.8 The anatomically aligned TKA externally rotated more than the mechanically aligned TKA.

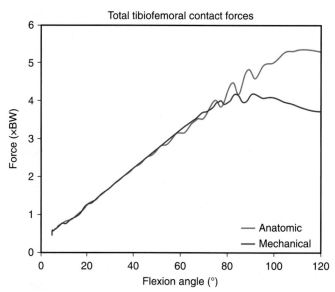

FIG 19.9 The anatomically aligned TKA had maximum tibiofemoral forces of approximately 5.3 × BW, whereas the mechanically aligned TKA had maximum force of approximately 4.2 × BW.

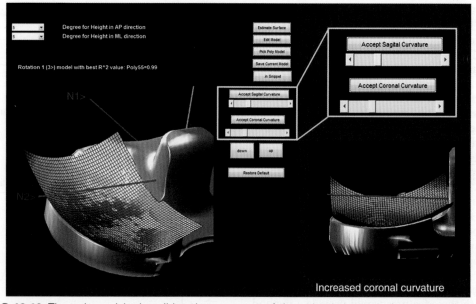

FIG 19.10 The polynomials describing the curvature of the polyethylene can be easily adjusted to generate new designs to evaluate.

- Forward modeling versus inverse modeling
  - Forward modeling uses muscle forces as inputs and computes motions. This approach is ideal for developing a theoretical knee simulator.
  - Inverse modeling uses known motions as inputs and computes forces. The motions are typically derived from motion capture systems or fluoroscopic methods.
- Rigid body models versus finite element analysis
  - Rigid body models assume materials do not deform to allow for faster computation.

- FEA captures the deformable nature of a body. This is computationally expensive, so many models look at a smaller region of interest.
- A forward model could be developed to act as a theoretical simulator of the knee. Such a model needs to use a controller to compute muscle forces while being able to analyze a wide variety of implant types.

The references for this chapter can also be found on www.expertconsult.com.

20

Contact Mechanics of the Human Knee

Adrija Sharma, Richard D. Komistek

Total knee arthroplasty (TKA) has evolved to be a very successful and reliable procedure reducing pain because of osteoarthritis, correcting deformities, and improving disability associated with other pathologic knee conditions.[30] The excellent outcomes of TKA, strong marketing by implant companies worldwide, and better patient education have encouraged surgeons to perform TKA surgeries on younger and culturally diverse patients who have increased activity demands that require increased magnitudes of knee flexion. New designs are being created with better and improved component sizing to improve the fit of the implants on the bones, which is believed to improve performance. It is universally accepted that the closer the implant mimics "normal knee" behavior, the better the patient's function will be.[5]

A TKA procedure inevitably and irreparably alters the complex geometry and soft tissue interactions occurring at the knee joint. To date, most TKA procedures require resection of one or both cruciate ligaments and loosening of the collateral knee ligaments for proper balancing. Moreover, the removed bone and meniscus are replaced with metal and plastic, respectively, whose properties are significantly different. Finally, TKA is always performed on nonnormal pathologic knees. As a result, differences in the contact mechanics observed after TKA compared to the contact mechanics of the normal knee must be expected. Studies of contact mechanics related to nonimplanted and implanted knees can be divided into two broad groups: (1) analysis of the movement of the femorotibial and patellofemoral articulations with flexion (kinematics) and (2) analysis of the forces and stresses acting on the surfaces that are in contact (kinetics). Kinematic analysis provides insight as to how successfully a TKA reproduces normal knee motion and directly affects patient outcomes. Kinetic analysis, on the other hand, is important for gaining a more in-depth understanding of implant longevity.

METHODS FOR STUDYING KNEE CONTACT MECHANICS

In vitro experimental testing protocols incorporating knee simulators, with or without the use of cadavers, are widely used in evaluating kinematics, studying the influence of soft tissues, and analyzing wear and longevity of nonimplanted and implanted knees.[29,38] Use of knee simulators represent a critical step in the design process of new TKAs. However, the standardized protocols that are used fail to simulate the actual operating conditions,[36] in which considerable intersubject variability exists both in terms of kinematics and kinetics, especially for TKA subjects.[27]

Invasive in vivo experimental techniques, including the use of fracture fixation devices, bone pins, minimally invasive halo ring pin attachments, and roentgen stereophotogrammetric analysis (RSA), have been found to provide high accuracy in kinematic measurements. Noninvasive in vivo methods, however, have superseded invasive techniques in popularity because of obvious ethical concerns. Currently, the most popular methods used for in vivo motion analyses are skin markers and medical imaging. Because of substantial relative movement of the skin over underlying osseous structures,[3] skin marker technology applying suitable correction measures, such as *artifact* assessment, the point cluster technique, and optimization using minimization, is used extensively when high-speed multibody movement must be tracked.[1] For slow-speed weight-bearing activities, the use of single-plane and bi-plane fluoroscopy[12,15,23,28] or open and closed magnetic resonance imaging (MRI) modalities,[11,13,14,19] coupled with two-dimensional to three-dimensional image registration techniques, have become the gold standards because of the low number of errors associated with these processes.

In vivo force measurements using telemetric knee implants have been reported and have provided invaluable insights into the kinetics of the implanted knee.[8,9,41] Because of the high costs involved in its development, telemetry still has not been used on a mass scale. Moreover, this technology is not feasible for studying normal knee joint forces. Therefore, computational modeling has always been a necessity for studying the contact forces occurring at the knee joint.[20] Because the lower limb is connected by many muscles, modeling the knee is inherently indeterminate in nature with more unknowns than equations. Therefore, reduction methods and optimization methods are used to obtain a solution.[27] In the optimization technique, the number of unknowns is greater than the number of equations that can be generated for the solution. Consequently, the process deals with the solution generated by the minimization of a suitably chosen objective function. However, there is still no consensus as to which objective function is physiologically most suitable. With optimization, you might possibly achieve a mathematically correct solution, but it may not be physiologically correct. The reduction technique, on the other hand, uses simplifying assumptions to reduce the complexity of the system. In this case the system remains determinate—that is, the number of unknowns is always made equal to the number of equations that can be generated to solve them. This method, therefore, generates a faster solution when compared with optimization, but only a certain number of unknown variables can be determined.

More recently, computed tomography (CT) and MRI-based techniques have been used to study contact areas and pressures in the normal knee.[4,25,38] Contact stress and strain variations are extensively studied using computational techniques. The use of linear and nonlinear finite element analysis with biofidelic models segmented out of CT and MRI scans has been the most popular method for studying behavior in the normal knee and in TKAs.[10,18] Because TKA components have regular geometry and the contact variation is elliptical in nature, faster contact algorithms using hertz contact, elastic foundation models, modified elastic foundation models, and explicit finite element analysis have also been used.[15,17,31] Computational methods have also tried to create virtual wear simulators using adaptive finite elements[21] and elastic foundation models coupled with a damage algorithm.[16]

NORMAL KNEE MOTION

The kinematics of the normal knee is complex. The tibiofemoral articulation has six degrees of freedom,[5] but only three of these motions are more dominant in the knee—flexion-extension, internal-external rotation, and anterior-posterior translation. Abduction-adduction, medial-lateral translation, and superior-inferior translation might occur, but are minimal in magnitude compared to the other three motions. At full extension to very early stages of flexion (<10 degrees), the femur is internally rotated with respect to the tibia.[12,14] In weight-bearing deep knee bend and squatting exercises, with the increase in flexion, the femur starts to roll with slip on the tibia in the posterior direction (posterior femoral rollback) and the femur externally rotates with respect to the tibia (Fig. 20.1).[19,24,28] The external rotation of the femur with respect to the tibia with increasing flexion occurs as the lateral condyle moves more posteriorly than the medial condyle. The highest rates of axial rotation have been found to occur from full extension to 30 degrees of flexion.[11,33] At this flexion range, the medial contact point translates posteriorly, mainly because of the change in the shape of the medial condyle.[32] Above 30 degrees of flexion, the knee enters the active functional arc and the axis of rotation crosses the centers of the almost circular posterior articular

surfaces of both femoral condyles. Because the medial collateral ligament is shorter and tighter than the lateral collateral ligament, in this phase, the medial contact point is relatively immobile and moves slightly in both the anterior and posterior direction, allowing the lateral condyle to move considerably posterior relative to the medial condyle. Consequently, the longitudinal rotation of the femur occurs at about an axis passing closer to the medial condyle. At very high ranges of flexion (>140 degrees), thigh-shank contact sets in and influences the tibia to move anteriorly with respect to the femur. This causes both femoral condyles to move considerably posterior with respect to the tibia, and the lateral femoral condyle can reach the posterior edge of the tibial plateau (see Fig. 20.1).[39,40]

Axial rotation of the femur with respect to the tibia is a critical factor in patellofemoral mechanics, allowing the patella to track along the anatomic trochlear groove of the femur.[26] In the normal knee, the patella always maintains contact with the femur.[22,38] From full extension to 90 degrees of flexion, there is a single region of contact between the femur and patella. However, at flexion angles greater than 90 degrees, the contact areas divide into two separate regions with medial tilting of the patella and contacts with the odd facet at approximately 135 degrees of flexion. The most dominant motion in the patella is its flexion in the sagittal plane, which increases with the flexion of the femorotibial joint. This motion causes the patellofemoral contact locations to travel superiorly with respect to the patella.[13,35]

NORMAL KNEE FORCES

During a weight-bearing deep knee bend, normal knee flexion is mainly driven by the extensor mechanism, primarily by the moment generated by the quadriceps muscles. The variation of the quadriceps force with knee flexion is characterized by three distinct regions: (1) 0 to 90 degrees of flexion, in which the force generally increases; (2) 90 to 120 degrees of flexion, in which the force reaches a peak; and (3) beyond 120 degrees, when the force starts to decrease.[35] Because the femorotibial and

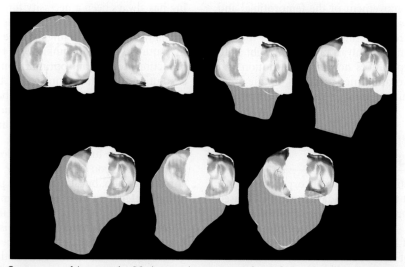

FIG 20.1 Sequence of images in 30-degree increments from full extension to maximum knee flexion (top: 0 to 90 degrees; bottom: 120 to 174 degrees) highlighting the contact kinematics of a sample normal knee subject. Regions in red are closer to the femoral condyles than regions in blue. The blue points indicate the location of the contact points.

patellofemoral contact forces are highly correlated with the force in the quadriceps, a similar variation in their patterns with respect to knee flexion is also observed. The moments generated by the quadriceps muscles are a function of the moment arm (perpendicular distance from the rotational center of the femoral condyles to the line of action of forces), cross multiplied by the force generated in the muscle.[6] So, for the same total moment, an increase in the moment arm is reflected by a decrease in the force, and vice versa. The moment arm of the quadriceps muscle depends on the location of the femoral condyles and the angle of the quadriceps with respect to the tibia. As flexion increases, there is a decrease in the angle of the quadriceps with respect to the tibial plateau, causing the moment arm to decrease (Fig. 20.2). However, with increasing flexion, the femorotibial condyles also move posteriorly, tending to increase the moment arm (Fig. 20.3). Thus, the two effects can offset each other, causing the force to increase from 0 to 90 degrees. In the flexion range of 90 to 120 degrees, the quadriceps muscle wraps around the femur and therefore its angle, with respect to the tibial plateau, remains relatively constant. As a result, the moment arm is always increased because of the posterior movement of the femoral condyles causing the forces in the quadriceps and the femorotibial contact forces to decrease (see Fig. 20.3). At very high flexion angles, the onset of thigh-calf contact reduces knee contact forces considerably.[40]

COMPARISON OF TOTAL KNEE ARTHROPLASTY AND NORMAL KNEE MOTION AND FORCES

Although flexion greater than 160 degrees has been reported for normal knees,[39] most modern high-flexion TKAs are designed for a maximum flexion of about 155 degrees[2] because they are always used in nonnormal pathologic knees, in which the maximum flexion observed in normal knees is generally not expected. Various clinical and design factors have been seen to affect postoperative flexion, but the consistent amount of maximum knee flexion reported for any modern TKA is within the range of 90 to 120 degrees. Even in the common flexion ranges, the in vivo kinematics of TKAs is different than in normal knees.[37] Some of the differences include the following:
1. Incidence of reduced posterior translation or paradoxical anterior slide of the femoral lateral condyle with respect to the tibia.

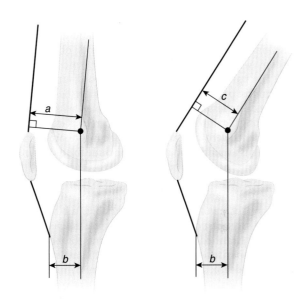

FIG 20.2 As the knee flexes from full extension, for the same location of the femoral condyles (distance *b*), the moment arm of the quadriceps moment arm decreases (length *c* < length *a*).

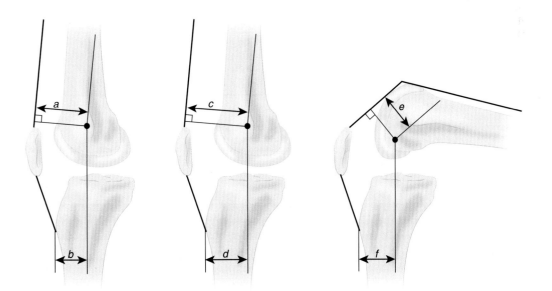

FIG 20.3 Left and middle: For the same flexion angle, as the femoral condyles move posteriorly (length *d* > length *b*), the quadriceps moment arm increases (length *c* > length *a*). Right: Beyond 90 degrees of flexion, the quadriceps wrap around the femur. The relative angle between the femur and the quadriceps does not change with flexion once wrapping starts. Under this condition, the quadriceps moment arm (length *e*) is influenced only by the location of the femoral condyles (length *f*).

2. Posterior translation of the femoral medial condyle comparable in magnitude to the translation of the lateral condyle leading to low axial rotation.

3. Reverse axial rotation patterns, in which the femur rotates internally relative to the tibial component with increase in flexion.

4. Incidence of condylar lift-off, in which one of the condyles separates and loses contact.

5. Incidence of patellar separation (patella losing contact with the femur), patellar dislocation, and abnormal patellar tracking.

An analysis was conducted to study the difference in the contact kinematics in TKA patients who do and do not achieve high flexion.[34] The kinematics of 250 patients, obtained using fluoroscopy while performing a deep knee bend activity, was studied. The patients were divided into two distinct nonoverlapping groups: patients with maximum weight-bearing flexion of 95 degrees or less (Group 1) and patients with maximum weight-bearing flexion of 110 to 130 degrees (Group 2). The selected patients were implanted with the most common types of TKA designs available today, which include fixed-bearing and mobile-bearing posterior stabilized (PS) knees and fixed-bearing, posterior cruciate–retaining (PCR) knees with symmetrical condyles and asymmetrical condyles. To restrict the variability and effect of confounding variables, a blocked stratified random sampling design was used where the percentage of patients in a stratified group was the same for both groups. Statistical comparisons were performed at full extension and at 30, 60, and 90 degrees of flexion, which were common to both groups. The analysis revealed that in the high-flexion group (Group 2), the anteroposterior (AP) positions of the medial and lateral femoral condyles with respect to the femur were always significantly more posterior than in the group that exhibited lower flexion (Table 20.1). The amount of AP translation, axial orientation, and amount of axial rotation of the femoral component with respect to the tibia were not found to be different across the two groups (Table 20.2).

A second analysis was conducted to compare the femorotibial contact forces in 50 patients from Group 1, 50 patients from Group 2, and 30 subjects having normal knees. The validated computational model as described by Sharma et al.[35] was used. Normal knee flexion up to 130 degrees was studied to remove any effects of thigh-calf contact, which the model does not take into account. Although there was considerable overlap between the two groups, the patients from Group 2 tended to exhibit a lower total femorotibial contact force than those from Group 1 at the common flexion ranges (Fig. 20.4). The variability of the axial femorotibial contact forces was found to be significantly higher in the TKAs than in the normal knees (Fig. 20.5). Some TKA patients experienced maximum forces comparable to those of the normal knee, but at higher flexion angles the magnitude of the contact forces for the normal knees was significantly lower than observed in the TKA patients. The average maximum axial contact forces observed was around 3.0 body weight (BW) for TKA patients who could flex their knees beyond 110 degrees and around 2.4 BW for normal knee subjects. The medial side experienced higher contact forces compared to the lateral side. The contact forces in the AP direction

TABLE 20.1 Means and Standard Deviations of Lateral and Medial Anteroposterior Femoral Condylar Locations and Axial Orientation[a]

Flexion (Degrees)	LAP (mm)			MAP (mm)			ORT (DEGREES)		
	Group 1	Group 2	p-Value	Group 1	Group 2	p-Value	Group 1	Group 2	p-Value
0	−4.2 ± 2.9	−5.4 ± 3.3	0.0009[b]	−4.0 ± 3.1	−4.9 ± 3.5	0.002[b]	0.2 ± 4.3	0.8 ± 6.1	0.4247
30	−5.8 ± 2.8	−7.0 ± 3.0	0.0004[b]	−4.8 ± 2.8	−5.7 ± 3.6	0.0018[b]	0.9 ± 5.1	1.7 ± 6.2	0.2548
60	−5.6 ± 3.1	−6.7 ± 2.9	0.0026[b]	−3.4 ± 3.2	−4.2 ± 3.7	0.0036[b]	2.6 ± 5.0	3.4 ± 5.9	0.2969
90	−6.0 ± 3.2	−7.4 ± 2.7	0.001[b]	−2.9 ± 2.8	−3.7 ± 3.3	0.0026[b]	3.8 ± 5.9	4.7 ± 6.3	0.2609

[a]From full extension to 90 degrees flexion across the two groups.
[b]Indicates that the means are statistically different ($p < 0.05$) across the two groups.
LAP, Lateral anteroposterior femoral condylar locations; MAP, medial anteroposterior femoral condylar locations; ORT, axial orientation.
Locations—anterior, positive; posterior, negative; Orientations—external, positive; internal, negative.
Modified from Sharma A, Dennis DA, Zingde SM, et al: Femoral condylar contact points start and remain posterior in high flexing patients. J Arthroplasty 29:945–949, 2014.

TABLE 20.2 Means and Standard Deviations of Lateral and Medial Anteroposterior Femoral Condylar Translations and Axial Rotation[a]

Flexion (Degrees)	LTRANS (mm)			MTRANS (mm)			AXROT (DEGREES)		
	Group 1	Group 2	p-Value	Group 1	Group 2	p-Value	Group 1	Group 2	p-Value
0-30	−1.6 ± 2.4	−1.6 ± 2.5	0.5137	−0.8 ± 2.2	−0.8 ± 2.4	0.5074	0.7 ± 3.3	1.0 ± 3.2	0.2404
30-60	0.2 ± 2.3	0.4 ± 2.2	0.2892	1.4 ± 2.6	1.5 ± 2.8	0.4240	1.7 ± 3.2	1.6 ± 3.5	0.5866
60-90	−0.3 ± 2.2	−0.8 ± 2.4	0.3236	0.2 ± 2.4	0.5 ± 2.7	0.3417	0.7 ± 3.0	1.4 ± 3.2	0.2343
0-90	−1.7 ± 3.5	−2.0 ± 3.2	0.4389	1.2 ± 2.4	1.1 ± 3.2	0.5649	3.6 ± 4.5	4.0 ± 5.0	0.2775

[a]From full extension to 90 degrees flexion across the two groups. No statistical differences were observed between the two groups.
AXROT, Axial rotation; LTRANS, lateral anteroposterior femoral condylar translations; MTRANS, medial anteroposterior femoral condylar translations.
Rotations—external, positive; internal, negative; Translations—anterior, positive; posterior, negative.
Modified from Sharma A, Dennis DA, Zingde SM, et al: Femoral condylar contact points start and remain posterior in high flexing patients. J Arthroplasty 29:945–949, 2014.

were significantly lower in the normal subjects than in the TKA subjects at any flexion angle (Fig. 20.6). The locations of the femoral condyles were found to be highly correlated with the contact forces (correlation coefficient = 0.86). At high flexion angles, the normal knee condyles remained more posterior when compared with the TKA subjects and, as a result, experienced smaller force magnitudes.

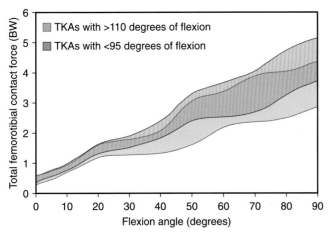

FIG 20.4 Range of maximum and minimum forces observed at the common range of flexion (0 to 90 degrees) in the two TKA groups. The TKA patients who achieved greater than 110 degrees of flexion tended to have lower magnitudes of femorotibial contact forces than the TKA patients who achieved a maximum flexion less than 95 degrees.

COMPARISON OF TOTAL KNEE ARTHROPLASTY CONTACT KINETICS

In the normal knee, stability is provided by the ligaments and joint capsule. For a TKA, however, laxity and stability are balanced by the ligaments that remain and the conformity between the femoral and tibial inserts. The bearing surfaces used in TKA designs do not replicate the normal knee surfaces anatomically, which represents a trade-off between the ability to accommodate normal kinematics and yet have sufficient conformity to reduce stresses, enhancing longevity. There are many knee implants on the market today that have shown excellent long-term results. In this section, we compare the kinetic performance of six different implants to have a general idea of the in vivo contact areas and stresses experienced by TKAs. There are three PS designs: (1) the Sigma Fixed Bearing PS (Sigma FB PS; DePuySynthes, Warsaw, IN), (2) the Sigma Rotating Platform PS (Sigma RP PS; DePuySynthes, Warsaw, IN), and (3) the Legacy PS Fixed Bearing (Legacy PS; Zimmer, Warsaw, IN) designs. The remaining three designs are of PCR type and all are manufactured by Zimmer Inc.: (1) the Nexgen PCR Fixed Bearing (Nexgen PCR), (2) the NKII Congruent PCR Fixed Bearing (NKII Congruent PCR), and (3) the NKII UltraCongruent PCR Fixed Bearing (NKII UltraCongruent PCR) designs. Comparisons were carried out for a weight-bearing deep knee bend activity. While all the PS designs have symmetrical condyles, all the PCR designs have asymmetrical condyles to facilitate femoral rollback. The Nexgen PCR has a slightly larger lateral condyle compared to its medial condyle. The NKII series has bigger medial condyles compared to their lateral condyles. The NKII UltraCongruent has a more conforming polyethylene

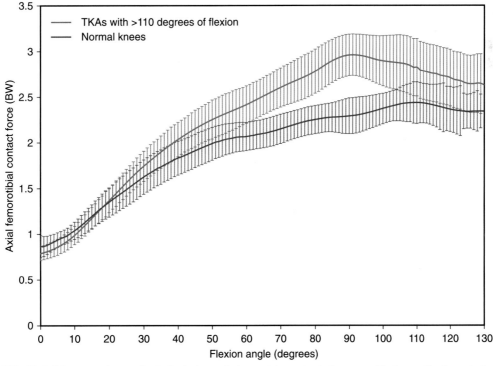

FIG 20.5 Mean and standard deviation of the axial contact forces with knee flexion at the common flexion range (0 to 130 degrees). The normal knee subjects experienced smaller magnitudes and smaller variability in the femorotibial contact forces when compared with the TKA patients, especially as flexion angles increased.

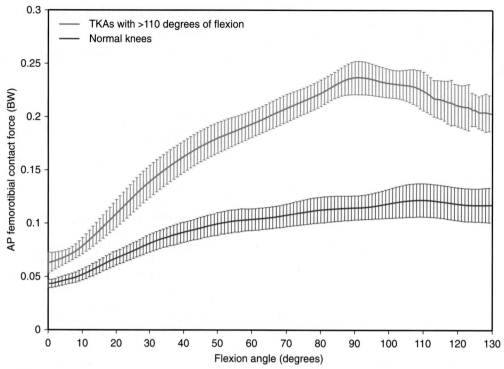

FIG 20.6 Mean and standard deviation of the AP contact forces with knee flexion at the common flexion range (0 to 130 degrees). The normal knee subjects experienced significantly lower forces throughout the flexion cycle compared to the TKA patients.

design compared to the NKII Congruent design. All designs incorporate a femoral component with multiple radii (radius decreasing with increasing flexion) in the sagittal plane. In the Sigma RP PS design, the polyethylene insert can rotate axially with respect to the tibial component and has a much more conforming and constrained femoropolyethylene articulating surface in the coronal plane compared with the Sigma FB PS design.

Because all these implants incorporate similar materials, the contact areas and contact stresses are mainly influenced by three factors: (1) the radii of the femoral condyles and the polyethylene bearing mating surfaces, (2) the relative position and orientation of the femoral component on the polyethylene bearing, and (3) the contact forces acting on the respective condyles, which influence the amount of deformation of the surfaces. The femorotibial contact forces were in a similar range for all implants. The Sigma RP PS design was able to maintain higher contact areas on both the medial and lateral condyles when compared with the Sigma FB PS design (Fig. 20.7). This is probably a result of the more conforming femoropolyethylene articulating geometry coupled with the capability of the polyethylene to rotate, which ensures that more of the femoral surface always stays in contact. For the Sigma FB PS and the Sigma RP PS designs, the contact areas had a tendency to decrease with flexion. This behavior was much more distinct for the lateral condyle. For the medial condyle, however, this area-decreasing behavior is probably compensated by increased deformation caused by an increase in the force acting on the medial side with the increase in flexion. The other TKAs did not exhibit this trend, however, probably because of differing femoral J-curve

radii in these designs. Only the NKII Congruent PCR design showed a significant increase in the contact areas with increasing knee flexion. The average contact stresses on both condyles increased with an increase in flexion (Fig. 20.8). The medial contact stresses were found to be higher than the lateral contact stresses, consistent with the observation that retrieved TKA implants exhibit more medial wear.[7] Although the contact stresses in the TKAs are significantly larger than the contact stresses reported for normal cartilage, it is encouraging to note that the TKAs are able to maintain contact sufficient to keep the average contact stresses below the yield strength of polyethylene, which is around 20 MPa to 25 MPa.[17]

CONCLUSION

Posterior movement of the femoral condyles causes a decrease in the force generated by the quadriceps. This translates to lower femorotibial contact forces and lesser constraint to movement, which could thereby affect the amount of knee flexion achieved. The contact forces in normal knees and TKAs are significantly different at higher flexion ranges, so designing TKAs in which the femoral condyles always remain posterior and move posteriorly with flexion (lateral condyle more posterior compared to the medial condyle to increase axial rotation) might be a key ingredient in successful future TKA designs. Conformity in the femoropolyethylene articulation seems to help implant longevity by reducing contact stresses and thereby wear. However, suitable care must be taken to provide sufficient laxity in the design to avoid increasing the forces acting on the design, which would then adversely affect the contact stresses that it experiences.

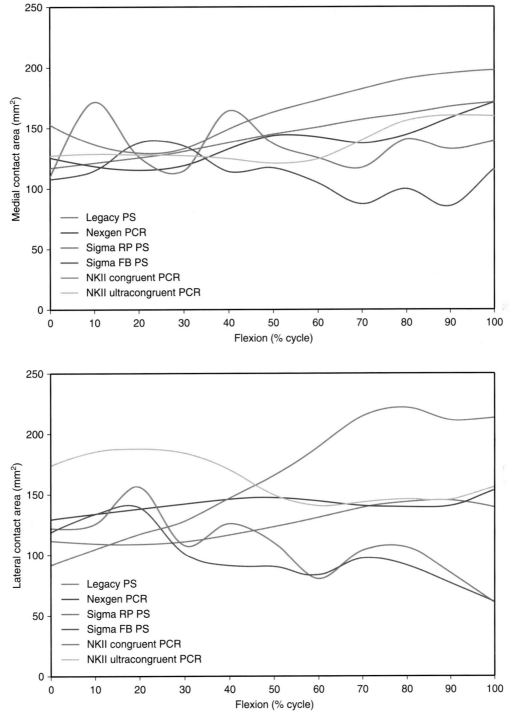

FIG 20.7 Average medial and lateral contact areas experienced in the TKA designs. The contact areas can exhibit a high amount of variability with flexion as it is a function of the design, orientation of the geometries, and contact forces. *PCR*, Posterior cruciate–retaining; *PS*, posterior stabilized.

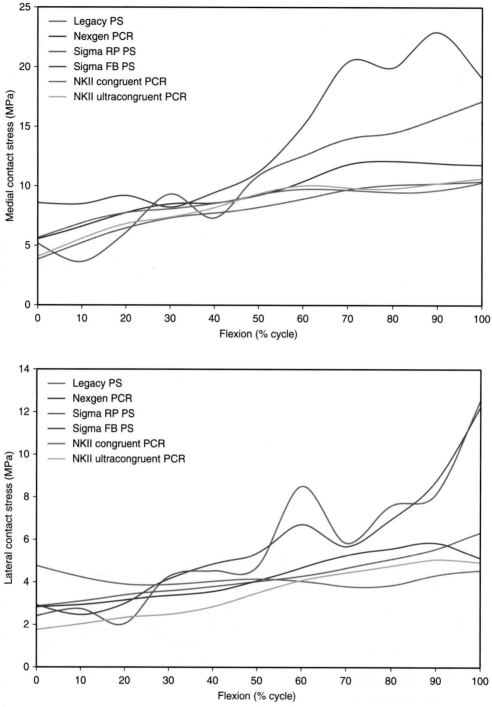

FIG 20.8 Average medial and lateral contact stresses experienced in the TKA designs. Contact stresses increase with flexion and the medial side experience larger magnitudes compared to the lateral side.

KEY REFERENCES

1. Andriacchi TP, Dyrby CO, Johnson TS: The use of functional analysis in evaluating knee kinematics. *Clin Orthop Relat Res* 410:44–53, 2003.
2. Argenson JN, Scuderi GR, Komistek RD, et al: In vivo kinematic evaluation and design considerations related to high flexion in total knee arthroplasty. *J Biomech* 38:277–284, 2005.
5. Blaha JD, Wojtys E: Motion and stability of the normal knee. In Scott WN, editor: *Insall & Scott surgery of the knee* (vol 1), ed 4, New York, 2005, Churchill Livingstone, pp 227–239.

6. Browne C, Hermida JC, Bergula A, et al: Patellofemoral forces after total knee arthroplasty: effect of extensor moment arm. *Knee* 12:81–88, 2005.
8. D'Lima DD, Patil S, Steklov N, et al: Tibial forces measured in vivo after total knee arthroplasty. *J Arthroplasty* 21:255–262, 2006.
11. DeFrate LE, Sun H, Gill TJ, et al: In vivo tibiofemoral contact analysis using three-dimensional MRI-based knee models. *J Biomech* 37:1499–1504, 2004.
17. Halloran JP, Easley SK, Petrella AJ, et al: Comparison of deformable and elastic foundation finite element simulations for predicting knee replacement mechanics. *J Biomech Eng* 127:813–818, 2005.

20. Komistek RD, Kane TR, Mahfouz M, et al: Knee mechanics: a review of past and present techniques to determine in vivo loads. *J Biomech* 38:215–228, 2005.

21. Laz PJ, Pal S, Halloran JP, et al: Probabilistic finite element prediction of knee wear simulator mechanics. *J Biomech* 39:2303–2310, 2006.

22. Leszko F, Sharma A, Komistek RD, et al: Comparison of in vivo patellofemoral kinematics for subjects having high-flexion total knee arthroplasty implant with patients having normal knees. *J Arthroplasty* 25:398–404, 2010.

29. McEwen HM, Barnett PI, Bell CJ, et al: The influence of design, materials and kinematics on the in vitro wear of total knee replacements. *J Biomech* 38:357–365, 2005.

35. Sharma A, Leszko F, Komistek RD, et al: In vivo patellofemoral forces in high flexion total knee arthroplasty. *J Biomech* 41:642–648, 2008.

34. Sharma A, Dennis DA, Zingde SM, et al: Femoral condylar contact points start and remain posterior in high flexing patients. *J Arthroplasty* 29:945–949, 2014.

38. Walker PS, Haider H: Characterizing the motion of total knee replacements in laboratory tests. *Clin Orthop Relat Res* 410:54–68, 2003.

40. Zelle J, Barink M, De Waal Malefijt M, et al: Thigh-calf contact: does it affect the loading of the knee in the high-flexion range? *J Biomech* 42:587–593, 2009.

The references for this chapter can also be found on www.expertconsult.com.

21

In Vivo Mechanics and Vibration of the Knee Joint

Ian M. Zeller

Knee joint injuries are among the most prevalent musculoskeletal problems, and there are a number of potential reasons for these injuries. In younger adults, sports tend to be a major cause of injury, whereas arthritic degeneration, such as rheumatoid arthritis and osteoarthritis, tend to affect older adults. Traumatic injuries acquired as young adults tend to exacerbate degenerative injuries later in life. To restore function and quality of life, many patients elect to undergo a total knee arthroplasty (TKA). There are currently more than 150 TKA designs on the market using principles developed by physicians and engineers to simulate the geometry and function of a healthy knee joint.[7] All of these designs collectively tend to have four main differences, which are (1) condyle geometry, (2) bearing mobility, (3) ligament preservation versus substitution, and (4) fixation technique.[35]

Evaluating these various designs in human subjects is inherently difficult because all measurements must be noninvasive to limit interference with joint function. Because cadaver tests fail to adequately simulate in vivo joint conditions,[23] researchers are constantly striving to develop novel methods for indirectly measuring joint mechanics in vivo. These methods have been used to evaluate the normal knee and justify design protocols of TKAs.

X-rays, computed tomography (CT), and magnetic resonance imaging (MRI) are common imaging techniques for discerning joint condition; however, they typically detect gross injuries and are unable to identify early-stage pathology. Arthroscopy overcomes the insufficiencies of the imaging modalities mentioned earlier, yet the procedure itself is semi-invasive. For this reason, there is a need for the development of a noninvasive evaluation technique with the ability to diagnose joint conditions in the early-stage onset of disease. One such promising technology involves the analysis of vibration signals from the knee joint during activities of daily living. Further developments of this technology may one day provide physicians with the information to expand treatment options prior to a TKA and eventually phase out the procedure altogether. Therefore while discussing knee joint mechanics, a discussion of these innovative assessment techniques becomes imperative. The aim of this chapter is to provide the reader with background related to knee joint kinematics and kinetics, along with an investigation into the use of vibrational signals as a diagnostic tool.

KNEE KINEMATICS: MOBILE OR FIXED, RETAINING OR SACRIFICING, AND PERSONALIZED OR PATIENT MATCHED?

Kinematics is the study of the pure motions and can be used to describe and understand the movements of the knee. There are several techniques that have been used to determine both in vivo and in vitro kinematics for normal and implanted knees. These invasive methods include cortical pins and roentgen stereophotogrammetric analysis. Noninvasive methods include skin marker analysis[1] and fluoroscopy-based model reconstruction. This section will focus on kinematics from fluoroscopic evaluation because it is both accurate and noninvasive.

In vivo fluoroscopic studies of the normal knee have shown that knee kinematic patterns are primarily determined by the condylar geometry of the articulating surfaces and the surgical accuracy of aligning these components. In addition, those studies have revealed what is referred to as the screw-home mechanism, in which the lateral condyles experience substantially more posterior motion than the medial condyle throughout flexion.[8]

Engineers and surgeons collaborate in an effort to develop TKA systems that reproduce more normal-like kinematic knee function. Fluoroscopic studies have documented that many implant designs demonstrate kinematics that are less predictable and less reproducible following a TKA procedure. Numerous kinematic variances from normal knee kinematic patterns have been demonstrated, including paradoxical anterior femoral translation during deep knee flexion, reverse axial rotational patterns, and femoral condylar liftoff.[12]

Anterior femoral translation during deep knee flexion occurs when the femoral component slides anteriorly during deep flexion rather than rolling posteriorly. One of the consequences is the anteriorization of the flexion axis, leading to posterior impingement of the components and/or soft tissue and a reduction in the quadriceps moment arm, resulting in reduced quadriceps efficiency. In addition, anterior sliding of the femoral component on the tibial polyethylene surface risks accelerated polyethylene wear. Some TKAs have shown the tendency to produce axial rotation opposite of the normal knee. This rotation risks patellofemoral instability by lateralizing the tibial tubercle and increasing the Q angle during deep flexion. Because of reduced posterior femoral rollback (PFR) of the lateral femoral condyle, maximum knee flexion is also reduced.[11]

Despite these limitations, TKAs have provided good midterm to long-term survivability; however, the question on which type of implant configuration provides the best postsurgical outcome is still a cause for debate. Bearing mobility is one such area of contention. The mobile-bearing implant was designed to reduce contact stress (thereby reducing wear) and to recreate more normal-like knee kinematics. Although in vitro studies have shown reduced wear with the use of a mobile-bearing implant,[17,18] in vivo metrics (such as kinematics, clinical outcomes, and survivability between fixed- and mobile-bearing implants) have produced similar results. A study conducted by

Post et al.[32] did not find any basis to justify one design over the other. Clinical success and long-term survivorship were found to be mainly dependent on component placement accuracy, and Post et al. concluded that the best result is achieved when the surgeon is comfortable with a design and can implant that design consistently. Studies have compared the performance of the mobile and fixed configurations in the same patient and concluded that the patient does not demonstrate any difference in terms of range of motion, knee scores, and survivorship.[3,22,33,35] Pagnano et al.[29] conducted a study on 240 rotating-platform TKAs, finding that patellar tracking was not improved. A multicenter study conducted by Wasielewski et al.[43] on 527 mobile-bearing TKAs found that 12% of the knees exhibit more than 10 degrees of axial rotation during a deep knee bend (DKB) activity and almost half the knees analyzed experienced less than 3 degrees of axial rotation. Rotational parameters were also found to be comparable with results reported for fixed-bearing TKAs by Dennis et al.[11] LaCour et al., in a 10-year follow-up study, documented that overall rotation of the mobile bearing component remained with the femoral component throughout flexion and this finding is retained long term.[24]

Retaining or substituting the posterior cruciate ligament is another area of importance in TKA design. Numerous studies have shown that certain cruciate-retaining (CR) total knee designs exhibit paradoxical femoral sliding instead of posterior femoral rollback, which decreases clinical weight-bearing flexion.[8] This paradoxical anterior sliding is not seen in posterior-stabilized (PS) TKAs. A study comparing PS TKAs with CR TKAs with asymmetrical condyles found that the CR designs exhibit lesser medial PFR; both designs achieve similar amounts of lateral PFR. Proponents of the CR design suggest that the PFR seen in PS TKAs originates from the guided motion when by the cam-post engages; this leads to higher rates of implant failure because of cam-post wear. Bourne and Baré[6] in their discussion of failure of the cam-post mechanism found

substantial differences among cam-post mechanisms between implant types; they suggested that the cam-post mechanism does not always engage as designed. They also concluded that the cam-post mechanism may result in increased wear; however, this analysis was limited to implants with varus-valgus constraints.

In a study performed to estimate cam-post engagement during a DKB activity for 10 knees with a fixed-bearing bicruciate-stabilizing (BCS) design and 9 knees with a high-flexion mobile-bearing PS design. In vivo, weight-bearing knee kinematics are reported for the participants while they perform a DKB activity under fluoroscopic surveillance. The three-dimensional kinematics are recreated from the fluoroscopic images using a previously published three-dimensional to two-dimensional registration technique.[26] Four metal beads are embedded into the polyethylene insert prior to the replacement surgery to determine the polyethylene insert location and orientation for the mobile-bearing design. Images from full extension to maximum flexion are analyzed at 10-degree intervals, thus recreating the three dimensional kinematics, leading to a better understanding of the cam-post mechanism. The distance between the interacting surfaces is monitored throughout flexion, and the predicted contact map is calculated. The mechanism is considered engaged when the minimum distance between the cam and post surfaces becomes zero.

This method has also been used to compare the cam-post mechanics for BCS and fixed bearing PS TKA designs. It is important to note that the BCS TKA design has both an anterior cam-post mechanism, which remains engaged at full extension and disengages in early flexion, as well as a posterior cam-post mechanism that disengages in full extension and engages deeper in flexion. This analysis focuses exclusively on the posterior cam-post mechanism. With respect to the BCS design, the cam-post engagement varied among patients, with the average flexion for engagement being 34.0 degrees (Fig. 21.1) and a

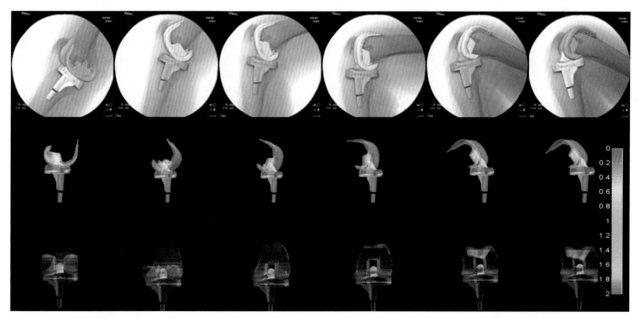

FIG 21.1 A three-dimensional to two-dimensional registration technique was used to determine three-dimensional knee kinematics for the bicruciate-retaining fixed-bearing TKA *(top)*. The cam-post interaction is monitored in the sagittal plane *(middle)*, and the distance map is displayed on the tibial post *(bottom)*.

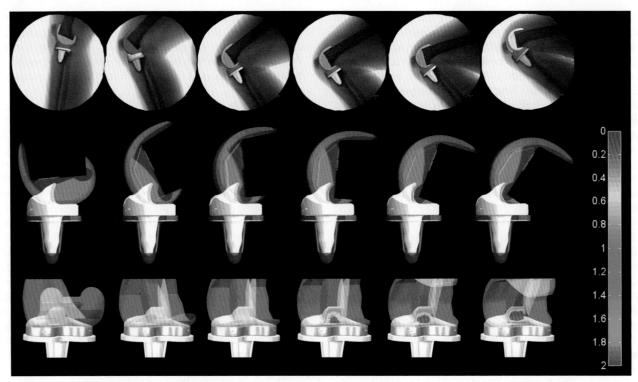

FIG 21.2 A three-dimensional to two-dimensional registration technique was used to determine three-dimensional knee kinematics for the mobile-bearing PS TKA *(top)*. The cam-post interaction is monitored in the sagittal plane *(middle)*, and the distance map is displayed on the tibial post *(bottom)*.

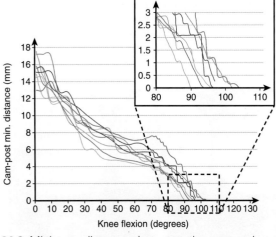

FIG 21.3 Minimum distances between the cam and post for mobile-bearing subjects were calculated during DKB activity.

highly variable range of 15 to 68 degrees of flexion. The typical contact pattern for most subjects shows initial contact with the tibial post medially, with the contact location moving centrally and superiorly with increasing knee flexion. For the mobile-bearing PS design the cam-post interaction is found to be very consistent among subjects (Fig. 21.2), and the stabilizing cam-post mechanism engages in deeper flexion (between 90 and 105 degrees). After the two components engage, they remain in contact until maximum flexion is achieved (Fig. 21.3). Unlike the fixed-bearing BCS design, the contact between the cam and post for the mobile-bearing PS design is located centrally on the

post at all times when engaged. This behavior is believed to be because of the mobility of the polyethylene insert, which rotates axially in accord with the rotating femur. Because the posterior surface of the mobile-bearing post remains parallel to the surface of the femoral cam, contact stresses on the polyethylene tibial post are more evenly distributed. Decreasing contact forces can increase the longevity of the implant. Such loading conditions are more difficult to replicate for a fixed-bearing TKA, in which external rotation of the femoral component may cause the cam-post mechanism to engage more medially. This increases the edge loading on the polyethylene, as was seen with the BCS design. Because the mobile insert ensures that the cam and post are parallel to each other, contact between them occurs centrally, hence reducing the chances of asymmetrical loading conditions, as seen in the fixed-bearing design. The results from this study are in accordance with the findings of Bourne and Baré[6] cited earlier and also suggest that mobile-bearing PS designs may have an advantage when compared with their fixed-bearing counterparts in terms of long-term survivability.

In addition to bearing mobility and ligament retention, advances in imaging and manufacturing technology have led to commercially available personalized TKA designs. Most TKA designs have a wide array of sizes and variants that are chosen to best match the patient. Personalized TKAs replicate a patient's individual femoral and tibial geometric features, and the design rationale is that doing so will allow for a better reconstruction of the mechanical axis and ultimately lead to more normal kinematics. Studies are currently under way to evaluate the mechanics of the personalized TKA, and early results are promising with respect to the ability to replicate kinematics similar to the normal knee.[31]

KNEE KINETICS: WHAT HAVE WE FOUND?

There are three important results that can arise from the determination of vivo forces and torques: (1) the performance of new designs can be predicted, (2) surgical procedures can be simulated to better predict and optimize clinical outcomes based upon varying surgical parameters, and (3) loading mechanisms contributing to degenerative joint disease can be investigated, with modifications or interventions to reduce these pathological effects.[22] The in vivo force studies related to the knee joint are divided into two broad categories: telemetry and mathematical modeling.

Telemetry

Because of its ability to report very accurate, real-time measurement of resultant forces in six degrees of freedom, telemetry has gained wide-scale credibility and approval in the research community.[41] The first reported case of measuring tibiofemoral forces via an instrumented implant in a TKA patient was in 2006 by D'Lima et al.[13] In this study, comprising three patients, each patient was implanted with a custom-made telemetric implant (Zimmer, Warsaw, Indiana). Forces at the tibiofemoral interface were assessed during lunge and chair-rise activities. All three patients experienced higher forces during the lunge activity, which ranged from 1.7 to 2.77 times body weight (BW), with the peak force occurring between 27% and 82% of the cycle. For chair rising and sitting, all patients revealed two peaks in net force. One peak (average, 1.83 times BW) was found at the early part of chair rising (between 11% and 20% of the cycle), whereas another peak (average, 1.61 times BW) was found at a late part of the cycle (78% to 83%). Patient-specific force distribution on both condyles was almost equal for the lunge activity, with both condyles experiencing almost equal forces. For the chair-rising activity, it was seen that the lateral condyle experienced higher force ratios (from 61.7% to 74.2% of total force) when compared with the medial condyle. Another study conducted by the same authors[14] assessed tibiofemoral forces for the same patient group while performing several activities of daily living, such as walking, bicycling, and exercising on an elliptical trainer. They found that during level walking, the knee experiences forces from 1.8 to 2.5 times BW. These forces are similar to those experienced by subjects walking comfortably on a treadmill. During the bicycling activity, the forces peaked at 1.03 times BW. Patients experienced higher forces while exercising on the elliptical trainer, with the mean peak tibial force being 2.24 times BW.

Mathematical Modeling

One of the primary restrictions with the use of telemetry is that implantation of the device is not feasible across different TKA designs that are commercially available. Data reported in studies thus far have been limited to very small patient groups, and expanding to larger patient populations will take substantial resources and time. Telemetry is also limited in that it is only effective at determining forces for knees with implanted devices. For these reasons, mathematical modeling techniques have been developed as an alternative theoretical methodology to calculate knee joint forces. There are two main strategies for mathematical modeling techniques: (1) the use of optimization techniques to solve an indeterminate muscle force system[39] and (2) the use of a reduction method that minimizes the number of muscle force unknowns to keep the system solvable. The premise for the reduction technique is that the number of equations of motion must be equivalent to the number of unknown quantities.[22,35,36]

Lundberg et al.[25] has developed a parametric model to determine tibiofemoral contact forces for TKA patients during level walking. The peak force reported was 3.3 times BW, with a maximum range of ±0.5 times BW (at 67% stance) for normal forces and a maximum range of ±0.82 times BW (at 76% of stance) for resultant forces. These results were very similar to published data pertaining to optimization techniques determining knee joint forces. Although the mediolateral force distribution was also found to correlate with that of other studies,[2,20,21,37] calculated forces were higher when compared with those reported for a similar activity using telemetry.

Komistek et al.[23] applied the reduction technique and used a fluoroscopy-driven inverse model based on Kane's method of dynamics. They reported that the maximum force acting between the femur and tibia for a healthy female subject having a normal knee is 1.7 to 2.3 times BW, depending mainly on walking speed. Using a similar approach, Sharma et al.[36] assessed tibiofemoral forces for subject with either a PS or CR high-flexion TKA while performing DKBs. They found that forces for each type of implant increase with increasing flexion and the medial condyle force was always higher than the lateral condyle force. To check for the amount of error, the model was also compared with data obtained from a fixed-bearing telemetric implant. The results showed that for the telemetric implant, the maximum force on the medial side was 1.9 times BW experienced at 90 degrees of flexion and 2.2 times BW at 105 degrees for the lateral side. The model predicted 1.89 times BW (at 89 degrees) and 2.05 times BW (at 101 degrees) for the medial and lateral condyles, respectively. Another study[35] by the same group analyzed five patients with a fixed-bearing TKA and five patients with a mobile-bearing TKA during the DKB activity finding that tibiofemoral force for both types of implants is similar in nature and magnitude. As in the previous study, they found that the force distribution is uneven between the medial and lateral condyles, with the medial condyle always having higher forces than the lateral condyle. The average medial tibiofemoral force varied from 0.5 times BW at full extension to 2.72 times BW at full flexion for the mobile-bearing subjects, whereas for the fixed-bearing subjects the medial force varied between 1.04 times BW at full extension to 2.73 times BW at full flexion. On the lateral condyle the medial force varied from 0.34 to 0.91 times BW for mobile-bearing subjects and from 0.43 to 0.92 times BW for fixed-bearing subjects. These results are consistent with reported data from telemetric devices under similar conditions.

KNEE VIBRATION DATA: THE FUTURE OF DIAGNOSIS?

One promising noninvasive method to provide information regarding the joint condition for use in early diagnosis is through the analysis of knee sound signals during ambulation. The first suggestion of knee joint sound as a viable diagnostic tool was reported by Heuter in 1885.[19] Seventeen years later, Blodgett[5] reported on auscultation of the knee with particular attention to sounds of apparently normal joints, the change in sounds with repetitive motion, and reproducibility over several days. He found that there was an age-related increase of sound and the relative absence of sound when an effusion was present.

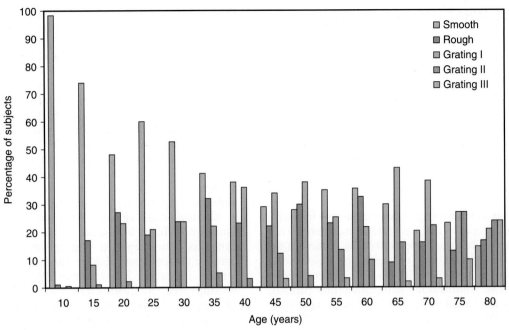

FIG 21.4 In 1929 Walters examined 1600 knee joints and found a steadily ascending ratio of all forms of audibility with increasing age. The vertical axis represents the percentage of subjects with rough grating noise levels (I, II, or III). (From Walters C: The value of joint auscultation. *Lancet* 1:920–921, 1929.)

Bircher[4] in 1913 reported that each type of meniscal injury emitted a distinctive sound signal. In 1929 the idea that knee sound was related to age was expanded (Fig. 21.4), and it was hypothesized that these sounds related to joint condition.[42]

Using a cardiophone, Steindler[38] recorded joint angles, and for the first time filtering was used to remove noise and improve the quality of the sound signal. He classified the joints based on pitch, amplitude, and sequence of the sounds, which in many cases were correlated with pathology demonstrated by operative findings. In 1953 Peylan[31] reported on a study of 214 patients with several types of arthritis, using regular and electronic stethoscopes. Although ultimately unsuccessful, this was the first attempt to distinguish between different types of arthritis. In 1961 Fischer and Johnson[16] first showed that sound signals could be heard in rheumatoid arthritis prior to visible radiographic changes. A good understanding of the nature of the knee joint signals, their diagnostic potentials, and the problems encountered in practice was later published by Mollan et al.[27,28] They were the first to use accelerometers instead of microphones or cardiophones to analyze the knee, and it was shown that this reduces skin movement artifact and ambient noise reduction.

The analysis of the sound signals collected by researchers has been very much dependent on advances in technology. In early studies sounds could only be heard and were analyzed qualitatively. Advances in signal processing have allowed for statistical analysis of the signal parameters, substantially increasing the power of the signal analysis. Such techniques as the short-time Fourier transforms and wavelet transform have become very effective means of evaluating components of signals. The advantage of using the wavelet transform is that it enables signals to be locally characterized in both time and frequency domains simultaneously. This enables the use of kinematic patterns to be used as aids in classification among the various groups and may also be a confirmation tool of which signal patterns based on certain pathologies can be validated. Along with pattern classification techniques, wavelet transforms have become the norm for determining the pathologic significance of knee sounds.

To eliminate the subjectivity in the diagnosis process, many pattern recognition techniques have been used to automate the diagnostic process. Fundamentally pattern recognition methods all work similarly. Feature vectors, which often consist of statistical parameters such as mean, deviation, and quantile, are first extracted from the original signal data. Supervised methods can then be used to compare those extracted features to datasets with known results, and using statistics the likelihood of a particular outcome can be determined. This is a common principle for determinant functions and neural network algorithms, which retroactively analyze performance to "learn" and better predict outcomes from data. Alternatively, unsupervised methods, such as clustering, can also be used to classify patterns using natural partitions of similar features.[15] In 2006 Umapathy and Krishnan[40] presented a technique using wavelet packet decomposition and a modified local determinant-based algorithm to analyze the vibration signals and identify the highly discriminatory basis functions for classifying results. Other techniques reported in the literature include pattern classification of features, such as acoustic power, analysis of the mean power, and median frequency.[9,10] Use of the matching pursuit time-frequency distribution method and least squares (autoregressive, all-pole, or linear prediction) modeling methods are also techniques that have been fairly successful.[34]

These pattern recognition techniques have accuracies from 85% to 91% when diagnosing knee condition as "normal" or "arthritic." To be useful as a reliable diagnostic technique, the first challenge that is faced is to increase this accuracy. Although most studies have concentrated on determining the onset of cartilage degeneration in a healthy knee, to be an effective diagnostic technique comparable to radiography and MRI, the level of disease determination has to be found in other areas. These would include isolation of vibrating frequencies for various soft tissue damage conditions, such as ligament ruptures, meniscal injuries, and maltracking of the patella. Apart from the determination of these diseases, early detection is just as important. Unless these challenges are met, the use of knee joint vibroarthrography signals will not be as effective of a diagnostic tool as existing imaging and arthroscopic methods.

An initial study was conducted on 76 normal, degenerative, and implanted knees to investigate whether it is possible to determine some of these conditions. The objective of this study was to assess and determine if differences could be detected between normal and degenerative knee joints based exclusively on vibration data. Patients with normal knees and well-functioning TKAs were analyzed under in vivo conditions using video fluoroscopy and vibration sensors while performing normal daily activities. The data capture setup consisted of video cameras, triaxial accelerometers, signal conditioner, data acquisition system, force plate, and synchronization trigger (Fig. 21.5).

Two triaxial accelerometers were attached to the lateral and medial epicondyles of the femur while two additional accelerometers were each attached to the patella and tibia tuberosity, respectively. Using a two-dimensional to three-dimensional registration technique, three-dimensional joint kinematics were obtained. For the vibration data, several statistical parameters were used to create feature vectors for pattern classification. Signals were also converted to audible sound and correlated with three-dimensional kinematics. There was a noticeable difference in the sound signals between the healthy, arthritic, well-functioning TKA and failed TKA (Fig. 21.6). Subjects who did not undergo fluoroscopic surveillance (degenerative [arthritic] knees and failed TKAs) were asked to complete a detailed questionnaire that was completed by the surgeon at the intrasurgery evaluation (primary or revision), which schematically distinguished the area and level of damage to the tibiofemoral interface (Fig. 21.7). Frequency analysis demonstrated that specific frequencies were in a similar range for all groups, but the magnitudes and variations were different for TKA and nonimplanted knees. Successful determination was possible between normal knees with and without articular cartilage damage, up to an accuracy level of 86%. This finding is very similar to results from Rangayan and Wu.[34] It was seen that in cases in which the surgeon had reported unicompartmental damage to the tibiofemoral interface, the signals obtained from the two accelerometers were quite dissimilar (Fig. 21.8), allowing for the potential for locating joint damage. The possibility of correlating conditions in the knee, such as condylar liftoff, cam-post engagement, and ligament damage, are currently under investigation. These results suggest that it may be possible to use vibration signals to determine various knee joint conditions; however, it will take the research community many years before such a technique will be competitive with currently used radiation and arthroscopy techniques.

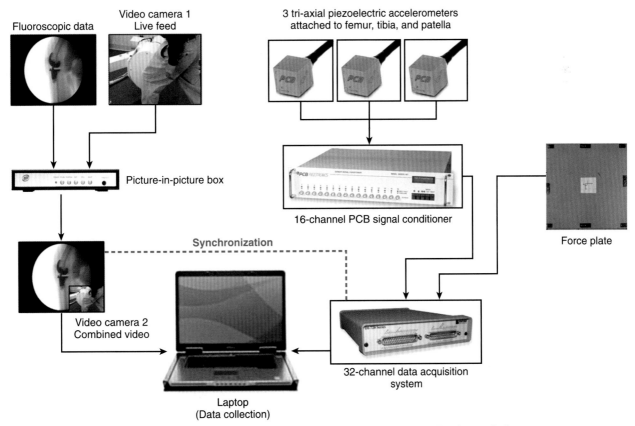

FIG 21.5 Schematic diagram for the vibroarthrography data collection technique.

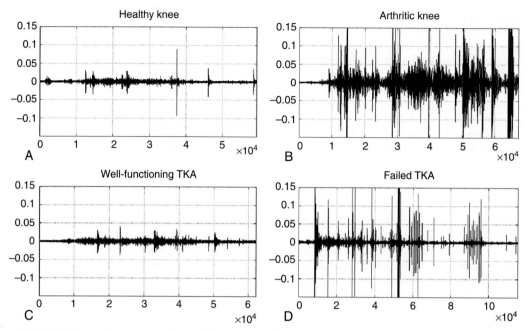

FIG 21.6 Vibroarthrograms reflect differences in vibrations between healthy (A) and arthritic (B) knees, as well as between well-functioning (C) and failed (D) TKAs.

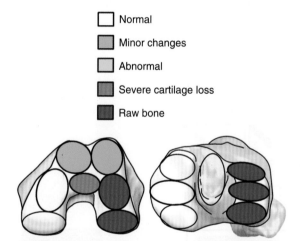

FIG 21.7 Intrasurgery evaluation sheet for sample patient, distinguishing the area and level of damage to the tibiofemoral interface.

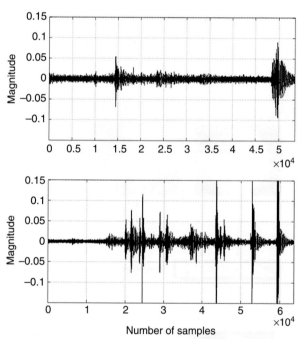

FIG 21.8 Filtered vibration signals from the medial *(top)* and lateral *(bottom)* femoral accelerometers, depicting the difference in vibration data for the sample patient in Fig. 21.7.

KEY REFERENCES

6. Bourne RR, Baré JV: Failure in cam-post in total knee arthroplasty. In Bellemans J, Ries MD, Victor JKM, editors: *Total knee arthroplasty: a guide to get better performance*, Heidelberg, 2005, Springer, pp 90–95.

8. Cates HE, Komistek RD, Mahfouz MR, et al: In vivo comparison of knee kinematics for subjects having either a posterior stabilized or cruciate retaining high-flexion total knee arthroplasty. *J Arthroplasty* 23:1057–1067, 2008.

11. Dennis DA, Komistek RD, Mahfouz MR, et al: A multicenter analysis of axial femorotibial rotation after total knee arthroplasty. *Clin Orthop Relat Res* 428:180–189, 2004.

12. Dennis DA, Mahfouz MR, Komistek RD, et al: In vivo determination of normal and anterior cruciate ligament-deficient knee kinematics. *J Biomech* 38:241–253, 2005.

13. D'Lima DD, Patil S, Steklov N, et al: In vivo knee moments and shear after total knee arthroplasty. *J Biomech* 40:S11–S17, 2007.

14. D'Lima DD, Steklov N, Patil S, et al: In vivo knee forces during recreation and exercise after knee arthroplasty. *Clin Orthop Relat Res* 466:2605–2611, 2008.

23. Komistek RD, Kane TR, Mahfouz MR, et al: Knee mechanics—a review of past and present techniques to determine in vivo loads. *J Biomech* 38:215–228, 2005.

34. Rangayan RM, Wu Y: Analysis of vibroarthrographic signals with features related to signal variability and radial-basis functions. *Ann Biomed Eng* 37:156–163, 2009.

35. Sharma A, Komistek RD, Ranawat CS, et al: In vivo contact pressures in total knee arthroplasties. *J Arthroplasty* 22(3):404–415, 2007.

36. Sharma A, Komistek RD, Scuderi GR, et al: High-flexion TKA designs—what are their in vivo contact mechanics? *Clin Orthop Relat Res* 464:117–126, 2007.

37. Shelburne KB, Torry MR, Pandy MG: Contributions of muscles, ligaments, and the ground-reaction force to tibiofemoral joint loading during normal gait. *J Orthop Res* 10:1983–1990, 2006.

40. Umapathy S, Krishnan S: Modified local discriminant bases algorithm and its application in analysis of human knee joint vibration signals. *IEEE Trans Biomed Eng* 53:517–523, 2006.

41. Varadarajana KM, Moynihana AL, D'Lima DD, et al: In vivo contact kinematics and contact forces of the knee after total knee arthroplasty during dynamic weight-bearing activities. *J Biomech* 41:2159–2168, 2008.

43. Wasielewski RC, Komistek RD, Zingde SM, et al: Lack of axial rotation in mobile-bearing knee designs. *Clin Orthop Relat Res* 466:2662–2668, 2008.

The references for this chapter can also be found on www.expertconsult.com.

22

Does Strain in the Patella Change After Total Knee Arthroplasty? A Finite Element Investigation of Natural and Implanted Patellae

Clare K. Fitzpatrick, Mark A. Baldwin, Azhar A. Ali, Peter J. Laz, Paul J. Rullkoetter

Patellar fracture and anterior knee pain remain as significant complications following total knee replacement (TKR). In several TKR studies reported in the literature the average incidence of anterior knee pain was 12%.[12] Long-term, large-cohort studies have reported patellar fracture rates of 0.68%, 1.14%, 3.8%, and 5.2% in TKR populations involving 12,424, 1494, 4583, and 8530 knees, respectively.[5,14,20,23] Even at these relatively low incidence rates, the number of patients experiencing these complications is significant, especially considering the growing number of TKRs performed worldwide. A wide variety of patellar fracture types and locations have been reported.[5,9,23] Fracture type classification includes transverse, vertical, avulsion, and comminuted, with fracture location reported as 40% superior or midbody and 30% inferior pole by Goldberg et al.[9] and as 28% superior, 18% inferior, 23% comminuted, 13% vertical, 11% transverse midbody and 6% medial or lateral margin by Ortiguera and Berry.[23]

Treatment of patellar fracture varies considerably from case to case. A substantial proportion of patellar fractures are asymptomatic and are identified only radiographically upon routine follow-up. Others present with anterior knee pain, swelling, reduced range of motion, catching, locking or giving way of the joint, and/or difficulty with daily activities[5,9] and may require bracing, open reduction, internal fixation, component revision, or partial or total patellectomy.[7] Revision surgeries have been reported with poor outcomes, including high rates of complication (50%) and reoperation (42%).[23] Goldberg et al.[9] described unsatisfactory outcomes in 13 of 18 (72%) knees that underwent revision for patellar fracture. Keating et al.[14] reported a deep infection rate of 45% of patellar fractures treated operatively.

Given the number of occurrences and the high rate of complication with revision procedures, patellar fracture represents a significant concern affecting comfort and functionality for a substantial number of patients. If the patient subset at risk for patellar fracture or anterior knee pain can be identified preoperatively, alternative treatments (eg, selection of a specific implant design, altered component placement, an unresurfaced patella) can be applied, and this may reduce the rate of complications. Meding et al.[20] investigated patient and surgical factors associated with increased risk of patellar fracture, identifying a body mass index greater than 30, male gender, lateral reticular release, and a large patellar component size as risk factors.

Dalury and Dennis[6] reported postoperative patellar resection thickness and asymmetrical patellar resection as important contributing factors to patellar fracture.

Previous studies have measured strain in the patella, using strain as a measure of risk for patellar fracture and component loosening.[18,29,33] In these experimental cadaveric studies, anterior surface strain was measured using a uniaxial strain gauge in specimen sample sizes of between 8 and 20 knees. A strain gauge can provide a localized measure of bone strain but does not fully characterize the strain distribution throughout the volume of bone. For example, Lie et al.[18] measured compressive anterior cortex strain in full extension and hypothesized that this would result in corresponding tensile strain on the posterior resected surface.

Subject-specific finite element (FE) analyses have been used to determine bone strain distributions in the hip, femur, and tibia and have been applied to assess fracture risk, evaluate fixation, and predict bone remodeling.* If accurate results are the goal, it is important to account for the varying material properties of bone as a function of density. Objectives of this study were (1) to develop subject-specific FE models of the patellofemoral (PF) joint during deep flexion, including density-mapped material properties from computed tomography (CT) scan data; (2) to quantify differences in bone strain distribution under natural and implanted conditions; and (3) to assess the consistency of distributions across multiple specimens. An understanding of bone strain distributions under natural and implanted conditions can provide insight into important factors (geometry, bone density) and may allow preoperative identification of at-risk patients.

MATERIALS AND METHODS

Specimen-specific FE models for eight male subjects were developed from CT and magnetic resonance imaging (MRI) scans of cadaveric knees. Femoral, tibial, and patellar bone and cartilage were reconstructed from MRI data, and patellar bone geometry was extracted from CT data. Eight-noded hexahedral meshes of articular cartilage were semiautomatically generated from the segmented geometries using custom-scripted

---

*See references 10, 17, 26, 28, 30, 31.

coordinate data extraction and mesh morphing techniques.[2] A convergence study was performed to determine an appropriate element size for the patellar bone mesh. Tetrahedral meshes with element edge length of 1.25, 1, and 0.8 mm were compared. Differences in average strain (per unit volume) between the coarsest and finest mesh were less than 0.03% in natural and implanted models. Perillo-Marcone et al.[25] reported an element size comparable with the slice thickness of CT images to be sufficient for mesh convergence; they recommended an element size of 1.4 mm for convergence of the Young modulus, along with stress and risk results with a CT slice thickness of 1 mm. CT slice thickness for specimens in the current study varied from 0.5 to 1 mm. Based on slice thickness, computational efficiency, and minimal differences between 1 mm and finest mesh, an average element edge length of 1 mm was determined to appropriately represent the heterogeneity captured by CT data. Patellar bones were meshed using four-noded tetrahedral elements, such that natural and implanted patellae shared an element subset (Fig. 22.1A). The shared anterior element set ensured that muscle load could be applied through a common extensor mechanism in both models, eliminating potential differences in load application. Average numbers of elements in natural and implanted patellae were 140,000 and 85,000, respectively.

Two model representations were developed for each specimen: a natural model with bone and cartilage and an implanted model with a size-matched domed patellar button, a femoral component, and a tibial insert. Articular cartilage ($E = 12$ MPa, $v = 0.45$)[21] and the patellar component ($E = 572$ MPa, $v = 0.45$)[11] were modeled as fully deformable. In the natural model, patellar cartilage nodes were equivalenced with the posterior patellar bone to facilitate load transfer to the bone. In the implanted model, TKR components were positioned under the guidance of an orthopedic surgeon, and an intermediate cement layer ($E = 3400$ MPa, $v = 0.3$) was modeled between the patellar bone and button. Nodes were equivalenced between the button and the cement and between the cement and the resected patellar bone surface. For computational efficiency, femoral and tibial bones, in addition to femoral and tibial components, were modeled as rigid bodies using triangular surface elements.

Patellar strain is dependent not only on geometry and loading and contact mechanics but also on material properties

of the bone. To account for specimen-specific bone material properties, mapped material properties of the patellar bone were extracted from CT data using BoneMat (Biomed Town, Bologna, Italy) (see Fig. 22.1B).[32] Calibration of CT data to correlate Hounsfield units (HUs) with apparent density (ρ) was performed using a linear relationship taken from the literature.[24] Several studies have derived empirical relationships between bone density and mechanical properties.[22,24] The power law for the Young modulus, $E = 1990\rho^3$.[46] As proposed by Keller[15] was applied in this analysis. The nonlinear nature of the density-elasticity relationship ensures that different properties will be obtained depending on whether the Young modulus for the element is calculated before or after averaging over the element. In a comparative study with experimentally obtained data, Taddei et al.[32] reported that transforming HU values into Young's modulus values prior to averaging over the element was found to improve strain prediction accuracy compared with prior algorithms, which averaged HU values and then transformed them to modulus values. Hence this material mapping algorithm was adopted for the current study and was applied using BoneMat (version 3).

Each natural and implanted model was incorporated into an FE model of the isolated PF joint, which included two-dimensional (2D) fiber-reinforced membrane representations of the extensor mechanism and PF ligaments (Fig. 22.2).[1] An attachment site for each of the patellar ligament vasti, the rectus femoris, and the medial and lateral PF ligaments was defined on the surface of the patellar bone. Each node in the attachment site was rigidly beamed to its closest ligament fiber to physiologically transmit the ligament or muscle load to the patellar bone. A 1000 N ramped load was distributed among the heads of the quadriceps muscle as follows: vastus intermedius, 20%; vastus lateralis longus, 30%; vastus medialis longus, 15%; vasti lateralis obliquus, 10%; vasti medialis obliquus, 10%; and rectus femoris, 15%; these values are proportional to their physiologic cross-sectional areas as measured experimentally by Farahmand et al.[8] Prior to flexion a 300-N load was applied to the quadriceps and was held constant to bring the PF articular surfaces into contact. The quadriceps load was then linearly ramped to 1000 N over a 120-degree simulated deep knee bend.

Maximum and minimum principal strains in the patella were quantified throughout the flexion cycle. Strain distributions

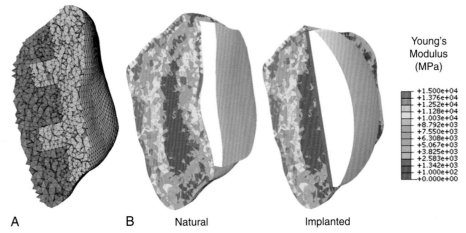

A   B   Natural   Implanted

Young's Modulus (MPa)

+1.500e+04
+1.376e+04
+1.252e+04
+1.128e+04
+1.003e+04
+8.792e+03
+7.550e+03
+6.308e+03
+5.067e+03
+3.825e+03
+2.583e+03
+1.342e+03
+1.000e+02
+0.000e+00

FIG 22.1 (A) Tetrahedral mesh of patellar bone for natural *(both light and dark elements)* and implanted *(dark elements only)* models. (B) Patellar bone with mapped material properties in natural and implanted models.

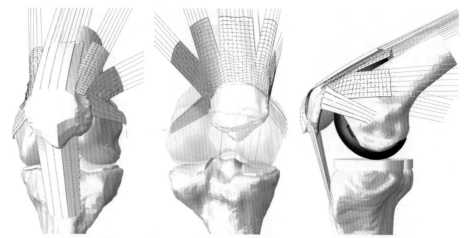

FIG 22.2 Anterior view of the natural PF model, including vasti, rectus femoris, patellar ligament, and PF constraint structures *(left)*; posterior view of the natural PF model shown with transparent femoral bone and cartilage *(center)*; and sagittal view of the implanted PF model during flexion.

throughout the bone volume were compared between natural and implanted conditions. Because peak maximum or minimum strain may occur in a very small localized region and may not provide an appropriate comparison, evaluations of a highly strained volume were performed, representing the bone volume experiencing strain above a specific threshold level. A threshold strain level of 0.5% was selected for comparison between natural and implanted cases. Bayraktar et al.[3] and Kopperdahl and Keaveny,[16] after measuring principal strains in trabecular and cortical bone, reported yield strains in the region of 0.6% to 1%. In addition, patellar bone volume was divided into four discrete regions: superior, medial, lateral, and inferior, centered at the midpoint of the patellar component. Strains in elements adjacent to the pegs of the patellar button were also compared with corresponding elements in the natural case. Strain levels and highly strained volumes in these regions were compared between implanted and natural cases. Finally, relationships between strain and the physical dimensions of the patella were investigated to determine whether strain correlated with size measurements that could be extracted preoperatively from x-rays.

RESULTS

Distributions of strain were obtained throughout the volume of the patellar bone for both natural and implanted cases. Regions of bone experiencing high strain were evaluated in terms of a highly strained volume (experiencing strains above 0.5%), and the location of this volume was compared between natural and implanted conditions. The primary mechanism of strain in the patella, particularly with increasing flexion, was compression of the articular surface, as anterior patellar ligament and quadriceps attachment sites served to increase the bending moment about the patella. The percentage of highly strained bone volume in compression was on the order of 3 to 4 times larger than the percentage of highly strained bone in tension across subjects.

Bone strain distributions throughout the patellar bone volume demonstrated variation both between subjects and between natural and implanted conditions (Fig. 22.3). Strain was relatively consistent throughout early flexion (<40 degrees)

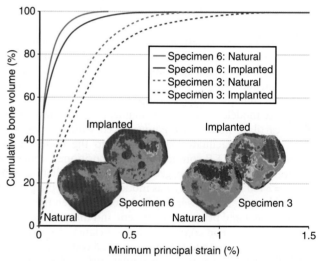

FIG 22.3 Distribution of bone strain throughout the patella with respect to bone volume for two specimens, indicating the percentage of bone volume below a particular minimum principal strain value. *Inset,* Minimum principal strain distribution along the resection plane for natural and implanted conditions.

and subsequently increased with increasing flexion in both natural and implanted conditions (Fig. 22.4). When highly strained volumes were compared between natural and implanted conditions throughout flexion, differences were found to be negligible in early flexion (<40 degrees) but became statistically significant ($p < 0.05$) in deeper flexion (see Fig. 22.4). At maximum flexion, an average increase of 190% in highly strained volume was noted after implantation (range, 20.5% to 465%). Only two specimens, which had the highest natural strain, showed little change (<30%) in comparison with the implanted case (Fig. 22.5).

Visual inspection of strain throughout the bone volume revealed that strain location, as well as magnitude, changed between natural and implanted conditions. Peak compressive principal strains among natural specimens were primarily

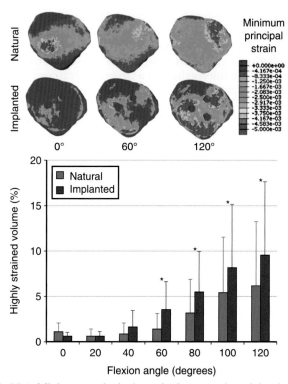

FIG 22.4 Minimum principal strain in natural and implanted specimens through flexion for a representative subject, shown along the plane of the patellar resection *(top)*. Mean (and standard deviation) highly strained volume of natural and implanted specimens throughout flexion *(bottom)*. Statistically significant differences ($p < 0.05$) represented by *.

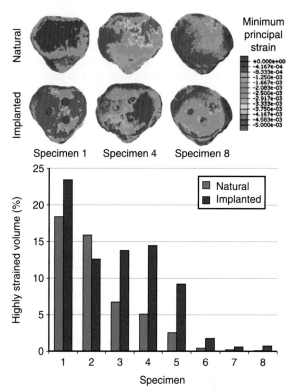

FIG 22.5 Minimum principal strain at 120 degrees flexion in three representative specimens (natural and implanted), shown along the plane of the patellar resection *(top)*. The highly strained volume in the natural and implanted cases for all eight specimens (ranked in order of decreasing natural highly strained volume) at 120 degrees flexion *(bottom)*.

noted in the softer cancellous bone underlying the contact patch in the proximal portion of the patella; however, in the implanted specimens these strains were focused medially, around the component pegs and at the distal nose of the patella. Upon quantitative comparison of strain distributions between regions, bone adjacent to the component pegs showed a larger highly strained volume in the implanted case (9.3%) than in the natural case (7.3%); however, this finding was not statistically significant. Comparison of quadrants (superior, inferior, medial, and lateral) showed that the natural specimens had an even highly strained volume distribution medially-laterally but substantially ($p = 0.09$) larger highly strained volume superiorly than inferiorly. However, the implanted specimens had an even highly strained volume distribution superiorly-inferiorly, with larger highly strained volume medially than laterally. Comparison between natural and implanted cases revealed that the medial region displayed the largest difference in highly strained volume ($p < 0.05$). The highly strained volume increased, on average, from 6.5% to 13.7% as the result of implantation. The inferior and lateral quadrants showed smaller increases in highly strained volume from 2.8% to 7.1% and from 6.4% to 9.6%, respectively, whereas the highly strained volume of the superior quadrant decreased slightly from 8.4% to 6.6% (Fig. 22.6).

A correlation coefficient of 0.85 was found between highly strained volumes of natural and implanted specimens. The highly strained volume for each subject was compared with

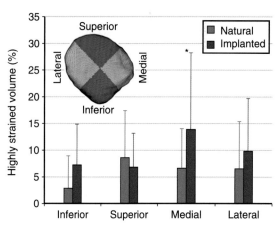

FIG 22.6 Mean (and standard deviation) highly strained volume of natural and implanted cases for all eight specimens separated into four regions. Statistically significant differences ($p < 0.05$) represented by *.

preoperative and postoperative patellar thickness and volume to determine correlations between these measurements. The strongest relationship was found between the implanted highly strained volume and the volume of remaining bone ($r = -0.74$). Weaker correlation was noted between postoperative patellar thickness and the implanted highly strained volume ($r = -0.61$).

DISCUSSION

Subject-specific FE models of the PF joint, including mapped material properties of the patellar bone, were developed for a series of specimens. These models were used to compare strain magnitude and distribution patterns between natural and implanted conditions. A significant increase in strain magnitude was predicted in the implanted case compared with the natural case, along with differences in the location of the most highly strained bone.

In this analysis the same loading conditions and soft tissue properties were applied across specimens. Despite elimination of potential variability in these parameters, wide variation in strain magnitude was observed between specimens; highly strained volumes ranged from 0.1% to 18.3% among natural specimens and from 0.5% to 23.4% in implanted specimens at 120 degrees flexion (Table 22.1). Although subject-specific geometry and material properties are substantial factors in intersubject variability, this variability may also be attributable in part to the generic HU-density relationship applied in this analysis. However, because the same density mapping was applied to each natural and implanted pair and because this study focused on performance of a comparative analysis between natural and implanted conditions, subtle differences in CT protocol between specimens would have minimal effect on reported results.

When natural and implanted specimens were compared, implantation was seen to result in an increase in the percentage of bone above a 0.5% strain threshold of approximately 200%. In general, this was a proportional increase, relative to the natural condition, with strong correlation ($r = 0.85$) between natural and implanted highly strained volumes. Ideally, post-TKR strain could be estimated from easily measurable preoperative parameters. A reasonably strong inverse relationship was found between implanted highly strained volume and bone volume ($r = -0.74$). This suggests that post-TKR patellar strain may be predicted with reasonable accuracy on the basis of knowledge of preoperative patellar geometry, aiding in the identification of those patients at higher risk of patellar fracture. However, a larger number of specimens may be necessary to validate this relationship.

Along with changes in strain magnitude, this analysis identified differences in the location of the highly strained volume of bone after TKR. The bone region around the component pegs showed an increase in strain in the implanted condition; however, this difference was smaller than anticipated. In this analysis, perfect bonding was assumed between the cement layer and the patellar bone. Janssen et al.[13] demonstrated that

ideal cement-bone bonding decreases deformation at the interface. A more realistic representation of cement-bone interaction may alter the strain distribution in this area. Comparison of strain between quadrants showed that the superior region in the natural condition exhibited a larger highly strained volume than the implanted condition. The natural femur, with a longer sulcus groove than the femoral component, plus geometric congruency between patellar and femoral cartilage, ensures that the natural patella maintains more superior and expansive contact with the femur in deep flexion than the implanted knee (Fig. 22.7A). The geometry of the patellar component resulted in smaller distinct medial and lateral contact patches located approximately at midheight of the patellar component, leading to a more even distribution of strain between superior and inferior compartments of the implanted knee. Contact pressure was slightly higher laterally than medially in the implanted specimens, but this did not explain the larger highly strained volume in the medial compartment. However, when the distribution of material properties in the patellar bone was evaluated, bone in the medial compartment was found to be significantly softer ($p < 0.005$) than bone in the lateral compartment (average Young's modulus was 2.6 and 3.7 GPa in the medial and lateral regions, respectively), accounting for the medial-lateral distribution of strain in the implanted condition (see Fig. 22.7B). This is representative of early postoperative conditions, before bone modeling has had a chance to occur. The medial-lateral distribution difference was not observed in the natural condition, and it is hypothesized that the denser cortical bone present on the articular surface of the natural patella offered some stress shielding to the lower modulus underlying cancellous bone in the medial compartment, providing a more even distribution of strain throughout the entire bone volume.

The current study is subject to limitations caused by simplification of loading conditions and physiologic representations and lack of directly comparable experimental strain data to validate FE strain predictions. Therefore this analysis is primarily a comparative study between natural and implanted conditions rather than a prediction of absolute magnitude of bone strain. To produce reliable comparisons between conditions, the model must reproduce physiologically reasonable PF mechanics. The fidelity of the kinematics of the isolated PF model has been assessed by Baldwin et al.[1] by comparing PF kinematics of the FE model versus experimental kinematic data from cadaveric subjects. PF contact pressure and area were compared with in vivo and in vitro measurements reported in the literature and were found to fall within the reported range,[4,19,27] although the magnitude of these values is dependent on the loading conditions used—large variability was measured in studies that

TABLE 22.1 Bone Volume, Highly Strained Volume, and 95th Percentile Strain Value for Natural and Implanted Conditions for Each Specimen

	SPECIMEN							
	1	2	3	4	5	6	7	8
Bone volume, natural patella, ×10³ mm³	19.2	19.4	21.4	22.4	21.8	18.9	23.1	22.7
Bone volume, resected patella, ×10³ mm³	10.0	10.9	12.5	14.1	12.8	12.2	16.5	16.3
Highly strained volume, natural, %	18.3	15.8	6.7	5.0	2.6	0.4	0.2	0.1
Highly strained volume, implanted, %	23.4	12.5	13.7	14.4	9.2	1.8	0.6	0.8
95th percentile strain, natural (dimensionless)	0.85	0.72	0.56	0.53	0.44	0.18	0.09	0.28
95th percentile strain, implanted (dimensionless)	1.31	0.82	0.82	0.94	0.64	0.35	0.10	0.39

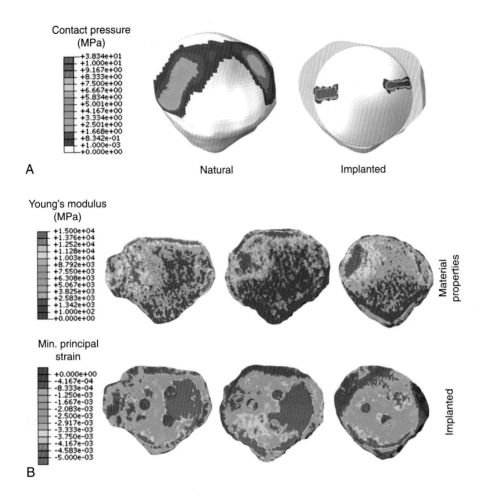

FIG 22.7 (A) Typical patellofemoral contact patch at 120 degrees flexion in natural *(left)* and implanted *(right)* models. (B) Mapped material properties and corresponding minimum principal strains in implanted conditions shown for three representative specimens along the plane of the patellar resection.

applied subject-specific loading conditions.[4] In the implanted case, FE-predicted femoral component–patellar button contact mechanics was compared with Tekscan (Tekscan Inc., South Boston, Massachusetts) measurements taken from experiments in quasistatic loading conditions at 30-degree intervals throughout flexion. FE-predicted peak contact pressure and area fell to within 10% of experimental data. Given the agreement between PF mechanics of the computational model and reported kinematic and contact mechanics, the force transmitted to the patellar bone in the FE model is physiologically reasonable. The material mapping algorithm applied here has been compared with experimental measurements in 13 strain gauge locations for a series of loading conditions, with a regression coefficient of 0.79 reported.[32] Hence, the analysis in this study provides an effective platform for relative comparison between natural and implanted PF joints. Thus far, implanted specimens have been assessed with components in neutral alignment only; however, the analysis described here is an ideal computational platform from which the influence of component alignment and intraoperative variability on patellar strain can be investigated; experimental assessment of this would not be feasible.

An understanding of the mechanisms of strain in TKR and of the relationship between preoperative and postoperative patellar strain may aid in identifying those patients at greatest risk for patellar fracture or anterior knee pain. Altered component placement or revised component designs could potentially reduce the incidence of patellar fracture in this at-risk group.

ACKNOWLEDGMENTS

This study was supported in part by DePuy Synthes, Inc.

KEY REFERENCES

1. Baldwin MA, Clary C, Maletsky LP, et al: Verification of predicted specimen-specific natural and implanted patellofemoral kinematics during simulated deep knee bend. *J Biomech* 42:2341–2348, 2009b.
4. Besier TF, Draper CE, Gold GE, et al: Patellofemoral joint contact area increases with knee flexion and weight-bearing. *J Orthop Res* 23:345–350, 2005.
5. Chun KA, Ohashi K, Bennett DL, et al: Patellar fractures after total knee replacement. *AJR Am J Roentgenol* 185:655–660, 2005.
7. Dennis DA: Periprosthetic fractures following total knee arthroplasty. *Instr Course Lect* 50:379–389, 2001.
9. Goldberg VM, Figgie HE, 3rd, Inglis AE, et al: Patellar fracture type and prognosis in condylar total knee arthroplasty. *Clin Orthop Relat Res* 236:115–122, 1988.

12. Helmy N, Anglin C, Greidanus NV, et al: To resurface or not to resurface the patella in total knee arthroplasty. *Clin Orthop Relat Res* 466:2775–2783, 2008.

14. Keating EM, Haas G, Meding JB: Patella fracture after post total knee replacements. *Clin Orthop Relat Res* 416:93–97, 2003.

16. Kopperdahl DL, Keaveny TM: Yield strain behavior of trabecular bone. *J Biomech* 31:601–608, 1998.

20. Meding JB, Fish MD, Berend ME, et al: Predicting patellar failure after total knee arthroplasty. *Clin Orthop Relat Res* 466:2769–2774, 2008.

23. Ortiguera CJ, Berry DJ: Patella fracture after total knee arthroplasty. *J Bone Joint Surg Am* 84:532–540, 2002.

30. Reuben JD, McDonald CL, Woodard PL, et al: Effect of patella thickness on patella strain following total knee arthroplasty. *J Arthroplasty* 6:251–258, 1991.

31. Schileo E, Taddei F, Cristofolini L, et al: Subject-specific finite element models implementing a maximum principal strain criterion are able to estimate failure risk and fracture location on human femurs tested in vitro. *J Biomech* 41:356–367, 2008.

34. Wulff W: Incavo SJ: The effect of patella preparation for total knee arthroplasty on patellar strain: a comparison of resurfacing versus inset implants. *J Arthroplasty* 15:778–782, 2000.

The references for this chapter can also be found on www.expertconsult.com.

23

Wear Simulation of Knee Implants

Louise M. Jennings, Raelene M. Cowie, Claire L. Brockett, John Fisher

Wear simulation testing of knee replacements allows the influence of various design and condition variables on the wear performance to be examined in a controlled environment. One million cycles is considered to represent a full year in vivo; however, this value is conservative for younger and more active patients, who may achieve over 2 million steps per year. This chapter examines the progression of experimental and computational knee simulator studies, a Stratified Approach for Enhanced Reliability (SAFER) approach to simulation, and the influence of bearing design, material, and kinematic input on the wear performance of the replacement knee.

INTRODUCTION TO WEAR SIMULATION

There are now many different bearings and surgical approaches for total knee replacement (TKR), manufactured from an increasing variety of materials (eg, varied degrees of cross-linkage in polyethylene). There is a need for rigorous in vitro simulator studies to compare the effects of bearing design and material on the function and wear performance of the TKR. Historically, simple configuration tribological tests, such as pin on plate or pin on disk, provided a platform for defining the wear properties of a material under defined cyclic loading and motion patterns. However, the outcomes of these studies do not always correlate with the clinical performance of the same material. A major challenge in the laboratory is to produce simulations that provide clinically relevant data and predictions of future clinical performance. A further consideration is the role that computational predictions can play in a combined experimental and computational approach to assessing the preclinical performance of knee replacements. Computational modeling can support the in vitro experimental design and selection of appropriate test conditions and provide additional insight and understanding that cannot be gleaned from experimental studies alone, such as the contact stresses and cross-shear, providing that the computational models have been adequately experimentally validated.

Numerous factors affect the in vivo performance of a TKR, including the bearing design, material, lubrication, component position, patient loading and activity, and joint kinematics. Therefore, the performance of knee replacement bearings should be assessed in a physiologic simulator designed to replicate the in vivo conditions as closely as possible so that interactions among all these variables may also be assessed.[5] This is challenging, given the range of conditions to which knee replacements are subjected in vivo. Current studies have predominantly focused on simulating standard gait, whereas more recently a wider envelope of conditions is beginning to be more widely considered in line with the SAFER approach.[12,21] The SAFER approach accounts for variations in surgical delivery, variations in kinematics, variations in the patient population, and degradation of the biomaterials technology, as well as combinations of all these different conditions. Testing under such a wide portfolio of stratified conditions cannot be achieved using experimental simulation alone because too many experimental simulations are needed. A new computational modeling approach has been recently developed that can be combined with the experimental approach.[1,2] The computational model uses a new complex wear law for polyethylene that accounts for a range of input variables, including variations in wear area, contact stress, cross-shear, and sliding distance. This information has been incorporated into finite element analysis wear prediction models for the knee, which have been experimentally validated under specific walking conditions. Computational models must always be experimentally validated for points at the extreme range of conditions, so that the computational models fall within an experimentally validated envelope.

Several different knee wear simulators have been developed both academically[8,28,38] and commercially,[24] and there are significant differences in the function and control of the simulators. Most current simulators use six degrees of freedom, four of which are actively controlled—axial load, anterior-posterior motion, internal-external rotation, and flexion-extension (Fig. 23.1). The remaining two degrees of freedom, abduction-adduction and medial-lateral displacement, tend to be free to move passively or, in some simulators, are fixed. Two hypotheses for the control of motion in the anterior-posterior and internal-external rotational directions have been proposed, and both are defined in standards: force control (International Organization for Standardization [ISO] 14243-1)[19] and displacement control (ISO 14243-3).[20]

The stability of a knee replacement in vivo is determined by a combination of the geometry of the implant and the natural soft tissues surrounding the joint. The relative contribution varies in different patients. Force-controlled simulator studies often use spring elements to represent the motion constraints that are created by the soft tissues in vivo.[9] The rationale for using force control suggests that it generates the most representative kinematics and provides a better indication of the mechanical behavior of a specific design. A simple linear spring cannot represent the complex force displacement relationships found in soft tissues. The geometry of the implant also dictates its resistance to motion, and therefore the tensioning of the springs may not highlight the effect of geometric

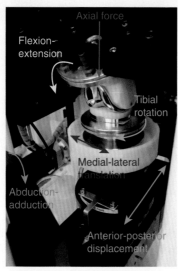

FIG 23.1 Degrees of freedom in a knee wear simulator.

differences between bearings when testing under force control. Under displacement control, the actual movements are directly controlled and provide a more repeatable set of motion conditions and wear; the machine force is limited, which prevents the knee replacement from experiencing excessive kinematics and ensures that the implant is not driven outside the geometric constraints.[5]

It is believed that the bearing type may dictate the appropriate test conditions. Because of differences in test conditions, implants studied, and simulator setup, it has been difficult to directly compare the two modes. However, studies involving identical implants tested in the same simulator, under load or displacement control, have been reported and have shown that similar levels of anterior-posterior translation occurred under force and load control. A low-conforming, fixed-bearing study in which rotation and anterior-posterior translation were controlled by force or displacement, also showed similar magnitudes of internal-external rotation, but the phase of the motion within the gait cycle differed significantly. The volumetric wear under load control was significantly higher than under displacement control. Low-conformity bearings and cruciate-retaining implants may undergo excessive displacement under load control testing.[35] Conversely, high-conformity bearings, tested under displacement control, may be driven to excessive displacement, which would not occur physiologically, and therefore experience very high stress. Moderately conforming bearings under both load and displacement control have been shown to generate equivalent wear volumes.[23] There are obvious merits to both test hypotheses, depending on the design philosophy of the implant. Wear simulation studies should be conducted to produce clinically relevant kinematic profiles and wear data, and there is merit in simulation systems that have the flexibility to adopt both approaches to control on the anterior-posterior and rotation motion axes.[5]

Furthermore, it is important to note that the current international standards, regardless of force and displacement control, describe a single set of idealized standard gait conditions for a standard patient in whom the prosthesis has been implanted with perfect surgical technique and under a single activity.

EFFECT OF INPUT KINEMATICS ON BEARING WEAR

Early wear simulator studies of TKR produced very low wear rates, which was related to the input kinematics used for the simulations. It has been shown that the magnitude of anterior-posterior displacement and internal-external rotation has a significant effect on the wear of the polyethylene bearing. A standard displacement-controlled simulator study might use an anterior-posterior displacement of 0 to 10 mm and an internal-external rotation of ±5 degrees to re-create the motion within the natural knee (high kinematics). A 50% reduction in anterior-posterior displacement, while maintaining a ±5-degree rotation, has been shown to result in a twofold reduction in mean wear rate[22] in fixed-bearing knees. Reducing the internal-external rotation to ±2.5 degrees while maintaining the 0- to 5-mm displacement resulted in a fourfold reduction in wear compared with high-kinematics studies. Removal of the internal-external rotation or the anterior-posterior displacement decreased the wear rate by an order of magnitude.[24] A shorter anterior-posterior displacement results in a reduced sliding distance and therefore a reduced polyethylene surface area subjected to wear. However, the significant change in wear resulting from reduced rotation and displacement is caused by a change in the cross-shear on the surface of the bearing. A reduction in rotation reduces the cross-shear, therefore reducing the exposure of the polyethylene to wear in the strain-softened direction. An increase in internal-external rotation results in an increased frictional force transverse to the sliding distance and therefore increases the wear in a fixed-bearing knee.

Lift-off of the femoral condyles from the tibial bearing has been shown in vivo through fluoroscopic studies. One experimental study investigated the effect of lift-off on the wear performance of fixed and mobile TKRs by examining inserts with similar contact geometry.[22] Condylar lift-off was achieved in the study by application of a rotation moment to the abduction-adduction axis to create 1 mm of lateral condyle lift-off during each gait cycle. A significant increase in wear rate was measured for fixed and mobile bearings, and it was notable that the reduced wear rates observed in the mobile knees compared with the fixed knees under standard gait conditions were not seen under lift-off. There was no significant difference between the wear rates of the bearings under lift-off conditions. The uneven loading of the insert during lift-off caused a medial-lateral shift, increasing the cross-shear on the medial condyle and increasing the wear. This study showed lift-off to have a significant impact on the wear rate of the bearing; however, this test had lift-off during every cycle and the clinical translation of this research would depend on the frequency of lift-off in vivo.

INFLUENCE OF BEARING DESIGN ON IN VITRO WEAR PERFORMANCE OF KNEE REPLACEMENTS

A wide variety of knee replacements are clinically available, which can be subdivided into two groups, fixed-bearing knees and mobile-bearing knees. In addition, designs may vary on the degree of conformity between the ultra–high-molecular-weight polyethylene (UHMWPE) insert and the femoral bearing. Unicompartmental knee replacements (UKRs) are also becoming increasingly popular clinically. In vitro wear simulator testing, under defined loading and motion conditions, can demonstrate the effect of bearing design on the wear performance of a knee replacement.

Comparison of Mobile and Fixed Bearings

Fixed-bearing knees have a UHMWPE insert that clips or pushes into the tibial tray. Because the insert is fixed, it cannot move relative to the tibial tray and therefore all motion occurs on the superior surface of the insert at the articulation with the femoral bearing (Fig. 23.2A). Two types of mobile bearings exist: (1) those that allow anterior-posterior translation and internal-external rotation of the UHMWPE insert with respect to the tibial tray and (2) rotating platform bearings, which permit rotation only at the insert–tibial tray interface (see Fig. 23.2B). The rotating platform mobile bearing translates a complex input motion into simple uniaxial motions by decoupling the motion; linear motion parallel to the flexion-extension axis occurs on the superior surface and unidirectional rotational motion occurs on the inferior surface of the UHMWPE insert[37] (see Fig. 23.2B).

Polyethylene molecules align preferentially in the principal direction of sliding (anterior-posterior), causing strain hardening, which increases wear resistance in this direction. However, this causes strain softening in the direction transverse to sliding, resulting in reduced wear resistance.

In the fixed-bearing knee, multidirectional motion introduced through the internal-external rotation of the knee causes increased cross-shear, which increases the polyethylene wear. Decoupling the motion at the knee through a rotating platform implant creates unidirectional motion at the superior and inferior interfaces, and reduced cross-shear and reduced wear rates compared with the fixed bearing.[27] More recent studies have also shown lower wear rates of the mobile-bearing designs compared with fixed bearings; however, these did not show significant differences because of the inherent variability in the simulation systems used.[16,37]

Effect of Conformity of the Contact

Historically, the main cause of failure in knee replacement was delamination, reported both clinically and experimentally. Delamination is a form of structural fatigue and is increased if stress levels are high or if the mechanical properties of the UHMWPE are poor. The former type of polyethylene, which was gamma-irradiated in air, was prone to oxidative degradation, a reduction in mechanical fatigue properties, and resulting delamination. To address the poor mechanical properties of polyethylene following oxidative degradation, knee replacement design tended toward higher conformity to reduce stress levels and decrease the risk of delamination. However, improvements in materials and sterilization techniques in the last decade, which substantially reduce degradation of the properties of UHMWPE, have resulted in considerable advancement in the wear performance of total fixed-bearing knee replacements. In particular, the introduction of UHMWPE with superior and stabilized mechanical properties has allowed less conforming designs to be investigated again. Historically, experimental wear studies of fixed-bearing knee replacements have shown reduced wear with less conformity,[3,10] but have not shown significant effects, most likely because of conformity changes being relatively small. More recently, studies examining the effect of conformity contrasted curved fixed inserts with completely flat inserts manufactured from identical UHMWPE material. A significant reduction in surface wear was reported under a range of test conditions representative of the clinical envelope for the flat design, with a low-medium level of cross-shear.[15] This reduction in surface wear has since been further supported by a combined experimental and computational study in which wear was shown to decrease with a decreasing level of conformity for four levels of conformity—curved, lipped, partial flat, and custom-made flat—for both conventional and moderately cross-linked UHMWPE.[1] However, it should be noted that less conforming fixed bearings will require suitable soft tissue constraint and therefore would not be a suitable low-wearing option for all patients.[13]

Unicompartmental Knee Replacements

UKRs are becoming an increasingly popular surgical intervention for the treatment of osteoarthritis when only one compartment of the knee requires replacement. The in vitro experimental wear study approach has been to set up pairs of medial and lateral unicompartmental knees anatomically side by side in the same study. Studies of both fixed- and mobile-bearing UKR designs[6,25] have shown higher wear on the medial bearing compared with the lateral. A study comparing the spherical Oxford mobile unicompartmental bearing with the low conformity Sigma HP PK fixed unicompartmental bearing reported

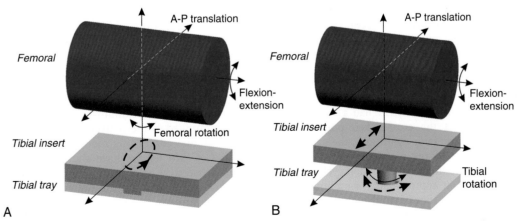

FIG 23.2 (A) Schematic of a fixed-bearing TKR. (B) Schematic of rotating platform mobile-bearing TKR.

lower wear rates for the lower conforming Sigma HP PK fixed unicompartmental bearing,[6] consistent with studies of low conforming TKRs and confirming the relationship of decreasing surface wear with decreasing conformity. The combined wear for the medial and lateral bearings of the lower conforming Sigma HP PK fixed unicompartmental bearings was significantly lower than the wear of a comparable fixed-bearing TKR.

WEAR PERFORMANCE OF NEW MATERIALS

Comparison of Standard Ultra–High-Molecular-Weight Polyethylene With Cross-Linked Materials

Early failures of TKR were attributed to high stresses and the oxidation of the polyethylene caused by the sterilization method. Sterilization using gamma radiation removes hydrogen from the molecule, breaking the polymer chains to create free radicals. Gamma sterilization in air makes oxygen available to combine with these radicals, resulting in oxidative degradation. In the absence of oxygen, these radicals recombine or form cross-linkages; therefore, more recent sterilization methods, such as gamma sterilization of bearings in a vacuum foil pouch (gamma vacuum foil [GVF]), have removed the oxygen. The length of shelf aging appears to have an effect on the extent of degradation; one study examined the effect of aging on the oxidation and wear performance of tibial inserts.[39] Two groups of inserts, both of the same design and identical GUR 1020 UHMWPE material, gamma-sterilized in air, were studied, one with a shelf life of 1 year and the other with a shelf life of 7 years. Assessment of oxidation showed the 7-year samples to have a significantly higher oxidative index value; the peak value was found at approximately 1 mm below the surface of the bearing insert. During wear simulator studies, subsurface cracking was noted on some of the 7-year bearings from 1 million cycles, with further cracking and evidence of delamination after the completion of 5 million cycles. The delamination and crack damage observed on these inserts was comparable to the failures seen in vivo.

Cross-linked polyethylene was introduced in TKRs following clinical and experimental success in total hip replacements. Cross-linkage occurs in polyethylene through exposure to radiation and cross-linked materials resist multidirectional wear. However, cross-linkage also reduces material toughness, so there is a balance between increasing wear resistance and preventing bearing fragility. During the cross-linking process, free radicals are produced, which have already been noted as a cause of oxidative degradation. Therefore, after radiation cross-linkage, the material is often remelted to remove these free radicals and make the material oxidatively stable. Several studies have shown a significant reduction in wear rate for cross-linked polyethylene material compared with standard polyethylene under standard test conditions.[7,14,30] Studies on aggressively aged polyethylene, representative of 5 years of shelf aging, showed that the conventional polyethylene had a significantly higher oxidative index than the cross-linked polyethylene. Furthermore, under wear-simulator conditions, the aged conventional polyethylene showed the formation of subsurface cracks on the inserts at approximately 0.5 million cycles, which progressed to delamination at approximately 4 million cycles. The aged cross-linked material showed no damage at 5 million cycles and was tested in 10 million cycles, with no evidence of cracking or delamination.[30] Moderate or medium levels of cross-linking are now being used routinely in the knee. Because

a high level of cross-linking can itself reduce the mechanical properties and toughness of the material, it is important in the knee to avoid the high levels of cross-linking that are more commonly found in the hip.

Because of the issues of reduced mechanical properties and toughness in highly cross-linked polyethylene, alternative methods of achieving oxidative stability have been investigated that attempt to maintain both the enhanced wear performance of highly cross-linked polyethylene and the mechanical properties of conventional polyethylene. This includes the introduction of vitamin E in the polyethylene; the antioxidative effect of vitamin E preserves the crystallinity of the material.[32] In the limited number of experimental wear simulation studies that have been carried out, the initial findings are promising. Vitamin E–stabilized UHMWPE tibial inserts have shown an improved wear performance compared to conventional polyethylene under standard test conditions[36] and when the polyethylene has been artificially aged.[18,29] More simulator studies and biologic and cytotoxic studies are required to fully assess antioxidant polyethylene.

Studies of New Materials

Although metal bearings (mainly cobalt-chrome-molybdenum [CoCrMo]) articulating with a conventional or cross-linked polyethylene insert are common and well-established materials for knee replacement, experimental research has also investigated alternative bearing materials. Alternative polymeric materials, such as polyurethane or carbon fiber–reinforced (CFR) polyetheretherketone (PEEK), have been examined experimentally in a unicondylar knee replacement configuration.[33,34] Polyurethane was selected because it is a compliant material, hypothesized to mimic the natural joint more accurately. These studies showed low wear rates for the material, although the bearing consisted of a polyurethane tibial component articulating with a CoCrMo femoral bearing; hence, there was no interaction between the polyurethane and a metallic tibial tray, which may have resulted in higher wear. However, the mechanical properties of the polyurethane construct are critical, as is the long-term stability of the material, and it is important to consider both these factors more fully in the development of solutions involving polyurethane.[4] The CFR-PEEK material was selected as a potential bearing because it has been shown to have a lower volumetric wear rate than UHMWPE in experimental studies of total hip replacement. Experimental studies of a highly conforming mobile unicondylar knee replacement showed reduced wear compared with a conventional UHMWPE bearing, highlighting this material as a potential alternative for UHMWPE in this low-contact stress situation.[33] However, there is concern about the use of CFR-PEEK in a high-contact stress application such as a low conforming or malaligned TKR where the material has exhibited high wear rates.[17]

Alumina- and zirconium-based ceramic bearings have also been examined as alternative materials for the femoral component. Studies contrasting monolithic alumina ceramic femurs with CoCrMo femurs have shown significant reductions in volumetric wear rates with ceramic bearings,[26,31] but further work is needed to confirm these findings. The toughness of ceramic remains a concern for manufacturing more complex geometries of femoral components, and has significant cost implications and complexities relating to the design of fixation interfaces. There is also interest in the use of a surface coating or treatment that can be oxidized as a hard surface layer on the femoral component, such as zirconium. This has been shown to reduce polyethylene wear in one simulator study.[11] However, extensive studies in other laboratories have not been reported.

SUMMARY

Experimental and computational wear simulation has enabled further development in the design progression of knee replacements through examining the influence of a variety of factors, such as design and material, on the wear performance of the bearing. This chapter has highlighted that rotating platform mobile-bearing knee replacements have shown reduced wear compared with conventional designs of fixed-bearing knees because of a decoupling of complex motions, resulting in lower-wearing unidirectional motion at both insert interfaces. However, recent research into fixed-bearing knees has shown that a reduced conformity can considerably reduce the wear to rates similar to those of the rotating platform mobile-bearing knee. Improved sterilization techniques have reduced the risks of subsurface cracking and delamination associated with oxidative degradation of polyethylene, and moderately cross-linked polyethylene can further reduce surface wear in fixed-bearing knees.

Simulation studies have shown the progress made toward low-wear options for TKR. However, this chapter has also illustrated the significant differences observed in wear rates under different kinematic conditions, indicating the importance of reviewing the test methodology when comparing wear rates from different studies. Although studies to date have examined conventional and novel materials and designs under representative gait conditions, progress in simulation proceeds toward developing new experimental and computational techniques to assess knee replacements throughout a wider range of functional activities and variations in surgical positioning to enhance their safety and reliability.

KEY REFERENCES

5. Barnett PI, McEwen HMJ, Auger DD, et al: Investigation of wear of knee prostheses in a new displacement/force-controlled simulator. *Proc Inst Mech Eng H* 216:51–61, 2002.

13. Fisher J, Jennings LM, Galvin AL, et al: 2009 Knee Society Presidential Guest Lecture: polyethylene wear in total knees. *Clin Orthop Relat Res* 468:12–18, 2010.

15. Galvin AL, Kang L, Udofia I, et al: Effect of conformity and contact stress on wear in fixed bearing total knee prostheses. *J Biomech* 42:1898–1902, 2009.

16. Grupp TM, Kaddick C, Schwiesau J, et al: Fixed and mobile bearing total knee arthroplasty. Influence on wear generation, corresponding wear areas, knee kinematics and particle composition. *Clin Biomech (Bristol, Avon)* 24:210–217, 2009.

19. International Organization for Standardization: Implants for surgery—wear of total knee-joint prostheses. Part 1. Loading and displacement parameters for wear-testing machines with load control and corresponding environmental conditions for test, 2009, ISO 14243-1 <http://www.iso.org/iso/catalogue_detail.htm?csnumber=44262>.

20. International Organization for Standardization: Implants for surgery—wear of total knee-joint prostheses. Part 3. Loading and displacement parameters for wear-testing machines with displacement-control and corresponding environmental conditions for test, 2014, ISO 14243-3 <http://www.iso.org/iso/home/store/catalogue_ics/catalogue_detail_ics.htm?csnumber=56649>.

22. Jennings LM, Bell CJ, Ingham E, et al: The influence of femoral condylar liftoff on the wear of artificial knee joints. *Proc Inst Mech Eng H* 221:305–314, 2007.

24. Johnson TS, Laurent MP, Yao JQ, et al: Comparison of wear of mobile and fixed bearing knees tested in a knee simulator. *Wear* 255:1107–1112, 2003.

25. Laurent MP, Johnson TS, Yao JQ, et al: In vitro lateral versus medial wear of a knee prosthesis. *Wear* 255:1101–1106, 2003.

27. McEwen HMJ, Barnett PI, Bell CJ, et al: The influence of design, materials and kinematics on the in-vitro wear of total knee replacements. *J Biomech* 38:357–365, 2005.

30. Muratoglu OK, Bragdon CR, Jasty M, et al: Knee-simulator testing of conventional and cross-linked polyethylene tibial inserts. *J Arthroplasty* 19:887–897, 2004.

35. Schwenke T, Orozco D, Sneider E, et al: Differences in wear between load and displacement control tested total knee replacements. *Wear* 267:757–762, 2008.

39. Young SK, Keller TS, Greer KW, et al: Wear testing of UHMWPE tibial components: influence of oxidation. *ASME J Tribol* 122:323–331, 2000.

The references for this chapter can also be found on www.expertconsult.com.

24

Knee Wear*

John H. Currier, Douglas W. Van Citters

Wherever there exists relative motion between two materials in contact with one another, there will be wear. It is the inevitable outcome of the mechanical, and occasionally chemical, interaction between surface asperities on two articulating bodies. Wear in total knees is no different; debris will be generated and volume will be lost from at least one of the contacting materials. The important clinical questions therefore concern the amount of debris produced, the size of the particles, and volume loss from the bulk that is sufficient to adversely affect the macroscopic mechanical environment. Answering these questions will give an indication of the potential biologic and biomechanical implications for the patient.

It is impossible to generate a meaningful answer to these questions without first understanding the system and clinical history of wear in total knee arthroplasty. This chapter will therefore introduce the field and the context in which the current literature should be considered through general observations taken from knee wear studies. Three such observations are presented to help guide the reader in more fully appreciating the clinical wear literature:

1. Wear and damage can be distinct phenomena in knee devices.
2. Quantitative measurement of true wear in knees is challenging because good reference data are difficult to obtain, more difficult than for hips.
3. Design and system selection can have as much of an effect on wear as the materials selected for the bearing surfaces.

WEAR AND DAMAGE

Damage and *wear* are terms often used interchangeably in the evaluation of tibial insert performance, but there is an important distinction in knees. Polyethylene wear is frequently cited

as the cause of device failure and revision by surgeons who contribute devices to retrieval laboratories. Wear refers to the quantified loss of material from a surface and can occur through abrasion, adhesion, or fatigue. Abrasive or adhesive wear, occurring on the backside and articular surfaces of tibial inserts, results in fine particle generation. Fatigue failure (cracking or delamination) is often secondary to oxidation and can result in large amounts of material removal, potentially altering the kinematic function of the device or causing catastrophic failure. Because the clinical impact of each process (abrasion or adhesion versus fatigue) can be different, understanding and maintaining a distinction of the terms is important.

Components of Wear

Scratching and Pitting. Deformation of tibial inserts by scratching and pitting, which often reflect damage but not wear, can be visually striking, yet represent only superficial surface changes in the polyethylene. This type of damage is almost ubiquitous on clinical retrievals and can result from third-body debris such as cement, residual bone fragments, or loose porous-coating beads. Scratched and pitted surfaces look damaged, but the damage may be only cosmetic (Fig. 24.1).

Scratched and pitted surfaces have been reproduced in laboratory simulations of the knee environment in the absence of material removal. Atwood et al.[4] demonstrated reproducible scratching and pitting of polymer pins in an oscillating pin-on-flat experiment. Of note, the damage and characteristic skipping marks observed in retrieval studies were not only reproduced on the polyethylene pins, but clinically comparable scratching was apparent on the cobalt-chromium-molybdenum (CoCrMo) counterface. This damage occurred when bone cement and bone debris from cutting were introduced into the articulation.

The ability of a softer material to scratch a harder material is documented elsewhere in the tribology literature.[46,75] In knees, the result is a scratch running in the direction of the predominant motion. It is well documented that counterface roughness and scratching can have dramatic effects on the wear rates of polymer bearings, depending on the degree of crossing motion encountered by the system.[39] Therefore, in vivo scratching of metallic femoral components is important to monitor when evaluating tibial wear.

Fatigue Failure. Fatigue failure occurs in all types of gamma-sterilized tibial inserts, regardless of design, material, or method of fabrication (molded or machined; Fig. 24.2).[20] The incidence of fatigue failure increases with time in vivo as oxidation and cycles of use increase. Higher initial oxidation means fewer cycles before failure. Hence, devices that were gamma-sterilized

*Acknowledgments: We especially appreciate the work of the many surgeons who dedicated time and effort to collaborating with the Dartmouth Biomedical Engineering Center Implant Retrieval Laboratory by sending retrieved devices. Without their commitment to this enterprise of continuing study and improvement, none of this work would be possible.

We also gratefully acknowledge the leadership and teachings of Professor John P. Collier, Director of the Dartmouth Biomedical Engineering Center (DBEC) for Orthopaedics. He has been the leader and an integral part of each investigation carried out at the DBEC laboratory over the past three decades. We also thank Dr. Michael B. Mayor for his ongoing dedication to the study and documentation of implant retrievals. The studies on which this chapter is built are combined efforts by all the faculty, researchers, and graduate students of the DBEC.

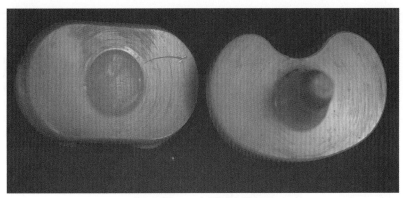

Scratching on LCS tibial insert
retrieved after 19 years (left),
Sigma rotating platform at 1 week (right)

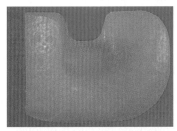

Standard gamma-nitrogen insert
(in vivo 3.2 years)

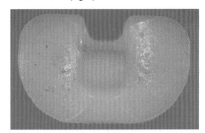

Highly cross-linked insert
(in vivo 1.5 years).

FIG 24.1 Scratching and pitting are common on retrieved knee bearings and often represent visible damage, but not loss of material in the form of debris. Improvements to polyethylene, such as cross-linking, do not prevent scratching or pitting caused by third-body debris. (A) Scratching on an LCS tibial insert retrieved at 19 years *(left)* and a Sigma RP retrieved at 1 week *(right)*. (B) Gamma–nitrogen barrier packaged insert at 3.2 years. (C) HXL polyethylene insert at 1.5 years. *LCS*, Low-contact stress.

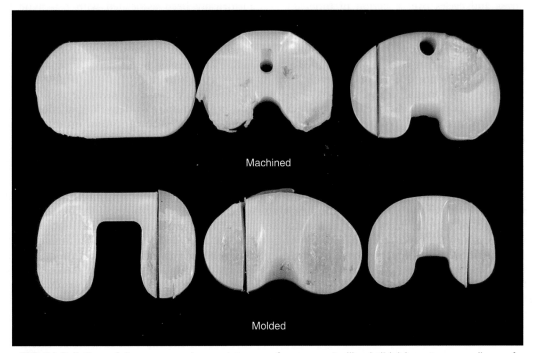

FIG 24.2 Fatigue failure occurs in most types of gamma-sterilized tibial inserts, regardless of design, material, or method of fabrication—machined *(top row)* or molded *(bottom row)*.

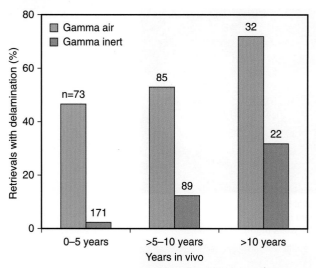

FIG 24.3 Incidence of fatigue failure in tibial bearings increases with time in vivo as oxidation and cycles of use increase. Higher initial oxidation means fewer cycles before failure. However, even gamma barrier–sterilized inserts eventually oxidize and are therefore subject to fatigue over the longer term. (From Berry DJ, Currier BH, Mayor MB, Collier JP: Gamma-irradiation sterilization in an inert environment: a partial solution. *Clin Orthop* 470(7):1805–1813, 2012.)

in air failed after shorter in vivo durations if they were first stored on the shelf. More recent findings have shown that even gamma barrier–sterilized inserts eventually oxidize and therefore are subject to fatigue over the longer term (Fig. 24.3).[7]

From a clinical perspective, it is difficult to predict when a device will fail because of fatigue mechanisms. Whereas most industrial fatigue life calculations only need to account for the distribution of stress and cycles over a period of time, the orthopedic engineer needs to be cognizant of the changes in material properties and the magnitude of stresses as a function of time. It is difficult, if not impossible, to gauge this for an individual patient, and fatigue failure is therefore identified as being more likely to happen once a component reaches a threshold oxidation value.[7,22] Although perhaps an oversimplification of the complex chemical-mechanical system, using such threshold values has helped researchers predict failure for long-duration retrievals.

Retrieved gamma air– and gamma barrier–sterilized tibial bearings show articular surface fatigue failure. This fatigue failure is driven by the oxidation of ultra–high-molecular-weight polyethylene (UHMWPE) and the resulting decrease in mechanical properties.[7] It is important to note that the debris released from these types of failed surfaces is not necessarily biologically active. Analyses of the functional biologic activity of wear debris have demonstrated a much stronger biologic response to debris in the submicrometer size range.[40,43] Debris from a device that fails through fatigue failure is orders of magnitude larger, often several millimeters in size.

The mechanism of UHMWPE debris generation has been well characterized in the literature.[†] It is generally understood

that oxidation, and therefore reduction of mechanical properties, happens at a faster rate below the exposed surface of a tibial bearing. This is independent of whether the material is exposed to oxygen on the shelf or to oxidizing species in the body.[7,22] In most knee designs, complete conformity is avoided to allow for femoral translation and rotation relative to the tibia. As a result, the nonconforming tibiofemoral contact sets up a stress environment in which the maximum contact stress is developed below the contact surface. Although the maximum subsurface oxidation and subsurface stress are not related to each other, they exist at approximately the same depth. This coincidental colocation allows for a mechanical situation in which cracks can nucleate and propagate to the surface from a depth of about 1 mm. If the cracks propagate immediately to the surface, 1-mm-dimension polyethylene pieces will spall off the device. If the cracks first propagate parallel to the surface before turning toward the articular region, even larger debris will be generated.

Current generation cross-linked UHMWPE formulations are designed to be resistant to oxidation and thereby avoid the colocation of applied stress and degraded material that has commonly led to fatigue failure of earlier tibial bearing materials. As will be covered later in this chapter, current retrieval studies are focused on monitoring these new bearing materials to investigate the effects of long-term exposure to the in vivo environment.

Adhesive and Abrasive Wear. Adhesive and abrasive wear is the process whereby small particles of bearing material are generated at the contact surface and become fine debris. This fine-particle generation is driven by abrasion and adhesion rather than by oxidative degradation. Adhesive and abrasive wear is an inevitable result of all intended articulations (Fig. 24.4); however, it can be easily masked by contact fatigue failure whereby large flakes of material are delaminated and removed.

Fine particulate debris from adhesive/abrasive wear has historically been associated with osteolytic response in hip arthroplasty. In hips, where adhesive/abrasive wear predominates, wear rates of 0.1 mm/year are thought to be sufficient to cause osteolysis.[33,65] The principal mechanism leading to bearing failure in knees has historically been contact fatigue damage on the articular surface.[42,53,86]

However, because contact fatigue failure is addressed by efforts to minimize oxidative degradation of the polyethylene, more attention is being focused on the backside wear of knee inserts. It has been recognized that in modular knee bearings, backside wear mechanisms of abrasion and burnishing can produce small debris particles of the size implicated as the cause of osteolysis.[63,87] Other studies have documented the effect of backside wear on the locking mechanisms for different modular knee systems.[16,66,73]

Adhesive and abrasive wear has been extensively studied over the last three decades, and a thorough discussion of the proposed mechanism is beyond the scope of this chapter. Currently the most widely accepted theory of adhesive and abrasive wear is that the stresses induced during multidirectional articulation orient the polyethylene molecules and, through strain hardening, improve wear behavior in one direction.[67,84] If stresses are applied to this oriented material through crossing motion, as observed in the hip and to a lesser extent in the knee, the directionally oriented polymer wears quickly because of what is termed a *strain-softening effect*.[34,85]

[†]References 34, 38, 49, 51, 67, and 84.

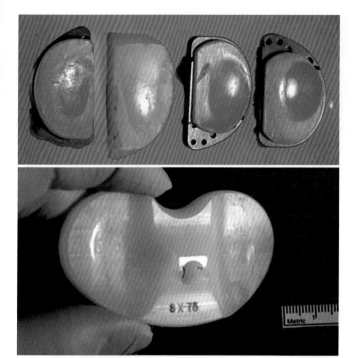

FIG 24.4 (A) Retrieved unicondylar tibial inserts (in vivo 1 to 4.8 years) illustrate articular surface wear. (B) Anatomic graduated component (AGC) (Biomet, Warsaw, IN) gamma-barrier insert, 9.5 years in vivo, showing articular surface abrasive/adhesive wear, but having minimal oxidation and no fatigue damage.

Cross-linking has been known to reduce wear in vitro and in vivo.[5,52,57,69,80] It is theorized that the primary mechanism for this phenomenon is a reduction of the plastic deformation of the near-surface polyethylene, as well as the strengthening of intermolecular bonds. For example, Edidin et al.[34] have shown that cross-linked polyethylene possesses a shallower plastic deformation zone. Muratoglu et al.[58] have shown wear resistance to be highly correlated with cross-link density, and Wang[84] has modeled the phenomenon with similar results.

Adhesive and abrasive wear is also common on the backside of fixed-bearing modular knees of many designs and types of locking mechanism (Fig. 24.5). With adhesive and abrasive wear, appearances can be deceiving, and this highlights the importance of the distinction between damage and wear (Fig. 24.6). It is therefore imperative that the researcher quantify material removal, rather than simply qualify the appearance of a surface.

Quantifying Wear

Retrieval studies have allowed the detailed assessment of all aspects of knee-bearing inserts and provide the opportunity for quantitative measurement of wear, provided that appropriate unworn reference surfaces are present and original dimensions are available. Knee inserts, by nature of their complex geometry, lack the intradevice reference frame provided by the spherical geometry of a hip implant. It has become clear that accurate and reliable wear data would be greatly enhanced by the inclusion of fiducial marks or wires embedded at known locations at manufacture of the bearings. In the absence of such

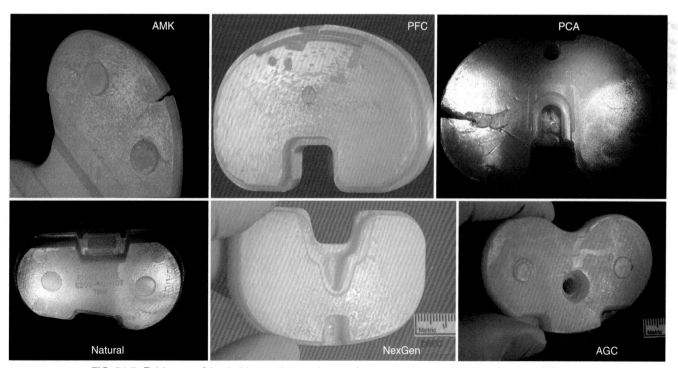

FIG 24.5 Evidence of backside motion and wear is common on retrievals of many different modular fixed-bearing knee designs. The insert-tray relative motion indicated by the patterns and backside wear features is most often rotational motion. Torque from the femoral component is not effectively resisted by arc-shaped peripheral capture rims, or by centrally located locking mechanisms.

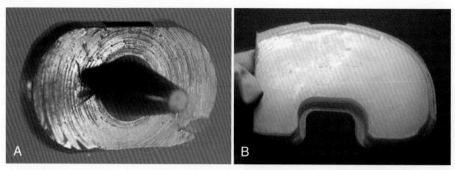

FIG 24.6 With knee wear, appearances can be deceiving, as evidenced by this pair of retrievals. (A) A scratched and pitted LCS insert in vivo 12.8 years, with measured backside wear of 267 mm³. (B) A much smoother, less damaged appearance of a PFC insert in vivo 11.8 years, with estimated backside wear of 1742 mm³.

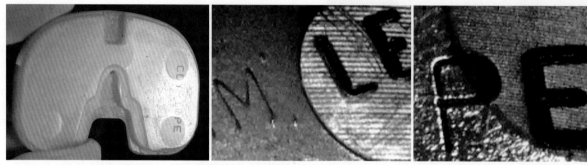

FIG 24.7 Extrusions, or pegs, on the backsides of knee inserts often appear in correspondence to screw holes in tibial trays. They may result from plastic creep of the material or as unworn plateaus of polyethylene remaining after the surrounding material was worn away, or a combination of the two. The different mechanisms have different implications regarding the generation of debris.

references provided by the manufacturers, deformation in knee inserts is ambiguous. An instructive example of this is the presence of so-called pegs, or extrusions of polyethylene, on the backside surfaces of inserts (Fig. 24.7). They can be interpreted as cold flow of an unsupported area of thin polyethylene, which would not entail loss of material, or they can be interpreted as polyethylene remaining after the surrounding material was worn away. The two interpretations have different implications regarding debris and its clinical impact.

Damage and wear on the articular (top side) of knee inserts have been documented in numerous studies. Cracking and delamination caused by oxidative fatigue of the polyethylene have been the primary modes of insert failure.[7,22,60] It is evident that wear has occurred because material has been delaminated and removed in relatively large pieces. However, accurately quantifying the amount of material lost is challenging. Gravimetric methods are not useful with retrievals because reference weights are not known. Geometry on the top-side surfaces of knee inserts is complex, consisting almost entirely of curved surfaces with sweeps and blends between them, usually with no reliable datum surface from which depths can be measured. Surface scanning and coordinate measuring machine metrology have been used with some success,[44,61,72] but warping of the inserts from extended in vivo duration and from the process of retrieval can far exceed the dimensional changes caused by wear, especially those from adhesive and abrasive wear.

A number of methods have been used to quantify the amount of material lost because of insert wear, ranging from gauging the depth of stamped manufacturer labels to laser surface scanning and computed tomography of bearings. A progression of published studies that report estimated in vivo wear rates for knee bearing inserts and the methods used are summarized in Table 24.1.

There are some notable general findings that can be taken from this group of studies. The measured wear rates of tibial bearings in terms of depth penetration ranges from 0.03 to 0.09 mm/year, and for the studies of larger series the rate narrows to 0.04 to 0.07 mm/year. Wear rate tends to be higher when calculated for short implantation time. This may reflect a bedding-in period and it likely also reflects measurement error and part thickness variation in the rate calculation with short time divisors. Reported wear rates of mobile bearings tend to be lower than fixed bearings. Damage rating based on visual appearance does not correlate to quantified material lost. When there is a wear bias, it is greater on the medial side. When distinguishable, backside wear is a significant contributor to total wear in fixed-bearing and mobile-bearing inserts. However, backside surfaces of mobile bearings do not incur more rapid wear than do fixed inserts.

Many modular knee designs use a peripheral capture mechanism that follows the curve of the anterior aspect of the tibial plateau. This locking geometry is not well suited to resist the

TABLE 24.1　Summary of Studies Reporting Quantitative Wear of Knee Bearings

Study	Bearing Type	Implant	N	In Vivo Avg Months (Range)	Assessment Method	Wear Rate	Notes/Findings
Argenson and O'Connor[1]	MB Uni	Oxford	23	39 (12–108)	Dial gauge measurement, NI inserts for reference	0.026–0.043 mm/year	Highly congruent; gamma-sterilized poly
Plante-Bordeneuve and Freeman[68]	FB	Freeman-Swanson	27	65 (45–80)	Dial gauge measurement, known design thickness	0.025 mm/year	Aberrant wear components omitted from average
Sanzén et al.[76]	FB	PCA	158	84 (58–116)	Plane radiographs	0.15 mm/year OA 0.08 mm/year RA	Rates estimated from group averages
Psychoyios et al.[70]	MB uni	Oxford	16	72 (10–154)	Dial gauge measurement, known design thickness	0.036 mm/year	Impingement had a big impact on wear rate
Benjamin et al.[6]	FB	AMK+PFC Synatomic	24 9	68 (9–132)	Through-thickness measurement Laser scan for volume Visual rating of damage pattern (1–6)	0.35 mm/year 794 mm³/year n/a	Wear rates decreased with duration
Lavernia et al.[54]	FB	PCA	28	74 (28–35)	Thickness measurement, NI used as reference	0.127 mm/year	Wear rate correlated to duration in this postmortem study
Collier et al.[14]	MB	LCS-MB	50	82	Dial gauge measurement	0.05 mm/year	Through-thickness measurement gave total wear estimate
Conditt et al.[17]	FB	AMK	15	91 (36–146)	Linear laser scans of backside, 3D computer reconstruction for vol.	138 mm³/year	Significantly more wear medially
Mayor et al.[56]	FB	PFC			Insert thickness compared to design drawings; backside wear reported	0.05 mm/year 99 mm³/year	Greater backside wear posterior and medial
Crowninshield et al.[18]	FB	NexGen	43	33 (2–80)	Visual rating of damage modes (0–3) Profilometry of engraved lettering	n/a 4.1 µm/year	Damage modes: no correl. w/ duration Backside wear has partial association with duration.
Kop and Swarts[50]	MB RP	AP Glide LCS	10 7	31 (10–51) 36 (9–70)	CMM, with math. reconstruction of unworn surfaces Visual rating of damage modes (0–3)	0.09 mm/year 80 mm³/year n/a	Same rates for both designs and no medial-lateral wear bias
Atwood et al.[3]	RP	LCS	100	41 (2–170)	Through-thickness measurement Backside surface only measurement	0.09 mm/year 0.06 mm/year	High initial wear rate, lower long-term rate; no medial-lateral bias 59% had <2-year duration
Engh et al.[37]	FB MB	AMK LCS-MB	31 23	32 (1–141) 29 (1–102)	Through-thickness measurement on n = 12 Visual rating of damage modes (0–3)	0.047 mm/year 0.048 mm/year n/a	Surface damage did not reflect material lost
Currier et al.[24]	FB	PFC & Sigma	220	127 (2–226)	Dimensional measurement, design drawings used as reference	0.038 mm/year	Backside-only wear
Van Citters et al.[82]	FB	NexGen	60	27 (0.1–86)	Through-thickness measurement Short duration (<10 mo) reference	0.05 mm/year	Conventional and XL poly showed similar wear rates
Kendrick et al.[47]	MB	Oxford Uni	47	101 (13–200)	Measured bearing thickness	0.07 mm/year	Highest wear with extra-articular impingement
Currier et al.[23]	MB	Sigma RP	76	34 (0.4–105)	Dial gauge thickness with design dimension from manufacturer as reference	0.023 mm/year	Wear is total through-thickness; no medial-lateral bias
Kendrick et al.[48]	MB	Oxford Uni	13	251 (206–311)	Radiostereometric analysis, component edge detection for insert thickness	0.022–0.070 mm/year	Lower total penetration rate seen for Phase 2 bearing design
Berry et al.[8]	FB RP	Sigma Sigma RP	218 94	65 (2.1–179) 39 (0.4–124)	Through-thickness and backside measurement Backside wear volume calculated Through-thickness measurement	0.07 mm/year total 0.02 backside; 44 mm³/year 0.04 mm/year	FBs: Medial wear bias; wear rate increases with duration RPs: No medial wear bias; wear rate does not increase with duration No wear difference between CR and PS inserts in either design
Teeter et al.[79]	FB	Genesis II	16	32 (0.5–86)	Micro-CT; NI inserts as control	0.049 mm/year	Total thickness deviation Duration <1 year excluded
Engh et al.[36]	FB MB	Sigma LCS + Sig RP	12 12	52(13–107) 53(12–108)	Micro-CT with matched NI controls	74 mm³/year 43 mm³/year	Backside wear is 5% of total on RP, 24% on FB; net wear is 69% of penetration
Rad et al.[72]	FB	NexGen	54	65	Laser scanning; mathematical reconstruction of original surface	0.16 mm/year 31 mm³/year	Articular surface wear only, no backside wear included.

3D, 3-Dimensional; *AMK*, anatomic modular knee; *AP*, anteroposterior; *CMM*, coordinate measuring machine; *CR*, cruciate retaining; *CT*, computed tomography; *FM*, fixed bearing; *LCS*, low contact stress; *MB*, mobile bearing; *NI*, never implanted; *OA*, osteoarthritis; *PCA*, porous-coated anatomic; *PFC*, press-fit condylar; *PS*, posterior stabilized; *RA*, rheumatoid arthritis; *RP*, rotating platform; *XL*, cross-linked.

torque applied to the insert by the femur by rotation under loaded flexion, and a centrally located locking mechanism is not effective at resisting tibiofemoral rotation. As backside wear progresses, the tightness of fit of the capture mechanisms is compromised. As a result, the locking geometry becomes less effective and allows more relative motion, which in turn promotes further wear. This progression of motion and wear is evident with even qualitative visual assessment of knees of a variety of designs (see Fig. 24.5). Efforts to devise locking mechanisms that better resist torque and geometries that are not progressively degraded by the observed backside wear patterns appear to be warranted.

FACTORS INVOLVED IN KNEE WEAR

Conformity

A notable observation from the study by Mayor et al.[56] is that backside wear had a strong dependence on the articular geometry of the insert. One of the three bearing geometries of the implant series studied is relatively flat in the anteroposterior (AP) plane and that geometry stands apart, with significantly lower wear penetration and wear rate than the other two more conforming insert designs. One implication of this finding is that torque transmitted to the insert by the femoral component can be a primary driver of backside motion and wear of the insert. This effect was confirmed in a study by Schwarzkopf et al. (Fig. 24.8).[77]

Retrieved inserts from posterior-stabilized knees frequently show damage that can affect the strength and failure resistance of the bearing, and also shed light on tibiofemoral alignment and articulation. Posterior-stabilized knee bearings with a post-and-cam mechanism are designed for contact of the femoral component on the posterior aspect of the post. The anterior facet and top of the post are generally not designed to incur significant contact and wear with normal knee articulation. A study by Puloski et al.[71] looked at retrievals of four different knee designs at an average of 3 years in vivo. They found damage

on 40% of the surface areas of posts, and damage to the anterior and lateral aspects of the posts was frequent and notable. Of the retrievals in that study, 30% had severe post damage and gross loss of polyethylene.

A retrieval study by Currier et al.[27] reported that 41% of retrievals of three commonly used posterior-stabilized knee designs show impingement damage across the anterior face of the post; deformation of the anterior corners of the posts and of the top crest of the posts occurred in 86% of those retrievals (Fig. 24.9). Whereas impingement was seen most frequently on the posterior face of the posts in all designs, the frequency in other zones indicates that tibiofemoral contact extends beyond the expected articulation of the cam against the posterior face of the post. Impingement across the anterior face of posts can be caused by hyperextension, knee instability, subsidence of the femur into the tibia with progressive articular wear, or a combination of these factors. The distinction between impingement uniformly across the anterior of the post and impingement at the anterior corners of the post helps distinguish rotation from simple hyperextension. More rotational impingement gives rise to a bow-tie appearance on the anterior surface of the post.

Tibiofemoral rotation to the design limit of the post-and-cam mechanism occurs frequently and with sufficient force to plastically deform the post in rotation. It is not uncommon for posterior stabilized insert retrievals to show permanent torsional deformation of the post (Fig. 24.10).

Cement

The role of cement in exacerbating wear of knee inserts is poorly understood, in large part because of a lack of uncemented retrievals that can be quantitatively assessed. Cementless fixation of knee components was inspired by the success of cementless hip arthroplasty and the failure of many cemented knees. Reliable ingrowth of the femoral and patellar components was generally achieved, but ingrowth of the tibial trays was far less frequently observed in retrievals.[13] Examination of many different types of designs made it clear that secure initial fixation was the key to ingrowth. The addition of porous-coated pegs and the use of screws dramatically improved the likelihood of well-fixed tibial components.

Paradoxically, as the problems with these systems were identified and solved, improvements in cemented fixation were leading many clinicians back to cemented designs. There were advances in cement mixing techniques and increased consistency and quality among batches.[41,45,55] Furthermore, these less technically demanding installations used devices that were less expensive than porous-coated components.

A study that looked at the backside surface wear of cemented versus cementless knees, controlled for knee design, including articular geometry, showed a significantly lower wear rate in the cementless group (Fig. 24.11).[25] That study further reported that 86% of the uncemented knee inserts had no discernible locking mechanism wear. This comparative study concluded that cement debris may play a larger role in the wear of tibial inserts than previously thought and that cementless fixation in knees has the potential to reduce insert wear significantly.

Tibial Tray

An important design objective of modular knee arthroplasty devices is to allow intraoperative flexibility and ease of bearing replacement. The intent in so-called fixed-bearing knees has been to lock the insert securely onto the metal tray so that

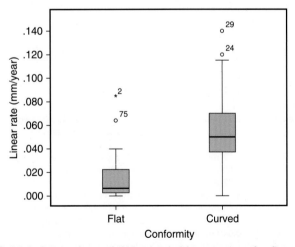

FIG 24.8 Comparison of linear backside wear rate for flat and curved inserts, indicating that the more conforming inserts incur more backside wear, likely owing to more effective transmission of torque from the femoral component. (From Schwartzkopf R, Scott RD, Carlson EM, et al: Does increased topside conformity in modular total knee arthroplasty lead to increased backside wear? *Clin Orthop* 473(1):220–225, 2015)

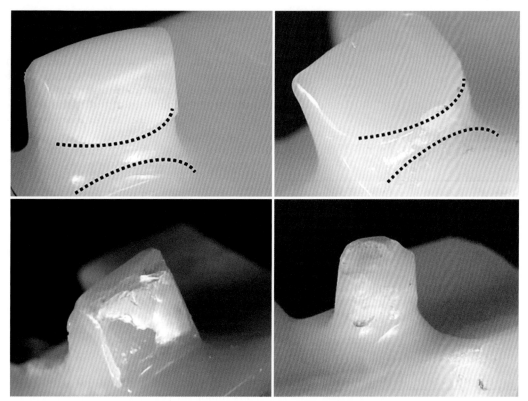

FIG 24.9 Studies of retrieved posterior-stabilized knees with tibial posts have reported that impingement and notable material loss occurs frequently on the anterior and lateral aspects of posts, and even more frequently on the anterior corners, resulting in the bow-tie wear pattern.

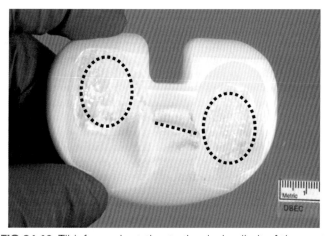

FIG 24.10 Tibiofemoral rotation to the design limit of the post-and-cam mechanism occurs frequently and with sufficient force to plastically deform the post in rotation. This retrieval shows malalignment in its articular wear pattern and a 10-degree permanent rotational deformation of the post.

relative motion of the components in vivo is prevented. However, despite the robustness of the insert-to-tray locking mechanism or its design, it is not practical in engineering terms to entirely eliminate relative motion at the interface between the components under in vivo loads. The metal tray and the UHMWPE insert have large differences in material properties that will govern relative motion under load. Moreover, any wear of the

backside surface of knee inserts in modular fixed bearings can degrade the mechanisms that lock the inserts onto the base plates.[16,35,66,73]

Studies of knee devices have documented that modular knees designed as fixed bearings are in fact not fixed in place, but move and experience abrasive wear. Parks et al.[66] performed an important in vitro study measuring the multidirectional motion of tibial inserts in tray locking mechanisms with clinically relevant loads. Studies of retrievals from several centers have documented marked wear of UHMWPE caused by relative motion.[15,35,56,60,64] Although this relative displacement is often termed *micromotion*, it is clear that the impact of this motion can be a significant amount of wear debris.

Cast, Machined, and Grit-Blasted Trays. Historically, most tibial trays were cast from a titanium-vanadium-aluminum (Ti-6V-4Al) alloy, and were usually manufactured with a rough (nonpolished) surface against which the insert was mated. These nonpolished tray surfaces readily show stippling marks, which clearly indicate a rotational motion pattern of inserts in their trays (Figs. 24.12 to 24.14). The rotational pattern tends to confirm that torque applied by the femoral component is the main driver for the backside micromotion. Dennis et al.[31,32] published a series of studies based on fluoroscopic analyses of knees that document axial rotation of healthy nonimplanted knees and knees with implants of a variety of designs. Although normal knees have shown the most relative rotation, implanted knees also undergo significant rotation (eg, >8 degrees) and associated femoral translations. The maximum rotation occurs at deepest knee flexion, when the load on the bearing is high.

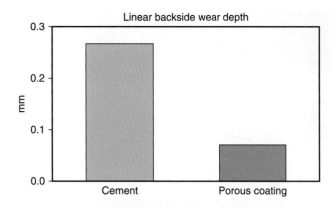

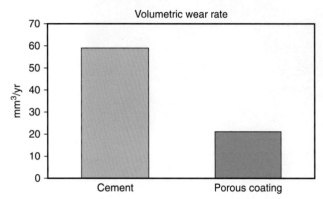

FIG 24.11 The presence of cement is shown to be a significant factor in backside wear of knee inserts. In a study of PFC fixed-bearing knees, controlling for the effect of articular geometry, those knees with cement fixation on the tibia or femur or both showed significantly more backside wear and a higher backside wear rate than knees with uncemented fixation of the femoral and tibial components.[25]

The concurrence of greatest relative motion and high load leads to high wear.

The stippling marks are sites where debris particles have caused wear with cyclic shifting of the insert (see Fig. 24.13). The debris that facilitates this tray stippling and the corresponding inverse marks on the polyethylene inserts can be from a number of sources—bone cement, porous-coating beads, bone chips, steel from surgical tools and instruments, and abrasive compounds used in device manufacturing.

Metal debris resulting from the generation of tray stippling marks can affect knee performance in at least two ways. First, the debris can exacerbate the wear process by being an abrasive medium on any surface where it resides or to which it migrates. Second, the breakdown of metal debris particles can contribute to metal ion concentration in the joint space and circulatory system.

Polished Trays. The incorporation of a polished metal tray surface aims to address the problem of backside wear of knee inserts. Fixed-bearing knee retrievals having a polished metal tray do not, in general, show the stippling marks seen on unpolished trays, but stippling has been seen in some cases on cemented polished trays (Fig. 24.15). Assessment of the effect of a polished tray in reducing insert wear requires a direct comparison of the clinical wear performance of a polished tray with a control series having an unpolished tray of the same knee design. Such a comparison was reported by Berry et al. and showed a significantly lower backside wear rate for inserts against polished CoCr trays (0.006 mm/year) than for inserts against grit-blasted titanium alloy trays (0.02 mm/year).[8]

Although the comparison offered by the Berry study had relatively short implantation times for the newer polished tray design, a follow-up of those series indicates that the lower wear rate of the polished tray has been maintained out to 6 years (Fig. 24.16).[81]

MOBILE-BEARING KNEES

Mobile-bearing knee retrievals open up an entirely new arena of observations on bearing damage, bearing wear, and in vivo kinematics. Mobile-bearing knees are an appealing alternative to fixed-bearing knees in that they address the problems of loosening of the tibial tray and of rotational malalignment. A potential disadvantage of mobile bearings, however, is the addition of the backside insert-tray interface, which is a wear surface of relatively large area. The wear performance of this additional articular surface is critical in how mobile bearings perform in terms of generating polyethylene wear debris and associated osteolysis.

The first mobile-bearing knee was the Oxford unicompartmental knee replacement, and early reports of wear measurements were published by its developers. Argenson and O'Connor,[1] in 1982, reported on a series of 23 retrieved Oxford bearings with in vivo durations of 1 to 9 years and found an overall penetration rate of between 0.026 and 0.043 mm/year, depending on the method used to calculate it. A later study on a small series out to 13 years confirmed a wear rate of 0.036 mm/year.[70] These knee bearings were all sterilized by gamma radiation and were therefore subject to oxidation and associated contact fatigue. However, being a highly congruent implant at all flexion angles, high contact stresses were avoided and loss of material through fatigue failure was not widely seen.

Studies that include larger series of retrievals and draw comparisons with fixed-bearing knee retrievals help in evaluating the performance of mobile bearings in the context of other designs. A retrieval study reported by Collier et al.[14] looked at a series of 192 mobile-bearing retrievals and compared them with a cohort of 619 fixed-bearing devices. In that study, the most commonly stated reason for retrieval of all devices was pain, more than 40% in both series, with no difference between fixed- and mobile-bearing retrievals. The second most common reason for retrieval in the fixed-bearing series was loosening, and here the mobile bearings performed significantly better, with an 8% incidence compared with 19% for fixed bearings. Mobile bearings also had a significantly lower incidence of patellar wear-through or fracture, which indicates that at least in that retrieval series, the lack of rotational constraint in the device was not detrimental to the patella. The results would tend to indicate that the ability of the devices to self-align was beneficial in terms of patellar damage and wear. A more detailed quantitative wear analysis of a mobile-bearing series was done by Atwood et al.,[3] which looked at 100 low contact stress (LCS) rotating platform (RP) knee retrievals (DePuy Orthopaedics). Wear measurements were made on the top articular surface (flexion interface) and backside (rotation interface) independently, using embedded marker wires as a reference. The total wear penetration, as determined by insert thickness change, decreased within the manufacturing tolerance but was

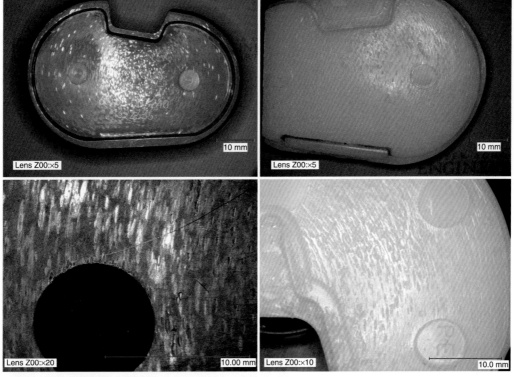

FIG 24.12 Rotational motion patterns seen on backside interfaces from nonpolished trays result from arc marks on the polyethylene insert and stippling marks on the tray surface. These marks are sites at which debris particles have caused wear with cyclic shifting of the insert in the tray.

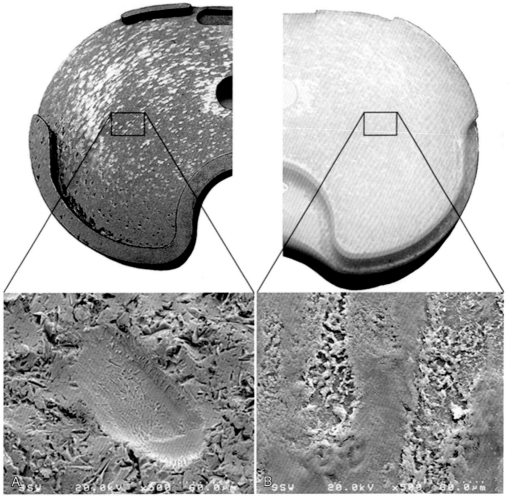

FIG 24.13 Scanning electron microscopy imaging of titanium alloy tray stippling (A) and corresponding arc marks in the poly insert (B). (From Brandt et al.[10])

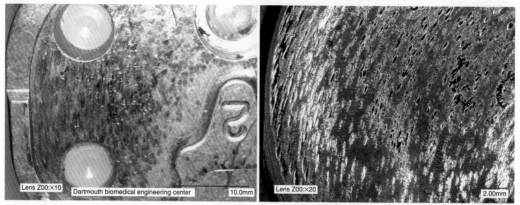

FIG 24.14 Nonpolished titanium alloy surfaces readily show a rotational motion pattern of the insert in the tray.

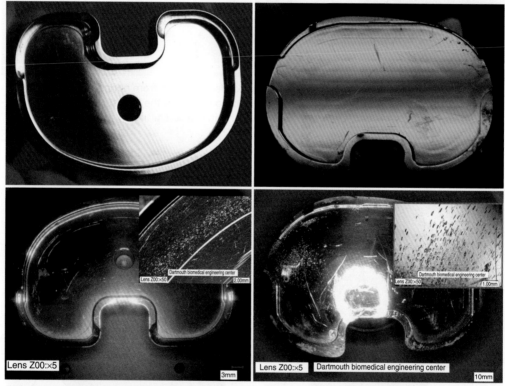

FIG 24.15 Fixed-bearing knee retrievals having a polished metal tray do not in general show the extent and frequency of stippling marks seen on unpolished trays; however, stippling can occur on cemented polished trays: polished CoCr *(left)* and polished titanium alloy *(right)*.

statistically identifiable. The average rate of wear on the rotation surface (backside) was 0.06 ± 0.2 mm/year (Fig. 24.17). More than 50% of the bearings in this series were in vivo less than 2 years, resulting in an overall distribution heavily weighted toward short durations. A subsequent study of another RP design showing longer-term follow-up reported an average total through-thickness wear rate of 0.027 mm/year (Fig. 24.18).[23]

The wear of the RPs in both series mentioned previously was determined to be uniform across the rotation surface. This is in contrast to studies on the press-fit condylar (PFC)[19,56] and NexGen knees,[83] which found that in these fixed-bearing designs, the backside surface typically wears unevenly.

This may reflect a bedding-in period and also likely reflects measurement error and part thickness variation in the rate calculation with short time divisors. For mobile bearings, the wear rate displays evidence of a bedding-in period[30,78] more strongly than that seen in fixed bearings (see Figs. 24.17 and 24.18 compared to Fig. 24.16). This may be indicative of contamination of the joint space with third-body particles during implantation that migrated to the mobile bearing articulating surfaces; these were the retrievals that wore quickly and had to be revised sooner.

Statistical analysis has shown that the damage ratings do not correlate with the quantitative wear measurements.[26,37] This

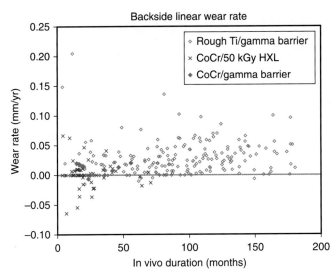

FIG 24.16 Linear backside wear rate of polished CoCr Sigma knees compared with an entire retrieval series of unpolished Ti-V-Al trays in the same design. The inserts from the polished tray knees have a significantly lower wear rate. The wear rate in the long-term series appears to be increasing with time in vivo. The increasing backside wear rate is consistent with the observation that locking mechanisms wear over time, leading to positive feedback between insert motion and insert wear. *HXL*, highly cross-linked.[81]

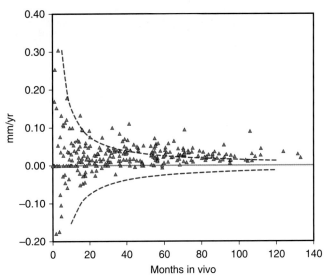

FIG 24.18 Wear rate (composite wear) for Sigma RPs versus duration in vivo. The average for all inserts is 0.027 mm/year. The dotted lines represent the imputed wear rate if the as-manufactured thickness of an insert falls at the low end of the part tolerance *(upper envelope)* or the high end of the part tolerance *(lower envelope)*.[23]

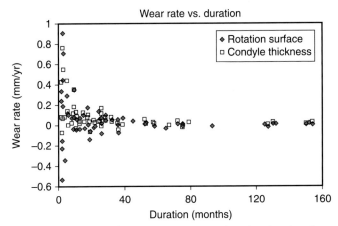

FIG 24.17 Calculated wear rate versus duration in vivo for a series of LCS RP knee inserts. The data are presented for the rotation surface (backside) and for the articular surface and backside surface combined (total condyle thickness change). The average backside wear rate on the rotation surface was 0.06 ± 0.2 mm/year. The backside wear rate for inserts in vivo greater than 24 months was 0.02 mm/year. (From Atwood SA, Currier JH, Mayor MB, et al: Clinical wear measurement on low contact stress rotating platform knee bearings. *J Arthroplasty* 23:431–440, 2008.)

result confirms that a worn appearance of the polyethylene does not indicate a large amount of material loss and again highlights the distinction between damage and wear. Retrievals of mobile bearings have demonstrated that severe damage to the articular surfaces arises within the first few months after implantation and can be indistinguishable from damage on a long-term knee

(Fig. 24.19). Detailed surface profilometry can be used to show that many damage features on mobile bearing backside surfaces are formed by plastic deformation rather than material removal. Machining marks are often found continuing without interruption through relatively deep pits and grooves (Fig. 24.20). The raised surfaces around damage features that are formed during plastic deformation of the material are subsequently worn down and/or plastically deformed downward to make the surface flatter and smoother over time. These raised features, such as the rims around pits and the raised edges of scratches, appear to bear much of the backside contact, perhaps shielding the surrounding backside surface area from loaded articulation. A characteristic common to most RP backside surfaces is evidence of unidirectional (ie, rotational) motion almost exclusively, with little to no cross-shear articulation or radial migration of debris (Fig. 24.21). This unidirectional motion and the polished CoCr tray counterface are likely important factors in the low wear rates reported for RP inserts, despite large articular surfaces, extensive motion, and clearly evident damage features.[3,23]

HIGHLY CROSS-LINKED POLYETHYLENE IN KNEES

The application of highly cross-linked (HXL) polyethylene in knee bearings has followed behind its application in hip bearings because the rolling-sliding contact of the knee does not provide the compelling rationale for reduced abrasive and adhesive wear seen in hips. If the problem of polyethylene oxidation and associated loss of mechanical properties is adequately addressed, the most common failure mode of knee bearings is eliminated.

Knee simulator studies have consistently shown marked improvement in adhesive and abrasive wear performance of

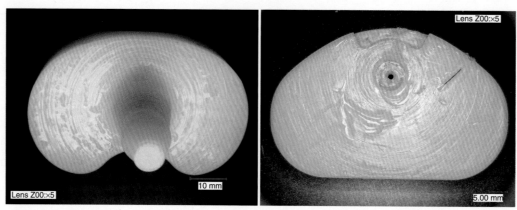

FIG 24.19 Retrieved mobile bearings demonstrate that severe damage to the articular surfaces can arise within the first few months after implantation: 9.5-year RP retrieval *(left)*, 14-month MBT retrieval *(right)*.

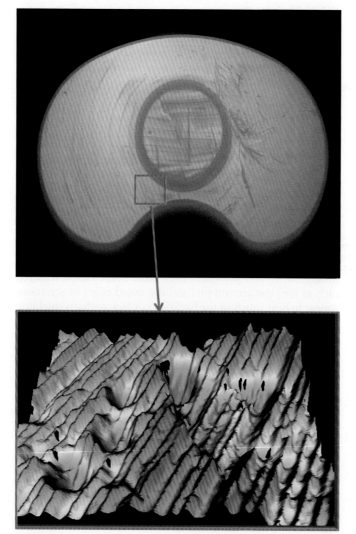

FIG 24.20 On mobile bearings, indentations from debris particle embedment often have preserved machining marks, indicating plastic deformation rather than material removal.

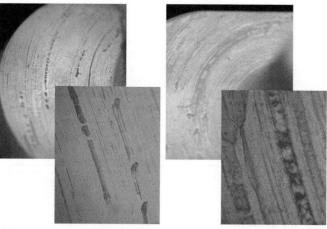

FIG 24.21 A characteristic common to most RP backside surfaces is evidence of unidirectional (ie, rotational) motion almost exclusively, with little to no cross-shear articulation or radial migration of debris. This is seen on porous-coated *(left)* and cemented knees *(right)*.

HXL knees relative to non–cross-linked counterparts,[‡] and most manufacturers offer HXL options in knee bearings. Studies of in vivo wear rates of HXL knees are few and the follow-up period is short in the results that have been presented. Recent results presented at Orthopaedic Research Society (ORS) in 2015 indicate that the wear rate of HXL polyethylene is trending lower compared to conventional polyethylene in three different tibial insert designs; however, the improvement is not statistically significant for any of the HXL materials at mean follow-up periods ranging from 28 to 55 months.[29] A more extensive comparison of clinical performance of HXL inserts compared to a matched cohort of conventional polyethylene inserts is offered by Currier et al.[21] There is no difference in measured wear rate of the two materials out to in vivo duration greater than 9 years (Fig. 24.22). These findings indicate that there are additional factors influencing in vivo wear of tibial inserts that are not fully accounted for in wear simulators and in computer modeling of wear.[69]

---

‡References 2, 11, 12, 40, 59, and 62.

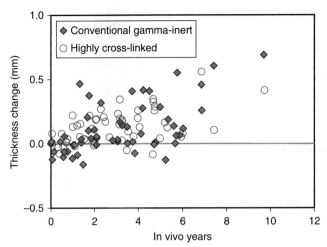

FIG 24.22 No statistically significant difference is seen in thickness change (wear) versus in vivo duration for HXL *(open circles)* and conventional gamma-N₂ sterilized *(solid diamonds)* tibial inserts. *HXL,* Highly cross-linked. (From Currier BH, Currier JH, Franklin KJ, et al: Comparison of wear and oxidation in retrieved conventional and highly cross-linked UHMWPE tibial inserts. *J Arthroplasty* 30(12):2349–2353, 2015.)

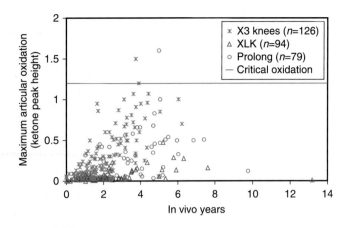

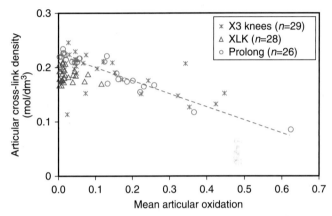

FIG 24.23 HXL materials in the knee have been shown to oxidize in the body at a rate indistinguishable from that of conventional gamma-barrier sterilized material *(left).*[28] Cross-link density of HXL material has been shown to decrease as it oxidizes.[74]

Additional findings of recent retrieval studies point to in vivo changes in HXL polyethylene that have the potential to significantly impact wear performance.[21,28] HXL materials in the knee are shown to oxidize in the body at a rate indistinguishable from that of conventional gamma-barrier sterilized material (Fig. 24.23). It is important to note that oxidation of polyethylene bearings was the root cause of susceptibility to fatigue damage in earlier generation gamma-sterilized inserts, as detailed earlier in this chapter. Furthermore, the cross-link density of the HXL material is shown to decrease as it oxidizes (see Fig. 24.23),[74] and it is the cross-link density of the polymer that produces its higher resistance to abrasive and adhesive wear. So although the early clinical wear data temper the high expectations based on simulator wear studies of HXL knee inserts, the unexpected finding of in vivo oxidation gives pause and bears close monitoring as follow-up times lengthen.

The articular surfaces of HXL polyethylene components can present the appearance of deformation and damage at least as great as conventional polyethylene, even with little to no wear. A qualitative study was published by Muratoglu et al.[63] comparing the articular and backside damage on HXL and conventional polyethylene tibial inserts. They found no difference in damage score between the two groups. Routine inspection of retrieved tibial inserts shows ample evidence of plastic deformation of the articular bearing surfaces, as well as pitting from debris indentation (Fig. 24.24). Studies by different groups have shown that much of this surface deformation is recoverable via the shape memory property of the polymer (Fig. 24.25).[60,62,83]

SUMMARY

No document written about retrieval studies is complete without acknowledgment of the limitations inherent in retrieval analysis. The implants that retrieval scientists have the opportunity to analyze are not representative of the overall population. By their nature, retrievals are generally failed devices. As the installed base of knee implants continues to grow into the millions, and the number of knee revisions grows to more than 60,000 per year, the sum of all retrieved devices submitted for analysis is a fraction of a percentage of those that are explanted.[9] It is impossible to extrapolate accurately based on this small and potentially biased sample; one can only identify phenomena.

As a result, the present discussion of knee wear has been put in the context of some key points that provide a framework for recognizing and comparing the wear trends that surgeons, engineers, and other medical professionals observe in knee performance:

- Wear and damage can be distinct processes in knee devices, and that distinction is very important with regard to the clinical impact of phenomena seen in these devices. Appearances can be deceiving with regard to wear.
- Quantitative measurement of true wear in knees is challenging because good reference data are difficult to obtain, especially in comparison to the data available for hips. Good fiducial points for wear measurement are rare and their implementation should be encouraged. In studies in which knee wear has been successfully quantified, it has been found that so-called fixed-bearing knees are seldom fixed, but in fact show bearing motion in the tibial trays, with resulting wear on the backsides. Mobile-bearing knees that eliminate crossing motion by allowing backside articulation tend to

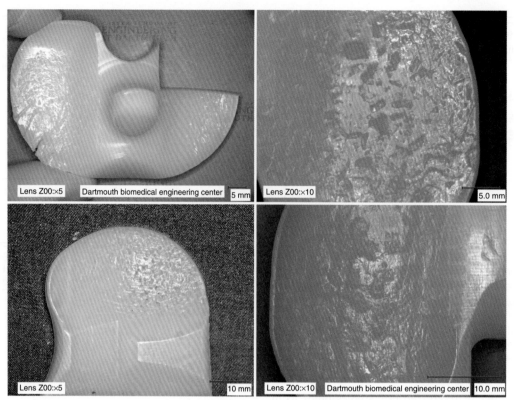

FIG 24.24 Routine inspection of retrieved HXL tibial inserts shows ample evidence of plastic deformation of the articular bearing surfaces, as well as pitting from debris indentation. HXL tibial inserts from four different manufacturers are shown here.

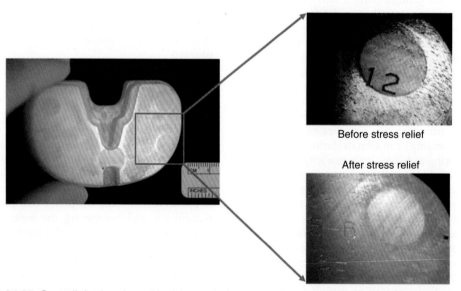

Before stress relief

After stress relief

FIG 24.25 Cross-linked and remelted insert before and after thermal stress relief in a vacuum oven. Some dimensional change is recovered through the shape memory effect, although some dimensional change must be attributed to material loss.

wear less. Polished tibial trays substantially reduce backside wear.

• The wear and damage observed in knee retrievals can convey important information about knee design and clinical inputs. For example, knee implants transmit substantial rotational torque to the tibial components, which results in damage and wear. Insert backside wear, when quantifiable, often exhibits more wear posteriorly and medially, reflecting the application of stress and tibiofemoral rotation under loaded flexion. Impingement on the posts of posterior-stabilized knee retrievals offers evidence that knees are aligned so that they commonly go into hyperextension.

This chapter on knee wear is based on the findings of careful analyses of retrieved devices that have been in clinical service.

Such an emphasis does not diminish the substantial effort and resources that have been, and continue to be, applied to in vitro testing and wear simulation of knee devices. In vitro wear testing is a critical part of the design process for new devices and of the process for obtaining regulatory approval to implant those devices. However, the most valid test of a joint arthroplasty device is by the patient. Weaknesses or shortcomings that arise in clinical service merit careful attention because they represent this, and they appropriately supersede test results and expectations based solely on laboratory studies by those developing and manufacturing the devices as part of their business. Historically, many shortcomings of arthroplasty devices were not foreseen and have been revealed only through retrieval studies. These studies should remain an integral part of documenting the successes of joint arthroplasty and guiding ongoing improvements.

KEY REFERENCES

3. Atwood SA, Currier JH, Mayor MB, et al: Clinical wear measurement on low contact stress rotating platform knee bearings. *J Arthroplasty* 23:431–440, 2008.

7. Berry DJ, Currier BH, Mayor MB, et al: Gamma-irradiation sterilization in an inert environment: a partial solution. *Clin Orthop* 470(7):1805–1813, 2012.

8. Berry DJ, Currier JH, Mayor MB, et al: Knee wear measured in retrievals: a polished tray reduces insert wear. *Clin Orthop* 470(7):1860–1868, 2012.

15. Conditt MA, Ismaily SK, Alexander JW, et al: Backside wear of modular ultra-high molecular weight polyethylene tibial inserts. *J Bone Joint Surg Am* 86:1031–1037, 2004.

17. Conditt MA, Thompson MT, Usrey MM, et al: Backside wear of polyethylene tibial inserts: mechanism and magnitude of material loss. *J Bone Joint Surg Am* 87A(2):326–331, 2005.

21. Currier BH, Currier JH, Franklin KJ, et al: Comparison of wear and oxidation in retrieved conventional and highly cross-linked UHMWPE tibial inserts. *J Arthroplasty* 30(12):2349–2353, 2015. <http://dx.doi.org/10.1016.j.arth.2015.06.014>.

22. Currier BH, Currier JH, Mayor MB, et al: In vivo oxidation of gamma-barrier-sterilized ultra-high-molecular-weight polyethylene bearings. *J Arthroplasty* 22:721–731, 2007.

23. Currier JH, Mayor MB, Collier JP, et al: Wear rate in a series of retrieved RP knees. *J ASTM Int* 8(3):172–184, 2011.

31. Dennis DA, Komistek RD, Mahfouz MR, et al: A multicenter analysis of axial femorotibial rotation after total knee arthroplasty. *Clin Orthop* 428:180–189, 2004.

32. Dennis DA, Komistek RD, Mahfouz MR, et al: Mobile-bearing total knee arthroplasty: do the polyethylene bearings rotate? *Clin Orthop* 440:88–95, 2005.

35. Engh GA, Lounici S, Rao AR, et al: In vivo deterioration of tibial baseplate locking mechanisms in contemporary modular total knee components. *J Bone Joint Surg Am* 83:2001, 1660–1665.

37. Engh GA, Zimmerman RL, Parks NL, et al: Analysis of wear in retrieved mobile and fixed bearing knee inserts. *J Arthroplasty* 24(Suppl 6):28–32, 2009.

48. Kendrick BJ, Simpson DJ, Kaptein BL, et al: Polyethylene wear of mobile-bearing unicompartmental knee replacement at 20 years. *J Bone Joint Surg Br* 93(4):470–475, 2011.

64. Noble PC, Conditt MA, Thompson MT, et al: Extraarticular abrasive wear in cemented and cementless total knee arthroplasty. *Clin Orthop* 416:120–128, 2003.

66. Parks NL, Engh GA, Topoleski LD, et al: The coventry award. Modular tibial insert micromotion. A concern with contemporary knee implants. *Clin Orthop* 356:10–15, 1998.

The references for this chapter can also be found on www.expertconsult.com.

25

The Asian Knee

Rajesh N. Maniar, Tushar Singhi, Parul R. Maniar

INTRODUCTION

Five decades of knee arthroplasty in the Western world have seen periodic modifications in implant design and technique to suit and match the requirements of the white population. The past two decades have seen an unprecedented surge in the demand for this surgery in Asian populations. In Asian populations knee arthroplasty is being performed using the same implants as in the Western world. With experience, a number of characteristics of the Asian knee that are distinctly different from the knees of white populations have been brought to the fore.

This chapter presents the scientific data and knowledge gained so far, with regard to the demographic differences, kinematic differences, and morphologic differences related to the knee and studied across Asian populations. The chapter also discusses their impact on the surgery of knee arthroplasty and their outcome. Lastly, it points to future directions to address the Asian knee characteristics and optimize its arthroplasty results.

DEMOGRAPHIC DIFFERENCES

Asians are more prone to knee osteoarthritis (OA) than that of the hip. The Asian hip to knee OA ratio is 1:9 as compared with 1:2 or 1:3 in white populations.[32,51] In patients undergoing knee arthroplasty the incidence of metabolic syndrome (body mass index (BMI) >30 kg/m^2, hypertension (HT), diabetes mellitus (DM) and hypercholesterolemia), which is a known risk factor of OA, was found to be 2 times higher in Asian compared with white populations.[39] Asian male to female ratio of knee OA is 1:4, as compared with a ratio of 1:1.5 in white populations.[129] It has been interestingly found that if OA was diagnosed on radiologic criteria alone, no significant difference in male to female prevalence remained in both populations.[129] In China and India, prevalence of OA in rural populations is reported as almost double to that in the urban population.[36,45]

Asian populations living in Western countries presented for total knee arthroplasty (TKA) at a stage when their knee function had deteriorated to a level much worse than that presented by white populations.[38,60] In our practice, one-third of Asian patients approach with severe deformities and late presentations (Fig. 25.1), usually with medial tibial defect in varus deformity. We prefer to treat the larger defects with autologous bone grafting, using a unique technique involving compression across the interface.[87]

DIFFERENCES IN BONE QUALITY

Bone Mineral Density

Asian populations have been found to have the lowest peak bone mineral density (BMD), the highest being in the Afro-Caribbean population, followed by white populations.[111,112,126,127] BMD in Indian women may be up to 25% to 30% lower than American-European scores.[94,111]

Vitamin D Deficiency and Rickets

In many Asian countries, vitamin D deficiency has been found to be rampant.[95] Vitamin D deficiency is the cause of rickets in children and osteomalacia and osteoporosis in adults. Genu varum or genu valgum has been described as the most common deformity in patients with rickets.[8,144] Varus knee is the main manifestation of osteomalacia.[149]

One study has reported that a 4% to 6% increase in varus alignment increased the loading in the medial compartment by up to 20%.[138] Such increased stress on the articular cartilage could lead to degenerative changes.[57] One other study found malalignment to be a risk factor for development of OA.[17] Varus deformity as a causative factor for OA needs to be evaluated further. However, a systematic review has shown that after OA has set in, a malaligned knee joint is more susceptible to progression of the OA.[138]

We recommend obtaining vitamin D blood levels in all Asian patients and treating any deficiency preoperatively. In our patients we have noted vitamin D–deficient patients showing poor Western Ontario and McMaster Universities (WOMAC) scores.[87a]

CULTURAL DIFFERENCES

The one trait distinctive of cultural activities across Asia is the requirement for the knee to go into deep flexion. Asian toilet facilities require a squatting position, prayer positions for Hindus and Buddhists involve sitting on the floor in a cross-legged position, a prayer position of Muslims entails kneeling in the *Namaz* position, the tea ceremony of Chinese involves kneeling in a different posture, and formal sitting in Japanese entails kneeling in the *seiza* position (Fig. 25.2). The popular yoga practice in Asia and certain Indian dance forms require the knee and many other joints to go into deep flexion and hyperextension. These activities cannot be overlooked because

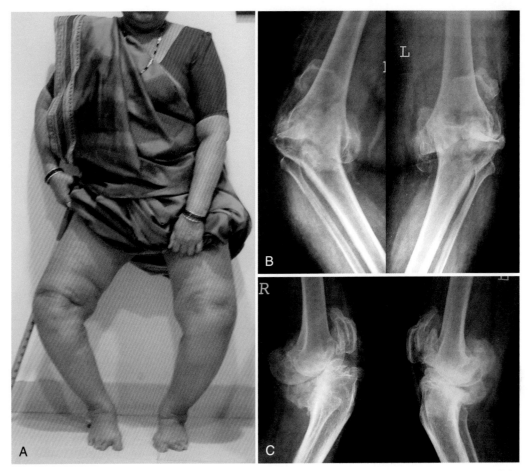

FIG 25.1 Clinical photograph (A) and radiographs (B and C) of a 52-year-old lady with severe OA knees with varus deformity of greater than 10 years' duration.

they are performed from early childhood and often several times a day.

KINEMATICS

Kneeling

Kneeling probably is the most common floor-based activity performed across the world. There are various forms of kneeling. White populations kneel with lesser hip and knee flexion compared with kneeling in *seiza*—a Japanese formal sitting position—or *Namaz*—a Muslim prayer position (see Fig. 25.2A to C and Table 25.1). These different forms of kneeling involve differences in the position of the ankle and torso.

Kinematic studies in knees of white populations have shown that with increasing flexion, there is posterior roll-back of the femoral contact point on the tibia and the lateral condyle excursion is far greater than medial condyle, so much so that in the final phase of deep flexion the lateral condyle slides off posteriorly from its contact on the tibial condyle.[68,69,75] There is also a subtle but definite and important difference in this movement between white and Japanese populations. In the Japanese the lateral condyle was found to have similar excursion as in the white population study, but the medial condyle remained much more stable with little excursion.[75] Other biomechanical studies have shown that repetitive kneeling can damage the cartilage and menisci in the natural knee, and the increased tibiofemoral

TABLE 25.1 Range of Movements in Different Floor-Based Deep Flexion Activities[10,47,158,159]

Parameters	Full Squatting	Cross-Legged Sitting	Kneeling (*Namaz, Seiza*)
Hip flexion	95° ± 27°	80°-101°	67°-119°
Knee flexion	157° ± 6°	130°-142°	144°-158°
Ankle plantar flexion	58° ± 14°	Minimal	32°-37°

contact pressures can lead to polyethylene wear in the implanted knee.[52,73]

Kneeling kinematics after TKA have been studied to follow normal knee kinematics, although it was observed that knee flexion angles were smaller and patella showed sagittal plane tilting.[1,12,134]

Cross-Legged Sitting

Cross-legged sitting, also known as the tailor or lotus posture (Fig. 25.1D), involves a complex combination of movements of the hip, knee, and ankle joints.[62,158] At the hip there is flexion (80 to 101 degrees), abduction (30 to 57 degrees), and external rotation (36 to 52 degrees); at the knee joint there is flexion (130

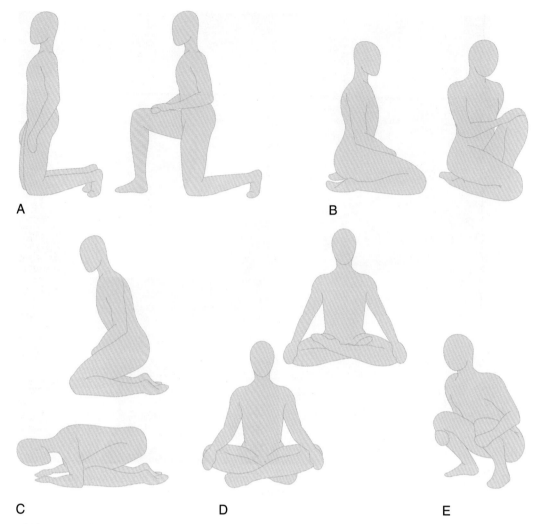

FIG 25.2 Different floor-based activities depicted—(A) kneeling (single leg and both legs), (B) *seiza* (single leg and both legs), (C) *Namaz* position, (D) cross-leg sitting (standard and lotus position), (E) squatting position. Illustrations by Kruttika Sequeira.

to 142 degrees) and internal rotation (17 to 34 degrees), and at the ankle there is minimal planter flexion assumed for this posture.

Cross-legged posture in Eastern culture is most frequently assumed while sitting on the floor, which means that it also entails getting into the posture from standing position and rising back into the standing position from the floor. Alternatively, this posture can be assumed on a higher surface, such as a bed or platform, which does not demand the additional maneuver of having to descend and ascend to or from the floor.

Squatting

Squatting is a resting postural complex that involves hyperflexion at the hip and knee joints, and hyperdorsiflexion at the ankle and subtalar joints (see Fig. 25.2E and Table 25.1). Squatting is an age-old posture assumed commonly for toilet facilities in India and other Asian countries. Even after knee OA sets in, squatting continues to be undertaken, especially in rural areas, out of necessity to use the toilet facility. A modified semi- or half-squat position may sometimes be adopted as a compromise. Squatting and partial squatting is also commonly performed as part of yoga, dance, and exercise. Apprehension exists in allowing this activity post-TKA for fear of increased stress on

the polyethylene and implant fixation, which could affect the long-term survival. A study by Nakamura et al. concluded that deep flexion did not affect the long-term durability of one high-flex ceramic implant.[110] In addition, a report by Mizu-Uchi concluded that squatting exerts forces 2.2 to 2.3 times the body weight, which is actually equivalent to that in walking.[70,102] Similarly Thambyah found that tibiofemoral contact force in squatting was not much different than in walking.[140] Indeed the ground reaction force was reported to be higher in walking than in squatting. On the other hand, they found that the tibiofemoral shear force, which is directed posteriorly in normal walking, becomes directed anteriorly in squatting.[140] It was also observed that the descent and ascent from a squatting position lead to higher contact forces.[29] These factors would have bearing on the stresses and fixation of tibial implant when squatting is undertaken after TKA.

Yoga and Dance

Yoga and Asian classical dance forms involve a combination of postures at the hip, knee, and ankle for which deep knee flexion is crucial (Fig. 25.3) along with hyperextension.

The kinematic differences seen in deep flexion, floor-based activities result in higher stresses on the ligaments and soft

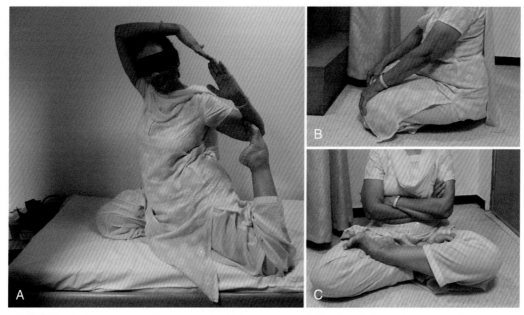

FIG 25.3 Patient performing yoga positions 5 years following left total knee replacement. (A) Mayuraasan, (B) Padmasan, and (C) Vajrasan.

tissues and increased contact forces across the knee joint. Kneeling has been shown to be most strenuous for the patellofemoral joint after TKA.[55] In addition, kinematics of deep knee flexion in squatting are shown to be different than other floor-based activities.[79]

MORPHOLOGICAL DIFFERENCES

Both tibiae and femurs in Asians are morphologically very different from white individuals. Measurements of their dimensions have been performed intraoperatively or radiologically on x-rays or computed tomography (CT) scan or in cadavers. This partly explains the variability in measurement seen among different Asian populations.

MECHANICAL AXIS

The mechanical axis (MA) of the lower extremity is a straight line of 180 degrees, passing through the centers of the femoral head, knee joint, and ankle joint. The line joining the femoral head center to the top of the intercondylar notch (ie, the femoral MA) and the line joining the proximal tibial center to the center of the ankle (ie, the tibial MA) are taken to be in one straight line. In recent times, investigators have reported that the femoral and tibial MAs are not in a straight line, but in the vast majority, they are found to be in a few degrees of varus. The extent of varus is shown to be significantly different in Asian and white populations (Table 25.2).[53,58,125,133]

Whether orienting TKA implants to recreate the MA in a few degrees of varus would improve functional outcome and patient satisfaction is currently under investigation.

MORPHOLOGY OF FEMUR

Femoral Size

Femoral size is expressed as the anteroposterior (fAP) and mediolateral (fML) diameters of the cut surface, which is

TABLE 25.2 Mechanical Axis: Variations in Young Adults of Different Populations

Population	MA Average (SD)	MA ACCORDING TO GENDER Male	Female
White[53]	0.55° (±0.33°)	0.94° (±0.42°)	0.16° (±0.52°)
White[34]	2° (±3.6°)	2.4° (±3.7°)	1.8° (±2.3°)
Chinese[137]	2.2° (±2.7°)	2.2° (±2.7°)	2.2° (±3°)
Indian and Korean[125]	2.4° (±2.6°)	—	—
Iranian[58]	1.5°	2.5° (±3°)	0.7° (±3°)
Japanese[53]	1.64° (±0.43°)	—	—
Indian[33]	2.2° (±3.6°)	—	—

MA, Mechanical axis; *SD*, standard deviation.

generally measured at 9 mm from the distal point of medial femoral condyle and perpendicular to the MA. fAP is measured from the posterior edge of the lateral condyle to the anterior-most cortex on the lateral side. fML is measured along the surgical epicondylar axis. In most studies the femoral size in Asians is smaller than in white populations (Table 25.3). This is related to the smaller height of Asians, and the dimensions of the lower femur are known to be proportional to the height. In addition, the femoral size in females is smaller than in males (see Table 25.3).

Femoral Shape

The femoral cut surface is more complex, with five separate surfaces. Commonly used parameters for shape include the following:
1. Condylar aspect ratio is the ratio of fML to fAP.
2. Trochlear aspect ratio is the ratio of the trochlear width to fAP. Trochlear width has been measured differently, either at the anterior margin of the cut anterior chamfer or at the transition point of the condyle to trochlea.

TABLE 25.3   Femoral Morphology: Cut Surface Sizes

Study	Ethnicity	ANTEROPOSTERIOR DIAMETER (mm)		MEDIOLATERAL DIAMETER (mm)	
		Male	Female	Male	Female
Mensch and Amstutz[100]	White	66.3	60.8	82.1 ± 4.7	76.8 ± 2.6
Lonner et al.[80]	White	62.27	56.32	76.9	67.49
Yue et al.[155]	White	67.5 ± 3.6	59.7 ± 2.6	86.0 ± 5.6	76.4 ± 4.0
	Asians	65.0 ± 2.8	58.8 ± 2.5	82.6 ± 3.6	72.8 ± 2.6
Li et al.[76]	White	59.6 ± 3.2	55.4 ± 2.8	74.6 ± 3.9	65.4 ± 1.4
	Chinese	56.5 ± 2.5	52.8 ± 2.6	72.7 ± 3.8	64.4 ± 2.6
Ho et al.[50]	Chinese	63.7		70.2	
Cheng et al.[22]	Chinese	66.6 ± 2.4	61.0 ± 24.6	74.4 ± 2.9	66.8 ± 3.11
Kwak et al.[71]	Koreans	46.2	41.5	74.4	65.9
Ha and Na[43]	Koreans	66.3	60.8	74.8	68.2
Lim et al.[78]	Koreans	59.0 ± 4.1	58.4 ± 3.1	81.5 ± 5.7	76.7 ± 3.7
Chung et al.[25]	Koreans	67.2	61.1	76.1	67.9

TABLE 25.4   Femoral Morphology: Aspect Ratio

Study	Ethnicity	Knees	NUMBER OF PATIENTS (KNEES)		ASPECT RATIO		Decreasing ML Dimension for Increasing AP Dimension	Female Sizes Smaller and Narrower
			Male	Female	Male	Female		
Ho et al.[50]	Chinese	OA	13	57	1.09 ± 0.06		Yes	—
Kwak et al.[71]	Koreans	Normal	50 (100)	50 (100)	1.61	1.59	Yes	—
Yue et al.[155]	White	Normal	20 (20)	16 (16)	1.28 ± 0.07	1.28 ± 0.06	Yes	Yes
	Chinese	Normal	20 (20)	20 (20)	1.27 ± 0.03	1.24 ± 0.04		
Mahfouz et al.[82]	White	Normal	(500)	(340)	1.41	1.36	—	Yes
	Asians	Normal	(40)	(40)	1.56	1.5		
Chung et al.[26]	Koreans	OA	50	975	1.13	1.11	Yes	Yes
Li et al.[76]	White	Normal	79	48	1.25 ± 0.05	1.18 ± 0.05	Yes	Yes
	Chinese	Normal	61	87	1.29 ± 0.04	1.22 ± 0.05		
Ishimaru et al.[56]	Japanese	OA	40 (40)	40 (40)	1.62 ± 0.15	1.43 ± 0.12	Yes	Yes
Yan et al.[150]	Chinese	Normal	50 (100)	50 (100)	1.06	1.03	Yes	Yes

OA, Osteoarthritis; *ML,* mediolateral; *AP,* antero-posterior.

Condylar aspect ratio (fML to fAP) is the most commonly used parameter. Its values are widely variable among studies (Table 25.4); some have reported it lower in Asian knees, others have reported it lower in knees of white individuals. It is understood that the condylar aspect ratio decreases with increasing fAP diameter, and it is lesser in females compared with males (see Table 25.4). The trochlear aspect ratio also decreases with increasing fAP diameter, but its gender difference is insignificant.[150] Yan et al. report that the gender difference in aspect ratio is most significant at the distal surface (condylar aspect ratio), and it reduces gradually toward the proximal trochlea (trochlear aspect ratio).[150]

Femoral shape mismatch may result in overhang or underhang of the prosthesis. Overhang can cause anterior knee pain, decreased range of motion (ROM) and altered patellofemoral kinematics.[20,83] Underhang can cause increased postoperative blood loss and early implant loosening.[114] Studies have shown that overhang of more than 3 mm produces clinical symptoms, but the precise degree of underhang that would result in clinical implications is not known.[83]

During surgery, if downsizing is performed to prevent mediolateral overhang, it could increase the flexion space, causing instability in flexion, or if the distal femoral cut is increased, it could cause the joint line to migrate proximally.[13]

Chung et al. studied 1025 TKAs in Koreans and reported that only 30% of knees had their condylar widths within 2 mm of the implanted prosthesis, 9% had condylar overhang, and 60% had underhang.[25] The gender difference showed that condylar overhang was seen in 10% of female knees versus 2% in male knees. Condylar underhang was seen in 59% of female knees and 89% of male knees. In addition, only 30% of knees had their trochlear width within 2 mm of the implant, 38% had trochlear overhang, and 32% had trochlear underhang. There was no gender difference seen in trochlear overhang or underhang. It was noted that trochlear overhang was present more in smaller sized knees, whereas underhang was more frequent in large knees. This suggests the need for more prosthesis sizes, varying the mediolateral dimensions for the same fAP diameter.

Dai et al. evaluated six different implant designs for the fit of the femoral component. The study population was composed of 135 white, 74 Indian, and 68 Korean patients.[30] They reported the least incidence of overhang (<8%) in two designs that had more sizes in the ML diameter for the same fAP diameter. There was no case of downsizing, but the incidence of underhang in these two designs was greater than 90% and higher than the other four designs. They concluded that prosthetic size variability would reduce the incidence of improper fit of femoral component.

Kim et al. similarly reported that with a standard prosthesis the femoral component was closely matched in 80 knees (58.0%), overhung in 14 knees (10.1%), and undercovered the cut bone in 44 knees (31.9%). In those with a gender-specific prosthesis, it was closely matched in 15 knees (10.9%), it under-covered the cut bone in 123 knees (89.1%), and none showed overhang.[63]

Current implants have the same aspect ratio for all sizes. Smaller Asian knees have comparatively higher aspect ratios, and the corresponding need for higher aspect ratios in small-size implants must be assessed.

Femoral Rotation

Femoral rotation is judged by different parameters, with no consensus on the best method. The parameters are the following:

1. The posterior condylar axis is the line joining the most posterior points of the medial and lateral femoral condyles. Erosion of the condyles in arthritis makes the reliability of this axis questionable.
2. The clinical epicondylar axis is the line joining the most prominent points of the medial and lateral femoral epicondyles.
3. The surgical epicondylar axis is the line joining the most prominent point on the lateral epicondyle to the middle of the sulcus on the medial epicondyle. Most researchers agree that this is the best line to judge femoral rotation.[15,27,116]
4. The Whiteside line is the line drawn from the apex of the intercondylar notch to the deepest point of the patellar groove.[11] Erosion of anterior aspects of the condyles in OA could compromise its reliability.[107,116]
5. The posterior condylar angle is the angle between the posterior condylar axis and surgical epicondylar axis. Griffin's study on normal knees in a white population has given this angle to be 3 degrees.[42]
6. The condylar twist angle is the angle between the posterior condylar axis and clinical epicondylar axis.[154]

Other angles include the angle between the line perpendicular to the Whiteside line and (a) with the surgical epicondylar axis or (b) with the posterior condylar axis.

7. The femoral component rotation is generally set according to the surgical epicondylar axis, by rotating the component 3 to 4 degrees to the posterior condylar axis.[42] If the posterior condylar angle is different from 3 to 4 degrees, as is known to happen in osteoarthritic knees, the femoral rotation will fail to be according to the epicondylar axis. Many researchers suggest taking all three axes (posterior condylar, surgical epicondylar, and Whiteside axis) into consideration before doing the femoral component rotation.[7,97,101,107,114]

Studies on knees of Japanese, Chinese, and Indian populations have demonstrated increased external rotation of the surgical epicondylar axis, as high as 9 degrees (Table 25.5) from the posterior condylar axis, as compared with white populations. Thus in Asian knees, if the cut is taken considering the posterior condylar axis alone, it could result in internal rotation. Internal rotation can lead to patellar maltracking, lateral retinacular pain, and flexion-extension gap-balancing problems.[5,9,14] External rotation can lead to excess bone removal from the posterior medial femoral condyle and balancing issues.[107] If the cut is taken according to the surgical epicondylar axis, it would lead to more bone being removed from the posteromedial femoral condyle compared with the posterolateral femoral condyle. Yip et al.[152] coined the analogy of "mountain and a mole" to describe this occurrence for the surgeon who is unaware of the racial differences and is suddenly faced with a bigger resected posteromedial femoral condyle (Fig. 25.4).

In absence of a definite conclusion, we recommend that all three axes (posterior condylar, surgical epicondylar, and Whiteside axis) be taken into consideration, along with the wear on femoral surfaces, before deciding on the femoral rotation.

Femoral Bowing

Coronal Femoral Bowing. The incidence of lateral bowing of the shaft in Asians is reported to be as high as 44% to 88% (Table 25.6). Parameters used to judge femoral bowing include the following:

1. The femoral bowing angle is the angle between the line connecting midpoints of the proximal femur and the line connecting midpoints of distal femur (Fig. 25.5). A negative angle indicates varus or lateral bowing and a positive angle indicates valgus or medial bowing.
2. Femoral condylar tilt angle: Femoral bowing orients the femoral condyles in varus/valgus position. The mechanical femoral joint angle (MFJA) is first determined. It is the lateral angle between the mechanical femoral axis and the distal femoral joint line. This MFJA subtracted from 90 degrees gives the femoral condylar tilt angle, which is normally 3 degrees of valgus. Negative angle denotes varus or lateral bowing and positive angle denotes valgus or medial bowing.

The mean angle of femoral bowing in different Asian studies varies from −1.6 to −5.4 (see Table 25.6). More importantly, the high range of variation (9.1 to −23 degrees) points to the severe degree of femoral bowing seen in a large number of patients (see Table 25.6).

Femoral bowing does not allow insertion of the intramedullary rod accurately along the anatomic axis. Rather, it follows the distal femoral axis. An erroneously or incompletely inserted intramedullay rod can result in an erroneous femoral cut and consequent varus alignment of the prosthetic component (Fig. 25.6). Some authors thus suggest considering the angle between the MA and distal femoral shaft axis instead of the anatomic axis for the femoral cut, which is likely to give a better aligned cut.[104] Alternately, short or thin rods may have to be used. One study has reported a 9-degree angulation of the distal femoral jig compared with the normal 5 degrees of angulation to achieve the femoral cut perpendicular to the MA in more than 20% of patients.[104] Yau et al. showed that in patients with more than 2 degrees femoral bowing, if a fixed angle of 5, 6, or 7 degrees for distal jigs was followed, it resulted in malalignment in 31%, 31%, or 34% of patients, respectively.[151] This is significantly more malaligned than in an unbowed femur, in which 5, 6, or 7 degrees of angle oriented jigs showed malalignment in only 3%, 0%, or 11% of patients, respectively.[151] Marco Polo et al. in their study on 185 female Korean patients showed a positive correlation of preoperative femoral bowing and varus condylar orientation with postoperative femoral component and limb alignment.[92] They showed that use of computer navigation in a separate group of 182 knees significantly reduced the number of outliers and produced better coronal femoral component alignment. Outliers were found to have inferior postoperative function scores. Another surgical problem with femoral bowing occurs with the placement of the femoral stem in primary or revision TKA. It could cause a long stem to fracture or result in impingement symptoms postoperatively.

Sagittal Femoral Bowing. Sagittal femoral bowing is a new parameter under recent research. It is expressed as the angle

TABLE 25.5 Femoral Morphology: Rotation Parameters

Study	Ethnicity	Type of Study	Age Mean (Range)	Number Patient (Knees) M/F	Posterior Condylar Angle in Degrees Mean (Range)	Condylar Twist Angle	Whiteside-Epicondylar Angle	Whiteside-Posterior Condylar Axis	Gender Difference
Mantas et al.[91]	White	Cadaveric study	43 (17-89)	19 (38) 14/5	—	M 4.4 F 6.4	—	—	—
Berger et al.[15]	White	Cadaveric study	—	(75)	M 4 F 5.2	—	—	—	—
Arima et al.[11]	White	Normal femur	Not specified	—	5.7	—	<90	93.1	—
Griffin et al.[42]	White	MRI study	42.8 (11-87)	104 (–) 41/63	3.11 (0-8.2)	—	—	—	None
Nagamine et al.[107]	Japanese	CT scan of FT OA knees	66.4	26 (27) –/–	—	6.2	89.9	93.9	—
		CT scan of PF OA knees	67.6	14 (17) –/–	—	6.4	88.7	94.9	—
		CT scan of normal knees	50.2	40 (40) 0/40	—	5.8	87.7	93.54	—
Yoshino et al.[154]	Japanese	CT scan of OA knees	75.5 (49-89)	48 (96) 10/38	3.0 (–)	6.4	—	—	—
Takai et al.[132]	Japanese	CT scan of normal knees	63.5 (51-81)	11 (19) 3/8	—	6.8	—	—	—
		CT scan of OA knees	75.7 (57-92)	22 (39) 3/19	—	6.3	—	—	—
Yip et al.[152]	Chinese	Cadaveric study	78 (17-94)	41 (82) 68/14	M 5.1 (1.7-9.7) F 5.8 (2.5-8.8)	—	—	97 (90.6-103.2)	Yes
Mullaji et al.[105]	Indian	CT scan of normal knees	31 (26-40)	50 (100) 42/8	5 (1.3-9.1)	—	90.8 (83.2-98.8)	95.8 (89-104.2)	None[a]
Sun et al.[131]	Chinese	CT scan of OA knees	68.9 (58-80)	32 (62) 2/30	2.36 (0-7.5)	—	—	—	—

[a]Female patients less in number.

F, Females; FT, femorotibial; M, males; OA, osteoarthritic; PF, patellofemoral; CT, computed tomography; MRI, magnetic resonance imaging.

TABLE 25.6 Femoral Morphology: Bowing Parameters

Author	Ethnicity	OA/N	Numbers (M/F)	Age in Years (Range)	Femoral Bowing Angle in Degrees Mean (Range)	% PATIENTS WITH BOWING MEAN (RANGE) ANGLE OF BOW — Medial	Lateral	Total	Femoral Condylar Orientation Angle	% Of Patients With Abnormal Orientation Angle
Nagamine et al.[106]	Japanese	OA	133 0/133	69.9 (50-89)	-2.2 (-3.5 to 11)	—	—	—	—	—
Yau et al.[151]	Chinese	OA	101 10/43	67 (45-81)	-1.6 (-19.7 to 9.1)	18% 4.4 (2.4-9.1)	44% 5.3 (2.1 to 19.7)	62%	—	—
Mullaji et al.[104]	Indian	N	25 25/0	32 (21-39)	-0.4	—	—	—	3.1	—
		OA	167 0/167	66.9 (49-85)	-3.6 (-13 to 0)	—	—	—	-0.1	—
Lasam et al.[92]	Koreans	OA	367 0/367	69 (50-88)	-5.4 (-23 to 6)	—	88%	—	-2.6 (-14 to 7)	80.4% varus orientation
		N	60 0/60	65.9 (50-85)	-3 (-16 to 4)	—	76.7%	—	1.1 (-4 to 7)	21.7% varus orientation

N, Normal; OA, osteoarthritis.

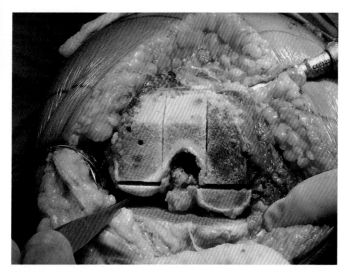

FIG 25.4 "Mountain and mole" appearance resulting from greater excision of bone from the posteromedial femoral condyle-Intraoperative photograph of an Indian TKA. On navigation, surgical epicondylar axis was externally rotated 8 degrees to the posterior condylar axis.

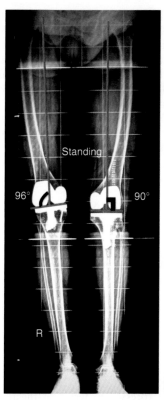

FIG 25.6 Radiographs of a patient with significant lateral femoral bowing. Right side operated with conventional technique and left side using navigation. Right side demonstrating varus femoral orientation because of standard 5-degree cut. Left side demonstrating femoral implant placed perpendicular to MA.

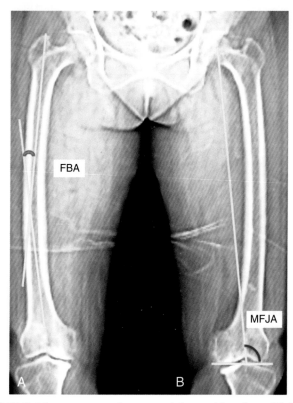

FIG 25.5 Measurements for coronal femoral bowing—(A) FBA and (B) femoral condylar orientation. *FBA*, Femoral bowing angle; *MFJA*, mechanical femoral joint angle.

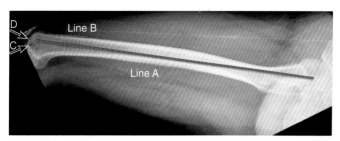

FIG 25.7 Radiograph showing measurements for femoral sagittal bows. *Line A*, MA of femur; *line B*, distal femoral anterior cortical axis; *point C*, highest point of intercondylar notch; *point D*, 1 cm anterior to point C.

between the sagittal MA and distal femoral anterior cortical axis. Sagittal MA, although interpreted differently in different studies, is most commonly taken as the line joining the center of the femoral head to a point, 1 cm anterior to the highest point of the intercondylar notch, as seen on the lateral knee radiograph (Fig. 25.7).[26] The distal femoral anterior cortical axis is the line joining two points on the distal femoral anterior cortex at a fixed distance from the distal most point of the femoral condyle (see Fig. 25.7).[26,135] Some authors have instead used the distal femoral medullary axis, which is the line joining the midpoints of the medullary canal in the distal third of femur.[26]

Tang's study on 100 Chinese knees reported a mean angle of 9.4 degrees, ranging from 6 to 16.7 degrees. They studied the femur in three divisions and showed that the distal third of the femur was more bowed than the middle and proximal third. They also reported greater bowing of the distal third in rheumatoid arthritis and in short-stature patients.[135] Chung et al. studied 200 Korean knees scheduled for TKA and reported a mean angle of 3 degrees, ranging from 1 to 8.5 degrees.[26]

These previous studies suggest a widely variable range of the sagittal femoral bowing angle. Surgically, it would predispose to an anteriorly tilted intramedullary rod, which would lead to the femoral component placement in extension or notching of the anterior femoral cortex or even supracondylar fracture.[118,123,124,135] If one uses short intramedullary rod then femoral component may become flexed. This may lead to post impingement against the anterior margin of the intercondylar box which would limit the range of extension and enhance the polyethylene wear.[113,115,117]

MORPHOLOGY OF TIBIA

Tibial Size

Tibial size is expressed in terms of anteroposterior (tAP) and mediolateral (tML) diameters. It is measured at the resection level, 4 to 8 mm from the top of the less-affected tibial plateau in a plane perpendicular to the tibial MA.* All studies have uniformly reported smaller tAP and tML in Asian knees compared with white populations (Table 25.7). The male knees have larger tibial dimensions than female knees in both Asian and white populations.[82,155]

Tibial Shape

Tibial shape is expressed in terms of the tibial aspect ratio, which is the ratio of tML to tAP. The comparison of tibial aspect ratio between Asian and white populations is widely variable in different reports (Table 25.8). This could partly be because of the differing measurement techniques. In addition, all available reports have considered the aspect ratio of small and large knees together for comparison between Asian and white populations.[76,82,155] It is important to consider that most Asian knees are smaller in size (see Table 25.7); it is observed that these smaller-sized knees in Asians have a significantly higher tibial aspect ratio.[22,72,76,155] Thus studies performed separately for small knees are needed for comparison between Asian and white populations.

*See references 22, 43, 72, 76, 78, 100, 142, 155.

Current implants have been designed to match the tibial aspect ratio of the knees of white populations. Asian surgeons experience that these implants fail to provide adequate coverage of the tibial plateau in Asian knees and may cause overhang or underhang. Overhang can lead to a painful knee because of soft tissue irritation and tendinitis.[72] Underhang can cause increased postoperative bleeding, subsidence, and loosening.[18,54,145] To prevent overhang in the mediolateral direction, if undersizing was performed, it resulted in the tibial surface remaining uncovered in the anteroposterior direction. The uncovered surface, if covered by polyethylene wear particles, could induce osteolysis. In addition, the tibial medial condyle being larger than the lateral condyle poses an asymmetrical surface for cover.[49,100,146] Thus there was development of asymmetrical and anatomic tibial base plates to improve tibial cover.

Shah's study compared the percentage of tibial coverage with four symmetrical tibial trays versus an asymmetrical tray in Indian patients.[121] He concluded that the asymmetrical tray provided more coverage than the symmetrical ones. He also showed that the tibial coverage with the symmetrical trays was more than 80%. Earlier studies in white populations have

TABLE 25.7   Tibial Morphology: Cut Surface Sizes

Study	Asian	ANTEROPOSTERIOR DIAMETER (mm)		MEDIOLATERAL DIAMETER (mm)	
		Male	Female	Male	Female
Mensch and Amstutz[100]	White	54.3	46.0	80.3	70.1
Yue et al.[155]	Asian	41.5	37.3	75.2	66.2
	White	45.0	39.3	78.7	69.0
Li et al.[76]	Chinese	49.6	44.2	77.2	69.1
	White	49.5	45.2	79.4	70.2
Uehara et al.[142]	Asian	53.8	46.6	83	71.7
Kwak et al.[72]	Koreans	48.2	43.3	76.1	67.6
Cheng et al.[22]	Chinese	51.3	45.7	76.4	68.8
Ha and Na[43]	Koreans	66.3	60.8	74.8	68.2
Lim et al.[78]	Koreans	52.7	45.7	80.6	70.0

TABLE 25.8   Tibial Morphology: Aspect Ratios

Study	Ethnicity	Knees	TIBIAL ASPECT RATIO		Gender Differences
			Males	Females	
Uehara et al.[142]	Japanese	Osteoarthritic	1.54	1.54	—
Kwak et al.[72]	Korean	Normal	1.58	1.56	—
Cheng et al.[22]	Chinese	Normal	1.49	1.51	Yes M > F
Yue et al.[155]	White	Normal	1.75	1.76	—
	Chinese	Normal	1.82	1.78	—
Mahfouz et al.[82]	White	Normal	1.4	1.37	Yes M > F
	Asians	Normal	1.33	1.42	Yes F > M
Mori et al.[103]	Japanese	Osteoarthritic	—	1.48	—
Li et al.[76]	White	Normal	1.61	1.54	Yes M > F
	Chinese	Normal	1.56	1.56	Yes M > F

TABLE 25.9 Tibial Morphology: Alignment Parameters

Study	Ethnicity	Subject	Sex	Numbers	Mean Varus Angle in Degrees Between Mechanical and Anatomic Axis	% Of Patients With Tibia Vara	Mean Tibial Plateau Inclination Angle (Range)
Ko et al.[67]	Chinese	OA	M	20 patients	−1.95 (0 to 5)	54%	—
		OA	F	52 patients	−1.73 (0 to 9)		—
Nagamine et al.[106]	Japanese	OA	F	133 patients	—	—	−7.2
Tang et al.[137]	Chinese	N	M	25 patients	—	—	−4.9
		N	F	25 patients	—	—	−5.4
Yoo et al.[153]	Koreans	OA	M (29) / F (138)	167 patients (246 knees)	−0.7 (−4 to 3)	71.1%	
Yau et al.[151]	Chinese	OA	M (10) /F (43)	101 knees	0.6 (8.4 to −8.5)	20% (32% if both vara and valga included)	—
Mori et al.[103]	Japanese	OA	F	74 patients (90 knees)	0.6 (−1 to 2.1)	>83%	
Lasam et al.[92]	Korean	OA	F	367 patients	—	—	−8.3 (−19 to 3)
		N	F	60 patients	—	—	−5.4 (−13 to 1)

N, Normal; OA, osteoarthritis; F, female; M, male.

shown that implants with symmetrical trays that were successful in the long term had 80% to 85% of tibial cover.[145] Further studies can evaluate this amount of tibial coverage in Asian knees with different implants.

Tibial Rotation

Proposed landmarks to judge tibial rotation include posterior tibial margin, tibial tuberosity, midsulcus of tibial spine, medial margin of patellar tendon, femoral transepicondylar axis, and ankle-foot axis.[†] In white individuals the medial one-third of the tibial tuberosity being perpendicular to the femoral transepicondylar axis is accepted as the best landmark. In Asians the upper end of the tibia exhibits more external rotation (ie, the tibial shaft exhibits more intorsion).[108,131] This is accentuated when there is associated varus or valgus.[108,131] Thus the tibial tubercle is an unreliable landmark to judge tibial rotation in Asians.[108,131] If it is used for judging rotation, a mismatch between femoral and tibial component would ensue, leading to anterior knee pain and also an intoeing gait after TKA.[108,131]

Depending on the landmarks used for rotation of the tibial base plate, the tibial aspect ratio to be matched also changes. If this is not considered, the tibial cut surface may remain uncovered. Martin's study revealed that for maximal coverage of the tibial cut surface, the tibial plate (with respect to the tibial tuberosity axis) had to be malrotated in more than 95% of knees with symmetrical trays and in 28% to 52% knees with asymmetrical trays.[93] In most of these knees the tibial plate had to be internally malrotated for better coverage. Excessive internal malrotation can be counterproductive; it can lead to patellar maltracking, pain, intoeing gait, compromised function, and early failure.[5,14]

Tibia Vara

MA of tibia is taken as parallel to the anatomic axis because the angle between them is only 2 degrees in normal knees. Unlike white individuals, Asians generally present with tibia vara; its

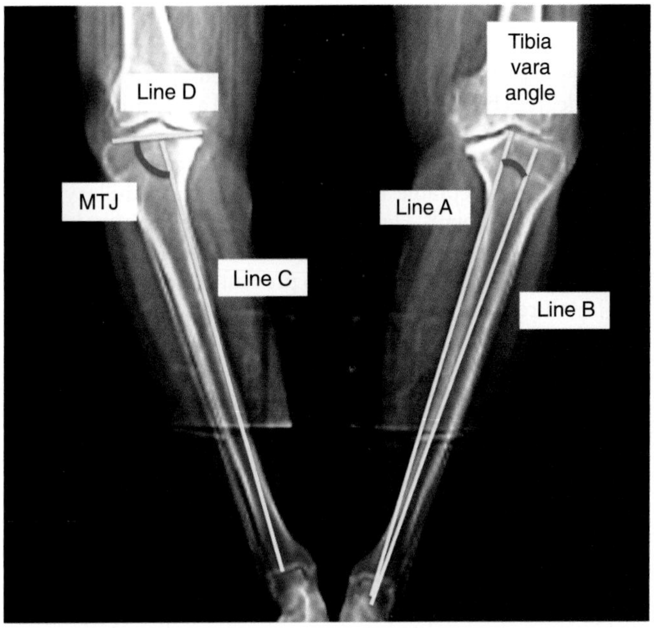

FIG 25.8 Radiograph showing calculation of tibia vara angle and tibial plateau inclination angle. Line A, MA of tibia; line B, anatomic axis of tibia; line C, MA of tibia; line D, tibial joint line. MTJA, Mechanical tibial joint angle.

reported incidence varies from 20% to 83% (Table 25.9). In tibia vara, the anatomic axis shifts to emerge lateral to the tibial eminence, causing the angle between the two axes to exceed 2 degrees. The MA can no longer be considered parallel to the anatomic axis.[67,98,136,153] Tibia vara is measured in the following ways:

1. Tibia vara angle: The angle between the anatomic and MA of tibia (Fig. 25.8).
2. Tibial plateau inclination angle: First the mechanical tibial joint angle between the tibial MA and the tibial joint line is calculated (see Fig. 25.8). Then the tibial plateau inclination

---

[†]See references 4, 6, 15, 19, 28, 31, 141.

value is calculated by subtracting mechanical tibial joint angle value from 90 degrees. Negative values indicate varus inclination, whereas positive values indicate valgus.

In a knee with tibia vara, applying a symmetrical base plate perpendicular to the anatomic axis would result in lateral overhang, because of the center of the base plate being displaced lateral to the center of the cut tibial surface. To prevent the lateral overhang, if a smaller base plate is used, it would result in uncovering of the cut surface medially and in the anteroposterior direction.[103]

Second, tibia vara poses a problem in getting a tibial cut with intramedullary technique. The tibial cut (ideally 90 degrees to the MA) is based upon inserting a long intramedullary rod, exactly parallel to the anatomic axis of the tibia. In tibia vara using this technique, the tibial cut would fail to be at 90 degrees to the MA because the long rod inserted parallel to the anatomic axis no longer is in alignment with the MA. In a study of 72 Chinese patients Ko et al. showed that a long rod could be inserted only in 46% patients because of tibia vara.[67] In the rest a short rod had to be used. They evaluated the tibial cut made on the basis of the long rod radiologically. They reported that an ideal tibial cut, 90 degrees to the MA, was obtained only in 18% patients, whereas an acceptable cut of greater than 90 degrees ±2 was obtained in 82% patients. In patients with the short rod, none obtained an ideal cut and 41% patients had unacceptable cuts. No patient who showed an angle of more than 2 degrees between the mechanical and anatomic axis could obtain an acceptable cut.

In a study on 93 Chinese lower limbs Yau et al. reported 40% potentially unacceptable tibial cuts with intramedullary technique in bowed tibia.[151] He suggested doing preoperative long leg x-ray in all patients to judge alignment and the use of extramedullary jigs/computer navigation to prevent unacceptable cuts.

The third surgical problem with tibial vara happens in patients in whom a stem is to be used either for primary or revision arthroplasty. The anatomic axis of the tibia does not always pass through the center of the tibial plateau and an offset stem is required, if the tibial plate is to be centralized on the cut tibial surface to provide proper cover. Studies in white populations have concluded that the anatomic axis exits the tibial plateau anteromedial to the center of the tibial plateau and an anteromedially offset stem should be used.[48,146,147] However, in Asians the anatomic axis exits the tibial plateau anterolaterally and an anterolaterally offset stem should be used.[67,98,136] This problem was highlighted in two separate studies that recommended to keep a wide range of offset stems available.[136,153] We suggest that a preoperative long leg x-ray should be performed in all patients before TKA to judge the proper alignment and an extramedullary jig should be used to cut the tibiae. Computer navigation would be of added value, and many studies have shown extremely good postoperative alignment in Asian knees with tibia vara, with its use.[23,86,157]

MORPHOLOGY OF PATELLA

Patellae in Asians are smaller and thinner than in white populations.[64] This is a reflection of smaller-sized bones in Asians.

A study from Japan indentified that a thin residual patella is a risk factor for patellar fracture post TKA. They found a statistically significant difference ($p = 0.01$) in the mean patellar thickness in patients who did not suffer patellar fracture (12.2 ± 1.6) as against those who developed patellar fracture (10.4 ±

1.8).[61] Other studies have also implicated the thin residual patella as a risk factor for occurrence of fracture.[119] A Korean study showed that patients with residual patellar thickness of less than 12 mm recorded poor WOMAC pain scores.[64]

Our practice is to resurface the patella in every TKA. We recommend leaving at least 12 mm of residual patellar thickness to prevent any risks. We suggest that along with patellar resurfacing, lateral retinacular release can be used to enhance the patellar tracking, which reduces the stresses on soft tissues, thus reducing the incidence of postoperative patellofemoral symptoms, while facilitating higher flexion.[90] In our practice we have reported a significantly lower incidence of patellofemoral symptoms with a high-flex implant, compared with that reported by other investigators.[3,88]

OUTCOME IN ASIAN TOTAL KNEE ARTHROPLASTY

Functional Results

Asian patients presenting for TKA are unequivocally concerned whether the artificial knee implant would allow them to perform the movements they need for their high-flexion activities and secondly whether such actions would be harmful to their artificial implants' survival.

Results have shown significant improvement in postoperative function scores in several studies across different Asian populations.[‡] These results are also comparable to the reports from white populations and comparable in males and females.[41] The results concur in terms of pain relief, correction of deformity, achieving ROM, and stability. However, current scores used to evaluate functional outcome in Asians do not evaluate their floor-based activities. Despite late presentation, significant deformity, and morphologic differences, results in Asians are gratifying. In our practice, 30% of cases are severely deformed knees (>15 degrees varus); we have successfully used standard posterior-stabilized implants in 95% of cases and resorted to more constrained implants in only 5% cases (Fig. 25.9).

Traditionally surgeons in Asia advise patients against undertaking such high-flexion postures. The past decade has seen an upsurge in the refinement in surgical techniques and implant designs to achieve high flexion and also to make it safer. Design focus was on improving the contact area in deep knee flexion, by increasing the height of the posterior condyles of the femur, increasing the height of the posterior lip of the tibial liner, and increasing the contact area in post and cam mechanism (for posterior-stabilized knees). The surgical technique is focused on managing flexion-extension space, removing posterior osteophytes adequately, ensuring appropriate posterior tibial slope and tibial femoral rotation, avoiding patellofemoral overstuffing, and ensuring central tracking for the patella.

Many studies report improved flexion with newer implants. Many studies also report equal or comparable flexion between standard and high-flex design, suggesting that improved surgical techniques rather than implant design made the difference.[84,99,120,130] Few studies have reported floor-based functional outcome in Asian patients.[§] Their results are variable and difficult to compare across different populations. A Korean study showed that patients achieving maximum flexion of more than 135 degrees had a better functional WOMAC score.[64] In our

---

‡See references 59, 81, 85, 88, 89, 124, 128, 130, 139.
§See references 2, 37, 44, 66, 85, 88, 89, 148.

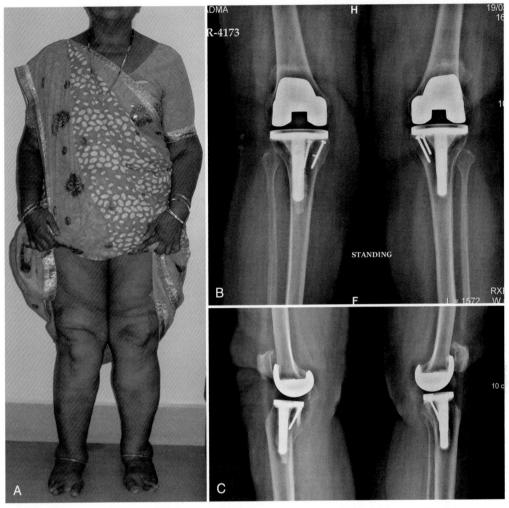

FIG 25.9 Ten-year postoperative clinical photograph (A) and radiograph (B and C) of the same patient shown in Fig. 25.1.

studies, we found that post TKA, 53% to 57% patients could assume the cross-legged posture on the floor and a greater number (67% to 81%) could do this on a higher surface.[85,88]

Other studies have shown that there is a poor correlation between subjective and objective outcome.[21,96] Matsuda concluded that most patients did not report symptoms, but they experienced difficulty with activities of daily living after TKA.[96] They showed that avoiding varus alignment and achieving better ROM appear to be important for increasing patient satisfaction and meeting expectations. The Korean knee score, a new evaluation system for patients with a floor-based lifestyle, was developed and validated in 2013.[65] More reports using such scoring methods for Asian activities are needed.

It has clearly emerged that many patients undertake floor-based activities post TKA (Fig. 25.10), even with standard implants (Fig. 25.11). It is understood that the most important determinant for good postoperative flexion is the level of preoperative flexion to begin with.[16] And this is well retained in most Asian patients despite their late presentation and significant deformity.

There are two studies that have raised concern of early loosening of the femoral implants of one specific high-flex design in the early follow-up period.[24,44] They found that

patients who achieved high flexion had a higher femoral revision rate at 3 to 4 years. Many other reports on high-flex designs have not shown such a trend.[74,88]

Whether high-flexion activity promotes early loosening of femoral component was also studied by Zelle et al.[156] In finite element models (FEMs) during deep flexion (ROM >120 degrees), tensile and shear stress were shown to be concentrated at the implant-cement interface beneath the proximal part of the anterior flange. They concluded that the interface beneath the anterior flange was not predicted to fail in the normal flexion range (ROM ≤120 degrees), whereas in further knee flexion the prediction became 2.2%. Beyond 140 to 145 degrees of flexion the thigh-calf contact reduced the knee forces and interface load, and thus the failure risk was reduced. Based on the greater critical stresses at the femoral fixation site between 120 and 145 degrees of flexion, they concluded that the femoral component has a higher risk of loosening at high-flexion angles.

Another study from the same laboratory in the Netherlands showed that in femoral fixation, the cement-bone interface is more prone to failure than the cement-implant interface. Furthermore, they showed that this risk can be significantly reduced by preparation of the anterior cortex before cementing by

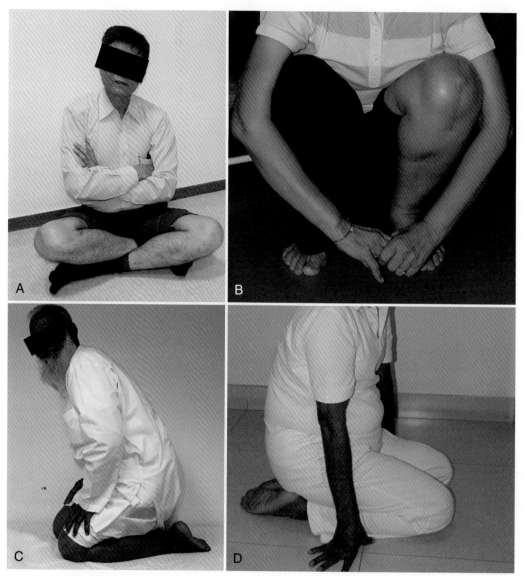

FIG 25.10 Photographs showing different floor-based activities being performed. (A) Cross-leg sitting [10 years post TKA], (B) squatting [8 years post TKA], (C) *Namaz* position [6 years post TKA], (D) *seiza* position [7 years post TKA].

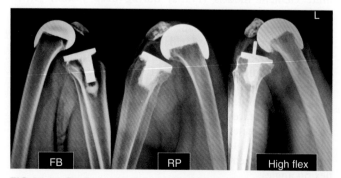

FIG 25.11 Radiograph of three different patients showing deep knee flexion with different implant designs. *FB*, Fixed bearing; *RP*, rotating platform.

drilling of holes behind the anterior flange. This improved the interface strength, reducing the failure rate from 31.3% to 2.6%.[143]

Few available studies reporting on long-term outcome of TKA and unicondylar implants in Asian knees show that survival of implants appears similar to white populations.** More studies are needed for better and specific evaluation.

Areas of Dissatisfaction

Studies report that 8% to 15% of Asian patients are dissatisfied with their TKA outcome.[35,66,139] Studies have also correlated restricted high-flexion activites to patient dissatisfaction post TKA.[109,122] A Japanese study found that inability to do squatting

---

**See reference 16, 59, 77, 81, 124, 128.

was one of the activities of daily living that correlated with patient dissatisfaction post TKA.[66]

Some studies report that patients who wanted to and could not kneel post TKA because of pain or discomfort were inclined critically toward quality of life and toward perceived success of the TKR procedure.[46,122] Discomfort and pain on kneeling were related to either the scar in front of the knee, which could take up to a year to mature, or related to patellofemoral articulation. A study found that patients who were unable to kneel had a larger area of sensitivity than patients who could kneel ($p = 0.002$).[46]

Kim et al. reported that the top five severe functional disabilities in Koreans post TKA were difficulties in kneeling, squatting, sitting with legs crossed, sexual activity, and recreational activities. The top five in order of perceived importance were difficulty in walking, using a bath tub, working, recreational activities, and climbing stairs. They also found that 88% patients who were dissatisfied with their replaced knees were inclined to perceive functional disabilities in high-flexion activities to be more important than satisfied patients.[66]

Gella et al. studied that the AP dimension of distal femur in Asians was significantly different than white populations preoperatively.[40] After being implanted with existing implants designed for white individuals, it became similar to dimensions for white populations. This limited the postoperative flexion and resulted in patient dissatisfaction, according to them.[40]

FUTURE

To meet the exponential increase in demand for TKA in Asian patients, the future should be directed toward addressing the Asian knee differences we have discussed and adapting to meet their specific function requirements post arthroplasty. First, performance of deep flexion activities should be adequately researched to find their role in the development and progression of OA. A greater understanding of how high flexion post TKA can be achieved and translated into deep flexion, floor-based activities would help to develop appropriate implant designs and surgical techniques. Implant sizes, geometry, and material would be required to match the Asian anatomy and bone quality. Specific studies on Asian populations with more standardization of methodology are needed toward achieving these targets. Next, performance of deep flexion activities post TKA must be evaluated for their impact on long-term survival of the implants. For this, evolving appropriate scoring methods to grade functional results specific to the Asian way of life would be needed. Lastly, these developments must bear in mind the cost factor if TKA is to reach the large majority of Asians.

KEY REFERENCES

22. Cheng FB, Ji XF, Lai Y, et al: Three dimensional morphometry of the knee to design the total knee arthroplasty for Chinese population. *Knee* 16(5):341–347, 2009.

25. Chung BJ, Kang JY, Kang YG, et al: Clinical implications of femoral anthropometrical features for total knee arthroplasty in Koreans. *J Arthroplasty* 30(7):1220–1227, 2014.

30. Dai Y, Scuderi GR, Penninger C, et al: Increased shape and size offerings of femoral components improve fit during total knee arthroplasty. *Knee Surg Sports Traumatol Arthrosc* 22:2931–2940, 2014.

66. Kim TK, Kwon SK, Kang YG, et al: Functional disabilities and satisfaction after total knee arthroplasty in female asian patients. *J Arthroplasty* 25(3):458–464, 2010.

76. Li P, Tsai TY, Li JS, et al: Morphological measurement of the knee: race and sex effects. *Acta Orthop* 80:260–268, 2014.

85. Maniar RN, Gupta H, Singh A, et al: Five- to eight-year results of a prospective study in 118 arthroplasties using posterior-stabilized rotating-platform knee implants. *J Arthroplasty* 26(4):543–548, 2011.

88. Maniar RN, Singhi T: High-flex rotating platform knee implants: two- to 6-year results of a prospective study. *J Arthroplasty* 27(4):598–603, 2012.

93. Martin S, Saurez A, Ismaily S, et al: Maximizing tibial coverage is detrimental to proper rotational alignment. *Clin Orthop* 472:121–125, 2014.

96. Matsuda S, Kawahara S, Okazaki K, et al: Postoperative alignment and ROM affect patient satisfaction after TKA. *Clin Orthop* 471(1):127–133, 2013.

103. Mori S, Akagi M, Asada S, et al: Tibia vara affects the aspect ratio of tibial resected surface in female japanese patients undergoing TKA. *Clin Orthop* 471:1465–1471, 2013.

131. Sun T, Lu H, Hong N, et al: Bony landmarks and rotational alignment in total knee arthroplasty for chinese osteoarthritic knees with varus or valgus deformities. *J Arthroplasty* 24(3):427–431, 2009.

140. Thambyah A: How critical are the tibiofemoral joint reaction forces during frequent squatting in Asian populations? *Knee* 15(4):286–294, 2008.

145. Wernecke GC, Harris IA, Houang MTW: Comparison of tibial bone coverage of 6 knee prostheses: a magnetic resonance imaging study with controlled rotation. *J Orthop Surg* 20(2):143, 2012.

151. Yau WP, Chiu KY, Tang WM, et al: Coronal bowing of the femur and tibia in Chinese: its incidence and effects on total knee arthroplasty planning. *J Orthop Surg* 15(1):32–36, 2007.

156. Zelle J, Janssen D, Van Eijden J, et al: Does high-flexion total knee arthroplasty promote early loosening of the femoral component? *J Orthop Res* 29(7):976–983, 2011.

The references for this chapter can also be found on www.expertconsult.com.

26

Mobile Fluoroscopy: Determination of Natural, Unrestricted Knee Motion

William R. Hamel, Richard D. Komistek

INTRODUCTION

Over the past two decades, fluoroscopy has been used as a tool to perform in vivo analysis of postoperative total joint replacement (TJR) results, primarily knees. The fluoroscope digital images frames when computationally combined with three-dimensional (3D) graphical models of the joint implants allow the 3D kinematics of the implanted joint motion to be revealed. Furthermore, the concept of inverse dynamics can then be used to calculate the actual forces occurring (eg, between the femur and tibia in the case of a knee joint).[3] Such information is useful in understanding the detailed in vivo kinematics of a TJR surgical result, including the resulting force system, which has particular relevance to the performance of the joint interface materials (eg, polyethylene wear).

Conventional C-arm fluoroscopes have been used to capture in vivo skeletal movement during activities, such as deep knee bends, chair rises, and walking on treadmills. C-arm fluoroscopes are static, or nonmoving devices, such that the recorded images are susceptible to blurring because of the relative motion of the joint features with respect to the field of view of the imaging sensor. In addition, because the imaging sensor is fixed, the field of view is limited to the sensor's size and often is not able to record all of the desired aspects of a particular activity. In some cases human operators have been used on either side of the C-arm to physically maneuver the unit such that the field of view approximately follows the subject's motion.

The concept of mobile fluoroscopy is about relieving the constraints associated with fixed C-arms by creating a robotic-type of fluoroscope that is capable of "tracking" a human subject during natural activities. Each person's musculoskeletal system is unique and displays unique motion details. A key aspect of mobile fluoroscopy is the capabilities to evaluate implant kinematics and kinetics while a subject is engaging their full musculoskeletal system through natural motion activities.

This chapter discusses the goals and requirements one can envision for the ideal mobile fluoroscope capable of imaging hip, knee, and ankle joints. Other research in mobile fluoroscopy from around the world will be touched upon, but with the specific capabilities and clinical results obtained with the tracking fluoroscope system (TFS) at the University of Tennessee, Knoxville, being the focal point.[2] Potential future directions in mobile fluoroscopy are summarized.

MOBILE FLUOROSCOPY CONCEPTS

Goals

Ideally a mobile fluoroscope is a device that allows one to image a particular skeletal joint or feature during any type of normal activity, such as walking or climbing stairs. In the context of joint arthroplasty a mobile fluoroscope should provide clear in vivo images of a particular skeletal joint of interest during natural movements that fully involve the subject's musculoskeletal system, thus providing meaningful data regarding the postoperative performance of the artificial joint. From a technical perspective this means that the mobile fluoroscope must have kinematic capabilities (eg, range of motion, speeds, and accelerations that are consistent with normal human movements). A robot can be thought of as a machine that uses sensors, controls, motor actuators, and mechanical structures to achieve desired 3D motion. The largest industrial application of robots today is in the automotive industry in which they are used to do a multitude of tasks that are essentially positioning various types of tools in 3D space (eg, spot-welding body frame parts together). A mobile fluoroscope is a robot in the same sense, but with the challenge of dynamically aligning the line of sight of the x-ray and image sensor on the skeletal joint of interest during natural movements. This is quite challenging because of the motion complexities, speeds, and accelerations.

Basic Functions

TJR is routinely performed for shoulder, hip, and knee joint repair and reconstruction. Some ankle procedures also involve implants and stabilizing fasteners. This discussion will focus on knees, hips, and ankles. Mobile fluoroscopy for shoulder joints is a much different challenge than for leg joints but involves the same basic functional concepts.

Let us begin by using walking in a straight line as the activity in which we would like to capture a series of fluoroscope frames for the in vivo analysis. The first function that must be achieved is following the subject's overall movement, which can be thought of as tracking the aggregate motion of their torso. The second function is tracking the relative motion of the leg joint of interest, which moves forward and backward and up and down relative to the torso during walking. The leg moves significantly with respect to the torso during walking, particularly at higher speeds. The horizontal range is dependent on the person's size and walking speed and can be as much as a meter.

The vertical motion range is on the order of 10 to 20 cm. Because the leg motion pivots at the hip, the relative motion at the knee is substantially less than the ankle. The up and down knee motion is more in the 4 to 8 cm range, and the back and forth motion is 7 to 12 cm but again very dependent on body size and walking speed. The hip motion is the smallest and is in the range of a few centimeters in both the vertical and horizontal motions. Detailed values for these gait motion ranges are well documented across the full range of body sizes and gender in numerous anthropometry datasets.

Anthropometry data can be used as well to quantify relative torso and leg motion for other interesting maneuvers (that engage the musculoskeletal system differently), such as chair rises, deep knee bends, stair ascent and descent, and ramp ascent and descent.

For walking activity the mobile, or robotic, fluoroscope must be able to sense and follow the person's body movement and simultaneously sense and follow, or track, the joint of interest, be it the hip, knee, or ankle. Sensing and tracking the joint of interest are the functions that are essential to ultimately keeping the fluoroscope line of sight aligned with the joint, the line of sight being the axis between the centers of x-ray generator and the x-ray imaging device. If these functions are performed perfectly, when one observes the resulting fluoroscope image stream, the knee joint for example will appear to be fixed in the center of the image while the femur and tibia bone segments move back and forth according to the gait motion, even though the subject has walked through a number of gait cycles. In a sense, it is as if the analyst is able to ride along with the joint during the in vivo analysis. The technical challenge is creating a machine that can mobilize the necessary equipment with sufficient power to accurately follow the skeletal joint of interest during dynamic movements. It turns out that this is a formidable technical challenge in terms of the current state of the art in robotics and fluoroscopy.

Tracking Fluoroscope System

We will now use the details of the mobile fluoroscope system developed in the Center for Musculoskeletal Research at the University of Tennessee, termed the TFS, as a basis for further discussion.[4,5] The current TFS is a second-generation patented design that began in 2007. To date, TFS-II has been used in extensive knee and hip TJR clinical studies.

The creation of the TFS began with a very basic assessment of general concepts. It was at this stage that it was recognized that the machine could be built as a self-contained mobile device using existing mobile robotics technology versus a fixed-in-place concept similar to large x-ray or computed tomography (CT) machines. The current TFS is battery powered, untethered, and omnidirectional. Diagnostic data are transmitted using a dedicated wireless local area data network. All of the TFS components can be transported through conventional doorways such that the system has the same portability of any laboratory diagnostic equipment.

The TFS concept is depicted in Fig. 26.1. Subject total body motion tracking is accomplished by sensing the distance and contour of the upper torso using dual laser range scanners. The computer control system uses this information to keep the distance between the mobile platform and the subject constant, thus following the subject as he or she walks, by varying the speed of the platform drive motors. The laser range scanners also provide the profile of the torso, which is used to infer the direction that the subject is turning, left or right.

The relative motion of the leg with respect to the torso is accommodated by vertical and horizontal servo actuators located on side wings. The right side actuators position the x-ray generator, and the left side actuators position the imaging sensor, in this case a high-resolution solid-state flat panel. The side actuator systems are slaved to one another such that the line of sight of the x-ray beam always follows the center of the imaging sensor. Two methods are used to control the line of sight such that it dynamically tracks the joint of interest. The preferred method (does not require that the subject wear any type of markers) is the concept of visual servoing, in which computer image processing is used to identify the location of the joint in each fluoroscope image frame, which in general will vary slightly from one frame to the next. Note that the TFS-II fluoroscope can provide images up to 87 frames per second, so this process is occurring very fast in comparison to the subject's motion speed. The visual servo control is analyzing and making

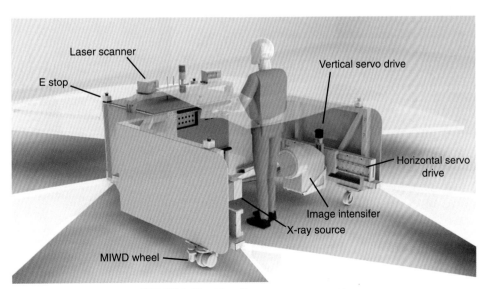

FIG 26.1 Tracking fluoroscope concept.

corrections for the joint motion as fast as every 12 milliseconds. Visual servoing depends on the frame images being of sufficient quality for reliable image processing results. In some test conditions, such as hip studies with high body mass index subjects, image contrast is not sufficient and requires the use of external target markers for the x-ray tracking or supplemental visual tracking using an additional digital camera. These three joint tracking modes assure that any subject can be diagnostically imaged.

The joint images are stored on onboard computers and transmitted to the control station via the dedicated wireless local area network. Lab technicians can view the results in real time, and all data are stored for the subsequent in vivo analysis.

The TFS is an active machine operating in the proximity of the subject. It has a fully independent safety system that monitors the subject's position relative to the machine and the integrity of the x-ray tracking system. In the event of a subsystem malfunction or actuation of a trip signal by the radiation technician or other test personnel, the system is de-energized safely in a matter of milliseconds.

Figs. 26.2 to 26.4 are photographs of the actual TFS-II that is currently being used in clinical studies for a number of TJR manufacturers.

Diagnostic Modes of Operation

The omnidirectional motion capabilities of the TFS mobile platform are essential to its ability to image hip, knees, and ankles regardless if the joint of interest is on the left or right side. Knees are normally done with mediolateral x-ray

exposures, and because of the nature of the x-ray projection form the source, the best images are obtained with the joint interest adjacent to the imaging sensor. As shown in Fig. 26.4, when doing left side knees the subject faces/walks away from the robot, and when doing right side knees the subject faces into the machine. Therefore left and right side knee imaging requires that the TFS track in opposite directions. Right and left ankles would have the same tracking motions.

Hip imaging is very different because the x-ray exposures must be performed in the anteroposterior directions because of the pelvic area hard tissues effects. As with knees, the highest quality images are obtained with the subject closest to the imaging sensor. Hip testing configurations are shown in Figs. 26.5 and 26.6. Note that the TFS-II must translate in directions that are 90 degrees to that of knee and ankle testing. In this case, right and left hips can be performed in the same direction, but if necessary the left hip direction can be 180 degrees from the right hip direction. The cutouts in the rear chassis and the left and right side wings of the TFS-II allow for the incorporation of ramps, chairs, or other walkover structures into the test protocol.

Currently our test protocols have all involved straight-line subject motions. However, it should be noted that the TFS-II mobile platform is capable of tracking any subject motion, such as turning motions or other changes of direction. This type of test motion may be useful in sports and military diagnostic applications.

Other Mobile Fluoroscope Systems

In terms of open publications, we are aware of the work of a group at ETH Zurich that has a machine for knee tracking during stair descents and straight-line walking. Studies are included in the PhD dissertation by Foresti.[1]

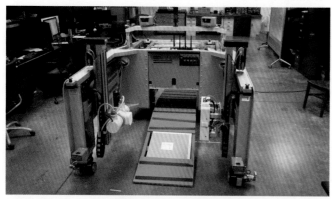

FIG 26.2 TFS II front view.

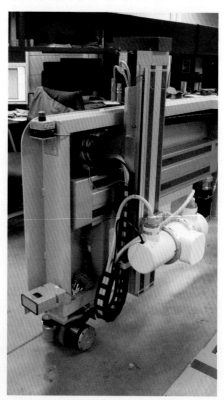

FIG 26.4 TFS II right side wing and x-ray actuators.

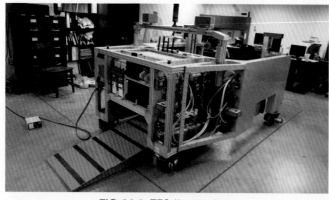

FIG 26.3 TFS II rear view.

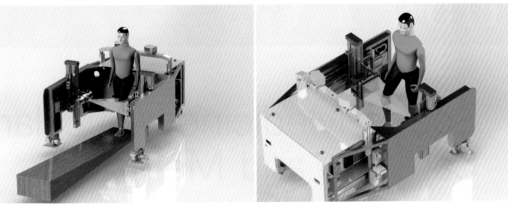

FIG 26.5 Diagnostic modes of operation. The omnidirectional motion capabilities of the TFS mobile.

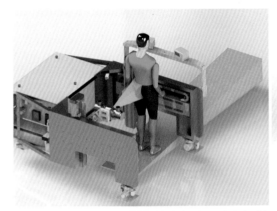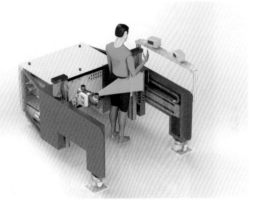

FIG 26.6 Left and right hip diagnostic configurations.

Future Directions

At this stage, mobile fluoroscopy is essentially a research tool being used in the study of orthopedic joint implant designs and in vivo kinematics and kinetics. The continual advancements in solid-state electronics and computer technologies will allow such machines to acquire higher resolution images faster in the future. This may open new opportunities to image patient maneuvers that are presently not possible. For example, a machine that could image athletes during extreme motions, such as jumping, landing, and fast turns, may very well be possible. In addition, there are several new research avenues that can extend the clinical value of the mobile fluoroscopic images in the TJR-type studies. Biplanar fluoroscopy can be integrated into the existing TFS concept and provide 3D imaging directly, potentially speeding up and enhancing the in vivo analysis. Although it may be a bit more futuristic, it may be possible to create the equivalent of CT scans of a joint of interest, by spinning the mobile fluoroscope about a patient standing in a fixed position.

Some initial conceptual research has been performed regarding shoulder and cervical spine imaging. A supplementary robot manipulator-type device with a miniaturized x-ray and imaging detector pair is not out of the realm of feasibility. The motion dexterity of the robot manipulator would facilitate the 3D motion that is common to the shoulder and upper body, especially in such motions as golf swings. Such capabilities would open the types of in vivo studies currently being performed on hips and knee to shoulder arthroplasty as well.

SUMMARY

Work on the notion of mobile fluoroscopy was begun approximately a decade ago. The technology has progressed to the point that in vivo studies of hip and knee implants and natural knees during normal and continuous walking activities are being performed routinely. The new diagnostic tools, which allow the full engagement of a subject's musculoskeletal system, are providing new insights into postoperative performance of implant designs. Continued developments will allow more realistic and complex test protocols that provide diagnostic methods not presently possible. Video recordings of typical tracking fluoroscope operation can be seen at *www.expertconsult.com*.

ACKNOWLEDGMENTS

We acknowledge the contributions of our many graduate student research assistants over the years while we were developing and refining the TFS. Their hard work and creativity have been essential.

The references for this chapter can also be found on www.expertconsult.com.

Sports Medicine: Articular Cartilage and Meniscus

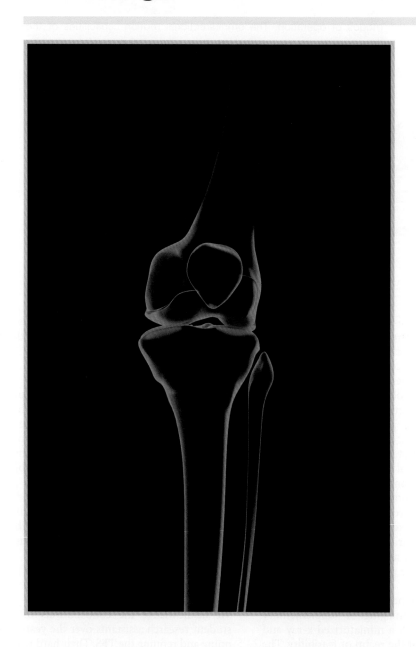

27

Articular Cartilage: Biology, Biomechanics, and Healing Response

Constance R. Chu, Grace Xiong, Thomas P. Andriacchi

Articular cartilage is a remarkable tissue with a unique functional architecture that supports multiplanar motion under a wide variety of loading conditions. In the absence of injury, and when allowed to function within its "zone of homeostasis,"[35] human articular cartilage can provide a lifetime of pain-free motion.[13] However, all too frequently, premature tissue failure occurs as a result of trauma, disease, or altered loading.[9] Although articular cartilage has limited capacity to heal injuries that compromise the articular surface resulting from increased fibrillation friction and shear stress,[23,57] new data support an ability to recover from subsurface injuries.[24,27] It is important for orthopedic surgeons to understand the basic science of articular cartilage in health, as well as in response to injury and disease, so to apply new concepts of preosteoarthritis,[26] functional tissue engineering, and precision medicine toward improving and maintaining joint health to support a lifetime of healthy movement.

BIOLOGY AND STRUCTURE

Articular cartilage can be thought of as a tissue where the three main components of water, collagen, and proteoglycans (PGs) are arranged in an intricate fashion to provide incredible functional characteristics. The tissue functions under extreme loading conditions, yet it is composed primarily of water. It is also aneural and avascular, properties that likely contribute to the mechanical durability of the tissue but also hamper protective and reparative processes. Although proportionately thicker in human knees than the stifle joints of even the largest modern quadrupeds,[25,38,56] articular cartilage is an incredibly thin tissue uniquely organized to provide extremely low-friction surfaces, permitting multiplanar motion that can resist or transmit repetitive tensile, shear, and compressive forces.[13,15,93] In the absence of injury or disease, articular cartilage can remain intact and functional throughout life, although factors such as trauma and obesity can accelerate cartilage degeneration.[8,40] As an avascular tissue, it also routinely survives for several days after donor death, and even longer with proper preservation.[18,33,65]

Because of differential functional needs, articular cartilage varies in cellularity and thickness within the same joint and between different joints, reflecting the sensitivity of knee cartilage to kinematic changes as a result of the local mechanical environment being associated with functional loading.[7,10,50] However, it consists of the same basic components and anisotropic structure throughout all joints. Grossly, human articular cartilage appears as a smooth, homogeneous tissue approximately 1 to 5 mm thick (Fig. 27.1). When probed, healthy cartilage is firm, resists deformation, and is smooth and slick. Diseased cartilage is soft, deforms when probed, feels rough, and may contain visible surface disruptions ranging from increased surface porosity with fine fibrillations to deep fissures, clefts, and full thickness cartilage loss.

The composition and matrix structure of articular cartilage varies with depth from the surface and has been traditionally divided into four structural zones.[15,73,77] The matrix composition has additionally been characterized into three regions based on distance from the chondrocyte.[45] This precise arrangement of tissue components provides specific mechanical properties for the tissue as a whole.[93]

Chondrocytes

Chondrocytes, which are the cells in articular cartilage, synthesize matrix components and respond to a variety of mechanical and biochemical stimuli to regulate cartilage homeostasis.[51] Despite these important roles, chondrocytes account for just a small fraction of articular cartilage tissue (1% of volume).[13] Chondrocytes are derived from pluripotential mesenchymal stem cells (MSCs) that differentiate into chondroblasts and mature chondrocytes during growth and development.[51,89] Articular cartilage is avascular; thus chondrocytes must derive nutrition and oxygen from the synovial fluid by diffusion and must meet energy requirements through glycolysis.[5] Chondrocytes within healthy, mature articular cartilage are individually surrounded by an extracellular matrix and form few cell-to-cell contacts (Fig. 27.2A).[13] Despite this isolated arrangement, chondrocytes are able to respond to a variety of mechanical and biochemical signals.[89]

Chondrocytes differ in size, shape, and metabolic activity in the different structural zones, but all cells contain endoplasmic reticulum and Golgi apparatus for matrix synthesis.[5,51] Chondrocytes synthesize the two major articular cartilage macromolecules—type II collagen and aggrecan—and organize the structure of the matrix.[13] Specific interactions between chondrocytes and the extracellular matrix are poorly understood, but the ability to detect and respond to a variety of mechanical and biochemical factors by the chondrocyte is vital for matrix synthesis and maintenance of tissue homeostasis. A few mechanisms have been discovered, including the presence of binding proteins (integrins)

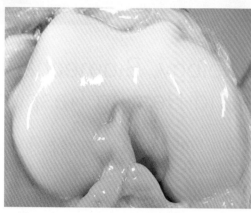

FIG 27.1 Gross Image of Articular Cartilage on the Femoral Condyle of a Healthy 20-Year-Old Female This image displays the smooth, homogeneous surface appearance of normal articular cartilage.

and osmotically sensitive ion channels on the cell surface of chondrocytes.[55,89]

Development and maintenance of the chondrocyte phenotype is an important research topic because current and future treatments for articular cartilage damage include implantation of stem cells and chondrocytes into defects.[16,42,54,61,83] To maintain chondrocyte cell phenotype, in vitro study of chondrocytes has shown that proliferation and expansion of chondrocytes in monolayer results in loss of cell phenotype and subsequent synthesis of type I collagen. However, culture conditions that include high cell density, cell-to-cell contact, and a three-dimensional environment appear to restore or maintain the chondrocyte phenotype assessed by cellular morphology and the production of type II collagen.[89] Receptors for growth factors such as transforming growth factor-β (TGF-β), fibroblast growth factor (FGF), and insulin-like growth factor-1 (IGF-1) have been identified on chondrocytes and appear important for production of cartilage matrix proteins.[89] A range of other molecules such as oxygen and common injectable anesthetics has been shown to impact chondrocyte metabolism and viability.[11,19,32] As an avascular tissue, chondrocytes are adapted to low oxygen tensions yet are typically cultured at higher oxygen tensions. Given that sustained hypoxia in vitro increased type II collagen gene expression and PG synthesis,[32] oxygen tensions should ideally be taken into account when chondrogenesis is desired in ex vivo applications.

Already few in number, the loss of chondrocytes adversely affects the ability of the remaining chondrocytes to adequately maintain matrix integrity. Rapid loss of articular cartilage, or chondrolysis, has been attributed to depletion of chondrocytes below a critical threshold, resulting from sustained administration of local anesthetics using pain pumps.[12] A one-time dose of local anesthetics such as bupivacaine or lidocaine has been reported to be toxic to human chondrocytes in vitro in a dose- and time-dependent manner.[20,22,48] In vivo work also showed chondrocyte loss after a single injection of 0.5% bupivacaine and that substantial chondrocyte loss after monoiodoacetate injection led to full thickness cartilage loss within a short period of time.[19] Further research will continue to shed light on the complex interactions of biochemical and mechanical factors on chondrocyte and articular cartilage health.

Extracellular Matrix

Articular cartilage (90%) is predominantly composed of the extracellular matrix, which consists of fluid and macromolecules.[13] The porosity of the zonal structure of the matrix determines its interaction with fluid and thus is responsible for determining the mechanical properties of the cartilage.[70,73] The main functions of the matrix are to resist tensile and shear forces through the arrangement of collagen fibrils, and to resist compressive forces through alteration in hydrostatic pressure.[36,53,60]

Tissue Fluid. Water is the largest component of the extracellular matrix (80% of articular cartilage by weight).[13] The fluid component of articular cartilage also includes high concentrations of cations, gases, and small proteins. The volume of water present in articular cartilage depends on the concentration and organization of the macromolecules—specifically, the distribution and relationships between PGs and the collagen network. The size, electronegativity, and concentration of PGs varies between cartilage zones, contributing to differences in water concentration, porosity, and permeability of the tissue.[77] Throughout joint movement, water continually moves into and out of the cartilage to aid in distribution of compressive forces and lubrication of the cartilage surface.[53,60]

Macromolecules. The macromolecules of the extracellular matrix include collagens (60% dry weight), PGs (25% to 35%), and noncollagenous proteins and glycoproteins (15% to 20%).[13] Type II collagen fibrils provide structural integrity and tensile and shear strength to the articular cartilage.[15,64] PGs, mainly aggrecan, attract water and provide resistance to compression.[77] The noncollagenous proteins and glycoproteins help bind chondrocytes to the matrix, stabilize matrix macromolecules, and assist in regulation of matrix homeostasis.[13]

Collagens. An exceedingly complex and incompletely described network of collagen fibrils contributes materially to the volume, shape, tensile, and shear strength of articular cartilage. Although multiple collagen types including II, VI, IX, X, and XI are present,[67] type II collagen accounts for 90% of the collagen in articular cartilage.[13] Type II collagen is composed of three alpha chains, which intertwine into a triple helix. These helices covalently cross-link in a lateral array to form collagen fibrils.[76] Levels of type II collagen are highest in the superficial zone and decrease in concentration with increasing depth from the surface (see Fig. 27.2A and B).[75] The collagen fibril network restrains the PGs in the matrix and prevents swelling of the cartilage to greater than 450 mOsm when water flows into the tissue.[70,82] This allows for the creation of high tissue pressure, which is vital for resistance of compressive forces.

Under physiologic conditions, type II collagen metabolism is slow and fibrils have a half-life of years. In the early stages of cartilage degeneration, degradation of collagen fibrils is observed.[62] Enzymes called matrix metalloproteinases (MMPs) are thought to contribute to this degradation, specifically collagenases and aggrecanases. Collagenases mediate cleavage of type II collagen.[62] Antibodies to specific neoepitopes on these fragments can be detected by synovial fluid, serum, or urine assays and are being studied for use as potential biomarkers of early cartilage degradation.[28,37,62]

Other collagen types are less prevalent but perform important functions, including stabilization and regulation of type II collagen fibrils. Type IX collagen forms cross-links along the

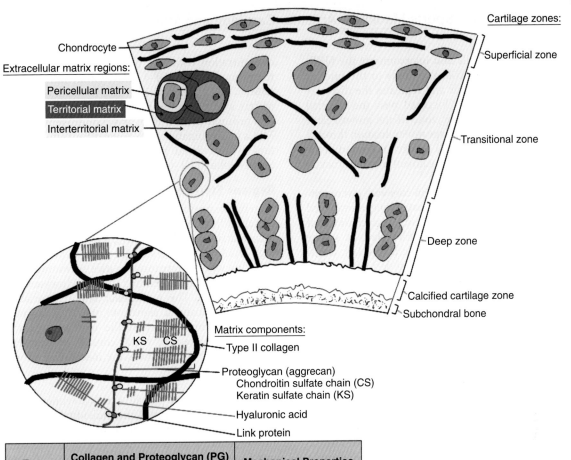

Zone	Collagen and Proteoglycan (PG) Composition and Organization	Mechanical Properties
Superficial	• High level parallel collagen fibrils • High (H$_2$O) • Low level PG	• Collagen resists tensile and shear forces • High fluid flow/exudation lubricates joint in response to compression and large matrix consolidation
Transitional	• Moderate level oblique collagen fibrils • Moderate (H$_2$O) • High levels PG	• Collagen resists shear compression • High PG creates hydrostatic pressure resisting compression with low fluid flow/exudation and moderate matrix consolidation
Deep	• Low level perpendicular collagen fibrils • Low levels (H$_2$O) • Very high levels PG	• High PG levels resist compression via creation of hydrostatic pressure resisting compression with very little fluid flow and little matrix consolidation

Compressive force   H$_2$O   H$_2$O

H$_2$O → H$_2$O   Exudation of water and compression of matrix

Compressive force   H$_2$O

H$_2$O   Small fluid flow and moderate compression of matrix

Compressive force

Very little fluid flow and small matrix compression

B

FIG 27.2 (A) Schematic of articular cartilage matrix regions and structural zones. The three matrix regions depicted with increasing distance from the chondrocyte are, respectively, pericellular, territorial, and interterritorial. The matrix regions are present in all zones but are depicted in only one area in the schematic. As described, chondrocyte morphology and organization vary between zones. Collagen fibril concentration and organization also vary between zones. The superficial zone is marked by high collagen content and parallel organization. Transitional zone is marked by moderate collagen content and oblique orientation. The deep zone is marked by low collagen content and vertical orientation. *Inset,* A chondrocyte is surrounded by the type II collagen fibril network and PGs. (Aggrecan molecules are shown with keratin and CS GAG chains on a HA backbone. The aggrecan molecules are bound to collagen by link protein.) (B) Table and schematic of composition, organization, and mechanical properties of articular cartilage zonal layers.

surface of type II collagen fibrils and interconnects the fibrils with PG aggregates.[67] Type XI collagen binds to the interior structure of type II collagen fibrils and regulates the diameter of the fibrils. Type X collagen is localized near the calcified cartilage zone and the hypertrophic zone of the growth plate and is thought to contribute to cartilage mineralization through calcium-binding properties.[67] Type VI collagen is located in the pericellular matrix and aids in the attachment of chondrocytes to the extracellular matrix.[45]

Proteoglycans. PGs consist of a protein core with glycosaminoglycan (GAG) side chains.[67] GAGs consist of long unbranched polysaccharide chains containing repeating disaccharides of amino sugars with negatively charged carboxylate or sulfate groups.[66] Specific GAGs include hyaluronic acid (HA), chondroitin sulfate (CS), keratan sulfate (KS), and dermatan sulfate (DS).[67] The major PG (90% of mass) in articular cartilage is aggrecan.[34] Aggrecan has many CS and KS side chains and noncovalently associates with an HA backbone to form aggregates (see Fig. 27.2A). HA is a long-chain nonsulfated GAG capable of binding a large number of aggrecan molecules. Link protein, a glycoprotein, stabilizes the association between HA and each aggrecan molecule.[67]

Aggrecans play a key role in generating hydrostatic pressure. The negatively charged aggrecans attract cations, increasing the osmolality of the tissue. Water is then attracted into the tissue, decreasing the osmolality.[82] Hydrostatic pressure created by the interaction of collagen, PGs, and water provides stiffness to the cartilage to absorb compressive mechanical loads without damage to the matrix. Displacement of water from PGs during compression of the superficial zone of matrix lubricates the joint.[93]

Similar to collagen, degradation of aggrecan is observed in early cartilage degeneration, and aggrecanases are thought to contribute.[9,34] Aggrecan synthesis and degradation can also be measured by antibodies to specific neoepitopes on fragments by synovial fluid or serum assays. Inhibitors of aggrecanases are being investigated for potential treatments for cartilage degeneration.[41]

Smaller PGs include decorin, fibromodulin, and biglycan.[67] The function of each PG is related to the specific core protein and GAG chains that it contains. Decorin contains DS side chains and is located at the surface of type II collagen fibrils. It is thought to inhibit the lateral growth of fibrils and contributes to their organization and stabilization. Fibromodulin has KS side chains and binds type II collagen fibrils, providing stabilization. Biglycan contains DS side chains, binds TGF-β, and interacts with type VI collagen in the pericellular matrix.[67] Expression of smaller PG changes within zones and with mechanical stress likely contributes to cell stabilization and signaling through interaction with other proteins.[13,67]

Noncollagenous proteins and glycoproteins. The matrix contains many additional proteins that represent a small volume of the tissue.[13] Cartilage oligomeric matrix protein (COMP), anchorin, and fibronectin function to bind chondrocytes to the matrix.[93] COMP binds to chondrocytes in the territorial matrix.[46] Anchorin binds to chondrocyte surface protein, anchoring chondrocytes to collagen fibrils.[93] Fibronectin is an adhesion molecule expressed on the surface of chondrocytes.[52] Ongoing research is investigating the roles of these proteins, with COMP showing promise as a biomarker of cartilage degradation in early osteoarthritis (OA).[37,62]

Other proteins include growth factors and cytokines, which bind to chondrocyte receptors, altering rates of matrix synthesis and degradation. Effects of these proteins depend on their concentration, cofactors, type of target cell, and number of cell receptors. TGF-β, IGF-1, FGF, bone morphogenetic protein (BMP), and platelet-derived growth factors (PDGFs) stimulate matrix synthesis and proliferation.[89] TGF-β, FGF, and PDGFs also promote proliferation and chondrogenic differentiation of MSCs in combination with many other factors. Matrix degradation is stimulated by interleukin-1 (IL-1), tumor necrosis factor-alpha (TNF-α), and MMPs.[86]

Regions Surrounding the Chondrocyte

Matrix composition and organization vary with distance from the chondrocyte. Three regions have been identified: pericellular matrix, territorial matrix, and interterritorial matrix (see Fig. 27.2A).[13] The pericellular matrix directly surrounds the chondrocyte; the territorial matrix surrounds the pericellular matrix and assists in binding the chondrocyte cell membranes to the matrix. The pericellular and territorial regions also transmit mechanical signals to the chondrocytes when the matrix deforms.[45] Most of the matrix is contained in the interterritorial region, which consists of collagen fibrils and PG aggregates and provides the mechanical properties of the cartilage.[77]

Pericellular Matrix. In all cartilage zones, the pericellular matrix directly surrounds the individual chondrocyte. Chondrocyte cell membranes attach to the rim of the pericellular matrix covering the cell surface. This region contains many PGs and proteins, including type VI collagen, decorin, and fibronectin.[45] This region contains little to no fibrillar collagen. The function of this region is not fully understood, but it serves to regulate the microenvironment of the chondrocyte. The presence of type VI collagen defines this region and anchors the chondrocyte cell membrane to the matrix.[45]

Territorial Matrix. The territorial matrix surrounds the pericellular matrix, forming clusters of chondrocytes. In the deep zone, the territorial matrix surrounds each column of chondrocytes. In this region, thin collagen fibrils adhere to the pericellular matrix and form fibrillar baskets around the cells.[62] This region confers some protection to chondrocytes from damage during joint loading.[77]

Interterritorial Matrix. Most of the matrix is contained in the interterritorial region. PGs are abundant in this region.[77] Compared with the other two regions, the interterritorial region possesses the largest-diameter collagen fibrils and is responsible for the mechanical properties of the cartilage.[77] The orientation of the collagen fibers in this region varies with depth from the surface, as described in the section describing the zonal structure of articular cartilage.[94]

Many advances have been made in the knowledge of articular cartilage biology, but many more questions remain, including questions related to the factors involved in regulation of matrix homeostasis and formation of the zonal structure of articular cartilage.

Zones

In addition to specific matrix regions, articular cartilage is anisotropic, with the composition, organization, and mechanical properties of the tissue varying with depth from the surface.[15,72,94] Four zones have been described, moving from the surface to the subchondral bone, respectively. They are the superficial zone, transitional zone, deep zone, and the zone of calcified cartilage (see Fig. 27.2A and B).[67] Each zone has unique chondrocyte morphology, arrangement of type II collagen fibers, and levels of PGs and water. This structure reflects the different mechanical properties predominating in each zone.[15,72,94]

Signals regulating the development and maintenance of the zonal structure of articular cartilage remain unknown and in need of additional research.[73] When bovine articular chondrocytes isolated from different zones were subjected to oscillatory loads, tensile loading was found to stimulate PG synthesis in both superficial zone and deep zone chondrocytes.[84] These data suggest that synthesis and organization of the matrix by chondrocytes are partially dependent on the mechanical environment.[84] More complete understanding of the anisotropic structure and signaling of articular cartilage are needed for development of functionally competent cartilage constructs and for induction of appropriate cartilage reparative responses to improve treatment of chondral injuries.

Superficial Zone. The superficial zone, the thinnest zone, consists of two layers.[13] The top layer is a clear film called the lamina splendens, which contains no cells, little polysaccharide, and few collagen fibrils. The main layer consists of flattened ellipsoid, densely packed, and horizontally arranged chondrocytes that synthesize a matrix with high collagen and low PG content.[13,93,94] Superficial zone chondrocytes also produce lubricin, which is important to boundary lubrication of articular cartilage.[85] The thick collagen fibrils are arranged parallel to the surface, although orientation and deformation patterns vary according to cartilage strain distributions (see Fig. 27.2A).[10] The abundance and parallel organization of collagen to the joint surface permits the superficial zone to provide strength to resist tensile and shear forces.[60] The high concentration of water and lubrication by factors such as lubricin also provides lubrication and resistance to compression.[53,85] Compromise of this layer, resulting from injury or in early cartilage degeneration, results in acute loss of matrix integrity as well as increased permeability, surface roughness, and decreased resistance to tensile forces. This leads to softening and increased loading for the remainder of the cartilage matrix, and progressive tissue degeneration.[15]

Transition Zone. The transitional zone is the largest zone and functions to resist shear and compressive forces.[15,60] The chondrocytes are spheroidal and synthesize matrix with larger-diameter collagen fibrils oriented obliquely to the surface into rotational arches (see Fig. 27.2A).[13,75] This arrangement allows the fibers to resist shear forces.[53] The higher PG and the lower water content of the matrix compared with the superficial zone permit increased compressibility and thus shock absorption and load distribution.[93]

Deep (Radial) Zone. The deep zone is of intermediate thickness and functions to resist compressive forces.[93] The chondrocytes are spheroidal, are arranged in vertical columns perpendicular to the surface, and synthesize the matrix with the greatest amount of PG (see Fig. 27.2A).[13,75] The collagen fibrils are the largest in diameter and are arranged vertically to resist compression, provide stiffness, and anchor the cartilage to the subchondral bone.[74] Removal of the deep vertical fibrils increases the tensile strain in the superficial fibrils and compromises attachment to the subchondral bone.[15]

Calcified Cartilage Zone. The thin calcified cartilage zone between the deep zone and subchondral bone anchors the cartilage to the bone via type X collagen. The tidemark is located in this zone and is the boundary between calcified and uncalcified cartilage.[13]

BIOMECHANICS

Normal Cartilage Response to Loading

The composition and structure of the articular cartilage extracellular matrix creates a low-friction surface capable of sustaining a wide range of static and dynamic mechanical loads. The coefficient of friction is estimated at a remarkably low 0.002 in synovial joints[30] and allows the tissue to withstand millions of loading cycles each year.[93] The precise functional architecture of cartilage gives the tissue its biomechanical properties: the superficial zone consisting of parallel collagen fibrils and high collagen levels resists tensile and shear forces, the transitional zone consisting of oblique collagen fibrils and high PG levels resists shear and compressive forces, and the deep zone consisting of perpendicular collagen fibrils and high PG levels resists compressive forces (see Fig. 27.2B).[13,15,64,77,93] Normal movement results in peak static stresses reaching 3.5 MPa, occurring over a long duration (5 to 30+ minutes) and resulting in compressive strains of 35% to 45%. Peak dynamic stresses reaching as high as 20 MPa (3000 lb per square inch) occur during extremely short durations (<1 second) and lead to compressive strains of 1% to 3%.[15,53,93]

Resistance to compressive loading is a function of the level of PGs and interaction with the collagen fibril network. In response to compression, cartilage exhibits biphasic viscoelastic properties: the solid matrix deforms, increasing the contact area and decreasing stress, and the tissue fluid is exuded and redistributed, lubricating the surface and decreasing friction.[15,81,92] Fluid pressurization provides the main strength of cartilage to resist compressive loads.[36,81] PGs have a large negative charge owing to the carboxylate and sulfate groups of GAGs. This high fixed negative charge density attracts mobile cations, generating increased osmolality.[36,66,82] Water is attracted to the tissue, decreasing osmolality and generating high fluid pressure. The collagen fibril network restrains the PG, preventing swelling and maintaining high fluid pressure.[70,82] The deep zone provides the most resistance to compressive load via deformation of its solid matrix. The high PG content and low permeability of the deep zone trap water, creating a high fluid pressure.[81,93] Distribution of compressive loads minimizes stress on subchondral bone, chondrocytes, and other matrix zones.

In addition to different types of stresses (tensile, shear, compressive), physiologic movement creates mechanical stresses of different magnitudes, durations, rates, and frequencies. A critical yet unknown level and pattern of mechanical stress are needed to maintain the normal balance of matrix homeostasis.[35,59,64,72] Simplifying these complex interactions, static compression suppresses matrix synthesis, whereas dynamic loading stimulates matrix synthesis.[43,72]

Static compression, even within the physiologic range, inhibits matrix synthesis, downregulating gene expression and synthesis of type II collagen and aggrecan and increasing expression of MMPs.[43,72] Similarly, both immobilization and excessive loading (high magnitude or long duration) result in decreased matrix synthesis.[93] Decreased levels of PG decrease the ability of the tissue to resist compressive forces, increasing the susceptibility of tissue to microdamage. Loss of PG caused by immobilization appears to be reversible on remobilization of the joint, but excessive loading often results in irreversible chondrocyte death and surface disruptions.[88]

On the contrary, dynamic loading increases synthesis of collagen type II and aggrecan and increases expression of tissue inhibitors of metalloproteinases (TIMPs), enzymes that counteract MMPs.[7] Moderate exercise is reported to increase PG synthesis and cartilage stiffness, but the specific type, intensity, duration, and frequency necessary to produce these beneficial changes are difficult to define.[64,93] The effects of these different variables on matrix homeostasis and details of the mechanosignaling processes are not well understood and require further research.

Alterations in Loading Patterns

Despite the ability of cartilage to withstand large variations in stress and compression, large or sustained changes to joint biomechanics can disrupt homeostasis, exceed cartilage compensatory mechanisms, and initiate development of OA. Measurable differences in structure, thickness, and biochemistry[4,14,29] exist in load-bearing regions and are correlated to forces typically experienced by the joint during motion.[2,50] For example, cartilage thickness mapping shows that areas of higher loading during normal walking have thicker cartilage,[2,49] and it has also been shown that the collagen organization[10] as well as cartilage biology vary with regional loading.[7] It has been suggested that these regional variations in healthy cartilage properties occur during development as an adaptation to individual loading patterns that occur during ambulation.[3,15] Although this type of adaptive response of cartilage to local loading conditions helps maintain homeostasis and cartilage health,[1,35] the limited adaptive capacity of mature articular cartilage renders the joint vulnerable to altered kinematic patterns during ambulation that can occur later in life as a result of conditions such as aging or soft tissue injury, such as anterior cruciate ligament (ACL) injury. In skeletally mature individuals, kinematic changes, particularly when repeated ambulatory loading shifts to regions less adapted to handle such loads, may therefore initiate OA development.[2] In particular, the sensitivity of the knee to kinematic changes[68,69] that results from ACL injury has been suggested as a factor in the occurrence of premature OA in this population. Changes to joint loading patterns may be the consequence of joint injuries such as ACL tears and intra-articular fractures, or from more gradual changes as a result of obesity or aging.[8]

DAMAGE PATHWAYS AND HEALING RESPONSE

Cartilage injuries can be divided into three general categories based on visible depth of injury: (1) cell and matrix damage without visible surface changes; (2) cartilage disruption with visible fibrillations, fissures, flaps, or defects; and (3) visible cartilage and subchondral bone disruption. Each injury type has a different healing response dependent on the degree of matrix disruption, the viability of the chondrocytes, and whether the injury involves the subchondral bone.[13]

Articular cartilage has limited capacity to heal, resulting from lack of a blood supply and the paucity of chondrogenic progenitor cells available to migrate to the injury site and mount an adequate repair response.[13] Cartilage injuries can

occur through biochemical means such as heightened inflammation and degradation resulting from systemic conditions such as rheumatoid arthritis and obesity or locally from injections or infection. Mechanical injuries, including a single load of great magnitude or repetitive joint overloading of lesser magnitude exceeding the homeostatic envelope of the tissue, are common and can potentiate risk for further cartilage degeneration.[17,35,78,79]

New research focuses on delineating potentially reversible preosteoarthritic states where cartilage overload has occurred yet the joint surface remains intact,[24,26] as well as improving the functional capacity of efforts to enhance and improve the repair of focal articular cartilage defects. There is additionally increasing emphasis on a systems based approach to maintenance of cartilage health and prevention of OA.[1,17] Under this new paradigm, cartilage disease and progression to OA reflect a combination of biological, structural, and biomechanical factors (Fig. 27.3).[1,17] As such, degenerative cartilage lesions reflect disease processes acting upon the entire joint, rather than only localized to the articular cartilage.[17]

Cell and Matrix Damage

Chondrocytes and articular cartilage matrix can be damaged by numerous factors inclusive but not limited to high impact loading, cumulative lower level tissue overload, biochemical factors, and changes related to aging and declining health.[15,78,79] Low-level tissue injury reflected primarily by turnover of the PG components likely occurs as a normal consequence of joint loading and can be restored by chondrocyte matrix synthesis.[13] Injuries resulting in transection or weakening of the collagen network result in measurable acute changes to the matrix[6,23,27,63] and may be irreparable if they involve the articular surface[23] or require longer periods to heal.[24,27] If the damage involves significant chondrocyte death, spontaneous repair to damaged tissue is limited and results in rapid and progressive matrix degeneration, even chondrolysis.[19] If chondrocytes are diseased or killed and not able to synthesize the new matrix, the damaged matrix loses PG, which results in decreased ability to resist mechanical forces. If the joint is subjected to the same or greater loads, the degenerative process accelerates with eventual progression to OA.[47] Furthermore, following impact injury, studies report increased joint tissue expression of proteins involved in cartilage degradation (TNF-α, IL-1, and MMPs).[7] The development of techniques such as biomarkers to detect this early damage to chondrocytes and the matrix is important for understanding the natural history of this largely "invisible" early disease and to further advance early treatment options with true disease modifying potential.[28,31]

Partial Thickness Cartilage Disruption

Without access to the vascular system, visible damage to the cartilage surface that does not extend into the subchondral bone does not initiate an effective reparative response.[13] Transient proliferation of chondrocytes near the edges of the defect has been observed, but the cells are trapped within the dense matrix and are unable to effectively proliferate and migrate into the defect to mount a repair response.[47,71] The cells briefly increase synthesis of type II collagen and PG, but the altered joint milieu and mechanics result in chondrocyte apoptosis and cessation of matrix synthesis.[43,78] Damage to the superficial zone disrupts the collagen network and increases the

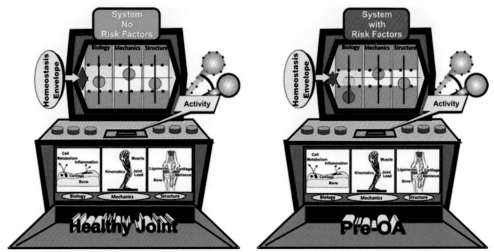

FIG 27.3 Systems View of Osteoarthritis Pathogenesis as a Combination of Biological, Structural, and Mechanical Factors In a preosteoarthritic state, the risk of developing subsequent osteoarthritis (OA) can be thought of in a probability, "slot-machine" analogy. The likelihood of developing OA in response to repeated activity is reflected by the degree of risk reflected in each of the contributing components. (From Chu CR, Andriacchi TP: Dance between biology, mechanics, and structure: a systems-based approach to developing osteoarthritis prevention strategies. *J Orthop Res* 33[7]:940, 2015.)

permeability of the matrix, thereby decreasing the ability of the matrix to resist tensile and compressive loads.[4] This results in increased stress in the matrix and subchondral bone, with eventual progression to OA.[58]

Cartilage and Subchondral Bone Disruption

Cartilage injuries penetrating the subchondral bone gain access to the vascular system and can elicit a reparative response.[13] This response includes formation of a hematoma, a fibrin clot, an inflammatory response, and migration of MSCs from the bone marrow.[39,44,47,54] Although the force required to produce a fracture of the subchondral bone is severe and also causes chondrocyte death and matrix damage, the reparative response results in formation of a fibrocartilage of variable quality within 6 to 8 weeks.[40,71] Fibrocartilage cells appear similar to fibroblasts; the matrix consists mainly of type I collagen and is different in composition and structure compared with normal cartilage.[71] Penetration of the subchondral bone induces a reparative response, but the synthesized fibrocartilage does not have the same composition, structure, and mechanical properties as normal articular cartilage.[39] Current research in cartilage repair emphasizes improving the structural, biochemical, and functional characteristics of the repair tissues.

Cartilage Homeostasis and Recovery in "Preosteoarthritis"

Mechanisms of damage may lead to a subclinical state of "preosteoarthritis," where cartilage and joint homeostasis is altered and OA risk is elevated, but where irreversible cartilage loss and OA have not yet developed.[17,26] Although cartilage damage heightens the risk for OA, new data show that articular cartilage with an intact surface retains some capacity for self-healing and recovery.[24,27] In injury models where the articular surface remains intact, early structural damage can be visualized by use of more sensitive magnetic resonance imaging (MRI) techniques

such as dGEMRIC, T1rho, or ultrashort echo-time enhanced T2* mapping (UTE-T2*).[27,90,91] Damage to the structural integrity of the deep zones of cartilage is evident; however, reversal of these changes suggestive of healing can be seen 2 years following anterior cruciate ligament reconstruction (ACLR) (Fig. 27.4).[27] Facilitating native pathways of cartilage healing after joint injury or abnormal mechanical loading prior to breakdown of the articular surface therefore has the potential to prevent or delay progression to OA.

FUTURE DIRECTIONS

Major challenges to the development of treatments for visible damage to articular cartilage include maintenance of cells with chondrocyte phenotypes, restoration of the functional structure of cartilage, and integration of repair tissue with the surrounding matrix.[73,89] Research into the mechanical and biochemical factors necessary to develop tissue-engineered cartilage repair and regeneration strategies continues and includes techniques to augment the in situ reparative response following injuries or techniques such as microfracture that access the bone marrow. Current research is also investigating potential chondroprotective agents, such as MMP inhibitors, growth factors, and cytokines, to reduce matrix damage and stimulate repair responses in surface intact articular cartilage.[21,41,80,87] The goal is development of a treatment aimed at addressing preosteoarthritis, with restoration of normal articular cartilage structure and function. Identification and staging of preosteoarthritic disease states will be crucial to facilitating cartilage and joint healing prior to onset of irreversible degenerative changes and presents a key new frontier in the approach to cartilage injury and repair. The latest research uses a systems-based approach to delineating reversible preosteoarthritic states, with the goal of maintaining cartilage and joint health to prevent the development of OA.

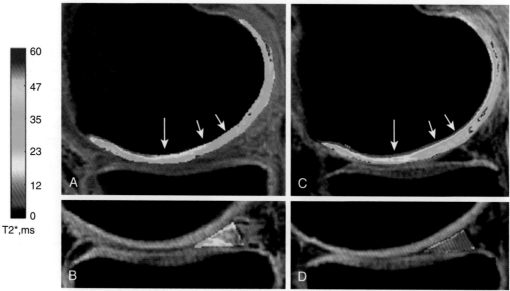

FIG 27.4 UTE-T2* mapping shows deep tissue meniscus and articular cartilage structural changes in a post-ACLR model that cannot be seen on conventional MRI. *Left*: UTE-T2* maps of articular cartilage deep tissue *(A, arrows)* and meniscus (B) of a subject after ACL tear, showing a mottled pattern that was higher than seen in uninjured controls. *Right*: UTE-T2* maps of the articular cartilage *(C, arrows)* and meniscus (D) of the same subject 2 years after anatomic ACL reconstruction. The return of the laminar pattern and low signal (shown in *red*) is comparable to uninjured controls. (B and D, from Chu CR, Williams AA, West RV, et al: Quantitative magnetic resonance imaging UTE-T2* mapping of cartilage and meniscus healing after anatomic anterior cruciate ligament reconstruction. *Am J Sports Med* May 8, 2014. Epub ahead of print.)

KEY REFERENCES

17. Chu CR, Andriacchi TP: Dance between biology, mechanics, and structure: a systems-based approach to developing osteoarthritis prevention strategies. *J Orthop Res* 33:939–947, 2015.
20. Chu CR, Izzo NJ, Coyle CH, et al: The in vitro effects of bupivacaine on articular chondrocytes. *J Bone Joint Surg Br* 90:814–820, 2008.
24. Chu CR, Millis MB, Olson SA: Osteoarthritis: from palliation to prevention: AOA critical issues. *J Bone Joint Surg Am* 96:e130, 2014.
40. Furman BD, Olson SA, Guilak F: The development of posttraumatic arthritis after articular fracture. *J Orthop Trauma* 20:719–725, 2006.
41. Glasson SS, Askew R, Sheppard B, et al: Deletion of active ADAMTS5 prevents cartilage degradation in a murine model of osteoarthritis. *Nature* 434:644–648, 2005.
44. Gudas R, Kalesinskas RJ, Kimtys V, et al: A prospective randomized clinical study of mosaic osteochondral autologous transplant versus microfracture for the treatment of osteochondral defects in the knee joint in young athletes. *Arthroscopy* 21:1066–1075, 2005.
47. Hunziker EB, Kapfinger E: Repair of partial-thickness defects in articular cartilage: cell recruitment from the synovial membrane. *J Bone Joint Surg Am* 78:721–733, 1996.
54. Magnussen RA, Dunn WR, Carey JL, et al: Treatment of focal articular cartilage defects in the knee. *Clin Orthop* 466:952–962, 2008.

79. Szczodry M, Coyle CH, Kramer SJ, et al: Progressive chondrocyte death after impact injury indicates a need for chondroprotective therapy. *Am J Sports Med* 37:2318–2322, 2009.
81. Thomas GC, Asanbaeva A, Vena P, et al: A nonlinear constituent based viscoelastic model for articular cartilage and analysis of tissue remodeling due to altered glycosaminoglycan-collagen interactions. *J Biomech Eng* 131:101–112, 2009.
83. Van Assche D, Staes F, Van Caspel D, et al: Autologous chondrocyte implantation versus microfracture for knee cartilage injury: a prospective randomized trial, with 2-year follow-up. *Knee Surg Sports Traumatol Arthrosc* 18:486–495, 2010.
89. Wescoe KE, Schugar RC, Chu CR, et al: The role of the biochemical and biophysical environment in chondrogenic stem cell differentiation assays and cartilage tissue engineering. *Cell Biochem Biophys* 52:85–102, 2008.
93. Wong M, Carter DR: Articular cartilage functional histomorphology and mechanobiology: a research perspective. *Bone* 33:1–13, 2003.
94. Youn I, Choi JB, Cao L, et al: Zonal variations in the three-dimensional morphology of the chondron measured in situ using confocal microscopy. *Osteoarthritis Cartilage* 14:889–897, 2006.

The references for this chapter can also be found on www.expertconsult.com.

28

Articular Cartilage Injury and Adult Osteochondritis Dissecans: Treatment Options and Decision Making

Justin W. Griffin, Phillip Locker, Nicole A. Friel, Brian J. Cole

Osteochondritis dissecans (OCD) is a pathologic process in which the subchondral bone and the overlying articular cartilage detach from the underlying bony surface.[10,40,55] The disease results in subchondral bone loss and destabilization of the overlying articular cartilage, leading to separation and increased susceptibility to stress and shear.[43] Fragmentation of both cartilage and bone leads to early degenerative changes and loss of function in the affected compartment. The true cause is unknown but is likely related to repetitive microtrauma, acute traumatic incident, ischemia, an ossification abnormality, or endocrine or genetic predisposition.[2,39,53]

The prevalence of OCD is estimated at 15 to 30 cases per 100,000, most frequently occurring in the knee, with medial femoral condyle (MFC) involvement in 80% of cases, lateral femoral condyle in 15%, and patellofemoral in 5%.[27,35] The lateral aspect of the MFC is the classic site of the OCD lesion. In addition to the knee, OCD has the propensity of occurring in the elbow, wrist, and ankle.[2,10,55]

OCD is divided into juvenile (JOCD) and adult (AOCD) forms.[9] The distinction between JOCD (open growth plates) and AOCD (closed growth plates) may be important in treatment and prognosis. JOCD often resolves with nonoperative management and has a much better prognosis compared with AOCD, which, once symptomatic, can follow a progressive, unremitting course.

Nonoperative treatments for symptomatic cases are rarely an option because of the inherent poor regenerative capacity of articular cartilage. Thus, cases of AOCD usually require surgical intervention, such as loose body removal, drilling, internal fixation, marrow stimulation, autologous chondrocyte implantation (ACI), or osteochondral autograft/allograft transplantation, to replace the damaged cartilage. In advanced cases, joint replacement may be the only feasible solution.

PRESENTATION

A patient with an OCD lesion complains primarily of pain and swelling of the affected joint, which can be triggered by physical activity. In the presence of a loose body, mechanical symptoms such as clicking, popping, and locking may accompany the primary complaints.

On physical examination, patients present with tenderness overlying the OCD region. Patients often present with an antalgic gait. If the OCD lesion is present in the classic location, the lateral aspect of the MFC, the patient will ambulate with the affected leg in relative external rotation (Wilson sign) to decrease contact of the lesion with the medial tibial eminence. Joint effusion, decreased range of motion, and quadriceps atrophy are also variably present, depending on the severity and duration of the lesion.[20,42]

Patellar OCD most often presents with patellofemoral pain, followed by swelling. Feelings of a loose body, locking, or giving way, or episodes of patellar subluxation, may also be noted. On examination, patients have retropatellar crepitus or pain and effusion.

IMAGING

Unfortunately, none of the physical findings observed during the examination can be used specifically to diagnose OCD; therefore confirmatory x-ray, magnetic resonance imaging (MRI), or computed tomography (CT) scans are required. Plain x-ray films should include standard anteroposterior, flexion weight-bearing anteroposterior (tunnel view), lateral, and Merchant views (Fig. 28.1). Flexion weight-bearing anteroposterior in addition to standard anteroposterior allows better visualization of lesions along the posterolateral aspect of the MFC.[26] Radiographic images of patients with AOCD show a lesion that typically appears as an area of osteosclerotic bone, with a high-intensity line between defect and epiphysis.

MRI is the mainstay in the diagnosis of OCD lesions and is the most informative imaging modality in the preoperative workup of OCD. Specifically, the quality of bone edema, subchondral separation, and cartilage condition are evaluated before treatment.[1] MRI can reliably indicate lesion size, location, and depth, providing insight into a patient's knee condition (Fig. 28.2). MRI images are assessed according to the criteria presented in the following list. Meeting one of the four criteria offers up to 97% sensitivity and 100% specificity in predicting lesion stability.[15,16,20,43]

- Thin, ill-defined, or well-demarcated line of high signal intensity, measuring 5 mm or more in length at the interface between the OCD lesion and underlying subchondral bone.
- Discrete rounded area of homogeneous high signal intensity, 5 mm or more in diameter beneath the lesion.
- Focal defect with an articular surface of the lesion with a width of 5 mm or more.
- High signal intensity line traversing the articular cartilage and subchondral bone plate into the lesion.

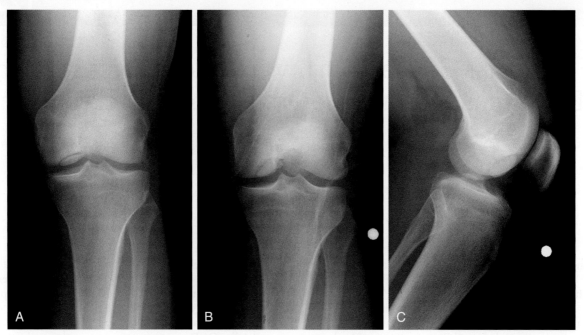

FIG 28.1 Radiograph of an Osteochondritis Dissecans (OCD) Lesion in the Classic Location of the Lateral Aspect of the Medial Femoral Condyle (MFC) (A) Standard anteroposterior. (B) Flexion weight-bearing anteroposterior. (C) Lateral.

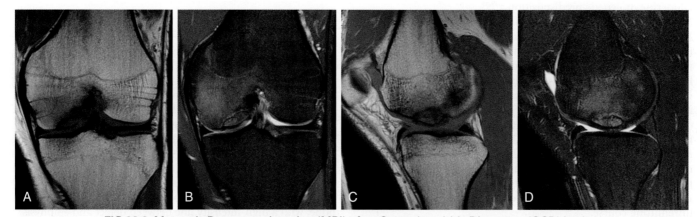

FIG 28.2 Magnetic Resonance Imaging (MRI) of an Osteochondritis Dissecans (OCD) Lesion at the Lateral Aspect of the Medial Femoral Condyle (MFC) Anteroposterior T1-weighted (A) and T2-weighted (B) views. Sagittal T1-weighted (C) and T2-weighted (D) views.

Furthermore, OCD lesions can be classified by MRI findings according to whether the lesion is attached, partially attached, or completely detached from the parent bone[37,43,49] (Table 28.1). Other imaging modalities such as CT scans are also used, which can be greatly beneficial in revealing the exact location and extent of the lesion.

Although the role of diagnostic imaging of OCD has been established, its usefulness in postoperative assessment is uncertain. Imaging has the advantage over second look arthroscopy by being noninvasive and able to appreciate subchondral structures; however, prognostic capabilities have yet to be reliably produced. Windt et al. performed a systematic review of 32 articles that assessed MRI imaging as a predictor of clinical outcome, and only nine found a positive correlation. In these studies, magnetic resonance observation of cartilage repair

tissue (MOCART) was used to assess cartilage condition.[14] It is the consensus of the American Academy of Orthopaedic Surgeons that patients treated surgically for OCD that remain symptomatic should be further examined and/or imaged.[13]

CAUSE, NATURAL HISTORY, AND PROGNOSIS

The definitive cause of OCD has yet to be established. A number of factors may contribute, such as repetitive microtrauma, acute stress and injury, restricted blood supply, endocrine abnormalities, and genetic predisposition.[2,39,53] Physical trauma is thought to be one of the major contributory factors in the development of OCD. Repetitive trauma to the joint leads to redundant healing, interrupting the blood supply to subchondral bone and possibly leading to avascular necrosis.[13] In adults, high-impact

TABLE 28.1 Magnetic Resonance Imaging Staging for Evaluation of Osteochondral Fracture[27,33,38]

Stage	Magnetic Resonance Imaging Findings
0	Normal
I	Signal changes consistent with articular cartilage injury, without disruption, and with normal subchondral bone
II	High-grade signal intensity; breach of the articular cartilage with a stable subchondral fragment
III	Partial chondral detachment with a thin high-signal rim (on T2-weighted images) behind the osteochondral fragment, representing synovial fluid
IV	Loose body in the center of the osteochondral fragment or free in the joint space

sports such as soccer, basketball, football, and weightlifting may put the athlete at higher risk of developing OCD. Endocrine abnormalities affecting calcium and phosphorus homeostasis or anomalies of bone formation can compromise the blood supply to subchondral bone and progress to avascular necrosis. Recent reports have suggested a genetic predisposition to OCD.[39]

Most AOCD cases arise from established but untreated or asymptomatic JOCD. However, many patients with AOCD present with a history of knee pain that began when they had open physes. These cases probably represent JOCD that did not heal and evolved to AOCD. An exception to this progression is JOCD that heals spontaneously; however, such lesions usually are not present in the classic location, which is the lateral aspect of the MFC.[13,55] AOCD may also arise de novo.[9,21]

The natural history of untreated OCD is poorly defined. Neither the literature nor our experience allows us to definitively determine whether untreated OCD has a higher likelihood of progressing to symptomatic degenerative joint disease (DJD) in the future. Linden performed a long-term retrospective follow-up study on patients with OCD of the femoral condyles, with an average follow-up of 33 years after initial diagnosis.[36] The author concluded that OCD occurring prior to closure of the physes (JOCD) does not lead to additional complications later in life, but patients who manifest OCD after closure of the physes (AOCD) develop osteoarthritis 10 years earlier than the normal population. In contrast, Twyman et al. evaluated 22 knees with JOCD and found that 50% had some radiographic signs of osteoarthritis at an average follow-up of 34 years.[56] The likelihood of developing osteoarthritis was also found to be proportional to the size of the area involved. The authors believe that lateral femoral condyle OCD has a poorer prognosis, but not all of these cases will become symptomatic over time, despite radiographic changes.

NONOPERATIVE TREATMENT

The ideal goal of conservative treatment is to attain lesion healing, which occurs more often before physeal closure. Stable OCD lesions in young patients have a favorable prognosis when treated initially with nonoperative treatment. Nonoperative treatment options include modified activity with decreased weight-bearing, anti-inflammatory medications, and management of patient symptoms. Traditional nonoperative treatment consists of an initial phase of knee immobilization with partial weight bearing to prevent repeated microtrauma lesions. Once the patient is pain free, weight bearing as tolerated is permitted, and a rehabilitation program emphasizing knee range of motion and low-impact strengthening exercises ensues. The goal is to promote healing in the subchondral bone and prevent chondral

separation. X-rays are usually taken 3 months after the start of nonsurgical therapy to assess the status of the lesion and the condition of the subchondral bone. If the lesion reveals adequate healing, patients are allowed to gradually return to activities; if no change is observed, x-ray assessment is repeated in 3 months.

SURGICAL TREATMENT

Surgical options are considered more often than not for AOCD because articular cartilage presents with an inherent poor ability to repair itself. Surgical options include loose body removal, drilling of the subchondral bone, internal fixation of the fragment, microfracture, osteochondral autografting and allografting, and ACI.[9,19,21,43] The overall goal of such intervention is to enhance the healing potential of the subchondral bone, fix the unstable fragment, and replace damaged bone and cartilage with implantable tissue.

The type and extent of surgery necessary for OCD depend on the patient's age, characteristics of the lesion (quality of articular cartilage; size of associated subchondral bone; and shape, thickness, and location of the lesion), diagnostic information provided by MRI and arthroscopy, and preference of the operating surgeon. The author's preferred algorithm for treatment of OCD lesions is shown in Fig. 28.3.

Positioning, Examination Under Anesthesia, and Diagnostic Arthroscopy

All patients are placed supine, with the leg supported by a standard thigh holder and the knee flexed at 90 degrees. The affected extremity is prepared and draped to the proximal thigh to ensure easy access to the knee. Examination under anesthesia assesses range of motion and ligamentous integrity. Lesions on the surfaces of the femoral condyle can usually be accessed using an arthroscopic approach. Standard portals are used and accessory portals are added when needed to improve visibility. More challenging locations, such as the patella and tibial plateau, may require an arthrotomy for better visualization and treatment.

A complete diagnostic arthroscopic evaluation of the structures in each compartment is performed. When the lesions are identified, a probe is used to determine the stability of the fragment (Fig. 28.4). Guhl's intraoperative classification is defined by cartilage integrity and fragment stability[25] (Table 28.2).

Loose Body Removal

When the fragment is comminuted, avascular, deformed, or otherwise irreparable, fragment removal is an isolated treatment option.[3] In cases involving chronic symptomatic lesions, fibrous tissue may impede anatomic reduction and adequate healing. In addition, the fragment may be associated with

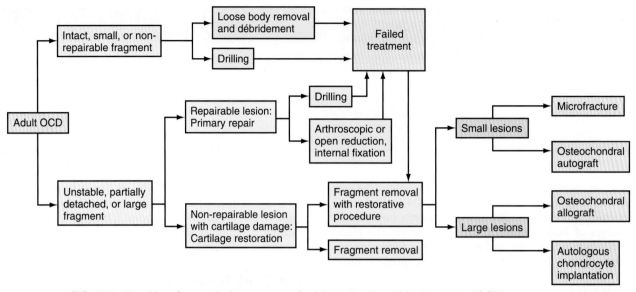

FIG 28.3 Algorithm for surgical treatment of adult osteochondritis dissecans (OCD).

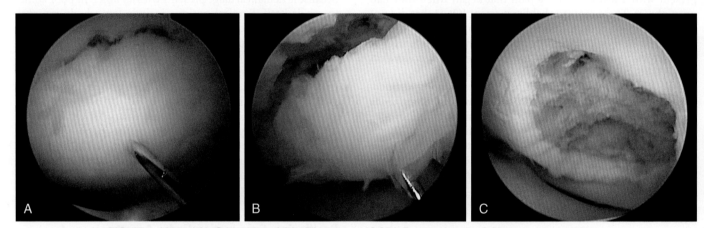

FIG 28.4 Unstable Osteochondritis Dissecans (OCD) Fragment (A) OCD lesion palpable at arthroscopy. (B) Palpation reveals unstable lesion. (C) Subchondral bone following removal of the OCD lesion.

TABLE 28.2	Guhl's Classification[18]
Stage	**Arthroscopic Findings**
I	Normal
II	Fragmentation in situ
III	Partial detachment
IV	Complete detachment, loose body present

only small amounts of subchondral bone with limited ability to heal.

Although OCD lesions should be reduced, stabilized, bone grafted, or restored when possible, patients with small or non-weight-bearing lesions may have good outcomes with isolated loose body removal. Ewing and Voto showed 72% satisfactory results in patients treated with fragment excision with or without drilling or abrasion.[19] A recent study showed successful outcomes in 8 of 9 patients treated with loose body removal alone for small (<2 cm²) AOCD lesions.[50] These results, however, are controversial and may pertain only to short-term outcomes.

Anderson and Pagnani excised OCD fragments in 11 patients with JOCD and 9 patients with AOCD. At an average of 9 years postoperatively, five failures and six poor outcomes were reported, and equally disappointing outcomes were seen with JOCD and AOCD.[4] Similarly, Wright and coworkers had 65% fair or poor results at an average 8.9 years postoperatively in 17 patients treated with fragment excision and suggested the use of aggressive cartilage preservation techniques and avoidance of fragment excision.[58]

The senior author's preference following obligatory fragment excision is benign neglect with formal patient education as to the symptoms of an osteochondral defect. Exceptions to this might include lateral femoral condyle OCD that is relatively uncontained toward the popliteus, which have a higher frequency of associated secondary lateral meniscus pathology and tibial disease. Similarly, large weight-bearing lesions of the MFC that are asymptomatic following fragment removal may be indicated for early restoration, based on patient preferences following objective education as to the relative risks of treatment versus benign neglect.

REPARATIVE PROCEDURES

The goal of reparative procedures is to restore the integrity of the native subchondral interface and preserve the overlying articular cartilage.[42]

Drilling

As mentioned previously, disruption of the blood supply to the subchondral bone is thought to be an important factor in the development of OCD.[5] Thus, treatment incorporates creation of vascular channels to the affected region. Arthroscopic drilling can be used to generate such channels and is usually performed in young patients.[1]

This technique is performed using an antegrade or a retrograde approach. Antegrade drilling is performed from the joint space, through the articular cartilage, and into the subchondral bone. Lesions of the MFC can be drilled through an anterolateral or anteromedial portal, and lesions of the lateral femoral condyle are usually accessible through the anterolateral portal. If the lesion is not accessible via standard portals, accessory portals are created to obtain an orthogonal drilling angle.[5] Multiple holes are drilled using a Kirschner wire (K-wire), making certain to uniformly cover the lesion. The return of blood and fat droplets from the drilled region is used to confirm the depth of the penetration.

Antegrade drilling has the undesirable consequence of violating the articular cartilage surface, causing the violation to fill with fibrocartilage. Retrograde drilling, although more difficult, avoids damage to the articular cartilage. The drill enters behind the lesion and penetrates the bony fragment without violating the cartilage or entering the joint. C-arm visualization or the use of an anterior cruciate ligament (ACL) guide is necessary to avoid joint penetration or dislodgement of the OCD fragment.[32] Targeting a three-dimensional lesion under intraoperative fluoroscopy that supplies a two-dimensional image has proved to be technically challenging, with failure rates up to 20%. This has lead to the development of three-dimensional image-based navigation in hopes of better accuracy. In a pilot study, Citek et al. had 100% accuracy using ISO-C3d technology and reported enhanced picture quality compared to 2D fluoroscopy. The study, however, did not have enough statistical power to claim superior accuracy, but opened the door for future investigation and development.[1]

Overall, outcomes of OCD drilling are generally favorable, and patient age is the best prognostic factor. Younger patients who have undergone this procedure demonstrate higher levels of radiographic healing and favorable relief of symptoms.[5,8,18,31] Louisia et al. compared outcomes of JOCD versus AOCD, reporting radiographic healing in 71% of JOCD cases and only 25% in adult AOCD cases.[38] Edmonds et al. evaluated the use of retrograde intraepiphyseal drilling in patients with stage I or II Guhl's classification and found that 75% of the 59 patients had 100% radiographic healing. Functional improvements were also noted, with a return to activity in 2.8 months and a mean healing time of 11.9 months.[2]

It is our opinion that drilling should be used when the defect is stable to palpation, despite MRI evidence of fluid behind the fragment, indicating biologic instability. When possible, drilling is performed through the intercondylar notch (ie, adjacent to the posterior cruciate ligament [PCL] femoral origin for OCD of the MFC) or along the lateral nonarticulating border of the distal femur using a 0.45-mm K-wire. When no gross ballotable instability is noted, we often place one or two bioabsorbable compression screws that are buried deep to the level of the subchondral plate (BioCompression Screw; Arthrex, Inc., Naples, Florida). With any evidence of instability, we make every effort to "hinge" the lesion open to expose the base, which is often covered in fibrovascular scar tissue.

Arthroscopic or Open Reduction and Internal Fixation

AOCD lesions that have become detached from the subchondral bone may present with articular cartilage flaps or loose bodies that require fixation.[43] Fixation is advised for symptomatic unstable lesions, provided that the lesion has sufficient subchondral bone to provide support for the fixation system. A cartilage flap, sometimes referred to as a *hinged lesion*, can be fixed using pins and screws. Unstable "trap door" lesions, which are partially elevated off the subchondral bone, require bed fixation, which can be achieved using microfracture awls to restore/improve blood supply, followed by fixation.[47]

Internal fixation can be achieved using a variety of fixation devices, as well as bone pegs and osteochondral grafts.[11,22] Internal fixation devices include cannulated screws, metal pins/K-wires, and bioabsorbable pins. The method of fixation is based largely on surgeon preference.

Constant thread pitch (AO) and variable thread pitch (Herbert, Acutrak) cannulated screws allow for compression across the lesion. AO screws, available in varying sizes, must be placed below the articular surface to avoid damage to the opposing articular surface. Variable pitch Herbert (partially threaded) and Acutrak (fully threaded) screws have a headless design that allows excellent compression of the fragment into the defect bed. Some surgeons bury the head of these screws, so as to allow early range of motion and prevent subsequent damage to the opposing tibial surface. However, it is the author's preference to use variable pitch metal screws and remove them at 8 weeks postoperatively to assess for healing and to avoid the consequences of fragment collapse, which can lead to prominent hardware. Bioabsorbable screws have been recommended by some to avoid removal, but questions remain as to the degree of compression they provide and the fact that they remain in situ for a prolonged time before enzymatic breakdown occurs.[28]

Before screw placement, unstable lesions are opened to expose the sclerotic bed. If necessary, lesions on the lateral aspect of the MFC may require superficial release of PCL fibers to expose the lateral margin of the lesion.[22] Cartilage at the lesion site is hinged open, the undersurface is débrided and curetted, and microfracture awls are used to stimulate bleeding from the subchondral bone. To place a screw, a guide wire is drilled through the fragment into the femoral condyle. The guide wire is then overdrilled and the screw is placed, compressing the fragment into the bed (Figs. 28.5 and 28.6). Another option is retrograde fixation, which most often is used for OCD lesions of the patella. Screws are placed from behind the lesion through the subchondral bone and into the bony portion of the fragment. Accurate screw placement is crucial for the success of this procedure and often involves the use of intraoperative fluoroscopy. Following any OCD procedure with internal fixation, the knee should be ranged to ensure that the screw head does not abrade the opposing surface.

K-wires and metal pins are advantageous because of their ease of insertion and availability in the operating room. However, K-wire use is limited because K-wires do not provide

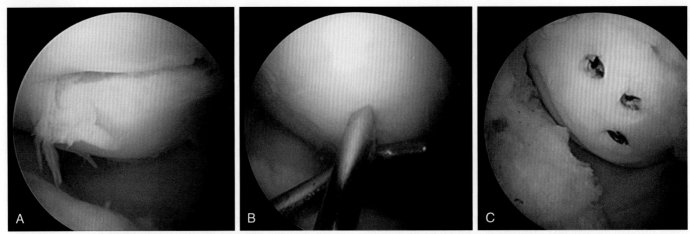

FIG 28.5 Arthroscopic Reduction, Internal Fixation of the Osteochondritis Dissecans (OCD) Fragment (A) Unstable fragment. (B) Fragment reduction and pin placement. (C) Fixation with metallic compression screws.

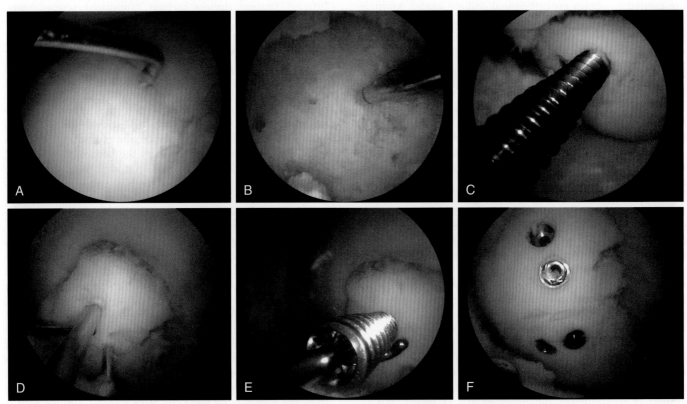

FIG 28.6 (A) Unstable osteochondritis dissecans (OCD) fragment palpable at arthroscopy. (B) Débridement and microfracture of the subchondral bone. (C) Screw placement for fixation. (D) Evaluation of reduced fragment. (E) Placement of additional screws to provide further compression and rotational stability. (F) Final fixation of two large fragments, each with two screws.

compression, may break or bend, and can migrate from the osteochondral fragment.

Bioabsorbable pins, both smooth and barbed, offer adequate fixation when a smaller device is used without the need for removal. Pins are placed by an anterograde method, and the small-head or headless pin can be impacted beneath the surface. Bioabsorbable pins have the disadvantages of implant fracture and foreign body reaction, resulting in aseptic synovitis. In

addition, they provide minimal compression across the defect junction.

In general, unless the lesion is very small, at least two fixation points are used to ensure compression and rotational stability. Screws are tightened until the fragment is compressed, but overtightening should be avoided to prevent fracture of the osteochondral fragment. All devices with a prominent head should be recessed beneath the cartilage surface to avoid further

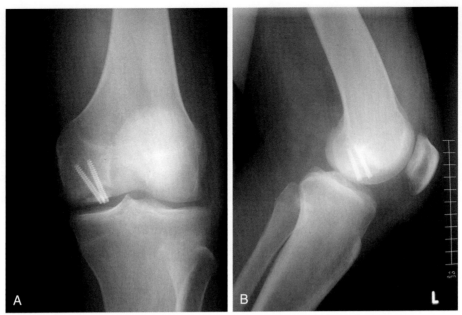

FIG 28.7 Anteroposterior (A) and lateral (B) views of an osteochondritis dissecans (OCD) lesion after screw fixation. Note that the screws are placed in the center of the lesion and are recessed below the cartilage surface.

injury to the juxtaposing cartilage (Fig. 28.7). As mentioned previously, nonabsorbable screws often require a second procedure for hardware removal; this affords the opportunity for a second look at the lesion site to verify healing.[43]

Large, displaced fragments should be augmented with bone grafting. After the base of the lesion has been examined, and débridement and penetration of the lesion bed have been performed with microfracture awls, the fragment still may not sit congruently within the defect site. Cancellous autograft can be harvested from Gerdy's tubercle on the ipsilateral limb. The bone graft is impacted into the defect site, and reduction of the fragment is reassessed until adequate reduction is achieved. Alternatively, small dowels of bone can be harvested arthroscopically using small-diameter instrumentation from the osteochondral autograft transfer systems. Once adequate reduction is achieved, the fragment is held in place with provisional K-wires until appropriate final fixation is achieved, as described previously. Osteochondral plugs help provide fixation and bone grafting across the lesion.

Postoperatively, all patients who have undergone arthroscopic or open reduction and internal fixation (ORIF) may heel-touch weight bear and, when available, may use continuous passive motion (CPM) machines for 4 to 6 hours per day.

Favorable outcomes have been reported after internal fixation of OCD fragments using absorbable and nonabsorbable screws. A study of Herbert compression screw fixation yielded 13 of 15 normal knees based on International Knee Documentation Committee (IKDC) clinical scoring, including 6 out of 8 in skeletally mature patients.[41] Kouzelis et al. treated patients with grade III and IV osteochondral lesions using reverse drilling and Herbert screw fixation and reported 90% normal or almost normal results using IKDC scoring.[32] Magnussen et al. reported healing in 92% of patients undergoing ORIF of grade IV OCD lesions, including healing in all seven skeletally mature patients.[40] Similarly, Pascual-Garrido et al. reported satisfaction in 13 of 15 AOCD cases treated with arthroscopic reduction internal fixation.[50]

Similar outcome scores have been reported with the use of bioabsorbable screw, nail, and pin fixation. Nakagawa et al. used fixation with bioabsorbable poly-L-lactide (PLLA) pins and showed 100% union and a clinical score of good (4/8) or excellent (4/8) in all patients.[48] Good and excellent clinical results were also achieved in all eight patients undergoing fixation with PLLA nails for OCD.[17] Weckstrom et al. compared bioabsorbable nails and pins in 30 patients with AOCD and showed significantly better fixation with nails (73% good to excellent) versus pins (35% good to excellent), suggesting that the barbs and the head of the nail allow for increased compression and rigid fixation.[57] There have been reports of questionable efficacy and complications associated with using bioabsorbable screws. Millington et al. experienced 6 out of 18 knees with unstable fragments that failed to fully unionize. Additionally, they noted screw back-out and breakage in 2 out of 11 knees.[3]

A new area of research is the use of a "hybrid fixation" for treatment of unstable OCD. This surgical approach includes filling the cartilage defect with an anterior tibial tuberosity autograft, using countersunk metal screws to fix the fragment, and filling in any gaps with 4.5 mm autograft osteochondral plugs obtained from the trochlea. Postoperative treatment included a non–weight-bearing protocol and screw removal after 3 months. This technique has an advantage over using traditional bone plugs or mosaicplasty by ensuring complete articular surface coverage. Limited outcome data have been published, but in a pilot study by Lintz et al., improved pre- to postoperative Hughston scores (of 2 to 4) and postoperative Lillois patellofemoral and IKDC subjective scores (of 78 and 70, respectively) were reported.[4]

Summary of Authors' Preferred Reparative Treatment Method

The method of fixation is based largely on the surgeons' preference, because no specific treatment has produced far superior outcomes. We prefer two to three partially threaded cannulated

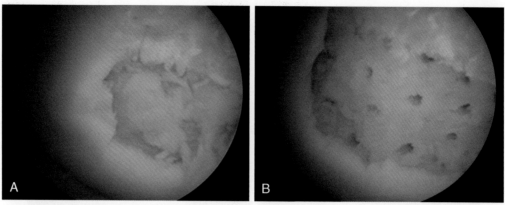

FIG 28.8 (A) Osteochondritis dissecans (OCD) lesion of the femoral condyle. (B) Treatment with microfracture.

screws with a second-look arthroscopy to remove the hardware and verify defect healing at 6 to 8 weeks. Bioabsorbable screws are also an option, especially when only one screw is needed for adequate stabilization of a macroscopically stable lesion, as is often seen with the early diagnosis and treatment of JOCD.

RESTORATIVE PROCEDURES

Restorative procedures attempt to replace damaged articular cartilage with hyaline or hyaline-like tissue.[34] These techniques should be considered as the next option if reparative treatments have failed and the patient presents with recurrent joint effusion, pain, and reduced range of motion. Multiple restorative techniques can be used for the treatment of OCD; however, the treatment algorithm should start with the least invasive options and progress to more invasive options.

Marrow Stimulation (Microfracture)

Microfracture involves production of tiny fractures in the subchondral bone, allowing an influx of pluripotent stem cells from the marrow into the defect site and forming a superclot. The presence of pluripotent cells allows differentiation and results in the production of fibrocartilage.[54] Microfracture is indicated in patients with a small, localized cartilage defect, typically measuring less than 4 cm^2 (Fig. 28.8). Postoperatively, rehabilitation requires 6 weeks of non–weight bearing, with use of CPM for 6 hours a day.

Gudas et al. randomized 50 patients with grade 3 or 4 lesions to be treated with either microfracture or osteochondral autograft transplantation (OAT) for their OCD. Both groups showed functional and objective improvements up to 4.2 years, after which the microfracture group had significant reductions in outcomes. These individuals still maintained overall improvements compared to preoperative evaluations. The microfracture group also showed a positive association between International Cartilage Repair Society (ICRS) results and lesion size, with lesions smaller than 3 cm^2 having significantly better outcomes.[5]

Gudas et al. randomized patients with posttraumatic, symptomatic full-thickness cartilage lesions (56%) and OCD lesions (44%) to treatment with microfracture or OAT. Clinical outcomes were significantly worse for the microfracture group, and the authors noted that whether treated with microfracture or OAT, patients with OCD had worse outcomes than those with

full-thickness cartilage defects.[24] Another similarly conducted study by Knutsen et al. randomized femoral condyle (28% with OCD lesions) cartilage defects to treatment with microfracture or ACI. Both groups demonstrated satisfactory results in 77% of patients at 5 years, with younger patients having better results in both groups. Overall, microfracture should be considered as a first-line treatment, especially in the setting of fragment removal with shallow defects that are relatively small. Whether fragment removal and microfracture fare better than fragment removal alone is not known, and we know little about which OCD lesions are optimal for initial microfracture treatment.[30]

Osteochondral Autograft Transplantation

In situations where the underlying subchondral bone integrity cannot support microfracture, OAT can be considered. The OAT procedure involves transplantation of osteochondral tissue from a low-weight-bearing region, such as the area just above the intercondylar notch or the lateral edge of the trochlea, with insertion of the plug into the defect.[52] A single autograft plug is preferred for defects smaller than 1 cm^2; however, some authors perform mosaicplasty with multiple smaller plugs for larger defects.

Good clinical results have been reported with osteochondral autografts. Miniaci and Tytherleigh-Strong have reported normal postoperative knee scores at 18 months for all 20 OCD patients (11 immature and 9 mature) treated with OAT, used as a biologic splint placed through the unstable fragment into the defect bed. In addition, radiographic evidence obtained 6 months postoperatively demonstrated adequate healing.[46] Outerbridge used osteochondral plugs taken from the ipsilateral lateral patella to treat patients with large osteochondral defects. The authors noted that all patients had increased function, and 81% returned to a high level of function. However, use of OAT is limited to small lesions because of limited supplies and donor site morbidity.

Emre et al. performed a retrospective analysis on 152 patients who had a mosaicplasty on grade III and IV cartilage lesions: 146 of the patients reported good to excellent results and improved Lysholm scores at a mean follow-up of 18.2 months. Factors associated with poorer prognosis were age, gender, lesion size, and concomitant intra-articular injuries. The author used backward regression analysis to create an equation predicting final follow-up Lysholm scores to aid in clinical decision making, 93.4 − [0.2 (age of patient) + 0.8 (lesion size) + 0.9

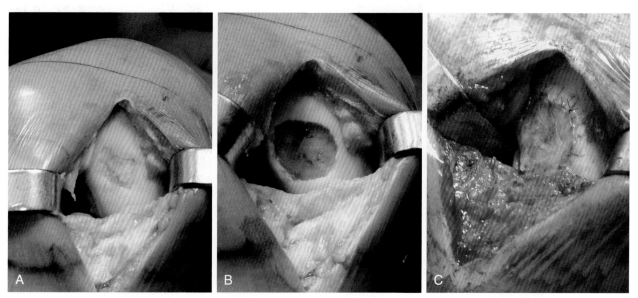

FIG 28.9 (A) Lesion at the lateral aspect of the medial femoral condyle (MFC). (B) Lesion prepared for autologous chondrocyte implantation (ACI). (C) Completed ACI.

(localization) + 2.8 (presence of associated intraarticular injuries)].[6]

Autologous Chondrocyte Implantation

With limited supplies and donor site morbidity associated with the OAT procedure, treatment for larger lesions requires a different technique. ACI is ideal for large, isolated osteochondral defects measuring up to 10 cm². This two-step procedure involves an initially healthy chondrocyte biopsy, performed arthroscopically with tissue extracted from the non–weight-bearing intercondylar notch region. Extracted cells are expanded in vitro over 4 to 6 weeks and then are reimplanted at the lesion site. At the time of implantation, defect preparation involves débridement of the calcified cartilage base and creation of vertical walls of healthy cartilage. A patch, periosteal, or synthetic collagen membrane is attached to the perimeter using absorbable sutures. The edges are sealed using fibrin glue, and in vitro cultured cells are injected beneath the patch[14,45] (Fig. 28.9). As with microfracture, 6 weeks of non–weight bearing postoperatively and CPM are indicated for both OAT and ACI.

Peterson and colleagues evaluated 58 patients (60% JOCD and 40% AOCD) who underwent an ACI procedure. At a 2- to 10-year follow-up, the authors reported the presence of repair tissue at the lesion site, with good to excellent clinical outcomes in 91% of patients.[51] As noted previously, Knutsen et al. reported 77% satisfactory results in patients with femoral condyle lesions treated with ACI.[30] In a large population of patients undergoing ACI, including 24% with OCD lesions, Bentley and associates reported 88% good to excellent outcomes based on clinical assessment.[7] Krishnan et al. performed ACI using a collagen membrane to treat 37 OCD patients (27 JOCD and 9 AOCD).[33] Among patients with juvenile-onset OCD, 91% good to excellent outcomes were achieved in patients treated before skeletal maturity, compared with 77% in those treated after skeletal maturity, suggesting that early treatment is optimal. Furthermore, adult-onset OCD patients had 44% good to excellent outcomes, and better clinical outcomes were seen in those with smaller (<6 cm²) lesions.

Defects deeper than 8 to 10 mm can still be treated with ACI, but concomitant or staged bone grafting is recommended. Prior to bone grafting, drilling through the bed following débridement allows appropriate blood flow into the defect, ensuring subsequent bone graft incorporation. When bone grafting is performed as a primary procedure in an effort to stage definitive treatment with ACI, most surgeons wait a minimum of 6 months to allow bone graft incorporation. Alternatively, a bilayer collagen membrane (periosteal "sandwich" technique) can be used without the need to stage the ACI.[6,12] A layer of periosteum or collagen membrane is used to seal the bone graft, and it is fixed with 6-0 Vicryl suture. A second layer is placed on top of the first and is similarly sewn; this is followed by injection of cultured cells between the two layers. Limited experience with this technique has been documented. Bartlett and associates reported three excellent results, one good, and one fair in five patients treated using ACI with a bilayer collagen membrane with bone graft.[6]

Because of the two-step nature of an ACI treatment, the chondrocyte implantation is typically done if the first line treatment done with the biopsy fails. ACI efficacy as a secondary treatment for OCD lesions was researched by the senior author and showed promising results. Forty of the patients enrolled in the Study of the Treatment of Articular Repair (STAR) had OCD and at least one previous failed procedure. Of the 40, 85% had successful treatment at 48 months with improved knee injury and osteoarthritis outcome score (KOOS) in pain, symptoms, sports and reaction ability, activities of daily living, and knee-related quality of life.[7]

Osteochondral Allograft

Large OCD lesions may also be treated with osteochondral allograft (OA) transplantation.[23] The OA graft provides the ability to resurface larger and deeper defects with mature hyaline cartilage and addresses the underlying subchondral bone deficiency, which is a hallmark of OCD. The donor tissue is generally fashioned in a cylindrical plug matching the diameter of the initial lesion (Fig. 28.10). To ensure proper fixation,

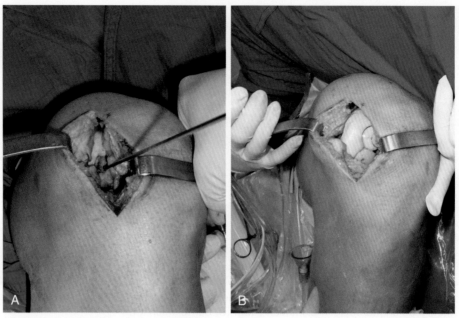

FIG 28.10 (A) Large osteochondritis dissecans (OCD) lesion of the femoral condyle. (B) Treatment with two osteochondral allograft plugs.

bioabsorbable compression screws or headless variable pitch titanium screws can be used. Postoperative rehabilitation is similar to that used following OAT or ACI.

It has been reported that fresh OA graft transplantation provides good to excellent clinical outcomes with long-term follow-up. Garrett presented a series of AOCD lesions of the femoral condyle, reporting 94% clinical success at a mean follow-up of 3 years.[21] McCulloch et al., in 25 patients with full-thickness defects, including six OCD lesions, presented an 84% success rate.[44] In a large study of 66 OCD lesions in 64 patients, treatment with a fresh OA yielded good to excellent results in 72% of patients. Overall, treatment of OCD with an OA graft can result in subjective improvement in 75% to 85% of patients, as supported by long-term follow-up.[29]

These positive results were further supported by Chalal et al., who did a systematic review of 19 studies with 644 knees, 30% with OCD cause, and found an overall satisfaction rate of 86%. Additionally, there was a relatively low complication rate and failure rate, 2.4% and 18% respectively, even with heterogeneity in allografts used and patient demographics.[8]

Other Frontiers

Advances in our understanding of articular cartilage physiology have lead to novel approaches in treating OCD. Kon et al. previewed what the future may hold for OCD patients by treating 62 knees with five newly developed techniques. They compared massive osteochondral autologous transplantation, bone-cartilage paste graft, second-generation autologous chondrocyte implantation plus bone graft, biomimetic osteochondral scaffold, and bone marrow–derived cell transplantation and found improvements in global mean IKDC and EuroQol visual analogue scale (EQ-VAS) at 5.3 years of follow-up.[9]

Biomimetic osteochondral scaffolding is an aspect that has been further researched since the previously mentioned study. The aim of this technology is to address the pitfalls of other cartilage transplant treatments—namely, the required two

surgeries in the ACI and limited donor cartilage available in OA and OATs. In biomimetic scaffolding, the cartilage defect is filled with a tissue that is engineered with a type 1 collage-hydroxyapatite nanostructure. The three-dimension structure is designed to replicate healthy osteocartilaginous tissue. The top layer is a smooth surface of hydroxyapatite nanocrystals on top of type 1 collagen. Below is a layer with both type 1 collagen plus hydroxyapatite. The deepest layer contains primarily mineralized hydroxyapatite with some type 1 collagen. Similar to Kon, Delcogliano and researchers reported increased EQ-VAS scores as well as Tenger Activity Scores at 2 year follow-up. Additionally, MRI analysis revealed 80% of the lesions had completely filled defects.[10] Filardo et al. also observed improved clinical outcomes 2 year postoperatively, with no correlation of lesion size to prognosis.[11]

Another one-step cartilage repair treatment that is being further researched is the use of bone-marrow-derived cells. This technique takes advantage of the multipotent mesenchymal stem cells that are present in the patient's bone marrow that have the ability to differentiate into chondrocytes and osteocytes. This procedure is done in three steps, with the first step being to obtain 120 mL of the patient's venous blood prior to surgery to create 6 mL of a platelet rich fibrin gel. During the operation, a needle is used to aspirate 60 mL of bone marrow from the posterior iliac crest into a calcium-heparin solution. Once the marrow is processed intraoperatively by removing plasma and erythrocytes, followed by being centrifuged, an arthrotomy is done and the concentrate is injected into a hyaluronic acid membrane that is in the cartilage defect. Following the procedure, the patient is restricted from weight bearing for a month. This technique has shown to improve clinical outcome measures, and histologic analyses of patients 1 year postoperatively revealed the deep layers having a proteoglycan-rich matrix and type II collagen throughout the sample.[12] This technique takes advantage of the mesenchymal stem cells that are present in bone marrow.

CONCLUSIONS

AOCD of the knee is a challenging problem that results in poor outcomes without surgical intervention once patients present with symptoms. Timely diagnosis can prevent compromise of the articular cartilage and can maximize the successful outcome of restorative procedures. Several surgical treatments have been used to treat OCD lesions. Reestablishment of the joint surface by improving blood supply via drilling or internal fixation is the primary goal of osteochondral fragment preservation. When the symptomatic fragment is not suitable for preservation, cartilage restoration techniques should be considered as an option. The overall goal for the treatment of AOCD lesions is to relieve pain, restore function, and prevent development of secondary osteoarthritis.

KEY REFERENCES

1. Adachi N, Deie M, Nakamae A, et al: Functional and radiographic outcome of stable juvenile osteochondritis dissecans of the knee treated with retroarticular drilling without bone grafting. *Arthroscopy* 25:145–152, 2009.
3. Alford JW, Cole BJ: Cartilage restoration, Part 2: techniques, outcomes, and future directions. *Am J Sports Med* 33:443–460, 2005.
6. Bartlett W, Gooding CR, Carrington RW, et al: Autologous chondrocyte implantation at the knee using a bilayer collagen membrane with bone graft: a preliminary report. *J Bone Joint Surg Br* 87:330–332, 2005.
14. Day JB, Gillogly SD: Autologous chondrocyte implantation in the knee. In Cole BJ, Sekiya JK, editors: *Surgical techniques of the shoulder, elbow, and knee in sports medicine*, Philadelphia, 2008, Saunders Elsevier, pp 559–566.
22. Gomoll AH, Flik KR, Hayden JK, et al: Internal fixation of unstable Cahill Type-2C osteochondritis dissecans lesions of the knee in adolescent patients. *Orthopedics* 30:487–490, 2007.
24. Gudas R, Stankevicius E, Monastyreckiene E, et al: Osteochondral autologous transplantation versus microfracture for the treatment of articular cartilage defects in the knee joint in athletes. *Knee Surg Sports Traumatol Arthrosc* 14:834–842, 2006.
29. Kang RW, Gomoll AH, Cole BJ: Osteochondral allografting in the knee. In Cole BJ, Sekiya JK, editors: *Surgical techniques of the shoulder, elbow, and knee in sports medicine*, Philadelphia, 2008, Saunders Elsevier, pp 549–557.
32. Kouzelis A, Plessas S, Papadopoulos AX, et al: Herbert screw fixation and reverse guided drillings, for treatment of types III and IV osteochondritis dissecans. *Knee Surg Sports Traumatol Arthrosc* 14:70–75, 2006.
34. Lewis PB, McCarty LP, 3rd, Kang RW, et al: Basic science and treatment options for articular cartilage injuries. *J Orthop Sports Phys Ther* 36:717–727, 2006.
43. McCarty LP III: Primary repair of osteochondritis dissecans in the knee. In Cole BJ, Sekiya JK, editors: *Surgical techniques of the shoulder, elbow, and knee in sports medicine*, Philadelphia, 2008, Saunders Elsevier, pp 517–526.
44. McCulloch PC, Kang RW, Sobhy MH, et al: Prospective evaluation of prolonged fresh osteochondral allograft transplantation of the femoral condyle: minimum 2-year follow-up. *Am J Sports Med* 35:411–420, 2007.
50. Pascual-Garrido C, Friel NA, Kirk SS, et al: Midterm results of surgical treatment for adult osteochondritis dissecans of the knee. *Am J Sports Med* 37(Suppl 1):125S–130S, 2009.
51. Peterson L, Minas T, Brittberg M, et al: Treatment of osteochondritis dissecans of the knee with autologous chondrocyte transplantation: results at two to ten years. *J Bone Joint Surg Am* 85(Suppl 2):17–24, 2003.
52. Rabalais RD, Swan KG, Jr, McCarty E: Osteochondral autograft for cartilage lesions of the knee. In Cole BJ, Sekiya J, editors: *Surgical techniques of the shoulder, elbow, and knee in sports medicine*, Philadelphia, 2008, Saunders Elsevier, pp 539–548.
54. Steadman JR, Rodkey WG, Briggs KK: Microfracture technique in the knee. In Cole BJ, Sekiya JK, editors: *Surgical techniques of the shoulder, elbow, and knee in sports medicine*, Philadelphia, 2008, Saunders Elsevier, pp 509–515.

The references for this chapter can also be found on www.expertconsult.com.

29

International Experience With Autologous Chondrocyte Implantation With Periosteum (Autologous Chondrocyte Implantation) Including Scaffold Guided Techniques and Tissue Engineered Matrix Support

Lars Peterson, Haris S. Vasiliadis

Articular cartilage is a unique tissue with no vascular, nerve, or lymphatic supply. The lack of vascular and lymphatic circulation may be one of the reasons why articular cartilage has such a poor intrinsic capacity to heal. There is no inflammatory response to tissue damage unless there is involvement of subchondral bone in the damaged area. Subsequently, there will be no macrophage invasion to phagocytose and remove the damaged and devitalized tissue and, furthermore, no migration of cells with repair capacity into the damaged area. The chondrocyte itself, encapsulated in its own matrix, is incapable of migrating and repopulating the damaged area.

Chondral injuries that penetrate down to subchondral bone will not heal but may progress to osteoarthritis over time by enzymatic degradation and mechanical wear. Osteochondral injuries that penetrate subchondral bone into trabecular bone with bleeding will result in inflammatory repair tissue filling the lesion with fibrocartilage produced by mesenchymal stem cells or fibroblasts. Unfortunately, the quality of the fibrocartilage repair tissue has been shown to not be able to withstand mechanical wear over time, and the fibrocartilage may degenerate and the lesion progress to osteoarthritis.[8,22]

Good results can be achieved with treatment of severe osteoarthritis of the knee by total joint replacement in older patients. However, this treatment exposes the patients to an increasing risk of potentially serious complications and also has a limited duration of life, finally demanding a revision surgery. Total knee arthroplasty burns the bridges to any other treatment options and is considered the last treatment option, indicated only for severe cases in elderly patients. In young and middle-aged patients, however, there is no optimal treatment for chondral injuries. The spectrum of treatment alternatives for articular cartilage defects in young and middle-aged patients can range from simple lavage and débridement, drilling, microfracturing, and abrasion to osteochondral grafting and autologous chondrocyte implantation (ACI).

The optimal healing of an articular cartilage injury should consist of regeneration with tissue identical to hyaline cartilage; however, repair of chondral injury involves filling with tissue not identical to hyaline cartilage (ie, fibrocartilage). The repair tissue should be able to fill and seal off the defective area with good adhesion to subchondral bone and complete integration to surrounding cartilage. It should be able to withstand mechanical wear over time and gradually be included in the natural turnover of normal cartilage, thus providing a variable duration of symptomatic relief.[8]

The functional unit of articular cartilage includes not only the different layers of cartilage but also subchondral and trabecular bone. Any treatment technique that interferes with subchondral and trabecular bone may not be able to restore the functional unit of cartilage, especially its shock-absorbing function.

Techniques that affect the subchondral bone plate include abrasion, arthroplasty, multiple drilling, and microfracture. All these techniques may result in stiffening of subchondral and trabecular bone and thereby promote osteophytes' formation underneath the repair tissue.[24,41] Osteochondral grafting may affect the subchondral and trabecular bone as the osseous part of the plug has to undergo resorption, revascularization, remodeling, and healing to the surrounding bone. Periosteal and perichondrial grafting also affect subchondral bone by drilling and abrading the subchondral bone plate.

Chondrocyte implantation does not violate subchondral or trabecular bone. On the contrary, for success with this technique, bleeding from subchondral bone should be avoided so that fibroblasts or stem cells are not introduced and result in fibroblastic repair tissue.[6]

HISTORICAL BACKGROUND OF AUTOLOGOUS CHONDROCYTE IMPLANTATION (TRANSPLANTATION)

In 1965 Smith was successful in isolating and growing chondrocytes in culture for the first time.[13] Epiphyseal chondrocytes grown in culture were injected into tibial articular defects in the rabbit knee but did not show any significant repair.

In 1982, experimental work started at the Hospital for Joint Diseases–Orthopedic Institute in New York to design an experimental rabbit model using articular chondrocytes isolated and grown in culture for implantation into a defect made in the patella and covered with a periosteal flap. The idea was to use

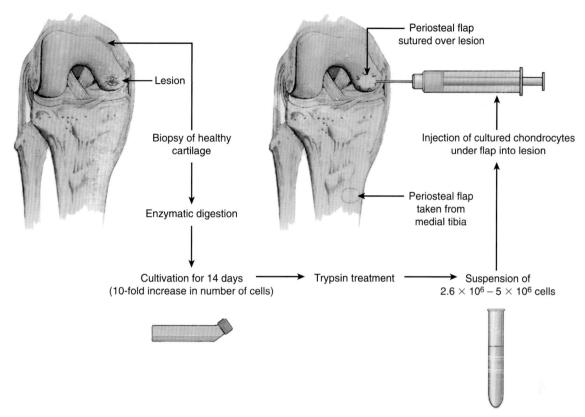

FIG 29.1 Diagram of the autologous chondrocyte implantation procedure.

articular chondrocytes because they are the only cells committed to form hyaline cartilage.

The initial results of ACI in this rabbit model were presented in 1984 and showed hyaline-like cartilage filling 80% of the patellar defect. No significant filling was seen in the control side, where the defect was treated with periosteal cover, but no cells.

Since 1984, extensive animal studies have been ongoing at the University of Göteborg, Sweden. The results from New York were confirmed and improved.

In 1985, work started on transferring the cell-culturing technique to human chondrocytes, and in 1987 the first ACI (or "transplantation," as first named) was performed in the human knee at the Department of Orthopaedics, University of Göteborg, after approval by the Ethical Committee of the Medical Faculty of the University of Göteborg (Fig. 29.1).

A pilot study of 23 patients with 39 months' follow-up reported in the *New England Journal of Medicine* in October 1994 showed that of the 16 patients who underwent femoral condyle procedures, 14 had a good or excellent result. Eleven of 15 biopsy specimens showed hyaline-like cartilage. Of the seven patients who underwent ACI of the patella, however, only two good or excellent results were achieved, and one biopsy specimen showed hyaline-like cartilage.[6]

Since 1987, more than 1600 patients have been operated on in Gothenburg, Sweden, and since 1995, more than 400 surgeons have performed ACI on more than 25,000 patients outside Sweden.

The clinical results from Sweden have been reported at the American Academy of Orthopaedic Surgeons in 1996, 1997,

1998, 2000, 2001, 2002, 2003, and 2004, while the long-term results of 10 to 20 years after the ACI were first presented at the International Cartilage Research Society (ICRS) meeting in 2009.[34,40]

INDICATIONS FOR AUTOLOGOUS CHONDROCYTE IMPLANTATION

ACI is indicated in patients between 15 and 55 years old with symptomatic, full-thickness, Outerbridge or ICRS grade III to IV cartilage injuries of the knee with a diameter larger than 10 mm up to an area of 10 to 16 cm^2 (Fig. 29.2). The location of the defect should be on the femoral or patellar articular surface and should be accessible for implantation via open arthrotomy. Only grade I to II Outerbridge or ICRS classification changes on the reciprocal articular surface should be included.

Osteochondritis dissecans of the medial or lateral femoral condyles with an unstable fragment, separated but attached flap, or empty bed is also an indication for ACI (Fig. 29.3).

Bipolar chondral injuries (ie, osteoarthritis) are undergoing investigational studies and could be considered a salvage procedure or a relative indication at present. A recent long-term follow-up study shows good results 10 to 20 years after the implantation, even for large bipolar lesions, where ACI has been performed as a salvage procedure.[34,40] There is evidence to support that ACI is indicated even for large bipolar lesions, delaying or even postponing the total knee arthroplasty. A definite decision regarding the indication is made during arthroscopic evaluation.

CLINICAL EVALUATION

A thorough history of symptoms, trauma, or repetitive loading is important, as well as a careful record of previous surgery. Clinical examination, including signs of local tenderness, swelling, range of motion, and crepitation, is performed.

Varus and valgus deformities are assessed, and patella malalignment, maltracking, or instability is evaluated. Clinical testing of ligament instability is performed.

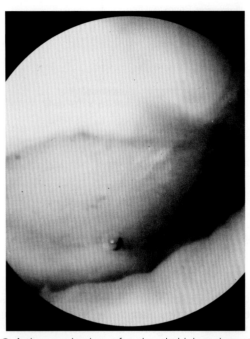

FIG 29.2 Arthroscopic view of a chondral injury down to bone on the medial femoral condyle, an indication for autologous chondrocyte implantation.

BACKGROUND FACTORS TO CONSIDER

An understanding of the optimal environment for survival of the repair tissue in the short and long term is of utmost importance. Varus or valgus malalignment should be evaluated on standing x-ray films of the knee in the extended position and 45 degrees of knee flexion. Additional information could be achieved through examining the hip, knee, and ankle axis on long, standing x-ray films. Varus or valgus deformity should be corrected. Magnetic resonance imaging (MRI) could be helpful to evaluate the articular cartilage injury and condition of the subchondral bone in more detail, as well as the status of the menisci. Previous meniscus surgery should be assessed, and after total or subtotal meniscectomy, meniscal transplantation should be considered.

Instability should be evaluated clinically and any instability should be corrected. Osseous defects deeper than 8 to 10 mm should be considered for autologous bone grafting and chondrocyte implantation. MRI could be a helpful tool to evaluate any bone pathology.

ARTHROSCOPIC EVALUATION— CARTILAGE RETRIEVAL

Under general or spinal anesthesia, complete stability testing of the knee is performed and the results compared with those on the healthy side. A complete examination of the knee joint should be performed, including visualization and probing of the articular cartilage surfaces, synovial lining, menisci, and cruciate ligaments, and the presence of any fragment or loose body should be identified. Undiagnosed pathology may be critical to the outcome of surgery. The cartilage injury is visualized, probed, and assessed for depth, size, and location. The opposing articular surface should be assessed and should be normal or have only fibrillation or superficial fissuring (Outerbridge or ICRS grade I to grade II). The defect should be evaluated regarding containment and shouldering. An uncontained lesion extends into the synovial lining of the joint. It could be

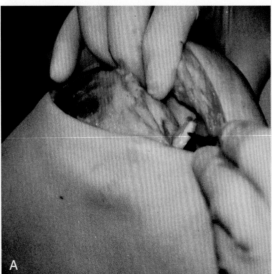
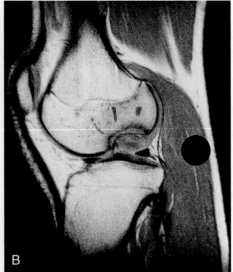

FIG 29.3 (A) Arthrotomy of a right knee with osteochondritis dissecans of the lateral femoral condyle and an avulsed but attached flap, an indication for autologous chondrocyte implantation. (B) Magnetic resonance image showing a deep osseous defect on the lateral femoral condyle.

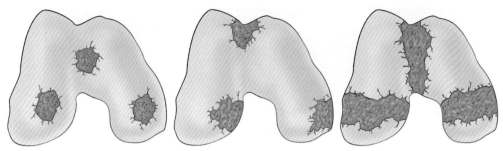

FIG 29.4 Schematic drawing showing containment of defects. The *left* drawing shows contained defects; the *middle* drawing, unilateral uncontained defects extending to the synovial lining; and the *right* drawing, bilateral uncontained defects.

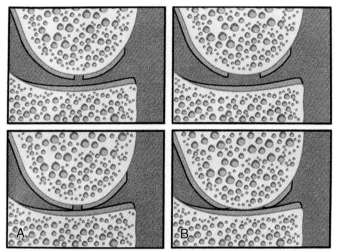

FIG 29.5 (A) Shouldered defects are usually smaller than 10 mm and are contained. (B) Unshouldered defects are larger. During weight bearing, the center of the defect is in contact with the opposing articular surface.

unilateral or bilateral, for example, extending from the synovial lining of the articular surface of the medial femoral condyle into the synovial lining of the intercondylar notch (Fig. 29.4).

A shouldered defect is a defect surrounded by normal cartilage in which the bone in the center of the defect is not in contact with the opposing articular surface. An unshouldered defect is so large that in a weight-bearing position the subchondral bone in the center of the defect is in contact with the opposing articular surface (Fig. 29.5). During arthroscopy, the proposed implantation is evaluated regarding different possibilities of the surgical approach, the intended amount of débridement, the extent of shouldering, containment of the defect, and so on.

Meniscal lesions should be treated at this time, but only after harvesting cartilage for cell culture. Cartilage fragments and loose bodies should be removed before harvesting the cartilage.

No or only gentle débridement of the injury should be performed at this time. When the specifics of the indication have been fulfilled, cartilage is harvested from the upper medial or upper lateral femoral condyle on minor weight-bearing areas (Fig. 29.6). It could also be harvested from the intercondylar notch. In 98% of our cases, cartilage is harvested from the upper medial femoral condyle. With a curette, three to four slices of cartilage 3 to 4–10 mm should be taken down to subchondral

bone on the upper medial femoral condyle.[8] Approximately 200 to 300 mg of articular cartilage is required for enzymatic digestion and cell culturing. The harvesting area should extend to the synovial lining to allow fibrous as well as synovial ingrowth for covering the harvest area. In more than 2000 patients who have had cartilage removed for cell culturing, no complications or late symptoms have occurred from the donor site. Optimal harvesting of cartilage is of greatest importance for the success of cell culturing, and optimal cell quality is necessary for the best possible result of this procedure.

CELL CULTURING

The retrieved cartilage is transferred to the cell culture lab in a sterile tube containing 0.9% NaCl. Upon the arrival, the cartilage is mechanically minced into smaller pieces (1 mm of diameter) and washed in medium supplemented with antibiotics (gentamicin sulfate, amphotericin B, L-ascorbic acid, and glutamine). Then it is subjected to overnight collagenase digestion, allowing isolation of the chondrocytes. The chondrocytes are then cultured in DMEM/F12 (Dulbecco's Modified Eagle Medium) with 10% autologous serum supplement and antibiotics. Primary cultures are performed in 25 cm² flasks incubated in 7% CO_2 in air at 37°C. After 1 week, the cells are trypsinized and passed into bigger culture flasks (75 cm²), where they are cultured for an additional week. Two weeks after the culture begins, the cells are trypsinized again, washed, counted, and resuspended in 0.3 to 0.4 mL of implantation medium, in a tuberculin syringe, to a treatment density of 30 million cells/mL. A second surgery is performed for the implantation of the cells into the cartilage defect area.

SURGICAL PROCEDURE— CHONDROCYTE IMPLANTATION

Chondral Lesions

The patient is placed under general or spinal anesthesia. With a tourniquet-controlled bloodless field, a minor parapatellar incision is made. The joint is opened and the injury assessed. For a good surgical technique, it is important to obtain good access to the defect, and the arthrotomy might need to be adjusted accordingly (Fig. 29.7). The patella may have to be dislocated in the case of implantation to multiple femoral or patellar lesions.

Clinical and radiological assessment has to be performed prior to the surgery, revealing a potential indication for a realignment procedure. A realignment procedure is then scheduled

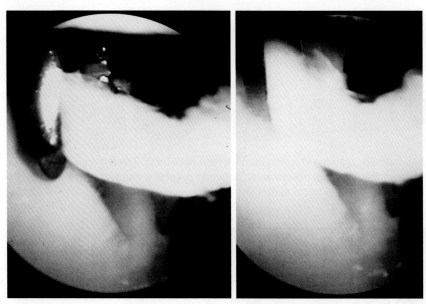

FIG 29.6 Arthroscopic views showing harvesting of articular cartilage from the upper medial femoral condyle with a curette (*right*).

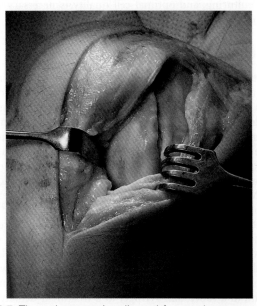

FIG 29.7 The arthrotomy is adjusted for good exposure of the defect.

in patients with patella lesions and patellofemoral malalignment or instability. Tibial or femoral osteotomies are also performed when needed, in cases of excessive varus or valgus deformity, for the protection of the implanted area. Corrective operations (osteotomy, reconstruction of extensor mechanism, anterior cruciate ligament [ACL] reconstruction), were performed before the implantation of the cells. In case of tibial osteotomy, medial transfer of the tibial tuberosity, or ACL graft fixation, the fixation is performed at the end of the procedure before the implantation of the cells.

Excision and Débridement of the Lesion. The cartilage lesion area is assessed, incised, and debrided with a curette down to the subchondral bone and until reaching healthy cartilage

in the periphery of the defect. Radical excision is the key to success. The resulting lesions should be as circular or oval as possible. If the lesion is not contained by healthy cartilage, it is better to leave a 3- to 4-mm rim of acceptable cartilage than to have the lesion border bone or synovium. Gentle débridement of the excised area is performed down to subchondral bone but without causing any bleeding. If bleeding occurs, an epinephrine sponge or a drop of fibrin glue can stop it. The excised defect is then measured in its longest diameter and longest perpendicular diameter. The defect should be shaped as geometrically as possible. A template of sterile aluminum foil or paper is used to model the exact size of the defect (Fig. 29.8).

Harvesting of the Periosteal Flap. Through a separate incision on the upper medial aspect of the tibia below the pes anserinus, the periosteum is dissected free of fascia, fat, and fibrous tissue. Even passing vessels should be dissected off the flap. Measure the intended periosteal flap, or use the template to create the exact size and form. Oversize the periosteal flap by adding 1 to 2 mm to the periphery of the intended flap. Incise the periosteum and use a sharp elevator to remove the periosteal flap. Use small movements to avoid rifts in the periosteum (Fig. 29.9). Mark the side of the periosteum to be able to identify the cambium layer. Saline is used to keep the periosteal flap moist. The periosteal flap should be as thin as possible and transparent to achieve more volume in the defect and allow the cells to spread and expand. The thinner the periosteal flap, the less risk for hypertrophy, fibrillation, or other complications.

Suturing of the Periosteal Flap. Anchor the periosteal flap in four corners with the cambium layer facing the inside of the bone of the defect. Then adapt the periosteum to the surrounding cartilage by placing 6-0 resorbable suture at 4- to 6-mm intervals. Insert the suture to a depth of at least 5 to 6 mm to avoid cutting the cartilage. The intervals between the suture are sealed with fibrin glue. An opening in the upper part of the defect is left for injection of the cells.

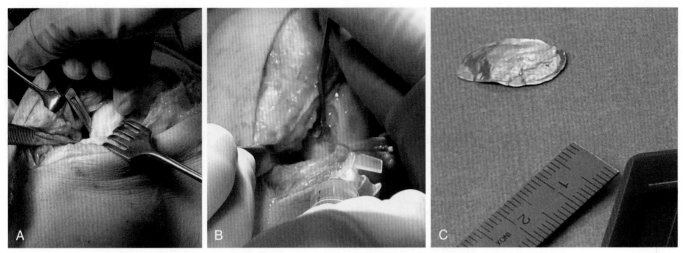

FIG 29.8 All damaged or undermined cartilage is excised (A) and carefully débrided (B). A template of the defect is made from sterile aluminum foil (C).

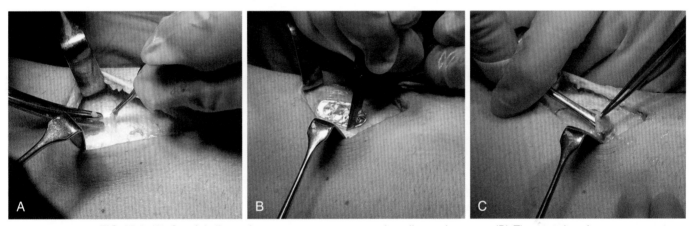

FIG 29.9 (A) Careful dissection to get access to good-quality periosteum. (B) The template is used for determining the correct size and form of the periosteal flap. (C) With careful technique the flap is removed.

Before injecting the cells, check that there is no leakage by introducing a soft catheter with a syringe into the defect. Inject saline slowly into the defect and check for any leakage. Then aspirate the saline and inject the cells into the defect, starting distally and withdrawing the syringe proximally as the cells are injected. Close the injection site with suture and fibrin glue (Fig. 29.10).

One surgical technique uses collagen I-III scaffold and Hyalograft as alternatives to the periosteal flap. Colagen I-III scaffold and Hyalograft have been used in our clinic since 2005. When using collagen I-III the sizing is important. Use the template to cut the scaffold as you would do for the periosteum in the first generation ACI, then inject the cell suspension on the rough surface intended to face the subchondral bone.

Osteochondral Lesions
(Osteochondritis Dissecans)

When treating osteochondritis dissecans by ACI, one must be attentive to the depth of the defect. If the bony defect is shallower than 6 to 8 mm, the lesion is treated the same way as a chondral lesion. Gently débride the sclerotic bottom of the

defect, but be careful to not cause bleeding. The cartilage is incised and débrided to vertical edges of healthy cartilage. Cover the defect with a periosteal flap, seal, and check for leakage. Then implant the chondrocytes and close the last opening.

If the bony defect is deeper than 6 to 8 mm, ACI is not enough, and concomitant autologous bone grafting is needed ("sandwich technique"). Start by abrading the sclerotic bottom of the defect to spongy bone and undercut the subchondral bone plate. Use a 2-mm bur and drill multiple holes into the spongy bone. The cartilage is débrided to healthy cartilage with vertical edges. Then harvest cancellous bone for grafting of the bony defect. If the bony defect is small, use bone from the tibial or femoral condyle, but if the defect is larger, bone has to be harvested from the iliac crest. Pack the bone from the bottom up and try to shape the bone graft to the contour of the condyle.

Harvest a periosteal flap to cover the bone graft at the level of subchondral bone, with the cambium layer facing the joint. Anchor it with horizontal or mattress sutures placed into the cartilage or through small drill holes in the subchondral bone plate, and use fibrin glue under the flap for fixation to the bone

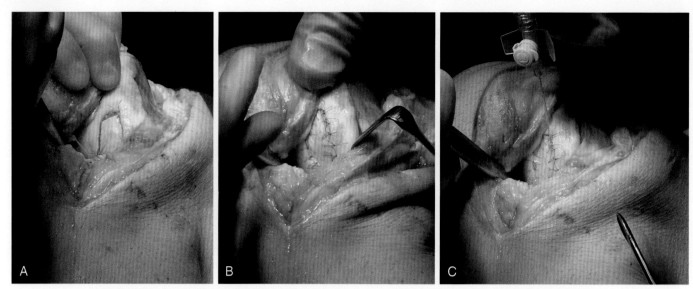

FIG 29.10 (A) The periosteal flap is first anchored with a suture in each corner. (B) The flap is then sutured to the cartilage rim. (C) The integrity of the chamber under the flap is tested with an injection of saline.

graft. This technique will avoid bleeding into the cartilage defect. Another periosteal flap is harvested and sutured to the cartilage edges, with the cambium layer facing the defect. Use fibrin glue to seal the intervals between the sutures. Test for a watertight seal with a gentle saline injection. If no leakage is present, aspirate the saline and inject the chondrocytes. Close the last opening and seal with fibrin glue (Fig. 29.11).

CONCEPT OF OPTIMAL ENVIRONMENTAL CONDITIONS FOR SHORT- AND LONG-TERM SURVIVAL OF REPAIR TISSUE

Over the years, it has become obvious when dealing with ACI and concomitant procedures that it is mandatory to create optimal local environmental conditions for the short- and long-term survival of the repair. Malalignment and instability will need corrective surgery for a good result. Procedures such as ACL reconstruction or high tibial osteotomy may be performed at the same time as the biopsy specimen is harvested. Otherwise, they could be done concomitant with the implantation. Pathological mechanics in the joint reduces the chance of successful repair. Patellar lesions are often related to a maltracking or unstable patella, and the patella must thus be realigned or stabilized for good healing. Stabilizing procedures may include anteromedialization and distalization of the tibial tuberosity, lateral release, proximal medial soft-tissue shortening (medial patelofemoral ligament [MPFL] and vastus medialis oblique [VMO]), and trochleaplasty (if it is dysplastic). In patients with trochlear and patellar lesions, especially large and uncontained ones, unloading with ventralization of the tibial tuberosity should be considered. A torn ACL is reconstructed after the cartilage lesion is débrided and covered with periosteum but before the chondrocytes are injected. To unload the transplanted area when a varus or valgus deformity is present, a high tibial or distal femoral osteotomy is performed. When these corrective surgeries are performed, a brace limiting range of motion to 0 to 60 degrees is used postoperatively for 3 weeks, and for

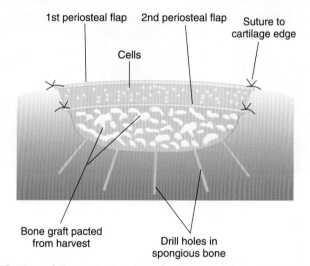

FIG 29.11 Schematic drawing of the sandwich procedure with layers of transplanted bone, periosteal flap, chondrocytes, and periosteal flap.

the following 3 weeks, range of motion is limited to 0 to 90–120 degrees. In patients with previous total or subtotal meniscectomy, meniscus allograft implantation should be considered.

POSTOPERATIVE TREATMENT

The patient is given antibiotic and thrombotic prophylaxis for 48 hours. Six to 8 hours after surgery, a continuous passive motion machine is used with a range of motion of 0 to 40 degrees. Range of motion is allowed the day after surgery, as well as isometric quadriceps training. Weight bearing is limited during the first weeks. Depending on the size, location, and containment of the lesion and concomitant procedures, weight-bearing ranges from loading to the pain threshold for 6 weeks, loading with 30 to 40 lb for 8 weeks, and then gradually increased weight bearing for another 6 weeks. Cycling on a stationary bike with low resistance could be started when the patient has reached 90 to 100 degrees of knee flexion. When full weight bearing is achieved, long-distance walking with increasing distances is encouraged. Swimming is allowed, as well as wet vest training, when the wounds are healed. Cross-country skiing, in-line skating, or outdoor skating if the patient is used to these techniques can be allowed when full weight bearing has been achieved. Running is not allowed until 9 months.

Return to professional sports is permitted after individual assessment, including overall clinical and functional tests and arthroscopic evaluation with the indentation test and probing to determine the hardness and condition of the repair tissue.

It is important to inform the patient about the healing process, starting with cells in a suspension changing to cotton-like tissue in the first 2 to 3 months and gradually maturing to a rubber-like tissue within 6 months. Continuous maturation with hardening is an ongoing process and is stimulated by gradually increased weight bearing, as well as motion. Such maturation will continue for 12 months or longer. The return of proteoglycans in the repair area and the cartilage in general can be assessed by a delayed gadolinium enhanced MRI of cartilage (dGEMRIC), showing normalization of proteoglycan concentration at 9 to 12–15 months postoperatively.[12]

RESULTS OF AUTOLOGOUS CHONDROCYTE IMPLANTATION: LONG-TERM SWEDISH EXPERIENCE

Since October 1987, more than 2000 patients have undergone ACI in Gothenburg, Sweden. Several follow-up studies have been published since.[32,33] In our latest study, in 2009, we present 224 patients evaluated 10 to 20 years after the ACI.[34]

The current follow-up evaluation has been performed 12.8 years from the time of implantation (range 10 to 20 years). Average age of the patients was 33.3 years (range 14 to 62) at the time of the ACI.

Seventy-four percent of the patients had isolated cartilage lesions, whereas 26% had multiple lesions. Forty patients had two lesions, 12 patients had three lesions, and 4 patients had more than three lesions. The location of the lesion varied; 52% had an isolated lesion on a femoral condyle, 22% had isolated patellar or trochlear lesion, 10% had kissing lesions, and 16% had multiple but not kissing lesions. The mean size of lesions per patient was 7 cm^2 (range 1 to 27 cm^2), whereas the mean size per lesion was 5.2 cm^2 (range 1 to 16 cm^2).

Concomitant procedures with ACI were performed mainly because of ligamentous insufficiency. Forty-six had an ACL reconstruction, with 42 having it at the same time with the ACI and 4 prior to ACI. Twenty-one patients had a high tibial osteotomy before or during the ACI, 5 had a reconstruction of a collateral ligament, and 2 had a posterior cruciate ligament (PCL) reconstruction. One in three patients (37%) had a previous operation before ACI that involved shaving or drilling of the subchondral bone of the lesion area. Thirty-four percent (76/224 patients) had a history of meniscal lesion and partial or total meniscectomy before or during the ACI. Sixty-six percent (148/224 patients) did not have meniscal involvement, at least until the implantation.

Patients were evaluated with the use of multiple functional scales and activity scores. The results that are reported mainly concern the injury locations considered an indication for ACI.[34,40]

Indentation tests were also performed in previous studies to measure the stiffness of the repair tissue, and biopsy tissue was harvested for analysis of microscopic appearance and biochemistry.[30] Indirect measurement of glycosaminoglycans of the repair tissue has been performed with dGEMRIC technique.[12,41]

Isolated Injury to the Femoral Condyle

Fifty-two patients with isolated femoral lesions were evaluated. Forty-one of the lesions were located on the medial condyle and 11 on the lateral, with the size per lesion exceeding between 0.6 and 14 cm^2 (average 4.9 cm^2). The patients' age at the time of surgery was 35.5 years (range 17 to 62).

Forty-seven patients (90%) responded that they benefitted from the treatment and would do the operation again. Thirty-six of the patients (69%) thought that they were the same or improved comparing to the previous years.

The average Tegner-Wallgren score was 8 (range 2 to 14), and 37 patients (84%) had a score of 6 or more. The average Lysholm score was 60.1 (range 46 to 81) before surgery and 72.6 (range 25 to 96) 10 to 20 years postoperatively. The overall Brittberg-Peterson score was 65.9 preoperatively (range 31 to 107), while being 38.4 (range 3 to 102.8) postoperatively, thus also suggesting an overall improvement in the quality of life and knee function. Noyes score was 5.4 (range 1 to 9), while Knee injury and Osteoarthritis Outcome Score (KOOS) was 77.3 for pain, 65 for symptoms, 83.1 for ADL, 45.1 for sports, and 51 for quality of life.

Femoral Condyle Lesions With ACL Reconstruction

Forty-six patients had a femoral condyle lesion and also an ACL reconstruction. In 42 cases, the ACL reconstruction was performed at the time of implantation, while in 4 cases the patients had been reconstructed earlier. Thirty-seven patients had a lesion on the medial femoral condyle and 13 on the lateral. Thirty-seven had an isolated femoral condyle lesion, while the remaining 9 had from 2 to 4 lesions (6 with 2 lesions, 2 with 3, and 1 patient with 4 lesions).

The average size of medial femoral condyle lesions was 4.5 cm^2 (range 1.2 to 10) and of the lateral was 4.6 cm^2 (range 2.4 to 10.5). The average age at the time of the implantation was 31.1 years (range 17.5 to 50.5).

Thirty-four of the patients evaluated their current status to be better or the same compared to previous years, and 41 of them (91.1%) would do the operation again.

The Tegner-Wallgren score was 8.1 (range 3 to 15), and the Lysholm was 69.2 (34 to 100). Total Brittberg-Peterson was 41.1 (range 2 to 103.4) and Noyes was 5.2 (range 1 to 9). KOOS was 72.8 for pain, 67.5 for symptoms, 81.3 for ADL, 41.1 for sports, and 48.2 for the quality of life. Preoperative values for Tegner-Wallgren and Lysholm were 7.2 and 59.1, respectively; the value for Brittberg-Peterson (total) was 56.3.

Osteochondritis Dissecans of the Femoral Condyle

Twenty-six patients with osteochondritis dissecans were evaluated in the study as of 2009. All of the lesions were isolated. Fifteen of those were located on the medial femoral condyle—9 on the lateral and 2 on the patella. Average size was 6.2 cm^2

(range 1 to 12). The average age was 26.8 years at the time of the implantation (range 15.7 to 52.4).

Twenty-one of the patients (81%) replied that they were better or the same compared to the previous years. Twenty-five (96.2%) would do the operation again.

The Tegner-Wallgren score was 8.6 in the latest follow-up (range 5 to 13). Twenty-four of the patients had a Tegner-Wallgren score equal or larger than 6. The mean Lysholm score was 67.4 (range 31 to 95). Preoperatively, Tegner-Wallgren was 6.4 (range 1 to 9) and Lysholm was 56.2 (range 13 to 85). The total Brittberg-Peterson score was 38.6 (range 2.7 to 99), while being 51.8 (range 9.4 to 104) preoperatively. Noyes score was 5.7 (3 to 9), and KOOS was 78 for pain, 65.2 for symptoms, 85.6 for ADL, 46.9 for sports, and 54.3 for quality of life.

Arthroscopic Assessment and Biopsies

In our previous follow-up study, arthroscopic assessment was performed for 46 patients. Macroscopic evaluation of the defect area showed a maximal defect score of 12 points. Isolated femoral condyle injuries in 20 patients showed an average of 10.3 points. Isolated femoral condyle lesions plus ACL reconstruction had an average score of 10.9 points and, with osteochondritis dissecans, an average score of 10.5 out of 12 maximum, which is complete filling of the defect until total integration to the surrounding cartilage and a normal surface. Biopsy samples were harvested and judged by unbiased scientists, and 80% showed hyaline-like cartilage (Fig. 29.12).[30]

Indentation Test of Repair Tissue

In the study of 2002, the indentation test with an arthroscopic probe showed no significant difference in stiffness between normal articular cartilage and hyaline-like repair tissue in the transplanted area. Patients with fibrous tissue in the repair area had a significant decrease in stiffness when compared with normal cartilage and the repair tissue of hyaline-like cartilage.[30]

Immunohistochemical Analysis

Twenty-two biopsy specimens were taken from both repair tissue ($n = 19$) and healthy cartilage ($n = 3$). Analysis was done

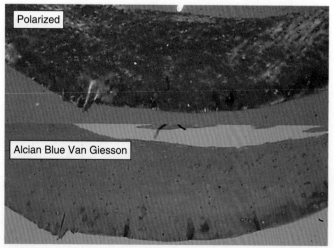

FIG 29.12 Biopsy specimen from repair tissue 9 years after autologous chondrocyte implantation.

in blinded fashion and involved the content of type I and II collagen, cartilage oligomeric matrix protein, and aggrecan. Hyaline-like repair tissue had characteristics similar to those of normal articular cartilage, whereas fibrous repair tissue differed in all analyzed parameters (Table 29.1).

Complications

There were no serious complications, no infections, no chronic synovitis, and no thrombosis. The reoperation rate was 5%. The main complications were periosteal hypertrophy with a clicking or crepitating sensation, sometimes with swelling early in the postoperative period. Most of these symptoms disappeared with time and continued rehabilitation. If symptoms remained, patients were treated arthroscopically by débridement of the hypertrophic periosteum or fibrillation (Fig. 29.13). This complication had no impact on the long-term result. A few patients sustained partial delamination of the grafted area, with or without a new trauma episode. These patients were treated by reimplantation of autologous chondrocytes and achieved good and excellent results.

Evaluation With Delayed Gadolinium Enhanced MRI of Cartilage

Thirty-six knees in 31 patients were assessed 9 to 18 years after treatment with ACI.[41] All patients had isolated lesions—27 on a femoral condyle, 1 on the trochlea, and 8 on the patella. The knees were evaluated with the dGEMRIC technique. Measurement of the concentration of gadolinium compounds on MRI T1 sequences (T1 mapping) provides information regarding the concentration of glycosaminoglycans in the normal cartilage or the repair tissue at the cartilage lesion area.

The quantity of proteoglycans in the repair tissue was found equal to the surrounding cartilage. That indicates an equal quality of the transplant and surrounding cartilage and thus a successful coverage of the defect area. This study shows that 9 to 18 years after the ACI, the cartilage defect area is restored in most of the cases.

Long-Term Durability

Fifty of 61 patients with femoral condyle injuries had good or excellent results after a 2-year follow-up. Fifty-one of these patients still had good or excellent result 5 to 10 years postoperatively, with an average follow-up of 7.4 years. Ten to 20 years after the implantation, 74% of the patients felt better or in the same status compared to previous years. Ninety-two percent were satisfied and would do the ACI again. Lysholm, Tegner-Wallgren, and Brittberg-Peterson scores were improved compared to the preoperative values. These outcomes indicate

TABLE 29.1	Immunohistochemical Analysis Comparing Normal Cartilage with Hyaline and Fibrous Repair Tissue		
	Normal Cartilage	Hyaline Repair	Fibrous Repair
Collagen type I	$- \rightarrow +$	$\rightarrow +$	$++ \rightarrow +++$
Collagen type II	$+++$	$++ \rightarrow +++$	$-$
Cartilage oligomeric matrix protein	$+++$	$++ \rightarrow +++$	$+ \rightarrow ++$
Aggrecan	$+++$	$++ \rightarrow +++$	$+ \rightarrow ++$

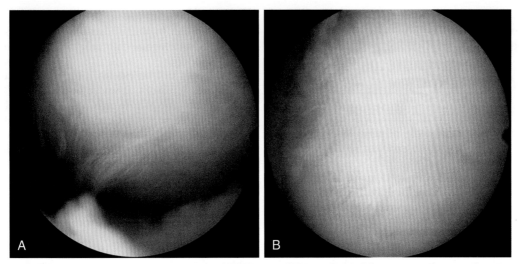

FIG 29.13 (A) Complication consisting of fibrillation of the periosteal flap 1 year after autologous chondrocyte implantation of the medial femoral condyle. (B) After débridement of the superficial fibrillation of the periosteal flap. The fibrillation did not have any impact on the long-term results.

high durability of the repair tissue after ACI. This is also indicated by the evaluation of the repair tissue, performed with biopsies or the dGEMRIC technique.

According to the 10 to 20 years follow-up, the improvement of patients was similar irrespectively of the number or size of lesions or regardless if the patients had a previous history of ACL reconstruction. Moreover, the average final values of the Lysholm, Tegner-Wallgren, and Brittberg-Peterson score were statistically not different among patients with single or multiple lesions or between patients with or without a previous or concomitant meniscal or ACL reconstruction surgery.

Shaving or drilling of the cartilage lesions before the ACI did not seem to affect the clinical improvement, in the medium-term (3 years) or final (10 to 20 years) follow-up. However, patients with preexisting bone surgeries (shaving or drilling) showed a deterioration ($p = .06$) of Lysholm score between medium- and long-term follow-up. The long-term evaluation with dGEMRIC revealed that lesions that had been previously treated with bone marrow stimulating surgeries (microfractures, drilling) had a higher incidence of intralesional osteophytes.

This evidence suggests that previous bone marrow stimulating surgeries may affect the long-term durability of ACI repair tissue.

Results of ACI in High Competitive Athletes

The high-level competitive athlete is a special category of patients, in the sense that they need a fast recovery to the preinjury level and a long lasting good clinical result that will allow them to continue a successful career. This patient group is also characterized by the high incidence of cartilage lesions, often accompanied by other concomitant knee injuries or findings (meniscal tear, ACL rupture, varus knees, etc.). Half of the athletes treated with an ACL reconstruction demonstrated a concomitant cartilage lesion,[25,35] whereas in the National Football League, or NFL (American football), eight cartilage injuries were reported annually for 14 consecutive years.[7]

According to the systematic review of Harris et al, ACI resulted in a high possibility for full recovery to sports

(78%)—much higher than MF (59%). Osteochondral Autograft Transfer System (OATS) seem to provide a comparative recovery rate, offering also a relatively faster return.[17] Similar outcomes have been found by another systematic review of Mithoefer et al.[25] However, it seems that ACI repairs tissues better, with a high recovery rate, and provides a recovery to the preinjury level, proven by durable positive clinical outcomes. Continued sports participation at the preinjury level was seen in 96% of ACI treated patients, whereas in only 52% of MF and 52% of OAT patients.[25] This clearly suggests a better repair tissue after treatment with ACI.

CARTILAGE REGISTRY REPORT

All patients treated by ACI in the United States and Europe are monitored in a registry outcome study. In a cohort of patients with both single ($n = 28$) and multiple lesions ($n = 11$) on the medial and lateral condyles and the trochlea with a 72-month follow-up, the modified Cincinnati Knee Rating Scale went from 3.15 preoperatively to 6.93 at 72 months. Eighty-two percent of the patients had functional improvement.

A cohort of 15 patients with multiple lesions and a minimum of 60 months' follow-up were evaluated with the modified Cincinnati Knee Rating Scale for overall patient evaluation, pain, and swelling. All parameters increased. The overall patient evaluation category increased from 2.73 to 7.53, pain from 2.80 to 7.33, and swelling from 3.73 to 7.47, and the overall condition was improved in 93% of patients.

Complications

No infections have been reported since the start of the study in 1995. Adverse events or complications were reported by 5.8% after implantation, and 2.9% had a complication considered to be at least possibly related to the autologous cultured chondrocytes. The most frequently reported adverse events are hypertrophic tissue at the repair site, intra-articular adhesions, superficial wound infection, hypertrophic synovitis, and postoperative hematoma.

Both the clinical results and the complications were on the same level as the Swedish results.

TISSUE ENGINEERED MATRIX SUPPORT USING MEMBRANES, CARRIERS, SCAFFOLDS, AND GELS IN AUTOLOGOUS CHONDROCYTE IMPLANTATION

TISSUE ENGINEERED MATRIX SUPPORT

The first generation ACI with the use of periosteum has been performed since 1987, with good to excellent results for most treated patients.

However, the procedure is technically demanding, requiring a suturing of the periosteum on the healthy cartilage and also to avoid any leakage of the injected suspension of chondrocytes. It also requires an open arthrotomy for the implantation with an additional incision for the harvesting of the periosteum. In addition to that, it has been reported by other authors that an increased rate of periosteal hypertrophies needed a second arthroscopy.

There is currently an increasing interest in the development of new materials and technique of ACI that could overcome the limitations and difficulties of first generation ACI and further improve and perfect the regeneration of hyaline articular cartilage. Remarkable progress has been achieved in the development of supportive materials (scaffolds, membranes, etc.) for the initial support for the repair tissue, also allowing to some extent arthroscopic technique for delivery of the cells in smaller and contained lesions.

Resorbable membranes have been used to replace the periosteum, but also as carriers with cells seeded onto the membrane for delivery into the defect. Different techniques for fixation of the membranes are also under development. Membranes made of collagen and type I/III of porcine origin are used, as well as synthetic material fex polyglycolic–polylactic acids with resorption times of about 6 to 12 weeks. Cells are also cultured in collagen membranes and in tridimensional scaffolds of esterified hyaluronic acid, with a resorption time of about 4 months. Chondrocytes are grown for 3 weeks in the scaffold and can, in smaller defects, be delivered arthroscopically and fixed by press fit technique.

Membranes and scaffolds provide a bed for the seeding and culturing of cells in two- or three-dimensional cultures. The aim is to reduce the intraoperative time and postoperative morbidity, avoiding the harvesting and use of periosteum. Scaffold guided ACI is still a two-stage operation; however, it may be faster, easier, and hopefully with less complications for the patient. The mechanical and functional properties of the scaffolds could also contribute to the viability, differentiation, and matrix production of the cells. However, the mechanical properties are not specified or regulated (eg, the friction coefficient of the joint-facing surface or the stiffness in comparison to normal surrounding cartilage). Longer resorption times may be required for mechanical support of the tissue during the rehabilitation for earlier return to work and sports.

What Is the Optimal Scaffold?

The ideal scaffold has to fulfill several requirements in terms of safety, material features, and regenerative properties.

First of all, it has to be safe for the patient, being noncarcinogenic and biocompatible without causing any inflammatory or immune reaction. It has to have the ability of being effectively sterilized without losing its biomechanical properties. The scaffold when implanted has to be free of live tissue (except from the autologous chondrocytes) or heterologous biologic material.

It should not be cytotoxic for the cells seeded or for the surrounding tissues. It must be capable of supporting and holding the cells. Those cells have to stay viable, be effectively attached to the scaffold, and be mechanically supported so as not to spread into the joint cavity after the implantation; however, the scaffold has to be permeable to allow the diffusion of factors that promote cellular production of the extracellular matrix.

The mechanical support should be applied until the cells start producing extracellular matrix. Then, the ideal scaffold has to start being gradually reabsorbed and be substituted by the hyaline (like) matrix produced by the cells.

The structure of the scaffold has to be effectively reproducible. Finally, it has to be easily transferred and handled by the surgeon so to be effectively applied on the defect area. The possibility of a less invasive but still effective fixation technique allows for transarthroscopic implantation, limiting the postoperative morbidity caused by an open incision.

Matrix Induced Autologous Chondrocyte Implantation. Autologous periosteum has been used as coverage for the implanted chondrocytes (first generation ACI with periosteum, ACI-P). The use of porcine type I/III collagen membranes in medicine led to the development of matrix-induced ACI (MACI, Verigen AG, Leverkusen, Germany). The chondrocytes are seeded on the MACI type I/III collagen membrane before implantation. The membrane is fixed by fibrin glue, resorbable pins, or additional sutures on the cartilage defect area. This aims to provide and stabilize the cells in the cartilage defect area, seeded on the bilaminate collagen membrane. Thus, the membrane is used as a carrier for delivering of the cells into the cartilage lesion. At present, the cells are seeded to the membrane and cultured for 48 hours before implanted in smaller lesions using arthroscopic technique and fixation with fibrin glue or resorbable pins. More than 7000 patients have been treated with MACI since 1998. However, the method has yet to be validated with long-term clinical studies. Only a few cohort studies have been performed with promising results.

MACI has shown clinical efficacy 3 years after implantation (range 2 to 5 years), but the number of participants in this cohort study was low.[4] Gigante et al. report a significant improvement of all measured clinical scores 3 years after the treatment of patellofemoral lesions with distal realignment of patella and MACI.[11] However, it was not clear from that study whether the improvement was the result of patellofemoral realignment or the treatment of cartilage lesion. Another recent study has demonstrated the ability to generate hyaline-like cartilage as early as 6 months after MACI.[42] Two randomized control trials with MACI have been published. Basad et al. report significantly better outcomes compared to microfracture, while the study of Bartlett et al. shows no differences compared to ACI-C, 12 months after the surgery.[2,3] A comparative study between ACI-C and MACI did not show any great differences in clinical results, histology or hypertrophy of the graft, or reoperation rate, showing an incidence of graft hypertrophy of 9% in each group.[2]

There is still limited literature to support the efficacy of MACI and its superiority over other treatment options for large

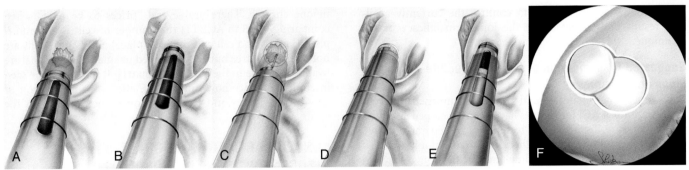

FIG 29.14 A variable diameter (6.5 to 8.5 mm) delivery device with a sharp edge is used to evaluate the size of the defect (A and B). A circular area with regular margins for graft implantation is prepared with a specially designed cannulated low-profile drill (C). The delivery device is then filled with a hyaluronic acid patch, which is transported and positioned in the prepared area (D and E). The graft is pushed out of the delivery device and precisely positioned within the defect where it remains tightly adhered to the subchondral bone (E and F). Because of the physical adhesive characteristics of the graft, no fibrin glue or sutures are used to fix the implant.

full thickness cartilage defects. More studies are needed, with better quality and longer follow-up.

The term MACI has been improperly used in the literature for any scaffold (ie, matrix) induced ACI technique. However, MACI is an established brand name, and any other use of that term can easily lead to misunderstandings. Therefore, we support the use of tissue engineered matrix support (TEMS) for the methods that use three-dimensional matrices as scaffolds for the culturing and seeding of cells.

Collagen-Covered Autologous Chondrocyte Implantation, (Chondro-Gide, Restore). Collagen type I/III membranes of porcine origin have also been used instead of the periosteal patch to cover the cartilage lesion area (Chondro-Gide, Geistlich, Wolhausen, Switzerland, or Restore, DePuy, Warsaw, Indiana, and MACI, Genzyme, Cambridge, Massachusetts).[16,38] Chondro-Gide is a porcine derived bilayer collagen type I/III. It consists of a porous layer of collagen fibers in a loose open weave arrangement that favors cell invasion and attachment and a compact membrane layer with a smooth surface, which is cell occlusive. The aim of using CACI is to reduce the operative time and a second incision for the periosteal harvest. It also may reduce the periosteal hypertrophy that has been reported from about 26% to about 5%.[15,16,38] Chondro-Gide can be seeded with cells and fixed by fibrin glue, but this still needs to be done via an arthrotomy.[37] Only short-term results have been reported.

Three-Dimensional Scaffolds for Autologous Chondrocyte Implantation. In third-generation techniques, chondrocytes are cultured in three-dimensional matrices (scaffolds) such as hyaluronic acid (Hyalograft C, Fidia Biopolymers Inc., Abano Ternme, Italy) in a three-dimensional culture before implanting in the cartilage defect area.[21,23]

Until recently, a number of third-generation ACI techniques were available in the EU, providing scaffolds with cultured chondrocytes embedded. However, the standards of the European Medicinal Agency (EMA) were implemented in 2012, and none of these techniques are currently on the market, as they have not been authorized by the European Commission. For similar reasons, the US Food and Drug Administration (FDA) has also not authorized any of these products in the US market. This situation is still under progress and awaiting newer and better basic-science preclinical studies, randomized controlled clinical trials, and/or better documentation in order for such products to regain the license and again find the way to medical application.

Therefore, the following refers to hyaluronic acid scaffolds, and it should be taken under consideration, provided that no such product is currently in clinical practice. There is evidence showing that hyaluronic acid is a potentially ideal molecule to be used in tissue engineering in cartilage repair, given its multifunctional involvement in cartilage homeostasis.

Hyalograft C was a three-dimensional hyaluronan-based scaffold made of HYAFF 11, a benzyl ester of hyaluronic acid with 20 μm fibers. Autologous chondrocytes harvested from the patient were expanded in vitro and then seeded in a three-dimensional culture onto the scaffold. They were cultured in the scaffold for 3 weeks prior to arthroscopic implantation into small contained cartilage defects with a press-fit technique.[14,26] The Hyalograft C constructs could be implanted into the lesion without the need of periosteal of collagen membrane coverings, avoiding suturing to the surrounding cartilage, thus limiting the operative time and simplifying the procedure (Fig. 29.14). Several studies provided the first medium-term clinical results, which were promising for the treatment of cartilage lesions. A prospective study of Kon et al. presented a superiority against microfracture up to 5 years postoperatively.[21] Marcacci et al. reported an improvement in 91.5% of the treated patients 2 to 5 years postoperatively, while Nehrer et al. showed a significant improvement even 7 years after the treatment.[23,27] Gobbi et al. found a significant improvement in both objective and subjective International Knee Documentation Committee (IKDC) scores 24 months after the treatment with Hyalograft C for cartilage defects of the patellofemoral joint.[13] There was also limited evidence from the histological evaluation of the repair tissue, showing a relatively high rate of hyaline-like specimens, with increased glycosaminoglycans (GAG) content.[13,23,39] However, larger studies of higher quality (mainly randomized control trials [RCSs]) and longer follow-up are needed to confirm the currently available results and to determine the long-term efficacy of the technique.

Suggested Classification of Anterior Cruciate Ligament Techniques

Following the new materials and techniques launched, different classifications of ACI techniques have been developed and used in the literature. Typically, ACI techniques are separated in two or three generations. However, there is not a commonly accepted classification, especially regarding the clarification of second and third generations.

Therefore we suggest the use of the following classification and terminology:

First generation ACI: ACI as first described in 1994, with the use of the autologous periosteal membrane as a patch for the covering of chondrocytes' suspension.[6]

Second generation ACI: ACI with TEMS of animal tissue origin (bovine or porcine collagen or others) or chemically synthesized matrix support (polyglucolic.polylactic acids or others) used either as membranes (eg, Chondrogide) or as cell carriers (eg, MACI).

Third generation ACI: ACI with three-dimensional TEMS of animal or chemical origin used as scaffolds for growing and delivering chondrocytes into the joint (eg, Hyalograft-C).

ALTERNATIVES TO AUTOLOGOUS CHONDROCYTE IMPLANTATION. USE OF CHONDRAL TISSUE FOR CARTILAGE REGENERATION

As described previously, ACI is a technique using autologous chondrocytes, aiming to regenerate the cartilage in lesion areas. The increased costs of the cell culturing and the fact that ACI is a two-stage operation has limited some widespread application and appeal of this approach. Therefore several other methods and/or techniques have been introduced, some of them based on the main concept of ACI, which is the regeneration of the cartilage based on the autologous chondrocytes.[10]

MINCED CARTILAGE AUTOGRAFT CARTILAGE AUTOGRAFT IMPLANTATION SYSTEM

The use of the Cartilage Autograft Implantation System (CAIS; DePuy/Mitek) aims to perform an implantation of autologous cartilage pieces in a scaffold construct. The technique includes harvesting of autologous healthy cartilage from limited weight bearing area of the knee just as in the ACI. A unique device is then used to mince this cartilage into small pieces, of 1 to 2 mm of diameter. After this, the device disperses the pieces onto a biodegradable scaffold. This scaffold usually consists of an absorbable copolymer foam of 35% polycaprolactone and 65% polyglicolic acid, reinforced with at polydioxanone mesh. Bioglue can be used to secure the scaffold in the lesion area. Similar to the third generation ACI, this scaffold aims to keep the cartilage pieces (instead of cells) in place and to facilitate the matrix regeneration.

An advantage of this technique is that everything, both the cartilage biopsy/retrieval and the implantation, are performed in one surgery. There are several "prices to be paid" when comparing CAIS to ACI: (1) the number of cells is not multiplied (because no cell culture takes place) and (2) the cells are not completely free but are entrapped in small pieces of mature hyaline cartilage in the extracellar matrix. It remains to be seen in clinical practice how much CAIS affects the production of new proteoglycans and the formation of new hyaline in the lesion area.

MINCED CARTILAGE ALLOGRAFT, JUVENILE ALLOGENEIC TISSUE (DENOVONT)

Although the use of allografts has been used since a long time ago, this has been done mainly in the form of large osteochondral allografts retrieved from adult donors. This method aims more to reconstruct bone-cartilage lesions in tumors and severe intra-articular fractures than to regenerate the cartilage itself.

Newer techniques aim to provide the lesion area with minced allogeneic cartilage. *DeNovo* NT (natural tissue graft) is a particulated juvenile cartilage implant used for the repair of articular cartilage damage. It consists of particulated cartilage pieces taken from juvenile donors. They are implanted in the cartilage lesion area and stabilized with bioglue. These minced pieces, which are part of this bioglue/allogeneic cartilage tissue-construct that fills the lesion area, potentially act like cells, producing hyaline cartilage.

This technique is similar to CAIS, with some important differences. No cartilage retrieval is necessary here because the minced cartilage is already provided in small packages. This saves time and also prevents postoperative morbidity because no cartilage retrieval from the patient is necessary. In addition, there is no limit to the amount of cartilaginous chips to be used—only the size and depth or lesion. Theoretically, the possibility of larger amount of tissue is provided; thus the increase of chondrocytes' density in the repair tissue would result in a better cartilage repair. Juvenile cells also have a theoretical advantage in cartilage formation compared with adult tissue.[1] On the other hand, the tissue implanted in DeNovo is not autologous but allogeneic.

INTERNATIONAL EXPERIENCE WITH AUTOLOGOUS CHONDROCYTE IMPLANTATION

Ochi et al. have done interesting research with autologous chondrocytes evenly distributed and transplanted in a collagen gel. Twenty-eight knees in 26 patients treated with chondrocytes in collagen gel (covered with a periosteal patch sutured to the defect) were monitored for at least 25 months. The treatment resulted in significant improvement in the Lysholm score. Pain and swelling were reduced in all patients, and locking was not present in any patient postoperatively. Arthroscopic assessment indicated that 26 knees had a good or excellent outcome.[28]

From Australia, Hart and Henderson et al. have confirmed the Swedish results in medium-term follow-up.[18]

From different centers in Europe, short- to medium-term results of ACI have been reported.[9]

Pavesio et al. and Marcacci et al. published promising short-term results on arthroscopic ACI with the use of Hyalograft C, a hyaluronic acid derivative.[23,29]

Guillen et al. reported good to excellent short-term results with type I collagen membranes. Nehrer et al. have also shown promising results with matrix-assisted chondrocyte implantation.[26]

Prospective randomized studies with short and medium-term results have been published by Knutsen et al.,[19,20] with comparison between ACI and microfracture as well as by Bentley et al.,[5] who randomized between ACI and mosaicplasty. Promising clinical results are presented, but the follow-up is too short to draw any conclusions regarding which technique is better suited for the lesions treated.[36]

FUTURE INDICATIONS

In young patients with multiple lesions (two or more in one joint) or bipolar lesion (ie, bone-to-bone articulation), it is possible to try ACI. In treating this patient group, it is of utmost importance to address background factors such as ligament instability, varus/valgus deformity, total/subtotal meniscectomy, bony defects in osteochondritis dissecans or after fracture, or patellar malalignment or instability.

It is important that the surgeon have optimal access to the defects, especially in the posterior part of the femur and the tibia. For that, you may need to detach the anterior insertion of the meniscus and its capsular insertion to the tibia. If this is not enough to reach the posterior part of the defect, the second step is to incise behind the collateral ligament. If that is not acceptable, do not hesitate to take down the collateral ligament from the femoral epicondyle with a bone block measuring 2×2 cm^2, and then you can open the joint to achieve excellent access to the posterior part of the tibia and femur.

Postoperative rehabilitation is longer in young early osteoarthritic patients (bipolar lesions), especially those who undergo concomitant procedures. Usually, we recommend partial weight bearing with 20 kg for 8 weeks and then progressively increased weight bearing up to full weight bearing at 4 months.

Patients with multiple lesions and a minimum of 3 years' follow-up had 84% good or excellent results. Those with bipolar tibial-femoral lesions had 75% good or excellent results, and patients with bipolar patellar-femoral lesions had 75% good or excellent results.

OTHER JOINTS

ACI has been used in the ankle joint with osteochondritis dissecans, as well as for cartilage and in lesions in the hip, shoulder, elbow, and wrist. In principle, this technique can be used in any joint with a localized articular cartilage lesion or osteochondritis dissecans.

The longest follow-up in the talus is now longer than 8 years, and the results are good in 80% of cases. The approach to medial or lateral localized injuries in the talus usually mandates a medial or sometimes a lateral osteotomy for optimal surgical access to the defect.[31]

The hip has been operated on in six young patients with osteochondritis dissecans or chondral lesions on the caput femoris. The shoulder has been operated on in three cases, in two with lesions of both the glenoid and the head of the humerus. The results seem promising in other joints, but we need more patients and longer follow-up for establishing these indications.

Further data collection and long-term results are needed before indications for these joints can be approved.

SUMMARY

Clinical experience with ACI is now longer than 28 years. Isolated articular cartilage injuries on the femoral condyles show good to excellent results in 90% of cases. Treatment of osteochondritis dissecans produces good-to-excellent results in 89% of cases. No serious complications have occurred, and a low number of adverse reactions have been reported. Biopsy specimens have shown hyaline-like cartilage in 80% of cases, and indentation tests have not indicated any significant difference between the indentation stiffness of hyaline-like repair tissue and normal surrounding cartilage. MRI enhanced gadolinium studies at 8 to 18 years have shown normal proteoglycan concentration, indicating chondrocyte function in the implanted areas.

The results from the Swedish study have been confirmed by Cartilage Repair Registry data, with the longest follow-up being 6 years, and by data from Boston and Atlanta, with the longest follow-up being 14 years. In the United States, more than 20,000 operations have been performed since 1995, and worldwide over 40,000 operations have been performed.

Promising results emerge from several new techniques using scaffolds and membranes as carriers, or to grow the cells in before implantation with arthroscopic techniques. Research on different cell types to be used is ongoing, along with how to safely use growth factors in the clinical work. We are moving forward to simplify and optimize the regeneration of articular cartilage.

KEY REFERENCES

2. Bartlett W, Skinner JA, Gooding CR, et al: Autologous chondrocyte implantation versus matrix-induced autologous chondrocyte implantation for osteochondral defects of the knee: a prospective, randomised study. *J Bone Joint Surg Br* 87:640–645, 2005.

5. Bentley G, Biant LC, Carrington RW, et al: A prospective, randomised comparison of autologous chondrocyte implantation versus mosaicplasty for osteochondral defects in the knee. *J Bone Joint Surg Br* 85:223–230, 2003.

6. Brittberg M, Lindahl A, Nilsson A, et al: Treatment of deep cartilage defects in the knee with autologous chondrocyte transplantation. *N Engl J Med* 331:889–895, 1994.

13. Gobbi A, Kon E, Berruto M, et al: Patellofemoral full-thickness chondral defects treated with second-generation autologous chondrocyte implantation: results at 5 years' follow-up. *Am J Sports Med* 37:1083–1092, 2009.

16. Gooding CR, Bartlett W, Bentley G, et al: A prospective, randomised study comparing two techniques of autologous chondrocyte implantation for osteochondral defects in the knee: periosteum covered versus type I/III collagen covered. *Knee* 13:203–210, 2006.

18. Henderson IJ, Tuy B, Connell D, et al: Prospective clinical study of autologous chondrocyte implantation and correlation with MRI at three and 12 months. *J Bone Joint Surg Br* 85:1060–1066, 2003.

21. Kon E, Gobbi A, Filardo G, et al: Arthroscopic second-generation autologous chondrocyte implantation compared with microfracture for chondral lesions of the knee: prospective nonrandomized study at 5 years. *Am J Sports Med* 37:33–41, 2009.

24. Minas T, Gomoll AH, Rosenberger R, et al: Increased failure rate of autologous chondrocyte implantation after previous treatment with marrow stimulation techniques. *Am J Sports Med* 37:902–908, 2009.

30. Peterson L, Brittberg M, Kiviranta I, et al: Autologous chondrocyte transplantation: biomechanics and long-term durability. *Am J Sports Med* 30:2–12, 2002.

32. Peterson L, Minas T, Brittberg M, Lindahl A: Treatment of osteochondritis dissecans of the knee with autologous chondrocyte

transplantation: results at two to ten years. *J Bone Joint Surg Am* 85(Suppl 2):17–24, 2003.

33. Peterson L, Minas T, Brittberg M, et al: Two- to 9-year outcome after autologous chondrocyte transplantation of the knee. *Clin Orthop* (374):212–234, 2000.

34. Peterson L, Vasiliadis HS, Brittberg M, Lindahl A: Autologous chondrocyte implantation: a long-term follow-up. *Am J Sports Med* 38:1117–1124, 2010.

40. Vasiliadis HS, Concaro S, Brittberg M, et al: Autologous chondrocyte implantation: 10–20 years follow up. Paper presented at the 8th World Congress of the International Cartilage Repair Society, Miami, FL, May 23–26, 2009.

41. Vasiliadis HS, Danielson B, Ljungberg M, et al: Autologous chondrocyte implantation in cartilage lesions of the knee: long-term evaluation with magnetic resonance imaging and delayed gadolinium-enhanced magnetic resonance imaging technique. *Am J Sports Med* 38:943–949, 2010.

The references for this chapter can also be found on www.expertconsult.com.

30

Osteochondral Autograft Transplantation

Yonah Heller, James R. Mullen, Nicholas A. Sgaglione

INTRODUCTION

The treatment of symptomatic focal articular cartilage defects continues to present a clinical dilemma for many orthopedists. Surgical approaches to this problem can be categorized into those that attempt to resurface focal defects through tissue repair or regeneration and those that reconstitute articular cartilage surfaces through transplantation of intact osteochondral grafts. The former includes repair strategies, such as marrow stimulation, and cell-based therapies, such as implantation of chondrocytes expanded *ex vivo*. The results of these resurfacing procedures have been associated with tissue repair predominated by fibrocartilage, which has been shown to have inferior wear characteristics compared to hyaline tissue.[77] Osteochondral autograft plug transfer (OAT) involves the direct transplantation of osteochondral segments from less loaded regions of cartilage to areas with symptomatic focal defects. Despite concerns of donor site morbidity and limited availability, this method has been demonstrated to reliably restore native hyaline cartilage architecture and the underlying subchondral bone.

Early work on autologous hyaline cartilage transplantation to the femoral or tibial condyles involved direct transfer of patellar osteochondral grafts. First described using a pedunculated patellar graft by d'Aubigné in 1945, Campanacci et al. published a case series of 19 patients who underwent free patellar graft trasfer.[15] The indications primarily included giant cell tumors and involved resection of almost the entire osteochondral segment of the patella followed by screw fixation to either the tibial or femoral condyle. Attempts to restore native articular cartilage contour were made through careful orientation of the patellar graft, but obvious donor-recipient mismatches were observed. Overall results were noted to be successful; however, decreased range of motion was found to be the primary postoperative complaint.

Later reports described the transfer of autogenous osteochondral fragments for treatment of osteochondritis dissecans (OCD) of the knee. Yamashita et al. in 1985 described two patients who underwent graft harvest from the superomedial femoral trochlea in a region which "in extension was in contact with neither patella nor meniscus."[112] Donor sites were filled with iliac crest bone graft, and all segments were fixed using orthogonal mini-cancellous screws. Second-look arthrotomy for screw removal revealed macroscopically intact hyaline cartilage with mild irregularities at the graft-native tissue interface. Slight surface contour irregularities were noted at both donor and graft sites, but with negligible clinical sequelae. Outerbridge et al. in 1995 described the transfer of an osteochondral graft from the lateral facet of the patella to repair a large osteochondral defect in the ipsilateral femoral condyle in 10 patients.[85] A manual press-fit technique was used for graft fixation. Preoperative and postoperative function was assessed using the Cincinnati knee score, with an average improvement from 43 points (range 24 to 64) to 93 points (range 79 to 100). All patients were satisfied with the procedure, in which 70% were able to resume full, unrestricted activity. Success was offset by increased patellofemoral pain and progression of degeneration of the medial facet of the patella. Second-look arthroscopy revealed solid graft fixation and intact surface hyaline cartilage.

Current OAT procedures benefit from improvements in technique and instrumentation. Although the principle of restoration of hyaline cartilage by direct transfer of less significantly loaded areas of articular cartilage remains unchanged, the use of smaller grafts decreases donor site morbidity and allows for more limited exposure. Improvements in surgical technique have resulted in more predictable success rates and fewer complications, with greater attention focused on restoring native articular cartilage topography. Indications for resurfacing have also expanded, with more defined pathoetiology and precise approach in regard to site, size, and geometry of pathologic sites. In this chapter, we review the current approach to OAT, including indications, technical considerations, pearls and pitfalls, postoperative regimens, and clinical results.

INDICATIONS

Numerous treatment algorithms have been proposed for the management of articular cartilage lesions.[18,94,101] Smaller lesions (<10 mm) are typically managed with simple débridement, citing the limited increase in biomechanical loading and rim stresses around the edges of the defect.[36] Primary treatment options typically include marrow stimulation techniques such as microfracture, which has been shown to provide good symptomatic relief and restoration of function in defects with perimeter well-defined edges and good containment.[78,105] However, recent studies have raised concerns regarding the durability of the fibrous/fibrocartilagenous repair tissue.[77] Larger lesions (surface area >200 mm^2) and those with defects extending into subchondral bone represent a more complex scenario that microfracture and/or débridement may not adequately be able to treat. In general, the literature has shown good initial results after microfracture up to 18 to 24 months, but multiple studies examining longer term data have shown that outcomes deteriorate with time, with worsening pain and decreased activity as little as 1 to 3 years after surgery.[35,49,50,51]

Osteochondral autograft transplantation is indicated for the management of focal nondegenerative articular cartilage lesions of the medial or lateral femoral condyles, the trochlear groove, and patella. The optimal size of pathologic lesions that may be successfully treated range from 10 to 25 mm diameter lesions to 150 to 250 mm² area lesions.[17,70] Overall, optimal lesion size indicated for treatment includes symptomatic lesions that are 50 to 250 mm². Smaller OCD lesions and osteochondral fractures represent a good indication for OAT because restoration of both the surface hyaline and underlying subchondral bone can be addressed. A variation on the typical OAT procedure has also been described for the treatment of unstable OCD lesions. Rather than conventional hardware fixation, single or multiple osteochondral plugs may be used as biological pegs to secure OCD lesions following débridement and backfill of underlying fibrous tissue.[75,79] Age is a consideration, and patients younger than 50 years old with an absence of degenerative pathology may be indicated for OAT, depending on the quality and availability of donor tissue. OAT has also shown success in patients with malalignment, in which patients undergo concomitant high tibial osteotomy. Minzlaff et al. showed a mean Lysholm score increase of 33 points, representing a significant improvement compared to preoperative scores, in which patients had an average varus malalignment of 4.7 degrees, corrected to 4 degrees of valgus in most cases. The visual analog scale (VAS) pain score decreased by a mean of 4.8 points, and 93% of the patients were satisfied with the results of the operative procedure. Mean survival rates were 95.2% at 5 years, 93.2% at 7 years, and 90.1% at 8.5 years after surgery.[76] Other important factors to be considered when defining treatment indications include compliance with postoperative weight-bearing restrictions and recovery.

TECHNICAL CONSIDERATIONS

In 1982, Lindholm et al. reported on a series of animal model experiments in rats, where different strategies were taken toward reconstituting medial femoral condyle defects.[66] Fixation of a loose osteochondral fragment with a bone peg or tissue adhesive was studied in conjunction with the use of either fresh frozen allografts or autogenous grafts harvested from the lateral femoral condyle. The authors concluded that precise reconstruction of the articular surface was essential, as failures were observed if joint surface congruity was inadequate. Subsequent studies have expanded on our understanding of the factors influencing outcomes from OAT. These include topography, contact pressures, fill pattern, depth of insertion, graft harvest, and graft insertion. Although advances in instrumentation and surgical techniques are essential and important, challenges still remain and several technique-related resurfacing factors must be addressed.

Topography

In 1991, Ateshian et al. described an analytical stereophotogrammetry technique through which the articular surface topography and cartilage thickness of the knee joint was mapped (Fig. 30.1).[3] This technique involved estimating three-dimensional (3D) coordinates of points on an object using measurements made in two or more photographic images taken from different positions. Using this technique, the precise 3D topography of the cartilage surfaces of various diarthrodial joints were obtained. In a later study, Bartz et al. described a

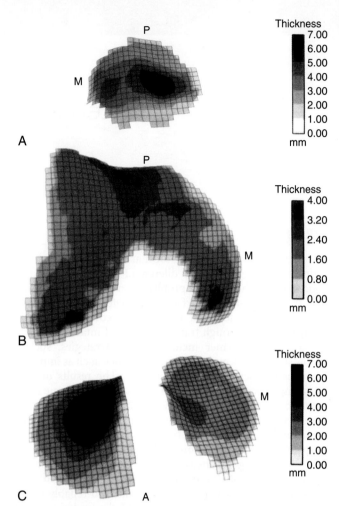

FIG 30.1 Grayscale of cartilage thickness superimposed on the topographic map of (A) patellar, (B) femoral, and (C) tibial articular surfaces. *A,* Anterior; *M,* medial; *P,* proximal. (From Ateshian GA, Soslowsky LJ, Mow VC: Quantitation of articular surface topography and cartilage thickness in knee joints using stereophotogrammetry. *J Biomech* 24(8):766–768, 1991, Fig. 6.)

method for computerized matching of the surface hyaline topography of donor and recipient sites for OAT, allowing for an analysis of which commonly used donor site is best matched to a specific defect recipient site.[8] The authors concluded that cartilage defects in the weight-bearing regions of the medial and lateral femoral condyles are best treated with grafts taken from the most inferior parts of the superomedial and superolateral borders of the trochlea (Fig. 30.2). Similarly, lesions in the saddle-shaped trochlea may be addressed with grafts from the intercondylar notch.[1] More recently, Nishizawa et al. reported on 3D laser scanning techniques and found the central trochlea to more accurately match the anterior femoral condyle, whereas peripheral trochlear donor sites were more congruent with the posterior femoral condylar recipient site (Figs. 30.3 and 30.4).[84]

It has been proposed that matching of cartilage thickness between donor and recipient sites is important to avoid subchondral step-off, which may result in a better loading response.[108] Although no biomechanical or animal studies have proven this to be the case, the structural composition of cartilage and the means by which contact pressures are distributed support this theory. Hydrostatic pressures within

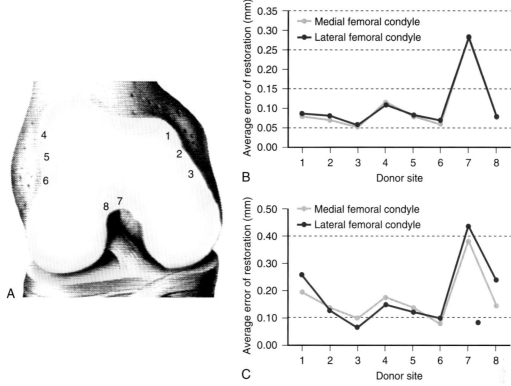

FIG 30.2 Surface topography measurements and calculations of topographic mismatch to a central weight-bearing defect in the medial femoral condyle for the eight most common OAT donor sites (A). (B) Average errors of restoration of surface topography for a 6 mm defect with osteochondral autograft plugs from each of the regions in (A). (C) Average errors of restoration of surface topography for an 8 mm defect. (From Bartz RL, Kamaric E, Noble PC, et al: Topographic matching of selected donor and recipient sites for osteochondral autografting of the articular surface of the femoral condyles. *Am J Sports Med* 29(2):209–210, 2001, Figs. 4, 6, and 7.)

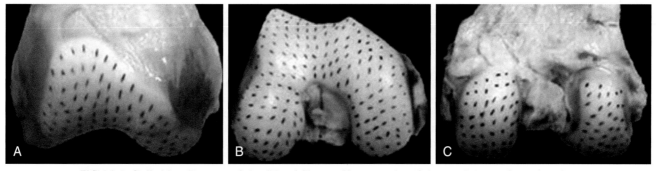

FIG 30.3 **Split Line Pattern of the Distal Femur** Photographs of the cartilage surface showing split lines created with a dissecting needle dipped in India ink. (A) Anterior view, (B) distal view, (C) posterior view. (From Below S, Arnoczky SP, Dodds J, et al: The split-line pattern of the distal femur: a consideration in the orientation of autologous cartilage grafts. *Arthroscopy* 18(6):615, 2002, Fig. 3.)

cartilage and the rate of increase with joint loading can be expected to vary with different cartilage thicknesses. Studies have shown that cartilage thickness is correlated with local joint load, with central condylar thickness up to 3.65 mm compared to as little as 0.22 mm in the sulcus terminalis.[106] Typical graft sites measure 1.2 to 1.6 mm in cartilage thick-

ness compared to condylar thicknesses in the 1.6 to 2.0 mm range.

The concept of split line orientation of surface cartilage should also be taken into consideration when the goal of more precise osteochondral autografting is preferred. In 1898, Hultkrantz demonstrated a distinct orientation of the collagen fibers

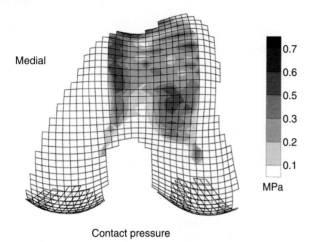

FIG 30.4 Grayscale of typical patellofemoral contact pressures superimposed on the topographic map of the distal femur. (From Ahmad CS, Cohen ZA, Levine WN, et al: Biomechanical and topographic considerations for autologous osteochondral grafting in the knee. *Am J Sports Med* 29(2):203, 2001, Fig. 2.)

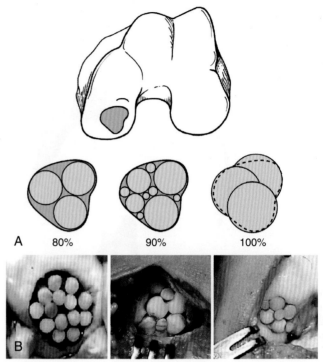

FIG 30.5 Filling Pattern for a Complex Lesion (A) Arrangement of osteochondral autograft plugs within a defect to achieve 80%, 90%, and 100% coverage. Note the different sizes of plugs used as well as the trimming of plugs to achieve greater coverage. (B) Representative photos demonstrating mosaic filling of large, complex lesions. (From Hangody L, Rathonyi GK, Duska Z, et al: Autologous osteochondral mosaicplasty. Surgical technique. *J Bone Joint Surg Am* 86-A(Suppl 1):68, 2004, Fig. 5.)

along the articular cartilage surface, postulating that this was related to directional variation in stiffness and strength. In 1925, Benninghoff further described the microarchitecture of articular cartilage to include collagen fibers oriented perpendicular to the joint surface in the deep layer, with parallel orientation superficially. Below et al. mapped the split line pattern of articular cartilage at the distal femur, demonstrating a characteristic pattern of collagen fiber orientation (see Fig. 30.3).[9] Although this may have no significant clinical effect, it is a theoretical concern that deserves consideration.

Contact Pressures

Contact pressures of the patellofemoral articulation have been examined by several investigators.[1,29,102] Simonian et al. reported that commonly used donor sites along the periphery of the femur at the patellofemoral joint and within the intercondylar notch are not completely free of joint loading forces. Ahmad et al. quantified a patellofemoral contact map exhibiting the differences in contact pressures at various sites along the distal femur, showing lowest contact forces at the superomedial border of the femur as well as along the most inferior part of the intercondylar notch (see Fig. 30.4). Garretson et al. measured contact pressures under two different loads through the entire range of knee motion. Although contact pressures were noted to be lower along the medial condyle, there were no significant differences along the far medial or far lateral edges of the distal femur. The authors concluded that harvesting of grafts from the medial femoral flare may have less impact on patellofemoral biomechanics, but limitations exist because the medial condyle is narrower and more sloped than the lateral condyle. The authors recommended that grafts 5 mm in diameter or smaller should be harvested from the medial femoral flare and larger grafts should be harvested from the lateral femoral flare. Overall consensus indicates that all articular surfaces bear some load; however, the edges of the medial and lateral flares bear the least force during patellofemoral articulation and may represent an optimal surface match contour for condylar lesions. Depending on the size of the recipient site and the number and size of

donor plugs needed, individualized strategies for harvesting may be devised with the underlying goal of minimizing alterations in patellofemoral biomechanics.

Fill Pattern

Depending on the size and pattern of the lesion, different technical strategies for coverage may be used. Smaller lesions can be covered with a single donor graft, depending on condyle size and topography. Larger lesions may require multiple grafts. Biomechanical studies of osteochondral defects in cadaveric knees demonstrated increased rim stress concentration in defects 10 mm or greater in diameter.[36] Smaller defects did not demonstrate significant load redistribution. Therefore complete fill of an osteochondral defect is not required for adequate reconstitution of lesions. Hangody et al. illustrated that multiple osteochondral plugs can be arranged to fill a large defect (Fig. 30.5).[43] Given the limited nature of donor plugs as well as the biomechanical considerations outlined previously, defects are typically tiled with multiple plugs of different sizes with fibrous fill in the intervening gaps. It has been proposed that gaps between osteochondral plugs be filled with hyaline-like tissue, but there is no evidence that this additional measure results in appreciably improved outcomes.[45]

In 2006, Burks et al. demonstrated that incomplete fill of a larger lesion better preserves the femoral condyle contour than untreated or bone-grafted defects.[14] Using an ovine model, a 6 mm plug was placed in the center of a 10 mm defect. While surrounded by fibrous tissue, this method better preserved the articular surface and contour compared to unfilled defects. Hyaline cartilage was noted in the central plug, and histologic evaluation was significantly higher in incompletely filled defects than in unfilled defects.

Depth of Insertion

Early concerns over subsidence of osteochondral plugs led to recommendations that osteochondral autograft plugs be placed slightly proud. In 2001, Pearce et al. performed a study on sheep comparing grafts placed flush with the joint surface and 2 mm proud.[90] Contrary to the authors' hypothesis, grafts placed proud showed poor bony incorporation, evidenced by surrounding fibroplasia and chondroplasia consistent with hypertrophic nonunion attributed to micromotion or shear of the grafts. The grafts placed flush with surrounding cartilage revealed good alignment and continuity, with interstices filled by well-attached repair tissue. In a subsequent series of biomechanical studies, Koh et al. studied contact pressures in elevated and countersunk osteochondral plugs placed in porcine knees, as well as grafts inserted at an angle with surface asymmetry.[56,57] Contact pressures were markedly elevated (roughly 50% increase in peak pressure) in grafts placed as little as 0.5 or 1 mm above the surface. Countersunk grafts exhibited approximately 10% increases in peak pressures when compared with grafts that were completely congruent. Interestingly, these countersunk graft still experienced less peak pressure than defects that were left unfilled (20% increase). Similarly, angled grafts placed with any part of the graft protruding above the surrounding cartilage resulted in significant increases in peak contact pressures, whereas those placed partially countersunk were similar to plugs placed orthogonally and flush. These results were corroborated in a case series by Nakagawa et al.[81] Clinical outcomes and second-look arthroscopy were compared in five patients following OAT; two had proud grafts and three had countersunk grafts. Patients with proud grafts complained of catching sensation about 4 months postoperatively as well as occasional knee pain. Second-look arthroscopy showed fibrillation and fissuring around the grafts. Patients with countersunk grafts reported no clinical symptoms and exhibited fibrocartilaginous tissue overlying the grafts with a smooth joint surface. Although the ideal osteochondral plug placement is flush with surrounding cartilage, there is far greater tolerance for plugs placed slightly countersunk as opposed to elevated. Any prominence of the transferred tissue results in significant elevation of contact pressures and may result in toggling, clefting, and perimeter breakdown of the graft with degradation of the transplanted cartilage.

Graft Insertion

Fixation of osteochondral autograft plugs is achieved through a press-fit technique. Donor harvester trephines are 1 mm larger than the recipient harvester tubes. Additionally, recipient sockets are prepared 2 mm shallower than the depth of the graft, allowing for better accuracy when seating grafts flush with surrounding cartilage. This method allows for all-arthroscopic delivery of grafts as well as arrangement of several grafts within a single defect bed. Several investigators have studied the effects of different parameters on graft stability. Kock et al. compared push-in forces for different lengths of plugs, as well as the effect of matching the donor to the recipient plug depth.[53] They found that longer plugs (>12 mm) were more stable when unmatched

to the recipient site depth because of higher frictional forces along the edge of the graft. In contrast, donor plugs that matched the recipient site depth (eg, those that contacted the base of the prepared defect) were more stable when shorter lengths were used. Kordás et al. found that grafts with larger diameters withstood greater push-in forces but that multiple grafts regardless of arrangement (row vs. circle) were less stable than individual plugs.[59] Similarly, overlap of multiple plugs with breach of interplug native bone (socket wall) was found to decrease stability.[38] It is hypothesized that this decreased stability may be related to less adjacent native articular cartilage and bone available to buttress the graft. Dilation of the recipient bed has been described as a means of obtaining an optimal press-fit. Shorter dilation lengths allow for more of a taper fit between the donor plug and recipient site. Similarly, slight oversizing of donor plugs relative to recipient sites increased stability by compensating for the extraction blade width. In a rabbit model, Makino et al. demonstrated increased stability and better preservation of cartilage thickness when grafts oversized by 1 mm relative to the recipient site were used.[69] Similarly, using a goat model, Kock et al. showed a significantly lower graft subsidence tendency in "bottomed" versus "unbottomed" osteochondral plugs.[52]

One disadvantage to the press-fit technique is the force required for graft impaction. Several studies have documented a decrease in chondrocyte viability following impaction, although the clinical relevance has yet to be determined.[7,12,37,111] Lower forces used to gently seat plugs into well-matched recipient sites may be benign, whereas the markedly increased forces required to compress a graft that would otherwise be left proud may adversely affect chondrocyte viability.[88] In this regard, minimizing impaction forces are of paramount importance to the viability and longevity of the transplanted, viable cartilage tissue.

Graft Harvest

Harvesting of osteochondral autografts has also been a focus of several studies, with emphasis on cell viability. Evans et al. reported superiority of manual punches over power trephines, with inadvertent skidding, ragged cartilage edges, and separation of cartilage from subchondral bone seen in the latter.[25] Chondrocyte viability was also decreased when power trephines were used for graft harvest. Duchow et al., in a study of pull-out strengths using porcine osteochondral autografts harvested using a manual punch, noted that plugs extracted by levering of the plug were less stable than those extracted by turning of the punch.[22] They also noted that failure loads were significantly lower in 10 mm long plugs compared to those 15 mm or 20 mm long. Moreover, repeated insertion and extraction led to decreased stability. The cutting profile of manual punches affected chondrocyte survival, with subtle compression of the articular cartilage resulting in a perimeter marginal zone of death.[46,47]

A critical concept in graft harvest is perpendicularity.[20] Although this may be achieved either through an open or arthroscopic approach, it is critical to harvest grafts that are orthogonal to the articular surface.[50] This allows for improved articular congruity in addition to more precise restoration of the condylar bevel and radius of curvature, which is of particular importance in defects requiring multiple plugs. In 2011, Epstein et al. compared open versus arthroscopic approach to graft harvest in a cadaveric model using magnetic resonance imaging (MRI) to assess graft perpendicularity. A significant difference favoring a mini-open approach for medial supracondylar ridge graft gravest was demonstrated, whereas all other donor site areas showed no statistical difference in perpendicularity with regard to approach.[23] Donor site morbidity remains a technical concern when considering OAT.

Early reports used iliac crest cortical bone grafts to fill lesions following graft harvest. Similar fill using the bone remaining from recipient site preparation using a trephine cutting technique has been documented by reversing the orientation of the "pathologic" bone dowels and inserting the "bone grafts" into the harvest site defects.[80] In a canine model, Feczkó et al. in 2003 compared several biodegradable materials for donor site filling, including hydroxyapatite, carbon fiber, polyglyconate-B, compressed collagen, and polycaprolactone.[27] On second-look arthroscopy and histologic evaluation, compressed collagen yielded the best fibrocartilage coverage of the harvest site defects. Several commercially available composite bone graft substitute polymer plugs are now available and have been used to fill donor site defects (OsseoFit, Kensey Nash Corp., Exton, Pennsylvania).[99] Espregueira-Mendes et al. reported on the use of tibio-fibular joint grafts for treatment of OCD lesions, in which no donor site, radiographic, or clinical complications were noted postoperatively.[24]

In cases where osteochondral plugs are transferred from the knee to other areas of the body, special attention must be paid to potential differences in cartilage thickness of donor and recipient sites. Using MRI cartilage mapping, Schub et al. showed that the thinnest area of harvestable knee cartilage is located in the posterior pole of the medial femoral condyle and distal-most anterior-lateral femoral condyle, which integrate best with more distant articular recipient sites in the body, such as the elbow.[97] In general, donor site morbidity has not been a major area of concern when harvesting bone plugs from the knee for OAT procedures in more distant sites of the body, such as the elbow and talus. In an effort to better define the confounding effect of the resurfacing procedure in association with the harvesting, a series of 43 patients undergoing talar OAT procedures were reported on by Baltzer and Arnold. In this study, the authors found that harvested plugs from the ipsilateral supero-lateral condyle of the knee showed a low overall donor-site morbidity rate, with knee discomfort that disappeared by 6 months postsurgery.[5]

PEARLS AND PITFALLS

Many of the complications associated with OAT are directly attributable to technical pitfalls. Hemarthrosis has been reported, which may be reduced by filling the donor site and placing a postoperative drain.[43] Another donor site morbidity issue includes donor site collapse secondary to the convergence of the defect base of adjacent harvest site defects. Avoiding such collapse can be attained by maintaining a 1- to 2-mm spread between harvest sites and preserving adequate space from the edge of the condyle. Additionally, the surgeon must always be mindful of the natural convergence of the individual graft bases resulting from the curvature of the condylar surface. Graft failure may occur for a number of reasons. Impaction forces, which have been proven to affect cellular viability, can be minimized by careful matching of the recipient site and the donor plug depth. While already incorporated into several commercial systems, optimization of the difference between plug diameter and recipient bed diameter to allow for good press-fit without excessive force is important. Careful removal of donor plugs

limits collateral damage to surrounding cartilage. Similarly, meticulous handling of the donor plug from the osseous side minimizes microtrauma to the graft cartilage surface, which can affect chondrocyte viability. OCD lesions and other bony defects extending into subchondral bone may require longer grafts or adjunctive bone grafting methods. In cases where multiple grafts are used, minimizing step-off between grafts and also relative to the surrounding cartilage will decrease surface fibrillation and edge-loading of grafts.

POSTOPERATIVE REGIMEN

Originally, the standard postoperative regimen involved initial protection from weight bearing, followed by gradual transition to weight bearing. However, recent articles have shown benefits to immediate weight bearing without detrimental effects. In 2014, Kosiur and Collins examined the effect of postoperative weight-bearing status on outcomes and complications after OAT for small defects less than 1 cm. Results showed no difference in cartilage repair outcomes, while demonstrating a statistically significant reduction in deep vein thrombosis and arthrofibrosis in the weight-bearing as tolerated group.[60] Nevertheless, if a more conservative postoperative approach is taken, immediate early range of motion is instituted with limited joint loading. Non-weight-bearing generally lasts 3 weeks and is followed by gradual advancement. Postoperative stiffness (particularly in the setting of hemarthrosis) may be prevented by early range of motion, and continuous passive motion (CPM) machines may be useful. However, CPM has not been definitively shown to affect outcomes.[26] Active physical therapy includes patellar mobilization, stretching, and progressive strengthening beginning with isometrics. Subsequent proprioceptive neuromuscular re-education occurs, with conditioning including swimming, leg press, and closed chain kinetic exercises. Normal daily activity can be achieved at 8 to 10 weeks, but progression to high demand sports may be delayed for as long as 6 months.

RESULTS

Several case series and more recent prospective randomized trials with long-term follow-up have been reported, all with generally positive results. Measures include validated outcome scores, such as the Knee Injury and Osteoarthritis Outcome Score (KOOS), International Cartilage Repair Society (ICRS) cartilage repair histological assessment score, International Knee Documentation Committee (IKDC) score, Lysholm scores, Modified Hospital for Special Surgery Score (HSS Score), modified Cincinnati score, and subjective activity level assessments using Tegner scores, as well as radiologic measures, including magnetic resonance observation of cartilage repair tissue (MOCART). Second-look arthroscopy and histological analysis of biopsy samples also provide objective evidence of structural articular cartilage resurfacing. Table 30.1 summarizes the results from a variety of Level IV case series. Hangody et al. documented data from a 17-year prospective multicenter study including 354 mosaicplasties. These mosaicplasties involved 187 medial femoral condyles, 74 lateral femoral condyles, 16 tibial plateaus, 18 patellas, and 8 trochlea. Good to excellent results were achieved in 91% of femoral condyle lesions, 86% of tibial plateaus, and 74% of patellofemoral lesions. This long-term study showed improved assessment scores across the board,

TABLE 30.1 Level IV Case Series Reports of Osteochondral Autograft Plug Transfer Procedures

Authors	Study Arm	Number	Age	Scoring System		Location	Size (cm²)
Ulstein KSSTA 2014[109]	MFx	11	31.7	Lysholm	Preop: 48.2 Follow-up: 69.7	10 MFC 1 LFC	2.6
Level II—Therapeutic	OAT	14	32.7		Preop: 49.2 Follow-up: 62.6	10 MFC 2 LFC 2 Trochlea	3
Gudas Arthroscopy 2013[31]	MFx	34	31.2	Tegner	Preop: 2.7 Postop 6.9 at 3 years	All MFC + ACL	2.7
Level II—Therapeutic	Debride	34	33.5		Preop: 2.5 Postop 6.2 at 3 years		2.9
	OAT	34	32.4		Preop 2.5 Postop 7.1 at 3 years		3.1
Bentley JBJS-BR 2012[11] Level 1	ACI	58	30.9	Cincinnati	Excellent 28 Good 7 Fair 6 Poor 2	24 MFC 13 LFC 1 Trochlea 20 Patella	4.41
	OAT	42	31.6		Excellent 4 Good 5 Fair 4 Poor 2	29 MFC 5 LFC 1 Tib Plat 5 Patellar	3.99
Gudas AJSM 2012 Level 1[32]	MFx	29	24.3	ICRS	Preop MFx-ACD: 64.8 ± 1.7 MFx-ACD: 78.2 ± 1.4 at 10 years Preop MFx-OCD: 50.9 ± 2.4 MFx-OCD: 73.9 ± 1.5 at 10 years		2.77
	OAT	28	24.6 ± 6.54		Preop OAT-ACD: 61.3 ± 1.7 OAT-ACD: 92.9 ± 1.45 at 10 years Preop OAT-OCD: 50.9 ± 1.8 OAT-OCD: 87.5 ± 1.3 at 10 years		2.8
Lim CORR 2012[65] Level II—Therapeutic	MFx	30	32.9	Lysholm	Preop: 51.2 ± 6.2 Postop 85.6 ± 6.8 at 5 years	23 MFC 7 LFC	2.77
	ACI	18	25.1		Preop 53.2 ± 7.2 Postop 84.8 ± 5.5 at 5 years	13 MFC 5 LFC	2.84
	OAT	22	30.4		Preop 52.4 ± 6.4 Postop 84.8 ± 6.1 at 5 years	19 MFC 3 LFC	2.75
Gudas JP 2009[34] Level I—Therapeutic	MFx	22	14.09	ICRS Functional and objective	19/22 Excellent/Good at 1 year 12/19 Excellent/Good at 4.2 years	20 MFC 2 LFC	3.17
	OAT	25	14.64		23/25 Excellent/Good at 1 year 19/23 Excellent/Good at 4.2 years	21 MFC 4 LFC	3.2
Dozin Clin J Sport Med 2005[21] Level II—Therapeutic	ACI	22	29.6	Lysholm	<60 (failure): 1 60-90 (partial success): 5 90-100 (complete success): 10 Lost to f/u: 6	14 MFC 2 LFC 6 Patella	2
	OAT	22	27.9		<60 (failure): 0 60-90 (partial success): 2 90-100 (complete success): 15 Lost to f/u: 5	12 MFC 3 LFC 7 Patella	1.9
Gudas Arthroscopy 2005, KSSTA 2006[33,35] Level Ia— Therapeutic	MFx	29	24.3	HSS	77 preop 83 at 12 months 82 at 24 months 91 at 36 months	23 MFC 6 LFC	2.8
	OAT	28			78 preop 88 at 12 months 91 at 24 months 91 at 36 months	25 MFC 3 LFC	2.8
Bentley JBJS—BR 2003[11] Level II—Therapeutic	ACI	58	30.9	Cincinnati	>80 (excellent): 40% 55-79 (good): 48% 30-55 (fair): 12% <30 (poor): 0%	24 MFC 13 LFC 20 Patella 1 Trochlea	4.66
	OAT	42	31.6		>80 (excellent): 21% 55-79 (good): 48% 30-55 (fair): 14% <30 (poor): 17%	29 MFC 5 LFC 5 Patella 2 Trochlea 1 LTP	

Continued

TABLE 30.1		Level IV Case Series Reports of Osteochondral Autograft Plug Transfer Procedures—cont'd						
Authors	**Study Arm**	**Number**	**Age**	**Scoring System**			**Location**	**Size (cm²)**
Horas JBJS 2003[45] Level II—Therapeutic	ACI	20	31.4	Lysholm	24.9 preop 27.55 at 3 months 45.75 at 6 months 57.50 at 12 months 66.75 at 24 months		17 MFC 3 LFC	3.86
	OAT	20	35.4		28.45 preop 27.95 at 3 months 53.45 at 6 months 68.25 at 12 months 72.70 at 24 months		16 MFC 4 LFC	3.63

ACI, Autologous chondrocyte implantation; *ACL,* anterior cruciate ligament; *CSE,* cartilage standard evaluation form; *HTO,* high tibial osteotomy; *HSS,* Hospital for Special Surgery scoring system; *ICRS,* International Cartilage Repair Society; *IKDC,* International Knee Documentation Committee; *JOA,* Japanese Orthopaedic Association; *KSS,* Knee Society for pain and mobility score; *KOOS,* Knee injury and osteoarthritis outcome score; *LFC,* lateral femoral condyle; *LTP,* lateral tibial plateau; *MCL,* medial collateral ligament; *MFC,* medial femoral condyle; *MFx,* microfracture; *OAT,* osteochondral autograft plug transfer; *OCD,* osteochondritis dissecans; *PCL,* posterior collateral ligament; *ROH,* removal of hardware; *QOL,* quality of life; *VAS,* visual analog scale.

including the HSS, Lysholm, Cincinnati, and ICRS scores.[39] After publishing his short-term and medium-term results, Solheim et al. evaluated his long-term follow-up data. This study showed significant improvement in the Lysholm score (49→72), as well as decreased pain VAS (58→33) at 10 to 14 year follow-up.[104] This trend among sites within the knee has been reported by other groups as well, with greatest success uniformly achieved in the treatment of femoral condyle lesions. Other prognostic factors include age, with patients older than 45 years faring less well than younger patients.

Several prospective randomized controlled studies have compared OAT to microfracture and autologous chondrocyte implantation (ACI) (Table 30.2). In 2003, Bentley et al. conducted a Level I therapeutic study that reported on 100 patients (mean age 31.3 years, range 16 to 49 years) who were randomized to ACI versus OAT.[10] Most lesions were posttraumatic, with a mean defect size of 4.66 cm². Cincinnati scores were good to excellent in 88% of ACI versus 69% of OAT patients, and second-look arthroscopy at 1 year showed good to excellent articular cartilage resurfacing in 82% of ACI versus 34% of OAT patients. However, this study was technically limited because the authors placed the osteochondral autograft plugs slightly prominent to allow contact during normal movement and to "ensure that nutrition was maintained by loading and by the passage of fluid through the articular cartilage." Subsequent work has shown that plugs placed prominently fare worse, with micromotion resulting in possible nonunion and differential loading of the articular surface resulting in fibrillation and early degeneration of the graft.

In 2005, Gudas et al. published a Level I study randomizing 60 patients (mean age 24.3 years, range 15 to 40 years) to either microfracture or OAT who were competitive athletes at the regional or national levels.[33] Clinical improvement was seen in both groups, but good-to-excellent results were achieved in 96% of OAT patients versus 52% who had undergone microfracture. HSS and ICRS scores were significantly better in patients treated with OAT compared to microfracture at 12, 24, and 36 months after surgery. Ninety-three percent of OAT patients and 52% of microfracture patients returned to sports activities at the preinjury level at an average of 6.5 months (range 4 to 8 months). MRI findings revealed similar success with joint surface congruity achieved in 94% of patients

following OAT versus 49% following microfracture. Repair tissue thickness appeared the same as surrounding cartilage in 68% of the OAT group, compared to 18% of the microfracture group. Of note, only all-arthroscopic procedures were included in this study.

In 2003, Horas et al. conducted a Level II therapeutic study that compared 40 patients (mean age 33.4 years, range 18 to 44 years) who underwent ACI or OAT.[45] Lesions ranged from 3.2 to 5.6 cm² in area (mean 3.75 cm²). Postoperative Lysholm scores were higher in patients treated with OAT compared to ACI at 6, 12, and 24 months. However, Meyers and Tegner activity scores were equivalent 2 years after treatment. The biopsy at 2 years showed consistent fibrocartilage with localized areas of hyaline-like regenerative cartilage near the bone following ACI, compared to intact hyaline cartilage that cannot be differentiated from surrounding native cartilage following OAT. However, this study failed to achieve greater than 80% follow-up. In a prospective randomized trial comparing OATs versus microfracture in 2012, Gudas et al. published 10-year follow-up data on the previously mentioned group of 60 athletes. Three to 10 years after OAT or microfracture procedures, patients had lower ICRS and Tegner scores. However, both groups still had significant clinical improvement over preoperative ICRS scores at 10-year follow-up, with significantly better results detected in the OAT group. There were 15 failures (26%), including 14% of OAT and 38% of the microfracture treatment groups. Twenty-five percent of patients from the OAT group versus 48% of the microfracture (MF) group had radiographic evidence of Kellgren-Lawrence grade I osteoarthritis at 10 years. The ICRS and Tegner scores of younger athletes (<25 years at time of surgery) remained significantly higher compared with older patients with 75% of the OAT group and 37% of the microfracture group, maintaining the same preinjury physical activity level.[32]

In general, patients fared well following OAT procedures, with significant increases in knee function and satisfaction. Complications included hemarthrosis, loosening of plugs, fibrous overgrowth, graft subsidence, and donor site morbidity. Careful attention to technique is critical because many complications can be directly attributed to user error. It is difficult to isolate morbidity from graft harvest in the setting of baseline knee pathology. Several studies in which OAT was performed in other joints, including talar dome, capitellum, and femoral

TABLE 30.2 Controlled Trials Comparing Osteochondral Autograft Plug Transfer to Alternate Techniques

Authors	N	Age (year)	Follow-Up	Scoring System	Subjective	Complications	Location	Size
Atik Bull HJD 2005[4]	12	38	4 years (2-8)	Lysholm 56->86	85% pain free	Slight joint effusion	9 MFC 1 LFC 1 Patella	Up to 5 plugs
Barber Arthroscopy 2006[6]	36	43	48 months (24-89)	Lysholm 44->84 Tegner 5 at f/u	—	—	27 MFC 9 LFC	1.9 plugs
Braun Arthritis Res & Ther 2008[13]	33	34.3	66.4 months (46-98)	Lysholm 49->86	27/33 return to sports 31/33 satisfied, would redo	—	27 MFC 6 LFC	5 cm^2 (6.2)
Chow Arthroscopy 2004[17]	30	44.6	45.1 months (24-63)	Lysholm 43.6->87.5	83.3% exc/good	Hematoma	28 MFC 2 LFC	2.2 plugs
Gaweda Int Orthop 2006[30]	19	25.5	24 months	Marshall 36.3->46.2 (vs. 40.7->47.1)	—	Joint effusion Decreased ROM	19 Pat	—
Figueroa Knee 2011[28]	10	20.2	37.3 months (24-70)	Lysholm 73.8->95 IKDC 93.6	100% exc/good	No documented postop complications due to OAT procedure	10 Pat	1.2 cm^2
Hangody AJSM 2010[39]	354	24.3	9.6 years (2-17)	HSS 67->89 Lysholm 64->93 Cincinnati 5.8->8.7 ICRS 63%->89%	Fem 91% exc/good Tib 86% exc/good Pat 74% exc/good	5% Don site disturb 8% Painful hemorrhage 2 Septic arthritis 3 Thromboembolic	187 MFC 74 LFC 16 Tib 18 Pat 8 Troch	2.5 cm^2
Hangody Injury 2008[44]	967			HSS, Cincinnati, Lysholm, ICRS	Femoral 92% exc/good Tibial 87% exc/good Troch/pat 74% exc/good	Persistent pain, 4 deep infections, 56 hemarthroses, 4 VTE	789 Fem 147 Pat-fem 31 Tib	—
Hangody KSSTA 1997[41]	44	30	25.1 months (12-54)	HSS 67-100 (94.2) Preop 62.2	Aborted mosaicplasty vs. abrasion arthroplasty due to HSS score difference	3 Hematomas	25 MFC 15 LFC 4 Both	—
Hangody Orthopedics 1998[42]	57	31.4	48.7 months (36-56)	HSS 64-100 (90.7)	54 return to normal activity	2 Hematomas	25 MFC 22 LFC 8 Patella	1-8.5 cm
Hangody J Sports Traumatol 1998	55	23.1	29.5 months (12-62)	HSS 67-100 (89)	51 return to normal activity	4 Hematomas	24 MFC 27 LFC 4 Patella	5.1 cm^2
Jakob CORR 2002[48]	52	33	37 months (24-56)	Improvement in ICRS	93% no/slight limitations 52% incr sports activity 88% satisfaction/would redo	Catching/locking 4 Graft failures (re-op)	—	4.9 cm^2
Karataglis Knee 2005[49]	36	31.9	36.9 months (18-73)	Tegner 1-8 (3.76) ADL/KOOS 18-98 (72.3)	86.5% improvement 18 return to sports	—	18 MFC 8 LFC 7 Trochlea 4 Patella	2.73 cm^2
Klinger KSSTA[51]	21	29	39 months (32-62)	Lysholm 62->90 Tegner 3.9>6.1	—	2 Hematomas	21 MFC	3.5 cm^2
Katani J Ortho Surg 2003[61]	16	64.9	67 months (28-111)	JOA: preop 68.1 (60-75)- >88.8 (80-100)	—	—	—	—
Kock Acta Orthopaedic 2010	13	33	49 months (31-65)	Lysholm 64-77 (p < .05) Cincinnati 67-78 (p < .09) Tegner 2.4->3.4 (p < .03)	—	12/13 Retropat crepitus	10 MFC 3 LFC	7.5-12.9 mm
Krusche-Mandl Osteoarthritis Cartilage 2012[62]	9	49	7.9 years (7.7-8.2)	IKDC 77.0 Lysholm 90. VAS 1.0	—	—	6 MFC 3 LFC	2.7 cm^2

Continued

TABLE 30.2 Controlled Trials Comparing Osteochondral Autograft Plug Transfer to Alternate Techniques—cont'd

Authors	N	Age (year)	Follow-Up	Scoring System	Subjective	Complications	Location	Size
Lahav J Knee Surg 2006[63]	16		40 months	KOOS: Pain 80.6, Symptoms 53.6, ADL 93.4, Sports 65.3, QOL 51.0 (6-88) IKDC 68.2	Would re-do 86%	—	—	—
Laprell Arch Orthop Trauma Surg 2001[64]	35	26	8.1 years (6-12)	CSE/ICRS 12-I, 14-II, 3-III	Subj incr in activity levels	Hemarthrosis 13; numbness 16	—	1.1-2.4 cm²
Ma Injury 2004[68]	18	29	42 months (24-64	Lysholm 47.5->92.4 Tegner 2.22->6.11	11 excellent 5 good 2 fair	Fibrillation in tib-plat OAT	11 MFC 5 LFC 2 LTP	4.1 cm²
Marcacci AJSM 2007[70]	30	29.3	7 years	IKDC: 7A, 16B, 4C, 3D at 7 years 11A, 12B, 4C, 3D, at 2 years IKDC subjective: 34.8->71.7	2 years: 22 return to sports same level 4 return to sports lower level 7 years: 7 same level, 14 lower level	3 failures tx with ACI	17 MFC 13 LFC	1.9 cm²
Marcacci Artthroscopy 2005[71]	37	29.5	24-48 months	IKDC: 78.3% exc/ good 14-A, 15-B, 5-C, 3-D	27 return to sports at same level 5 lower level	2 failures (insuff graft integration)	23 MFC 14 LFC	2.1 cm²
Marcacci Orthopedics 1999[72]	13	31	61.5 months (13-141)	Cincinnati: 3 excellent/8 good Swedish: 4 excellent/8 good Lysholm: 8 excellent/4 good IKDC: 4 excellent/8 good	—	1 flexion deform/stiff	11 MFC 1 LFC 1 LFC + LTP	1.5-3 cm²
Miniaci Arthroscopy[75]	20	14.3	3.4 years (2-6)	Preop IKDC: 0-A, 5-B, 8-C, 7-D Postop: 19-A, 1-B at 24 months	—	—	19 MFC 1 LFC	4.1 plugs
Outerbridge CORR 2000[86]	16	27	7.6 years (2-14.6)	Cincinnati: 35->85	100% improved function 81% high level of function	5 re-op due to pain, detach in 1 meniscus tear in 1 3 normal	10 MFC 8 LFC	4.5 cm²

ACI, Autologous chondrocyte implantation, *ADL,* activities of daily living; *HSS,* Hospital for Special Surgery scoring system; *ICRS,* International Cartilage Repair Society; *IKDC,* International Knee Documentation Committee; *KOOS,* Knee injury and Osteoarthritis Outcome Score; *LFC,* lateral femoral condyle; *LTP,* lateral tibial plateau; *MFC,* medial femoral condyle; *OAT,* osteochondral autograft plug transfer; *ROM,* range of motion; *VTE,* venous thromboembolic event.

head, document significant morbidity to the knee following graft harvest.[2,93] In multiple cases, knees that were asymptomatic prior to graft harvest developed some degree of impairment postoperatively. This morbidity may be independent of patient age or the size and number of grafts taken.[89] Although this may be an important consideration in OAT harvest for other joints, the morbidity associated with graft harvest in the same knee is usually offset by improvements achieved through the OAT procedure itself.

GROSS MORPHOLOGY AND HISTOLOGY

Examination of articular surfaces following OAT during second-look arthroscopy has generally shown good incorporation of the graft. Articular surfaces consistently show good restoration of surface congruity with fibrous fill at the periphery of grafts (Fig. 30.6). Probing of grafts demonstrates some fibrillation or fraying of cartilage edges (Fig. 30.7), but more often grade I chondromalacia or better appearance of the articular cartilage surface.

Several detailed reports of postoperative histological analysis of OAT resurfacing have been described. These include biopsies taken at second-look arthroscopy as well as entire joint surfaces resected during total knee arthroplasty.[45,54] In all cases, a persistent cleft is seen in the cartilage layer between transplanted osteochondral segments and neighboring tissue (Fig. 30.8A). However, good integration at the osseous level is seen, with reconstitution of articular cartilage topography (see Fig. 30.8B-D). Two studies examining OAT performed in rabbits with concomitant use of platelet-rich plasma (PRP) showed significantly higher mean modified ICRS histological scores and graft integration scores compared to OAT alone.[33,103]

IMAGING

MRI has emerged as the gold standard with which to noninvasively monitor and evaluate structural outcomes and congruity of cartilage resurfacing procedures. (Fig. 30.9). This is in part because of superior soft tissue contrast, direct multiplanar capabilities, and lack of ionizing radiation.[91] Several different

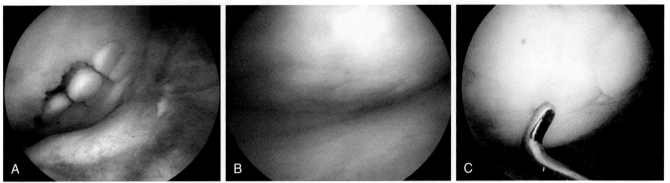

FIG 30.6 Arthroscopic Views of Defect Repair Using Osteochondral Autograft Plug Transfer
(A) Arrangement of multiple 5.5 mm diameter osteochondral autograft plugs to restore a 3.5 cm^2 OCD lesion of the lateral femoral condyle. (B) Second-look at 3 years shows complete restoration of joint surface congruence with no evidence of fibrillation or degeneration. (C) Second-look arthroscopy 1 year after OAT of a medial femoral condyle defect. Probing of the repair tissue shows good alignment with the surrounding healthy articular cartilage as well similar firmness. (From Gudas R, Stankevicius E, Monastyreckiene E, et al: Osteochondral autologous transplantation versus microfracture for the treatment of articular cartilage defects in the knee joint in athletes. *Knee Surg Sports Traumatol Arthrosc* 14(9):837, 2006. Fig. 2; Hangody L, Fules P: Autologous osteochondral mosaicplasty for the treatment of full-thickness defects of weight-bearing joints: 10 years of experimental and clinical experience. *J Bone Joint Surg Am* 85-A(Suppl 2):31, 2003, Fig. 10.)

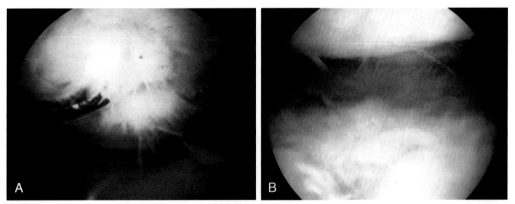

FIG 30.7 Arthroscopic Views of Defect Repair Using Osteochondral Autograft Plug Transfer
(A) Second-look arthroscopy at 2 years following mosaicplasty of the medial femoral condyle shows fibrillation of the osteochondral plugs and incomplete filling of the spaces between them. (B) Second-look arthroscopic view of lateral tibial surface after 26 months shows an uneven surface and degenerative changes with fibrillation. (From Bentley G, Biant LC, Carrington RW, et al: A prospective, randomised comparison of autologous chondrocyte implantation versus mosaicplasty for osteochondral defects in the knee. *J Bone Joint Surg Br* 85(2):226, 2003. Fig. 6; Ma HL, Hung SC, Wang ST, et al: Osteochondral autografts transfer for posttraumatic osteochondral defect of the knee-2 to 5 years follow-up. *Injury* 35(12):1290, 2004, Fig. 3.)

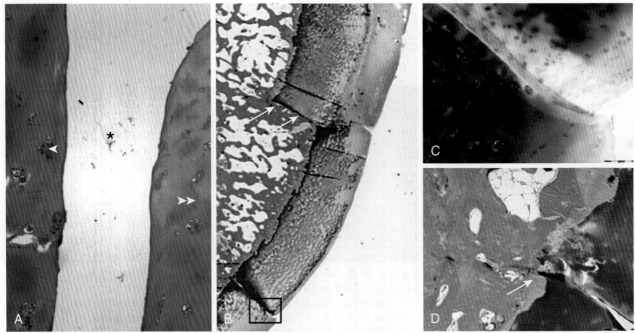

FIG 30.8 (A) Histological appearance of a biopsy specimen taken 22 months after osteochondral transplantation. A cleft (*) remains between the native cartilage *(single arrowhead)* and the osteochondral transplant *(double arrowhead)* in the cartilage layer (toluidine blue; original magnification, ×200). (B) Histological appearance of three adjacent plugs at the recipient site. Note adequate restoration of the joint surface *(black box)* with hyaline cartilage and the relative deep placement of one plug *(white arrows)* (Masson's trichrome; ×12.5). (C) Enlargement of boxed area in (B). Note cluster formation of chondrocytes at the boundary of each plug and less staining, indicating loss of proteoglycans (toluidine blue; ×100, bar = 200 μm). (D) Enlargement of dotted boxed area in (B). Note reconstruction of the tidemark *(arrow)* at the transition zone, a clearly visible fissure between the two cartilage plugs and full incorporation of the plugs in the subchondral bone (Masson's trichrome; ×100, bar = 200 μm). (From Horas U, Pelinkovic D, Herr G, et al: Autologous chondrocyte implantation and osteochondral cylinder transplantation in cartilage repair of the knee joint. A prospective, comparative trial. *J Bone Joint Surg Am* 85-A(2):190, 2003. Fig. 6; Kock N, van Susante J, Wymenga A, Buma P: Histological evaluation of a mosaicplasty of the femoral condyle-retrieval specimens obtained after total knee arthroplasty—a case report. *Acta Orthop Scand* 75(4):507, 2004, Fig. 2.)

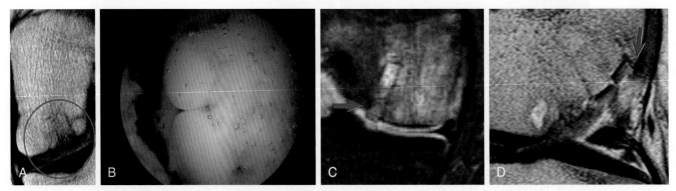

FIG 30.9 Contouring (A) Clinical photo showing plug congruence and (B) on MRI. (C and D) Incongruence of plugs on MRI *(red arrows)*.

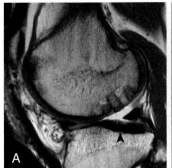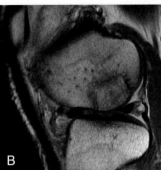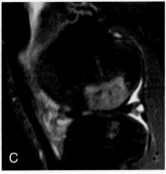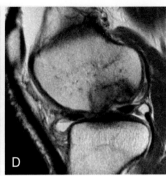

FIG 30.10 (A) Sagittal cartilage-sensitive magnetic resonance image of the knee in a 21-year-old man treated with mosaicplasty for a large osteochondral defect of the lateral femoral condyle. There is restoration of the radius of curvature using multiple plugs. Note the thinning of cartilage over the more posterior plugs and the fibrillation of cartilage over the tibial plateau *(arrowhead)*. Sagittal cartilage-sensitive magnetic resonance image of the knee (B) in a 17-year-old boy, 7 months after mosaicplasty for OCD using a fresh osteochondral allograft. There is intact cartilage over a graft that is slightly proud. A corresponding fat-suppressed magnetic resonance image (C) demonstrates intense bone marrow edema pattern in the graft. A sagittal magnetic resonance image obtained 6 months later (D) demonstrates interval collapse and fragmentation of the allograft, with debris in the posterior recess of the joint. (Modified from Potter HG, Foo LF: Magnetic resonance imaging of articular cartilage: trauma, degeneration, and repair. *Am J Sports Med* 34(4):670–671, 2006, Figs. 16 and 17.)

techniques have been developed for cartilage-specific imaging. Potter and Foo reported on several studies where diagnostic MRI was compared to arthroscopically visualized articular surfaces.[92] They concluded that fat-suppressed fast spin echo (FSE) imaging results in the least interobserver variability as well as the highest sensitivity and specificity. This technique allows for differential contrast between fluid, subchondral bone, and meniscus. Moreover, based on different levels of water sequestration, one can differentiate between articular cartilage, fibrocartilage, and synovial fluid. This provides valuable information regarding structural restoration and repair, including viability of the repair site, tissue fill volume, surface congruence, status of underlying subchondral bone, and perimeter integration (Fig. 30.10). Additional cartilage-specific sequences have been reported, including T1 rho-weighted fast spin-echo, T1 3D gadolinium-enhanced MRI of cartilage (dGEMRIC), gradient refocused acquisition in the steady-state and iterative decomposition of water and fat with echo asymmetry and least-squares estimation (GRASS-IDEAL), isotropic 3D steady-state free precession (SSFP), and driven equilibrium Fourier transform. These imaging methods, which can assess the physiologic status of the tissue, are promising but await further validation in advance of clinical application.

Assessment of collagen organization within the extracellular matrix can be used to provide information regarding the ultrastructural composition of cartilage. T2 relaxation time mapping has been shown to correlate with specific regions of cartilage.[83] Collagen is highly organized in the deep (radial) zone of cartilage, with fibers oriented perpendicular to the articular surface, resulting in low T2 values. In the transitional zone, collagen fibers have a more random orientation and correspondingly increased T2 values. The superficial zone consists of fibers oriented in a more ordered fashion parallel to the joint surface, which also have shorter T2 values. This detailed information allows identification of cartilage defects as well as

monitoring of postoperative integrity of cartilage resurfacing (Fig. 30.11).[55,83]

Several investigators have reported on the correlation between postoperative MRI and clinical measures. The MOCART and 3D MOCART grading systems have been described (Table 30.3), but reports have shown mixed correlation with clinical outcomes.[58,107] In particular, the significance of bone marrow edema following OAT is unclear because several studies have noted persistence of edema as long as 3 years postoperatively.[67,82] This edema does not correlate with knee pain and may represent normal remodeling following graft transfer. Similarly, MR findings consistent with osteonecrosis do not necessarily bear clinical relevance. Longer-term data showed increasing MOCART and 3D MOCART scores during the initial 2 years following surgery, with either plateauing or slight decreased scores measured in years 2 to 7. There was an association found between clinical and MOCART scoring parameters.[113] *Ex vivo* MRI with contrast of articular cartilage following OAT in a patient who subsequently underwent total knee arthroplasty showed direct correlation between histology and MRI. Although the prognostic significance of such findings is unknown, the MR images were able to identify differences in cartilage thickness as well as level of integration of subchondral bone. It remains to be seen whether specific examination of plugs for signs of common complications will have greater clinical relevance.

FUTURE DIRECTIONS

OAT has been clinically described and available for longer than 20 years. Despite its reported success in restoring focal articular cartilage defects, it remains a narrowly defined surgical option. Several factors are responsible for this—most notably, donor site morbidity, technical challenges, and learning curves. As more sophisticated biomaterials are developed and validated

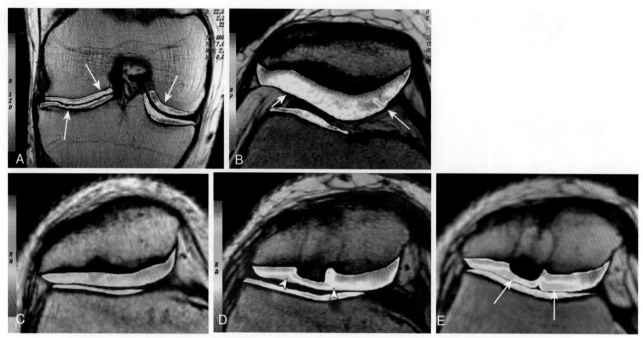

FIG 30.11 (A) Quantitative T2 map demonstrates prolongation over the central portion of the lateral tibial plateau, as well as over the inner margin medial and lateral femoral condyles *(arrows)*. (B) Quantitative MRI in a 25-year-old woman with patellofemoral pain and normal radiographs. Axial quantitative T2 map, color coded according to relaxation times stratified from 10 ms *(red)* to 90 ms *(blue)*, demonstrates a discrete fissure yielding prolonged T2 values in the central portion of the medial facet *(long arrow)*. Also of note is global prolongation of T2 values without the superficial 75% of the lateral patella facet *(short arrow)*, consistent with lateral facet overload. (C-E) Corresponding axial T2 relaxation time maps in an 18-year-old patient with a patellar autologous osteochondral plug. The color maps are coded to capture T2 values ranging from 10 to 90 ms, with orange/red reflecting the shorter values and green/blue reflecting longer T2 values. Before surgery (C), expected focal T2 prolongation is seen at the site of the full-thickness cartilage defect. The adjacent cartilage demonstrates normal color stratification. Four months after surgery (D), the repair cartilage maintains color stratification of normal cartilage. The repair-native interface and adjacent cartilage, however, demonstrate T2 prolongation *(white arrowheads)*. Sixteen months after surgery (E), marked and more diffuse T2 prolongation is demonstrated over the repair and adjacent cartilage *(white arrows)*. The opposite cartilage also demonstrates similar prolongation of T2 values, compared with before. (Modified from Koff, MF, Potter HG: Noncontrast MR techniques and imaging of cartilage. *Radiol Clin North Am* 47(3):498–499, 2009. Figs. 5 and 6; Nho SJ, Foo LF, Green DM, et al: Magnetic resonance imaging and clinical evaluation of patellar resurfacing with press-fit osteochondral autograft plugs. *Am J Sports Med* 36(6):1107, 2008, Fig. 4.)

in clinical trials, donor site morbidity may be minimized. Adjuvant therapy, such as catabolic inhibitors, joint cytoprotective agents, and PRP may improve the environment in which chondrocytes subjected to transplantation and impaction loads are able to recover. Smyth et al. studied the effect of PRP and hyaluronic acid (HA) on the histological results of autologous osteochondral transplantation in a rabbit model. After undergoing a lateral femoral condyle osteochondral autograft, the rabbits were injected with PRP, HA, PRP+HA, or saline control. Modified ICRS scores were found to be significantly different in the PRP group compared to the saline group (18.2 + 2.7 vs. 13.5 + 3.3 p = .002). Similarly, the PRP + HA group showed significantly improved ICRS scores (17.9 + 2.6 vs. 14.0 + 3.3 p = .006). In contrast, HA alone or the addition of HA to PRP did not prove to have significant impact on the histologic scoring.[103]

Computer-assisted navigation may improve the precision of graft harvesting and implantation, as well as aiding in restoration of the native articular surface contours. In a cadaveric study, Di Benedetto et al. showed computer navigation allows for permanent visualization of the angle of recipient-site preparation, depth of the donor and recipient plug, and the angle of graft insertion at the recipient site, which allows for greater precision and reproducibility.[19] Remaining issues include further examination of cartilage thickness mismatch and its effects, which is most notably seen in OAT of patellar defects.

SUMMARY

OAT has been demonstrated to be a successful method of restoring symptomatic focal articular cartilage defects in the knee.

TABLE 30.3 Cartilage Repair Tissue Assessment: Grading and Point Scale

Variables

1. Degree of defect repair and filling of the defect
   Complete (on a level with adjacent cartilage)
   Hypertrophy (over the level of the adjacent cartilage)
   Incomplete (under the level of the adjacent cartilage; underfilling)
   >50% of the adjacent cartilage
   <50% of the adjacent cartilage
   Subchondral bone exposed (complete delamination or dislocation and/or loose body)
2. Integration to border zone
   Complete (complete integration with adjacent cartilage)
   Incomplete (incomplete integration with adjacent cartilage)
   Demarcating border visible (split-like)
   Defect visible
   <50% of the length of the repair tissue
   >50% of the length of the repair tissue
3. Surface of the repair tissue
   Surface intact (lamina splendens intact)
   Surface damaged (fibrillations, fissures, and ulcerations)
   <50% of repair tissue depth
   >50% of repair tissue depth or total degeneration
4. Structure of the repair tissue
   Homogen
   Inhomogen or cleft formation
5. Signal intensity of the repair tissue
   Dual T2-FSE
   Isointense
   Moderately hyperintense
   Markedly hyperintense
   3D-GE-FS
   Isointense
   Moderately hypointense
   Markedly hypointense
6. Subchondral lamina
   Intact
   Not intact
7. Subchondral bone
   Intact
   Edema
   Granulation tissue, cysts, sclerosis
8. Adhesions
   No
   Yes
9. Synovitis
   No synovitis
   Synovitis

FSE, Fast spin echo.
From Marlovits S, Striessnig G, Resinger CT, et al: Definition of pertinent parameters for the evaluation of articular cartilage repair tissue with high-resolution magnetic resonance imaging. *Eur J Radiol* 52(3):313, 2004.

Best results have been seen in isolated lesions of the femoral condyles, with trochlear, patellar, and tibial lesions showing less predictable success. Traditional size constraints have indicated OAT for lesions that are 50 to 250 mm^2, but individual factors such as patient age, condyle size, concomitant knee pathology (including malalignment), and patient expectations and goals may influence the decision-making process. As long-term studies reveal more regarding the durability of fibrocartilage, OAT may prove a more appropriate management strategy for symptomatic focal osteochondral defects in the younger or high-demand patient. Meticulous attention to technique is essential; careful review of the literature reveals higher failure rates when recipient site plug positioning is suboptimal. Histological evaluation of OAT resurfaced sites reveals incorporation of grafts at the subchondral level but no integration at the articular cartilage level. Although the literature favors second-look arthroscopy, advances in articular cartilage-specific MRI imaging techniques may allow for more accurate, noninvasive monitoring of structural surgical outcomes, which have also been shown to correlate with clinical outcomes.

A continued and seemingly unavoidable limitation of OAT is the availability of donor tissue. Although certain regions of the knee experience higher relative demand than others, studies have shown that no areas are free from contact. As the indications and demand for treating more complex lesions expand, donor site availability will become the rate-limiting factor. Improved strategies for filling of donor sites may limit the morbidity associated with harvest.

Hybridization methods and carrying out OAT with other procedures, such as microfracture, bone graft substitutes, scaffolds, or other biologics, may play a role in maximizing the usefulness of donor plugs. In light of several other strategies aimed at reconstituting articular cartilage defects, it remains to be seen whether the long-term benefits of restoring native hyaline cartilage outweigh donor site morbidity. However, current evidence demonstrates that with stringent indications, meticulous techniques, and comprehensive attention to donor harvest sites, OAT can result in successful outcomes in active patients with symptomatic focal articular cartilage defects of the knee.

The references for this chapter can also be found on www.expertconsult.com.

31

Osteochondral Allograft Transplantation

Michael R. Boniello, Samuel P. Robinson, Kevin F. Bonner

Articular cartilage defects present a challenging clinical problem for orthopedic surgeons. The limited healing capacity of cartilage has led to the development of various treatment options for symptomatic defects. Currently available techniques with at least midterm published outcome reports include marrow-stimulating techniques (subchondral drilling, microfracture), autologous osteochondral transfer (osteochondral autograft transfer system [OATS]; mosaicplasty), autologous chondrocyte implantation (ACI), and osteochondral allograft transplantation. Each of these techniques has potential benefits and limitations. Resulting repair tissue and clinical outcomes may be variable with some of these techniques; as a consequence, the optimal treatment of many defects is controversial. Treatment algorithms have been proposed that take into account patient and lesion factors, but thus far these algorithms have not been validated.[*]

The use of fresh osteochondral allografts has a fairly extensive clinical history, extending over three decades.[†] Allograft transplantation is currently gaining in popularity owing to increasing appreciation that it reliably restores viable hyaline cartilage when compared with alternative treatment options for larger defects.[8] Although logistic issues are inherent in obtaining allografts, including waiting for an appropriate graft, the procedure itself is not technically demanding in most cases. Fresh allografts are most useful in treating large chondral or osteochondral lesions (>2 cm²), such as those seen with osteochondritis dissecans, trauma, osteonecrosis, and selected cases of degenerative arthrosis. However, allografts may also be an optimal revision option for even smaller defects following other prior failed cartilage resurfacing procedures in younger patients in whom arthroplasty options are undesirable. With the increased appreciation that some marrow-stimulating procedures may detrimentally affect the integrity of the important underlying subchondral bone architecture, and thus may jeopardize revision cellular procedures, osteochondral grafts may play an even greater role in the future.[40,41,68]

Patients and physicians have an interest in biologic resurfacing solutions for chondral or osteochondral injury in an effort to postpone or prevent arthroplasty procedures. Because most biologic resurfacing procedures are performed in younger individuals, most resurfacing options should realistically be considered a bridging procedure to improve pain and function until the patient is a more appropriate arthroplasty candidate.

BASIC SCIENCE

The long-term success of osteochondral allografts is dependent on preservation of the hyaline cartilage surface, healing of the osseous base to the host bone, and maintenance of structural integrity during the remodeling process.[83] Investigators have shown that chondrocyte viability is paramount in maintaining the normal extracellular architecture of hyaline cartilage and in preventing the development of degenerative joint disease, but the acceptable degree of chondrocyte viability required is unknown at this time.[44,81] Although nonviable cartilage will appear grossly normal for a period of time, it will not maintain its histologic, biochemical, or biomechanical properties. As a result, the cartilage will fibrillate, develop clefts, and erode over time.[44,81]

Freezing of articular cartilage, although attractive in terms of decreasing immunogenicity and allowing storage, causes chondrocyte cell death to a variable degree with current preservation methods.[80,87] Although up to 90% of isolated chondrocytes are able to survive the freezing process, freezing of chondrocytes embedded within their matrix has not been nearly as successful.[10,72,79,80,87] This discrepancy is believed to result from poor penetration of cryopreservative, unequal rate of cooling, and high water content within the extracellular matrix.[80,87] Because cryopreservation techniques have not been shown to preserve an acceptable degree of cartilage viability, fresh allografts are considered the mainstay for allograft transplantation of articular cartilage.[27,33,77] However, whether or not the transplantation of fresh viable osteochondral grafts avoids a degenerative course superior to that of frozen grafts is a topic of ongoing controversy.[44,88] It is important to note that current "fresh" allografts are actually refrigerated (not frozen) for a time prior to implantation, in contrast to historical fresh allografts, which were transplanted much closer to the time of procurement.[53]

Immune compatibility testing and postoperative immunosuppression are not required with osteochondral allograft transplantation despite the fact that chondrocytes and subchondral bone have been shown to have immunogenic potential.[50-52,76] Chondrocytes are surrounded by a matrix that isolates them from the host immune cells and makes them relatively "immunologically privileged."[17,37] Although donor cells within the osseous component are immunogenic, their immunogenicity is muted and probably is not clinically significant in most patients because the cells are nonviable.[15,28] When an osteochondral allograft is implanted into a host bed, a local inflammatory response is stimulated by the surgical trauma and the graft itself.[84] This response is believed to peak between the second and

---

[*]References 7, 11, 25, 58, 67, and 71.
[†]References 4, 9, 15, 16, 37, and 54.

third weeks and is primarily directed against the bone constituent of the graft that contains the marrow elements and other immunogenic elements.[82] Therefore, pulse lavage of the bone just before implantation is recommended in an attempt to cleanse the graft and remove unbound antigenic blood and marrow elements. After the initial response, the inflammatory reaction may burn out or may persist for up to 18 months.[19,84]

In general, the osseous component of osteochondral allografts retains its structural integrity and is replaced with host bone via creeping substitution over a period of years depending on the size.[18,35,64,69] If the nonviable bony trabeculae cannot withstand mechanical stresses during the remodeling process, subchondral microfracture, collapse, and fragmentation may occur. Based on our understanding of the remodeling process and the stresses placed on grafts before completion of this process, it is somewhat surprising how relatively infrequently this occurs clinically. One potential benefit of minimizing the donor graft depth is a theoretical decrease in remodeling time.

Although cartilage matrix, glycosaminoglycan content, and biomechanical properties are not initially altered, percent chondrocyte viability, viable cell density, and metabolic activity have been found to progressively decrease over time following procurement.[‡] Fresh osteochondral allografts harvested within 24 hours of donor death and preserved at 4°C have been shown to maintain up to 100% chondrocyte viability at 4 days.[20,30,79] Contemporary allograft storage techniques preserve reasonably high chondrocyte viability with a significant decline in survival after 15 to 20 days.[‡] By 44 days, chondrocyte viability falls to approximately 67%.[74] Malinin et al. showed in a primate model that osteoarticular allografts transplanted after 21 days of storage underwent more severe degenerative changes than allografts that had been stored for less than 21 days.[57] Although increased cell viability is certainly optimal, acceptable chondrocyte viability appropriate for clinical implantation is controversial. This is a result of reports of successful clinical outcomes and favorable histologic biopsy analysis of grafts implanted 4 to 6 weeks following procurement.[29] Because of concerns related to infections, fresh osteoarticular allografts are currently stored hypothermically for a minimum of 14 days to allow serologic and microbiologic testing. After this time, grafts theoretically should be transplanted as soon as possible to optimize chondrocyte viability.

Research continues regarding the optimal media composition for maximal preservation of chondrocyte viability while in cold storage.[75,85] Recently, studies using proprietary media and storage techniques have shown promise, like the Missouri Osteochondral Allograft Preservation System (MOPS).[26] A study using this proprietary media showed a 90% chondrocyte viability at 60 days of preservation at room temperature, compared to the standard media's 56% viability for the same duration of storage.[38] Other studies have investigated the effects of proton supplementation, Etanercept-enriched media, and growth factor-enriched media, all endorsing an increased allograft viability with prolonged storage times.[31,55,85,95]

Long-term chondrocyte viability following osteochondral allograft transplantation has been shown in multiple biopsy and retrieval reports.[§] Researchers have biopsied transplants at various time intervals following the index procedure. Williams

et al. found 82% chondrocyte viability at 4-year follow-up with no significant immune reaction to the cartilage or the bone within the allograft.[92] Davidson et al. reported no significant detectable differences in graft versus native cartilage cell density or viability.[29] Grafts were stored for 4 to 6 weeks before transplantation and were biopsied at a mean of 40 months postoperatively. Jamali et al. confirmed that actual implanted donor chondrocytes were the source of cell viability by showing that female chondrocytes were still viable 29 years following transplantation into a male recipient.[46] This potential for long-term survival supports the use of osteochondral allografts in an attempt to maintain extracellular matrix and thus prevent long-term articular degeneration within the graft.

INDICATIONS

At this time, it is unknown why some chondral or osteochondral lesions are asymptomatic, whereas others cause significant morbidity.[90] Because we do not understand the natural history of most chondral lesions, surgery is typically indicated only for the treatment of symptomatic lesions. Debate continues regarding the treatment of asymptomatic full-thickness defects found at the time of surgery performed for other primary procedures (eg, anterior cruciate ligament reconstruction), but that discussion is beyond the scope of this chapter. The objectives of any biologic resurfacing procedure, including fresh allograft transplantation, are pain relief and functional improvement. Although our goal is the prevention of progressive joint deterioration and subsequent need for arthroplasty, most biologic resurfacing is performed in younger individuals with long life expectancies. Realistically, these biologic procedures should be considered a bridging procedure to improve pain and function until the patient is a more appropriate arthroplasty candidate.

Fresh osteochondral allografts are most useful in treating large chondral or osteochondral lesions (>2 cm), such as those seen with osteochondritis dissecans, trauma, osteonecrosis, and selected cases of degenerative arthrosis in young patients in whom arthroplasty options are undesirable. Allografts can also be used in a salvage procedure following failed cartilage resurfacing procedures. Patients with localized, unipolar, traumatic, nondegenerative, chondral lesions, osteochondritis dissecans, or osteonecrosis are believed to be optimal candidates for fresh osteochondral allografting and have obtained the best results.[8,17,37] Relatively focal nonacute chondral lesions, which tend to be degenerative in nature, may also benefit from allograft transplantation in the appropriate setting. However, results are often dependent on the status of the surrounding articular surface, and whether or not the underlying mechanical and physiologic factors that contributed to the initial chondral loss continue. Patients with associated pathology are more likely to benefit from a concomitant procedure, such as an unloading osteotomy or a meniscus transplant, in an effort to delay the progression of degeneration.

Primary treatment with an osteochondral autograft or allograft is often the optimal treatment when there is significant subchondral bone involvement of greater than 5 to 10 mm.[17,25,67] The authors tend to favor osteochondral autograft (smaller lesions) or allograft (moderate to larger lesions) for any defect with subchondral bone involvement. Fresh osteochondral allografts are well suited for these types of lesions because they can restore the subchondral plate, in addition to hyaline cartilage.

---

‡References 1, 5, 57, 70, 74, 91, and 93.
§References 34, 42, 46, 62, 65, and 92.

An absolute contraindication to an osteochondral allograft transplant is active infection. Patients who are of appropriate age and activity level for prosthetic replacement are typically not considered good candidates. Associated grade III or IV kissing lesions of the tibiofemoral or patellofemoral articulation are generally considered a relative contraindication.[8] Malalignment, ligamentous instability, and meniscal insufficiency must be addressed before or at the time of the resurfacing procedure.[37] Patients with inflammatory arthropathy, crystal-induced arthropathy, diffuse significant synovitis or are significantly immunosuppressed are also relative contraindications. The effects of altered bone metabolism that result from long-term steroid use or smoking have not been studied, although we generally consider this a contraindication.

PROCUREMENT, SCREENING, AND STORAGE

Allograft tissue should be obtained from an accredited tissue bank that adheres to the guidelines established by the American Association of Tissue Banks (AATB) and the US Food and Drug Administration (FDA).[2,89] Graft procurement should be carried out within 24 hours of death under strict aseptic conditions and processed within 72 hours per AATB guidelines.[2,4,6,39] Donors are screened for risk of disease transmission, including detailed medical and social history for risk factors of exposure to human immunodeficiency virus (HIV), hepatitis B, and hepatitis C.[3,89] The FDA previously mandated titers for HIV-1 and HIV-2 antibody, hepatitis B surface antigen, hepatitis core antibody, hepatitis C antibody, human T-lymphocyte virus 1 antibody, HIV p24 antigen, and the rapid plasma reagin test for syphilis. Beginning in 2005, all AATB-accredited tissue banks were required to perform nucleic acid testing (NAT) for HIV-1 and the hepatitis C virus to further reduce the window period associated with conventional (enzyme immunoassay [EIA] method) donor screening antibody or antigen tests.[12]

One of the issues of greatest concern surrounding the use of fresh allograft material is the risk of infectious organism transmission, including viral and bacterial disease. Current tissue bank processing and donor screening reduce the risk of disease transmission to very low levels, although the exact risk estimate is unknown for fresh osteochondral allografts.[3,12-14,86] Not all cases are detected, and surveillance systems have not been designed to define the true incidence of these infections. In 1995, based on reports in the literature, the incidence of infection was estimated to be 0.02% from approximately 20,000 organ transplants per year, and 0.0004% from approximately 900,000 allografts per year.[22] In 2007, AATB-accredited tissue banks distributed just over 1.1 million musculoskeletal allografts. Most of these were processed grafts, which went through proprietary washing and sterilization. Only approximately 2200 of the distributed grafts were classified as osteochondral allografts.[12] Heightened awareness among clinicians and improved diagnostic tests have enhanced the detection of tissue-associated infection.

The risk of bacterial transmission from contaminated fresh allograft tissue is of greater concern compared with processed nonviable grafts because cytotoxic cleansing treatments cannot be used. One case report describes a fatal bacterial infection following implantation of a fresh osteochondral allograft contaminated with *Clostridium*.[49] A subsequent investigation by the Centers for Disease Control and Prevention identified 26 potential patients with allograft-associated infection: 13 with *Clostridium* species and 14 associated with a single processing agency.[49] Malinin et al. found that 64 of 795 consecutive donors of musculoskeletal tissue (8.1%) had *Clostridium* contamination.[47,56] They also found that the risk of *Clostridium* contamination increased with the length of time between donor death and allograft harvest. In addition to a review of the medical records, cultures of tissue, donor blood, and donor blood marrow are used as screening tools to limit the risk of transmitted bacterial infection.[59,60] Episodes of allograft-associated infection in the past decade have improved awareness, enhanced our understanding of the problem, and may decrease this risk in the future.

Harvested tissues are typically stored in antimicrobial solutions at temperatures just above freezing. Screening tests (except final fungal cultures) typically are not completed for approximately 14 days from the time of procurement; thus grafts are not released until at least that time. Although debate is ongoing regarding reasonable cell viability and graft expiration to optimize graft usefulness, most tissue banks currently consider fresh, hypothermically stored osteoarticular grafts expired at a maximum of 42 days from procurement.

PREOPERATIVE PLANNING

Confirming that the patient is an appropriate candidate for a fresh allograft is important before tissue is ordered. This can often be accomplished with high-quality magnetic resonance imaging (MRI), in addition to weight-bearing radiography (Fig. 31.1A and B). When concern arises about whether a patient is a candidate for an allograft, we typically perform a diagnostic arthroscopy to evaluate the lesion of interest, as well as the remainder of the knee. If the patient had a recent arthroscopy performed elsewhere, arthroscopic pictures, operative reports, and radiographic studies are often sufficient. Long-alignment films are required if malalignment is in question to determine whether associated malalignment necessitates a concurrent unloading osteotomy.

Obtaining an acceptable donor graft from an AATB-accredited tissue bank is a key component of the procedure. Size matching from an appropriately screened donor is the main criterion for obtaining an acceptable osteochondral graft. Graft size is measured radiographically. Anteroposterior (AP) and lateral radiographs with magnification markers placed at the patient's joint can be used to calculate dimensions (Fig. 31.2A-C). Care must be taken to allow for appropriate correction of magnification error. A match is considered acceptable at ±2 mm; however, significant variability in anatomic morphology may be noted. Differences between men and women may be particularly apparent. Larger defects typically require more precise graft matches to optimize articular congruity. However, when an osteoarticular plug or dowel technique (mega-OATS) is used, a same-size or larger donor surface is often acceptable. Accepting a smaller donor for a large graft is not recommended. Wait times for an acceptable graft vary and can be lengthy and frustrating for patients. It is common to send measurements to several trusted AATB-certified tissue banks in an effort to increase the odds for procuring a compatible graft within a reasonable time frame.

SURGICAL TECHNIQUE

Before anesthesia is administered, the osteochondral allograft should be examined to confirm the adequacy of the size match

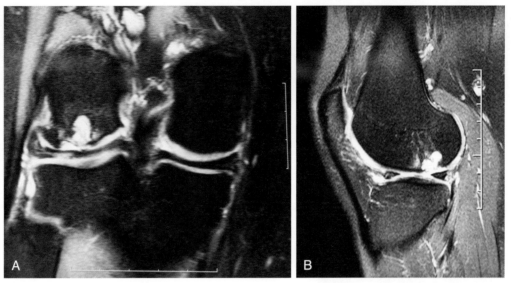

FIG 31.1 (A and B) Coronal and sagittal T2-weighted MRI shows an osteochondral lesion of the distal lateral femoral condyle.

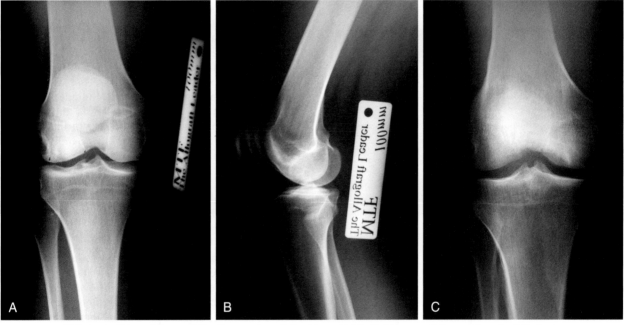

FIG 31.2 AP and Lateral Radiographs of the Knee With Evidence of Osteochondral Pathology Magnification markers are present. (A and B) AP and lateral radiographs of an osteochondral lesion of the lateral femoral condyle. (C) AP radiograph of an osteochondral lesion of the medial femoral condyle.

and the quality of the tissue (Fig. 31.3). Allograft tissue is soaked in a normal saline/antibiotic solution and is kept safe on a back table, which is set up with the allograft workstation. The patient is positioned supine on the operative table with a tourniquet on the proximal thigh. A leg holder is valuable for accessing the lesion by positioning the leg at between 70 and 100 degrees of knee flexion. Alternatively, a sandbag may be taped on the table to help keep the knee flexed to an optimal position. In most cases, we perform a diagnostic arthroscopy before making the arthrotomy, to assess the remainder of the joint and confirm that the patient is a good candidate for the procedure.

This procedure is typically performed through a medial or lateral arthrotomy. The extent of exposure varies depending on the position and magnitude of the lesion. Exposure for a typical osteochondritis dissecans lesion on the lateral side of the medial femoral condyle is more extensile in that the patella will be retracted farther laterally to allow access to the lesion. Eversion of the patella typically is not necessary unless a patellar lesion is the focus of the procedure. More central or peripheral lesions often can be treated through a more limited approach. Because high degrees of knee flexion are required to access very posterior lesions, the patella can compromise access to these areas of the

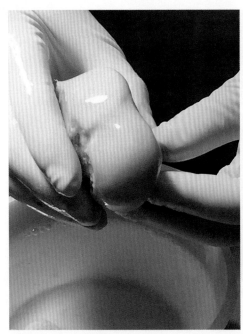

FIG 31.3 Inspection of the procured fresh allograft.

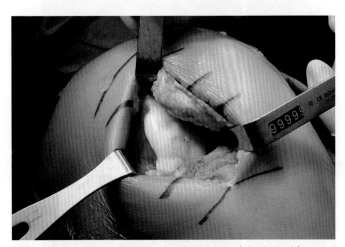

FIG 31.4 Exposure of osteochondral lesion of the lateral femoral condyle through lateral parapatellar arthrotomy.

articular surface. A more extensile proximal parapatellar, mid-vastus, or subvastus approach is often helpful in mobilizing the patella. If needed, a tibial tubercle osteotomy can be performed to enhance exposure, although this is typically not necessary.

In cases where the lesion is posterior or very large, the meniscus may need to be taken down at the meniscocapsular junction and may be repaired as part of the closure. Larger bulk allografts may require more extensive exposure. For a typical condylar lesion, retractors are placed medially and laterally, including one in the notch, to retract the patella and gain exposure to the joint (Fig. 31.4). The knee is flexed or extended until the lesion is exposed through the arthrotomy site. Once visualization is achieved, the lesion is inspected and palpated to determine its depth, size, and margins.

The two most commonly used techniques for the preparation and implantation of osteochondral allografts are the press-fit plug technique and the shell graft technique. Each technique has advantages and disadvantages. The press-fit plug technique

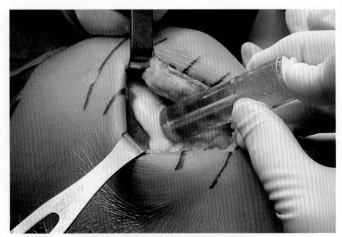

FIG 31.5 Sizing of the lesion for proposed dowel graft.

is similar in principle to OATS and is optimal for contained condylar lesions between 15 and 35 mm in diameter. This technique is certainly the most commonly used in practice. In most cases, a stable press fit is achieved, and additional fixation is not required. One disadvantage of this technique is the sacrifice of adjacent areas of normal cartilage and bone to convert the lesion into a circular recipient defect. In addition, limitations on where the circular coring system can be used have been identified; specifically, tibial, large uncontained patellar lesions, and far posterior condylar lesions are not conducive to this technique. The large plug transplant technique may also be used for contained patellar and trochlear lesions, but these areas can be technically more challenging because of the topography of the articulation. Shell grafts, on the other hand, have the advantages of minimizing normal cartilage and bone sacrifice and accommodating cartilage lesions of the tibia and patella and many trochlear lesions. Disadvantages of shell grafts include technical difficulty and less inherent graft stability, thus typically requiring the need for fixation.

Press-Fit Plug Allograft Technique

Several proprietary instrumentation systems are currently available for the preparation and implantation of press-fit plug allografts between 15 and 35 mm in diameter. Although the authors of this chapter describe only one of the instrumentation systems in the technique section, most systems are similar. The size of the proposed graft is determined by using a sizing dowel to cover as much of the defect as possible while limiting the sacrifice of normal tissue (Fig. 31.5). Sometimes a lesion is more amenable to the use of two overlapping cylindrical plugs (termed the "snowman" or "MasterCard" configuration). Once the sizing dowel is in the appropriate position, a guide wire is driven several centimeters into the center of the lesion (Fig. 31.6). It is important that the guide wire be drilled perpendicular to the curvature of the articular surface.

An appropriately sized cannulated scoring reamer is used initially over the guide pin to cut through just the articular cartilage and create a sharp circumferential edge (Fig. 31.7A). A cannulated coring drill is used to ream the subchondral bone and create the recipient site (see Fig. 31.7B and C). Debate continues regarding optimal reaming depth. Proper preparation of the lesion will result in a healthy, bleeding bone recipient site; therefore, the depth of the preparation will depend on the quality of the subchondral bone. Without bone involvement, the recipient site should be in the range of 6 to 10 mm deep, which typically translates into 3 to 8 mm of bone preparation. A trend toward reaming less and having only 3 to 6 mm of bone on the donor plug has been noted. The benefits of creating a shallower defect include less bone sacrifice, increased interface bone density, and less bone volume to incorporate and remodel over time. Potential negatives include the theoretical loss of stability from the circumferential press fit (less depth) and increased reliance on an exact depth match, which may be more technically difficult. The effects of these issues on short- and long-term outcomes are currently unknown. In cases of bone loss, reaming needs to advance slowly until a healthy recipient bone bed is achieved.

Before the guide pin is removed, debris is removed from the recipient site, and the cannulated dilator is placed into the defect. The dilator not only makes delivery of the graft easier but allows preliminary recipient site measurements. The guide pin is removed, and precise depth measurements are made in all four quadrants of the recipient site. The corresponding anatomic location of the recipient site is identified and marked with a surgical marker on the graft (Fig. 31.8), which is secured onto the commercially available workstation (Fig. 31.9). The 12 o'clock position on the future donor plug is marked to ensure

proper orientation once removed. The workstation contains a mobile coring reamer guide, which needs to be secured in such a way that the coring reamer will harvest the graft from the appropriate anatomic location (see Fig. 31.9A-C). Placing the original sizing dowel down the guide and letting it rest perpendicular on the articular cartilage will greatly assist in properly securing the mobile guide. The appropriately sized coring reamer can be used to core out the graft (Fig. 31.10). Once the graft has been removed, depth measurements from each quadrant of the recipient site are marked. A graft clamp, which serves as a cutting guide, is used to secure the articular side of the graft by lining up the depth marks with the guide edge (Fig. 31.11). The graft is cut with an oscillating saw and is trimmed with a rasp to the appropriate thickness in all four quadrants (Fig. 31.12A and B). Care must be taken to ensure that the thickness of the graft precisely matches the prepared defect. The leading edges are chamfered to facilitate graft insertion. Just before insertion, the graft is copiously irrigated with pulse lavage to remove donor marrow elements. The dilator is again inserted into the recipient site to ease the insertion of the graft and prevent excessive impact loading on the articular surface (Fig. 31.13).

The graft is inserted by hand in the appropriate orientation and is gently tamped into place until it is flush with

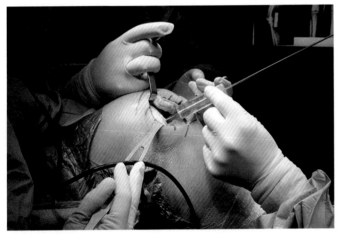

FIG 31.6 Using a commercially available sizing guide, a guide wire is placed in the center of the osteochondral lesion. The guide wire is placed perpendicular to the articular surface.

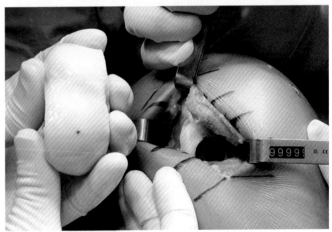

FIG 31.8 The corresponding anatomic location of the recipient site is identified on the graft.

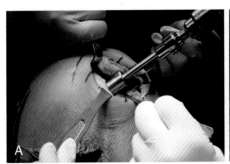 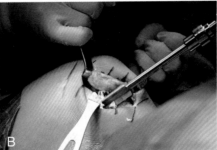 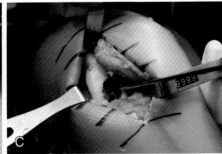

FIG 31.7 Reaming the Recipient Site Over the Guide Wire (A) Initially, a scoring reamer is used to create a sharp edge on the adjacent articular cartilage. (B) Next, the appropriately sized reamer is advanced into the subchondral bone to create the recipient site. (C) Prepared recipient site bordered by healthy, bleeding subchondral bone.

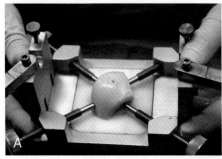
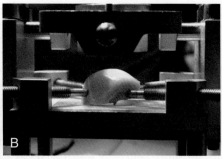
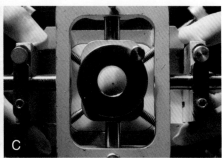

FIG 31.9 A commercially available allograft workstation is used to secure the graft (Arthrex, Naples, FL). (A) Allograft secured on workstation. (B) Mobile coring reamer guide secured overtop of allograft on workstation. (C) View from above of the mobile coring reamer guide secured overtop of allograft on workstation.

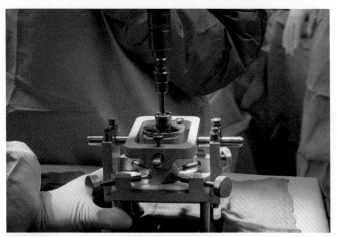

FIG 31.10 The osteochondral graft is harvested with a coring reamer.

the surrounding cartilage (Fig. 31.14A-C). Care is taken to minimize impact loading of the allograft during insertion, because this has been shown to cause chondrocyte death.[48,73] The articular congruity is matched as perfectly as possible. The graft should not be left proud in any areas relative to the recipient cartilage. Small edge mismatches can be débrided with a No. 15 blade if needed. Countersinking and surface mismatches greater than 1 mm from the surrounding joint surface are not acceptable. If the graft does not fit properly, the recipient site or the graft itself is refashioned carefully. When necessary, a threaded pin can be placed centrally to remove the graft. Once the graft is seated, the need for additional fixation is determined. Rarely in the authors' practice do press-fit dowel plugs require additional fixation. If the graft is large and uncontained, fixation may be necessary. The knee is brought through a complete range of motion to confirm that the graft is stable. The wound is copiously irrigated, and a routine closure is performed.

Shell Allograft Technique

The cartilage defect is identified through the previously described arthrotomy, and the circumference of the lesion is marked with a surgical pen. An attempt is made to create a geometric shape that will be amenable to hand crafting of the graft and minimizing the sacrifice of normal cartilage. A No. 15 blade is used to cut around the lesion, and sharp ring curettes are used to remove all tissue inside this border. With a motorized 4.0-mm burr and

sharp curettes, the defect is débrided to a depth of 4 to 5 mm. A foil template can be used to achieve a precisely sized graft. A large piece of foil from suture packs can be manually fashioned over the articular cartilage of the involved compartment. The foil is manually pressed into the defect while the foil mold of the surrounding bone is maintained. The mold of the defect is cut out of the foil and is confirmed to be a precise match with the lesion. The foil template is placed over the matched allograft and is used to outline the corresponding area on the donor graft. This demarcated cartilage is used as a guide for meticulous preparation of a shell of osteochondral allograft, with 4 to 5 mm of subchondral bone remaining.

In the authors' experience, the graft should be slightly oversized initially and bone and cartilage carefully removed as necessary to provide appropriate fitting. This takes multiple trials and an abundance of patience. If deeper bone loss is seen within the defect, more bone can be left on the graft and/or the defect can be grafted with cancellous bone before graft insertion. The graft is meticulously modified until it is flush with the articular surface (Fig. 31.15). Once the graft has been seated, graft stability can be determined. Typically, graft fixation is required.

An alternative shell graft technique, which may be technically easier than the procedure just described, uses a saw blade to make a cut similar to those made in unicompartmental or total knee arthroplasty. The depth of the resection is measured, and a graft is fashioned from the matching donor site. Sites that typically benefit from this method include the tibial plateau, patella, and trochlea. These types of shell grafts require fixation with compression screws or bioabsorbable devices.

POSTOPERATIVE MANAGEMENT

Intravenous antibiotics are discontinued after the first 24 hours postoperatively. The authors advocate the avoidance of nonsteroidal antiinflammatory drugs (NSAIDs) for the first 6 to 8 weeks to optimize bone-to-bone healing. Deep venous thrombosis (DVT) prophylaxis is controversial and variable based on patient-specific factors. The authors' preference is to typically use aspirin 325 mg PO BID for most patients. Postoperative radiographs are performed routinely after the procedure to assess graft-host integration. Postoperative MRI is not performed routinely as persistent high T2 signal abnormalities within and adjacent to the graft site are very common, and the clinical significance of such phenomena is unknown.

Postoperative rehabilitation is based on the size, location, stability, and containment of the graft, as well as concomitant

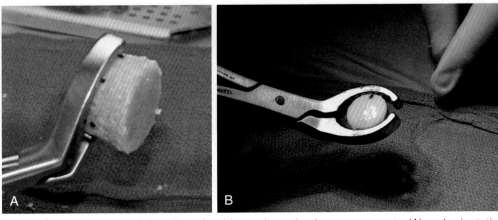

FIG 31.11 Preparation of the allograft with quadrant depth measurements (A) and orientation marks on the cartilage (B).

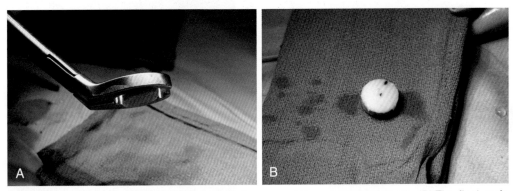

FIG 31.12 (A) The graft is cut with an oscillating saw at the appropriate depth. (B) The final graft is ready for implantation.

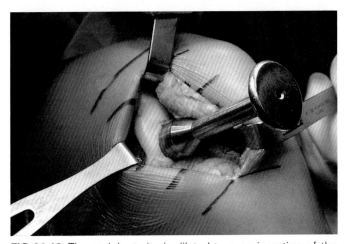

FIG 31.13 The recipient site is dilated to ease insertion of the graft and prevent excessive impact loading on the articular surface.

procedures. Early postoperative management focuses on controlling pain and swelling while working on range of motion. This includes the use of a continuous passive motion (CPM) machine, starting in the immediate postoperative period. Extended CPM use is desirable but is not required. Alternatively, a low-resistance stationary bike can be used. Patients are generally allowed full range of motion, unless prohibited by concurrent reconstructive procedures such as meniscal repair

or transplantation. Patellofemoral grafts or shell grafts with less inherent stability may require limitations in range of motion.

Weight bearing is assessed on the basis of the size and stability of the graft. Smaller and inherently more stable grafts may start toe-touch weight bearing immediately for the first 6 weeks and then may progress to weight bearing as tolerated beyond that point. When concern arises regarding the stability of a plug graft, and in essentially all cases of tibiofemoral shell grafts, we are conservative with the use of a non–weight-bearing regimen for the first 6 to 8 weeks. Isolated patellofemoral grafts can often bear weight as tolerated with a brace locked in extension. In these patients, weight bearing is progressed slowly at 6 to 8 weeks as tolerated over a 4- to 6-week period. However, high patellofemoral force activities are avoided for months if not indefinitely depending on the setting.

For most press-fit dowel grafts, braces may be used to help protect the extremity until quadriceps strength returns. When grafting involves the patellofemoral joint, braces are locked in extension for ambulation for the first 6 to 8 weeks. In patients undergoing large shell or bipolar tibial-femoral grafting, an unloader brace may be used to prevent excessive stress on the grafted surfaces.

The postoperative strengthening and rehabilitation program is dictated on the basis of graft stability, current understanding of allograft healing, symptoms, and evidence of radiographic incorporation. Typically, patients are started on a quadriceps strengthening program. At 4 weeks, patients are allowed closed-chain exercises such as cycling. Strengthening of the lower

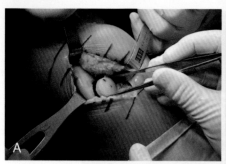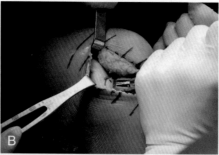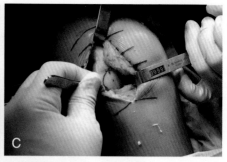

FIG 31.14 (A) The graft is inserted by hand in the appropriate rotation and (B) is gently tamped into place. (C) The osteochondral allograft in its final position (press-fit plug technique).

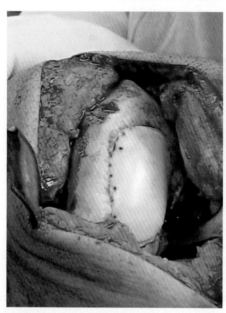

FIG 31.15 Photograph of shell allograft after implantation for a medial lesion.

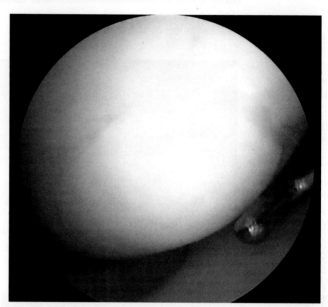

FIG 31.16 Arthroscopy photograph of fresh, refrigerated, osteochondral allograft plug of the medial femoral condyle 7 years postoperatively. The graft is well incorporated with maintenance of the hyaline cartilage.

extremity continues with a focus on hamstring and quadriceps, using an isometric program and avoidance of open-chain exercises. When it is believed that functional rehabilitation has been completed appropriately, patients are able to return to recreation and sports 4 and a half to 12 months after surgery. Patients are generally cautioned about excessive impact loading of the allograft, particularly for larger grafts.

RESULTS

Similar to other cartilage resurfacing procedures, the results of fresh or prolonged refrigerated osteoarticular allografts are variable, depending on defect location, origin of the lesion, status of the surrounding articular cartilage and meniscus, degree of bipolar disease, patient age, and alignment. In general, focal, post-traumatic, well-shouldered femoral condylar defects and osteochondritis dissecans of the medial femoral condyle tend to have the best outcomes in clinical practice and in the literature (Fig. 31.16). Certainly, other lesions can also do well in this often challenging patient population. Although the results are far from optimal, outcomes with osteoarticular grafts

compare favorably with those of other biologic resurfacing options in the treatment of larger defects. The following is a summary of work by authors who have reported from large centers with vast allograft experience.

Chahal et al. undertook a systematic review of osteochondral allograft outcomes, which included 19 studies, 644 knees in total with a mean defect size of 6.3 cm², and a mean follow-up period of 58 months.[23] The most common indications for surgery were from post-traumatic causes (38%), followed by osteochondritis dissecans (30%), osteonecrosis (12%), and idiopathic causes (11%). Sixty-five percent of patients had little to no arthritis at follow-up, and the short-term complication rate averaged 2.4% with a frank failure rate of 18%. Overall the subjective satisfaction rate among patients was 86%. Of the 19 studies included, 11 used radiographic endpoints, and at 1 year postoperatively, 86% allografts showed radiographic healing of the graft to the host bone. Survival of the medial and lateral femoral condyle allografts was shown to be between 91% and 95% at 5 years and between 74% and 76% at 15 years. Tibial plateau allografts revealed the poorest survival outcomes, showing 95% survival at

5 years, but only 46% at 20 years. Definition of "failure" varied among the studies, ranging from fragmentation to reoperation to total knee arthroplasty. There were only two reported cases of deep infection in this group. As expected, success was higher in unipolar grafts versus bipolar grafts. Emmerson et al. reported a series of individuals with osteochondritis dissecans of the femoral condyle treated with fresh osteochondral allografts.[32] This series included 66 knees in 64 patients with average follow-up of 7.7 years (range, 2 to 22 years). In this series, the size of the lesions varied, and the average size was 7.5 cm[2]. Of 65 knees available for follow-up, 47 (72%) were rated good or excellent; 7 (11%) were rated fair; and 1 (2%) was rated poor. Ten patients (15%) underwent reoperation. The average clinical score improved from 13.0 preoperatively to 16.4 postoperatively on the Merle d'Aubigné-Postel (18-point scale) ($p < .01$). Subjective knee function improved from a mean of 3.4 to 8.4 on a 10-point scale ($p < .01$).

Chu et al. reported on 55 consecutive knees undergoing osteochondral allografting.[24] This study evaluated patients with a variety of diagnoses, including traumatic chondral injury, avascular necrosis, osteochondritis dissecans, and patellofemoral disease. Of 55 procedures, 43 were unipolar replacements, and 12 were bipolar resurfacing replacements. Among these knees, 42 of 55 (76%) were rated good to excellent, and 3 of 55 (5%) were rated fair. It is important to note that 84% of knees that underwent unipolar femoral grafting were rated good to excellent, and only 50% of knees with bipolar grafts achieved good or excellent status. No realignment osteotomies were reported in this series. Many patients who underwent unipolar replacement were allowed to return to recreational and competitive sports. McDermott et al. reported on fresh osteochondral allografts implanted within 24 hours of harvest.[64] In this study, patients with a unifocal traumatic defect of the tibial plateau or femoral condyle had a 75% success rate after an average follow-up of 3.8 years. Patients with osteoarthritis and osteonecrosis fared worse, with failure rates of 58% and 79%, respectively.

Ghazavi et al. reported on 126 knees in 123 patients with post-traumatic lesions of the distal femur at an average follow-up of 7.5 years.[39] Eighty-five percent of patients were rated as successful, whereas the remaining procedures failed. Factors related to failure included age over 50 years, bipolar defects, malalignment, and workers' compensation cases. Aubin et al. later reported on the long-term results of these same allografts.[4] Kaplan-Meier survivorship analysis showed 85% graft survival at 10 years and 74% survival at 15 years. Patients with surviving grafts had Hospital for Special Surgery (HSS) scores of 83 points at 10-year follow-up. Radiographic analysis revealed that 52% of knees had moderate to severe arthritis at latest follow-up.

Garrett reported on his experience with the use of fresh osteochondral allografts with press-fit and large shell techniques in the treatment of osteochondritis dissecans.[36,37] Six patients had undergone concomitant correctional osteotomy for angular malalignment of 5 degrees or greater. Patients were counseled to refrain from running and jumping sports postoperatively. Of 113 patients with follow-up ranging from 1 to 18 years, 103 (91%) reported that they were free of pain, stiffness, and swelling.[36] All 10 failures resulted from fragmentation of the graft. McCulloch et al. found 84% patient satisfaction in 25 consecutive patients who had undergone fresh, refrigerated, osteochondral allografting for the treatment of localized osteochondral defects of the femur. At an average of 3 years of follow-up, 79% of knees were functioning at the same level as unaffected knees.[63] Radiographically, 88% of the grafts had incorporated with the host bone surrounding the defect. Average International Knee Documentation Committee (IKDC) scores in this population improved from 29 preoperatively to 58 at follow-up. Williams et al. reported on 19 patients with an average age of 34 years who were treated with fresh stored allografts implanted an average of 30 days following procurement (range, 17 to 42 days).[94] Mean lesion size was 602 mm[2], and average follow-up was 48 months. MRI was used to assess the grafts at an average of 25 months following implantation. Activities of daily living scale score increased from a baseline of 56 to 70 at the time of final follow-up. The mean Short Form-36 score increased from a baseline of 51 to 66 at the time of final follow-up. Normal articular cartilage thickness was preserved in 18 implanted grafts. Allograft cartilage signal properties were isointense relative to normal articular cartilage in 8 of the 18 grafts. Osseous trabecular incorporation of the allograft was complete or partial in 14 patients and poor in 4 patients. Complete or partial trabecular incorporation positively correlated with Short Form-36 scores at the time of follow-up.

LaPrade et al. studied 23 consecutive patients who underwent osteoarticular grafting of focal articular cartilage defects of the femoral condyle using refrigerated grafts that were implanted an average of 20.3 days (range, 15 to 28 days) following procurement.[53] At an average follow-up of 3 years, investigators found an increase in mean IKDC score from 52 points to 68.5 points with good osseous incorporation into host bone. No graft failures were noted in this group. Davidson et al. reported on 67 patients treated with massive osteoarticular allografts of the distal femur.[29] Grafts were stored in a cell culture medium at 4°C for 4 to 6 weeks before transplantation. Mean IKDC scores improved from 27 preoperatively to 79 postoperatively ($p = .002$). Ten knees underwent second-look arthroscopic evaluation and biopsy at a mean of 40 months (range, 23 to 60 months) after implantation. Mean graft and native cartilage cellular density and viability were not statistically different. Jamali et al. described the outcomes of 20 knees in 18 patients who were treated with fresh osteochondral allografting of the patellofemoral joint.[45] Bipolar grafting of the trochlea and the patella was performed in 12 patients, and isolated patellar lesions were treated in 8 patients. Five failures occurred, but the remaining knees showed improvement from 11.7 to 16.3 on an 18-point scale after surgery. Radiographically, four patients had no evidence of patellofemoral arthritis, and six patients had only mild arthrosis.

Gracitelli et al. compared the outcomes of primary versus secondary allograft transplantation, the latter being defined as allograft transplantation in the setting of a failure of a primary procedure such as marrow stimulation.[41] The scores on the 18-point scale increased 3.9 points from 12.7 to 16.6 in the primary transplantation group, and 3.2 points from 12.9 to 16.2 points for the secondary transplantation group ($p = .46$). The IKDC pain score decreased from 6.2 to 2.4 in the primary group, compared to the secondary group, which had a decrease from 5.4 to 2.6. The primary transplantation group overall had fewer reoperations (11/46) compared to the secondary transplantation reoperation rate (20/46), $p = .04$. The primary transplantation group had a lower satisfaction rate of 87% compared to the secondary transplantation satisfaction rate of 97%. The graft failure rate was 11% in the primary transplantation group, and

15% in the secondary transplantation group ($p = .53$). Both groups had equivalent survivorship rates (87.4% and 86% for primary and secondary, respectively).

Meric et al. reported the survivorship of 48 bipolar osteochondral allografts to be 64.1% at 5 years.[66] Twenty-two of these knees failed, requiring revision surgery or total knee replacement. Of the remaining 26 knees, the mean IKDC pain score improved from 7.5 to 4.7 ($p = .021$), and the mean IKDC function score improved from 3.4 to 7.0 ($p = .001$). The 18-point score improved from 12.1 to 16.1 ($p \leq .001$), with 88% of the patients scoring 15 or better, and the Knee Society Function (KS-F) score improved on average from 70.5 to 84.1 ($p = .071$).

In a retrospective study, Raz et al. described the outcomes for unipolar allografting performed for posttraumatic osteochondral defects and osteochondritis dissecans with a defect size larger than 3 cm in diameter and 1 cm in depth.[78] Survivorship of these grafts was 91% at 10 years, 84% at 15 years, 69% at 20 years, and 59% at 25 years. Thirteen of the 58 knees required revision, 3 underwent graft removal, 9 were converted to TKA, and 1 required multiple débridements, eventually requiring an above-knee amputation. Grafts surviving at 15 years had a score of 86 on the HSS scale ($p = .004$).

COMPLICATIONS

The most common complications after any knee arthrotomy include quadriceps inhibition, DVT, arthrofibrosis, synovitis, persistent knee pain, and superficial or deep surgical wound infection. Allograft-related complications include graft-related infection transmission, delayed graft union or nonunion, graft fragmentation and collapse, graft subsidence, and inflammatory-mediated pain. When present, most of these complications are treated in keeping with general practice guidelines. Some complications that are specific to allograft transplantation warrant specific discussion.

Local infection following the implantation of a fresh osteochondral allograft is rare, but its consequences can be devastating. It is critical to differentiate deep infection from superficial infection with the use of physical examination findings and joint aspiration. Although deep infection following allograft implantation is more likely related to the surgical procedure than to graft transmission, management of the infection, once recognized, is the same.[22] Deep infections involving the allograft need to be addressed immediately and aggressively. Death in the immediate postoperative period has resulted from implantation of a contaminated fresh osteochondral graft.[21] The authors recommend removal of the allograft in the setting of a deep infection because the tissue may be the source of infection, or the donor bone may serve as a nidus for a deep surgical infection. Patients considering fresh osteochondral allograft transplant need to be informed preoperatively of the infection risk and counseled to look for signs of infection before the time of discharge from the hospital.

Although delayed union and nonunion are always possible, problems with donor-host bone healing are actually rare. This complication is more common in larger bulk allografts or in the setting of compromised bone at the recipient site. Complete healing occasionally may take a more extended period of time and may alter the postoperative activity level. MRI or computed tomography (CT) may assist in diagnosis in the setting of clinical suspicion, but these are not necessarily performed as part of routine follow-up after surgery.[94]

Graft fragmentation or collapse is a complication that may occur months to years after surgery.[36] Fragmentation and collapse of nonvascularized allograft bone is a much more common cause of graft failure than problems with the cartilage component of the allograft. In fact, cartilage-related complications of the allograft are rare in short- to medium-term follow-up. Patients with graft fragmentation or collapse typically present with new-onset pain or mechanical symptoms. Radiographs may show graft fragmentation or collapse, joint space narrowing, cyst formation, or mixed sclerotic regions. MRI typically shows areas of graft collapse and edema. However, care must be taken in interpreting postoperative allograft MRI images because even asymptomatic, well-functioning osteochondral allografts may demonstrate significant signal abnormalities.

Allograft subsidence can be a unique problem after this procedure. According to some reports, many grafts subside by 1 to 3 mm, but up to 30% may subside up to 4 to 5 mm.[61] Other authors have not regarded subsidence as a significant problem.[94] As long as frank collapse does not occur, most of these patients are relatively asymptomatic and can be observed.[61] Whether from subsidence, fragmentation, or collapse, individual patient and specific graft considerations must be taken into account when treatment options for a failed osteochondral allograft are evaluated. In some cases, it is not unreasonable to expect a successful result from repeat fresh allograft transplantation. When degenerative arthritic changes prohibit revision allograft transplant, and when symptoms warrant intervention, unicompartmental or total knee arthroplasty is often the best salvage option.

Persistent pain following graft implantation may be multifactorial; therefore, it may be difficult to elucidate the specific cause. Clearly, failure because of progressive chondrosis and pain is a common end point for many patients with chondral lesions. This may occur with or without osteochondral grafting. Although not considered a direct complication of surgery in most cases, it is the most common cause of persistent pain and a poor outcome. Some patients with pain beyond what is considered "normal" have a low-grade inflammatory reaction related to the transplanted graft. An immune response to fresh osteochondral allografts has been observed in some individuals, as shown by the development of anti–human leukocyte antigen (HLA) antibodies.[82] It has recently been shown that there is an increase in immunogenic reactions as graft sizes increase, and the data suggested that there is a possibility of worse clinical outcomes with this increased immunogenicity, however more investigation is warranted.[43] Histologic evaluation of failed fresh allografts has not revealed evidence of immune-mediated rejection.[69] Although immunosuppression is not required, a subset of patients may produce a more significant inflammatory reaction, which may be an underlying cause of low-grade discomfort and pain. At this time, however, this hypothesis is without scientific evidence, and additional study is required.

CONCLUSIONS AND RECOMMENDATIONS

Cartilage and osteochondral injuries in young active individuals who are not candidates for arthroplasty procedures present a challenge to orthopedic surgeons. Symptomatic smaller lesions can often be treated successfully with alternative approaches such as débridement, microfracture, or autograft transfer procedures. However, when clinical failure occurs in this setting, revision with a fresh allograft can often lead to a successful outcome. These authors have found this to be especially true following marrow-stimulating techniques in high-activity individuals. Larger chondral or osteochondral defects (>2 cm^2) often benefit from osteochondral allograft transplantation as the primary treatment. Although ACI may also be a reasonable option in some patients, these authors have found fresh allografts to yield more reliable results on the femoral condyle and tibia, and as a result, currently consider the use of ACI only for the patellofemoral compartment.

Significant advantages and disadvantages are associated with the use of allograft tissue. Advantages when compared with alternative treatment options include lack of donor site morbidity, the ability to treat large defects including associated subchondral bone deficiency or pathology, and the ability to reliably restore viable hyaline cartilage. Disadvantages include supply issues and costs and the logistics of delivering an aseptic, size-matched graft with a high percentage of viable chondrocytes. Many clinical and basic scientific studies support the theoretical foundation and efficacy of osteochondral allograft transplantation. The surgical technique for most femoral condyle lesions is fairly straightforward with large dowel instrumentation systems. Other techniques are more demanding but can still be used with success. Enhanced understanding and advances in graft procurement and storage, refinement of indications, and progress made in surgical techniques should continue to improve clinical outcomes in this challenging patient population.

KEY REFERENCES

4. Aubin PP, Cheah HK, Davis AM, et al: Long-term follow up of fresh femoral osteochondral allografts for posttraumatic knee defects. *Clin Orthop* 391(Suppl):S318–S327, 2001.

17. Bugbee WD: Fresh osteochondral allografting. *Oper Tech Sports Med* 8:58–162, 2000.

24. Chu CR, Convery FR, Akeson WH, et al: Articular cartilage transplantation—clinical results in the knee. *Clin Orthop* 360:159–168, 1999.

25. Cole BJ, Farr J: Putting it all together. *Oper Tech Orthop* 11:151–154, 2001.

29. Davidson PA, Rivenburgh DW, Dawson PE, et al: Clinical, histologic, and radiographic outcomes of distal femoral resurfacing with hypothermically stored osteoarticular allografts. *Am J Sports Med* 35:1082–1090, 2007.

37. Garrett J, Wyman J: The operative technique of fresh osteochondral allografting of the knee. *Oper Tech Orthop* 11:132–137, 2001.

42. Gross AE, Kim W, Las Heras F, et al: Fresh osteochondral allografts for posttraumatic knee defects: long-term followup. *Clin Orthop* 466:1863–1870, 2008.

45. Jamali AA, Emmerson BC, Chung C, et al: Fresh osteochondral allografts: results in the patellofemoral joint. *Clin Orthop* 437:176–185, 2005.

53. LaPrade RF, Botker J, Herzog M, et al: Refrigerated osteoarticular allografts to treat articular cartilage defects of the femoral condyles: a prospective outcomes study. *J Bone Joint Surg Am* 91:805–811, 2009.

57. Malinin T, Temple HT, Buck BE: Transplantation of osteochondral allografts after cold storage. *J Bone Joint Surg Am* 88:762–770, 2006.

63. McCulloch PC, Kang RW, Sobhy MH, et al: Prospective evaluation of prolonged fresh osteochondral allograft transplantation of the femoral condyle: minimum 2-year follow-up. *Am J Sports Med* 35:411–420, 2007.

64. McDermott AG, Langer F, Pritzker PH, et al: Fresh small-fragment osteochondral allografts: long term follow-up study on first one hundred cases. *Clin Orthop* 197:96–102, 1985.

74. Pearsall AW, 4th, Tucker JA, Hester RB, et al: Chondrocyte viability in refrigerated osteochondral allografts used for transplantation within the knee. *Am J Sports Med* 32:125–131, 2004.

92. Williams SK, Amiel D, Ball ST, et al: Analysis of cartilage tissue on a cellular level in fresh osteochondral allograft retrievals. *Am J Sports Med* 35:2022–2032, 2007.

94. Williams RJ, 3rd, Ranawat AS, Potter HG, et al: Fresh stored allografts for the treatment of osteochondral defects of the knee. *J Bone Joint Surg Am* 89:718–726, 2007.

The references for this chapter can also be found on www.expertconsult.com.

32

Articular Cartilage Repair With Bioscaffolds

Brian Chilelli, Jack Farr, Andreas H. Gomoll

The presumed ultimate goal of articular cartilage restoration is to recreate normal hyaline cartilage at the site of a cartilage defect. Currently, this has only been achieved through osteochondral transfer, noting that limitations of autograft and allograft implants preclude widespread use. Although hyaline-like tissue properties may be demonstrated using cell therapy alone, the tissue lacks the natural stratification of normal hyaline cartilage. As with most bodily tissues, the natural structure serves a distinct purpose: efficiency of resources and energy, function (low coefficient of friction, dispersal of loads to underlying bone both spatially and temporally), and durability. If the goal is to restore these articular cartilage characteristics, all aspects of normal hyaline cartilage must be addressed: basilar integration with bone and calcified cartilage, marginal integration, filling of the defect level to the surrounding normal cartilage walls, and natural stratification duplicating the variability of the morphology and density of chondrocytes, as well as the regional differences in the extracellular matrix (ECM). To achieve these goals, one approach is to use a scaffold to influence the cells. There are many variations on this theme, ranging from the most basic scaffold, the fibrin clot that occurs with any marrow stimulation procedure, to three-dimensional multiphasic (osteochondral promoting) scaffolds, with chondrocytes seeded and cultured in a stratified manner.[7,24,37,57]

Scaffolds used in cartilage defect repair techniques are often categorized by their structure (eg, monophasic, biphasic, multiphasic) and whether they are with or without cells. As an alternative terminology, the term *scaffolds without cells* may replace the term *cell-free scaffolds*. The basis for this is to highlight that although the scaffolds are cell-free at the time of implantation, they are thought to function by providing a structural guidance for endogenous pluripotential cells. Therefore, these techniques may be better categorized as scaffolds populated with migrated host cells or scaffolds populated with exogenous cells; these exogenous cells may range from acutely harvested minced autograft cartilage, stored particulated allograft, or cultured chondrocytes seeded at surgery or grown on the scaffold. Part I of this chapter is a review of the basic scientific aspects of the scaffolds used to restore articular cartilage—that is, in theory, what is the best scaffold? Part II outlines the currently available scaffolds, those in clinical use and those in preclinical development.

PART I: SCIENTIFIC BASIS FOR DESIGN CONSIDERATIONS OF BIOSCAFFOLDS

Cartilage, like most other tissues, is composed of two components: the ECM, made up of various macromolecules and water, and the cells contained within the ECM, which produce and maintain the former. Cartilage repair requires restoration of both components to produce a tissue that is biomechanically and biochemically able to withstand the demands of repetitive joint loading without early degeneration and failure. In addition, as an organ, the joint is composed of and depends on the integration and interplay of various building block materials. Without transgressing into a discussion of the interaction of the menisci, ligaments, capsule, synovium, and cartilage, it is necessary to couple cartilage with the underlying bone. Without complete basilar integration through the calcified cartilage layer, a supposedly perfect cartilage construct will fail through delamination. Classic cell-based approaches, such as microfracture (marrow stimulation) and autologous chondrocyte implantation (ACI), rely on a cellular component to produce ECM, thus filling the lesion and achieving basilar and marginal integration. These procedures require activity restrictions to protect the immature tissue and are associated with long recovery times and complex postoperative rehabilitation, mainly because of the slow production and maturation of the ECM component by the cells. Many current and future approaches have the objective of modifying the classic cell-based techniques through the addition of bioscaffolds, with the goal of simplifying the surgical technique, decreasing postoperative restrictions on the patient, expediting recovery and return to full activity, and improving outcomes.

Scaffold Requirements

Scaffold function can generally be divided into two roles: cell delivery and structural support for cell migration or stratification with composite maturation. The former uses the scaffold as a carrier substrate to help deliver cells into the defect and maintain them in situ until the new cartilage construct can achieve marginal and basilar integration. Theoretically, after the scaffold has fulfilled its purpose, it could be removed or, more realistically, resorb on its own. This function is comparatively simple, with the demands in terms of mechanical properties being minimal, and therefore a number of materials have been found to be suitable for this, including the fibrin clot from microfracture, fibrin glue, alginate or agarose, collagen, hyaluronic acid (HA), and artificial polymers, such a polylactic acid (PLA) and polyglycolic acid (PGA) and their modifications.[55]

The second role, to act as a support structure during cell and ECM maturation, is far more complex and may require more advanced engineering to produce a scaffold that optimizes the physical and biochemical structure of the ECM while providing adequate porosity to allow cell invasion and growth (Table 32.1).[35] The ideal scaffold should allow early or even immediate

TABLE 32.1 Desirable Attributes for Bioscaffolds Used in Cartilage Repair

Structure and Chemistry	Mechanical Properties, Strength, and Integrity	Clinical Application
Biocompatible synthetic vs. naturally derived	Mechanical properties comparable to hyaline cartilage	Preformed intraoperatively vs. custom shape or contour vs. injectable
Porosity-permeability—optimal porosity with three-dimensional architecture	High porosity (does not apply to gel-type scaffolds)	Ease of intraoperative handling and fixation
Optimized geometry to regenerate native matrix (ECM) orientation	Composite structure with varying properties throughout its thickness	Delivery attributes—arthroscopic (air or liquid) vs. miniopen vs. formal open
Resorption without local or systemic adverse effect vs. benign particulate breakdown scavenging	Biocompatible	Chondral vs. osteochondral defects
Resorption temporal profile follows new cartilage deposition	No toxic degradation products	Reproducibility
Surface chemistry (protein absorption-deposition, enabling cell adhesion, migration, and outgrowth)	Assists in cell and tissue differentiation; resorbable	Regulatory approval pathway and final indications cost, value

ECM, Extracellular matrix.

weight bearing; thus, it would require mechanical properties strong enough to protect the cells while at the same time not being so stiff as to completely shield the cells from all stresses, which are important signals for tissue maturation. The scaffold should provide secure fixation and enhance basilar integration with the subchondral bone and circumferential integration with the surrounding cartilage. To allow cell growth, the scaffold must consist of a system of interconnected pores; the material should be hydrophilic to ease cell seeding, penetration, and adhesion. Furthermore, certain modifications can improve cell adhesion to a scaffold, such as the binding of adhesion ligands to the scaffold material. It should slowly resorb with time, at a pace that allows gradual replacement through host tissue, and this process should not generate degradation products that are toxic or inflammatory.

Basic Science

The following section will review basic aspects and concepts, including the physical and biologic characteristics of bioscaffolds for cartilage repair. More specific information on individual membranes currently in clinical practice or under development will be provided in the second part of this chapter.

Physical Characteristics

Mechanical strength. Mechanical characteristics of hyaline cartilage vary with the joint in question, as well as the specific location within the respective joint. A bioscaffold allowing early or even immediate weight bearing is desirable and should closely mirror the mechanical properties of hyaline cartilage until it has been replaced by mature repair tissue. The scaffold functions to protect the growing tissue while ensuring an appropriate level of physiologic loading to enhance the reparative process,[65] an effect first described by Pauwels,[68] who recognized the influence of physical stimuli on cell differentiation pathways of mesenchymal stem cells.

Elasticity (Young's modulus) of human hyaline cartilage has been reported as between 1 and 20 MPa, depending on the layer and location, several orders of magnitude lower than that of immature (1000 MPa) or cortical (17,000 MPa) bone.[43] It appears from computer modeling that an inhomogeneous three-dimensional scaffold with higher stiffness in the superficial layer, which gradually decreases toward the base of the defect, might be best suited to encourage cartilage, rather than fibrous tissue, regeneration. This theory has been substantiated by findings of

a tensile modulus 6 to 20 times higher in the superficial regions than in the deeper regions, whereas permeability demonstrated a reverse distribution, increasing with increasing depth. The higher stiffness at the surface better protects the immature tissue from the high shear forces experienced at this level, and the lower stiffness at the base allows sufficient strain rates to encourage chondrogenic differentiation.

Structure. Studies have investigated effects of the overall three-dimensional structure of scaffolds on cells and tissue production. Although chondrocytes attach and grow even on flat nonphysiologic surfaces (two-dimensional growth, such as in a Petri dish), they gradually dedifferentiate into a more fibroblastic phenotype with increased type I collagen production. Conversely, chondrocytes maintain their spherical appearance when grown in three-dimensional culture, such as open-pored scaffolds or alginate beads, and matrix production is improved quantitatively and qualitatively with increased type II collagen.[57] Cartilage ECM consists of a mesh of collagen fibers 10 to 140 nm in diameter,[75] and studies have demonstrated improved cell adherence to fibers of submicron size.[94] Many studies have therefore investigated the use of spun or woven nanofibers of various materials for use in bioscaffolds.[34]

A system of interconnected open pores facilitates cell seeding of bioscaffolds to produce a three-dimensional structure. The normal pore area of hyaline cartilage has been reported as 5 to 33 nm,[74] but this is not directly comparable to the requirements of a bioscaffold. The former reflects the size of a lacuna, but pores in a bioscaffold need to be large enough to allow cell seeding, penetration, and proliferation, followed by production of ECM. However, increased pore size beyond a threshold value has been demonstrated to decrease attachment for a variety of cells, whereas increased specific surface area (a measure of overall porosity) was found to have a positive effect.[63] In general terms, a material porosity of 80% to 90% has been found to be beneficial in terms of quantity and quality of regenerated tissue.[36] In addition to pore size, which allows cell migration, the nanostructure of the material must allow cell adherence during migration.

Biologic Characteristics

Biocompatibility. More commonly an issue with synthetic bioscaffolds, biocompatibility refers to tissue reactivity toward the implanted material. Biocompatibility can be improved by surface modification of the material to improve cell adhesion;

for example, the wettability of hydrophobic polymers, such as the polyesters PGA and PLA, can be improved by gas plasma treatment to polymerize specific monomers to the scaffold surface.[66] Biomolecules can also be attached, such as arginine-glycine-aspartic acid (RGD), and interact with integrin receptors to anchor the cell cytoskeleton to the ECM.[82] However, even within the group of biologic scaffold materials, such as collagen and HA, subtle variations exist that influence cell adhesion. In a review of several collagen membranes, type II collagen appeared to be better suited to enhance cell attachment than type I collagen membranes.[29,45]

Degradation. Generally a concern with artificial scaffold materials, degradation products seen during absorption can lead to foreign body reactions and inflammatory responses. For example, both PGA and PLA degradation through hydrolytic cleavage of ester bonds can result in acidic by-products[91] that have been implicated in foreign body and other inflammatory reactions. Buffer substances can be added to influence the rate of resorption as well as the acidity of degradation products.

Bioactivity. Ideally, a bioscaffold will not only provide mechanical support but guide the cells contained within to produce a better repair tissue. Attaching growth factors to the scaffold material has been investigated by several authors, who reported a shift to a more hyaline-like appearance of regenerated cartilage after the addition of various factors, including the bone morphogenic protein (BMP), insulin-like growth factor (IGF), and transforming growth factor (TGF) families.[3]

Summary of Desired Scaffold Attributes. An ideal bioscaffold should provide a mechanically stable environment for cells, either delivered with the membrane or absorbed from the local environment—for example, after microfracture. The scaffold should be strong enough to allow early weight bearing while conducting sufficient stress to the cells to encourage differentiation and production of a hyaline cartilage–like ECM. The scaffold should resorb over time without residual degradation products, and the resorption time should be timed to coincide with tissue maturation. Bioactive substances such as ligand factors to improve cell attachment, and growth factors that aid in cell differentiation, may be bound to the scaffold material to produce a better or more rapid repair tissue. At this time, various types of bioscaffolds are being actively explored, but no approach has been demonstrated to be clearly superior to others, and significant changes will evolve as these are brought into clinical practice.

PART II: SCAFFOLDS IN DEVELOPMENT

Part I of this chapter established the scientific basis for the use of scaffolds in the repair of articular cartilage defects of the knee. However, at the time of this writing, none are clinically available in the United States. Although the list of desirable attributes for an articular cartilage repair scaffold represents realistic goals, attempting to achieve all the attributes in one scaffold remains elusive.[87] As with all aspects of medicine, if there was a true best method or best scaffold, then all physicians would adopt that single technique. However, in this relatively new field, the reality is that many approaches remain under evaluation[11] because none has provided the stated end goal—to produce a truly stratified hyaline cartilage, with full basilar and marginal integration implanted, using a minimally invasive technique with minimal inconvenience to the patient and cost

to society. Nevertheless, from the viewpoint of demand matching, the laudable but possibly unobtainable stated goal may not be necessary for many knee lesions. Consider that many first-generation cartilage repair techniques appear to work satisfactorily in up to 70% of patients. Therefore, the goal may need to be restated using a patient function and pain perspective, and not a histologic perspective. That is, the cartilage repair goal may be the most cost-effective and acceptably durable treatment for a specific patient and specific cartilage lesion, rather than a fully integrated hyaline cartilage. This on-the-ground clinical approach should not deter basic science research, but illustrates the difference between preclinical results and clinical applications. It is important to keep both the patient and the patient's knee in mind while exploring the newer scaffold cartilage repair options.[60]

The first clinical application of a scaffold for knee cartilage repair was reported in 1999 by Behrens.[6] The two-stage technique was an extension of the original ACI. After an autologous biopsy was cultured, the chondrocytes were seeded onto a porcine collagen I-III scaffold (Chondro-Gide, Geistlich Biomaterials, Wolhusen, Switzerland) and allowed to grow on the scaffold before implantation. It was termed *matrix-associated autologous chondrocyte implantation* (MACI; Vericel, Cambridge, Massachusetts). Shortly after the first application of MACI, Hyalograft C (Anika Therapeutics, Bedford, Massachusetts) was introduced in 1999. The product was first developed by Fidia Advanced Biopolymers Laboratories (Padova, Italy) and was an esterified derivative of HA, known as Hyaff-11.[59] Like the two-stage MACI, the autologous cartilage was harvested from the patient, followed by expansion and seeding onto the scaffold, where they are allowed to grow. Both of these three-dimensional scaffolds have been shown to improve the maintenance of a chondrocyte-differentiated phenotype when compared with two-dimensional culturing. These initial biodegradable polymers have been joined by several other seeded, cultured scaffold applications. In addition, these scaffolds allowed arthroscopic implantation in certain regions of the knee, typically the femoral condyles and trochlea, which was not possible with first-generation ACI. Because this is a rapidly changing field, our goal here is to show current scaffold applications in a general sense, with the understanding that the initiated reader will review current literature and conference presentations before making any clinical decisions. In addition, it is necessary for the reader to fully understand the regulatory process in his or her respective country, because allowed clinical use may vary over time.

As an overview, it is important to re-emphasize that not all cutting-edge cartilage techniques use scaffolds. Understanding the importance of marrow stimulation, osteochondral autograft, and allograft as stand-alone techniques, the subset of cell therapies may be classified as follows: (1) cells alone, (2) scaffolds without cells at time of implantation (host cell source), (3) scaffolds with seeded cells, and (4) scaffolds with seeded and cultured cells. This section will focus only on those applications using scaffolds.

Scaffolds Without Cells at Time of Implantation (Host Cell Source)

Autologous Matrix-Induced Chondrogenesis. Autologous matrix-induced chondrogenesis (AMIC) is a porcine collagen I-III matrix (Chondro-Gide) that is applied over the defect immediately following microfracture. This scaffold is thicker than the original one used in MACI, to allow potential filling of a full bottom to top defect. The goal is to provide a matrix that allows host cells to migrate into the scaffold and have an environment that improves the chondrogenesis from that of marrow stimulation alone.[28,39]

Matrix-Modulated Marrow Stimulation. This system uses BST-CarGel (Piramal, Mumbai, India), which is a mixture of chitosan (structural component of crustacean shells) liquid and autologous blood (1:3 ratio) to form a viscous material (in situ polymerized hydrogel) implanted into marrow stimulation prepared defects (microfracture or drilling).[33,54] It has intrinsic cytocompatibility and is completely biodegradable. The construct allows both reinforcement of the clot and impedance of clot retraction.[10] The cationic charge of the chitosan increases the adhesiveness of the mixture to cartilage lesions, potentially allowing longer clot residency. This maintenance of critical blood components above the marrow access holes common to these subgroups of scaffolds may allow a more optimal tissue repair process, noting that in this case, the chitosan has some intrinsic ability to stimulate wound repair.[77] In a level I randomized control trial, Stanish et al. compared BST-CarGel to microfracture for symptomatic focal lesions of the femoral condyles.[83] Their results revealed similar clinical benefits and safety at 12 months but greater lesion filling and superior repair tissue quality in the BST-CarGel group. More recently, all-arthroscopic techniques have been described utilizing microfracture in combination with BST-CarGel.[86]

Matrix-Modulated Marrow Stimulation

GelrinC. GelrinC (Regentis Biomaterials, Or-Akiva, Israel) is an in situ biodegradable photopolymerized hydrogel made from polyethylene glycol diacrylate (PEG-DA) covalently conjugated to a structural backbone of separated, denatured, disulfide-reduced fibrinogen chains. The scaffold (Fig. 32.1) is for use in conjunction with marrow stimulation techniques for the local repair of damaged cartilage and bone. It fills discontinuities across a focal cartilage defect and may include bone. The degradation of this implant is controlled and mediated by protease activity on the fibrinogen moieties and by hydrolysis

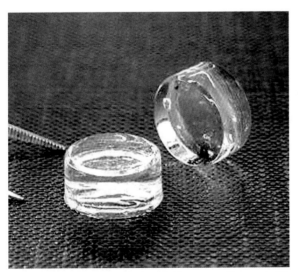

FIG 32.1 In Situ Implant, GelrinC (Courtesy Regentis Biomaterials, Or-Akiva, Israel.)

of the PEG. This allows a longer time frame (when compared with degradation of blood clot alone) for formation of tissue at the repair site, with implications that this altered temporal sequence will allow for more mature repair tissue—in the case of cartilage, more hyaline-like than fibrocartilage. This may allow functional tissue to fill the space occupied previously by the implant. The scaffold completely degrades within 6 to 12 months. The major degradation products are PEGylated peptides, amino acids, and PEG, and have been shown to be nontoxic to chondrocytes, bone, and the body.[69,72]

Chondrotissue. Chondrotissue (BioTissue AG, Zurich, Switzerland) is a PGA-hyaluronan implant.[79] The scaffold is immersed with autologous serum or platelet-rich plasma (PRP) and implanted into full-thickness articular cartilage defects pretreated with microfracture. Human serum is used as a chemoattractant and efficiently recruits mesenchymal progenitors. Chondrogenic differentiation of progenitor cells on stimulation with hyaluronan was demonstrated by Erggelet et al.[19] and Wakitani et al.[93] The Chondrotissue implants are secured in place with fibrin glue or bioresorbable fixation implants such as Smart Nails (ConMed Linvatec Italy, Milano, Italy). Initial studies have demonstrated this technique to be safe and effective.[17,67,78,98] At an average follow-up of 5 years, Siclari et al. reported increased knee injury and osteoarthritis outcome score (KOOS) scores compared to preop that reached statistical significance.[80] Additionally, 20 out of 21 patients underwent magnetic resonance imaging (MRI) and had complete lesion fill.

Biologic adhesive and photopolymerized hydrogel with microfracture. ChonDux (Biomet, Warsaw, Indiana) combines a biologic adhesive and photopolymerized hydrogel with microfracture.[74] The biologic adhesive is a processed chondroitin sulfate that bonds with defect cartilage and defect base to aid in bonding the hydrogel in the defect. The hydrogel is a combination of PEG and HA; it aids in the retention of the marrow stimulation elements, is conducive to chondrogenesis, and potentially reduces fibrosis tissue production.[7,9] ChonDux is not commercially available, and clinical trials have been terminated.

Multiphase Scaffold to Fill Osteochondral Defect. There are many experimental models using a multiphase scaffold to address the bone and cartilage component of an osteochondral defect, as detailed by Lynn et al.[58]

TruFit synthetic implants. One biphasic scaffold plug option is the TruFit plug (Smith & Nephew Endoscopy, Andover, Massachusetts; Fig. 32.2). This is entirely synthetic and is designed to mimic the physical and mechanical properties of cartilage and bone. It is composed of POLYGRAFT (Smith & Nephew Endoscopy), a porous hydrophilic material comprised of an 85:15 poly(D,L-lactide–coglycolide) copolymer (PLDG), PGA fibers, calcium sulfate (bone phase only), and a trace amount of surfactant. PGA reinforcement fibers improve the early structural integrity of the scaffold and provide a mechanically stable environment for possible cell migration and tissue repair.[76] The superficial phase is malleable to allow contouring with the adjacent articular surface after implantation. Calcium sulfate in the bone phase resorbs in the first several months, releasing calcium ions, which may enhance osteoconductivity.[25] The material of the scaffold degrades in approximately 6 to 9 months[81] by hydrolysis of ester linkages into lactic and glycolic acids, which are metabolites of the Krebs cycle and have very minimal toxicity. There are few outcome studies following implantation of TruFit plugs, but there is concern regarding

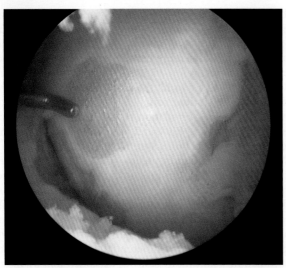

FIG 32.2 TruFit Bgs Plug After Arthroscopic Placement
(From Cole BJ, Gomoll AG: Biologic joint reconstruction: alternatives to arthroplasty. Thorofare, NJ, 2009, Slack.)

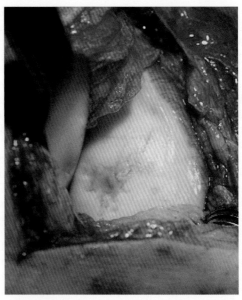

FIG 32.3 Femoral condyle chondral defect. (Courtesy Vericel and Dr. Leela Biant.)

durability of the implants and long-term outcome. Joshi et al. followed 10 patients treated with TruFit CB plugs for patellofemoral defects and reported 8 out of 10 patients complaining of pain and swelling at 18 months follow-up.[40] The reoperation rate for implant failure at final follow-up was 70%. As a result, the authors concluded that they do not recommend TruFit synthetic implants for osteochondral patellar defects in active patients. A recent systematic review found no data available to support the use of TruFit plugs for osteochondral defects, compared to conservative treatment or other cartilage techniques.[90] Smith & Nephew no longer offers the TruFit plug for cartilage repair use.

MaioRegen. MaioRegen is an osteochondral biomimetic scaffold (Fin-Ceramica Faenza, Faenza, Italy), which has a porous, three-dimensional, composite trilayered structure, mimicking the osteochondral unit.[89] Each layer is separately synthesized using an atelocollagen aqueous solution (1%) in acetic acid, isolated from the equine tendon.[23] The layer that promotes cartilaginous tissue consists of type I collagen and has a smooth surface. The intermediate layer (tide mark–like) consists of a combination of type I collagen (60%) and HA (40%), whereas the bone-specific layer consists of a mineralized blend of type I collagen (30%) and HA (70%). In an Italian study, 37 patients treated with MaioRegen demonstrated statistically significant improvement in International Knee Documentation Committee (IKDC) and Tegner scores from initial evaluation to the 2- and 5-year follow-ups.[49] The MRI evaluation showed improvement in the magnetic resonance observation of cartilage repair tissue (MOCART) score and complete filling of cartilage in 78.3% of the lesions.

Chondromimetic. Chondromimetic (Tigenix, Leuven, Belgium) is a biphasic, porous, resorbable implant that contains the biocompatible and resorbable materials collagen and glycosaminoglycan, with calcium phosphate added to the bone layer phase of the dual-layer porous implant.[58] The scaffold is rehydrated with sterile fluids and autologous blood products in an effort to optimize its biologic effectiveness through cell infiltration and tissue regeneration.

Agili-C. Agili-C (CartiHeal [2009] Ltd., Israel) is a rigid biphasic, biodegradable implant. The bone phase of the implant is composed of calcium carbonate in aragonite crystalline form. The cartilage phase is a composite of modified aragonite and HA. The implant promotes adhesion, proliferation, and differentiation of bone marrow mesenchymal stem cells. It can be implanted in a single-step open or arthroscopic procedure. Promising results have been documented using a caprine model with 12-month follow-up.[50] Clinical studies are limited to one case report, but further studies are in development. The implant is not available in the United States.

Other scaffold plug options that are currently only for osseous fill include Osseofit Kensey (Kensey Nash, Exton, Pennsylvania[44]) and OsteoSponge and OsteoSponge filler (Bacterin International, Belgrade, Montana[4]).

Composite Bone Allograft Plug

CR-Plug. The CR-Plug (RTI Biologics, Alachua, Florida; Fig. 32.3) is a composite bone allograft plug that consists of cancellous bone covered with a thinner layer of demineralized bone. Although demineralized bone has been shown to allow for the formation of hyaline-like cartilage in animal models,[26,96,100] this allograft implant is being promoted by the manufacturer as a bone void filler. Demineralized bone provides a scaffold for cell migration, and the growth factors inherent to bone are retained even after demineralization. At the time of implantation, the firmness of the demineralized bone is similar to hose cartilage. A pilot study was terminated early because of a potential change in the regulatory pathway for allografts used in cartilage repair. It is not currently available for clinical use.

Polymer Scaffold

Aseed Scaffold. The Aseed Scaffold[14] (Coloplast A/S, Humlebaek, Denmark) is composed of a methoxypolyethyleneglycolpoly(l,d[lactide]-co-glycolide), (MPEG-PGLA) polymer. The scaffold has a thickness comparable to that of human cartilage. The scaffold is cut to fit the defect and secured by fibrin glue. Its canal-like design allows for host cells to integrate into the scaffold fully, with the goal of augmenting the outcome of marrow stimulation alone.

Scaffolds With Seeded Autologous Cells (Single-Stage)

Autologous Chondrocyte Transplant, Collagen Patch–Seeded. An autologous chondrocyte transplant (ACT), collagen patch–seeded, is a standard ACI cell suspension seeded onto a collagen patch immediately before implantation. After several minutes, the cells have adhered sufficiently for implantation. The advantage over conventional cultured chondrocytes on scaffolds is that no cells are discarded, as noted by Steinwachs.[85]

Cartilage Autograft Implant System. In a cartilage autograft implant system (CAIS; DePuy Mitek, Raynham, Massachusetts), autologous cartilage is minced arthoscopically by a custom harvester into 1- to 2-mm pieces. These pieces are uniformly dispersed by a custom device onto a synthetic scaffold (35% polycaprolate [PCL], 65% PGA and polydiaxonone [PDS] mesh) where they are fixed on the scaffold with fibrin glue. The minced cartilage scaffold construct is implanted and fixed with bioabsorbable staples during the same surgery through a miniarthrotomy.[21,27] In a prospective clinical safety trial, 29 patients with focal articular cartilage defects were randomized to either microfracture or CAIS.[13] The IKDC score of the CAIS group was significantly higher compared with the microfracture group at 12 and 24 months follow-up, and there was a difference in the number of adverse effects. A phase III trial of CAIS versus microfracture in the United States was terminated as a result of slow enrollment. Building upon the earlier success of minced autograft, Foldager's group reported on successful clinical outcomes with "autograft cartilage chips," as well as a mini-pig study.[12] Commercially, a mechanical mincer system (Revielle, Exactech, Gainsville, Florida) is being studied, where the minced cartilage is fixed in defects with bone marrow aspirate concentrate (BMAC) and fibrin glue. This is as an offshoot of the Taiwanese prospective randomized clinical study of BiPhasic Cartilage Repair Implant (BiCRI, Exactech Taiwan, Ltd.), in which minced cartilage in absorbable cylinders are implanted. The Taiwan study is a phase III clinical trial comparing BiCRI to marrow stimulation for the treatment of focal chondral defects.

Cell Replacement Technology

Instruct products. Cell replacement technology (CRT) instruct products (CellCoTec, Bilthoven, The Netherlands) consist of a cell processor, a mechanically functional scaffold, and reusable surgical instrumentation.[96] In the operating room, autologous cartilage is harvested and bone marrow is aspirated. Chondrocytes are then isolated and mixed with the bone marrow aspirate and seeded onto a rehydrated scaffold. This is performed during a single, minimally invasive surgical procedure. Advantages may include a comparatively short rehabilitation time because of the use of a mechanically functional scaffold.[62]

Scaffolds With Seeded Allogenic Cells (Single-Stage)

Cord Blood Stem Cells With Hyaluronan. Cartistem (Medipost, Seoul, Korea) contains mesenchymal stem cells derived from umbilical cord blood and added to an HA scaffold. The product is implanted at the site of a marrow stimulation prepared defect. Safety and efficacy has been confirmed following the completion of Phase III trials in Korea. It has been approved

for phase I/IIA clinical trials at select institutions within the United States.

Engineered Juvenile Cartilage With Fibrin Adhesive. Revaflex (ISTO Technologies Inc., St. Louis, Missouri; previously DeNovo ET) is an in vitro–grown three-dimensional hyaline-like cartilage tissue containing viable cultured juvenile allograft chondrocytes, which create their own ECM.[61] This construct is lifted from a plastic mesh, and thus only the cell-formed matrix is implanted. It has been promising in both animal and human models that juvenile cartilage possesses superior chondrocytic activity, higher cell density, and increased healing potential over adult cartilage.[1,56] The cultured juvenile chondrocytes are cryopreserved in a large tissue bank. Prior to implantation, the cells are thawed and cultured in a serum- and scaffold-free process to produce a hyaline-like cartilage graft, which is applied to a prepared chondral defect with a fibrin adhesive.[32] A phase III trial comparing Revaflex to microfracture is in the early planning stages.

Scaffolds With Cells Cultured on or Within a Scaffold (Two-Stage)

Seeded With Autologous Chondrocytes

Matrix-associated autologous chondrocyte implantation. MACI (Vericel; Fig. 32.4) is an autologous chondrocyte that is expanded, seeded onto a type I-III collagen membrane, and cultured. It is then implanted with suture or fibrin glue. A number of clinical reports from studies performed outside the United States have reported similar efficacy to ACI, with a lower complication rate.[5,38,101] Saris et al. conducted a randomized controlled trial with 2-year follow-up comparing matrix-associated autologous chondrocyte implantation (MACI) to microfracture.[70] There were 144 patients included in the study, with a mean lesion size of 4.8 cm^2. The outcomes assessed included KOOS scores, knee-related quality of life, and repair tissue quality based on histology/MRI. Their conclusion was that for cartilage defects greater than 3 cm^2 in size, treatment with MACI was both statistically and clinically better than

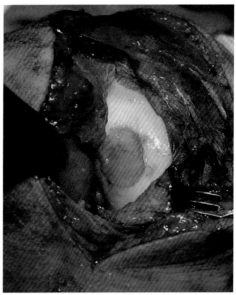

FIG 32.4 Treatment with the MACI membrane. (Courtesy Vericel and Dr. Leela Biant.)

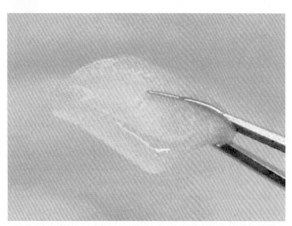

FIG 32.5 NeoCart This autologous hyaline neocartilage implant is ready for transplantation (Courtesy Histogenics, Waltham, MA.)

microfracture with similar structural repair tissue and safety. The product has recently been withdrawn from the market for commercial reasons, but the safety and efficacy has not changed. The marketing authorization has been suspended following the closure of the European manufacturing site in Denmark. The suspension is in effect until a new manufacturing site is registered.

CartiGro. CartiGro ACT[88] (Stryker, Montreux, Switzerland) is similar to MACI but is currently using a different (thicker) scaffold (Chondro-Gide; Geistlich Biomaterials, Switzerland) porcine I/III onto which cells (CartiGro ACT) are cultured. Since 2000, CartiGro has been implanted in more than 800 patients.[11]

NeoCart. NeoCart (Histogenics, Waltham, Mass; Fig. 32.5) is a three-dimensional bovine collagen scaffold seeded with expanded autologous chondrocytes, which are then grown on the scaffold in hydrostatic bioreactor and implanted with proprietary bioadhesive (greater adherence than fibrin glue).[16,95] The use of a bioreactor with cyclic pressurization attempts to recreate conditions in the knee, with the goal of promoting the chondrocytes to synthesize glycoproteins.[84] Initial studies have confirmed safety of the procedure and associated it with greater clinical efficacy compared to microfracture at 2 years after treatment.[15,16] Currently a phase III trial is being conducted in the United States.

CaReS and CartiPlug. CaReS and CartiPlug (ArthroKinetics, Boston, Massachusetts) are autologous chondrocytes seeded onto three-dimensional collagen type I gel. The diameter and thickness of the transplant can be chosen individually, depending on the nature of the defect. The cells are isolated from the patient's biopsy, mixed with the collagen gel, and after the complete gelling and 2 weeks of culture in the patient's serum cultivation medium, the chondrocyte-loaded gel is available for transplantation. The transplantation is performed by a mini-open technique using a thin layer of fibrin glue. A prospective multicenter study of 116 patients treated with CaReS resulted in encouraging midterm results with significant functional improvement and improved pain levels.[71] The product is not available in the United States.

Hyalograft C. Hyalograft C (Anika Theraputics, Bedford, Massachusetts) is a hyaluronan-based biodegradable polymer (HYAFF-11) scaffold with a nonwoven three-dimensional structure. It is 20 μm thick and is seeded with expanded

autologous chondrocytes, which are grown on the scaffold for 2 weeks. The construct is implanted by miniarthrotomy or arthroscopically. Several studies have documented favorable clinical results following implantation of Hyalograft C.[22,31,47,48,51] However, Anika Therapeutics elected to withdraw Hyalograft C from the market in 2013, and therefore it is no longer available for use. The current application of the product involves seeding the HYAFF-11 scaffold with BMAC and applying it to a prepared chondral defect.[30] In addition, there are plans to initiate a randomized control trial for the use of the Hyaff-11 membrane in conjunction with marrow stimulation in the United States.

Bioseed C. Bioseed C (BioTissue Technologies, Freiburg, Germany) is a polyglactin poly-*p*-dioxanon fleece with a standard size of 2 × 3 cm^2 or 2 × 1 cm^2. Autologous chondrocytes are expanded ex vivo and then loaded on a 2-mm thick porous scaffold using a fibrin glue to distribute the cells, providing a three-dimensional environment and securing the bioengineered tissue.[18,41,42] Several studies have demonstrated improved clinical outcomes following treatment with Bioseed C.[20,52,53,64] However, Zeifang et al. found no difference in efficacy between full-thickness chondral defects treated with the original periosteum covered ACI, compared to those treated with Bioseed C.[99]

Cartipatch. Cartipatch (TBF Tissue Engineering, Bron, France) consists of autologous chondrocytes that are implanted on a hydrogel composed of agarose and alginate. This hydrogel is of vegetal origin (ultrapurified agarose-alginate suspension [GelForCel; TBF Tissue Engineering]). It is mixed with an isolated autologous cell suspension and can be modulated at 37°C into complex shape implants, which solidify at approximately 25°C. Matrix elasticity improves handling.[2,46,73] Advantages of this technique include the ability of the implant to mold to the shape of the defect, and theoretically the product results in a more even distribution of chondrocytes within the scaffold. In a phase II prospective multicenter trial, Selmi et al. reported on 17 patients who were followed for 2 years following the Cartipatch procedure.[73] There was a statistically significant increase in IKDC score, from a mean of 37 preoperatively to 77.8 at final follow-up. Histological analysis revealed hyaline-like or mixed hyaline-fibrocartilage repair tissue, with complete integration to the subchondral bone in 11 of 13 patients.

Novocart 3D. Novocart 3D (TETEC Tissue Engineering Technologies, a B Braun Company, Reutlingen, Germany) is an autologous chondrocyte implanted onto a collagen-based biphasic scaffold. A specific, protective, dense layer was developed to cover the collagen sponge to prevent synovial cells from invasion and improve the mechanical properties of the scaffold. The transplantation is performed by a mini-open technique using a dedicated instrumentation. For the fixation of the graft, resorbable mini-pins can be used.[46] Zak et al. evaluated 23 patients clinically and radiographically 24 months following transplantation with Novocart 3D.[97] The authors reported statistically significant improvement in all outcome scores (IKDC, KOOS, Noyes, Tegner activity scale, and VAS (visual analog scale)), except KOOS-symptoms. The MRI evaluation was favorable, with a mean MOCART score of 73.2 and a mean 3D MOCART score of 73.4. A pivotal study randomized with microfracture is recruiting patients in the United States currently.

BioCart Cartilage Regeneration System implant. The BioCart Cartilage Regeneration System implant (ProChon, Ness Ziona, Israel; Fig. 32.6) uses a fibrin scaffold, which is a natural homologous biopolymer (constituting part of the normal scaffold of wound healing) and is copolymerized with hyaluronan

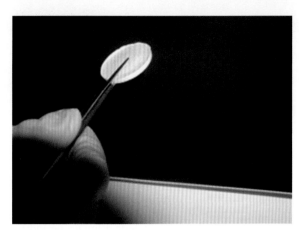

FIG 32.6 BioCart—dry, lyophilized, fibrin–HA three-dimensional bioscaffolds with interconnection pores ranging from 10 to 50 μm. (Courtesy ProChon Biotech, Ness Ziona, Israel.)

to produce a matrix that serves as a three-dimensional scaffold for chondrocyte transplantation. Pore sizes range from 10 to 15 μm. The scaffold degrades almost completely in 3 to 4 weeks. The degradation products of fibrin are fragments of polypeptides produced when the protein is broken down by the enzyme plasmin. Hyaluronan is degraded by a family of enzymes called hyaluronidases. The degradation products of hyaluronan are oligosaccharides and very low-molecular-weight hyaluronan, which are known to exhibit proangiogenic properties. The scaffold is seeded and cultured with chondroctyes that have been in the presence of the fibroblast growth factor (FGF2v), which allows a more robust chondrocytic phenotype and matrix production, with a lower number of passages.[92]

KEY REFERENCES

1. Adkisson HD, Martin JA, Amendola R, et al: The potential of human allogeneic juvenile chondrocytes for restoration of articular cartilage. *Am J Sports Med* 38(7):1324–1333, 2010.
12. Christensen BB, Foldager CB, Jensen J, et al: Autologous dual-tissue transplantation for osteochondral repair: early clinical and radiographical results. *Cartilage* 6(3):166–173, 2015.
15. Crawford DC, DeBerardino TM, Williams RJ, 3rd: NeoCart, an autologous cartilage tissue implant, compared with microfracture for treatment of distal femoral cartilage lesions: an FDA phase-II prospective randomized clinical trial after two years. *J Bone Joint Surg Am* 94(11):979–989, 2012.
49. Kon E, Filardo G, Di Martino A, et al: Clinical results and MRI evolution of a nano-composite multilayered biomaterial for osteochondral regeneration at 5 years. *Am J Sports Med* 42:158–165, 2014.
50. Kon E, Filardo G, Shani J, et al: In vivo animal study and clinical outcomes of autologous atelocollagen-induced chondrogenesis for osteochondral lesion treatment. *J Orthop Surg Res* 10:82, 2015.
56. Liu H, Zhao Z, Clarke RB, et al: Enhanced tissue regeneration potential of juvenile articular cartilage. *Am J Sports Med* 41(11):2658–2667, 2013.
70. Saris D, Price A, Widuchowski W, et al: Matrix-applied characterized autologous chondrocytes versus microfracture: two-year follow-up of a prospective randomized trial. *Am J Sports Med* 42(6):1384–1394, 2014.
86. Steinwachs MR, Waibl B, Mumme M: Arthroscopic treatment of cartilage lesions with microfracture and BST-CarGel. *Arthrosc Tech* 3(3):399–402, 2014.

The references for this chapter can also be found on www.expertconsult.com.

33

Management of Failed Cartilage Repair

Eric C. Makhni, Maximilian A. Meyer, Brian J. Cole

INTRODUCTION

Despite advances in biologic and surgical treatment options for patients with focal cartilage defects of the knee, there remains a high clinical failure rate following treatment. This number approaches 25% in many clinical series.[3,12,14,19] After failure of articular cartilage repair, patients may complain of persistent pain, inability to return to activity or sport, or experience a progression of degenerative joint disease. Failure may be secondary to numerous factors, including neglected comorbidities, patient-specific factors, the lesion, or even the technical management of the initial condition. To successfully manage patients with failed cartilage repair, the clinician must first identify the underlying reason for failure, as well as the various modalities for treatment.

The goal of this chapter is to present the reader with the most common reasons for failure following commonly used cartilage procedures (microfracture, autologous chondrocyte implantation [ACI], and osteochondral autograft or allograft). The chapter will also review common history and physical exam findings in patients with prior failed cartilage surgery, as well as treatment algorithms and techniques in managing these complex patients.

Risk Factors for Failure

Early versus Late Failure. Failure may occur in the early or late period following initial cartilage surgery. Factors responsible for early failure include technical error in management (Fig. 33.1), failure of biology (graft incorporation), patient noncompliance with postoperative precautions/protocols, or trauma. Late failures may also result from failure of graft incorporation or maturation, the indolent progression of underlying disease, progression of additional untreated pathology (ie, limb malalignment or additional cartilage defects), or breakdown of initial repair construct. Notably, patients may fail to achieve symptom relief either initially or after a period of symptom quiescence, and there may not be obvious graft site deterioration. These clinical scenarios must be critically evaluated for additional comorbidities that can contribute to compartmental overload and persistence or a return of clinical symptoms.

Failure Following Prior Microfracture. Clinical failure rates following microfracture have ranged from 11% to 23% at 5 years[5,7,14] and up to 38% at 10 years[9] (Fig. 33.2). The cause of failure has been highlighted by a recent systematic review by Mithoefer et al.[18] Patient-related factors include elevated body mass index (BMI) of greater than 30 kg/m^2, age greater than 45 years, and higher preoperative activity scores. Lesion-related factors associated with failure include a longer period of pre-surgical symptoms (>12 months) and lesions that were larger than 2 cm^2 to 4 cm^2. In a different review of Level I and II studies, Goyal et al.[7] reported satisfactory outcomes following microfracture in younger patients and those with lower activity levels. However, they also reported disease progression 5 to 10 years following treatment.

Failure Following Autologous Chondrocyte Implantation. Rates of failure following ACI have been reported to range from 19% to 23% at 5 years follow-up (Fig. 33.3).[3,14,19] Patient-specific factors contributing to failure include increased BMI and increased physical activity levels,[2,13] as well as female gender and prior surgery. This is particularly relevant in patients with prior microfracture, where failure rates of subsequent treatment with ACI have been demonstrated to increase.[17,20] From a technique perspective, use of a periosteal patch during ACI has been shown to cause reoperation because of graft hypertrophy (as opposed to cellular membrane use).[6] Biologic failure commonly manifests as graft hypertrophy, delamination, and incomplete incorporation/growth.

Failure Following Osteochondral Autograft/Allograft Transplantation. As with microfracture and ACI, both patient-specific as well as technical considerations contribute to failure risk in patients undergoing surgery. Preliminary evidence suggests that younger age may lead to improved outcomes, whereas other factors, such as BMI, gender, prior surgical history, and graft characteristics, may not play a predictive role.[15,21] It is our experience that technical considerations regarding proper graft implantation are of the utmost importance in minimizing risk for failure following osteochondral autograft/allograft transplantation. We recommend that recipient sites be filled completely, to minimize likelihood of cyst formation, and also recommend using minimal force during graft impaction (and thereby minimizing likelihood of chondral cell injury) and not allowing the plug to be greater than 1 mm proud compared to its surrounding cartilaginous levels.[2,4] Plugs that are placed greater than 1 mm proud have been shown to contribute to early failure, as these plugs experience increased contact pressures that lead to adverse mechanical outcomes.[2,16] Finally, in lesions that are greater than 4 cm^2, evidence supports the use of ACI over that of microfracture and osteochondral autograft transplantation.[10]

CLINICAL EVALUATION

Clinical evaluation of the patient with a failed cartilage surgery involves gaining not only a comprehensive understanding of the

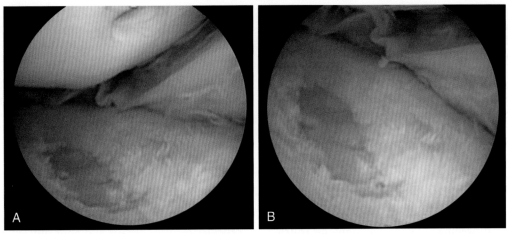

FIG 33.1 Patient with osteochondritis dissecans previously treated with Bioscrew fixation, now presenting with persistent knee pain. (A) Arthroscopic assessment after removal of protruding screw that had caused disruption of tibial cartilage. (B) This patient was subsequently treated with microfracture.

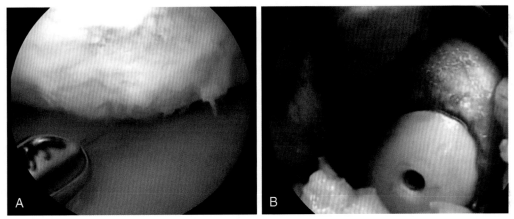

FIG 33.2 (A) Arthroscopic imaging of a 32-year-old man with osteochondritis dissecans on the medial femoral condyle that was previously treated with microfracture. (B) This patient was treated with osteochondral allograft transplantation and has had full return to athletic activity at 2 years follow-up.

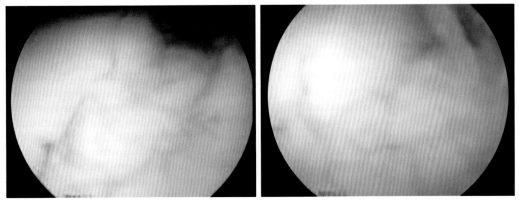

FIG 33.3 Arthroscopic imaging of failed autologous chondrocyte implantation at the junction of the medial femoral condyle and trochlea.

patient's presenting symptoms and relevant physical exam findings but also his/her detailed past surgical and treatment history. Understanding the pathology identified at index treatment through review of the operative notes and pictures, inquiring as to the specifics of the postoperative rehabilitation (ie, weight-bearing restrictions, passive range of motion, etc.) and the course of symptom changes over time, is particularly helpful in making subsequent decisions regarding further management. Additional diagnostic workup, such as preoperative and current imaging, may also aid in establishing an optimal treatment plan.

History

The workup of any patient with a known or suspected cartilage syndrome begins with an assessment of the chief complaint. Cartilage lesions may cause a variety of symptoms, including pain (with or without swelling), mechanical symptoms (catching, locking), or symptoms of malalignment or instability when in conjunction with other pathologies. These symptoms may prevent the patient from obtaining a desired level of activity or performance during sport.

Similar to patients with a primary focal cartilage defect, pain is most often the patient's chief complaint, which is aggravated by certain positions or activities. Pain at the ipsilateral joint line is often associated with a condylar injury that can be aggravated by weight-bearing activities. Joint line pain caused by meniscal deficiency may be difficult to discern from symptoms caused by a focal cartilage defect. However, a previous history of even a partial meniscectomy may heighten the surgeon's awareness to the possibility of functional meniscal deficiency causing or contributing to continued symptoms. Patients presenting with pain in the anterior compartment of the knee may be suffering from a trochlear or patellar lesion, which can be aggravated by activities that increase patellofemoral contact pressure, such as stair climbing or squatting. In addition to pain, patients may also report activity-related effusions in the knee.

Prior attempts at treatment should be reviewed with the patient. If prior surgeries have been performed, the timing and type of surgery, type of rehabilitation that followed, and whether the patient experienced a period of symptomatic relief postoperatively should be thoroughly discussed preoperatively. In addition, nonsurgical management such as oral medications, injections, bracing, physical therapy, and lifestyle modification should also be discussed as an important part of the patient's prior treatment. Finally, all attempts should be made to obtain comprehensive treatment records from initial management, including relevant diagnostic (pre and posttreatment) and intraoperative images. Understanding the physical characteristics of the lesion (eg, size, shape, and location) is useful for surgical planning.

Physical Examination

The physical examination of a patient with a symptomatic cartilage lesion begins with observation of the patient's gait and body habitus. Gait evaluation may reveal any antalgia caused by pain or weakness, malalignment, or a varus or valgus thrust associated with ligament insufficiency or clinical malalignment. The physician should also observe and measure any associated quadriceps atrophy and effusions, and determine the location of any previous surgical incisions.

Palpation of bony and soft tissue structures about the knee may provide some insight into the location of the patient's symptoms, associated conditions such as meniscal deficiency, or

presence of a subtle effusion. Patients with chondral injuries of the condyle typically present with ipsilateral joint line pain or tenderness directly over the presumed defect area. Meniscal injury or deficiency may also present similarly to condylar pain with joint line tenderness; however, the pain is occasionally appreciated more posteriorly. Patellofemoral lesions may have pain and crepitus in the anterior compartment. Patellar tilt and glide should be evaluated for tightness of the lateral retinaculum and potentially neglected patellar instability. Finally, range of motion should be assessed in both knees, noting limitation in range and/or flexion contractures.

Identification of associated pathology is critical to the successful outcome of revision and complex articular cartilage restoration. As noted, persistent instability, malalignment, or meniscal deficiency is often a cause of premature failure of articular cartilage repairs and poor outcomes. Stability of the anterior cruciate ligament (ACL), posterior cruciate ligament (PCL), medial collateral ligament (MCL), as well as the lateral collateral ligament (LCL) and posterolateral complex, should be a routine part of any knee examination.

Imaging

Standard radiographs for cartilage injury should include bilateral knees in at least three views: anteroposterior (AP) weight-bearing view; non-weight-bearing, 45-degree flexion lateral view; and axial (Merchant) view of the patellofemoral joint. Additional views include a 45-degree flexion posteroanterior (PA) view, which may be useful to identify subtle joint space narrowing. A full-length alignment view of the affected and unaffected limb may help evaluate the mechanical axis and associated varus or valgus malalignment (Fig. 33.4). A computed tomography (CT) scan may be useful to assess the patellofemoral joint and the associated tibial tubercle-trochlear groove (TT-TG) distance.[1,22] This measurement is particularly useful in patients with patellar instability when associated with chondrosis. Magnetic resonance imaging (MRI) scans are often used in the preoperative assessment of previously failed cartilage repair procedures. They provide a detailed assessment of lesion size, depth, quality of subchondral bone, and presence or absence of bony fractures. MRI may also confirm the presence of associated ligamentous, meniscal, or other soft tissue pathology. Symptomatic patients may demonstrate persistent edema and fissuring at the site of prior cartilage repair surgery (Fig. 33.5). Finally, if there is any uncertainty regarding the precise morphology and location of the lesion, the patient may require a diagnostic arthroscopy and detailed assessment of the lesion and other cofactors that might be contributing to their symptoms (such as additional cartilage lesions or meniscal deficiency).

TREATMENT ALGORITHM

Treatment of failed cartilage lesions depends on both lesion characteristics and the nature of the prior surgical attempt. The goal for all patients, however, is to ensure that any compartment at risk is adequately off-loaded and supported. This entails realignment (high tibial osteotomy, distal femoral osteotomy, or tibial tubercle osteotomy) surgery for underlying varus or valgus deformity or off-loading the patellofemoral joint and meniscal allograft transplantation in settings of deficient meniscus. In patients with ACL deficiency (or other ligamentous deficiency), along with malalignment and cartilage defect, we

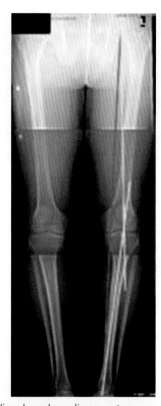

FIG 33.4 Standing long-leg alignment x-rays. The mechanical axis of the extremity is represented by the *red line*, from the center of the femoral head to the center of the talus. This patient has an obvious varus deformity to the lower extremity. The desired correction for this patient is just beyond neutral. This angle is calculated by a line drawn from the center of the femoral head to the desired correction level at the joint line and a second line from the center of the talus to the same correction point at the joint line *(yellow)*.

will often stage the treatment according to the primary complaint. (Patients with instability will undergo ligament reconstruction first, whereas those with pain will undergo unloading procedure and cartilage treatment first.) When realignment surgery is indicated, we will correct to neutral alignment if there is no evidence of degenerative disease in the diseased compartment; however, if there are arthritic changes, we will slightly overcorrect beyond neutral. When considering patients who require multiple procedures (eg, high tibial osteotomy along with meniscus transplantation and osteochondral allografting), we prefer to stage the procedures in patients who are older and less active. In these cases, any realignment or off-loading surgery will be performed first to assess if there is any satisfactory relief that may preclude performing subsequent procedures. Finally, patients who have progression of disease from focal lesions to more diffuse disease may no longer be candidates for cartilage restoration procedures.

Our preferred algorithm for failed cartilage treatment depends on the location, characteristic, and prior treatment of the affected lesion. Additionally, the presence or absence of suchondral edema on MRI also plays a significant role when considering treatment options (Fig. 33.6). In patients with prior failed surface treatment or marrow stimulation procedures, with no evidence of subchondral edema in their MRI, we will consider performing ACI if the lesion is between 2 and 3 cm^2 in size. Otherwise, our preference is to perform an osteochondral procedure in the revision setting. For lesions that are 1 cm^2 in size, we will perform osteochondral autograft transplantation (except in the patellofemoral joint, where we do not perform this procedure in the revision setting, although some authors have achieved success with this procedure). In larger lesions, namely those that are 2 cm^2 or larger and with associated subchondral edema on MRI, our preference is to perform osteochondral allograft (OA) procedure rather than a mosaicplasty or osteochondral autograft procedure (Fig. 33.7).

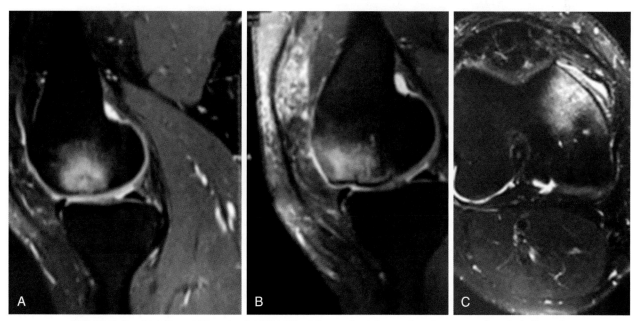

FIG 33.5 Sagittal (A and B) and axial (C) MRI of the patient 6 months after osteochondral allograft transplantation, presenting with continued knee pain and effusions. High signal regions correspond to subchondral edema causing symptoms.

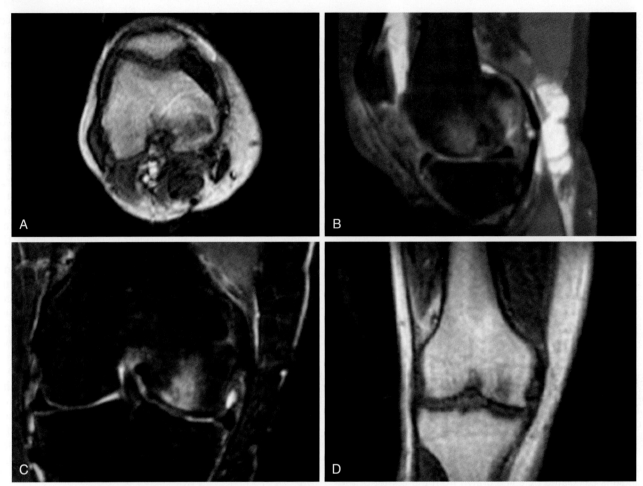

FIG 33.6 Axial (A), sagittal (B), and coronal (C and D) MRI of same patient in Fig. 33.2, who had a failed microfracture for previous osteochondritis dissecans of the medial femoral condyle.

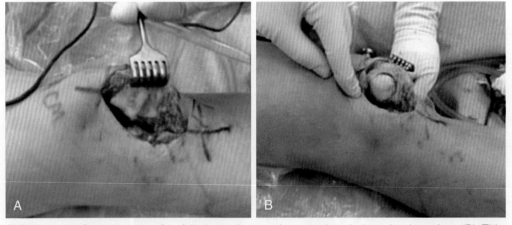

FIG 33.7 (A) Gross image of a failed patellar autologous chondrocyte implantation. (B) This patient was treated with revision osteochondral allograft transplantation and is doing well at 1 year follow-up.

Similarly, for all other patients with larger lesions following failed treatment, and when there is bony involvement (edema on MRI), our main revision procedure is osteochondral allograft. This has also been used with "kissing lesions" of the patellofemoral joint (eg, lesions on the patella that interact with lesions on the femoral condyle [Fig. 33.8]). In patients with persistent symptoms despite prior osteochondral allograft, treatment depends on the integrity of the graft. If intact, we will typically not revise the graft and instead perform a débridement or treat nonoperatively.

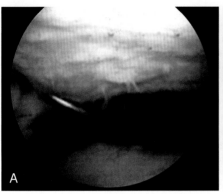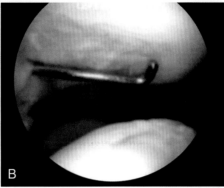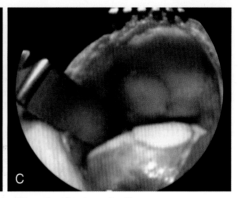

FIG 33.8 (A and B) A "kissing lesion" that was previously treated with microfracture in the trochlea and DeNovo in the patella. (C) Revision osteochondral allograft transplantation yielded excellent functional outcomes in this patient at 1 year postoperatively.

REHABILITATION

Rehabilitation protocols vary according to the procedure(s) performed. In general, patients are placed in a hinged knee brace postoperatively and advised to use a continuous passive motion machine for 4 to 6 weeks for up to 6 hours/day. Patients who have a revision procedure on the femoral condyle or required an osteotomy with their revision procedure are protected with partial weight bearing and often use a postoperative hinged unloader brace (TROM Adjuster, DonJoy, Carlsbad, California). Rehabilitation of a revision procedure performed on the PF compartment allows for weight bearing as tolerated, with a knee brace locked in extension, as long as the tibial tubercle osteotomy is not performed at that time, which would also require a period of protected weight bearing. The goals of early rehabilitation are increased range of motion, patellar mobilization, quadriceps sets, isometrics, and proximal core strengthening. Six to 12 weeks postoperatively, patients begin to focus on a functional strengthening program. At about 3 months postoperatively, patients are advanced to muscular endurance with progressive running activities, advanced closed-chain strengthening, and plyometrics.

RESULTS FOLLOWING REVISION CARTILAGE SURGERY

Several recent studies have reported on clinical outcomes in patients undergoing treatment for prior failed cartilage surgery of the knee. Increased failure rates have been reported in patients undergoing ACI following failed marrow stimulation procedure.[19,20] Minas et al. reported a failure rate of 26% in these patients (29 failures in 111 joints), compared to an 8% (17 of 214) failure rate in patients who had no prior treatment.[17] Other studies, however, have reported slightly higher success rates in patients treated with ACI in the revision setting. These include use of ACI following failed treatment for adult osteochondritis dissecans (85% success),[3] as well as in patients undergoing ACI as a revision procedure (76% success in 126 patients).[23]

Outcomes following osteochondral allograft following prior marrow stimulation have also been reported. Gracitelli et al.[8] recently reported on the outcome of 92 knees undergoing osteochondral allograft (46 as a primary procedure and 46 as a revision following prior marrow stimulation). Although the revision group ultimately experienced a higher reoperation rate (44% vs. 24%), there was no ultimate difference in functional scores or survivorship (with both groups experiencing improvement). However, there is evidence that indicates revision osteochondral allograft may not be as effective as primary osteochondral allograft. Horton et al.[11] reported on a series of 33 patients who underwent revision osteochondral allograft with an overall failure rate of 39% (with an overall 10 year survival of 61%).

CONCLUSION

In conclusion, management of the patient with failed cartilage surgery remains challenging. To effectively manage these patients, the clinician must have a thorough understanding of risk factors and mechanisms of failure following the index procedure. In formulating a treatment plan, all patient comorbidities should be considered and addressed, including weight, mechanical alignment, and associated ligamentous or meniscal deficiencies. In considering these factors, along with characteristics and detailed treatment history of the symptomatic lesion, the clinician may then be able to formulate a treatment plan. Finally, care should be given to adequately counsel the patient regarding outcomes and expectations following surgery, especially in cases of failed initial treatment.

KEY REFERENCES

2. Chahal J, Thiel GV, Hussey K, et al: Managing the patient with failed cartilage restoration. *Sports Med Arthrosc* 21(2):62–68, 2013.
3. Cole BJ, DeBerardino T, Brewster R, et al: Outcomes of autologous chondrocyte implantation in study of the treatment of articular repair (STAR) patients with osteochondritis dissecans. *Am J Sports Med* 40(9):2015–2022, 2012.
5. Gobbi A, Karnatzikos G, Kumar A: Long-term results after microfracture treatment for full-thickness knee chondral lesions in athletes. *Knee Surg Sports Traumatol Arthrosc* 22(9):1986–1996, 2014.
6. Gomoll AH, Probst C, Farr J, et al: Use of a type I/III bilayer collagen membrane decreases reoperation rates for symptomatic hypertrophy after autologous chondrocyte implantation. *Am J Sports Med* 37(Suppl 1):20S–23S, 2009.
7. Goyal D, Keyhani S, Lee EH, et al: Evidence-based status of microfracture technique: a systematic review of level I and II studies. *Arthroscopy* 29(9):1579–1588, 2013.

8. Gracitelli GC, Meric G, Briggs DT, et al: Fresh osteochondral allografts in the knee: comparison of primary transplantation versus transplantation after failure of previous subchondral marrow stimulation. *Am J Sports Med* 43(4):885–891, 2015.

9. Gudas R, Gudaite A, Pocius A, et al: Ten-year follow-up of a prospective, randomized clinical study of mosaic osteochondral autologous transplantation versus microfracture for the treatment of osteochondral defects in the knee joint of athletes. *Am J Sports Med* 40(11):2499–2508, 2012.

11. Horton MT, Pulido PA, McCauley JC, et al: Revision osteochondral allograft transplantations: do they work? *Am J Sports Med* 41(11):2507–2511, 2013.

13. Jungmann PM, Salzmann GM, Schmal H, et al: Autologous chondrocyte implantation for treatment of cartilage defects of the knee: what predicts the need for reintervention? *Am J Sports Med* 40(1):58–67, 2012.

14. Knutsen G, Drogset JO, Engebretsen L, et al: A randomized trial comparing autologous chondrocyte implantation with microfracture. Findings at five years. *J Bone Joint Surg Am* 89(10):2105–2112, 2007.

15. Levy YD, Gortz S, Pulido PA, et al: Do fresh osteochondral allografts successfully treat femoral condyle lesions? *Clin Orthop* 471(1):231–237, 2013.

17. Minas T, Gomoll AH, Rosenberger R, et al: Increased failure rate of autologous chondrocyte implantation after previous treatment with marrow stimulation techniques. *Am J Sports Med* 37(5):902–908, 2009.

18. Mithoefer K, McAdams T, Williams RJ, et al: Clinical efficacy of the microfracture technique for articular cartilage repair in the knee: an evidence-based systematic analysis. *Am J Sports Med* 37(10):2053–2063, 2009.

20. Pestka JM, Bode G, Salzmann G, et al: Clinical outcome of autologous chondrocyte implantation for failed microfracture treatment of full-thickness cartilage defects of the knee joint. *Am J Sports Med* 40(2):325–331, 2012.

23. Zaslav K, Cole B, Brewster R, et al: A prospective study of autologous chondrocyte implantation in patients with failed prior treatment for articular cartilage defect of the knee: results of the Study of the Treatment of Articular Repair (STAR) clinical trial. *Am J Sports Med* 37(1):42–55, 2009.

The references for this chapter can also be found on www.expertconsult.com.

34

Osteochondritis Dissecans of the Knee in the Young Patient

Matthew D. Milewski, Carl W. Nissen, Kevin G. Shea

Osteochondritis dissecans (OCD) of the knee continues to be a challenging pathology in the young patient in terms of pathogenesis and treatment. A current working definition of OCD states it is a focal, idiopathic alteration of subchondral bone with risk for instability and disruption of adjacent articular cartilage that may result in premature osteoarthritis.[30] Despite its relative low incidence, OCD of the knee has been a vexing problem for orthopedic providers, and the American Academy of Orthopaedic Surgeons have sought to address diagnosis and treatment considerations with Clinical Practice Guidelines (CPGs).[19,20] Although these CPGs exposed many of the inadequacies in the current literature for clear evidence-based treatment for OCD of the knee, these CPGs have served as goals for future research endeavors to improve diagnosis and treatment of this condition.

HISTORY

Paget first described the OCD condition in the late 19th century as a "quiet necrosis" of the bone.[81] However, Konig later named the condition OCD, believing it results from an inflammatory process.[58] This was later rejected by Konig himself and universally is thought to not be a result of an inflammatory process, but the misnomer has remained over time.[6] Although the term OCD has persisted in the orthopedic literature, it has been largely replaced by the term osteochondrosis in the basic science and veterinary literature.

EPIDEMIOLOGY

A recent study in a major managed care system identified the incidence of OCD of the knee in patients aged 6 to 19 years of age as 9.5 per 100,000 children, overall.[54] However, there was a 3.3 times increased risk of OCD in the patients 12 to 19 years old compared with those 6 to 11 years old. In addition, male patients had a 3.8 times greater risk of OCD compared with females. Seven percent of patients had bilateral lesions in this series, but other series have suggested bilaterality of OCD may occur in between 14% and 30% of cases[38,49,57,69,74] (Fig. 34.1). Overlap with some atypical variants in ossification may account for some variation in terms of incidence.[37] In terms of lesion location, medial femoral condyle lesions accounted for 64% of cases, lateral femoral condyle accounted for 32% of cases, and the patella, trochlear groove, and tibial plateau represented less than 4% of cases. This more recent data has location data that closely matches classic studies in the 1970s.[62]

PATHOPHYSIOLOGY

The pathophysiology and cause of OCD of the knee continues to be idiopathic. Multiple different theories have been considered and embraced in the past. Konig's initial inflammatory theory still has been rejected.[6,33] Other main causes have included trauma, overuse, and genetic and vascular causes. There is a possible link between OCD of the lateral femoral condyle and discoid meniscus, with possible abnormal meniscal function leading to overload of the subchondral bone cartilage in this compartment.[24,44,91] Various other theories have been proposed, including links to embolism, ossification abnormalities, patient height, endocrine function, and Osgood-Schlatter disease, but these have not been as well supported.[33,74,86,87,90]

Trauma and repetitive injury have been popular causes for OCD of the knee. Fairbank suggested the typical medial femoral condyle lesion resulted from internal tibial torsion, causing the tibial spine to repetitively impact on the medial femoral condyle.[33] However, this mechanism does not account for lesions in other areas of the knee.[49,74] Repetitive microtrauma could lead to stress fractures in the subchondral bone that is potential susceptible in terms of its vascular supply.* However, direct trauma has also only been reported in some series in 21.2% to 46% of patients with OCD and possibly in as little as 10% of young patients with OCD lesions.[2,14,45,103] It has been theorized that young athletically active children are more susceptible,[28,33,45,49,103] but even this theory has been questioned as to whether these patients are more or less active than their unaffected peers.[74]

Genetic links have been postulated for a familial form of OCD with an autosomal dominant inheritance[43,73,80,84,92] (Fig. 34.2). In contrast, Petrie along with Hefti and colleagues have conducted studies that showed a low rate of family members having associated OCD lesions.[45,83] Multiple epiphyseal dysplasia can also have a similar appearance to familiar OCD.[22,86,87] A variety of animal models have been examined to look at genetic causes of OCD.[7,68] Goat, bovine, and equine models are known, and osteochondrosis is the leading cause of lameness in horses and leg weakness in pigs. PTH1R has been identified as a strong candidate gene for OCD in equine and bovine models and shows involvement in pathways that mediate cartilage to bone transition during endochondral ossification and growth plate maturation.[7]

*References 2, 12, 14, 16, 48, and 59.

These animal models have also led to increased and renewed interest in the vascular causes of OCD lesions. It has been postulated that an area of vascular failure occurs within the subchondral bone and cartilage and has been identified in the bovine model using high resolution computed tomography (CT) and magnetic resonance imaging (MRI) scans and then confirmed with histological section.[79] Some of these animal lesions, particularly the bovine lesions, may resolve spontaneously. Further study of these animal models, particularly in experimental models, is needed to better define the cause and help guide treatment options.

HISTORY AND PHYSICAL EXAM

The presentation of young patients with OCD has a wide range of symptoms. Unfortunately, the presentation can often be

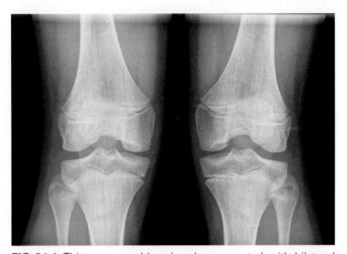

FIG 34.1 Thirteen-year-old male who presented with bilateral knee pain and radiographic evidence of bilateral medial femoral condyle lesions.

benign, with the patient often having symptoms for some time even with occasional activity related pain; they may lack swelling or mechanical symptoms that would normally alert families and clinicians to intra-articular pathology. The patient may limp occasionally and have symptoms that would be similar to more common knee problems of young athletes, such as patellofemoral syndrome.

On physical exam, unless chondral irregularities or displaced fragments are present, the exam is also benign. Tenderness to palpation may be present over the medial femoral condyle. Wilson described a maneuver that now bears his name in which the tibia, medially rotated with the knee flexed to 90 degrees, is then extended to elicit pain that may be relieved by lateral rotation.[101] However this test has more recently been found to be positive in only 25% of cases with a known OCD lesion.[23]

DIAGNOSTIC IMAGING

Because the history and physical exam findings for OCD can often be benign, initial radiographic evaluation is key to making and confirming this diagnosis. Anteroposterior, lateral, sunrise, and notch views are important for evaluation. Some lesions may be missed unless the sunrise and notch views are obtained. Bilateral views have been advocated for initial evaluation, since there has been reported to be a 14% to 30% rate of bilateral lesions.[38,49,57,69,74] Normal ossification variants can mimic OCD lesions, and bilateral radiographs can help aid in making these distinctions.[11,37] Lower limb alignment films may also be useful once the diagnosis of OCD has been made, as alignment may play a role in the origin and treatment of OCD lesions.[37,50] Left hand radiograph for bone age staging is also appropriate in young patients, so that one is able to document the appropriate skeletal maturity, as this can change treatment options. A multicenter research group has recently identified specific radiographic features for the diagnosis and prognosis of knee OCD lesions.[98] These features include location, growth plate maturity, size along with progeny (or

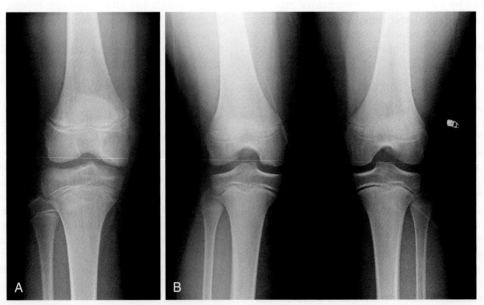

FIG 34.2 (A) Twelve-year-old female with right knee pain, found to have a medial femoral condyle OCD lesion; (B) 13-year-old male (brother) presented 1 year later with right knee pain and found to have a similar medial femoral condyle OCD lesion.

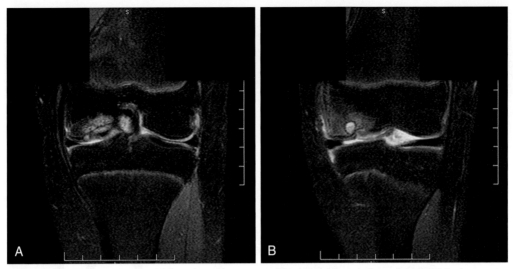

FIG 34.3 (A) Thirteen-year-old female with an unstable medial femoral condyle OCD lesion; note the cyst-like structure (B).

lesion) bone fragmentation, displacement, boundary, central radiodensity, and contour. Further studies will need to define the most reliable specific radiographic features that correlate with prognosis and healing.

Historically, a bone scan has been recommended by Cahill et al. to determine the healing status of the lesion and to rule out normal ossification variants.[12,15,16] Few centers, if any, use bone scans routinely now, because of the availability of MRI. CT scans have been recommended by Cepero et al. in evaluating the extent and location of OCD lesions in young patients, particularly if they have trouble staying still for an MRI, but this does pose the increased risk of radiation exposure.[18]

MRI has become the imaging modality of choice after initial radiographs have been obtained for the evaluation of OCD lesions and may be more useful for evaluating the articular cartilage integrity, subchondral bone status, and assessing stability of a particular lesion. De Smet et al. defined four criteria for instability of OCD lesions in adults on MRI, with 97% specificity and 100% sensitivity.[25] These four criteria included a hyper-intense signal seen on T2 sequences at the fragment-femur interface, adjacent focal cystic (high signal intensity) areas, a focal defect in articular cartilage (>5 mm), and a hyper-intense signal line equal to fluid that traverses both articular cartilage and subchondral bone. Kijowski et al. refined the previously mentioned MRI criteria for instability in juvenile patients.[55] Their criteria included a rim-like hyperintense signal equal to joint fluid, with a second deeper linear margin of low signal and multiple sites of discontinuity of subchondral bone. These criteria yielded 100% sensitivity and specificity for instability in juvenile patients. They also found multiple cyst-like foci or a single cyst-like focus greater than 5 mm in size was highly specific for instability (100%) but had low sensitivity (25% to 38%) (Fig. 34.3). Further studies will be needed to assess not just instability features at initial diagnosis but also potential for healing.

TREATMENT

A variety of treatment options are available for OCD of the knee, depending on the patient's age, stability, location, and size of the lesion. The goals of treatment of OCD of the knee in the young patient is to save the native bone/cartilage progeny fragment if possible, ultimately prevent early onset osteoarthritis through early detection, prompt initial treatment, recognize signs of instability, and design interventions to facilitate lesion healing or salvaging lesions not amenable to healing. There are unfortunately few high quality high-level evidence studies to guide the treatment of OCD of the knee.

INITIAL MANAGEMENT

Younger patients, particularly those with open physes, have a better potential for healing.[3,99] Some studies have suggested that medial femoral condyle OCD lesions have a better prognosis for healing.[36,96] Initial conservative management for the young patient with open physes and stable lesions as defined on initial imaging is generally recommended. Wall and colleagues developed a nomogram to help predict the potential for healing in this young population.[99] Age, lesion size, and the presence of mechanical symptoms could predict healing with conservative treatment in approximately two-thirds of patients. There is no consensus in the literature in regard to how best to treat patients conservatively. Healing has been reported in up to 50% of OCD lesions in young patients at an average of 10 months, with activity restrictions but not mobility or weight bearing restrictions.[12,14,16] In contrast, other studies have reported good to excellent results with bracing or casting,[38,85,99] and there remains no consensus on the exact methods for conservative treatment.[19,20,45]

SURGICAL TREATMENT

Indications for surgical intervention in the treatment of OCD of the knee in young patients is reserved for those patients that have symptomatic, stable lesions and have shown no progressive healing on imaging after a minimum of 3 months of appropriate nonoperative treatment, along with those patients that present with an unstable or displaced lesion.[19,20,57] Untreated, unstable lesions can be a precursor to osteoarthritis at a young age and require prompt treatment.[12,13] Goals of surgical

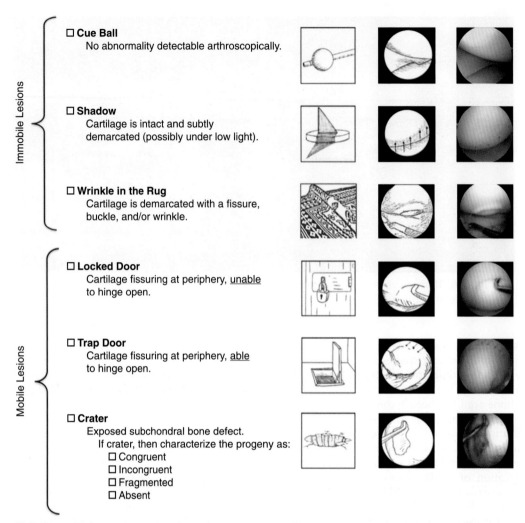

Immobile Lesions

☐ **Cue Ball**
No abnormality detectable arthroscopically.

☐ **Shadow**
Cartilage is intact and subtly demarcated (possibly under low light).

☐ **Wrinkle in the Rug**
Cartilage is demarcated with a fissure, buckle, and/or wrinkle.

Mobile Lesions

☐ **Locked Door**
Cartilage fissuring at periphery, <u>unable</u> to hinge open.

☐ **Trap Door**
Cartilage fissuring at periphery, <u>able</u> to hinge open.

☐ **Crater**
Exposed subchondral bone defect.
If crater, then characterize the progeny as:
    ☐ Congruent
    ☐ Incongruent
    ☐ Fragmented
    ☐ Absent

FIG 34.4 ROCK Arthroscopy Classification. (From Carey JL, 3rd, Wall EJ, Shea KG, et al: Reliability of the ROCK osteochondritis dissecans knee arthroscopy classification system—multi-center validation study. *Am J Sports Med* 44(7):1694–1698, 2016. Fig. 34.1.)

intervention include an assessment of lesion stability at the time of arthroscopy, stabilization of the lesion, restoration or improvement in lesion blood supply, and subchondral bone/cartilage restoration or replacement as salvage if needed.

Assessment of stability at the time of arthroscopy is crucial to understanding the stability of the lesion and to help guide treatment. Multiple grading systems and classifications have been described, but none of the prior systems have been rigorously assessed for inter- and intra-rater reliability.[†] Recently, a multicenter research group has developed and validated an arthroscopic classification system[17] (Fig. 34.4).

Surgical treatment options for OCD of the knee involve several different goals, each with different techniques. These goals including drilling to stimulate or incite a vascular healing response to the avascular subchondral bone; fixation to stabilize loose subchondral bone and articular cartilage; bone grafting when needed to support articular cartilage contour, stability, and vascularity; and when needed, salvage of the articular cartilage and subchondral bone with biologic replacements.

Drilling of OCD lesions of the knee in young patients is designed to stimulate a healing response by disruption of the sclerotic margin and introduction of biologic factors from adjacent healthy cancellous bone.[46] It is indicated for lesions found to be stable at the time of arthroscopy in skeletally immature patients that have failed conservative treatment. Drilling of stable lesions has been reported to produce high rates of healing.[1,9,29,42,46]

Three main techniques are available for drilling: transarticular, retroarticular, and notch drilling.[46] The advantage of transarticular drilling includes direct visualization of the lesion while drilling to ensure adequate spacing and coverage of the lesion, with the disadvantage being disruption of the articular surface with the drill holes. Generally, small smooth K-wires are used in this technique, with either a 0.062- or 0.045-inch wire with about 6 to 10 passes of the wire to uniformly cover the lesion with several millimeters of separation between the drill passes.[5,56]

Retroarticular drilling has the advantage of not disrupting the articular cartilage surface, allowing for more passes, and may allow better access for posteriori lesions surface but has several disadvantages, including being more technically challenging and requiring fluoroscopic guidance and the requisite

---

[†]References 21, 32, 41, 51, 52, 77, and 90.

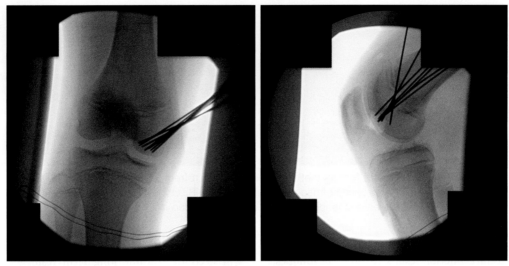

FIG 34.5 Fluoroscopic images of a 12-year-old female that failed conservative treatment for a medial femoral condyle OCD lesion and was found to be stable at arthroscopy and underwent retroarticular drilling.

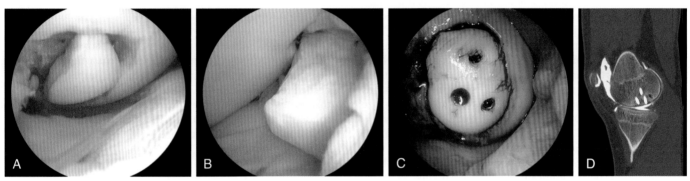

FIG 34.6 Sixteen-year-old male with right knee unstable OCD (A and B) treated with open reduction internal fixation and bone grafting (C). CT arthrogram (D) shows near complete osseous union and slight thinning of articular cartilage prior to screw removal.

radiation exposure[46] (Fig. 34.5). It is also possible to miss the progeny bone with this technique. Gunton et al. reviewed several studies using retroarticular drilling and found an 86% healing rate at 5.6 months.[42] Retroarticular drilling with retroarticular bone grafting has also been described and is technically demanding and not as widely used.[61,64]

Drilling through the intercondylar notch is similar to transarticular drilling, except the point of pin entry is through the bare area of the notch and thus doesn't violate the articular cartilage surface.[53] The disadvantages of this technique relate to the fact that only a portion of some larger lesions will be accessible through the notch. It can often be combined with other techniques to optimize drilling coverage and spread while minimizing articular cartilage disruption.

Fixation is generally indicated for unstable but salvageable OCD lesions (Fig. 34.6). A variety of different fixation devices and techniques have been described.[39,55a] Metal variable-pitch and cannulated screws have been used for years and have the advantage of reliable compression but may necessitate removal later to prevent iatrogenic joint damage if the metal screw becomes prominent through the articular cartilage.[59,93,102] They also may interfere with postoperative imaging, and thus, titanium options may be preferred over stainless steel screws. Biodegradable pins/rods have been used in the past

and more recently evolved into biodegradable screws.[27] The advantages include rigid fixation that obviates the need for hardware removal and does not interfere with secondary MRI imaging postoperatively. The disadvantages include breakage of the device, difficulty with insertion at times, loss of fixation, formation of cystic lesions around the screws, and possible foreign body immune response.[26,35,88,95] Biologic fixation techniques have also been used for the fixation of OCD lesions of the knee. Miniaci and Tytherleigh-Strong used autogenous osteochondral grafting (mosaicplasty) with excellent results, but this is a technically demanding procedure that requires a graft long enough to pass through the lesion and into normal subchondral bone.[70] Navarro and colleagues have described a technique for fixation using autologous "bone sticks" from the proximal tibia, with satisfactory results in 90% of cases.[76] Overall, the literature supports fixation of salvageable OCD lesions with good to excellent results, using a variety of fixation strategies and techniques.

Although salvage of native cartilage and bone has been shown to have better results than excision,[4,40,66,75,94] some lesions cannot be salvaged, and alternative treatment options are necessary in these circumstances. Microfracture or marrow stimulation techniques have been used in the treatment of OCD lesions, but the depth of bone loss makes this technique more

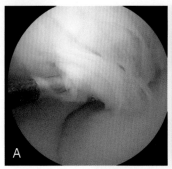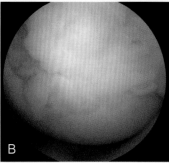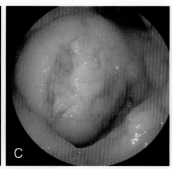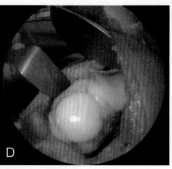

FIG 34.7 Fourteen-year-old female that failed previous microfracture for a large medial femoral condyle OCD lesion. Arthroscopy images are shown in A–B. Open arthrotomy is shown in C. Twenty-five millimeters osteochondral allograft has been placed in D.

challenging. In a small prospective series, microfracture has been shown to produce inferior results to other techniques, including osteochondral autograft transplantation (OAT).[40] In addition, it is important to consider not only the deficient articular cartilage issue with unsalvageable OCD lesions but also the deficient subchondral bone. Therefore, it is important for surgeons treating these lesions to have strategies in place to rebuild the subchondral bone in addition to "resurfacing" the articular cartilage surface. OAT has been a popular technique for addressing unsalvageable OCD lesions, as it addresses both the deficient articular cartilage and subchondral bone. It has shown good clinical results in small to medium sized lesions and defects.[40,70,71] Results seem to deteriorate when lesion size exceeds 6 cm^2.[47,100] OAT has also been combined with screw fixation with good results.[63] Limitations to this technique include the size limits, as mentioned previously, along with donor site morbidity. However, donor site morbidity has been reported to not be as significant in younger patients.[78]

Fresh frozen osteochondral allografts represent another salvage technique (Fig. 34.7). The advantages of this technique include no donor site morbidity, and this can be used for large lesions as needed. Disadvantages include concerns about lack of bone integration between graft and host, host immune response, and chondrocyte viability after transplantation. Multiple authors have shown good results, using these allografts for posttraumatic cartilage defects of the knee.[10,67,89] Two studies have examined fresh osteochondral allograft for large OCD lesions with Emmerson et al., showing 5 year survivorship at 91%.[31,65] Further studies will need to confirm the long term results of these early reports for osteochondral allografts in young patients with large defects from unsalvageable OCD lesions.

Autologous chondrocyte/cartilage implantation (ACI) is another salvage technique for OCD of the knee. The advantages of this technique include use of the patient's own chondrocytes, along with long-term data showing good survivorship and clinical results in osteochondral defect treatment.[‡] The disadvantages include the cost along with need for a second surgery for the biopsy of the chondrocytes. It is also important to know that subchondral bone also needs to be replaced or built up to support the implanted chondrocytes. Initial complications associated with periosteal flap overgrowth have improved with new collagen matrices. Good outcomes have been shown at midterm time points for ACI in the treatment of specifically OCD lesions of the knee, with better results being correlated with younger patients and smaller lesions.[34,60,82] Further studies will need to examine long term results—particularly those associated with new matrix associated ACI treatment strategies and techniques in the treatment of unsalvageable knee OCD lesions in young patients.

CONCLUSION

OCD is a focal, idiopathic alteration of subchondral bone with risk for instability and disruption of adjacent articular cartilage that may result in premature osteoarthritis. Further research is needed to better define the exact cause and pathophysiology of this condition. Well-designed multicenter trials and prospective cohorts are needed to evaluate the various treatment options and strategies for this condition.

KEY REFERENCES

12. Cahill BR: Osteochondritis dissecans of the knee: treatment of juvenile and adult forms. *J Am Acad Orthop Surg* 3:237–247, 1995.
14. Cahill BR, Ahten SM: The three critical components in the conservative treatment of juvenile osteochondritis dissecans (JOCD). Physician, parent, and child. *Clin Sports Med* 20:287–298, 2001.
16. Cahill BR, Phillips MR, Navarro R: The results of conservative management of juvenile osteochondritis dissecans using joint scintigraphy. *Am J Sports Med* 17:601–606, 1989.
38. Green WT, Banks HH: Osteochondritis dissecans in children. *J Bone Joint Surg Am* 35:26–64, 1953.
55a. Kocher MS, Czarnecki JJ, Andersen JS, et al: Internal fixation of juvenile osteochondritis dissecans lesions of the knee. *Am J Sports Med* 35:712–718, 2007.
74. Mubarak SJ, Carroll NC: Juvenile osteochondritis dissecans of the knee: cause. *Clin Orthop* 157:200–211, 1981.
75. Murray JRD, Chitnavis J, Dixon P, et al: Osteochondritis dissecans of the knee; long-term clinical outcome following arthroscopic debridement. *Knee* 14:94–98, 2007.
82. Peterson L, Minas T, Brittberg M, et al: Treatment of osteochondritis dissecans of the knee with autologous chondrocyte transplantation: results at two to ten years. *J Bone Joint Surg Am* 85:17–24, 2003.
85. Pill SG, Ganley TJ, Milam RA, et al: Role of magnetic resonance imaging and clinical criteria in predicting successful nonoperative treatment of osteochondritis dissecans in children. *J Pediatr Orthop* 23:102–108, 2003.
99. Wall EJ, Vourazeris J, Myer GD, et al: The healing potential of stable juvenile osteochondritis dissecans knee lesions. *J Bone Joint Surg Am* 90:2655–2664, 2008.
103. Yoshida S, Ikata T, Takai H, et al: Osteochondritis dissecans of the femoral condyle in the growth stage. *Clin Orthop* 346:162–170, 1998.

‡References 8, 34, 60, 72, 82, and 97.

The references for this chapter can also be found on www.expertconsult.com.

35

Secondary, Spontaneous, and Postarthroscopy Osteonecrosis of the Knee: Diagnosis and Management

Eric J. Strauss, Brandon J. Erickson, Charles Bush-Joseph, Bernard R. Bach, Jr.

Defined as the in situ death of a segment of bone, osteonecrosis occurs secondary to a compromise in osseous blood supply. Although more commonly seen affecting the femoral head, osteonecrosis of the knee has the potential to progress to irreversible changes, causing significant symptomatology, disability, and pain. This disease process may eventually require operative intervention. In addition to the secondary osteonecrosis (also termed *avascular necrosis* [AVN]) associated with corticosteroid exposure, alcohol consumption, sickle cell disease, and other common predisposing factors, two other types of osteonecrosis of the knee have been described: spontaneous osteonecrosis of the knee (SPONK) and osteonecrosis in the postoperative knee (ONPK).

First described in 1968 by Ahlback et al.,[3] SPONK has been recognized as a distinct clinical entity, with the potential to cause significant morbidity.[39,63] In contrast to cases of secondary osteonecrosis, SPONK tends to affect a different patient population, mainly older female patients, with a different pattern of bony involvement. More recently, osteonecrosis of the knee following arthroscopic surgery has been described, most commonly following arthroscopic meniscectomy. Initially reported by Brahme et al.[14] in 1991, ONPK has also been noted to occur subsequent to anterior cruciate ligament reconstruction and chondroplasty procedures.[10,24,58]

This chapter will review the current knowledge of these entities, describing their clinical and radiographic presentation, hypothesized cause, strategies for management, and clinical outcomes.

SPONTANEOUS OSTEONECROSIS OF THE KNEE

SPONK is a disorder of uncertain cause, classically described as a focal lesion occurring in the medial femoral condyle of a patient in the fifth or sixth decade of life, with women affected almost 3 to 5 times as commonly as men.* Typically, patients present with the sudden onset of severe pain, localizing to the medial aspect of the knee just proximal to the joint line. Although a traumatic cause has been implicated in SPONK, only a minority of patients recall a specific injury that precipitated their symptoms. In the acute phase of the disease, patients will often report pain with weight-bearing activities localized to the involved area of the knee and an increase in the severity of their pain at night. Depending on the stage of the lesion and its size, this acute-phase pain will either gradually resolve (often within 6 to 10 weeks) or become chronically debilitating.

Clinical Evaluation

Examination of the affected knee in the acute phase of SPONK, typically the first 6 to 8 weeks following symptom onset, will demonstrate a small to moderate effusion, with limitation of range of motion secondary to pain and associated muscle spasm. Palpation will often elicit a localized area of tenderness over the involved area, typically noted as the medial femoral condyle, just proximal to the joint line in the flexed knee. Although the medial femoral condyle is most commonly affected in spontaneous osteonecrosis of the knee, lesions involving the medial tibial plateau, the lateral femoral condyle, and rarely, the patella have also been reported in the orthopedic literature.† Identifying the area of maximal tenderness to palpation can serve as a guide to localizing the involved area. Patients with SPONK have been shown to have concomitant medial meniscal tears, often involving the meniscal root, and may have meniscal findings on examination. Ligamentous examination of the affected knee is typically normal in cases of SPONK.

Causes

Similar to the proposed mechanisms associated with osteonecrosis of the femoral head, two main causes have been suggested in the pathogenesis of SPONK—traumatic and vascular. With most affected patients being older women (typically in the sixth decade of life) with osteoporotic bone, some believe that SPONK develops as a consequence of microfractures occurring in weak subchondral bone secondary to minor trauma.[40] It has been suggested that following an episode of trauma to the knee, fluid enters the intercondylar region, filling the potential space created by the subchondral microfractures in the femoral condyle.[9,33,70] This fluid increases the intraosseous pressure in the area, leading to focal osseous ischemia and eventual necrosis. Researchers have questioned this theory as the mechanism of SPONK. Mears et al.[43] performed histopathologic evaluation of specimens

---

*References 3, 8, 34, 39, 63, and 70.

†References 8, 21, 22, 34, 40, 41, 57, 63, and 70.

taken from 24 patients diagnosed with SPONK and found that only 1 patient had evidence of bone necrosis. Of the specimens in this study, 75% had demonstrable osteoporosis, implying that osteonecrosis is more of a secondary phenomenon following insufficiency fracture, rather than the primary inciting mechanism of the disease. Others have supported the insufficiency stress fracture theory as the cause of SPONK, believing that when bony necrosis develops, it occurs as a consequence of physiologic resorption and remodeling following fracture.[34,55,67] This often occurs in older postmenopausal women.

Where a vascular cause continues to be the dominant theory for osteonecrosis of the femoral head, with up to 75% of affected patients showing evidence of an underlying thrombophilia or coagulopathy, these predisposing factors have yet to be consistently demonstrated in patients with SPONK.[32,39] In the hip, many believe that the presence of a coagulation disorder, including resistance of activated protein C, low tissue plasminogen activator activity, and hypofibrinolysis, causes intraosseous venous occlusion that culminates in the hypoxic death of bone. Evaluation of the coagulation profiles of patients affected with SPONK is necessary to determine whether this mechanism is present in the pathogenesis of the disease. Glueck et al. evaluated six patients with thrombophilia (four of whom had concurrent hypofibrinolysis) and stage II SPONK who were treated with enoxaparin to prevent subchondral collapse and progression to arthritis and found that no one progressed to joint collapse or severe arthritis. Four patients were asymptomatic at 15.1 years follow-up, one improved on rivaroxaban after failing enoxaparin, and one had residual pain at 2.25 years. All patients required assistive devices for ambulation prior to treatment, compared to no one following treatment. Although this is a small series of patients, the results suggest that testing for thrombophilia and/or hypofibrinolysis in patients with SPONK may allow directed treatment with anticoagulation.

The presence of a medial meniscal tear has been proposed as a potential third cause behind the development of SPONK.[52,56] Case series have identified medial meniscal tears in 50% to 78% of patients with SPONK, with a recent series by Robertson et al.[65] noting that tears, specifically in the area of the meniscal root, coexisted with spontaneous osteonecrosis in 24 of their 30 patients (80%). They theorized that in older patients with osteoporotic bone, discontinuity of the medial meniscus results in loss of hoop stress distribution in the medial compartment, increasing the load experienced in the femoral condyle and potentially predisposing patients to the development of subchondral insufficiency fracture. No study to date has proven a causal relationship between meniscal tears and SPONK, although there certainly appears to be a positive association.

Radiographic Evaluation and Staging

Cases of suspected SPONK should be initially evaluated with a plain, weight-bearing x-ray series of the knee, including an anteroposterior, 45-degree flexion posteroanterior, lateral, and skyline or Merchant views. Early in the disease process, plain x-rays may fail to identify any abnormalities, despite the presence of significant symptomatology. As the condition progresses, plain film findings may include a radiolucent lesion with a surrounding sclerotic halo in addition to subtle flattening of the involved femoral condyle (Fig. 35.1). In advanced cases, with significant subchondral collapse, secondary degenerative changes may be evident, with loss of joint space, sclerosis in the medial tibial plateau, and osteophyte formation (Fig. 35.2).

Several staging systems have been described for SPONK, based on plain radiographs.[2,39,63,70] In the four-tiered system described by Koshino,[36] stage I disease is defined as incipient, with patients reporting pain with activity; however, plain x-rays are negative for pathology. In stage II SPONK, or the avascular stage, a round to oval subchondral lucency in the weight-bearing area is present, with associated increased density in the surrounding femoral condyle. Subchondral collapse heralds stage III SPONK. During the collapse or developed stage of disease (stage III), x-rays demonstrate a sclerotic halo bordering the radiolucent lesion. Further subchondral collapse with associated development of arthritic changes in the affected compartment defines stage IV disease.

Aglietti et al.[2] have modified the Koshino staging system to include five stages of disease. In stage I, the x-rays are normal in appearance.[39] Subtle flattening of the affected femoral condyle characterizes stage II SPONK, which indicates the potential for subsequent collapse. Stage III describes the characteristic radiolucent lesion with a circumferential sclerotic border, and stage IV disease is heralded by an increase in the size of the sclerotic halo as the subchondral bone begins to collapse. Stage V SPONK includes continued subchondral collapse, with the development of associated secondary degenerative changes.

Prognostic implications can be made based on the plain x-ray appearance of the lesion, primarily based on its overall size or percentage of the condyle that is involved. The width of the lesion can be measured on the anteroposterior view, with those measuring less than 1 cm classified as small and those more than 1 cm classified as large.[3,50,70] In many of the early studies of SPONK, the area of the lesion within the condyle was used to predict which cases would progress to severe degenerative arthritis.[40,51] Cases in which the lesion was less than 2.5 cm² were unlikely to progress, whereas those with an area more than 5 cm² were considered to have a poor prognosis. Another useful plain x-ray measurement is the ratio of the width of the lesion compared with the overall width of the femoral condyle on the

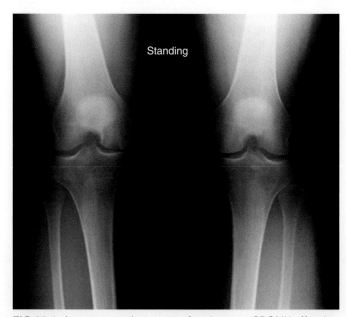

Standing

FIG 35.1 Anteroposterior x-rays of early stage SPONK affecting the right medial femoral condyle developing in a 67-year-old man.

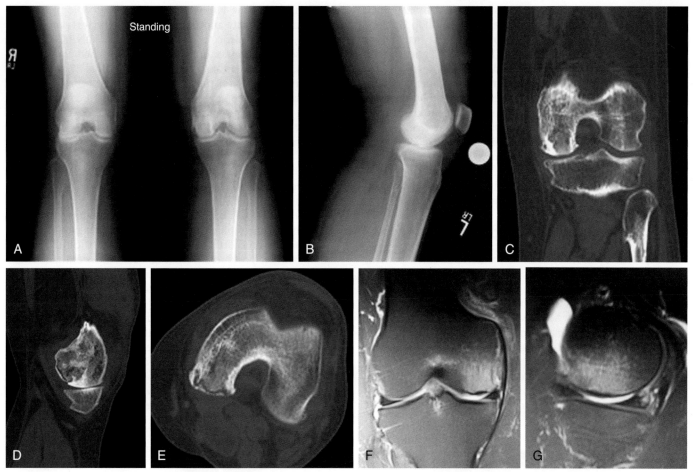

FIG 35.2 (A-G) Anteroposterior and lateral x-rays and CT scan cuts depicting late-stage SPONK with collapse and associated degenerative changes in a 71-year-old male patient who went on to require total knee arthroplasty. Coronal and sagittal T2 MRI slices demonstrating SPONK of the medial femoral condyle in a 64-year-old female patient.

anteroposterior view to obtain a percentage of the condyle that is involved.[2,7] This measure is not affected by differences in magnification of the view and has been shown to correlate with prognosis. Studies have demonstrated that good outcomes were common in lesions with a size ratio less than 0.45, whereas those with a ratio more than 0.5 typically progress to severe degenerative arthritis.[39] A recent long-term population study found that 0 of 10 (0%) patients with lesions of less than 0.2 required surgery, while 6 of 7 (85.7%) patients with lesions greater than 0.4 required some form of surgery during the follow-up period.

In both the hip and the knee, magnetic resonance imaging (MRI) has become the standard imaging modality for the detection of osteonecrosis. MRI is both sensitive and specific for the evaluation of SPONK, often demonstrating more extensive involvement than was evident on plain radiography.[‡] T1-weighted imaging in cases of SPONK shows a discrete low-signal area, often surrounded by an area of intermediate signal intensity. A serpiginous low signal line is often present at the margin of the lesion, delineating the necrotic area from the adjacent area of bone marrow edema. T2-weighted images typically show high signal intensity at the lesion edge, in the

region of the bone marrow edema. Some have suggested using gadolinium-enhanced MRI for the evaluation of cases of SPONK. The addition of gadolinium is believed to provide information on the extent of osseous activity and turnover at the edges of the lesion, with enhanced adjacent activity believed to be a positive prognostic sign indicative of healing potential.

Clinical Course

The course and prognosis of patients with spontaneous osteonecrosis of the knee are dependent on the size and stage of the lesion. Most patients present with a similar history and physical examination. Pain is often severe at symptom onset and is present with weight bearing, with a typical increase in severity at night, and has a significant impact on the patient's daily activities. The intense pain associated with the acute phase of SPONK may last up to 6 weeks, at which point the extent of the patient's symptoms divides them into two main groups.[39] Those who will have a satisfactory outcome will typically report improvement in their pain and intermittent swelling after the 6-week time point, although mild symptoms with activity may continue for up to 12 to 18 months. These patients most commonly have smaller lesions evident on imaging studies, with lesions usually less than 20% to 40% of the width of the involved femoral condyle. Despite significant improvement in their

‡References 12, 14, 39, 61, 69, and 70.

symptoms and the ability to resume normal daily activities, most patients with SPONK will eventually develop osteoarthritic changes in the involved compartment. Insall[29] has reported that at 2-year follow-up, almost all patients with osteonecrosis of the knee have evidence of at least grade I osteoarthritis, with joint space narrowing. Patients whose symptoms fail to improve after 6 weeks tend to follow a more relentless and progressive disease course. They are more typically those with large lesions encompassing more than 50% of the width of their femoral condyle. These patients, in the poor prognosis group, often never report improvement in their knee function or extent of pain. Serial imaging will often demonstrate a rapid progression with collapse and the subsequent development of degenerative changes in the affected compartment.

OSTEONECROSIS IN THE POSTOPERATIVE KNEE

First reported by Brahme et al.[14] in a series of seven patients who developed radiographic evidence of osteonecrosis following the arthroscopic treatment of meniscal pathology, ONPK has been recognized as a rare but significant complication of arthroscopic surgery.[58,70] Many early case reports describing this entity found it subsequent to arthroscopic meniscectomy, leading it to be referred to as postmeniscectomy osteonecrosis of the knee. However, more recently, osteonecrosis lesions have been noted to occur following other arthroscopic procedures, including chondroplasty and anterior cruciate ligament reconstruction—hence the current name of ONPK.[10,24,31]

Considering the large number of arthroscopic procedures performed annually and the relatively few reports of cases of ONPK, the prevalence is low.[31] At present, ONPK following arthroscopic meniscectomy has been described in 9 clinical studies, including a total of 47 patients.[58] In all 47 cases, postoperative MRI demonstrated evidence of osteonecrosis that was not present in preoperative imaging studies. In contrast to the patient population typically affected by SPONK, ONPK tends to affect slightly younger patients (mean, 58 years; range, 21 to 82 years), with an equal gender distribution (23 women and 24 men).[70]

In these 47 patients, lesions of ONPK predominantly affect the medial femoral condyle (39 [82%]), followed by the lateral femoral condyle (4), lateral tibial plateau (2), and medial tibial plateau (1). In each of the reported cases, osteonecrosis developed in the geographic location of the patient's pathology and arthroscopic procedure, with none arising in the contralateral compartment postoperatively (Fig. 35.3). Concomitant chondral lesions in the region of the meniscal tear were reported to exist in 65% of patients who went on to ONPK, with chondromalacia of the medial compartment noted to exist in 33 of these 47 published cases. One further study reported 5 cases of OPNK but did not give enough clinical data about the patients to list along with the previously mentioned 47 patients.

In patients who develop osteonecrosis of the knee following arthroscopic surgery, symptoms of pain, swelling, and limited range of motion may persist or even worsen postoperatively, despite the fact that an adequate resection of their meniscal tear

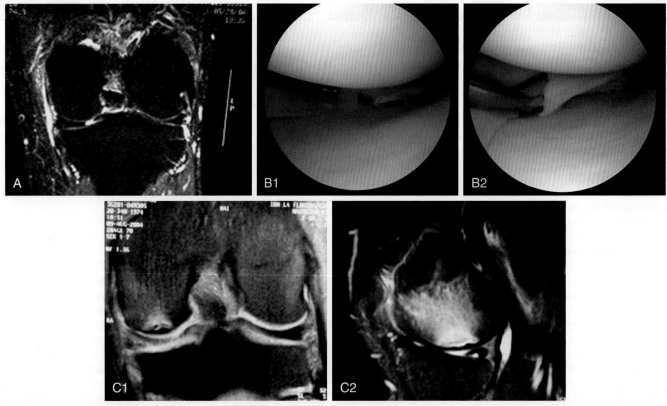

FIG 35.3 (A) Preoperative MRI scan demonstrating medial meniscal tear with no evidence of pathology affecting the medial femoral condyle. (B) Intraoperative arthroscopic images demonstrating radial tear of the posterior horn of the medial meniscus. (C) Postoperative MRI scan demonstrating changes within the medial femoral condyle indicative of ONPK.

was performed.[24,31,53,58] Cases of persistent or worsening symptoms after knee arthroscopy need to be considered for the possibility of an evolving osteonecrosis lesion, a diagnosis that needs to be distinguished from SPONK, bone marrow edema syndrome, and a recurrent meniscal tear.

Clinical Evaluation

Patients with ONPK typically report continued or increased pain in the medial aspect of their knee postoperatively. Examination of the affected knee will often demonstrate a small to moderate effusion with limitation of range of motion secondary to pain and associated muscle spasm, similar to what was seen preoperatively. Palpation will elicit localized tenderness over the medial joint line and medial femoral condyle, provided the lesion is located in this region. The ligamentous examination will often be normal.

Cause

At present, the exact cause of ONPK has yet to be fully elucidated. Similar to the previously described correlation of meniscal tears with the development of spontaneous osteonecrosis of the knee, some believe that altered knee biomechanics following meniscectomy are responsible for the pathogenesis of the disease.[53,58,68] Previous studies have shown that approximately 50% of joint compressive forces are transmitted through the meniscus in extension and up to 85% of the load in 90 degrees of knee flexion.[4] Partial meniscectomy increases tibiofemoral contact pressures in the treated compartment, potentially leading to subchondral insufficiency fractures from altered load transmission. Histopathologic evaluation of specimens from cases of ONPK have supported this theory, demonstrating evidence of subchondral insufficiency fractures, with bony necrosis present distal to the fracture site.[67] A corollary to the insufficiency fracture theory of ONPK is the possibility that overly aggressive postoperative rehabilitation contributes to the development of this condition. In an attempt to restore function, rapid resumption of weight-bearing activities and exercise are often started within days of the operative procedure. It is possible that if aggressive therapy is resumed prior to bony remodeling in response to the altered load distribution that occurs postmeniscectomy, insufficiency fractures may develop.

Others have hypothesized that the pathologic articular cartilage in the affected compartment has increased permeability to arthroscopic fluid.[58,62] This increase in fluid permeability may also occur following the instrumentation of the articular surface, during shaving chondroplasty, or with inadvertent contact of arthroscopic instruments with the femoral condyle during meniscectomy. Influx of arthroscopy fluid may cause subchondral edema and subsequent osteonecrosis from increased intraosseous pressure. Localized osteoarticular injury from the use of a laser or radiofrequency probe during the arthroscopic procedure has been described as a third potential cause of ONPK.[23,27,37,70] It has been proposed that direct thermal injury or injury from photoacoustic shock from these instruments induces an inflammatory response, leading to bony edema, increased local intraosseous pressure, and eventual osteonecrosis, although this has yet to be proven.

Radiographic Evaluation and Staging

In the early stages of osteonecrosis in the postoperative knee, because the disease is primarily one of bone marrow, plain x-rays are of limited value in the initial workup. Although the bone scan will often be positive in cases of ONPK, with a high level of sensitivity for changes in local osseous vascularity, its specificity and spatial resolution are poor. The diagnosis of ONPK is dependent on MRI findings of the affected joint, with two specific criteria that need to be filled: the absence of osteonecrosis on preoperative MRI performed 4 to 6 weeks after the onset of symptoms and a time association between the arthroscopic procedure and the development of a suspicious bone marrow edema pattern on postoperative MRI scans.[31,52,58,59]

To distinguish cases of ONPK from those of SPONK, the preoperative MRI must be normal with respect to the condition of the bone and bone marrow of the medial and lateral femoral condyles and medial and lateral tibial plateaus. However, it is important to acknowledge that in the early stages of spontaneous osteonecrosis of the knee, MRI of the affected knee may be devoid of findings; this is described as the window period of SPONK, between symptom onset and MRI evidence of signal changes. Most authors have reported using a period of 4 to 6 weeks following the development of symptoms as sufficient time for radiographic evidence of SPONK to be present.[31,58] This is largely based on an animal study by Nakamura et al.,[54] in which MRI changes developed in all specimens by 4 weeks following surgically induced femoral head osteonecrosis. The distinction between SPONK and ONPK may not be possible with imaging studies performed prior to this 4- to 6-week time point of symptom onset.

A temporal association between the arthroscopic procedure and postoperative MRI signal changes must be present for the diagnosis of ONPK to be made. In the nine clinical studies, reporting cases of osteonecrosis in the postoperative knee, the mean time between arthroscopy and MRI establishing the diagnosis of ONPK was 18 weeks (range, 3 to 176 weeks).[58] This criterion is more difficult to assess and qualify, because bone marrow edema commonly occurs following arthroscopic knee procedures. In a study of 93 patients with a mean age of 36.6 years undergoing arthroscopic meniscectomy, Kobayashi et al.[35] found that 34% had MRI evidence of bone marrow edema in the operative compartment within 8 months of their procedure. Although it may be related to the age of the patients in this study, none progressed to ONPK.

MRI performed in the early stages of ONPK will demonstrate a nonspecific large area of bone marrow edema in the femoral condyle, ipsilateral to the prior meniscectomy, with heterogenous signal present on T2 imaging. By 3 months postoperatively, the extent of edema typically decreases, and MRI findings in cases of ONPK are similar to those seen in cases of SPONK, with T1 imaging showing a discrete low-signal area surrounded by an area of intermediate signal intensity. A line of low signal is often present at the margin of the lesion, delineating the necrotic area from the adjacent area of bone marrow edema. T2 images will typically show a high signal intensity at the lesion edge, in the region of the bone marrow edema. As the lesion progresses to its final stages, bone sequestration may be present, with a surrounding high signal rim, along with condylar flattening and the possibility of loose body development.[6,58]

Clinical Course

Review of the 47 reported cases of ONPK shows that 93.6% (44 of 47) had permanent lesions evident on MRI or progressed to irreversible stages of disease. Of these cases, 17 required additional operative intervention, with 9 undergoing total knee arthroplasty, 6 having repeat arthroscopy, and 2 treated with high tibial osteotomy.

In contrast to the correlation of clinical course and prognosis with the size of the lesion in SPONK, this correlation has been less reliable in cases of ONPK. Rapid progression of disease occurred in five of seven cases of ONPK, with a mean lesion size of 40% of the width of the femoral condyle in a series by Johnson et al.,[31] but a similar series by Muscolo et al.[53] found a mean lesion size of 24%. From the available data, it appears that in susceptible patients, even those with small areas of postoperative bone marrow signal changes have the potential to progress to osteonecrosis. Further study of cases of osteonecrosis in the postoperative knee is required in an effort to identify useful factors for predicting prognosis.

COMPARISON OF SPONTANEOUS OSTEONECROSIS OF THE KNEE, OSTEONECROSIS IN THE POSTOPERATIVE KNEE, AND SECONDARY OSTEONECROSIS OF THE KNEE

During the evaluation of patients with suspected SPONK or ONPK, the treating orthopedic surgeon must also consider other potential causes of osteonecrosis affecting the knee. In contrast to cases of SPONK or ONPK (in which patients tend to be older, have isolated, unilateral joint involvement, and no identifiable risk factors for disease), secondary osteonecrosis or AVN occurs in a younger patient population (≤45 years), tends to affect multiple condyles simultaneously, and is bilateral in approximately 80% of affected patients. Additionally, patients with secondary osteonecrosis of the knee have involvement of other sites, including the femoral head (in 90% or more of cases) and proximal humerus with a history of risk factors for AVN[22] (Table 35.1).

In the early stages, patients with secondary osteonecrosis often present with the gradual onset of a traumatic, mild, bilateral knee pain.[70] The location of the pain may vary depending on the number, size, and distribution of the necrotic foci, with most patients reporting symptoms on both the medial and lateral aspects of their knees. In addition to coincident symptoms in their hips and shoulders, most patients with secondary osteonecrosis have identifiable risk factors for disease, including corticosteroid exposure, alcohol consumption, sickle cell disease, and systemic lupus erythematosus (Box 35.1). Compared with the small focal disease seen in cases of SPONK and ONPK, the radiographic workup of patients with secondary osteonecrosis of the knee will typically identify large lesions involving multiple sites within the femoral condyles and tibial plateaus (Fig. 35.4). Secondary osteonecrosis lesions within the knee are pathologically similar to those in SPONK and ONPK and tend to progress to collapse, eventually requiring operative intervention.

TREATMENT OPTIONS

Various treatment options are available for the management of cases of secondary osteonecrosis, SPONK, and ONPK. These range from nonoperative and pharmacologic treatment to joint-preserving operative procedures and ultimately joint arthroplasty. Because these diseases are relatively rare, a validated treatment algorithm has yet to be developed, and management is taken on a case-individualized basis.

TABLE 35.1 **Comparison of Spontaneous Osteonecrosis and Osteonecrosis in the Postoperative Knee With Secondary Osteonecrosis**

Parameter	Secondary Osteonecrosis of the Knee (AVN)	SPONK, ONPK
Affected patient population, age (year)	≤45	≥55-60
Onset of symptoms	Gradual	Acute
Bilateral disease	>80%	<5%
Number of lesions	Multiple foci present	One focus
Lesion size	Large	Small
Location of lesion	Multiple sites within femoral condyles and tibial plateaus	Typically, medial femoral condyle
Other sites of disease	Femoral head (>90%) and proximal humerus	Rare
Identifiable risk factors	Present	Absent

AVN, Avascular necrosis; *ONPK,* osteonecrosis in the postoperative knee; *SPONK,* spontaneous osteonecrosis of the knee.
Adapted from Mont MA, Ragland PS: Osteonecrosis of the knee. In Scott WN (ed): Insall & Scott surgery of the knee, ed 4, Philadelphia, PA, 2006, Churchill Livingstone, pp 460–480.

BOX 35.1 **Risk Factors for Secondary Osteonecrosis**

Alcoholism
Caisson's disease
Chemotherapy
Coagulopathies
Corticosteroids
Cushing's syndrome
Diabetes
Familial thrombophilia
Gaucher's disease
Gout
Hyperlipidemia
Inflammatory bowel disease
Liver disease
Organ transplantation
Pancreatitis
Pregnancy
Radiation
Renal disease
Sickle cell disease (and other hemoglobinopathies)
Smoking
Systemic lupus erythematosus (and other connective tissue disorders)
Tumors

Nonoperative Treatment and Pharmacologic Therapy

Nonoperative Management. Once a lesion is identified, an attempt at nonoperative management is often undertaken. Protected weight bearing with crutches, coupled with analgesics and anti-inflammatory medication, is the mainstay of nonoperative treatment. Typically, the restrictions on weight bearing are maintained for a 4- to 8-week period. As the patient's symptoms improve, a resumption of normal activities of daily living, as well as the use of physical therapy for quadriceps and hamstring strengthening, is allowed.

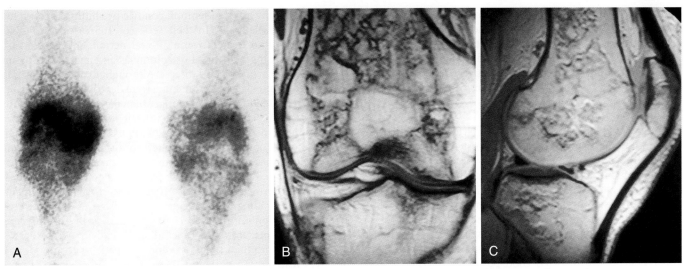

FIG 35.4 Bone scan (A) and coronal (B) and sagittal (C) MRI cuts demonstrating a case of secondary osteonecrosis affecting the distal femur and tibial plateau in a 33-year-old man with a history of corticosteroid exposure. (From Mont MA, Ragland PS: Osteonecrosis of the knee. In Scott WN [ed.]: Insall & Scott surgery of the knee, ed 4, Philadelphia, PA, 2006, Churchill Livingstone, pp 460–480.)

Secondary to their large size and occurrence in a young, active patient population, nonoperative management of cases of secondary osteonecrosis tends to fair poorly. In a series of 248 knees in 136 patients with secondary osteonecrosis of the knee, Mont et al.[46] have reported successful outcomes (Knee Society score ≥80 and no surgical intervention) in only 20% of the 41 knees treated, with protected weight bearing and analgesic medication at a mean of 8 years of follow-up.

In contrast to Mont et al. experience with secondary osteonecrosis, good to excellent results have been reported for cases of SPONK following nonoperative management if the lesion size is small (<20% to 40% of the width of the femoral condyle).[8,39,50] In a series of 79 cases of medial femoral condyle SPONK, Lotke et al.[40] reported that 32 of 36 patients (88.9%) with stage I disease had resolution of their symptoms after a period of protected weight bearing and analgesic treatment. In this series, only one patient with stage I disease went on to require total knee arthroplasty. Similar good results of nonoperative treatment were reported by Yates et al.[69] in their series of 20 cases of stage I SPONK. Resolution of the lesion was evident on follow-up MRI in 19 of 20 patients at a mean of 8 months (range, 3 to 18 months). As the lesion size and stage increases, the success of nonoperative treatment for cases of SPONK becomes less reliable, with most authors reporting a slow relentless progression to degenerative arthritis. Based on the available data, it appears that the nonoperative treatment of cases of ONPK is less successful in improving patient symptoms, functional outcome, and lesion resolution. Of the 47 reported cases in the orthopedic surgery literature, 3 patients (6.4%) had improvement in the MRI appearance of their lesion following 6 weeks of protected weight bearing.[58]

In an effort to reduce the weight-bearing forces experienced at the site of an osteonecrotic lesion and protect the weakened subchondral bone from collapse, an unloader brace may be used as part of a nonoperative management approach. Although there are little data in the orthopedic surgery literature to support their use in cases of secondary osteonecrosis, SPONK,

or ONPK, unloader braces have been shown to be useful for patients with symptomatic varus gonarthrosis. In an evaluation of 11 patients with medial compartment osteoarthritis, Lindenfeld et al.[38] have found that a valgus-producing unloader brace reduced the adduction moment experienced at the knee during gait, leading to a 48% reduction in pain scores and a 79% increase in function during activities of daily living. Similar benefits to unloading the medial compartment with a valgus-producing brace were reported by Draganich et al.[19] in their study of 10 patients with varus gonarthrosis. They found that both off-the-shelf and custom unloader braces significantly reduce knee pain and stiffness while improving functional scores compared with an unbraced state. Specific studies evaluating patients with osteonecrosis are required, but by reducing the adduction moment at the knee and the joint forces experienced in the medial compartment, unloader braces may protect lesions of the medial femoral condyle, potentially improving symptoms and allowing for successful healing.

Pharmacologic Treatment. Little has been published on the pharmacologic treatment of osteonecrosis of the knee, with most of the data extrapolated from the literature on femoral head osteonecrosis. Available medical treatment options include bisphosphonates, vasodilators, statins, and anticoagulants. As stable analogues of pyrophosphate, bisphosphonates function to promote bone formation via a reduction of osteoclast activity.[26,60] Alendronate has shown efficacy in relieving pain and reducing the incidence of collapse in cases of femoral head osteonecrosis.[1,15,16] However, Meier performed a double-blind, placebo-controlled randomized controlled trial to evaluate the effect of 12 weeks of ibandronate on clinical and radiographical outcomes of SPONK in 30 patients. The authors found no benefit of ibandronate over placebo in regards to pain score and radiologic grading. All patients did receive oral diclofenac (70 mg), calcium carbonate (500 mg), and vitamin D (400 IU). Hence, it does not appear that bisphosphonates offer any added benefit for patients with SPONK over oral anti-inflammatory medications. Attention has also been given to vasodilators such as iloprost[5,18,44] and anticoagulants such as enoxaparin[28] as potential disease-modifying agents in early stage, precollapse osteonecrosis. Further study is required to determine whether these medical interventions will effectively alter the clinical course in cases of secondary osteonecrosis, SPONK, and ONPK.

Surgical Management

Arthroscopic Débridement.
The use of arthroscopic débridement in the management of secondary osteonecrosis, SPONK, and ONPK has limited applications. Because the primary pathology is intraosseous, arthroscopic débridement has little likelihood of altering the course of the disease process; however, it may lead to symptomatic improvement in patients in whom mechanical symptoms are present secondary to unstable chondral fragments or loose bodies. In a series of five cases of SPONK treated with arthroscopic débridement and chondroplasty, Miller et al.[45] have reported good postoperative outcomes in four of five patients at a mean follow-up of 31 months, with Hospital for Special Surgery (HSS) knee scores improving from 52 to 82. Other authors have reported on open debridement and placement of autologous iliac crest concentrated bone marrow osteoprogenitor cells, with good results at 5 years. However, the natural history and progression of the osteonecrosis lesions in these patients was not altered by the arthroscopic procedure.

Some authors have reported performing arthroscopic retrograde drilling (through the articular cartilage layer to reach the lesion site) for cases of SPONK or ONPK.[17] Although retrograde drilling may stimulate revascularization within the lesion, the potential for damage to the intact articular surface and the difficulty associated with localizing the focus of the lesion accurately in the precollapse stage makes antegrade drilling (toward the articular surface without violating the cartilage layer) and core decompression more attractive treatment options.

Core Decompression.
Relief of elevated intraosseous pressure via extra-articular drilling has been used frequently in early-stage, precollapse cases of osteonecrosis of the femoral head with variable results. Core decompression as a treatment for osteonecrosis of the knee was first described in 1989 by Jacobs et al.[30] in their series of 28 patients. They reported good results in their stage I and II cases (7 patients) and in 52% of their stage III cases. Mont et al.[49] reviewed their experience with core decompression in 47 knees in patients with secondary osteonecrosis and reported good to excellent results in 72% at a mean follow-up of 11 years. More recently, in a series of 16 patients with a mean age of 64 years, Forst et al.[25] found that core decompression provided symptom relief and successful healing (normalization of bone marrow signal on MRI) in 15 stage I cases and 1 stage II case of SPONK at 3-year follow-up.[39] Based on their findings, they recommended core decompression as a useful treatment option for early stage osteonecrosis of the knee (Fig. 35.5). However, it is important to note that these studies lacked control groups, with the possibility that these cases of early stage disease might have improved without intervention.

High Tibial Osteotomy.
Appropriately selected patients with SPONK or ONPK may be managed with a high tibial osteotomy as a joint-preserving treatment option.[20,39,63] Typically reserved for younger active patients, high tibial osteotomy can function

to offload the affected femoral condyle by shifting the weight-bearing axis laterally. In their series of 105 cases of SPONK diagnosed and treated over a 20-year period, Soucacos et al.[66] reported using high tibial osteotomy as an effective treatment for patients with stage III disease. Although no details regarding the technique or patient outcome were described, better results were reported for patients younger than 65 years and for lesions less than 50% of the width of the femoral condyle in size. Koshino,[36] in a study of 37 cases of SPONK managed with high tibial osteotomy, with or without a concomitant drilling–bone grafting procedure, has found that the outcomes are best when the combined procedures were performed and the mechanical axis was corrected to at least 10 degrees of valgus alignment. Follow-up radiographic evaluation in this series demonstrated that the lesion improved in 17 patients and resolved completely in 13 patients. In a study including 10 patients with SPONK managed with high tibial osteotomy (6 patients) or nonoperative treatment (4 patients), Marti et al.[42] found that patients treated with high tibial osteotomy had a higher incidence of improvement in the appearance of their lesion on follow-up MRI (83% vs. 25%) and a higher incidence of symptom improvement (100% vs. 50%). Johnson et al.[31] reported two cases of ONPK treated with high tibial osteotomy, one performed 8 months and the other 10 months after the index arthroscopic medial meniscectomy; however, clinical outcome and follow-up were not described. Takeuchi et al. performed an opening wedge high tibial osteotomy with concurrent lesion curettage and retrograde drilling in 30 patients with SPONK. At 40 months, the authors found significant improvements in knee clinical outcome scores without any issues with nonunion or implant failure.

The use of high tibial osteotomy for cases of secondary osteonecrosis of the knee is typically not recommended secondary to the multifocal nature of this variant of disease, with most patients having bicondylar femoral involvement and coincident lesions present within the tibial plateau.

Knee Arthroplasty.
For patients in whom joint-preserving treatments fail to provide symptomatic improvement and in those with large or advanced lesions, knee arthroplasty is the finite treatment of choice. Depending on patient factors, lesion characteristics, and condition of the remainder of the joint, unicompartmental knee arthroplasty (UKA) or standard total knee arthroplasty (TKA) may be used.[39,63] Unicompartmental arthroplasty is an effective treatment method for those with disease isolated to a single femoral condyle or tibial plateau, with the benefit of preserving the patient's bone stock and functioning cruciate ligaments. For cases of secondary osteonecrosis and extensive cases of SPONK or ONPK in patients with evidence of degenerative change in the contralateral compartment or patellofemoral joint, tricompartmental replacement is a better treatment option.

In a series of 31 patients with a mean age of 36 years whose secondary osteonecrosis was treated with total knee arthroplasty, Mont and Hungerford[47] reported good to excellent results in 55% of their cases at a mean follow-up of 8.2 years. Of patients in this study, 37% required revision for aseptic loosening and 10% developed deep infection. Bonutti et al.[13] have reported the outcome of arthroplasty in 19 patients with osteonecrosis in the postoperative knee, with 4 patients undergoing UKA and 15 undergoing TKA. At a mean follow-up of 62 months, 18 patients had a good or excellent outcome based on

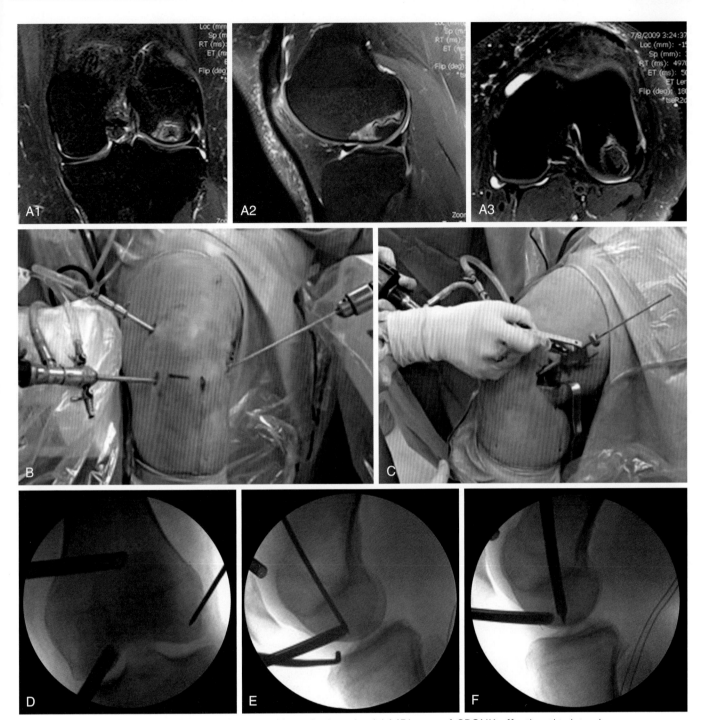

FIG 35.5 (A) Preoperative coronal, sagittal, and axial MRI cuts of SPONK affecting the lateral femoral condyle. (B-F) Arthroscopy-assisted, fluoroscopic-guided core decompression of the lateral femoral condyle.

Knee Society score (mean, 92; range, 60 to 100). Data on TKA for cases of osteonecrosis of the knee have demonstrated good outcomes, but in the long term, they do not appear to function as well as TKA performed for cases of osteoarthritis. In a series of 32 knees with SPONK of the medial femoral condyle, Ritter et al.[64] have reported results inferior to those seen in a comparison group treated for osteoarthritis. Patients treated for SPONK had worse pain relief (82% vs. 90%) and a higher incidence of revision surgery (17% vs. 0%) compared with the osteoarthritis

patients. Similar results were reported by Bergman and Rand[11] in their series of 36 cases of osteonecrosis of the knee managed with TKA. Good to excellent results were reported to occur in 87% of the study of patients at a mean of 4 years of follow-up. Whereas implant survivorship at 5 years was predicted to be 85%, with revision surgery defined as the endpoint, survivorship was predicted to be 68% when moderate or severe pain was used as the endpoint. It was theorized that if foci of osteonecrosis exist in the supporting subchondral or metaphyseal bone, persistent pain may complicate the outcome of TKA. Other studies have shown better outcomes of TKA for cases of SPONK. In a series of 32 TKAs performed in 30 patients, of which 8 were done as treatment of SPONK, Mont et al. reported excellent results with a Knee Society score of 98 at a mean of 108 months postoperatively.[48] Similarly, Bruni et al. evaluated 84 patients following UKA for isolated medial compartment SPONK at 10 years after surgery and found an implant survivorship of 89%.

SUMMARY AND CONCLUSIONS

Secondary osteonecrosis, spontaneous osteonecrosis of the knee, and osteonecrosis in the postoperative knee are clinical entities that have the potential to cause significant morbidity in affected patients. In addition to the knowledge about the patient population at risk, classic presentation, and imaging characteristics, the treating physician needs to maintain a high index of suspicion for these disorders, as early diagnosis and treatment may allow for improved clinical outcome. Continued study of patients with SPONK and ONPK is needed in an effort to identify specific risk factors that predispose certain patients to their development. In the future, it is possible that pharmacologic intervention and alterations in postarthroscopy rehabilitation protocols in susceptible patients may alter the course of disease for those who develop SPONK and ONPK.

KEY REFERENCES

17. DeFalco RA, Ricci AR, Balduini FC: Osteonecrosis of the knee after arthroscopic meniscectomy and chondroplasty: a case report and literature review. *Am J Sports Med* 31:1013–1016, 2003.

20. Duany NG, Zywiel MG, McGrath MS, et al: Joint-preserving surgical treatment of spontaneous osteonecrosis of the knee. *Arch Orthop Trauma Surg* 130(1):11–16, 2010.

21. Ecker ML: Spontaneous osteonecrosis of the distal femur. *Instr Course Lect* 50:495–498, 2001.

22. Ecker ML, Lotke PA: Spontaneous osteonecrosis of the knee. *J Am Acad Orthop Surg* 2:173–178, 1994.

24. Faletti C, Robba T, de Petro P: Postmeniscectomy osteonecrosis. *Arthroscopy* 18:91–94, 2002.

31. Johnson TC, Evans JA, Gilley JA, et al: Osteonecrosis of the knee after arthroscopic surgery for meniscal tears and chondral lesions. *Arthroscopy* 16:254–261, 2000.

34. Kattapuram TM, Kattapuram SV: Spontaneous osteonecrosis of the knee. *Eur J Radiol* 67:42–48, 2008.

42. Marti CB, Rodriguez M, Zanetti M, et al: Spontaneous osteonecrosis of the medial compartment of the knee: a MRI follow-up after conservative and operative treatment, preliminary results. *Knee Surg Sports Traumatol Arthrosc* 8:83–88, 2000.

46. Mont MA, Baumgarten KM, Rifai A, et al: Atraumatic osteonecrosis of the knee. *J Bone Joint Surg Am* 82:1279–1290, 2000.

49. Mont MA, Tomek IM, Hungerford DS: Core decompression for avascular necrosis of the distal femur: long term followup. *Clin Orthop Relat Res* 334:124–130, 1997.

52. Muscolo DL, Costa-Paz M, Ayerza M, et al: Medial meniscal tears and spontaneous osteonecrosis of the knee. *Arthroscopy* 22:457–460, 2006.

58. Pape D, Seil R, Anagnostakos K, et al: Postarthroscopic osteonecrosis of the knee. *Arthroscopy* 23:428–438, 2007.

65. Robertson DD, Armfield DR, Towers JD, et al: Meniscal root injury and spontaneous osteonecrosis of the knee: an observation. *J Bone Joint Surg Br* 91:190–195, 2009.

67. Yamamoto T, Bullough PG: Spontaneous osteonecrosis of the knee: the result of subchondral insufficiency fracture. *J Bone Joint Surg Am* 82:858–866, 2000.

70. Zywiel MG, McGrath MS, Seyler TM, et al: Osteonecrosis of the knee: a review of three disorders. *Orthop Clin North Am* 40:193–211, 2009.

The references for this chapter can also be found on www.expertconsult.com.

36

Healing of Knee Ligaments and Menisci

Ian D. Hutchinson, Seth L. Sherman, Arielle J. Hall, Scott A. Rodeo

Muscles, ligaments, and menisci complement the bony architecture of the knee and allow for normal kinematics throughout the range of motion. Ligaments are critical to the static stability of the knee joint. The menisci serve to guide the femoral condyles in their articulation with the tibial plateau and distribute the weight more evenly. Structural damage to the ligaments or menisci can result in altered joint kinematics and joint forces, ultimately leading to degenerative changes in the knee. Therefore, it is imperative to restore homeostatic balance within the knee through preservation of the meniscus and through ligament healing, repair, or reconstruction.

It is the purpose of this chapter to review the basic science aspects of ligament and meniscal healing, as well as the biology of current repair and reconstructive strategies, to provide a fundamental basis for optimized care, including the advancement of treatment strategies for these injuries.

LIGAMENTS

Structure and Function

Anatomy and Biochemistry. Ligaments are fibrous bands that span two or more bones and are critical to the static stability of the knee joint.[62] All ligaments are composed of densely organized, fibrous connective tissue consisting of mainly water and type I collagen (approximately 70% to 90% of dry weight).[74] Water is attracted into the extracellular matrix of the ligament by negatively charged proteoglycans, including decorin sulfate, chondroitin sulfate, and keratin sulfate (less than 1% of dry weight). This accounts for the ligament's rate-dependent response to mechanical load, or viscoelasticity.

Collagen is responsible for the ligaments characteristic form and tensile strength. Collagen molecules orient along the long axis of the ligament to form fibrils.[74] Ligaments contain a bimodal distribution of collagen fibril diameters. There is a group of fibrils between 40 and 75 µm in diameter and a second group between 100 and 150 µm in diameter.[50,62] The fibrils are grouped into fibers that range from 1 to 20 µm in diameter, which are then grouped into fascicles from 360 to 1500 µm in diameter. The collagen in ligaments contains stable and unstable collagen cross-links and has a characteristic crimp pattern.

Other components of the extracellular matrix of ligaments include types III, IV, V, and VI collagen (3% to 90% of dry weight), elastic fibers, including elastin, fibrillin, and microfibrillar-associated glycoprotein (usually less than 5%), and a small percentage of noncollagenous proteins, including fibronectin, laminin, thrombospondin, and tenascin.[62]

Fibroblasts are the dominant cell type in ligaments, responsible for forming and maintaining the extracellular matrix.

Other cell types present include endothelial cells, peripheral nerve cells, and tissue mast cells.[62] Compared with tendons, ligaments are more metabolically active.[51] Intrinsic ligament fibroblasts possess plump nuclei and have a higher DNA content compared with tenoblasts. The higher metabolic activity in ligaments may be the result of a functional need for more rapid adaptation.

The normal ligament insertion site into bone is a highly specialized tissue that functions to transmit complex mechanical loads from soft tissue to bone.[74] Ligaments, in general, have two distinct types of insertion sites: direct and indirect.[146] The femoral insertion of the anterior cruciate ligament (ACL) is an example of a direct insertion site. At a direct insertion site, the ligament often enters the bone directly at a right angle to the bony surface. This transition contains four distinct zones—ligament, unmineralized fibrocartilage, mineralized fibrocartilage, and bone (Fig. 36.1). Cartilage-specific collagens including types II, IX, X, and XI are found in the fibrocartilage of the insertion site, with collagen X playing a fundamental role in maintaining the interface between mineralized and unmineralized fibrocartilage.[65,132] Proteoglycans are also abundant in the fibrocartilaginous region of the insertion site, probably functioning to decrease stress concentration at the insertion.

An example of an indirect insertion is the tibial insertion of the medial collateral ligament (MCL). At this insertion site, collagen fibers blend with the periosteum, which are then anchored to bone via Sharpey's fibers. These Sharpey's fibers are obliquely oriented to the long axis of the bone, securely anchoring the ligament into bone and conferring mechanical strength (Fig. 36.2).[74]

Finally, the somatosensory function of the ACL is becoming more recognized; the intact ACL contains mechanoreceptors capable of detecting changes in tension that facilitate somatosensory feedback regarding the direction, speed, and acceleration of knee joint motion during dynamic activities.[45,46] It is estimated that 1% of the ACL is composed of neural elements, and these are most concentrated in the subsynovial layer of the synovium that enfolds the ACL at the insertion sites.[90,158] The ACL is primarily innervated by Ruffini receptors but also contains Pacinian corpuscles, Golgi tendon organs, and free nerve endings.[76,79,158,212] Innervation of the ACL comes from the posterior articular nerve; however, afferent fibers have also been demonstrated in the medial and lateral articular nerves.[90] Pitman et al. have demonstrated the neuroreceptive function of the ACL by recording scalp somatosensory evoked potentials (SSEP) following intraoperative stimulation of the ACL using electrodes in nine patients.[140]

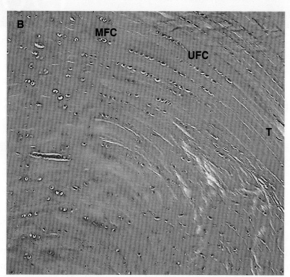

FIG 36.1 Normal tendon to bone direct insertion site of the rabbit ACL. Note the four zones—tendon *(T)*, unmineralized fibrocartilage *(UFC)*, mineralized fibrocartilage *(MFC)*, and bone *(B)*. (From Gulotta LV, Rodeo SA: Biology of autograft and allograft anterior cruciate ligament reconstruction. *Clin Sports Med* 26:509–524, 2007.)

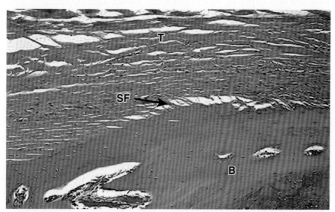

FIG 36.2 Normal tendon to bone indirect insertion site of the rabbit MCL with Sharpey's fibers. *B,* Bone; *SF,* Sharpey's fibers; *T,* tendon. (From Gulotta LV, Rodeo SA: Biology of autograft and allograft anterior cruciate ligament reconstruction. *Clin Sports Med* 26:509–524, 2007.)

Biomechanics and Function

The biomechanical characterization of a healing ligament is based on two elements, functional testing and tensile testing. Functional testing determines the contribution of the ligament to knee kinematics as well as the in situ forces of the ligament in response to external loading conditions. Tensile testing assesses the structural properties of the bone-ligament-bone complex and the material properties of the ligament substance.[199,201]

There are four basic aspects of ligament mechanical functional testing. These include laxity, stiffness, strength, and viscoelasticity.[62] Failure or overload of these functions may result in ligamentous injury and loss of critical joint-stabilizing properties of the ligament (Fig. 36.3). Healing of a ligament may be assessed using these parameters as outcome measures for success.

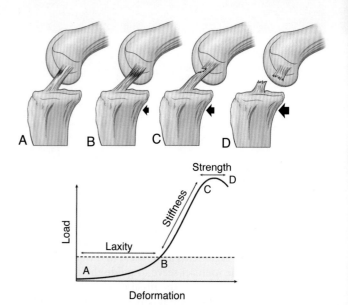

FIG 36.3 Schematic and graphic descriptions of laxity, stiffness, and strength. (From Frank CB: Ligament healing: current knowledge and clinical applications. *J Am Acad Orthop Surg* 4:74–83, 1996.)

Laxity refers to the displacement of bones to which a ligament is attached from an anatomic position to a position in which the ligament takes up load. It is a function of both joint position and direction of load.[62] Structurally, the laxity of a ligament is partly a function of number of fibers recruited by a specific movement and the orientation of these fibers to resist displacement.

Stiffness is the amount of load required to displace the bones to which a ligament is attached. The more load required, the stiffer the ligament-joint complex. Stiffness is also a function of fiber recruitment, with stiffer ligaments having more fiber recruitment. In injured or damaged ligaments, either fibers are not recruited or those recruited are not as stiff as normal ligament fibers.[139]

Strength refers to the maximum tensile load that a bone-ligament-bone complex can withstand before it fails. Failure load is a function of both the number of fibers that tighten within a ligament, and the quality of those fibers. The direction of applied force during ligament testing also influences the structural and mechanical properties. Applying the force in the direction of the ligament will recruit a greater proportion of fiber bundles and thus result in higher forces.[30] Therefore, load direction is a critical determinant of ligament strength.

Viscoelasticity refers to the ability of tissues to respond to repeat loading by altering length or load over time. Variations can account for as much as 10% changes in ligament length and up to 60% to 70% of changes in ligament loads under physiologic conditions. Creep is a viscoelastic property in which there is an increase in ligament length that occurs over time when the ligament is subjected to a constant load (Fig. 36.4). Another property, load or stress relaxation, occurs when a load decreases over time when a ligament is held at a specific deformation.

Tensile testing provides information on the strength and quality of healing tissue and allows comparisons with intact ligaments. Two sets of information can be obtained from

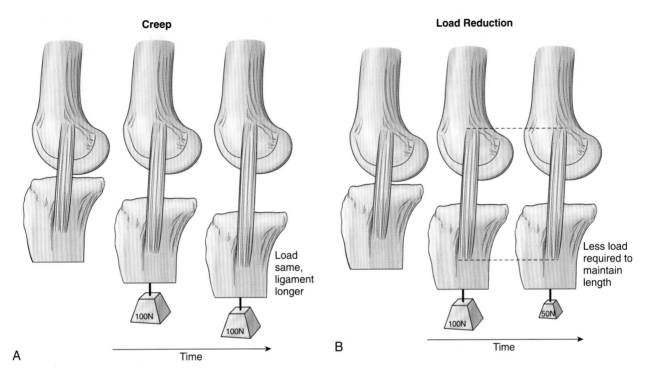

FIG 36.4 The Viscoelastic Properties of Ligaments (A) Creep is the increase in the length of a ligament that occurs over time when a ligament is subjected to a constant load. (B) Load relaxation is the decrease in load that a ligament experiences over time when it is held at a specific deformation. (From Frank CB: Ligament healing: current knowledge and clinical applications. *J Am Acad Orthop Surg* 4:74–83, 1996.)

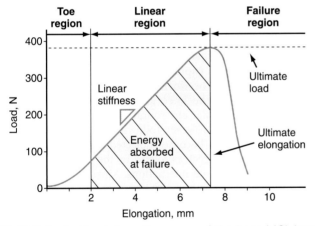

FIG 36.5 Typical load-elongation curve of the bone-MCL-bone complex. (From Woo SL, Vogrin TM, Abramowitch SD: Healing and repair of ligament injuries in the knee. *J Am Acad Orthop Surg* 8:364–372, 2000.)

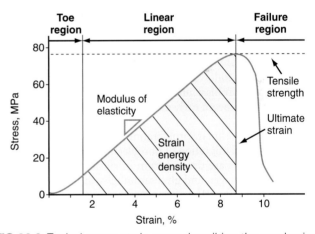

FIG 36.6 Typical stress-strain curve describing the mechanical properties of the MCL midsubstance. (From Woo SL, Vogrin TM, Abramowitch SD: Healing and repair of ligament injuries in the knee. *J Am Acad Orthop Surg* 8:364–372, 2000.)

uniaxial tensile testing. The load-elongation curve demonstrates the structural properties of the bone-ligament-bone complex, and the stress-strain curve demonstrates the material properties of the ligament substance (Figs. 36.5 and 36.6).[200] Both curves demonstrate characteristic toe, linear, and failure regions. In the initial low-stiffness toe region, elongation of a ligament occurs because of straightening of the crimp pattern.[30] With further load, there is increasing recruitment of ligament fiber bundles. The slope of the linear region reflects the stiffness of the ligament or ligament complex. Structural properties that

are evaluated with the load-elongation curve include linear stiffness, ultimate load, and energy absorbed at failure. The stress-strain curve provides information on modulus of elasticity, tensile strength, ultimate strain, and strain energy density.

Biology of Ligament Injury and Healing

Ligament healing involves the restoration of the structural integrity of the tissue following an injury. The ability of an injured ligament to heal is affected by a number of variables, including the site and severity of the injury, presence of injury to other ligaments with resultant instability patterns, various intrinsic factors (eg, age, circulation status), type of treatment initiated, and degree of immobilization and rehabilitation after injury.[200] Knowledge of the basic science of ligament injury and healing is instrumental in making informed treatment decisions in a clinical setting.

Age-Related Changes in Ligament and Ligament Degeneration. The structural and mechanical properties of ligaments change with skeletal maturation.[6,162] In the setting of open physes, ligaments often fail by bone avulsion, whereas ligaments fail in the midsubstance in the skeletally mature. Structural and mechanical properties of ligaments are also positively correlated with age; specimens from younger donors demonstrate superior properties compared with specimens from older donors.[187] Water content, as well as rate of collagen synthesis, decreases with age in both the MCL and ACL in a rabbit model.

The gross and microscopic changes of ligament degeneration can occur in acute and chronic settings. Following acute, full-thickness ligament disruption, an initial inflammatory response occurs whether the ligament is intra-articular or extra-articular. As an example, the torn ends of an acutely ruptured ACL rapidly involute. These changes are related to an increase in collagenase activity, apparently in response to local cell damage.[4] Chronic degeneration of a ligament is uncommon, but when it occurs, several histologic changes are involved, including collagen fragmentation and mucoid degeneration.[159]

Healing of Extra-Articular Ligaments. Extra-articular healing proceeds in three phases: (1) inflammation, (2) cellular and matrix proliferation, and (3) remodeling.[54,198] During phase I, a fibrin clot forms at the injury site. Potent vasodilators are released, including histamine and serotonin. There is infiltration of inflammatory cells and phagocytosis of necrotic debris by macrophages, followed by proliferation of capillary endothelial buds and fibroblast proliferation near the end of phase I. These fibroblasts begin early matrix synthesis. This early matrix is disorganized.[103]

Matrix and cellular proliferation are characterized by a proliferation and migration of fibroblasts to the site of injury.[103] Proliferating cells are derived from intrinsic and extrinsic cell populations. Collagen and glycosaminoglycan (GAG) synthesis is upregulated. Type III collagen, formed in the initial healing period, is eventually removed and replaced by type I collagen. The mechanical strength of the repair tissue begins to increase as the new matrix is deposited.

There is a relative decrease in cellularity and vascularity during the remodeling phase of healing. There is an increase in collagen density and a gradual decrease in the content of collagen type III. Collagen fibrils gradually become organized along the axis of the ligament. Collagen cross-linking and posttranslational modifications occur during this phase and result in increased tensile strength. Collagen fibril diameters and collagen cross-links remain abnormal for at least 1 year after ligamentous injury.[104,126] Alpha smooth muscle actin containing fibroblasts, or myofibroblasts, may be responsible for tensioning the ligament during the remodeling phase of healing.[54]

There is increased matrix synthesis and cellularity seen throughout the entire ligament (not just at the injury site) during the healing phase. Near the end of the remodeling phase, the uninjured area of the ligament returns to normal cellularity

TABLE 36.1   Differences Between Normal Ligaments and Scars

Normal (Uninjured) Ligaments	Ligament Scars
Collagen aligned	Collagen disorganized
Collagen densely packed	Defects between collagen fibers
Large collagen fibrils	Small collagen fibrils
Mature fiber cross links	Immature cross links
Primarily collagen type I (<10% type III)	More collagen type III
Small proteoglycans	Some large proteoglycans
Other components minor	Excesses of other components
Low cell density	Increased cell density
Low vascularity	Increased vascularity

From Frank CB: Ligament healing: current knowledge and clinical applications. *J Am Acad Orthop Surg* 4:74–83, 1996.

and matrix organization, whereas scar tissue persists at the injury site.[77,108] A few early studies noted apparent ligament regeneration, but subsequent studies have shown that although normal ligament strength may recover in some cases, this is not because of formation of true ligament tissue.[61,199] Although the strength and stiffness of the collateral ligaments have been restored to 40% to 90% of normal values in animal studies, only about 30% to 70% of the material properties are restored. This scar tissue has inferior material properties compared with normal ligament matrix. It is weaker and creeps more than normal ligament and is also associated with an increased concentration of minor collagens (types III, V, and VI), decreased collagen cross-links, and an increased amount of glycosaminoglycans (Table 36.1).[86]

Anterior Cruciate Ligament Injury and Healing Response. In adults, most ACL ruptures occur in the midsubstance of the ligament. It may be worth considering that although the ACL resides within the knee joint, it is insulated from the biological intra-articular environment by an investing layer of synovial membrane. However, following ACL rupture, the torn ends of the ligament become subjected to the intra-articular environment with direct exposure to the synovial fluid and homeostatic joint tissue interactions. Murray and co-workers found that following rupture, the human ACL undergoes four histological phases: inflammation, epiligamentous regeneration, proliferation, and remodeling.[123] Immediately following injury, the initial hemarthrosis results in inflammation that creates a hostile environment for ligament healing. The torn ends of the ACL are not in contact, and a fibrin clot does not form between the ends of the injured ligament to act as a scaffold for subsequent repair.[124] In addition, following knee injury, there is upregulation of urokinase plasminogen activator (uPA) production by synoviocytes; uPA converts the inactive plasminogen molecule present in synovial fluid into its active form, plasmin.[152] Ultimately, plasmin degrades fibrin and disrupts stable clot formation at the tear site, and the lack of such provisional scaffold is believed to be disadvantageous to all intra-articular soft tissue healing (including ACL and meniscus).[123,125,174] They also observed the formation of an alpha-smooth muscle actin-expressing synovial cell layer on the surface of the ruptured ends of the ligament and postulate that it is this layer that may inhibit a healing response following ACL injury and direct repair because of retraction of the ends of the ruptured ligament. For these reasons, the ACL rarely heals following rupture. Therefore, ACL reconstruction is the preferred treatment for patients with symptomatic knee instability.

Biologic Differences Between Anterior Cruciate Ligament and Medial Collateral Ligament Healing. In direct contrast to the findings in ACL injuries, both clinical experience and animal studies of MCL injuries have indicated a relatively good, but seldom perfect, healing response.[61,94,97] Numerous studies have examined the mechanisms accounting for the different healing potentials of the ACL and MCL.[5] Multiple factors account for the differences, including ligament ultrastructure, local environment, and cellular properties. The primary factor appears to be the presence of a fibrin clot that bridges the ends of the torn ligament and serves as a provisional scaffold following MCL injury. There are differences in fibril diameter, fibril diameter distributions, and subfascicular area fractions. MCL fibril diameters are larger and the subfascicular area fraction is higher in the MCL, indicating more densely packed fibrils.[6] Cellular metabolism may also play a role in healing potential. MCL fibroblasts proliferate more rapidly than ACL fibroblasts in vitro and they have differential response to growth factors. There are also differences in cellular response to various chemotactic agents, such as cytokines. ACL and MCL cells demonstrate differential mitogenic, chemotactic, and matrix synthetic responses to mechanical load. There is increased expression of specific integrins on the cell surface of MCL fibroblasts in the healing MCL, as compared with minimal integrin expression in the healing ACL cells. Messenger RNA for procollagen expression is also higher in the healing MCL compared with the healing ACL.

Biomechanical factors may also play a role in the ability to heal. The ACL contributes to knee stability in multiple directions, whereas the MCL primarily restrains valgus rotation. Therefore, a ruptured MCL receives some protection from other structures, such as the ACL and capsule, and may not be subjected to the same forces that could impede ACL healing.[200] The ACL may not be able to accommodate the multidirectional demands so as to allow healing.[201] Knowledge of the in vivo ligamentous loads would help determine the optimal load and amount of strain to optimize ligament healing.

Combined Ligamentous Injuries. The prognosis for combined ACL-MCL injuries is generally worse than for single-ligament injuries, regardless of selected treatment modality.[64,88,200] Although the clinical treatment of these combined injuries remains controversial, evidence from recent animal models may assist in clinical decision making with regard to optimization of ligament healing potential.

Rabbit and canine models have studied the effects of ACL deficiency on the healing of the injured MCL. In these models, knees with untreated combined injury demonstrated increased valgus laxity and significant reduction in the tissue quality of the healed MCL.[201] In contrast, another rabbit study demonstrated that reconstruction of the ACL combined with nonoperative full weight bearing and mobilization of the MCL leads to successful MCL healing.[202] Studies of ACL reconstruction combined with MCL repair have demonstrated improved structural properties and functional testing of the MCL in the short term, with no biochemical or biomechanical difference versus nonoperative MCL treatment after 52 weeks.

Patient-Related Systemic Factors. The healing response of ligaments is affected by a variety of endocrine or metabolic abnormalities, systemically or locally. Systemic factors include diabetes mellitus and its effect on the circulatory system, insulin deficiency, and alteration of collagen synthesis and cross-linking, and the effect of various changes in the endocrine system on the ultimate load of the repaired ligament, and the rates of collagen and glycosaminoglycan synthesis or degradation.[184] Local factors, such as poor circulation or infection, impede the proliferation of cells and prolong the inflammatory phase of healing.[200]

Treatment of Ligamentous Injuries

Immobilization Versus Controlled Motion and Exercise. Rehabilitation of an injured ligament often depends on whether there is joint instability associated with the injury. Stable joints may be treated with immobilization for varying time periods, followed by exercise protocols to gain motion and strength. Unstable joints may additionally be treated with specific bracing techniques or surgical intervention. The effects of proper techniques in rehabilitation on patient outcome have been studied in several areas. Injured ligaments have abnormal proprioception, and training regimens may improve this. Supervised rehabilitation of postural and balance training may reduce the number of re-injuries in the ankle and play a role in injury prevention.[91] Joint position sense (JPS) in ACL-deficient knees is impaired. Although knee stability can improve with exercise therapy, there may be no improvement in JPS.[34] The role of JPS in the stability of ACL-deficient knees remains unclear.[70]

Postoperative rehabilitation contributes greatly to the success of ACL reconstruction. Early joint motion is beneficial for reducing pain, improving articular cartilage nutrition, and minimizing scar formation that limits joint motion. Functional sports agility programs during the early rehabilitation period after ACL reconstruction are well tolerated and beneficial to overall outcome.[164]

Aggressive rehabilitation programs that involve contraction of the dominant quadriceps muscles have now become popular. Closed kinetic chain exercises (foot fixed against a resistance) are the mainstay of rehabilitation of ACL-insufficient or ACL-reconstructed knees. Some authors have suggested that open- and closed-chain exercises can be modified to minimize the risk of applying excessive strain on the ACL graft and of excessive patellofemoral joint stress.[50,57] However, open kinetic chain exercises (foot not fixed against a resistance) may result in increased anterior-posterior knee laxity compared with the normal knee.[111] The relationship between rehabilitation exercises and the optimum mechanobiology of the healing ACL graft is not completely understood. However, it is becoming clear that immediate, high-strain graft loading may compromise early tendon to bone interface healing in the bone tunnels, as demonstrated in a controlled loading rat model of ACL reconstruction.[135]

Bracing. Functional knee braces provide a protective strain-shielding effect on the normal ACL when anterior shear loads and internal rotation torques are applied to the knee in non-weight-bearing and weight-bearing conditions.[22] However, this protective effect is at loads that are less than those seen in normal walking. Future studies should strive to determine the actual loads transmitted across the knee and ACL graft strain

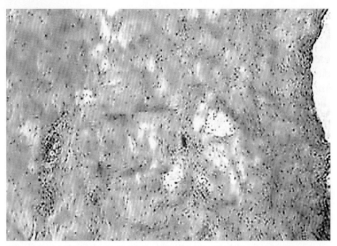

FIG 36.7 Histology of intra-articular graft ligamentization in a rabbit ACL reconstruction. The graft has been repopulated by the host cells. (Courtesy Dr. David Amiel, University of California, San Diego, CA.)

during various rehabilitation exercises and relate these to the healing response of the knee and ACL graft.[21]

Electrical and Mechanical Stimulation. Electrical stimulation has been shown to enhance the repair of biologic tissues such as bones and tendons. The use of direct current yielded improvements in maximum rupture force, energy absorbed, stiffness, and laxity in the rat MCL.[108] In addition, low-intensity pulsed ultrasound (LIPUS) with stimulation at 30 mW/cm^2 of energy has recently been applied to ligament-to-bone healing with some success. Animal models have demonstrated accelerated healing of the intra-articular ACL and extra-articular MCL, with the regenerated interface more closely resembling the native insertion.[181,191] The mechanism by which this is achieved is not fully understood, but LIPUS treatment is believed to promote cellular proliferation of osteoblasts and fibroblasts, upregulation of bone morphogenetic proteins, and enhancement of angiogenesis and protein synthesis at the repair site.[47,107,109,176,178]

Intra-Articular Ligament Reconstruction

Tendon graft biology. When surgical intervention is indicated for the treatment of a damaged ligament, a tendon graft is often used for the reconstruction. The tendon is placed in a new biologic and mechanical role. There is a gradual biologic transformation of tissues that are transplanted to an intra-articular environment, such as in ACL reconstruction. This process has been termed *ligamentization* (Fig. 36.7).[5] This gradual biologic transformation of the transplant begins with graft avascular necrosis. The intrinsic graft cells do not survive transplantation to the new environment. Cell necrosis occurs over the first 3 weeks. This is followed by cellular repopulation, which occurs prior to revascularization of the ligament. Repopulating cells appear to be derived from synovium and obtain their nutrition by synovial diffusion. Other possible sources of repopulating cells include mesenchymal stem cells, marrow cells, blood cells, and cells from the residual ACL stump.[90,123] It is also possible that there is a surviving subset of cells in the graft, although this is less likely. The eventual phenotype of the repopulating cells is not known. It is not known whether these cells assume the

phenotype of normal ACL cells. These cells remain metabolically active for a prolonged period of time during the healing process of intra-articular ligament grafts.

The revascularization phase begins 6 to 8 weeks following graft transplantation.[5] Vascular synovial tissue forms around the graft. New blood supply to the graft is derived from the fat pad, tibial remnant, and posterior synovial tissues. Growing capillary buds are seen histologically. Revascularization progresses from the periphery to the central portion of the graft.

Matrix synthesis occurs in the ligament graft following cellular repopulation and revascularization.[5] Over time, the collagen and glycosaminoglycan content of the graft becomes similar to a normal ligament.[26] Similarly, the collagen crimp pattern and reducible cross-link profile becomes more like that of a normal intra-articular ligament, as compared with the extra-articular tendon graft. However, there is a persistent abnormal unimodal distribution of small-diameter collagen fibrils in the graft. There is variable return of the pyridinoline collagen cross-links. Type III collagen also has been found to remain elevated for a variable period of time following graft transplantation. These persistent abnormalities in collagen cross-links, collagen type, and collagen fibril diameter probably contribute to the inferior biomechanical properties of the graft.

The last phase in the graft incorporation process is the remodeling phase.[5] There is a gradual decrease in cellularity and vascularity and an increase in matrix organization. This process occurs for a minimum of 1 year following graft transplantation.

Graft attachment site biology. Surgical reconstruction of a ligament relies on attachment of the grafted tendon to bone. Tendon to bone healing occurs by the formation of a fibrovascular interface tissue between the tendon and bone. In this way, the tendon becomes anchored to the bone. There is gradual reestablishment of collagen fiber continuity between the tendon and bone. Some animal studies have demonstrated direct collagen fiber continuity between the tendon and bone (Sharpey's fibers), whereas other studies have demonstrated formation of a fibrocartilage interface between tendon and bone.[146,147] The concomitant bone formation is generally an intramembranous process. The attachment strength gradually increases as collagen fiber continuity improves.

Bone plug healing, such as seen in bone-tendon-bone ACL reconstructions, involves incorporation of the bone plug into the bone tunnel over a 12-week period.[5] The original insertion site of the patellar tendon may remain histologically normal. The comparative strength of the healed tendon to bone attachment versus the healed bone plug attachment is unknown.

Healing of a tendon graft in a bone tunnel, as is required in ACL reconstruction using semitendinosus tendon, begins with the formation of a fibrovascular interface tissue between the tendon and bone.[146] There is progressive bone ingrowth into this interface tissue, with gradual reestablishment of an indirect type of insertion by intramembranous bone formation. The increase in strength of the healing tendon to bone attachment correlates well with the progressive bone ingrowth and maturation of the interface (Figs. 36.8 and 36.9).

Healing of tendon to the surface of bone also occurs by bone ingrowth into the fibrous interface tissue that forms between the tendon and bone.[154] In a larger animal model (goats), an indirect insertion forms, whereas studies in smaller animals have demonstrated formation of a direct insertion. Further study is required to determine the basic cellular mechanism of

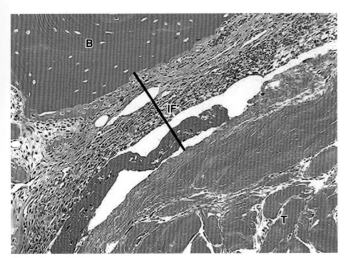

FIG 36.8 Tendon to bone interface after ACL reconstruction with a tendon graft in a rabbit at 1 week. Note the fibrovascular interface (scar) tissue between the tendon and the bone. *B*, Bone; *IF*, interface tissue; *T*, tendon. (From Gulotta LV, Rodeo SA: Biology of autograft and allograft anterior cruciate ligament reconstruction. *Clin Sports Med* 26:509–524, 2007.)

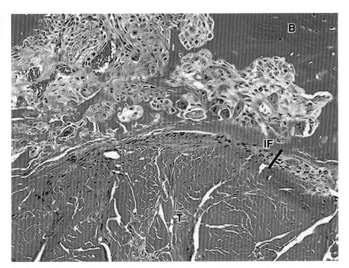

FIG 36.9 Tendon to bone interface at 2 weeks. Note the decrease in interface tissue at 2 weeks. *B*, Bone; *IF*, interface tissue; *T*, tendon. (From Gulotta LV, Rodeo SA: Biology of autograft and allograft anterior cruciate ligament reconstruction. *Clin Sports Med* 26:509–524, 2007.)

tendon to bone healing. Studies have demonstrated that bone morphogenetic protein-2, a potent osteoinductive agent, can augment tendon healing in a bone tunnel.[147]

Finally, remnant incorporation has been proposed to enhance healing of the ACL graft at the aperture, and promote graft ligamentization and reinnervation. Systematic reviews analyzing the clinical impact of remnant incorporation remain inconclusive in the context of global knee function in shorter-term follow-up (<4 years), where conventional ACL techniques are performing adequately.[24,137] In addition, repair of the aperture to the graft has been associated with a decreased degree of bone tunnel widening, although clinical outcome remained unchanged in the short term.[210] There is no doubt that immediate potential

complications of inaccurate tunnel placement, impingement, and the potential for development of a Cyclops lesion may deter some surgeons away from this remnant incorporation, but medium- to long-term studies are necessary in this area to assess the impact of potential biological, biomechanical, and somatosensory advantage on knee joint health and locomotion.

Biological Augmentation of Ligament Healing

Point of Care Biological Augmentation. Although basic science studies have demonstrated positive effects of platelet-rich plasma (PRP) on graft healing and integration following ACL reconstruction in the preclinical setting, these observations have yet to be translated in clinical studies with regard to overall outcome or improved ACL graft ligamentization.[10] Clinical studies are more likely to be confounded by the variability in both preparation and application of PRP. A recent systematic analysis by Andriolo et al. identified marked heterogeneity in PRP augmentation studies for ACL reconstruction. Examining the current evidence regarding the efficacy of PRP in this setting, their findings suggested more benefit on intra-articular graft remodeling and reducing subjective anterior knee pain at the donor site following bone-patellar tendon-bone ACL reconstruction. The cumulative evidence examining the use of PRP to enhance graft-tunnel interface development is less robust, and overall, concomitant PRP administration with ACL reconstruction was not associated with clear clinical benefits in the short term.[10]

Regarding partial ACL tears, Seijas et al. presented a retrospective review of return to play in 19 professional soccer players who received plasma rich in growth factors (PRGF) using the Endoret preparation technique.[161] The patients received a 4 mL injection in the intact posterolateral bundle during arthroscopy and 6 mL into the joint space. In this study, PRGF treatment resulted in normalization of knee stability using the KT-1000 in all cases; 95% (18/19) were able to return to their previous level of play at mean of 16 weeks.

Silva et al. investigated the effect of autologous bone marrow-derived stem cell concentrate on bone-to-tendon healing at the femoral graft interface using magnetic resonance imaging (MRI) in a prospective randomized study of 43 patients (including 20 controls).[166] ACL reconstruction was undertaken using hamstring grafts; in the intervention group, bone marrow aspirate concentrate from the anterior iliac crest was injected within the portion of the graft destined for the femoral tunnel, with the remaining injected directly into the tunnel itself. MRI did not detect any differences between groups with respect to signal to noise ratio at the graft-tunnel interface, and this was correlated by a single postoperative biopsy from each group. Of note in this study, (1) there was no characterization of the aspirate or concentrate for the examined patients; (2) postoperative timing of the MRI was not described; and (3) the postoperative rehabilitation included immediate full weight bearing and full range of motion (crutches for 3 to 4 weeks and no brace) and closed-chain exercises were started immediately. There is currently very little information available about the optimal rehabilitation protocol following the use of PRP in this setting.

Growth Factors. Growth factors such as epidermal growth factor (EGF), basic fibroblast growth factor (bFGF), acidic fibroblast growth factor (aFGF), platelet-derived growth factor BB (PDGF-BB), and transforming growth factor beta (TGF-β) are currently being evaluated for their effects on fibroblast proliferation, matrix synthesis, and cell migration. Animal models have shown that TGF-β is a good promoter of matrix synthesis, whereas PDGF-BB, EGF, and bFGF are positive mitogens on fibroblasts of the ACL and MCL.[156,200] Investigators have demonstrated the possibility that growth factors can enhance the in vivo healing of injured ligaments.[104,197] In one rabbit model, high doses of PDGF delivered with a fibrin sealant led to significant increases in the structural properties of the femur-MCL-tibia complex.[87]

Future Directions in Ligament Healing

Basic science research is actively exploring methods to improve the quality of healing ligament tissue and to find novel ways to accelerate and enhance the healing process. Advances in the fields of molecular biology, cell biology, and biochemistry may have applications to the ligament healing process.[200] These approaches include innovative biologic and bioengineering techniques using growth factors, gene transfer therapy, cell therapy, scaffolding materials, and mechanical stimuli.[25]

Gene Transfer. Gene transfer technology has been developed to design and enhance delivery vehicles for growth factors. Controlling and regulating the expression of proteins within a host cell will enable researchers to administer treatments over a prolonged period of time.[200] Although further studies are required, preliminary studies have shown positive effects on collagen fibril diameter and distribution, as well as significant increases in mechanical properties using gene transfer techniques.[129]

Cell Therapy. The concept of cell therapy is that implantation of pluripotent or genetically manipulated cells can enhance the repair of ligaments via a paracrine effect or by direct participation in the repair response.[200] Both in vivo and in vitro studies have already demonstrated that mesenchymal stem cells are capable of differentiating into many cell types involved in ligamentous healing. A study by Watanabe et al.[193] has demonstrated the ability of donor bone marrow cells to migrate to the area of MCL injury after transplantation. Cell therapy may lead to new methods of treatment for ligament injuries in the future, with candidate cells derived from the fat pad, blood vessels, periosteum, and patellar tendon currently under investigation.[89]

Integrated Tissue Engineering Approaches. Biologic scaffolds offer the potential to accelerate ligament and tendon healing and regeneration. One example of this approach is the use of porcine small intestine submucosa. Research has shown that this submucosa can be modified in vitro by seeding marrow stromal cells on the scaffold and by applying cyclic stretching to increase cell alignment. When applied in vivo, the tissue-engineered scaffold could potentially accelerate the healing process.[25] Further research is needed in this area before these scaffolds gain widespread clinical applications.

Bioenhanced ACL repair using a bioactive scaffold (a collagen platelet composite) was proposed by Murray and Fleming as a new potential treatment for ACL injury.[121,122,189] In a porcine model, they demonstrated significant advantages over traditional ACL suture repair; structural properties of the bioenhanced ACL repairs were equivalent to those of conventional ACL reconstruction. Collagen forms a co-polymer with fibrin and prevents accelerated intra-articular degradation, providing a structural matrix and a vehicle for endogenous growth factors.

Preclinical models have also suggested that bioenhanced ACL repair can minimize posttraumatic osteoarthritis after ACL injury and reconstruction.[122]

Recent interest has developed in stem/progenitor cells that characteristically express CD34 surface markers that are found in the human ACL following injury.[115] CD34 positive progenitor cells are abundant in blood vessels and have high proliferation and multilineage differentiation potentials, including the potential to migrate to the site of ACL injury.[205] To achieve direct delivery of these cells to the graft and tendon-bone interface within the tunnel, Mifune et al. developed a cell sheet–wrapped tendon graft in the rat model.[118] They observed that ACL-derived CD34 cell sheet transplantation resulted in enhanced ACL reconstruction healing at the bone-tendon interface in the tunnels and on global graft maturation.

In an attempt to regenerate the ACL and its insertions, Spalazzi et al. developed a degradable triphasic scaffold, modeled after the native stratified ligament insertion site and customized to the resident cell populations and graded mechanical properties.[170] The interconnected poly-lactic-co-glycolic acid (PLGA) scaffold consisted of three distinct phases: Phase A (PLGA 10:90 mesh), designed to support fibroblast proliferation and ligament formation; Phase B (sintered PLGA 85:15 microspheres), designed as the interface region for fibrochondrocyte proliferation; and Phase C (sintered PLGA 85:15 and 45S5 bioactive glass composite microspheres), designed for bone formation. Following encouraging in vitro studies, in vivo studies were performed on a subcutaneous athymic rat model where the triphasic scaffold supported multilineage cellular interactions as well as tissue infiltration and abundant matrix production.[169] Of note, controlled phase-specific matrix heterogeneity was reproducibly induced on the scaffold. Cell seeding demonstrated a positive effect on native cell infiltration and matrix production that corresponded to increased mechanical properties in the cell-seeded groups compared to the acellular controls.

MENISCI

Structure and Function

The menisci of the knee are C-shaped wedges of fibrocartilage interposed between the condyles of the femur and tibia. They are actually extensions of the tibia that serve to deepen the articular surfaces of the tibial plateau to accommodate the condyles of the femur better. The peripheral border of each meniscus is thick and convex and attached to the joint capsule, whereas the inner border tapers to a thin, free edge.[192] The proximal surfaces of the menisci are concave and in contact with the condyles of the femur; their distal surfaces are flat and rest on the tibial plateau (Fig. 36.10).

The medial meniscus is somewhat semicircular in form, approximately 3.5 cm in length and considerably wider posteriorly than anteriorly. The anterior horn of the medial meniscus is attached to the tibial plateau in the area of the anterior intercondylar fossa, anterior to the ACL (Fig. 36.11). The posterior fibers of the anterior horn merge with the transverse ligament, which connects the anterior horns of the medial and lateral menisci.[192] The posterior horn of the medial meniscus is firmly attached to the posterior intercondylar fossa of the tibia between the attachments of the lateral meniscus and posterior cruciate ligament. The periphery of the medial meniscus is attached to the joint capsule throughout its length. The tibial

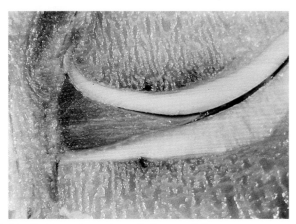

FIG 36.10 Frontal section of the medial compartment of a human knee illustrating the articulation of the menisci with the condyles of the femur and tibia. (From Warren R, Arnoczky SP, Wickiewicz TL: Anatomy of the knee. In Nicholas JA, Hershman EB [eds]: *The lower extremity and spine in sports medicine*, St Louis, MO, 1986, CV Mosby, p 657.)

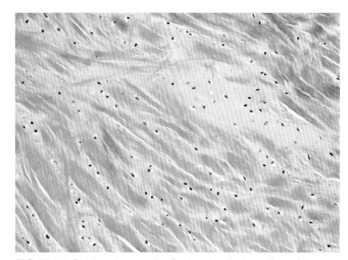

FIG 36.12 Photomicrograph of a longitudinal section of human meniscus showing the histologic appearance of meniscal fibrocartilage (hematoxylin-eosin, ×100).

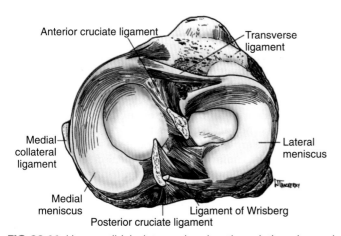

FIG 36.11 Human tibial plateau showing the relative size and attachments of the medial and lateral menisci. (From Warren R, Arnoczky SP, Wickiewicz TL: Anatomy of the knee. In Nicholas JA, Hershman EB [eds]: *The lower extremity and spine in sports medicine*, St Louis, MO, 1986, CV Mosby, p 657.)

portion of the capsular attachment is referred to as the coronary ligament. At its midpoint, the medial meniscus is more firmly attached to the femur and tibia through a condensation in the joint capsule known as the deep MCL.

The lateral meniscus is more circular in shape and covers a larger percentage of the articular surface of the tibial plateau than the medial meniscus does. The anterior and posterior horns are approximately the same width (see Fig. 36.11). The anterior horn of the lateral meniscus is attached to the tibia anterior to the intercondylar eminence and adjacent to the attachment of the ACL, with which it partially blends.[192] The posterior horn of the lateral meniscus is attached posterior to the intercondylar eminence of the tibia, anterior to the posterior horn of the medial meniscus. In addition to this posterior attachment to the tibia, two ligaments may run from the posterior horn of the lateral meniscus to the medial femoral condyle, passing in front of or behind the origin of the posterior

cruciate ligament. These attachments are known as the anterior meniscofemoral ligament (ligament of Humphrey) and the posterior meniscofemoral ligament (ligament of Wrisberg). Although there is no attachment of the lateral meniscus to the lateral collateral ligament, it has a loose peripheral attachment to the joint capsule.

Histologically, the meniscus is a fibrocartilaginous tissue composed primarily of an interlacing network of collagen fibers interposed with cells (Fig. 36.12).[13] The predominant type of collagen in the meniscus is type I, but types II, III, and V are present as well.[117] Although other components, such as proteoglycans, glycoproteins, and water, also contribute to the makeup of the extracellular matrix of the meniscus, it is the specific orientation of the collagen fibers that appears to be most directly related to the function of the meniscus. Although the principal orientation of the collagen fibers is circumferential, a few small, radially oriented fibers appear on both the femoral and tibial surfaces of the menisci, as well as within the substance of the tissue. It is theorized that these radial fibers act as ties to provide structural rigidity and help resist longitudinal splitting of the menisci as a result of overcompression (Fig. 36.13).[28] Tissakht and Ahmed[186] have measured the tensile modulus in the radial and circumferential directions in the human meniscus. Their study showed that the meniscus is much stronger and stiffer in the circumferential direction than the radial direction, and the low circumferential shear strength is thought to be at least partly responsible for the occurrence of longitudinal tears.[7,211]

Subsequent light and electron microscopic examinations of the menisci have revealed three different collagen framework layers—a superficial layer composed of a network of fine fibrils woven into a mesh-like matrix; a surface layer just beneath the superficial layer composed, in part, of irregularly aligned collagen bundles; and a middle layer in which the collagen fibers are larger, coarser, and oriented in a parallel, circumferential direction (Fig. 36.14).[28,203] It is this middle layer that allows the meniscus to resist tensile forces and function in transmission of load across the knee joint. When an axial load is applied to the knee joint, the meniscus is compressed, but because of its wedge-shaped structure and firm anterior and posterior

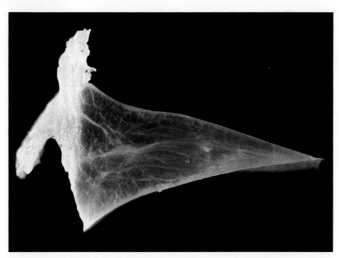

FIG 36.13 Cross-section of a lateral meniscus showing the radial orientation of fibrous ties within the substance of the meniscus. (From Arnoczky SP, Torzilli PA: The biology of cartilage. In Hunter LY, Funk FJ Jr [eds]: *Rehabilitation of the injured knee*, St Louis, MO, 1984, CV Mosby, p 148.)

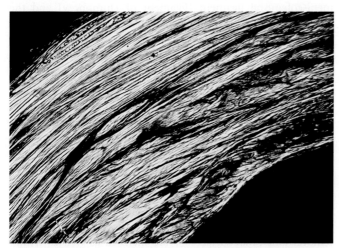

FIG 36.14 Photomicrograph of a longitudinal section of a meniscus under polarized light demonstrating the orientation of the coarse, deep, circumferentially oriented collagen fibers.

attachments to the tibia, it is displaced away from the joint center, resulting in tensile stress (hoop stress) in the circumferential collagen fibers.[180] There are significant regional variations in the circumferential tensile strength and stiffness, with lower values in the posterior two-thirds of the medial meniscus than in the anterior or the lateral meniscus.[58] These variations are probably because of differences in collagen fiber ultrastructure because the variations in material properties are not correlated with differences in biochemical composition.[186]

The exact biomechanical and biological roles of the meniscus in knee joint health and intra-articular homeostasis are not fully understood; however, it is clear that meniscectomy (partial or total) is associated with premature or accelerated knee joint degeneration. Roos et al. observed a relative risk of 14 (increasing prevalence of 1400%) of osteoarthritic knee degeneration at 21 years post meniscectomy.[151] Fairbank[53] originally described radiographic changes after meniscectomy

that included narrowing of the joint space, flattening of the femoral condyle, and formation of osteophytes. Biomechanical studies have demonstrated that the medial meniscus transmits 50% of the joint load in the medial compartment, whereas the lateral meniscus transmits 70% of the joint load in the lateral compartment.[37] At least 50% of the compressive load of the knee joint is transmitted through the meniscus in extension, which increases to approximately 85% of load transmission in 90 degrees of flexion. In a meniscectomized knee, the contact area is reduced by approximately 50%.[2,66] This reduction significantly increases mean and peak stresses, resulting in articular damage and degeneration. Partial meniscectomy has also been shown to increase contact pressure significantly.[19] In an experimental study, resection of as little as 15% to 34% of the meniscus increased contact pressure by more than 350%.[160] Thus, even partial meniscectomy does not appear to be a benign procedure.*

Another proposed function of the meniscus is that of shock absorption, although this has been disputed in biomechanical literature.[9] Rather, it is less controversial to recognize that the biphasic nature of the meniscus contributes load dissipation in a similar manner to articular cartilage at articular surfaces. As a biphasic structure, the meniscus is composed of a fluid phase (the interstitial water) and solid phase (collagen, GAGs, and the other matrix proteins).[171] The collagen network and GAGs form a porous, permeable solid matrix. Interstitial fluid flow and solid matrix deformation during loading cause the meniscus to act as a viscoelastic material. Articular cartilage demonstrates the same biomechanical characteristics, albeit with intrinsic depth-dependent variation based on a differential amount of proteoglycans and varied collagen fiber orientations.

The menisci are thought to contribute to knee joint stability and overall joint conformity.[106,112] The menisci serve to increase congruity between the condyles of the femur and tibia. The superior concave and inferior flat surface of the meniscus conforms to the femoral and tibial condyles, and the wedge shape of the meniscus contributes to its function in joint stabilization. Medial meniscectomy in the ACL-intact knee has little effect on anteroposterior motion; however, in the ACL-deficient knee, medial meniscectomy results in an increase in anterior tibial translation of up to 58% at 90 degrees of flexion.[3,105,136] These findings support the concept that medial meniscal transplantation should be considered at the time of reconstruction of the ACL in the medial meniscus–deficient knee.

The lateral meniscus also plays a role in joint stability. Cadaveric studies demonstrate that the lateral meniscus has a role in control of anterior tibial translation of the lateral tibial plateau during the pivot shift in the ACL-deficient knee.[127] This contrasts with the role of the medial meniscus, which functions more during straight anterior tibial translation testing (Lachman test).

The joint conformity provided by the menisci may promote the viscous hydrodynamic action required for fluid-film lubrication. This function assists in the overall lubrication of the articular surfaces of the knee joint. Water may be extruded into the joint space during compressive loading, aiding in joint lubrication.[14,141] The meniscus may also aid in articular cartilage nutrition by helping maintain a synovial fluid film over the articular surface and by compressing synovial fluid

---

*References 8, 36, 41, 55, 101, and 155.

into articular cartilage.[58] However, the exact contribution of the meniscus to joint lubrication has yet to be fully elucidated.

Finally, the menisci may provide proprioceptive feedback for joint position sense. Neural elements are most abundant in the outer portion of the meniscus, particularly types I and II nerve fibers. The anterior and posterior horns of the meniscus are innervated with mechanoreceptors that may play a role in proprioceptive feedback during extremes of motion.[49,98] These mechanoreceptors are thought to be part of a proprioceptive reflex arc that may contribute to dynamic, functional stability of the knee and may interact with similar somatosensory elements in the capsule and ligaments.[14]

In summary, the proposed functions of the menisci include load bearing, joint stability, lubrication, and proprioception. Loss of the meniscus, partially or totally, significantly alters these functions and predisposes the joint to degenerative changes. Because acute traumatic tears of the meniscus usually occur in young (13- to 40-year-old) and active individuals, the need to preserve the meniscus, and thus minimize these degenerative changes, is of paramount importance.[13] The development of techniques to salvage the meniscus have all but replaced traditional total meniscectomy in the treatment of many meniscal lesions. Although partial meniscectomy may be the only option for some inner, avascular tears, research into new techniques of meniscal repair may eliminate even partial meniscectomy and the undesirable consequences of loss of this important structure.

Biology of Meniscal Injury and Healing

Thomas Annandale was credited with the first surgical repair of a torn meniscus in 1883.[11] It was not until 1936, when King published his classic experiment on meniscus healing in dogs, that the actual biologic limitations of meniscus healing were set forth. King[99] demonstrated that for meniscus lesions to heal, they must communicate with the peripheral blood supply. Enhancing vascularity at or near the site of meniscal injury has remained a major focus in the techniques of surgical repair. In addition, advances in cellular and molecular biology now allow researchers to investigate the role of specific growth factors and cytokines in the cellular response to injury. Further application of these findings will continue to suggest means of enhancing meniscal repair.

Vascular Anatomy of the Meniscus. The vascular supply to the medial and lateral menisci of the knee originates predominantly from the medial and lateral genicular arteries (inferior and superior branches).[15] Branches from these vessels give rise to a perimeniscal capillary plexus within the synovial and capsular tissues of the knee joint. The plexus is an arborizing network of vessels that supply the peripheral border of the meniscus about its attachment to the joint capsule (Figs. 36.15 and 36.16). These perimeniscal vessels are oriented in a predominantly circumferential pattern, with radial branches being directed toward the center of the joint (Fig. 36.17). Anatomic studies have shown that the degree of peripheral vascular penetration is 10% to 30% of the width of the medial meniscus and 10% to 25% of the width of the lateral meniscus.[42] The middle genicular artery, along with a few terminal branches of the medial and lateral genicular vessels, also supplies vessels to the menisci through the vascular synovial covering of the anterior and posterior horn attachments. These synovial vessels penetrate the horn attachments and give rise to smaller vessels that enter

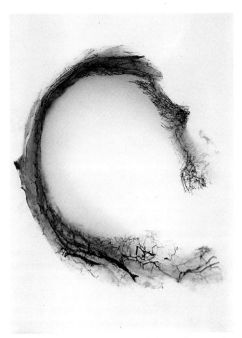

FIG 36.15 Superior aspect of a medial meniscus after vascular perfusion with India ink and tissue clearing with a modified Spalteholz technique. Note the vascularity at the periphery of the meniscus, as well as at the anterior and posterior horn attachments. (From Arnoczky SP, Warren RF: Microvasculature of the human meniscus. *Am J Sports Med* 10:90–95, 1982.)

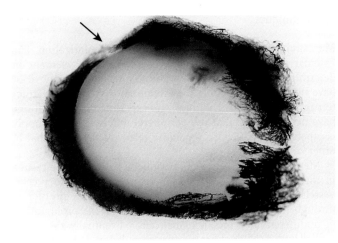

FIG 36.16 Superior aspect of a lateral meniscus after vascular perfusion with India ink and tissue clearing with a modified Spalteholz technique. Note the absence of vascularity at the posterior lateral aspect of the meniscus (*arrow*). This is adjacent to the popliteal hiatus. (From Arnoczky SP, Warren RF: Microvasculature of the human meniscus. *Am J Sports Med* 10:90–95, 1982.)

the meniscal horns for a short distance and end in terminal capillary loops.

A small reflection of the vascular synovial tissue is also present throughout the peripheral attachment of the medial and lateral menisci on the femoral and tibial articular surfaces.[15] This synovial fringe extends for a short distance over the peripheral surfaces of the meniscus and contains small, terminally

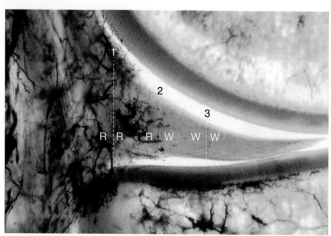

FIG 36.17 A 5-mm-thick frontal section of the medial compartment of a human knee (Spalteholz preparation). Branching radial vessels from the perimeniscal capillary plexus penetrate the peripheral border of the medial meniscus. *RR*, Red-red zone; *RW*, red-white zone; *WW*, white-white zone. (From Arnoczky SP, Warren RF: Microvasculature of the human meniscus. *Am J Sports Med* 10:90–95, 1982.)

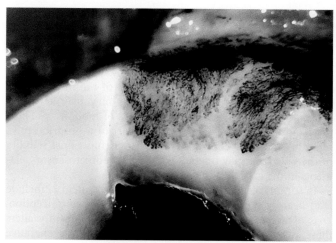

FIG 36.18 A meniscus 6 weeks after the creation of a radial lesion. Fibrovascular scar tissue has filled the defect, and vascular proliferation from the synovial fringe can be seen. (From Arnoczky SP, Warren RF: The microvasculature of the meniscus and its response to injury: an experimental study in the dog. *Am J Sports Med* 11:131–141, 1983.)

looped vessels. Although the synovial fringe is adherent to the articular surfaces of the menisci, it does not contribute vessels to the meniscus per se. The clinical significance of these fringe vessels lies in their potential contribution to the reparative response of the meniscus, as seen in synovial abrasion techniques.

Meniscal Healing Is Dependent on Zonal Vascularization. The vascular supply of the meniscus is the essential element in determining its potential for repair. This blood supply must have the ability to support the inflammatory response characteristic of wound repair. Clinical and experimental observations have demonstrated that the peripheral meniscal blood supply is capable of producing a reparative response similar to that in other connective tissue.[16,82]

Meniscal injury within the peripheral vascular zone results in the formation of a fibrin clot, rich in inflammatory cells. Vessels from the perimeniscal capillary plexus proliferate through this fibrin scaffold, accompanied by the proliferation of undifferentiated mesenchymal cells.[16] Eventually, the lesion is filled with a cellular fibrovascular granulation tissue that glues the wound edges together and appears to be continuous with the adjacent normal meniscal fibrocartilage.[31] Increased collagen synthesis within the granulation tissue slowly results in a fibrous scar (Fig. 36.18). The exact phenotype of the cells that initiate and regulate the healing process is unknown. Like other connective tissues, the lesion heals with scar tissue that likely has inferior material properties. For example, the tensile strength of the healed lesion did not reach the strength of normal meniscus even by 12 to 16 weeks in one animal study.[14] Furthermore, the long-term histologic and biomechanical characteristics of the reparative tissue are unknown.

Experimental studies have shown that radial lesions of the meniscus that extend to the synovium are completely healed with fibrovascular scar tissue by 10 weeks (Fig. 36.19).[16,31] Modulation of this scar into normal-appearing fibrocartilage, however, requires several months. Further study is required to

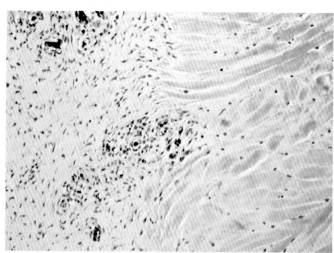

FIG 36.19 Photomicrograph of the junction of the meniscus and fibrovascular repair tissue at 10 weeks (hematoxylin-eosin, ×100). (From Arnoczky SP, Warren RF: The microvasculature of the meniscus and its response to injury: an experimental study in the dog. *Am J Sports Med* 11:131–141, 1983.)

delineate the biomechanical properties at each stage of this repair process.

The ability of meniscal lesions to heal has provided the rationale for the repair of peripheral meniscal injuries, and a number of reports have demonstrated excellent results after primary repair of peripheral meniscal injuries.[35,43,44,116,149] Follow-up examination of these peripheral repairs has revealed a process of repair similar to that noted in experimental models.

When examining injured menisci for potential repair, lesions are often classified by the location of the tear relative to the blood supply of the meniscus and the vascular appearance of the peripheral and central surfaces of the tear (see Fig. 36.17).[12] The so-called red-red tear (peripheral capsular detachment) has a functional blood supply to the capsular and meniscal side of

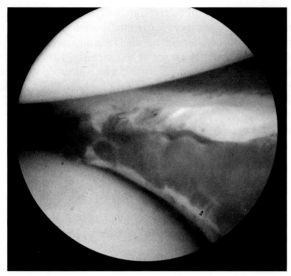

FIG 36.20 Arthroscopic view of a peripheral tear in a human meniscus. Note the vascular granulation tissue present at the margin of the lesion. This is classified as a red-white tear. Also note the proliferation of the synovial fringe over the femoral surface of the meniscus. (From Arnoczky SP, Torzilli PA: The biology of cartilage. In Hunter LY, Funk FJ Jr [eds]: *Rehabilitation of the injured knee*, St Louis, MO, 1984, CV Mosby, p 148.)

the lesion and obviously has the best prognosis for healing. Red-white tears (meniscus tears through the peripheral vascular zone) have an active peripheral blood supply; however, the central (inner) surface of the lesion is devoid of functioning vessels (Fig. 36.20). These lesions have sufficient vascularity to heal by the aforementioned fibrovascular proliferation. White-white tears (meniscus lesions completely in the avascular zone) are without blood supply and theoretically cannot heal. However, as discussed later, specific meniscal repair enhancement techniques have been developed to address tears in the white-white zone.

Meniscal Tissue Degeneration. Intrinsic meniscal degeneration begins around 30 years of age, progresses with age, and occurs in both men and women and in active and inactive subjects.[131] Histologic analysis demonstrates mucinous degeneration, hypocellularity, and loss of normal collagen fiber organization.[195] The cause of such changes is unknown, but may reflect recurrent chronic microtrauma to the meniscus. Studies in animals have demonstrated that following ACL transection, the menisci undergo alterations in their extracellular matrices, including an increase in water content.[1,117] An initial decrease in the concentration of GAGs has also been observed following ACL transection. However, in joints with chronic ACL insufficiency, the concentration of GAGs was found to increase substantially. This reflects a remarkable ability of meniscal fibrochondrocytes to replenish the lost GAGs.

Degenerative meniscal tissue is believed to have a poorer potential for healing.[14] Careful attention should be paid to the appearance and consistency of the meniscus at the time of surgery. Although preservation of the meniscus may be more important in a knee with axial malalignment, the rate of healing may be lower because of concomitant degenerative changes.[75]

Meniscal Repair

Indications. Based on the established important functions of the meniscus and the clinical results of meniscectomy, most clinicians try to preserve the meniscus via repair whenever possible. Although the treatment of meniscal tears should be individualized (based on tear and patient characteristics), the most commonly accepted criteria for meniscal repair include the following: (1) a complete vertical longitudinal tear longer than 10 mm in length; (2) a tear within the peripheral 10% to 30% of the meniscus or within 3 or 4 mm of the meniscocapsular junction; (3) a peripheral tear that can be displaced toward the center of the plateau by probing, thus demonstrating instability; (4) the absence of secondary degeneration or deformity; (5) a tear in an active patient; and (6) a tear associated with concurrent ligament stabilization.

Although it is most critical to perform meniscal repair on young patients in an attempt to decrease the eventual articular cartilage wear of a meniscectomized knee, meniscal repair can also be successful in older patients.[32] Well-vascularized longitudinal red-red tears and red-white tears are ideal for repair and also have the highest rate of healing. Stable longitudinal tears (<1 cm in length) and partial-thickness tears often remain asymptomatic or heal without suturing.[163] Although degenerative tears and radial tears can also be repaired, the function of a repaired meniscus has yet to be proved.

The onset of degenerative change has been linked to the amount of meniscus removed.[8] Large bucket handle tears as seen in young active patients would require a large portion of the meniscus to be removed if not repaired. In these younger patients, meniscal repair is often extended into the white-white (avascular) zone by using the vascular enhancement techniques discussed later. A poorer prognosis in a meniscectomized knee has also been associated with varus alignment and ACL deficiency, so meniscal repair should similarly be considered in these situations when possible.[29,55] In addition, decreased healing rates are seen in ACL-deficient knees, so any instability of the knee should also be addressed.[119,183]

Biological Augmentation of Meniscal Repair. The desire to preserve meniscal tissue has led to efforts to extend the region of viable meniscal repair to the central, avascular portion of the meniscus (white-white tears).[12] Experimental and clinical observations have shown that these lesions are incapable of healing under usual circumstances and have provided the rationale for partial meniscectomy.[15,99] In an effort to extend the level of repair into these avascular areas, techniques have been developed to provide vascularity to these white-white tears, as well as to enhance the repair of red-white tears. Such techniques include débridement, creation of vascular access channels, trephination, use of synovial pedicles, and synovial abrasion. Also discussed will be the use and delivery of growth factors to promote meniscal healing and the role of mechanical load on healing of meniscal repairs. Finally, innovations in gene therapy and tissue engineered menisci will be explored.

Vascular access channels and trephination. The creation of vascular access channels (VACs) was one of the early techniques used to extend the vascular response into the avascular zone of the meniscus.[15,82] The premise of this technique is to create full-thickness channels connecting the avascular lesion to the peripheral vasculature of the meniscus. Experimental studies in animals have demonstrated that lesions in the avascular portion of the meniscus, when connected to the peripheral vasculature by means of a full-thickness VAC, heal through the proliferation of fibrovascular scar tissue from the VAC into the tear (Fig. 36.21). VACs can allow for an extensive influx of vessels into a white-white tear, but they also cut across the predominantly circumferential orientation of the collagen fibers of the meniscus. This disruption in collagen architecture may adversely affect the function of the meniscus, especially if the VAC is carried out through the peripheral rim of the meniscus. Consequently, the original VAC technique has not been used extensively in the clinical situation.

The technique of trephination was introduced as a means of creating a pathway for vascular migration without imparting

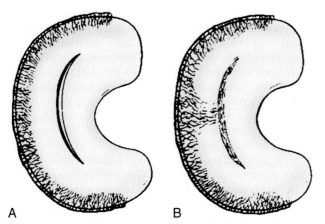

FIG 36.21 Schematic drawing showing the concept of connecting a lesion in the avascular portion of the meniscus with the peripheral blood supply through the use of a vascular access channel. (A) Tear in an avascular zone. (B) Vascular proliferation through an access channel. (From Arnoczky SP, Warren RF: The microvasculature of the meniscus and its response to injury: an experimental study in the dog. *Am J Sports Med* 11:131–141, 1983.)

significant damage to the collagen architecture of the meniscus.[148] In this procedure, a series of horizontally oriented trephinations are made with a hypodermic needle (18-gauge needle or larger) through the peripheral aspect of the meniscal rim to produce a series of bleeding puncture sites, which provide an avenue for vascular ingrowth. This modification of the VAC technique minimizes the damage done to the collagen architecture of the meniscus but still allows for the influx of a vascular response. Initially developed in an animal model, clinical application of this technique has been described with and without the use of sutures.[208,210] In the first clinical report of trephination, this technique was used to treat incomplete lesions in the peripheral and middle third of the meniscus.[60] Although a 90% success rate was reported in this series, there was no control group with which to compare the specific efficacy of the technique. More recently, controlled studies have found trephination alone to be successful in treating stable meniscal lesions; it has also been identified as a means of augmenting traditional suture repair.[165,206]

Synovial pedicles (flaps) and abrasion. An additional approach to extend the vascular supply to an avascular meniscal tear involves the use of a synovial pedicle or flap. In this technique, a pedicle of the highly vascular synovial tissue immediately adjacent to the peripheral attachment of the meniscus is rotated into the avascular lesion and sutured in place. Although animal experiments using this technique suggest excellent potential for augmenting repairs in the white-white zone of the human meniscus, there is a paucity of clinical research in this area, possibly because of the technical difficulties in adapting synovial pedicle use to an arthroscopic approach.[67,69]

Synovial abrasion is a technique in which the synovial fringe of the femoral and tibial surfaces of the meniscus is abraded with a rasp to stimulate a proliferative response (Fig. 36.22). During the normal repair process of peripheral lesions, a vascular pannus develops from the synovial fringe and extends over the femoral and tibial surfaces of the meniscus (see Fig. 36.18). The combination of this vascular response with the peripheral meniscal blood supply provides support for the repair process.

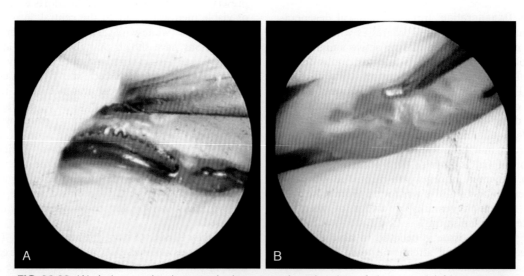

FIG 36.22 (A) Arthroscopic photograph demonstrating abrasion of the synovial fringe on the surface of the meniscus with a rasp. (B) Arthroscopic photograph taken 8 weeks after synovial abrasion demonstrating a vascular pannus extending into a white-white tear. (Courtesy Dr. Charles Henning.)

Because the vascular pannus observed in the repair process is often extensive, it was theorized that stimulation of the synovial fringe could accentuate this response and help extend it into avascular or marginally vascularized areas.[13,82] The ability of synovial abrasion to enhance the healing potential of tears in avascular areas of the meniscus has been demonstrated in several animal models.[134,145] Clinical application of synovial abrasion alone, as well as in conjunction with other enhancement techniques (including trephination and fibrin clot), has been shown to be effective in treating stable or partial-thickness meniscal tears.[82,165] Additionally, the efficacy of synovial abrasion and the simplicity of the surgical technique have led to recommendations for its use in augmenting suture repairs.[20,81,157]

Marrow-stimulating techniques. Cannon and Vittori[33] have found that meniscal healing rates improve from 53% to 93% when the repair is performed in conjunction with ACL reconstruction. Shelbourne and Heinrich's long-term follow-up[164] of lateral meniscal tears left in situ at the time of ACL reconstruction has demonstrated 96% normal or near-normal results. These clinical findings suggest that blood and marrow elements may produce a milieu bathing the healing meniscus, thus providing essential mitogenic and chemotactic elements. There may also be a beneficial effect from the slower rehabilitation protocol when meniscus repair is done with concomitant ACL reconstruction.[92] Assuming that the cytokines and growth factors in the blood and marrow elements introduced into the knee after notchplasty and tunnel drilling in ACL reconstruction are responsible for the improved repair rates, there would be a theoretical advantage to reproducing the presence of blood and marrow elements during meniscal repair in an ACL-intact knee. Microfracture of the intercondylar notch has been proposed as a means of re-creating the hemarthrosis present after ACL reconstruction in the hope of improving meniscal repair outcomes.[63] Although this adjunct procedure is relatively easy to execute and associated with limited additional risk, its efficacy has not been explored in the literature.

Growth factors. Recent emphasis has been directed toward applications of cell and molecular biology to promote meniscal healing and regeneration. Numerous growth factors have been identified as signaling molecules that control mitogenic behavior and differentiation of cells. These growth factors have been used on meniscal cells to test their effects on the healing of tears or defects, as well as their effects on extracellular matrix synthesis in tissue and cell culture (Table 36.2). Cells from the peripheral part of the meniscus have an increased ability to synthesize collagen in cell culture, compared with cells derived from the inner part of the meniscus.[173] There are other differences in cellular physiology between the cells in the inner and outer regions of the meniscus, including the responsiveness to growth factors and cytokines. Webber et al.[194] have tested the effect of fibroblastic growth factor (FGF) and human platelet lysate (PL), both of which were found to stimulate proliferation of meniscal cells. TGF-β increased proteoglycan synthesis of fibrochondrocytes from all different regions of the meniscus in a dose-dependent manner.[38,182] Spindler et al.[172,173] have demonstrated that the cells in the inner, central region of the tissue are much less responsive to platelet-derived growth factor-AB (PDGF-AB) than the cells in the peripheral portion of the tissue. Conversely, Bhargava et al.[23] have demonstrated that at optimal concentrations, PDGF-AB, hepatocyte growth factor (HGF), and bone morphogenetic protein-2 (BMP-2) are equally effective in stimulating DNA synthesis in cells isolated from

TABLE 36.2 Effects of Various Growth Factors on Meniscal Tissue

Type	In Vitro or In Vivo (Animal)	Cell Source	Result
FGF[6]	In vitro	Rabbit	Stimulates proliferation
Human PL[6]	In vitro	Rabbit	Stimulates proliferation
ECGF[62]	Dog	No	Improves healing in cylindrical defect
ECGF[60]	Dog	No	Increases short-term healing in tears
PDGF-AB[54]	In vitro	Ovine	Affects mitogenic response from outer third of meniscus
TGF-β[53]	In vitro	Ovine	Increases proteoglycan synthesis
Hyaluronic acid[59]	Rabbit	No	Increases rate of healing in a cylindrical defect
TGF-β[52]	In vitro	Human	Increases proteoglycan synthesis
PDGF-AB[55]	In vitro	Bovine	Stimulates cell migration, increased DNA synthesis
HGF[55]	In vitro	Bovine	Stimulates cell migration, increased DNA synthesis
BMP-2[55]	In vitro	Bovine	Some cell migration, increased DNA synthesis
IGF-1[55]	In vitro	Bovine	Some cell migration
IL-1[55]	In vitro	Bovine	Some cell migration
EGF[55]	In vitro	Bovine	Some cell migration
Hyaluronan[58]	Rabbit	No	Stimulate collagen remodeling in peripheral zone

HGF, Human growth factor.
From Sweigart MA, Athanasiou KA: Toward tissue engineering of the knee meniscus. *Tissue Eng* 7:111–129, 2001.

different zones of the meniscus. BMP-2 and insulin-like growth factor-1 (IGF-1) stimulated the migration of fibrochondrocytes from the middle zone by 40% to 50%. This study also reported that interleukin-1 (IL-1) and EGF stimulated migration of meniscal cells. Other studies have reported that hyaluronan and hyaluronic acid increased healing in a cylindric meniscal defect and stimulated collagen remodeling in the peripheral zone.[168,179] Endothelial growth factor (ECGF) was reported to accelerate healing of an allograft to the joint capsule.[128] Hashimoto et al.[78] have tested the effect of ECGF on a cylindric defect in the canine meniscus and found that defects that contained both the fibrin sealant and ECGF have the best healing. In vivo, both fibroblastic growth factor-2 (FGF-2) and connective tissue growth factor (CTGF) have demonstrated enhancement of meniscal repair in a rabbit model; surprisingly, delivery of vascular endothelial growth factor (VEGF) in an attempt to promote vascularization of the tear did not show an advantage in a sheep model.[80,100,130]

Point of care biological augmentation. The increasing use of biologics—for example, blood clot, fibrin, PRP, and platelet-rich fibrin (PRF)—has benefited from specific growth factor studies where cell behavior in controlled stimuli is more easily assessed. Thus, the compositional characterization of biologics is essential to interpreting their effects; it is also becoming apparent that the growth factor profiles in biologics may be

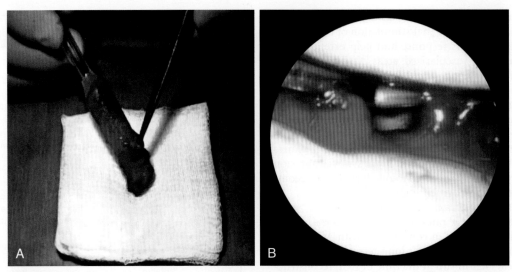

FIG 36.23 (A) Fibrin clot precipitated onto the surface of a glass syringe barrel. (B) Arthroscopic photograph of a fibrin clot being sutured into a meniscal tear. (From McAndrews PT, Arnoczky SP: Meniscal repair enhancement techniques. *Clin Sports Med* 15:499–510, 1996.)

customized to an extent in their preparation.[93,102,177] Earliest developments investigated the use of a fibrin clot to induce and support a healing response in the avascular portion of the meniscus. An in vitro study has shown that when meniscal fibrochondrocytes are exposed to growth factors normally found in a blood clot, the cells demonstrate a marked increase in proliferation and matrix synthesis.[194] An in vivo study in animals has demonstrated that when a defect in the avascular portion of the meniscus is filled with a fibrin clot, the defect is able to heal with connective tissue similar to that seen in normal meniscal repair.[17] Approximately 50 to 60 mL of whole blood is obtained from the patient and placed in a sterile glass beaker. Then, with the sintered glass barrel from a 20-mL glass syringe, the blood is stirred gently until a fibrin clot is precipitated on the surface of the barrel (Fig. 36.23). This process usually takes between 3 and 5 minutes. The consistency of the clot formed in this manner is similar to that of wet chewing gum and is capable of holding sutures placed through its substance. Although use of the fibrin clot technique in white-white tears has been limited, clinical studies have suggested improved healing rates in red-white meniscal tears in which a fibrin clot was used.[83,84] These findings have been substantiated again recently by Jang et al., who augmented arthroscopic inside-out repair with autologous fibrin clots and reported a success rate of 95% in 41 meniscus tears (19 radial tears, 12 longitudinal tears in the red-white zone, 7 transverse, and 3 oblique).[96] In addition, Ra et al. investigated the efficacy of arthroscopic inside-out repair in with fibrin clot placed in situ with radial tears.[143] At 30 months, there were improvements in clinical scores (Lysholm score and IKDC subjective knee score from 65 ± 6 and 57 ± 7 to 94 ± 3 and 92 ± 3, respectively). Objectively, radiographic healing was demonstrated in 11 of 12 MRIs, and second-look arthroscopy showed healing of the meniscus lesion in 6 of 7 cases.

The use of PRP is another potential way to provide growth factors to the area of an avascular meniscal lesion, but in greater concentrations than possible in a normal fibrin clot. PRP is defined as a platelet concentration of at least 1,000,000 platelets/µL in 5 mL of plasma.[114] This represents a threefold to fivefold increase in concentration over normal circulating platelet numbers. PRP contains increased concentrations (above normal circulating plasma levels) of several growth factors, including PDGF, TGF-β, EGF, and IGF-I.[153,196,198] Ishida et al. reported a preclinical study of the effects of PRP on meniscal tissue regeneration using a gelatin hydrogel.[95] In their study, PRP was prepared using a double spin technique and characterized; platelet counts and growth factor compositional analyses were recorded and compared to platelet poor plasma (PPP), revealing significantly more PDGF-BB, TGF-β1, and VEGF in the PRP. In vitro, a positive effect of PRP on cell viability/proliferation and matrix production (sulfated GAG) was demonstrated using cells from the inner two-thirds of the meniscus. In addition, gene expression analysis revealed no difference in Type I collagen expression with significant up-regulation of biglycan and decorin and down-regulation of aggrecan expression in the PRP treated cells. The in vivo study arm, focused on the delivery of PRP to the tear interface using a cross-linked, lyophilized gelatin hydrogel (incorporated and incubated for 1 hour). Experimental groups included PRP, PPP, and control (phosphate buffered saline) for the treatment of a 1.5-mm defect in the anterior inner two-thirds of the meniscus in a skeletally mature rabbit model. Using a semi-quantitative histological repair scoring system, there was an increased tissue bonding, fibrochondrocyte number, and glycosaminoglycan matrix in the PRP group compared to PPP and the control at 4, 8, and 12 weeks. Furthermore, there was significantly increased tissue regeneration in the PRP group at 12 weeks. In addition, the PPP and control groups were seen to have a more fibrous repair with relatively decreased GAG staining.

There is a relative paucity of literature reporting the effect of PRP on clinical outcomes in meniscal repair. Griffin et al. report a study that assessed the usefulness of PRP in arthroscopic meniscal repair (without ACL reconstruction) at a minimum follow-up of 2 years.[73] Their results did not show any differences in reoperation or clinical outcome scores; however, the study was admittedly underpowered, making definitive conclusions difficult to derive. In addition, Pujol et al. presented a case control study of 34 consecutive patients who had an open repair of horizontal meniscal tears extending into the avascular zone with and without PRP augmentation.[142] Interestingly, they observed a positive significant difference in magnetic resonance (MR) radiographic healing status in the PRP group; however, this did not correlate with clinical outcome scores (Knee Injury and Osteoarthritis Outcome Score [KOOS], IKDC scores) at approximately 30 months postoperatively. Although positive trends in both clinical outcome scores for the PRP groups were seen, these only achieved significance for the KOOS pain and sports parameters.

A corollary to the use of a fibrin clot or PRP is the proposed use of synthetic fibrin glue. The fibrin adhesive, which is formed by combining various factors in the normal clotting cascade (fibrinogen, thrombin, $CaCl_2$, and factor XIII) with an antifibrinolysate (aprotinin), has been used in other surgical applications to hold biologic tissues in approximation. Although the adhesive property of fibrin glue is superior to that of a natural fibrin clot, the synthetic material lacks the biologically active growth factors normally found in the clot. Thus, although it may be able to hold wound edges in apposition more securely than a natural fibrin clot can, it has not been shown to play an active role in stimulating the repair process.[27]

Knee joint loading and mechanobiology. There is little guidance available regarding the effect of knee joint (and tear) loading and range of motion on meniscal healing. One study using a dog model has found that cast immobilization of repaired meniscal lesions in the vascular zone of canine menisci resulted in a decrease in collagen formation after 10 weeks of immobilization, compared with nonimmobilized controls.[48] An experimental study in rabbits has found that immobilization of the normal meniscus results in diminished matrix permeability and degenerative changes in the deep layers of the meniscus.[133] The adverse effect of such immobilization was associated with a significant reduction in blood flow compared with the nonimmobilized joint.[24] In clinical situations, a period of joint immobilization may be necessary for initial postoperative protection of articular tissues, but normal mobility of the joint should be restored as soon as possible to promote joint homeostasis. In fact, in vitro mechanobiology studies are beginning to characterize the role of mechanics in meniscal healing, with current literature suggesting that tensile strain on fibrochondrocytes may reduce inflammatory factors and increase GAG and collagen production.[59,60] However, harnessing the anabolic effects of loading in the acute phase may be hampered by proinflammatory cytokines in the postinjury joint milieu, in addition to concerns for early tear interface healing.[62]

Future Directions for Meniscal Healing: Cells, Gene Therapy, and Integrated Tissue-Engineered Solutions

Research is currently ongoing into methods to enhance meniscus healing and to regenerate meniscus tissue (see Fig. 36.5). Recent studies have demonstrated the ability to transfect meniscal fibrochondrocytes with relevant genes using gene therapy techniques, suggesting that bioactive factors could be delivered to the meniscus by transferring growth factor genes to meniscal cells.[52,71,72,85,113] Tissue engineering techniques using absorbable polymer scaffolds seeded with cells and growth factors are also being explored as a means of healing meniscus lesions, as well as potentially regenerating meniscus tissue.[†] In addition, the use of scaffolds and hydrogels to augment meniscal repair seeks to

provide a three dimensional (3-D) matrix across the tear while acting as a vehicle for cells, growth factors and biologics.[92] This was explored clinically by Piontek et al., who describe a novel all-inside tear wrapping technique outside the repair with a collagen membrane.[139] Mesenchymal stem cells (MSCs) have been explored as a potential cell source to facilitate meniscal repair and regeneration with and without scaffold/hydrogel carriers. Combining a hyaluronan scaffold seeded with undifferentiated MSCs in the rabbit model, Zellner et al. noted superior meniscal repair compared to a precultured prochondrocytic MSC group; this finding suggests the potential of MSC to exert a potential paracrine function at the repair site in addition to providing a pluripotent cell source.[204] Meanwhile, Moriguchi et al. observed enhanced healing of avascular tears in the miniature swine model using scaffold-free tissue-engineered constructs derived from synovial mesenchymal stem cells.[120]

Vangsness et al. recently reported on a randomized double-blind controlled study investigating the safety of intra-articular injection of allogenic MSCs into the knee 7 to 10 days following partial meniscectomy. The ability to stimulate meniscus regeneration and the effects on osteoarthritic changes in the knee were investigated.[188] There were 55 patients across seven institutions, with each randomized to three treatment groups, including (1) injection of 50 million allogeneic MSCs, (2) injection of 150 million MSCs, (3) a control group receiving a sodium hyaluronate vehicle alone. Patients were followed out to 2 years with longitudinal MRI and clinical assessment. Using an a priori threshold of 15% of meniscal volume, there was significantly increased meniscus volume in 24% of patients who received 50 million cells and in 6% of patients who received the higher dose (150 million cells); no volumetric increase was seen in the control group. In patients with osteoarthritic changes, MSC administration was associated with improvements in visual analog scale (VAS) pain scores. Finally, no ectopic tissue formation was observed nor clinically important safety issues encountered.

Recent emphasis in meniscal research has been directed toward applications of molecular biology to promote meniscal regeneration. Gene transfer has emerged as a new approach for growth factor delivery.[52] Several investigators have demonstrated the ability to transfer specific genes into meniscal chondrocytes using retroviral and adenoviral vectors.[72,85,113] Goto et al.[71] have implanted an adenoviral suspension with a fibrin clot into experimentally created canine and lapine meniscal lesions. They demonstrated successful delivery with gene expression lasting for the 3-week duration of the experiment. In the same study, they observed successful transgene expression 6 weeks after transplantation of retrovirally transduced cells into meniscal defects. In addition, Zhang et al. investigated the usefulness of overexpressing the human IGF-1 gene in delivered bone marrow stromal cells to an anterior horn, avascular zone meniscal tear (goat model).[208] Their findings support enhanced histological repair using this approach, compared to the control and non-manipulated stromal cells.

The future ability of gene therapy to treat meniscal injuries depends on precise identification of appropriate growth factors and finding the most effective means for gene delivery. Understanding the appropriate length of time for gene expression and finding a means to control levels of gene expression are important.[72] Future research in gene therapy will also focus on methods to accelerate meniscal allograft healing and enhance bioengineered meniscal tissue.

---

†References 39, 40, 68, 110, 138, and 175.

ACKNOWLEDGMENTS

We acknowledge the contributions of Matthew J. Crawford, Julie A. Dodds, and Steven P. Arnoczky from the previous edition of the chapter.

KEY REFERENCES

3. Allen CR, Wong EK, Livesay GA, et al: Importance of the medial meniscus in the anterior cruciate ligament-deficient knee. *J Orthop Res* 18:109–115, 2000.

8. Andersson-Molina H, Karlsson H, Rockborn P: Arthroscopic partial and total meniscectomy: a long-term follow-up study with matched controls. *Arthroscopy* 18:183–189, 2002.

14. Arnoczky SP, McDevitt CA: The meniscus: structure, function, repair, and replacement. In Buckwalter JA, Einhorn TA, Simon SR, editors: *Orthopaedic basic science*, Rosemont, IL, 2000, American Academy of Orthopaedic Surgeons, pp 531–545.

36. Chatain F, Adeleine P, Chambat P, et al: A comparative study of medial versus lateral arthroscopic partial meniscectomy on stable knees: 10-year minimum follow-up. *Arthroscopy* 19:842–849, 2003.

37. Cole BJ, Carter TR, Rodeo SA: Allograft meniscal transplantation. Background, techniques, and results. *J Bone Joint Surg Am* 84:1236–1250, 2002.

63. Freedman KB, Nho SJ, Cole BJ: Marrow stimulating technique to augment meniscus repair. *Arthroscopy* 19:794–798, 2003.

74. Gulotta L, Rodeo SA: Basic science aspects of ACL: graft healing, vascularity, microscopic anatomy. In Bach BR Jr, editor: *ACL surgery:* *how to get it right the first time and what to do if it fails*, Thorofare, NJ, 2010, Slack.

116. McCarty EC, Marx RG, DeHaven KE: Meniscus repair: considerations in treatment and update of clinical results. *Clin Orthop* 402:122–134, 2002.

123. Murray MM, Martin SD, Martin TL, et al: Histological changes in the human anterior cruciate ligament after rupture. *J Bone Joint Surg Am* 82(10):1387–1397, 2000.

136. Papageorgiou CD, Gil JE, Kanamori A, et al: The biomechanical interdependence between the anterior cruciate ligament replacement graft and the medial meniscus. *Am J Sports Med* 29:226–231, 2001.

138. Peretti GM, Caruso EM, Randolph MA, et al: Meniscal repair using engineered tissue. *J Orthop Res* 19:278–285, 2001.

155. Scheller G, Sobau C, Bulow JU: Arthroscopic partial lateral meniscectomy in an otherwise normal knee: clinical, functional, and radiographic results of a long-term follow-up study. *Arthroscopy* 17:946–952, 2001.

164. Shelbourne KD, Heinrich J: The long-term evaluation of lateral meniscus tears left in situ at the time of anterior cruciate ligament reconstruction. *Arthroscopy* 20:346–351, 2004.

165. Shelbourne KD, Rask BP: The sequelae of salvaged nondegenerative peripheral vertical medial meniscus tears with anterior cruciate ligament reconstruction. *Arthroscopy* 17:270–274, 2001.

200. Woo SL, Vogrin TM, Abramowitch SD: Healing and repair of ligament injuries in the knee. *J Am Acad Orthop Surg* 8:364–372, 2000.

The references for this chapter can also be found on www.expertconsult.com.

37

Arthroscopic Meniscal Resection

Tristan Camus, Yair D. Kissin, W. Norman Scott, Fred D. Cushner

Once considered a functionless structure, the menisci are now known to provide several crucial functions in the knee, including lubrication, proprioception, shock absorption, and force transmission, thereby alleviating the contact pressures on articulate cartilage. Meniscal integrity in the anterior cruciate ligament (ACL)-deficient knee is of particular importance because the menisci significantly improve joint stability.[24] Our improved understanding of the function of the meniscus, as well as advances in orthopedic surgical techniques, has shifted the management of meniscal pathology toward tissue preservation, rather than resection. Current research has focused on the improvement of meniscal repair, and meniscal transplantation techniques, in an effort to preserve normal joint anatomy and biomechanics. In many circumstances, however, meniscal injury is unsuitable for repair or transplantation, and may therefore require partial resection. This chapter reviews the indications, techniques, and consequences of meniscal resection.

The menisci consist of circumferential and radial fibers, which distribute hoop stresses and shear stresses, respectively. There is a linear relationship between the extent of meniscectomy and increased contact pressures in the knee. Partial meniscectomy by as little as 10% has been shown to increase contact pressures in the knee by 65%, and total meniscectomy by 235%.[2,23] Lateral meniscectomy was associated with inferior postoperative outcomes when considering knee function, Lysholm scores, activity level, repeat surgeries, and instability.[33] The lateral compartment is less conforming than the medial compartment, and loss of the meniscus on the lateral side may lead to an increased amount of instability and resultant force transmission to the articular cartilage, causing the increased degeneration and the poor outcomes observed.[31] Maintenance of as much meniscal tissue as possible is therefore essential in decreasing overall contact stresses across the knee joint. However, the menisci are mostly avascular structures, as illustrated in landmark work done by Arnoczky and Warren, which has helped our understanding of the limited healing potential of torn meniscus.[10]

Vascular supply is crucial to meniscal healing. The medial, lateral, and middle geniculate arteries provide the major vascularization to the inferior and superior aspects of each meniscus. The premeniscal capillary network arises from branches of these arteries. Only 10% to 30% of the meniscal borders receive direct blood supply. The lateral meniscus has less capsular attachment than the medial meniscus, and thereby has less perfusion. The remaining portion of each meniscus (70% to 90%) receives nourishment by diffusion from the synovial fluid. The zones of the menisci are therefore described in relation to

this limited blood supply; the red-red in the well-perfused periphery, red-white in the middle, and white-white in the avascular rim. Tears within 3 mm of the meniscosynovial junction, are considered vascular and potentially repairable, but those larger than 5 mm from this junction are considered avascular and generally irreparable. It is for this reason that most meniscal tears approached surgically undergo resection rather than repair (Fig. 37.1).[1,18]

The radiographic abnormalities associated with meniscectomy have long since been described, and include joint space narrowing, osteophyte formation, and condylar squaring.[11] Many long-term studies with greater than 10 year follow-up have shown progressive arthritis in the surgical knee compared to the unaffected side. Although postmeniscectomy radiographic changes do not always correlate with poor clinical outcomes, most of these long-term studies have concluded that meniscectomy accelerates the onset and severity of arthritis.[12,13,30]

As previously discussed, meniscal tears can be classified by the location of the tear in relation to the blood supply and healing potential (Fig. 37.2). Meniscal tears are also classified according to the tear pattern. Tears can be vertical, both longitudinal or radial, horizontal, or they can be complex. Complex displaceable tears consist of parrot beak, flap, and bucket handle tears (Fig. 37.3). In addition to vascularity and pattern, the chronicity of the tear and associated injuries also play an important role in classification and treatment. Acute tears less than 3 weeks old are more amenable to repair, whereas chronic and degenerative tears are less likely repairable. Associated injuries, such as ACL tears, also affect the management of meniscal tears. The incidence of concomitant meniscal tears varies considerably, ranging from 16% to 82% in acute ACL tears, and up to 96% in chronic ACL tears.[17] In acute ACL injuries, the lateral meniscus is more commonly involved, whereas the medial meniscus is typically involved in chronically ACL-deficient knees.[17] It has been shown that the results of ACL reconstruction are worse in knees requiring meniscectomy, and therefore earlier repair of acute ACL tears is recommended to avoid the development of unrepairable meniscal pathology.

Several patient-related factors to consider in the management of meniscal tears are age, activity level, ability to comply with physical therapy, and body mass index (BMI). Young athletes have a higher success rate with meniscal repair procedures than older, more sedentary patients. Partial meniscectomy requires less cooperation with physical therapy from the patient, and therefore an inability to participate in a more stringent

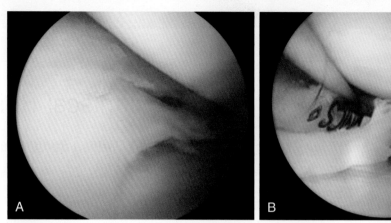

FIG 37.1 (A) Flap tear of the medial meniscus in the avascular zone. (B) Resection of the tear with a mechanical shaver.

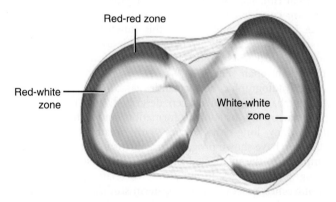

FIG 37.2 Classification of meniscal tears according to location. Red-red zone (outer third, vascularized), red-white zone (middle third), and white zone (inner third, avascular).

rehabilitation protocol may make resection a better choice than repair. Finally, patients with elevated BMIs (variably defined in the literature as >30) have inferior results with meniscal resection compared to their counterparts with normal BMIs, often as a result of concurrent arthritis or other obesity-related pathology in the knee; therefore patients with elevated BMIs should be counseled preoperatively about the difference in expected outcome.[14,31]

Recent research, most notably by Sihvonen et al., has demonstrated that degenerative medial meniscus tears, even in the absence of co-existing arthritis, do not benefit from arthroscopic meniscectomy.[31,34] Other studies have found similar findings in patients with coexisting osteoarthritis (OA), showing no difference in outcomes between patients undergoing surgery and rehabilitation versus those undergoing rehabilitation alone).[19,20,27] It is therefore important to distinguish the type of tear and the extent of concurrent knee pathology existing in patients with meniscal injury prior to undertaking arthroscopic resection.

According to the American Board of Orthopaedic Surgery, arthroscopic meniscal resection, code 29881, heads the list of the Current Procedural Terminology (CPT) codes in the candidate case submissions for Part II of the orthopedic certification examination. Medial meniscal tears, code 836.0, and lateral meniscal tears, code 836.1, are in the top three ICD-9 codes submitted for the examination as well.[16,26]

CLINICAL ASSESSMENT

Meniscal tears are common. In one cadaver study, 73% of specimens had meniscal pathology.[29] The detection of meniscal tears in asymptomatic knees on magnetic resonance imaging (MRI) is high. In a recent study, 91% of symptomatic knees had meniscal tears by MRI, but so did 76% of matched control knees.[4] In another study of healthy volunteers with no knee symptoms, 13% of those younger than age 45 years and 36% of those older than age 45 years had meniscal tears by MRI.[6] In patients with radiographic signs of OA, more than 60% of patients were found to have meniscal tears on MRI scans, regardless of the presence or lack of symptoms. In knees without radiographic evidence of OA, meniscus tears were seen in 23% of asymptomatic knees.[9,15,37]

MRI should therefore only be used to confirm the clinical suspicion of a tear, rather than to screen for tears. The MRI findings alone should never be used in isolation to guide treatment, but must always be correlated with the clinical history, and the physical exam findings. Many patients present to the orthopedic surgeon with positive MRI scans, having never undergone radiographs of the knee or even an appropriate physical examination. Occasionally, a weight-bearing radiograph is sufficient to diagnose and determine a treatment plan for a patient, thereby making MRI unnecessary. An acute injury with subsequent mechanical symptoms rather than a vague spontaneous onset of symptoms, along with findings of joint line tenderness and rotatory pain, with provocative tests such as the McMurray, Apley grind, and Thessaly tests, are likely to correlate with symptomatic meniscal tears.[32]

Once a symptomatic meniscal tear has been diagnosed, the surgeon must carefully select treatment based on sound clinical judgment. Not all meniscal tears require surgical intervention, as many tears become asymptomatic with a course of activity modification, physical therapy, and nonimpact strengthening.[36] Those that fail nonoperative measures are indicated for surgery, which usually involves arthroscopic partial resection or repair, and occasionally transplantation. Although this chapter will deal mainly with resection, the final choice between repair and partial resection is made at the time of surgery, on careful assessment of the tear. Indications for repair include longitudinal tears in the red-red zone, tears between 1 and 4 cm in length, meniscocapsular junction and red-white zone tears, and radial tears extending into the red-red zone.[21]

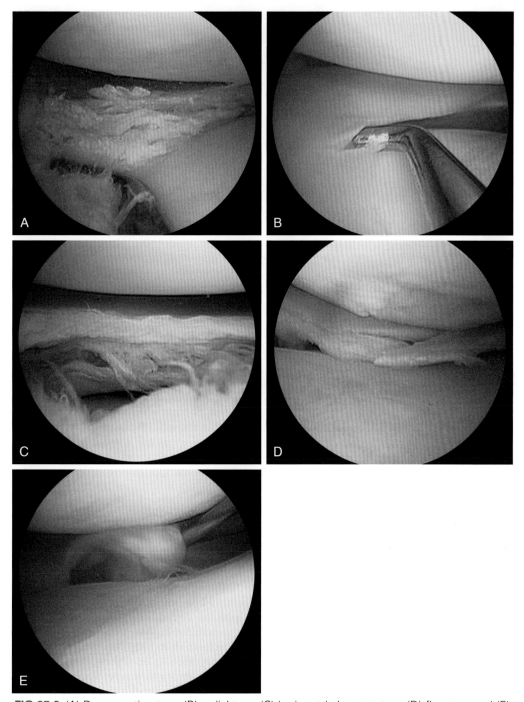

FIG 37.3 (A) Degenerative tear, (B) radial tear, (C) horizontal cleavage tear, (D) flap tear, and (E) parrot-beak tear.

Preoperative counseling is crucial to fully explain the associated risks of surgery. The surgeon must identify the patient's expectations of the operation and align those expectations with the anticipated outcome. The postoperative course should be discussed in great detail, including the unlikely possibility that symptoms may not resolve or even worsen.

Once the decision has been made to proceed with arthroscopic surgery, the procedure should be performed as quickly as possible to avoid further articular cartilage damage resulting from unstable meniscal flaps (Fig. 37.4). Rarely, a delay of several weeks is necessary to allow for a decrease in swelling and to regain a functional range of motion of the knee.

SURGICAL TECHNIQUE

The goals of arthroscopic partial meniscectomy are to identify the extent of tear and any other pathology, determine that the tear is irreparable, resect meniscal fragments to a stable rim, create a smooth border of remaining functional meniscus, and treat any other pathology identified.[5]

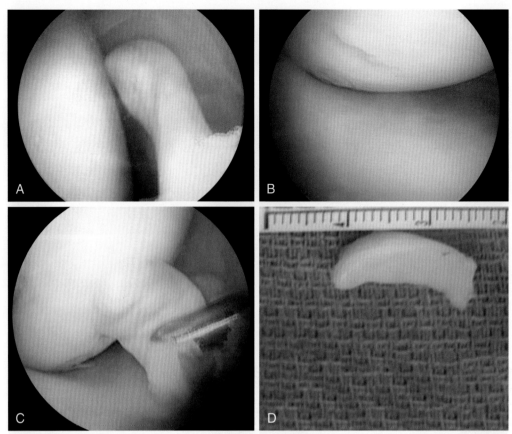

FIG 37.4 Unstable chronic lateral meniscus tear with fragment causing articular indentation of lateral femoral condyle. (A) Unstable, flipped meniscal fragment. (B) Articular indentation from entrapment. (C) Removal of the meniscal fragment. (D) Meniscal tear after removal.

Metcalf et al. have provided general guidelines for arthroscopic resection that apply to most resectable meniscal lesions: (1) All mobile fragments that can be pulled past the inner margin of the meniscus into the center of the joint should be removed. (2) The remaining meniscal rim should be smoothed to remove any sudden changes in contour that might lead to further tearing. (3) A perfectly smooth rim is not necessary because the meniscus is proven to remodel. (4) The probe should be used repeatedly to gain information about the mobility and quality of the remaining rim. (5) The meniscocapsular junction and the peripheral meniscal rim should be protected. This maintains meniscal stability and is vital in preserving the load transmission properties of the remaining meniscus. (6) To optimize efficiency, both manual and motorized resection instruments should be used. Manual instruments allow for more controlled resection, whereas motorized instruments remove loose debris and smooth frayed fragments. (7) In uncertain situations, more rather than less intact meniscal rims should be left to avoid segmental resection, which essentially results in a total meniscectomy.[26]

The patient is positioned for standard knee arthroscopy, and the procedure can be done on an outpatient basis under general, regional, or in certain circumstances, local anesthesia. A pneumatic tourniquet can be used but is not mandatory, and flow can be obtained with a pump or gravity. The patient is positioned supine on the operating room table with a lateral post to aid in obtaining valgus stress during the procedure or with the leg placed in a circumferential leg holder. An experienced

assistant can be helpful in positioning the limb in appropriate degrees of flexion and extension and varus or valgus to aid in the surgeon's visualization, but iatrogenic injury to the collateral ligaments can occur with overly aggressive force and must be avoided.

Most meniscal work can be done using a standard 30-degree arthroscope, but some surgeons also use a 70-degree arthroscope for visualization of the posterior corners of the knee. A standardized, systematic evaluation of the knee should be performed at each procedure to avoid missing pathology that may need to be addressed, as well as to identify normal intact structures in a reproducible fashion (Fig. 37.5). Portal placement is essential; although most meniscal work is done through the anteromedial portal and is visualized through the anterolateral portal, anterior portions of the medial meniscus may be approached by switching portals, or by using accessory portals,[28] to avoid causing chondral damage with arthroscopic instruments.

The two-portal technique for standard arthroscopy appears to allow an earlier return of quadriceps strength and function and faster return to work and activities compared with the three-portal technique.[35] The menisci should be probed on the superior and inferior surfaces to assess the presence and extent of damage, and displaceable tears can be brought into the field of view to plan resection (Fig. 37.6). It is also critical to run the articular rim beneath the menisci with the probe because this may reveal hidden flaps of the meniscus that would not otherwise be seen (Fig. 37.7). Visualization of the posterior

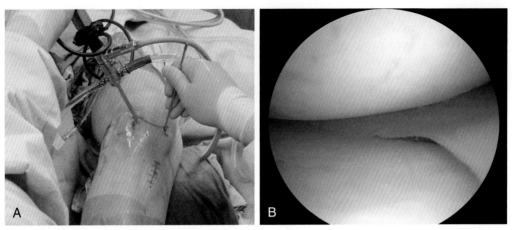

FIG 37.5 (A) Standard positioning for arthroscopic view of medial meniscus. (B) Arthroscopic view of lateral meniscus.

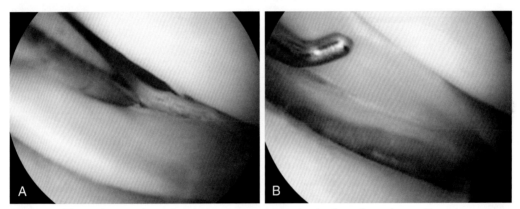

FIG 37.6 The arthroscopic probe demonstrates a tear in the lateral meniscus. Superior surface (A) and inferior surface (B) of the meniscus.

medial corner of the knee, which lies between the posterior collateral ligament (PCL) and medial femoral condyle, commonly referred to as the Gillquist view (Fig. 37.8), is essential to assess the meniscocapsular attachment of the posterior horn of the medial meniscus. This is also where a flipped segment of the meniscus can be missed and mistakenly left untreated if not detected (Fig. 37.9).

Most medial meniscal resection is carried out with an upbiter and lateral meniscal resection with a straight biter. Curved and 90-degree biters may also be useful for contouring certain tears. The mechanical shaver is then used to smooth the resected edges of the tear and rid the knee of debris (Fig. 37.10).

Posterior root tears of both the medial and lateral meniscus pose a difficult problem, especially in patients with tight collateral ligaments and those with an associated ACL tear (Fig. 37.11). Posteromedial meniscal root avulsions have been associated with 3 mm of meniscal extrusion, and extrusion of 3 mm has been linked to substantially increased articular cartilage loss and osteophyte formation. Historically, meniscectomy has been used to manage these tears, but given the results of recent studies, repair is becoming the standard of care for posterior root avulsions. Not all patients, however, are candidates for repair. The criteria for repair include age younger than 50, with no significant OA (less than Outerbridge grade 3), joint-space narrowing, or malalignment.[22] Patients who do not meet

these criteria require resection. To aid in resection, the biter may need to be inverted when resecting the posterior horn of the lateral meniscus because the instrument jaw excursion may commonly be limited by the tibial spines. If performing a simultaneous ACL reconstruction, completing a notchplasty prior to meniscectomy may allow easier access to this region of the lateral meniscus. The posterior horn of the medial meniscus may be accessed best by placing the knee in slight flexion and external rotation. However, with an ACL-deficient knee, the knee may shift and thereby close down the posteromedial corner. A skilled assistant's help may be necessary to provide a posterior drawer force on the knee to obtain access in this situation.

Bucket handle tears are commonly encountered and require careful assessment. Tears that can be reduced must be assessed for stability and reparability. The aforementioned criteria for meniscal repair should be applied.[21] If it is determined at the time of surgery that the tear is irreparable, then it should be resected (Fig. 37.12).

One efficient method of resecting a bucket handle tear begins by using an arthroscopic scissor to detach the posterior limb of the tear; the low profile of the scissor allows easy access to a tight area without damaging surrounding articular cartilage. The next step involves near-complete detachment of the anterior limb of the tear using a scissor or biter. Alternatively, the

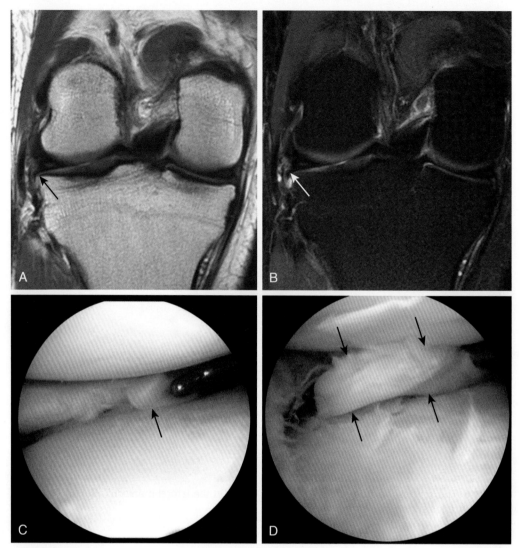

FIG 37.7 (A and B) Coronal magnetic resonance images demonstrating complex flap tear. (C and D) Arthroscopic images of complex flap tear identified by use of the probe.

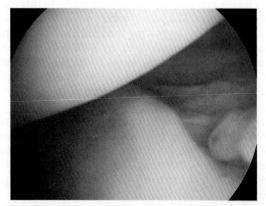

FIG 37.8 Visualization of the posterior medial corner of the knee, which lies between the PCL and medial femoral condyle. This is commonly referred to as the Gillquist view.

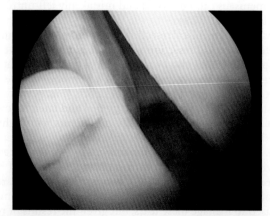

FIG 37.9 Gillquist view with a flipped posterior horn medial meniscal fragment.

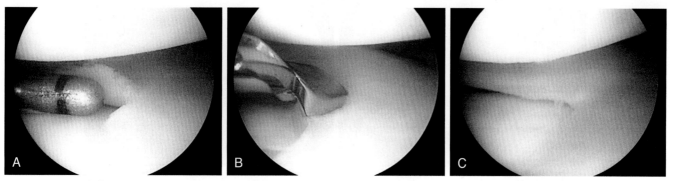

FIG 37.10 (A) Arthroscopic image of shaver to smooth resected meniscal border. (B) Use of biter to remove torn meniscus. (C) View of stable, smooth border following partial meniscectomy.

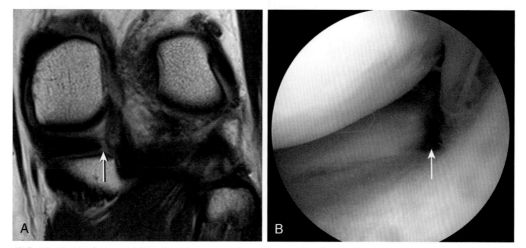

FIG 37.11 (A) Coronal MRI showing posterior root meniscal tear. (B) Corresponding arthroscopic image of posterior root tear.

posterior rim may be partially detached, and the anterior rim completely detached. The final step is grasping the torn segment of meniscus and completing the detachment by applying a twisting motion to pull the remnant out of the knee in its entirety. The portal may need to be enlarged, depending on the size of the resected segment (Fig. 37.13). Alternatively, a spinal needle can be introduced into the knee to stabilize the torn segment in the intercondylar notch as the limbs are detached. An arthroscopic shaver is then used to smooth down the areas where the tear was resected.

The overall principle of meniscal resection is to remove only the torn meniscal tissue while maintaining as much intact meniscus as possible, especially peripherally, and avoiding iatrogenic injury to the surrounding intact meniscus and articular cartilage. Repeated passes of hand and motorized instruments can risk injury to the articular cartilage, and small-diameter and curved instruments may be useful for avoiding such injury. Maintenance of a stable rim of intact meniscus, free of edges from where a new tear could theoretically propagate, is the final objective of meniscal resection (Fig. 37.14).

It is important to record clear pictures or video of the procedure to review these images with the patient in the postoperative period. This allows the surgeon to provide better explanations of the arthroscopic findings in terms of meniscal pathology or extent of articular cartilage damage to provide a reasonable expectation for recovery.

POSTOPERATIVE COURSE AND COMPLICATIONS

Typically, arthroscopic meniscectomy is performed as an outpatient procedure, with patients discharged the day of surgery. Complications such as infection, bleeding, neurologic injury, deep vein thrombosis, pulmonary embolism, and compartment syndrome are rare, but they must not be overlooked. Patients with American Society of Anesthesiologists (ASA) classification greater than 3, diabetes, or pulmonary disease are at increased risk of adverse events following arthroscopy,[3] and the decision to undergo meniscectomy should be carefully reviewed in these patients. Complications specific to the procedure are also rare but include iatrogenic damage to articular cartilage, damage to the collateral ligaments, inadequate or over-resection of meniscus, and failure to recognize and treat other pathology in the knee.

A home exercise program emphasizing range of motion and nonimpact strengthening is usually implemented to help the patient regain function. Given the correlation between meniscectomy and the development of OA, recent research has focused upon the kinematic differences in knees with partial

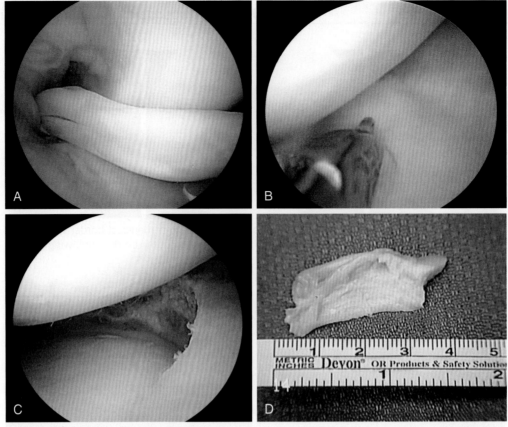

FIG 37.12 (A) Bucket handle meniscus tear, displaced in the intercondylar notch. (B) Reduced bucket handle tear. (C) Resected bucket handle tear, to smooth, stable border. (D) Remnant of resected meniscus.

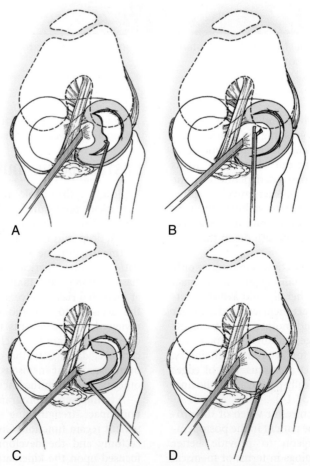

FIG 37.13 (A) Displaced bucket handle tear. (B) Reduction of bucket handle tear. (C) Partial detachment. (D) Completion of detachment and removal through arthroscopic porthole.

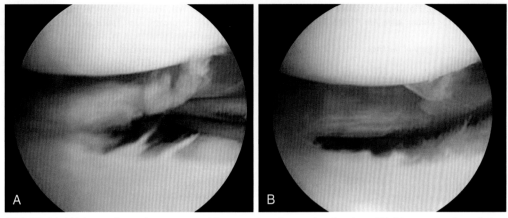

FIG 37.14 (A) Lateral meniscus tear with central or free-edge fraying. (B) After resection of the torn portion of the meniscus.

meniscectomies, and the mechanical component in the pathway to joint degeneration, using strength and muscular activation parameters in an attempt to improve rehabilitation of the affected knee.[8]

Studies have shown that 82% of patients can expect to return to sedentary work within 1 week, and only 4% of patients report knee-related activity restriction at 20 weeks.[25] There are essentially no restrictions following meniscal resection, other than those mediated by pain and swelling, which can differ tremendously among patients. Return to sports occurs once range of motion, strength, and perceived confidence in the knee have returned to normal.

Outcomes of Partial Meniscectomy

Given that the meniscus is as a crucial load-bearing structure, optimizing contact area and minimizing contact stress, meniscal resection is not without consequence, having been proven to accelerate the onset of OA. Load transmission of hoop tension through the circumferential fibers is critical, further emphasizing the importance of maintaining a peripheral meniscal rim. Radial tears of the meniscus at the posterior roots eliminate hoop tension, altering tibiofemoral contact mechanics in a way similar to total meniscectomy because of meniscal extrusion. Tears just posterior to the midcoronal plane also have a worse prognosis because of the resultant increase in tibial rotation that causes higher contact pressures and theoretically an increased risk of OA.[8] Review of recent literature shows that patient age and gender have no significant association with any clinical or radiographic outcome variables at up to 15 years postoperatively.[7] Patients with bucket handle tears had faster return to sports and underwent fewer revision surgeries than those with flap tears, which potentially reflects the increased difficulty involved in successfully resecting a flap tear. In comparing the outcomes of medial and lateral meniscectomies, there was no statistically significant difference in medial versus lateral meniscectomy overall. Patients with ACL-deficient knees had worse outcomes than patients with stable knees. The best radiographic results following medial meniscectomy occurred in valgus knees rather than varus knees. The amount of meniscal tissue removed affected outcome because patients with less than 50% of their meniscal rim remaining had worse radiographic changes at 12 years than those with greater than 50% remaining. The degree of OA at the time of meniscectomy is also directly related to outcome because increased modified Outerbridge cartilage scores at the time of surgery are correlated with poorer physical results at 12 years.[10]

CONCLUSION

The standard of care for meniscal tears has shifted toward tissue preservation, including repair, and transplantation. Nevertheless, most meniscal tears are irreparable because of their size, type, or lack of vascularity, and therefore they often require partial resection. The surgeon must carefully assess the patient both clinically and intraoperatively before making the decision to resect rather than repair a tear. Once the decision to resect has been made, careful surgical technique must be used to fully resect injured tissue, while attempting to preserve as much of the peripheral meniscal rim as possible and avoid iatrogenic damage to the knee. Optimal outcome is only achieved with proper patient selection and communication, to best align patient expectations with expected results.

KEY REFERENCES

1. Arnoczky SP, Warren RF: Microvasculature of the human meniscus. *Am J Sports Med* 10:90–95, 1982.
7. Burks RT, Metcalf MH, Metcalf RW: Fifteen-year follow-up of arthroscopic partial meniscectomy. *Arthroscopy* 13:673–679, 1997.
9. Englund M, Guermazi A, Gale D, et al: Incidental meniscal findings on knee MRI in middle-aged and elderly persons. *N Engl J Med* 359:1108–1115, 2008.
10. Fabricant PD, Jokl P: Surgical outcomes after arthroscopic partial meniscectomy. *J Am Acad Orthop Surg* 15:647–653, 2007.
13. Fauno P, Nielson AB: Consequences of arthroscopic meniscal resection. *Ugeskr Laeger* 155:3388–3390, 1993.
14. Ford GM, Hegmann KB, White GL Jr, et al: Associations of body mass index with meniscal tears. *Am J Prev Med* 28:364–368, 2005.
15. Fritz RC: MR imaging of meniscal and cruciate ligament injuries. *Magn Reson Imaging Clin N Am* 11:283–293, 2003.
16. Garrett WE Jr, Swiontkowski MF, Weinstein JN, et al: American Board of Orthopaedic Surgery Practice of the Orthopaedic Surgeon: Part-II, certification examination case mix. *J Bone Joint Surg Am* 88:660–667, 2006.
20. Kirkley A, Birmingham TB, et al: A randomized trial of arthroscopic surgery for osteoarthritis of the knee. *N Engl J Med* 359:1097–1107, 2008.

23. Lee SJ, Aadalen KJ, Malaviya P, et al: Tibiofemoral contact mechanics after serial meniscectomies in the human knee. *Am J Sports Med* 34:1334–1344, 2006.

32. Scott WN, editor: *Insall & Scott surgery of the knee*, ed 4, New York, NY, 2006, Churchill Livingstone.

33. Shelbourne KD, Heinrich J: The long-term evaluation of lateral meniscus tears left in situ at the time of anterior cruciate ligament reconstruction. *Arthroscopy* 20:346–351, 2004.

35. Stetson WB, Templin K: Two- versus three-portal technique for routine knee arthroscopy. *Am J Sports Med* 30:108–1111, 2002.

37. Zanetti M, Pfirrmann CW, Schmid MR, et al: Patients with suspected meniscal tears: prevalence of abnormalities seen on MRI of 100 symptomatic and 100 contralateral asymptomatic knees. *AJR Am J Roentgenol* 181:635–641, 2003.

The references for this chapter can also be found on www.expertconsult.com.

38

Arthroscopy-Assisted Inside-Out and Outside-In Meniscus Repair

Eduard Alentorn-Geli, J.H. James Choi, Joseph J. Stuart,
Dean C. Taylor, Claude T. Moorman III

INTRODUCTION

Meniscal tears are an extremely common injury in the athletic and general population and an important cause of knee disability. The treatment of these injuries depends on a constellation of factors, mainly related to the clinical presentation, tear pattern, and location of the injury. There are two main clinical presentations of these injuries: acute meniscal tear in the setting of a previously healthy tissue (young athlete) or a chronic tear (or acute chronic), which occurs in previously degenerated tissue (general population). The most commonly observed tear patterns are vertical longitudinal, horizontal cleavage, radial, oblique, flap tears, bucket handle, or complex tears. These injuries can be located in the anterior horn, body of meniscus, posterior horn, or the root, and involve the medial meniscus, the lateral meniscus, or both. The location of the injury can also be described according to the meniscus vascularity: red-red zone (peripheral third, closest to the capsule), red-white zone (central third), and white-white zone (most central third of the meniscus).

Meniscal tears can be treated nonoperatively or surgically. Many meniscal tears can be treated nonoperatively, especially in degenerative-type tears. The most important factor in deciding the most appropriate treatment is the symptomatology. Meniscal tears with less pain and no mechanical symptoms (clicking, catching, or locking) may respond to rest, activity modification, anti-inflammatory medications, physical therapy, or cortisone injections aimed to decrease intra-articular inflammation. More symptomatic tears or those unresponsive to conservative treatment may be treated surgically. There are several surgical options for the treatment of meniscal injuries: partial meniscectomy, meniscal repair, meniscal implants (for partial meniscal defects with adequate meniscal rim), or meniscal transplants (for complete meniscal absence). Partial meniscectomy has been associated with increased risk of osteoarthritis at 10- to 20-year follow-up, compared with normal controls in some series.[16,27] However, lower rates of osteoarthritis have been noted in patients in whom smaller portions of meniscus were removed.[10,25] It is thus desirable to pursue treatment options that preserve or restore functional meniscal tissue. Although it has not been shown that meniscal repair results in complete restoration of joint kinetics or functional meniscal tissue, some long-term studies have shown better clinical outcomes and less joint space narrowing following meniscal repair than following partial meniscectomy.[39,43,57] Therefore, if surgical treatment is indicated, meniscal repair should be attempted whenever possible. There are several options for meniscal repair: trephination, inside-out or outside-in sutures, or all-inside devices. This chapter is focused on the surgical treatment of meniscal tears through meniscal repair using the arthroscopy-assisted inside-out and outside-in meniscus repair techniques.

INDICATIONS

The first step in the treatment of meniscal tears is to decide which injuries may benefit from surgical treatment and, if so, which injuries have a better chance of healing after repair. The types of meniscal injury patterns with better chances of healing include acute tears with nondegenerated meniscus tissue (especially if operated in the acute setting), located in the red-red zone (meniscal rim less than 4 mm); vertical longitudinal tears; bucket handle tears; certain large flap tears; tears in young patients; injuries in a stable knee; or meniscal repairs associated with concomitant anterior cruciate ligament reconstruction.* Complex degenerative tears are more difficult to repair and generally heal less reliably.[23] Although radial tears have been traditionally considered unamenable to repair given poor chances of healing,[23] successful results have also been reported with meniscal suture in this tear pattern.[15,40,53,58] Finally, patient factors play a large role in determining whether meniscal repair should be performed, because outcomes are generally poorer in older patients and those with articular cartilage degeneration. One must also consider the significantly increased healing time required after meniscal repair when compared with partial meniscectomy and the willingness and ability of the patient to comply with required postoperative restrictions.

The indications for outside-in meniscal repair have evolved in the recent years. Although this repair technique was not initially indicated for lateral meniscus tears to avoid the risk of injury to the peroneal nerve,[56] the indications have been expanded now to include injuries to either the medial or lateral meniscus. The principal indications for the outside-in technique include tears of the anterior horn or anterior half of the body of the meniscus and meniscal tears in small knees to avoid risk of cartilage damage with the inside-out cannulas

---

*References 5, 12, 14, 36, 46, 50, 52, and 55.

(pediatric population).[55] The use of this technique for tears in the far posterior horn may increase the risk of damage to neurovascular structures and decrease the healing rate.[53] The indications for inside-out meniscal repair are less restricted, but the ideal scenario for inside-out meniscal repair is a vertical longitudinal or bucket handle tear in the red-red zone or red-white zone in a previously healthy meniscal tissue in the setting of a young patient with a stable knee.

SURGICAL TECHNIQUE FOR MENISCAL REPAIR

The general principle for meniscal repair includes the preparation of the tear with synovial abrasion, which induces peripheral bleeding in an attempt to promote migration of undifferentiated mesenchymal cells that would help in the healing of the meniscus. Then the meniscus can be repaired with sutures (placed outside-in or inside-out) or all-inside devices (discussed elsewhere in this book). The repair of meniscal tears through trephination has also been described.[19] This method attempts to create vascular channels through the induction of holes in the avascular portions of the meniscus.

Inside-Out Technique

Inside-out techniques remain the standard for meniscal repair by many surgeons yielding reproducible, solid fixation of tears in the posterior and middle thirds of the meniscus.[13,46,56] This technique requires the combination of arthroscopy to pass the sutures through the appropriate place in the meniscus and an approach to the knee to catch the needles and avoid damage to neurovascular structures. This procedure is therefore slightly different for the medial and lateral meniscus. Both share in common that the procedure begins with arthroscopic inspection of the joint, identification of meniscal tears, and determination of whether repair is appropriate. If an appropriate tear is identified, an accessory incision is made then, depending on the location of the tear. The procedure can be done as outpatient surgery and with general or regional anesthesia. The patient is positioned lying supine, and it must be ensured that circumferential access to the affected knee is possible. The surgeon must also ensure that the leg can be moved from extension to flexion (at least 90 degrees) and from valgus and semiflexion (for medial meniscus) to figure-of-four (for lateral meniscus).

Medial Meniscal Tear. The repair of the medial meniscus through an inside-out technique requires an accessory posteromedial incision. A longitudinal 3-cm skin incision just posterior to the medial collateral ligament is created with one-third of the incision above the joint line and two thirds below the joint line (Fig. 38.1). The pes anserine fascia (PA) is identified and split, retracting the medial hamstring tendons posteriorly (Fig. 38.2). This allows visualization of the medial head of the gastrocnemius muscle and protects the vulnerable infrapatellar branch of the saphenous nerve posteriorly (Fig. 38.3). The medial head of the gastrocnemius is dissected free from the posteromedial joint capsule and retracted posteriorly with a spoon or popliteal retractor (Fig. 38.4). The spoon or retractor is used to protect the neurovascular structures from getting damaged by the needles passing from inside to outside the joint. The tear is visualized through the arthroscope and an arthroscopic rasp is used to roughen the edges of the tear (Fig. 38.5). The arthroscope is usually placed in the anteromedial portal, and a cannula is passed into the anterolateral portal and directed toward the

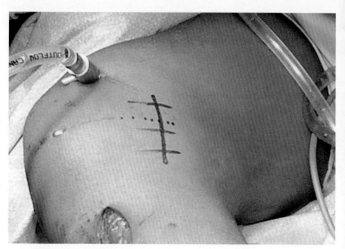

FIG 38.1 The posteromedial accessory incision for meniscal repair has been marked, posterior to the superficial medial collateral ligament extending one-third above and two-thirds below the joint line *(dashed line)*.

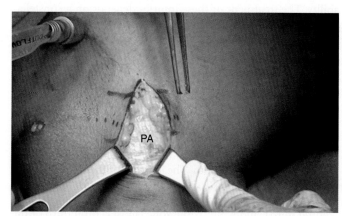

FIG 38.2 The incision has been taken through skin and subcutaneous fat to the PA fascia. *PA,* Pes anserine.

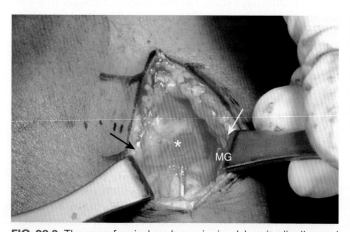

FIG 38.3 The pes fascia has been incised longitudinally, and the anterior portion *(black arrow)* has been retracted forward. The posterior portion along with the medial hamstring tendons *(white arrow)* have been retracted posteriorly. The medial head of the gastrocnemius *(MG)* is also being retracted posteriorly, revealing the underlying posteromedial joint capsule *(*)*.

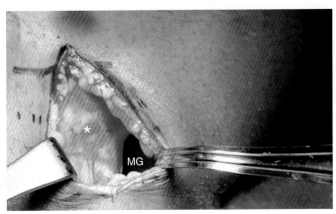

FIG 38.4 The gastrocnemius muscle *(MG)* has been retracted posteriorly behind the spoon, isolating the joint capsule *(*)*.

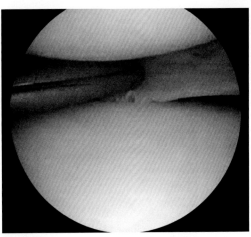

FIG 38.6 A long flexible needle is directed through a cannula, through the meniscus tear and out through the posteromedial capsule.

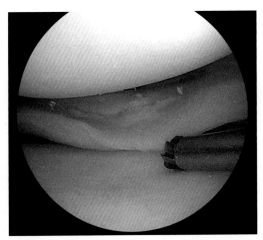

FIG 38.5 An arthroscopic rasp to be used to roughen the edges of the tear prior to repair to facilitate healing.

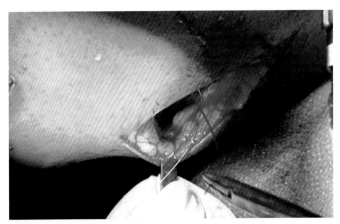

FIG 38.7 A second needle is passed through the meniscus and pulled out of the posteromedial incision in the same manner. The suture connecting the two needles forms a vertical mattress suture and reduces the meniscus tear.

tear for needle passage. Alternatively, the arthroscope can be placed in the anterolateral portal, and the anteromedial portal can be used for needle passage. The working portal will be elected depending on the location of the tear. Cannuli of different curvatures are available to facilitate access to any portion of the posterior and middle thirds of the meniscus. A long flexible needle with attached 2 to 0 or 0 nonabsorbable suture is passed through the cannula, across the meniscus tear, and out through the posteromedial capsule (Fig. 38.6). The sutures should be placed sequentially in a posterior to anterior fashion. An assistant ensures capture of the needle by the spoon and guides the needle out of the accessory incision. The procedure is repeated with a second needle attached to the other end of the suture, completing a vertical mattress suture (Fig. 38.7). If more than one suture is required, they are generally placed in an alternating manner, 3 to 5 mm apart, on the femoral and tibial surfaces of the meniscus to reduce the meniscus appropriately. After passing all sutures, they are tied sequentially in a posterior to anterior direction (Fig. 38.8). It is important to tie the sutures with the knee near full extension, because tying them in 90 degrees of flexion could tether the posteromedial capsule and limit knee extension or break the sutures when the patient extends the knee.[6,29]

Lateral Meniscal Tears. The repair of the lateral meniscus through an inside-out technique requires an accessory posterolateral incision. A longitudinal 3-cm skin incision is made on the posterolateral knee just posterior to the fibular collateral ligament centered over the joint line (Fig. 38.9). Flexion of the knee helps displace the neurovascular structures further posteriorly to reduce the risk of injury. The interval between the iliotibial band (ITB) and biceps femoris (BF) tendon is developed (Fig. 38.10) until the lateral border of the lateral head of the gastrocnemius is visualized (Fig. 38.11). The lateral gastrocnemius is dissected off the posterolateral capsule, and a spoon or popliteal retractor is placed anterior to the tendon, effectively protecting the neurovascular structures located posteriorly and medially (Fig. 38.12). With the arthroscope in the anterolateral portal, zone-specific cannuli can then be used as described to place vertical mattress sutures in the torn lateral meniscus from posterior to anterior and again alternating the upper surface and under surface of the meniscus. The repair of tears in certain locations may be facilitated by switching the arthroscope to the anteromedial portal and working through the anterolateral portal. After passing all sutures, they are again tied in a posterior

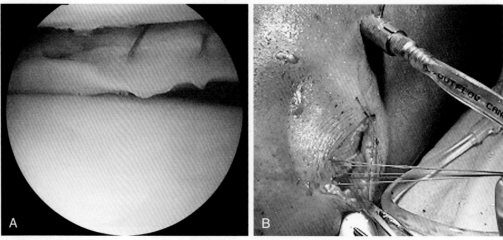

FIG 38.8 (A) Additional sutures are placed in the same manner, reducing the tear. (B) After all are placed, they are tied sequentially from posterior to anterior, with the knee in approximately 20 degrees of flexion.

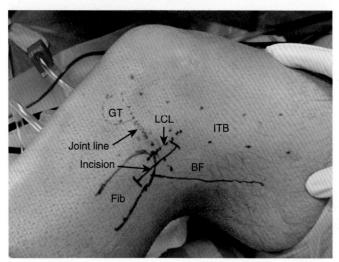

FIG 38.9 The posterolateral accessory incision has been marked, posterior to the LCL and spanning the joint line. GT, the ITB, and BF have been labeled. *BF,* Biceps femoris; *GT,* Gerdy's tubercle; *ITB,* iliotibial band; *LCL,* lateral collateral ligament.

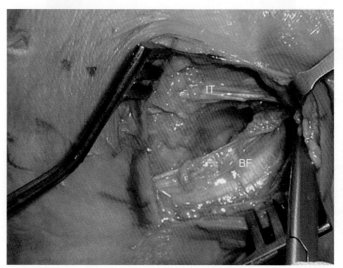

FIG 38.10 The incision has been taken down through skin and subcutaneous tissue. The interval between the ITB anteriorly and the BF posteriorly has been separated. The common peroneal nerve lies posterior to the biceps femoris. *BF,* Biceps femoris; *IT,* iliotibial band.

to anterior direction.[6,29] Care should be taken to avoid catching the popliteus tendon or the lateral collateral ligament (LCL) with the sutures.

Outside-in Technique

There are several variants of the outside-in technique, but all share in common the use of a spinal needle through which either the final suture or a shuttle suture is passed after penetrating the meniscus. After identification and preparation of the tear, the arthroscope is used to transilluminate the skin and localize the tear (Fig. 38.13). A spinal needle is introduced through the skin and across the meniscus tear (Fig. 38.14). A wire suture shuttle is then advanced through the needle and into the joint, where it is retrieved out of an anterior portal (Fig. 38.15). The suture to be used in the repair is passed through the loop in the wire and pulled out through the meniscus (Fig. 38.16). A second needle is placed relative to the first needle in

such a manner as to make a vertical mattress stitch, and a wire is pulled through this needle and out through the anterior portal in the same manner (Fig. 38.17). The other end of the suture is passed through the wire (Fig. 38.18). Pulling this suture out through the meniscus completes the construct (Fig. 38.19). After the sutures are secured inside the knee, a small incision is made between the two sutures' exit sites. The plane between the capsule and the subcutaneous tissue should be bluntly developed, and the sutures are tied together over the capsule, reducing the tear. Alternatively, two spinal needles can be initially passed through the meniscus and the skin incision created between both needles to reduce the risk of inadvertently cutting the sutures. If additional sutures are required, they can generally be placed through the same incision.

Numerous alternative methods have been described, allowing placement of sutures in a standard vertical mattress configuration. In the suture shuttle method, two sutures are passed into

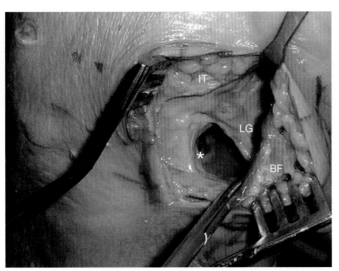

FIG 38.11 Spreading the ITB and BF allows visualization of the LG, inserting into the distal femur. The posterolateral joint capsule (*) is visible. *BF,* Biceps femoris; *IT,* iliotibial band; *LG,* lateral head of the gastrocnemius.

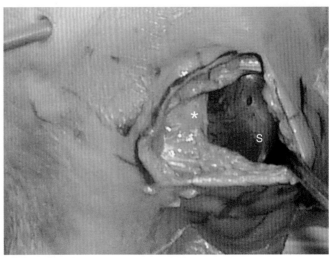

FIG 38.12 The lateral head of the gastrocnemius has been elevated off the joint capsule, and a spoon *(S)* has been placed in the incision, retracting the gastrocnemius and biceps posteriorly, protecting the common peroneal nerve. The joint capsule (*) is now easily visualized.

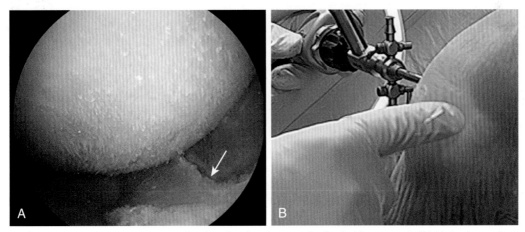

FIG 38.13 (A) A meniscus tear is visualized arthroscopically *(white arrow).* (B) Light from the arthroscope is used to mark the approximate location of the tear on the outside of the knee.

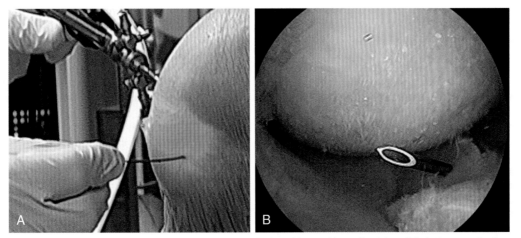

FIG 38.14 (A) A spinal needle is passed through the skin and into the joint. (B) Arthroscopically, the needle is seen crossing the meniscus tear.

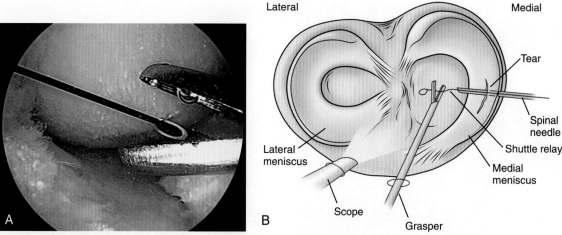

FIG 38.15 (A) A wire is passed through the needle and retrieved into an anterior portal. (B) Line drawing from superior perspective demonstrating wire loop retrieval.

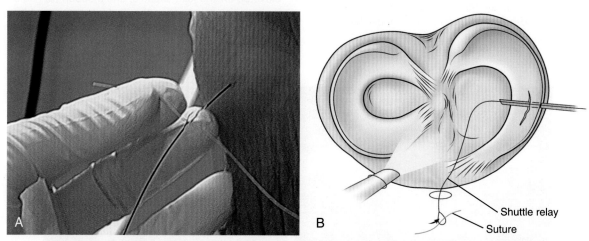

FIG 38.16 (A) Suture to be used in the repair is threaded through a loop in the wire and pulled into the joint and through the meniscus tear as the needle is removed. (B) Line drawing from superior perspective demonstrating suture passed through the wire loop.

the joint through two spinal needles and retrieved through an anterior portal. They are tied together with a square knot. The knot is then pulled back through the meniscus and out of the skin by traction on either suture, resulting in a standard vertical mattress suture. Passage of the knot through the meniscus can be difficult and is facilitated by tying a smaller dilator knot in one suture prior to tying the square knot and pulling this knot through the meniscus first.[44]

Alternatively, specific devices have been developed to facilitate this repair method, including a shuttle relay that can be passed through the second needle instead of suture. Suture from the first needle is then passed through the shuttle relay, which is withdrawn along with the second needle. This technique obviates the need to pull a knot through the meniscus and avoids extracting suture from anterior portals, where soft tissue could become entrapped.[44] The same technique can be used with a wire loop stylet that is passed through the spinal needle to retrieve the second suture.

Another technique involves passing suture through one needle and retrieving it anteriorly as described previously, tying a three- or four-throw mulberry knot, and then pulling the suture back into the joint against the meniscus, reducing the

tear.[35,56] If this method is used, the second needle should be directed to the opposite surface of the meniscus from the first to reduce and secure the repair appropriately. However, this technique does not result in the creation of true vertical mattress sutures and may have inferior strength; also, there may be concerns for chondral abrasion because of protruding knots facing the cartilage.

As noted, the outside-in technique is frequently used to repair tears in the anterior horn or anterior half of the body of the meniscus. We have found this technique to be particularly useful when used in association with an all-inside technique on large meniscal tears extending anteriorly from the posterior third of the meniscus. One can use an all-inside technique to address the posterior extent of the tear and then repair the anterior portion with an outside-in technique (Fig. 38.20). This hybrid technique can be used to stabilize even the largest tears rapidly.

BIOMECHANICAL TESTING

In recent years, a considerable amount of research has focused on the biomechanical properties of meniscal repair techniques

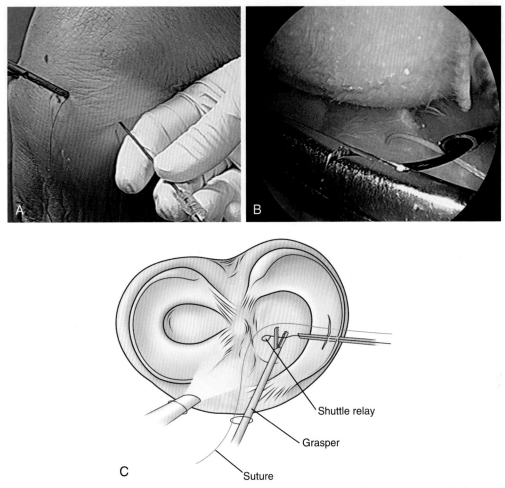

FIG 38.17 (A) A second needle is passed in such a way that a vertical mattress suture is formed. (B) The wire is again retrieved via an anterior portal. (C) Line drawing from superior perspective demonstrating the placement of a second spinal needle and wire for suture retrieval.

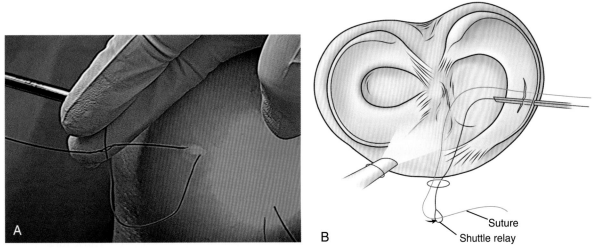

FIG 38.18 (A) The other end of the suture is passed through a loop in the suture. (B) Line drawing from superior perspective demonstrating the other end of the suture passing through the wire loop.

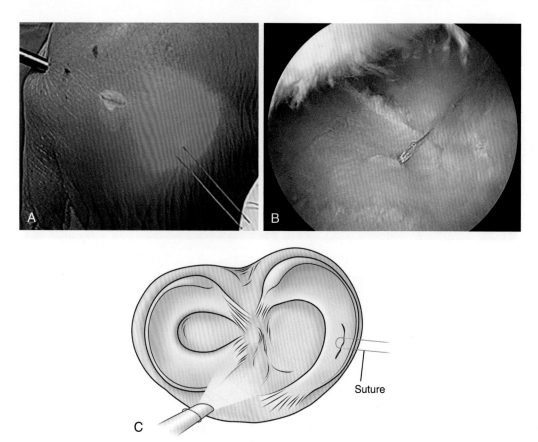

FIG 38.19 (A) The wire and suture are again pulled through joint and through the meniscal tear. (B) Pulling on the two sutures reduces the meniscus tear. (C) Line drawing from superior perspective demonstrating the completed repair.

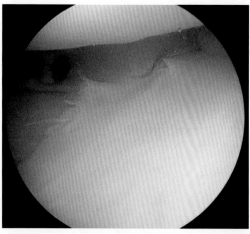

FIG 38.20 Hybrid meniscal repair technique. All-inside fixation is used for the posterior portion of the meniscal tear, and an outside-in technique is used for the anterior extent of the tear.

and constructs. A recent systematic review and meta-analysis involving 41 publications compared the biomechanical properties of meniscal repair through inside-out/outside-in techniques versus all-inside devices.[11] This study demonstrated that meniscal repair through inside-out/outside-in had higher load to failure and stiffness compared to techniques all-inside techniques.[11] It was also observed that vertical mattress configuration had better load to failure compared to horizontal construct.

Other studies have further demonstrated that the vertical mattress sutures with increased inclination angles (angles between the horizontal and the direction of the suture from the meniscal to the capsule attachments) had higher load to failure compared to decreased inclination angle (where sutures across the meniscus are close to the horizontal).[17] Most of the studies used 0 polydioxanone (PDS), 2 to 0 OrthoCord, and 0 Ethibond for the meniscal suture. It was concluded that meniscal suture through inside-out or outside-in techniques remains the standard of treatment for meniscal tears. It should be noted that almost all of the included studies dealt with vertical longitudinal tears (and some bucket handle tears). Therefore, these results can only be applied for this type of tear. In addition, it is likely that a comparison between sutures and second-generation devices would only demonstrate similar results.[41,45]

Although a repair with good or excellent biomechanical properties is not necessarily associated with healing and better clinical outcomes, it seems reasonable to think that a surgeon may want to aim for a strong construct in meniscal repair. It has been demonstrated in an animal model that all-inside devices had inferior meniscal healing results compared to inside-out techniques.[26]

Some studies have evaluated the biomechanical properties of the repair of radial tears.[†] Presently, there is not enough evidence at this point to conclude that inside-out/outside-in meniscal sutures have better biomechanical properties compared to all-inside devices for radial tears.[2]

[†]References 7, 9, 24, 31, 34, and 38.

RESULTS

The relative advantages and disadvantages of each technique are summarized in Table 38.1. Overall, there are data to support good clinical outcomes with both inside-out and outside-in techniques.[30,55] Numerous case series have demonstrated excellent clinical and functional outcomes after inside-out meniscal repair of longitudinal tears in young patients and elite athletes in the mid- and long-term follow-up.[32,37,51] In fact, it was observed that the repair of meniscal injuries through inside-out technique was chondroprotective in the mid- and long-term follow-up of young individuals.[37,51] The inside-out meniscal repair has also demonstrated good clinical outcomes, adequate return to sports rate, and healing rates in lateral meniscus radial tears extending into the capsular zone with or without the addition of a fibrin clot.[3,21,40] In general, it has been observed that lateral meniscus, tears involving small peripheral rims, tears repaired in association with anterior cruciate ligament reconstruction, and acute tears have better chances of healing and successful outcomes.[30]

The inside-out and all-inside repairs for isolated meniscal tears were compared in a systematic review.[20] The study involved 19 publications, and it was reported that there were no clinical differences in clinical failure rate or subjective outcome between both repair methods. In general, a clinical failure of 17% can be expected with meniscal repair through the inside-out technique (19% for the all-inside technique).[20] The authors observed more nerve symptoms associated with the inside-out and more implant-related complications (soft tissue irritation, swelling, and implant migration or breakage) associated with the all-inside technique.[20] In a different study, it was demonstrated that the inside-out and outside-in techniques had higher healing rates (95% and 100%, respectively) compared to all-inside technique.[22] The healing rate may be related to the tear pattern or the association of anterior cruciate ligament reconstruction.[20] In fact, it has been observed that the failure rate of inside-out or outside-in meniscal repair is higher in isolated repairs, compared to tears repaired in association with anterior cruciate ligament reconstruction.[18]

There is less research specifically conducted for the outside-in meniscal repair, but most of the available studies have demonstrated good healing rates and clinical outcomes.[55] Studies have demonstrated a failure rate of 12% and improved clinical and functional outcomes (International Knee Documentation Committee [IKDC] and Lysholm scores) at both the short- (minimum 2 years) and long-term (mean of 12 years) follow-up after meniscal repair through the outside-in technique with or without anterior cruciate ligament reconstruction.[1,48] In general, the outside-in technique allows excellent healing rates (84% to 100%)[22,36,55] and good clinical outcomes (77%) after applying an accelerated rehabilitation program.[33,55] The chances of failure with outside-in meniscal repair are higher in anterior cruciate ligament-deficiency knee,[36] or tears of the posterior horn of the medial meniscus, compared to lateral meniscus tears or tears in the anterior or middle portion of the medial meniscus.[54,55]

REHABILITATION OF MENISCAL REPAIR

The rehabilitation process of meniscal tears treated by surgical repair may take up to 8 months. An adequate rehabilitation process is crucial to ensure adequate success of the repair. The first phases of rehabilitation are aimed to protect the integrity of the repair, avoiding disuse changes in bone and soft tissue, and restoring and preserving knee range of motion. Biomechanical studies have suggested that loading of the knee in extension helps reduce longitudinal tears, whereas loading in flexion and tibial torsion produce stresses on the meniscus likely to be detrimental to healing.[8,28,42,49] A significant amount of research has focused on the safety of accelerated rehabilitation protocols. Shelbourne et al.[47] and Barber[4] have compared patients placed in accelerated rehabilitation protocols that included immediate, full weight bearing with patients placed in conservative rehabilitation protocols that restricted range of motion and weight-bearing status for 6 weeks after inside-out suture repair. No statistically significant differences in failure rates were noted in either study, with failure rates ranging from 9% to 19%.[6,47] Both studies noted a more rapid return to full range of motion with the accelerated protocols, but no differences in final range of motion were noted. Similar results have been reported when allowing patients undergoing concurrent ACL and meniscal repair to progress with standard ACL rehabilitation protocols.[33]

In general, patients are permitted to partially weight bear as tolerated using crutches and wearing the knee brace locked in extension. During the first month it is important to work on regaining full extension and increasing the quadriceps tone through isometric exercises. The knee flexion should be strictly limited to 90 degrees. During the second month, the brace may be unlocked at all times, including with deambulation, and completely removed at 6 weeks postoperatively. Complete weight bearing may be allowed at 6 weeks postoperatively, and the brace should be removed, provided that the patient has adequate quadriceps tone and absence of limping. Knee flexion should progress to unrestricted motion. After the second month, the aim should be to increase muscle tone of the lower extremity, achieve normal gait, and gain complete range of motion by the end of the third month. After the third month, the aim should be to further increase muscle strength, add jogging, and later in time (around 4 to 5 months postoperatively), add more demanding exercises and sport-specific drills. The return to

TABLE 38.1 Advantages and Disadvantages of Repair Techniques

INSIDE-OUT TECHNIQUE		OUTSIDE-IN TECHNIQUE	
Advantages	Disadvantages	Advantages	Disadvantages
Quickly pass many sutures with preloaded needles	Requires a significant accessory incision	Relatively rapid	Facilitated by the use of a shuttle relay (increased cost)
Easy passage of braided sutures without a shuttle relay	Increased time in surgery	Easy access to anterior two-thirds of meniscus	Not useful for tears of the posterior third of the meniscus
Protection of neurovascular structures for posterior horn tears	Requires capable assistance	Can easily place sutures in any desired orientation	Difficult to pass braided suture without a shuttle relay

sport in athletes is expected around 6 to 8 months postoperatively if the patient has symmetric strength and function for the quadriceps and hamstring for both legs, is able to raise from a full squat position, and has no effusion or quadriceps atrophy.[29,55] In cases of repair of radial tears, the rehabilitation process should not be accelerated. The patient is allowed to only perform touch-down weight-bearing for 2 to 4 weeks with the knee brace locked in extension.[55] Weight-bearing, range of motion, and strengthening are progressively advanced only after the first 4 weeks.[55]

CONCLUSIONS

Meniscal tears are common injuries, and because of the inherent functions of the menisci, the tissue should be preserved whenever possible. Meniscus repair is more frequently successful in acute, vertical longitudinal peripheral (red-red zone) tears in younger patients. Concurrent ACL reconstruction enhances meniscal healing, but any residual ligamentous instability is detrimental. Vertical mattress sutures placed using an inside-out technique remain the standard. Care must be taken to protect vulnerable vascular structures when using these techniques. Tears that extend more anteriorly in the meniscus are amenable to repair with an outside-in technique, particularly augmenting an inside-out or all-inside technique used posteriorly (hybrid technique). Recent studies have demonstrated the effectiveness and safety of accelerated rehabilitation protocols after meniscal repair.

ACKNOWLEDGMENTS

The authors would like to give special thanks to Dr Robert A. Magnussen and Dr Richard C. Mather for their excellent contribution to the fifth edition version of this chapter, upon which this new version was built.

KEY REFERENCES

4. Barber FA: Accelerated rehabilitation for meniscus repairs. *Arthroscopy* 10:206–210, 1994.
11. Buckland DM, Sadoghi P, Wimmer MD, et al: Meta-analysis on biomechanical properties of meniscus repairs: are devices better than sutures? *Knee Surg Sports Traumatol Arthrosc* 23:83–89, 2015.
14. Cannon WD, Vittori JM: The incidence of healing in arthroscopic meniscal repairs in anterior cruciate ligament-reconstructed knees versus stable knees. *Am J Sports Med* 20:176–181, 1992.
22. Hantes ME, Zachos VC, Varitimidis SE, et al: Arthroscopic meniscal repair: a comparative study between three different surgical techniques. *Knee Surg Sports Traumatol Arthrosc* 14:1232–1237, 2006.
30. Johnson D, Weiss WM: Meniscal repair using the inside-out suture technique. *Clin Sports Med* 31(1):15–31, 2012.
36. Morgan CD, Wojtys EM, Casscells CD, et al: Arthroscopic meniscal repair evaluated by second-look arthroscopy. *Am J Sports Med* 19:632–637, 1991.
43. Rockborn P, Messner K: Long-term results of meniscus repair and meniscectomy: a 13-year functional and radiographic follow-up study. *Knee Surg Sports Traumatol Arthrosc* 8:2–10, 2000.
46. Scott GA, Jolly BL, Henning CE: Combined posterior incision and arthroscopic intra-articular repair of the meniscus. An examination of factors affecting healing. *J Bone Joint Surg Am* 68:847–861, 1986.
52. Tenuta JJ, Arciero RA: Arthroscopic evaluation of meniscal repairs. Factors that effect healing. *Am J Sports Med* 22:797–802, 1994.
55. Vinyard TR, Wolf BR: Meniscal repair: outside-in repair. *Clin Sports Med* 31(1):33–48, 2012.
56. Warren RF: Arthroscopic meniscus repair. *Arthroscopy* 1:170–172, 1985.

The references for this chapter can also be found on www.expertconsult.com.

39

All-Inside Arthroscopic Meniscal Repair

Megan M. Gleason, F. Winston Gwathmey, Jr., David R. Diduch

The meniscus contributes several key functions to the knee, including joint stability,[34] shock absorption and load transmission,[14] proprioception,[18] and articular cartilage nutrition.[21] In 1948 Fairbanks showed the long-term morbidity of meniscectomy as it relates to the formation of osteoarthritis.[20] Loss of meniscal volume with meniscectomy is shown to increase peak pressures and mean contact pressures between tibia and femur,[1] leading to the formation of degenerative joint changes.[2,4] The size and location of meniscal tears are also important. The lateral meniscus bears approximately 70% of the tibiofemoral contact pressure, whereas the medial meniscus accounts for 40%.[51] Tears involving the posterior root of the medial meniscus behave similarly to complete medial meniscectomy in biomechanical studies because of extrusion and, if repaired, restore normal contact pressures.[3] Therefore, under appropriate circumstances, meniscal repair is preferred to meniscectomy.

Techniques of meniscal repair have evolved over time and include outside-in, inside-out, and all-inside repairs. Although the inside-out vertical mattress repair, in which suture is passed through the meniscal tear and tied over the capsule, remains the gold standard for treatment, several all-inside devices have seen increased use over recent years. These devices may offer reliable repair of the meniscus with decreased surgical time, decreased technical difficulty, and minimal risk to neurovascular structures.

INDICATIONS FOR ALL-INSIDE MENISCAL REPAIR

The indications for inside-out meniscal repairs also apply to all-inside repairs. However, complete bucket handle tears in which several sutures are required may be a relative contraindication. Unfortunately, not all meniscal tears are suitable for repair and subsequent healing. Although magnetic resonance imaging (MRI) may aid in predicting which tears will be amenable to repair versus meniscectomy, the final surgical plan is often made during arthroscopy. It is important to consider possible meniscal repair in your surgical plan and inform patients appropriately.

The meniscus is 70% water and 30% organic material (primarily type I collagen) and is a relatively avascular tissue. Arnoczky and Warren[6] studied the microvascular perimeniscal plexus on the periphery of the meniscus, supplied by the medial and lateral geniculate arteries (Fig. 39.1).

This plexus forms short capillaries that extend from the periphery inward, extending 10% to 30% of the meniscal width medially and 10% to 25% of the meniscal width laterally.[6] The remaining meniscus receives its nutrition through synovial diffusion. The popliteal hiatus in the lateral compartment also creates a relatively hypovascular area in the posterior lateral meniscus.

DeHaven classified meniscal tears in the peripheral 3 mm as vascular (also referred to as the red-red zone), whereas those more than 5 mm from the meniscocapsular junction are considered avascular (white-white zone), and those in between as variable (red-white zone) (Fig. 39.2).[17] Tears in the vascular periphery of the meniscus have the best ability to heal, whereas tears in the central white-white zone demonstrate poorer healing rates and are less amenable to repair.[28]

In addition to location, meniscal tear orientation and complexity must also be considered. Longitudinal vertical tears, bucket handle tears, and meniscocapsular separations are most amenable to repair. Side-to-side sutures may be placed peripherally in the red-red zone of radial tears in an attempt to preserve a peripheral rim and hoop stresses (Fig. 39.3).

Tears longer than 4 cm in length are typically considered unstable and less amenable to healing, whereas tears shorter than 1 cm are generally stable.[12] Radial tears tend to be avascular, given their central location; however, they may extend into the periphery and be amenable to fixation.[37] Longitudinal tears may be more amenable to fixation than horizontal tears, given the orientation of collagen bundles (Fig. 39.4).

Improved results are seen with meniscal repairs performed less than 6 weeks from initial injury.[41,48] Degenerative tearing usually represents chronic damage from an ongoing degenerative process and may be best treated by partial meniscectomy. Tears with increasing complexity may also be better managed with partial meniscectomy. These include tears with horizontal cleavage planes or multiple flaps.[46] Oblique undersurface tears can also be complex with decreased likelihood of healing as they often extend from the vascular to avascular zone.

Patient factors also played an important role in determining appropriate candidates for meniscal repair. Younger patients tend to heal more effectively,[9] and it is more important to preserve the meniscus to limit the eventual onset of osteoarthritis. Meniscal repair has been shown to be more successful in the setting of a concurrent anterior cruciate ligament (ACL) reconstruction.[12,41] Lateral meniscus tears are more commonly found with acute ACL tears, whereas medical meniscus tears are often seen in ACL-deficient knees secondary to instability. All-inside techniques are likely to do well in the setting of concurrent ACL reconstruction, as opposed to isolated meniscal repairs. Furthermore, meniscal healing rates are typically lower in an ACL-deficient knee,[26] and therefore repair may be contraindicated if the ACL is not also reconstructed. Finally, meniscal repair

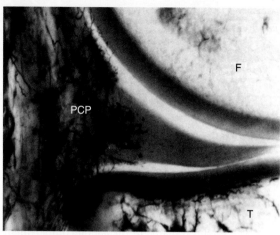

FIG 39.1 Microvasculature of the Meniscus A perimeniscal capillary plexus supplied by the medial and lateral genicular arteries perfuses the periphery of the meniscus. The remaining central portion of the meniscus is essentially avascular and has limited healing potential. *F*, Femur; *PCP*, perimeniscal capillary plexus; *T*, tibia. (From Arnoczky SP, Warren RF: The microvasculature of the human meniscus. *Am J Sports Med* 10(2):90–95, 1982.)

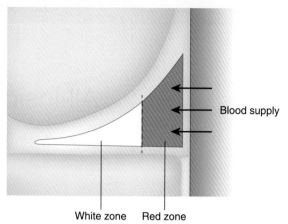

FIG 39.2 Meniscal zones (red-red, red-white, white-white). (Modified from Tudor F, McDermott ID, Myers P: Meniscal repair: a review of current practice. *Orthopaed Trauma* 28(2):88–96, 2014.)

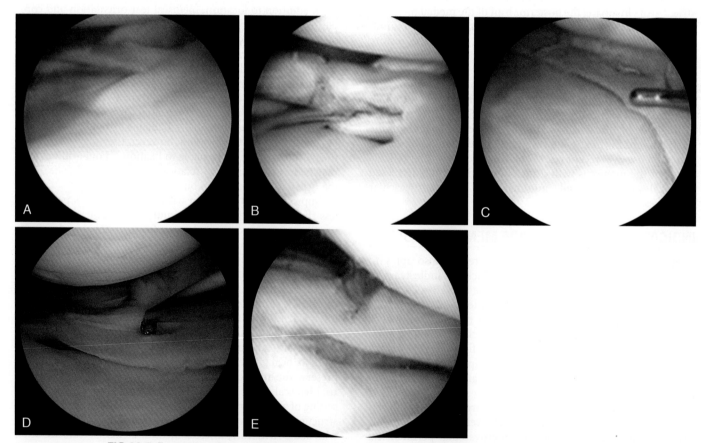

FIG 39.3 Examples of meniscal tears amenable to fixation. (A), (B) and (D) Longitudinal meniscal tears; (C) and (E) Peripheral vertical meniscal tears.

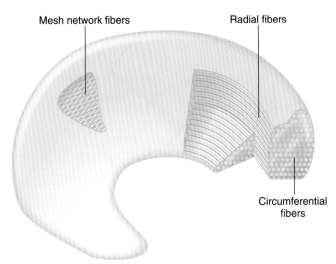

Mesh network fibers   Radial fibers

Circumferential
fibers

FIG 39.4 Meniscal collagen fiber organization. (From Bullough PG, Munuera L, Murphy J, et al: The strength of the menisci of the knee as it relates to their fine structure. *J Bone Joint Surg Br* 52B:564–567, 1970.)

requires a patient willing to comply with a prolonged rehabilitation course as opposed to resection.

TECHNIQUES

The technique and devices used for all-inside meniscal repair have evolved over the past three decades, with the goal of improving the strength of the repair, reducing morbidity, decreasing surgical time, and improving the ability to fix posterior horn tears. Regardless of the device used, an intact meniscal rim is required to anchor the repair. Injuries associated with meniscocapsular separation are best treated with alternative means because the all-inside devices are not currently equipped to adequately repair such an injury.

First-Generation All-Inside Repairs

The first generation of all-inside repair, described by Morgan in 1991, used curved suture hooks to pass sutures across the meniscus from the posterior knee.[40] This required accessory posterior portals, which presented a risk to neurovascular structures, and was technically challenging. This technique has largely been abandoned in favor of newer devices.

Second-Generation All-Inside Repairs

The second generation of all-inside meniscal repair used technique-specific devices, such as the T-Fix (Smith and Nephew, Andover, MA), to pass sutures across the tear and anchor it peripherally. This was achievable through anterior arthroscopic portals without the need for accessory posterior portals and therefore less risk to neurovascular structures. The T-Fix consisted of a polyethylene bar attached to a braided polyester suture. The bar was deployed through a sharp cannula to capture the peripheral meniscus or capsule. Adjacent sutures were then tied with arthroscopic knots on the meniscal surface. The device confirmed that it was possible and safe to repair the meniscus by deploying an anchor across the tear and into the periphery of the meniscus and/or capsule. However, the suture knots were a potential source of chondral abrasion and could not be tensioned after placement. Early results were encouraging,[19]

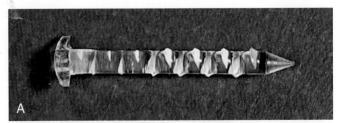

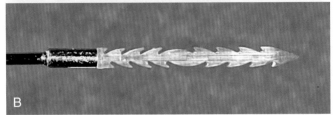

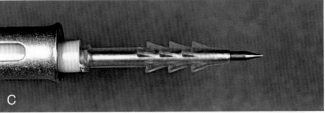

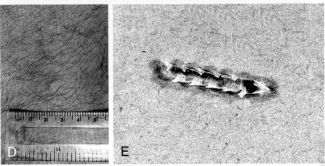

FIG 39.5 Example of Meniscal Arrows and Associated Complications (A) Meniscus Arrow (ConMed Linvatec, Utica, NY). (B) Meniscal dart (Arthrex, Naples, FL). (C) BioStinger (ConMed Linvatec, Utica, NY). Device migration has been reported with rigid all-inside meniscal repair devices. (D) This patient complained of a painful nodule that developed at his knee joint line after meniscal repair. (E) Exploration of the nodule revealed a broken meniscal arrow that was excised. (A to C from Stärke C, Kopf S, Petersen W, Becker R: Meniscal repair. *Arthroscopy* 25:1033–1044, 2009; D and E from Bonshahi AY, Hopgood P, Shepard GJ: Migration of a broken meniscal arrow: a case report and review of the literature. *Knee Surg Sports Traumatol Arthrosc* 12:40–51, 2004.)

but the T-Fix was replaced by new devices (third generation) that were easier to use and offered more compression across the repair.

Third-Generation All-Inside Repairs

The third-generation meniscal repair technique used rigid bioabsorbable devices, including arrows, screws, darts, and staples (Fig. 39.5A-C).

The most commonly used device was the Meniscal Arrow (ConMed Linvatec, Utica, NY). The rigid implant, often made of poly-L-lactic acid (PLLA), remained intact for up to 12 months and slowly absorbed over 2 to 3 years. The Meniscal

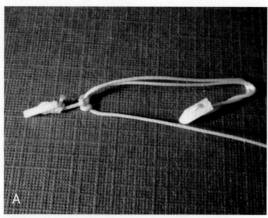
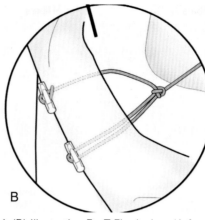

FIG 39.6 (A) Fourth-generation all-inside meniscal repair.(B) Illustrative FasT-Fix device. (A from Barber FA, Schroeder FA, Oro FB, et al: FasT-Fix meniscal repair: mid-term results. *Arthroscopy* 24:1342–1348, 2008; B from Smith & Nephew: *Meniscal repair with FasT-fix suture system.* Andover, MA, 2008, Smith & Nephew Endoscopy.)

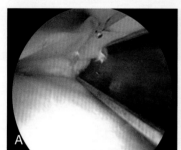
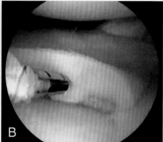
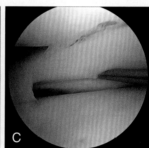
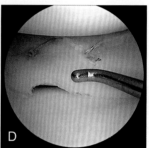

FIG 39.7 FasT-Fix clinical images. (A) A skid is introduced into the knee to protect the femoral condyle and tibial plateau as the FasT-Fix is passed toward the meniscal tear. (B) The FasT-Fix needle penetrates the meniscal tissue for deployment of the first anchor. (C) The FasT-Fix needle is passed into the undersurface of the meniscus tissue.(D) FasT-Fix sutures may be tied in a horizontal or vertical mattress configuration.

Arrow had excellent early results, with 90.6% healing at 2 years[23]; however, these results rapidly declined, with only 71.4% success rate in the same patients at 6 years.[33] Kurzweil et al. reported an overall failure rate of 28% with the Meniscus Arrow at average follow-up of 54 months; in isolated meniscus repairs without concurrent ACL reconstruction, the failure rate was up to 42%.[32] In addition to failure of the meniscal repair, the Meniscal Arrow has also been associated with adverse effects, including transient synovitis, inflammatory reaction, cyst formation, device failure, device migration, and chondral damage.*

The introduction of any rigid material into the knee joint poses a risk for chondral damage. Complications of the third-generation arrows, if placed too proud or the device loosened or migrated prior to dissolving, included significant chondral damage, such as grooving in the femoral condyle.[39] Because of poor long-term outcomes and numerous potential complications, the rigid third-generation devices are rarely used nowadays.

Fourth-Generation All-Inside Repairs

The fourth-generation all-inside meniscal repair devices were designed to address the shortcomings of the third-generation

devices, including the inability to tension the repair. There are several devices on the market, including the FasT-Fix (Smith and Nephew, Andover, MA) and Omnispan (Depuy Mitek, Raynham, MA). These devices are suture based and lower profile and allow for variable compression and re-tensioning across the meniscal tear.

The FasT-Fix is composed of two 5-mm suture anchors connected by a nonabsorbable polyester suture with a pretied slipknot. Another version of the FasT-Fix, the Ultra FasT-Fix, consists of polyetheretherketone (PEEK) anchors with ultra–high-molecular-weight polyethylene (UHMWPE) sutures (Ultrabraid) to improve strength and ease of use. The suture and anchors are loaded into a straight or curved passer with a depth-limiting sleeve. This allows for adequate insertion of the anchor while minimizing risk of damage to the neurovascular structures; a depth of 12 to 13 mm is usually sufficient and safe. The passer is carefully introduced into the joint through the anterior portal, and the first anchor deployed. The inserter is then withdrawn from the meniscus but maintained in the joint. The inserter is then passed again, in either a horizontal or vertical mattress, and the second anchor is deployed. The pretied slipknot is advanced with a push-pull technique to apply variable compression across the tear (Figs. 39.6 and 39.7D).

One of the primary advantages of the FasT-Fix is the ability to place the suture-based device in a vertical mattress

*References 5, 11, 27, 31, 38, 47, and 49.

configuration, as is the technique for inside-out meniscal repair. Traditionally a vertical mattress suture is superior over horizontal mattress sutures; however, some studies have shown no significant difference in load-to-failure when using high-strength suture material.[8] Complications include technical difficulty in positioning the device posteriorly, misfires, device breakage, anchor pull-out, and tangled sutures.

The Omnispan device also allows for all-inside meniscal repair with vertical mattress sutures. It is composed of two PEEK backstop anchors with a UHMWPE suture for mattress configurations. Because the slip knot is on the periphery at one of the backstops, no knot rests on the surface of the meniscus.

All-Suture All-Inside Repair

Although the fourth-generation devices have proven successful in meniscal repair, further advancements have been made in repair techniques. The NovoStitch (Ceterix, Fremont, CA) and Meniscal Scorpion (Arthrex, Naples, Florida) are all-inside suture-based devices that use a vertical pass through the meniscus to encircle the tear (Figs. 39.8 and 39.9A-C).

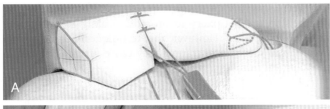
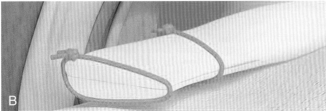

FIG 39.8 Ceterix Novostitch illustrative images. (A) Repair of radial meniscal tear and meniscal root repair. (B) Circumferential compression stitch. (Courtesy Ceterix Orthopaedics, Fremont, CA).

These devices allow for repair of meniscal tears while avoiding the need to incorporate the capsule and minimizing the risk to nearby neurovascular structures. Circumferential suture fixation provides more uniform compression across the edges, leading to perpendicular tension across the tear. This optimizes the coaptation forces, thereby providing the best mechanical environment for healing.[50] The all-suture, all-inside devices may be used for vertical or radial tears, lateral meniscus tears at the popliteal hiatus, horizontal cleavage tears, or root tears.[45]

CLINICAL RESULTS

Although we are surgically able to mend the meniscus with suture, healing must occur to sustain the repair. Meniscal repairs have been shown to heal more reliably when performed with concurrent ACL reconstructions. A retrospective study looking at meniscal repair using FasT-Fix (Smith and Nephew, Andover, MA) showed a 14.5% failure rate with concurrent ACL surgery and 27% failure rate with delayed reconstruction.[35] However, a study looking at FasT-Fix repairs from 1999 to 2007 followed 75 repairs and found a 16% failure rate at 5 years, with no difference in failure rate with or without concurrent ACL reconstruction.[10] A case series looking at meniscal repair using FasT-Fix, outside-in, or hybrid technique with subsequent computed tomography (CT) arthrography showed similar results with no significant difference in healing between meniscus repair alone and meniscus repair with ACL reconstruction.[43] Failure in these studies was defined as subjective function of the postoperative knee and/or need for revision surgery for meniscectomy or revision repair. Meniscal repairs in the setting of ACL reconstruction may heal well given the favorable biologic milieu; however, a stable repair appears to be equally as important to the healing process.

A biomechanical study by Rosso et al. in 2014 compared the FasT-Fix (Smith and Nephew, Andover, MA) and the Omnispan (Depuy Mitek, Raynham, MA) devices with corresponding suture controls in cyclic load to failure. The Omnispan had the highest load-to-failure and was stronger and stiffer; the inside-out vertical mattress suture fixation had a higher load-to-failure than the FasT-Fix.[44]

All-suture, all-inside meniscal repair is thought to have several advantages over the fourth-generation devices. The

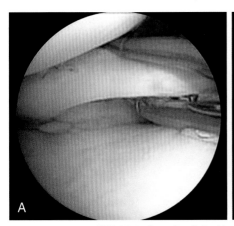
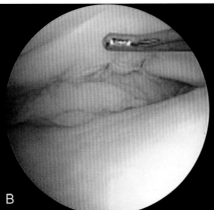
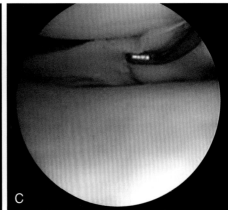

FIG 39.9 Ceterix clinical images. (A) Upper and lower jaws of Ceterix NovoStitch device (Fremont, CA) are deployed to allow for passage of suture. (B) Undersurface of meniscus following Novostitch repair (C) Peripheral meniscal repair using Novostitch.

fixation does not require crossing the meniscocapsular junction, which is critical in fixation of posterior horn tears, as well as lateral meniscus tears at the popliteal hiatus. The method of suture deployment may also allow for better configuration of sutures, depending on the morphology of the tear. A biomechanical study using porcine menisci showed the Ceterix Novostitch (Fremont, CA) was comparable to suture-based inside-out repair in load-to-failure, and similar to the FasT-Fix all-inside repair in regards to displacement during cyclic loading.[36] Although this device shows promise, long-term studies are needed for further assessment. One unique use of the NovoStitch may be for repair of radial tears. Zhang et al. showed a decrease in tibiofemoral contact pressures in cadaver menisci following repair of radial tears; these findings were comparable to inside-outside repairs.[54]

COMPLICATIONS

There are a number of complications that can arise with the use of all-inside meniscal repair devices, ranging from arterial injury to chondral abrasion. The most concerning complications include damage to the nearby neurovascular structures. Although the traditional inside-out repair is also plagued with potential neurovascular complications, the all-inside repairs show increased risk of damage to the popliteal artery, especially with fixation of posterior tears. A cadaver study by Cohen et al. showed that the passing needles of all-inside repair devices come within millimeters of the popliteal artery when performing repairs of the posterior horn of the meniscus.[13] Another cadaver study by Cuellar et al. looked at the distance from the posterior horn of the lateral meniscus to the popliteal artery and peroneal nerve. They found the safest position for fixation using the FasT-Fix device is with the knee in 90 degrees of flexion, with the distance to critical structures decreasing with extension of the knee.[16]

Earlier-generation meniscal repair devices were fraught with complications involving chondral abrasion from the devices themselves, suture knots, or loose bodies. Although this is still an area of concern, the newer-generation meniscal repair devices have reduced the incidence of these complications. Regardless, all-inside meniscal repairs should be gently challenged after fixation to evaluate for loose bodies, disengaged anchors, or undertensioned sutures.

Finally, the failure of meniscal repair may result in persistent or worsening symptoms. Failure of repair is often difficult to evaluate with traditional imaging, sometimes necessitating the use of MR arthrography to detect unhealed or re-torn menisci or chondral injuries.[25] Repeat or "second-look" arthroscopy is the best means to re-evaluate the meniscus and allows for revision repair or meniscectomy. Postoperative arthrofibrosis may require a return to surgery for lysis of adhesions or manipulation under anesthesia.[25]

ADJUNCTS TO HEALING

In addition to restoring the meniscal structure, meniscal repair also requires the appropriate biologic environment. Various techniques have been implemented to augment healing, including maximizing the proinflammatory cytokines and growth factors thought to promote healing.

Rasping or meniscal abrasion at the site of the tear promotes a healing response via the expression of cytokines.[42] An arthroscopic rasping device is introduced into the meniscus tear and used to mechanically stimulate the torn meniscal edges and promote expression of growth factors for neovascularization (Fig. 39.10).

Trephination involves using a spinal needle to create vascular channels to the periphery to promote healing and stimulate fibrochondrocytes.[53] However, this technique is controversial because the mechanical trauma may cause further damage to the meniscal infrastructure.

A fibrin clot is constituted from fibrin and platelets and is derived from autologous blood. It is placed in the tear to serve both a structural and biologic function. A dog model showed healing in avascular meniscal tears augmented with clot.[7] Henning at al. showed improvement in failure rate seen with clot and repair as compared with repair alone (Fig. 39.11).[29]

Platelet-rich plasma (PRP) is also derived from autologous blood that is spun down to concentrate platelets. Given the multitude of growth factors in platelets, it is thought to promote healing when activated by such agents as thrombin or calcium chloride.[15] However, a retrospective study comparing isolated meniscal repairs with and without PRP showed no significant difference in outcome scores; unfortunately, this study was underpowered, and more research needs to be performed to verify the utility of PRP (Fig. 39.12).[24]

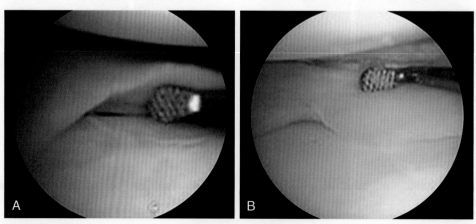

FIG 39.10 Rasping of meniscus prior to repair. (A) Undersurface tear and (B) peripheral tear.

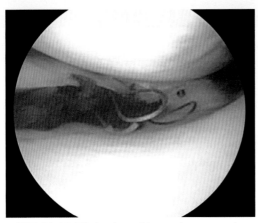

FIG 39.11 Fibrin clot with meniscus repair.

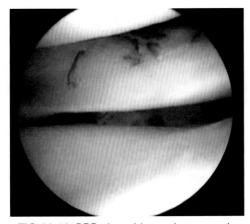

FIG 39.12 PRP clot with meniscus repair.

Tissue engineering, namely the use of biologic structural scaffolds and stem cells, is an area of important ongoing research in meniscal repair. A variety of materials are under investigation, including collagen-based, hyaluronic acid–based, polyglycolic acid (PGA) and polylactic-co-glycolic acid (PGLA) scaffolds. A study looking at meniscal tears in the avascular zone of rabbits showed healing with fibrocartilage-like tissue when filled with a hyaluronan/collagen composite matrix and stem cells and meniscal-like tissue when filled with the same composite and mesenchymal stem cells.[52] An in vitro study by Freymann et al. showed meniscal-derived stem cell proliferation in three-dimensional (3D) cultures in the presence of hyaluronic acid and human serum, resulting in meniscal matrix formation.[22] More research is necessary; however, current studies show great promise for avascular meniscal repair.

POSTOPERATIVE REHABILITATION

The biomechanics of the knee show increased pressure on the meniscus with weight bearing in flexion and posterior translation of femoral condyles relative to tibia when moving from extension to flexion. This can cause significant stress on the meniscal repair, possibly leading to failure before the meniscus has adequate time to heal. The postoperative protocol is critical to healing, and it is important to confirm the patient's ability and willingness to comply with the restrictions.

The patient should maintain toe-touch weight bearing on the operative extremity and avoid knee flexion during weight bearing until quadriceps function returns. Weight bearing in complex extension may be paradoxically favorable to compress a longitudinal tear pattern but contraindicated with repairs of radial tears. A hinged brace can help to gradually progress flexion while providing additional support. Given the increased strain on the meniscus with deep flexion, the patient is instructed to avoid squats and excessive tibial internal and external rotation for at least 4 months. Studies also recommend avoidance of athletics that requires running or cutting for at least 4 months.[30]

SUMMARY

Meniscal repair, when possible, is the preferred means to manage meniscal injury. Total and partial meniscectomies have been shown to result in early osteoarthritis of the knee, which can be especially detrimental in the young athletic patient population.

Factors that portend good results with meniscal repair include location and type of tear, young age of patient, concomitant ACL reconstruction, and unstable tears. With the current devices available, all-inside meniscal repair is an excellent option if a vertical mattress suture pattern can be obtained. Given the longitudinal orientation of the collagen bundles within the meniscus, vertical mattress fixation allows for added strength and stability with suture tensioning perpendicular to the collagen. Horizontal mattress sutures are tensioned parallel to the collagen bundles, resulting in mechanically inferior fixation. When repair with a vertical mattress pattern is possible, the all-inside repair is comparable to the gold-standard inside-out technique, with less morbidity and decreased surgical time. When vertical mattress patterns are not possible because of tear configuration or location or the inability to appropriately position the device, inside-out repair remains the preferred method of fixation.

Healing of the meniscus following repair may be augmented with rasping, fibrin clot, and other promising adjuncts. This is an important area of future research and may assist in healing the relatively avascular meniscal tears. At this time, postoperative rehabilitation is still an important component of healing. Avoidance of deep flexion in weight bearing will decrease the strain on the repair and likely lead to improved outcomes.

The references for this chapter can also be found on www.expertconsult.com.

40

Meniscal Allograft Transplantation

Kostas Economopoulos, Thomas R. Carter, Anikar Chhabra

Our understanding of the function of the meniscus has evolved over the past half century. Historically, the meniscus was considered a vestigial remnant of leg muscle that could be removed without any harmful effect.[75] Our views of the meniscus changed when Fairbanks[25] reported the importance of the meniscus in the protection of articular cartilage of the knee and described the radiologic changes that occur following meniscectomy. Currently, every attempt at preserving the meniscus is made; however, meniscal repair or a partial meniscectomy is not always possible, and total meniscectomy may be the only available option. Meniscal allograft transplantation has become a viable option for patients who develop pain following total or near total meniscectomy. The first meniscal allograft was associated with complete knee transplantation over a century ago.[49] In 1984, Milachowski et al.[52] performed the first modern meniscal allograft transplantation in humans. Since the first meniscal transplantations, our techniques have improved and transitioned from open procedures to arthroscopy-assisted procedures. Cvetanovich et al. reported an estimated 3295 meniscal transplants being performed between 2007 and 2011.[21] The number of meniscal transplants performed each year continues to increase, making it important for the orthopedic surgeon to understand the indications, complications, multiple techniques, and results of this procedure.

MENISCAL ANATOMY AND FUNCTION

Anatomy

Menisci are fibrocartilaginous biphasic structures containing solid and fluid phases. Water makes up roughly 75% of the meniscus and collagen fibers, and a small amount of proteoglycans and cells make up the other 20% to 25%. Collagen makes up between 60% and 95% of the dry weight of the meniscus, with type I collagen constituting 90% of the collagen and types II, III, V, and VI, contributing a small amount to the dry weight of the meniscus. The solid phase also contains proteoglycans, which are covalently attached to negatively charged glycosaminoglycans. The charged extracellular matrix allows water to bind, leading to a slower flow of water through the meniscus. The biochemical makeup of the meniscus allows it to serve several functions.

The structural orientation of the collagen fibers is related to its function. Collagen fibers are primarily oriented in a circumferential manner. Radially oriented fibers function as ties for the circumferentially oriented fibers and resist longitudinal splitting of the meniscus. During axial loading, the femoral condylar surfaces displace the menisci radially because of their concave wedge shape. The menisci convert axial load into tensile strain. Because menisci are anchored anteriorly and posteriorly, this displacement generates circumferential hoop stress that resists extrusion of the menisci from between the femoral condyle and tibial plateau. Biomechanical studies have shown that the meniscus is 100 times stronger and stiffer in the circumferential direction compared with the radial direction. The low circumferential shear strength is believed to be in part responsible for the occurrence of longitudinal tears.[64]

The menisci are relatively avascular, especially in the inner third of their body. The limited peripheral blood supply mainly comes from the lateral and medial genicular arteries. A perimeniscal capillary plexus within the synovial and capsular tissues of the knee joint arises from these feeding vessels. In the adult, vascular penetration is 10% to 30% of the width of the medial meniscus and 10% to 25% of the width of the lateral meniscus.[6] Because the menisci are predominantly avascular, nutrition to the meniscus must be derived through diffusion or mechanical pumping.

Knowledge of the meniscal anatomy, in particular bony attachment sites, is imperative when performing meniscal transplantation. The menisci form a semilunar wedge-shaped structure that fills the void created by the incongruous femoral condyle and tibial plateau. The medial meniscus is an oval-shaped fibrocartilaginous structure covering almost 30% of the medial tibial plateau. The anterior and posterior horns of the medial meniscus are further apart than the anterior and posterior horns of the lateral meniscus. The anterior horn of the medial meniscus is a flat fan-shaped structure that inserts in line with the medial tibial eminence 6 to 8 mm anterior to the anterior cruciate ligament (ACL) tibial insertion. The insertion site is under the patellar fat pad at the junction of the medial tibial plateau and anterior tibia, and often requires anterior fat pad débridement for good visualization. Landmarks demarcating the bony insertion of the anterior horn of the medial meniscus include the anterior border of the ACL tibial insertion, articular margin of the anteromedial tibial plateau, and anterior intercondylar fossa.[41] The anterior horn of the medial meniscus is often also secured by the intrameniscal ligament, which connects to the anterior horn of the lateral meniscus. The posterior horn of the medial meniscus inserts directly anterior to the tibial insertion of the posterior cruciate ligament (PCL), on the downslope of the posterior intercondylar fossa, behind the posterior horn insertion of the lateral meniscus. The PCL, medial tibial spine, and articular margin of the posteromedial tibial plateau serve as arthroscopic landmarks for the insertion of the posterior horn of the medial meniscus.

The lateral meniscus covers approximately 50% of the lateral plateau and has a more circular shape compared with the medial meniscus. The insertion site of the anterior horn of the lateral meniscus is directly anterior to the lateral tibial spine and adjacent to the tibial insertion of the ACL. Arthroscopic landmarks include the anterior half of the ACL tibial insertion, lateral tibial spine, and articular margin of the anterolateral tibial plateau. The posterior horn of the lateral meniscus inserts directly posterior to the lateral tibial spine, adjacent and anterior to the insertion of the posterior horn of the medial meniscus. Arthroscopic landmarks identifying the insertion of the posterior horn of the lateral meniscus include the posterior border of the ACL tibial insertion, lateral tibial spine, and articular margin of the posterolateral tibial plateau.[41]

Compared with the lateral meniscus, the medial meniscus is firmly attached to the peripheral structures and has less anteroposterior mobility. In flexion, the medial meniscus has only up to 5 mm of translation, compared with 11 mm of the lateral meniscus. The medial meniscus has several peripheral attachments, including the coronary ligaments anteriorly, joint capsule and medial collateral ligament centrally, and joint capsule posteriorly. The popliteus interrupts the posterior capsular attachments of the lateral meniscus, and there are no attachments to the lateral collateral ligament.

Function

The meniscus serves several important functions in the knee, including load bearing, shock absorption, joint stability, and joint lubrication. During weight bearing, the meniscus experiences several stresses, including tensile, compressive, and shear stresses. The medial meniscus transmits 50% of the joint load of the medial compartment, whereas the lateral meniscus transmits 70% of the joint load of the lateral compartment. This increases to 85% of the joint load when the knee is flexed to 90 degrees.[1] Radin et al.[62] have demonstrated that these loads are well distributed when the menisci are intact. Total medial meniscectomy leads to 50% to 70% decreased contact area and an increase in contact stress of 100%.[30,43] Because the lateral meniscus carries a higher proportion of the joint load due to the surface area, a lateral meniscectomy leads to a significantly higher increase in contact force compared with a medial meniscectomy. Total lateral meniscectomy leads to a 40% to 50% decrease in contact area and an increase in contact force of 200% to 300% compared with the intact meniscus.[7]

The biphasic nature of the meniscus allows it to function as shock absorber. Interstitial fluid flow and solid matrix deformation during loading cause the meniscus to act as a viscoelastic material, leading to creep and stress relaxation. Knees with an intact meniscus have a 20% higher shock absorption capacity compared with knees that do not have intact menisci.[82] In addition to their other functions, the menisci also play an important role in enhancing joint stability.[47] Medial meniscectomy in the ACL-intact knee has little effect on anteroposterior motion, but in the ACL-deficient knee, it results in an increase in translation of almost 60% at 90 degrees of flexion. Force on the medial meniscus increases by 52% in extension and 197% at 60 degrees of flexion in the ACL-deficient knee.[3] The conformity created by the meniscus promotes the viscous hydrodynamic action required for fluid film lubrication. This lubrication assists in the overall lubrication of the articular surfaces of the knee joint.[64] The multiple functions of the meniscus depend on their microstructure and macrostructure, both of which can be addressed by meniscal transplantation.

NATURAL HISTORY OF THE MENISCUS-DEFICIENT KNEE

In 1948, Fairbanks[25] described the changes that occur in the knee following meniscectomy, including ridge formation, narrowing of the joint space, and flattening of the femoral condyles. These changes lead to alterations in the biomechanics of the knee joint. Cox et al.[20] have studied the effects of partial and total meniscectomy in dogs. Partial meniscectomy led to less severe degenerative changes, with the degree of degeneration directly related to the amount of meniscus resected. In dogs with total meniscectomy, the degree of degenerative change was directly related to the amount of missing fibrocartilage. It was concluded that the knee menisci function to protect the articular cartilage from degenerative damages. McGinty et al.[51] have compared the outcomes of patients undergoing total and partial meniscectomy. Using the Fairbank criteria, they found that patients with partial meniscectomy have less narrowing of the joint line compared with patients with a total meniscectomy. They identified early radiographic degenerative changes in 62% of 89 patients treated with total meniscectomy, compared with 36% of 39 patients treated with partial meniscectomy. Because the lateral meniscus carries a higher percentage of the load force of the knee, degenerative changes generally progress more rapidly in the lateral compartment following lateral meniscectomy.[40,87]

BIOLOGY OF THE TRANSPLANTED MENISCAL ALLOGRAFT

Several characteristics of the meniscus make it optimal tissue to transplant. First, meniscal tissue elicits a minimal immune response. Immune reactions have been described in 1.3% of transplants reported in the literature.[72] Ochi et al.[56] placed fresh meniscal allograft in the subcutaneous tissue of mice and evaluated their immune response. They detected no specific antibodies in the serum throughout the 24-week period after grafting. They concluded that in mice, fresh meniscus was not immunogenic. Although the normal meniscus consists of relatively few chondrocytes embedded in an extracellular matrix, it also contains class II and ABH-positive endothelial cells and class II-positive synovial cells.[46] These antigens are present at the moment of transplantation and could evoke an immune response in the host that would modulate the results of meniscal allografting. Rodeo et al.[65] have performed an immunologic study that identified class I and II human leukocyte antigens (HLAs) on frozen meniscal allografts. Twenty-eight deep frozen and nonirradiated samples were evaluated. Overall, 9 of 12 specimens contained immunoreactive cells, including B lymphocytes or cytotoxic T cells in the meniscus or synovial tissue. No frank immunologic rejection was identified. The immune response to the meniscal allograft does not seem to affect the clinical outcome of the transplantation.

The primary functions of the meniscus can be accomplished, even if the structure is devoid of live cells. The meniscus is for the most part acellular, and most of its function is derived from its structure. The fate of the meniscal cells that accompany the meniscal allograft is unknown. Arnoczky et al.[4] have studied the cellular repopulation of deep-frozen meniscal allografts.

TABLE 40.1	**Graft Preservation Techniques**			
	PRESERVATION TECHNIQUE			
Parameter	**Fresh**	**Cryopreserved**	**Fresh-Frozen**	**Freeze-Dried (Lyophilization)**
Viable cells	Yes	Yes	Acellular	Acellular
Method of maintenance	Lactated Ringer's solution at 4°C	Controlled freezing process	Stored at −80°C	Vacuum freezing
Duration of maintenance	7 days	10 years	Up to 5 years	Indefinite
Advantages	Donor cell preservation and minimal disruption of meniscal integrity	Main collagen framework maintained	Low cost	Low cost

The menisci appeared to be repopulated with cells that originated from the adjacent synovium; however, the central core of the meniscus remained acellular. There was also loss of collagen orientation in the superficial layer of the meniscus. The structural remodeling associated with the cellular repopulation of deep-frozen meniscal allografts may make the transplanted meniscus more susceptible to injury. Jackson et al.[37] have used DNA probes to determine the fate of donor fibrocytes following meniscal transplantation. The results of this study demonstrated that host cells rapidly repopulate the transplanted meniscus. There is no evidence that these new cells will maintain the extracellular matrix of the meniscus on a long-term basis. Similarly, DeBeer et al.[22] have shown that human cryopreserved meniscal allograft donor cells arc 95% replaced by host cells 1 year after transplantation. Wada et al.[84] have noted that frozen meniscal allografts show collagen remodeling coincident with revascularization and cellular repopulation. Types I and III procollagen mRNA levels were elevated, representing active remodeling. These data indicate the adaptation of the repopulating cells from the host to the frozen allograft at 26 weeks after transplantation. In the goat model, Jackson et al.[38] have shown the proteoglycan concentration to be decreased in the meniscal allograft. They also noted that transplanted menisci undergo gradual, incomplete revascularization, with new capillaries derived from the capsular and synovial attachments. Our understanding of meniscal biology following transplantation has improved, but further research is necessary to answer several unanswered questions.

GRAFT PREPARATION AND DISEASE TRANSMISSION

Prevention of disease transmission with meniscal transplantation begins with careful donor screening. Transmission of human immunodeficiency virus (HIV) with frozen connective tissue allografts is estimated to be 1 in 8 million.[10] Blood and tissue from the donor are sampled at the time of graft harvest and remain in quarantine while being tested for hepatitis B and C, syphilis, and HIV. Tissue is procured within 12 hours of death for fresh grafts or within 24 hours if the body is stored at 4°C. Grafts are processed by débridement, pulsatile ultrasonic washing, and use of ethanol to denature proteins. Beginning in early 2005, HIV and hepatitis C screening were performed using direct nucleic acid testing by the polymerase chain reaction (PCR) assay. This method decreases the window that these viral infections can be missed, from 4 to 6 weeks down to 10 days.[11] Harvesting is done in a sterile fashion or

a clean nonsterile environment and secondarily sterilized. Secondary sterilization methods include the use of ethylene oxide, gamma radiation, or chemical means. Negative effects to the meniscal allograft have been reported with secondary sterilization. Gamma radiation at the level required to eliminate viral DNA may adversely affect the material properties of the meniscus.[77] Yahia and Zukor[86] have shown that exposure to more than 2.5 mrad of gamma radiation negatively affects the mechanical properties of collagen-containing tissues. Because 3 mrad of gamma radiation are recommended to eliminate HIV DNA, gamma radiation is not recommended. Ethylene oxide has been discontinued because of reports of graft failure and synovitis. Ethylene chlorohydrin, a by-product of ethylene oxide, has been found to induce synovitis in musculoskeletal allografts.[38]

The optimal method for meniscal graft preservation has yet to be determined. Currently, there are four primary preservation methods, including fresh, cryopreserved, fresh-frozen (deep-frozen), and freeze-dried (lyophilization; Table 40.1).

Fresh graft preservation leads to logistic issues for transplantation. The short period of time to size and perform serologic testing properly makes finding a suitable recipient difficult. Because of these issues, fresh grafts are rarely used in clinical practice today. The question still remains whether fresh graft is superior to grafts preserved using the three other methods. Good results have been reported in patients transplanted with fresh grafts. Verdonk[79] has found intact grafts of all 40 transplanted meniscal allografts using follow-up magnetic resonance imaging (MRI). One of the benefits of using a fresh graft includes viable cells present in the graft, which may be important in cartilage transplantation. However, Jackson et al.[37] have shown that donor DNA in the transplanted meniscus was entirely replaced by host DNA at 4-week follow-up. The importance of viable cells in the meniscal transplant remains to be determined.

Cryopreservation has provided a useful alternative to fresh grafts in terms of safety and function. The graft is thawed in the operating room just prior to surgery. Arnoczky et al.[5] have shown that the material properties of transplanted cryopreserved allografts in dogs are similar to those of normal menisci after 6 months. Cell viability ranging between 5% and 54% has been described in the literature. Gelber et al.[31] have shown that meniscal cryopreservation does not alter the meniscal ultrastructure or the biomechanical properties. Fabbriciani et al.[24] reported no difference in appearance or healing between meniscal allografts that were cryopreserved and those that were deep frozen. The expense and difficulty of this process, along with the uncertainty of donor cell viability, have decreased the popularity of this preservation process.

Fresh-frozen meniscal preservation is a simpler and less expensive method than cryopreservation. Deep freezing has been shown to destroy viable cells of connective tissue and to denature histocompatibility antigens, making frozen allografts less likely to provoke an immune response.[9] Milachowski et al.[52] have reported shrinkage in one of five deep-frozen grafts by MRI. At 48 weeks, deep-frozen grafts showed little revascularization or remodeling but good preservation.

Due to the detrimental effects of lyophilization, it is not recommended for processing meniscal allografts.[9] Milachowski et al.[52] have reported shrinkage in 9 of 10 lyophilized and gamma-sterilized allografts. All lyophilized allografts were remodeled and completely revascularized at 48 weeks. The same group of patients was reviewed 14 years postoperatively.[85] Second-look arthroscopy and MRI showed shrinkage of the lyophilized grafts. Gelber et al.[31] have evaluated the collagen meniscal architecture of excised meniscal transplants at the time of total knee replacement. They found the fibrils in frozen meniscal allografts to be of smaller diameter and in more disarray compared with nonfrozen controls. These findings may explain the shrinking associated with this type of preservation.

INDICATIONS AND CONTRAINDICATIONS FOR MENISCAL TRANSPLANTATION

The indications for meniscal transplantation continue to evolve as long-term clinical results become available. Currently, meniscal transplantation is an accepted procedure for patients with meniscus-deficient knees. The goal of meniscal transplantation is to reduce pain and prevent progression of arthritis. Consideration of meniscal transplantation should only be entertained when nonsurgical measures to control pain have been exhausted, including activity modification, antiinflammatories, injections, and unloading bracing. Some research suggests meniscal transplantation only after 6 months of conservative treatment have been attempted and failed.[34,39,69] With concurrent ACL reconstruction, earlier meniscal transplantation may improve clinical outcomes.[33,47,69] Veltri et al.[78] have suggested the ideal meniscal transplantation candidate to be skeletally mature, younger than 50 years, post-total or subtotal meniscectomy, with a ligamentously stable knee or planned stabilization, no evidence of malalignment, and minimal arthrosis. Although they used 50 years old as the upper age limit in patients with minimal arthritis, this is controversial because physiologic age is more accurate than absolute age.[57]

Outerbridge published a classification of cartilage lesions associated with chondromalacia patellae in 1961 (Table 40.2).[57] This classification system has been modified to describe articular cartilage lesions seen at the time of arthroscopy. It can be used to classify the patient's arthrosis to determine whether he or she is a candidate for meniscal transplantation. Garret,[29] Noyes et al.,[54] and Cole et al.[17] have demonstrated improved results in meniscal transplantation in patients whose degenerative changes are Outerbridge grade I or II. Patients with Outerbridge grade III or IV degeneration levels had less predictable outcomes. No studies were able to define whether the poor results found in patients with advanced degenerative changes were caused by the degenerative disease itself or associated knee malalignment.

TABLE 40.2	Outerbridge Classification
Grade	**Features**
Original Description[a]	
I	Softening and swelling of the cartilage
II	Fragmentation and fissuring less than 1 inch in diameter
III	Fragmentation and fissuring greater than 1 inch in diameter
IV	Erosion of cartilage down to bone
Currently Accepted Description	
I	Softening
II	Partial-thickness fissures
III	Full-thickness fissures
IV	Exposed subchondral bone

[a]Initial description was based on macroscopic changes of the patella. This system was modified to describe arthroscopic changes in the articular cartilage.

Another critical factor in determining a successful candidate is the mechanical alignment of the knee. Malalignment is defined as valgus or varus asymmetry between 2 and 4 degrees compared with the contralateral knee, or the mechanical axis falling into the affected meniscus-deficient compartment on weight-bearing films. Meniscal transplantation in a malaligned knee causes abnormal pressure on the meniscal allograft, resulting in impaired vascularization, degeneration, and failure of the graft.[63] In cases of malalignment, meniscal transplantation is contraindicated until a concurrent corrective osteotomy is performed. Cameron and Saha[12] have reported 85% good results in patients undergoing meniscal transplantation and corrective osteotomy. It remains to be determined whether the osteotomy or the meniscal transplantation led to clinical improvement.

Meniscal transplantation can be considered for patients with concomitant ACL instability. Garret[29] has reported significantly improved KT-1000 arthrometer results for ACL reconstruction when performed in combination with medial meniscal allograft transplantation compared with a group of patients who underwent ACL reconstruction only, with persistent medial meniscal deficiency.

The primary absolute contraindication to meniscal transplantation is advanced arthrosis of the meniscus-deficient knee. Most researchers consider previous infection in the knee, inflammatory arthritis, neuropathy, and evidence of osteonecrosis as contraindications to meniscal allograft transplantation.[53] Obesity is a relative contraindication to surgery because of the increased force across the joint, leading to an increased failure rate. The indications and contraindications for meniscal transplantation will continue to evolve as long-term results become available. A summary of indications and contraindications is listed in Table 40.3.

PREOPERATIVE CONSIDERATIONS

Evaluation

The key to successful meniscal transplantation includes patient selection and appropriate preoperative evaluation. The operative report of all previous surgeries should be reviewed. In addition, any available intraoperative photographs can be used to determine the extent of articular damage and degeneration, along with the status of the remaining meniscus. If previous arthroscopic pictures are not available, and appropriateness for

TABLE 40.3	Contraindications to Meniscal Transplantation
Contraindication	**Features**
Absolute	Advanced arthritis
	Joint space narrowing
	Femoral flattening
	Osteophytes
	Outerbridge grades III and IV changes
	Joint incongruity
Relative	Malalignment
	Focal chondral defects
	Ligament instability
	Obesity
	Rheumatoid arthritis
	Gout
	Immune compromise
	Metabolic disease
	Infection
	Lack of commitment to postoperative restrictions

meniscal transplant is unknown, diagnostic arthroscopy is indicated to determine the degree of meniscus loss and arthrosis.

The preoperative physical examination should include gait inspection, stance, and the ability of the patient to get in the squatting position. Prior incisions should be evaluated. Palpation of the joint line, McMurray's test, knee range of motion, presence of effusion, and muscle strength and wasting should all be evaluated. The examination must include a thorough ligamentous evaluation and definition of axial alignment of the limb. Patient compliance should be gauged throughout the evaluation.

Radiograph studies should include weight-bearing, 45-degree flexion posteroanterior, Merchant, and weight-bearing lateral views using magnification markers for sizing. Long-leg alignment radiographs are imperative to evaluate lower limb mechanical alignment. MRI is important for determining the status of the hyaline cartilage, subchondral bone, and menisci.

Graft Sizing

Good clinical outcomes following meniscal transplantation rely on selection of an appropriately sized meniscal allograft. The tolerance of size mismatch in knees undergoing meniscal transplantation is not known. Although too small a meniscal allograft does lead to uneven contact forces, more meniscus is not always better. The meniscus must be properly sized for optimum reduction of contact pressures. Dienst et al.[23] have shown that oversized lateral meniscal allografts lead to greater forces across the articular cartilage, whereas undersized allografts result in normal forces across the articular cartilage but greater forces across the meniscus. They concluded that grafts within 10% of the native meniscus were able to reproduce contact mechanics close to the intact state. Huang et al.[36] have found increased contact pressures when allografts did not match the native menisci. The greatest predictor of differences in contact pressure was the difference in the width of the menisci. It was concluded that protocols used to select allografts should focus on cross-sectional parameters to match the native meniscus.

Sizing of allografts is done using plain radiography, computed tomography (CT), or MRI or by making direct measurements. The use of the contralateral knee in patients with prior meniscectomy has been described to help sizing. However, Kim et al.[44] have shown that there is variability in meniscal size between opposite knees. The most commonly used method for sizing today is plain radiographs. Pollard et al.[60] have found that the meniscal width equals the distance (coronal) from the peak of the tibial eminence to the periphery of the tibial metaphysis on anteroposterior films. Medial meniscal length is 80%, and lateral meniscal length is 70% of the measured sagittal length of the tibial plateau on the lateral radiograph. Measurement error averaged 7.8% by these parameters. Axial CT scans can size the meniscus without concern for rotation or magnification. However, the patient must endure a much larger load of radiation. Shaffer et al.[71] have compared the accuracy of plain x-rays and MRI for preoperative sizing of meniscal allografts. Overall, MRI was slightly more accurate than plain radiography; however, only 35% of the menisci measured with MRI were within 2 mm of the actual meniscal size. Carpenter et al.[13] have compared the accuracy of MRI with both plain radiograph and CT in estimating the size of the meniscal allograft. MRI was found to be the most accurate for meniscal height but consistently underestimated the anteroposterior and mediolateral sizes. Prodromos et al.[61] have compared MRI with plain radiography in estimating the appropriately sized meniscal allograft. They concluded that human knee menisci are bilaterally symmetric in size and that direct MRI measurement of the contralateral intact meniscus predicts actual meniscal size better than estimation of size indirectly from measurement of the tibial plateau on which it is located. They proposed contralateral MRI meniscal measurement as a new gold standard to size menisci before transplantation. Although plain radiographs are currently the gold standard, it appears that MRI techniques are improving and will probably be the study of choice for determining meniscal allograft size.

SURGICAL TECHNIQUES

Several techniques have been described for meniscal allograft transplantation. The main differences between the techniques include open versus arthroscopically assisted, soft tissue fixation versus bony fixation, and bone plug versus bone-bridge.[72] Initial studies discussing meniscal transplantation described open techniques; however, arthroscopy-assisted techniques have become more popular. Both techniques have shown equivalent outcomes, but the arthroscopic approach decreases surgical morbidity, avoids collateral ligament injury, and promotes early rehabilitation.[12,14,30,52,76] Regardless of the technique used, the most important factor in successful meniscal transplantation is appropriate sizing and anatomic placement of the transplanted meniscus.[17] Although it is technically easier to anchor the meniscus with soft tissue alone, bone promotes improved load transmission and provides more normal biomechanics of the transplanted meniscus.[2,16,59] There remains debate whether bone plugs or bone-bridge is the optimal method for meniscal transplantation. The bone plug method is primarily used in the medial meniscus, where the anterior and posterior horns of the meniscus are separated by greater than 1 cm. Bone plugs allow for minor modifications in the final position of the meniscal horn position, which is useful because of some variation in meniscal horn anatomy.[8,45] Because the distance between the meniscal horns in the lateral compartment is 1 cm or less, use of bone plugs presents the risk of tunnel communication, which may compromise fixation.[41] Lateral meniscal transplantation is typically performed using a bone-bridge technique, in which the two horns of the meniscus are maintained on the same bone block. Proponents of the bone-bridge technique cite ease of insertion and maintenance of the anatomic relationship of the anterior and posterior horns.[19,26] Regardless of the technique used, care must be taken to size the allograft properly and securely fix it to its anatomic anterior and posterior horn footprints along with the capsule peripherally.

Patient Positioning and Initial Evaluation

Once general anesthesia is induced, appropriate prophylactic antibiotics are given. A thorough examination under anesthesia is performed on all patients to determine the stability and range of motion of the knee. A tourniquet should be placed as high as possible on the thigh, but not inflated. Depending on surgeon preference, the operative leg may be placed in a cushioned leg holder or unsupported in the supine position. Visualization of the posteromedial or posterolateral corner is important for medial or lateral allograft transplantation, respectively, facilitating inside-out repair. The contralateral leg should have thromboembolic deterrent (TED) hose and sequential compression devices (SCDs) placed to prevent deep venous thrombosis (DVT). Once the patient is prepped and draped, a diagnostic arthroscopy should be performed to confirm meniscal deficiency and evaluate the status of the articular cartilage and ligaments. The remaining body of the involved meniscus is débrided to a 1- to 2-mm synovial rim, which leaves a vascular source to help graft healing. The anterior and posterior horn attachments are initially preserved to serve as guide points for drilling the tibial tunnels if the bone plug technique is planned. In the lateral compartment, the meniscal rim anterior to the popliteus tendon can often be saved.

Bone Plug Technique

Graft Preparation. The appropriate graft size and side should be confirmed before preparing the meniscal allograft. If the size or side of the meniscal allograft is incorrect, the procedure should be abandoned until the appropriate allograft is available. The allograft will be delivered as a meniscus on a hemi tibial plateau or a complete tibial plateau. The allograft is thawed in warm saline. Once thawed, the first step in preparing the allograft is to remove all ligament tissue from the graft periphery. The anterior and posterior horn insertion sites should be isolated. Preparation of the posterior bone plug begins by placing a guide pin in the center of the attachment site of the posterior horn at roughly a 60-degree angle. A collared pin is then placed through the hole in the center of the posterior horn insertion. A coring reamer is placed over the collared pin, creating a bone plug measuring 6 to 8 mm. The posterior bone plug should be beveled to make insertion easier. The top of the posterior horn of the meniscus is marked with a marking pen for orientation. Preparation of the anterior bone plug is performed in the same manner. A guide pin is placed through the anterior horn of the meniscus. Compared with preparation of the posterior bone plug, the guide wire is placed more antegrade for the anterior bone plug. A collared pin is placed over the guide wire in the center of the anterior horn insertion site, and a 9- to 10-mm reamer is used to create the bone plug. Two 2-0 nonabsorbable Ethibond sutures are passed retrograde through each bone plug, creating sutures that can be passed through the tibial tunnel for proper allograft placement. When the sutures are passed through the bone plug, the suture should include the root in a whipstich

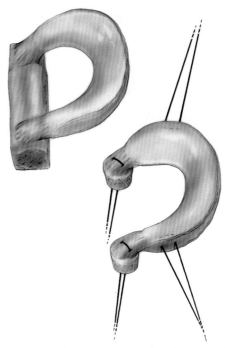

FIG 40.1 Nonabsorbable sutures are placed retrograde through the bone plugs. Guide sutures are preinserted into the posteromedial and anterior portions of the allograft.

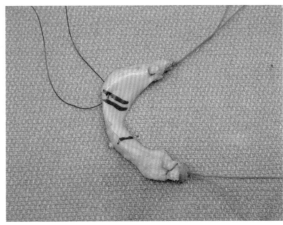

FIG 40.2 A traction suture is placed at the junction of the posterior and middle thirds of the allograft to facilitate the introduction of the meniscus.

fashion to secure the horn and bone better. If this is not done, the chance of the sutures breaking out of the bone is increased (Fig. 40.1). A traction suture to facilitate the introduction of the meniscus is created by placing a 0 polydioxanone suture (PDS) at the junction of the posterior and middle thirds of the meniscus (Fig. 40.2). The anterior aspect of the posterior bone plug is marked with a sterile ink marking pen to assist in orientation.

Preparation of the Recipient Bed. Starting just adjacent to the tibial tubercle, the posterior tibial tunnel is made by placing a guide pin into the anatomic posterior horn attachment of the old meniscus. A tibial tunnel is drilled over the guide wire to a diameter of 9 mm (Fig. 40.3). If ACL reconstruction is to be

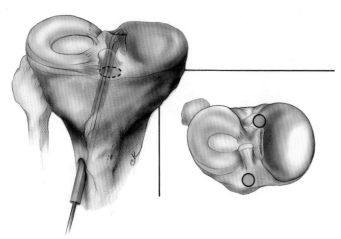

FIG 40.3 The posterior tibial tunnel is created by drilling over a guide pin that has been placed through the footprint of the native posterior horn attachment.

done, this posterior tunnel is brought out through the lateral side of the tibia so that it will diverge from the ACL tibial tunnel. The rim of this tunnel is smoothed, and any remaining posterior horn meniscal tissue is removed. A limited notchplasty of the medial femoral condyle is performed, if necessary. At least 8 mm of opening adjacent to the PCL in the femoral notch is needed to pass the posterior osseous portion of the graft.[55]

Meniscus Implantation. The tourniquet is inflated for the first portion of implantation. The exposure is similar to a posterior horn inside out meniscus repair technique. A 3-cm vertical posteromedial incision is made just posterior to the superficial medial collateral ligament. The fascia anterior to the sartorius is incised and the pes anserinus muscles are retracted posteriorly. The plane between the semimembranosus tendon and capsule is established. Blunt dissection is used to separate the medial aspect of the gastrocnemius tendon and posteromedial aspect of the capsule. A 3-cm anteromedial incision is created just medial to the patellar tendon. The posterior bone plug with attached meniscus is passed through the anteromedial arthrotomy, along with the secondary meniscal body suture (Fig. 40.4). The secondary meniscal body suture is passed out through the posteromedial approach. The knee is then flexed to 90 degrees for best visualization. The posterior attachment guide wire is retrieved, and the sutures attached to the posterior bone are passed. To assist in passage of the posterior bone portion of the graft, the knee is flexed to 20 degrees, and a maximum valgus load is placed on the knee. Pulling on the posteromedial suture and using a blunt instrument helps reduce the meniscus into its proper anatomic location. The knee can be flexed and extended to assess meniscal fit and displacement.

A guide pin is then passed through the insertion site of the anterior horn footprint. A 9-mm tunnel is reamed over the guide pin. A Houston suture passer is passed up the anterior tunnel, and the sutures on the anterior bone plug are captured and brought down the anterior tunnel. The bone plug is press-fit into the anterior tunnel using a tamp. The sutures attached to the anterior and posterior bone plugs are tied to each other over an anterior bone-bridge or button.

The anterior arthrotomy is closed and peripheral attachment of the meniscus is performed by passing sutures arthroscopically. An inside-out technique is used to attach the periphery

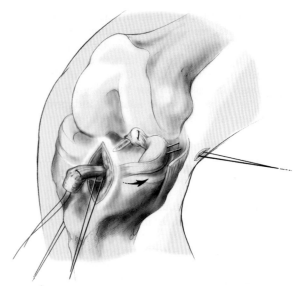

FIG 40.4 The posterior bone plug is passed through the anteromedial arthrotomy with the assistance of the secondary meniscal body suture.

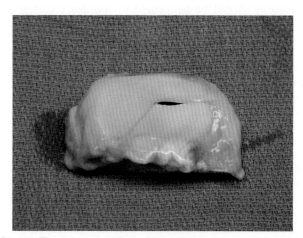

FIG 40.5 The meniscal allograft block is thawed and inspected. The anterior and posterior horns are then identified and marked.

of the meniscus to the capsule. Eight to 10 vertically placed 2-0 nonabsorbable mattress sutures are placed from posterior to anterior using standard inside-out technique. The sutures should be placed superiorly and inferiorly, with constant tensioning of the meniscus from posterior to anterior. After final inspection with the knee in flexion and extension, the remaining wounds are closed in typical fashion.

Bone-Bridge Technique

Graft Preparation. Following thawing and inspection of the meniscal allograft block, the attachment sites of the anterior and posterior horn are identified on the bone block (Fig. 40.5). Using an oscillating saw, the bone-bridge is cut to a width of 7 mm, a height of 1 cm, and a length of 35 mm. Care must be taken not to detach the anterior or posterior horn from their bony attachment. A rasp that is used to create the slot in the tibia can be used to template the bone-bridge. A meniscal bridge sizing jig is used to establish the definitive width of the box at 7 to 8 mm. The bone-bridge should loosely fit through the sizing jig

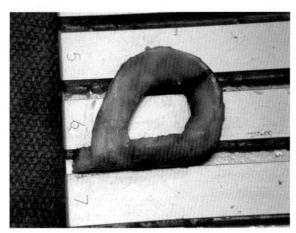

FIG 40.6 A sizing jig is used to confirm that the bone-bridge will loosely pass through the created slot.

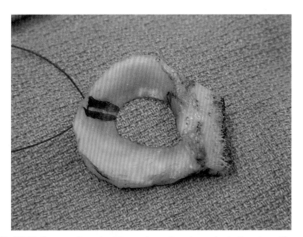

FIG 40.7 A nonabsorbable suture is placed at the junction of the posterior and middle thirds of the allograft meniscus. The suture will assist in meniscal placement.

(Fig. 40.6). A 0 PDS is placed at the junction of the posterior and middle thirds of the meniscus to function as a reduction suture, which will be used for meniscal placement (Fig. 40.7).

Tibial Preparation. The remaining meniscus is trimmed down to a 1- to 2-mm rim until punctuate bleeding occurs. The remnants of the anterior and posterior horns are left to act as footprints and assist in graft placement. A 3-cm anterolateral arthrotomy is made adjacent to the patellar tendon. A spinal needle may be used to create a reference line with the anterior and posterior horns. Electrocauterization is used to mark the correct center of the anterior and posterior horn attachment sites. A superficial reference line is created between the two horns, initially using an arthroscopic shaver and then a 4-mm burr. The reference slot should bury the 4-mm burr and be parallel to the sagittal slope of the tibial plateau. A depth gauge is used to determine whether the slot is level by placing the hook of the depth gauge over the posterior cortex. An insertion pin is placed through a drill guide parallel to the tibial plateau in the sagittal plane. The pin should not penetrate the posterior cortex to protect the neurovascular bundle. The drill guide is removed and a cannulated 7- or 8-mm reamer is used to drill over the guide pin. The reamer can be followed arthroscopically as it passes through the provisional

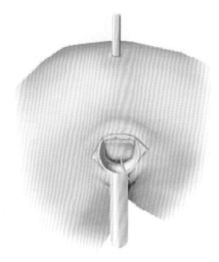

FIG 40.8 The meniscus is peripherally attached to the postero-lateral capsule using long, flexible, nitinol needles passed through the accessory posterolateral incision.

slot. A 7- or 8-mm box cutter is gently impacted into the provisional slot to the level of the posterior cortex. The slot is smoothed out using a 7- or 8-mm bone rasp.

Allograft Implantation. The exposure is similar to a posterior horn inside out lateral meniscus repair. A 3-cm posterolateral accessory incision is made and centered behind the lateral collateral ligament. The interval between the biceps tendon insertion and iliotibial band is identified and incised. Dissection is performed anterior to the biceps femoris to prevent injury to the peroneal nerve. Sharp dissection allows the lateral head of the gastrocnemius to be freed from the posterior capsule at the joint line. Care must be taken not to extend the dissection too far proximally to avoid entering the joint. A capsular repair will be necessary if this does occur. Blunt dissection is used to enlarge the space between the posterolateral capsule and lateral head of the gastrocnemius. A popliteal retractor is then placed behind the lateral meniscal bed. A single-barrel zone-specific cannula for an inside-out suture technique is placed through the medial portal and is used to advance a long, flexible, nitinol suture-passing pin through the knee capsule site at the junction of the posterior and middle thirds of the meniscus. The pin should exit out through the accessory posterolateral incision (Fig. 40.8). The proximal end of the nitinol pin is then withdrawn through the arthrotomy site. The traction suture is placed through the loop of the nitinol pin, and the sutures are withdrawn through the accessory incision. The meniscus is inserted through the anterolateral arthrotomy. The bone-bridge is aligned with the recipient slot by gently pulling on the reduction suture. The meniscus is properly captured by the tibiofemoral articulation by cycling the knee. Final fixation of the bone-bridge in the slot is performed by placing an interference screw on the far side of the bone block (Fig. 40.9).

The periphery of the meniscus is fixed to the capsule using 8 to 10 vertically placed 2-0 nonabsorbable mattress sutures. The sutures are placed from posterior to anterior using a standard inside-out technique. Sutures are placed on both the dorsal surface and undersurface of the meniscus for more anatomic attachment. The sutures are tied with the knee in full extension

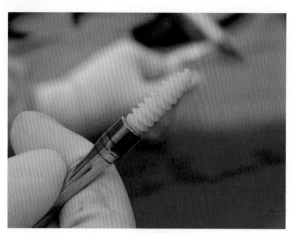

FIG 40.9 An interference screw is used for final fixation of the bone-bridge in its slot.

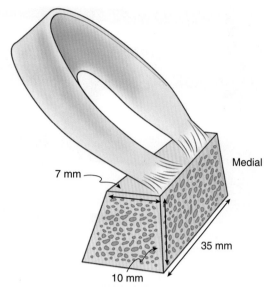

FIG 40.10 The dovetail bone block is prepared into a trapezoidal shape measuring $7 \times 10 \times 35$ mm³.

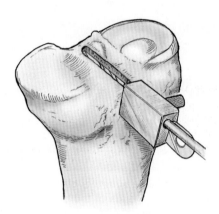

FIG 40.11 A drill guide and drill are used to create an initial bone slot that will eventually be formed into a trapezoid-shaped bone slot.

as to not over-capture the meniscus. If tied in flexion, the sutures can pull through at the extremes of motion. Arthroscopic visualization of the meniscus is helpful for confirming appropriate placement of the meniscus while the sutures are tied.

The bone-bridge technique is a technically demanding procedure, with several pitfalls. One of the technical problems is caused by the anatomy of the anterior horn insertion site on the tibia. The meniscal insertion site is 8 to 9 mm, whereas the bone-bridge is typically only 7 mm wide. To deal with this problem, the anterior portion of the bone-bridge is cut slightly wider than the rest of the bridge to accommodate for the widened insertion site. Another situation that may be encountered while performing the bone-bridge technique is avulsion of the insertion site of the meniscus. If this occurs, a no. 2 Ethibond suture can be placed through the substance of the meniscus and then passed through the bone-bridge using a Kirschner wire (K wire) or free needle. The meniscus is anchored down to the bone by tying the two ends of the Ethibond together. If bone fracture occurs, a K wire can be used as an internal splint during introduction of the meniscus. The interference screw can be used to fix the fracture once it is in its final position and the K wire is removed. If the fracture is not amenable to repair, the bone-bridge can also be converted to a double bone plug allograft.

Dovetail Technique

The dovetail technique attempts to simplify graft preparation with a time-saving series of cuts preparing the bone component of the graft to sit securely in a semitrapezoidal recipient slot created in the tibia. A matching semitrapezoid-shaped recipient slot created in the tibia with a series of step drills, rasps, and dilators matches the bone block preparation.

Allograft preparation begins with trimming off excess soft tissue so that the anterior and posterior horns can be easily identified. The allograft tibial plateau is cut to the desired anteroposterior length. Using the trapezoidal rasp for tibial slot preparation, an outline of the dovetail bone block is drawn on the end of the bone plug. Using an oscillating saw, the bone plug is fashioned into a trapezoid-shaped bone-bridge, with the vertical wall on the medial side and the angled wall on the lateral side (Fig. 40.10).

The tibial slot is created by initially burring a shallow trough between the anterior and posterior horns of the meniscus. To determine the AP depth of the tibial plateau, an osteotome is advanced to the posterior cortex following the path of the previously created trough. Using drill guides, drills are used to create an initial slot (Fig. 40.11). Trapezoidal rasps and dilators are used to create a trapezoidal slot in which the trapezoidal bone-bridge is placed (Fig. 40.12). A tamp may be used to position the bone block into the slot. The knee is brought into a figure-of-four position to open the lateral compartment, making the passage of the trapezoidal bone-bridge easier. The posterior horn must clear the femoral condyle before the bone plug will set fully against the posterior cortex.

Soft Tissue Technique

An alternative technique to bony fixation procedures is a soft tissue–only technique. The graft is prepared similar to the bone plug method; however, the bone plugs are removed from the allograft. Transosseous tunnels are drilled and the graft is passed in a similar manner to the bone plug method with conventional ACL guides. No. 2 braided nonabsorbable sutures secure the

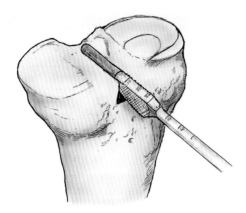

FIG 40.12 A trapezoid-shaped rasp is used to smooth out the bone-bridge slot.

graft after it is passed through the transosseous tunnels to their anatomic insertion sites. Fixation is performed over a bone-bridge or over a button. The remaining meniscal allograft is then secured with the use of arthroscopic inside-out suture techniques.

COMBINED TECHNIQUES

Meniscal Transplantation With Anterior Cruciate Ligament Reconstruction

Meniscal transplantation with ACL reconstruction can be performed together in combined injuries, particularly in cases of failed ACL surgery secondary to total or subtotal medial meniscectomy. Standard femoral and tibial tunnels are drilled and prepared before meniscal allograft insertion. Autograft or allograft tissue can be used for ACL reconstruction, depending on patient and surgeon preference, but allograft tissue use in this situation is increasing in an attempt to decrease donor site morbidity. The tibial tunnel often encroaches on the bone used for the trough for the meniscus, so care must be taken while drilling the tunnel.[68] When using the medial double-plug technique, the soft tissue and osseous portions of the transplantation are performed first.[17] The tibial tunnel for the ACL reconstruction is drilled slightly more medially than usual to avoid communication between the tibial tunnel and the tunnel for the posterior horn of the meniscus. Caution must be taken when using a trough technique for a medial meniscal allograft in combination with ACL reconstruction because the anterior and posterior horns of the native medial meniscus are often in line with the ACL, which can lead to ACL damage or encourage potential medialization of the horn attachments. When performing a bone-bridge technique for lateral meniscal transplantation, the tibial trough is created and the meniscal graft placed before the tibial tunnel for the ACL is drilled. To avoid the lateral slot, the tibial tunnel for the ACL is drilled slightly distally and medially.

Meniscal Transplantation With High Tibial Osteotomy

High tibial osteotomy (HTO) should be performed in combination with meniscal transplantation in patients with axial malalignment. Similar to HTO performed for isolated medial compartment arthritis, the HTO in combination with meniscal transplantation should correct the knee to just past neutral to

unload the affected limb. It is important to correct the alignment to the mechanical axis of the opposite tibial spine, not into the opposite compartment as done with treatment of unicompartmental arthritis. Most researchers recommend using an opening medial osteotomy to create a valgus correction rather than a closing lateral osteotomy. All soft tissue and osseous portions of the meniscal transplantation are completed before proceeding with the tibial osteotomy. Fixation of the graft is performed once the osteotomy is completed. The osteotomy should be performed as distally as possible to avoid interference with the meniscal transplant tunnel or trough. Fluoroscopy is appropriate when placing the proximal screw to avoid the previously placed tunnels or trough. Rigid fixation of the osteotomy is recommended because the tibia is under great stress to place the meniscal graft.

Articular Cartilage Procedure With Meniscal Transplantation

Preoperative planning is important when considering performing a combined meniscal transplantation with articular cartilage procedure. Typically, all the steps of the meniscal transplant are performed first, followed by the chondrocyte transplantation. This sequence helps avoid inadvertent damage to the chrodral procedure.

RESULTS

Results of meniscal allograft transplantation reported in the literature are difficult to interpret because of the small number of patients in the studies, the heterogeneous population of patients studied, lack of outcome measure evaluation of the allografts, and validity of methods used. Few studies are available describing the outcome of an isolated medial or lateral meniscus transplantation. Multiple studies with concurrent procedures of ACL reconstruction, tibial osteotomy, and chondral resurfacing have been performed. However, a lack of unified outcome measures for meniscal transplantation makes interpretation of the current literature difficult. Current studies use several knee outcome measures to evaluate meniscal transplantation, including the Lysholm, modified Hospital for Special Surgery (HSS), International Knee Documentation Committee (IKDC), Tegner, and Cincinnati scores; Western Ontario and McMaster Universities (WOMAC) Osteoarthritis Index; and Knee Injury and Osteoarthritis Outcome Score (KOOS).[58] Long-term results are now available, allowing us to better evaluate the efficacy of meniscal transplantation in decreasing pain, improving patient function, and presumably slowing the progression of arthritis.

Short-term studies of meniscal transplant uniformly show good results over the initial 2- to 3-year period. Milachowski et al.[52] have reported their early results on 22 patients with at least 14 months of follow-up. All patients underwent simultaneous ACL reconstruction in addition to meniscal transplantation. Second-look follow-up at 3 years showed meniscal shrinkage, which was thought to be secondary to freeze-drying the graft. In the entire series of 22 patients, there were only three failures that required removal (one fresh-frozen graft and two freeze-dried grafts). Generally, the fresh-frozen grafts were found to have a more normal gross appearance than the freeze-dried grafts. Noyes et al.[55] have reported their results of 40 meniscal transplantations in 38 knees. Concomitant procedures such as osteochondral autograft and ACL reconstruction did not

TABLE 40.4 **Summary of Short-Term Results[a]**

Study	Follow-Up (Month)	No. of Allografts	Combined Procedures	Results
Milachowski et al.[52]	14	22	All combined with ACL reconstruction	Three failures by second-look arthroscopy
Cameron and Saha[12]	31	67	21 isolated, 5 ACL, 34 HTO, 7 HTO + ACL	58 successful (92%)

ACL, Anterior cruciate ligament; *HTO,* high tibial osteotomy.
[a]Up to 3 years.

TABLE 40.5 **Summary of Intermediate Results[a]**

Study	Follow-Up	No. of Allografts	Combined Procedures	Results
Cole et al.[18]	36 months	31	16 ACI, 15 osteochondral allograft	48% (60% ACI, 36% OCA normal or almost normal by IKDC score)
Garrett[30]	2-7 years	43	7 isolated, 24 ACL, 13 HTO	35 of 43 (81%) successful
van Arkel and de Boer[76]	2-5 years	23	—	Three failures
Carter[14]	48 months (mean)	51	—	45 of 51 (88%) successful
Sekiya et al.69	3.3 years (mean)	32	—	96% of patients thought their overall function improved following surgery
Stollsteimer et al.[73]	40 months (mean)	23	—	13 of 23 normal or almost normal IKDC scores
Kim[b]	58 months (mean)	14	—	Modified Lysholm score increased from 71.4 preoperatively to 91.4 postoperatively
Verdonk et al.[80]	7.2 years (mean)	100	13 HTO	Modified HSS scores improved from 60.1 to 88.6
Noyes et al.[55]	40 months	38		89% successful
McCormick[50]	59 months	200	60% concomitant procedures	95% allograft survival at 5 years

ACI, Autologous chondrocyte implantation; *ACL,* anterior cruciate ligament; *HSS,* Hospital for Special Surgery; *HTO,* high tibial osteotomy; *IKDC,* International Knee Documentation Committee; *OCA,* osteochondral allograft.
[a]3 to 10 years.
[b]From Kim JM, Bin S: Meniscal allograft transplantation after total meniscectomy of torn discoid lateral meniscus. *Arthroscopy* 22:1344–1350, 2006.

increase the rate of complications. It was concluded that meniscal transplantation is supportive for reducing pain and increasing function in the short term. Short-term results (2 to 3 years) are summarized in Table 40.4.

Medium-term follow-up appears to maintain the improvement in pain and function following meniscal allograft transplantation. Cole et al.[18] have reported on 44 meniscal transplants in 39 patients with a minimum 2-year follow-up. They found that patients demonstrated statistically significant improvements in standardized outcome surveys and visual analog scale (VAS) pain and satisfaction scores. They concluded that meniscal transplantation alone or in combination with other reconstructive procedures shows reliable improvements in knee pain and function over the first 2 years. Van Arkel and de Boer[76] reported their results of 23 isolated meniscal transplantations with a follow-up of 2 to 5 years. The three unsuccessful results were caused by detachment of the graft from the capsule, leading to graft failure. Second-look arthroscopy was performed on 12 of the transplants at different time periods following transplantation. Five of the 12 menisci showed detachment from the capsule. The study concluded that lack of revascularization caused by malalignment of the knee led to graft failures. Verdonk et al.[80] has reported that the cumulative survival rates at 10 years were 74.2% for the medial meniscus and 69.8% for the lateral meniscus following transplantation.

Sekiya et al.[69] have also reported intermediate results of isolated lateral meniscal transplantation. There was no signifiant difference in joint space narrowing between the transplanted

lateral meniscus and contralateral lateral compartment. Stollsteimer and coworkers[73] have shown that clinical results continue to be favorable at an average of 40 months postmeniscal transplantation. On average, the allograft was 63% the size of the native meniscus. Although the patients reported good results following the procedure, allograft shrinkage was a concern. Kim et al.[44] have reviewed 14 meniscal allografts performed in patients with a total or near-total meniscectomy for torn discoid lateral menisci. All patients showed improvement in their symptoms, and Lysholm scores increased from 71.4 preoperatively to 91.4. Secure peripheral integration into the capsule was seen in all patients on MRI scans. It was determined that meniscal allograft transplantation after total meniscectomy for torn discoid lateral menisci could be a reasonable option for symptomatic patients. McCormick et al. reported their results of 200 patients undergoing meniscal transplantation at a mean follow-up of 59 months.[50] Thirty-two percent of the patients returned to the operating room (OR) for subsequent procedures, including 59% requiring meniscal débridement. Almost 5% of the patients required revision meniscal transplantation or total knee replacement. The group reported a 95% survival rate of the graft at a 5-year mean follow-up. Those patients undergoing secondary procedures following the primary procedure had an 88% survival rate at 5 years but were at a higher risk for failure. Results of medium-term follow-up (3 to 10 years) are summarized in Table 40.5.

The results of meniscal allograft transplantation after 10 years are less conclusive. von Lewinski and coworkers[83] have reported

TABLE 40.6 Summary of Long-Term Results[a]

Study	Follow-Up	No. of Allografts	Combined Procedures	Results
Hommen et al.[35]	141 months (mean)	22	—	35% failure rate
von Lewinski et al.[83]	20 years	5	5 ACL	2 normal IKDC scores, 2 abnormal, 1 severely abnormal
Getgood et al.[32]	10 years	48	OCA	69% survival
Carter et al.[15]	10 years	41	11 isolated, 26 ACLs, 2 osteotomy, 1 ACL/osteotomy and 1 MCL	83% survivorship; 10 year IKDC score 70.1 compared to preop value of 50.6
Kazi et al.[42]	15 years	86	86 osteotomy	71% survival; 17% required debridement of the graft

ACL, Anterior cruciate ligament; MCL, medial collateral ligament; OCA, osteochondral allograft.
[a]Longer than 10 years.

on Milachowski's original cohort of patients at 20-year follow-up. The radiologic results revealed clear degenerative changes with long-term follow-up after the meniscal transplantation, although some patients were doing well regarding the subjective and clinical results at the 20-year follow-up examination. Using MRI, Hommen et al.[35] have reported a 25% failure rate of medial meniscal transplantation and 50% failure of lateral transplantation at an average of 141 months. Of 15 patients in the study with postoperative radiographs, 10 showed narrowing of the involved tibiofemoral compartment. Although meniscal transplantation improved knee pain and function, the average knee function was fair at long-term follow-up. Carter reported his 10 year results following 41 meniscal transplantations.[15] Eighty percent of the patients noted improvement in symptoms at 10-year follow-up. Graft survivorship at 10 years was 83%. Verdonk et al. also reported their long-term results of 42 meniscal transplants.[81] A Knee Society Score (KSS) score revealed a significant improvement in pain and function at the final follow-up at a minimum of 10 years. Radiologic evaluation showed no further progression of joint space narrowing in 13 of 32 patients. MRI analysis showed no progression of cartilage degeneration in 6 of 17 patients evaluated. Seven cases were converted to total knee arthroplasty, with an overall failure rate of 18%. Long-term follow-up studies (>10 years) are summarized in Table 40.6.

The results of combined ACL and meniscal transplantation show good short- and intermediate-term results. Graf et al.[33] reported on eight patients undergoing concomitant ACL reconstruction and medial meniscal transplantation, with an average follow-up of 9.7 years. Of the eight patients, six were extremely pleased with their knee function and were active in recreational sports. They concluded that the addition of the knee-stabilizing procedure improved the outcomes of the eight patients. Rueff et al.[67] compared the 5-year outcomes of patients undergoing primary ACL reconstruction and either meniscal transplantation or meniscal repair–partial meniscectomy. At 5 years, the pain levels of the meniscal allograft group were similar to the meniscal repair–partial meniscectomy group.

Short- and intermediate-term results are also available for combined meniscal transplantation with articular cartilage repair. Farr et al.[27] have studied 36 patients undergoing combined meniscal allograft transplantation and femoral condyle autologous chondrocyte implantation (ACI), with a minimum of 2-year follow-up. Statistically significant improvements in the standardized outcomes surveys, VAS score, and satisfaction were reported. It was noted that the improvements were less than the literature-reported outcomes of either procedure performed in isolation; however, the results are promising for the combined pathology. Of the 36 patients, eight patients had kissing chondral defects secondary to previous meniscectomy; significant improvement was seen in six of these eight patients at 1 year. Each patient was able to lead an active lifestyle and five maintained the improvement at a mean follow-up of longer than 3 years. Rue et al.[66] have reported on 16 patients undergoing combined meniscal allograft transplantation with ACI and 15 patients undergoing combined meniscal transplantation with osteochondral allograft (OCA). These studies showed good initial results of combined meniscal transplantation with chondral allograft. Getgood[32] reviewed 48 patients with combined OCA and meniscal allograft transplantation. The 5-year survivorship was 78% for the meniscal allograft transplantation and 73% for the OCA, with survivorship dropping to 69% and 68% for the meniscal allograft transplantation and OCA, respectively, at 10 years. The overall success rate of concomitant meniscal allograft transplantation and OCA was comparable, with reported results for either procedure in isolation. Stone et al. evaluated 119 meniscal allograft transplantations performed concurrently with articular cartilage repair in 115 patients.[74] The study had a mean follow-up of almost 6 years, with 20.1% failing at a mean of 4.6 years. The survival of the transplant was not affected by gender, severity of cartilage damage, axial alignment, degree of joint space narrowing, or whether the transplant was medial or lateral.

The importance of correct axial alignment has been well described in the literature. Cameron and Saha[12] described 63 meniscal transplantations, with 34 of these performed in combination with a valgus HTO, varus HTO, or varus distal femoral osteotomy to correct for preoperative malalignment. Of the patients undergoing combined osteotomy and meniscal transplant, 29 (85.3%) attained good to excellent results. Verdonk et al.[81] presented the clinical, radiologic, and MRI outcomes of the menisci and articular cartilage of 42 meniscal transplantations at a minimum 10-year follow-up. Patients undergoing HTO and medial meniscal transplantation showed better modified HSS scores than patients undergoing medial meniscal transplantation alone at the final follow-up. Fairbanks's changes remained stable in 9 of 32 knees (28%). Long-term results showed no significant difference in the survival of the allograft with or without osteotomy and transplantation.[42] These results show encouraging trends in pain relief and function following meniscal transplantation combined with osteotomy.

The short- and intermediate-term results of meniscal transplantation indicate decreased pain and improved function in the treated knee. Scrutiny of these studies shows considerable variability in indications, type of graft, surgical technique, presence of concomitant surgery, duration of follow-up, and outcome evaluation. The long-term results begin to show degenerative changes and shrinkage of the allograft; however, most patients continue to have decreased pain and improved function. Current studies show a mutually beneficial effect of combined meniscal transplantation with other procedures such as ACL reconstruction, HTO, or cartilage restoration. It is evident that these procedures work synergistically and do not increase the complication rate when performed together. Long-term studies are necessary to determine the durability of the grafts and status of arthritis in these patients.

COMPLICATIONS

Complication rates associated with meniscal transplantation range from 10% to 50% in the literature. Graft tearing is the most common complication encountered with meniscal transplantation. Tears of meniscal allograft are approached the same way as tears in the native meniscus are treated, including meniscal repair if possible or partial meniscectomy. Matava[49] performed a systematic review of meniscal transplantation and identified 45 tears in 547 patients, for a tear rate of 8.2%. Allograft tears led to reoperation in 25% of Graf et al.[33] patients and 26% of Stollsteimer et al.[73] subjects. Infection and immune reactions are uncommon complications following meniscal transplantation. Cameron and Saha[12] have reported wound infections in 2 of 67 transplanted knees. Both were treated by antibiotics and resolved. Stollsteimer et al.[73] have described 1 of 22 patients who developed a pyogenic infection requiring removal of the meniscal allograft. Matava[49] reported only three studies specifically describing a postoperative immune response. No reports of HIV transmission have been described in the literature from the use of allografts. Other complications that may occur with meniscal transplantation include loss of graft fixation, hemarthrosis, synovitis, and arthrofibrosis. Complications associated with meniscal transplantation are summarized in Box 40.1.

POSTOPERATIVE REHABILITATION

Postoperative rehabilitation following meniscal allograft transplantation is similar to the protocols followed after meniscal repair (Box 40.2). Rehabilitation following meniscal transplantation consists of five phases. Phase I consists of the first 6 weeks following surgery and includes bracing and 50% weight bearing. Pain control, quadriceps strengthening, and full extension are the primary goals of this phase. Phase II consists of full weight bearing, with encouragement of full range of motion. Pivoting, twisting, hopping, jumping, and running are not allowed. Months 3 to 4 make up phase III. Progress to open- and

closed-chain resistance exercises takes place during this phase, including isokinetic exercises. Phase IV occurs during months 4 to 6; the patient continues to progress with strengthening and flexibility, along with single-leg squats and light jogging. Sport-specific drills and plyometrics occur during phase V, 6 months postoperatively. There is no consensus regarding the timing of return to athletic activities.

CONCLUSION

Meniscal allograft transplantation is an increasingly popular treatment for young symptomatic patients with meniscus-deficient knees. The ideal candidate for the procedure is a patient who is physiologically young; has a stable, well-aligned knee, with minimal arthritis; and is complaining of focal pain on the meniscal deficient side of the knee. Meniscal allograft transplantation should be considered as an accepted operation for these patients and only used once other conservative measures have been exhausted. Many techniques have been described for performing the transplantation, and much debate continues about which technique is superior. The important guidelines

---

BOX 40.1   Complications

Graft tearing
Infection and immune reaction
HIV transmission
Loss of graft fixation
Hemarthrosis
Synovitis
Arthrofibrosis

HIV, Human immunodeficiency virus.

BOX 40.2   Rehabilitation Protocol

Phase I: 0-4 Weeks
- Brace 0-90 degrees for 4 weeks postoperatively
- 50% weight bearing for 4 weeks postoperatively
- Wean off crutches beginning 4 weeks postoperatively
- Limit flexion to 90 degrees until 4 weeks postoperatively
- Pain, edema control, patellar mobilizations
- Quadriceps sets, hamstring co-contractions at multiple angles
- Straight leg raise in brace at 0 degree until quadriceps can maintain knee locked
- Heel slides in brace
- Obtain full extension

Phase II: 4-b12 Weeks
- Stationary bike with seat high; lower as tolerated
- Leg press with 50% BW maximum
- Leg extensions with ROM restrictions, high volume, light weight
- Leg curls with ROM restrictions, high volume, light weight
- Full weight bearing
- No pivoting, twisting, hopping, jumping, running
- Encourage full ROM
- Normalize gait mechanics

Phase III: 3-4b Months
- Progress open-, closed-chain resistance exercises
- Isokinetic exercises
- Treadmill forward and retro walking
- Single-leg stance for proprioception
- Cardiovascular fitness
- Slide board—initially short distance; increase as tolerated
- Manage patellofemoral signs and symptoms

Phase IV: 4-6b Months
- Continue and progress strengthening and flexibility
- Single leg squats
- Plyometrics (4 months)
- Light jogging on treadmill (4 months)

Phase V: 6+ Months
- Sport-specific drills
- Plyometrics

BW, Body weight; *ROM,* range of motion.

for successful meniscal replacement include bony fixation and anatomic replacement of the anterior and posterior horns. Typically, the bone plug technique is used for medial meniscal replacement because the anterior horns are separated by a larger distance compared with the lateral meniscal horns. Because the lateral meniscal horns are separated by 1 cm or less on average, a bone-bridge technique is recommended. Clinical trials have shown favorable outcomes for cryopreserved or fresh-frozen allografts. Negligible rates of disease transmission because of careful procurement and sterilization protocols have been reported in the literature. Mid- and long-term reports have demonstrated predictable improvements in pain, swelling, and knee function following meniscal allograft transplantation. Despite these results, there is minimal evidence that meniscal transplantation restores meniscal function. Further long-term studies are necessary to determine the efficacy of meniscal transplantation in slowing down the degenerative process that occurs with meniscal deficiency.

KEY REFERENCES

17. Cole BJ, Cater TR, Rodeo SA: Allograft meniscal transplantation. *J Bone Joint Surg Am* 84:1236–1250, 2002.

23. Dienst M, Greis PE, Ellis BJ, et al: Effect of lateral meniscal allograft sizing on contact mechanics of the lateral tibial plateau: an experimental study in human cadaveric knee joints. *Am J Sports Med* 35:34–42, 2007.

27. Farr J, Rawal A, Marberry KM: Concomitant meniscal allograft transplantation and autologous chondrocyte implantation: minimum 2-year follow-up. *Am J Sports Med* 35:1459–1466, 2007.

33. Graf KW Jr, Sekiya JK, Wojtys EM: Long-term results after combined medial meniscal allograft transplantation and anterior cruciate ligament reconstruction: minimum 8.5-year follow-up study. *Arthroscopy* 20:129–140, 2004.

35. Hommen JP, Applegate GR, Del Pizzo W: Meniscus allograft transplantation: ten-year results of cryopreserved allografts. *Arthroscopy* 23:388–393, 2007.

49. Matava MJ: Meniscal allograft transplantation: a systematic review. *Clin Orthop* 455:142–157, 2007.

58. Packer JD, Rodeo SA: Meniscal allograft transplantation. *Clin Sports Med* 28:259–283, 2009.

65. Rodeo SA, Seneviratne A, Suzuki K, et al: Histological analysis of human meniscal allografts. A preliminary report. *J Bone Joint Surg Am* 82:1071–1082, 2000.

68. Sekiya JK, Elkousy HA, Harner CD: Meniscal transplant combined with anterior cruciate ligament reconstruction. *Oper Tech Sports Med* 10:157–164, 2002.

72. Sohn DH, Toth AP: Meniscus transplantation: current concepts. *J Knee Surg* 21:163–172, 2008.

80. Verdonk PC, Demurie A, Almqvist KF, et al: Transplantation of viable meniscal allograft. Survivorship analysis and clinical outcome of one hundred cases. *J Bone Joint Surg Am* 87:715–724, 2005.

81. Verdonk PC, Verstraete KL, Almqvist KF, et al: Meniscal allograft transplantation: long-term clinical results with radiological and magnetic resonance imaging correlations. *Knee Surg Spots Traumatol Arthrosc* 14:694–706, 2006.

83. von Lewinski G, Milachowski KA, Weismeier K, et al: Twenty-year results of combined meniscal allograft transplantation, anterior cruciate ligament reconstruction and advancement of the medial collateral ligament. *Knee Surg Sports Traumatol Arthrosc* 15:1072–1082, 2007.

85. Wirth CJ, Peters G, Milachowski KA, et al: Long-term results of meniscal allograft transplantation. *Am J Sports Med* 30:174–181, 2002.

The references for this chapter can also be found on www.expertconsult.com.

41

Synthetic Meniscal Substitutes and Collagen Scaffold for Meniscal Regeneration

Ian D. Hutchinson, Patrick G. Marinello, Suzanne A. Maher, Arielle J. Hall, Seth L. Sherman, Scott A. Rodeo

The menisci function within the knee joint to distribute load, enhance lubrication, and deliver joint congruency and stability. Macroscopically, the menisci are wedge-shaped fibrocartilaginous structures that circumscribe the peripheral joint margins of the medial and lateral compartments, conforming to the articular surfaces of the tibia and femur. Each meniscus has anterior and posterior insertions to the tibia that serve to counter extrusive forces and transmit "hoop stresses" generated in the circumferentially oriented collagen fibers during axial loading. In addition, the coronary ligament serves as a continuous peripheral attachment at the joint line; there also is continuity with the capsular tissue and the medial collateral ligament fibers for the medial meniscus.[28,42] At a microstructural level, the menisci are composed of an inhomogeneous anisotropic arrangement of type I collagen fibers combined with proteoglycans, glycoproteins, and elastin.[4] Adding to its biological complexity, the composition of meniscal tissue is zone dependent. In the inner, avascular zone, the composition of the matrix is closer to hyaline cartilage (increased glycosaminoglycan [GAG] and collagen type II), and meniscal cells resemble articular chondrocytes. However, at the peripheral vascularized zone, the tissue is more type I collagen rich with less GAG, and meniscal cells are more fibroblast-like.[40]

The meniscus develops in utero as a fully vascularized and relatively homogenous tissue, and during childhood through to skeletal maturity, there is peripheral regression of vascularization coincident with gradual changes in inner zone tissue composition and increasing biomechanical demands.[15] Given this gradual development of meniscal tissue, it is not surprising that successful regeneration and restoration of function has been challenging. To achieve the desired characteristics of meniscal tissue, ideally a meniscal scaffold would incorporate the following characteristics: (1) provide a matrix amenable to tissue ingrowth and cellular infiltration (pore-size and inter-connectivity) while maintaining a near native compressive stiffness to exert a profibrochondrogenic biophysical effect; (2) be able to withstand the complex loading environment of the knee joint during tissue regeneration; and (3) facilitate zonal tissue regeneration sensitive to the cellular and matrix variations between the vascular and avascular zones.

Meniscal substitutes and scaffolds are indicated, where available, to restore meniscal tissue volume and to improve functional outcomes in patients with symptomatic meniscal deficiency following partial meniscectomy. It is important to note that all of the currently available meniscal scaffolds in clinical use or under clinical investigation require an intact peripheral rim to prevent meniscal extrusion and stable root attachments for secure implant fixation. In addition, the meniscal substitute, NUsurface, also requires an intact medial meniscal rim for containment. Therefore, meniscal allograft transplantation (MAT) remains the only therapeutic option for patients with peripheral meniscal rim deficiency, inadequate meniscal root tissue, or for patients undergoing total meniscectomy in a symptomatic compartment. In this chapter, we will discuss the emergence of clinically available meniscal scaffolds and substitutes placing particular emphasis at this time on collagen meniscus implant (CMI) that has been recently restored as a clinical option in the United States. Actifit (polyurethane scaffold) is discussed as a clinically available scaffold in Europe. NUsurface is introduced as a free-floating medial meniscal substitute undergoing clinical trials in Europe and Israel. We will conclude with a brief update and commentary on recent developments in tissue engineering approaches and concepts regarding meniscal scaffolds and substitution at the preclinical level.

OVERVIEW OF MENISCAL SCAFFOLDS

Meniscal scaffolds may be derived from extracellular matrix (ECM) (eg, collagen, GAG, hyaluronan) or synthetic materials. These acellular, porous scaffolds are implanted within in the knee joint without cells with the intention of being populated by matrix-generating cells from the peripheral meniscal rim, vasculature, and/or synovium. The CMI is an example of an ECM constituent scaffold and is now available for clinical use in both Europe and the United States. Actifit is a synthetic polyurethane-based scaffold that is only currently available in Europe. In this section, we will review the basic science that led to the development of these scaffolds; CMI is afforded an extended review of the indications for its use, method of implantation, and postoperative care, given its availability for use in the United States.

COLLAGEN MENISCAL IMPLANT

In December 2008, the US Food and Drug Administration (FDA) approved the first collagen-based meniscal implant for commercial use in the United States, known as Menaflex

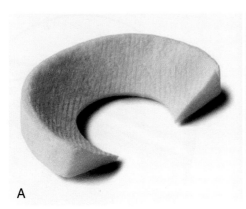
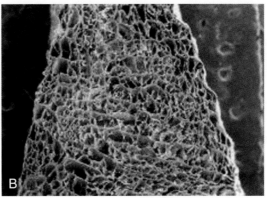

FIG 41.1 (A) Collagen meniscal implant (CMI), Menaflex (RenGen Biologics). (B) Scanning electron micrograph of a cross-section of the collagen meniscal implant, Menaflex. (From Stone KR, Steadman JR, Rodkey WG, Li ST: Regeneration of meniscal cartilage with use of a collagen scaffold. Analysis of preliminary data. *J Bone Joint Surg Am* 79(12):1770–1777, 1997.)

(ReGen Biologics, Franklin Lakes, New Jersey). It was available in the United States from December 2008 until it was withdrawn in October 2010, for reasons not related to its clinical performance.[43] The collagen meniscal scaffold was reapproved for use by the FDA in March 2015, and reintroduction to the clinical arena in the United States is expected using the name CMI (Ivy Sports Medicine GmbH, Gräfelfing, Germany).

CMI is manufactured from type I collagen harvested from bovine Achilles tendon (Fig. 41.1). The harvested tendon is washed, the collagen fibers are isolated and purified using sequential chemical treatments and organic solvents, and the purified collagen fibers are swollen in the presence of equal quantities of hyaluronic acid and chondroitin sulfate. GAGs are added and the resulting compound is co-precipitated by the addition of ammonium hydroxide. The collagen fibers and associated extracellular components are then dehydrated and manually oriented in a mold. The resulting structure is lyophilized and sterilized by gamma irradiation. The end product is an acellular scaffold intended to support cell migration and de novo tissue growth from existing meniscal tissue, the synovium, and synovial fluid.[56] The CMI can be trimmed to match the specific dimensions of a patient's meniscal defect. The resulting implant has the tensile strength to support attachment of the implant to a rim of the native meniscus with sutures and immediately withstand the sheer and compression forces within the knee joint, while maintaining a porous matrix to allow tissue regeneration. The CMI has been studied in humans to replace partial meniscal defects of the medial and lateral meniscus. In Europe, both medial and lateral implants are available for surgical implantation, whereas in the United States, only the medial implant is currently available for use.

Pathway to Clinical Use

Although the clinical use of CMI has been limited in the United States because of regulatory issues, it has been available in Europe for well over 10 years. CMI development involved almost two decades of research and consequently its performance in vitro and in vivo has been studied extensively.[48,49,54–56] The construct has been shown to support cellular ingrowth and to encourage tissue regeneration in many small and large

animal models. Stone et al.,[55] for example, have evaluated CMI in a canine model. An 80% subtotal resection of the medial meniscus was created, and the defect was then treated with the collagen-based scaffold. The investigators found that the implant was compatible with meniscal fibrochondrocyte ingrowth and concluded that it could induce regeneration of the meniscus in the mature dog.

Clinical Indications

In the United States, CMI is indicated for use in individuals who have symptomatic medial meniscus deficiency. This may be offered in the acute setting for an irreparable meniscus tear following partial or subtotal meniscectomy, or in the subacute or chronic setting for patients with symptomatic postmeniscectomy syndrome. Medial and lateral CMI implantation has been successfully achieved in Europe for both acute and chronic lesions. Meniscus specific indications include an intact peripheral rim to prevent meniscal extrusion and stable root attachments to allow for secure time-zero scaffold fixation. Correction of knee malalignment, instability, and treatment of focal cartilage lesions should be performed concomitantly (ie, realignment osteotomy, anterior cruciate ligament (ACL) reconstruction, cartilage restoration, respectively) or as part of a staged treatment regimen alongside CMI. Contraindications to CMI include uncorrected knee alignment, ligamentous instability, untreated focal high grade ipsilateral compartment cartilage lesion, total or subtotal meniscectomy (devoid of peripheral rim and/or stable meniscal roots), X-ray evidence of moderate to severe joint space narrowing, global arthritis, and increased body mass index (BMI).

Surgical Technique, Postoperative Care, and Rehabilitation

CMI is implanted arthroscopically and is currently available in three sizes: medial meniscal scaffold (7.5 mm and 9 mm) and lateral (9.5 mm). The meniscus is débrided to the vascular zone and, using a customized measuring device, an implant is chosen for the specific defect. Standard inside-out, outside-in, and all-inside suturing techniques have been described to secure the implant. A posteromedial incision is used for placement of a posterior retractor when using the inside-out suture technique. Before the implant is inserted (Fig. 41.2), a temporary suture is

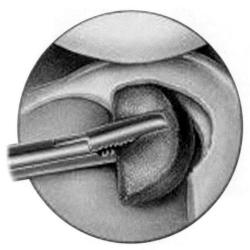

FIG 41.2 Illustration depicting insertion of the collagen meniscal implant. (From Stone KR, Steadman JR, Rodkey WG, Li ST: Regeneration of meniscal cartilage with use of a collagen scaffold. Analysis of preliminary data. *J Bone Joint Surg Am* 79(12):1770–1777, 1997.)

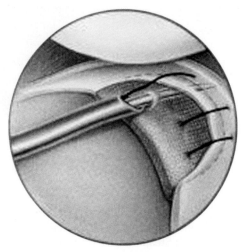

FIG 41.4 Illustration depicting suturing of the collagen meniscal implant. (From Stone KR, Steadman JR, Rodkey WG, Li ST: Regeneration of meniscal cartilage with use of a collagen scaffold. Analysis of preliminary data. *J Bone Joint Surg Am* 79(12):1770–1777, 1997.)

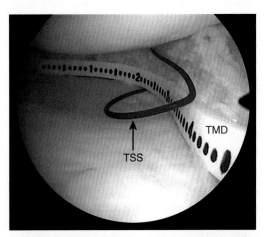

FIG 41.3 Following the partial meniscectomy, the size of the meniscal defect was measured using specific instrumentation. The numbers on the Teflon measuring device (TMD) represent centimeters, and the hash marks represent millimeters. The temporary stay suture (TSS; *arrow*) can be used to guide the TMD and stabilize the collagen meniscus implant (CMI) during suture fixation. The TSS is removed after the CMI has been sutured to the meniscus rim. (From Rodkey WG, DeHaven KE, Montgomery WH 3rd, et al: Comparison of the collagen meniscus implant with partial meniscectomy. A prospective randomized trial. *J Bone Joint Surg Am* 90:1413–1426, 2008.)

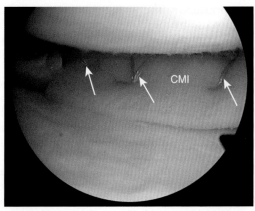

FIG 41.5 After the collagen meniscus implant (CMI) was delivered into the joint, it was sutured to the host meniscus remnant with nonabsorbable sutures *(white arrows)* and an inside-out technique. (From Rodkey WG, DeHaven KE, Montgomery WH 3rd, et al: Comparison of the collagen meniscus implant with partial meniscectomy. A prospective randomized trial. *J Bone Joint Surg Am* 90:1413–1426, 2008.)

placed in the midlesion and oriented to capture the CMI once introduced. The implant is introduced via the ipsilateral working portal using a specially designed delivery cannula and subsequently guided by the initial suture, which serves to lasso and temporarily secure the meniscal implant. Vertical mattress sutures are placed to secure the implant to the rim of the existing meniscus. The implant is secured to the anterior and posterior horn of the existing meniscus via horizontal mattress sutures (Figs. 41.3 and 41.4). Use of 2-0 nonabsorbable sutures is recommended. After the implant is properly secured to the existing meniscal tissue, the initial temporary suture is removed

and the newly placed meniscal implant is checked for fixation integrity (Fig. 41.5).[49]

The postoperative rehabilitation protocol is designed to limit excessive loads on the implant prior to tissue ingrowth. Immediately following implantation, the knee is placed in a knee brace locked in full extension and kept non-weight-bearing for 6 weeks. Knee motion is started immediately postoperatively with flexion limited to 60 degrees for the first 4 weeks and 90 degrees for the following 2 weeks. After 6 weeks, the brace is unlocked, the patient is allowed to be fully weight bearing, and physical therapy starts and continues until 6 months postoperatively, at which point the patient resumes normal activities. These are general guidelines; the protocol and timeframes for progression of activities will vary based on the individual patient's progress.[49]

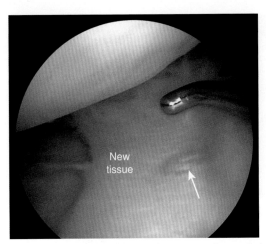

FIG 41.6 One-year second-look arthroscopy showed that the collagen meniscus implant (CMI) had been replaced by new tissue. One of the sutures can still be seen *(arrow),* although it is covered by synovial tissue. The probe demonstrates the approximate interface between the new tissue generated by the CMI and the host meniscus rim. (From Rodkey WG, DeHaven KE, Montgomery WH 3rd, et al: Comparison of the collagen meniscus implant with partial meniscectomy. A prospective randomized trial. *J Bone Joint Surg Am* 90:1413–1426, 2008.)

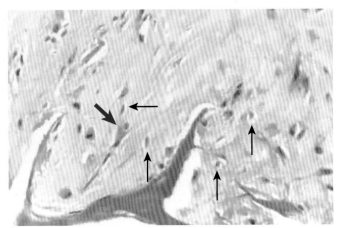

FIG 41.7 In this biopsy specimen, obtained at 1 year, the collagen meniscus implant (CMI) appears to provide a scaffold for meniscus-like fibrochondrocytic matrix production by the host. The CMI was integrated into this tissue as it was assimilated and/or resorbed *(large purple arrow).* Cells that appear to be meniscal fibrochondrocytes *(small black arrows)* are noted to be surrounded by lacunae, suggesting that they are viable and active cells (hematoxylin and eosin, ×100). (From Rodkey WG, DeHaven KE, Montgomery WH 3rd, et al: Comparison of the collagen meniscus implant with partial meniscectomy. A prospective randomized trial. *J Bone Joint Surg Am* 90:1413–1426, 2008.)

Clinical Outcomes

Most of the early clinical trials were conducted by the developers of the device, starting with an initial study focused on the feasibility of implantation.[56] A subsequent study was used to assess its short-term clinical effectiveness.[49] These two studies corresponded with the phase I and II clinical trials as required by the FDA, which led to a multicenter, multisurgeon prospective randomized trial[48] in which 311 patients from 16 centers and 26 surgeons were divided into two cohorts, acute and chronic injury, to determine the effectiveness of the CMI. Patients were randomized to receive a CMI implant or to undergo a partial meniscectomy (considered the standard of care). Inclusion criteria were age 18 to 60 years, presence of an acute irreparable medial meniscus tear (acute group), or failed previous meniscectomy (chronic group). Patients were excluded if they had posterior cruciate ligament (PCL) insufficiency, an abnormal mechanical axis, and/or a significant chondral lesion. Of these 311 patients, 157 were allocated to the acute study arm (75 CMI treatment, 82 controls) and 154 were allocated to the chronic study arm (85 CMI treatment, 69 controls). No patients were lost in the acute arm follow-up, and three patients were lost in the chronic group, allowing for final analysis of 308 patients.

The defect size for the CMI implanted patients was recorded at the time of surgery and was reassessed via arthroscopy at 1 year after the index surgery (Fig. 41.6). A significant increase in the amount of meniscus tissue in the experimental group was found in the acute and chronic groups. This suggested that the meniscal implant provided a significant contribution of new tissue surface area when compared with the control, which was assumed to have no new growth.[2,7,36] A needle biopsy taken of the scaffold showed fibrochondrocyte-like cells residing within lacunae, which is suggestive of matrix generation (Figs. 41.7 and 41.8). Remnants of the scaffold (10% to 25% of the initial area)

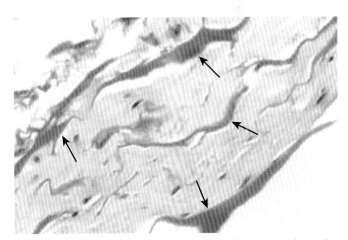

FIG 41.8 In this biopsy specimen, obtained at 1 year, it can be seen that most of the collagen meniscus implant (CMI) has been resorbed or assimilated into the new matrix. The *arrows* point to darker staining structures that are remnants of the CMI (hematoxylin and eosin, ×100). (From Rodkey WG, DeHaven KE, Montgomery WH 3rd, et al: Comparison of the collagen meniscus implant with partial meniscectomy. A prospective randomized trial. *J Bone Joint Surg Am* 90:1413–1426, 2008.)

were seen in the biopsy specimens, but most of the scaffold had been reabsorbed and replaced with meniscus-like tissue. At the junction between the matrix and the native meniscal rim, there was evidence of vascular infiltration into the site of scaffold implantation. There were no obvious inflammatory infiltrates or evidence of adverse immune response.

Clinical outcome scales included the visual analogue pain (VAS) score, the Lysholm score, and the patient self-assessment

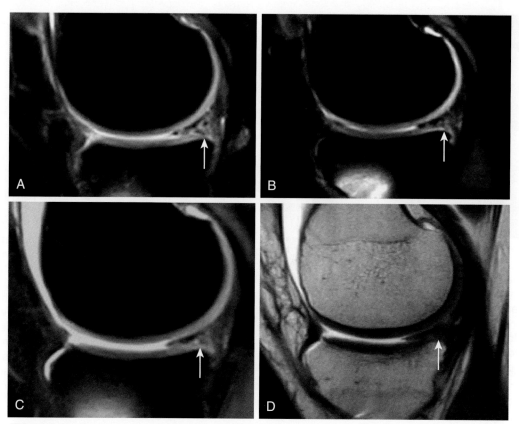

FIG 41.9 (A) Examination at 6 months. Collagen meniscus implant (CMI) size is identical to that of the normal meniscus, type 3 *(arrow)*. The sagittal images obtained with fat-suppressed T2/DP show an inhomogeneous and marked increase in signal intensity, type 1 *(arrow)*. (B) Same patient as in (A); follow-up at 12 months. On the T2/DP-weighted sagittal images with fat suppression, scaffold size is type 3 *(arrow)*, but signal intensity is reduced compared with the previous examination; signal characteristics are type 2 *(arrow)*. (C) Same patient, follow-up at 24 months. Scaffold size is still type 3 *(arrow)*, but signal intensity is reduced with respect to the examination at 12 months; signal characteristics are type 3 *(arrow)*. (D) Same patient, follow-up at 24 months. On the spin-echo (SE) T1-weighted sagittal images obtained after intra-articular injection of contrast material, CMI size is type 3 *(arrow)*. The implant has integrated, and there is no infiltration of contrast agent. (From Genovese E, Angeretti MG, Ronga M, et al: Follow-up of collagen meniscus implants by MRI. *Radiol Med* 112:1036–1048, 2007.)

score; all scores increased in the treatment and control groups in both the chronic and acute arms of the study as a function of time. Patients in the chronic group who were treated with the CMI were able to regain more of their preinjury activity when compared with the control (partial meniscectomy) cohort as measured by the Tegner index, which was considered a primary benefit of the CMI implant.

This study has several weaknesses, including a relatively short follow-up time of 5 years, the unblinded nature of the index procedure, and reliance on subjective patient satisfaction scores.[48] In addition, radiologic outcomes of the implanted collagen matrix were not provided. Overall, this longitudinal, randomized, prospective, controlled study supported the previous findings and demonstrated de novo tissue formation at the site of scaffold implantation. However, the function of the newly formed tissue and its ability to protect the adjacent cartilage from degeneration over the long term remains unknown.

Genovese et al.[25] examined the radiologic outcomes (magnetic resonance imaging [MRI] and magnetic resonance [MR] arthrography) of CMI in 40 patients at 6, 12, and 24 months

postoperatively (Figs. 41.9 to 41.11). The implant position, signal intensity, and incorporation into the host tissue were assessed; these MRI diagnostic criteria have since been widely applied to assess meniscal scaffolds. A progressive reduction in the signal intensity of the regenerating tissue was found, indicating gradual tissue incorporation and maturation. There was a strong hyperintense signal in 80% of the implants at 6 months, whereas only 35% of the implants imaged at 12 months had a hyperintense signal. None of the implants showed normal meniscus signal intensity at 6 or 12 months; however, at 24 months, approximately 27% of the patients showed characteristics similar to those of the normal meniscus. A limitation of the study was the inability to determine chondral damage.

Bulgheroni et al.[12] followed 34 patients who underwent placement of a CMI for medial meniscal deficiency out to a minimum of 5 years. Evaluation included Lysholm II and Tegner activity scores, as well as plain radiographs, traditional MRI, and MR arthrography. The Lysholm and Tegner scores were significantly improved when compared with the preoperative status. Radiological analysis demonstrated that the chondral

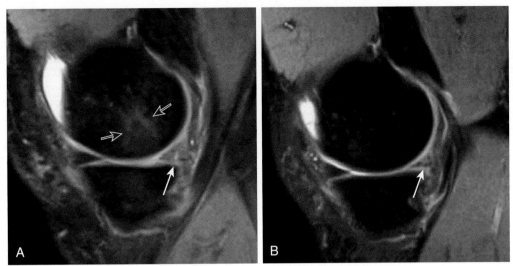

FIG 41.10 (A) Examination at 6 months. In the T2/DP sagittal images with fat suppression, collagen meniscus implant (CMI) size is type 3, and the signal intensity has inhomogeneously increased, reaching type 1 *(white arrow)*. The femoral condyle bone marrow shows an area with edema and interstitial hemorrhage identified by its high signal *(empty white arrows)*. (B) Same patient, follow-up at 12 months. The complex size has decreased to type 2 *(white arrow)*, but the CMI size has decreased to type 2 *(white arrow)*. CMI signal intensity is reduced compared with the previous examination and is now type 2 *(white arrow)*. In comparison with the examination at 6 months, the bone marrow edema and interstitial hemorrhage have completely resolved. (From Genovese E, Angeretti MG, Ronga M, et al: Follow-up of collagen meniscus implants by MRI. *Radiol Med* 112:1036–1048, 2007.)

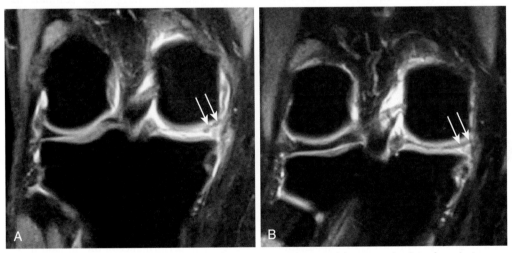

FIG 41.11 On the T2/DP-weighted and fat-suppressed coronal images, the interface between the prosthetic meniscus and native meniscus is indicated by a sharp hyperintense line at both 6 *(white arrows* in A) and 12 *(white arrows* in B) months. (From Genovese E, Angeretti MG, Ronga M, et al: Follow-up of collagen meniscus implants by MRI. *Radiol Med* 112:1036–1048, 2007.)

surfaces of the medial compartment where the implant was fixed did not show any further progression of chondral degeneration when compared with the patient's preoperative status. The MRI signal generated by the CMI gradually decreased over the 5-year follow-up period, suggesting progressive tissue maturation. Contracture of the meniscal implant (shrinkage) was also observed but this did not seem to be detrimental to clinical outcomes.

Long-term longitudinal studies (>10 years) have been available in the clinical literature since 2011, derived exclusively from European experiences with CMI. The first long-term prospective controlled study came from Zaffagnini et al., who followed 33 nonconsecutive male patients (mean age 40 years) for a minimum of 10 years.[64] In their study, implantation of a meniscal scaffold was compared to partial meniscectomy; the patient decided on the treatment strategy. Clinical outcome measures and weight-bearing radiographs were undertaken preoperatively and at latest follow-up. In addition, longitudinal MRIs used the Yulish score to assess cartilage status, and scaffold morphology and integration was assessed using the Genovese score. Compared to partial meniscectomy, CMI implantation resulted in significantly lower VAS for pain and higher objective International Knee Documentation Committee (IKDC) and Tegner index scores. There was no significant difference in Lysholm score. Radiographically, there was significantly less medial joint space narrowing in the scaffold group and no significant difference in Yulish scores during the study period. Regarding tissue regeneration and scaffold morphology, Genovese scores remained constant between 5 and 10 years; at 10 years, there were 11 patients with a myxoid degeneration signal, 4 had a normal signal (with reduced size), and 2 patients had no recognizable implant. Monllau et al. published a therapeutic case series of medial CMI implantation from Spain of 25 patients at minimum follow-up of 10 years with a more heterogeneous patient population (20 males, 5 females; mean age 29.2 years).[41] In their study, 80% of patients underwent the procedure at the time of meniscectomy, and the remaining patients presented with symptomatic postmeniscectomy medial compartments. At 10 years, the Lysholm score remained significantly improved from the preoperative score (persisting from the first year of follow-up), and patients remained satisfied with the procedure. Radiographs demonstrated minimal joint narrowing and MRI using the Genovese criteria demonstrated smaller implants than expected, with 67% of patients categorized as group 2 and 21% categorized as group 3 (corresponding to a normal meniscus). Finally, the failure rate was 8% (2/25) with both patients undergoing medial MAT.

Accounting for concomitant procedures, Bulgheroni et al. compared the long-term outcomes of patients who underwent ACL reconstruction with CMI implantation compared to partial medial meniscectomy in a retrospective, comparative study at mean follow-up of 9.6 years.[11] There were 17 patients in each group, and patient demographics were matched; the timing of surgery was further categorized into acute (<6 months) and chronic (>6 months). They observed significant improvements in clinical outcomes scores (Lysholm, Tegner, and IKDC) compared to preoperative scores in all groups; there were no differences between the experimental groups for clinical or radiographic measures. Of note, the chronic ACL reconstruction group that underwent CMI implantation had lower VAS pain scores at latest follow-up. After acute ACL reconstruction, patients with CMI showed better arthrometric scores. Linke et al. compared the clinical results of combined CMI implantation and high tibial osteotomy (HTO) and HTO alone (n = 30 in each group) at 3 months, 1 year, and 2 years postoperatively.[38] They did not find a significant difference between both groups at a 2-year follow-up, suggesting, not surprisingly, that realignment has the overwhelming effect on symptoms in the varus knee. Long-term follow-up results in this patient group will be important to assess for any additional chondroprotective effect of CMI.

Focusing on lateral implantation, Zaffagnini et al. reported a 2-year prospective single arm multicenter study from European centers.[63] Clinical outcome scores for function and pain during rest, routine, and strenuous activities were charted in the context of patient satisfaction scores and functional questionnaires for 43 patients (mean age 30 ± 12 years). Multiple regression was applied to identify outcome predictors. The results

suggested that functional improvements began at 6 months and continued through 12 months for strenuous activities. Pain was significantly improved at latest follow-up, with 58% of patients returning to full activity and 95% of patients satisfied with the procedure. Serious adverse effects related to the scaffold occurred in 7% of patients corresponding to an 89% survival probability at 2 years. Finally, increased BMI, concomitant procedures, and chronicity of symptoms appeared to negatively affect outcome.

Meanwhile, there is a growing body of histological data to characterize the tissue regeneration within the CMI scaffold in vivo. Biopsies of implanted scaffold have shown new blood vessels and collagen fibrils and progressive replacement of CMI with immature collagen.[44,50,56] Using electron microscopy, Reguzzoni et al. further characterized tissue regeneration by describing parallel lacunae walls with collagen fibrils, blood vessels, and fibroblast-like cells.[44] At the 5-year mark, Steadman and Rodkey observed fibrocartilage and organized ECM in all patients that they biopsied; importantly, there was no evidence of infection, inflammation, or immune reaction.[54]

POLYURETHANE SCAFFOLD (ACTIFIT)

Actifit (Orteq Sports Medicine, London) is a porous, biodegradable, aliphatic polyurethane with a porosity of 80% and pores ranging in size from 150 to 355 µm (Fig. 41.12).[27] Approved for use in Europe since 2008, it is currently being assessed by the FDA. A considerable body of work has been published on the development, characterization, and in vivo performance of the porous scaffold, including its initial preclinical testing as a total meniscal replacement by Tienen et al.[57,58] and Welsing et al.[61] In a dog model, the scaffold was fully integrated with newly formed tissue and did not elicit an adverse foreign body reaction at 24 months. As a total meniscus replacement, the scaffold did not prevent degeneration of the articular cartilage of the tibial plateau, likely attributed to inadequate fixation. More recently, its use as a partial meniscal replacement scaffold has been explored, with indications that the scaffold can effectively transmit loads in the knee after implantation.[9]

The clinical indications for the use of the Actifit implant are similar to those of CMI. Actifit is used to restore meniscal volume in patients with partial/subtotal meniscectomy with remaining intact horns and peripheral meniscal rim. Verdonk et al. reported the first prospective, single-arm, multicenter, proof-of-principle study to determine the clinical efficacy, safety, and performance of the implant in 52 patients at 2 years minimum follow-up. The irreparable partial meniscal defects were in either compartment (34 medial and 18 lateral), with 88% of patients having undergone 1 to 3 previous surgeries on the index meniscus.[29,60] They observed tissue growth into the scaffold in 36 of 42 subjects using dynamic contrast-enhanced MRI (DCE-MRI) at 6 months. At 12 months, second-look arthroscopy demonstrated tissue ingrowth in all subjects, and in 10 of 33 subjects, the meniscal lesion was completely filled. Biopsies showed that the regenerative tissue was composed of type I collagen, fibroblasts, and fibrochondroblast-like cells (Figs. 41.13 and 41.14). Importantly, no evidence of articular cartilage damage related to the presence of the implant was found, and stable or improved International Cartilage Repair Society (ICRS) cartilage grades were observed in 92.5% of patients between baseline and 24 months. The 2-year reoperation

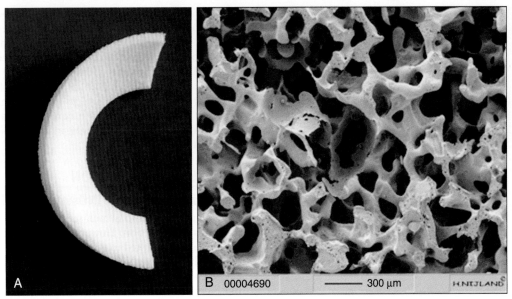

FIG 41.12 (A) The Actifit implant. (B) Microscopic view demonstrating the porosity of the polyurethane material. The average porosity is 80%, with pores ranging in size from 150 to 355 μm.

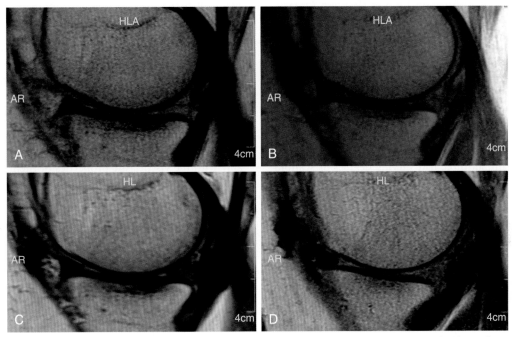

FIG 41.13 Magnetic Resonance (MR) Images of Actifit Implant. (A) 1 week postimplantation. (B) 3 months postimplantation. (C) 12 months postimplantation. (D) 24 months postimplantation. (Courtesy Dr. Rene Verdonk.)

rate was 17% in this study and was mainly attributed to the procedure by the authors. Reoperation was more common on the lateral side, and 7% of failures were attributed to the scaffold where procedural deficits were not involved, presenting with knee pain and effusion. A smaller study of 10 patients by Efe et al. reported similar findings, with general clinical improvement and lack of serious adverse side effects, synovitis, or signs of joint injury/inflammation in the operated compartment at 1 year.[18] Similarly, Kon et al. described improvement in pain and functional symptoms in a similar cohort of 18 patients at 2 years

without adverse side effects.[35] Bulgheroni et al. reported similar clinical outcomes at 2 years, and arthroscopic biopsies revealed a bifringent scaffold with an amorphous, heterogeneous matrix with spindle like fibroblasts and bulging fibrochondrocyte-like cells at 4 months.[10] Later biopsies demonstrated more organized tissue, with some biopsies demonstrating chondrocyte-like arrangement, all coincident with grade 2 Genovese MRI signal intensity.

Regarding concomitant procedures, Gelber et al. investigated the use of medial Actifit implantation during opening wedge

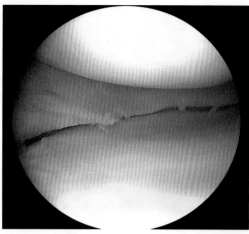

FIG 41.14 Arthroscopic appearance at 12 months postimplantation. (Courtesy Professor Johan Bellemans, Leuven, Belgium.)

HTO for medial meniscus deficient varus knees in a prospective comparative study (40 men and 20 women, median age of 51 years). At a mean follow-up of 31.2 months, patients treated with realignment osteotomy and meniscectomy demonstrated superior improvement in functional scores (Western Ontario Meniscal Evaluation Tool [WOMET], IKDC, and VAS) compared to patients with concomitant implantation of a medial Actifit.[23] Patients were satisfied equally with both procedures.

Bouyarmane et al. reported a multicenter study focused on the use of Actifit in chronic, symptomatic postpartial meniscectomy lateral compartments.[8] Fifty-four patients (37 males/17 female, mean age 28 years) were followed, and significant improvements in VAS, IKDC, and all Knee Injury and Osteoarthritis Outcome Score (KOOS) subscores were demonstrated at 2 years. Three patients (5.5%) underwent reoperation for pain; all three had varying degrees of scaffold tears, of which two responded to partial débridement. Finally, Gelber et al. evaluated the influence of articular chondral injury on the Actifit MRI, using the Genovese criteria in 54 patients at a mean follow-up of 39 months.[24] The presence of an increased degree of chondral injury using the ICRS cartilage score was associated with worse morphological MR characteristics and smaller size of the scaffold, likely because of the unfavorable biomechanical environment in the setting of chondral lesions; neither MR signal intensity (all Genovese type 2) nor short-term functional outcomes were affected by the degree of chondral injury. It is also worth noting that concomitant procedures were warranted in 69.5% of patients in this study, including ACL reconstruction and HTO, PCL reconstruction (one case), and microfracture.

COMPARISON OF EARLY CLINICAL RESULTS OF MENISCAL SCAFFOLDS

Most studies describing the early clinical outcomes of both meniscal scaffolds (CMI and Acitfit) are derived from the similar centers of excellence in Europe. Thus, there may be an intrinsic element of reproducibility and comparability with regard to patient selection, concomitant procedures, surgeon experience, rehabilitation, and outcome analysis (clinical, arthroscopic, and radiological) when comparing early experiences with both scaffolds. However, there is only one study that describes the outcome of both scaffolds together from Spencer et al., who treated both medial and lateral meniscal defects with either CMI (12 patients) or Actifit (11 patients).[53] During second look arthroscopy at 1 year, the Actifit group appeared to demonstrate earlier filling of the defects; however, overall clinical outcome scores at a mean of 19.1 months was satisfactory and comparable for both treatment groups. The current literature also supports this observation with equivocal clinical results from both scaffolds in the short term, in anticipation of long-term Actifit studies.

MENISCAL SUBSTITUTION

Nondegradable Implant (NUsurface Meniscal Implant)

For patients with subtotal meniscectomy, MAT remains the standard treatment option. However, as a regenerative procedure, MAT is usually limited to younger patients (<50 years) because of the diminished biological capacity of the intra-articular environment with advancing age.[17] NUsurface is a freely floating polycarbonate urethane meniscal implant (NUsurface, AIC, Memphis, Tennessee) developed to substitute for medial meniscus tissue in the symptomatic, deficient compartment of middle-aged patients. NUsurface approximates the shape of a discoid meniscus and requires an intact peripheral rim of meniscal tissue for containment within the medial compartment; the nonanchored design and pliable nature of the device facilitate its implantation through a mini-arthrotomy. The implant was investigated in the preclinical setting using a sheep model and found to exert some chondroprotective effects, albeit with additional tibial attachment at the insertions and Kevlar reinforcement.[66] In addition, application of finite element models to the existing design supports its potential to approximate native loading in the meniscus deficient compartment.[66] Biomechanical characterization of the material properties of NUsurface implants during repetitive loading compares favorably with the viscoelastic properties of the natural meniscus.[52] A subsequent study evaluated the long-term wear performance of this device by simulating loading for a total of 5 million gait cycles (Mc), approximating 5 years of in-vivo loading (International Organization for Standardization [ISO]-14243 loading conditions).[19] Five implants were tested and remained in good condition during the simulation with an average gravimetric wear rate of 14.5 mg/Mc; volumetric changes in reconstructed μ-CT scans point to an average wear rate of 15.76 mm³/Mc (18.8 mg/Mc). In addition, particles isolated from the lubricant had average diameter of 15 μm. In addition, a recent pilot study of kinematic implant behavior was undertaken by Verdonk et al. using an open MRI in three patients.[17] Results suggested that femoral rollback and tibiofemoral contact were not impacted by the implant, and there were only differences in the anteroposterior motion of the implant compared to the native meniscus within an arc of motion from 0 to 120 degrees of knee flexion.

The Verifying the Effectiveness of the NuSurface System (VENUS) clinical study is a multicenter, prospective randomized, interventional clinical trial to test the hypothesis that the NUsurface implant is superior to the nonsurgical standard of care (nonsteroidal anti-inflammatory drugs [NSAIDs], physical therapy, intra-articular steroid, and intra-articular hyaluronic acid). Currently recruiting in Europe and Israel, the patient population is age 30 to 75 years with longer than 6 months history of a painful meniscus deficient medial compartment.

PRECLINICAL ADVANCES IN MENISCAL SCAFFOLDS AND SUBSTITUTES

Although not yet used clinically, resorbable hyaluronic acid–based scaffolds combined with polycaprolactone were designed by Chiari et al.,[14] with pores ranging in size from 200 to 300 μm. Two types of meniscal implants were designed, one indicated for total meniscal replacement and one for partial meniscal replacement. The total meniscal implant was augmented with circumferential polylactic acid fibers that protruded from the anterior and posterior horns of the implant to facilitate attachment to the tibial plateau. The partial meniscal implant was augmented with a polyethylene terephtalate net, which provided attachment sites for the sutures used to secure the implant to the remaining native meniscal tissue in a sheep model. On the basis of 6-week follow-up data, it was found that for both total and partial meniscal replacement, the implants incorporated well into the native synovium and did not cause any adverse reactions. Gross and histologic inspection confirmed the presence of new tissue ingrowth in the total meniscal replacement implant and adhesion to the native meniscus in the partial meniscal replacement. Extrusion of the implant, primarily in the posterior area of the joint capsule, was reported, leading to some concern about the mechanical strength of the attachment sites. In the sheep model, Kon et al. tested the same scaffold material for total meniscus replacement, and their results suggested that preseeding with autologous chondrocytes at the time of implantation had a positive effect on meniscal tissue formation.[34]

Replacing the entire meniscus with a synthetic nondegradable functional implant that can carry and distribute the load without damaging the articular surfaces of the joint has been a long-standing goal in the field of musculoskeletal soft tissue research. However, finding the optimal combination of synthetic materials to allow for a wear-resistant functional substitute has been difficult, with the result that no synthetic implant is clinically available as yet. Nondegradable hydrogels, such as polyvinyl alcohol (PVA), have been suggested as suitable meniscal substitute materials because of their high water content, low coefficient of friction, and stability when implanted. In small animal models, PVA-based total meniscal replacements demonstrated an ability to protect cartilage and remain intact for periods of up to 12 months.[33] PVA-based implants were also followed for up to 12 months in an ovine model and, at 2 months postoperatively, the implants demonstrated an ability to protect the knee joint from degeneration as compared with the meniscectomized knee.[32] At 4 months, however, the tibial plateau was significantly more degenerated when compared with that of the allograft-implanted group, with degenerative changes particularly evident on the peripheral region of the tibial plateau. By 12 months, radial tears in the posterior aspect of the implant were evident. These studies highlight the challenges of designing a substitute that can withstand the rigorous mechanical environment of the knee.

Seeded meniscal scaffolds were investigated by Kang et al.,[31] who developed a meniscal scaffold consisting of polyglycolic acid (PGA) fiber meshes cross-linked with poly(lactic-co-glycolic acid). The scaffold was seeded with allogenic rabbit meniscal cells, cultured in vitro for 1 week, and then transplanted in the rabbits following medial meniscectomy. At 10 weeks, neovascular tissue formation and tissue growth were observed, demonstrating the feasibility of using allogenic cells to form a transplantable seeded scaffold into the knee. Angele et al.[3] implanted a hyaluronan–bovine collagen composite scaffold seeded with marrow-derived mesenchymal stem cells (MSCs) into a rabbit model and found increased tissue ingrowth in cell-seeded scaffolds when compared with the acellular controls. Cristino et al.[16] seeded MSCs onto a hyaluronic acid–based scaffold (HYAFF 11, Fidia Advanced Biopolymers, Abano Terme, Italy). In addition, Fisher et al. developed a multilamellar MSC seeded nanofibrous construct composed of bovine MSCs seeded into a poly-(ε-caprolactone) scaffold with fibers aligned in either one direction or circumferentially.[22] Cell infiltration and collagen formation occurred independent of fiber alignment, and a newly formed collagenous matrix followed the direction of the scaffold fibers with varied stiffness.

Finally, a significant advance in the regeneration of complex meniscal tissue was demonstrated by Lee et al., who produced a polycaprolactone 3D printed, anatomically correct meniscal scaffold capable of spatiotemporally delivering human connective tissue growth factor (CTGF) and transforming growth factor–β3 (TGFβ3) from microparticles as biochemical cues to endogenous progenitor cells to drive zone specific regeneration in an acellular scaffold.[37] In a sheep model, the functionalized scaffold resulted in endogenous cells regenerating the meniscus with zone-specific matrix phenotypes: primarily type I collagen in the outer zone, and type II collagen in the inner zone, reminiscent of the native meniscus. Spatiotemporally delivered CTGF and TGFβ3 also restored inhomogeneous mechanical properties in the regenerated sheep meniscus.

SUMMARY

Although promising, the clinical usefulness of meniscal implants as a point of care option remains in its infancy. Ultimately, the ability of a construct to withstand physiologic loads and aid in knee joint stability will remain a crucial part of the product design process for both degradable and nondegradable solutions.[39] Prospective, randomized controlled clinical trials are warranted to assess the long-term efficacy of meniscal scaffolds, whereas regression analysis will aid to identify the factors that impact outcome and will help define the optimal operative candidates and guide patient expectations. Meanwhile, it is becoming evident that increased BMI (>25 kg m^{-2}), multiple concomitant procedures, and chronicity of the meniscal lesions have a negative effect on outcomes. It will also be important to carefully interpret the clinical significance of early and preliminary data; developing thresholds of minimal differences in pain and outcome scores to power future multicenter studies should be encouraged. In addition, the application of biological augmentation strategies to enhance meniscal regeneration in meniscal substitutes is eagerly anticipated.

In conclusion, replicating the complex structure and function of the meniscus in scaffolds or substitutes is challenging. Defining realistic goals for meniscal implants in specific patient populations may be the key to success as therapeutic options expand in this space; identifying a spectrum of patient needs (eg, meniscal tissue regeneration with prolonged chondroprotection, acute symptom alleviation, temporization of early joint degeneration) will encourage complimentary approaches to meniscal restoration using substitutes.

KEY REFERENCES

4. Arnoczky S, McDevitt C: The meniscus: structure, function, repair, and replacement. In Buckwalter J, Einhorn T, Simon S, editors: *Orthopaedic basic science: biology and biomechanics of the musculoskeletal system*, Rosemont, IL, 2000, American Academy of Orthopaedic Surgeons, pp 532–545.

25. Genovese E, Angeretti MG, Ronga M, et al: Follow-up of collagen meniscus implants by MRI. *Radiol Med* 112:1036–1048, 2007.

32. Kelly BT, Robertson W, Potter HG, et al: Hydrogel meniscal replacement in the sheep knee: preliminary evaluation of chondroprotective effects. *Am J Sports Med* 35:43–52, 2007.

42. Mow V, Flatow E, Ateshian G: Biomechanics. In Buckwalter J, Einhorn T, Simon S, editors: *Orthopaedic basic science: biology and biomechanics of the musculoskeletal system*, Rosemont, IL, 2000, American Academy of Orthopaedic Surgeons, pp 135–180.

44. Reguzzoni M, Manelli A, Ronga M, et al: Histology and ultrastructure of a tissue-engineered collagen meniscus before and after implantation. *J Biomed Mater Res B Appl Biomater* 74:808–816, 2005.

48. Rodkey WG, DeHaven KE, Montgomery WH 3rd, et al: Comparison of the collagen meniscus implant with partial meniscectomy. A prospective randomized trial. *J Bone Joint Surg Am* 90:1413–1526, 2008.

49. Rodkey WG, Steadman JR, Li ST: A clinical study of collagen meniscus implants to restore the injured meniscus. *Clin Orthop* 367:S281–S292, 1999.

51. Scotti C, Pozzi A, Mangiavini L, et al: Healing of meniscal tissue by cellular fibrin glue: an in vivo study. *Knee Surg Sports Traumatol Arthrosc* 17:645–651, 2009.

54. Steadman JR, Rodkey WG: Tissue-engineered collagen meniscus implants: 5- to 6-year feasibility study results. *Arthroscopy* 21:515–525, 2005.

55. Stone KR, Rodkey WG, Webber R, et al: Meniscal regeneration with copolymeric collagen scaffolds. In vitro and in vivo studies evaluated clinically, histologically, and biochemically. *Am J Sports Med* 20:104–111, 1992.

56. Stone KR, Steadman JR, Rodkey WG, et al: Regeneration of meniscal cartilage with use of a collagen scaffold. Analysis of preliminary data. *J Bone Joint Surg Am* 79(12):1770–1777, 1997.

The references for this chapter can also be found on www.expertconsult.com.

Sports Medicine: Ligament Injuries

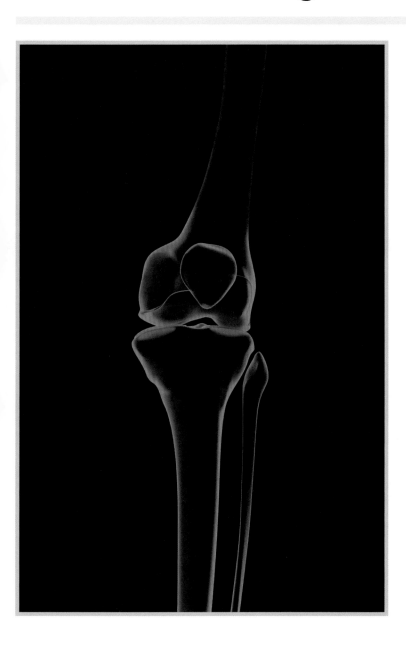

42

Classification of Knee Ligament Injuries

Kristopher D. Collins, Craig S. Radnay, Christopher A. Hajnik, Giles R. Scuderi, W. Norman Scott

Given the extensive investigation of ligamentous injuries of the knee, it is essential that a standardized, valid, reproducible, and universally accepted classification system be adopted.

Effective systems of classification necessitate agreement on both the meaning and appropriate use of terms to describe abnormal knee kinematics, such that there is no ambiguity. Furthermore, clinical examination findings, operative findings, and anatomic studies must be correlated in an attempt to clarify the classification of these injuries. By reviewing the current and classic literature, this chapter discusses the relationship of knee anatomy and kinematics, defines terms, and attempts to classify knee ligament injuries in an understandable fashion.

RELATIONSHIP OF CAPSULAR AND LIGAMENTOUS STRUCTURES

Understanding the relationship of the surrounding capsular and ligamentous structures is critical to defining stability of the knee.

Medial Structures

Hughston et al.,[36] Warren and Marshall,[90,91] and LaPrade et al.[48] have clearly described the supporting structures on the medial side of the knee (Fig. 42.1). These structures include the medial collateral ligament (MCL) and the posteromedial capsular ligament, termed the posterior oblique ligament. Dynamic support is supplied to the medial compartment by the medial head of the gastrocnemius and the semimembranosus tendon with its aponeurosis, the oblique popliteal ligament. Brantigan and Voshell[10] have described the MCL as having vertical and oblique portions that behave differently as the knee flexes. The parallel anterior fibers of the superficial medial ligament are arranged around the axis of flexion allowing tension to remain constant throughout the arc of motion. Posteriorly, the oblique fibers of the superficial ligament blend with the deeper layer within the posteromedial corner to form the posterior oblique ligament, which relaxes in flexion (Fig. 42.2).

Recent cadaveric experiments have confirmed the biomechanical role of each of the medial supporting elements. Robinson et al.[70] confirmed that the superficial MCL is the main resistor to valgus stress across the arc of knee motion. The superficial MCL remained tight throughout knee range of motion. Conversely, the posterior medial capsule is lax while the knee is in flexion. As the knee extends, the posterior medial capsule becomes tight resisting 32% of the valgus moment in full extension. The deep MCL was found to provide secondary restraint with no change in valgus laxity, provided the superficial MCL was intact. Griffith et al.[33] found that the superficial MCL

has the greatest load response with valgus and external rotation torques. The distal division of the MCL showed a change in the load response dependent on knee flexion angles, whereas the proximal division shows no difference in load response throughout the tested flexion angles. The posterior oblique ligament was found to have the greatest load response with internal rotation near extension, but as the knee is brought into flexion, the superficial MCL takes on a larger role in resisting internal rotation. In a second study by Griffith et al.,[32] it was found that the proximal superficial MCL was the primary stabilizer to valgus stress, and the distal division of the superficial MCL serves as the primary stabilizer to external rotation at 30 degrees of flexion. Again, the posterior oblique ligament was found to be a primary stabilizer to internal rotation stress in concert with the distal division of the superficial MCL. The deep MCL was found to be important for internal rotation stability in a flexion-dependent manner.

Although these previous qualitative assessments are useful in developing an understanding of medial-sided knee injuries, LaPrade et al.[48] have made a quantitative assessment of the medial structures of the knee. Claiming that the layered approach is not helpful for surgical exposure, because it often leads to an oversimplification of structures with frequent inaccuracies regarding ligamentous attachment sites, they sought to verify the relationships of medial knee structures to pertinent osseous anatomy through cadaveric dissection. They confirmed that the medial epicondyle lies anterior and distal to the adductor tubercle. They also consistently recognized a third, previously undescribed osseous prominence, which lies distal and posterior to the adductor tubercle, near the attachment depression of the medial gastrocnemius tendon. They labeled this new structure the gastrocnemius tubercle and noted that the posterior oblique ligament attachment was actually closer to this structure than the adductor tubercle.

The superficial MCL is the largest medial knee structure, measuring between 10 and 12 cm in length. Its femoral attachment lies slightly proximal and posterior to the medial epicondyle.[48] There are two distinct tibial attachments. Proximally, it attaches to the soft tissues directly over the anterior arm of the semimembranosus. Distally, it attaches to posteromedial tibia approximately 6 cm from the joint line.

The posterior oblique ligament has been recognized as a posterior medial capsular thickening (Fig. 42.3). It is made up of superficial, central, and capsular arms, with the central arm forming the largest component of this structure. The central arm contributes most fibers for femoral attachment and adheres to the medial meniscus as it merges distally with the posteromedial capsule.[48]

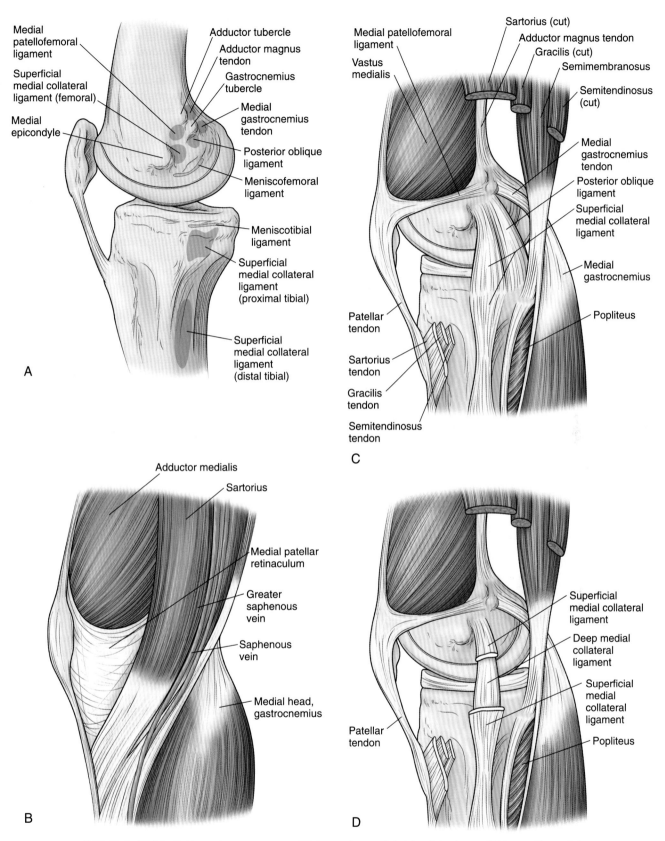

FIG 42.1 (A) Medial knee bony anatomy. (B) Layer 1, medial side of the knee. (C) Layer 2, medial side of the knee with the medial collateral ligament and posterior oblique ligament. (D) Layer 3, medial side of the knee. (Redrawn from LaPrade RF, Engebretsen AH, Ly TV, et al: The anatomy of the medial part of the knee. *J Bone Joint Surg Am* 89:2000, 2007.)

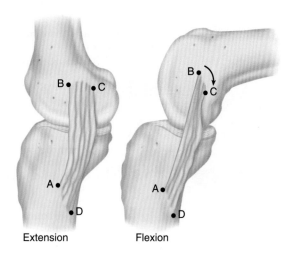

Extension   Flexion

FIG 42.2 Medial collateral ligament in flexion and extension. (From Scott WN [ed]: *The knee*, St Louis, MO, 1994, CV Mosby.)

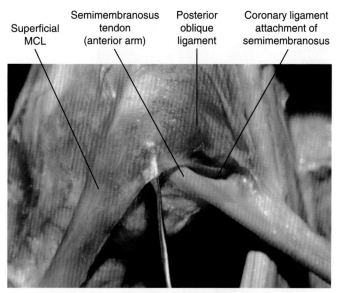

Superficial MCL · Semimembranosus tendon (anterior arm) · Posterior oblique ligament · Coronary ligament attachment of semimembranosus

FIG 42.3 Oblique fibers of the superficial medial collateral ligament blend with the posterior oblique ligament. Note the coronary ligament attachment from the anterior arm of the semimembranosus. (From Detterline A, Babb J, Noyes FR: Medial and anterior knee anatomy. In Noyes FR (ed): *Noyes' knee disorders*, ed 2, Philadelphia, PA, 2017, Elsevier. Fig. 1.6.)

A subsequent study by Wijdicks et al.[93] has concluded that the attachments of medial ligamentous structures could be correlated to the location of osseous landmarks seen on plain radiographs. This may aid in pre- and intraoperative assessment of surgical repairs and reconstructions of these structures.

Lateral Structures
The lateral supporting structures have been described by Hughston et al.[37] and Seebacher et al.[73] (Fig. 42.4). The lateral collateral ligament (LCL) is the major static support to varus stress, whereas the iliotibial tract provides both dynamic and static support. Terry et al.[84] have investigated the roles of the iliotibial tract, iliopatellar band, and iliotibial band as dynamic and static stabilizers of the lateral side of the knee.

The posterolateral corner is composed of the LCL, popliteus aponeurosis, popliteofibular ligament (PFL), and posterolateral capsule. Although these individual static structures have often been grouped together as the arcuate ligament complex, other studies have highlighted their individual importance (Fig. 42.5). Together, their function is augmented by the dynamic effects of the biceps femoris, popliteus, and lateral head of the gastrocnemius.[5]

On the femoral side, the LCL attaches to a small depression between the lateral epicondyle and supracondylar process, and it attaches distally to the posterior aspect of the fibular head.[12,49] The popliteus originates from the posteromedial aspect of the proximal tibia, courses intra-articularly, and inserts anterior and distal to the LCL attachment. Its function in providing dynamic stability to the lateral meniscus is controversial—countering views on its role in retraction and protection of the meniscus have been espoused.[77,87,88] The PFL arises from the myotendinous junction of the popliteus and inserts on the fibular styloid process. It provides an important restrain to external rotation.[50]

Anterior Cruciate Ligament
The anterior cruciate ligament (ACL; Fig. 42.6) is the primary structure that controls anterior displacement in the unloaded knee. The anatomic and functional aspects of the ACL have undergone extensive investigation.[56-58,83] For reconstruction purposes, the focus has often centered on the relationship of the ligament to osseous landmarks. On the femoral side, the anterior border of the ACL is a bony ridge on the medial wall of the lateral femoral condyle, commonly referred to as the resident's ridge.[69] On the tibial side, the ACL posterior border lies at a ridge between the medial and lateral intercondylar tubercles at the base of the tibial eminence.

The ACL has been described as a single ligament, with different portions taut throughout the range of motion (ROM).[6] In investigating the functional anatomy of the ACL, Odensten and Gillquist[65] found no anatomic separation of the ligament into different bundles. However, they did confirm that the ligament is twisted through 90 degrees, and that both the length[47,85,88,89] and tension[27] of different fibers in the ligament change as knee flexion occurs. Therefore, they believe that there are different functional portions of the ACL.[92] Based on this concept of different functional portions of the ACL, Girgis et al.[29] have divided the ACL into anteromedial and posterolateral bands. Amis and Dawkins[3,4] have supported this multifascicular structure of the ACL with division into two bundles. The two bundles are defined by their tibial insertion with an anteromedial and posterolateral bundle. The anteromedial and posterolateral bundles originate from the proximal and distal ACL origin of the femur. Amis and Dawkins[3,4] found that the fiber bundles were not isometric; the anteromedial bundle lengthens and the posterolateral bundle shortens during flexion (Fig. 42.7). These changes in fiber length correlate with their changing participation in total ACL action as the knee is flexed. Because of this, an isolated anteromedial bundle rupture will have a greater effect on the anterior drawer test, and an isolated posterolateral bundle rupture will have a greater effect on the Lachman test.[4,27] The posterolateral bundle also plays an important role in resisting external and internal rotation.[4,14,94]

Tibial rotation is better resisted by a combination of capsular structures, collateral ligaments, the joint surface, and meniscal geometry, whereas the cruciates play only a secondary role.[3,4,63]

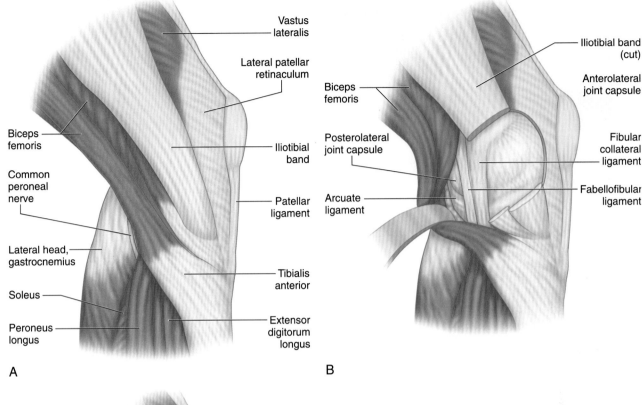

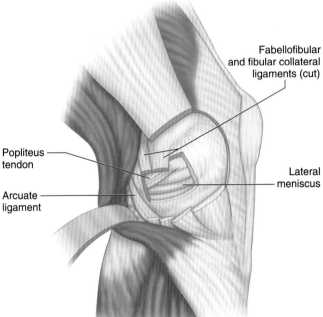

FIG 42.4 (A) Layer 1, lateral side of the knee. (B) Layer 2, lateral side of the knee with the lateral collateral ligament. (C) Layer 3, lateral side of the knee with the arcuate complex. (From Scott WN: *Ligament and extensor mechanism injuries of the knee: diagnosis and treatment*, St Louis, MO, 1991, Mosby Year Book.)

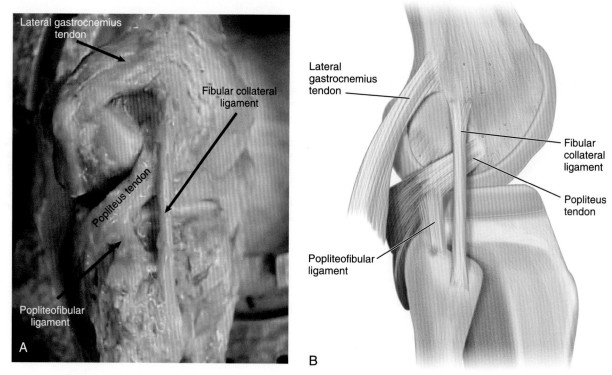

FIG 42.5 Image (A) and illustration (B) of the anatomy of the posterolateral corner and the relationships of individual structures to each other. (From LaPrade RF, Ly TV, Wentorf FA, et al: The posterolateral attachments of the knee: a qualitative and quantitative morphologic analysis of the fibular collateral ligament, popliteus tendon, popliteofibular ligament, and lateral gastrocnemius tendon. *Am J Sports Med* 31:854–860, 2003.)

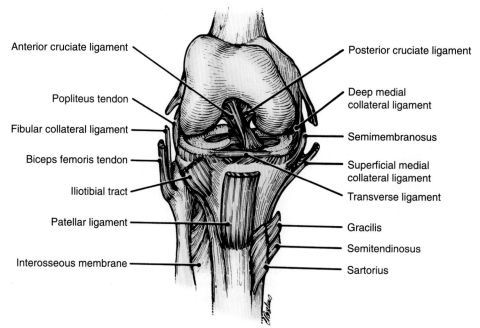

FIG 42.6 The anterior cruciate ligament has been described as a single ligament with different portions taut throughout the range of motion. (From Scott WN: *Ligament and extensor mechanism injuries of the knee: diagnosis and treatment*, St Louis, MO, 1991, Mosby Year Book.)

However, recent evidence suggests a larger role for the ACL in rotational stability if both bundles remain functionally intact.[14] Despite this, the MCL is anatomically better suited than the ACL and has the mechanical advantage to control torsion or laxity because its attachments are further removed from the axis of tibial rotation.[76] The MCL will provide significant resistance to the anterior drawer test only after the ACL is gone, and when both ligaments are lost, the knee will exhibit large tibial

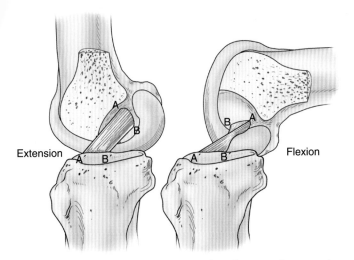

FIG 42.7 Diagram of the anterior cruciate ligament in extension and flexion. Note that in extension the posterolateral bulk is taut, whereas in flexion the anteromedial band is tight and the posterolateral bulk is relatively relaxed. (From Girgis FG, Marshall JL, Al Monajem ARS: The cruciate ligaments of the knee joint: anatomical, functional and experimental analysis. *Clin Orthop* 106:216, 1975.)

excursions and response to anterior force if it is unchecked by muscle action. Injuries to the medial structures further compromise anterior stability when they accompany ACL injuries.[80]

Posterior Cruciate Ligament

The posterior cruciate ligament (PCL; Fig. 42.8) is believed to be the most important of the knee ligaments because of its cross-sectional area, tensile strength, and location in the central axis of the knee joint.* Its position provides 95% of the total resistance to posterior displacement of the tibia. Both James et al.[42] and Kennedy et al.[46] have shown that the tensile strength of the PCL is almost twice that of the ACL. Hughston et al.[36] have described the PCL as the fundamental stabilizer of the knee because it is located in the center of the knee joint and functions as the axis about which the knee moves in flexion and extension, as well as in rotation.

The PCL prevents posterior translation at all angles of flexion.[13,26,35] Patients who have an isolated injury of the PCL may maintain fairly good function of the knee.[25] Gollehon et al.[30] have found that isolated sectioning of the PCL produces increased posterior translation of the tibia at all degrees of flexion of the knee, with the greatest increase occurring from 75 to 90 degrees. Absence of the PCL has no effect on primary varus or external rotation of the tibia as long as the LCL and capsular structures are intact.

Like the ACL, the PCL is a continuum of fascicles, with different portions being taut throughout ROM. The anterior portion, which forms the bulk of the ligament, tightens in flexion, whereas the smaller posterior portion tightens in extension

---

*References 13, 15, 17, 18, 39, and 40.

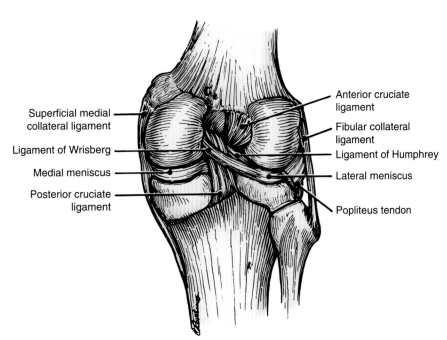

Superficial medial collateral ligament
Ligament of Wrisberg
Medial meniscus
Posterior cruciate ligament
Anterior cruciate ligament
Fibular collateral ligament
Ligament of Humphrey
Lateral meniscus
Popliteus tendon

FIG 42.8 The posterior cruciate ligament is an important ligament because of its cross-sectional area, tensile strength, and location in the central axis of the knee joint. (From Scott WN: *Ligament and extensor mechanism injuries of the knee: diagnosis and treatment*, St Louis, 1991, Mosby Year Book.)

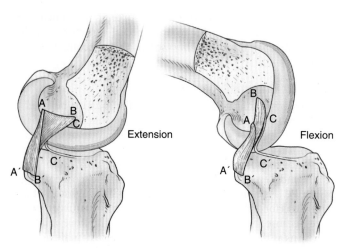

FIG 42.9 Posterior cruciate ligament. In flexion, the bulk of the ligament becomes tight, whereas in extension it is relaxed. (From Girgis FG, Marshall JL, Al Monajem ARS: The cruciate ligaments of the knee joint: anatomical, functional and experimental analysis. *Clin Orthop* 106:216, 1975.)

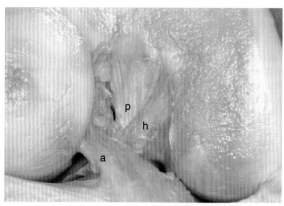

FIG 42.10 Close-up of an anatomic specimen seen from the anterior aspect demonstrating the relationship of the ACL (a), ligament of Humphrey (h), and PCL (p) from anterior to posterior in the intercondylar notch.

(Fig. 42.9).[6] The PCL originates from the posterior part of the lateral aspect of the medial femoral condyle and inserts on the posterior surface of the tibia. The femoral footprint consists of a medial intercondylar ridge at its proximal border and a medial bifurcate ridge that occasionally divides the two functional bundles.[24] The insertion reaches approximately 1 cm below the articular surface in a nonarticular area that Jacobsen[41] has termed the intercondylaris posterior. Tajima et al.[81] have further investigated the tibial insertion site and noted that the insertions of its two bundles are located in different planes, with a change in slope between them. Lying anterior to the PCL and connecting the posterior horn of the lateral meniscus to the medial femoral condyle is the ligament of Humphrey (Fig. 42.10). The ligament of Wrisberg passes posterior to the PCL to attach on the PCL. The ligaments of Humphrey and Wrisberg (Fig. 42.11) are so intimately related that early authors described them as separate portions of a single ligament.[54] Clancy et al.[15] have noted that the meniscofemoral ligament may serve as a secondary stabilizer in a posterior cruciate-deficient knee. The

presence of these structures may account for the absence of posterior drawer in isolated PCL tears.

KINEMATICS

In classifying knee ligamentous instabilities, it is important that the terms be clearly understood and used in a lucid and universally accepted manner. The terms in the literature should be specific to define positions of the knee, motions of the knee, and ligamentous injury. Noyes et al.[64] have taken the time to review the literature and define terms that are in common orthopedic usage.

Position

Position refers to the orientation of the tibia with respect to the femur and determines the tension in each of the ligaments and supporting structures. Dislocation is a term indicating a complete noncontact position of both the tibia and femur or the patellofemoral joint. Dislocations of the knee are classified by the final tibial position—anterior, posterior, medial, lateral, or rotary.[52] Subluxation is defined as an incomplete partial dislocation and does not have limits.

Motion

Motion is the process of changing position and describes the displacement between the starting and ending points. Displacement is the change in position and is described according to 6 degrees of freedom, a combination of three translations and three rotations. Translation is the parallel displacement of a rigid body or, in the case of the knee joint, the tibia, with respect to the femur. Translation of the tibia is composed of three independent components or translational degrees of freedom—medial lateral translation, anteroposterior translation, and proximal distal translation. Rotation describes motion or displacement about an axis and, in the knee, has 3 degrees of freedom—flexion-extension, internal-external rotation, and abduction-adduction. Range of motion is defined as the displacement that occurs between the two limits of movement for each degree of freedom. There is an ROM for each of the translational and rotational degrees of freedom. For motions other than flexion-extension, ROM generally depends on the angle of knee flexion. The limits of motion are defined as the extreme positions of movement that are possible in each of the 6 degrees of freedom. Injury to the ligamentous and osseous structures about the knee alters the limits of motion. By convention, the limits of flexion and extension are described relative to the neutral position or extension of 0 degrees, with flexion described in positive terms and hyperextension in negative terms. Coupled displacement concerns motion in 1 or more degrees of freedom that is caused by a load applied in another degree of freedom. The amount of coupled rotation depends on where the force is applied to the tibia or on whether the center of rotation is constrained or allowed to move freely. An example is the internal rotation that results when an anterior load is applied to the tibia.[26] When assessing ligamentous stability, motion of the knee joint may occur freely or be constrained, based on the integrity of the ligamentous structures. The ligaments determine the constraint of the knee joint. Elongation or stretching of the ligament limits joint motion and is also supported by compressive joint contact forces that act in an opposite direction. Two ligaments are required to limit translation and rotation—one for each direction. A

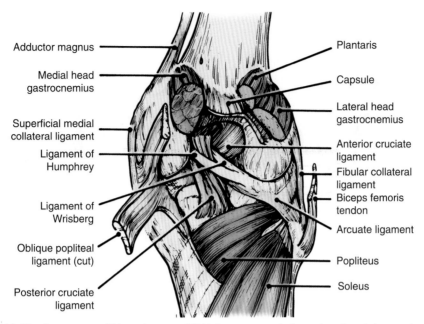

Adductor magnus

Medial head gastrocnemius

Superficial medial collateral ligament

Ligament of Humphrey

Ligament of Wrisberg

Oblique popliteal ligament (cut)

Posterior cruciate ligament

Plantaris

Capsule

Lateral head gastrocnemius

Anterior cruciate ligament

Fibular collateral ligament

Biceps femoris tendon

Arcuate ligament

Popliteus

Soleus

FIG 42.11 The ligaments of Humphrey and Wrisberg are so intimately related that early authors described them as separate portions of a single ligament. (From Scott WN: *Ligament and extensor mechanism injuries of the knee: diagnosis and treatment*, St Louis, MO, 1991, Mosby Year Book.)

single ligament alone is unable to resist rotation. If the motion is unconstrained, the tibia displaces into its maximum position. Most clinical tests performed on the knee, however, are constrained.

The force that displaces the knee has three properties, an orientation or line of action, a sense (forward or backward) along its line of action, and a magnitude. The effect of a force depends on all three of its properties and its point of application. The moment causes an angular or rotational acceleration and has three properties, an orientation or line of action, a sense (clockwise or counterclockwise) about its line of action, and a magnitude. When indicating the moment of the knee joint, it is essential that the axis of rotation be defined.

Laxity

Laxity is a term used to describe the looseness of the joint, which can be normal or abnormal. To avoid confusion, it is better to measure the amount of displacement in millimeters of translation and rotation. The differences between the involved and uninvolved knee should also be reported clearly. Instability is characterized by increased or excessive displacement of the tibia caused by a traumatic injury.

CLASSIFICATION OF LIGAMENT INJURIES

Several terms have been used to describe an injury to a ligament.

Sprain

A sprain is an injury to a joint ligament that stretches or tears ligamentous fibers but does not completely disrupt the ligament. In the handbook Standard Nomenclature of Athletic Injuries,[1] sprains are characterized on the basis of indirect evidence of ligament injury, including the history, symptoms, and physical examination (Fig. 42.12). A first-degree sprain is a tear involving a minimal number of fibers of a ligament, with localized tenderness and no instability. A second-degree sprain tears more ligamentous fibers, with slight to moderate abnormal motion. In a third-degree sprain, there is a complete tear of the ligament, with disruption of fibers and demonstrable instability. Third-degree sprains are further subdivided as follows: grade I, less than a 0.5-cm opening of the joint surfaces; grade II, a 0.5- to 1-cm opening of the joint surfaces; and grade III, a rupture larger than a 1-cm opening. Rupture of a ligament implies complete tearing of the ligament, with concomitant loss of function. Because a ligament may undergo a complete tear but still retain continuity between displaced fibers, it is the loss of function (resistance to displacement) that defines a tear, not the property of continuity.[64] Deficiency of a ligament implies that the ligament is absent or that there is loss of function, such as when the ligament still exists but is stretched and nonfunctional.[59]

Instability

The most elaborate classification system of knee ligament instability was developed by Hughston et al.[36,37] and the American Orthopaedic Society of Sports Medicine Research and Education Committee in 1976.[2] This classification system attempts to describe the instability by the direction of tibial displacement and, when possible, by structural deficits. The classification of knee ligament instability is based on rotation of the knee about the central axis of the PCL. All rotatory instabilities indicate subluxation about the intact PCL. Once the PCL is damaged, the instability is designated as straight instability, which indicates subluxation or translation without rotation around a central axis. The subluxation hinges on the intact MCL or LCL.

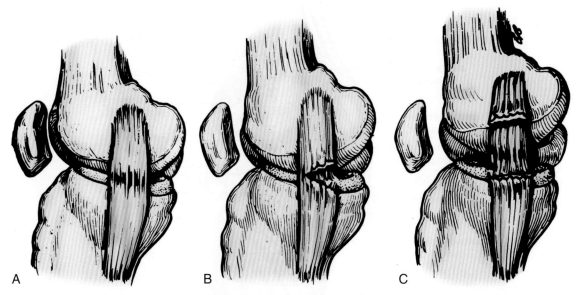

FIG 42.12 Sprains have been characterized on the basis of ligament injury: first-degree (A), second-degree (B), and third-degree (C) sprains. (From Scott WN: *Ligament and extensor mechanism injuries of the knee: diagnosis and treatment.* St Louis, MO, 1991, Mosby Year Book.)

Rotatory Instability. Rotatory instability can be classified as anteromedial, anterolateral, posterolateral, posteromedial, or combined (Fig. 42.13).[71] Combined instability is not as clearly defined as rotatory or straight instability.

Anteromedial rotatory instability. External tibial rotation plus anterior translation is manifested as anteromedial rotatory instability, which causes the medial tibial plateau to subluxate anteromedially on the medial femoral condyle.[38] This motion implies disruption of the medial capsular ligament, MCL, posterior oblique ligament, and ACL.[44,45,79] The medial meniscus is considered an important stabilizing structure and may also be injured.[68] On clinical examination, the abduction stress test result is positive, with abnormal excess opening of the medial joint space at 30 degrees, along with positive anterior drawer and Lachman test results.

Anterolateral rotatory instability. This instability results in excessive internal tibial rotation and anterior subluxation, which implies disruption of the lateral capsular ligament, the arcuate complex, and the ACL. The iliotibial band may be damaged to a varying degree, with most of the injury occurring to the deep fibers, which are attached to the posterior cortex of the lateral femoral condyle. Clinical examination reveals positive results for an adduction test at 30 degrees of flexion and for the anterior drawer, Lachman, and pivot-shift tests. The anterior drawer test result with the tibia rotated externally will be negative because the tibia will not be able to rotate internally. The radiographic presence of a Segond fracture implies an avulsion fracture of the attachment of the anterior oblique band of the lateral capsule from the tibia. This finding, associated with a tear of the ACL, is pathognomonic for anterolateral rotatory instability.[72]

Posterolateral rotatory instability. This instability is apparent when the lateral tibial plateau rotates posterior to the lateral femoral condyle.[9,16,37] The pathologic condition involves tears of the PFL, popliteus tendon, and LCL, with possible injury to the biceps tendon. The PCL is not torn and is the axis on which the knee rotates. The patient may be observed walking with a lateral thrust.

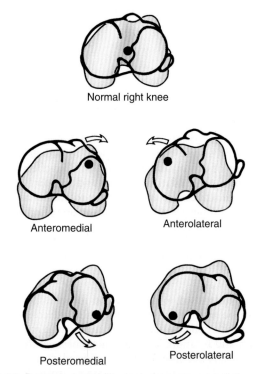

FIG 42.13 Rotatory instability includes anteromedial, anterolateral, posteromedial, and posterolateral instability, which are described in terms of abnormal tibial rotation. (From Scott WN: *Ligament and extensor mechanism injuries of the knee: diagnosis and treatment,* St Louis, MO, 1991, Mosby Year Book.)

On examination, numerous specific tests to help diagnose injuries of the posterolateral corner of the knee have been described; most should be performed with any posterior subluxation of the knee reduced.[17] The posterior drawer test should be performed at 30 and 90 degrees of flexion. If posterior translation, varus rotation, and external rotation are increased

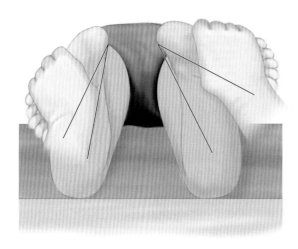

FIG 42.14 The prone external rotation test, which is performed at both 30 and 90 degrees of knee flexion. Forceful external rotation is exerted by the examiner, and the amount of external rotation is measured by comparison of the axis of the medial border of the foot with the femur. (From Veltri DM, Warren RF: Isolated and combined posterior cruciate ligament injuries. *J Am Acad Orthop Surg* 1:70, 1993.)

at 90 degrees but are normal at 30 degrees, a tear of the PCL should be suspected. With posterior translation, increased at 30 degrees but normal at 90 degrees, posterolateral injury should be assumed. Combined injury should be suspected if posterior translation, varus rotation, and external rotation are increased at all degrees of flexion. The dial test (tibial external rotation test) is best done with the patient prone at both 30 and 90 degrees of flexion (Fig. 42.14). Increased external rotation at 30 but not 90 degrees is characteristic of injury to the posterolateral corner; increased external rotation at both angles suggests injury to both the PCL and the posterolateral corner. The posterolateral external rotation test is performed with the knee flexed 30 and 90 degrees, with components of posterior and external force applied to the proximal end of the tibia while palpating for posterolateral tibial subluxation. Again, subluxation at 90 degrees implies injury only to the PCL; subluxation at both 30 and 90 degrees suggests injury to both the PCL and posterolateral corner. Veltri and Warren[88] have reported that the most useful tests for the diagnosis of posterolateral knee injury are the dial test at 30 and 90 degrees of flexion and the varus stress test at 0 and 30 degrees of flexion.

Posteromedial rotatory instability. This instability is manifested by posterior rotation of the medial tibial plateau on the medial femoral condyle. It implies disruption of the MCL, the medial capsular ligament, the posterior oblique ligament, the ACL, and the posteromedial capsule. There may be stretching or major injury to the semimembranosus tendon. The PCL is intact. Hughston et al.[36] do not believe that posteromedial rotatory instability occurs if the PCL is intact because the tightening of the PCL that accompanies internal rotation would prevent this type of instability. If the PCL is disrupted, there would be no fixed axis of rotation, and the instability would be straight posterior.

Combined anteromedial and anterolateral rotatory instability. This instability results in simultaneous anterior subluxation of the medial and lateral tibial plateaus. It implies injury to the

medial and lateral supporting structures, along with a tear of the ACL. Medially, the injury involves the middle third of the medial capsular ligament, the posterior oblique ligament, and the MCL. Laterally, there is a tear of the middle third of the lateral capsular ligament, the iliotibial band, and the short head of the biceps. Clinically, the knee demonstrates positive results for the anterior drawer, Lachman, pivot-shift, and abduction stress tests at 30 degrees of flexion; the results of the adduction stress test at 30 degrees are equivocal.

Combined anterolateral and posterolateral rotatory instability. This instability is the result of disruption of all of the lateral capsular ligaments, with or without a tear of the iliotibial band. Although the ACL is torn, the PCL remains intact. There is a high incidence of lateral meniscal tears. On clinical examination, results of the adduction stress test are markedly positive, along with positive results for the Lachman and anterior drawer tests.

Combined anteromedial and posteromedial rotatory instability. This instability occurs when all the medial and posteromedial structures, including the semimembranosus complex, are torn along with an injury to the ACL. The PCL is intact.

Straight Instability. The four types of straight instability are medial, lateral, posterior, and anterior.

Straight medial instability. This instability is caused by disruption of the medial supporting structures, including the MCL, middle third of the medial capsular ligament, and the posterior oblique ligament. Although the ACL is usually torn, Hughston[36] has noted that the PCL must be torn for straight medial instability to exist. This opinion is not held by all clinicians; some investigators believe that the PCL may not be disrupted. Because the axis of rotation is the LCL, the clinical examination will demonstrate medial joint space opening with an abduction stress test at 30 and 0 degrees. If the ACL is torn, the anterior drawer result will be positive in all three rotational positions. With a torn PCL, the posterior drawer result is positive.

Straight lateral instability. This instability is the result of a tear of the lateral supporting structures and the PCL, with an axis hinging on the MCL. It is manifested by a lateral opening with an adduction stress test in the fully extended position. The injury involves disruption of the lateral capsular ligament, the LCL, the arcuate complex, and the PCL. Clinically, the adduction stress test result is positive at 30 and 0 degrees, but the degree of opening depends on the level of injury to the iliotibial band. The posterior drawer result is positive in the neutral position and will show increased translation with the knee rotated externally. If there is an ACL tear, the anterior drawer and Lachman test results will be positive. The pivot-shift result may not be positive if there is an injury to the iliotibial band.

Straight posterior instability. This instability occurs in patients with isolated injury to the PCL. Although there might be injury to the arcuate ligament and the posterior oblique ligament, the MCL, LCL, and ACL are intact. On examination, the knee demonstrates a posterior drop-back of the tibia without evidence of rotation. Whereas the posterior drawer test result is markedly positive, medial, lateral, and anterior test results are negative.

Straight anterior instability. This instability is the result of disruption of the ACL and is demonstrated by a positive result of the anterior drawer test in neutral rotation with an equal amount of medial and lateral subluxation. There is no evidence

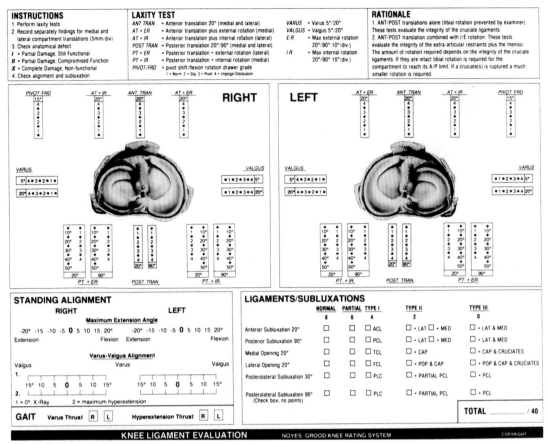

FIG 42.15 The knee ligament evaluation form used in the Noyes-Grood rating system. (From Noyes FR, Grood ES: Classification of ligament injuries: why an anterolateral laxity or anteromedial laxity is not a diagnostic entity. *Instr Course Lect* 36:185, 1987.)

of rotational displacement. In contrast, Hughston et al. defined straight instability as an injury to the PCL and related supporting structures, with loss of the central axis of rotation. Therefore, they did not regard straight anterior instability as an injury to the ACL, but rather as an injury to the PCL. With this in mind, Hughston et al.[36,37] claimed not to have encountered any anterior displacement great enough to rupture the PCL without also rupturing the MCL and LCL.

Noyes and Grood Rotatory Instability Model.

Noyes and Grood[34,62,63] have maintained that the terms for rotatory instability, as discussed earlier, are imprecise and do not represent a specific definable motion or set of motions. An almost infinite number of combinations of joint motion actually exist and can occur, depending on the abnormalities in any of 1, 2, or 3 of the degrees of freedom. Accurate diagnosis requires knowledge of precise abnormalities and biomechanical data as to which ligaments limit the use of motion. As a result of such information, they developed the bumper model of the knee. They found this model to be useful in understanding how the ligaments and capsular structures limit anterior and posterior translation and internal and external rotation.

Noyes and Grood developed a knee ligament evaluation form (Fig. 42.15). The clinician examines and tests the knee for integrity of the primary and secondary ligament restraints. It is important to select a laxity test to diagnose a specific ligament injury. The extent of damage to each structure is reported as

follows: I, partial damage, still functional; II, partial damage, compromised function; and X, complete damage, nonfunctional. The assessment of the functional capacity of the injured ligaments and capsule is only an approximation. Ultimately, it is necessary to quantitate the damaged structures. In the bumper model, the bumpers do not represent exact ligament structures; instead, they represent the final restraints to tibial motion, with summation of the effect of the ligament, menisci, and capsular structures.

Type I motion is described as normal, and there are three clinically identifiable types of anterior knee subluxation that can occur after a rupture of the ACL. Noyes and Grood[34,62,63] have recommended performing the anterior drawer and Lachman tests in a neutral position without rotation for initial evaluation of the ACL. The anterior drawer test is then repeated with internal and external rotation to determine the maximum excursion of the lateral and medial tibiofemoral compartments to provide information on the laxity of the extra-articular ligamentous restraints. The results of the laxity tests are indicated on the evaluation form first by recording the amount of central subluxation and, second, by indicating the amount of translation of the medial and lateral compartments when tibial rotation is added. The clinical significance of identifying these three types of anterior subluxation rests in their different natural histories and treatment programs. Type II subluxation is characterized by tight extra-articular structures; the amount of anterior and lateral tibial translation is only slightly increased.

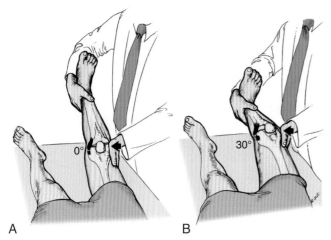

FIG 42.16 (A) Valgus stress in extension tests the medial collateral ligament and the posteromedial capsule. (B) Stress in 30 degrees of flexion tests only the medial collateral ligament. (From Tria AJ Jr, Klein KS: *An illustrated guide to the knee*, New York, NY, 1992, Churchill Livingstone.)

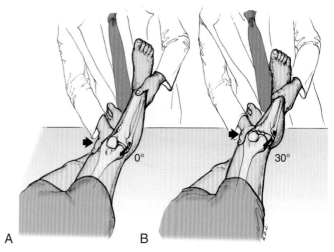

FIG 42.17 (A) Varus stress in extension tests the lateral collateral ligament and the posterolateral capsule. (B) Stress in 30 degrees of flexion tests only the lateral collateral ligament. (From Tria AJ Jr, Klein KS: *An illustrated guide to the knee*, New York, NY, 1992, Churchill Livingstone.)

Type III subluxation consists of anterior subluxation with increased translation of the medial and lateral tibial compartments. The translation of the lateral tibial compartment will be greater because of associated increases in the internal rotation units. Type IV anterior subluxation indicates gross subluxation with increased translation of the medial and lateral compartments. As the degree of subluxation increases, the axis of rotation is shifted medially outside the joint.

The final diagnosis of a ligament defect must be made in precise anatomic terms; in cases of partial disruption or after healing occurs, the clinician must analyze the remaining functional capacity of the ligaments. It has been suggested that identifying these types of anterior subluxation has clinical significance because each carries a different prognosis. Type II subluxation, characterized by tight extra-articular structures, and has a better prognosis than that of types III and IV subluxation; ACL reconstruction is recommended.[62] With type IV subluxation, it is important to restore the associated damaged ligamentous structures, especially the lateral extraarticular structures.

DETERMINATION OF KNEE LIGAMENT INSTABILITY

The joint motion assessed on clinical examination determines the classification of knee ligament instability. It is important that the objective findings on the clinical examination correlate with the pathologic knee motion and allow standardized classification of knee ligament instability. Clinical findings have been substantiated by biomechanical studies.

Ligament Injury Tests
Valgus Stress Test. This test should be performed first on the normal extremity for later comparison. The involved knee is flexed to 30 degrees, and a gentle valgus stress is applied to the knee, with one hand placed on the lateral aspect of the thigh and the other hand grasping the foot and ankle (Fig. 42.16). Placing the hip in relative extension helps relax the hamstring

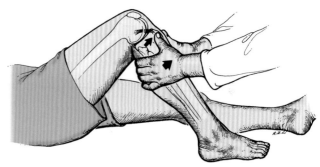

FIG 42.18 The anterior drawer test is performed with the knee flexed to 90 degrees and with anterior force applied to the proximal end of the tibia. (From Tria AJ Jr, Klein KS: *An illustrated guide to the knee*, New York, NY, 1992, Churchill Livingstone.)

musculature. The valgus stress test must also be performed with the knee in full extension or in the amount of recurvatum present in the opposite uninvolved limb. The degree of opening of the medial side of the knee should be quantified, graded, and recorded.

Varus Stress Test. This test is similar to the valgus stress test. The varus stress test is carried out with the knee in full extension and in 30 degrees of flexion. The degree of lateral opening should be quantified, graded, and recorded (Fig. 42.17).

Anterior Drawer Test
The hip is flexed to 45 degrees, with the knee flexed to 80 to 90 degrees (Fig. 42.18). The examiner sits on the table and, using the buttocks, stabilizes the patient's foot. The examiner places his or her hands about the upper part of the tibia and palpates the hamstrings to make sure that they are relaxed. The examiner then gently pulls and pushes the proximal portion of the tibia in a to-and-fro manner. The test is performed in neutral,

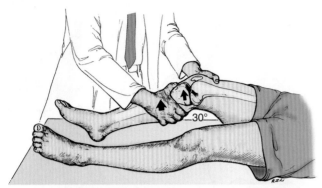

FIG 42.19 The Lachman test is performed in 30 degrees of flexion with anterior force exerted on the proximal end of the tibia. (From Tria AJ Jr, Klein KS: *An illustrated guide to the knee*, New York, NY, 1992, Churchill Livingstone.)

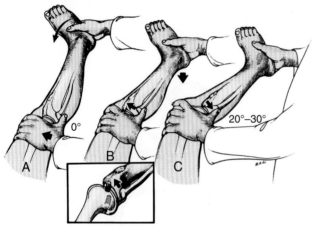

FIG 42.20 The pivot-shift test begins with the knee in full extension (A) and applies internal rotation (B) and valgus stress (C) to demonstrate anterolateral subluxation. (From Tria AJ Jr, Klein KS: *An illustrated guide to the knee*, New York, NY, 1992, Churchill Livingstone.)

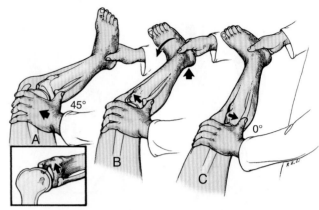

FIG 42.21 (A) The Losee test begins with the knee in flexion but externally rotates the foot. Valgus stress is applied (B), and the tibia is internally rotated as the knee is extended (C). (From Tria AJ Jr, Klein KS: *An illustrated guide to the knee*, New York, NY, 1992, Churchill Livingstone.)

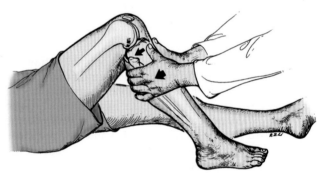

FIG 42.22 The posterior drawer test is performed in 90 degrees of flexion with posterior force applied to the proximal end of the tibia. (From Tria AJ Jr, Klein KS: *An illustrated guide to the knee*, New York, NY, 1992, Churchill Livingstone.)

internal, and external rotated postures of the foot. The degree and type of anterior drawer should be reported.

Lachman Test. This test has become the standard examination for evaluating the integrity of the ACL and is used to assess anterior knee laxity and stiffness, with the knee in about 30 degrees of flexion (Fig. 42.19). In this position, an anterior drawer is applied to the proximal part of the calf, at which time the examiner perceives displacement of the tibia and assesses the end point stiffness.[43] The slightest increase in anterior displacement of the tibia would be considered a positive test result when compared with the contralateral knee. End point stiffness should be clearly documented.

Pivot-Shift Test. The pivot-shift test[28] (Fig. 42.20) and the Losee test[52] (Fig.42.21) demonstrate anterior subluxation and reduction of the tibia, with the knee in flexion-extension from 10 to 40 degrees as a result of ACL disruption. Patients with an MCL disruption or previous iliotibial tract surgery may have less dramatic findings on physical examination.[20]

Posterior Drawer Test. The standard test to assess the PCL has been the posterior drawer test. The knee is flexed to 90 degrees, and posterior force is exerted on the tibia in an attempt to sublux it posteriorly in relation to the femur (Fig. 42.22). Before initiating the test, to avoid a potential false-negative examination finding, it is important to ensure that the tibia rests at its normal anatomic position approximately 1 cm anterior to the femoral condyles. A grade III posterior drawer in addition to more than 10 mm of posterior tibial translation on stress radiographs has been shown to represent a combined PCL and posterolateral corner injury.[74] A posterior Lachman test result has also been described for acute PCL injuries (Fig. 42.23). The knee is held in 30 degrees of flexion, and the tibia is forced posteriorly. Any motion in this direction correlates with a tear of the PCL.[86]

Quadriceps Active Test. A knee with chronic PCL deficiency may demonstrate posterior sag when the knee and hip are flexed to 90 degrees. To perform the 90-degree quadriceps active test, the clinician sits beside the examining table, with the patient's knee flexed to 90 degrees at eye level (Fig. 42.24). The foot is stabilized by the clinician, and the patient is asked to slide her

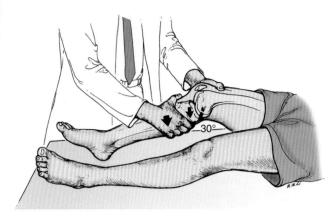

FIG 42.23 The posterior Lachman test applies posterior force to the proximal end of the tibia with the knee flexed 30 degrees. (From Tria AJ Jr, Klein KS: *An illustrated guide to the knee*, New York, NY, 1992, Churchill Livingstone.)

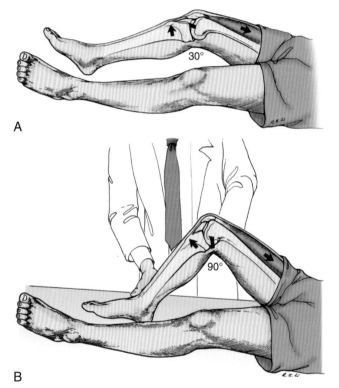

FIG 42.24 Quadriceps active test for the anterior cruciate ligament in 30 degrees of flexion (A) and for the posterior cruciate ligament in 90 degrees of flexion (B). (From Scott WN [ed]: *The knee*, St Louis, MO, 1994, CV Mosby.)

or his foot gently down the table. The clinician's hand prevents the foot from moving forward, thereby allowing anterior translation of the tibia, which occurs when the tibia is posteriorly subluxated secondary to PCL disruption.

Reverse Pivot-Shift Test. This test is used to diagnose injuries to the posterolateral ligament complex. The clinician supports the patient's limb with a hand under the heel, with the knee in full extension and neutral rotation (Fig. 42.25). A valgus stress is

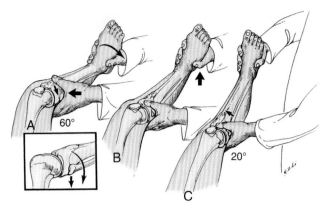

FIG 42.25 (A) The reverse pivot-shift test begins with the knee flexed and the tibia externally rotated. (B and C) The knee is then extended and posterolateral capsular laxity demonstrated. (From Tria AJ Jr, Klein KS: *An illustrated guide to the knee*, New York, NY, 1992, Churchill Livingstone.)

applied and the knee is flexed. In a positive test, at about 20 to 30 degrees of flexion, the tibia will rotate externally, and the lateral tibial plateau will subluxate posteriorly and remain in this position during further flexion. When the knee is then extended, the tibia reduces. In the standard pivot-shift test, the tibia is subluxated anteriorly in early flexion and reduces between 20 and 40 degrees of flexion. In the reverse pivot-shift test, the tibia is initially reduced, and then the lateral tibial plateau posteriorly subluxates at 20 to 30 degrees of flexion. In a patient with a combined ACL and posterolateral ligament complex injury, one may observe the tibia go from anterior subluxation to a reduced position and then to a posterior subluxated position.[20] A knee with a posterolateral injury should be tested at 0 to 30 degrees of flexion for maximum primary posterior translation and at 75 to 90 degrees of external rotation for minimum translation. A knee in which an isolated PCL injury is suspected should be tested at 75 to 90 degrees of flexion for maximum primary posterior translation and at 0 to 30 degrees for minimum translation. In an isolated PCL injury, no change should be expected in primary external rotation. If both the posterolateral structures and PCL are ruptured, there will be a substantial increase in primary posterior translation, external rotation, and varus rotation at all angles of flexion of the knee, as compared with an intact knee or one in which either structure has been injured in isolation.[30]

Ligament Testing Devices Used in Classification

It is important that the classification of ligament injuries be precise and that the clinician understand the remaining functional capacity of the ligaments. Difficulties still remain in the evaluation of these injuries, and it is anticipated that newer diagnostic devices will provide detailed information to enable the clinician to determine the different types of instability under defined loading conditions.

In the 1980s, several ligament testing devices were developed in an attempt to quantitate anteroposterior displacement of the knee joint objectively.[†] The variability in subjective clinical

---

[†]References 19, 23, 24, 55, 66, 67, and 75.

TABLE 42.1 Lysholm Scale

Parameter	Finding	Score	Parameter	Finding	Score
Limp	None	5	Pain	None	25
	Slight or periodic	3		Inconstant and slight during strenuous activities	20
	Severe and constant	0		Marked during or after walking >2 km	10
Support	None	5		Marked during or after walking <2 km	5
	Stick or crutch needed	2		Constant	0
	Weight bearing impossible	0	Swelling	None	10
Locking	None	15		After strenuous activities	6
	None, but catching sensation present	10		After ordinary activities	3
	Occasional	6		Constant	0
	Frequent	2	Squatting	No problem	5
	At examination	0		Slight problem	4
Stairs	No problem	10		Not beyond 90 degrees of knee flexion	2
	Slight problem	6		Impossible	0
	One step at a time	3			
	Impossible	0			
Instability	Never	25			
	Rarely during athletic activities	20			
	Frequently during athletic activities	15			
	Occasionally during daily activities	10			
	Often during daily activities	5			
	Every step	0			

Adapted from Lysholm J, Gillquist J: Evaluation of knee ligament surgery results with special emphasis on using a scoring scale. *J Sports Med* 10:150, 1982.

grades given to many testing maneuvers makes it difficult to compare injuries and clinical results. Objective quantitative ligament testing devices provide the opportunity to more accurately compare populations of patients. The pathologic anteroposterior motion of cruciate ligament injuries can be diagnosed with the KT-1000 arthrometer (MEDmetric, San Diego, California). Daniel et al.[23] have reported that 97% of 120 normal subjects tested with the KT-1000 arthrometer demonstrated less than a 3-mm right-left difference, whereas the right-left difference was 3 mm or greater in 90% of 33 patients with an acute ACL injury with the manual maximum test. Miyasaka et al.[58] have found that use of the KT-1000 arthrometer and quadriceps active tests helped them diagnose a PCL injury with high accuracy. In another study, 40 of 41 patients with documented PCL rupture were found to have pathological laxity by this method.[21] Objective quantification of knee laxity in ACL and PCL injury with instrumented testing is useful. Daniel et al.[22] have shown that 96% of patients with an arthroscopically confirmed tear of the ACL had a maximum manual KT-1000 test result, with more than 3-mm side-to-side difference. It has been suggested that further quantitative reporting should include 89 N, maximum manual, compliance index, and side-to-side difference because variations in testing parameters have been noted.[7] There are pitfalls and limitations with the use of current instrumented testing devices. Bach et al.[8] found that the KT-1000 is useful only for anteroposterior translation because it does not allow assessment of rotational or varus-valgus instability. The clinical applicability of the Genucom computerized system appears to be limited by variability in measurements of knee laxity.[31] The problem is that this device assumes that the change in stiffness of the soft tissues can be accurately predicted from one angle of flexion of the knee to another. However, major variations in the effect of the position of the knee are expected between subjects and even between repeated examinations of the same individual.

Objective quantitation of knee laxity in ligamentous injuries is an important diagnostic adjunct. Testing devices that objectively measure laxity permit the clinician to evaluate the injured or postsurgical knee and predict the functional outcome. In a prospective study, Daniel et al.[22] have shown that the early KT grade is a predictor of the late KT grade.

KNEE LIGAMENT RATING SYSTEMS

In the course of developing knee ligament rating systems, investigators have attempted to correlate function and clinical findings. Although universal acceptance has not been achieved, several rating systems have been popularized. The Lysholm scale[53] (Table 42.1) is based solely on the patient's subjective evaluation of function, with no weight given to objective findings. In an effort to rate a patient's level of function, Tegner and Lysholm[82] have developed a knee activity assessment that questions patients about their participation in sports and work (Table 42.2). Twenty-five years after their introduction, the Lysholm score and Tegner activity scale have demonstrated acceptable responsiveness and psychometric parameters as patient-administered scores.[11]

Because it is important to include objective clinical findings with the level of activity, Noyes et al.[61] designed the Cincinnati knee rating system that uses subjective and objective criteria (Table 42.3). The subjective criteria include a system rating scale, assessment of function, and sports rating scale. Objective testing includes ROM, the presence of crepitus, KT-1000 testing, and a radiographic review. The scale includes a scheme for a final rating of excellent, good, fair, or poor. Although these rating systems have gained regional or institutional acceptance, the American Orthopaedic Society of Sports Medicine and its European equivalent, under the auspices of the International Knee Documentation Committee, have published a knee ligament injury evaluation form (Fig. 42.26).

TABLE 42.2   Tegner and Lysholm Activity Scales

Level	Type of Sport or Activity	Example(s)
10	Competitive sports	Soccer—national or international level
9	Competitive sports	Soccer—lower divisions
		Ice hockey
		Wrestling
		Gymnastics
8	Competitive sports	Bandy
		Squash or badminton
		Athletics (eg, jumping)
		Downhill skiing
7	Competitive sports	Tennis
		Athletics (eg, running)
		Motocross or speedway
		Handball or basketball
	Recreational sports	Soccer
		Bandy or ice hockey
		Squash
		Athletics (eg, jumping)
		Cross-country track finding (orienteering), both recreational and competitive
6	Recreational sports	Tennis or badminton
		Handball or basketball
		Downhill skiing
		Jogging at least five times weekly
5	Work	Heavy labor (eg, construction, forestry)
	Competitive sports	Cycling
		Cross-country skiing
	Recreational sports	Jogging on uneven ground at least twice weekly
4	Work	Moderately heavy work (eg, truck driving, scrubbing floors)
	Recreational sports	Cycling
		Cross-country skiing
		Jogging on uneven ground at least weekly
3	Work	Light work (eg, nursing)
	Competitive and recreational sports	Walking on rough forest terrain
2	Work	Light work
		Walking on uneven ground
1	Work	Sedentary work
		Walking on uneven ground
0	Sick leave or disability pension because of knee problems	

Adapted from Tegner Y, Lysholm J: Rating systems in evaluation of knee ligament injuries. *Clin Orthop* 198:43, 1985.

TABLE 42.3   Cincinnati Knee Rating System

A. ASSESSMENT OF FUNCTION

Activity	Function	Points
Activities of Daily Living		
Walking	Normal, unlimited	40
	Some limitations	30
	No more than 3-4 blocks possible	20
	Less than 1 block with cane or crutch	0
Stair climbing	Normal, unlimited	40
	Some limitations	30
	No more than 11-30 steps possible	20
	No more than 1-10 steps possible	0
Squatting, kneeling	Normal, unlimited	40
	Some limitations	30
	No more than 6-10 possible	20
	No more than 0-5 possible	0
Sports Activities		
Straight running	Fully competitive	100
	Some limitations, guarding	80
	Run half-speed, definite limitations	60
	Not able to do so	40

Continued

TABLE 42.3 Cincinnati Knee Rating System—cont'd

A. ASSESSMENT OF FUNCTION

Activity	Function	Points
Jumping, landing on affected leg	Fully competitive	100
	Some limitations, guarding	80
	Definite limitations, half-speed	60
	Not able to do so	40
Hard twisting, cutting, pivoting	Fully competitive	100
	Some limitations, guarding	80
	Definite limitations, half-speed	60
	Not able to do so	40

B. SYMPTOM RATING SCALE

Symptoms	Activities	Points
None	Able to do strenuous work, sports with jumping and hard pivoting	10
With strenuous work, sports	Able to do moderate work, sports with running, turning, and twisting	8
With moderate work, sports	Able to do light work, sports with no running, twisting, or jumping	6
With light work, sports	Able to perform activities of daily living alone	4
Frequent and limiting	Activities of daily living produce moderate symptoms	2
Constant and not relieved	Activities of daily living produce severe symptoms	0

C. SPORTS ACTIVITIES RATING SCALE

Level	Participation	Motion	Sport	Points
I	4-7 days/weeks	Jumping, hard pivoting, cutting	Basketball, volleyball, football, gymnastics, soccer	100
		Running, twisting, turning	Tennis, racquetball, handball, baseball, ice hockey, field hockey, skiing, wrestling	95
		No running, twisting, jumping	Cycling, swimming	90
II	1-3 days/weeks	Jumping, hard pivoting, cutting	Basketball, volleyball, football, gymnastics, soccer	85
		Running, twisting, turning	Tennis, racquetball, handball, baseball, ice hockey, field hockey, skiing, wrestling	80
		No running, twisting, jumping	Cycling, swimming	75
III	1-3 times/months	Jumping, hard pivoting, cutting	Basketball, volleyball, football, gymnastics, soccer	65
		Running, twisting, turning	Tennis, racquetball, handball, baseball, ice hockey, field hockey, skiing, wrestling	60
		No running, twisting, jumping	Cycling, swimming	55
IV	None	No problems with activities of daily living	40	
		Moderate problems with activities of daily living	20	
		Severe problems with activities of daily living (uses crutches, full disability)	0	

D. SCHEME FOR FINAL RATING

Signs	Excellent	Good	Fair	Poor
Pain	10	8	6-4	2-0
Swelling	10	8	6-4	2-0
Partial giving way	10	8	6-4	2-0
Full giving way	10	8	6-4	2-0
Walking	40	30	20	0
Stairs or squatting (choose lower score)	40	30	20	0
Running	100	80	60	40
Jumping	100	80	60	40
Hard twists, cuts, pivots	100	80	60	40
Effusion (mL)	Normal	<25	26-60	>60
Lack of flexion (degrees)	0-5	6-15	16-30	>30
Lack of extension (degrees)	0-3	4-5	6-10	>10
Tibiofemoral crepitus[a]	Normal	—	Moderate	Severe
Patellofemoral crepitus[a]	Normal	—	Moderate	Severe
Anterior displacement (KT-1000; mm)	<3	3–5	6	>6
Pivot-shift test, joint space narrowing	Negative	Slip	Definite	Severe
Medial tibiofemoral (radiographs)[b]	Normal	Mild	Moderate	Severe
Lateral tibiofemoral (radiographs)[b]	Normal	Mild	Moderate	Severe
Patellofemoral (radiographs)[b]	Normal	Mild	Moderate	Severe
Functional testing (limb symmetry, %)[c]	85-100	75-84	65-74	<65

Adapted from Noyes FR, Barber SD, Mangine RE: Bone-patellar ligament-bone and fascia lata allografts for reconstruction of the anterior cruciate ligament. *J Bone Joint Surg Am* 72:1125, 1990.

[a]Moderate indicates definite fibrillation and cartilage abnormality of 25 to 50 degrees; severe, cartilage abnormality of more than 50 degrees.
[b]Moderate indicates narrowing of less than half the joint space; severe, more than half the joint space.
[c]Use an average of at least three one-legged hop-type tests.

THE SEVEN GROUPS	THE FOUR GRADES				GROUP GRADE (see footnotes)			

	A: normal	B: nearly normal	C: abnormal	D: sev. abnorm.	A	B	C	D
1 Patient subjective assessment								
On a scale of 0 to 3 how did you rate your pre-injury activity level?	☐ 0	☐ 1	☐ 2	☐ 3				
On a scale of 0 to 3 how did you rate your current activity level?	☐ 0	☐ 1	☐ 2	☐ 3				
If your normal knee performs 100%, what percentage does your operated knee perform?	_____ %				☐	☐	☐	☐

2 Symptoms

(Grade at highest activity level known by patient)

	I Strenuous activities	II Moderate activities	III ADL/Light activities	IV ADL problems	A	B	C	D
Pain	☐	☐	☐	☐				
Swelling	☐	☐	☐	☐				
Partial giving way	☐	☐	☐	☐				
Full giving way	☐	☐	☐	☐	☐	☐	☐	☐

3 Range of motion Flex/Ext: Index side: __ / __ / __ Opposite side: __ / __ / __

					A	B	C	D
Lack of extension (from zero degrees)	☐ <3°	☐ 3–5°	☐ 6–10°	☐ >10°				
Δ Lack of flexion	☐ 0–5°	☐ 6–15°	☐ 16–25°	☐ >25°	☐	☐	☐	☐

4 Ligament examination

					A	B	C	D
Δ Lachman (25° flex) (manual, instrumented, x-ray)	☐ 1 to 2 mm	☐ 3 to 5 mm	☐ 6 to 10 mm	☐ >10 mm				
Endpoint: ☐ firm ☐ soft	☐ firm		☐ soft					
Δ Total a.p. transl. (70° flex)	☐ 0 to 2 mm	☐ 3 to 5 mm	☐ 6 to 10 mm	☐ >10 mm				
Δ Post. sag in 70° flex	☐ 0 to 2 mm	☐ 3 to 5 mm	☐ 6 to 10 mm	☐ >10 mm				
Δ Med. joint opening (valgus rotation)	☐ 0 to 2 mm	☐ 3 to 5 mm	☐ 6 to 10 mm	☐ >10 mm				
Δ Lat. joint opening (varus rotation)	☐ 0 to 2 mm	☐ 3 to 5 mm	☐ 6 to 10 mm	☐ >10 mm				
Pivot shift	☐ neg.	☐ + (glide)	☐ ++ (clunk)	☐ +++ (gross)				
Reversed pivot shift	☐ equal	☐ glide	☐ marked	☐ gross	☐	☐	☐	☐

5 Compartmental findings

					A	B	C	D
Crepitus patellofemoral	☐ none		☐ moderate	☐ severe				
Crepitus medial compartment	☐ none		☐ moderate	☐ severe				
Crepitus lateral compartment	☐ none		☐ moderate	☐ severe (palpable & audible)	☐	☐	☐	☐

6 X-ray findings

					A	B	C	D
Med. joint space narrowing	☐ none		☐ <50%	☐ >50%				
Lat. joint space narrowing	☐ none		☐ <50%	☐ >50%				
Patellofemoral joint space narrowing	☐ none		☐ <50%	☐ >50%	☐	☐	☐	☐

7 Functional test

					A	B	C	D
Δ One leg hop (% of opposite side)	☐ 100–90%	☐ 90–76%	☐ 75–50%	☐ <50%	☐	☐	☐	☐
Final evaluation					☐	☐	☐	☐

Footnotes:
• Group grade: The lowest grade within a group determines the group grade.
• Final evaluation: The worst group determines the final evaluation.
• In a final evaluation all 7 groups are to be evaluated; for a quick knee profile the evaluation of groups 1–4 are sufficient.

FIG 42.26 International Knee Documentation Committee knee rating system. (From the International Knee Documentation Committee: knee ligament injury and reconstruction evaluation. In Aichroth PM, Dilworth Cannon WD Jr [eds]: *Knee surgery: current practice*, New York, 1992, Martin Dunitz/Raven Press, p 760.)

KEY REFERENCES

11. Briggs KK, Lysholm J, Tegner Y, et al: The reliability, validity, and responsiveness of the Lysholm score and the Tegner activity scale for anterior cruciate ligament injuries of the knee. *Am J Sports Med* 37:890, 2009.

14. Chhabra A, Starman JS, Ferretti M, et al: Anatomic, radiographic, biomechanical, and kinematic evaluation of the anterior cruciate ligament and its two functional bundles. *J Bone Joint Surg Am* 88(Suppl 4):1, 2006.

32. Griffith CJ, LaPrade RF, Johansen S, et al: Medial knee injury: part 1, static function of the individual components of the main medial knee structures. *Am J Sports Med* 37:1762, 2009.

33. Griffith CJ, Wijdicks CA, LaPrade RF, et al: Force measurements on the posterior oblique ligament and superficial medial collateral ligament proximal and distal divisions to applied loads. *Am J Sports Med* 37:140, 2009.

34. Grood ES, Noyes FR: Diagnosis and classifications of knee ligament injuries: biomechanical precepts. In Feagin JA Jr, editor: *The crucial ligaments*, New York, NY, 1987, Churchill Livingstone, p 245.

36. Hughston JC, Andrews JR, Cross MJ, et al: Classification of knee ligament instabilities: the medial compartment and cruciate ligaments. *J Bone Joint Surg Am* 58:159, 1976.

37. Hughston JC, Andrews JR, Cross MJ, et al: Classification of knee ligament instabilities: the lateral compartment. *J Bone Joint Surg Am* 58:173, 1976.

48. LaPrade RF, Engebretsen AH, Ly TV, et al: The anatomy of the medial part of the knee. *J Bone Joint Surg Am* 89:2000, 2007.

49. LaPrade RF, Ly TV, Wentorf FA, et al: The posterolateral attachments of the knee. *Am J Sports Med* 31:854–860, 2003.

50. LaPrade RF, Tso A, Wentorf FA: Force measurements on the fibular collateral ligament, popliteofibular ligament, and popliteus tendon to applied loads. *Am J Sports Med* 32:1695–1701, 2004.

53. Lysholm J, Gillquist J: Evaluation of knee ligament surgery results with special emphasis on using a scoring scale. *J Sports Med* 10:150, 1982.

62. Noyes FR, Grood ES: Classification of ligament injuries: why an anterolateral laxity or anteromedial laxity is not a diagnostic entity. *Instr Course Lect* 36:185, 1987.

64. Noyes FR, Grood ES, Torzilli PA: Current concepts review: the definition of terms for motion and position of the knee and injuries of the ligaments. *J Bone Joint Surg Am* 71:465, 1989.

70. Robinson JR, Bull AM, Thomas RR, et al: The role of the medial collateral ligament and posteromedial capsule in controlling knee laxity. *Am J Sports Med* 34:1815–1823, 2006.

82. Tegner Y, Lysholm J: Rating systems in evaluation of knee ligament injuries. *Clin Orthop* 198:43, 1985.

94. Zantop T, Herbort M, Raschke MJ, et al: The role of the anteromedial and posterolateral bundles of the anterior cruciate ligament in anterior tibial translation and internal rotation. *Am J Sports Med* 35:223, 2007.

The references for this chapter can also be found on www.expertconsult.com.

43

Sports Knee Rating Systems and Related Statistics

Christopher M. Kuenze, Joe Hart

PATIENT-REPORTED KNEE RATING SCALES AND RELATED STATISTICS

Outcomes following orthopedic injury are typically determined via physical exam or other objective assessments completed by a physician or medical professional. Patient-reported outcomes (PRO) in the form of survey-style questionnaires are a fixture in the orthopedic literature, because they enable tracking of a diverse compliment of outcomes from the perspective of the patient following injury and/or surgery. These instruments are designed to ask a series of pertinent questions and quantify the values on a scale that can be compared across the entire population and prospectively over time. The challenge with PROs is selecting the most appropriate instrument to measure the outcome of interest in a reliable and valid manner. Instruments can be used as a consistent outcome in single or multisite prospective databases. They can be used to compare outcomes over short or long periods of time (eg, before and after surgery) or to determine the natural history of injuries or disease processes. These instruments can also be used to compare patient groups, treatments, surgical techniques, other medical therapies, and so forth. PROs may be designed to evaluate general quality of life or can be region specific or injury specific. For example, an instrument to evaluate knee function after anterior cruciate ligament (ACL) reconstruction may ask questions about ambulation, pain with kneeling, or confidence in cutting during sports, whereas an outcomes instrument to evaluate outcomes following shoulder injury may ask questions about overhead motion, ability to lift objects during activities of daily living, or pain with throwing.

PRO are ubiquitous within studies aimed at determining the success or failure of treatment following orthopedic injury; however, they should also be considered as one of many tools used to understand outcomes and guide treatment decision making in the clinical environment. In this chapter, PRO instruments that are commonly used for persons with knee pathologies or a history of knee surgery will be identified and discussed. In addition, a review of basic statistical concepts will help explain how these instruments can be used to test hypotheses relevant to the practice of orthopedic surgery.

SELECTING APPROPRIATE SELF REPORT OUTCOME INSTRUMENT INSTRUMENTS

Familiarity with the characteristics and supporting evidence for PROs is essential when making decisions about which PRO is most appropriate for a given clinical question or patient population. To ensure successful integration of PROs into the clinical and research environments, a given scale should reliably and accurately represent the patients' condition while detecting changes in self-reported condition resulting from changes in disease or injury state. A great deal of time and thought are required to develop a series of questions that will be provocative enough to accurately represent the patients' condition and be sensitive to subtle changes in the condition of the patient. It is important to note that PROs are developed in a systematic manner that requires the input of content experts and comprehensive testing to establish the validity and reliability of the individual questions as well as the instrument as a whole in each patient population of interest. Relevant instruments for which validity and reliability statistics have been reported via well-designed research studies should be considered first.

GLOBAL OUTCOMES AND QUALITY OF LIFE SCALES

The Short Form 36 Item Form

The 36 Item Short Form (SF-36) is a common general health questionnaire used in health science research that includes 36 questions about general health status. This generic general health scale is not specific to a disease or pathology and therefore allows for wide ranging comparisons across patient populations.[52] This scale is also available in a shorter 12 item form, known as the SF-12, which shares all 12 of its items with the SF-36. Both the SF-12 and SF-36 have been shown to be reliable and valid when administered in several languages both in person and via telephone and are easily compared to previously established normative values.[26,53] Recent research[17,52,53] has shown that these scales are most reliable when administered in individuals between the ages of 18 and 75, and the SF-12 may be more appropriate when used in studies with large sample sizes. Currently, these scales have been used widely in research involving knee and hip osteoarthritis (OA), ACL reconstruction, patellofemoral pain syndrome, and other sports injury populations.[23,27,48,49]

The SF-36 and SF-12 scales consist of eight subscales (physical function, role-physical, bodily pain, general health, vitality, social functioning, role-emotional, and mental health) that allow for individual scoring as well as calculation of a physical and mental composite score.[52,53] Composite and subscale scoring is based on a scale of 0 (worst health) to 100 (most healthy). The SF-36 has shown better specificity (Table 43.1) and is less likely to experience floor and ceiling effects in injured populations, whereas the SF-12 offers easier scoring and a shorter amount of time for administration.[52,53,57] Most commonly, this scale is used in combination with a more region- or injury-specific scale to

TABLE 43.1 **Summary of Common Patient-Reported Outcome Measures Used in the Clinical and Research Environments**[18]

Scale	Common Uses	Specific Populations	Scale Range (Total Score)	MCID (Units)	MDC (Units)
SF-36	Well-being	Severe knee OA[2]	0-100 points	7.8	
Tegner activity rating[50]	Physical activity level	All populations	0-10 levels	Not reported	1.0
Marx activity scale[32]	Physical activity level	ACL injury	0-16 points	Not reported	9.9
VAS[11,51]	Pain	Knee injury and OA	0-100 mm	19.9-20.0	
IKDC[21]	Knee related function	ACL injury, PCL injury, meniscus injury, articular cartilage injury, PF pain	0-100 points	3.19-16.7	6.7-20.5
Cincinnati knee scale[3]	Knee related function	ACL injury, PCL injury, meniscus injury, articular cartilage injury, PF pain, tibial osteotomy	0-100 points	14.0-26.0	27.5
KOOS[43]	Knee related function	Knee OA, ACL injury, meniscus injury, cartilage injury	0-100 points	Not reported	Symptoms = 9.9-24.3
				Not reported	Pain = 11.8-29.0
				Not reported	ADL = 11.9-31.5
				Not reported	Sports = 12.2-70.0
				Not reported	QOL = 14.2-34.0
WOMAC[5]	Knee related function	Rheumatoid arthritis, Knee OA	0-100 points	Pain = 7.5-17.5	Pain = 14.4-16.2
				Function = 5.89-8.1	Function = 10.6-15.0
				Stiffness = 6.3-18.8	Stiffness = 22.9-30.6
				Overall = 11.5	Overall = 10.7-15.3
Lysholm scale[30]	Knee related function	ACL injury, PCL injury, meniscus injury, articular cartilage injury, PF pain	0-100 points	10.1	8.9-15.8

ACL, Anterior cruciate ligament; *ADL,* activities of daily living; *IKDC,* International Knee Documentation Committee; *MCID,* minimal clinically important differences; *MDC,* minimal detectable change; *OA,* osteoarthritis; *QOL,* quality of life measure; *PCL,* posterior cruciate ligament; *PF,* patellofemoral; *VAS,* visual analog scale.
This table includes populations of interest, scale of the instrument, the range of MCID across patient populations, and the range of MDC reported. The MCID value indicates the magnitude of the difference (whether the difference is an improvement or deterioration in outcome) that is necessary to be interpreted as a clinically important change (eg, a difference of 11.5 points, based on a 100-point scale). The MDC describes the magnitude of change that must occur for the instrument to confidently detect the difference.

allow for a more global assessment of a patient's general health status in conjunction with region specific function through the use of another outcome instrument.

Global Rating of Change

The global rating of change (GROC) scale is a basic PRO that allows for simple tracking of patient outcomes by determining how much better or worse the patient is feeling after an injury, treatment, or surgery. The GROC scale can have multiple forms. One commonly used GROC form consists of one item: a 15-point scale ranging from patients reporting they feel a great deal better (positive values) to a great deal worse (negative values). A score of zero means the patients perceived no change in their condition.[15,40]

Scoring of the GROC varies throughout the literature. In many cases, a value of −7 is assigned to the descriptor of greatest decrement, whereas a value of +7 is assigned to the descriptor of greatest improvement.[15,40] This system of scoring allows for easy comparison of patient reported changes over time with regard to function, symptoms, or affective outcome measures. Use of the GROC can be modified based on the question asked. For example, a patient can provide a GROC score when asked, "How would you rate your outcome following your shoulder surgery?" This scale can be used for a variety of conditions and patient populations to prospectively track improvement following injury or surgery. The primary strength of the GROC is its ability to provide an overall (global) understanding of how a patient perceives the outcome following their injury/condition/procedure.

Currently, this rating scale is most commonly used in research involving surgical interventions, knee OA, and patellofemoral pain.[11,39] Although this scale allows for an easy comparison over time, it is generally combined with a region or pathology specific scale, like the SF-36 and SF-12, to provide a more comprehensive review of patient outcome.[46] Currently, no minimal clinically important differences (MCID) have been established for this scale in patients with knee pathology because of the wide scope of populations and injury severities represented.

Visual Analog Scale

The Visual Analog Scale (VAS) is possibly the most easily understood and widely used pain rating scale in clinical research and clinical practice. Although there are many iterations of this scale, the concept remains consistent throughout. Patients are asked to place a mark intersecting a 100-mm line with two polar descriptors—for example, "no pain" at the low or "0" end of the scale and "worst imaginable pain" on the high or "100" end of the scale. The distance (in mm) from one end of the scale (the zero point or the point representing no pain) is then measured to represent the subjective level of pain perceived by the patient. VASs can also be used in an alternative form in which patients are asked to identify a number from 0 to 10 that represents their current level of perceived pain at a specific time or during an activity.[13] This form of VAS is considered to be more patient friendly as a result of the ease of completion; however, it may limit the sensitivity to change over time. In many cases, more than one VAS can be used to better characterize the pain or other symptoms experienced by the patient. These scales include such questions as current pain, worst pain in the previous 24 hours, worst pain during work-related activity, average pain over the previous 24 hours, least pain in the previous 24 hours, and so forth.[13] Although these are representative of some commonly used scales, the questions used can easily be altered to better fit both the patient population and pathology being studied.

The VAS has been shown to be valid and reliable in many forms throughout the literature and in many cases is commonly used as a gold standard when attempting to validate a new assessment instrument.* Sensitivity is highly variable depending on the structure of the scale used, the question of interest, and the population in which the measurement is taken. Although this flexibility and ease of application is a strength of the VAS, it may be difficult to establish clear cutoff points for patient improvement or clinically important scores within a specific patient population. Currently, MCID have been established in patients with knee OA (19.9 mm), hip OA (15.3 mm), and anterior knee pain (20.0 mm), indicating that a change of that magnitude would represent a clinically meaningful change (see Table 43.1).[11,51]

The VAS has been used as a framework for knee-specific outcomes scales. For example, the Knee Disorders Subjective History,[13] which is constructed using a series of VAS, has been used to characterize function following knee joint injury or surgery. This scale involves 28 questions about knee joint function during specific activities. For example, the question, "Do you feel grinding when your knee moves?" is rated on a 10-point scale ranging from " none" to "severe"; the question, "Is your knee stiff?" is rated on a 10-pont scale ranging from "none" to "I can barely move my knee because of stiffness." In this case, questions can be scored individually or combined for a total score.

The ACL Quality of Life Measure (ACL-QOL)[33] is another outcome measure that incorporates scores from a series of VASs (100 mm lines with polar descriptors) for 31 total questions. Scores for each question are combined to form a single score on a 100% scale where 100% indicates highest function/quality of life in ACL deficient patients. The scale is divided into subsections that ask specific questions about symptoms and physical complaints (4 questions), work-related concerns (4 questions), recreational activities and sports participation or competition (12 questions), lifestyle (6 questions), and social and emotional (5 questions). ACL deficient patients reporting a low score on this scale have been found to be more likely to go on to have reconstruction surgery as compared to patients who reported a higher score.[33]

Tegner Activity Rating

The Tegner Activity Rating was developed in 1985 as a patient reported score describing typical daily activities. This scale offers patients the choice of 10 distinct levels of physical activity participation, ranging from disability as a result of injury to elite athletics. The patient provides a rating (values are from 0 to 10, 10 indicating the highest level of activity) for both current level of activity and the level of activity prior to injury.[50] The available ratings are broken into four distinct regions, with a rating of 0 corresponding to disability as a result of knee

problems, 1 to 5 representing levels of work related activity and recreational sport, 6 to 9 representing competitive and higher levels of recreational and organized/competitive sports, and 10 representing the highest and most elite international or professional level competitive sport.[50] These levels, depending on the population of interest, may not adequately represent the spectrum of daily function and activity and therefore may not allow for clear comparison between patients. In practice, this scale is commonly associated with the Lysholm score and can allow for a reasonable characterization of patient activity levels, especially when measured in a preinjury physically active population. Currently, this scale has been shown to be valid and reliable in patients with meniscal injury, patellar instability, and ACL injury.[6,7,38] In patients with ACL injury, a minimal clinically important change of 1.0 has been established.[7] This suggests that a change in activity rating following ACL injury of at least one point needs to be met in order for the change to be considered clinically important. When the scale is used for young patients involved in high levels of activity, it is important to note that transitions from the higher ratings (competitive-elite sports) to lower levels (work and recreational activity) may reflect the natural course of time as an athlete graduates from competitive sports and begins to pursue other professional or life interests. Whether or not this change is a result of injury or other noninjury-related factors is a potential confounder to this score. Alternatives to this scale that may be more appropriate in the recreationally active or nonelite athletic population include the International Physical Activity Questionnaire[9] and the Marx Activity Scale.[8]

KNEE SPECIFIC OUTCOMES SCALES

International Knee Documentation Committee Subjective Knee Evaluation Form

The International Knee Documentation Committee Subjective Knee Evaluation Form (IKDC) was developed as a standardized assessment tool for knee injury and treatment. It was first published as a patient reported outcome measure in 1993 and revised to its current form in 1997. This scale is knee specific but allows for measurement of subjective outcomes regarding a variety of pathologies. Currently, the IKDC includes 18 total items regarding symptoms (7 items), general function (2 items), and sport activities (9 items).[20] Patients are encouraged to complete all of the included items; however, scoring is possible as long as 16 of 18 items are completed. Following completion, the scores are converted to a 100-point scale, with 100 representing the best possible score and highest knee function.[20] The strength of this rating scale lies in the diversity of items regarding both patient reported knee joint symptoms and function during activities that specifically involve the knee joint (walking, jogging, stair climbing, etc.), which allows for a better representation of the limitations or improvements that may be expected in a variety of populations and pathologies.

The IKDC has been shown to be both reliable and valid for a variety of pathologies, including ACL injury, meniscal injury, articular cartilage injury, patellofemoral pain, and knee OA.[1,19,21] Normative values have been established to allow for easy comparison of healthy and pathologic populations. A minimally important difference of 11.5 points has been suggested but has not been validated in all pathological populations (see Table 43.1).[21] The IKDC scale is available in several languages

---

*References 11, 13, 28, 37, 38, 39, 44, and 51.

and can be completed in less than 10 minutes. The IKDC represents a clear and concise assessment tool for knee related research that can be applied across pathologies and population characteristics.

Western Ontario and McMaster Universities Osteoarthritis Index

The Western Ontario and McMaster Universities Osteoarthritis Index (WOMAC) was developed to assess symptoms and function in patients with lower extremity OA. This scale is composed of 24 items divided among three subscales: pain (5 items), stiffness (2 items), and function (17 items). Each item asks the patient to provide a categorical or Likert rating (none, mild, moderate, severe, or extreme) in response. Each item is scored and combined in total or within each subscale and normalized to a 100-point scale where a score of 100 represents no symptoms and a score of 0 represents the worst symptoms.[45,57] The WOMAC is most commonly used for assessing changes in outcomes related to OA in the older adult population but has been used more broadly to measure change in symptoms and subjective outcomes in a spectrum of knee injuries.[4]

The WOMAC has become the most widely reported subjective outcome measure for patients with lower extremity OA and has been shown to be valid, reliable, and sensitive to change over time.[4] Minimal clinically important difference has been established as 9.1 points in the knee OA population indicating that total WOMAC score. This difference has also been calculated when the WOMAC is compared with the SF-36 in a rehabilitation population, with a 12% change from baseline was considered to be clinically important.[2] This value has not been validated in other populations but may act as a benchmark for comparison within the population of patients with OA. The WOMAC, which is currently available in several languages and several methods of administration, has been shown to take an average of 10 to 15 minutes to complete.[56,57] Although the WOMAC has several strengths and weakness, its prevalence in the knee and hip OA literature makes it an important consideration when assessing subject OA outcomes.

Knee Injury and Osteoarthritis Outcome Scale

The Knee Injury and Osteoarthritis Outcome Scale (KOOS) was first published in 1998 and was developed as a patient reported instrument to assess subjective opinion regarding their knee injury. As the name implies, this scale was designed for use in patients with knee OA and aptly includes the pain, stiffness, and function sections of the WOMAC scale, which allows for easy comparison of KOOS and WOMAC scores. More recently, this scale has been more broadly used in patients with knee injuries, which may result in posttraumatic OA.[42,45] The KOOS consists of 42 items divided within 5 subscales: pain (9 items), symptoms (7 items), function in daily living (17 items), knee related quality of life (4 items), and function in sport and recreation, which are scored on a 5 point Likert scale.[42,45] After completion, each subscale is normalized to a 100-point scale where a score of 100 represents no symptoms and a score of 0 represents the worst possible symptoms.[42,45] Although commonly done, a combination of these subscales is not recommended because each subscale has a variable number of items. The KOOS generally requires 10 to 15 minutes to complete and is available in several languages.

Validity and reliability of the KOOS has been established in patients following ACL reconstruction, partial meniscectomy,

tibial osteotomy, and when measuring the effects of posttraumatic OA.[12,42,44,45,55] It has been reported that a change of 8 to 10 points on a transformed subscale score may represent the minimal clinically important difference.[42] The KOOS has been shown to be most sensitive to change in young active populations, with greatest responsiveness on the function in sport and recreation, and knee related quality of life subscales. Despite this fact, the KOOS has been used in the literature in wide range of ages (18 to 78 years old) and levels of physical activity. Reference values for the healthy population across diverse age and gender characteristics are available and allow for easy comparison between healthy and pathologic populations.

Kujala Anterior Knee Pain Scale

The Kujala scale or Anterior Knee Pain Scale (AKPS) is a patient reported knee specific scale that was developed in 1993 for patients with anterior knee pain. This 13-item scale contains questions related to symptoms reported by patients both at rest and during specific functional tasks including walking, running, jumping, squatting, sitting for long periods of time, and stair climbing. Each item in the AKPS includes specific responses from which the patient can choose, each of which is assigned a point value to allow for easy scoring. The AKPS is based on a 100-point scale, with a score of 100 representing pain free function and a score of 0 representing the presence of maximal pain and worst function.[28]

The AKPS has been shown to be valid and reliable in differentiating the difference in severity of anterior knee pain as well as the effect of treatment on anterior knee pain. Sensitivity of this scale has been shown to be good to excellent in most cases, with the exclusion of differentiating between patients with repetitive patellar dislocation and those with one-time dislocations.[38] This may be a result of the lack of questions relating to the progression of the patient's condition and instead the exhaustive focus on the effects the condition has on daily symptoms and function (see Table 43.1).[24,47,54] In all cases, these differences were reported as improvements over time or following treatment. The AKPS is a widely used scale both clinically and in clinical research for monitoring longitudinal changes in patient reported symptoms and function and should be considered when attempting research regarding anterior knee or patellofemoral pain.

Other Common Scales

There are several other commonly used scales for various assessments of knee symptoms and functions. The Cincinnati Knee Rating Scale[34-36] assesses knee symptoms as well as functional activity to allow for assessment of six subscales scores as well as a 100 point composite score. The scale is a mixed survey which incorporates both clinician and patient reported scores and is most commonly used for assessment following ACL injury and ACL reconstruction.[34-36] Although it is considered to be comprehensive, it has only been partially validated.

Similar to the Cincinnati Knee Rating Scale, the Lysholm Knee Scale[6,7,25] is widely used for assessment of knee ligament injury and surgical outcomes. This scale consists of eight items (limp, support, stair climbing, squatting, instability, locking, catching, pain, and swelling) that are weighted and scored on a 100-point scale. The Lysholm Scale has been validated for several knee pathologies and is commonly combined with activity scales in an effort to achieve a comprehensive assessment of knee function.[6,7,25]

The ACL Quality of Life Scale[33] is a 32-item scale specifically designed as an outcome measure for chronic ACL deficiency. The 32 items are divided among 5 subscales (symptoms and physical complaints, work-related concerns, recreational activities and sport competition, lifestyle, and social and emotional function) and transformed to a 100-point scale. This scale has been shown to be valid and reliable, and may have some value in predicting which patients may eventually require surgical intervention.[33]

Finally, the Hospital for Special Surgery (HSS) Knee Score[14] was developed as an assessment for total knee replacement outcomes. The HSS Knee Scale is based on a 100-point scale, divided into seven categories.[14] This scale uses both patient and clinician reported outcomes and has been shown to be both valid and reliable when assessing patients with knee replacements.

COMMON STATISTICAL CONCEPTS IN OUTCOMES RESEARCH

Outcome scores can be used to describe the distribution and severity of disease, to assess responsiveness to treatments, and to test specific hypotheses related to outcomes research. Epidemiology is the study of the distribution/frequencies and determinants of injury and/or disease. Common measures of frequency include prevalence and incidence; common measures of association include relative risks (RRs) and odds ratios (ORs) (Table 43.2).

Prevalence and Incidence

Prevalence is calculated as the proportion of individuals within a population that have an outcome of interest now—or at a particular point in time. Prevalence values are calculated as the number of existing cases of disease or injury divided by the total population identified as at risk. Alternatively, incidence is the proportion of new cases of an outcome or disease within a specific time interval. Therefore, to calculate incidence, a follow-up period or time interval should be established. Absolute risk is a derivative of incidence, where the number of new occurrences of disease or injury over a period of time is divided by the total number of patients at risk. For example, if 6 of 100 patients undergoing ACL reconstruction report poor subjective outcomes at a 6-month follow-up evaluation, the absolute risk for poor outcome is 6% (6/100).

Relative Risk and Odds Ratio

RR is used to compare the incidence of injury or disease between two cohorts of patients. RR is calculated as the incidence of injury or disease in one group divided by the incidence of injury

TABLE 43.2	Common Epidemiologic Measures and Their Interpretation	
Measure	**Calculation**	**Interpretation**
Prevalence	$\dfrac{\text{\# Existing instances of outcome}}{\text{Total population at risk}}$	The proportion of individuals within a population who exhibit an outcome of interest
Incidence	$\dfrac{\text{\# New instances of outcome}}{\text{Total population at risk}}$	The proportion of new instances of an outcome of interest within a specific time interval
Absolute risk	$\dfrac{\text{\# New outcomes (incidence)}}{\text{Total population at risk}}$	The proportion of the population of interest that are at risk for developing the outcome of interest
Relative risk	$\dfrac{\text{Incidence in an exposed group}}{\text{Incidence in an unexposed group}}$	1.0: Risk/odds of outcome is identical between groups
>1.0: Risk/odds of outcome is greater in exposed vs. unexposed group <1.0: Risk/odds of outcome is less in exposed vs. unexposed group		
Odds ratio	$\dfrac{\text{Probability of outcome in an exposed group}}{\text{Probability of an outcome in an unexposed group}}$	
Specificity	True negatives/total patients without disease	Of all patients who *do not* have the disease or outcome of interest, the proportion who tested negative. Specific clinical tests have high true negative and low false positive rates.
Sensitivity	True positives/total patients with disease	Of all patients who have the disease or outcome of interest, the proportion who tested positive. Sensitive clinical tests have high true positive and low false negative rates.
Positive predictive value	True positives/total patients with positive test result	Proportion of patients with a positive test result who were correctly diagnosed
Negative predictive value	True negatives/total patients with negative test result	Proportion of patients with a negative test result who were correctly diagnosed.
Positive likelihood ratio	Sensitivity/(1−specificity)	Example: (+)LR = 5; a positive test indicates that the patient is 5-times more likely to have the outcome of interest than a patient with a negative result
Negative likelihood ratio	(1−sensitivity)/specificity	Example: (−)LR = 0.2; a negative test will be present in only 2 out of every 10 patients who actually have the outcome of interest.

LR, Likelihood ratios.

or disease in another group. Groups can be defined as a cohort of patients who were exposed to risk or an intervention. For example, RR could be used to compare the incidence of symptomatic OA in patients with and without a history of ACL reconstruction. RR values range from 0 to infinity and are interpreted relative to a value of 1.0. RR equal to 1.0 indicates that the incidence of the outcome of interest is identical in the exposed and unexposed groups. RR less than 1 indicates an inverse relationship, or decreased risk in the exposed group and a RR greater than 1 indicates increased risk among patients in the exposed group (group presented in the numerator of the RR calculation). When comparing a treatment (exposed) versus a control group for a particular outcome of interest, an RR of 0.5 indicates that treated patients have $\frac{1}{2}$ the risk for developing the outcome of interest, whereas an RR of 2.5 indicates a $2\frac{1}{2}$ times increased risk of developing the outcome of interest when in the treatment group. Because RR values are calculated from incidence rates (requiring a follow-up period), they are most appropriate for prospective cohort studies or clinical trials.

Odds can be calculated as the proportion of patients with an injury, disease, or outcome of interest divided by the proportion of patients who do not have the injury, disease, or outcome of interest. ORs compare odds in a group of patients who have been exposed to a particular risk factor or treated in an intervention study with a cohort of patients who were not exposed to either the risk factor or the treatment. ORs are more commonly used in retrospective studies, and the interpretation of an OR is similar to the interpretation of an RR in most cases.

Reliability, Validity, Accuracy, and Precision

Reliability is concerned with the reproducibility of a measure, whereas validity describes the ability of a measure, test, or instrument to effectively represent truth and reality. Accuracy describes the ability of a test or measure to differentiate between positive (+) and negative (−) diagnoses. Therefore, accuracy of a particular diagnostic test or outcome instrument can be calculated by dividing the number of times the test correctly diagnosed the disease of interest with a positive result (true positives) added to the number of times the test correctly determined the absence of a disease with a negative result (true negatives) divided by the total number of patients in a given study (Table 43.3). Precision describes the repeatability of a test result with multiple testing. (Is the test yielding similar scores/results when the same specimen/patient is tested on multiple occasions?)

Sensitivity, Specificity and Likelihood Ratios

Sensitivity, specificity, positive, and negative predictive values can be calculated from a contingency table (see Table 43.3). Sensitivity describes the ability to detect true positive test results, where specificity describes the ability to detect true negative test results (see Tables 43.2 and 43.3). When a highly sensitive (Sn) test is negative (N) (high sensitivity), it is good for ruling OUT an injury (mnemonic: SnNOUT). When a highly specific (Sp) test is positive (P) (high specificity), the test is good for ruling IN an injury or disease (mnemonic: SpPIN).

Likelihood ratios (LR) are calculated from sensitivity and specificity. Positive LR describes the impact of a positive examination finding (clinical test) on the probability that a disease exists: (+)LR = sensitivity/(1 − specificity). Negative LR describes the impact of a negative clinical test on the probability that the disease is present: (−)LR = (1−sensitivity)/specificity.

TABLE 43.3 Effectiveness of Diagnostic Tools Can Be Measured by Constructing a 2×2 Contingency Table That Compares the Outcome of a Specific Diagnostic Test Versus a Gold Standard

	Disease Present (+)	Disease Absent (−)	
Diagnostic test (+)	True positives	False positives	a
Diagnostic test (−)	False negatives c	True negatives d	b

[a]Positive predictive value = True positives/total patients with positive test result.
[b]Negative predictive value = True negatives/total patients with negative test result.
[c]Sensitivity = True positives/total patients with disease.
[d]Specificity = True negatives/total patients without disease.
In a person who has the disease or outcome of interest, a positive diagnostic test will indicate a "true positive," whereas a negative diagnostic test will indicate a "false negative." Likewise, in a person who does not have the disease or outcome of interest, a positive test result will indicate a "false positive," whereas a negative diagnostic test will indicate a "true negative."

Receiver operating characteristic (ROC) curves are graphical representations of the relationships between sensitivity and specificity, where the sensitivity value is plotted on the vertical axis and 1−specificity is plotted on the y-axis. The area under the ROC curve is an estimate of the overall diagnostic value of a given test. When the area under the ROC curve equals 1.0, the test has perfect diagnostic value. An area of 0.5 indicates the diagnostic value of a particular test is no better than random guessing.

Hypothesis Testing Using Outcomes Data

Outcomes data or dependent variables that are collected during a research study can be patient reported (as described earlier in this chapter) or objective (measured by an instrument or other device). The data can be summarized with descriptive statistics including the mean (arithmetic average), median (value dividing data set into equal halves), and mode (most commonly occurring data value). Data distributions are presented as histograms to visualize these descriptive statistic concepts. When a dataset is normally distributed, the mean, median, and mode are the same value (Fig. 43.1).

Data collected from a patient, subject, specimen, and so forth can be classified as continuous or categorical. Continuous data such as height, weight, time, age, and so forth have an infinite number of possible values. In contrast, categorical or discrete data can be binary (yes/no, failure/success, satisfactory/unsatisfactory, gender), ordered (severities—mild, moderate, severe; outcome—excellent, good, fair, poor) or unordered (race). Categorical data have a discrete number of possible values, and therefore the most commonly reported descriptive statistic for categorical data is the mode.

Confidence intervals (CI) quantify the precision of a mean or another statistic such as an OR or RR. CIs take into account the variability and sample size used to calculate the statistic of interest (Fig. 43.2). A 95% confidence interval describes a range of data values around a sample statistic (mean, OR, RR) where there is 95% certainty that the actual value representative of the entire population lies somewhere within the calculated upper and lower limits of the CI. CIs can provide an estimate of the variability of sample data; hence they can estimate the precision

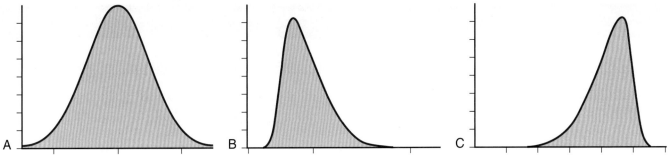

FIG 43.1 (A) Histogram showing a graphical depiction of tabulated data frequencies—the data are normally distributed; therefore, the mean, median, and mode are the same value. Examples of non-normally distributed data are (B) skewed to the right *(positive skew)* and (C) skewed to the left *(negative skew).*

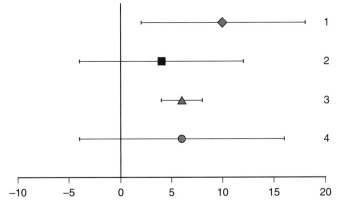

FIG 43.2 Confidence Intervals Quantify the Precision of a Mean or Another Statistic Such as an Odds Ratio or Relative Risk. A 95% confidence interval describes a range of data values around a sample statistic (mean, OR, RR) where there is 95% certainty that the actual value representative of the entire population lies somewhere within the calculated upper and lower limits of the CI. In this example, (1) Represents a measure with a mean of 10 in which there is 95% confidence that the true value of the outcome measure falls between 2 and 18. Although not precise, there is high confidence of a positive finding. (2) Represents a mean of 4 and identical precision to the measure in example 1. In this case, the CI crosses 0 indicating that a positive or negative finding may be possible. (3) Represents a mean of 6 with a confidence interval spanning from 4 to 8, which may represent a more precise measurement as compared to example 4, despite an identical mean estimate. (4) Represents a mean of 6 with a confidence interval spanning -4 to 16, which is indicative of a less precise measurement as compared to example 3, despite an identical mean estimate.

of the measure. Furthermore, CIs present accuracy of the test statistic to represent reality. CIs that are large have poorer precision and are less likely to be accurate. Small CIs have better precision and are more likely to be accurate.

Parametric and Nonparametric Inferential Statistics

Inferential statistics attempt to generalize findings from a representative sample to the entire population. Inferential statistics can be divided into parametric statistics and nonparametric statistics. Parametric tests use the mean and standard deviations

when comparing groups or identifying associations and are best suited for normally distributed continuous data. Nonparametric statistical tests use medians and ranks and are therefore more powerful alternatives when data are not normally distributed because they are less sensitive to outliers (more robust), or when sample sizes are low. The goal of inferential statistics is to estimate parameters (descriptors of the entire population), and therefore, statistical tests should be parametric if possible (Table 43.4).

Statistical Tests for Comparing Two Groups

If a research study proposes to compare two groups of data, whether they are paired or independent, the *t*-test is appropriate. There are two basic types of *t*-tests. Paired *t*-tests are used to compare data from paired samples or data collected from the same person. The independent samples *t*-test is used to compare continuous data between two independent groups. The nonparametric equivalent to the paired samples *t*-test is the Wilcoxon signed rank test, the nonparametric equivalent to the independent samples *t*-test is the Mann-Whitney U test.

Statistical Tests for Comparing More Than Two Groups

If a research study proposes to compare three or more groups, an analysis of variance (ANOVA) is the appropriate inferential statistical test. The ANOVA can be used to compare three or more independent groups of data. For example, an ANOVA could be used when comparing PRO among patients treated with treatment A, treatment B, and treatment C. When comparing data collected from the same subjects (at multiple time points, for example), the repeated measures ANOVA is appropriate. An advantage of the ANOVA model is the ability to control for other variables that may influence an outcome within a specific group or at a specific time point. When a confounding factor exists and influences the outcome of a study, an analysis of co-variance (ANCOVA) is appropriate. An example would be a case in which one group was significantly older than the other groups in a given study. The nonparametric equivalent for the ANOVA is the Kruskal-Wallis Test; Friedman's test is a nonparametric test similar to the repeated measures ANOVA.

Post Hoc Tests

Specific between group comparisons are necessary after a statistically significant (ie, $p \leq .05$) ANOVA or F-test to determine the exact characteristics of group differences. The

TABLE 43.4   Summary of Common Patient Reported Outcome Measures Used in the Clinical and Research Environments[18]

Scale	Common Uses	Specific Populations	Scale Range (Total Score)	MCID (Units)	MDC (Units)
SF-36	Well-being	Severe knee OA[2]	0-100 points	7.8	
Tegner activity rating[50]	Physical activity level	All populations	0-10 levels	Not reported	1.0
Marx Activity Scale[32]	Physical activity level	ACL injury	0-16 points	Not reported	9.9
VAS[11,51]	Pain	Knee injury and OA	0-100 millimeters	19.9-20.0	
IKDC[21]	Knee related function	ACL injury, PCL injury, meniscus injury, articular cartilage injury, PF pain	0-100 points	3.19-16.7	6.7-20.5
Cincinnati Knee Scale[3]	Knee related function	ACL injury, PCL injury, meniscus injury, articular cartilage injury, PF pain, tibial osteotomy	0-100 points	14.0-26.0	27.5
KOOS[43]	Knee related function	Knee OA, ACL injury, meniscus injury, cartilage injury	0-100 points	Not reported	Symptoms = 9.9-24.3
				Not reported	Pain = 11.8-29.0
				Not reported	ADL = 11.9-31.5
				Not reported	Sports = 12.2-70.0
				Not reported	QOL = 14.2-34.0
WOMAC[5]	Knee related function	Rheumatoid arthritis, knee OA	0-100 points	Pain = 7.5-17.5	Pain = 14.4-16.2
				Function = 5.89-8.1	Function = 10.6-15.0
				Stiffness = 6.3-18.8	Stiffness = 22.9-30.6
				Overall = 11.5	Overall = 10.7-15.3
Lysholm Scale[30]	Knee related function	ACL injury, PCL injury, meniscus injury, articular cartilage injury, PF pain	0-100 points	10.1	8.9-15.8

This table includes populations of interest, scale of the instrument, the range of minimal clinically important differences across patient populations and the range of minimal detectable change reported. The MCID value indicates the magnitude of the difference (whether the difference is an improvement or deterioration in outcome) that is necessary to be interpreted as a clinically important change. For example, a difference of 11.5 points (based on a 100-point scale). The minimal detectable change (MDC) describes the magnitude of change that must occur for the instrument to confidently detect the difference.

p-value associated with the ANOVA test only indicates that a difference exists somewhere between the groups compared. In the hypothetical example provided, post hoc tests would be used to compare outcomes among (1) treatment groups A and B, (2) treatment groups A and C, and (3) treatment groups B and C. Each of these post hoc tests would have an associated p-value indicating the presence of a statistically significant difference (ie, if the p-value is 0.05 or less). Examples of common post hoc tests are Tukey, Sidak, Dunnet, Scheffe, and so forth.

Statistical Tests for Categorical Data

The Chi-square test and Fisher exact test are appropriate when data are categorical. For example, when comparing patient outcomes (good, fair, poor) between treatment A and treatment B, these tests would be appropriate. A statistically significant test is interpreted, in the example given previously, that a relationship between outcome and treatment exists. Constructing a contingency table to evaluate frequencies would aid in interpreting the relationship. The Fisher exact test may be used when sample sizes are low or when the number of occurrences in one of the "categories" (eg, only one person with treatment B had a poor outcome) is small.

Statistical Tests for Describing Relationships

Correlations describe the strength of a relationship between two variables. A Pearson product moment correlation coefficient (r) is used to correlate two arrays of continuous, normally distributed data. The value of a correlation coefficient can range from −1 to 0 to +1. Values closer to + or −1 indicate stronger relationships. Values closer to 0 indicate weaker relationships. Positive correlation coefficients represent direct relationships. Positive correlations indicate a relationship where patients who score high on one scale tend to also score high on the other scale. Correlation coefficients that are negative indicate indirect relationships where patients who score high on one scale tend to score low on another scale. Although several interpretations of the magnitude of a correlation coefficients have been proposed, a common method describes the strength of a correlation coefficient that is less than 0.33 to be "weak," between 0.33 and 0.66 as "moderate," and greater than 0.66 as "strong."

Spearman Rho is the nonparametric equivalent to the Pearson correlation coefficient and is appropriate for non-normally distributed or categorical data. Both correlation coefficients have associated p-values that describe whether the coefficient represents a true relationship (ie, $p = .05$ or less) or is a result of chance ($p > .05$).

Probability Values and Statistical Error

Test statistics are typically reported with an associated probability value (p-value) that helps researchers interpret the test statistics as being "statistically significant" or "statistically nonsignificant." This decision is made based on an arbitrary decision regarding an acceptable rate of committing a Type I error. In statistics, a Type I error is the probability of being wrong when concluding that a relationship among test variables exists (ie, observing differences when in truth there are none). As a matter of tradition, we typically accept this type of error 5% of the time or less. Therefore, if the *p*-value is less than or equal to 0.05, we conclude a statistically significant relationship. The correct interpretation of *p*-values less than or equal to 0.05 is that the observed relationship or difference is most likely not a result of chance. Conversely, a *p*-value greater than 0.05 indicates that observed differences or relationships likely resulting from chance alone, and not resulting from the hypothesized differences or relationships. The *p*-value is influenced by the variability of the data, the number of subjects from which data was collected, and the magnitude of the differences between groups. It is most difficult to observe statistically significant differences if data variability is high, if the number of subjects is low, and/or if the magnitude of difference is minimal.

Minimal Clinically Important Differences

Descriptive and inferential statistics are among the many tools in the researchers' toolbox to describe study data and highlight group differences and/or relationships. Typically, the *p*-value associated with a particular statistical test is used to determine whether a statistical difference or relationship is statistically significant (ie, likely not a result of chance when the *p*-value is 0.05 or less). When interpreting study data, it is important to not only consider statistical test findings and *p*-values that describe statistically significant relationships but also determine the clinical importance or meaningfulness of the observed differences or relationships. The concept of MCID has been described as a difference in outcome score in a clinical research study that a patient perceives as beneficial or that would necessitate a change in treatment.[10,16,22] For example, small differences/changes that are observed in a clinical research study (or clinical trial) that are statistically significant may or may not be large enough to result in a benefit to patients. Therefore, both statistical significance and/or clinical importance should be considered when drawing conclusions from study data.

MCID values can be calculated using a distribution approach, anchor approach, and expert opinion approach.[31] In the distribution approach, CI are calculated and compared between groups. If there is no overlap among the ranges of the CI from two independent groups, then the difference is said to have reached a clinically important difference. The anchor method for determining the MCID is to compare the changes detected with a particular outcomes instrument with an existing validated "gold standard."[41] This will allow development of a 2X2 contingency table and calculation of specificity, sensitivity, and other statistics described earlier in this chapter. Finally, the expert opinion method of determining MCID takes into consideration input from patients or expert health care professionals.

The MCID should not be confused with the minimal detectable change (MDC), which is a statistical estimate of the smallest change that can be detected by a given measure or patient reported outcome. Although many of the components required to calculate the MDC are similar to those used to calculate the MCID, the MDC is purely a comparison of the clinical or research finding to the inherent error present when using a specific measurement tool. For example, if a 2-degree change in active knee extension range of motion was assessed using a goniometer, when compared to the MDC which has been established as 8.2 degrees, the clinician should have low confidence that a measurable change actually occurred.[29] The MDC can be calculated in a number of ways; however, most commonly it is derived from the standard error of the measurement tool as estimated over multiple days. The MDC is an extremely important statistic to be considered when evaluating changes in clinical findings and, when combined with the MCID, enables the clinician or researcher to have the highest confidence in their findings.

Another way to interpret study differences is to calculate an effect size. Effect sizes measure the magnitude of a treatment effect. These statistics not only describe the mean difference between treatment groups but also account for data variability. To calculate an effect size, the difference between treatment groups is divided by the standard deviation; therefore, if data are highly variable, then the estimated effect size will weaken. Effect sizes range in value from 0 to infinity, where values closer to zero indicate no treatment effect and are interpreted as stronger as the value increases. Although there are different ways to interpret the magnitude of effect sizes, one common method is to consider effect sizes less than 0.2 "small"; less than 0.5 are considered "medium," and 0.8 and higher are considered "large."

In summary, the MCID value describes the minimum difference that needs to be observed following a treatment for the change to be considered clinically meaningful or important. The MCID values can be used to determine the minimum necessary reduction or improvement in outcome score to be considered clinically important.

KEY REFERENCES

8. Cameron KL, Peck KY, Thompson BS, et al: Reference values for the Marx Activity Rating Scale in a young athletic population: history of knee ligament injury is associated with higher scores. *Sports Health* 7(5):403–408, 2015.

18. Irrgang J: Summary of clinical outcome measures for sports-related knee injuries: final report, 2012, Baltimore, AOSSM Outcomes Task Force, pp 1–391.

31. Make B: How can we assess outcomes of clinical trials: the MCID approach. *COPD* 4(3):191–194, 2007.

41. Romero L, Nieuwenhuijse M, Carr A, et al: Review of clinical outcomes-based anchors of minimum clinically important differences in hip and knee registry-based reports and publications. *J Bone Joint Surg Am* 96(Suppl 1):98–103, 2014.

57. Wright RW: Knee injury outcomes measures. *J Am Acad Orthop Surg* 17(1):31–39, 2009.

The references for this chapter can also be found on www.expertconsult.com.

44

Medial Ligamentous Injuries of the Knee: Acute and Chronic

Ian Power, Gehron Treme, Robert C. Schenck, Jr.

ANATOMY AND BIOMECHANICS

Sound treatment rationales and reproducible reconstruction results require a working knowledge of the structures of the medial side of the knee. Several studies have made useful contributions to the current understanding of the anatomy and biomechanics of these structures.

The anatomic study by Warren and Marshall provides the basis for knowledge of the medial side of the knee.[53] In their classic paper the authors described medial knee anatomy using a spatial concept of three distinct layers (Fig. 44.1). Layer 1 consists of the crural fascia of the knee and is present from the patella anteriorly to the popliteal fossa posteriorly. The sartorius fascia is found in this layer and blends with the crural fascia anteriorly as it attaches to the tibia. The gracilis (G) and semitendinosus tendons are found between layers 1 and 2.

Layer 2 is the superficial medial collateral ligament (SMCL), which, in the absence of scarring, can be easily identified deep to the G and semitendinosus tendons after the crural fascia is incised. In a quantitative study, LaPrade et al. found that the superficial MCL (sMCL) attached to the femur an average of 3.2 mm proximal and 4.8 mm posterior to the medial epicondyle (Fig. 44.2).[32] The tibial attachment of the SMCL has two divisions, with the proximal division attaching to soft tissue and the distal division attaching directly to the posteromedial tibia. The vertically oriented fibers of the SMCL blend with more obliquely oriented fibers in the posterior portion of the knee capsule and semimembranosus insertion at the posteromedial corner (PMC) (Fig. 44.3). This blending of tissue planes forms the posteromedial capsular pouch enveloping the medial femoral condyle.

The third and final layer of the knee consists of the knee joint capsule. The capsule thickens from anterior to posterior and a distinct component of the capsule deep to the SMCL represents the deep medial collateral ligament (dMCL), which has meniscofemoral and meniscotibial attachments but no attachment to the overlying SMCL.[32] Recently the nomenclature describing the structures of the PMC have become better defined in the orthopedic literature.[27,32,44] The posterior oblique ligament (POL) has been identified as a thickening of the posterior medial capsule in this region, and its importance in medial stability has become increasingly recognized. The POL attaches proximal and posterior to the attachment site of the SMCL on the femur. The previously described oblique portion of the SMCL is now recognized as the POL. The POL has a superficial, central, and capsular arm, with the central arm being the

most robust of the three and the primary portion of the POL that should be repaired or reconstructed with medial injuries (Fig. 44.4). The PMC is further reinforced by contributions from the semimembranosus and its sheath through multiple attachments.

In contrast to the anatomic nomenclature, little debate exists regarding the biomechanical role of the medial knee structures. Robinson et al. found that the anterior aspect of the SMCL remained taught throughout motion, whereas the PMC consistently loosened in flexion and tightened in full extension and internal rotation.[44] Griffith et al. demonstrated that both divisions of the SMCL serve as primary restraints to valgus load and external rotation with the degree of knee flexion affecting the load response.[21] In addition, the POL serves as a restraint to internal rotation and valgus at and approaching full extension and exhibits a flexion-dependent reciprocal role in resistance to internal rotation with the SMCL. In a second biomechanical study, Griffith et al. further defined the primary static stabilizers of the knee.[20] The authors found that the proximal division of the SMCL serves as the primary stabilizer to valgus stress, the distal division of the SMCL as the primary stabilizer to external rotation at 30 degrees of flexion, and that, when viewed as a single functional unit, the SMCL serves as a primary restraint to valgus and internal rotation at all flexion angles and to external rotation at 30 degrees of flexion. The primary restraints to internal rotation were the POL and distal SMCL division at all flexion angles. In addition, they found that the dMCL had important contribution to flexion dependent internal rotation stability. Wijdicks et al. found that these relationships and load values changed with sequential cutting of structures, demonstrating the intricate load-sharing properties of the medial knee structures.[55]

DIAGNOSIS

As with any injured extremity, examination of the knee with a suspected medial side injury should follow a standard stepwise process. A thorough history can frequently lead the examiner to suspect a medial collateral ligament (MCL) injury. Asking the patient to describe the injury can be a useful way to extract valuable information. Isolated MCL injuries occur with a valgus moment across a flexed knee and may occur in a contact or noncontact situation. Rotational mechanisms more commonly result in multiple ligament damage.

Inspection of knee alignment and the soft tissue envelope can give clues to the severity of the injury. A hemarthrosis raises

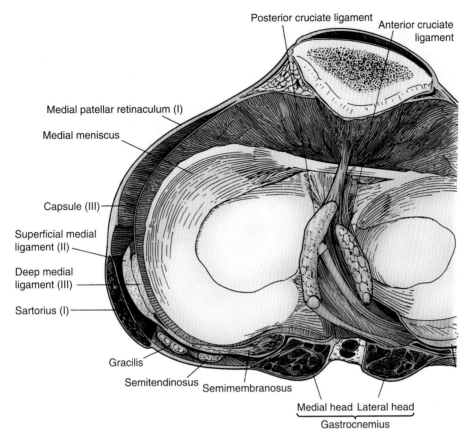

FIG 44.1 Cross-section of the knee demonstrating the layering concept as described by Warren and Marshall. Note the sartorius fascia, SMCL, and dMCL, with the pes tendons between layers 1 and 2. (From Radnay CS, Silver SG: Medial ligament injuries of the knee. In Scott WN [ed]: *Insall and Scott surgery of the knee*, ed 4, Philadelphia, 2006, Churchill Livingstone.)

suspicion of intra-articular involvement, as opposed to localized swelling usually seen with isolated MCL injury. Depending on the acuity, bruising can also be seen along the medial side of the knee. The patient's neurovascular status should be evaluated and documented, particular in the case of suspected multiligament injury. Patients with an MCL injury will typically have pain along the expanse of the ligament with a point of focal maximal tenderness depending on the point of rupture. Although frequently challenging secondary to patient discomfort, a standard cruciate exam and evaluation of the lateral structures should always be completed. In the acute situation, resting the flexed knee on a pillow improves patient tolerance to the ligamentous examination and improves the quality of information obtained. The amount of joint line opening with valgus stress at 0 and 30 degrees determines the grade of the MCL injury. Comparison is made to the uninjured knee with less than 5 mm of increased opening, indicating a grade I injury, 5 to 10 mm grade II, and more than 10 mm grade III. Placing a finger along the joint line and comparing to the uninjured knee helps to quantify the amount of joint line opening. The quality of the endpoint should also be recorded. Increased laxity in full extension is indicative of injury to the POL and often indicates a combined ligament injury, most commonly an anterior cruciate ligament (ACL) tear. Fetto found an 80% incidence of combined ligament injury with grade III MCL tears.[14] Attention should also be paid to rotational instability. The PMC complex limits internal rotation of the knee and

increased rotational motion should raise suspicion of injury to this structure. Increased external rotation has been primarily attributed to lateral side and PCL injury. However, Griffith et al. demonstrated that the SMCL serves as primary restraint to ER, and this should be considered during that portion of the exam.[20] Use of visual inspection of the tibia during external rotation will help to determine if the increased external rotation is related to medial or lateral injury. Injury to the medial structures will result in the anteromedial tibia rotating anteriorly, whereas the posterolateral tibia will effectively fall away when increased external rotation results from a lateral injury. Often with multiligamentous injuries an examination under anesthesia is needed to determine the degree of functional integrity for collateral ligaments.

IMAGING

Initial imaging examination should begin with standard radiographs. With acute or subacute injury, standard anterior to posterior, lateral, and sunrise patella views are obtained with special attention given to the potential for fracture and to joint malalignment, indicating multiligament injury. Widening of the joint space on non–weight-bearing films is frequently seen in the multiligament injured knee. The chronically injured knee should have a full complement of weight-bearing radiographs with the addition of a Rosenberg view to assess the amount of joint wear resulting from the chronic injury. Long cassette

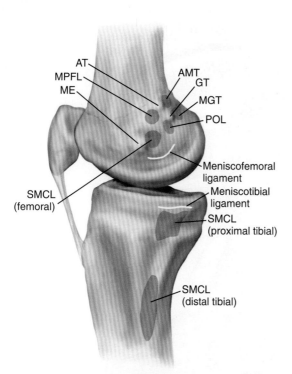

FIG 44.2 Illustration of the femoral osseous landmarks and attachment sites of the main medial knee structures. *AMT,* Adductor magnus tendon; *AT,* adductor tubercle; *GT,* gastrocnemius tubercle; *ME,* medial epicondyle; *MGT,* medial gastrocnemius tendon; *MPFL,* medial patellofemoral ligament; *POL,* posterior oblique ligament; *SMCL,* superficial medial collateral ligament. (Reprinted with permission from LaPrade RF, Engebretsen AH, Ly TV, et al: The anatomy of the medial side of the knee. *J Bone Joint Surg Am* 89(9):2000, 2007.)

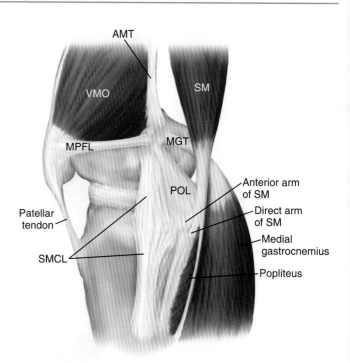

FIG 44.3 Illustration of the main medial knee structures (right knee). *AMT,* Adductor magnus tendon; *MGT,* medial gastrocnemius tendon; *MPFL,* medial patellofemoral ligament; *POL,* posterior oblique ligament; *SM,* semimembranosus muscle; *SMCL,* superficial medial collateral ligament; *VMO,* vastus medialis obliquus muscle. (Reprinted with permission from LaPrade RF, Engebretsen AH, Ly TV, et al: The anatomy of the medial side of the knee. *J Bone Joint Surg Am* 89(9):2000, 2007.)

standing radiographs help to define joint alignment, which may be critical in determining options for reconstruction. Stress radiography may be used to confirm the diagnosis of a medial side injury, to quantify the amount of laxity compared with the uninjured knee, and to monitor results of reconstruction or repair after surgery.

Magnetic resonance has become an invaluable tool to assess the medial ligamentous structures and can define the location and quality of the MCL injury (Figs. 44.5 and 44.6). In addition, magnetic resonance imaging (MRI) allows for evaluation for meniscal lesions, osteochondral injury, or damage to other ligaments. Distal avulsion of the MCL with displacement superficial to the pes tendons, similar to a Stener lesion in the thumb, may indicate a need for operative repair. Rubin et al. compared MRI findings with findings at the time of surgery and noted respective diagnostic sensitivity and specificity of 94% and 99% for ligament and meniscal damage with an isolated injury.[45] These values decreased to 88% and 84%, respectively, when two or more structures were damaged. In addition, Rasenberg et al. noted a high degree of agreement between instrumented grading of MCL injury to grading by MRI.[42] Miller et al. noted that trabecular microfractures occurred in 45% of patients with isolated MCL tears and that all of these injuries resolved in 2 to 4 months on follow-up imaging.[37] The information found with MRI should be correlated with the history and physical exam

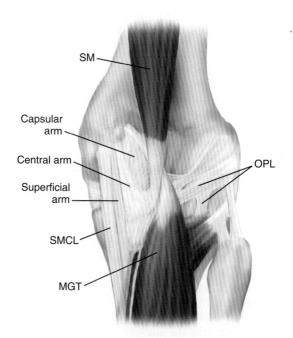

FIG 44.4 Illustration of the three arms of the posterior oblique ligament (posteromedial aspect, right knee). *MGT,* Medial gastrocnemius tendon; *OPL,* oblique popliteal ligament; *SM,* semimembranosus muscle; *SMCL,* superficial medial collateral ligament. (Reprinted with permission from LaPrade RF, Engebretsen AH, Ly TV, et al: The anatomy of the medial side of the knee. *J Bone Joint Surg Am* 89(9):2000, 2007.)

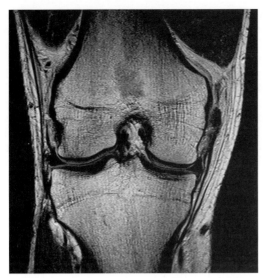

FIG 44.5 Coronal MRI of a proximal MCL rupture.

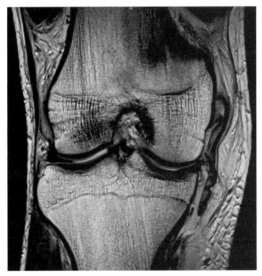

FIG 44.6 Coronal MRI of a distal MCL rupture.

to determine the extent of injury and develop an appropriate plan of care for the patient.

Ultrasonography is a less expensive imaging modality that can be used to identify intact and injured medial knee structures, including deep and superficial MCL, POL, and semimembranosus structures and attachments. Drawbacks include need for a skilled technician to perform the exam and interpretation, making it less common at this time.[7]

TREATMENT

Brace Wear

Prevention of MCL injuries has been studied extensively. The use of prophylactic knee braces (PKBs) to protect the medial knee structures is commonly used in collegiate down linemen. Several studies have shown that PKBs decrease strain on the MCLs.[6,15,16] Surrogate modeling in vitro testing demonstrates that bracing decreases forces across the MCL by 20% to 30%, with custom bracing providing improved protection over off-the-shelf versions.[6] Though these models have been validated,

obvious limitations exist when comparing a surrogate knee model loaded in an in vitro setting with the athlete's knee injured during competition.

Similar to laboratory testing, clinical studies have demonstrated some limited protective benefit to PKBs in certain sporting populations.[1,2,49] Sitler et al. analyzed the effects of prophylactic knee bracing on knee injury in West Point cadets playing full-contact American football.[49] The incidence of MCL injuries was decreased in braced defensive players compared with unbraced controls. However, severity of injury was not affected by brace wear. In addition, in a study sponsored by the Big Ten football conference, Albright et al. demonstrated that linemen, linebackers, and tight ends were at highest risk for MCL injury, bracing consistently decreasing injury rates both at practice and in games.[2] The linebacker and tight end groups were less likely to wear PKBs, citing the concern for performance limitation in the brace.

Well-documented performance effects of prophylactic knee bracing exist. Styf et al. showed that intramuscular pressures increased with brace wear and raised the potential for early muscle fatigue as a result.[51] Greene et al. demonstrated that some braces worn to protect against knee injury might result in decreased speed and agility.[19] With a trade-off in protection for performance, a decision must be made as to which athletes benefit most from prophylactic bracing.[38] The most common practice is for PKB use in offensive and defensive down linemen with skill position players opting to perform without braces.

ISOLATED MEDIAL COLLATERAL LIGAMENT INJURY

Injury to the MCL results in a robust healing response because of its blood supply, relatively wide surface area, association with other secondary stabilizers, and extra-articular location. These factors contribute to the well-documented ability of the MCL to heal without the need for surgical repair or reconstruction. In the absence of injury to secondary stabilizers, particularly the ACL, acute MCL injuries will heal with rare exception. In a rabbit model, Frank et al. showed that MCL injuries at the proximal or distal insertion sites were slower to heal than those seen for midsubstance disruption.[17]

The mainstay of treatment of isolated MCL injuries has long been nonoperative with an expectation of good outcomes.* Lundberg and Messner reported patients treated nonoperatively with grade I or II MCL injury can expect good return of function, normal to near-normal stability, and no increased risk of osteoarthritis at 10-year follow-up.[35] The authors felt that exclusion of additional ligament injury, namely ACL injury, was imperative to successful treatment of these injuries. Indelicato et al. followed 21 athletes for a mean of 46 months with isolated grade III MCL injuries nonoperatively and demonstrated 95% good and excellent results.[28] The average return to full-contact sport was 9.2 weeks after injury for the group, and all athletes with remaining college eligibility returned to play football. Holden et al. treated 51 football players with grade I and II MCL injuries nonoperatively, with 80% of the players returning to sport in an average of 21 days.[26] The 20% of players who failed to complete the rehabilitation were found to have previously unrecognized associated injury to the ACL and/or the medial

---

*References 9, 26, 28, 29, 35, 43, and 52.

meniscus. The authors stressed that truly isolated injury to the MCL could be treated nonoperatively with an expectation of good functional results and that vigilance is required to detect other potential injuries because their presence consistently compromised results of rehabilitation. Jones et al. reported on 24 high school football players with isolated grade III MCL injuries treated nonoperatively.[29] Twenty-two of the 24 athletes returned to football in an average of 34 days.

Although no standardized rehabilitation protocol for isolated MCL injury exists, several basic tenants of treatment are typically used. First, the knee is stabilized in a brace to protect against a second valgus insult. Bracing may also improve pain control and allow the injured athlete to more actively participate in the rehabilitation program. Second, early motion and weight bearing is encouraged and improves the rate and quality of the healing response.[52] Third, quadriceps and hamstring strengthening are started early in the process to prevent deconditioning and optimize the function of the knee's dynamic stabilizers. The decision to allow athletes to return to play is dictated by their pain level, functional improvement, and stability on exam. In a prospective study of athletes with grade III MCL injuries, Reider et al. instituted a functional rehabilitation program that adhered to these principles.[43] At 5-year follow-up the mean Hospital for Special Surgery knee score was 45.9, and the authors thought that the functional, nonoperative treatment of these injuries with functional rehabilitation produced results as good as surgical treatment or immobilization without the treatment-related morbidity of those two approaches.

COMBINED INJURIES

Anterior Cruciate Ligament and Medial Collateral Ligament

Although recommendations for the treatment of isolated MCL injuries have been well established, the appropriate treatment of patients with combined ACL and MCL injuries continues to evolve. The ACL acts as a secondary stabilizer to valgus stress in the knee and, as such, contributes to the innate healing potential of the MCL, when intact. Similarly, an intact MCL improves healing of a reconstructed ACL. Loss of a functional ACL has been shown to diminish the capacity of the MCL to heal with nonoperative treatment.[57] Bates et al. demonstrated in a kinetic cadaver study with vertical jump simulation that the isolated ACL provides more stability to anterior and medial forces, as well as flexion, abduction, and adduction torque than the isolated MCL, suggesting the first priority should be reconstructing the ACL.[3] Similarly, Zhang et al. demonstrated that simultaneous combined reconstruction showed improved valgus, anteromedial, and anteroposterior stability at 2-year follow-up.[61]

Some concerns have been raised regarding residual laxity in valgus after ACL reconstruction and the effects this may have on the reconstructed knee. Zaffagnini et al. compared the immediate postoperative stability of combined ACL/MCL injuries treated with reconstruction of both ligaments or reconstruction of the ACL injury only. The authors found that addressing the ACL alone led to greater immediate postoperative laxity than did reconstruction of both ligaments.[59] These findings initially raised concerns for abnormal stresses across the ACL graft that might compromise outcomes in knees treated with ACL reconstruction and nonoperative treatment of the grade II MCL injury. A subsequent study by Zaffagnini with minimum 3-year follow-up showed no significant valgus laxity

and no difference in AP stability or other parameters. Similarly the outcomes literature has not consistently shown residual valgus laxity if the ACL is successfully reconstructed in the acute phase after motion is regained.[†]

Despite these findings, there are some patients with acute ACL/MCL injuries who have persistent valgus laxity at the time of ACL reconstruction. Grant et al. advocated for patients with ACL and MCL tears to undergo braced, nonoperative treatment of the MCL while regaining motion prior to ACL reconstruction. For those failing to heal the MCL with persistent valgus instability, concomitant reconstruction could take place when the ACL was reconstructed.[18]

In a prospective randomized trial evaluating knee range of motion and quadriceps power, Halinen et al. compared two treatment groups of knees with combined ACL/MCL injuries.[22] In group 1, patients were treated with early ACL reconstruction and MCL repair, whereas group 2 received ACL reconstruction only. Both groups regained acceptable knee motion and quadriceps strength, but the knees in group 2 saw both variables return more quickly. In a second portion of this study, the authors followed these patients for a mean of 27 months and evaluated both subjective and objective outcomes measures.[23] No differences were seen in motion, power, instrumented stability, Lysholm, or International Knee Documentation Committee (IKDC) scores. The authors recommended nonoperative treatment of combined injuries when the ACL was reconstructed acutely after return to full motion had been achieved.

Noyes and Barber-Westin demonstrated that operative treatment of the medial structures in ACL/MCL injuries resulted in an increased rate of flexion loss and patellofemoral pain.[41] They recommended nonoperative treatment of the MCL with early reconstruction of the ACL. Shelbourne and Porter found similar results with acute ACL reconstruction and nonoperative MCL treatment.[48] They stated that residual laxity at the MCL tended to be asymptomatic and that outcomes for ACL reconstruction alone with this combined injury pattern were similar to that for ACL reconstruction for an isolated ACL tear. Finally, Hillard-Simbell recommended that patients with combined ACL/MCL injuries could be treated with ACL reconstruction only.[25] In addition, the authors compared patients with combined ACL/MCL injuries treated with ACL reconstruction only with a group of patients treated with ACL reconstruction for an isolated ACL tear, finding no differences between the groups with respect to laxity, return to sport, functional limitation, strength, or one-legged hop testing for distance.

Less has been written on combined ACL/MCL injuries in the pediatric patient. Sankar et al. reported on 12 patients with this injury pattern and found similar results to that in the adult literature.[46] Patients had similar outcomes and return to sport with ACL reconstruction alone compared with ACL reconstruction in patients with isolated ACL injury. Again, the authors recommended nonoperative treatment of MCL injuries if the ACL injury is reconstructed acutely.

COMBINED MULTILIGAMENT INJURY AND KNEE DISLOCATIONS

The existing orthopedic literature is much less clear regarding the most effective treatment of those knees with medial-sided

---

[†]References 22, 23, 25, 39, 46, 48, and 60.

injury in association with a multiligament disruption. The combination of the relative rarity of the injury, the heterogeneity of injury patterns, treatment approach and technique, and associated medical and trauma issues make clarification of this condition difficult and elusive. A literature review by Kovachevich et al. found no consensus with regards to reconstruction or repair of the medial structures, although patients had good results with both approaches.[31] No direct comparison has been done of nonoperative treatment and operative reconstruction, and most of the information we have on this condition has been gleaned from reports on treatments of knee dislocation with multiple patterns and frequently multiple techniques. Stannard recommended treating medial and posteromedial instability, and medial instability in knee dislocations with allograft or autograft reconstruction in all cases, with good results.[50]

Treatment protocols vary among surgeons. Some surgeons prefer early reconstruction/repair of all injured ligaments, some prefer to brace for 4 to 6 weeks to regain motion and reconstruct the cruciates alone if valgus stability is restored, others prefer to address the MCL and PCL acutely and reconstruct the ACL if needed later, whereas some reconstruct or repair the collaterals and address the cruciates in a delayed fashion. Although final results seem to be similar with all approaches, note should be made that a risk of arthrofibrosis exists with early reconstruction or repair of all structures.[40,47,54]

In a study of multiligamentous knee injuries with 2- to 10-year follow-up, Fanelli and Edson reported on outcomes of operative and nonoperative treatment of combined ligament injuries with MCL involvement with reconstruction of the cruciates.[10] Fifteen patients in the study had injury to the MCL, with seven treated with surgical reconstruction and eight treated in a brace. All patients treated operatively and seven of eight patients treated nonoperatively had normal valgus testing at 30 degrees of flexion. In a later study, 44 out of 127 bicruciate injuries with medial and/or lateral reconstructions were evaluated at 5 to 22 years (mean: 10 years); 41 of 44 (93%) had returned to preinjury level or one Tegner grade below baseline, and 10 of 43 (23%) had developed osteoarthritis. There was an overall loss of some flexion but no flexion contractures.[11,12]

TECHNIQUE

Although some authors advocate repair of the medial stabilizing structures, many surgical techniques for medial collateral reconstruction exist, with many being evolutions of the technique originally described by Bosworth.[5] Bosworth described a transplantation of the semitendinosus tendon (ST) beneath a fascial, periosteal, and cortical flap at the femoral attachment of the MCL. The tendon is left attached both proximally and distally. The Bosworth technique has been modified to detach the tendon proximally and secure it to the femur at the MCL origin, with the remaining portion of the graft secured to the tibia distally. An important distinction between modern reconstructions and the original technique described by Bosworth and modified by others involves the tibial attachment of the SMCL graft. The graft must be secured within the fiber footprint of the native SMCL as opposed to the site of attachments of pes anserine tendons. This ensures that the graft runs along the course of the native ligament and avoids anterior placement. Grafts placed anterior to the SMCL attachment risk limiting knee flexion and/or loss of valgus stability as the

patient regains motion. Anatomic single- and double-bundle techniques have also been described using free tendon grafts.[4,13] In a cadaver study, Feeley et al. tested four reconstruction options, including single-bundle reconstruction, the Bosworth technique, a double-bundle technique, and the modified Bosworth reconstruction.[13] The authors found that the modified Bosworth and anatomic double-bundle techniques provided better stability to valgus stress and external rotation at 0 and 30 degrees of flexion. As the anatomy of the PMC has become better defined, attention has been turned to reconstructing its functional components, namely the POL. Because of this, there is some discussion as to the best site of attachment for the posterior limb of the reconstruction. Support exists for routing the posterior limb beneath the direct head of the semimembranosus, through a posterior tibial tunnel, or directly onto the proximal SMCL tibial attachment.[30,34,58] Laprade et al. advocate for an anatomic SMCL and POL reconstruction using two separate free grafts rather than creating a sling for POL, with good short-term follow-up.[33] Dong et al. describe a triangular reconstruction from a single femoral site with two tibia attachments to reconstruct SMCL and POL.[8] In addition, the POL may be imbricated at the time of SMCL reconstruction.[36] All techniques have yielded similar results clinically. Intraoperative and postoperative confirmation of anatomic placement may be confirmed radiographically on a lateral x-ray, using the intersection of the posterior cortical line and Blumensaat line.[24,56]

AUTHORS' PREFERRED TREATMENT

We treat isolated MCL injuries nonoperatively with full-time brace wear and a functional rehabilitation program. Immediate weight bearing is encouraged, with active and passive range of motion started as soon as the patient tolerates it. A full-length brace is used for the first 2 to 4 weeks then converted to a short-hinged knee brace for another 6 weeks or through the completion of the current season, if applicable. Athletes are allowed to return to sport after they demonstrate restoration of valgus stability at 0 and 30 degrees of flexion, full range of motion, and successful completion of sport-specific functional rehabilitation. Time to return to play depends on the degree of injury, the athlete's recovery, and the sport/position involved with typical return times between 4 and 6 weeks after injury. Exceptions to the nonoperative treatment of isolated MCL injuries include large bony avulsions identified on radiographs, Stener-type lesions of the distal MCL, and patients with persistent functional valgus instability after nonoperative treatment.

Regardless of MCL injury grade, most acute ACL/MCL combination injuries are treated with isolated ACL reconstruction after range of motion has been reestablished. Patients with persistent valgus laxity, particularly in extension, after motion is regained and medial structures are allowed to heal are treated with ACL and MCL reconstruction. In both cases, standard post-ACL reconstruction rehabilitation is followed with the exception of continued brace wear similar to that for an isolated MCL injury for a total of 3 months. For chronic ACL tears with residual valgus instability, we recommend simultaneous reconstruction of the ACL and MCL. We prefer to address ACL/PCL/MCL injuries with reconstruction of all injured ligaments after range of motion has been regained. The cruciate ligaments are reconstructed initially and the functional integrity of the MCL is then assessed.

SURGICAL TECHNIQUE

We reconstruct the SMCL with an anatomic single-bundle (ASB) technique and pants-over-vest imbrication to address the POL and PMC. Depending on concomitant procedures and availability, a doubled ST autograft, ST and G autograft, or ST/G allograft is used. A medial incision is used, creating full-thickness skin flaps. The sartorious fascia is identified and incised, allowing for harvest of the ST and G. The fascial incision is sharply carried proximally, exposing the SMCL. The grafts are prepared on the back table. Each tendon is cut to 18 cm and each end stitched with no. 2 nonabsorbable sutures. The prepared graft is then secured on the back table, covered with a moist lap sponge until needed. The femoral landmarks are identified, and the POL is visualized. A longitudinal capsular incision is made along the posterior aspect of the SMCL (Fig. 44.7). Care is taken to avoid damaging the meniscus. With the knee in 10 to 15 degrees of flexion, a pants-over-vest imbrication is completed using several no. 2 nonabsorbable sutures and reinforced with a final running suture over the top of the repair (Fig. 44.8 and 44.9). Care is taken to tie these sutures with knee flexed no more than 10 to 15 degrees to avoid a postoperative flexion contracture.

The femoral tunnel is marked in its anatomic location just proximal and posterior to the medial epicondyle. The prepared grafts are then used to locate the site for the tibial tunnel (Fig. 44.10). This location should be 4 to 6 cm distal to the joint line, within the fiber footprint of the SMCL, and allow for 25 mm

of graft within the tibial tunnel and at least 25 mm of graft in the femoral tunnel.

A short guide pin is advanced into the tibia to, but not through, the lateral cortex (Fig. 44.11). An 8-mm cannulated drill is used to drill a blind tunnel 25 mm in length. A long Beath pin is drilled bicortically starting at the femoral insertion of SMCL, aiming anterior and proximal, ending up outside the skin. An 8-mm tunnel is then drilled to, but not through, the lateral cortex and is typically approximately 55 mm in length. The Beath pin is used to pull a passing suture through the femoral tunnel. The bone tunnel is meticulously cleaned of

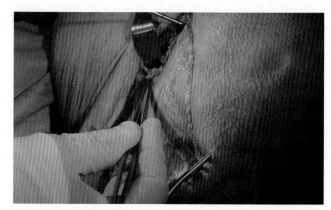

FIG 44.9 Imbrication will be oversewn with a running no. 2 nonabsorbable suture.

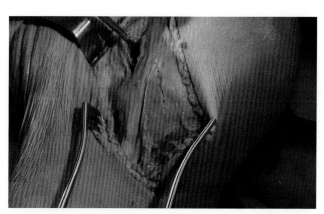

FIG 44.7 Longitudinal capsular incision posterior to the SMCL.

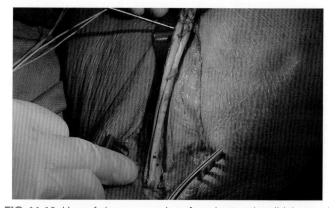

FIG 44.10 Use of the prepared graft to locate the tibial tunnel distal to the joint line.

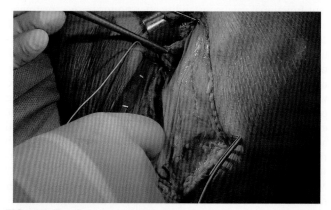

FIG 44.8 Pants-over-vest imbrication with no. 2 nonabsorbable suture.

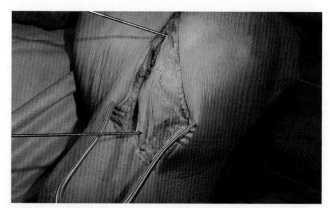

FIG 44.11 Short guide pin in the tibia, just touching the lateral cortex.

soft tissue with electrocautery to allow easy passage of the graft. The inferior limb of the graft is secured to the tibia with an 8 × 23 mm polyetheretherketone (PEEK) screw with biotenodesis technique (Arthrex, Naples, Florida), and then the suture is tied over the screw for backup fixation (Fig. 44.12). The femoral graft is then passed into the femoral tunnel and tensioned with the knee in 30 degrees of flexion and varus stress. It is fixed with a 9 × 23 mm PEEK screw (Fig. 44.13). The femoral end of the graft is reinforced with a single no. 2 nonabsorbable suture to the soft tissue around the tunnel. The tibial end of the graft is sewn to the residual SMCL starting 1 cm below the joint line and extending down to the tibial tunnel (Fig. 44.14).

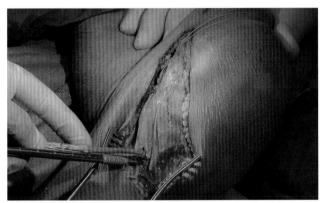

FIG 44.12 Biotenodesis technique fixation of tibial limb of graft with PEEK screw.

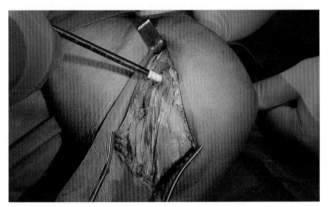

FIG 44.13 Femur fixation with PEEK screw.

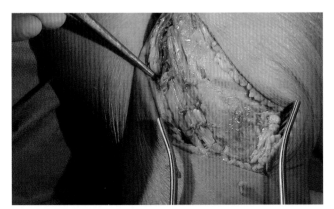

FIG 44.14 Graft sewn to residual SMCL on tibial side of joint line.

Postoperative rehabilitation consists of 2 weeks of touch-down weight bearing in a long leg brace in full extension. Progression is then allowed for full range of motion and advancing weight bearing as tolerated while braced in extension for the first 6 weeks. The brace is discontinued after 6 weeks and standard return to activity and rehabilitation used as dictated by other ligament injuries involved.

KEY REFERENCES

3. Bates NA, Nesbitt RJ, Shearn JT, et al: Relative strain in the anterior crucial ligament and medial collateral ligament during simluated jump landing and sidestep cutting tasks. *Am J Sports Med* 20(10):1, 2015.

13. Feeley BT, Muller MS, Allen AA, et al: Biomechanical comparison of medial collateral ligament reconstructions using computer-assisted navigation. *Am J Sports Med* 37(6):1123, 2009.

18. Grant JA, Tannenbaum E, Miller BS, et al: Treatment of combined complete tears of the anterior cruciate and medial collateral ligaments. *Arthroscopy* 28:110, 2012.

21. Griffith CJ, Wijdicks CA, LaPrade RF, et al: Force measurements on the posterior oblique ligament and superficial medial collateral ligament proximal and distal divisions to applied loads. *Am J Sports Med* 37(1):140, 2009.

23. Halinen J, Lindahl J, Hirvensalo E, et al: Operative and non-operative treatments of medial collateral ligament rupture with early anterior cruciate ligament reconstruction: a prospective randomized study. *Am J Sports Med* 34(7):1134, 2006.

28. Indelicato PA, Hermansdorfer J, Huegel M: Nonoperative management of complete tears of the medial collateral ligament of the knee in intercollegiate football players. *Clin Orthop* 256:174, 1990.

31. Kovachevich R, Shah JP, Arens AM, et al: Operative management of the medial collateral ligament in the multi-ligament injured knee: an evidence based systematic review. *Knee Surg Sports Traumatol Arthrosc* 17(7):823, 2009.

32. LaPrade RF, Engebretsen AH, Ly TV, et al: The anatomy of the medial side of the knee. *J Bone Joint Surg Am* 89(9):2000, 2007.

38. Najibi S, Albright JP: The use of knee braces. Part 1: prophylactic knee braces in contact sports. *Am J Sports Med* 33(4):602, 2005.

43. Reider B, Sathy MR, Talkington J, et al: Treatment of isolated medial collateral ligament injuries in athletes with early functional rehabilitation. A five-year follow-up study. *Am J Sports Med* 22(4):470, 1994.

44. Robinson JR, Sanchez-Ballester J, Bull AM: The posteromedial corner revisited. An anatomical description of the passive restraining structures of the medial aspect of the human knee. *J Bone Joint Surg Br* 86(5):674, 2004.

52. Thornton GM, Johnson JC, Maser RV, et al: Strength of medial structures of the knee joint are decreased by isolated injury to the medial collateral ligament and subsequent immobilization. *J Orthop Res* 23(5):1191, 2005.

53. Warren LF, Marshall JL: The supporting structures and layers on the medial side of the knee: an anatomical analysis. *J Bone Joint Surg Am* 61(1):56, 1979.

60. Zaffagnini S, Bonanzinga T, Marcheggiani Muccioli GM, et al: Does chronic medial collateral ligament laxity influence the outcome of anterior cruciate ligament reconstruction? A prospective evaluation with a minimum three-year follow-up. *J Bone Joint Surg Br* 93-B:1060, 2011.

61. Zhang H, Sun Y, Han X, et al: Simultaneous reconstruction of the anterior cruciate ligament and medial collateral ligament in patients with chronic ACL-MCL lesions: a minimum 2 year follow-up study. *Am J Sports Med* 42:1675, 2014.

The references for this chapter can also be found on www.expertconsult.com.

45

Fibular Collateral Ligament and the Posterolateral Corner

Robert F. LaPrade, Chase S. Dean, Jason M. Schon, Jorge Chahla

Although less commonly injured than the cruciate ligaments or the medial knee ligament complex, injuries to the fibular collateral ligament (FCL) and posterolateral corner (PLC) account for a significant portion of knee ligament injuries.[34] Associated PLC injuries provide a potential source of residual instability following anterior cruciate ligament (ACL) and posterior cruciate ligament (PCL) reconstruction and can lead to reconstruction graft failure.[14,29,30] A high index of suspicion is necessary when initially evaluating the injured knee to detect these sometimes occult injuries. Furthermore, a diligent physical examination and a comprehensive review of radiographic studies are necessary to identify these injuries. The purpose of this chapter is to review the anatomy and clinically relevant biomechanics of the FCL and PLC. Nonoperative and operative treatment options will be presented, as well as the postoperative rehabilitative protocol and potential complications.

ANATOMY

An understanding of the complex anatomy of the lateral aspect of the knee is required prior to performing a physical examination, reviewing the radiographic images, or embarking on a complex reconstruction. We will review the major components of the lateral knee ligament complex, as well as their insertions and actions (Fig. 45.1).

Fibular Collateral Ligament

The FCL is the primary stabilizer to varus stress of the knee.[10,11,33] The femoral attachment of the FCL is in a small bony depression 1.4 mm proximal and 3.1 mm posterior to the lateral epicondyle.[27] At its femoral origin, the cross-section of the FCL is 0.48 cm². As the FCL travels distally to its attachment on the fibular head, the cross-sectional area decreases slightly to 0.43 cm². The FCL fibular attachment site is 8.2 mm posterior to the anterior margin of the fibular head and 28.4 mm distal to the tip of the fibular styloid. The FCL occupies 38% of the width of the fibular head at its attachment; the average length of the FCL is 69.6 mm.[27]

Popliteus Tendon

The popliteus muscle courses proximolaterally from its distal insertion on the posteromedial tibia. It becomes tendinous in the lateral third of the popliteal fossa and becomes intra-articular as it courses deep to the FCL. The cross-section of the popliteus tendon (PLT) at its femoral insertion is 0.59 cm².[27] Its proximal insertion is along the proximal half of the popliteal sulcus and is always anterior (18.5 mm on average) to the insertion of the

FCL femoral attachment (Fig. 45.2). The tendinous portion of the popliteus is approximately 55 mm in length.

Popliteofibular Ligament

The popliteofibular ligament (PFL) originates from the musculotendinous junction of the popliteus muscle and inserts 38 degrees from the vertical in a distolateral direction onto the posterior surface of the fibular styloid.[22] It has two divisions (Fig. 45.3), anterior and posterior. The posterior division is larger at its fibular attachment site (3 vs. 6 mm, respectively).[27] The PFL provides an important restraint to external rotation.[33]

Lateral Gastrocnemius Tendon and Fabellofibular Ligament

The lateral gastrocnemius tendon originates along the supracondylar process of the distal femur. This attachment is found 13.8 mm posterior to the femoral attachment site of the FCL (see Fig. 45.1).[27] Because it is less frequently injured than the other structures of the posterolateral knee, it can serve as an important landmark during surgical reconstruction. As the lateral gastrocnemius tendon courses distally, it becomes inseparable from the lateral capsule, just proximal to the fabella. The fabella (Latin for "little bean") is a sesamoid bone that is found within the lateral gastrocnemius tendon in 30% of individuals.[16] If not fully ossified, a cartilaginous analogue is found approximately 66% of the time.[16] The fabellofibular ligament is a thickening of collagen that extends vertically from the fibular styloid to the fabella. It is the distal edge of the capsular arm of the short head of the biceps femoris. It courses between the biceps and gastrocnemius tendons.

Biceps Femoris Tendon: Long and Short Heads

The two heads of the biceps tendon provide important stabilization of the lateral knee complex. The main tendon of the long head of the biceps femoris divides approximately 1 cm proximal to the fibular head into direct and anterior arms.[27] The direct arm inserts onto the posterolateral aspect of the fibular head and is the more important of the two. The anterior arm has a small insertion site on the more distal and anterior fibular head before most of the tendon continues on as a broad fascial aponeurosis over the anterior compartment of the leg (Fig. 45.4). The anterior arm forms a bursa as it passes superficial to the FCL and the interval between the direct arm and the anterior arm, which provides a crucial access point to the FCL during reconstruction. The long head of the biceps tendon is also an important anatomic landmark for identification of the peroneal

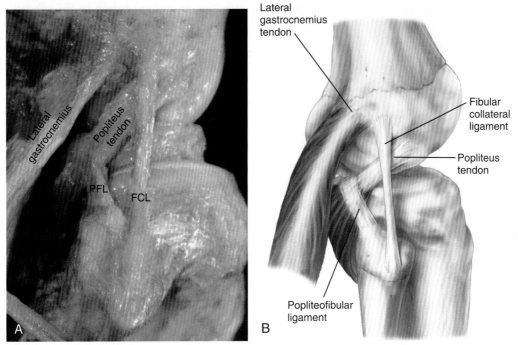

FIG 45.1 (A) Lateral knee dissection showing the fibular collateral ligament, popliteofibular ligament, popliteus tendon, and lateral gastrocnemius tendon. (B) Drawing of lateral knee dissection. (From LaPrade RF, Ly TV, Wentorf FA, Engebretsen L: The posterolateral attachments of the knee. A qualitative and quantitative morphologic analysis of the fibular collateral ligament, popliteus tendon, popliteofibular ligament, and lateral gastrocnemius tendon. *Am J Sports Med* 31:854–860, 2003.)

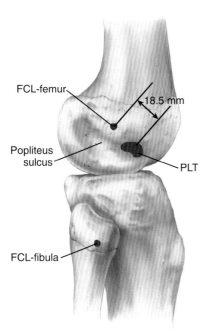

FIG 45.2 Drawing of the Attachment Sites of the Insertions of the PLT and FCL The PLT inserts on average 18.5 mm anterior to the FCL on the femur. *FCL,* Fibular collateral ligament; *PLT,* popliteus tendon. (From LaPrade RF, Ly TV, Wentorf FA, Engebretsen L: The posterolateral attachments of the knee. A qualitative and quantitative morphologic analysis of the fibular collateral ligament, popliteus tendon, popliteofibular ligament, and lateral gastrocnemius tendon. *Am J Sports Med* 31:854–860, 2003.)

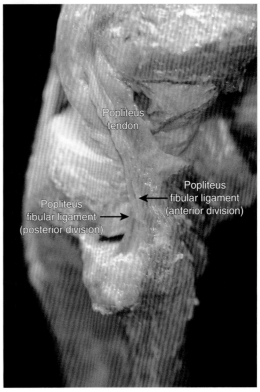

FIG 45.3 Photograph of a cadaveric dissection of a left knee showing the popliteus tendon, fibular collateral ligament, and anterior division and posterior division of the popliteofibular ligament.

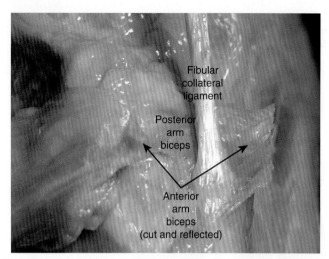

FIG 45.4 Anatomic image of cadaveric dissection demonstrating the anterior and posterior arms of the biceps femoris fibular insertion and their relation to the fibular collateral ligament.

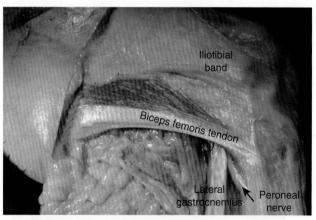

FIG 45.5 Cadaveric dissection photograph of a lateral knee dissection showing the iliotibial band (ITB), biceps femoris tendon, lateral gastrocnemius, and peroneal nerve *(right knee)*.

nerve, which lies slightly posterior in the distal aspect of the tendon (Fig. 45.5).

The short head of the biceps tendon also divides into two main segments that attach along the posterolateral aspect of the knee. The main insertion is along the lateral aspect of the fibular styloid, medial to the direct arm attachment of the long head. The other main insertion, the anterior arm of the short head of the biceps tendon, passes deep to the FCL and inserts on the tibia just posterior to Gerdy's tubercle. At this point, the anterior arm of the short head of the biceps tendon blends with the meniscotibial ligament, a thickening of the lateral capsule that attaches the capsule to the meniscus and tibia. This capsular arm of the short head of the biceps tendon courses proximally until it joins with the lateral gastrocnemius tendon and posterolateral capsule.

Iliotibial Band

The iliotibial band (ITB) is the most superficial layer of the lateral aspect of the knee. Its broad superficial layer is the first structure encountered deep to the subcutaneous tissues and covers a significant portion of the lateral knee (see Fig. 45.5). The ITB inserts at Gerdy's tubercle, along the anterolateral aspect of the tibia. The other components of the ITB includes an anterior expansion known as the iliopatellar band, a deep layer that blends with the lateral intermuscular septum, and a capsulo-osseous layer that attaches to the tibia just posterior and proximal to the main attachment at Gerdy's tubercle.[50]

Lateral Capsular Thickenings

The meniscofemoral and meniscotibial ligaments are capsular connections of the meniscus to the femur and tibia, respectively. The coronary ligament is an attachment of the lateral meniscus to the joint capsule. This helps anchor the lateral meniscal root posteriorly. The anterolateral ligament (ALL) is a lateral capsular thickening that originates posterior and proximal to the FCL and lateral femoral epicondyle and courses anterodistal inserting on the anterolateral tibia approximately midway between the center of Gerdy's tubercle and the anterior margin of the fibular head, anterior and proximal to the anterior arm of biceps femoris.[17] A Segond fracture is a bony avulsion injury of the ALL at its tibial insertion.[3,17]

CLINICALLY RELEVANT BIOMECHANICS OF THE POSTEROLATERAL KNEE

The structures of the lateral knee and PLC provide the primary restraint to varus stress of the knee[10,11] as well as posterolateral rotation of the tibia relative to the femur.[33] These structures are also important secondary stabilizers to anterior and posterior tibial translation when the cruciate ligaments are torn.[19] We will next review these static and dynamic stabilizers with regard to the stresses experienced by the knee.

Varus Stress

The FCL is the primary restraint to varus stress across the knee. Cutting studies have demonstrated that selective sectioning of the FCL results in an increase in varus opening.[10,11] In cutting series in which the FCL was left intact, varus stability remained preserved. Another sectioning study reported that the PLT functions as a minor primary varus stabilizer of the knee.[36] The PFL, ITB, lateral gastrocnemius tendon, and short and long heads of the biceps tendon, as well as the cruciate ligaments, are secondary restraints to varus force; their contributions have been noted after sectioning of the FCL.[19,36]

External Tibial Rotation

The FCL and popliteus complex are the primary restraints to tibial external rotation.[33] Several studies have demonstrated that sectioning of the FCL, PFL, and PLT results in increased tibial external rotation, which is most prevalent at approximately 30 to 40 degrees of knee flexion.[45]

Just as the FCL and popliteus complex act as a secondary restraint to the PCL in resisting posterior tibial translation, the PCL acts as a secondary restraint to prevent external rotation of the tibia on the femur.[19] Because of this relationship, combined PCL and PLC injuries are particularly unstable under external rotation forces.

Internal Tibial Rotation

The ACL is the primary stabilizer to internal rotation of the tibia at low flexion angles, and its contribution decreases as knee flexion increases to 90 degrees. The ALL is a primary stabilizer working synergistically with the ACL to provide increasing resistance to internal rotation as the knee flexes to 90 degrees.[44] Recent biomechanical studies have reported that the contribution of the ALL during internal rotation increases significantly with increasing flexion (above 35 degrees), whereas that of the ACL decreases significantly.[44] The PLT has a small, yet significant contribution to internal rotatory stability of the knee.[36] The FCL and the other PLC structures are secondary restraints to internal rotation. Their contribution becomes better appreciated in the ACL–deficient knee.

Anterior Tibial Translation

The ACL is the primary restraint to anterior tibial translation.[49] Additionally, the PLT also provides minimal contribution to anteroposterior (AP) stabilization near extension.[36] In knees with an intact ACL, the lateral ligament complex does not provide significant restraint to anterior tibial translation. However, in an ACL-deficient knee, the structures of the PLC provide an important secondary anterior translation stabilization role.[30] This is particularly true during the first 40 degrees of knee flexion.

Posterior Tibial Translation

The PCL is the primary restraint to posterior tibial translation, but the structures of the PLC also play a primary role in preventing posterior translation of the tibia on the femur.[10] This contribution is noted most in full extension and at lower degrees of flexion.[11,49] The contribution of the PLC increases in PCL-deficient knees, in which the PLT appears to contribute the most to secondary stability.[13]

INJURIES TO THE FIBULAR COLLATERAL LIGAMENT AND POSTEROLATERAL CORNER

Mechanism of Injury

A direct blow to the medial (particularly the anteromedial) knee is a common mechanism of injury to the FCL and PLC, although noncontact hyperextension and noncontact varus stress injuries have also been well described.[32] Only 40% of PLC injuries are sports-related.[45] Motor vehicle accidents, falls, and other high-energy trauma compose a significant portion of these injuries. Usually, injuries to the PLC are associated with ACL or PCL tears, whereas only approximately 25% of PLC injuries are isolated.[31,34]

History and Physical Examination

Patients usually highlight a discrete event in regard to the onset of their knee injury. However, in the chronic setting, previous surgeries and a prolonged time since the injury may make the details of the actual injury less clear.

Common symptoms include pain, subjective side-to-side instability (near extension), difficulty with stairs or uneven ground, swelling, and ecchymoses. A varus thrust gait is sometimes noted. Patients may also report paresthesias in the peroneal nerve distribution, as well as a foot drop. It has been reported that common peroneal nerve injury can be seen in up to one-third of PLC injuries.[32,49]

A complete history, including details of the accident, subsequent injuries, previous surgeries, and other associated injuries should be ascertained. Furthermore, a review of the patient's past medical history (including problems with

bleeding, clotting, or anesthesia), medications, tobacco use, and goals regarding return to sports and activities should be obtained.

A detailed physical examination is an important and required component of a patient's evaluation. A patient's gait should be assessed (when possible) for evidence of a varus thrust during the initiation of the stance phase.[7] The alignment of the limbs should be evaluated and the skin examined for any evidence of penetrating trauma, open wounds, or ecchymoses. A detailed neurovascular examination with diligent recording of distal pulses, as well as muscle grading of ankle dorsiflexion, plantar flexion, inversion, and eversion strength, is also completed. Sensory examination of the distal extremity is performed with attention to the dorsum of the foot, which is supplied by the superficial peroneal nerve, and to the first web space, which is supplied by the deep peroneal nerve.

A detailed examination of the knee is then performed with active and passive range of motion measurements. Stability examination of the ACL is performed using a Lachman and pivot shift test, whereas stability of the PCL is performed using the posterior drawer test. The patella is evaluated for evidence of chronic or acute subluxation or dislocation. Palpation is performed along the deep infrapatellar bursa, Gerdy's tubercle, pes anserine bursa, and patellar tendon attachment on the inferior pole of the patella. The structures of the PLC are then palpated, with specific attention to any tenderness along the femoral attachment of the FCL and PLT and at the fibular head. Tibiofemoral joint stability is then assessed. Specific tests to assess for PLC injuries are presented in the following sections.

Varus Stress Test. With the knee in full extension and at 30 degrees of flexion, the femur is stabilized to the examination table with the examiner's hand (Fig. 45.6). A varus force is

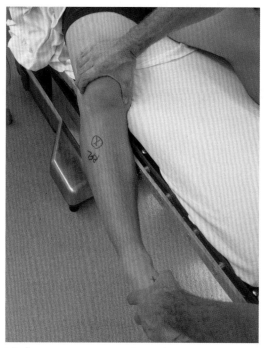

FIG 45.6 A varus stress test is performed by stabilizing the femur with the examiner's right hand and palpating the lateral joint line. The other hand provides a varus stress to the ankle. The test is performed at 0 and 30 degrees.

applied through the patient's ankle. The lateral knee joint line is palpated by the examiner's finger (with the hand that is stabilizing the knee), and the amount of lateral compartment gapping is assessed. All stability examinations should be graded on the amount of opening (as compared with the contralateral side) and firmness of the endpoint. Opening of the lateral compartment with the knee flexed to 30 degrees indicates an injury to the FCL and possibly to the secondary stabilizers of the PLC. The knee is then brought up to full extension; if the stability is restored, an isolated injury to the FCL is presumed. If the varus instability persists in full extension, a combined FCL, PLC, and cruciate ligament injury is assumed.

Dial Test. The dial test measures external rotation of the tibia relative to the femur. The test is performed in the prone or supine position. The femur is fixed with one hand (in a reduced position) while the ankle and foot are externally rotated (Fig. 45.7). This is done with the knee flexed to 30 degrees. An increase of more than 10 degrees of external rotation compared with the uninvolved side suggests an injury to the PLC.[11] The knee is then flexed to 90 degrees. Because of its role as an important secondary stabilizer, a knee with an intact PCL will see a decrease in external rotation. If at 90 degrees there is an increase in external rotation, as compared with 30 degrees, a combined PLC and PCL injury is presumed. A sequential sectioning study by Bae et al.[2] demonstrated increased external rotation following sectioning of at least three ligaments of the PCL and PLC complex. It was cautioned that the dial test might not be sufficiently sensitive to identify one- or two-ligament injuries.

External Rotation Recurvatum Test. In the external rotation recurvatum test, the patient assumes a supine position, with the knees and hips extended. The big toe is grasped and the leg lifted from the table with gentle pressure applied to the proximal knee (Fig. 45.8). The height of the heel in centimeters or degrees of hyperextension of the knee is recorded and compared with the contralateral side. A wide variation of the sensitivity of this test has been reported. Recently, LaPrade et al.[26] evaluated this

test and found it to identify less than 10% of injuries in a series of 134 patients with PLC injuries. However, in their study, a positive external rotation recurvatum test predicted a combined ACL and PLC injury.

Posterolateral Drawer Test. The posterolateral drawer test is performed in the same position as the conventional drawer test, with the patient supine and the knee flexed to 90 degrees with the foot stabilized flat on the table by the examiner. With the examiner's fingers grasping the femoral condyles, a posteriorly directed force is applied with the tibia in external rotation. An increase in translation with external rotation as compared with the contralateral normal knee suggests an injury to the PLC.

Reverse Pivot Shift. The reverse pivot shift is performed by positioning the patient supine with the knee flexed near 90 degrees. While palpating the joint line, a valgus load is applied across the knee and an external rotation force is applied to the tibia. The knee is then slowly extended while maintaining valgus stress and external rotation. Reduction of the previously subluxated lateral tibial plateau at approximately 35 to 40 degrees of flexion is a positive result. This reduction is the result of the ITB function changing from knee flexor to knee extender with extension.[32] Regarding PLC injuries, a positive reverse pivot shift has been reported to have a positive predictive value of 68% and a negative predictive value of 89%.[32,45] It is always important to compare the results with the contralateral knee because the test has been reported to be positive in 35% of normal knees.[6]

Imaging
Plain Radiographs. Standing AP and lateral radiographs of the knee should be obtained, as well as a bent knee patellofemoral view. Radiographs are frequently normal in acute injuries. The

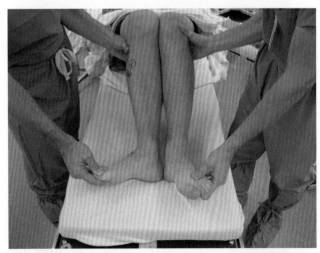

FIG 45.7 The dial test evaluates for external rotation of the tibia on the femur. It is performed at 30 and 90 degrees. Here, a positive dial test at 90 degrees is shown on the patient's right side. This suggests a combined posterolateral corner and posterior cruciate ligament injury.

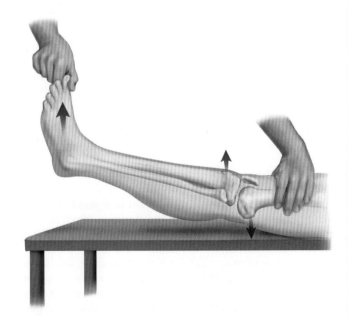

FIG 45.8 Drawing of the External Rotation Recurvatum Test The femur is fixed to the examination table, and the patient's leg is lifted by the big toe. Increase in recurvatum through the knee as compared with the uninjured side is considered a positive test. (From LaPrade RF, Ly TV, Griffith C: The external rotation recurvatum test revisited. *Am J Sports Med* 36:709–771, 2008.)

presence of Segond fractures[21] (Fig. 45.9), tibial spine avulsions, or fibular head fractures or avulsions (arcuate sign[37]; Fig. 45.10) may be visualized. A standing long-leg AP alignment radiograph is highly recommended for chronic PLC injuries because malalignment should be assessed and corrected if present prior to or at the time of surgical reconstruction (Fig. 45.11).

Stress Radiographs. Varus and posterior stress radiographs are also an important component of the radiographic workup of a patient with a suspected FCL or PLC injury (Fig. 45.12).[15,23,47] Varus stress radiography is helpful to definitively characterize the severity and resultant laxity from PLC injury and reveals information not available from alternative imaging.[12] Contralateral knee stress films are obtained for comparison. Varus stress radiographs have been shown in cadaveric sectioning studies to be sensitive, reproducible, and correlate with the magnitude of underlying injury.[23,49] LaPrade et al.[23] have demonstrated that sectioning of the FCL results in 2.7 mm of increased lateral gapping with varus stress and that sectioning of the entire PLC allows 4.0 mm of increased lateral gapping. Combined injuries to the PLC and PCL should be suspected when posterior drawer testing demonstrates more than 12 mm of posterior translation of the tibia.

Kneeling posterior stress radiography is a highly dependable technique for evaluating posterior knee instability and displacement. However, accuracy is dependent on reproducible patient positioning, consistent radiography technique, and usage of reliable landmarks for measurements. It has been determined that displacement measurements made from kneeling stress radiographs demonstrate high interobserver and intraobserver reliability.[15]

Magnetic Resonance Imaging. Magnetic resonance imaging (MRI) is an important diagnostic tool for evaluating the structures of the PLC, especially in acute injuries. Both T1- and T2-weighted MRI series provide important information regarding the structures involved and extent of injury. Coronal and sagittal series should be obtained. The sensitivity and specificity

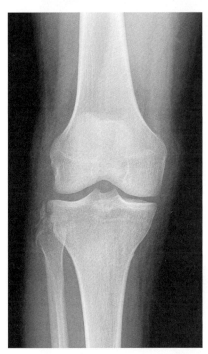

FIG 45.9 AP radiograph of the knee demonstrating a Segond fracture of the lateral tibial plateau.

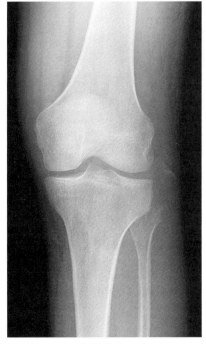

FIG 45.10 AP radiograph of the knee demonstrating a fracture of the fibular head *(arcuate sign)*.

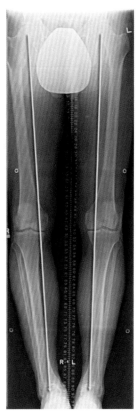

FIG 45.11 Long-leg standing AP radiograph demonstrating varus malalignment, as indicated by the mechanical axis of the limb visualized medial to the medial tibial spine.

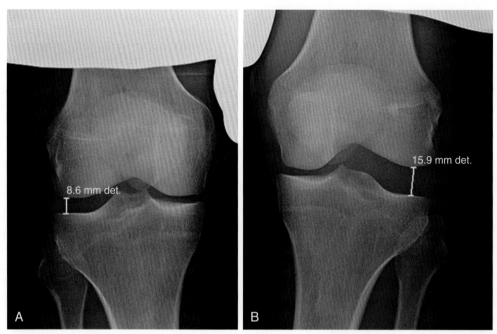

FIG 45.12 (A) Stress radiographs of the uninjured *(right)* knee demonstrate 8.6 mm of lateral compartment opening of the knee. (B) Stress films of the patient's contralateral injured *(left)* knee demonstrates a 15.9-mm opening, resulting in a side-to-side difference of 7.3 mm, indicative of a complete PLC grade III injury.

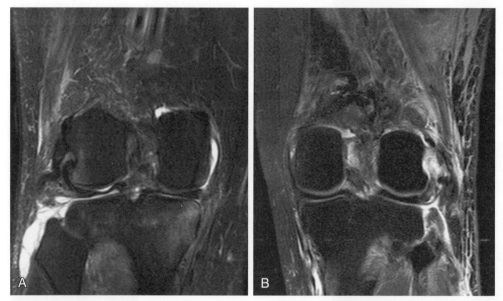

FIG 45.13 (A) Coronal T2-weighted MRI image of a right knee demonstrating an avulsion of the fibular collateral ligament from its fibular attachment site. The popliteus tendon is visualized deep to the ruptured fibular collateral ligament. (B) Coronal T2-weighted MRI image of a left knee demonstrates avulsion of the femoral attachment of the popliteus tendon.

for identifying injuries to specific components of the PLC are high and over 90% for identifying injuries to the superficial layer of the ITB, anterior arm of the biceps femoris tendon, midthird capsular ligaments, and FCL (Fig. 45.13).[18] The reported diagnostic sensitivity of injuries to the popliteus femoral origin and fabellofibular ligament ranges from 80% to 90%. Only the PFL demonstrated sensitivity and specificity less than 80% (68.8% and 66.7%, respectively).[21] The cartilage, menisci, and cruciate ligaments should also be evaluated for

associated injuries. Although MRI is essential for evaluation of ligamentous injuries, it is often difficult to determine if surgical intervention is recommended when diagnosing partial PLC injuries. Varus stress radiography is supportive of MRI findings and contributes additional objective information regarding the clinical extent of injury.[12]

Diagnostic Arthroscopy. The intra-articular structures of the PLC can be visualized with arthroscopy. These include the

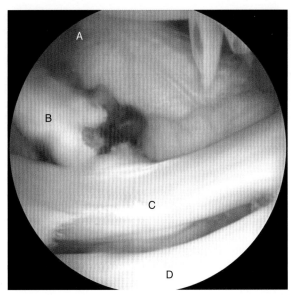

FIG 45.14 Arthroscopic Image of the Lateral Compartment of the Knee *(A)* Lateral femoral condyle; *(B)* popliteus tendon; *(C)* lateral meniscus; *(D)* lateral tibial plateau. The femoral and tibial articular surfaces are seen at the *top* and *bottom* of this figure. The lateral meniscus is seen traveling across the *center portion.* The popliteus tendon has been avulsed from its femoral insertion. Hematoma is seen along its course. A drive-through sign is shown by the increased lateral compartment gapping.

popliteal tendon's origin (Fig. 45.14), meniscofemoral ligament, coronary ligament of the lateral meniscus, and meniscotibial ligaments. LaPrade[18] has evaluated these structures arthroscopically and noted injuries to them in 33%, 37%, 73%, and 80% of knees with grade III PLC injuries, respectively. This study also confirmed that concomitant injuries are frequent, documenting ACL tears in 63% of knees, PCL tears in 23%, and lateral meniscus tears in 22%. Chondromalacia was noted in 23% of the procedures. A posterolateral drive-through sign (increased laxity of the lateral compartment) is performed by passing the arthroscope through the interval between the popliteal tendon and the lateral femoral condyle, and is an indirect indicator of an FCL and possibly a PLC injury.[18]

TREATMENT

Grade I and II injuries to the PLC can typically be treated nonoperatively.[45] Knee bracing with a knee immobilizer or hinged knee brace locked in full extension for 3 to 6 weeks is usually sufficient. Full weight bearing is commonly allowed, and passive and active prone knee flexion is performed to prevent stiffness. In more involved injuries, a course of protected weight bearing is sometimes prescribed. Stress radiographs are a reliable and reproducible method that can be used at the time of injury and prior to return to play to compare side-to-side differences.[15,36] After 3 to 6 weeks, sports-specific therapy is initiated and return to play can be considered once pain is absent and full range of motion, strength equal to the contralateral side, and clinical stability to varus stress testing are attained. Bracing can be continued after return to play, depending on the type of sport and the severity of the injury.

Grade III injuries to the PLC are best treated with surgery because symptomatic instability remains a significant risk.[45] In

combined PLC and ACL or PCL-injured knees, concurrent repair or reconstruction of the PLC is recommended because the PLC-deficient knee places significant stress on the newly reconstructed ACL or PCL graft, increasing the risk of graft failure.[14,29,30] The following will review the available treatments, including repair and reconstruction.

Repair

Intrasubstance repairs of the FCL and popliteus have been historically unsuccessful and therefore should not be performed. However, other structures of the PLC are amenable to intrasubstance repair. These include the coronary ligament of the lateral meniscus, meniscofemoral and meniscotibial ligaments, and fibers of the popliteomeniscal ligaments. Horizontal or vertical sutures are placed through these structures after adequate visualization has been achieved. We recommend using 0-0 braided, nonabsorbable suture for this. These sutures should be tensioned with the knee in full extension. Early range of motion up to 90 degrees is immediately allowed. Techniques have been described in which the avulsed ends of the popliteus and/or the FCL have been placed within a bone tunnel or tied down with suture anchors at the femoral origin. This recession technique uses an eyelet-passing pin for passage of sutures across the distal femur.[19,35] Prior to passage of the sutures, a 5-mm reamer is used to create a bone tunnel. The sutured ends of the FCL or popliteus are then placed into a Beath pin, which is advanced medially. The tendon is passed into the freshly drilled tunnel, and the passing suture is tied down medially over a cortical fixation device. The location of the starting point for the tunnel is at the anatomic origin of the involved structure.

A prospective cohort study by Stannard et al.[48] compared PLC repair with reconstruction. They reported that repair was inferior to reconstruction in the management of acute PLC injuries. They compared the use of a suture anchor and repair of damaged structures with a modified two-tailed reconstruction (discussed later). The reconstruction group fared better and had fewer failures (9% vs. 37%) than the repair group.

Reconstruction

Numerous posterolateral knee reconstructive techniques have also been described. These include nonanatomic and anatomic techniques. A biceps tenodesis theoretically reconstructs the FCL, although it does so nonanatomically.[46] This technique, initially described and popularized by Clancy,[4] redirects the biceps tendon, or a slip of the biceps tendon, from its distal attachment on the fibular head to a site along the distal lateral femur approximately 1 cm anterior to the origination of the FCL.[46] This technique requires harvesting 6 to 8 cm of biceps tendon and looping it over a screw and spiked washer.

The Stannard reconstruction technique (modified two-tailed reconstruction) is a nonanatomic reconstruction of the FCL, PFL, and PLT.[48] A tibialis anterior or tibialis posterior allograft is used. After exposure of the lateral knee, a bone tunnel is drilled along the PLT in an anterior to posterior direction. This tunnel will be the anchor point of one end of the allograft and approximates the tibial position of the PLT. The allograft is then advanced proximally over a previously placed screw at the reported isometric point of the lateral femoral condyle to re-create the popliteus. The allograft is then brought back inferiorly toward the fibular head and passed through a tunnel drilled in the fibular head. This arm of the allograft reportedly reconstructs the PFL. The allograft is passed in a posterior to anterior direction through the fibula and returned to the screw in the distal femur. This final arm re-creates the FCL. The screw and a spiked washer are advanced, and the graft is tensioned between 40 and 60 degrees of knee flexion.

Preferred Techniques

Fibular collateral ligament reconstruction. For isolated FCL injuries, we recommend reconstruction using a semitendinosus autograft. After harvesting the semitendinosus via a standard technique, attention is turned to the open reconstruction of the FCL.[5] An incision is made along the lateral knee over the lateral epicondyle, along the posterior border of the ITB. This is extended proximally and distally for approximately 10 cm. The common peroneal nerve is identified posteromedial to the biceps tendon, and an extensive neurolysis is performed both anteriorly and posteriorly. The nerve is then retracted from the surgical field to minimize the risk of iatrogenic nerve injury. A 1-cm longitudinal incision is made in the distal aspect of the long head of the biceps femoris tendon to access the biceps bursa, where the fibular FCL insertion can be found. Injuries to the FCL usually leave the midsubstance of the ligament intact, although functionally incompetent. A tag suture is placed into the FCL remnant just proximal to the fibular head, and gentle tension is applied to help identify the FCL femoral attachment (Fig. 45.15). The distal attachment of the FCL is then identified along the lateral aspect of the fibular head. A guide pin is placed through this depression with an ACL-targeting guide. The exit point of the guide pin is along the posteromedial downslope of the fibular head, distal to the insertion of the PFL (Fig. 45.16). Aiming too proximally can damage the attachment of the PFL. A 6-mm reamer is then used to create a tunnel.

Attention is then turned to the femoral FCL insertion, and the previously placed tag suture is tensioned again to identify the femoral FCL insertion. If the remnant FCL cannot be found, the proximal FCL attachment is identified using the landmarks as described by LaPrade et al. 1.4 mm proximal and 3.1 mm posterior to the lateral femoral epicondyle.[27] The ITB is then incised in line with its fibers aiming slightly anterior to the femoral attachment identified in the previous step (Fig. 45.17). Sharp dissection with a knife is performed to lift the FCL

femoral attachment site subperiosteally, which is slightly proximal and posterior to the femoral epicondyle. An eyelet-passing pin is placed through the center of the FCL femoral attachment site and directed anteromedially and approximately 20 to 30 degrees proximally across the femur to avoid damage to the trochlea and potential collision with ACL tunnels in cases where the ACL is reconstructed concurrently. A 6-mm tunnel is reamed to a depth of 25 mm and tapped with a 7-mm tap (Fig. 45.18). The previously tubularized graft is recessed into the femoral tunnel by pulling on the passing sutures and a 7 × 23 mm bioabsorbable screw is placed (Fig. 45.19). A tract is made deep to the superficial layer of the ITB, and passing sutures are used to place the graft into the fibular tunnel (Fig. 45.20). With the knee flexed to 20 degrees, a 7 × 23 mm bioabsorbable interference screw is implanted with tension applied to the graft and a gentle valgus force is applied to the knee to prevent any lateral compartment gapping (Fig. 45.21). After the screw is placed, the free end of the graft is trimmed. However, if bone quality is poor, the extra graft is continued posteriorly around the fibular head, between a split in the anterior arm of the biceps femoris and secured to itself using a nonabsorbable suture (Fig. 45.22).

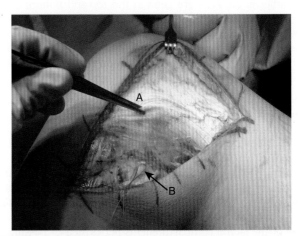

FIG 45.16 *(A)* The ITB is split in line with its fibers and reflected, demonstrating the femoral insertion of the fibular collateral ligament. *(B)* The stay suture is again visualized at the fibular insertion of the FCL.

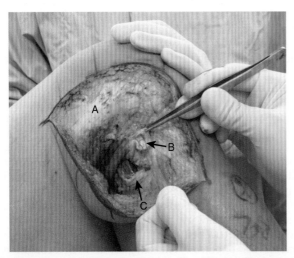

FIG 45.15 Lateral Knee Dissection The ITB *(A),* fibular collateral ligament *(B),* with a stay suture at its fibular attachment, and peroneal nerve *(C)* are visualized following neurolysis.

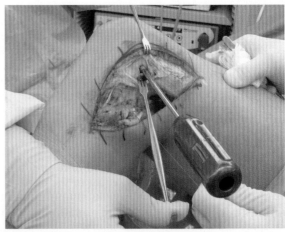

FIG 45.17 The femoral tunnel is tapped in preparation for placement of the graft and interference screw.

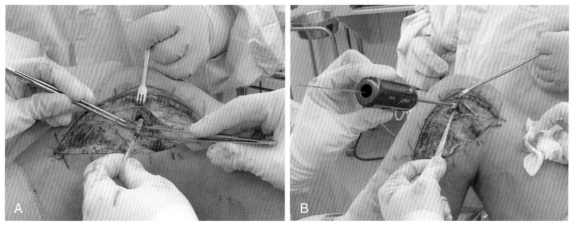

FIG 45.18 (A) The graft is placed within the femoral tunnel. (B) A bioabsorbable interference screw is placed to secure the graft.

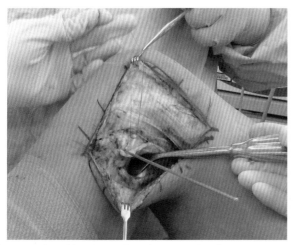

FIG 45.19 A guide pin is placed across the fibular tunnel. The pin is started at the anatomic insertion of the fibular collateral ligament.

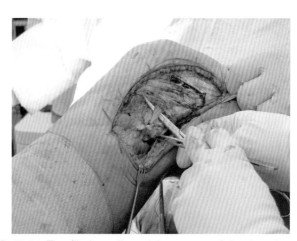

FIG 45.21 The fibular collateral ligament graft in place is seen deep to the hemostat. A valgus force is applied across the knee, the graft tensioned, and an interference screw placed within the fibular head.

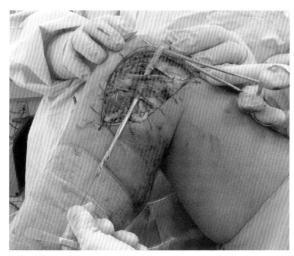

FIG 45.20 The graft is routed deep to the ITB.

Posterolateral corner reconstruction. When a PLC injury is present in addition to a FCL injury, we recommend an anatomic reconstruction of both the PLC and FCL. Described by LaPrade et al. in 2004,[25] this technique anatomically reconstructs the FCL, PT, and PFL. Following a lateral approach and peroneal nerve neurolysis, the attachment sites of the FCL on the lateral fibular head and the PFL on the posteromedial fibular head are identified. An ACL-cannulated guide is then used to drill a guide pin from the FCL attachment on the lateral aspect of the fibular head posteromedially to the PFL attachment site (Fig. 45.23). This is overreamed with a 7-mm reamer. The posterior tibial popliteal sulcus is then identified with direct palpation in the interval between the lateral gastrocnemius and soleus muscles. This marks the musculotendinous junction of the popliteus. With a retractor protecting the neurovascular structures, an ACL-cannulated guide is used to direct a guide pin from anterior to posterior (Fig. 45.24). The anterior location of the tibial tunnel is found between the tibial tubercle and Gerdy's tubercle at the so-called flat spot (Fig 45.25). The pin is over-reamed with a 9-mm reamer. The femoral attachment of the

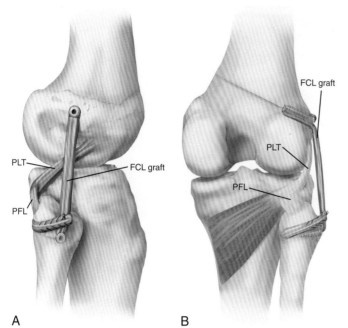

A   B

FIG 45.22 Drawing of lateral (A) and posterior (B) views of the anatomically reconstructed fibular collateral ligament (FCL graft). The free tail of the graft is brought around the posterior aspect of the fibular head and sutured to itself to provide an extra point of fixation. The popliteus tendon *(PLT)* and *PFL* are shown as well. (From Coobs BR, LaPrade RF, Griffith CJ, Nelson BJ: Biomechanical analysis of an isolated fibular [lateral] collateral ligament reconstruction using an autogenous semitendinosus graft. *Am J Sports Med* 35:1521–1527, 2007.)

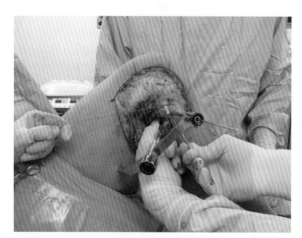

FIG 45.23 An ACL cannulated guide is used to place a guide pin for the fibular tunnel for the posterolateral corner reconstruction. The anatomic insertion of the fibula collateral ligament is the starting point. The guide pin should exit at the insertion of the popliteofibular ligament on the fibular styloid.

popliteus and the FCL are then identified. Eyelet pins are placed at their anatomic attachment sites and advanced anteromedially (Fig. 45.26). The distance between these two pins is measured and should be approximately 18.5 mm.[27] The lateral cortex is reamed for both pins (9 mm diameter) to a depth of 25 mm. An Achilles allograft is split lengthwise, and the tendon is tubularized. Two 9 × 20 mm bone blocks are fashioned.

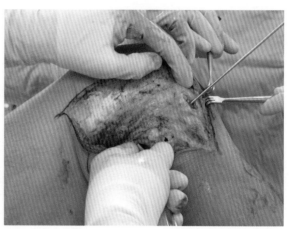

FIG 45.24 The guide pin is placed for the popliteus tunnel. This is drilled anterior to posterior, with the exit point at the popliteal sulcus on the posterior tibia. Retractors are placed to protect the neurovascular structures.

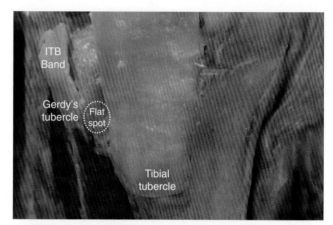

FIG 45.25 The anterior location of the tibial tunnel is identified between the tibial tubercle and Gerdy's tubercle at the so-called "flat spot" *(right knee)*.

Passing sutures in the bone blocks are used to reduce the bone blocks into the femoral tunnel and fixed with 7-mm cannulated interference screws (Fig. 45.27). The FCL graft is routed deep to the ITB (Fig. 45.28) and through the tunnel in the fibular head. A 7-mm biointerference screw is placed with the knee in 20 degrees of flexion, with a valgus force across the knee to reconstruct the FCL. The tail of the placed FCL graft is continued to the posterior tibial aperture of the popliteus tunnel, re-creating the PFL (Fig. 45.29). Both the popliteofibular graft (the continued free tail of the FCL graft) and the PLT graft are combined and routed through the tibial tunnel posteriorly to anteriorly and held in place with a 9-mm interference screw (Fig. 45.30). The knee is flexed to 60 degrees and an anterior force is placed across the tibia as the screw is advanced to complete the reconstruction (Fig. 45.31). An examination under anesthesia is then performed to verify graft stability. The remainders of the graft tails are cut and the wounds are closed in layers.

As with FCL reconstruction, we recommend initial identification of the common peroneal nerve distal to the posterior border of the biceps femoris tendon as part of any open PLC reconstruction. This allows for protection of the nerve during the surgical procedure and provides an opportunity for in situ

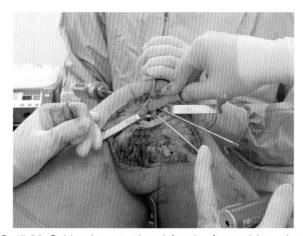

FIG 45.26 Guide pins are placed for the femoral insertion of the fibular collateral ligament and popliteus tendon reconstruction. The popliteus tendon inserts on average 18.5 mm anterior to the fibular collateral ligament. This figure shows both guide pins in place and a ruler confirming the appropriate relationship.

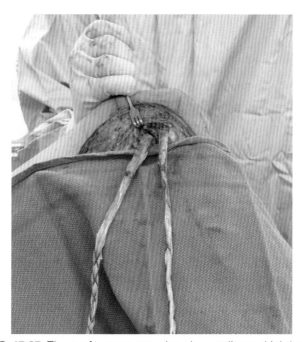

FIG 45.27 The grafts reconstructing the popliteus *(right)* and fibular collateral ligament *(left)* are shown after being placed within the femoral tunnel. These are held in place with interference screws.

neurolysis and decompression as it crosses the fascial bands of the lateral compartment.

Postoperative Management. Postoperatively, a knee immobilizer is worn and weight bearing is limited for 6 weeks following surgery. Quadriceps strengthening exercises including straight leg raises are initiated immediately postoperatively in the knee immobilizer only. At 1 to 2 weeks postoperatively, range of motion exercises are initiated. Closed-chain strengthening exercises are initiated at 6 weeks to help restore quadriceps strength. Hamstring strengthening is limited to avoid stressing the repair or reconstruction until at least 4 months postoperatively. Weight

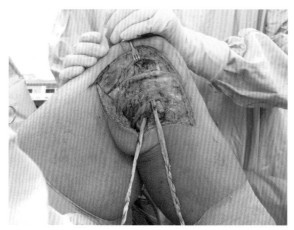

FIG 45.28 The grafts are routed into position. The fibular collateral ligament graft has been routed deep to the ITB and is now seen on the *right*. The popliteus graft is routed deep to the fibular collateral ligament graft and is now on the *left*.

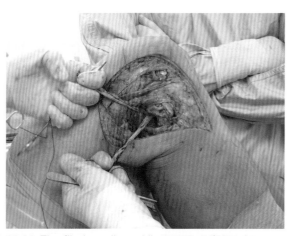

FIG 45.29 The fibular collateral ligament graft has been routed through the fibular tunnel. Valgus stress is applied to the knee, the graft tensioned, and an interference screw placed within the fibular head. The free tail is then continued to the posterior aspect of the tibia and combined with the popliteus graft, reconstructing the popliteofibular ligament.

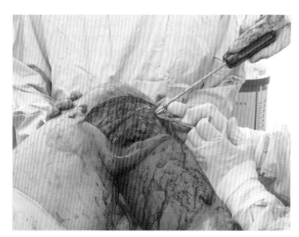

FIG 45.30 The grafts are combined and passed from posterior to anterior through the tunnel drilled in the proximal tibia. An interference screw is placed from anterior to posterior to fixate the grafts.

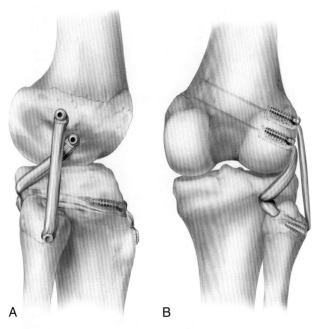

FIG 45.31 Drawings of the lateral (A) and posterior (B) knee demonstrating the fibular collateral ligament and posterior lateral corner reconstruction. (From LaPrade RF, Johansen S, Wentorf FA, et al: An analysis of an anatomical posterolateral knee reconstruction: an in vitro biomechanical study and development of a surgical technique. *Am J Sports Med* 32:1405–1414, 2004.)

bearing is slowly progressed, starting at 6 weeks. An exercise bike is added when enough knee flexion is present to allow for rotation of the pedals. Sport-specific training is initiated at 4 months, with a return to sports or activity allowed when normal knee range of motion and normal strength and stability comparable to the contralateral side have been achieved (frequently at 6 to 9 months, although not uncommon to take 12 months). Finally, the athlete should complete sport-specific therapy prior to returning to competitive athletics.

Biomechanical Validation. In 2007, Coobs et al.[5] biomechanically tested an isolated anatomic FCL reconstruction using an autogenous semitendinosus graft. In cases of isolated FCL injury, they found that this technique restored varus, external, and internal rotation to near normal stability.

In 2004, LaPrade et al.[25] demonstrated that the two-graft technique anatomically reconstructs the primary static stabilizers of the posterolateral knee and restores static stability, as measured by joint translation in response to varus loading and external rotation torque. There were no significant differences in varus translation between the intact and reconstructed knees at 0, 60, and 90 degrees of knee flexion. Moreover, there was no significant difference in external rotation between the intact and reconstructed posterolateral knees at any flexion angle.[25] In 2010 McCarthy et al.[41] published a follow-up study that biomechanically validated the necessity of anatomic reconstruction of the PFL to restore knee stability for this anatomic PLC reconstruction technique. Additionally, they reported that anatomic PLC reconstruction did not overconstrain the knee.

In 2010 LaPrade et al.[36] published a biomechanical analysis of the PLT, demonstrating its role as a primary static stabilizer

to external rotation. Anatomic reconstruction of the PLT was shown to significantly reduce external rotation in PLT deficient cadaveric knees.

Results. LaPrade et al.[31] reported that an anatomic FCL reconstruction using a semitendinosus graft at a mean 2-year follow-up resulted in improved patient outcomes and near-normal lateral compartment stability in patients with grade III FCL injuries. The modified Cincinnati score improved from 28.2 preoperatively to 88.5 postoperatively, and IKDC subjective outcome scores improved from 34.7 preoperatively to 88.1 postoperatively. Furthermore a 2015 study[43] reported that anatomic FCL reconstruction resulted in significant preoperative to postoperative improvements in mean Lysholm and WOMAC scores, median SF-12 physical component subscale scores, the median Tegner activity scale and postoperative patient reported outcome scores at an average of 2.7 years postoperatively.

Levy et al.[39] completed a systematic literature review of multiligament knee injuries and found that operative management provides improved outcomes compared with nonoperative management. They also reported that surgical management completed early (within 3 weeks) improves outcomes as compared with procedures performed after 3 weeks, and that reconstruction provides better outcomes than repair of PLC injuries. No recommendations were given with regard to the type of reconstruction (anatomic vs. nonanatomic). Furthermore, other studies regarding primary repair of acute PLC injuries have reported failure rates of approximately 40%.[38,48] A 2015 systematic review by Geeslin et al.[9] reported that acute repair of grade III PLC injuries with staged cruciate reconstruction was associated with a 38% failure rate, compared to a more robust reconstruction approach that simultaneously repaired cruciate and PLC injury, which resulted in only a 9% failure rate.

Yoon et al.[51] compared a lateral sling technique with an anatomic reconstruction and demonstrated improved Lysholm scores, and notably less varus and external rotation laxity in the anatomic reconstruction group. A prospective study by Geeslin and LaPrade[8] of 24 patients at an average follow-up of 2.4 years from anatomic reconstruction of acute PLC injuries, with or without concurrent cruciate injury, demonstrated significant improvement in all IKDC objective subscores. Additionally, the patients had significant improvement in side-to-side differences in lateral compartment gapping with varus stress radiographs (6.2 mm preoperatively and 0.1 mm postoperatively). The mean Cincinnati and IKDC subjective outcomes scores improved from 21.9 to 81.4 points and from 29.1 to 81.5 points, respectively. One concern regarding the anatomic reconstruction technique is its technically demanding nature.[40] High-quality studies with long-term follow-ups are needed to gain a better understanding of the outcomes of PLC reconstruction.

Chronic Posterolateral Corner Injuries

PLC injuries longer than 3 months duration are classified as chronic injuries. These injuries present specific challenges that are not always present in the management of acute injuries. When evaluating a chronic PLC injury, standing long-leg AP alignment radiographs are mandatory to evaluate the patient's alignment. The reconstructed FCL, PLT, and PFL will not tolerate any varus malalignment.[14,20,29] Varus malalignment is defined as being present when a line from the center of the femoral head

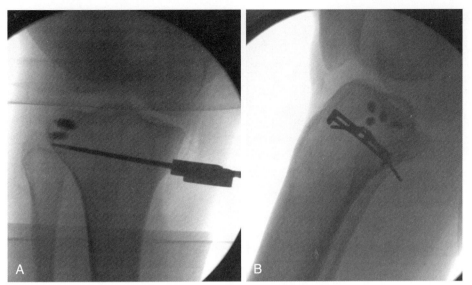

FIG 45.32 (A) AP intraoperative image of the guide pins for a proximal medial opening wedge osteotomy. There are suture anchors in place in the lateral proximal tibia from a prior failed lateral ligament reconstruction. (B) Lateral intraoperative radiograph of the knee showing guide pins in place for a proximal tibial opening wedge osteotomy. The final desired slope is approximated by the slope of the guide pins. Previously placed suture anchors are seen.

to the center of the ankle joint (the mechanical axis) falls medial to the tip of the medial tibial spine on a long-leg alignment radiograph.[1] When varus malalignment occurs, a corrective osteotomy must be performed prior to reconstruction. We recommend a proximal tibial medial opening wedge osteotomy. As compared with a lateral tibial closing wedge osteotomy, the medial opening wedge osteotomy has been biomechanically validated to decrease both varus motion and external rotation laxity.[20] Additionally, the opening wedge osteotomy has the theoretical benefit of tightening the posterior capsule.[28] Furthermore, an opening wedge osteotomy allows an opportunity for a biplanar osteotomy in the setting of a cruciate-deficient knee or in a knee with recurvatum or a flexion contracture. In a knee with a deficient ACL, the tibial slope should be decreased; in a knee with a deficient PCL, the tibial slope should be increased. Genu recurvatum can be addressed by increasing the tibial slope, and a flexion contracture at the knee can be addressed by decreasing the tibial slope.

Preferred Technique: Medial Tibial Opening Wedge Osteotomy for Chronic Posterolateral Corner Injury With Varus Malalignment.

The patient is positioned supine on a radiolucent table with a tourniquet around the upper thigh. A bump can be placed under the contralateral hip to improve exposure to the proximal medial tibia. A standard vertical incision is made midway between the tibial tubercle and posterior medial border of the tibia at the distal aspect of the tibial tubercle. The dissection is carried straight to the bone to avoid devascularization of the skin flaps. The distal aspect of the patellar tendon and superficial medial collateral ligaments are identified and protected. The dissection is continued posteriorly and a radiolucent retractor is placed to protect the neurovascular bundle. Another retractor is placed deep to the patellar tendon. Two guide pins are placed parallel to the joint line (in the coronal plane), just distal to the metaphyseal flare. In the sagittal plane, the guide pins approximate the desired tibial slope (Fig. 45.32).

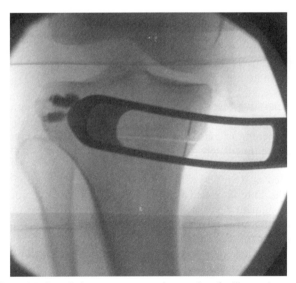

FIG 45.33 A radiolucent retractor is used to facilitate the osteotomy. An oscillating saw is used to perform the osteotomy. Note that the lateral cortex was not violated by the osteotomy.

An oscillating saw is used to osteotomize the medial cortex (Fig. 45.33). This is followed by osteotomes anteriorly and posteriorly, frequently checking the position with fluoroscopic imaging to avoid damaging the lateral cortex. A hinge of bone (approximately 1 cm in width) is maintained along the proximal lateral tibia. A spreader is used to distract the medial cortex until the desired correction is obtained. The spreader is left in place for approximately 5 minutes to allow for stress relaxation of the lateral cortex. A staple is placed laterally if propagation of the osteotomy occurs through the lateral cortex. A plate is fixed along the medial cortex, with two 4.5 mm cortical screws distally and two 6.5 mm fully threaded cancellous screws

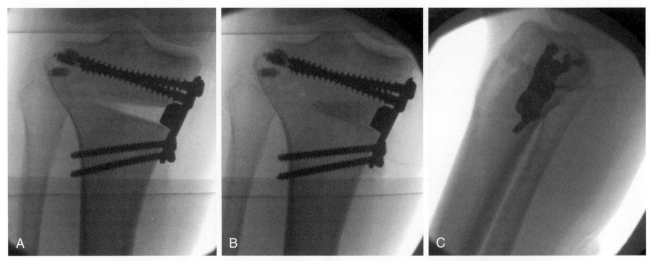

FIG 45.34 (A) A plate is placed across the osteotomy site and screws are placed proximally and distally to the osteotomy. The lateral cortex remains intact. (B) Bone graft or bone graft substitute is packed into the osteotomy site. (C) Lateral intraoperative radiograph demonstrating the bone graft as well as the medial plate and screw construct.

proximally (Fig. 45.34). A wide variety of osteotomy plates are commercially available. Autologous or allograft bone is placed into the osteotomy site under fluoroscopic guidance. We recommend the placement of a large Richards staple anteriorly while hyperextending the knee to prevent the breach from expanding postoperatively. The wound is closed in layers, and the knee is placed in an immobilizer.

Postoperative Management. A patient with a proximal tibial osteotomy is kept in a knee immobilizer for 8 weeks. Quadriceps strengthening exercises such as straight leg raises are recommended immediately postoperatively. Prone flexion and extension are initiated four times daily. Progressive weight bearing is initiated at 8 weeks, with a goal of full weight bearing at 3 months. Enteric-coated aspirin, 325 mg orally daily, or another anti-coagulant agent, as indicated, is initiated for deep venous thrombosis prophylaxis. Standing radiographs are obtained at 3 months and the alignment is reviewed. Complete healing is ensured prior to proceeding with PLC reconstruction (Fig. 45.35). We do not recommend this type of osteotomy for patients who use tobacco, given the risk of impaired soft tissue healing and delayed or nonunion. Gradual return to activities is then allowed. If instability persists, a staged reconstruction can be performed at the 6- to 9-month mark.

Results. An outcome study[24] of 54 patients with chronic PLC injuries who underwent anatomic reconstruction with an average follow-up of 4.3 years reported a significant improvement between preoperative and postoperative IKDC objective scores for varus gapping at 20 degrees, external rotation at 30 degrees, reverse pivot shift and single-leg hop. A systematic review of minimum 2-year outcomes following chronic PLC reconstruction by Moulton et al.[42] reported a 90% success rate of surgical management according to the individual investigators examination or stress radiographic assessment of objective outcomes. However, differences in study design and patient population prevented and quantitative comparison of surgical techniques.

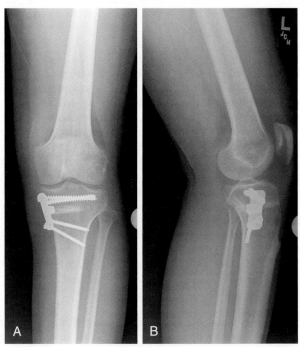

FIG 45.35 (A) Final AP radiograph of a healed proximal tibial opening wedge osteotomy. (B) Lateral radiograph of a healed proximal tibial opening wedge osteotomy.

Arthur et al.[1] have reviewed their results of valgus osteotomy for chronic PLC injuries. They found that 8 of 21 patients (38%) had sufficient improvement of knee function, such that subsequent PLC reconstruction was not necessary. High-velocity injuries and patients with concomitant cruciate injuries were more likely to proceed to a second-stage reconstruction compared to patients with low-velocity injuries and isolated PLC injuries.

Complications. Routine surgical complications such as infection and wound breakdown can be encountered. Preoperative evaluation of the skin and soft tissues should be performed to minimize this risk. Up to 30% of patients with a PLC injury demonstrate a peroneal nerve injury,[32,49] and there is also an iatrogenic risk of peroneal nerve injury at the time of surgery. Careful dissection is paramount to avoid injury to the peroneal nerve. Deep venous thrombosis is a risk following this procedure, and consideration for venous thromboembolism prophylaxis should be entertained. No data exist about the incidence of deep venous thrombosis following PLC reconstruction, although patients with a positive family history, smokers, or those on oral contraceptives warrant particular consideration of chemical prophylaxis. We routinely use enteric-coated aspirin, 325 mg orally daily, for 6 weeks. Graft failure or recurrent varus laxity is also reported. This complication is hopefully minimized by attention to graft choice, anatomic tunnel placement, and correction of existing malalignment and associated cruciate injury.

KEY REFERENCES

8. Geeslin AG, LaPrade RF: Outcomes of treatment of acute grade-III isolated and combined posterolateral knee injuries: a prospective case series and surgical technique. *J Bone Joint Surg Am* 93:1672–1683, 2011.

10. Gollehon DL, Torzilli PA, Warren RF: The role of the posterolateral and cruciate ligament in the stability of the human knee. A biomechanical study. *J Bone Joint Surg Am* 69:233–242, 1987.

11. Grood ES, Stowers SF, Noyes FR: Limits of movements in the human knee. Effect of sectioning the posterior cruciate ligament and posterolateral structures. *J Bone Joint Surg Am* 70:88–97, 1988.

18. LaPrade RF: Arthroscopic evaluation of the lateral compartment of the knees with posterolateral complex grade 3 complex knee injuries. *Am J Sports Med* 25:596–602, 1997.

19. LaPrade RF: *Posterolateral knee injuries: anatomy, evaluation, and treatment,* New York, NY, 2006, Thieme.

20. LaPrade RF, Engebretsen L, Johansen S, et al: The effect of a proximal tibial medial opening wedge osteotomy on posterolateral knee instability: a biomechanical study. *Am J Sports Med* 36:956–960, 2008.

22. LaPrade RF, Griffith CJ, Coobs BR, et al: Improving outcomes for posterolateral knee injuries. *J Orthop Res* 32:485–491, 2014.

23. LaPrade RF, Heikes C, Bakker AJ, et al: The reproducibility and repeatability of varus stress radiographs in the assessment of isolated fibular collateral ligament and grade III posterolateral knee injuries. An in vitro biomechanical study. *J Bone Joint Surg Am* 90:2069–2076, 2008.

24. LaPrade RF, Johansen S, Agel J, et al: Outcomes of an anatomic posterolateral knee reconstruction. *J Bone Joint Surg Am* 92:16–22, 2010.

25. LaPrade RF, Johansen S, Wentorf FA, et al: An analysis of an anatomical posterolateral knee reconstruction: an in vitro biomechanical study and development of a surgical technique. *Am J Sports Med* 32:1405–1414, 2004.

27. LaPrade RF, Ly TV, Wentorf FA, et al: The posterolateral attachments of the knee. A qualitative and quantitative morphologic analysis of the fibular collateral ligament, popliteus tendon, popliteofibular ligament, and lateral gastrocnemius tendon. *Am J Sports Med* 31:854–860, 2003.

31. LaPrade RF, Spiridonov SI, Coobs BR, et al: Fibular collateral ligament anatomical reconstructions: a prospective outcomes study. *Am J Sports Med* 38:2005–2011, 2010.

36. LaPrade R, Wozniczka JK, Stellmaker MP, et al: Analysis of the static function of the popliteus tendon and evaluation of an anatomic reconstruction: the "fifth ligament" of the knee. *Am J Sports Med* 38:543–549, 2010.

41. McCarthy M, Camarda L, Wijdicks CA, et al: Anatomic posterolateral knee reconstructions require a popliteofibular ligament reconstruction through a tibial tunnel. *Am J Sports Med* 38:1674–1681, 2010.

43. Moulton SG, Matheny LM, James EW, et al: Outcomes following anatomic fibular (lateral) collateral ligament reconstruction. *Knee Surg Sports Traumatol Arthrosc* 23:2960–2966, 2015.

The references for this chapter can also be found on www.expertconsult.com.

46

Anterior Cruciate Ligament Injuries and Reconstruction: Indications, Principles, and Outcomes

Russell M. Odono, William J. Long, W. Norman Scott

Injury to the anterior cruciate ligament (ACL) is the most common ligament injury in the knee and results in 129,000 to 200,000 reconstructions per year in the United States and 400,000 worldwide.[67,97,133] Greater participation in sporting and recreational activities by the general population continues to expose more individuals to the risk of ACL rupture. Because the experience of orthopedic surgeons with ACL injuries has expanded, the science and technique of ACL reconstruction has expanded as well. Numerous methods for reconstructing the ligament exist, including the use of patellar tendon autograft, quadriceps tendon autograft, hamstring tendons, and allograft material. The most extensive research has been performed on the use of patellar tendon autograft, and this technique remains the gold standard for ACL reconstruction.[77]

HISTORY OF ANTERIOR CRUCIATE LIGAMENT RECONSTRUCTION

Use of the central third of the patellar tendon to reconstruct a torn ACL was first described by Jones[82] to provide a more physiologic procedure than previously described. His technique involved transferring the patellar tendon with a patellar bone block to the intercondylar region of the femur while maintaining the distal attachment of the tendon to the tibial tubercle. Other authors subsequently modified Jones's technique by using the medial third of the patellar tendon.[5,54] Marshall et al.[99] described using the central third of the patellar tendon along with the prepatellar fascia and central portion of the quadriceps tendon. These modifications of Jones' technique also involved creating a more anatomic placement of the reconstructed ligament by passing it through a tibial tunnel, from the anterior aspect of the tibia to the normal tibial ACL insertion site, and leaving the distal attachment of the patellar tendon in place on the tubercle. The femoral side of the graft was passed through bone tunnels in the femur or over the top of the lateral femoral condyle and secured with sutures or staples. Clancy et al.,[44] in an effort to obtain bony union at the femoral fixation site, first described harvesting a block of patellar bone along with the proximal portion of the patellar tendon. They also described detaching the tibial origin of the graft along with a block of bone when the graft was found to be too short. The bone–patellar tendon–bone graft (BPTB) is now the gold standard in ACL reconstruction. Advantages of this type of autograft include its increased stiffness and energy to failure, as well as its ability to revascularize.[12] It has been shown that a 14- to 15-mm-wide BPTB graft has a mean strength that is approximately 168% that of a normal ACL.[117] Current graft widths are closer to 10 mm, but continue to possess greater tensile strength than a native ACL.[166] In addition, the BPTB autograft has a superior ability to achieve stable initial fixation as a result of the bone plugs providing bone-to-bone healing.

PREDISPOSING FACTORS AND ASSOCIATED INJURIES

Several studies have attempted to identify factors predisposing to ACL injury and have found an association between such injury and intercondylar notch stenosis.[92,157] Souryal and Freeman[156] prospectively examined 902 high school athletes and noted that athletes who sustained ACL tears had statistically significant stenosis of the intercondylar notch when compared with those who did not have such injuries. Harner et al.[74] compared 31 patients with noncontact, bilateral ACL injuries with 23 controls who had no history of knee injury. Computed tomography (CT) analysis of the lower extremities revealed that the width of the lateral femoral condyle was significantly larger in the injured knee group and was the predominant contributor to intercondylar notch stenosis. A recent meta-analysis concluded that a decreased notch width or notch width stenosis was a predisposition to ACL injury.[174] A study comparing notch width measurements in men and women, with and without ACL tears, revealed a narrower intercondylar notch width in women than in men, and a narrower width in patients with ACL tears than in controls.[144] MRI analysis of the contralateral uninjured knee in first time noncontact ACL injured patients demonstrated that decreased intracondylar notch width, increased thickness of the bony ridge at the anteromedial outlet of the femoral notch, and decreased ACL volume, increased the risk of suffering a noncontact ACL injury.[167] These results may enable identification of individuals at increased risk for unilateral and, in particular, bilateral ACL tears, which have an overall incidence of approximately 4%. In addition, this may be one of the factors responsible for the increased incidence of ACL tears in female athletes.

Much attention has been focused on the cause of ACL tears in women. Studies investigating injury rates noted that women sustain four to eight times the number of ACL injuries as men in the same sports.[11,28] Possible reasons for this discrepancy include extrinsic factors, such as muscle strength, and intrinsic factors, such as joint laxity, notch dimensions, increased convexity in the lateral articular compartment of the knee, and lower stiffness to applied load.[140,164] Beynnon et al.[23] found a 21.7% increase in risk for noncontact ACL injury in females for each degree of increase in lateral tibial plateau slope. Studies of genetic predisposition have linked the lack of CC genotype of the COL5A1 in women to increased rates of ACL injuries.[131]

Little objective evidence is currently available, however, to support a single hypothesis. The association between female athletes' menstrual cycle and ACL injuries has been examined.[24,122] More injuries than expected were noted during the preovulatory and ovulatory[169] phases of the cycle, when a surge in estrogen production occurs. This finding suggests that non-contact ACL tears in female athletes may be related in part to hormonal fluctuations, but the hormones responsible for the observed association have yet to be determined. A recent meta-analysis has concluded that neuromuscular training and strengthening can reduce the risk of ACL injury in female athletes, particularly those younger than 18 years of age.[172]

Associated injuries at the time of ACL tear affect surgical management and outcomes. Jumping versus nonjumping ACL injuries were reviewed in 263 patients. Injuries associated with a jumping mechanism exhibited a significantly higher rate of meniscal tears.[8,127] Postulating that anthropomorphic characteristics were associated with intra-articular injury at the time of ACL tear, Bowers et al.[31] reviewed their ACL database for height, weight, and body mass index (BMI). Increases in all three variables were associated with higher rates of associated intra-articular pathologies at the time of ACL reconstruction. It was thus hypothesized that by reducing weight and BMI, patients could reduce associated injuries and improve outcomes following ACL reconstruction.

INDICATIONS FOR RECONSTRUCTION

Identification of patients with an ACL injury can usually be made on the basis of the history and physical examination. Patients commonly describe a history of a deceleration injury, with or without contact, during maneuvers such as cutting and pivoting. Patients with this injury mechanism associated with an audible pop, severe pain, and significant swelling of the knee can be assumed to have a torn ACL. Physical examination confirms the diagnosis by demonstrating a positive pivot shift via the Lachman[163] or anterior drawer test of the injured knee as opposed to a contralateral normal knee (Fig. 46.1). A recent meta-analysis showed the Lachman to be the most specific test at 94% and the pivot shift to be the most sensitive test at 98%.[20]

After the acute phase of knee pain and swelling subsides, symptomatic patients complain of persistent instability and giving way of the knee, which can be associated with intermittent episodes of swelling. Once a torn ACL is diagnosed, one must decide whether to recommend nonoperative or operative treatment. Satisfactory results from conservative treatment of ACL tears have been reported.[60] McDaniel and Dameron[106] noted that 70% of patients with complete ACL tears treated conservatively return to strenuous sports. Similarly, Giove et al.[64] reported a 59% rate of return to sports activities after a program emphasizing hamstring strengthening. However, sports requiring sudden stopping and pivoting had the lowest rate of return to participation. Buss et al.[37] evaluated the results of conservative treatment of acute, complete ACL injuries in older, lower-demand patients. They noted that 70% of patients were able to continue with moderate-demand sports at an average follow-up of 46 months. They concluded that conservative treatment in this group of patients can be successful, despite a modest amount of residual instability. Grindem et al.[71] performed a prospective cohort study comparing surgical and nonsurgical treatments of ACL tears, and found little difference in function or strength at 2 years, but noted that those who elected to undergo surgery were more active in higher-level sporting activities.

Numerous other studies, however, have reported less successful outcomes of nonoperative treatment.[8,57,117,118,153] Noyes et al.[119] studied 103 athletically active patients an average of 5.5 years after ACL injury. Despite an initial return to sports activity by 82% of the participants, 55% sustained a significant reinjury within 1 year of the original injury and only 35% were

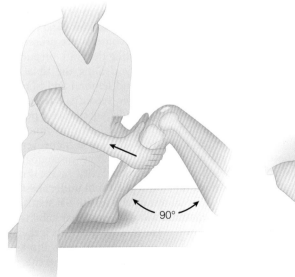

Anterior drawer test

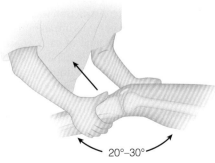

Lachman test

FIG 46.1 (A) Demonstration of the anterior drawer test with the knee at 90 degrees. (B) The Lachman test performed with the knee flexed at 20 to 30 degrees.

participating in strenuous sports at the most recent follow-up. Hawkins et al.[76] reported on 40 patients treated nonoperatively with an average follow-up of 4 years and noted 87.5% fair or poor results; only 14% of patients were able to return fully to unlimited athletic activity. Similarly, Barrack et al.[19] reported 69% fair or poor results after nonoperative treatment in an active naval midshipmen population. Daniel et al.[49] determined that the best predictor for later meniscal or ligament reconstruction surgery is total hours per year of levels I and II sports participation before injury. This observation highlights the fact that individuals who engage in demanding recreational or vocational activities do not respond well to nonoperative treatment of ACL injuries.

The decision to reconstruct an ACL tear should be based not only on the presence of symptomatic instability, but also on the lifestyle and activity level of the patient. In a prospective nonrandomized trial of an ACL reconstruction algorithm by Fithian et al.,[58] patients were categorized as low, medium, or high activity level and had reconstructions if they fell into the medium or high-level group. At an average 6.6-year follow-up, early reconstruction was associated with a reduced rate of knee laxity, symptomatic instability, late meniscal tears, and further surgery.

We do not use guidelines based on age in our practice because the more important factor is the overall level of activity. It is generally agreed that younger individuals have higher levels of activity, and therefore place greater demands on their knees. However, many older individuals are participating in higher levels of recreational sports and are doing so for longer periods. Consequently, age itself should not be a contraindication to ACL reconstruction. Plancher et al.[130] reported 97% good or excellent results after ACL reconstruction in patients older than 40 years at a mean follow-up of 55 months. All patients were satisfied with the procedure, and most were able to return fully to their sports activities, including tennis and skiing.

Symptomatic patients with a more sedentary lifestyle and those who are willing to modify their level of activity can be considered for nonoperative treatment, consisting of a supervised rehabilitation program. One option is to initially treat all patients with an ACL rupture nonoperatively and perform reconstruction on those for whom this form of treatment fails. This approach can involve several months of rehabilitation, followed by several more months if reconstruction is ultimately performed. We have found that most patients are unwilling to accept this amount of time away from their recreational activities; therefore, we recommend early reconstruction for symptomatic patients with greater lifestyle demands. When comparing early reconstruction versus rehabilitation and optional delayed reconstruction, early reconstruction was found to be less costly and more effective when considering an optimal societal healthcare delivery model.[103] The goal of early reconstruction in this patient population is to provide stability, which allows a return to previous activity levels without further damage to the knee, such as meniscal tears and arthrosis. The significant reinjury rates in nonreconstructed knees[58,118] emphasizes the potential sequelae of continued high levels of activity in patients with ACL injury.

In a review of 3475 patients in the Norwegian National Knee Ligament Registry undergoing ACL reconstruction between 2004 and 2006,[69] timing of reconstruction was examined for its relationship to meniscal tears and cartilage lesions. The odds of cartilage lesion increased by almost 1% for each month elapsed between injury and reconstruction. When examining secondary cartilage lesions in groups 0 to 3, 4 to 12, and longer than 12 months after injury, time to surgery longer than 12 months was found to be an independent predictor of significant articular injury.[132]

TIMING OF SURGERY

The timing of ACL reconstruction has been debated; however, no consensus has yet been reached regarding the ideal timing. Initial concern existed over reconstruction of the ACL during the early postinjury period because of the increased risk for arthrofibrosis and difficulty gaining full motion of the knee postoperatively. Shelbourne et al.[152] demonstrated a higher rate of arthrofibrosis in patients undergoing ACL reconstruction within the first week after injury than in those who underwent reconstruction 21 days or longer after injury. The same authors noted, however, that when an accelerated rehabilitation protocol was followed postoperatively, the rates of arthrofibrosis in the two groups were comparable. A meta-analysis showed that with modern surgical technique and an accelerated rehabilitation protocol, ACL reconstruction could be performed as early as 1 week after injury with no increased rates of stiffness.[90] Noyes and Barber-Westin[116] reported that 69% of knees with chronic rupture scored in the normal or very good range after reconstruction as compared with 100% of knees with an acute rupture. Other studies have also found earlier return to sporting activities and better clinical and laxity testing results in knees undergoing early reconstruction.[98] Hunter et al.[80] have shown that the use of modern arthroscopic surgical techniques and an aggressive rehabilitation protocol can yield results that are independent of the timing of surgery. We agree that the specific number of days after injury when the reconstruction should be performed is not as important as the preoperative condition of the knee. Criteria for successful results of ACL reconstruction are minimal or no swelling, good leg control, and full range of motion, including full hyperextension.[149]

SURGICAL TECHNIQUE

Arthroscopic reconstruction of a torn ACL with a BPTB autograft is our procedure of choice and is the technique described here. Steps of the reconstructive procedure include diagnostic arthroscopy, harvesting the graft, preparing the graft, performing the notchplasty, drilling the tibial and femoral tunnels, passing the graft, and femoral and tibial fixation of the graft. Before beginning the reconstructive procedure, however, the knee is examined under anesthesia. A positive Lachman test and pivot shift sign are sought on the injured knee as clinical evidence of a torn ACL. These maneuvers are repeated on the uninjured contralateral knee for comparison and to determine the degree of normal laxity in the knee for the individual patient. A positive pivot shift under anesthesia is the most sensitive clinical test of the functional status of the ACL because it demonstrates a loss of rotational stability imparted by an intact ligament.[16,94] The injured extremity is then prepared and draped in the usual sterile fashion after the application of a thigh tourniquet well above the operative site.

Diagnostic Arthroscopy

After inflation of the thigh tourniquet, the arthroscope is inserted into the knee through a standard lateral portal, and the ACL is visualized to confirm the injury. The ACL is most commonly torn from its proximal attachment on the femur, which results in a stump of tissue that is usually easily visualized through the arthroscope. At times, however, the appearance of the ACL can be deceiving. A torn ACL can become scarred to the surface of the posterior cruciate ligament (PCL) and give the erroneous impression of an intact ligament. Visualization of the ACL with the leg in the figure-of-four position enables adequate assessment of its proximal attachment site in these cases. This view clearly demonstrates absence of the ACL attachment to the femur in ACL-deficient knees. In cases where visualization is poor, a large persistent vertical septum is present, or synovitis obscures the ligament, we do not hesitate to make a second medial working portal, insert the full-radius resector, and remove this tissue.

Meniscal resection or repair can also be performed at the diagnostic examination or can be addressed during preparation of the graft. A second medial working portal is established if the menisci are addressed at this stage. Otherwise, the arthroscope is removed and attention is turned to the graft.

Graft Harvesting

The patellar and tibial tubercle landmarks are drawn on the skin and a vertical incision is made from the inferior pole of the patella to 1 cm medial to the tibial tubercle. Skin flaps are developed to identify the full width of the tendon and the paratenon is incised in line with the skin incision and reflected. A 9- or 10-mm catamaran blade is used to make the incision in the tendon from the patella to the tibial tubercle, with care taken to remain parallel to the tendon fibers. In general, no more than one third of the patellar tendon is used. The incision is carried proximally over the patella for a distance of 25 mm from the tendon insertion, and distally over the tibial tubercle, also 25 mm from the attachment site of the tendon. A small oscillating saw is used to cut bone plugs to a depth of approximately 8 mm. We apply a Steri-Strip at a 10-mm depth along the blade as a simple reference when performing these cuts. The bone plugs are then carefully removed with a curved osteotome.

We have examined the effect of graft diameter on postoperative knee stability by testing ACL-reconstructed knees with the knee ligament (KT) arthrometer after the use of a 9- or 10-mm-diameter graft.[66] The average time from surgery to KT arthrometer testing was 6.6 months, and at the time of testing, the average side-to-side difference for the 9-mm group was 1.02 mm. The average side-to-side difference for the group receiving 10-mm grafts was 1.14 mm. No significant differences between the two groups could be identified with regard to knee stability.

Graft Preparation

Excess soft tissue is first removed from the graft, and the diameter of the bone plugs is trimmed with a rongeur to the appropriate width of 9 or 10 mm. The plug from the tibial tubercle is prepared for placement in the femoral tunnel, where its anatomy and less curved geometry provide maximum bone fill. The edges of the plugs are rounded to permit smooth passage of the graft and the diameters are checked by passing the graft through a tunnel template of the correct size. Three drill holes are then made in the patellar bone plug and one in the tibial tubercle bone plug, followed by passage of no. 5 nonabsorbable suture through these holes (Fig. 46.2). The suture facilitates passage and tensioning of the graft. Finally, the total length of the graft is measured. In general, if the total length is between 92 and 97 mm, fixation with interference screws can be achieved.

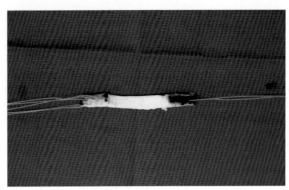

FIG 46.2 Completed preparation of a bone–patellar tendon–bone graft. Methylene blue ink is placed on the cancellous surfaces of the plugs to facilitate their orientation during graft passage.

Fixation with a screw and washer on the tibial side is usually required for grafts measuring outside this range.

Notchplasty

A second arthroscopic portal is made medial to the patellar tendon, if not done previously, as well as a superomedial inflow portal to improve visualization. The remnants of the ACL are then removed with an intra-articular punch and full-radius resector. The lateral wall of the intercondylar notch is cleared of soft tissue attachments, taking care not to injure the adjacent PCL. The motorized burr is then inserted into the medial portal and the notchplasty is begun. The amount of bone to be removed remains controversial and ultimately depends on intraoperative assessment by the surgeon.

Several studies have attempted to establish guidelines for assessing the adequacy of the notchplasty.[65,162] Odensten and Gillquist[121] noted an average maximum distance of 21 mm between the inner surfaces of the medial and lateral femoral condyles in 20 normal cadaver knees. As a result, they suggested that the notchplasty should restore the notch width to this diameter. Berg[21] has defined an adequate notchplasty on the basis of the notch width index[157] and stated that this index, which is the ratio of the intercondylar width to the total femoral condylar width at the level of the popliteal groove, should be at least 0.250 to prevent impingement of the graft. Howell et al.[79] described the relationship between the placement of the tibial tunnel and the required size of the notchplasty. A more anteriorly placed tibial tunnel requires up to 6 mm of bone removal from the intercondylar roof as compared with only minimal removal of bone for tunnels placed 2 to 3 mm posterior to the ACL tibial insertion site. Berns and Howell[22] further defined the requirements for notchplasty by determining the flexion angle at which the graft contacts the roof, with the use of a force transducer in cadaver knees. The angle at which contact occurs averages 12.8 degrees for knees with an eccentrically placed tibial tunnel and requires 4.6 mm of bone removal to achieve zero impingement. This angle of contact decreases to 4.1 degrees when the tibial tunnel is placed 4 to 5 mm posterior to the slope of the intercondylar roof and requires only 1.3 mm of bone removal to prevent impingement. We prefer a generous notchplasty, in which up to 6 mm of bone are removed from the anterior edge of the lateral wall of the notch to prevent any possible impingement on the graft (Fig. 46.3).

The effect of the extent of the notchplasty on the patellofemoral articulation has been investigated. Morgan et al.[111] measured the patellofemoral contact area and pressure after increasing degrees of notchplasty (3, 6, and 9 mm) and found no statistical difference among the groups. They concluded that routine notchplasty, including up to 9 mm, does not affect the patellofemoral articulation. Patellofemoral complications related to the size of the notchplasty have similarly not been a problem in our experience.

The notchplasty is continued posteriorly to the posterior edge of the lateral wall. It is important to identify and remove the resident's ridge to prevent inadvertent anterior placement of the femoral tunnel. This ridge is located at the level of the anterior border of the PCL. Therefore, care must be taken to extend the notchplasty posterior to this border. A hooked probe is useful in ensuring that the over-the-top position and posterior edge of the lateral wall have been reached. The surface of the lateral wall should be smooth, with no rough edges that could impinge on and abrade the graft.

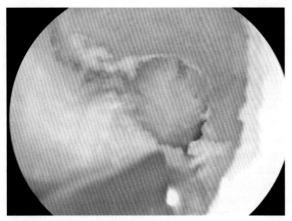

FIG 46.3 Arthroscopic view of a completed femoral notchplasty. The posterior edge of the notch roof must be visualized for correct femoral tunnel position.

Tunnel Placement

The choice of location for the tibial and femoral tunnels can have a significant effect on the outcome of ACL reconstructive surgery. Several studies have examined the effect of the tunnel site on graft impingement,[78,171] range of motion,[135] and overall clinical results.[84] It is recognized that anterior placement of the femoral tunnel is to be avoided to prevent excessive tightness of the graft and thus limit full knee flexion. Similarly, excessive anterior placement of the tibial tunnel may result in graft impingement and early failure. In an attempt to identify definitive landmarks for reproducible tibial tunnel placement, Morgan et al.[111] determined that the ACL central insertion point on the intercondylar floor averages 7 mm anterior to the anterior border of the PCL with the knee flexed to 90 degrees; therefore, this is the ideal location for the tibial tunnel.

We routinely set the tibial drill guide at 55 degrees. The guide tip is placed through the medial portal and positioned with the use of several landmarks, including the anterior border of the PCL, posterior border of the anterior horn of the lateral meniscus, and interspinous area of the tibial plateau. The tunnel is positioned to enable the graft to drape the PCL (Fig. 46.4). The starting point for the guide pin on the proximal end of the tibia is approximately one fingerbreadth medial to the tibial tubercle and two fingerbreadths distal to the medial joint line. After insertion of the guide pin, the tunnel is drilled with a reamer, and the intra-articular edges of the tunnel are smoothed with a rasp to prevent abrasion of the graft (Fig. 46.5). Attempts have been made to consistently produce the correct tibial tunnel length to prevent graft extrusion with tunnels that are too short, and to prevent difficult distal fixation and femoral tunnel placement with tunnels that are too long.[109] We have found, however, that this is not always accurate and may be altered by small variations in operative technique.[125]

Attention is then turned to the femoral tunnel. We use a transtibial technique for placement of this tunnel. The guide pin, which represents the center of the tunnel, is placed in the 1:30- to 2 o'clock position for the left knee or the 10 to 10:30 o'clock position for the right knee and 6 or 7 mm anterior to the over-the-top position, depending on whether a 9- or 10-mm

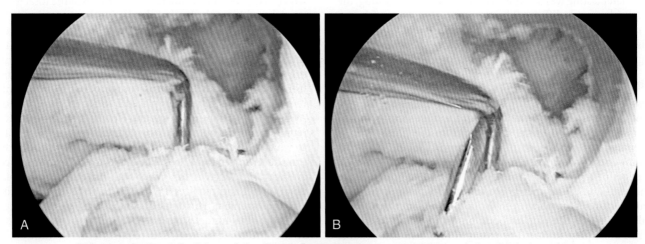

FIG 46.4 Optimal Position of the Tibial Guide (A) Proper positioning of the tibial pin guide adjacent to the posterior cruciate ligament. (B) The tip of the guide pin should be at the level of the posterior edge of the anterior horn of the lateral meniscus such that the graft will drape over the posterior cruciate ligament.

graft, respectively, is used (Fig. 46.6). The guide pin is inserted to a depth of 35 mm, or 1.5 inches, to ensure that there is room for the tunnel without violating the posterior cortex (Fig. 46.7). An indentation, or footprint, in the bone is made with the reamer by hand over the guide pin to confirm the correct position in relation to the posterior cortex. This also ensures that the posterior cortex is intact (Fig. 46.8). The tunnel is then reamed to 30 mm with the knee in a flexed position. The reamer is removed and the arthroscope is placed in the medial port to assess the integrity of the posterior cortex by visualizing the tunnel directly before passage of the graft (Fig. 46.9).

Testing for isometry can be performed at this point or just before committing to the femoral tunnel. Isometer readings are obtained to determine the position of the graft that will result in equal length and tension throughout a full range of motion. However, it has been shown that these readings may vary widely from the final graft isometry because of eccentric placement of the graft within the bone tunnels.[45] Additionally, because the normal ACL is nonisometric, intra-articular testing for isometry is not required if anatomic zones are maintained.[168]

GRAFT PASSAGE

A Beath pin is drilled through the femoral tunnel while maintaining the hip and knee in a hyperflexed position. This position allows the tip of the needle to be pushed through the soft tissues and exit the skin on the anterolateral aspect of the distal part of the thigh. The Beath pin is used to pull the suture in the femoral bone plug through the femoral tunnel. The graft is passed through the tunnels by grasping the sutures on either end of the bone plugs and pulling the graft into the joint. The graft is inserted so that the cancellous bone of the femoral plug is facing anterolaterally in the femoral tunnel (Fig. 46.10). This allows interference screw placement against the cancellous surface of the graft because insertion of a fixation screw on the cortical surface of the plug may lead to disruption of the ligamentous attachment. Tension is applied to the graft through manual pull on the bone plug sutures and the orientation of the graft is assessed (Fig. 46.11). The arthroscope is used to visualize the intra-articular side of the tibial tunnel to verify that the tibial bone plug does not enter into the joint. Assessment of graft clearance from the notch roof is performed at 15 degrees of flexion and in full knee extension (Fig. 46.12).

Graft Fixation

Kurosaka et al.[89] introduced the self-tapping interference screw, which demonstrated improved mechanical properties when compared with buttons or staples. Regardless of technique, failure occurred at the fixation site. Interference screw fixation demonstrated an increase in ultimate failure load and overall construct stiffness, which may potentiate earlier range of motion and accelerated rehabilitation.[56] Paschal et al.[126] compared fixation strengths between 9-mm interference screws and sutures tied over a cancellous screw and washer (post fixation) in porcine knees. Higher ultimate failure loads and less displacement of the bone graft were noted with interference screw fixation. Matthews et al.[104] found no difference in the force to failure of patellar tendon-bone grafts in cadaveric knees when comparing interference screw fixation with post fixation. They did note, however, that post fixation strength is dependent on the type of suture used; no. 5 nonabsorbable suture material provided optimal strength. Despite the conflicting biomechanical results, no studies to date have demonstrated any differences

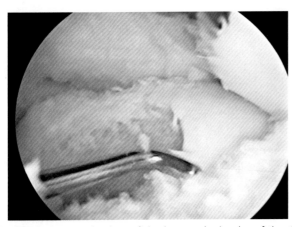

FIG 46.5 Arthroscopic view of the intra-articular rim of the tibial tunnel showing the relationship to the posterior edge of the anterior horn of the lateral meniscus (located at the tip of the probe).

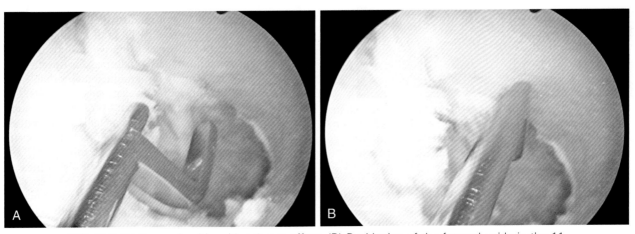

FIG 46.6 (A) Femoral guide with a 6-mm offset. (B) Positioning of the femoral guide in the 11 o'clock position for a right knee. The guide is placed in the 1 o'clock position for a left knee. Note that the posterior tip of the guide is in the over-the-top position on the femur.

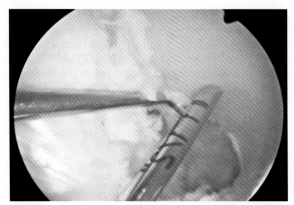

FIG 46.7 Femoral pin inserted to a depth of 1.5 inches.

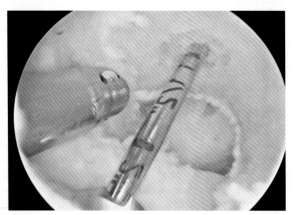

FIG 46.8 Initial reaming over the guide pin to create a femoral footprint. This allows visual inspection of the posterior rim to verify adequate wall thickness before completion of the reaming.

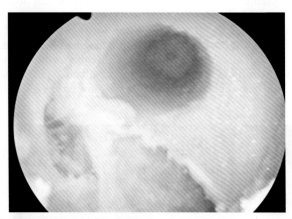

FIG 46.9 Arthroscopic view of a reamed femoral tunnel to confirm the integrity of the posterior wall. The distance between the posterior rim of the tunnel and the posterior edge of the notch roof should be approximately 2 mm.

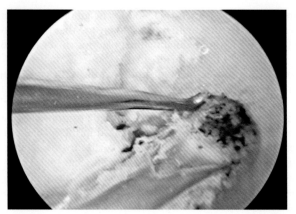

FIG 46.10 Passage of the femoral bone plug into the femoral tunnel, with the cancellous surface oriented superolaterally in the tunnel.

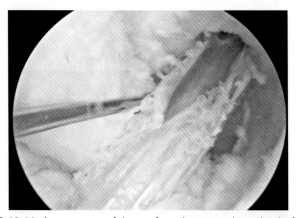

FIG 46.11 Appearance of the graft under manual tension before fixation.

in clinical outcome when comparing interference screw fixation with post fixation.

Absorbable interference screws have been introduced, and several studies have examined the biomechanical properties and clinical results of these screws versus standard metal interference screws.[81] Pena et al.[128] investigated the insertional torque

and failure load for metallic and absorbable interference screws in young and middle-aged cadaveric knees. They noted a higher mean insertional torque for the metal screws as well as a greater mean failure load. Other laboratory studies, however, did not demonstrate any differences between the two types of screws.[40,81] Caborn et al.[41] have compared the maximum load to failure of titanium alloy interference screws with that of absorbable screws in a human cadaveric model with the approximate physiologic strain rate of in vivo BPTB graft loading. No statistical differences were noted between the two groups in the failure mode or the maximum load to failure. A prospective study by Arama et al.[9] that compared titanium and absorbable screws at 5-year follow-up, showed equivalent clinical results.[100] Barber et al.[17] performed a randomized, prospective, multicenter comparison of bioabsorbable and metallic interference screws in 110 patients undergoing arthroscopic ACL reconstruction with patellar tendon autografts. At a minimum 12-month follow-up, postoperative Tegner and Lysholm scores and KT arthrometer maximum side-to-side differences were not statistically significant between the two groups. It was concluded that the absorbable screw is a reasonable alternative to the metal interference screw for bone plug fixation.

Potential problems with the use of interference screws include length mismatch in the tunnel, graft, and screw; divergence of the screw; graft fracture; and suture laceration.[13] Screw

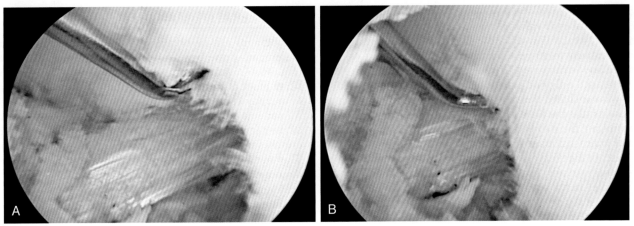

FIG 46.12 An arthroscopic probe is used to assess graft clearance from the roof of the notch with the knee in 30 degrees of flexion (A) and in the fully extended position (B). No impingement should occur in either position.

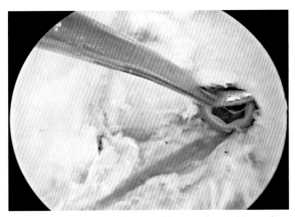

FIG 46.13 Fixation of the femoral bone plug with an interference screw. The screw should be fully seated with no protrusion from the rim of the tunnel into the joint.

divergence has been implicated in failure of graft fixation[104]; however, others have observed that screw divergence of less than 30 degrees does not appear to lead to early failure provided that intraoperative stability is noted.[53] Similarly, we examined the effect of divergence between the femoral interference screw and femoral bone plug.[141] Radiographs and KT-2000 values from 100 consecutive endoscopic autologous BPTB ACL reconstructions were reviewed at a minimum follow-up of 1 year. The mean anteroposterior divergence angle was 6.6 degrees (range, 0 to 32 degrees), and no association was found between the divergence angle and KT-2000 measurements.

The guide pin for the femoral interference screw should be inserted between the edge of the femoral tunnel and the cancellous surface of the bone plug in a direction parallel to the orientation of the graft. The interference screw is passed over the guide pin and advanced into the femoral tunnel. The screw should engage at least 75%, if not 100%, of the bone block (Fig. 46.13). A 7-mm interference screw is recommended if the bone plug–tunnel gap is 2 mm or less. A gap greater than 2 mm requires the use of a 9-mm screw.

Several studies have examined the effect of twisting the graft 90 to 180 degrees before fixation of the tibial plug in an attempt to reproduce the normal helicoid orientation of the ACL fibers.

In vitro studies noted enhanced isometry of the graft fibers,[52] improved graft strength,[46] and restoration of normal tibial rotation in relation to the femur[138] as a result of graft twisting. The clinical significance of these findings, however, remains unclear. Diduch et al.[51] have performed a prospective randomized study examining the clinical and arthrometric results of patients undergoing ACL reconstruction with and without pretwisting of the graft. They reported no clinical failures in either group and no statistically significant differences clinically or by arthrometry between the two groups. The study concluded that pretwisting of the graft has no short-term effect on knee laxity.

The precise amount of initial tension applied to the graft before fixation has not been determined. This has a direct effect on the stability of the knee because inadequate tension will lead to persistent instability, whereas excessive tensioning may lead to elongation of the graft or early fixation failure. Previous studies investigating graft tension concluded that excessive tightness may result in abrasion on the edges of the bone tunnels or the intercondylar roof; in addition, revascularization of these overly tight grafts may be impaired.[34,173]

Burks and Leland[35] noted that the tension applied to an ACL graft to obtain normal anteroposterior translation is dependent on the graft tissue; grafts that are not as stiff require more tension. They determined that 3.6 lb of tension applied to the knee at 20 to 25 degrees of flexion is required for patellar tendon grafts. Numerous studies have revealed that BPTB grafts are the stiffest construct with less postoperative laxity, with an initial 90 N graft tension providing improved stability without overconstraining the knee.[59,114,117]

In addition to the amount of tension, the position of the knee during application of the tension has also been investigated. Bylski-Austrow et al.[39] reconstructed cadaveric knees with a flexible cable and examined the effect of varying degrees of tension and knee position during tensioning. They noted that knees tensioned in 30 degrees of flexion were overconstrained and that this is independent of the initial tension used. Similarly, Melby et al.[107] reported overconstraint of reconstructed cadaveric knees when tensioned at 30 degrees of flexion. In addition, greater quadriceps force was necessary to achieve full extension as the graft tension increased, particularly when tensioned in 30 degrees of flexion. Nabors et al.[113] evaluated 57 patients after ACL reconstruction with a patellar tendon autograft in which the graft was tensioned by a maximal sustained one-handed pull on the tibial end, with the knee in full passive extension. At a minimum 2-year follow-up, the Lysholm score improved from 65 preoperatively to 90 postoperatively, the mean side-to-side difference on instrumented laxity testing was reduced from 7.6 to 0.8 mm, and only one patient had a postoperative contracture. It was concluded that tensioning of the graft in full extension ensures that the knee will come to full extension without compromising the stability of the knee. We use a similar technique of graft tensioning, in which a manual pull is exerted on the sutures in the tibial end of the graft so that there is no laxity in the suture strands. Fixation of the graft is then performed with the knee in full extension.

Fixation of the tibial plug is dependent on the length of the plug with respect to the extra-articular edge of the tibial tunnel. Interference screw fixation is used when the end of the plug is within 5 mm of the extra-articular edge of the tibial tunnel. The bone plug can be visualized in the tibial tunnel with the arthroscope to ensure that the interference screw is placed on the cancellous side of the bone plug. If the tibial plug is positioned more than 5 mm from the extra-articular tunnel edge (long or short), fixation is achieved by tying the sutures over a tibial post. We use a burr to create a trough in the anterior tibia distal to the tunnel. This allows the graft to sit flush against the tibia. The post screw is then placed at least 1 cm distal to the trough and a 6.5-mm partially threaded screw with a washer is placed in a unicortical fashion, for the post.

The functional adequacy of the graft is then tested by performing a manual Lachman test, directly visualizing the graft with the arthroscope to ensure no protrusion of bone intra-articularly, and probing the graft to verify proper tension throughout a range of motion. A bone graft is placed in the patella defect, followed by closure of the paratenon and skin in successive layers.

POSTOPERATIVE MANAGEMENT

Radiographs can be obtained in the recovery room to assess placement of the bone tunnels, if not done intraoperatively (Fig. 46.14). At the completion of the procedure, a femoral nerve block is placed by the anesthesiologist prior to returning to the recovery room. The knee is placed in a hinged knee brace. All patients are dismissed home on the day of surgery. Because of the nerve block, patients are instructed to use the brace and crutches until the block has resolved, usually within 24 hours. They are then permitted to mobilize without the crutches and discontinue the brace as they feel comfortable.

A continuous passive motion (CPM) machine is delivered to the home. Patients begin with 4 hours/day on the CPM, which may be split into two 2-hour sessions. Range of motion on the CPM machine starts at 0 to 60 degrees and is increased daily, as tolerated. The CPM machine is discontinued when full motion is obtained or when they are comfortable shifting to a stationary bike for active motion activities.

All patients undergo a standardized, supervised, postoperative rehabilitation protocol that focuses on immediate weight bearing and obtaining full range of motion, including early full extension. Rehabilitation of the knee is considered complete when equal quadriceps strength is achieved, which is defined as being within 10% of the strength of the contralateral uninjured leg by isokinetic testing. When this goal is attained, the patient may return to full activities, including return to sports.

COMPLICATIONS

Complications associated with ACL reconstruction can be classified as intraoperative and postoperative. Intraoperative complications include patellar fracture, incorrect tunnel placement, violation of the posterior cortex of the femur, graft fracture, and

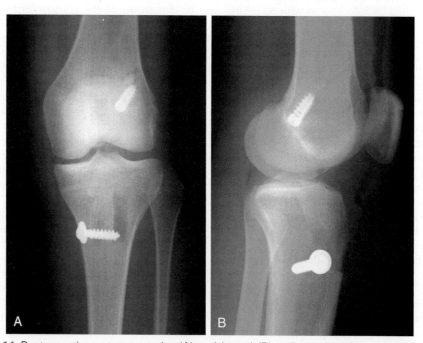

FIG 46.14 Postoperative anteroposterior (A) and lateral (B) radiographs after anterior cruciate ligament reconstruction showing correct placement of the bone tunnels. In this case, fixation of the femoral plug was achieved with an interference screw and the tibial plug was secured by tying sutures over a screw and washer.

suture laceration. Postoperative complications include patella fractures, quadriceps or patellar tendon avulsion, loss of motion, graft stretching and failure, patellofemoral symptoms, and quadriceps weakness.

Intraoperative Complications

Correct placement of the tunnels is crucial to the outcome of ACL reconstruction. Careful evaluation of the position of the guide pins before reaming can prevent erroneous tunnel placement. It is much easier to reposition the guide pin than to correct the position of a tunnel that has already been reamed. However, if a reamed tunnel is noted to be slightly malpositioned, the orientation of the graft plug and interference screw may compensate. For example, if the tibial tunnel is noted to be slightly anterior, placing the graft posteriorly and the screw anteriorly in the tunnel will effectively move the insertion site of the graft posterior to the center of the hole.[13] When there is gross malpositioning of the reamed tunnel, re-reaming of the tunnel in the correct position should be performed, followed by the use of a larger diameter interference screw and bone graft, if necessary, to achieve adequate fixation.

Violation of the posterior cortex of the femur can occur from inadvertently reaming too far into the femoral tunnel and not maintaining the femur in a flexed position during the reaming. When this complication occurs, fixation with an interference screw is no longer possible because the graft will be pushed out of the posterior aspect of the femur by the screw. Fixation with a screw and post on the lateral aspect of the distal end of the femur through a separate incision is necessary, or the traditional two-incision technique with a more anteriorly placed tunnel can be used.[36] This problem can be avoided by maintaining clear visualization during advancement of the reamer into the femoral tunnel and not exceeding 30 mm in the depth of insertion.

Graft fracture and suture laceration can be caused by inadequate space for the plug and screw in the tunnel. In this situation, as the screw is inserted, the graft becomes overly compressed and can fracture. A tight fit can also predispose to the screw engaging the sutures and causing laceration and loss of tension on the graft. Overreaming of the tunnels by 1 mm can prevent an overly tight fit of the interference screw. In addition, we routinely place a single suture in the end of the femoral bone plug and use an interference screw that is shorter than the length of the plug. This prevents the screw from reaching the suture and possibly causing laceration. On the tibial side, the screw should be inserted under direct visualization to avoid entangling the sutures. If laceration occurs at this end, the tibial plug can be passed into the joint and pulled through the patellar tendon defect and new holes can be drilled. The plug is then passed back into the joint and pulled through the tibial tunnel from inside-out. In the event of bone plug fracture, sutures can be placed in the end of the tendon with a Krackow-type stitch and tied over a screw and post.

Patella fracture after ACL reconstruction is infrequent, and the literature on this complication consists mostly of case reports.[43,105] Direct force and indirect force have been implicated in the cause of this fracture. Simonian et al.[155] suggested that an indirect force can result in different patellar fracture patterns, depending on the time elapsed from harvesting. They determined that stellate fractures can occur without direct injury in the early postoperative period (within 5 weeks). After this period, the fracture pattern is more likely to be transverse.

Fracture of the patella during graft harvesting can be avoided by not deepening the cuts more than 8 mm and by maintaining a 45-degree orientation of the sagittal saw blade to the perpendicular surface of the patella. The cuts should also not extend beyond the limits of the fragment to avoid a possible stress riser. In the event of an intraoperative patellar fracture, the patellar fragments should be rigidly fixed to facilitate early range of motion postoperatively.

Postoperative Complications

Despite initially good results after ACL reconstructive surgery, postoperative complications may occur that are detrimental to the long-term outcome. Fortunately, patellar and tibial avulsions are rare, but they are devastating when they do occur. Several case reports have documented this complication, with some occurring up to 6 years after the reconstructive surgery.[29,102] Nixon et al.[115] noted that the patellar tendon donor site, left open at the time of surgery, was histologically identical to normal tendon at 2 years. Others have shown that the ultrasound signal of the tendon returns to normal by 1 year.[1] This time frame may explain why most of these avulsions occur within the first 10 months after surgery.

Much attention has been focused on postoperative loss of motion after ACL reconstruction. This complication may result from preoperative, intraoperative, or postoperative factors. The presence of an effusion, limited range of motion, and concomitant ligamentous injuries of the knee preoperatively are factors that predispose to poor postoperative motion.[72,149] Intraoperative factors include erroneous tunnel placement and inadequate notchplasty. Anterior placement of the femoral tunnel results in overtightening of the graft and loss of full flexion (Fig. 46.15). Placement of the tibial tunnel too far anteriorly can result in impingement of the graft and lead to loss of full extension. Similarly, an inadequate notchplasty can also lead to extension

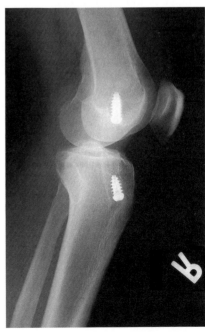

FIG 46.15 Lateral radiograph after anterior cruciate ligament reconstruction showing anterior femoral placement of the graft and interference screw.

loss secondary to impingement. Finally, postoperative immobilization and the rehabilitation protocol can have a significant effect on ultimate range of motion. Previous methods of cast immobilization after reconstruction and therapy emphasizing limited knee extension resulted in significant rates of postoperative arthrofibrosis. The trend toward limited or no immobilization and more aggressive rehabilitation has decreased these rates.[47,68,148] The concern over possible stretching and failure of the graft as a result of aggressive rehabilitation has not been realized. Histologic analysis of the patellar tendon autografts used for ACL reconstruction has revealed that the grafts undergo ligamentization over a period of months to years,[6,55,101] but that a necrotic stage may not occur and the grafts may be viable as early as 3 weeks postoperatively.[136]

The incidence of arthrofibrosis after ACL reconstructive surgery has decreased as postoperative rehabilitative protocols emphasizing early motion have been instituted. The cause of the arthrofibrosis may be poor patient motivation or compliance with the therapy regimen or other factors, such as incorrect bone tunnel placement or the development of reflex sympathetic dystrophy. Treatment of postoperative arthrofibrosis begins with recognition of the problem. Initial treatment with physical therapy should focus on stretching exercises and may also involve the use of static or dynamic braces to regain motion, particularly extension. Manipulation under anesthesia may be necessary if no significant improvement is noted with physical therapy alone. Manipulation is most effective if performed within the first 6 weeks after reconstructive surgery, and aggressive physical therapy must follow the manipulation to prevent recurrence. Adequate anesthesia with an indwelling epidural catheter can facilitate this early rehabilitation. If the manipulation is unsuccessful or it is longer than 6 weeks after surgery, arthroscopic or possibly open release of the adhesions will be required. Revision of the notchplasty may be needed at this time if scar tissue has developed in this area. Once again, aggressive physical therapy must follow any release to prevent recurrence. If the limited range of motion is a result of improper tunnel placement, revision of the tunnels will need to be performed to prevent recurrence.

Stretching of the graft results in recurrence of instability symptoms and a positive Lachman test on examination. This may occur acutely or gradually over time and may be the result of improper tunnel placement, inadequate tension at the time of the reconstruction, or loss of fixation. Treatment of this complication must start with determining the reason for the failure. Graft incompetence immediately postoperatively is most likely caused by inadequate tensioning at surgery. Tunnel-graft mismatch may result in incarceration of the plug in the tunnel and lead to fixation of the plug with laxity in the graft. Proper tunnel sizing and evaluation of graft tension after fixation is achieved should prevent this unnecessary complication. Early (within 6 weeks) acute failure indicates a loss of fixation of one of the plugs because this is the weak link in the construct until bony union occurs. Removal of the interference screw and insertion of a larger diameter screw or fixation with the screw-and-post technique are required. Improper tunnel placement can result in loss of motion, as noted, or stretching and failure of the graft. In the latter case, treatment consists of graft revision with correct tunnel placement.

The most common and persistent complication of ACL reconstruction may be postoperative patellofemoral pain. The exact cause of this problem has not been determined, but several studies have suggested that a relationship exists among persistent flexion contracture, patellofemoral pain, and quadriceps weakness. Sachs et al.[137] reported on 126 patients undergoing ACL reconstruction and noted a 19% rate of patellofemoral pain, which correlated positively with the presence of a flexion contracture. Similarly, Aglietti et al.[3] noted a 5% incidence of patellofemoral pain and a 20% incidence of patellofemoral crepitus without pain in 226 patients after ACL reconstruction. A positive correlation was found between patellofemoral symptoms and flexion and extension losses. Although some studies have suggested that the morbidity of the donor site in autologous patellar tendon reconstructions may contribute to patellofemoral pain,[165] Shelbourne and Trumper[150] have shown that the incidence of anterior knee pain is related more to failure to obtain full knee hyperextension. In their study, 602 patients who underwent ACL reconstruction, followed by a rehabilitation protocol emphasizing full knee hyperextension, were compared with 122 control patients with no history of knee injury. No differences in patellofemoral symptoms were found between the two groups. It was concluded that anterior knee pain can be prevented through a program of early motion and full knee hyperextension. No detrimental effects on stability of the knee from the hyperextension protocol have been noted, provided that precise location of the graft is achieved.

OUTCOMES

Early results of open reconstruction of the ACL were encouraging in terms of restoration of knee stability.[54,91,139] Marshall et al.[99] reported on 40 patients with an average follow-up of 22 months. Four patients were considered failures because of recurrent giving way in two, inability to return to sports in one, and persistent synovitis in one. Clancy et al.[44] reported good or excellent results in 94% of 50 patients at an average 33-month follow-up. None of the patients had any postoperative episodes of instability, and all but six were able to return to full sports activity. O'Brien et al.[120] reviewed 79 patients undergoing intra-articular ACL reconstruction with use of a free, nonvascularized autologous graft from the central third of the patellar tendon. Augmentation with an extra-articular lateral sling of iliotibial band was performed in 60% of the reconstructions. Episodes of giving way were eliminated in 95% of patients; however, nine were unable to return to previous activity levels, and 40% of those who did maintain previous levels of activity continued to wear a brace. Addition of a lateral sling had no effect on the outcome.

Despite these early results, persistent problems associated with ACL reconstruction became evident; these included flexion contracture, patellofemoral pain, limited range of motion, and quadriceps muscle atrophy, in addition to a prolonged rehabilitation period. Technological advances in orthopedic surgery have resulted in the emergence of arthroscopically assisted ACL reconstruction. This reduces the surgical morbidity associated with open reconstruction and facilitates rehabilitation and return to activity. Several studies have shown that when compared with open reconstruction, the arthroscopically assisted technique results in a decreased incidence of patellar symptoms, knee stiffness, and need for manipulation, with no difference in knee stability.[2,15,38] Current techniques of ACL reconstruction have evolved and now involve the use of a single-incision arthroscopic approach that reduces the surgical morbidity further and has been shown to yield consistently good results.[14,124,151] Despite concern with this newer technique regarding potential divergence of interference screw fixation, graft breakage, and posterior cortical violation, comparison studies between the single-incision and two-incision techniques have shown similar results in terms of outcome and complications.[10,73,142]

Harner et al.[73] prospectively compared patients undergoing the two-incision rear-entry technique for ACL reconstruction with another group undergoing the single-incision arthroscopic reconstruction technique. At an average follow-up of 35 months, no significant functional or radiographic differences were noted between the two groups. It was concluded that the single-incision technique yields reliable results, provided that tunnel placement and graft fixation were accurately performed, and that this technique is less invasive and more cosmetic. They also noted other potential benefits of this technique including less postoperative pain and therefore a faster rehabilitation period. Reat and Lintner[134] prospectively studied 30 patients with chronic ACL injuries. The patients were randomly assigned to undergo reconstruction with the one- or two-incision technique. At a mean follow-up of 17 months, no statistically significant differences were found between the two groups, including early postoperative pain and range of motion. It was concluded that the two techniques are interchangeable and that both should be familiar to surgeons because the two-incision technique allows for salvage of intraoperative loss of arthroscopic fixation of the femoral bone plug.

Sgaglione and Schwartz[142] retrospectively reviewed 90 patients who underwent ACL reconstruction with the endoscopic single-incision or arthroscopically assisted two-incision technique. Similar outcomes were noted in subjective, functional, and objective data for the two groups. Four cases of posterior cortical violation occurred in the endoscopic group; however, all of them occurred early in the series. A 33% rate of screw divergence in the endoscopic group versus 14% in the two-incision group was also noted, but no clinical differences in these patients and those with parallel screw placement were found.

George et al.[62] performed a systematic review of four prospective randomized controlled trials comparing two-incision (rear entry) with one-incision (all-endoscopic) techniques. There was no significant difference in objective test scores and outcomes. Crawford et al.[48] performed a systematic review of studies published between 1980 and 2012 with a minimum of 10-year follow-up, and concluded that 1 in 9 patients undergoing surgery will have a rerupture or clinical failure at long-term follow-up.

Several studies have reported on the longer-term follow-up of ACL reconstruction with autologous patellar tendon graft. Bach et al.[15] retrospectively reviewed the results of 97 patients 5 to 9 years after arthroscopically assisted ACL reconstruction with patellar tendon autograft. A manual maximum side-to-side difference of 3 mm or less was noted in 70% of the patients, and 82% had excellent or good results according to the modified Hospital for Special Surgery scoring system. In addition, all patients had a pivot shift result of 1+ or less, and no patient demonstrated clinical findings of chronic patella tendinitis. It was concluded that this technique of ACL reconstruction yields reliable stability and a high level of patient satisfaction. Shelbourne and Gray[145] reported on the 2- to 9-year follow-up of ACL reconstruction performed through a medial miniarthrotomy, followed by accelerated rehabilitation. A total of 1057 patients were prospectively monitored and objective data were available for 806 of these patients. The mean manual maximum KT-1000 knee arthrometer score was 2.0 mm; quadriceps muscle strength testing revealed 94% strength after acute reconstruction and 91% strength after chronic reconstruction. Patients were able to return to sports-specific activities at a mean of 6.2 weeks postoperatively and to athletic competition at full capacity at 6.2 months postoperatively. Otto et al.[124] retrospectively reviewed the 5-year results of 68 patients who underwent single-incision ACL reconstruction with patellar tendon autograft. Three patients experienced rerupture of their ACL grafts before the 5-year evaluation; of the remaining patients, 98% exhibited 5 mm or less of laxity on the Lachman test, and 77% were participating in level I or II activities according to the International Knee Documentation Committee (IKDC) score. Extension loss of more than 3 degrees was seen in 5% of the patients; however, the postoperative therapy regimen consisted of the use of a brace, which did not allow full extension for the first 4 weeks after reconstruction. It was concluded that this technique results in excellent stability of the knee and allows return to a high level of function, and that even better results are anticipated with newer postoperative therapy regimens. Mohtadi et al.[110] compared 330 patients in a prospective randomized clinical trial with patella tendon autograft, quadruple-stranded hamstring, and double-bundle hamstring tendon techniques. At 2 years they found that hamstring and double-bundle grafts had more reruptures when compared to BPTB.

When comparing surgical results, one must consider the postoperative rehabilitation protocol. Previous ACL reconstruction rehabilitation was characterized by periods of immobilization and non–weight bearing in casts. More recent protocols now emphasize early range of motion and full weight bearing, as tolerated, with or without brace support. These aggressive programs have been shown to restore range of motion, reduce patellofemoral complications, and hasten return to activities without compromising knee stability.[87,145,148] As a result, overall outcomes of ACL reconstruction have improved.

Gender differences have been noted with respect to predisposing factors to ACL injury, but outcome studies have also demonstrated a poorer outcome in women following reconstruction. Meta-analyses have demonstrated persistent laxity following reconstruction, with increased rates of postoperative pivot shift and decreased subjective and outcome scores, including Tenger and Lysholm scores, and decreased ability to return to sport in females.[26,161] Shelbourne and Gray[146] reported the rates of reinjury in 1415 patients at 5 years post reconstruction. They noted a similar rate of rerupture in the operative knee, but a significantly higher rate of rupture in the contralateral knee in women (7.8%) than in men (3.7%). The incidence of injury to either knee was associated with a younger age and higher level of activity.

A medium-term follow-up study by Spindler et al.[159] reviewed patients at an average of 5.4 years following reconstruction. Only 69% of patients (217 of 314) were available for follow-up. Predictors of poor outcome on multiple scales included the patient's recollection of hearing or feeling a pop at the time of the injury, a weight gain of more than 15 lb (6.8 kg), and no change in educational level since the surgery. Of note, there was a lack of association between the outcome and the occurrence or form of treatment of a meniscal tear or chondromalacia of the articular cartilage.

Anterior Cruciate Ligament Reconstruction and Development of Arthrosis

One concern that has existed since the advent of surgical reconstruction is whether stabilizing the knee reduces the risk of developing arthritis. There is still a lack of definitive evidence, but in a study by Louboutin et al.,[93] reconstruction of the ligament reduced the rate of developing osteoarthritis (OA) from 60% to 100% with untreated knees down to 14% to 26% with a normal medial meniscus, and 37% with a meniscectomy at 20 years following ACL reconstruction. A systematic review demonstrated low rates of OA at more than 10 years following reconstruction. When isolated ligament reconstruction was required, the rate of arthritis was 0% to 13%, but when a meniscectomy was performed, it rose to 21% to 48%. Louboutin et al. pointed out the nonuniform manner in which OA was determined in these studies.[122] Hart et al.[75] used single-photon emission computed tomography (SPECT) to determine the rates of arthritis at an average of 10 years following reconstruction in 31 patients, using the contralateral knee as a control. They found that 31% of patients had uptake; 13% of those were symptomatic and had a meniscectomy at about the time of reconstruction, but only one patient (7%) was symptomatic in the nonmeniscectomized knees. Oiestad et al.[123] prospectively followed 221 patients over 10 to 15 years, who had isolated ACL injury or combined ACL and meniscal and/or chondral injury. They found significantly higher prevalence of radiographic arthritis in the combined injury compared to the isolated injury, 80% and 62% respectively, yet no difference in symptomatic arthritis. In a review of 502 patients at a mean of 14.1 years postoperatively, another factor noted to be associated with more arthritis and pain was the loss of full extension following surgery.[146] Barenius et al.[18] looked at BPTB and hamstring ACL reconstructions 14 years postoperatively, and found a fivefold increased prevalence of osteoarthritis in the operative extremity when compared to the healthy contralateral extremity, with meniscectomy being a strong associating risk factor. They found no difference in rates of arthritis in BPTB or hamstring reconstructions, or time between injury and reconstruction.

Fifty-five patients with established medial knee arthritis and a chronic ACL tear underwent reconstruction and were followed at an average of 10 years by Shelbourne and Benner.[143] They concluded that reconstruction provides long-term pain relief and improves function. Two patients underwent osteotomy or total knee arthroplasty (TKA), and the importance of obtaining full motion postoperatively was noted. In the MOON and MARS study groups, Borchers et al.[30] observed 508 primary and 281 revision ACL reconstructions and found previous meniscectomies to be a significant risk factor for future chondral damage. Plancher et al.[130] also demonstrated excellent outcomes (97% good to excellent at 5.5 years) following ACL reconstruction in patients older than 40 years, many of whom had preexisting arthritis.

At the other end of the age spectrum, adolescent athletes also sustain ACL injuries to the knee. Concern exists regarding ACL reconstruction because of the possibility of growth and angular deformities following standard tunnel placement across an open physis. Traditionally, options included avoiding twisting or pivoting sports versus physical therapy, rehabilitation, and return to sport with or without a brace. Because of the increased demands in this age group, and unwillingness to modify activities to such an extent, surgical reconstruction has been proposed.

Reconstruction has been addressed in one of two ways—traditional tunnel positioning[7,86,147] or a modified physeal-sparing technique.[85] Both techniques demonstrate low complication rates without significant growth disturbance, indicating that successful reconstruction can be obtained in the adolescent athlete with open growth plates.

Graft Choice

Graft selection has remained a topic of discussion. In a prospective, randomized controlled trial (RCT) of a BPTB versus a two-strand hamstring graft at 3-year follow-up, the objective results of ACL replacement with a BPTB autograft were superior to those of replacement with a two-strand semitendinosus-gracilis graft with regard to knee laxity, pivot shift grade, and strength of knee flexor muscles. However, comparable results were noted in patient satisfaction, activity level, and knee function. Differing fixation techniques, and the fact that only two strands were used in the hamstring reconstructions, likely contributed to the poorer outcomes in this group.[25]

There have been a number of meta-analyses performed on graft selection and outcomes. The first combined nine RCTs and found the only differences to be a slight increase in arthrometer testing laxity with hamstrings, and more pain with kneeling in patents with patellar tendon grafts. It was concluded that graft type may not be the primary determinant in outcomes following ACL reconstruction.[158] A second meta-analysis was performed to explore outcome differences between the two graft sources, combining 14 studies with 1263 patients. This review demonstrated no significant difference in IKDC score and return to preinjury activity level. Of note, at latest follow-up, only 41% of BTB and 33% of hamstring graft reconstruction patients reported their knee as normal based on their IKDC score.[27] A more recent meta-analysis of randomized clinical trials comparing BPTB with hamstring autograft included six combined studies, with a total of 423 patients. Results demonstrated decreased instability on postoperative pivot shift testing with the use of BPTB reconstructions.[26]

Two review articles combined the results of smaller studies examining the results of autograft versus allograft for ACL reconstruction. The meta-analysis by Krych et al.[88] focused only on patellar tendon grafts, whereas the systematic review by Carey et al.[42] incorporated one study with hamstring grafts. When excluding one specific study with a sterilization method that compromised the graft, there were no differences in outcome scores, laxity, clinical failure rates, and return to sports. The authors did point out a significant limitation in these studies because none of the included studies were randomized.

Rates of ACL reconstruction were examined in a review of the state database for New York over a 10-year period from 1997 to 2006. These rates were used to extrapolate a national rate of approximately 105,000 ACL reconstructions in 2006. Observed trends included increasing rates (22%) over the 10-year time period and a 6.5% rate of surgery on either knee within 1 year following ACL reconstruction. Predictors of further surgery include female gender, other interventions in the knee at the time of ligament reconstruction, and treatment by a lower-volume surgeon.[96]

Through the work of Scandinavian ACL registries on more than 45,000 primary ACL reconstructions, the rate of revision surgery for BPTB versus hamstring autografts at 5 years was 2.8% versus 4.2%.[63] Following more than 12,000 primary ACL reconstructions between 2004 and 2012, the Norwegian registry found that those with a hamstring autograft had twice the risk of revision compared to BPTB autograft at 4-year follow-up, with age being the most important risk factor for revision.[129] Large registries in Norway, Sweden, and Denmark have continued to increase our understanding with respect to epidemiology, associated injuries, techniques, perioperative and postoperative protocols, and outcomes.[70]

NEW DIRECTIONS

Proponents of double-bundle reconstruction of the ACL have noted that it better re-creates the two-bundle anteromedial and posterolateral anatomy of the native ligament. Three recent RCTs compared single-bundle (SB) to double-bundle (DB) hamstring reconstructions. The first study randomized 68 patients into two equal arms. Results at a mean of 25 months indicated that DB ACL reconstruction via a four-strand semitendinosus tendon is superior to the SB technique with regard to anterior and rotational stability.[112] The second study of 70 patients at an average 18-month follow-up demonstrated a significant advantage in anterior and rotational stability as well as objective IKDC scores for four-tunnel DB ACL reconstruction compared with SB ACL reconstruction.[154] A third prospective RCT also examined 70 patients receiving an SB or DB hamstring graft for ACL reconstruction. At a minimum 2-year follow-up, DB ACL reconstructions showed better visual analogue scale (VAS) scores, less anterior knee laxity, and improved final objective IKDC scores than SB reconstruction.[4] Two recent meta-analyses comparing SB to DB hamstring reconstructions found that DB reconstructions demonstrated less anterior laxity using a KT-1000 arthrometer, better anterior and rotational stability, less anteroposterior (A-P) laxity, and higher IKDC objective scores.[50,170]

Other investigators have found no significant differences. This includes a meta-analysis by Meredick et al.[108] that combined the results of four RCTs and demonstrated no clinically significant differences in KT-1000 arthrometer or pivot shift testing. Another recent RCT of 50 male athletes reconstructed with an SB or DB technique was designed to investigate results in this high-demand subset of patients at a minimum 2-year follow-up. The SB group was reconstructed with a graft placed at a more horizontal position (10 or 2 o'clock) and it was believed that this may have contributed to the comparable results in the SB group because there were no differences in laxity, rotational stability, or outcome scores.[160]

Conversion to a DB technique also has implications for operative time and cost to the healthcare system. Brophy et al.[33] performed a cost-benefit analysis on this technique modification. They concluded that the DB technique has the potential to introduce considerable new expense into the procedure, and thus does not appear to be cost-effective at this time. These results have been criticized by proponents of the technique because of the limited scope of the comparisons and the short duration of clinical outcomes used for comparison in this review.[61]

A recent all-inside arthroscopic technique for ACL reconstruction has been described. This modification avoids the cortical disruption associated with standard tibial techniques and offers better cosmesis.[32] Lubowitz et al.[95] performed an RCT comparing the all-inside technique with ACL reconstruction with a full tibial tunnel at 2 years. They found no differences in IKDC, Knee Society Score (KSS), and SF-12 scores, narcotic

consumption, and tibial and femoral widening. They noticed significantly lower VAS pain scores for the all-inside technique. Further long-term studies are needed to further evaluate the efficacy of this technique.

It has long been known that the ACL provides more than simple mechanical restraint to the knee. A recent study comparing functional brain magnetic resonance imaging (MRI) scans noted central nervous system reorganization in several motor-related areas in patients with chronic ACL-deficient knees when compared with controls.[83] This may lead to further studies, and modifications of rehabilitation protocols, in an effort to address this nonmusculoskeletal aspect of ACL injuries.

CONCLUSION

The goal of ACL reconstruction is to restore stability of the knee without loss of motion and thereby allow patients to return to their preinjury level of function. The patellar tendon autograft has proved to be a reliable substitute for the native ligament and has yielded good long-term results. Refinements in surgical technique and postoperative therapy regimens have reduced complication rates and decreased recovery times after the procedure. Future challenges for ACL reconstruction are to decrease rates of injuries in athletes, improve surgical techniques, and further optimize rehabilitation protocols. Newly developed registries, similar to those in the arthroplasty literature, will provide increased objective outcome data that can be used to advance techniques.

ACKNOWLEDGMENTS

We thank Dr. Henrik Bo Pedersen for his valuable assistance in preparation of the illustrations in this chapter.

KEY REFERENCES

5. Alm A, Gillquist J: Reconstruction of the anterior cruciate ligament by using the medial third of the patellar ligament. *Acta Chir Scand* 140:289, 1974.
62. George MS, Huston LJ, Spindler KP: Endoscopic versus rear-entry ACL reconstruction: a systematic review. *Clin Orthop* 455:158, 2007.
66. Gotlin R, Cushner FD, Scott WN: Influence of graft diameter on knee stability: KT arthrometry study (unpublished data).
69. Granan LP, Bahr R, Lie SA, et al: Timing of anterior cruciate ligament reconstructive surgery and risk of cartilage lesions and meniscal tears: a cohort study based on the Norwegian National Knee Ligament Registry. *Am J Sports Med* 37:955, 2009.
70. Granan LP, Forssblad M, Lind M, et al: The Scandinavian ACL registries 2004-2007: baseline epidemiology. *Acta Orthop* 80:563, 2009.
77. Hospodar SJ, Miller MD: Controversies in ACL reconstruction: bone-patellar tendon-bone anterior cruciate ligament reconstruction remains the gold standard. *Sports Med Arthrosc* 17:242, 2009.
88. Krych AJ, Jackson JD, Hoskin TL, et al: A meta-analysis of patellar tendon autograft versus patellar tendon allograft in anterior cruciate ligament reconstruction. *Arthroscopy* 24:292, 2008.
93. Louboutin H, Debarge R, Richou J, et al: Osteoarthritis in patients with anterior cruciate ligament rupture: a review of risk factors. *Knee* 16:2394, 2009.
96. Lyman S, Koulouvaris P, Sherman S, et al: Epidemiology of anterior cruciate ligament reconstruction: trends, readmissions, and subsequent knee surgery. *J Bone Joint Surg Am* 91:2321, 2009.
111. Morgan CD, Kalman VR, Grawl DM: Definitive landmarks for reproducible tibial tunnel placement in anterior cruciate ligament reconstruction. *Arthroscopy* 11:275, 1995.

113. Nabors ED, Richmond JC, Vannah WM: Anterior cruciate ligament graft tensioning in full extension. *Am J Sports Med* 23:488, 1995.

119. Noyes FR, Mooar PA, Matthews DS, et al: The symptomatic anterior cruciate-deficient knee. Part I: the long-term functional disability in athletically active individuals. *J Bone Joint Surg Am* 65:154, 1983.

130. Plancher KD, Steadman JR, Briggs KK, et al: Reconstruction of the anterior cruciate ligament in patients who are at least forty years old. A long-term follow-up and outcome study. *J Bone Joint Surg Am* 80:184, 1998.

145. Shelbourne KD, Gray T: Anterior cruciate ligament reconstruction with autogenous patellar tendon graft followed by accelerated rehabilitation: a two- to nine-year follow-up. *Am J Sports Med* 25:786, 1997.

147. Shelbourne KD, Gray T, Wiley BV: Results of transphyseal anterior cruciate ligament reconstruction using patellar tendon autograft in tanner stage 3 or 4 adolescents with clearly open growth plates. *Am J Sports Med* 32:1218, 2004.

148. Shelbourne KD, Nitz P: Accelerated rehabilitation after anterior cruciate ligament reconstruction. *Am J Sports Med* 18:292, 1990.

150. Shelbourne KD, Trumper RV: Preventing anterior knee pain after anterior cruciate ligament reconstruction. *Am J Sports Med* 25:41, 1997.

The references for this chapter can also be found on www.expertconsult.com.

47

Bone-Patellar Tendon-Bone Autograft Anterior Cruciate Ligament Reconstruction

Robert A. Magnussen, Joseph P. DeAngelis, Kurt P. Spindler

INTRODUCTION

Although general indications for anterior cruciate ligament (ACL) reconstruction are discussed elsewhere in this text, it is important to review advantages and disadvantages of patellar tendon autograft reconstruction. Numerous recent high-level systematic reviews have shown both bone-patellar tendon-bone (BPTB) autograft and hamstring grafts (HGs) produce reliable ACL reconstruction results with few clinical outcome differences between the two.* Some recent registry data have suggested that BPTB autograft may be associated with lower failure risk,[15,25] but randomized controlled trials and other large prospective cohort studies have not confirmed these findings.[19,22] A systematic review of the one- versus two-incision BPTB autograft technique showed no reproducible difference in pain medication requirement, rehabilitation time, laxity, or other outcome measure.[13]

Advantages of a BPTB autograft technique
- Interference screw fixation provides immediate strength to allow aggressive early rehabilitation.
- Bone-to-bone graft healing leads to improved strength compared with tendon-to-bone healing in the early (less than 6 weeks) postoperative period.[32]
- Avoidance of injury to the hamstring musculature, the function of which is critical for certain explosive athletes (sprinters) and protective to the ACL.

Contraindications to BPTB autograft technique
- Patients requiring repetitive kneeling for recreational, occupational, or religious reasons: more anterior knee discomfort and pain with kneeling has been noted following patellar tendon graft harvest.[18,23,28,29,39]
- History of extensor mechanism rupture: the potential risk of patellar fracture, patellar tendon rupture, or avulsion has been described.[5,8]
- Small patellar tendon width (<25 mm), significant patellar tendinosis, or presence of a large Osgood-Schlatter ossicle: all may compromise graft strength.[4]

SURGICAL TECHNIQUE

Patient Positioning

The patient is positioned supine with a proximal thigh tourniquet in place, taking care to leave adequate room for an anterolateral incision on the femur, if needed. The foot of table is flexed beyond 90 degrees or removed, allowing the knee to bend to 90 degrees. The patient should be positioned so the thigh extends 3 to 4 inches beyond the edge of the table to avoid displacement of neurovasculature anteriorly and decrease the risk of injury. The contralateral leg should be padded to protect the common peroneal nerve and bony prominences from intraoperative compression. Much of the case, including notch preparation, tunnel drilling, and graft passage, is performed with the thigh resting on the operative table and the knee flexed to approximately 90 degrees.

Diagnostic Arthroscopy

The case begins with a systematic diagnostic arthroscopy. Each articular surface in the knee (patella, trochlea, medial and lateral tibial plateaus, and femoral condyles) should be inspected and graded. Treatment of unstable articular cartilage flaps, removal of loose bodies, and marrow stimulation techniques, such as microfracture or abrasion, should be performed prior to ACL reconstruction. Similarly, both menisci should be inspected and probed for tears. In general, small stable or partial tears should be left alone, with the decision to repair or excise the tear dependent on its location and orientation. Following documentation and treatment of any articular cartilage and meniscal injuries, ACL reconstruction proceeds.

Graft Procurement

There are many techniques for harvesting the BPTB graft from the extensor mechanism. General principles include atraumatic harvest, maintenance of solid bone-tendon attachment on either end of the graft, and careful preservation of remaining patellar tendon attachment sites on the tibia and patella. Careful harvest is critical in minimizing damage to articular surfaces of patella and trochlea, as well as the risk of patella fracture, patellar tendon rupture, and graft disruption.

The harvest can be approached either through a single longitudinal incision or two smaller transverse incisions. Because it provides easy visualization of the entire length of graft, a longitudinal incision is recommended. Using the anteromedial portal and tibial tubercle as landmarks, an incision is made from 1 cm proximal to the anteromedial portal to the tibial tubercle distally, incorporating the anteromedial portal. Making certain the incision extends distally to the inferior aspect of the tibial tubercle allows graft harvest and tibial tunnel drilling with a single incision. A scalpel is used through skin, dermis, and subcutaneous tissues until the transverse prepatellar fascia is encountered. Skin flaps are developed in the plane just superficial to this fascia, more laterally than medially. Use of an Army-Navy retractor should allow visualization of the entire patella proximally and 2.5 cm of the tibial tubercle distally.

The transverse fascia (peritenon) is divided longitudinally in the center of the patellar tendon from the superior pole of the patella distal to the tibial tubercle. Based on surgeon preference, this layer may or may not be closed after harvest. Dissection should be carried medially and laterally to expose the central portion of the patellar tendon (15 to 20 mm). If peritenon closure in not planned, it is important to avoid dissecting too far medially or laterally, causing fat pad herniation. The width of the tendon is measured with the knee flexed 90 degrees. The maximum width of BPTB graft is one-third of entire width of the patellar tendon. A 10-mm graft is standard in our practice because a typical patellar tendon measures 30 mm in width. For a 27-mm tendon, most would harvest a 9-mm graft and adjust tunnel size accordingly. Some authors recommended avoidance of patellar tendon harvest in patients with a tendon width of less than 25 mm[4]; however, Shelbourne et al. have left as little as 14 mm of patellar tendon following harvest without experiencing subsequent patellar tendon rupture (personal communication).

Following determination of tendon width and desired graft size, harvest begins. The tendinous portion of the graft is divided first. A scalpel is used with the knee flexed to 90 degrees to put tension on the patellar tendon. Care is taken to ensure the harvest is in line with the fibers of the patellar tendon. After the tendon is divided, the surgeon can mark the size of the anticipated rectangular bone blocks with electrocautery (Fig. 47.1). Bone plugs are generally between 20 and 25 mm in length and the same width as the graft. However, the length of the patellar block is adjusted to preserve a minimum of 1 cm of intact proximal patellar bone to avoid patella fracture.

Harvesting the patellar block should proceed with careful attention to detail to avoid iatrogenic compression injury of patellar or trochlear articular cartilage as the knee is in flexion during harvest. This goal is accomplished through the use of an oscillating saw with a narrow blade. Cuts should begin distally with cuts extending just through the anterior cortex of the patella to avoid injury to the deep surface. As the cuts are extended proximally, they should not exceed a depth of 6 to 7 mm. The cuts should be angled toward the center of the patella so the resulting bone block is trapezoidal. Thickness of the cortex varies by patient age and size and should be anticipated by the surgeon. Next, the proximal horizontal cut is completed with care taken not to extend the cut more medially or laterally than the respective vertical limbs. Failure to make the cuts square ("T-ing" the cuts) leads to stress risers and potential postoperative fracture (Fig. 47.2).

After the saw cuts are completed, a $\frac{1}{4}$-inch osteotome is gently tapped into the horizontal cut and two-finger pressure is used to elevate the block (Fig. 47.3). If only two-finger pressure is used, the bone block will not fracture. Work with osteochondral autografts has demonstrated that the vigorous tapping to inset plugs can generate chondrocyte death.[36] These data suggest avoidance of vigorous tapping on the patella during graft harvest.

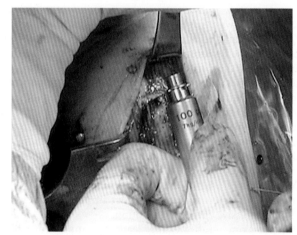

FIG 47.2 A small oscillating saw is used to cut the cortical bone of the patella, outlining the bone block. Care is taken not to "T" the cuts.

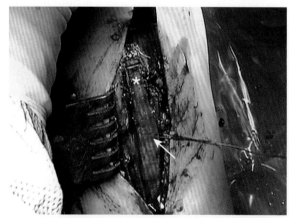

FIG 47.1 The patellar tendon has been divided sharply, and the desired size of the patellar bone block (*) has been marked with electrocautery. Notice the stitch securing the graft to the drape (arrow) to avoid accidently dropping it during harvest.

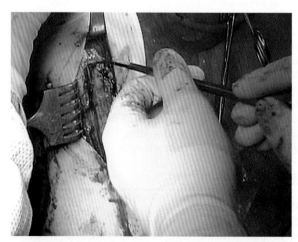

FIG 47.3 A $\frac{1}{4}$-inch osteotome is used in the transverse cut to free the bone block from its bed. Only "two finger" pressure should be used to avoid bone block fracture.

The tibial cut can be completed with either an oscillating saw or osteotome because there is no articular cartilage to injure with compression. Our preferred technique is to use ½-inch osteotomes for the vertical cuts and ¼-inch osteotomes for the distal horizontal cut (Fig. 47.4). When harvesting the tibial bone block, care must be taken to ensure that the proximal end is at the insertion of the patellar tendon into bone, not the proximal end of the tibia. If the surgeon does not carefully visualize this point, then a shorter than desired bone block can inadvertently be harvested. Again, two-finger pressure is used with an osteotome to lever the block out, avoiding bone block fracture. The shape of this bone block is generally more triangular than the patellar block to avoid damage to remaining tibial attachments.

To avoid inadvertent dropping of the graft on the floor, we recommend putting a stitch in the middle and securing it to the drapes during harvest. The patellar tendon defect is closed with interrupted, figure-of-eight, heavy, absorbable suture with knee flexed 90 degrees. Bone graft resulting from graft preparation is used to fill the patellar defect, with any remaining bone used for the tibial defect.

Graft Preparation

The graft is prepared on the back table. Extreme caution must be used to avoid damage to the tendon or bone blocks and avoid inadvertently dropping the graft on the floor and contaminating it. One way to prevent the tendon from falling on the floor is to leave the stitch that was in the tendon in place and secure it to the back table drape with a hemostat. In general, the goal during bone block preparation is to size the blocks to fit comfortably and snugly within the tunnels. The bone blocks are usually brought down to size to fit easily within their respective sizing sleeves with rongeurs. If a graft passer is to be used to pass the graft up into the femur, the bone block going into the femur should be downsized by 1 mm. Thus, if you plan to have a 10-mm tunnel and use a graft passer, you should size the femoral block to fit easily into a 9-mm sleeve. This will allow you to place the graft into the graft passer and slide it up through the tunnel with relative ease. For the tibial tunnel, the graft is sized to fit comfortably within a sleeve that is the same size as the tibia tunnel.

To pass the graft, the surgeon will need to place holes in the patellar and tibial bone block for sutures. If one is using a suture that could be cut by metallic screws or the metal taps required for bioabsorbable screws, one should consider placing the suture tunnels perpendicular to one another so one will remain intact even if the other is cut. The use of FiberWire or some other strong suture material that is not easily cut with any of the taps allows placement of both tunnels in the same direction—usually straight through the cortex. The size of the holes in the bone should be just large enough to pass the metal needle of the suture through it, and no larger, to minimize stress risers in the graft. After the graft is appropriately sized and the surgeon's suture of choice is placed into two bone blocks, the graft is rinsed with saline and placed in a moist saline-soaked sponge until needed (Fig. 47.5).

Notch Preparation and Consideration of Notchplasty

Significant disagreement exists among surgeons regarding the need to débride ACL remnants from the lateral wall of the notch, the need for and degree of notchplasty, and the amount of Hoffa fat pad that should be excised. Sufficient ACL tissue and fat pad should be débrided for the surgeon to accurately visualize appropriate entry points for the femoral and tibial tunnels (Fig. 47.6). Some surgeons prefer to preserve the residual ACL stump to aid in graft placement and potentially improve graft healing and proprioception,[6,14] whereas others débride all ACL tissue and rely on other landmarks. In all cases, but particularly if some native ACL stump is preserved, one must then ensure that there is no graft impingement in the notch at any

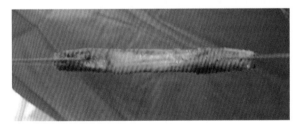

FIG 47.5 Prepared patellar tendon graft demonstrating placement of passing sutures through the shaped bone blocks.

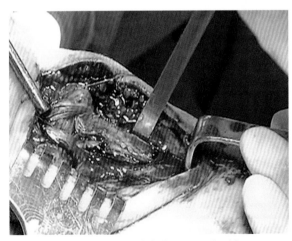

FIG 47.4 The tibial bone block is harvested with osteotomes.

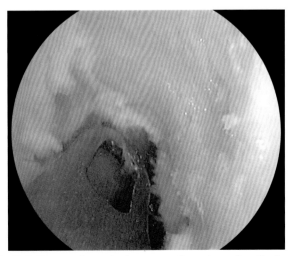

FIG 47.6 Prepared notch demonstrating clear visualization of the lateral wall and the posterior extent of the notch.

point in range of knee motion. A good rule of thumb is to be certain that one can easily place a 5.5-mm burr between the lateral wall of the notch and posterior cruciate ligament (PCL), with a few millimeters on either side. If the notch is too narrow for this maneuver to be performed, notchplasty should be considered. Notchplasty is generally performed anteriorly to posteriorly using a burr. The need for further notchplasty should be rechecked later in the procedure after the graft passer is placed through the tunnels. One should ensure that the graft passer slides easily without impingement through the full normal range of knee motion. Any impingement should be adjusted by further notchplasty.

Tibial Tunnel Preparation

The goal in tibial tunnel placement is to position the tunnel within the ACL footprint so that the graft will neither impinge anteriorly or laterally on the intercondylar notch in extension, nor wrap around the PCL in full flexion. Numerous anatomic landmarks have been described as references to aid in tunnel placement, including the posterior edge of the anterior horn of the medial or lateral meniscus or the anterior aspect of the PCL. Various commercial guides are available to reference off these structures. Placement can be checked prior to reaming by bringing the knee into full extension, following guide pin placement. Some surgeons prefer to leave behind sufficient stump of the ACL as to seal the tunnel after the graft is placed through, whereas others prefer to remove all residual ACL tissue to facilitate visualization. It is currently unknown which technique is most beneficial.

Our standard technique is to place the tibial targeting guide at an angle of 50 to 55 degrees and place it at the posterior edge of the anterior lateral meniscus, centered halfway between the PCL and the lateral wall of the notch (Fig. 47.7). Care should be taken when drilling this guide pin, to make sure the starting point is sufficiently distal on the tibia to leave a sufficient anterior bone bridge. The tunnel is generally placed at approximately the level of the tibial tubercle. Placing the starting point too far medial will result in damage to the pes anserine tendons, whereas starting too far lateral could damage the patellar tendon insertion.

After the guide pin is placed, the knee is brought into full extension to check the position as above. If the location is not acceptable, the pin can be moved with either a "Gatling gun" or 3- to 5-mm offset guides to the correct position. After the pin is appropriately placed, the tunnel is drilled to the appropriate size. A curette should be placed over the intra-articular end of the guide pin during drilling to avoid inadvertent pin migration during overdrilling. Care should be taken to avoid plunging with the drill as the PCL, the lateral wall of the notch, or the lateral femoral condyle could be damaged. The intra-articular mouth of the tunnel is then smoothed with rasps to avoid graft laceration on a sharp bony lip.

Femoral Tunnel Preparation

Femoral tunnel location has been the source of renewed interest in recent years. There is considerable debate as to how far down the lateral wall the center of tunnel should be. Using the clock-face method, recommendations range from 11 to 9 o'clock (right knee) or 1 to 3 o'clock (left knee). Classic teaching is to place the graft at the 10 o'clock (right knee) or 2 o'clock (left knee) position. Increased focus on anatomic placement has led numerous authors to recommend placement farther down the lateral of the notch.[7,9] It is believed that more horizontal graft can better restore rotational stability than vertical grafts.[21,24,30,35] Anteroposterior position of the femoral tunnel has been shown to influence graft isometry more significantly than mediolateral position in the notch.[17] Therefore excellent visualization is required to ensure the graft is not placed too anterior in the notch. The recommended position is 7-mm anterior to the "over-the-top" position at the back of the femoral notch when drilling a 10-mm tunnel (Fig. 47.8). There are three basic techniques frequently used to drill the femoral tunnel: transtibial, two-incision, and accessory medial portal.

Transtibial Technique. One technique for drilling the femoral tunnel involves drilling the femoral tunnel through the tibial tunnel. A guide pin is placed through the tibial tunnel in a retrograde manner and centered on the desired femoral tunnel location. Studies have demonstrated that it is very difficult to obtain anatomic femoral tunnels using this method.[27] The use

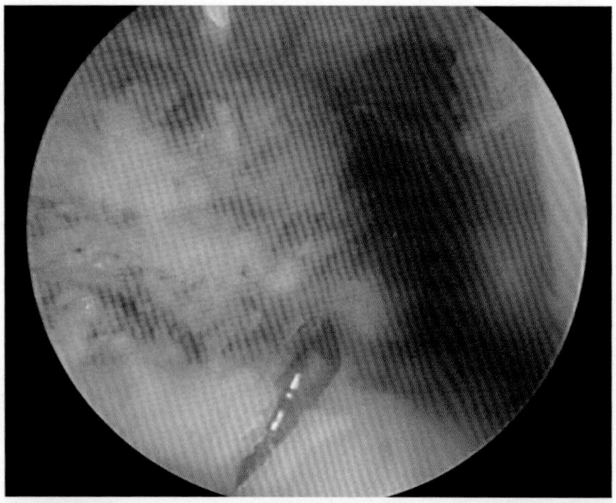

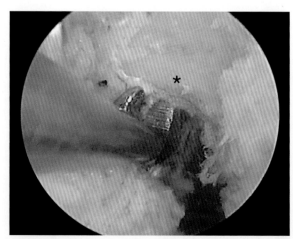

FIG 47.7 Appropriate placement of the tibial tunnel guidewire just posterior to the anterior horn of the lateral meniscus, centered between the PCL and the lateral wall of the notch.

FIG 47.8 A 7-mm offset guide demonstrating an appropriate entry point for the femoral tunnel into the notch (*).

of flexible reamers for the femoral tunnel may facilitate more anatomic femoral tunnel placement with this method. After the guide pin has been placed, one must check to ensure adequate posterior bone is present to avoid posterior wall blowout while drilling the tunnel. After the guide pin is appropriately placed, the femoral tunnel is overdrilled with the appropriately sized cannulated drill. The tunnel should be deeper than the bone block's length (usual tunnel depth is approximately 35 mm), but it is not necessary to penetrate the lateral cortex of the femur. After drilling, the drill and guide pin are removed and a rasp is used to smooth the sharp edges of the tunnel to avoid graft laceration. Advantages of this technique include its relative ease and efficiency, as well as the avoidance of an incision on the anterolateral femur.

Accessory Medial Portal Technique. The accessory medial portal technique for femoral tunnel placement was developed to solve the problem of vertical graft placement noted to occur frequently with a transtibial technique. After desired femoral tunnel position has been identified, the location of the accessory medial portal is determined by spinal needle localization. The portal should be placed so the spinal needle can easily touch the desired location of the tunnel in the notch without touching the medial femoral condyle. Hyperflexion of the knee is generally required to reach the desired tunnel entry point. A portal is created in the desired location, and the guide pin is drilled into the desired tunnel entry point via the portal. The pin site is then inspected to ensure adequate posterior bone is present to avoid posterior wall blowout during drilling.

The appropriately sized cannulated drill is then advanced over the guide pin and into the notch. Extreme caution must be used to avoid damage to the articular cartilage of the medial femoral condyle when advancing the drill toward the notch. The tunnel is then overdrilled to a depth exceeding the length of the bone block. The hyperflexed knee position and more horizontal graft position obtained with this technique generally lead to a shorter femoral tunnel than the transtibial technique, and it may be required to drill through the lateral cortex to obtain adequate tunnel length. The drill and guide pin are then carefully removed, again taking care to avoid damage to the articular surface of the medial femoral condyle.

Two-Incision Technique. The two-incision technique allows a wide range of femoral tunnel position without constraints by tibial tunnel or portal drilling. Ex vivo data have shown improved ability to reproduce the native femoral insertion of the ACL with an independent drilling technique than a transtibial technique.[1,20]

Numerous guide systems exist to facilitate drilling of the femoral tunnel in an outside-in manner. Our preferred guide system includes a stylus that enters the notch from the front via the anteromedial portal, with an adjustable aimer that extends anteriorly to the anterolateral thigh. With the arthroscope in the anterolateral portal, the hooked stylus of the guide is inserted through the anteromedial portal and centered over the desired intra-articular entry point of the tunnel (Fig. 47.9). The other end of the guide is positioned over the anterolateral thigh, and the drill sleeve is inserted to mark the entry point into the skin (Fig. 47.10).

The sleeve is removed, and a 2-cm incision is made parallel to the long axis of the femur, one-third proximal to and two-thirds distal to the skin mark. The incision is carried down

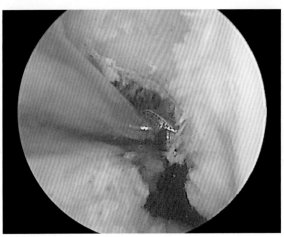

FIG 47.9 Femoral drill guide positioned in the notch and centered on the position marked with the 7-mm offset guide.

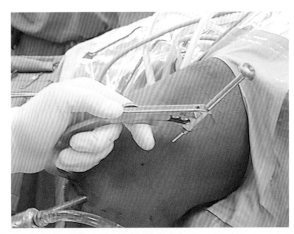

FIG 47.10 The opposite end of the femoral guide is centered over the anterolateral thigh to localize placement of the accessory anterolateral incision.

sharply to the iliotibial band, and tissue overlying the iliotibial band is cleared with a Cobb elevator. The iliotibial band is then incised anterior to the lateral intermuscular septum and parallel to its fibers. The vastus lateralis muscle is then swept anteriorly off the septum and lateral border of the femur. A Z knee retractor is placed along the anterior femur and used to pull the vastus lateralis anteriorly. The drill sleeve is again placed through the femoral drill guide and advanced to bone (Fig. 47.11). An entry position on the lateral femur is chosen, taking care that sufficient bone remains posteriorly to maintain the posterior wall of the femoral tunnel.

After ensuring that the intra-articular portion of the guide remains in the desired position, a 2-mm drill is drilled through the sleeve in an antegrade manner and advanced into the joint under arthroscopic visualization. The femoral drill guide and sleeve are then removed, leaving the 2-mm drill in place. The lateral femoral is again palpated to ensure that sufficient posterior bone remains. A cannulated drill is then used to overdrill the femoral tunnel in an antegrade manner, again under direct visualization (Fig. 47.12). Careful attention should be paid not to plunge. After the drills are removed, a curved rasp is used to clean out the intra-articular portions so there are no rough edges to abrade the graft. One should clean the lateral cortex to

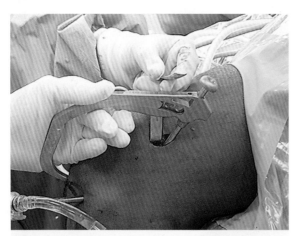

FIG 47.11 The anterolateral incision has been created and the drill guide advanced to bone on the anterolateral femoral metaphysis.

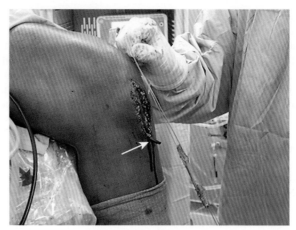

FIG 47.13 The bone-patellar tendon-bone graft ready for passage. The graft passer can be visualized protruding from the distal end of the tibial tunnel (arrow).

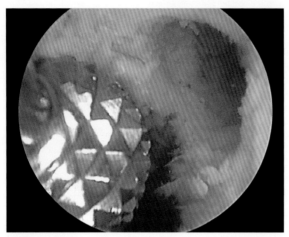

FIG 47.12 Completed femoral tunnel in the 2 o'clock position in the notch.

make sure there are no impinging soft tissues that could interfere with graft passage or interference screw placement.

Graft Passage

Regardless of drilling technique, grafts are generally passed from distal to proximal. The first step is to pull the sutures attached to the graft through the tunnels. With a transtibial or accessory medial portal technique, this is generally accomplished by drilling a beath pin through the femoral tunnel (either via the tibial tunnel or accessory medial portal) and out through the anterolateral thigh. If an accessory medial portal technique is used, one must then advance the beath pin into the knee joint and retrieve if through the tibial tunnel, using a grasper. The leading sutures for the graft are then placed through the beath pin and pulled through both tunnels (Fig. 47.13). With a two-incision technique, a commercially available graft passer can be passed through the femoral tunnel in a retrograde manner, pulled through the tibial tunnel using a grasper, and used to pull the graft's sutures through the tunnels. Alternatively, a free suture can be passed through the femoral tunnel, retrieved through the tibial tunnel, and used to pull the graft's sutures through the tunnels. Use of a suture passage device may facilitate passage of the suture through the femoral tunnel.

The graft is then passed through the tibial tunnel, into the knee joint, and up into the femoral tunnel. Passage should be performed under arthroscopic visualization. The most common cause of difficult passage is difficulty passing the proximal bone block into the femoral tunnel. Guiding the graft into the tunnel with a probe or hemostat via the anteromedial portal may be helpful. Bone block length of 20 mm may also allow easier passage of the graft. Another sticking point may be entry to the distal bone block into the tibial tunnel. This location should be checked if passage is difficult. If a graft passer is used, the femoral block of the graft (which has been downsized by 1 mm) is placed into the graft passer and brought up approximately 1 to 2 cm. This leaves the tibial block out of the graft passer because it is the same size as the tibial tunnel and would have difficulty fitting through the tunnel inside the graft passer. At this point the surgeon pulls the graft and the graft passer up through the tibial tunnel and into the femur. After the leading bone block has engaged the femoral tunnel, the plastic graft passer is completely removed and passage continues until the bone block is completely within the femur.

Graft Fixation

Fixation of patellar tendon autografts is most commonly performed with interference screws. Alternatively, buttons can be used proximally and sutures can be tied over a post, either proximal or distal. Interference screws (metal or bioabsorbable) are the most popular choice for fixation for several reasons. First, interference fixation is more rigid than button or post fixation because it is more apical and effectively shortens the graft. Second, tying over a post, at least on the tibia, has been associated with more postoperative hardware-related pain. Thus the technique presented here focuses exclusively on interference screws.

Regardless of the specific type of screw used, there are several principles that guide screw selection and placement. First, the screw should not be longer than the bone block to avoid damage to the graft as it moves during knee range of motion. Second, the screw should be inserted until it is flush with the cortex of the femur or the tibia so that it is secured in the most rigid bone and is not prominent. Third, the width of the chosen screw should be based on the gap size of between the bone block and the tunnel. If the size difference is 1 mm, a 7-mm screw is used.

If the gap is 2 mm, an 8-mm screw is used. If the gap is 3 to 4 mm, a 9-mm screw is used. Screw size can be modified based upon the relative "softness of bone," with a larger screw used for the same gap size in softer bone. Finally, some bioabsorbable screws require tapping, whereas others do not. This requirement depends on the specific type of screw and its mechanical properties. If a screw requiring tapping is to be used, it is wise to make sure that the sutures in the bone blocks are in a position such that they will not lacerate when tapping.

The femoral interference screw is generally placed first, with the technique dependent on the technique used in drilling the femoral tunnel. If a transtibial or accessory medial portal technique has been used, the femoral interference screw is placed from within the joint in a retrograde manner. First, a small awl is used through a medial portal to create a starting point for the screw between the graft and the edge of the tunnel. A guidewire is then placed via the medial or accessory medial portal into the tunnel next to the graft. A tap is used if needed, followed by insertion of the screw. The distal sutures on the graft should be held to ensure that the graft does not migrate proximally with screw insertion.

In a two-incision ACL reconstruction, the femoral interference screw is inserted from outside to inside in an antegrade manner. This technique eliminates the possibility that the tap or interference screw could cut the graft, as has been reported with retrograde interference screw placement.[2] A tap is used if needed, followed by insertion of the screw. It is critical to provide tension on the proximal sutures to avoid distal migration of the graft during screw placement.

After femoral fixation is achieved, the tibial screw can be secured under tension. The ideal tension is unknown at the present time. Some surgeons prefer to cycle the knee a few times prior to fixation; other people do not. Graft fixation can be performed in full extension or in 20 degrees of flexion. When fixing the tibial side, the tibia should be translated maximally posteriorly against the PCL. The tibial screw is then inserted with or without a guidewire. Care is again taken not to push the graft proximally into the tunnel because this error could result in a lax graft. After the graft is fixed, the knee should be ranged from hyperextension to 100 degrees, a Lachman test should be performed on the table, and the position and tension of the graft should be checked arthroscopically to ensure that no impingement occurs at any degree of flexion (Fig. 47.14).

Closure

After graft placement and fixation are satisfactory, the knee is rinsed and drained and all open incisions are irrigated. Bone graft is then placed in the patellar harvest defect, and any remaining graft is placed in the tibial defect. The patellar tendon is closed with interrupted, figure-of-eight, heavy, absorbable sutures with the knee bent at 90 degrees. The transverse fascia over the patellar tendon may be left open or closed; however, if one elects not to close the patellar tendon defect, it is recommended that this fascia be closed. The IT band can be closed with interrupted absorbable sutures or left open, according to surgeon preference. The skin is closed with inverted, absorbable, deep dermal sutures and a subcuticular running suture (Fig. 47.15). Drains are not routinely used during this procedure, and efforts should be made to maintain good hemostasis except for unavoidable bone bleeding.

Pearls

1. The key to obtaining a reproducible ACL reconstruction is to have adequate visualization of the notch and native femoral and tibial ACL attachments for placement of your femoral and tibial tunnels.
2. Excellent visualization of the patellar tendon is the key to an atraumatic harvest of the patellar tendon bone blocks. Care must be taken to avoid compression injury to the articular surfaces of the patella and trochlea and to avoid damage to the remaining tibial attachment of the patellar tendon to the tibia.
3. There are many commercially available guide systems and templates. The surgeon should be familiar with the nuances, strengths, and weaknesses of the guide system they choose so that they can confirm a reproducible anatomic tunnel position.
4. It is recommended that the patellar bone block be more trapezoidal in profile, which would reduce the depth of the harvest bone and potentially minimize any possibility of intra-articular violation or extra stress at the donor site. At the tibial site the graft should be more triangular, which maximizes the remaining bone deep to the medial and lateral portion of the remaining tendon so as to maintain a sturdy attachment.
5. Adequate confirmation of each step is required so that the optimal position and fixation are maintained. For example,

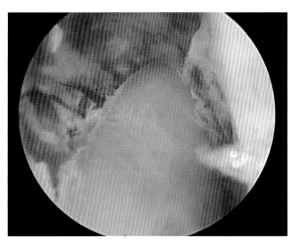

FIG 47.14 Completed ACL graft visualized in the notch.

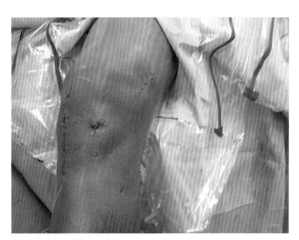

FIG 47.15 Closed incisions. The subcuticular closure allows for excellent cosmetic appearance of all incisions.

one should confirm the accurate position of guide pins for the femur and tibia. Second, one should confirm there is adequate lateral and posterior bone for the femoral tunnel. Third, one should confirm after drilling these tunnels that the intra-articular openings are chamfered and that the graft passer passes through the notch without impingement throughout range of motion. Fourth, after the graft is passed and fixed in the femur, isometry is checked. Fifth, after tibial fixation, stability is checked by a manual Lachman, as well as arthroscopic inspection for impingement and tension.

6. When placing either metal or bioabsorbable interference screws, the specific gap sizes of the tunnel, screw width and length, and fixation of the graft without twisting or pushing it into the tunnel are critical.

7. Finally, when harvesting the patellar bone block, at least 1 cm of proximal patella should be preserved and bone graft should be placed at the patella defect to provide complete healing of the patella and decrease the risk of iatrogenic patellar fracture.

Pitfalls

1. Adequate confirmation of the guide pins should be visualized arthroscopically, as well as through the incisions to make sure that the proper position is achieved and maintained. If not, these pins should be moved by various methods (Gatling gun or fixed parallel pin guides).

2. Notchplasty should be performed first when needed for visualization and later to avoid impingement.

3. Avoidance of intraoperative fracture of the patella or damage to the patellar block or patellar tendon requires meticulous attention to detail, the use of an oscillating saw, and gentle harvesting of the graft from the bone, as previously mentioned.

4. Graft fixation is achieved when the sutures are held, gap sizes are understood, and properly sized screws are inserted without pushing the bone block into the tunnel or rotating the block.

5. Prior to incision closure, consideration should be made for thorough irrigation of the open wounds to minimize potential for infection.

POSTOPERATIVE MANAGEMENT AND REHABILITATION

The goals after reconstructed ACL are to manage pain, decrease swelling, restore range of motion, gain quadriceps control and strength, participate in neuromuscular education, and engage in sport-specific retraining. Our practice is to allow immediate weight-bearing as tolerated on the operative extremity, with crutches used until the patient is able to walk without a limp. We do not currently use a brace following surgery, although bracing should be considered if patients undergo regional anesthesia that could lead to postoperative quadriceps weakness. Factors that modify the typical ACL reconstruction protocol include concurrent performance of meniscus repair or articular cartilage–stimulating procedures, such as microfracture. The rehabilitation protocol should be adjusted and should be in sync with the surgeon's operative technique, the rehabilitation specialist's skill, and patient factors, including age, compliance, and level of activity to which the patient plans to return. Randomized trials demonstrated the safety and efficacy of accelerated rehabilitation protocols following patellar tendon autograft ACL reconstruction.[33]

KEY REFERENCES

1. Abebe ES, Moorman CT, 3rd, Dziedzic TS, et al: Femoral tunnel placement during anterior cruciate ligament reconstruction: an in vivo imaging analysis comparing transtibial and 2-incision tibial tunnel-independent techniques. *Am J Sports Med* 37(10):1904–1911, 2009. PMID: 19687514.

2. Arciero RA: Endoscopic anterior cruciate ligament reconstruction: complication of graft rupture and a method of salvage. *Am J Knee Surg* 9(1):27–31, 1996. PMID: 8835026.

3. Biau DJ, Tournoux C, Katsahian S, et al: Bone-patellar tendon-bone autografts versus hamstring autografts for reconstruction of anterior cruciate ligament: meta-analysis. *Br Med J* 332(7548):995–1001, 2006. PMID: 16603564.

4. Busam ML, Provencher MT, Bach BR, Jr: Complications of anterior cruciate ligament reconstruction with bone-patellar tendon-bone constructs: care and prevention. *Am J Sports Med* 36(2):379–394, 2008. PMID: 18202298.

12. Gabler CM, Jacobs CA, Howard JS, et al: Comparison of graft failure rate between autografts placed via an anatomic anterior cruciate ligament reconstruction technique: a systematic review, meta-analysis, and meta-regression. *Am J Sports Med* 44:1069–1079, 2016. PMID: 25999439.

13. George MS, Huston LJ, Spindler KP: Endoscopic versus rear-entry ACL reconstruction: a systematic review. *Clin Orthop* 455:158–161, 2007. PMID: 17146361.

15. Gifstad T, Foss OA, Engebretsen L, et al: Lower risk of revision with patellar tendon autografts compared with hamstring autografts: a registry study based on 45,998 primary ACL reconstructions in Scandinavia. *Am J Sports Med* 42(10):2319–2328, 2014. PMID: 25201444.

19. Kaeding CC, Pedroza AD, Reinke EK, et al: Risk factors and predictors of subsequent ACL injury in either knee after ACL reconstruction: prospective analysis of 2488 primary ACL reconstructions from the MOON cohort. *Am J Sports Med* 43(7):1583–1590, 2015. PMID: 25899429.

20. Kaseta MK, DeFrate LE, Charnock BL, et al: Reconstruction technique affects femoral tunnel placement in ACL reconstruction. *Clin Orthop* 466(6):1467–1474, 2008. PMID: 18404292.

22. Li S, Chen Y, Lin Z, et al: A systematic review of randomized controlled clinical trials comparing hamstring autografts versus bone-patellar tendon-bone autografts for the reconstruction of the anterior cruciate ligament. *Arch Orthop Trauma Surg* 132(9):1287–1297, 2012. PMID: 22661336.

23. Liden M, Ejerhed L, Sernert N, et al: Patellar tendon or semitendinosus tendon autografts for anterior cruciate ligament reconstruction: a prospective, randomized study with a 7-year follow-up. *Am J Sports Med* 35(5):740–748, 2007. PMID: 17293471.

25. Maletis GB, Inacio MC, Funahashi TT: Risk factors associated with revision and contralateral anterior cruciate ligament reconstructions in the Kaiser Permanente ACLR registry. *Am J Sports Med* 43(3):641–647, 2015. PMID: 25548148.

30. Scopp JM, Jasper LE, Belkoff SM, et al: The effect of oblique femoral tunnel placement on rotational constraint of the knee reconstructed using patellar tendon autografts. *Arthroscopy* 20(3):294–299, 2004. PMID: 15007318.

31. Thompson J, Harris M, Grana WA: Patellofemoral pain and functional outcome after anterior cruciate ligament reconstruction: an analysis of the literature. *Am J Orthop* 34(8):396–399, 2005. PMID: 16187732.

33. van Grinsven S, van Cingel RE, Holla CJ, et al: Evidence-based rehabilitation following anterior cruciate ligament reconstruction. *Knee Surg Sports Traumatol Arthrosc* 18:1128–1144, 2010. PMID: 20069277.

The references for this chapter can also be found on www.expertconsult.com.

48

Anterior Cruciate Ligament Reconstruction With Hamstring Tendons

Leo A. Pinczewski, Lucy Salmon, Emma Heath

The evolution of anterior cruciate ligament (ACL) reconstructive surgery has been from open surgery to arthroscopy-assisted to current all-arthroscopic techniques. There are many surgical options, which involve graft choice, fixation, and surgical technique, for treating ACL injuries.

Graft options include hamstring tendon autograft, patellar tendon autograft, and allograft, both irradiated and sterile harvest. The ideal graft should be biologically active, easy to harvest with minimal donor site morbidity, have the strength of the native ACL, incorporate quickly, and allow rigid fixation to enable early mobilization and rehabilitation. Most surgeons prefer autograft because of ready availability, decreased cost, faster graft incorporation, and no risk of disease transmission associated with the use of allografts.[19,24,41] Historically, patellar tendon autograft was the gold standard; however because of both short- and long-term complications related to donor site morbidity,[*] hamstring tendon autografts have gained increased popularity. The quadriceps tendon has limited use as a graft option.

Biomechanical advantages of hamstring tendon grafts include increased strength, stiffness, and larger cross-sectional area for vascular ingrowth and ligamentization (Table 48.1).[42,86,116] In addition, we opine that the quadruple strand hamstring graft construct more accurately reproduces the ACL anatomy.

An understanding of the process of graft healing is required to manage the reconstructed ACL safely through the rehabilitation process. It is proposed that the ACL remodels through four phases; acute inflammatory, revascularization, cellular proliferation, and finally collagen remodeling.[22] This is referred to as ligamentization.[6] Most studies on graft healing have been conducted using animal models.[6,40,94] Few studies have examined the process of ligamentization in humans, and the true process is not completely understood.[22] Several authors have found, using core biopsy of traumatically failed hamstring autografts, that complete graft integration with the surrounding bone occurs, with the presence of Sharpey-like fibers as early as 6 to 12 weeks, with interference screw fixation.[85,89] Other biopsies of suspensory fixation methods have shown the graft to be enveloped with a layer of granulation tissue and that macroscopically and histologically show no direct connection between tendon graft and bone could be found. There are no neural elements in the reconstructed ACL,[8] and it would appear that a normal ligament never forms after ACL reconstruction.[37,75]

There have been several well-conducted prospective studies and meta-analyses comparing the results of hamstring and patellar tendon autografts. The results of these studies suggest that a functionally stable knee is achieved in more than 95% of patients with hamstring tendon or patellar tendon autograft ACL reconstructions.[35] The incidence of pain and osteoarthritis is higher with patellar tendon; however, graft reinjury rates, laxity, and activity level are higher with the hamstring tendon.[35,69,88] The most consistent difference between the two graft options in these studies is increased kneeling and anterior knee pain[†] and greater loss of postoperative extension[‡] with patellar tendon reconstructions. Over the short term the hamstring tendon graft has been associated with tendon discomfort for up to 6 to 8 weeks after surgery, weakness with high knee flexion, and greater anteroposterior (AP) laxity on clinical testing.[7,25,33] The issue of increased laxity is related to fixation, which has subsequently been resolved with alternate fixation devices. Over the long term the patellar tendon graft is associated with higher rates of radiographic degenerative change.[69] In studies in which fixation, surgical technique, and rehabilitation are standardized, the incidence of ACL graft rupture is equivalent with hamstring and patellar tendon autograft.[29,99,101,109] Other studies have shown long-term contralateral ACL rupture is three times more likely after patella tendon than hamstring tendon graft in ACL reconstruction.[69] It is generally well accepted that reconstruction of the ACL with hamstring tendon autograft is effective for restoring AP laxity to the knee, has good subjective outcomes, and allows a high proportion of patients to return to their desired activity level.

For immediate postoperative mobilization, the ACL graft-fixation construct should be strong enough to withstand the everyday forces required for walking and activities of daily living, which have been estimated to be up to 450 N.[45,49,81,86] There are currently a multitude of fixation options for hamstring tendon autografts. These can be classified into aperture and suspensory fixation, metal, and bioabsorbable materials, as well as plastic materials such as the PEEK screw which is described further below. There are several considerations when selecting a fixation device. Firstly, healing and maturation of the graft needs to be considered. The stages of rehabilitation also need to be considered. Studies on fixation devices and their biomechanical properties have been conducted on animal or cadaver models, and in vivo results differ. Commonly used fixation devices and their biomechanical properties are summarized in Table 48.2.

Aperture fixation with interference screws is commonly used in ACL surgery. Soft tissue interference screws with blunt threads were designed for hamstring tendon grafts to enable compression of the graft against the tunnel wall without graft damage. Improved initial soft tissue graft fixation strength can be achieved

---

[†]References 9, 29, 30, 34, 35, 68, 92, 95, 101, and 125.
[‡]References 2, 30, 32, 39, 54, and 90.

[*]References 31, 33, 96, 98, and 102.

TABLE 48.1   Biomechanical Characteristics of Various Anterior Cruciate Ligament Graft Types

Graft Type	Ultimate Tensile Load (N)	Stiffness (N/mm)	Cross-Sectional Area (mm^2)
Native ACL[126]	2160	242	50
10-mm patellar tendon autograft[125]	1784	210	45
Four-strand gracilis and semitendinosus hamstring tendon autograft[43]	4090	776	53

ACL, Anterior cruciate ligament.

with the use of a longer[15] and larger-diameter screw.[122] Proper graft-tunnel fit with the tunnel sized 0.5 mm larger than the graft diameter also improves fixation strength.[111] Nurmi et al.[87] have found that there is no difference in initial fixation strength between compaction and extraction drilling, using a porcine model. However, extraction drilling often leaves sharp bony edges, which can damage the graft on insertion, within the tunnel, and compaction drilling may still be beneficial to avoid graft damage and assist graft passage. Concentric or eccentric screw placement does not influence initial fixation properties.[103,105]

Suspensory fixation has been reported to result in an increased incidence of tunnel widening compared with aperture fixation.[12,48] The exact mechanism of this is unknown, but proposed reasons include a greater distance between the fixation point and tunnel aperture, leading to micromotion between the graft and bone. However, clinical studies have shown that there is no difference between aperture and suspensory fixation methods with respect to physical examination; instrumented testing; Lysholm, Tegner, and International Knee Documentation Committee (IKDC) scores.[72,106]

Graft fixation is also affected by bone mineral density.[15,20,45] The bone mineral density of the proximal tibia is lower than that of the distal femur. Corry et al.[25] have found that females undergoing ACL reconstruction with hamstring tendon autograft and that 7 × 25-mm interference screw fixation had increased postoperative laxity compared with their male counterparts; subsequently Hill et al.[47] demonstrated that supplemental tibial fixation with a staple successfully restored normal laxity but at the expense of increased kneeling pain at 2-year follow-up in females. Older patients are another subgroup of patients with decreased bone mineral density for whom supplemental tibial fixation may need to be considered. A longer and larger-diameter screw has been shown to be effective in increasing fixation strength.

There has been a recent trend toward using bioabsorbable fixation devices. Possible advantages of bioabsorbable devices include easier revision surgery, minimal interference with future imaging, such as magnetic resonance imaging (MRI),[45,83] and decreased risk of graft laceration during insertion of bioabsorbable interference screws.[16,127] Ultimately, the benefit of bioabsorbable screws is resorption of the device, with subsequent bony replacement of the device in the tunnel. Unfortunately, this has not consistently been the case in vivo. Those bioabsorbable screws that have resorbed rapidly have shown no evidence of new bone formation and frequent ganglia and cyst formation in the tunnels.[11,93,119] Other disadvantages of bioabsorbable

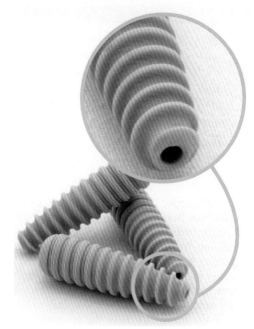

FIG 48.1 PEEK screw, an inert plastic screw allows for imaging of the fixation/graft interface.

devices include synovitis[13,36] and device breakage.[21] With current software and imaging techniques, the metal artifacts from titanium screws can largely be eliminated. If revision is required, a small, screw-shaped femoral defect is superior to a larger fibrous defect or a partly resorbed bioscrew with remnant material adhering to the tunnel wall. Despite the advances in imaging techniques, the fixation/graft interface is unable to be imaged with metal screws. PEEK screws have resolved this issue. The PEEK screw is composed of polyetheretherketone, or PEEK polymer. This screw is composed of an inert plastic and has been successfully used as an alternative to metal implants in orthopaedics since the late 1990's.[66a] Our current technique is to use PEEK interference screw fixation for hamstring tendon autografts (Fig. 48.1). Research has demonstrated a higher ultimate failure load with the PEEK screw compared with the RCI (Smith & Nephew, Cincinnati, OH) screw.[1] Signature Orthopaedics has found that the PEEK screw has 2 times the push-out strength as the titanium screw[28] furthermore, other research also demonstrated equivalent pull-out force.[121]

When assessing the outcome of ACL reconstruction, it is imperative to acknowledge that variations in the surgical technique and selection of patients have a direct effect on outcomes. The surgical technique described in this chapter, using the anteromedial portal and a four-strand hamstring tendon autograft, has been used in an ongoing prospective study of 200 patients with an isolated ACL injury since 1994. A summary of the 10-, 15-, and 20-year outcomes of this group is shown in Table 48.3.[90,100,115] Ongoing longitudinal assessment is continuing, and we are currently collecting the 20-year outcomes.[115]

Successful ACL reconstruction relies on anatomic placement of the graft. The ACL is intricately involved in knee kinematics, and proper graft placement is needed to ensure knee function and stability. Recreating a functional ACL graft requires both the graft within the tunnel and the tunnel itself to be in an anatomic position.

Corry et al.[25] have found a left- to right-sided difference in knee laxity measurement. It was hypothesized that this

TABLE 48.2 Commonly Used Fixation Options in Hamstring Tendon Anterior Cruciate Ligament Reconstruction

Implant	Manufacturer[a]	Type of Fixation (A or S)	Material	Ultimate Strength (N)	Stiffness (N/m)	Slippage Under Cyclic Load
Metal interference screw (BPTB)	—	A	—	559[67]	74[67]	—
Femoral devices						
RCI screw	Smith & Nephew	A	Ti	546[65]	68[65]	3.9 mm after 1500 cycles of 200 N[65]
PEEK (polyetheretherketone) screw	Signature Orthopaedics	A	PEEK Biocomposite	555[28]	70[28]	1.2 mm after 1500 cycles of 200 N[28]
BioScrew	ConMed Linvatec	A	PLLA	589[64]	66[66]	4.0 mm after 1500 cycles of 200 N[66]
Endopearl + BioScrew	ConMed Linvatec	A	PLLA	659[123]	42	—
Endobutton CL	Smith & Nephew	S	Ti	864[3] 1086[66]	79	1.75 mm after 100 sec of 250 N cyclic loading[3]; 3.9 mm after 1500 cycles of 200 N[66]
Cross pin	DePuy Mitek	S	Ti	35 mm: 1003 70 mm: 1604[23]	—	—
RigidFix (bioabsorbable cross pin)	DePuy Mitek	S	PLLA	639[128] 868[66]	226[128] 77[66]	6.02 mm after 100 sec of 250 N cyclic loading[3]; 3.7 mm after 1500 cycles of 200 N[66]
TransFix	Arthrex	S	Ti	1470	207	2.8 mm after 1000 cycles of 150 N[78]
Bio-TransFix	Arthrex	S	PLLA	746[3] 1492[78]	210[78]	1.4 mm after 100 sec of 250 N cyclic loading[3]; 2.6 mm after 1000 cycles of 150 N[78]
Bone mulch screw	Biomet	S	Ti	1112	115[66]	2.2 mm after 1500 cycles of 200 N[66]
Sutures tied over a 6.5-mm screw post	—	S	—	573[113]	18[113]	—
Tibial devices						
Intrafix	Mitek	A	Ti	1332[66]	223[66]	1.5 mm after 1500 cycles of 200 N[66]
WasherLoc	Biomet	S	Ti	975[66] 905[75]	87[66] 200[75]	3.2 mm after 1500 cycles of 200 N[66]; 0.6 mm at 250 N; 2.0 mm at 500 N[75]
AO washer-screw + sutures around screw post	Synthes	S	—	442[75]	60[75]	4.9 mm at 500 N
RCI screw	Smith & Nephew	A	Ti	350[75]	226[75]	1.8 mm at 150 N; 3.7 mm at 500 N[75]
BioScrew	Arthrex	A	PLLA	647[18] 612[66]	65[18] 91[66]	4.1 mm after 1500 cycles of 200 N
Double soft tissue staple	—	S	—	785[75]	118[75]	3.3 mm at 500 N[75]

A, Aperture; *BPBT*, bone-patellar tendon-bone; *PLLA*, poly-L-lactic acid; *S*, suspensory; *Ti*, titanium.
[a]Arthrex, Naples, Florida; Biomet, Warsaw, Indiana; DePuy Mitek, Raynham, Massachusetts; Synthes, West Chester, Pennsylvania.

difference is related to graft rotation during femoral screw insertion. With a standard screw, clockwise graft rotation occurs, leading to a posterior final graft position in left knees, but a relatively anterior final graft position in right knees. This was improved with the use of a reverse thread screw for right-sided ACL reconstructions.[82,98]

Improper tunnel placement is one of the most common, yet avoidable, reasons for early graft failure.[§] Single-incision

arthroscopic ACL reconstruction was introduced and popularized using transtibial femoral tunnel drilling.[80] When constrained by the tibial tunnel, proper placement of the femoral tunnel can be more difficult to achieve reproducibly and often results in vertical graft placement, leading to residual anterolateral rotatory instability.[10,46,60] This led to double-bundle techniques. Subsequent research has confirmed that lower, more anatomic, tunnel placement in the lateral femoral condyle results in increased rotational stability of the knee, with elimination of the pivot shift phenomenon.[43,56,59,71]

[§]References 4, 17, 26, 44, 55, 61, 78, and 107.

TABLE 48.3	10-, 15-, and 20-Year Outcomes of Isolated Anterior Cruciate Ligament Reconstruction[a]		
		Outcome	
Parameter	10-year	15-year	20-year
No. of patients reviewed	86/90	152	71
ACL graft rupture (%)	13	18	18
Contralateral ACL rupture (%)	10	9	10
Mean KT-1000 (mm)	1.6	1.6	1.0
Lachman grade 0 (%)	79	75	76
Grade 0 pivot (%)	86	86	90
Normal or nearly normal IKDC range of motion grade (%)	98	—	92
Lysholm median	89	93 (mean)	92
Patients able to hop >90% of contralateral limb (%)	80	—	77
No knee-related decrease in activity (%)	89	—	—
Overall IKDC grade A or B (%)	83	93	93
Grade A radiograph (%)	81	51	59

ACL, Anterior cruciate ligament; *IKDC,* International Knee Documentation Committee.
[a]Using four-strand hamstring tendon graft, interference screw fixation, and anteromedial portal.

The low anteromedial portal technique was first described by the senior author (LP) and has been used since 1989. It has gained popularity because of recognition of the importance of femoral tunnel placement as a by-product of double-bundle ACL reconstruction techniques.** The principle of the low anteromedial portal technique is drilling of the femoral tunnel independent of, and before, drilling the tibial tunnel, allowing the tunnels to be placed within their respective ACL footprints.[60,113,114] Another advantage of this technique is improved visualization. In the transtibial technique, after the tibial tunnel is drilled, the irrigation solution escapes through this tunnel, decreasing the intra-articular pressure and obscuring visualization required for femoral tunnel placement. It also allows improvement of graft/screw contact area because of collinearity of tunnel, graft, and screw, and therefore soft tissue fixation strength.

The key to successful femoral drilling via the anteromedial portal requires that the knee be flexed to 120 degrees at the time of drilling and screw insertion (Fig. 48.2). This helps to prevent posterior wall blowout.[44] A low central anteromedial portal, 1 cm proximal to the joint line, helps to prevent injury to the medial femoral condyle during femoral tunnel drilling and screw insertion[113] and allows an anterior orientation to the femoral tunnel.

Tunnel placement, assessed postoperatively with routine radiographs, is one of the greatest aids in ACL reconstructive surgery. The intended tunnel position is determined arthroscopically from intraoperative landmarks. The information that can be obtained from routine postoperative AP and lateral radiographs of the knee allows the surgeon to correlate perceived intraoperative tunnel placement to an objective measure and to learn the subtle variations in intraoperative anatomy between patients. Without this feedback, improvement in surgical technique is difficult.

**References 26, 44, 113, 114, and 128.

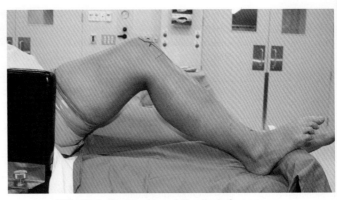
FIG 48.2 Positioning of the limb for surgery.

Successful results 7 and 15 years after surgery are strongly associated with the radiologic position of the tunnels.[14,90] The center of the femoral tunnel should be located 86% posteriorly along Blumensaat line, and on the AP view it should be at a distance of 43% lateral to the lateral femoral epicondyle. Anterior placement of the femoral tunnel is associated with adverse clinical outcomes as a result of excessive constraint, leading to loss of movement or elongation of the graft with cyclic loading. The tibial tunnel should be centered 48% posteriorly along the tibial plateau on the lateral radiograph. Placement of the tibial tunnel center 50% or more posteriorly is associated with loss of knee flexion and increased incidence of graft rupture. More anterior placement is associated with graft impingement and decreased range of motion. In the coronal plane, the tibial tunnel should be centered 47% across the width of the tibial plateau from the medial cortex. This correlates with the position of the medial tibial spine on AP x-ray. More lateral placement is associated with impingement of the graft, whereas medial placement will result in loss of flexion. The graft inclination angle should be measured from a 30-degree, weight-bearing posteroanterior radiograph. This angle is subtended by a line connecting the medial wall of the femoral tunnel and the medial wall of the tibial tunnel and a line perpendicular to the tibial plateau[91] (Fig. 48.3).

SURGICAL TECHNIQUE

Management of ACL injury involves preoperative, operative, and postoperative considerations. The surgical technique and its rationale described in this chapter have been used by the senior author (LP) in more than 10,000 hamstring tendon ACL reconstructions.

Timing of Surgery

It is now well accepted that ACL reconstruction should not be performed until the knee has recovered from the acute injury—after the effusion has resolved and almost full pain-free range of motion has been achieved. Early intervention should only be considered in the acutely locked knee caused by a displaced bucket-handle meniscal tear demonstrated on MRI scan; however most patients with fixed flexion deformity in an acute, first-time cruciate ligament injury have a medial ligament strain preventing terminal extension, rather than a bucket-handle tear of the meniscus.[57] It is not justifiable to perform an arthroscopic procedure because of loss of terminal extension in an acute injury of the knee, without an MRI scan to confirm that surgery

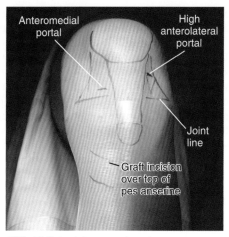

FIG 48.3 Incisions and surface anatomy.

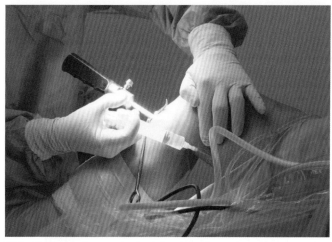

FIG 48.4 Local anesthetic injection along hamstring tendon track.

will be of benefit. Conversely, delaying ACL reconstruction more than 4 months from ACL injury is associated with higher incidence of meniscal and chondral damage.[110] Ideally, and particularly in young patients, ACL reconstruction should be performed after the acute symptoms have resolved and not delayed more than 5 months from injury.

Preoperative Considerations

The evolution of ACL reconstructive surgery, advent of day surgery, and anesthetic technique have resulted in this operation being an elective outpatient procedure. All patients receive antibiotic prophylaxis. The most common bacteria causing infection are coagulase-negative staphylococci and *Staphylococcus aureus*.[58,118] Coagulase-negative staphylococci are often resistant to first-generation cephalosporins but are susceptible to vancomycin. Accordingly, patients receive 1 g vancomycin and 2 g of a cephalosporin IV 1 hour prior to induction of anesthesia for prophylaxis against these common bacteria. We understand that this antibiotic regimen is controversial; however, using this antibiotic regimen, our infection rate has dropped to less than 0.1%. Furthermore, we wrap the graft in a vancomycin-soaked gauze after it is prepared. Vancomycin resistance has never been reported using the antibiotic in this manner.

Positioning and Examination. Following induction of anesthesia, the patient is positioned supine on the operating table, lying close to the edge of the table on the operative side. The knee is examined for range of motion and ligamentous stability with the Lachman, pivot shift, and anterior and posterior drawer tests and varus and valgus stability at 0 and 30 degrees of flexion; tests for posterolateral rotary instability as required. A tourniquet is placed high on the thigh, and a straight leg raise is performed to stretch the hamstring tendons. The tourniquet is then inflated after the limb is exsanguinated. The knee is positioned at 70 degrees of flexion using a footrest and a lateral thigh post (Fig. 48.4). The footrest is placed at the end of the operating table, which allows the surgeon to stand at the foot of the table to harvest the graft, rather than leaning over the limb toward the center of the table. This decreases surgeon postural morbidity.

Hamstring Tendon Harvest and Graft Preparation. A sound knowledge of the surface anatomy around the knee is imperative for successful graft harvest. The hamstring tendons insert at the pes anserine, 1 cm medial to the tibial tubercle and 1 to 3 cm distal to the tubercle. The gracilis and semitendinosus tendons are harvested through a 2-cm oblique incision centered over the pes anserine to decrease the incidence of injury to the infrapatellar branch of the saphenous nerve (Fig. 48.5). However, until a level of surgical comfort is achieved in harvesting the tendons, a vertical incision, which is extensile, should be used. Although this places the infrapatellar branch of the saphenous nerve at greater risk, it is preferable to an insufficient graft. A vertical skin incision is also recommended for patients in whom palpation of the tendons is difficult or for whom prior trauma or surgery may have created scar tissue about the pes anserine, making a difficult harvest. If palpation of the tendons is difficult, centering the incision three fingerbreadths below the joint line approximates the correct position.

Following incision of the skin and subcutaneous fat, a gauze is used to dissect the deep layer of the superficial fascia from the sartorial fascia. The gracilis and semitendinosus tendons are palpated, a 1-cm incision is made in the fascia, along the superior margin of the sartorius tendon, and Metzenbaum scissors are used to enlarge this fascial incision bluntly along the line of the sartorious tendon to expose the gracilis and semitendinosus tendons. Until both tendons are clearly and separately identified, neither tendon should be harvested, to ensure that the semitendinosus tendon is not mistaken for the gracilis tendon. This is also to ensure that there isn't inadequate harvest due to lack of attention to the vinculi. The gracilis tendon, being more proximal, can be hooked out of the subsartorial space with a right-angled forceps and is harvested first. It rarely has any significant vinculi. The tendon stripper applied to the tendon should be passed beyond the proximal tibia and then aimed at the muscle origin on the pubic symphysis. A tendon stripper that may be mechanically closed around an attached tendon is used (ConMed Linvatec, Largo, Florida). It is advanced to 22 cm and, by rotating the handle, the graft is amputated from its muscular attachment at this length. With the harvest of the gracilis tendon, the semitendinosus tendon is thus exposed and extreme care must be taken to identify all of its vinculi to prevent partial harvest of the tendon. The vinculi pass distally and medially from the body of the tendon toward the medial gastrocnemius fascia.

Using a right-angled forceps to hook around the tendon, providing distal traction, an arthroscopy probe is used to palpate its inferior and medial surface for vinculi. There are usually two vinculi along the semitendinosus tendon, one distally near its insertion and one more proximally.[117] Because the proximal vincula is not usually found more than 12 cm from the distal insertion into the tibia, it can be hooked and pulled out of the wound or divided close to the tendon, depending on its mobility. Another indicator that there are no more vinculi is the presence of a round tendon with mesotendon and visibility of its vascular supply. After the vinculi have been divided, the tendon stripper is applied and 22 cm of tendon is harvested, with the instrument aimed more laterally at the ischial tuberosity. Prior to amputating the tendons, 50 mL of local anesthetic solution (40 mL of 0.5% bupivacaine with adrenaline diluted in 100 mL of normal saline, corrected for weight or 1 mg/kg naropin diluted to 200 mL) is administered along the track of the tendon stripper through multiple percutaneous punctures using a 19-gauge spinal needle (Fig. 48.6). This provides significant postoperative pain relief from the graft harvesting.

The tendons are left attached distally at the pes anserine insertion while the graft is prepared (Fig. 48.7). Muscle tissue is meticulously removed from the tendons, as is the mesotendon tissue near its tibial insertion, which can cause ganglion formation if transplanted into the tibial tunnel. The free ends of the tendons are clipped together at a 22-cm length, folded over two no. 5 nonabsorbable leading sutures back to their tibial insertion, and then whipstitched using a no. 2 Vicryl absorbable suture over a length of 40 mm to form a four-stranded bundle. No. 1 dyed Vicryl is then used to suture 25 mm of tendon on the looped femoral end, which is then sized for diameter. A surgical pen is used to mark 30 mm from the end of the graft. The graft is left attached at its distal insertion wrapped in vancomycin-soaked gauze until it is passed through the joint. This eliminates the risk of losing the graft from the sterile field. Preconditioning of the graft is not performed.

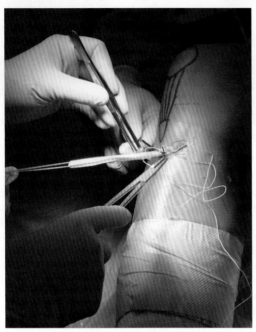

FIG 48.5 Graft preparation.

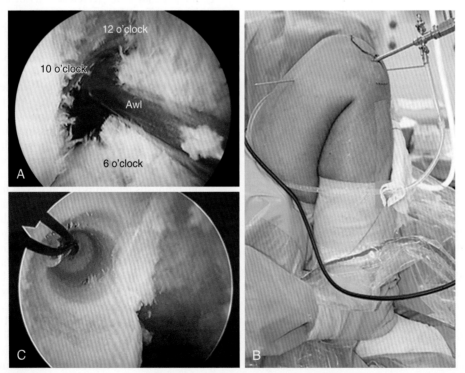

FIG 48.6 (A) Awl confirmation of femoral tunnel placement on lateral wall of intercondylar notch. (B) Beath pin inserted through the anteromedial portal, through the femoral tunnel, and exiting the lateral thigh with the knee in full flexion. (C) Femoral tunnel placement with reference to the posterior cortex of the lateral femoral condyle.

Arthroscopy and Notch Preparation. Proper portal placement facilitates surgery. A high anterolateral portal is made toward the top of the lateral triangle soft spot, adjacent to the lateral border of the patellar tendon. A low and central anteromedial portal is made 1 cm above the medial joint line over the anterior horn attachment of the medial meniscus (see Fig. 48.5), which allows anterior orientation to the drilling of the femoral tunnel. The position of this portal can be checked with a small-gauge needle to ensure that the anterior horn of the medial meniscus is avoided. Diagnostic arthroscopy is then performed, and any meniscal or chondral injuries are addressed prior to starting the reconstruction.

ACL reconstruction begins with the establishment of a field of view by dividing the ligamentum mucosum from the intercondylar notch, allowing the fat pad to retract anteriorly. The ACL stump is then débrided as close to the tibia as possible, and the lateral wall of the notch is exposed. Notchplasty is not performed, except in rare cases of chronic ACL deficiency with osteophytes overgrown in the notch. Notchplasty was popularized in the 1980s and 1990s to improve visualization and to avoid impingement.[62,97] However, with a high anterolateral viewing portal, the femoral ACL footprint can be visualized and anatomic placement of the graft will prevent impingement.

Exposure of the lateral wall begins at the most inferior, anterior aspect of the notch adjacent to the articular surface of the lateral femoral condyle. A curette is used in a curved, upward sweeping motion to remove the fibrous tissue and periosteum from the lateral wall to expose the femoral attachment of the ACL. The posterior border of the lateral intercondylar notch is confirmed visually and with an arthroscopic probe. It is critical to avoid mistakenly identifying resident's ridge as the posterior border that leads to anterior tunnel placement.

Tunnel Placement

Femoral Tunnel. The femoral tunnel for hamstring tendons is centered 5 mm anterior to the posterior capsular insertion into the lateral femoral condyle. This should be checked arthroscopically to be at the 10 to 10:30 clock position on the clockface in the right knee (2 to 2:30 clock position in the left knee). A 45-degree angled bone awl, inserted through the anteromedial portal and impacted into the center of the femoral tunnel site, provides an indication of the position of the proposed tunnel. The arthroscope is then withdrawn to view the lateral wall of the intercondylar notch, which should be aligned vertically along the 6 to 12 o'clock line. The position of the femoral tunnel, as indicated by the awl, can now be confirmed with reference to the roof of the intercondylar notch (see Fig. 48.2).

After the position of the femoral tunnel has been confirmed, the knee is fully flexed at least to 120 degrees and a bicortical femoral tunnel is drilled using a 4.5-mm drill. A 2.4-mm beath pin is introduced through the anteromedial portal, into the femoral tunnel, and out the anterolateral thigh (see Fig. 48.2). This allows for 2.1 mm of adjustment to fine-tune the final tunnel reaming. The femoral tunnel is then reamed to a 30-mm depth, using a cannulated RCI femoral stepped reamer (Smith & Nephew, Andover, Massachusetts), with a 10-mm aperture to accommodate the head of the screw and graft. The minimum tunnel diameter with a 6.5-mm graft is 7.5 mm with the use of a 7-mm screw. Otherwise, the tunnel should be reamed at a diameter 0.5 to 1 mm greater than the diameter of the graft, depending on the hardness of bone (Fig. 48.8). Care must be taken to avoid damage to the posterior cruciate ligament (PCL) and the femoral articular surfaces inserting the reamer during femoral tunnel reaming. With the knee still fully flexed, a doubled nylon suture is pulled through the anteromedial portal and out the lateral thigh, using the beath pin. It is then folded on itself and held taut using a hemostat on the anterolateral thigh. This will subsequently be used to pull the leading sutures of the graft.

The knee is then lavaged of the bony reamings, which tend to accumulate in the lateral and posterolateral compartments. These are a cause of persistent effusion in the postoperative period and are best removed.

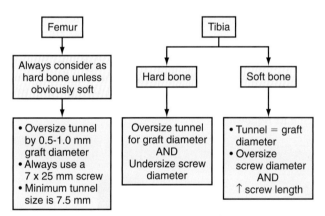

FIG 48.7 Algorithm for selection of interference screw size.

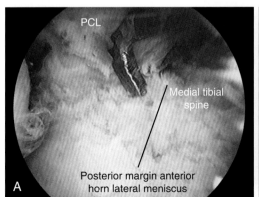
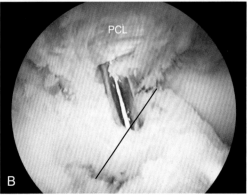

FIG 48.8 Tibial tunnel. (A) Elbow-aiming tibial guide placement. (B) Beath pin piercing PCL.

Tibial Tunnel

The knee is brought back to its resting position at 70 degrees of flexion. The tibial aperture in the joint should be centered at 5 mm (or half a tunnel diameter) medially along a line that joins the apex of the medial tibial spine to the posterior margin of the anterior horn of the lateral meniscus at its attachment to the tibia. This places the tibial aperture both medial and posterior in the native ACL footprint. It has been shown that placing the graft in the center of the tibial ACL footprint leads to graft impingement.[50] Furthermore, this medial tibial placement and lateral femoral placement creates an obliquity in the coronal plane that has been documented to better control rotary stability.[91] An elbow-aiming ACL tibial guide (Acufex, Smith & Nephew) is placed through the anteromedial portal. A 4.5-mm drill, centered in the tibial graft incision, is used first. A 2.4-mm beath pin is then introduced into the joint and held in place by piercing the PCL with the tip of the pin (Fig. 48.9). A 45-mm tibial tunnel is then drilled using the RCI tibial stepped reamer. The tibial tunnel is drilled at the same diameter as the graft diameter.

Passage of the Graft

With the knee flexed at 70 degrees, the hemostat on the lateral thigh securing the nylon suture is released and a grasping forceps is inserted through the tibial tunnel to bring the looped end of the nylon suture out the tibial tunnel. This nylon loop has now been passed through both tunnels and is used to pass the no. 5 lead sutures from the graft construct, first through the tibial tunnel and then into the femoral tunnel and out the lateral thigh. The tendons are carefully released from the pes anserine, and the graft is drawn through the joint up into the femoral hole up to the 30-mm mark on the graft.

Femoral Fixation

A guidewire is introduced through the anteromedial portal. The tip of the guidewire is placed at the femoral tunnel entrance between the anterior edge of the tunnel and the graft, and the knee is then flexed to 120 degrees to advance the guidewire to

its 25-mm mark between the bone and graft. A 7 × 27 PEEK RCI screw is used for almost all femoral fixations, with a reverse threaded screw used for right-sided femoral tunnels. The screw should be advanced 5 to 10 mm deep into the tunnel aperture, such that the head of the screw is not visible after the screwdriver is removed. The knee is then put through a range of motion, and the graft is checked to ensure that it does not impinge on the notch. Our algorithm for screw size selection is shown in Fig. 48.8.

Graft Tensioning and Tibial Fixation

The graft is tensioned following femoral fixation. With the knee in its resting position at 70 degrees of flexion, tension is applied to the four-stranded graft and its sutures at the external tibial aperture using a hemostat to wind up the sutures and graft exiting the tibial tunnel. A guidewire is then inserted between the graft and the posterior medial aspect of the tibial tunnel. While maintaining tension on the graft, a PEEK RCI screw is advanced until the screw captures the graft lightly. The knee is then slowly extended to full hyperextension, allowing any slippage of the bundles to occur, equalizing bundle tension. With the knee in full hyperextension, the screw is advanced up the tibial tunnel until the head is 5 to 10 mm up the tunnel. The hamstring graft is then divided 5 mm longer than the tunnel, allowing a plug of tendon tissue to fill the external tibial aperture, covering the screw head. This decreases blood and marrow leakage from the tibial tunnel initially and minimized cyst formation when bioabsorbable screws were used in the past.

The knee is put through a full range of motion, and restoration of stability is confirmed with the Lachman, pivot shift, and anterior drawer tests. The joint is irrigated and suctioned of any remaining debris, and the proximal lead sutures are removed from the lateral thigh puncture. After traction is applied to a lead suture and it is felt to have moved, it should be cut at the skin level, then extracted by pulling on its partner. This prevents a braided suture that has been in contact with the skin being dragged into the femoral tunnel through the hamstring graft during its removal.

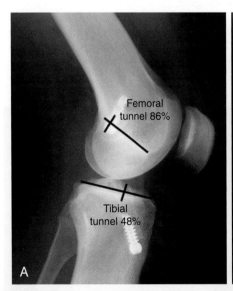 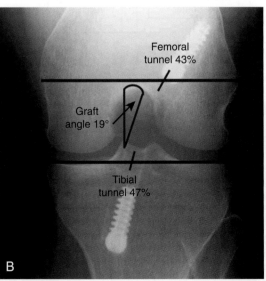

FIG 48.9 Recommended radiologic tunnel positions after ACL reconstruction. (A) Sagittal view. (B) Coronal view.

Closure

Skin closure is achieved using a subcuticular resorbable suture so that removal is not required. Local anesthetic, 50 mL (40 mL of 0.5% bupivacaine with adrenaline diluted in 100 mL of normal saline, corrected for weight) is infiltrated into the wounds, the surrounding soft tissues, and the vastus medialis muscle prior to closure. Studies have confirmed that intra articular injections can induce chondrocyte death. Furthermore, clinical experience is that capsular infiltration is far more effective than intra-articular injection for pain relief. A compression dressing is then applied.

POSTOPERATIVE MANAGEMENT

Immediate, full weight-bearing and joint motion are encouraged without the use of a brace. An accelerated rehabilitation program, as detailed in Table 48.4, is routinely used. Although initially described for use with patellar tendon autografts, equal success has been shown with this program in four-strand hamstring tendon autografts with rigid fixation.[51,52,73] The rehabilitation protocol is provided to the patient and treating physical therapist. Patients are recommended to attend physiotherapy, starting on postoperative day 1. A wound check is

TABLE 48.4 Rehabilitation Protocol Following Anterior Cruciate Ligament Injury and Hamstring Tendon Reconstruction

Stage	Aims	Goals	Treatment Guidelines
Prehabilitation	Prepare patient for surgery	Full range of motion Pain-free mobile joint Teach simple postoperative exercises	Operating on pain-free mobile joints minimizes complications. May take many months. Do not be pressured by patient into early surgery. Preprogramming postoperative rehabilitation is beneficial.
I: Acute recovery (day 1 to 10-14)	Postoperative pain relief and management of soft tissue trauma Wean off crutches and progress to normal gait.	Wound healing Manage graft donor site morbidity. ↓ swelling Restore full extension (including hyperextension). Establish muscle control.	↓ swelling and pain with ice, elevation, and cocontractions. Aim for full range of motion using active and passive techniques. Patella mobilizations. Gait retraining with full extension at heel strike. Return of coordinated muscle function encouraged with biofeedback. Begin quadriceps strengthening as static cocontraction with hamstrings, emphasizing vastus medialis oblique (VMO) control at various angles of knee flexion. Gentle hamstring stretching to minimize adhesions. Active hamstring strengthening begins with static weight-bearing cocontractions and progresses to active free hamstring contractions by day 14. Resisted hamstring strengthening should be avoided for at least 6 wk.
II: Hamstring and quadriceps control (2-6 wk)	Return patient to normal function. Prepare patient for stage III.	Develop good muscle control and early proprioceptive skills. If not done sooner, restore normal gait. Reduce any persistent or recurrent effusion.	Progress cocontractions for muscle control by ↑ repetitions, length of contraction, and more dynamic positions. Gradually introduce gym equipment (eg, stepper, leg press, minitramp). Hamstring strengthening progresses with ↑ complexity and repetitions; open chain hamstring exercises are commenced. Watch for hamstring strains. Low-resistance, high-repetition weights aim to ↑ hamstring endurance. Continue with intensive stretching exercises. Eccentric hamstring strengthening is progressed as pain allows at week 6.
III: Proprioception (6-12 wk)	Improve neuromuscular control and proprioception.	Continue to improve total leg strength. Improve endurance capacity of muscles. Improve confidence.	Progress cocontractions to more dynamic movements (eg, step lunges, half-squats). Proprioceptive work more dynamic (eg, lateral stepping, slide board). Can begin jogging in straight lines on the flat. Progress resistance on gym equipment (eg, leg press, hamstring curls). Solo sports (eg, cycling, jogging, swimming) are usually permitted with little or no restrictions. Open chain exercises commence (if no patellofemoral symptoms) 40-90 degrees, progressing to 10-90 degrees by 12 wk.
IV: Sport-specific (12 wk to 5 mo)	Prepare to return to sport	Incorporate more sport-specific activities. Introduce agility and reaction time into proprioceptive work. Increase total leg strength. Develop patient confidence.	Progress strength work. Proprioceptive work should include hopping and jumping activities and emphasize good landing technique; incorporate lateral movements. Agility work may include shuttle runs, ball skills, sideways running, skipping. Sport-specific activities (eg, tennis—lateral step lunges, forward and backward running drills; volleyball, basketball—vertical jumps)
V: Return to sport (5-6 m)		Return to sport safely and with confidence.	Continue progression of plyometrics and sport specific drills. Return to training and participating in skill exercises. Continue to improve power and endurance. Add PEP[a] program[38] to warmup to reduce further ACL injury. Complete PEP program for 30 consecutive days prior to return to sport.

ACL, Anterior cruciate ligament; *mo,* month; *wk,* week.
[a]*PEP,* Prevent injury, enhance performance.

performed at 7 to 10 days following surgery, and patients should be walking normally without support at this time. Routine follow-up is at 6 weeks and 6 months postoperatively. Patients report an inability to detect a difference in their knee joints and have regained full confidence during athletic activities by 18 months.

Routine radiographs are obtained at the first postoperative visit. Tunnel and screw position are scrutinized. Recommended radiologic positions of the tunnels in the coronal and sagittal views are shown in Fig. 48.3.[91]

Gilchrist et al.[38] have shown that ACL injury may be decreased with the implementation of a specific motor-retraining rehabilitation program which incorporates strengthening and plyometric and agility components.[38,84] Patients who suffer one ACL injury have a 33% incidence of rupturing their contralateral ACL or the graft.[115] The reported incidence of ACL rupture in a normal athletic population is 1.5% to 1.7% per year.[67,108] If one in three patients will sustain a further ACL injury following reconstruction, the addition of these programs to the rehabilitation of ACL-reconstructed patients to reduce this risk is a worthwhile consideration.

COMMON COMPLICATIONS AND THEIR TREATMENT

The common complications of ACL reconstruction using ipsilateral hamstring tendon autograft, treatment options, and strategies for prevention are shown in Table 48.5

SUMMARY

This technique of endoscopic ACL reconstruction through a low anteromedial portal, using a four-strand ipsilateral hamstring tendon autograft and aperture fixation allows the femoral and tibial tunnels to be made independently. It is advantageous with respect to allowing more anatomic placement of the graft within the native ACL footprints compared with transtibial procedures. It reliably reestablishes a stable joint and enables immediate weight bearing and accelerated rehabilitation. Although controversy still remains regarding the ideal graft and method of graft fixation, the goals remain as follows: in the short term, to ensure secure, anatomic graft placement, allowing immediate rehabilitation and a stable knee that permits return to sports; and in the

---

TABLE 48.5 Potential Common Complications of Anterior Cruciate Ligament Reconstruction

Intraoperative Complications	Reported Incidence (%)	Treatment Options	Preventive Strategies
Femoral tunnel blowout	1.2[5]	Suspensory fixation Outside-in femoral screw insertion	Deep knee flexion during femoral tunnel placement
Graft contamination (dropped graft)	1.0[5]	4% chlorhexidine gluconate soak[80]	Leave graft attached to proximal tibia until graft passage
Graft amputation	6.0[5]	Alternate graft Three-strand graft Suspensory fixation	Careful identification of all vinculi prior to graft amputation Harvest the gracilis tendon first to improve visualization of the semitendinosus
Screw tunnel divergence	0.6[5]	—	Use the anteromedial portal.
Bioabsorbable screw breakage	0.9[5]	Alternate fixation device	Use a titanium screw unless contraindicated
Significant graft rotation around screw during insertion	—	Remove screw and reinsert.	Tension the proximal and distal ends of the graft during screw insertion
Early Postoperative Complications			
Infection	0.14-1.7[119]	Varies according to severity and cultures	Use of antiseptic soap for 2 wk prior to surgery. Antibiotic prophylaxis, including vancomycin Larger medial portal to allow easy instrument passage
Loss of motion/stiffness (≥5 degrees at 4 wk)	25[77]	Aggressive physiotherapy; MUA if required	Appropriate surgical timing Anatomic graft placement Tension the graft in full hyperextension under axial compression Accelerate rehabilitation
Deep vein thrombosis	1.5[27]	Anticoagulant therapy	Immediate weight bearing and early mobilization
Pulmonary embolus	0.2[54]	Anticoagulant therapy	Immediate weight bearing and early mobilization
Late Postoperative Complications			
Tunnel widening	36-94,[105,121] depending on fixation	No known clinical implications	Aperture fixation
Cyclops lesion	2-3.6[91,77]	Arthroscopic excision of lesion	Anatomic graft placement Look for ACL stump remnant after graft placement
Traumatic graft failure	1.0/year[100]	Revision ACL reconstruction	Neuromuscular training program during rehabilitation
Contralateral ACL rupture	1.0/year[100]	ACL reconstruction	Neuromuscular training program during rehabilitation
Pretibial subcutaneous cyst	2[91]	Removal of tibial screw and ganglion	Filling of tibial aperture with remnant graft material

ACL, Anterior cruciate ligament; *MUA,* manipulation under anesthesia; *wk,* week.

long term, prevention of further intra-articular injury and osteoarthritis. Accurate placement of the ACL graft is crucial in obtaining a successful outcome after reconstruction.

KEY REFERENCES

1. Aga C, Rasmussen MT, Smith SD, et al: Biomechanical comparison of interference screws and combination screw and sheath devices for soft tissue anterior cruciate ligament reconstruction on the tibial side. *Am J Sports Med* 41(4):841–848, 2013.

14. Bourke HE, Gordon DJ, Salmon LJ, et al: The outcome at 15 years of endoscopic anterior cruciate ligament reconstruction using hamstring tendon autograft for 'isolated' anterior cruciate ligament rupture. *J Bone Joint Surg Br* 94-B(5):630–637, 2012.

22. Claes S, Verdonk P, Forsyth R, et al: The "ligamentization" process in anterior cruciate ligament reconstruction: what happens to the human graft? A systematic review of the literature. *Am J Sports Med* 39(11):2476–2483, 2011.

33. Feller JA, Webster KE: A randomized comparison of patellar tendon and hamstring tendon anterior cruciate ligament reconstruction. *Am J Sports Med* 31(4):564–573, 2003.

46. Harvey A, Thomas NP, Amis AA: Fixation of the graft in reconstruction of the anterior cruciate ligament. *J Bone Joint Surg Br* 87-B(5):593–603, 2005.

64. Kousa P, Järvinen TL, Vihavainen M, et al: The fixation strength of six hamstring tendon graft fixation devices in anterior cruciate ligament reconstruction. Part I: femoral site. *Am J Sports Med* 31(2):174–181, 2003.

91. Pinczewski LA, Lyman J, Salmon LJ, et al: A ten-year comparison of hamstring tendon and bone-patellar tendon-bone anterior cruciate ligament reconstructions. A controlled, prospective trial. *Am J Sports Med* 35(1):564–574, 2007.

92. Pinczewski LA, Salmon LJ, Jackson WF, et al: Radiological landmarks for placement of the tunnels in single-bundle reconstruction of the anterior cruciate ligament. *J Bone Joint Surg Br* 90-B(2):172–179, 2008.

98. Rue J-PH, Lewis PB, Parameswaran AD, et al: Single-bundle anterior cruciate ligament reconstruction: technique overview and comprehensive review of results. *J Bone Joint Surg Am* 90(Suppl_4):67–74, 2008.

101. Salmon LJ, Refshauge K, Russell V, et al: Gender differences in outcome after anterior cruciate ligament reconstruction with hamstring tendon autograft. *Am J Sports Med* 34(4):621–629, 2006.

111. Sri-Ram K, Salmon LJ, Pinczewski LA, et al: The incidence of secondary pathology after anterior cruciate ligament rupture in 5086 patients requiring ligament reconstruction. *Bone Joint J* 95-B(1):59–64, 2013.

The references for this chapter can also be found on www.expertconsult.com.

49

Anterior Cruciate Ligament Reconstruction With Central Quadriceps Free Tendon Graft

Harris S. Slone, John W. Xerogeanes

BACKGROUND

Although anterior cruciate ligament (ACL) reconstruction continues to be one of the most commonly performed knee surgeries worldwide, controversy still exists with regard to graft choice. Donor-site morbidity, failure rates, cosmesis, fracture, cost, and other concerns regarding commonly used grafts have precipitated investigation into alternative graft options. Recently, there has been an increased interest in quadriceps tendon autograft for ACL reconstruction,[5] although the graft has been successfully used for decades.[2] Anatomic, histologic, and biomechanical properties of the quadriceps tendon make it an ideal option for ACL reconstruction.[6] It is a versatile graft, which can be used with most modern surgical techniques and methods of fixation in accordance with surgeon preference. Minimally invasive surgical techniques have recently become popularized in conjunction with the development of specialized instrumentation, facilitating quick and easy harvest of the quadriceps tendon for ACL reconstruction.[7] The use of quadriceps tendon autograft for ACL reconstruction is supported by numerous studies, which demonstrate excellent clinical outcomes with low donor-site morbidity when compared to alternative graft options.[1,3,4,6]

PREOPERATIVE CONSIDERATIONS

Once the decision has been made to proceed with ACL reconstruction, one should assess the patient's age, avocations, demands, and expectations to determine which graft option is most appropriate. Full symmetric range of motion should be obtained prior to surgery, unless an associated injury precludes full motion. Physical therapy may be required to obtain motion, control swelling, and recruit the thigh and leg musculature preoperatively.

If an MRI has been obtained, the quadriceps tendon thickness can be evaluated for preoperative planning, and determination of a partial-thickness or full-thickness graft is needed. The tendon thickness is measured at the midsagittal point of maximal thickness of the tendon, 3 cm proximal to the proximal pole of the patella. Rarely will the quadriceps tendon thickness be inadequate for ACL reconstruction. In general, partial-thickness grafts are preferred; however, a full-thickness harvest should be planned if the patient has a tendon less than 6 mm thick. No functional difference has been observed between patients who have received partial- versus full-thickness harvests.

POSITIONING

Examination is performed after induction of general anesthesia. A tourniquet is applied to the operative thigh, and the operative leg is placed into a circumferential leg holder. This allows the knee to "rest" at 90 degrees of knee flexion, which facilitates graft harvest. The nonoperative leg is placed into a well-padded lithotomy leg holder. Following preparation and draping, an Esmarch bandage is used to exsanguinate the operative extremity and the tourniquet is inflated.

GRAFT HARVEST

Graft harvest can be performed before or after diagnostic arthroscopy and treatment of coexistent intraarticular pathology. In general, we prefer to start with graft harvest when the history, imaging, and examination under anesthesia are all consistent with ACL rupture. If graft harvest is performed after arthroscopic evaluation, it is important to drain the knee of arthroscopic fluid to minimize distention on the undersurface of the quadriceps tendon, which may increase the risk of inadvertent full-thickness perforation.

The proximal pole of the patella, vastus medialis obliquus (VMO), lateral patellar border, and medial patellar border are identified and marked with the knee flexed to 90 degrees. Gentle knee flexion and extension distinguishes the mobile lateral patellar border and the stationary lateral trochlear ridge. A 1.5- to 2-cm mark is placed extending from the midline of the proximal pole of the patella proximally in line with the femoral shaft (Fig. 49.1). Local anesthetic solution with epinephrine is injected at the planned incision site to the skin and subcutaneous tissue. Following skin incision, a wide ellipse of the subcutaneous tissue and fat is performed, which is critical to allow for visualization through the small incision. Distention of this tissue with previously injected local anesthetic makes it easier to excise. Overlying paratenon is excised, and a Ray-Tech sponge over a key elevator is used to remove any remaining overlying soft tissue over the anterior surface of the tendon. An Army-Navy retractor is placed at the proximal apex of the incision, and the arthroscope is inserted into the wound, with the fluid turned off (Fig. 49.2). If any crossing vessels overlying the tendon are identified, they should be coagulated with a radiofrequency (RF) device or electrocautery. The VMO, vastus lateralis musculature, and distal rectus musculature are identified (Fig. 49.3). The arthroscope is advanced proximally to the distal myotendinous junction of the rectus femoris. The light cord is then rotated and positioned to have the light shine through the anterior thigh skin. A mark is placed at this point or maximal trans-illumination (Fig. 49.4). A ruler is used to measure the distance from this mark to the proximal pole of the patella, providing the surgeon an estimate of potential graft length prior to harvest.

The Arthrex (Naples, Florida) quadriceps tendon harvest knife is a low-profile cutting device that allows the surgeon to pick a desired width and depth of graft harvest. For most patients, a blade width of 10 mm and depth of 7 mm is used. The knife is inserted into the incision and pressed firmly down on the anterior surface of the central portion of the quadriceps tendon. The knife is then advanced proximally incising the

quadriceps longitudinally, in the direction of the previously placed mark on the anterior thigh, which identifies the distal myotendinous junction of the rectus femoris (Fig. 49.5). Alternatively, an antigrade technique can be used, starting proximally at the point of trans-illumination and advancing distally with a "pull" type motion, although we have found the retrograde "push" motion more predictable. A 15-blade is used to carry the longitudinal incisions distally to the superior pole of the patella, tapering the end of the graft slightly, as distal graft diameter will be increased by 0.5 to 1 mm following suture for graft preparation. The depth of the harvest can be referenced based on the

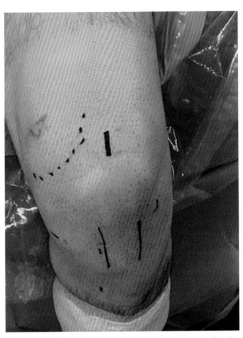

FIG 49.1 The knee is marked preoperatively.

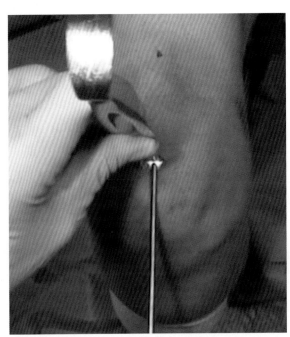

FIG 49.2 An Army-Navy retractor is placed at the proximal apex of the incision, and the arthroscope is placed into the wound with the fluid turned off.

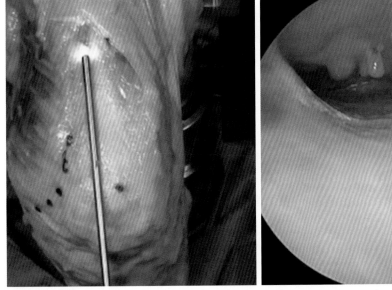

FIG 49.3 The VMO, vastus lateralis, distal rectus femoris tendon, and most proximal portion of the quadriceps tendon are identified.

depth of the longitudinal incision with the harvest knife (7 mm in most cases). The two longitudinal limbs are connected as the tendon is sharply dissected off of the patella. A small layer of fat exists between the distal quadriceps tendon and the underlying capsule, and deeper dissection should be avoided if a partial-thickness harvest is planned. Dissection is carried proximally in either a partial-thickness or full-thickness manner. An Alyss clamp can be placed on the tendon end to facilitate control of the graft during dissection, and Metzenbaum scissors can be used to dissect proximally.

Once 3 cm of tendon has been elevated, a looped suture is used to whipstitch the tendon, starting 2 cm from the patellar

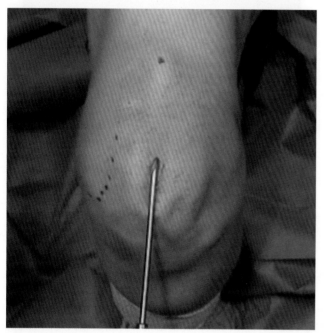

FIG 49.4 The point of maximal transillumination is marked on the anterior thigh.

end of the graft, placing four throws proceeding distally, and locking the last throw (by entering the tendon behind the last stitch) with the needle exiting the central portion of the tendon. The needle is left in place for further graft preparation once harvested. Further proximal dissection can be performed using Metzenbaum scissors with tendon on the sutures, if desired. The Arthrex (Naples, Florida) Quadriceps Tendon Stripper/Cutter device is used to strip the tendon until a desired length has been reached (ruler on the shaft of the device can be used for reference), and then cut the tendon proximally (Fig. 49.6). It is important to maintain firm tension on the sutures while the tendon is being stripped and cut. In general, a graft length of 7 cm is adequate for most patients undergoing anatomic ACL reconstruction (Fig. 49.7).

Following graft harvest, the arthroscope is reinserted (fluid off), and the harvest site can be evaluated for full-thickness rent if partial-thickness graft was planned. Areas of full-thickness harvest are closed with 0-Vicryl suture. A strip of gel foam can be placed into the harvest site. The subcutaneous layer is closed, and skin is closed according to surgeon preference. During the case, the surgeon should monitor the harvest site and thigh to ensure no excessive fluid extravasation.

GRAFT PREPARATION

A looped suture is again used to whipstitch the proximal side of the graft in a similar fashion, starting 2 cm centrally, placing four throws, and locking the last stitch, which exits the central portion of the graft. Usually, the smaller diameter end is used for the femoral side (most often the end dissected off the patella). The Arthrex Tightrope RT (Naples, Florida) is used for femoral fixation. The needle attached to the suture from previous whipstitch is passed through the loop of the Tightrope RT, and passed back into the central portion of the graft, exiting 5 mm away from the graft end. Three additional throws are placed, moving away from the end of the graft. The loop of suture is cut, leaving tails long enough to wrap around the graft, and then tied. The knot can be shuttled back into the central

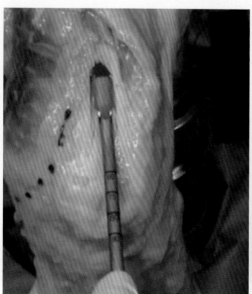

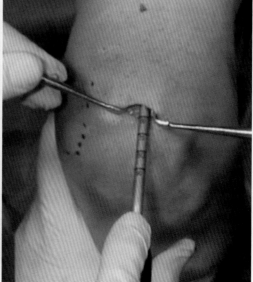

FIG 49.5 The triple-blade harvest knife is used to incise the quadriceps tendon.

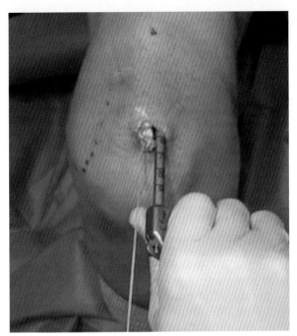

FIG 49.6 The stripper/cutter device is used for the final portion of the harvest.

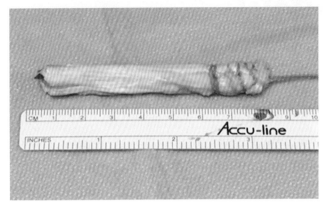

FIG 49.7 The quadriceps tendon graft is measured following harvest.

portion of the graft if desired. A whipstitch is placed in the tibial side, starting about 2 cm centrally, and four throws are placed working toward the end of the graft, locking the last stitch and exiting the central portion of the end of the graft.

TUNNEL DRILLING

Following treatment of any associated intraarticular pathology, the femoral and tibial tunnels are drilled. In the acute setting, the ACL soft-tissue stumps are useful landmarks for tunnel placement. In the chronic setting, the intercondylar ridge and bifurcate ridge can be used to identify the anatomic location for the femoral tunnel. We recommend the use of an accessory far medial portal, although we have found the retro-drill useful in certain settings including revision ACL reconstruction. It is critical to view the femoral side with the arthroscope in the anteromedial portal, regardless of which technique is used. Femoral sockets are drilled to 25 mm. A looped suture is placed for later graft passage. The tibial tunnel is marked in the center of the footprint, which is parallel to just anterior to the posterior aspect of the anterior horn of the lateral meniscus along the medial tibial eminence. Once the tibial guide pin is drilled, the knee can be extended, and the pin should correspond with the apex of the notch. A full-thickness tunnel is drilled in standard fashion.

GRAFT PASSAGE AND FIXATION

A hemostat is used to stretch the medial portal. A looped suture is placed retrograde up through the tibial tunnel. The looped sutures from the femoral tunnel and tibial tunnels are grabbed simultaneously and pulled out the accessory far medial portal to ensure no soft-tissue suture bridge is created. The graft is first passed into the femoral tunnel, leaving about 5 mm for final tightrope RT tightening. The graft is passed into the tibial tunnel, the knee is cycled with tension on the sutures, and tibial sutures are tied over a post with the knee in full extension. Final tightrope RT tightening is performed with the knee in full extension.

REHABILITATION

Postoperative principles of rehabilitation following quadriceps tendon ACL reconstruction are similar to alternative autografts. Full early motion, specifically terminal extension, should be emphasized. For isolated ACL reconstructions, we allow weight bearing once quadriceps function has returned. Most patients start in-line jogging around 3 months. We generally allow patients to return to sport between 7 and 9 months, following functional testing.

KEY REFERENCES

4. Lund B, Nielsen T, Faunø P, et al: Is quadriceps tendon a better graft choice than patellar tendon? A prospective randomized study. *Arthroscopy* 30(5):593–598, 2014.
6. Slone HS, Romine SE, Premkumar A, et al: Quadriceps tendon autograft for anterior cruciate ligament reconstruction: a comprehensive review of current literature and systematic review of clinical results. *Arthroscopy* 31(3):541–554, 2015.
7. Slone HS, Xerogeanes JW: Anterior cruciate ligament reconstruction with quadriceps tendon autograft. *JBJS Essent Surg Tech* 4(3):e16, 2014.

The references for this chapter can also be found on www.expertconsult.com.

50

Allograft Anterior Cruciate Ligament Reconstruction

Matthew J. Salzler, Jonathan A. Stone, Christopher D. Harner

Allograft usage in orthopedic operations has increased significantly over the past several decades.[23] Approximately 30% of the estimated 300,000 anterior cruciate ligament (ACL) reconstructions done annually are performed with an allograft, with some larger community-based registry data showing rates up to 41% for primary ACL reconstruction.[49,71,87] A variety of factors, including surgeon preference, technical difficulty, graft availability, and harvest site morbidity, have increased the popularity of allograft. These data persist despite evidence that allograft has higher failure rates in young patients.[32,61,86,114] In addition, a plethora of new data from several large prospective multicenter trials have helped to further refine the best surgical candidates for allograft usage. Understanding that allografts have their own unique risks and disadvantages that the surgeon and patient must consider and balance as part of the informed consent is critical in an era of evidence-based medicine.

ALLOGRAFT CONSIDERATIONS

Graft Options

ACL reconstruction using autograft patellar tendon was first described by Jones in 1963.[53] Nowadays patellar tendon autograft is considered the gold standard for ACL reconstruction.[108] Patellar tendon autograft offers high initial strength, earlier bone-to-bone healing, and proven success by a multitude of outcome studies.[1,6,20,24,74] However, despite being the gold standard graft choice, there are several disadvantages to autogenous patellar tendon harvest. These include anterior knee pain, patellar shortening, decreased range of motion, longer surgical time, infrapatellar fat pad fibrosis, patellar fracture, and patellar chondrosis.* Dynamic disadvantages of autograft patellar tendon harvest include decreased quadriceps strength, quadriceps inhibition, altered patellar alignment, and decreased active range of motion.[48,59,70]

Quadrupled hamstring autografts (semitendinosus and gracilis tendon autograft) have been shown to have the highest tensile strength and excellent clinical results.[42,115] In one community-based study in the United States, hamstring autograft is used in 30% of primary ACL reconstructions.[49] Another study from Denmark revealed an increase in use of hamstring tendon grafts for primary ACL reconstruction from 68% to 85% from 2005 to 2011.[95] However, disadvantages include decreased knee flexion and hip extension strength, which can be detrimental to athletes who rely on knee flexion strength beyond 90 degrees of flexion (eg, sprinters, wrestlers, gymnasts, martial arts practitioners).[48,103,110] In addition, the surgeon is dependent on patient autograft quality for reconstruction; decreased hamstring size has been correlated in some studies with higher risk of revision.[69] Furthermore, hamstring strength has been shown to be protective of ACL reconstruction by way of the ACL-hamstring reflex arc. Removing the semitendinosus and gracilis tendons results in disruption of this arc and a decrease in the protective effect of the hamstrings on the ACL graft.[11]

Quadriceps tendon autograft is also being used in some centers for ACL reconstruction. A systematic review of 14 studies suggests equivalent results between quadriceps tendon (with patellar bone plug) autograft and patellar tendon autograft.[104] After a 2-year follow-up, one study has found that kneeling pain is significantly less than with a bone-patellar tendon-bone (BPTB) autograft, but anterior knee pain in the two groups is similar.[60]

Because of the potential drawbacks of autograft ACL reconstruction with patellar tendon, hamstring, or quadriceps tendon, allograft ACL reconstruction is increasing in the United States and likely worldwide.[5,49,77,95,108] Advantages of an allograft include elimination of donor site morbidity, decreased surgical time, smaller incisions, lower incidence of arthrofibrosis, decreased postoperative pain, no loss of donor graft function, faster subjective recovery time, and predictable graft sizes.[23,35,54] Allograft options include patellar tendon, hamstring, anterior tibialis, posterior tibialis, Achilles, quadriceps tendon, and fascia lata. However, allograft drawbacks also exist, such as disease transmission, slower incorporation, possible immunologic reaction, finite supply, tunnel expansion, inferior biomechanical strength, cost, and possible increased postoperative laxity, decreased patient outcome scores, and increased failure rate in select patient populations.†

Graft Procurement and Sterilization

There are more than 150 individual tissue banks that provide allograft for surgical use. Most of these tissue banks are members of the American Association of Tissue Banks (AATB). Beginning in May 2005 and updated in January 2009, federal legislation was passed mandating that all United States tissue banks be subject to the US Food and Drug Association (FDA) "Good Tissue Practice" guidelines.[33] These guidelines specify a minimum standard for tissue procurement, as well as testing

---

*References 5, 12, 21, 27, 79, 80, 91, 92, and 103.

†References 40, 44, 46, 55, 56, 71, 86, 90, 93, 100, 102, 106, 112, and 114.

and processing, require periodic inspections of tissue bank facilities, and necessitate reporting adverse events to the FDA.[23,108]

Graft procurement begins with donor screening to eliminate donors who are at high risk for transmitting communicable diseases. This involves screening prior to death and evaluating cause of death. High-risk donors are eliminated; these include those who have a known communicable disease, show active signs of infection despite not having a diagnosis, or whose lifestyle places them at high risk for infection. Physical examination is the next step to assess the potential donor for high-risk behavior (eg, needle marks, skin findings). Third, blood tests and tissue cultures are taken from the potential donor to rule out an otherwise undetermined communicable disease. Required serologic tests include human immunodeficiency virus (HIV) types 1 and 2, hepatitis B, hepatitis C, and syphilis. The AATB-affiliated tissue banks also test donors for human T-cell lymphotropic virus (HTLV) types I and II. Certain tissue banks may accept positive bacterial cultures, relying on the sterilization process to eliminate the infection. Tissue banks that are part of the AATB require destruction of all tissue that demonstrates positive cultures for clostridia or group A streptococcus.[23] After these criteria are met and passed, the graft is suitable for procurement in the standard sterile surgical fashion. Each tissue bank has a specific time window for acceptable retrieval of graft tissue. After being obtained, the graft is placed in an antimicrobial solution and taken to the sterilization plant.

Sterilization is performed via two techniques, tissue irradiation and chemical processing. It has been found that high levels of irradiation (>25 kGy) can reliably inactivate HIV and spores. However, these same high levels of irradiation can be detrimental to the biomechanical properties of the graft itself.[41,58,89,100,108] A retrospective cohort study of the Kaiser Permanente ACL reconstruction registry examining the relationship between graft processing and graft type with regards to need for revision surgery identified radiation dosage greater than 1.8 Mrad to have statistically higher revision rates after 1 year.[111] In a meta-analysis of allograft versus autograft stability, irradiated grafts were found to have a statistically higher rate of increased laxity (arthrometric side-to-side measurement >5 mm) compared with nonirradiated grafts.[93] One randomized study by Sun et al.[107] compared BPTB autograft, irradiated (2.5 Mrad) BPTB allograft, and nonirradiated BPTB allograft in 99 patients. After evaluation at 31 months postoperatively, no statistically significant difference was found among the three groups with regard to IKDC functional and subjective evaluations, but a trend toward inferior outcome scores was noted in the irradiated group. KT-2000 testing found that only 31.3% of irradiated patients had less than a 3-mm side-to-side difference compared with 87.8% in the autograft group and 85.3% in the nonirradiated allograft group. Furthermore, graft failure in the irradiated group occurred in 34.4% of patients compared with 6.1% in the autograft group and 8.8% in the nonirradiated allograft group. Finally, graft irradiation was compared in a study evaluating irradiated (2 to 2.5 Mrad) versus nonirradiated Achilles allograft with regard to early failure.[96] At 6 months of follow-up, the nonirradiated group had a 2.4% graft failure rate compared with 33% failure rate in the irradiated group, a statistically higher failure rate that led the authors to cease using irradiated allografts for ACL reconstruction.

Thus most tissue banks now use lower dose irradiation, which inactivates most organisms but does not alter the strength of the graft. Low-dose radiation may not inactivate such viruses as HIV.[107] Various tissue banks will use different radiation dosages, and some banks have abandoned irradiating as a sterilization technique because of adverse effects on graft biomechanics. A meta-analysis comparing autograft to nonchemically nonirradiated allograft tissue showed no statistical difference between groups when looking at outcomes scores, Lachman, pivot shift testing, KT-1000, or failure rates.[64] Another systematic review of nine prospective and retrospective studies of autograft versus nonirradiated allograft found no statistical difference between graft failure rate, postoperative laxity, or functional outcomes in a cohort whose average age included patients in their late 20s and 30s.[75] Sun et al. published a prospective randomized study comparing autograft BPTB with nonirradiated allograft BPTB, with 5.6-year follow-up data.[109] No statistically significant difference was found other than shorter surgical time and longer postoperative fever for the allograft group (80 patients, average age 32.8 years) compared with the autograft group (76 patients, average age 31.7 years). These studies imply that nonirradiated allograft may be a reasonable alternative to autograft use for ACL reconstruction in certain patient populations.

Chemical processing involves a succession of cleansing, disinfection, and rinsing of the tissue to remove viable cells, lipids, and microorganisms. Penetration into the deepest parts of the tissue is the primary challenge in chemical sterilization. Various tissue banks have their proprietary chemical cleansing solutions, some of which have been associated with higher revision rates.[111] Tissue "sterility" (sterility assurance level) is defined by the tissue banking industry as $p < .000001$ that a viable microbe is not present in tissue after having undergone the sterilization process. After the sterilization process is complete, the graft is then frozen at $-70°C$ to $-80°C$ until surgery. Deep freezing has been shown to decrease the risk of graft rejection by causing cell necrosis and loss of immunogenicity.[35] Freezing of allograft tissue has led to variable results in biomechanical properties, with some studies suggesting no difference, whereas others demonstrating that freezing is detrimental to graft strength.[76,83] Deep freezing does not destroy HIV or the hepatitis C virus.

Tissue irradiation, chemical processing, and deep freezing have been found in some studies to result in decreased graft biomechanical strength. Because the procurement and sterilization protocols of tissue banks can vary, the surgeon and hospital should be well aware of the quality and techniques of tissue processing of the company that they choose to use as their source of graft tissue.

Infection

The risk of disease transmission is an important factor when weighing the options of allograft versus autograft ACL reconstruction. Possible infectious agents include HIV, hepatitis B, hepatitis C, HTLV, syphilis, aerobic bacteria, and anaerobic bacteria. With tissue banks adopting varying procedures on graft sterilization, the risk of disease transmission is also variable. The risk of HIV infection has ranged in the literature from 1 to 400,000 to 8,000,000, with a commonly quoted figure of 1 to 1,600,000.[5,14,15,23] The risk of hepatitis B and C virus infection has consistently been shown to be higher than that of HIV transmission. Bacterial infection is also a concern with regard to disease transmission with *Clostridium* spp. (a spore-forming anaerobe) being a common pathogen. In a Centers for Disease

Control and Prevention (CDC) study performed in 2002, 26 cases (18 used for ACL reconstruction) of allograft-associated bacterial infections were identified in approximately 1 million transplanted allografts. Half of these were found to be caused by *Clostridium* spp., with one death.[18] In another CDC study,[57] published in 2004, 70 cases of allograft-associated infection were reported; it was found that since 1995, 6 were caused by hepatitis C and none by HIV. Of these patients, 14 were found to have *Clostridium* infections.

Routine culture of allografts prior to implantation has yielded 4.8% to 9.7% positive cultures for bacterial organisms, but no clinical infection was correlated with these positive culture results.[17,39] Thus far, routine preimplantation cultures have not been recommended. Because tissue banks differ in their methods of sterilization, the surgeon should be familiar and comfortable with the tissue processing of the bank selected and be able to discuss possible infection transmission risks with patients as part of the informed consent.

Several recent papers have been published regarding risk factors for postoperative infection after ACL reconstruction. Brophy et al.[13] reviewed the Multicenter Orthopaedic Outcomes Network (MOON) database and found diabetes, as well as use of hamstring autograft, any allograft, or combined autograft plus allograft compared with BPTB autograft, to be associated with increased risk of infection. Body mass index (BMI) and smoking were not found to increase risk. Another study examined all primary ACL reconstructions performed at one institution over the course of 5 years, finding hamstring autograft but not allograft was associated with increased infection rates.[7] Finally, the Kaiser Permanente ACL reconstruction registry was reviewed and found hamstring autograft to have a higher incidence of infection compared with BPTB autograft and allograft. Overall infection rate was 0.48%.[72]

Graft Biology

Allograft incorporation and healing is critical to the success of ACL reconstruction. One commonly cited disadvantage of allograft usage for ACL reconstruction is slower and less extensive incorporation compared with autograft ACL reconstruction.[29] Allograft versus autograft ACL reconstruction has been compared from histologic, biomechanical, and radiographic perspectives. A sheep study[100,101] comparing native ACL, reconstructed soft tissue autograft ACL, and reconstructed soft tissue allograft ACL has suggested that allograft demonstrated delayed remodeling histologically at 6 and 12 weeks postoperatively. However, at 52 weeks the differences were less apparent. Biomechanically, allografts at 52 weeks demonstrated statistically significant anteroposterior (AP) laxity compared with autografts; this was not present at 6 and 12 weeks. Allograft healing was improved in a rabbit histologic study when the fresh frozen Achilles allografts were coated with mesenchymal stem cells compared with controls (Achilles allograft only).[105] Radiographically, BPTB allografts were found to have less revascularization by contrast-enhanced magnetic resonance imaging (MRI) at 1, 4, 6, and 12 months after surgery compared with BPTB autografts but were found to equalize at 18 months postoperatively. The authors suggested that revascularization is slower in BPTB allografts compared with BPTB autografts.[81] However, computed tomography (CT) imaging of BPTB bone plugs at 1 week, 2 months, and 5 months did not show a significant difference in bony incorporation of BPTB allograft versus BPTB autograft.[50,68]

For allograft ACL reconstruction to be successful, the graft must heal adequately in the bone tunnel. The intra-articular portion of the allograft must undergo the process of ligamentization in which the graft remodels to resemble the histology of a native ligament more closely.[40]

Soft tissue allografts must undergo tendon-to-bone tunnel healing. The native ACL insertion site is an example of direct insertion from tendon to bone. Four distinct histologically appreciable zones comprise this insertion site—tendon, unmineralized fibrocartilage, mineralized fibrocartilage, and finally bone. With soft tissue ACL reconstruction, this direct insertion site is not replicated. Rather, indirect insertion is relied on for soft tissue graft healing within the bone tunnel. Indirect insertion is naturally exemplified by other ligaments, such as the medial collateral ligament (MCL), which broadly inserts along the surface of the bone through fibers that travel obliquely from the long axis of the ligament to the long axis of the bone. These fibers, known as Sharpey fibers, are also seen histologically in ACL reconstruction with tendon grafts and correlate with the biomechanical properties of the graft insertion site.[36,40,98]

A number of strategies have been used to improve the strength and healing of the soft tissue graft within the bone tunnel. Creating a longer tunnel has been shown to increase the strength of the graft-tunnel interface, presumably by increasing the amount of contact between the graft and the bone.[94,116,117] Impregnating the graft with mesenchymal stem cells, as suggested earlier, has shown superior healing, as well as more normal tendon to bone insertion histology.[67,85,105] The application of bone morphogenic proteins to the graft has also been shown to increase bone formation around the graft, as well as graft pull-out strength.[78] Inhibition of osteoclast activity has been investigated with the use of osteoprotegerin (OPG). OPG-treated grafts in rabbits demonstrated greater bone formation and smaller sized bone tunnels around the graft.[30] Inhibiting degrading matrix metalloproteinases (MMPs) in rabbit allograft ACL reconstruction has shown more Sharpey fibers and a stronger load to failure.[25] The primary healing response after graft implantation involves the arrival of inflammatory cells facilitated by cyclooxygenase-2 (COX-2). Studies have shown that avoiding antiinflammatory medications, such as COX-2 inhibitors, allows the primary healing phase to proceed without chemical interruption. Some have cautioned against the use of nonsteroidal antiinflammatory drugs (NSAIDs) to prevent inhibition of the primary healing response.[22,40,84]

Compared with soft tissue grafts, which require soft tissue-to-bone healing within the osseous tunnel, BPTB grafts require bone-to-bone healing. This bone-to-bone healing is widely accepted as the strongest form of healing for ACL reconstruction. Histologic studies have demonstrated that the implanted bone plug demonstrates initial osteonecrosis and hypocellularity followed by revascularization, fibroblast invasion, and collagen synthesis, with subsequent rapid incorporation of the plug by surrounding bone.[26,52,88,113] These changes have been found to be similar in autograft versus allograft BPTB healing. Within 3 weeks, histologic incorporation is visible but still fragile. At 3 weeks after implantation the weakest point of a BPTB autograft remains the graft-tunnel interface. However, at 6 weeks, this interface has healed so that the site of graft failure is at the patellar tendon insertion into the bone plug.[40] Although some studies evaluating timing of incorporation have suggested no significant difference between autograft and allograft bone plugs, others have shown that allograft bone plugs require a longer time to incorporate and central portions of the plug may not incorporate at long-term evaluation.[10,50,51,73] Healing of the bone plug likely occurs from the end of the tunnel furthest from the influences of degradative enzymes in the synovial fluid.[10]

Ligamentization of the graft is the phase of graft incorporation in which the intra-articular portion of the graft undergoes changes that more closely resemble the histologic properties of a native ligament. Whether autograft or allograft, this process takes several months and undergoes a series of steps.[40,51] Similar to the initial events of bone plug incorporation, the ligamentous portion also undergoes an initial phase of avascular necrosis and acellularity. Despite being devoid of cells, the graft maintains its collagenous structure, which serves as a scaffold for subsequent steps—cellular repopulation, revascularization, and ligament maturation.[3,4] The timing of these steps, outlined in a rabbit model, has demonstrated that at 2 weeks, necrosis of the graft begins. At 4 weeks the graft is completely devoid of cellularity but the collagen scaffold remains intact. At 12 weeks, vascular proliferation and cellular repopulation are appreciated. At 6 months the cellularity of the graft is similar to that of a native ligament. Finally, at 9 months the graft is mature and histologically similar to a native ACL.[84] In humans, surface blood flow studies have suggested that after an initial period of increased flow, ACL allografts demonstrate normal surface blood flow at 18 months, implying the end of graft remodeling.[100]

RESULTS OF ALLOGRAFT ANTERIOR CRUCIATE LIGAMENT RECONSTRUCTION

Autograft ACL reconstruction has generally been accepted as the gold standard for ACL graft choice, providing optimal graft strength and healing. Nonetheless, the use of allograft ACL reconstruction is increasing because of disadvantages specific to autogenous graft harvest. There have been many studies comparing subjective and objective outcomes of allograft versus autograft ACL reconstruction, including multicenter prospective cohort studies, randomized controlled trials, and meta-analyses. Recent relevant studies are reviewed in this section.

A multitude of reviews have been performed on the MOON database, which began in 1993 and now includes 7 institutions, 17 surgeons, and more than 4400 patients registered to establish the largest prospective longitudinal ACL reconstruction cohort. Spindler et al.[106] examined 2- and 6-year follow-up of 448 patients with unilateral ACL reconstructions, both primary and revision, performed in 2002 from the MOON database with excellent follow-up (88% and 84%, respectively). Allograft was used 16% of the time and was derived from a variety of tissue banks using different sterilization techniques. Use of allograft was a predictor of worse IKDC and KOOS outcome scores. The authors recommend choosing autograft instead of allograft to improve long-term functional outcomes.

Hettrich et al.[46] examined the 2- and 6-year rates and predictors of subsequent surgery on 980 patients enrolled in the MOON trial from 2002 to 2003, of which 23% had allograft and 77% had autograft. Follow-up was 92% at both time points. Notably, 7.7% of patients underwent ACL revision on the ipsilateral extremity, with use of allograft (OR 2.33) and younger age at index surgery increasing the risk of subsequent surgery.

Kaeding et al.[56] examined risk factors for ipsilateral and contralateral ACL tears in the MOON cohort, with 2-year follow-up data on 2683 patients who had primary unilateral ACL reconstruction between 2002 and 2008, with 93%

follow-up. Risk of ipsilateral retear was associated with allograft use compared with BPTB autograft (OR 5.2), as well as decreasing age and higher preoperative Marx activity score.

Outside of the MOON cohort, Krych et al.[62] performed a meta-analysis of six prospective trials comparing 256 patients with BTPB autograft with 278 with BPTB allograft ACL reconstruction. Those in the allograft group were more likely to rerupture in comparison with those in the autograft group (OR 5.03) and more likely to have a hop test less than 90% of the contralateral nonoperated limb (OR 5.66). However, when irradiated and chemically processed grafts were excluded, there was no difference between the allograft and autograft groups with regard to graft rerupture, rate of reoperation, IKDC normal and near-normal scores, Lachman, pivot shift, and hop tests, patellar crepitus, or return to sport.

One study has prospectively evaluated autograft quadrupled hamstring tendon versus allograft quadrupled hamstring tendon without complete randomization.[31] A cohort of 37 autograft hamstring ACL reconstructions was compared with 47 allograft hamstring patients. No difference was found in Tegner, Lysholm, KT-1000, or IKDC scores at follow-up periods of approximately 1 year.

A noncomparative long-term outcome study evaluated 61 patients with a mean age of 20.9 years who underwent free tendon allograft ACL reconstruction.[82] Mean long-term follow-up of 11.5 years was compared with 2-year postoperative data in the same group of patients; of these, 87% of patients maintained a negative Lachman test result, whereas 85% of patients maintained a negative pivot shift test result. Mean KT-2000 laxity measurements were a 1.6-mm side-to-side difference at long-term follow-up and no more than 3 mm in 92% of patients. All patients except one assessed their knee as normal or near-normal by IKDC score. It was concluded that free tendon allograft ACL reconstruction affords knee stability for the long term. Another long-term follow-up study also found good clinical results (IKDC, Lysholm, Tegner, one-leg hop test) in 55 patients followed for a mean of 10 years after having undergone free tendon allograft ACL reconstruction.[2] Harreld et al.[45] have described self-reported patient outcomes at short-term (mean, 2.8 years) and long-term (mean, 7.8 years) follow-up after ACL allograft (mix of BPTB and free tendon allograft) reconstruction. No differences were found in the short-term group compared with the long-term group with regard to IKDC subjective evaluation or Knee Outcome Survey Activities of Daily Living Scale (KOS-ADLS) scores. However, there was a statistically significant decrease in the KOS-ADLS score in the long-term cohort, suggesting that over the long term, patients have a decreased perception of sporting activity knee function.

A prospective randomized multicenter trial performed between 2002 and 2006 compared 147 patients to autograft hamstring or fresh frozen, nonirradiated, nonchemically processed tibialis anterior allograft. Mean age was 33 years, and they report 69% 2-year follow-up. No statistical differences were seen in radiographic outcomes, stability measurements, and functional outcome scores between groups at minimum 2-year follow-up.[65]

Rihn et al.[97] have prospectively compared 39 irradiated (2.5 Mrad) BPTB allograft ACL reconstructions with 63 BPTB autograft ACL reconstructions, with an average follow-up of 50.4 months. It was found that both cohorts have similar IKDC scores and KT-1000 measurements. The authors conclude that irradiated BPTB allograft has results similar to those of BPTB autograft ACL reconstruction. Two other prospective BPTB allograft versus autograft prospective cohort studies have found equivalent functional outcomes, one at 25.6-month and another at 47.1-month follow-up.[9,63]

A large meta-analysis of 76 studies performed from 1998 to 2012 compared BPTB autograft to allograft with regard to patient satisfaction, return to preinjury activity level, and postoperative functional outcomes. Minimum follow-up was 2 years, and patient groups older than 40 or those that included workers' compensation programs were excluded. Overall rupture rates of 4.3% and 12.7% (OR 3.24) were reported for the autograft and allograft groups, respectively; 57.1% of autograft recipients returned to preinjury activity level compared with 68.3% of allograft recipients, which may reflect age and preinjury activity level. Subjective IKDC, Lysholm, and Tegner scores; single-legged hop; and KT-1000 measurements all were in favor of autograft. Return to preinjury activity level, overall IKDC score, pivot shift testing, and anterior knee pain rates were statistically in favor of allograft; however, the authors note that many studies removed allograft failures from pivot shift calculations. They conclude that autograft is the preferred graft in younger patients.[61]

In a retrospective comparative study, 111 patients who underwent primary ACL reconstruction with BPTB allograft between 1993 and 2005 were compared with 411 matched patients who received BPTB autograft during the same time period. Follow-up was a minimum of 2 years. Failure was defined as revision ACL reconstruction, 2 or greater Lachman (no endpoint), any pivot shift, and/or KT-1000 with greater than 4-mm difference. The allograft cohort was noted to be significantly older than the autograft cohort (average age: 28.1 vs. 22.2 years). Females were statistically more likely than males, as well as those with "chronic" injuries compared with "acute" injuries, to receive allograft. Preinjury Tegner activity scores were not different between groups. Allografts experienced a significantly higher rate of failure (24.4%) compared with autograft (10.7%). Postoperative Tegner scores were found to be higher in the autograft group. Decreasing age at surgery was found to be a predictor of failure. Interestingly, patients whose preoperative Tegner scores were low (0 to 5) were found to have the same rate of failure as those who received autograft at any preoperative Tegner score, whereas those whose preoperative Tegner score was high and received allograft had a 2.6 to 4.2 times higher chance of having a graft failure. The authors conclude that allograft should not be used in young patients with high preoperative Tegner activity scores.[8]

Prodromos et al.[93] performed a meta-analysis of 20 studies with allograft follow-up data and compared this with a previously published dataset on BPTB and hamstring autograft ACL reconstructions. The autograft group was found to have both a statistically higher level of normal stability (defined as arthrometric side-to-side difference of 0 to 2 mm) and a lower level of abnormal stability (difference of >5 mm). They note that abnormal stability often represents a graft failure.

Maletis et al.[71] reported on a retrospective cohort study of Kaiser Permanente ACL reconstruction registry examining association of graft type with risk of early aseptic revision. They note a 3.02-times increased risk of aseptic revision with allograft compared with BPTB autograft. In addition, for each year increase in age at the time of surgery, the risk of revision decreased by 7%.

Two systematic reviews have looked at large cohorts of patients without regard to age or activity level. One compiled eight studies, both prospective and retrospective, with greater than 24-month follow-up on all patients that showed no difference in outcome scores, instrumented laxity measurements, and failure rates between autograft and allograft patients.[16] Another review combined data of 31 prospective studies of autograft alone, allograft alone, and direct comparisons of graft types. Graft failure was 4.7 per 100 reconstructions for autograft versus 8.2 per 100 reconstructions for autograft, which did not reach statistical significance. Other measurements including instability, functional outcomes, and postoperative complication rates were not significant.[34] Another similar meta-analysis of 56 studies comparing autograft and allograft included patients with primary unilateral ACL reconstruction, mean age less than 41 years, and follow-up of at least 2 years. The only measurement to reach statistical significance was KT-1000 arthrometer testing, which favored autograft over allograft.[112] These studies exhibit the difficulty in extrapolating compiled data from large cohorts of dissimilar patient populations.

Several studies have looked specifically at young patients. One prospective cohort study of cadets at the U.S. Military Academy examined 120 cadets who had 122 ACL reconstructions prior to matriculation. Of these reconstructions, 61 were BPTB, 45 were hamstring autograft, and 16 were allograft. The cohort had an average age of 19 years and was felt to be homogenously active, as nearly all activities were standardized. There were a total of 20 reconstruction failures seen during the cadets' tenure. Cadets who had allograft reconstruction were found to be 7.7 and 6.7 times more likely to experience a graft failure compare to BPTB and all autografts, respectively.[86] Another study examined 73 primary ACL reconstructions in an adolescent cohort ages 11 to 18 years performed at a tertiary care pediatric hospital, with 38 patients receiving allograft and 35 patients receiving autograft. There was no statistical difference in age between groups. All allografts had less than 2.0 Mrad radiation as a sterilization process. Eleven (29%) failures were seen in the allograft group compared with 4 (11.4%) in the autograft group. Of the grafts that did not fail, there was no difference seen in functional outcome or rate of return to previous activity level. The authors note that although the risk for autograft failure appeared to decline by 24 to 48 months postoperatively, the rate of allograft failure continued in a more linear fashion.[32] Lastly, a meta-analysis of seven studies compared autograft versus allograft rates of failure. Inclusion criteria were patients less than 25 years of age or those with high activity level, defined as military personnel, patients with Marx score greater than 12, and collegiate and semiprofessional athletes. Mean age was 21.7 years. Pooled failure rates were 9.6% for autograft and 25.0% for allograft ($p < .00001$).[114] These studies suggest that allografts should be used with caution in a younger patient population.

Only recently have improved data been released regarding outcomes of allograft in revision ACL reconstructions. Similar to the MOON cohort, the Multicenter ACL Revision Study (MARS) cohort was designed to identify predictors of outcome in revision ACL reconstruction. At this time, there are 87 participating surgeons at 52 sites, 54% academic and 46% private practice, with more than 1200 enrolled patients. In one study examining the effect of graft choice on outcome using data from the MARS cohort, 1205 revision ACL reconstructions performed between 2006 and 2011 were reviewed for 2-year patient outcomes. Autograft was used in 48% of patients, allograft in 49%, and both in 3%. Autograft use was predictive of improved IKDC, and KOOS sports, recreation, and quality of life subscales. In addition, patients with autograft were 2.78 times less likely to sustain a graft rupture compared with those with allograft.[38] Another study also supports a similarly high use of allograft in revision ACL reconstruction with a reported rate of 50%.[28] In a worldwide panel of 34 sports medicine surgeons, 33.8% reported use of allograft in ACL revisions compared with only 13% for primary reconstructions.[77]

OPERATIVE CONSIDERATIONS

Choice of Surgical Technique

The senior author (CH) prefers to perform an anatomic ACL reconstruction, regardless of graft choice. It is believed that this is best done through femoral tunnel placement from the medial portal rather than the transtibial position.[99] It is preferable to avoid interference screws to allow circumferential healing of the graft within the tunnel. Graft fixation of choice is the EndoButton (Smith & Nephew, Andover, Massachusetts) for the femoral side and the graft tied over a post for the tibial side.

Patient Evaluation

Selecting the appropriate patient for ACL reconstruction begins with a thorough history and physical examination. This includes a full assessment of mechanism of injury, activity level, comorbidities, and expectations. Physical examination should include evaluation for other injuries about the knee, including meniscal, MCL, and posterolateral corner injuries. With regard to imaging, flexion weight-bearing plain radiographs are routinely used to evaluate for acute fractures, bony avulsions, status of the growth plate, and presence of arthritis. MRI scans are also obtained to confirm an ACL-deficient knee but more to evaluate for other injuries about the knee associated with the ACL tear, such as menisci, collateral structures, and articular cartilage. History, physical examination findings, and imaging studies are correlated to establish the complete diagnosis for each injured knee. Indications for ACL reconstruction include an active patient with episodic knee pain and subjective instability that correlates with an ACL-deficient knee on physical examination and MRI.

Prior to ACL reconstruction, the patient undergoes knee rehabilitation with the goal of full active range of motion, symmetric quadriceps strength, and a normal heel-to-toe gait. We prefer to familiarize our patients with the physical therapy protocol prior to surgery. On occasion, if a large knee effusion is hindering preoperative rehabilitation, an aspiration will be performed in the office. This rehabilitation process generally requires 3 to 6 weeks.

Approximately 5% to 10% of our patients will present with an ACL tear with an associated ligamentous injury. If an acute (<3 weeks) posterior lateral corner injury is present, we will repair the posterior lateral corner and stage the ACL reconstruction. If the patient presents with a concomitant MCL injury, we may delay surgery for 4 to 6 weeks, allowing the MCL to heal.

A thorough discussion regarding the nature of the patient's injury and possible surgical intervention, as well as the attendant risks, benefits, and alternatives, should take place with the patient. We think that this should only be performed by the surgeon ultimately responsible for the care of the patient. Only after the patient has a thorough understanding of all these considerations is he or she asked to sign the consent form.

Graft Selection

Graft choice for ACL reconstruction is influenced by patient age, activity level, gender, associated injuries, degree of laxity, and planned concomitant operations. As a general guideline, autografts are recommended for patients younger than 35 years because it is presumed that these patients are more active. Those older than 35 years are counseled about allograft tissue. We recommend BPTB autografts to all high-level athletes involved in cutting sports (eg, football, basketball, rugby), patients with a history of hamstring injury, and larger patients. With bone-to-bone healing, a more aggressive rehabilitation course may be taken. Hamstring autografts are recommended to most women because of better donor site cosmesis, unless their activity level dictates otherwise, and for augmentation in the young athlete. Allografts tend to be reserved for older athletes and most multiligamentous injury reconstructions. Only fresh frozen, nonirradiated allografts are used. Allograft BPTB is preferred for older athletes, but occasionally we will use tibialis anterior allograft in older women. In the setting of ACL augmentation, soft tissue allograft (eg, tibialis anterior) is more amenable to graft passage and requires smaller-diameter bone tunnels while allowing preservation of the remaining native bundle. In revision ACL surgery, a variety of grafts are used. BPTB and occasionally hamstring autografts are preferred. If these are unavailable, then BPTB allograft is preferred in most cases.

Anesthesia

Our preferred anesthesia for an ACL reconstruction involves a combined a femoral nerve block administered in the preoperative holding area. Intraoperatively, a general anesthetic with a laryngeal mask airway (LMA) can be used. Ultimately, anesthesia should be individualized taking into account the patient's comorbidities and preferences, as well as surgical team needs.

Examination Under Anesthesia. A thorough bilateral knee examination under anesthesia is performed after the general anesthetic is administered. For the ACL, we use the Lachman, anterior drawer, and pivot shift test and compare side-to-side differences. Discrepancies among these test results may signify an isolated bundle rupture amenable to augmentation. The results are considered along with previously collected data (ie, history, prior examination, and imaging studies) to confirm the diagnosis of an ACL tear.

Positioning and Setup

The patient is positioned supine on the operating table with the heels at the end of the table (Fig. 50.1). The surgical site is shaved appropriately with an electric razor, taking into consideration other procedures that may be necessary during the operation (eg, meniscal repairs). No tourniquet or leg holders are used. The operative leg is brought into neutral rotation by placing an appropriate sized bump under the ipsilateral buttock. A 10-pound sandbag is affixed to the table in a location that holds the leg flexed at 90 degrees of flexion. A side post is placed at the midthigh level to support the leg without assistance when the leg is flexed to 90 degrees. Bony prominences of the nonoperative leg are well padded to prevent pressure sores and peroneal nerve palsies. With the knee flexed to 90 degrees, anatomic landmarks are marked. Standard anterolateral and anteromedial portals are marked (see Fig. 50.1B). A 3-cm tibial tunnel incision is drawn on the anteromedial tibial surface. Proposed

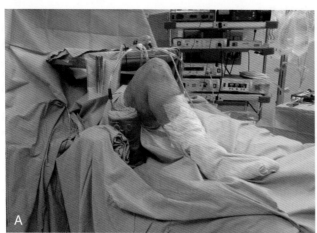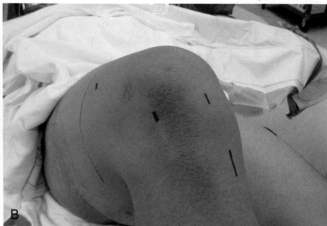

FIG 50.1 (A) Patient setup. The patient is positioned supine with a lateral leg rest and a bump holding the right knee at 90 degrees of flexion. (B) Incision. A tibial tunnel incision and standard anterolateral, anteromedial, and superlateral portals are shown on this right knee.

incisions for possible medial and/or lateral meniscal inside-out repairs are also marked. With the leg in extension, a standard anterolateral outflow portal is marked. All incisions are then infiltrated with 0.25% bupivacaine hydrochloride with 1:200,000 epinephrine. The surgical team then scrubs, allowing time for the local anesthetic and, more importantly, hemostatic agents to take effect. The limb is then prepped with alcohol and povidone-iodine (Betadine) and draped in a standard sterile fashion; chlorhexadine is used only if the patient has an iodine allergy. The inflow is connected to a pump while the outflow drains to gravity.

Arthroscopic Evaluation

Prior to thawing the allograft, a diagnostic arthroscopy is usually performed. If a repairable meniscal tear is encountered, we prefer to repair it using an inside-out suture technique. If a meniscal root tear is encountered, we prefer to repair these also through bone tunnels, as described by Harner et al.[43] With all meniscal repairs, we tie the suture after the graft is secured. Focal full-thickness articular injuries are initially managed at the time of ACL reconstruction with microfracture.

PROCEDURE

Graft Preparation

Once the graft has thawed, it is ready for preparation. With BPTB allograft preparation, the bone on either side of the tendon is trimmed to 20 mm in length by 10 mm in diameter (Fig. 50.2). The plug dimensions are verified by graft sizing tubes. The tendinous portion is trimmed to a 10- to 11-mm width and should be 45 to 55 mm in length. If the patient is shorter than 5 feet 6 inches, tendinous length of less than 45 mm is preferred. If the patient is taller than 6 feet, tendinous length of greater than 55 mm is preferred. The leading bone plug is tapered to facilitate graft passage. Two 1.5-mm holes are drilled into the tibial bone plug, from cancellous to cortical, at approximately 5 and 15 mm from the end. A no. 5 braided polyester nonabsorbable suture (Ethibond Excel, Ethicon, Somerville, New Jersey) is then threaded through each hole. An EndoButton CL BPTB (Smith & Nephew) is attached to the femoral bone plug. The appropriate loop size is determined for full bone plug length

to reside within the femoral tunnel. A mark is placed at the soft tissue to bone interface of the leading bone plug. The graft is then wrapped in a moist sponge to protect the graft from desiccation until the time of implantation.

For soft tissue allograft, anterior tibialis is our graft of choice. The graft is doubled over an EndoButton CL (Smith & Nephew). We generally use the shortest loop available (15 mm) to maximize the amount of graft material in the tunnel because this has been shown to maximize pull-out strength.[37] The free ends of the graft are individually whipstitched, and the graft is tensioned on a graft board. The graft is then wrapped in a moist sponge to protect the graft from desiccation until the time of implantation.

Notch Preparation

While the graft is being prepared, attention is turned to the femoral notch. The ACL tear pattern is evaluated. Partial tears in which a functionally intact bundle (anteromedial or posterolateral) may be treated differently are assessed, which may also explain physical examination irregularities. When possible, we prefer to attempt augmentation of an intact bundle with our graft. The torn portion of the ACL is removed with a shaver. With a complete tear, the femoral stump is totally removed to permit observation as far posteriorly in the notch as possible. We prefer to leave as much tibial stump as we can, removing only that which impairs visualization and graft passage. It a has been shown that maximal preservation of the tibial remnant enhances proprioceptive and vascular properties.[66] We do not think that a notchplasty is routinely necessary. If needed for visualization, a minimal (1- to 2-mm) notchplasty is performed for better visualization and/or to relieve graft impingement. The fat pad is left intact to prevent scarring, pain, and potential patella baja.

Tunnel Site Selection

Our goal is to make femoral and tibial tunnels in their anatomic positions. We believe that an anatomic femoral tunnel position is best achieved through the anteromedial portal because it allows us to place the femoral tunnel independently of the confines of the tibial tunnel. This technique may be used regardless of graft type, instrumentation, or fixation method.

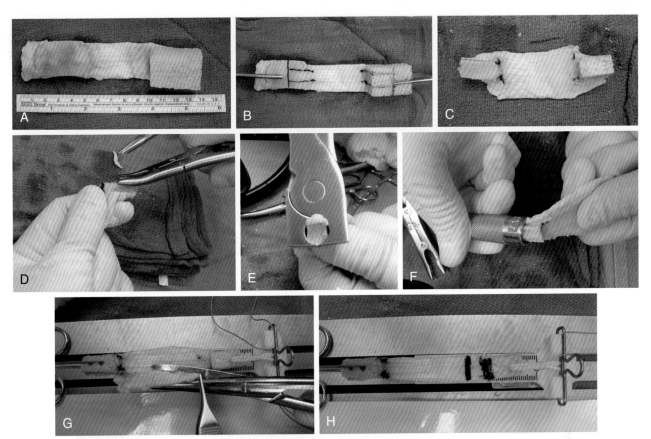

FIG 50.2 (A) Thawed bone-patellar tendon-bone allograft. (B) Projected bone plug markings (20 × 10 mm plugs). (C) Bone plugs cut with oscillating saw. (D) Rongeur used to size and taper plug. E, Compaction pliers used to finalize plug dimensions. F, Sizing tube to confirm plug size. G, Graft placed in tension to cut excess fibers that do not exhibit tension. H, Final graft construct.

Medial portal femoral tunnel preparation also allows for flexibility of tunnel creation, whether a single-bundle, double-bundle, or revision situation exists. Medial portal femoral tunnel preparation has been shown to decrease tunnel widening and minimize interference screw divergence.[15,19]

After the notch is prepared, the next step is to identify the femoral tunnel starting point. The center of the femoral footprint of the ACL is identified. This is typically 4 to 6 mm anterior to the posterior wall of the notch in the 10 o'clock (right knee) or 2 o'clock (left knee) position. Note that this is an approximation and that this footprint can vary based on ACL size and bony anatomy. A 30-degree awl is used to first identify the over-the-top position at the 10 o'clock or 2 o'clock location. The awl is then impacted into the bone approximately 6 mm anterior to this position (Fig. 50.3A). If the femoral footprint of the ACL is visible, the starting point should also acknowledge the position of the native ACL. Intraoperative fluoroscopy is used to confirm the starting position with the awl in place, with the goal of the starting point to be in the superoposterior quadrant of the lateral femoral condyle, with adequate distance between the awl and the back wall (see Fig. 50.3B).

Tibial Tunnel. After the femoral starting point is marked with the awl, anatomic tibial tunnel placement is accomplished with arthroscopic landmarks and fluoroscopic imaging. An elbow ACL tibial guide (Acufex, Smith & Nephew) is preferred (Fig.

50.4A). The point of the guide is placed at the intersection of the line made by the free edge of the anterior horn of the lateral meniscus (in the coronal plane) and the mid–medial half of the distance between the medial and lateral tibial spines (in the saggital plane). This point should also be in the mid to posterior half of the existing tibial stump, if available for confirmation (see Fig. 50.4B). The tip of the guide is held in place while the base of the guide is adjusted so that the bullet portion of the guide will contact the tibia midway between the anterior and medial crests of the tibia. The bullet of the guide is advanced, scoring the skin. A 2-cm skin incision is then made centered around the skin marking. The skin and subcutaneous tissues are sharply dissected until the tibial periosteum is encountered. A 3/32-inch Kirschner wire (K wire) is advanced through the bullet into the knee joint until it reaches the elbow portion of the guide. The guide is then disassembled and removed. The pin position is confirmed with respect to the above-mentioned landmarks (see Fig. 50.4C). The knee is brought to full extension to confirm that the graft will not impinge in extension. The pin position is evaluated on lateral and AP fluoroscopic imaging (Fig. 50.5). On the lateral view (with the knee fully extended) the pin should enter the tibial plateau at approximately the junction of the anterior and middle thirds of the plateau. In addition, it should be in line with the radiographic shadow, indicating the roof of the notch (Blumensaat line), with the knee flexed 90 degrees for BPTB allografts and 2 to 4 mm more

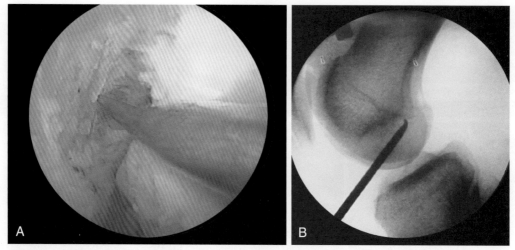

FIG 50.3 (A) Femoral starting point is marked with a pointed awl. Note the approximate 10 o'clock position for this right knee. (B) Femoral starting point confirmed on lateral fluoroscopy. Note the posterior and midcondylar position on the lateral femoral condyle, as well as the approximate 5-mm distance from the over the top position.

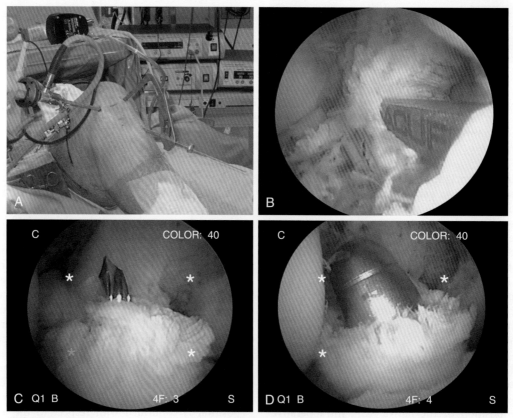

FIG 50.4 (A) External view of tibial elbow guide in right knee. The guide pin is passed with the knee in 90 degrees of flexion. (B) Tibial elbow guide placed in center of native anterior cruciate ligament (ACL) tibial insertion site for this right knee. (C) Arthroscopic view of tibial guide pin in right knee. Note the preservation of the ACL stump. (D) Arthroscopic view of tibial tunnel dilator after tibial tunnel underdrilled by 0.5 to 1.0 mm in right knee. Again, note preservation of the tibial stump.

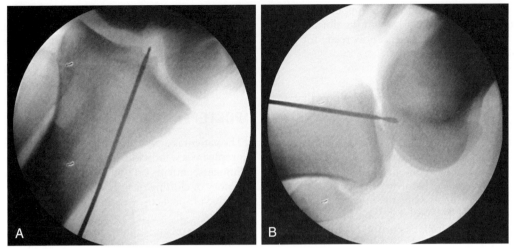

FIG 50.5 (A) Fluoroscopic anteroposterior view of tibial guide pin. Note that the guide pin emerges into the knee at the downslope of the medial tibial eminence. (B) Lateral fluoroscopic view of the tibial guide pin, taken with the knee in extension. Note that the pin is in line or slightly posterior to Blumensaat line, entering the knee in the anterior third of the tibial plateau.

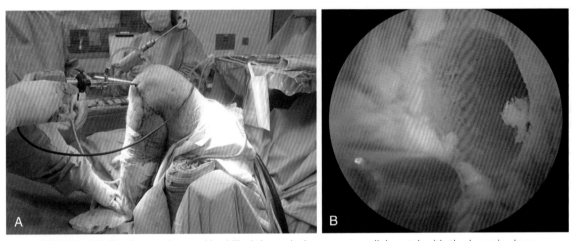

FIG 50.6 (A) The femoral tunnel is drilled through the anteromedial portal with the knee in deep flexion in this left knee. (B) Arthroscopic view of femoral tunnel in deep flexion in left knee.

posteriorly if a soft tissue graft is used. On the AP view the pin should emerge into the joint on the downslope of the medial tibial spine. If fluoroscopy demonstrates a slightly misplaced pin, a 3- or 5-mm tibial pin offset guide is used to fine-tune the pin placement. The tibial tunnel is then created with a cannulated compacting reamer 0.5 to 1.0 mm smaller than the graft size. Tunnel dilators are then used to dilate the tibial tunnel sequentially to the size of the soft tissue graft or 0.5 mm larger than the graft if using a BPTB allograft (see Fig. 50.4D). The final dilator is left in place, and again the knee is brought to extension to check for impingement of the dilator with the notch. If the graft impinges, an appropriate notchplasty is performed.

Femoral Tunnel. Attention is then returned to the femoral insertion site. Through the anteromedial portal, a ³⁄₃₂-inch K wire is introduced to the hole previously made by the awl. Once engaged in this hole, the knee is flexed to 120 degrees to improve visualization of the insertion site, prevent breaching the posterior cortex, increase tunnel length, and avoid risk to posterior neurovascular structures. The K wire is then impacted into the insertion site with the knee flexed to 120 degrees (Fig. 50.6A). A 1.0-mm undersized acorn reamer is advanced over the wire, taking care not to abrade the medial condyle or patella. If this proves to be difficult, a half-round reamer can be used with the smooth portion facing the at-risk cartilaginous surface until it is seated against the lateral condyle. The position of the drill is checked to confirm adequate distance from the back wall and desired trajectory. The drill is then advanced by hand to begin the footprint of the insertion site, reevaluated, and drilled by power to the depth mandated by the fixation technique. A shaver is introduced in the tunnel to remove the bone and soft tissue debris (see Fig. 50.6B). Dilators are next introduced through the anteromedial portal to dilate the tunnel to the size of the soft tissue graft (or 0.5 mm larger than the graft if using a BPTB allograft). Our fixation of choice is the EndoButton (Smith & Nephew). A 3.2-mm EndoButton drill is used to breach the lateral femoral cortex. A Beath pin with an affixed no. 5 Ethibond looped suture is then advanced through the drilled femoral tunnel, through the EndoButton drill track, and through the lateral thigh soft tissue. This looped Ethibond suture is then retrieved intra-articularly from the tibial tunnel. The Beath pin is left in place. The knee is now ready for graft passage.

Graft Passage

The knee is now flexed to 90 degrees. Passing sutures that are threaded through the two eyes of the EndoButton on the femoral side of the graft are placed around the Ethibond loop, which is now exiting the tibial tunnel. The Beath pin is then pulled from the lateral thigh and the passing sutures are delivered through the femoral tunnel and out the lateral thigh. One set of passing sutures is pulled (allowing the EndoButton to slant through the drilled tunnel) while the other set of passing sutures is intermittently pulled, only relieving their slack. If a BPTB allograft is used, the cancellous portion of the bone plug is anterior, allowing the graft to reside posteriorly in the tunnel. To facilitate graft passage, a right angle clamp can be used that acts as an intra-articular pulley to help to get an appropriate angle into the femoral tunnel. Also, with BPTB allografts, the bone plug can be gently impacted to encourage passage through the tunnel. Finally, the knee can be further flexed to help to ease passage of the graft. After the EndoButton has exited the cortex (determined by appropriate graft markings and confirmed by fluoroscopy), the EndoButton is flipped by applying tension to the lagging strand of the femoral passing sutures. Tension is placed on the tibial side of the graft to seat the EndoButton flush with the femoral cortex. Appropriate seating is also confirmed by fluoroscopy. With tension on the tibia-sided lead sutures, the graft is cycled to reduce creep within the graft. Graft isometry is also evaluated, as is impingement in extension.

Graft Fixation

We prefer tibial post fixation, regardless of graft type. A standard 4.5-mm large-fragment cortex screw with a washer is placed bicortically, approximately 5 to 10 mm distal to the tibial tunnel. When the far cortex is engaged but prior to final seating of the screw and washer, the two pairs of tibial lead sutures are individually tied around the post with the knee in 15 to 30 degrees of flexion. The screw is then fully seated. The graft is arthroscopically evaluated for tension and impingement (Fig. 50.7). Postoperative Lachman and pivot shift tests are repeated to confirm

reversal of preoperative findings. Final radiographs are taken to verify hardware placement and tunnel position (Fig. 50.8). The wounds are irrigated and closed in layers. A sterile dressing is applied. A cold therapy sleeve is placed over the dressing. A hinged knee brace is then centered over the joint line, locking the knee in full extension.

POSTOPERATIVE MANAGEMENT

The patient is discharged the same day. Deep venous thrombosis prophylaxis is individualized, depending on specific risk factors. Smokers, patients on oral contraceptives, patients with a family history of clotting disorders, and those with a previous DVT all receive prophylaxis. Rehabilitation follows a standard protocol in which full return to activity is expected by 6 to 12 months, depending on graft choice and patient-specific factors. We allow a longer time for allografts to incorporate.

In the first week after surgery, patients are allowed to bear weight with crutches, with the brace locked in full extension. A recent study has shown that brace wear does not affect pain or range of motion within the first 2 weeks after surgery, but we think that it protects the newly reconstructed graft and gives patients a feeling of safety.[35,47] Basic home exercises, including quadriceps sets, straight leg raises, and heel slides, are permitted out of the brace with the goal of achieving full extension and full flexion, and initializing return of quadriceps strength. The patient is seen in 1 week, and sutures are removed. Patients are sent to formal physical therapy after this visit. The added focus at this time is to begin gait training with the brace unlocked to practice a heel-to-toe gait. The goal at 1 month is full range of motion and a normal heel-to-toe gait. The brace is discontinued when this is confirmed at the second appointment, 1 month after surgery. Strengthening of the lower extremity is the subsequent focus, with gradually increasing light resistance training (eg, exercise bicycle, closed-chain low-resistance weights). At

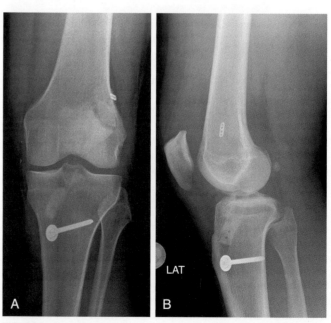

FIG 50.8 Postoperative anteroposterior (A) and lateral (B) x-ray demonstrating a well-positioned femoral EndoButton and tibial post in this left knee.

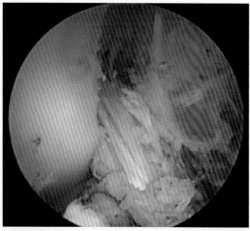

FIG 50.7 Final view of reconstructed anterior cruciate ligament with bone-patellar tendon-bone allograft in right knee.

the third postoperative visit (at 3 months after surgery), the patient should exhibit significant return of quadriceps and hamstring strength. More aggressive strengthening exercises are permitted, taking care to avoid open-chain knee extensions. The delicate decision is made at this time as to when the patient can begin in-line exercises, generally between 3 and 6 months. At 6 to 12 months from surgery, full return to sport is gradually permitted.

KEY REFERENCES

5. Baer GS, Harner CD: Clinical outcomes of allograft versus autograft in anterior cruciate ligament reconstruction. *Clin Sports Med* 26(4):661–681, 2007.

31. Edgar CM, Zimmer S, Kakar S, et al: Prospective comparison of auto and allograft hamstring tendon constructs for ACL reconstruction. *Clin Orthop* 466(9):2238–2246, 2008.

34. Foster TE, Wolfe BL, Ryan S, et al: Does the graft source really matter in the outcome of patients undergoing anterior cruciate ligament reconstruction? An evaluation of autograft versus allograft reconstruction results: a systematic review. *Am J Sports Med* 38(1):189–199, 2010.

38. Group M, Group M: Effect of graft choice on the outcome of revision anterior cruciate ligament reconstruction in the Multicenter ACL Revision Study (MARS) Cohort. *Am J Sports Med* 42(10):2301–2310, 2014.

40. Gulotta LV, Rodeo SA: Biology of autograft and allograft healing in anterior cruciate ligament reconstruction. *Clin Sports Med* 26(4):509–524, 2007.

41. Guo L, Yang L, Duan XJ, et al: Anterior cruciate ligament reconstruction with bone-patellar tendon-bone graft: comparison of autograft, fresh-frozen allograft, and gamma-irradiated allograft. *Arthroscopy* 28(2):211–217, 2012.

46. Hettrich CM, Dunn WR, Reinke EK, et al: The rate of subsequent surgery and predictors after anterior cruciate ligament reconstruction: two- and 6-year follow-up results from a multicenter cohort. *Am J Sports Med* 41(7):1534–1540, 2013.

56. Kaeding CC, Pedroza AD, Reinke EK, et al: Risk factors and predictors of subsequent ACL injury in either knee after ACL reconstruction: prospective analysis of 2488 primary ACL reconstructions from the MOON cohort. *Am J Sports Med* 43(7):1583–1590, 2015.

71. Maletis GB, Inacio MC, Desmond JL, et al: Reconstruction of the anterior cruciate ligament: association of graft choice with increased risk of early revision. *Bone Joint J* 95-B(5):623–628, 2013.

75. Mariscalco MW, Magnussen RA, Mehta D, et al: Autograft versus nonirradiated allograft tissue for anterior cruciate ligament reconstruction: a systematic review. *Am J Sports Med* 42(2):492–499, 2014.

95. Rahr-Wagner L, Thillemann TM, Pedersen AB, et al: Comparison of hamstring tendon and patellar tendon grafts in anterior cruciate ligament reconstruction in a nationwide population-based cohort study: results from the danish registry of knee ligament reconstruction. *Am J Sports Med* 42(2):278–284, 2014.

106. Spindler KP, Huston LJ, Wright RW, et al: The prognosis and predictors of sports function and activity at minimum 6 years after anterior cruciate ligament reconstruction: a population cohort study. *Am J Sports Med* 39(2):348–359, 2011.

109. Sun K, Tian SQ, Zhang JH, et al: Anterior cruciate ligament reconstruction with bone-patellar tendon-bone autograft versus allograft. *Arthroscopy* 25(7):750–759, 2009.

114. Wasserstein D, Sheth U, Cabrera A, et al: A systematic review of failed anterior cruciate ligament reconstruction with autograft compared with allograft in young patients. *Sports Health* 7(3):207–216, 2015.

115. West RV, Harner CD: Graft selection in anterior cruciate ligament reconstruction. *J Am Acad Orthop Surg* 13(3):197–207, 2005.

The references for this chapter can also be found on www.expertconsult.com.

51

Double-Bundle Anterior Cruciate Ligament Reconstruction

Zaneb Yaseen, Daniel Guenther, Sebastián Irarrázaval, Freddie H. Fu

Single-bundle anterior cruciate ligament (ACL) reconstruction has largely been a successful surgery over the past several decades, with satisfactory subjective patient outcomes in the short term.[5] However, some long-term studies have found significant sequelae of ACL injury and its reconstruction, with the development of early arthritic changes in a large percentage of patients. Pinczewski et al.[22] have reported arthritic changes at 10 years postoperatively in 39% of patients who underwent patellar tendon autograft ACL reconstruction. In addition, others have reported a subset of patients, between 30% and 40%, who have persistent instability or are unable to return to their previous level of activity.[2] These results compare favorably with nonoperative treatment of ACL injuries; however, potential areas for improvement obviously remain.

Over the past decade there has been an increase in interest in double-bundle ACL reconstruction. With the primary goals of re-creating the two functional bundles of the ACL and individualizing each surgical procedure, the double-bundle reconstruction was first described in the 1980s. Over the past decade the technique has gained popularity as a better understanding of the normal anatomy and biomechanics of the ACL has been achieved.

This chapter will explore the native anatomy and biomechanics of the ACL and the double-bundle reconstruction technique.

ANATOMY AND BIOMECHANICS

The ACL originates on the medial aspect of the lateral femoral condyle and runs obliquely to its insertion at the medial tibial eminence. It consists of two bundles, the anteromedial (AM) and posterolateral (PL) bundle (Fig. 51.1). The bundles are named according to their insertion on the tibia. The femoral origin of the AM bundle is located posterior and proximal to the PL bundle on the medial wall of the lateral femoral condyle. The bundles cross each other and the AM bundle inserts AM to the PL bundle on the tibia, with a close relationship to the anterior horn of the lateral meniscus. The femoral origin of the PL bundle is located anterior and distal to the AM bundle. The PL bundle inserts PL to the AM bundle on the tibia, with a close relationship to the posterior horn of the lateral meniscus. The bundles are covered by a thin membrane and separated by a distinct septum, containing vascular-derived stem cells.[17]

To help to identify each bundle, there are distinct bony landmarks that signify the anatomic extents of each bundle, as well as the ACL as a whole. On the femoral side the lateral intercondylar ridge (resident's ridge) is the anterior border of the ACL. This bony landmark runs from proximal to distal with the knee straight, and no cruciate fibers insert anterior to this point. The lateral bifurcate ridge, which is subtle but often present, separates the anterior portion of the AM bundle from the PL bundle.

On the tibial side the insertion varies and shape and size.[14,29] Medially the ACL inserts up to a bony ridge that is an anterior extension of the medial intercondylar tubercle.[25] Posteriorly no fibers extend beyond a ridge of bone at the anterior aspect of the tibial spine between the medial and lateral tibial intercondylar tubercles. The PL bundle lies just anterior to the insertion of the posterior horn of the lateral meniscus. The anterior and lateral borders are less well defined and consist of diffuse expansions.

With the knee in full extension, the AM and PL bundles are parallel. During knee flexion the AM bundles tighten and twists around the PL bundle. The AM bundle is the primary restraint against anterior tibial translation at 90 degrees of knee flexion. With increased internal or external rotation, the ACL tightens so that it may operate as a major restraint against rotational moments.[18] Most recent evidence suggest that both the AM and PL bundles behave synergistically to control anterior translation and rotational stability, with the AM bundle being more tight in flexion and the PL bundle being more tight in extension.[1,7,13,32,33] Disruption of the ACL changes knee kinematics significantly. The transfer of forces can be effective only if the joint is mechanically stable.[4] ACL deficiency leads to an increased anterior tibial translation and an increased internal tibial rotation.

Understanding the biomechanical function and insertional anatomy of the ACL highlights the importance of each bundle. This is critical to the correct application of the double-bundle technique.

PREOPERATIVE CONSIDERATIONS

Patient Evaluation

Patient evaluation begins with a thorough history and careful physical examination. The history and mechanism of injury should be explored because this can help to determine whether other ligamentous injuries may be present. Such symptoms as locking or catching may suggest meniscal injuries.

A complete physical examination is performed on both lower extremities for comparison. Visual inspection for gait, overall limb alignment, ecchymosis, joint effusion, and muscular atrophy is performed. Evaluation of range of motion (ROM) followed by palpation of the parapatellar region, joint line, and bony prominences aids in the diagnosis of the ACL tear and any concomitant pathology. Special tests, including the Lachman maneuver, pivot shift, anterior and posterior drawer, reverse pivot shift, McMurray, dial, and varus-valgus tests, may be difficult to perform in the acute setting but are crucial to a complete evaluation. The degree of anterior laxity can be also be quantified with the KT1000 arthrometer (MEDmetric, San Diego, California); a 3-mm or greater side-to-side difference is suggestive of an ACL injury.[26]

Prior to any surgical management, full motion must be obtained and swelling should be allowed to resolve. If a concomitant ligament injury occurs, such as injury to the medial collateral ligament, surgery can be delayed to allow for healing. However, if a displaced meniscus tear or unstable cartilage defect is noted, surgery is recommended more acutely.

Imaging

Plain radiographs are obtained and consist of weight-bearing extension and 45-degree flexion posteroanterior views. Non–weight-bearing, 45-degree lateral and axial (Merchant) views are also obtained. Standard magnetic resonance imaging (MRI) sequences are helpful for diagnosing the ACL tear, as well as any additional injuries and bone bruise pattern. Oblique coronal views, taken in the plane of the ACL, are helpful for visualizing the two bundles of the ACL (Fig. 51.2). Measurements are obtained from the sagittal MRI and include tibial insertion size and ACL angle, as well as quadriceps and patellar tendon thickness.

For cases involving revision ACL reconstruction, MRI or computed tomography (CT) with three-dimensional reconstructions can provide better detail of prior tunnel placement, degree of bone lysis, and tunnel expansion (Fig. 51.3). Long leg cassette x-rays can also be performed to evaluate for any limb alignment abnormalities.

Indications and Contraindications

Double-bundle reconstruction is indicated for those patients with acute ACL tears, persistent instability after single-bundle reconstruction, some cases with combined ligament or meniscal injury and ACL injury, or failure of nonoperative treatment. This typically includes athletes of all ages in cutting, jumping, or pivoting sports and patients with demanding employment, including manual labor or firefighting. Patients who have failed nonoperative treatment are also candidates. Those with a sedentary lifestyle or with lower-demand activities can possibly be treated nonoperatively.

Absolute contraindications to double-bundle reconstruction include tibial footprint size less than 14 mm, advanced degenerative changes (grade 3 or greater), infection, and patient noncompliance.[23] In patients with open physes or multiligament injuries, consideration should be made to performing a single-bundle reconstruction. Relative contraindications include a narrow notch and severe bone bruising over the lateral femoral condyle.

Regardless of type of reconstruction, each individual case requires an in-depth conversation between the treating surgeon and patient to develop an appropriate plan acceptable to both

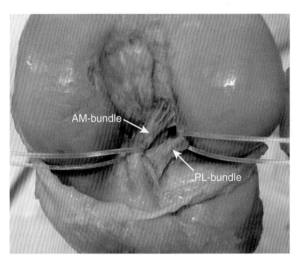

FIG 51.1 Cadaveric specimen showing the AM and PL bundles of the ACL. *AM,* Anteromedial; *PL,* posterolateral. (Reprinted with permission from Hofbauer et al.[9])

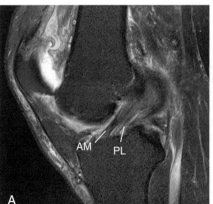
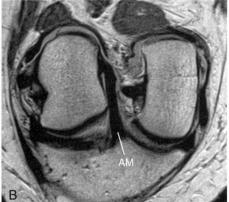
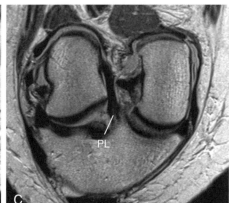

FIG 51.2 Magnetic Resonance Imaging of the Anterior Cruciate Ligament (A) T2-weighted sagittal ACL with *AM* and *PL* bundle. (B) Coronal oblique cut shows the *AM* bundle. (C) Coronal oblique cut shows the *PL* bundle. *AM,* Anteromedial; *PL,* posterolateral.

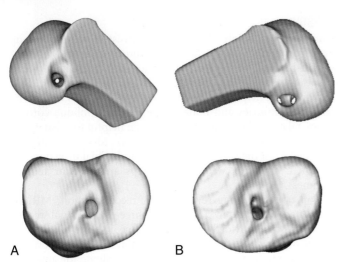

FIG 51.3 Three-dimensional CT scan of the femur and tibia after single-bundle ACL reconstruction (A) and double-bundle ACL reconstruction (B).

parties. All consent forms include the option of allograft tissue in case hybridization is required.

TECHNIQUE

The goal of double-bundle ACL reconstruction is to re-create the native anatomy. This requires a thorough evaluation and identification of the ligament insertion sites, which can be more time-consuming than in a single-bundle reconstruction but is necessary to optimize clinical outcomes.

Setup

As with all surgical procedures, the plan is reviewed and correct extremity is confirmed with the patient in the preoperative area. The patient is brought to the operating room, where the anesthetic of choice is administered. While under anesthesia, a thorough examination of both extremities is performed. Careful attention is paid to rotational instability.

At our institution, the nonoperative extremity is placed in a well-leg holder, which is padded to protect the peroneal nerve. A pneumatic tourniquet is placed proximally on the thigh of the operative extremity. The leg is then placed in an arthroscopic circumferential leg holder with the foot of the table dropped. Range of motion is verified to allow full extension and flexion beyond 120 degrees. Alternatively, the reconstruction can be performed without the leg holder as long as hyperflexion is possible. The leg is then prepped and draped in a sterile fashion. Prior to incision, a time-out is performed and the tourniquet is insufflated to 350 mm Hg after elevation of the extremity for 3 minutes. In addition, a portable fluoroscopy device is draped so that it can be used to confirm femoral fixation and in some cases to confirm guidewire position for either tunnel.

Graft Selection and Preparation

Both autograft and allograft options exist for the double-bundle reconstruction, and one must consider the patient's age, anatomy, prior surgical history, activities, and occupation when discussing this with the patient. Autograft is preferred for patients younger than 35 years and allograft for those older than 40.

Although allograft tissue eliminates donor site morbidity, one must counsel the patient regarding possible disease transmission, slow healing, and potentially higher failure rate.[16,29] If allograft is chosen, tibialis anterior or Achilles tendons are preferable because of the large diameter and length. If tibialis anterior is chosen, two grafts are obtained with at least 24 cm in length. After the graft diameters are determined (see later), each graft is trimmed so that its doubled-over diameter will be the desired size. Each soft tissue end is stitched with a strong nonabsorbable suture to facilitate graft passage and fixation. If Achilles allograft is used, the bone block is placed at the femoral insertion site.

Autograft options include hamstring and quadriceps tendon grafts. Hamstring grafts are harvested and prepared in standard fashion. However, because the diameters of the harvested hamstring tendons may be smaller than those required for the double-bundle reconstruction, the surgeon can hybridize the reconstruction with the addition of an allograft tendon.

Quadriceps graft is chosen after first examining the sagittal MRI to calculate tendon thickness, which should have a minimum thickness of 7 mm. A full-thickness, 11 mm–wide graft is harvested with or without bone block. This is detached as proximally as possible to maximize graft length. For an all soft tissue graft, at least 8 cm of tendon must be harvested. If a bone block is desired, a 20-mm-long and 10-mm-thick bone plug is harvested from the superior patella with care to not disrupt the cartilage surface. The soft tissue portion of the graft can be split and trimmed to provide the two bundles for reconstruction. However, with the bone plug, only one femoral tunnel is used, as will be described later.

Graft Preparation

Multiple fixation methods can be used for securing the ACL graft. The senior author of this chapter prefers closed-loop suspensory fixation. All soft tissue grafts were prepared first by securing the tissue ends with a no. 2 nonabsorbable braided suture. These were then folded in half over a closed-loop suspensory device. They are then tensioned to 15 lb to remove creep until they are ready for passage. The grafts are marked at the depth that the button will be able to exit the tunnel and flip into position. For grafts involving a bone block, the bone block is sized appropriately. Then, one small hole is drilled into the distal one-third of the block, and the fixed-loop device is secured. The soft tissue portion is split such that there is enough graft to reproduce the AM and PL bundles. The soft tissue ends are then secured using a nonabsorbable no. 2 suture.

Portal Establishment

A three-portal technique is used to visualize the ACL footprints properly. The anterolateral (AL) portal is established first, just lateral to the patellar tendon and superior to the inferior pole of the patella to avoid the infrapatellar fat pad.[23] The AM and accessory anteromedial (AAM) portals are established under direct visualization using an 18-gauge spinal needle. The AM portal is established along the medial border of the inferior patellar tendon or transtendinous such that the spinal needle is in line with the native ACL, taking care not to injure the intermeniscal ligament. Following the establishment of the AM portal, the shaver is introduced and some of the fat pad is removed to facilitate visualization. The AAM portal is established at the level of the joint line, approximately 1.5 cm medial to the AM portal. The spinal needle should pass safely above

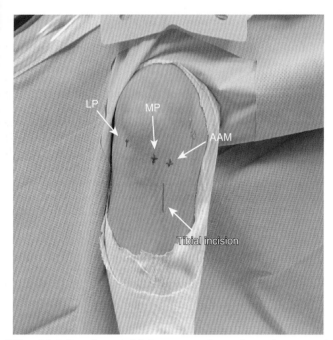

FIG 51.4 Portal establishment using the three-portal-technique—*LP*, AM portal, and *AAM* portal. *AAM*, Accessory anteromedial; *AM*, anteromedial; *LP*, anterolateral portal. (Reprinted with permission from Pombo et al.[23])

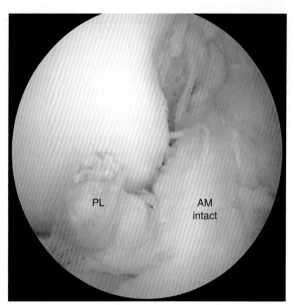

FIG 51.5 Complete tear of *PL* bundle of ACL, with *AM* bundle intact. *AM*, Anteromedial; *PL*, posterolateral.

the medial meniscus and reach the center of the femoral ACL footprint with enough space to allow for safe passage of instruments without risking damage to the medial femoral condyle as femoral tunnel drilling occurs from this portal (Fig. 51.4).

Defining the Rupture Pattern and Anterior Cruciate Ligament Footprints

After the diagnostic arthroscopy is completed, the ACL tear is carefully studied from each portal site to identify each bundle and the tear pattern (Fig. 51.5). The tibial and femoral footprints are then uncovered with the use of a thermal device on a very low setting. The bony anatomy of the lateral femoral condyle is helpful in locating the boundaries of each bundle (Fig. 51.6). After the footprints are identified, the length and width of the AM and PL bundle insertion sites on the tibia and femur are measured with an arthroscopic ruler (Fig. 51.7). The smaller insertion size for each bundle determines the graft size, and the grafts are prepared accordingly. In our experience the AM bundle typically measures 7 to 9 mm in diameter and the PL bundle typically measures 5 to 7 mm.[15] If the sizes are adequate (>14) and notch is not too narrow, it is safe to then proceed with double-bundle reconstruction (Fig. 51.8).

Tunnel Placement

For all soft tissue grafts, the sequence of events is as follows. The PL femoral tunnel is prepared first through the AAM portal. An awl is used to mark the center of the PL bundle femoral insertion. The insertion site is confirmed with the arthroscope through all three portals to appreciate all aspects of the planned tunnel placement. Next, a flexible guidewire is placed through the AAM portal to the marked center of the PL insertion and is advanced with the knee in hyperflexion. The pin is advanced through the femoral cortex and the skin. The length of the femoral tunnel is then measured. An ideal length should be 30

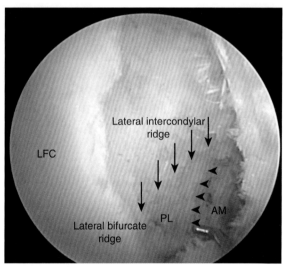

FIG 51.6 Marking of the femoral insertion sites (*AM* and *PL* bundles) with a thermal device. *Long arrows* depict the lateral intercondylar ridge (resident's ridge); *arrowheads* depict the lateral bifurcate ridge. *AM*, Anteromedial; *LFC*, lateral femoral condyle; *PL*, posterolateral.

to 40 mm, such that at least 20 mm of the graft can be in the tunnel and enough length can be left to allow the button to flip (approximately 7 mm). The knee can be taken out of hyperflexion. Tunnels that are too short may be because of inadequate flexion of the knee. The graft can be secured using a number of methods, including screw and washer or a polyethylene button. If a straight guidewire is used, it is important to keep the knee in the same amount of hyperflexion throughout all drilling and passage. The cannulated drill bit is then passed over the guidewire with care not to damage the medial femoral condyle. This is sized approximately 1 to 2 mm smaller than the graft diameter. The tunnel is then dilated by hand to the final dimension. The drill is advanced to the appropriate depth (in general approximately 27 mm), with care to preserve the lateral cortex.

Next, the tibial tunnels are addressed. This sequence is the same regardless of graft choice. A vertical 4- to 5-cm incision is made over the AM proximal tibial, approximately 2 cm distal from the joint line and 1 to 2 cm medial to the tibial tubercle. If hamstrings were harvested, the same incision is used for tibial drilling. The ACL guide, usually set to approximately 45 degrees, is then placed in the center of the PL bundle either via the AM or AAM portal. The guidewire is then advanced. The position is confirmed, and the ACL guide is then adjusted to approximately 55 degrees and placed in the center of the AM bundle. It is important to ensure that the start point for the guidewire is at least 1 to 1.5 cm away from the previously placed guidewire. The tunnels should not be allowed to converge. After the guidewires are appropriately placed, the knee is taken to full extension to ensure there will be no graft impingement. The wires are then overdrilled with cannulated reamers approximately 1 to 2 mm smaller than the graft diameter. The tunnels are then dilated by hand to the final diameter.

Finally, the AM femoral tunnel is prepared in a similar fashion to the PL femoral tunnel (Fig. 51.9).

In cases using a bone block, one femoral tunnel is drilled, but the insertion point is placed in the center of both footprints so that one anatomic tunnel can be drilled. The remainder of the steps are similar.

Graft Passage and Fixation

A beath pin with a looped suture attached is placed through the AAM portal into the femoral PL tunnel and brought out through the AL thigh. A suture-grasping device is placed through the tibial PL tunnel, and the suture is retrieved. A second beath pin is used for the AM bundle, and the suture is passed in a similar fashion. The PL bundle is passed first with arthroscopic guidance, and the button device is flipped on the lateral femoral cortex. The AM bundle is passed in a similar fashion. The flipped button is confirmed using portable fluoroscopy. Grafts with a bone block are pulled in through the AAM portal pulled into the femoral tunnel. The button device is flipped on the lateral femoral cortex. The sutures for the distal limbs are brought out through the appropriate tibial tunnel. Arthroscopy is used to visualize the position of the two bundles, and the knee is fully extended to confirm that there is no impingement. The knee is cycled approximately 15 to 20 times while holding tension on the distal suture limbs. The PL bundle is secured first with an interference screw in full extension. The

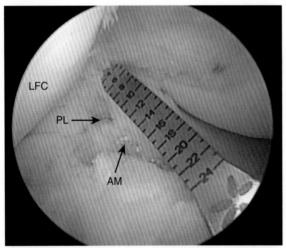

FIG 51.7 Measurement of the tibial insertion site of the ACL after marking with a thermal device. The insertion site measures 20 mm. *AM,* Anteromedial; *LFC,* lateral femoral condyle; *PL,* posterolateral.

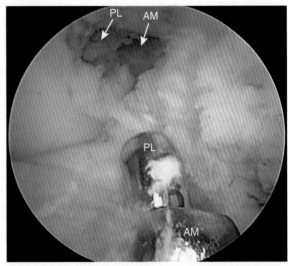

FIG 51.9 Views of femoral and tibial tunnels in double-bundle reconstruction with soft tissue graft. *AM,* Anteromedial; *PL,* posterolateral. (Reprinted with permission from Pombo et al.[23])

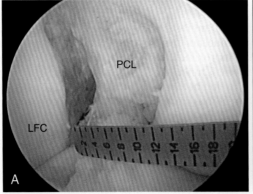

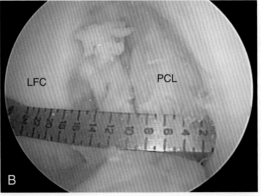

FIG 51.8 Measurement of the Intercondylar Notch   (A) Narrow notch measuring 12 mm. (B) Wide notch measuring 20 mm. *LFC,* Lateral femoral condyle.

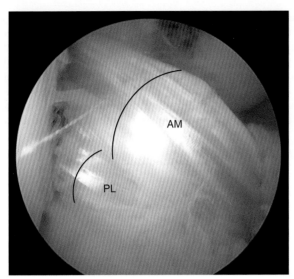

FIG 51.10 Anatomic double-bundle ACL reconstruction. Both grafts (*AM* and *PL* bundles) can be visualized. *AM,* Anteromedial; *PL,* posterolateral.

AM bundle is fixed in 30 degrees of flexion. Arthroscopy is again performed to verify graft position, and the knee is brought through a full ROM (Fig. 51.10). Images are obtained from each of the portal sites to confirm anatomic position. A Lachman exam is then performed to confirm stability. If there is residual laxity or a "pop" is experienced, the knee should be examined again and the grafts confirmed and redone if necessary. The wounds are copiously irrigated and incisions closed. The knee is then carefully padded and placed into a hinged knee brace locked in extension.

POSTOPERATIVE REHABILITATION

Patients are discharged home the same day with instructions to begin quadriceps sets and heel slides, if indicated, and remain in the brace locked in extension when ambulating and sleeping. Weight-bearing restrictions and motion depend upon any concomitant meniscal or chondral surgery. Patients generally follow up in 1 to 2 weeks from the surgery date. Postoperative rehabilitation programs are separated into five stages. Initially, particular attention is paid to minimizing inflammation, gaining full ROM (particularly extension), and brace use. Formal physical therapy begins at approximately 1 week. Full ROM should be obtained by 4 to 6 weeks after surgery. If patients struggle and cannot regain motion, then a manipulation under anesthesia can be considered between 8 and 12 weeks. Manipulations after that point have a higher risk of fracture.

After motion is achieved, the next milestones include discontinuation of the brace and crutches (when full extension without a lag has been achieved, typically by 6 weeks), stationary bike, leg press, double and single leg squats, lunges, and fast walking on treadmills. This usually lasts until approximately 16 weeks. Stage 2 begins when a patient is able to walk for 15 minutes without symptoms, perform 10 single leg squats for 45 degrees of flexion without balance, and be at least 4 months postoperative. Stage 2 includes introduction back to jogging when quadriceps strength is near normal. The patient continues to

work on proprioception, balance, and strengthening. Patients can progress to stage 3 when they are able to jog 2 miles without difficulty and perform leg press at greater than 85% to their contralateral side. This occurs around 6 to 8 months postoperatively and involves agility drills, such as lateral shuffling, forward/backward shuttle runs, carioca drills, and ladder drills. Advancement to stage 4 occurs after the patient is able to perform a leg press at 90% of the contralateral limb, 10 single leg squats to 60 degrees of knee flexion, and demonstrate no compensatory mechanisms during deceleration and agility drills. This occurs around 7 to 9 months, and at this point jumping begins. Initially, up and down jumps must be mastered, and then forward, side, and box jumps can be attempted. After the jumps have been mastered and there is good core, quadriceps, and pelvifemoral strength, they can progress to stage 5. This is achieved no earlier than 9 months postoperatively and involves gradual progression to single leg hops, sprinting, pivoting, and cutting activities. After the patient is cleared to full activity, the patient is offered a functional ACL brace initially if they return to a cutting activity.

POTENTIAL PITFALLS AND RECOMMENDATIONS

The potential pitfalls of double-bundle reconstruction are similar to the single-bundle technique. However, concern has been expressed regarding the potential injury to the lateral and PL structures, including the peroneal nerve, with drilling of the femoral PL tunnel. Several cadaveric studies have shown that this risk is minimal if the femoral tunnels are drilled in at least 120 degrees of flexion.[8,21]

There are several points that must be made to optimize surgical outcome and avoid potential mistakes. A high lateral portal is important to avoid poor visualization because of the fat pad. The medial portals should be done under direct visualization for placement above the medial meniscus and with adequate clearance to avoid damaging the medial femoral condyle.

It is important to maintain a good bone bridge between tunnels. When using all soft tissue grafts, marking the PL bundle with ink can help to maintain orientation during graft passage and graft fixation. If the harvested hamstrings are too small, then hybridization with allograft should be considered. It is important to visualize the femoral and tibial ACL insertions properly. This is accomplished by viewing through multiple arthroscopy portals and using the bony and soft tissue landmarks to accurately identify the insertion sites. By properly identifying the insertions, the anatomic location of the reconstruction can be identified and mismatching of the tibial and femoral tunnels can be avoided. Similarly, one should avoid referring to the reconstruction in the "o'clock" terminology. The femoral notch is a three-dimensional structure and to describe it using a two-dimensional process leads to nonanatomic placement of the reconstruction. Finally, one must properly restore the tension pattern in the two bundles of the ACL, as described. Nonphysiologic tensioning may lead to overtensioning or undertensioning at certain flexion angles, which could result in graft failure.[3]

RESULTS

The biomechanical results of the double-bundle reconstruction have been studied extensively in cadaveric and in vivo settings.

Woo et al.[31] have evaluated the single-bundle reconstruction in response to an anterior tibial and combined rotatory load in cadavers. Although the reconstruction was successful at limiting anterior translation, it was ineffective at providing stability to the combined load. A similar study evaluated both the single- and double-bundle reconstruction, with better biomechanical stability, particularly in rotatory testing, found in the double-bundle anatomic approach.[32] One possible benefit to better normalization of stability is an improvement in contact areas and stresses within the knee. Morimoto et al.[19] have evaluated the contact area and pressure in a normal knee; after single- and double-bundle reconstruction, they found that the single-bundle reconstruction resulted in a smaller contact area and higher contact pressures, whereas the double-bundle reconstruction approached that of the normal knee.

Comparison of single-bundle and double-bundle ACL reconstruction has been studied over the years. A Cochrane review examining the effects of double- versus single-bundle ACL reconstruction found some limited evidence that double-bundle ACL reconstruction has some superior results in objective measurements of knee stability and some protection on reinjury or new meniscal injury. Further randomized control trials are necessary to further delineate these findings.[30] An evidence-based study found that double-bundle ACL reconstruction showed better outcomes in rotational laxity, although functional recovery was similar between both techniques.[27] Järvelä et al.[10] have reported on the 2-year follow-up of a randomized controlled clinical trial comparing double- and single-bundle reconstructions. Rotational stability was best in the double-bundle group, with no significant difference in anterior stability. In addition, Fu et al.[6] conducted a 2-year prospective study and found that double-bundle reconstruction results in good restoration of joint stability with a normal or near-normal Lachman examination in 98% of patients and a normal pivot shift test in 94% of patients. Patient-reported measures were also promising, with scores similar to those reported for the single-bundle approach. The results of these two studies are similar to other reports in the literature.[11,12,20,24,28] However, despite objective evidence of improved rotational stability after double-bundle reconstruction, these studies fail to show significant differences in subjective measures. The reason for this remains perplexing but possibly relates to lack of knowledge regarding how these small differences affect the patient's interpretation of the outcome and the outcome measure's ability to detect these subtleties. Nevertheless, future long-term studies are required to determine the true benefits of the double-bundle reconstruction.

CONCLUSION

The past several decades have seen significant advances in the understanding of the anatomy and biomechanics of the ACL. Using this information, surgical techniques have been developed in an attempt to replicate better what is seen in dissection and in the laboratory. The double-bundle reconstruction is one such technique and has the potential to more accurately reproduce the native anatomy of the ACL. It is a complex procedure that should be performed only by those with an understanding of the anatomic approach and with advanced training. Although initial biomechanical and clinical reports appear promising, better evaluation tools and longer-term studies are required.

KEY REFERENCES

2. Biau DJ, Tournoux C, Katsahian S, et al: ACL reconstruction: a meta-analysis of functional scores. *Clin Orthop* 458:180–187, 2007.
3. Colvin AC, Shen W, Musahl V, et al: Avoiding pitfalls in anatomic ACL reconstruction. *Knee Surg Sports Traumatol Arthrosc* 17:956–963, 2009.
Ferretti M, Ekdahl M, Shen W, et al: Osseous landmarks of the femoral attachment of the anterior cruciate ligament: an anatomic study. *Arthroscopy* 23:1218–1225, 2007.
6. Fu FH, Shen W, Starman JS, et al: Primary anatomic double-bundle anterior cruciate ligament reconstruction: a preliminary 2-year prospective study. *Am J Sports Med* 36:1263–1274, 2008.
Gabriel MT, Wong EK, Woo SL, et al: Distribution of in situ forces in the anterior cruciate ligament in response to rotatory loads. *J Orthop Res* 22:85–89, 2004.
Jordan SS, DeFrate LE, Nha KW, et al: The in vivo kinematics of the anteromedial and posterolateral bundles of the anterior cruciate ligament during weightbearing knee flexion. *Am J Sports Med* 35:547–554, 2007.
14. Kopf S, Musahl V, Tashman S, et al: A systematic review of the femoral origin and tibial insertion morphology of the ACL. *Knee Surg Sports Traumatol Arthrosc* 17:213–219, 2009.
19. Morimoto Y, Ferretti M, Ekdahl M, et al: Tibiofemoral joint contact area and pressure after single- and double-bundle anterior cruciate ligament reconstruction. *Arthroscopy* 25:62–69, 2009.
20. Muneta T, Koga H, Mochizuki T, et al: A prospective randomized study of 4-strand semitendinosus tendon anterior cruciate ligament reconstruction comparing single-bundle and double-bundle techniques. *Arthroscopy* 23:618–628, 2007.
Petersen W, Zantop T: Anatomy of the anterior cruciate ligament with regard to its two bundles. *Clin Orthop* 454:35–47, 2007.
23. Pombo MW, Shen W, Fu FH: Anatomic double-bundle anterior cruciate ligament reconstruction: where are we today? *Arthroscopy* 24:1168–1177, 2008.
24. Prodromos C, Joyce B, Shi K: A meta-analysis of stability of autografts compared to allografts after anterior cruciate ligament reconstruction. *Knee Surg Sports Traumatol Arthrosc* 15:851–856, 2007.
25. Purnell ML, Larson AI, Clancy W: Anterior cruciate ligament insertions on the tibia and femur and their relationships to critical bony landmarks using high-resolution volume-rendering computed tomography. *Am J Sports Med* 36:2083–2090, 2008.
28. Siebold R, Dehler C, Ellert T: Prospective randomized comparison of double-bundle versus single-bundle anterior cruciate ligament reconstruction. *Arthroscopy* 24:137–145, 2008.
Zelle BA, Vidal AF, Brucker PU, et al: Double-bundle reconstruction of the anterior cruciate ligament: anatomic and biomechanical rationale. *J Am Acad Orthop Surg* 15:87–96, 2007.

The references for this chapter can also be found on www.expertconsult.com.

52

Anterior Cruciate Ligament Reconstruction via the Anteromedial Portal and Single-Tunnel, Double-Bundle Techniques

Benton E. Heyworth, Andrew Wall, Thomas J. Gill

ANTERIOR CRUCIATE LIGAMENT RECONSTRUCTION VIA THE ANTEROMEDIAL PORTAL

Use of the anteromedial portal (AMP) for establishment of the femoral tunnel in anterior cruciate ligament reconstruction (ACLR) surgery is an area of growing clinical and research interest. Femoral tunnel creation has traditionally been performed by placing instruments through the previously reamed tibial tunnel. Several studies* have suggested that use of the AMP eliminates the constraint in instrumentation positioning imposed by the transtibial (TT) technique, which can lead to the creation of a more vertical femoral tunnel or one with a nonanatomic aperture. The AMP is meant to allow for more anatomic, lower placement of the femoral tunnel and better re-creation of the native origins of the anteromedial (AM) and posterolateral (PL) bundles on the femoral condyle. The AM portal enables the surgeon to visualize and position the femoral tunnel independently of the tibial tunnel.[44] In addition, the AMP technique places the femoral tunnel more centrally in the anterior cruciate ligament (ACL) footprint.[16,49] However, some reports[3,21,32,34] have underscored the technical challenges and steep learning curve associated with application of the AMP technique. Complications that have been described include lateral femoral condyle back wall blowout, peri-ACL femoral fractures,[25,35] iatrogenic damage to the anterolateral cartilage of the medial femoral condyle (MFC), bending or breakage of the guide pin or beath pin, and difficulty with graft passage.

In addition, there are various difficulties associated with the AM portal technique, such as short femoral tunnels, graft length mismatch, inadequate femoral tunnel fixation, back wall blowout, neurovascular injuries, difficulties in visualization, and difficulties in determining socket depth.[32,44] Because the femoral tunnel angle is typically smaller, or less steep, than that used with the TT technique and because the tunnel is directed toward the lateral cortex rather than the anterior cortex of the distal femur, the length of the femoral tunnel is generally shorter. With the use of bone-patellar tendon-bone (BPTB) grafts, either autograft or allograft, shorter femoral tunnel length can cause the graft to be longer than the overall distance from the proximal extent of the femoral tunnel to the distal extent of the tibial tunnel on the anterior cortex of the tibia (ie, graft-length mismatch). Although this situation is rarely seen with the technique to be described, detailed preoperative planning can avoid this pitfall,[19] and several approaches can be used to address it when it occurs. Shortening of the bone plug lengths, seating the distal end of the femoral bone plug several millimeters deep to the aperture of the femoral tunnel, use of a free tibial bone block, and rotation of the tibial bone plug within the tibial tunnel are all acceptable, well-described techniques for addressing length issues and should be familiar to surgeons performing ACLR.[53,54]

When using soft tissue grafts, there are a number of options for femoral fixation. The growing popularity of the AMP technique and its shorter femoral tunnel has increased the demand for soft tissue fixation constructs with flexibility in length. For example, because the commonly used EndoButton CL (Smith & Nephew, Andover, Massachusetts) uses suspensory cortical fixation and the construct contains a continuous loop of suture (with a minimum length of 15 mm), shorter femoral tunnels may leave a relatively short or unsatisfactory amount of graft contained within the tunnel. Smith & Nephew has introduced a 10-mm suture loop length to help with shorter tunnel lengths. The newer EndoButton Direct (Smith & Nephew) device allows direct fixation of the graft onto the button, which maximizes the amount of graft in the femoral tunnel and may therefore be better suited for AMP techniques. The ACL Tightrope (Arthrex, Naples, Florida) is another suspensory fixation option for soft tissue grafts and allows the doubled-over end of the graft to be advanced to the most proximal aspect of the femoral tunnel. The Femoral Intrafix (DePuy Mitek, Raynham, Massachusetts) uses aperture fixation via a sheath and screw construct. Because it allows for separation of different portions of the graft, thereby replicating the two bundles,[17] the Femoral Intrafix represents the senior author's current implant of choice when using the AMP technique with soft tissue grafts. The AperFix femoral implant (Cayenne Medical, Scottsdale, Arizona) can also offer aperture fixation. However, AMP technique with this device requires a slightly larger portal because both the implant and all graft limbs must be passed through the portal and the smallest length of the implant is 29 mm, requiring a femoral tunnel length of at least 30 to 35 mm.

---

*References 3, 5, 7, 8, 10, 16, 20, 22, 42, and 49.

Here we describe our approach for creation of the AMP for ACLR with a BPTB graft and offer technical tips related to avoidance of common complications.

Technique

Creation of an appropriately located AMP is the most essential, primary step in ACLR surgery that uses the AMP technique (Fig. 52.1). Although some favor the use of an accessory AMP, we prefer instead to use a single AMP that is slightly more inferior to the standard portal in ACLR. The only exception to this approach is the need to perform a concomitant procedure that requires standard portal placement, such as meniscal repair, in which case two AMP portal incisions may be made. In this scenario the first portal is established 1 to 2 mm inferior to the inferomedial pole of the patella and the second, femoral tunnel–creating AMP is 1 to 2 mm superior to the superior rim of the tibial plateau. Arthroscopic visualization of AMP creation from a standard anterolateral portal (ALP) is advised to avoid damage to the anterior horn of the medial meniscus, given the relatively inferior position of the AMP. In addition, some surgeons have recommended a more medial position of the portal compared with the AMP placement typically used in ACLR. However, we have found that damage to the cartilage of the MFC can be a significant complication that is best avoided with AMP placement 2 to 3 mm medial to the medial edge of the patellar tendon.

Following standard diagnostic arthroscopy and débridement of the torn ACL, a notchplasty may be performed, but we have found this necessary only in the minority of cases with abnormally narrow notches, less than 15 mm in width. Given the relatively inferior position of graft placement on the femoral condyle, compared with traditional TT technique, graft impingement is rarely encountered. The posterior aspect of the soft tissue at the ACL footprint on the tibial surface is used as a landmark for tibial tunnel creation, in conjunction with the posterior aspect of the anterior horn of the lateral meniscus. We

prefer to completely débride the soft tissues and mark the center of the footprint with the electrocautery device or a small curette prior to insertion of a standard ACL guide. Following standard tibial tunnel reaming and use of the motorized shaver to eliminate bony debris, a reverse chamfer drill is used to smooth the posterior intra-articular edge of the tibial tunnel to prevent bony abrasion of the graft during cyclic knee flexion.

A similar approach as described for the tibial footprint is used to identify and mark the center of the femoral ACL footprint. The soft tissues are then completely débrided from the lateral wall of the intercondylar notch, while preserving the mark for the center of the footprint. An arthroscopic probe is used to identify the back wall of the femoral condyle definitively to avoid back wall blowout. The AMP is used to introduce the offset femoral guide and the guidewire as a unit past the MFC, just as Cain and Clancy[10] initially described introduction of the guidewire and reamer as a unit. The knee must be hyperflexed 110 to 120 degrees to allow the trajectory of the guidewire directly into the center of the femoral footprint. Alternatively, flexible guide pins and reamers have been introduced in an effort to avoid the need for hyperflexion, minimize articular cartilage damage on the MFC, and allow the length of the femoral tunnel to be maximized via a more proximally directed orientation. The guidewire is advanced to the level of the anterolateral femoral cortex and the offset guide is removed. A second guidewire is introduced through the AMP to the femoral footprint, just adjacent and parallel to the first, to allow for measurement of the approximate length from footprint to cortex to ensure adequate tunnel length. If insufficient tunnel length is anticipated, the angle of the guidewire can be altered to increase tunnel length or other techniques to address mismatch can be planned, such as slight shortening of one or both bone plugs, depending on the estimated length. The second guidewire is removed, and the reamer is then introduced into the notch under arthroscopic visualization, taking care to avoid damage to the MFC cartilage by the edges of the reamer.

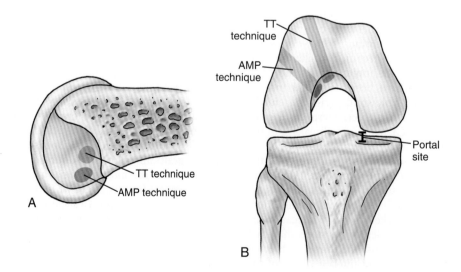

FIG 52.1 (A) In some knees, in which the anatomic footprint for the femoral tunnel cannot be reached using *TT technique*, or in certain revision cases, use of the *AMP* for guidewire and reamer advancement may allow for optimal tunnel position. (B) An anterior view of the knee demonstrates the angle of the femoral tunnel when the *AMP* is used to establish the tunnel, relative to the *TT technique*. *AMP,* Anteromedial portal; *TT,* transtibial.

Provided the angle of knee flexion is not changed and the trajectory of the guidewire is maintained, we have found the risk of damage to the cartilage or bending of the guidewire to be minimal. In addition, the 30-degree arthroscope may be replaced with a 70-degree arthroscope if adequate visualization of the femoral footprint cannot be achieved with instrumentation in the notch, although this is not necessary in most cases. The reamer is advanced 5 to 10 mm into the femoral ACL footprint and withdrawn slightly to allow for reassessment of the adequacy of the back wall, with a goal of 1 to 2 mm of intact posterior bone. The reamer is then advanced to the appropriate depth, which varies according to graft type and graft length. The guidewire-reamer unit is removed. A beath pin with a looped passing suture is introduced through the AMP into the notch, and the knee is again hyperflexed, with direct assessment of avoidance of contact between the beath pin and MFC before advancement into the femoral tunnel. The pin is passed through the skin of the anterolateral thigh. The loop of the passing suture is left in the notch, an arthroscopic grasper is introduced through the tibial tunnel, and the passing is suture brought out of the tibial tunnel.

Graft passage is performed in standard fashion, with free sutures on the femoral side of the graft having been fed through the looped passing suture. If a BPTB graft is used, an arthroscopic probe or grasper is used to orient the femoral bone block in the proper trajectory for smooth advancement into the femoral tunnel. Graft fixation is performed in standard fashion, with a femoral interference screw passed through the AMP over a nitinol wire. Care must be taken to advance the screw into the tunnel, with the knee in the same degree of hyperflexion that was used during femoral reaming. This avoids the complication of graft-screw divergence that has been reported for the AMP technique. Standard cycling of the graft and tibial interference screw fixation, with the knee in full extension and maximal manual traction on the graft, is then performed. A routine approach to wound closure is used.

Discussion

Use of the AMP in ACL reconstruction has the advantage of allowing for placement of a femoral tunnel in a more anatomic location than that seen with classic TT techniques. It can be particularly useful in revision surgery, in which the primary surgery may have involved placement of a more vertical femoral tunnel (eg, at 11:00 or 1:00 o'clock, if not higher). Not only can a vertical primary position be responsible for graft failure through re-tear or persistent rotational instability, but the more anatomic placement may be performed without significant primary graft or tunnel débridement, interference screw removal, or bone grafting. In addition, use of the AMP has gained interest because of the growing popularity in double-bundle surgery, in which a more complex tibial tunnel configuration may warrant great flexibility in femoral tunnel placement, as is afforded by the AMP technique.

Despite its advantages in revision or double-bundle procedures, use of the AMP may have its greatest role as a new standard technique in primary ACL reconstruction, given the increasingly recognized importance of femoral tunnel position on restoration of native knee kinematics.[17,55,59,60] In comparison with the TT procedure, the AM portal technique allows unconstrained femoral socket positioning.[44] It remains to be seen whether there is a significant difference in long-term degenerative joint changes and overall clinical outcome between AMP and TT techniques,[11,13] or whether the acute angle formed at the graft entrance to the femoral creates a "killer turn" that can lead to long-term graft damage. Despite the technical challenges associated with its use, complications can be avoided with a thorough understanding of the potential pitfalls and technical principles. Critical to success with AMP techniques are an understanding of native footprint anatomy, appropriate inferior AMP placement, introduction and advancement of instruments into the joint and notch under arthroscopic visualization, meticulous measurements of graft and tunnel length, and experience with appropriate flexion and hyperflexion angles of the knee for the different portions of the procedure. Although more clinical outcomes studies related to use of this technique are warranted, early, lower-level evidence, cadaveric studies, and descriptions of its technique have been favorable.[†]

The AMP has continued to grow in popularity, and we believe that it should become a technique familiar to all surgeons performing ACLR, especially in the revision setting. One approach favored by many surgeons for primary ACLR is creation of the tibial tunnel and assessment of potential femoral tunnel positioning through the TT tunnel. Because even minute variations in knee anatomy and tibial tunnel position can influence the ability to achieve anatomic placement of the femoral tunnel, this step allows for use of the AMP technique at this time if the TT approach does not allow for optimal graft placement. In the senior author's experience, an optimal femoral tunnel can often be achieved transtibially, and the TT approach can be used for the single-tunnel, single-bundle technique and the single-tunnel, double-bundle (STDB) technique, as will be described.

ANTERIOR CRUCIATE LIGAMENT RECONSTRUCTION VIA SINGLE-TUNNEL, DOUBLE-BUNDLE TECHNIQUE

Although a number of clinical outcomes studies have demonstrated good results using single-bundle ACLR,[2,38,46] several long-term studies have shown unsatisfactory rates of osteoarthritis and knee pain following this technique.[‡] Therefore double-bundle ACLR has gained increasing interest based on clinical and biomechanical evidence suggesting that reestablishment of the separate AM and PL bundles may more closely restore native knee joint stability, improved joint laxity, and kinematics.[§] However, double-bundle reconstruction techniques involving the creation of two tibial tunnels, and either one or two femoral tunnels, are more technically challenging, with longer operative times and more bone loss. This potentially increases complication rates and makes revision surgery more difficult. In addition, clinical and biomechanical studies have been performed that fail to demonstrate improved outcomes.[24,29,30,45,50]

Here we describe a technique of STDB ACLR that was developed in our laboratory. It takes advantage of the potential biomechanical advantage of separate AM and PL bundles while avoiding the technical challenges and pitfalls associated with the creation of two bony tunnels.

[†]References 5, 7, 18, 20, 28, 31, 32, and 52.
[‡]References 1, 23, 26, 39, 41, and 43.
[§]References 6, 12, 14, 15, 17, 29, 30, 33, 36, 37, 48, and 56-58.

Technique

Knee arthroscopy is performed through standard AM and ALPs to confirm the ACL tear, and the ACL remnant is débrided with a motorized shaver. A notchplasty is performed only if necessary. The lower extremity is then exsanguinated, and a thigh tourniquet is inflated to 280 mm Hg. The semitendinosus and gracilis tendons are harvested in standard fashion through a 2- to 3-cm incision in the skin overlying the pes anserinus insertion on the AM surface of the proximal tibia. The harvested grafts are pretensioned on a graft preparation board (DePuy Mitek), with 20 lb of force, while the tibial and femoral tunnels are prepared in standard fashion. If optimal anatomic positioning of the femoral tunnel cannot be achieved through a TT technique, an AMP technique is used to centralize the tunnel on the femoral ACL footprint, as described earlier.

Two different femoral fixation devices, with slightly different techniques, may be used to achieve an STDB soft tissue graft construct, depending on surgeon preference. The first STDB technique involves use of the Femoral Intrafix (DePuy Mitek) device. This has the dual advantage of aperture fixation using a femoral sheath and interference screw construct, while maximizing biologic healing, via compression of the graft against cancellous bone throughout the length of the tunnel. The semitendinosus and gracilis tendons are looped over a single strand of suture, and only the AM bundle is colored on the proximal end of the graft to identify the bundle easily. To achieve the desired anatomic position for the AM and PL bundles, a graft-positioning tool from the Intrafix set is used. The graft is placed in the fork of the positioning tool, with one bundle on either side of the fork. When the passing suture is used to pull the graft into the tunnel, the graft-positioning tool is advanced through the tibial tunnel until it reaches the aperture of the femoral tunnel, at which time the AM and PL bundles are rotated by rotating the positioning tool. When the desired positions of the

two bundles are achieved, the construct is then fully advanced into the femoral tunnel. The keel of a sheath trial is then placed between the strands to maintain the separation of the two bundles within the single tunnel. The femoral Intrafix sheath is then inserted into the tunnel, taking care not to alter the position of the two bundles. The graft is secured by the Intrafix screw into the sheath. Tibial tunnel fixation involves placement of the tibial Intrafix sheath with the AM and PL bundles placed in two opposite quadrants of the sheath at their anatomic insertion sites on the tibial plateau. A 40-N graft tension is applied to the graft while the tibial Intrafix screw is advanced with the leg in full extension.

An alternative STDB construct that may be used, provided that femoral tunnel length is adequate (>30 to 35 mm), is the AperFix (Cayenne Medical) femoral implant. In this technique the semitendinosus and gracilis tendons are passed through the device and looped to form four strands (Fig. 52.2B). Because the device allows for isolation of the separate tendons of the hamstrings, the two strands of the semitendinosus tendon are used to represent the AM bundle and the two gracilis tendon strands represent the PL bundle (Fig. 52.3A). The implant is passed through the tibial tunnel into the femoral tunnel. Before deployment, the two bundles are positioned inside the femoral tunnel in the native ACL bundle positions. The semitendinosus limbs of the graft construct are placed in a slightly deeper and higher position on the femoral condyle, with the knee in the flexed position, and the gracilis limbs of the graft construct are placed in an anteroinferior position on the femoral condyle. The implant is then deployed in standard fashion, with the deployment knob expanding the teeth of the implant into the femoral cancellous bone. With the graft now secured at the femoral end, the distal end of the graft is rotated by 90 degrees in a clockwise direction for the left knee (counterclockwise for the right knee), giving rise to the native anatomic relationship

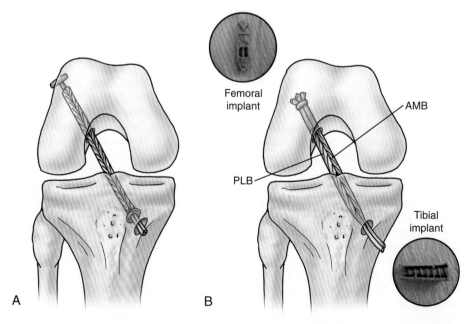

FIG 52.2 Schematic representation of single-bundle (A) and single-tunnel, double-bundle (B) anterior cruciate ligament reconstruction. *AMB,* Anteromedial bundle; *PLB,* posterolateral bundle. (From Gadikota HR, Seon JK, Kozanek M, et al: Biomechanical comparison of single-tunnel-double-bundle and single-bundle anterior cruciate ligament reconstructions. *Am J Sports Med* 37:962–969, 2009.)

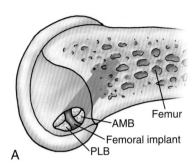
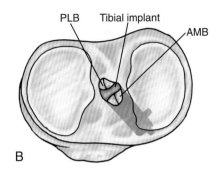

FIG 52.3 Schematic illustration of the femoral implant and separation of the two bundles in the femoral tunnel (A) and the tibial implant and separation of the two bundles in the tibial tunnel (B). *AMB,* Anteromedial bundle; *PLB,* posterolateral bundle. (From Gadikota HR, Seon JK, Kozanek M, et al: Biomechanical comparison of single-tunnel-double-bundle and single-bundle anterior cruciate ligament reconstructions. *Am J Sports Med* 37:962–969, 2009.)

of the AM and PL bundles as they pass into the tibial tunnel in the location of the ACL footprint (see Fig. 52.3B). This degree of rotation is based on the in vivo biomechanical study performed by Jordan et al.[27] that demonstrates approximately 80 degrees of ACL rotation as the knee flexes from 0 to 120 degrees. After cycling the knee five times, the graft is tensioned under maximal manual axial graft tension, with the knee in full extension, using the AperFix tensioning device. The graft is secured on the tibial side using the AperFix sheath and interference screw.

In either technique the skin incisions at the two portal sites are repaired using 4-0 monofilament sutures, and the incision at the tibial footprint is approximated at the deep dermal layer by 2-0 braided suture and then by a running subcuticular monofilament suture. The postoperative rehabilitation protocol involves 50% partial weight bearing with the use of crutches for the first 6 weeks. An unlocked hinged knee brace is used for weight bearing but removed for therapy, which includes the use of a continuous passive motion machine. Strength and stretching exercises are advanced according to standard post-ACL reconstruction principles.

Discussion

Although interest in double-bundle ACL reconstruction continues to grow, there is also increasing evidence that its purported advantages may not be replicated in clinical outcomes or patient satisfaction. Interestingly, a cadaveric study by Rue et al.[42] has demonstrated that a well-oriented, laterally angled tibial tunnel in single-bundle, single-tunnel surgery allows for re-creation of the femoral footprints of both the AM and PL bundles, bringing into question the need for double tunnels at all. A separate clinical study with 2-year follow-up[50] failed to show any difference in the functional outcomes of 2 cohorts of 19 patients undergoing single-bundle, single-tunnel versus double-tunnel, double-bundle reconstructions, respectively. A third clinical trial[29] showed improved rotatory laxity at 30 and 60 degrees flexion with double-bundle reconstruction but no difference in functional outcome after 2 years.

To date, few clinical studies have been published regarding the use of an STDB construct for ACL reconstruction. Caborn and Chang[9] have described their technique, in which a tibialis anterior allograft is folded over to replicate the AM and PL bundles, which are separated in single femoral and tibial tunnels and secured with interference screws. However, their technique

does not involve rotation of the graft limbs prior to tibial fixation, as described for our technique. Shino et al.[47] have described several alterations in the reaming for and positioning of a BPTB autograft, which therefore causes different portions of the graft to mimic the two bundles of the native ACL, but the authors do not support this interpretation with biomechanical or clinical data. Takeuchi et al.[51] have reported on a technique involving a bone-hamstring-bone composite graft, in which a bone block is removed from the tibia at the pes insertion, divided in two, and sutured to the ends of a standard hamstring autograft. This composite graft allows for separation of the limbs of the semitendinosus and gracilis autograft, similar to our technique. They reported ultimate fixation strength in their composite graft superior to that of a standard BPTB autograft.

Two biomechanical cadaveric studies from our institution have investigated the AperFix and Intrafix STDB techniques described earlier. In 2009 Gadikota et al.[15] showed that the STDB approach with the AperFix reduces anterior tibial translation at all flexion angles, compared with the ACL-deficient state. Interestingly, when compared with ACL-intact specimens, knees with STDB reconstructions showed comparable anterior tibial translation at low flexion angles but decreased translation at 60 and 90 degrees, suggesting slight overconstraint. However, the maximum difference was less than 3 mm in all cases. A second 2010 study investigating femoral interference screw fixation with soft tissue grafts demonstrated that the STDB technique restores anterior knee stability better when compared with a conventional single-bundle reconstruction.[17] The advantage of both techniques is that they represent technically simple methods of re-creating double-bundle anatomy without introducing many of the technical challenges and risk of complications inherent in the technique. A case study in 2015 by Heng et al. concluded that greater stress concentrations from the presence of multiple femoral tunnels and multiple cortical violations may increase the chances of peri-ACL femur fracture.[21] Back wall blowout may happen because, during extreme knee flexion, the socket will be parallel to the back wall of the intercondylar notch.[4,40,44]

KEY REFERENCES

5. Bedi A, Altchek DW: The "footprint" anterior cruciate ligament technique: an anatomic approach to anterior cruciate ligament reconstruction. *Arthroscopy* 25:1128–1138, 2009.

15. Gadikota HR, Seon JK, Kozanek M, et al: Biomechanical comparison of single-tunnel-double-bundle and single-bundle anterior cruciate ligament reconstructions. *Am J Sports Med* 37:962–969, 2009.

17. Gadikota HR, Wu JL, Seon JK, et al: Single-tunnel double-bundle anterior cruciate ligament reconstruction with anatomical placement of hamstring tendon graft: can it restore normal knee joint kinematics? *Am J Sports Med* 38:713–720, 2010.

18. Gavriilidis I, Motsis EK, Pakos EE, et al: Transtibial versus anteromedial portal of the femoral tunnel in ACL reconstruction: a cadaveric study. *Knee* 15:364–367, 2008.

20. Harner CD, Honkamp NJ, Ranawat AS: Anteromedial portal technique for creating the anterior cruciate ligament femoral tunnel. *Arthroscopy* 24:113–115, 2008.

32. Lubowitz JH: Anteromedial portal technique for the anterior cruciate ligament femoral socket: pitfalls and solutions. *Arthroscopy* 25:95–101, 2009.

42. Rue JP, Ghodadra N, Bach BR, Jr: Femoral tunnel placement in single-bundle anterior cruciate ligament reconstruction: a cadaveric study relating transtibial lateralized femoral tunnel position to the anteromedial and posterolateral bundle femoral origins of the anterior cruciate ligament. *Am J Sports Med* 36:73–79, 2008.

59. Zantop T, Diermann N, Schumacher T, et al: Anatomical and nonanatomical double-bundle anterior cruciate ligament reconstruction: importance of femoral tunnel location on knee kinematics. *Am J Sports Med* 36:678–685, 2008.

60. Zantop T, Herbort M, Raschke MJ, et al: The role of the anteromedial and posterolateral bundles of the anterior cruciate ligament in anterior tibial translation and internal rotation. *Am J Sports Med* 35:223–227, 2007.

The references for this chapter can also be found on www.expertconsult.com.

53

Complications of Anterior Cruciate Ligament Reconstruction

Brian E. Walczak, Samuel R.H. Steiner, Jason D. Archibald, Geoffrey S. Baer

Rupture of the anterior cruciate ligament (ACL) is one of the most common ligament injuries to the knee. More than 100,000 ACL reconstructions are performed each year in the United States. The goal of these procedures is to re-create a stable and functional knee joint that allows return to the level of activity prior to injury. Current arthroscopic techniques have success rates reported between 75% and 95%. However, as many as 5% to 10% of ACL reconstructions are revisions.[25] As with all surgical procedures there are inherent risks to the reconstruction of the ACL. Complications from ACL reconstruction can be viewed as intraoperative or postoperative. Intraoperative complications include malpositioned tunnels, improper tensioning, and failure of graft fixation. Postoperative failures include infection, arthrofibrosis, graft failure, and osteoarthritis (OA). The choice of graft also precludes an inherent set of complications, whether it is autologous bone-patellar tendon-bone (BPTB), autologous hamstring, or allograft.

INTRAOPERATIVE COMPLICATIONS

Tunnel Placement

Intraoperative complications often result from technical errors. Technical shortcomings are the cause of 60% to 77% of all ACL revision cases. These errors include nonanatomic tunnel placement, graft impingement, improper tensioning, and inadequate graft fixation. Proper positioning of the femoral and tibial tunnels is essential to successful reconstruction of the ACL. Among these intraoperative complications, improper femoral tunnel placement is the most common. In a report from the Multicenter ACL Revision Study (MARS) Group, 48% of revision cases were attributed to femoral tunnel malposition. It was the only cause of failure in one-quarter of all revisions,[65] specifically an anteriorly located femoral tunnel,[45] which leads to excessive strain during flexion and restricted range of motion. A femoral tunnel that is too vertically oriented (the 12 o'clock position) may control anteroposterior forces on the knee joint but will lack the rotational control of the native ACL.[74] A femoral tunnel located too posteriorly in the notch risks blowing out the posterior wall of the tunnel, which may compromise fixation of the graft. If this occurs, one may move from interference to suspensory fixation, or another option is to redrill the femoral tunnel using an outside-in technique. Jepsen et al.[43] randomized 60 patients undergoing ACL reconstruction to low or high femoral tunnel positions and found no difference in laxity at 25 and 70 degrees, but a significant increase was found in subjective knee stability in the group with low (2 o'clock

position) femoral tunnels. While drilling the femoral tunnel, one should attempt to recreate the anatomic attachment of the native ACL, whether it is through a transtibial, anteromedial, or retrodrill technique.[1]

The tibial tunnel is more forgiving than the femoral tunnel, but malpositioning can also lead to complications. The tunnel should be located just posterior to Blumensaat line when viewed on a lateral x-ray. When the tibial tunnel is drilled too anterior of the native footprint, the graft will impinge and likely fail. When too posterior, the graft becomes too vertical and loses rotational stability in the same fashion as the anteriorly drilled femoral tunnel.[57] Inderhaug et al. defined posterior drilled tunnels as being at or behind 50% of the anteroposterior diameter or the Amis and Jakob line (AJL) of the tibia. They found that posterior tibial tunnels had a significantly higher frequency of rotational instability and a worse subjective outcome compared with anteriorly placed tunnels.[39] Medial or lateral malpositioning of the tibial tunnel can lead to impingement, increased laxity, or chronic synovitis.[57,66] Studies have looked at the effects tibial reaming has on meniscal root attachments. LaPrade et al. examined the association of anterior meniscal injury during tibial reaming. The authors found a significant mean decrease in the attachment area and ultimate strength of the anterior lateral meniscus root after tibial reaming.[52] Avulsion of the anterior medial meniscus root has also been reported highlighting the importance of placing the tibial guide and reaming the tibia in the center of the ACL tibial footprint.[51]

Some complications regarding tunnel placement are inherent to the technique used for reconstruction. During ACL reconstructions using a double-bundle technique, one must avoid convergence of the two tunnels in the femur and tibia. This can be accomplished by measuring the footprint to ensure appropriate size, careful pin placement, avoiding tunnels greater than 9 mm in diameter, and potentially drilling tunnels using an outside-in technique. Several systems have been developed to help to prevent tunnel convergence. An anteromedial portal may be used to drill the femoral tunnels. Anteromedial drilling allows anatomic placement of the femoral tunnels that is independent of the tibial tunnels. If an anteromedial portal is used, care must be taken to avoid damage to the medial femoral condyle because the guide pin or reamer passes closely by the articular surface. We recommend careful visualization during creation of the anteromedial portal and the use of half-fluted reamers to help to avoid cartilage damage (Fig. 53.1). In addition, an anteromedial drilling technique may lead to shorter femoral tunnels than typically encountered with a transtibial

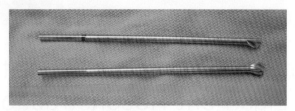

FIG 53.1 Half-fluted reamers may be used during femoral tunnel drilling from an anteromedial portal technique to prevent damage to the articular cartilage during drilling.

technique. Fixation strategies should be adjusted to ensure an adequate amount of graft within the femoral tunnel to allow graft integration.

Impingement of the graft is often caused by nonanatomic tunnel placement but can also result from oversized grafts and inadequate notchplasty. Impinging ACL grafts will deform with strain and will likely become lax or fail.[30] Abrasion of the graft on the lateral femoral condyle or intercondylar roof can cause chronic synovitis, ligament attenuation, and failure.[90] However, aggressive notchplasty may damage articular cartilage. A dog model demonstrated histopathologic changes at 6 months, similar to those of early degenerative arthritis in groups undergoing aggressive notchplasty.[53] Others have noted that although notchplasty may assist in visualization during arthroscopy, there does not appear to be a clinical difference in patients who did or did not receive a notchplasty during their ACL reconstruction.[71] Minimizing the notchplasty may reduce postoperative pain, bleeding, swelling, and potential notch regrowth.[26,73]

Patient factors may be a consideration when attempting to avoid surgical complications. Matsubara et al. found that single-bundle ACL reconstruction with the graft placed at the center of the footprint may reduce the risk of intercondylar roof impingement in hyperextensible knees and recommended cautiously considering the possibility of impingement in these patients after double-bundle ACL reconstruction.[61]

Graft Tension

Another complication of ACL reconstructions arises from improper tensioning of the graft. Inadequate tensioning creates a loose graft that will not re-create joint stability and kinematics. Overtensioning of the graft can lead to loss of motion, graft stretching, excessive stress on the articular cartilage, poor vascularity, and subsequent graft degeneration.[40,101] Failure to precondition a graft cyclically can decrease forces within the graft by 30% soon after fixation.[35] A review of the randomized controlled trials evaluating graft tension in ACL reconstructions using BPTB autograft and hamstring autografts found no statistically or clinically relevant differences in various graft tensions.[6] The amount of tension that should be applied to optimize outcome is unknown at this time.

Graft Contamination

Graft contamination caused by the graft being dropped onto the floor of the operating room is a rare but dangerous intraoperative complication, which can lead to early septic arthritis. Cooper et al.[20] investigated the incidence of positive cultures in dropped grafts in an operating room environment. Six of 10 grafts (60%) that were dropped on the floor for 3 minutes had a positive culture at 10 days. Three of 10 grafts (30%) that were dropped on the floor for 3 minutes and then soaked in sterile

saline containing bacitracin and polymyxin B for 15 minutes also had positive cultures at 10 days. Similarly, Molina et al.[64] harvested native ACLs during total knee arthroplasties, dropped them onto the operating room floor for 15 seconds and then cultured them. In this study, 29 of 50 specimens (58%) were found to have positive cultures. Grafts soaked in solutions exhibited drops in the positive culture rate: 12 of 50 (24%) in the povidone-iodine solution group, 3 of 50 (6%) in the antibiotic solution group, and 1 of 50 (2%, in broth only) in the chlorhexidine gluconate group. Although data regarding dropped grafts are limited, a survey of surgeons found that many recommend cleansing the graft and proceeding with the ACL reconstruction rather than harvesting a different autograft or switching to allograft.[40] A combination of chlorhexidine gluconate and triple antibiotic solution in sterile saline appears to be the most effective for preventing positive cultures.[34] The most effective way to prevent graft contamination caused by a dropped graft is clearly prevention. We recommend minimizing hand-offs during the reconstruction, clear communication between staff when the graft is being moved, and clamping the graft on the field.

Graft Fixation and Maturation

Until a graft has incorporated into the host bone tunnels, it is dependent on adequate fixation strength for stability. Current rehabilitation protocols emphasize early range of motion and strengthening, underscoring the need for stable fixation. One study has found no difference in clinical outcome among interference screws, whether they were metallic, titanium, or bioabsorbable.[26] Furthermore, good results have been found with soft tissue grafts when using EndoButton, femoral transfix, soft tissue screws, or a tibial-sided screw and washer. However, adjustable loop femoral suspension devices have been shown to lengthen under cyclic loads in the laboratory setting and reach clinical failure.[12] This lengthening is believed to be because of suture slippage into the adjustable-length loop.

BPTB grafts begin to incorporate between 6 and 12 weeks. At 16 to 24 weeks a normal bone-ligament junction forms. However, caution must be exercised in patients with low bone mineral density because interference screw fixation has low stiffness in osteopenic cancellous bone. This may necessitate switching to fixation based on cortical rather than cancellous bone. Cortical bone may also be used as backup fixation (eg, tie sutures around a screw and washer or a staple).

A graft goes through morphologic changes over time and becomes similar to a native ACL, a process termed *ligamentization*. This process consists of several steps, including necrosis (0 to 4 weeks), revascularization and cellular proliferation (4 to 12 weeks), and remodeling (3 to 6 months).[80] Arthroscopically collected samples of patellar tendon and hamstring ACL grafts taken at 6 and 12 months after ACL reconstruction have demonstrated the amount of collagen cross-linking in the ACL graft returns to the level of native ACLs within 1 year of reconstruction.[60] Ligamentization takes a longer period of time in allografts and hamstring autografts. Animal studies have shown a delay of revascularization and proliferation in allograft compared with autograft at 6 and 12 weeks of healing, whereas at 52 weeks the differences are less distinct.[34,79] Although labeled as ligamentization, the incorporated graft does not have the same physical properties of the native ACL. The collagen fibers of the graft are uniform in length and diameter, unlike the various fibers of the native ACL, which are able to distribute loads throughout the range of motion. Furthermore, there are different proportions of glycosaminoglycans and collagen-reducible cross-links. These can contribute to biologic failure of the graft.[30] The processes of graft incorporation and ligamentization should be taken into account when determining advances in rehabilitation, as well as return to sporting activities, to prevent an early failure of the graft.

POSTOPERATIVE COMPLICATIONS

Infection

Infection is a rare but devastating complication following ACL reconstruction. It can lead to the loss of articular cartilage and increase the risk of arthrofibrosis. Postoperative infections are typically classified as acute (<2 weeks), subacute (between 2 weeks and 2 months), or late (>2 months), with the majority occurring in the acute or subacute periods.[83] After being identified, infection should be treated with prompt arthroscopic irrigation and débridement. Broad-spectrum antibiotics should be initiated until a more culture-specific regimen can be identified. If still functional, the graft can often be maintained. Risk factors for infection include previous arthroscopic or open knee surgery, diabetes,[14] concomitant procedures,[46,88] and potentially being a professional athlete.[88] In a retrospective review of 3126 ACL reconstructions, Barker et al.[11] have identified 18 infections (0.58%). Infections occurred in 6 of 1349 allografts (0.44%), 7 of 1430 BPTB autografts (0.49%), and 5 of 347 hamstring autografts (1.44%). The most common organism was *Staphylococcus aureus*. The increased rate of infection in hamstring grafts was statistically significant. A higher risk of infection or need for graft removal was not seen with allografts. Another review in China demonstrated a similar rate of infection (0.52%) among 4068 patients over a 10-year period. Of these 21 infections 20 were autologous hamstring grafts and 1 was a patellar tendon allograft.[98] Katz et al.[48] have reviewed 801 reconstructions and found an infection rate of 0.75% (six patients). Their analysis showed that autograft (2 of 170) had twice the risk of infection compared with allograft (4 of 628), but this difference was not statistically significant ($p = 0.77$). In a series by Judd et al. all 11 of their infections were with hamstring autografts (193 patients), whereas no infections occurred with patellar tendon autografts (217 patients).[46] It is hypothesized if this is because of prominent hardware because surgeons in the study used a post and washer or if it is because of foreign body burden from suture placed in the hamstring autograft. In a review of 17 infections out of 2198 patients (0.8%) from the Multicenter Orthopaedic Outcomes Network (MOON) knee group, bone-tendon-bone autografts are associated with a lower risk of infection compared with other graft options.[14]

Follow-up of postoperative septic arthritis has shown equivocal objective and subjective results at approximately the 5-year period,[13] whereas other longer-term studies have shown diminished subjective, functional, and radiographic outcomes.[81]

Stiffness

Loss of motion is the most common complication after ACL reconstruction, occurring in 4% to 35% of cases.[29] The causes are often multifactorial, and the aforementioned complications can all contribute to joint stiffness. Other factors include prolonged immobilization, poor patient compliance, intercondylar notch scarring, capsulitis, cyclops lesion, and reflex sympathetic dystrophy.[17] Harner et al.[37] have retrospectively reviewed 244

ACL reconstructions for postoperative stiffness and found an incidence of 11.1%. Factors associated with loss of motion included acute reconstruction less than 1 month from injury, male gender, and concomitant medial collateral ligament (MCL) repair. Shelbourne et al.'s retrospective review[85] of 169 ACL reconstructions found that acute reconstructions are not associated with increased risk of arthrofibrosis (4%) when an accelerated postoperative rehabilitation program is followed. Loss of both extension and flexion is more common, with loss of extension thought to be more detrimental to function. A knee flexion contracture greater than 10 degrees prevents a normal gait and increases loads across the patellar femoral joint. Loss of flexion past 125 degrees interferes with activities of daily living, including sitting, stair climbing, and running. Historically, ACL reconstructions were initially immobilized, and motion was slowly advanced. This led to increased rates of arthrofibrosis. Current physical therapy protocols have emphasized early range of motion, which has decreased rates of stiffness without adversely affecting clinical outcomes.

Treatment of arthrofibrosis includes physical therapy and dynamic braces. A manipulation under anesthesia may aid in the recovery of motion, especially when performed within the first 6 weeks of the postoperative course. Arthroscopic lysis of adhesions or resection of a cyclops lesion may be necessary. Loss of motion resulting from technical errors (eg, misplaced tunnels) during the initial surgery may require revision ACL reconstruction. Administration of a tapered course of oral steroids in the early postoperative period for patients with decreased range of motion has also been described as a method to improve flexion by reducing inflammation and intra-articular scar formation.[75]

Extensor mechanism dysfunction is uncommon after ACL reconstruction but can play a role in the development of arthrofibrosis. Early postoperative rehabilitative protocols emphasize quadriceps strengthening. Deficits in quadriceps strength can often be found in up to 20% of patients at 6 months post ACL reconstruction.[72] Although the magnitude and incidence of quadriceps weakness decrease with time, its role in maintaining knee joint stability underscores the importance of early aggressive strengthening of this muscle group.

Graft Failure

Biologic graft failure may occur in the early postoperative course (first 6 months) before full incorporation and ligamentization. As noted, this is usually a result of an intraoperative technical error. Other causes of early graft failure include premature return to sports, infection, and graft insufficiency. Late graft failures occur in 5% to 10% of individuals who have returned to their preinjury level of activity.[36,44] Spindler et al.[89] have reviewed nine randomized controlled trials comparing patellar tendon and hamstring autografts. There was no significant difference in failure between the two choices of graft with an overall incidence of 3.6% and a minimum of 2 years of follow-up. Salmon et al.[77] followed 760 ACL reconstructions over a 5-year period. They reported a 6% risk of ACL graft rupture, as well as a 6% risk of contralateral native ACL injury, which was not affected by choice of patellar tendon or hamstring autograft.[50] Similarly, Wright et al.[101] have reported on data collected in the MOON cohort study. In their report 235 patients who underwent ACL reconstructions were followed up for 2 years. There were 14 ACL injuries, 7 in the contralateral knee (3%) and 7 in the reconstructed knee (3%). Although females are two to eight times more likely to tear their native ACL than their male counterparts, there does not appear to be any differences in failure rates of ACL reconstructions between males and females.[77] Data have suggested that allograft reconstructions may suffer from a higher failure rate compared with autograft.[38]

Arthritis

OA is a common postoperative disease complicating ACL reconstructions. Although the development of OA is known to be associated with ACL injury, clinical research continues to attempt to determine whether this is primarily related to the initial injury, associated damage to adjacent structures (eg, meniscus, cartilage, subchondral bone), surgical treatment, or continued participation in sport; this is an important area of clinical research.[5,10,58,67] What is more difficult to define is whether ACL reconstruction actually protects against the development of OA.

The risk of OA has been reported to be 50% after an ACL injury and as high as 70% when associated with a meniscal injury.[32] Keays et al.[49] followed 56 ACL reconstructions for 6 years after surgery and noted that meniscectomy and chondral damage are associated with a higher risk of tibiofemoral and patellofemoral arthritis. Øiestad et al.[70] have reviewed 7 prospective and 24 retrospective studies on the development of knee OA following ACL reconstruction. At 10 years follow-up, the prevalence of radiographic OA in isolated ACL injuries was 0% to 13% and higher with combined injuries (21% to 48%). They concluded that previous data overestimated the prevalence of OA after ACL reconstruction. No differences were seen in patients who were treated nonoperatively versus those who underwent ACL reconstruction, regardless of graft selection. Similarly Barenius et al. examined the risk of OA at 14-year follow-up.[10] In this randomized controlled trial comparing the risk of degenerative disease in patients who underwent ACL reconstruction using patellar tendon autograft and quadrupled hamstring autograft, the authors found no difference in the prevalence of OA between groups. However, they found a threefold increase in the prevalence of OA after ACL injury treated with reconstruction compared with the contralateral knee most frequently involving the medial compartment (57% vs. 18%, respectively). Initial meniscus resection was a strong risk factor for progression.

Murray et al. reviewed both the clinical and radiographic results of 114 patients who underwent bone-patella-bone autograft reconstruction.[67] At 13-year follow-up, the authors found worse subjective International Knee Documentation Subjective Knee Form (IKDC) outcome scores with associated chondral injury, previous surgery, return to sport, and worse radiologic grades in the ipsilateral medial compartment. Poor radiologic grades were principally associated with chondral and meniscal injury identified at the time of ACL reconstruction. Their results indicate that injuries to the cartilage and meniscus may be the main predictors of degenerative bone disease long-term.

More recently, Ajuied et al. published a meta-analysis reporting on the development and progression of OA after ACL injury.[5] Included studies had a minimum of 10-year follow-up. ACL injury was associated with a relative risk of 3.89 and 3.84 for the development of minimal and moderate-severe OA, respectively. Moreover, ACL-reconstructed knees were associated with almost a 1.5-fold decrease in the development of any grade of OA (relative risk 4.98 vs. 3.62). However, patients who underwent ACL reconstruction had more severe OA that the authors suggested may be influenced by return to sport.

GRAFT-SPECIFIC COMPLICATIONS

The choice of ACL graft carries an inherent set of complications, whether the surgeon uses patellar tendon autograft, hamstring autograft, or allograft.

Bone-Patellar Tendon-Bone Autograft

The BPTB autograft is considered the gold standard and is often the graft of choice in high-demand athletes. It is thought that the bone plug to bone tunnel healing occurs more quickly than soft tissue grafts.[40] Anterior knee pain is the most frequently noted complication associated with patellar tendon autograft. Sachs et al.[76] studied 126 patients who had undergone BPTB autograft ACL reconstructions and found patellofemoral pain in 19% of patients, which correlated positively with a flexion contracture. Aglietti et al.[3] reviewed their series of 226 patellar tendon ACL reconstructions and reported a 5% incidence of painful patellofemoral crepitus with pain and 20% with crepitus and no pain. In a review of nine randomized trials Spindler found a range of anterior knee pain between 13% and 43%, with no significant differences between hamstring and BPTB autografts.[89] However, all four studies that evaluated kneeling pain found significantly more pain in the patellar tendon groups (36% to 67% of patients).

Graft tunnel mismatch is an intraoperative complication that may occur when the BPTB graft is too long and less than 20 mm of the bone plug remains within the tibial tunnel, preventing effective use of interference screw fixation. This is more likely to occur when the patellar tendon is more than 50 mm.[84] Strategies to remedy this problem include recession of the graft further into the femoral tunnel, insertion of a bone plug into the tibial tunnel, and fixation at the tibia with a post and screw. Furthermore, the graft may be rotated to decrease the amount of mismatch. Rotation of 540 degrees will decrease length by 10%[97] and 630 degrees by 25%,[7] without any statistical difference in ultimate failure strength (Fig. 53.2). Furthermore, Barber[9] reported on 50 patients who underwent flipping of the bone plug 180 degrees onto the tendon to shorten the length of tendon between bone plugs. No significant complications were found at a mean follow-up of 28 months.

Patellar fractures following patellar tendon harvest are rare but have been reported in the literature. Tay et al.[93] have reviewed five case reports and eight series reports and found an incidence rate of 0.55%. These fractures may be direct, the intraoperative result of a technical error during the harvest, or indirect, occurring on average 11 weeks after the ACL reconstruction. They are usually stellate or transverse shaped. Many authors recommend primary bone grafting of the harvest sites intraoperatively to reduce the risk of fracture.[20] Lee et al.[54] have reviewed 1725 consecutive patients who underwent primary ACL reconstruction using a BPTB autograft and reported three complications related to harvest of the patellar tendon graft—one intraoperative fracture, one postoperative fracture, and one patellar tendon rupture. With a 0.2% acute complication rate, they concluded that the patellar tendon is a safe and viable choice of graft for ACL reconstruction.

The shape of the patellar tendon bone plugs affects the risk of fracture. Using a porcine model, Moholkar et al.[63] showed that the shape of the bone plug affects the risk of fracture. The

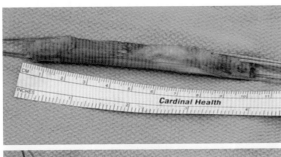

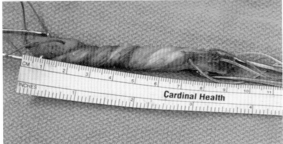

FIG 53.2 Graft tunnel mismatch can be a concern in patients with patella alta or a long patellar tendon. Twisting of the graft by 540 degrees can shorten the graft by 10% without weakening the reconstruction. (A) Patellar tendon graft prior to twisting. (B) Patellar tendon graft twisted 540 degrees, shortening the graft by over 1 cm to help correct for graft tunnel mismatch.

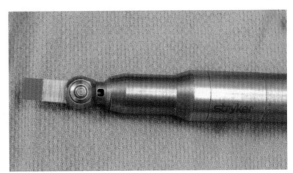

FIG 53.3 A Steri-Strip may be used to mark the saw blade at 1 cm to prevent overpenetration of the blade, reducing the risk for patellar fracture or cartilage damage.

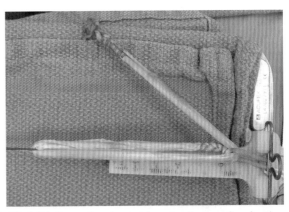

FIG 53.4 Tripling of a hamstring tendon graft of adequate length allows the creation of a graft with greater caliber than simply doubling over each graft. In this case, by tripling the semitendinosus tendon and doubling the gracilis tendon, the graft size was increased from 6.5 to 8.5 mm.

impact energy required to create a 1% probability of complete fracture was 7 J for a sharp-cornered defect, 17 J for a trapezoidal plug, 22 J for a sharp-cornered defect with a drill hole at the corner, 40 J for a round-cornered defect, and 49 J for a normal patella. They concluded that the use of a round-cornered patellar defect would reduce the risk of patellar fracture intraoperatively and postoperatively. DuMontier et al.[21] used a cadaveric model to demonstrate that the mean ultimate tensile strength of the patellar tendon after harvesting is not altered (2500 to 3000 N) whether the defect left in the patellar is circular, rectangular, or triangular. To avoid patellar fractures, it is recommended to avoid the primary use of osteotomes during harvest of the tendon. The graft should be located in the central portion of the patellar tendon. The bone plugs should be 25 mm or less in length and 10 mm or less in width. Two-thirds of the patellar depth should be preserved, and the bone plugs should be cut in a triangular or trapezoidal shape with the saw. Cross-hatching at the corners should be avoided. We use an oscillating saw with a Steri-Strip around the blade to mark 1 cm of depth and fill in the patellar defect with autologous bone graft in an attempt to reduce fracture risk and anterior knee pain (Fig. 53.3).

Hamstring Autograft

Hamstring autograft reconstructions have become more prevalent in the past decade. Initial concerns of inadequate strength of single- or double-stranded grafts have been addressed with the use of four-stranded semitendinosus and gracilis autografts. Current literature reveals few clinical differences in range of motion, isokinetic strength, laxity, or long-term results between hamstring and BPTB autografts.[89] A common complication seen in hamstring ACL reconstructions is intraoperative premature amputation of the gracilis or semitendinosus tendons, usually caused by an incomplete release of the tendon from the fascial bands. Solman and Pagnani[87] have documented up to

five accessory bands or insertions of the semitendinosus alone that must be mobilized prior to harvest. There is a consistent band to the medial head of the gastrocnemius approximately 5.5 cm proximal to the pes anserinus. Tuncay et al.[95] have studied the anatomy of the fascial band between the semitendinosus and gastrocnemius in 23 cadaveric knees. The mean width of the band was 2.6 cm, and the mean distance from the semitendinosus insertion to the fascial band was 7 cm. The size of the harvested hamstring tendons can be difficult to predict. If there is insufficient hamstring length, the surgeon may need to select an alternate graft. When the tendons have a small caliber but a long length, the grafts may be tripled to provide a graft of greater caliber (Fig. 53.4).

Another complication associated with hamstring tendon harvesting for ACL reconstruction is injury to the saphenous nerve, which is located between layers I and II and is at risk for injury when the tendon stripper is moved proximally. Sanders et al.[78] have reviewed the results of 164 patients who had undergone ACL reconstruction using hamstring autograft over a 4-year period. Of the patients surveyed, 74% reported postoperative sensory disturbance. Injury to the sartorial branch of the saphenous nerve (SBSN) and infrapatellar branch of the saphenous nerve (IPBSN) occurred in 32%, and isolated injury to the SBSN occurred in 23% and to the IPBSN in 19%. This was followed by an examination of the saphenous nerve anatomy in 11 cadavers. They found that the saphenous nerve is intimately associated with the gracilis over a span of 4.6 cm, between 7.2 and 11.8 cm proximal to its insertion. Placing the knee in a figure four position or knee flexion to 90 degrees will relax the saphenous nerve as it passes over the medial hamstrings and may reduce the risk of injury to the saphenous nerve.[71]

Another complication of hamstring tendon harvest for ACL reconstruction is hamstring weakness. Initial studies by Lipscomb et al.[56] demonstrated the mean strength of the hamstrings to be 99% of the contralateral leg after hamstring ACL reconstruction, a finding confirmed by others.[4,18] Later data raised questions regarding hamstring function after harvesting. Nakajima et al.[68] found decreased hamstring strength in deep flexion after ACL reconstruction. More recently, Tashiro et al.[92] randomly assigned 90 patients to gracilis and semitendinosus or semitendinosus alone ACL reconstructions. They found significant decreases in hamstring muscle strength at 70 degrees or more of flexion in both groups but less so in the semitendinosus only group. Similarly Gobbi et al.[33] prospectively followed a group of 97 patients who were also randomized to gracilis and semitendinosus hamstring or semitendinosus alone. They found no differences in clinical results and flexion and extension strength but found a significant deficit in internal rotation. It has been suggested by Adachi et al.[2] that although peak flexion torque and total work are not significantly altered by hamstring harvesting, the more hamstring tendons are harvested, the more peak torque angle is shifted to a shallower angle, which may explain weakness in deep flexion. Regrowth of the harvested hamstring tendons has been observed,[31] and magnetic resonance imaging (MRI) studies have correlated the extent of tendon regrowth with the amount of strength regained after hamstring harvest for ACL reconstruction.[91]

Both femoral and tibial tunnels widen in hamstring ACL reconstructions postoperatively.[55,69,82,100] Clatworthy et al.[19] have evaluated the incidence and degree of tunnel widening in a prospective series of 73 patients receiving a hamstring or patellar tendon autograft. Tunnel widening was evaluated with anteroposterior and lateral radiographs after validation with MRI. At a minimum 1-year follow-up the tunnel area for hamstring grafts was increased 100.4% in the femur and 73.9% in the tibia, whereas the tunnel area for BPTB grafts decreased 25% in the femur and 2.1% in the tibia. Despite these observations, no clinical significance has been correlated with tunnel widening in long-term studies. However, tunnel widening may pose a difficult problem in revision ACL reconstruction, requiring a two-stage reconstruction initially to treat the bone defects prior to proceeding with ACL reconstruction (Fig. 53.5).

Allograft Tissue

Allograft tissue has been advocated as an alternative to autograft tendons in ACL reconstructions secondary to shortened surgical times, less postoperative pain, and lack of donor site morbidity.[8,38] Complications associated with allograft ACL reconstructions include disease transmission and slower incorporation of the graft.

Viral transmission of human immunodeficiency virus (HIV) and hepatitis are among the most concerning diseases that may be transmitted through allograft use. Since a blood test for HIV has been available, there has been one transmission of HIV in 1985 through the surgical use of allograft tissue.[94] Since then, more than several million grafts have been implanted in the

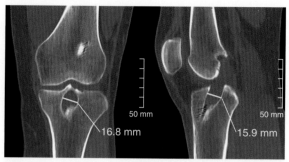

FIG 53.5 Tunnel dilation can pose a significant problem when approaching revision ACL reconstruction. In this case a two-stage reconstruction was undertaken to allow treatment of the significant bone defects prior to revision of the ACL reconstruction.

United States without a documented transmission of HIV.[86] With current serologic tests to screen donors and tissue processing and storage, the estimated risk of HIV transmission with connective tissue allografts is 1:8,000,00.[7] Two cases of hepatitis C transmission were reported in 1991, one of which occurred before a specific blood test for hepatitis C was available. A third case of hepatitis C transmission was reported by the Centers for Disease Control and Prevention (CDC) in 2002 in a patient receiving a patellar tendon allograft.[96] Freeze-dried grafts appear to have lower risk of viral transmission than fresh-frozen or frozen allograft tissue; however, freeze drying, ethylene oxide sterilization, and irradiation higher than 2.5 Mrad have been shown to decrease the biomechanical properties of the allograft.[40,62]

Bacterial infection is another complication that may occur following allograft ACL reconstruction. In 2002 the CDC reported on 26 cases of allograft-associated bacterial infections. Of these, 14 grafts had been processed by a single facility and 18 of the infections followed anterior cruciate reconstruction.[96] Between 1998 and 2003, 14 patients were infected with *Clostridium septicum* following musculoskeletal allograft implantation. This resulted in one death. The others were treated with hospitalization, intravenous antibiotics, and joint irrigation and débridement; 10 patients required removal of their allografts.[47] Other isolated bacterial species include gram-negative bacilli and *Streptococcus pyogenes*. The CDC has made specific recommendations regarding tissue processing to decrease the risk of microbial contamination. We recommend using an accredited tissue bank and reviewing their processing techniques.

There has been concern that allograft ACL reconstructions may have a higher failure rate than autograft reconstructions. Both autografts and allografts go through a similar process of ligamentization, as discussed earlier. The remodeling of allografts has been demonstrated to occur at a slower rate than in autografts.[41] Consequently, many surgeons will delay a patient's return to activity after allograft ACL reconstruction to allow the graft time to mature fully. Consistent with longer incorporation times, failure rates do appear to be higher in allograft reconstructions. Carey et al.[16] have performed a systematic review of nine studies comparing autograft and allograft anterior cruciate reconstructions. The short-tem clinical outcomes between both grafts did not differ significantly. Another systematic review by Foster et al.[24] analyzed the results from 31 prospective studies comparing autograft and allograft ACL reconstructions. Their meta-analysis found few statistical differences between the two graft choices. The graft failure rate was $4.7/100 \pm 0.5/100$ for autograft and $8.2/100 \pm 2.1/100$ for allograft. Although not statistically significant, this could represent a concerning trend. They concluded that the choice of graft had minimal effect on the clinical outcome for the patients. However, the authors in both of these reviews noted that the results are not stratified to control for patient age or activity level.

Edgar et al.[22] have prospectively compared identical quadrupled hamstring autografts with allograft constructs in 84 patients. The two cohorts were similar in age, acute or chronic nature of their ACL injury, and incidence of concomitant meniscal injuries. At a mean follow-up of 50 months, there were no differences in subjective or objective outcomes. Laxity did not appear to be increased in the allograft group. An additional review of prospective studies comparing autograft BPTB and allograft BPTB grafts was presented by Krych and colleagues.[50] Six studies met their inclusion criteria, including 256 autograft and 278 allograft patients. Allograft patients were more likely to rupture their graft than autograft patients (odds ratio, 5.03; $p = 0.01$). However, when irradiated and chemically processed grafts were excluded, no significant difference between the two groups was seen. More recent data presented from the MOON study at the American Orthopaedic Society for Sports Medicine (AOSSM) 2008 meeting in Orlando, Florida, showed an odds ratio of failure of 6.77 in allograft ACL reconstructions in 10- to 19-year-old patients when compared with autografts.[38]

MEDICAL COMPLICATIONS

Deep venous thrombosis (DVT) is a potentially life-threatening complication of ACL reconstruction that may lead to pulmonary embolism (PE). The American College of Chest Physicians has recommended that patients undergoing knee arthroscopy who do not have additional thromboembolic risk factors should use early mobilization alone as thromboprophylaxis.[28] The risk of DVT for routine arthroscopy is reported to be between 0.6% and 17.9%, depending on the diagnostic technique.[15,27] However, ACL reconstruction is often associated with longer operative times and has a theoretically higher risk. Marlovits et al.[59] prospectively followed 175 patients following ACL reconstruction who were randomized to enoxaparin or placebo for 20 days postoperatively. Of the enoxaparin group, 2.8% developed DVT as confirmed by magnetic resonance venography, compared with 41.2% of the placebo group. Risk factors for DVT were age older than 30 years and immobilization before surgery. No cases of PE were diagnosed in either group. Gaskill et al. reviewed 16,558 ACL reconstructions from the Department of Defense Medical Data Repository and identified 87 DVT (0.53%).[27] The odds of DVT increased in patients aged greater than 35 years, history of nicotine use, concomitant high tibial osteotomy, and concomitant PCL reconstruction. Nonsteroidal drug use was associated with decreased odds.

KEY REFERENCES

1. Abebe ES, Moorman CT, 3rd, Dziedzic TS, et al: Femoral tunnel placement during anterior cruciate ligament reconstruction: an in vivo imaging analysis comparing transtibial and 2-incision tibial tunnel-independent techniques. *Am J Sports Med* 37:1904–1911, 2009.

6. Arneja S, McConkey MO, Mulpuri K, et al: Graft tensioning in anterior cruciate ligament reconstruction: a systematic review of randomized controlled trials. *Arthroscopy* 25:200–207, 2009.

8. Baer GS, Harner CD: Clinical outcomes of allograft versus autograft in anterior cruciate ligament reconstruction. *Clin Sports Med* 26:661–681, 2007.

11. Barker JU, Drakos MC, Maak TG, et al: Effect of graft selection on the incidence of postoperative infection in anterior cruciate ligament reconstruction. *Am J Sports Med* 38:281–286, 2010.

16. Carey JL, Dunn WR, Dahm DL, et al: A systematic review of anterior cruciate ligament reconstruction with autograft compared with allograft. *J Bone Joint Surg Am* 91:2242–2250, 2009.

24. Foster TE, Wolfe BL, Ryan S, et al: Does the graft source really matter in the outcome of patients undergoing anterior cruciate ligament reconstruction? An evaluation of autograft versus allograft reconstruction results: a systematic review. *Am J Sports Med* 38:189–199, 2010.

26. Fu FH, Bennett CH, Ma CB, et al: Current trends in anterior cruciate ligament reconstruction. Part II. Operative procedures and clinical correlations. *Am J Sports Med* 28:124–130, 2000.

38. Harner CD, Lo MY: Future of allografts in sports medicine. *Clin Sports Med* 28:327–340, 2009.

43. Jepsen CF, Lundberg-Jenson AK, Faunoe P: Does the position of the femoral tunnel affect the laxity or clinical outcome of the anterior cruciate ligament–reconstructed knee? A clinical prospective, randomized, double-bind study. *Arthroscopy* 23:1326–1333, 2007.

50. Krych AJ, Jackson JD, Hoskin TL, et al: A meta-analysis of patellar tendon autograft versus patellar tendon allograft in anterior cruciate ligament reconstruction. *Arthroscopy* 24:292–298, 2008.

60. Marumo K, Saito M, Yamagishi T, et al: The "ligamentization" process in human anterior cruciate ligament reconstruction with autogenous patellar and hamstring tendons: a biochemical study. *Am J Sports Med* 33:1166–1173, 2005.

70. Øiestad BE, Engebretsen L, Storheim K, et al: Knee osteoarthritis after anterior cruciate ligament injury: a systematic review. *Am J Sports Med* 37:1434–1443, 2009.

77. Salmon L, Russell V, Musgrove T, et al: Incidence and risk factors for graft rupture and contralateral rupture after anterior cruciate ligament reconstruction. *Arthroscopy* 21:948–957, 2005.

89. Spindler KP, Kuhn J, Freedman KB, et al: Anterior cruciate ligament reconstruction autograft choice: bone-tendon-bone versus hamstring. Does it really matter? A systematic review. *Am J Sports Med* 32:1986–1995, 2004.

101. Wright RW, Dunn WR, Amendola A, et al: Risk of tearing the intact anterior cruciate ligament in the contralateral knee and rupturing the anterior cruciate ligament graft during the first 2 years after anterior cruciate ligament reconstruction: a prospective MOON cohort study. *Am J Sports Med* 35:1131–1134, 2007.

The references for this chapter can also be found on www.expertconsult.com.

54

Revision Anterior Cruciate Ligament Reconstruction

Shawn G. Anthony, Pramod B. Voleti, Riley J. Williams III

INTRODUCTION

Although primary anterior cruciate ligament (ACL) reconstruction is commonly a successful procedure, failure rates of 3% to 15% have been reported,[4,32] resulting in an estimated 10,000 to 20,000 revision ACL reconstructions performed annually.[47] The success of revision surgery relies on determining the etiology of failure for the primary operation. Potential causes of failure include recurrent trauma, premature return to activity, technical errors, insufficient treatment of concomitant injuries, loss of motion, and failure of graft incorporation.[13,16] The results of revision ACL reconstruction in the literature have been inferior compared with primary reconstructions.* Improved knowledge of ACL anatomy, knee kinematics, and surgical technique may allow patients undergoing revision ACL reconstruction to more reliably return to a high level of function.

ETIOLOGY

The goal of revision ACL surgery is to restore knee stability so as to maximize patient function and prevent further chondral and meniscal injury.[2] For revision ACL reconstruction to be successful, it is paramount to determine the underlying etiology leading to failure of the index reconstruction. At the time of revision surgery, the causative factors should be addressed to provide the optimal clinical result. The etiology of failure may be related to loss of motion, recurrent trauma resulting in a graft injury, or pain associated with articular cartilage damage, surgical error, or failure to treat concomitant pathology.†

Loss of Motion

Loss of motion is one of the most common and potentially debilitating complications following ACL reconstruction.[25] Extension loss is more commonly encountered and often less tolerated than flexion loss.[35] Postoperative motion loss may be attributed to multiple factors, such as limited preoperative range of motion, insufficient rehabilitation prior to reconstruction, tibial and femoral tunnel malposition, excessive graft tension, extensor mechanism scarring, arthrofibrosis, multiligamentous injury, and/or prolonged immobilization.[29] Early recognition of developing stiffness after surgery is necessary to provide the appropriate conservative or surgical intervention. Loss of motion after ACL reconstruction has been shown to be associated with development of radiographic arthritic changes,[43]

so correction of postoperative motion loss is of critical importance.

When revision surgery is indicated for motion loss, importance is placed on maximizing knee range of motion, decreasing inflammation, and improving muscle strength prior to the revision procedure. In addition, the cause of motion loss must be identified and addressed. Assessment for graft impingement, tunnel malpositioning, and arthrofibrosis can be ascertained by physical examination, diagnostic imaging, and intraoperative visualization. During the revision, a systematic evaluation of the knee allows for careful débridement of fibrotic structures through arthroscopic or open procedures.[37] When motion loss is significant, a staged revision reconstruction may be indicated.

Persistent Pain

Persistent pain after ACL reconstruction is often multifactorial. Articular cartilage loss, meniscal pathology, prominent hardware, neuromas, graft site morbidity, prolonged inflammatory response, painful scars, and infection are all potential causes of pain after ACL reconstruction. Often the exact source of pain is difficult to ascertain; however, selection of an optimal treatment plan relies on accurately determining the cause.

Recurrent Instability

Instability after ACL reconstruction can be divided into three categories: traumatic failure, atraumatic failure, and failure caused by graft malposition or fixation loss. Analysis of these categories of instability relies on patient history, physical examination, imaging, and careful review of the prior operative technique.

Patients with traumatic failure report a single traumatic event in a previously well-functioning stable knee. The mechanism is often the same as that occurring in a native rupture of the ACL. Instability that occurs in the early postoperative course may be the result of trauma to the ACL before full graft incorporation.[20,29] Returning to athletics before neuromuscular coordination and strength have returned may also leave the knee prone to recurrent injury.[20,23] Soccer players and adolescents have been identified as having an increased risk of revision surgery.[3] In most of these cases, the primary reconstruction was appropriately performed, and the same tunnels can be used for the revision. Important considerations include identification of the graft used for the primary reconstruction and appropriate graft selection for the revision procedure. Controversy exists regarding the ideal graft type for the revision procedure.[1,39]

Atraumatic failure of ACL reconstructions can occur for multiple reasons. Potential etiologies include failure of graft

---

*References 1, 6, 16, 38, 51, 56, and 57.
†References 12, 20, 23, 28, 34, and 53.

TABLE 54.1 Common Technical Errors and Results

Error	Result
Femoral tunnel malposition	Graft impingement and/or loss of extension
Anterior	Excessive graft length changes (tension in flexion)
Vertical	Rotational instability
Tibial tunnel malposition	Graft impingement and/or loss of extension
Anterior	Excessive graft length changes (tension in flexion)
Posterior	Excessive graft length changes (tension in extension)
Inadequate notchplasty	Graft impingement and/or loss of extension
Inadequate graft tensioning	Translational and/or rotational instability
Unrecognized ligament injury	Translational and/or rotational instability
Unrecognized chondral or meniscal injury	Persistent pain and/or mechanical symptoms
Poor fixation	Translational and/or rotational instability

biological integration, failure of bone healing, improper graft tension, or missed associated instabilities, such as persistent medial laxity or posterolateral corner deficiency.[‡] An increased lateral tibial posterior slope has also been associated with increased risk for early graft failure.[14] Determining the type of graft tissue used in the primary operation is important to avoid similar problems in the revision setting. For example, Singhal et al. reported unacceptably high reoperation rates with the use of allograft tibialis anterior tissue in patients under the age of 25 years.[46] Studies have also shown that exposure to high levels of gamma irradiation (4 Mrad) may weaken the structural properties of allograft tissue, leaving it prone to failure.[42] Tunnel widening may be present as a result of mechanical and/or biologic factors related to graft motion within the tunnel and release of inflammatory cytokines.[55] A thorough physical examination to assess for other instability patterns that can predispose to early ACL graft failure should be performed. Secondary causes of instability should be addressed at the time of revision to provide the best chance for an optimal outcome.

The third potential cause of recurrent instability is graft malposition or loss of graft fixation (Table 54.1). Errors in surgical technique related to tunnel placement and graft fixation are the most common cause of failure in ACL reconstruction.[20,23] The location of the previous tunnels should be assessed with preoperative imaging. Standard orthogonal views, magnetic resonance imaging (MRI) and computed tomography (CT) can be useful in fully investigating prior tunnel position. Graft malposition can occur on both the tibial and femoral side. Anterior femoral tunnel placement is the most common error.[53] Anterior femoral tunnel placement results in flexion deficits and early graft failure as a result of excessive tension and impingement in extension.[13] This error can occur when using an arthroscopic technique that does not adequately visualize the over-the-top position.[23] During revision surgery, a new tunnel may need to be placed posterior to the original anterior tunnel. If preexisting hardware is not impeding proper tunnel placement, it should be left in place so as to avoid creating a larger

defect. In addition, the use of the anteromedial portal along with flexible reaming instrumentation can facilitate femoral tunnel placement more posterior and inferior to index femoral tunnels that may have been created using the transtibial technique. When a posterior femoral tunnel position with femoral cortical compromise is identified as the cause for failure, the revision reconstruction can be performed using a two-incision, outside-in technique to create divergent tunnels. If this technique is not possible, a two-stage revision should be considered.

Central femoral tunnel position may result in a vertical graft that provides anteroposterior (AP) stability without rotational control.[10,33] This problem can manifest on physical examination with a negative Lachman examination but a positive pivot shift. If adequate bone stock remains, an appropriately positioned femoral tunnel should be created with either an endoscopic or a two-incision technique. Recent discussion on anatomic ACL reconstruction suggests placing the femoral tunnel lower on the intercondylar notch.[8,11,33] The use of an accessory anteromedial portal has been described as a means of drilling a more anatomic femoral tunnel site.[8,24] Independent drilling of femoral and tibial tunnels has been shown to outperform conventional transtibial drilling in a cadaver model.[48] However, Rue et al.[41] have shown that it is technically possible to create an obliquely oriented single-bundle femoral tunnel in the anatomic footprint through a tibial tunnel angled approximately 60 degrees from the proximal tibial joint surface. This correlates to a femoral tunnel approximately midway between the anteromedial and posterolateral bundle origins of the ACL.[41]

Errors in tibial tunnel placement can also lead to ACL graft failure. A tibial tunnel placed too anterior will result in graft impingement on the intercondylar notch in extension and early graft failure.[26,27] A posterior tibial tunnel may result in a vertical graft and loss of rotational control,[9] as well as excessive laxity in flexion and impingement on the posterior cruciate ligament. In cases of tibial tunnel malposition, an attempt can be made to drill a properly oriented tibial tunnel if adequate bone stock is present.[50] In a meta-analysis, Kopf et al.[30] reported that there is wide variability in the location of the femoral and tibial ACL footprints and stressed the importance of using anatomic landmarks when creating tunnels.

Loss of graft fixation is another potential cause for graft failure and recurrent anterior knee instability. Graft fixation loss may occur secondary to poor bone quality, screw breakage, screw divergence, graft damage during screw insertion or graft damage secondary to proud screw placement in situ (screw threads cutting graft in knee extension). Poor bone quality may necessitate supplemental revision techniques, such as compaction drilling or bone grafting. Additional fixation may be warranted on the femoral side, such as the use of a suspensory device, lateral screw post, or ligament button. On the tibial side a screw post, staple, or ligament button may be used. Whenever possible, an attempt at aperture fixation should be considered. Interference screws have been shown to be stronger than staples, suture fixation around a post, or soft tissue washer with screw fixation.[20,49] However, interference screws can be complicated by poor fixation in osteopenic bone, disruption of the bone plug, and transection of the graft.[20] If graft damage occurs during femoral screw placement, the graft can be reversed such that the tibial bone block is placed on the femoral side and soft tissue fixation techniques are used on the tibial side.

In cases in which the patient with a failed ACL expects to return to pivoting sports (soccer, lacrosse, basketball, American

---

[‡]References 20, 23, 28, 36, 38, and 51.

football), the authors encourage the consideration of a lateral iliotibial band tenodesis. This extra-articular procedure provides additional knee stability in the revision setting by reducing tibia internal rotation and anterior translation, leading to a higher percentage of patients with negative pivot shift test at long-term follow-up.[17,52] This supplemental procedure has demonstrated promise in protecting individuals undergoing revision ACL reconstruction from rerupture.[18]

PATIENT EVALUATION

A thorough history is important to gather complete information related to the patient's current symptoms and prior treatment course. The patient should be asked to describe the event that resulted in the initial ACL injury because this may provide clues to concomitant injuries. The length of time from injury to ACL reconstruction is important when discussing issues of motion loss or arthrofibrosis. When possible, review of the original operative report and arthroscopic images can elucidate the type of graft, fixation methods, concomitant procedures, and status of the articular cartilage and menisci. The patient's postoperative course should be evaluated regarding rehabilitation protocol, timing of return to high-demand activities, recurrent sensation of instability, signs of infection, and traumatic episodes that may have resulted in graft failure. Lastly, the patient's expectations and desired level of activity should be assessed.

Physical examination should begin with assessment of the patient's gait and overall limb alignment. Observation of skin color, signs of infection, and previous incisions is performed. Range of motion should be evaluated with particular attention to loss of extension. Quadriceps strength and circumference are compared with the contralateral limb to evaluate for muscle atrophy. The knee is evaluated for the presence of an effusion, prominent hardware, and joint line tenderness. Signs of patellar tendonitis and patellar mobility in the medial/lateral and superior/inferior planes are important to assess after prior bone-patellar tendon-bone reconstructions. A stability examination is performed, including anteroposterior drawer, Lachman, and pivot shift tests. Finally, the medial and lateral collateral ligaments and posterolateral corner are evaluated because failure to address pathology in these structures has been reported as a cause of early failure of ACL reconstruction.

Imaging begins with standard weight-bearing AP, lateral, Merchant, and 45-degree flexion posteroanterior (PA) views. The presence and location of hardware are noted. The femoral and tibial tunnels can be assessed for malposition and widening. Several radiographic methods of quantifying tunnel widening have been described.[15,31] The femoral tunnel is typically easier to assess on the AP view, and the lateral view better delineates the position of the tibial tunnel by using Blumensaat line as a reference.[27] The 45-degree flexion PA view allows for assessment of early loss of joint space.[40] If limb alignment is in question, standing full-length views are indicated. Bone loss can be accurately assessed using CT; we recommend the use of three-dimensional CT reconstructions for preoperative planning purposes.

MRI provides detailed information regarding the integrity of the graft, incorporation of bone plugs or bioabsorbable screws into the native bone, and status of articular cartilage, menisci, and surrounding ligaments. The presence of an effusion and bone marrow edema patterns can provide clues to the acuity of

the trauma and the degree of injury. Articular cartilage injury can be quantified using cartilage-sensitive MRI sequences.[44] MRI has also been used to calculate the cross-sectional area of the femoral and tibial tunnels to assess for tunnel widening.[19,45]

SURGICAL TECHNIQUES

Preoperative Planning

After the preoperative patient evaluation is complete and the cause of failure of the primary ACL reconstruction has been ascertained, revision ACL reconstruction can be performed. Proper preoperative planning is critical to anticipate challenges during the revision procedure. Many important factors should be considered when planning for revision procedures (Table 54.2). A methodical approach is necessary to account for each technical aspect of the case. Reviewing prior operative reports, arthroscopic images, and imaging studies provides valuable information as to surgical approach, hardware used, type of graft, and coexisting pathology at the time of the primary procedure.

The first step is to select the graft type to be used for the revision procedure. There are a number of graft tissue options available (Box 54.1). If allograft tissue was used for the primary procedure, use of ipsilateral autograft tissue is recommended because of the possibility of previous rejection of the allograft and/or presence of tunnel widening. The use of autograft tissue facilitates timely soft tissue graft healing to bone; this decreases the likelihood of late atraumatic recurrent knee instability in treated patients. The authors recommend the use of autograft tissue from the contralateral limb, if available, in the revision ACL setting. Several reports have found no difference in

---

TABLE 54.2 Technical Considerations in Planning Revision Anterior Cruciate Ligament Reconstruction

Parameter	Technical Consideration
Motion loss	Rehabilitation preoperatively and postoperatively; arthroscopic or open débridement
Limb malalignment	Prior osteotomy; concurrent high tibial osteotomy
Tunnel osteolysis	Débridement; bone grafting
Graft removal	Intact vertical graft; malpositioned incompetent graft; synthetic graft
Hardware removal	Location and need for removal based on location
Revision graft selection	Determine original graft used; autologous tissue options; allograft tissue options
Revision tunnel placement	Location and quality of bone
Graft fixation	Aperture versus suspensory fixation
Associated injuries	Meniscus, articular cartilage, collateral ligaments, posterolateral corner, capsule

---

BOX 54.1 Graft Sources

Autogenous	Allograft
(Ipsilateral, contralateral)	Bone-patellar tendon-bone
Bone-patellar tendon-bone	Hamstring
Hamstring (semitendinosus and gracilis)	Achilles tendon-bone
Quadriceps tendon-bone	Tibialis anterior

outcomes of revision surgery with autograft versus allograft tissue.[1,6,21] However, studies from the multicenter ACL revision study (MARS) group have found increased revision failures with the use of allograft tissue.[22] The primary advantages of allograft tissue are the absence of donor site morbidity and decreased operative time. Second, the large bone blocks available with Achilles tendon and bone-patellar tendon-bone allografts provide versatility in shaping the bone blocks to fill preexisting bone tunnels. It is important to note that allograft tissue runs the risk of disease transmission, increases cost, and recellularizes more slowly and less completely than autograft tissue.[39] As such, the authors recommend using autograft tissue when possible with either limb used as a donor source.

The next step is to identify potential problems related to existing tunnel malposition, tunnel widening, and hardware placement. Review of previous operative reports and radiographs allows for identification of the manufacturer and size of implants used in the primary reconstruction. Tibial hardware can often be removed directly through the previous anterior tibial incision. Removal of femoral hardware can present a more difficult challenge. In many cases, femoral screws may not need to be removed. If a two-incision or accessory anteromedial portal technique is planned, the divergent nature of the new femoral tunnel often avoids the existing femoral screw. In cases in which the previous femoral tunnel is placed too anterior, there is often room to drill the new femoral tunnel in the proper posterior position without obstruction from the existing hardware. Regardless of hardware position, it is important to have the appropriate screw drivers, staple extractors, and broken hardware removal sets available in case they are needed. When tunnel widening is present, the technique and potential instrumentation or bone graft needed to address the defect should be planned preoperatively to ensure availability. If a previous double-bundle reconstruction has been performed, the two tunnels may have eroded into one another and a larger bone defect may be present that needs to be addressed.

Anesthesia and Setup

The patient is placed on the operating table in the supine position. Regional anesthesia should be used whenever possible. Frequently, a combined spinal-epidural anesthetic with or without a femoral nerve block for postoperative pain management is administered. Routine use of antibiotic prophylaxis is recommended. After placement of a pneumatic tourniquet, the operative extremity is placed in a cradle leg holder or against a lateral post. Care should be taken to position the patient such that the knees fall below the distal break in the table. This position enables the bottom of the table to be dropped during surgery, allowing knee flexion. The ability to flex the knee greater than 90 degrees is of particular importance when using an anteromedial portal technique. Prior to sterile preparation of the extremity, an examination under anesthesia is performed and compared with the contralateral knee. Passive range of motion is measured with care to note any flexion or extension deficits. The integrity of the medial and lateral collateral ligaments is assessed in both full extension and 30 degrees of flexion. The posterolateral corner is assessed with external rotation at 30 degrees of knee flexion. It is important to recognize and address persistent varus, valgus, or posterolateral instability, because they are known causes of early ACL graft failure. The posterior cruciate ligament is assessed with the posterior drawer test, posterior sag, and external rotation at 90 degrees of knee

flexion. Finally, the integrity of the ACL is evaluated with both the pivot shift and the Lachman tests. The Lachman test assesses graft function in the anteroposterior plane, whereas the pivot shift test is used to evaluate rotational instability. The operative extremity is then prepped and draped in standard sterile fashion. Prior skin incisions are marked. A portable fluoroscopic image intensifier may be used during the case to assess tunnel placement and localize previous hardware.

Operative Technique

At the initiation of the procedure, a diagnostic arthroscopy is performed. The menisci are visualized and probed from posterior to anterior. The articular cartilage surfaces are evaluated, taking care to flex and extend the knee in each compartment so as to completely visualize the condyles. If there is concern for medial or lateral collateral ligament instability, then valgus or varus stress can be applied to the compartment with a 3-mm probe in place to measure the degree of opening. Concomitant meniscal, chondral, and ligamentous pathology should be addressed accordingly.

The previous ACL graft is then assessed in the intercondylar notch. In addition to direct visualization of the graft, a probe is used to assess graft tension. An arthroscopic Lachman test can also be performed. The attachment of the graft on the femur and tibia should be carefully scrutinized and probed.

After the decision is made to proceed with revision reconstruction, the existing graft is removed with a combination of arthroscopic biters, motorized shavers, and an electrocautery device. On the femoral side, the over-the-top position is identified, and the integrity of the back wall is assessed. If the patient has a narrow notch or visualization of the back wall is impeded, a revision notchplasty is performed. A notchplasty ensures that the revision graft does not impinge on the roof of the notch with the knee in extension. Next, the existing femoral tunnel and hardware are identified, and a decision is made whether the existing hardware needs to be removed. If a new tunnel can be correctly positioned without interference with the existing hardware, the hardware should be left in place to avoid creating a larger defect in the bone. However, if the hardware conflicts with proper femoral tunnel positioning, it should be removed.

The prior graft material is then removed from the tibial footprint site. The anatomic landmarks for proper tibial tunnel position are visualized, including the anterior edge of the posterior cruciate ligament, the tibial spines, and the posterior border of the anterior horn of the lateral meniscus. The existing tibial tunnel is evaluated to determine whether it can be used and whether existing hardware may interfere with tunnel placement. Next, the tibial tunnel entrance site is exposed most often through the previous tibial incision. Subperiosteal dissection is performed, and existing hardware is removed if necessary. A guide wire can be placed so as to optimize tunnel position prior to drilling (Fig. 54.1).

After preparation of the graft sites, there are four revision options available: (1) re-reaming existing tunnels, (2) drilling new tunnels that avoid existing ones, (3) drilling divergent tunnels, or (4) bone grafting and staged revision reconstruction.

The first option is to proceed with single-stage revision using the previously well-placed tunnels if bone stock is sufficient. If this option is chosen, the tunnels should be re-reamed to remove sclerotic bone and fibrous tissue to facilitate biologic graft incorporation. The procedure is then continued in a fashion similar to primary ACL reconstruction. Fixation on the femoral side is achieved most commonly with an interference screw. Secondary fixation can be provided using a lateral incision on the femur. After femoral fixation is complete, the graft is tensioned by cycling the knee to remove creep. The graft is visualized arthroscopically with the knee in full extension to confirm that there is no impingement on the femoral notch. Fixation on the tibial side is completed using an interference screw. Secondary fixation can be obtained with a suture anchor, soft tissue button, or staple. The Lachman and pivot shift tests should be performed after fixation to ensure the competency of the graft.

When existing tunnels were placed in a nonanatomic position and no significant tunnel widening is present, new anatomic tunnels can be drilled bypassing the previous tunnels and hardware. Multiple options are available to achieve anatomic tunnel placement, including transtibial, two-incision, and anteromedial portal techniques.

When tunnel widening is present, a third option is available. If the existing tunnels are anatomic and bone quality is good, the divergent tunnel or funnel technique can be used (Fig. 54.2). This technique recreates the original intra-articular footprint of the primary reconstruction while creating a bone tunnel with a new extra-articular orientation. The new orientation of this tunnel establishes a bone bridge for adequate fixation. If bone quality is poor, available fixation options include stacked interference screws, matchstick bone grafting, large bone plug–graft constructs, allograft dowels (Fig. 54.3), and structural bone void fillers.[4,5,7,54] In our experience, aperture fixation with metal interference screws should be used whenever possible given the

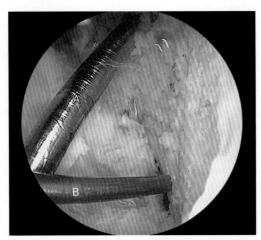

FIG 54.1 A guide wire is initially placed through the original tibial and femoral tunnels (transtibial technique). This wire placement is followed by a new guide wire placed through an accessory anteromedial portal for the femoral tunnel. Optimal position is then determined and this placement is selected for drilling.

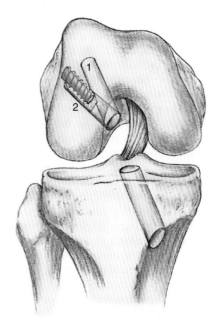

FIG 54.2 **The Funnel Technique** This technique is used for a widened but anatomically placed tunnel in which the aperture of the new tunnel remains unchanged but the angle and direction of the tunnel are new, thereby creating an anatomic tunnel in new bone stock. (From Bach BR Jr: Revision anterior cruciate ligament surgery. *Arthroscopy* 19(Suppl 1):14–29, 2003.)

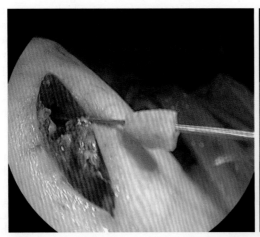

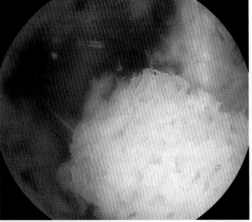

FIG 54.3 **Guided Bone Plug Placement Over a Guide Wire** This method can be used for grafting of the tibial (*left,* open view) and femoral tunnels (*right,* arthroscopic view). A new guide wire is placed prior to drilling of the new tunnel.

association of bioabsorbable screws and suspensory fixation with tunnel widening. However, suspensory fixation may be added as supplemental fixation, especially in the setting of posterior cortical compromise.

The fourth option is primary bone grafting of the tibial or femoral tunnels if widening is greater than 100% of the original tunnel width or approximately 16 to 20 mm in any dimension on preoperative imaging (Fig. 54.4). In addition, if placing an isometric, anatomic graft is not possible using the aforementioned techniques, primary bone grafting and staged reconstruction should be strongly considered. The widened tunnels require meticulous preparation with a focus on adequate débridement of the sclerotic tunnel rim and fibrous material within the tunnels. Primary bone grafting requires removal of all previous hardware prior to placing either morcellized iliac crest autograft or allograft bone chips in both the femoral and tibial tunnels. A large allograft bone dowel may also be fashioned to fill the defect. Other injectable bone substitutes, such as demineralized bone matrix and calcium phosphate, have also been used with success in this setting. Although these injectable forms offer the advantage of ease of arthroscopic placement, little data exist regarding their efficacy. Revision reconstruction should be staged at 3 to 4 months following bone grafting after sufficient consolidation has occurred (Fig. 54.5).

Rehabilitation

Although the goal of most patients is to return to full athletic activity, the first priority is to return to functional activities of daily living. The postoperative protocol is similar to that used for primary reconstruction, but it should be amended depending on the quality of fixation achieved at revision surgery and concomitant procedures performed.

For isolated revision ACL reconstruction using an allograft, our immediate postoperative protocol consists of partial weight bearing with the knee locked in extension. Early range of motion with an emphasis on achieving full extension is started immediately. At 6 weeks postoperatively, when the patient has demonstrated normal gait and sufficient quadriceps strength, the brace is discontinued and the patient is allowed to bear weight as tolerated. Straight-ahead jogging is allowed at 4 months, followed by sport-specific rehabilitation. Return to athletics is allowed at 6 months if the knee is stable on examination and quadriceps strength is 80% of the contralateral side.

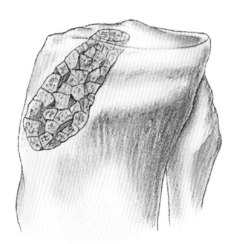

FIG 54.4 Tunnel widening greater than 100% (16 to 20 mm) or such that anatomic graft placement is not possible should be reconstructed in a staged fashion. Removal of all implants and débridement of old graft and fibrotic material within the tunnels should be followed by primary bone grafting of both tunnels. (From Bach BR Jr: Revision anterior cruciate ligament surgery. *Arthroscopy* 19(Suppl 1):14–29, 2003.)

CONCLUSION

As more ACL reconstructions are being performed, the demand for revision ACL reconstruction is increasing. Although studies have shown good outcomes with revision surgery, the results do not match those of primary ACL reconstruction. Revision ACL surgery is a technically demanding procedure, and meticulous preoperative planning and analysis of the cause for failure is necessary for a successful result. Associated pathology must be diagnosed and treated. To optimize outcome, graft selection, tunnel placement, and graft fixation must be carefully planned. Surgeons who perform revision ACL reconstruction procedures should be familiar with a variety of techniques and instruments available at their disposal for performing each of these steps.

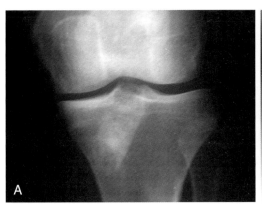
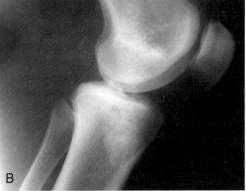

FIG 54.5 Anteroposterior (A) and lateral (B) projections following staged bone grafting of a widened tibial tunnel.

KEY REFERENCES

3. Andernord D, Desai N, Bjornsson H, et al: Patient predictors of early revision surgery after anterior cruciate ligament reconstruction: a cohort study of 16,930 patients with 2-year follow-up. *Am J Sports Med* 43(1):121–127, 2015.

6. Battaglia MJ, 2nd, Cordasco FA, Hannafin JA, et al: Results of revision anterior cruciate ligament surgery. *Am J Sports Med* 35(12):2057–2066, 2007.

7. Battaglia TC, Miller MD: Management of bony deficiency in revision anterior cruciate ligament reconstruction using allograft bone dowels: surgical technique. *Arthroscopy* 21(6):767, 2005.

12. Carlisle JC, Parker RD, Matava MJ: Technical considerations in revision anterior cruciate ligament surgery. *J Knee Surg* 20(4):312–322, 2007.

14. Christensen JJ, Krych AJ, Engasser WM, et al: Lateral tibial posterior slope is increased in patients with early graft failure after anterior cruciate ligament reconstruction. *Am J Sports Med* 43(10):2510–2514, 2015.

16. Denti M, Lo Vetere D, Bait C, et al: Revision anterior cruciate ligament reconstruction: causes of failure, surgical technique, and clinical results. *Am J Sports Med* 36(10):1896–1902, 2008.

22. Group M, Group M: Effect of graft choice on the outcome of revision anterior cruciate ligament reconstruction in the Multicenter ACL Revision Study (MARS) Cohort. *Am J Sports Med* 42(10):2301–2310, 2014.

31. Laxdal G, Kartus J, Eriksson BI, et al: Biodegradable and metallic interference screws in anterior cruciate ligament reconstruction surgery using hamstring tendon grafts: prospective randomized study of radiographic results and clinical outcome. *Am J Sports Med* 34(10):1574–1580, 2006.

32. Lind M, Menhert F, Pedersen AB: Incidence and outcome after revision anterior cruciate ligament reconstruction: results from the Danish registry for knee ligament reconstructions. *Am J Sports Med* 40(7):1551–1557, 2012.

38. Noyes FR, Barber-Westin SD: Revision anterior cruciate ligament reconstruction using a 2-stage technique with bone grafting of the tibial tunnel. *Am J Sports Med* 34(4):678–679, author reply 679–680, 2006.

39. Prodromos CC, Fu FH, Howell SM, et al: Controversies in soft-tissue anterior cruciate ligament reconstruction: grafts, bundles, tunnels, fixation, and harvest. *J Am Acad Orthop Surg* 16(7):376–384, 2008.

47. Spindler KP: The Multicenter ACL Revision Study (MARS): a prospective longitudinal cohort to define outcomes and independent predictors of outcomes for revision anterior cruciate ligament reconstruction. *J Knee Surg* 20(4):303–307, 2007.

50. Steiner ME, Murray MM, Rodeo SA: Strategies to improve anterior cruciate ligament healing and graft placement. *Am J Sports Med* 36(1):176–189, 2008.

56. Wright RW, Dunn WR, Amendola A, et al: Anterior cruciate ligament revision reconstruction: two-year results from the MOON cohort. *J Knee Surg* 20(4):308–311, 2007.

57. Wright RW, Gill CS, Chen L, et al: Outcome of revision anterior cruciate ligament reconstruction: a systematic review. *J Bone Joint Surg Am* 94(6):531–536, 2012.

The references for this chapter can also be found on www.expertconsult.com.

55

Revision Anterior Cruciate Ligament Surgery: One-Stage versus Two-Stage Technique

Cody L. Evans, Mark D. Miller, David R. Diduch

The number of primary anterior cruciate ligament (ACL) reconstructions performed annually in the United States continues to rise, from 87,000 in 1994 to 130,000 in 2006.[21] When extrapolated, this number rises to more than 200,000 annual reconstructions by 2015, reflecting both an increase in absolute number and procedures per capita. Following ACL reconstruction, the failure rate varies as a function of time: within 2 years of reconstruction the rate ranges from 2% to 5%,[9,13,36,38] whereas the failure rates at 10 and 15 years are 9% and 11%, respectively.[6,39] The Danish ACL registry reveals a 4.1% failure rate at 5 years.[20] The overall rate of revision ACL surgery is expected to climb in proportion to the growing number of primary reconstructions being performed. Applying the 4.1% revision rate from the Danish registry to the projected 200,000 annual reconstructions performed in the United States in 2015 yields a total of 8100 revision procedures required within the first 5 years of primary reconstruction, highlighting the expanding relevance of revision surgery.

As the need for ACL revisions increases, surgeons must be able to readily identify the causes of failure of the primary procedure and address them in a systematic fashion. Pitfalls must be recognized and avoided to optimize the success of the revision procedure. The accurate placement of femoral and tibial tunnels should not be compromised by the index tunnel placement.[12] Depending on the type and location of the fixation, the location and size of the existing tunnels, and the quality of the bone, the surgeon must be prepared to use a number of different techniques, including a staged approach, if indicated.

The revision surgery can be performed as a single procedure (one stage) or as two separate procedures (two stage), if necessary. The two-stage surgery ensures adequate healing of bone tunnels, which will then provide a good bed for fixation of the ACL graft without compromising the location of the bone tunnels.[32] However, this technique exposes the patient to the inherent risks of two surgeries and the hazards of an unstable knee while waiting for the graft to incorporate, causing meniscal injury or cartilage damage. An obvious advantage of the one-stage surgery is to avoid the need for a second surgery. For the technique to be successful, adequate bone quality is required, which allows placement of tunnels with acceptable size and location. If adequate bone is not available, the surgeon must have the ability to bypass existing tunnels or fill bone defects with adequate density and strength.[3,5,16,25,34]

Chapter 54 addressed the causes of ACL failure and the planning and decision making for revision surgery. One of the most challenging aspects of ACL revision surgery is how to deal with previous technical errors, methods of fixation, and tunnel widening. Old tunnels may be poorly positioned and interfere with new tunnel location, hardware may block the path of the new tunnel or fixation device, and an enlarged tunnel or large bone defect may jeopardize graft security and incorporation. This chapter presents a treatment algorithm based on different scenarios and describes the surgical techniques for one-stage and two-stage procedures.

In 2011 the Multicenter ACL Revision Study (MARS) cohort completed 2-year follow-up of 1205 patients undergoing revision ACL reconstruction from 2007 to 2009. Up to 8% of revisions in this cohort required bone grafting—either of the tibia or the femur—in a staged approach, because of dilation of bone tunnels.[23] Since the last edition of this text was published in 2011, new manuscripts based on data from the MARS cohort continue to shed light on the revision ACL population, a subset which has been, up to this time, represented in relatively low numbers in the US literature.

PREOPERATIVE WORKUP

Determining the cause of failure is crucial to achieving a successful outcome and avoiding a repeat failure. Historically, the most common cause of failure of the primary ACL reconstruction has been attributed to errors in surgical technique,[14,17,26,33] most commonly because of nonanatomic tunnel placement.[1,29,36] More recent studies have blurred the distinction between purely traumatic, technical, and biologic etiologies of graft failure; however technical error remains the most common surgeon-dependent factor contributing to failure.[23]

Poor tunnel location results in excessive changes in graft length, plastic deformation, and ultimately failure. It can occur on the femoral and tibial sides (one or both) and in the sagittal (too anterior or too posterior) and coronal planes (too vertical or too horizontal). Usually the femoral tunnel is nonanatomic. Specifically, it is usually placed too far anterior because the posterior femoral cortex is not adequately visualized (Fig. 55.1).[12,15] Other technical errors include improper graft tensioning, inadequate fixation, graft impingement, and failure to address unrecognized pathology.

Graft choice must be given special consideration in the revision setting. The use of allograft gains additional attention in this context because there may be insufficient autograft available, making allograft an attractive or necessary option. Previous work has suggested a higher incidence of graft failure in young, active patients receiving allograft for primary ACL reconstruction.[18] Similarly the MARS group was able to show that patients undergoing revision ACL reconstruction using autograft were 2.78 times less likely to sustain graft failure when compared with allograft.[23]

A thorough history and physical examination should be obtained, and a meticulous review of operative notes with details about previous hardware and location should be performed. Specific attention should be paid to the previous surgical technique, the type of graft used, and the type of fixation. Each of these factors may affect the revision procedure.

Posteroanterior (PA), lateral, sunrise, and lateral hyperextension radiographic views should be obtained to determine previous tunnel and hardware position, whether tunnel expansion has occurred, and whether any degenerative changes are present (Fig. 55.2). Consider standing views on a long cassette to determine the mechanical axis. If significant bony defects are present on the radiographs, a computed tomography (CT) scan is often beneficial in planning new tunnel placement and to help to determine whether bone graft or void fillers will be needed (Fig. 55.3). CT has been shown to be superior to plain radiography and magnetic resonance imaging (MRI) in identifying and measuring bone tunnels following reconstruction.[22]

The hospital or surgery center must have the necessary equipment and implants for the revision surgery (Fig. 55.4). Custom-sized allograft materials should be ordered in advance, if needed. Consider having soft tissue allografts in stock as a backup for unexpected occurrences. Achilles tendon allograft is also very useful in revision situations. A variety of sizes and types of bone graft should be readily accessible (Fig. 55.5). Specific instrumentation (if possible) or a universal screw removal set (Fig. 55.6) should be available to remove the previous hardware. It is also often useful to use fluoroscopic guidance to facilitate removing retained hardware or assist in tunnel placement, especially if one is attempting to bypass the previously placed hardware.

The patient must be appropriately counseled about the surgery and expected outcomes. The patient should have realistic goals and understand that the results of revision surgery are less predictable and generally less favorable.[4,7,33,36] Occasionally it is not possible to determine preoperatively whether a one- or two-stage procedure will be performed, and the patient should consent to the possibility of additional surgery if necessary.

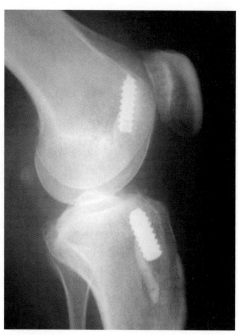

FIG 55.1 Lateral knee x-ray with excessive anterior femoral tunnel location.

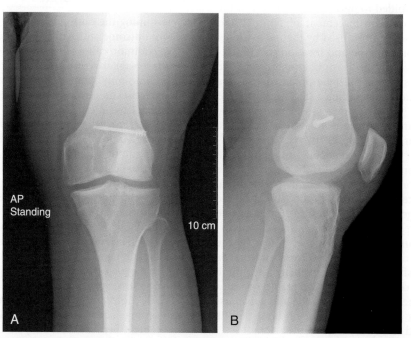

FIG 55.2 (A) PA and (B) lateral x-rays of the knee showing tunnel lysis and early degenerative changes.

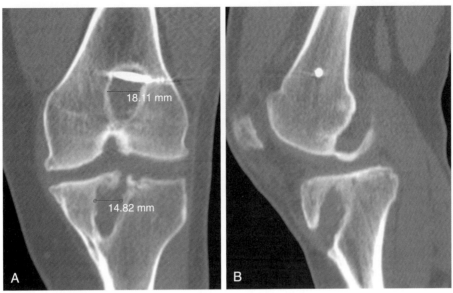

FIG 55.3 (A) Coronal and (B) saggital CT images showing femoral tunnel widening >18 mm and tibial tunnel widening >14 mm.

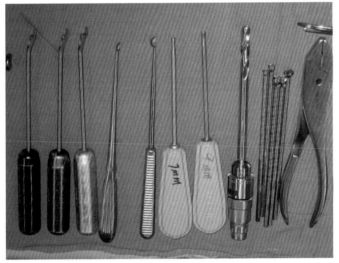

FIG 55.4 Revision ACL instrumentation set.

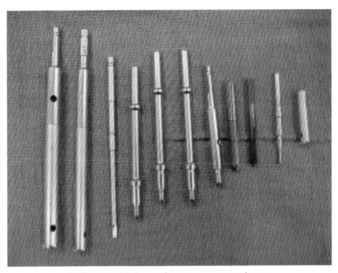

FIG 55.6 Universal screw removal set.

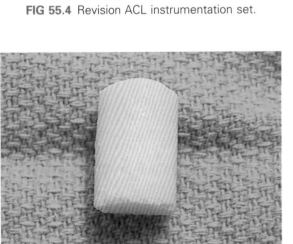

FIG 55.5 Cloward dowel cylindric bone allograft measuring 12 × 16 mm.

TREATMENT OPTIONS

The majority of revisions can be performed as a single procedure,[23,24] which is the preferred method because it avoids a second procedure and associated morbidity.[27] In general, there are four primary indications to proceed with a two-stage revision: (1) excessive bone loss that might limit graft fixation, (2) loss of joint motion (arthrofibrosis) requiring surgical intervention, (3) active joint infection that precludes placement of new hardware, and (4) severe malalignment requiring deformity correction. By far the most common indication for a staged procedure is tunnel widening.

One-stage surgery can usually be performed in the setting of adequate bone quality and tunnel placement, when the hardware is not in the way. In the ideal scenario the alignment of the initial tunnels is so malpositioned that the normal landmarks and bone stock will be preserved (see Fig. 55.1). If this is the case, the previous tunnels and hardware can simply be bypassed with new anatomically placed tunnels.[25] However, it is often not this simple.

Two-stage surgery should be considered for significant widening of the tunnels when tunnels are close but not ideal (causing an hourglass shape or tunnel confluence) and when an excessive amount of bone is removed during the hardware extraction process. Many authors suggest bone grafting and staged revision if the amount of cystic widening (or osteolysis) is greater than 15 mm.[1,15] The initial procedure involves removing the existing hardware and filling the bony defects with bone graft. Typically the bone graft is incorporated over a period of several months. Then, during the second stage, new tunnels can be drilled and the ACL revision procedure can be performed. Tunnel confluence is a problem wherein two independently drilled tunnels converge along their paths to create a single larger tunnel, compromising fixation if the defect is too large or by allowing for excessive translation of the graft at the joint line, the so-called windshield-wiper effect. A common scenario encountered in the revision setting is improper tunnel placement from use of a transtibial technique for the primary reconstruction.[19] Transtibial ACL reconstruction commonly results in a posteriorly placed tibial tunnel and an anterior and superiorly placed femoral tunnel. It is the posteriorly placed tibial tunnel that is most commonly problematic—especially in smaller knees—because placing a properly positioned tunnel risks creating a tunnel diameter that exceeds the limits of reliable graft fixation.[37]

If small or moderately sized bony defects are present, caused either by tunnel widening or from the removal of previous hardware, these must be addressed intraoperatively. Tunnel widening is a well-documented phenomenon felt to occur because of micromotion at the graft-tunnel interface and also because of possible immunologic rejection, most commonly with use of allograft.[37] Thus significant bone loss can occur even in properly positioned femoral and tibial tunnels, necessitating a grafting procedure to fill the defect. The defect can be filled with autograft plugs[8,28] or allograft dowels.[3,5] Other techniques use structural grafts, including bioabsorbable interference screws[2,16] or calcium phosphate cement,[34] to fill the void. These rigid bone void fillers allow new tunnels to be drilled anatomically (without compromising location) and the graft to be securely fixed in one procedure.

Paessler[28] has described a technique in which iliac crest corticocancellous autograft bone plugs can be used during a one-stage procedure. The iliac crest graft is harvested through a 2- to 3-cm incision, using a specialized harvesting tube. The trajectory for the tube harvester is marked with a Kirschner wire (K-wire) passed into the iliac crest. A harvesting tube is used that matches the diameter required for the corticocancellous plug, and the plug is removed with a removal device. The harvested plugs can then be inserted into the tunnel defects in an arthroscopic or open fashion.

To avoid the morbidity associated with harvesting bone graft from the iliac crest, Franceschi describes a technique[11] of harvesting graft from the safe zone of the tibial metaphysis. The safe zone, located between the anterior roots of the menisci and anterior to the ACL insertion and tibial articular cartilage, corresponds to the starting point of a tibial intramedullary nail. This area can be accessed through a patellar-splitting approach and may use a previous incision from a bone-patellar tendon-bone (BPTB) graft harvest. By using an Osteochondral Autograft

Transfer System (OATS) tube harvester (Arthrex, Naples, Fla) they were able to harvest a graft 1 mm larger than the size of the measured defect and then insert the graft arthroscopically via a press-fit technique. Follow-up CT scans at the 6-month mark confirmed graft incorporation and showed no evidence of fracture at the harvest site.

Said et al. describe a similar technique[31] of using the OATS tube harvester to obtain iliac crest autografts in a percutaneous fashion followed by impacting the grafts by use of the OATS instruments. This can be performed for femoral and tibial tunnel defects; however, there are potential pitfalls to keep in mind. First, the OATS harvester is available in a limited number of diameters, and the maximum obtainable graft length is 25 mm. Secondly, a backstop must be in place when grafting a tibial defect to prevent extrusion of graft material into the joint.

Battaglia and Miller[5] have recommended using cylindric bone allografts, or Cloward dowels, to fill bone voids (Fig. 55.7). The previous tunnel is aggressively débrided and reamed, and the corresponding sized dowel is inserted. The most common sizes are 12 mm in diameter by 25 to 35 mm in length, although up to 18-mm diameter dowels have been used successfully. A variety of different sized dowels must be available. This study noted that even with meticulous preoperative planning, the exact size of the defect is often difficult to predict.

A similar technique involves replacing an existing metal interference screw in the femoral tunnel with a bioabsorbable screw.[16] If the existing tunnel is partially overlapped by the new tunnel, the reamer can drill through the corner of the absorbable screw; the remaining screw fills the void and provides structural support. The stacked interference screw concept specifically refers to inserting a second interference screw, adjacent to the one providing structural support, to reinforce fixation.[2]

In a recent study by Vaughn et al.[34] the authors performed a cadaveric study to determine the load-to-failure of a BPTB graft placed after filling bone defects with calcium phosphate cement. They found that using standard fixation techniques and anatomically drilled tunnels, the load-to-failure of the reconstruction using the bone cement was not significantly different from that of the control group, a primary ACL reconstruction with standard interference screw fixation. However, although it has been shown that calcium phosphate bone cement is stronger than cancellous bone, this biomechanical study on cadavers did

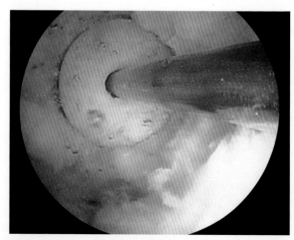

FIG 55.7 Bone allograft dowel insertion in bone defect.

not necessarily correlate to in vivo results. A significant question that remains is whether the cement would inhibit incorporation of the graft into bone.

A two-stage technique should also be considered in the setting of decreased range of motion (arthrofibrosis) following index ACL surgery. If there is a flexion contracture more than 5 degrees or a flexion loss more than 20 degrees, a manipulation under anesthesia, lysis of adhesions, and aggressive physical therapy should be performed to improve motion prior to revision.[15] In addition, a staged revision must be performed in the setting of an underlying infection. Obviously, the definitive reconstruction should be delayed until the infection is eradicated.

Thomas et al.[32] have advocated a two-stage procedure if the tibial tunnel from the index procedure would overlap the correctly placed new tibial tunnel either partially or fully. After débriding the old tunnel, bone was harvested from the iliac crest in the form of dowels and impacted in the tunnel. The femoral tunnel was not grafted because it was later drilled in virgin bone via a different technique (outside-in). A CT scan was obtained 4 months later to confirm adequate healing of the bone graft. A revision ACL procedure was then performed similar to a primary procedure.

The decision to perform one-stage or two-stage revision ACL surgery is complex and multifactorial. It must take into consideration technical factors from the previous surgery, such as tunnel location and previous graft type, and patient-dependent factors, such as activity level and bone quality. The following scenarios provide a treatment algorithm to facilitate the decision making process in a stepwise manner. The decision tree starts by first identifying whether the tunnels are in an acceptable location.

Acceptable Femoral and Tibial Tunnel Locations

Remove fixation?
- Yes
  - Easily performed without large defect
  - Difficult; metal cross pins may require overdrilling with a hollow drill, causing a large defect (see Fig. 55.2)
- No
  - Retain screw and drill through portion of screw to avoid complications of screw removal.[25]

Assess for large bone defect secondary to cystic widening or implant removal.
- Small to moderate (<15 mm; Fig. 55.8)
  - One-stage bone grafting with autograft or allograft
  - Structural graft
  - Bioabsorbable interference screws
  - Bone cement
  - Use Achilles or BPTB allograft with larger bone plug (rotate plug to fill defect).
- Large (>15 mm; Fig. 55.9): Bone grafting and staged **re**vision

  Drill tunnel.
- Endoscopic transtibial
- Two-incision outside-in technique
- Accessory medial port—divergent

  Graft fixation. Consider dual fixation if there is any question of bone quality (Fig. 55.10).
- Femoral side: Interference screw and lateral cortex (over the top) fixation (EndoButton, Smith & Nephew, Andover, Massachusetts)
- Tibial side: Interference screw plus post and washer or staple

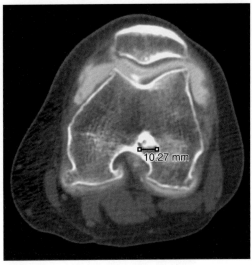

FIG 55.8 Axial CT image showing moderately sized femoral tunnel measuring approximately 10 mm.

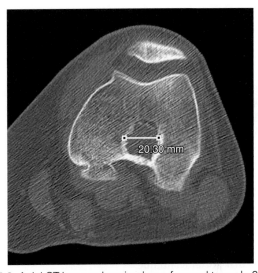

FIG 55.9 Axial CT image showing large femoral tunnel >20 mm.

Unacceptable Femoral Tunnel Location

Is hardware blocking new tunnel path?
- Yes; remove hardware.
- No; leave hardware in place.
  Femoral tunnel
- Cystic widening?
  - <15 mm; consider one-stage bone grafting.
  - >15 mm; consider two-stage revision with bone grafting.
- Consider surgical approach used at index procedure.
  - Transtibial? Consider accessory medial port drilling.
  - Two-incision? Use endoscopic technique to change trajectory and avoid hardware.
- Evaluate tunnel location.
  - Too anterior? (most common)
  More than one tunnel diameter?
- Bypass old tunnel and redrill new tunnel endoscopically.

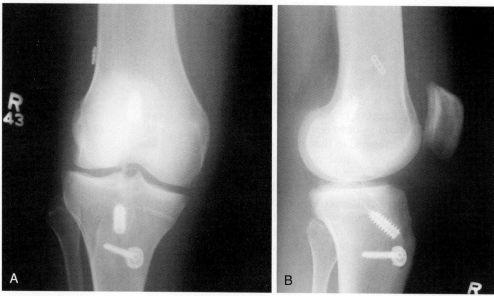

FIG 55.10 Postoperative (A) anteroposterior (AP) and (B) lateral x-rays with dual fixation of the femoral and tibial tunnels.

Less than one diameter? (hourglass shape or tunnel confluence)
- Hamstring graft with small diameter. Drill small tunnel posteriorly that fits without overlap.
- Simultaneous bone grafting
  - Autograft bone plug
  - Allograft bone dowel
  - Bioabsorbable interference screws
  - Bone cement
- Use Achilles or BTPB allograft with larger bone plug (rotate plug to fill defect).
- Bone grafting and staged revision
  - Too posterior? (usually with deficient posterior wall; Fig. 55.11)
  - Drill anatomic tunnel using two-incision or accessory medial portal technique.
  - Too vertical? (Fig. 55.12)
  - Drill tunnel from same starting point but at a different angle or orientation to create a new intact femoral tunnel (funnel or tunnel diversion concept[2]; Fig. 55.13)

Graft fixation: Consider dual fixation.

Unacceptable Tibial Tunnel Location

Is hardware blocking new tunnel path?
- Yes; remove hardware.
- No; leave hardware in place.
  Tibial tunnel
- Cystic widening?
  - <15 mm; consider one-stage bone grafting.
  - >15 mm; consider two-stage revision with bone grafting.
- Evaluate tunnel location (similar principles to femoral side). Too anterior?
- More than one diameter?
  - Drill new tunnel posterior to the original tunnel without removing fixation.
- Less than one diameter?

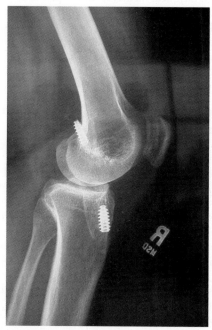

FIG 55.11 Lateral x-ray with penetration through the posterior femoral cortex with the interference screw.

- Expand existing tunnel until center is optimal position. Fill the void between the anterior wall and new graft with allograft bone, core reamings, structural graft, or BPTB allograft with large bone plug.
- Create new tibial tunnel with new extra-articular starting point that ends at the optimal intra-articular position.[7]
  Too posterior?
- More than one diameter?
  - Drill new tunnel anteriorly to the original tunnel without removing fixation.
- Less than one diameter?

- Expand existing tunnel until center is optimal position. Fill the void between the posterior wall and new graft with allograft bone, core reamings, and structural graft or BPTB allograft with large bone plug.
- Potential for tunnel overlap causing the graft to fall posteriorly into the old tunnel: Recommend bone grafting and staged revision.[7]

Graft fixation: Consider dual fixation.

SURGICAL PROCEDURES

One-Stage Technique

Perform examination under anesthesia and diagnostic arthroscopy.

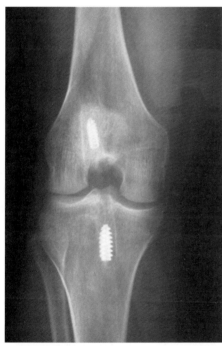

FIG 55.12 Anteroposterior (AP) x-ray with vertically oriented femoral and tibial tunnels.

- Débride the previous ACL graft.
- After the available landmarks are visible, a complete evaluation of the tunnel location is possible.
  Remove tibial interference screw (if necessary).
- The remaining tibial defect can be filled by packing it with bone graft from the drilling of the revised tunnel or allograft croutons.
- Consider replacing a metal interference screw with a bioabsorbable screw and drill through a portion of the screw.
  Insert guide pins for new femoral tunnel prior to hardware removal.
- If the previous interference screws can be bypassed with the new tunnels, simply drill the tunnel in standard fashion.[25]
- If the guide pin placement is satisfactory, with the retained hardware partially interfering with new tunnel placement, and it appears that adequate fixation can be obtained with the hardware in place, then drill through a portion of the retained hardware.[25]
  - Bioabsorbable interference screws are easily drilled through.
  - Metal screws and implants are typically made from softer alloys, making it possible to drill through a small portion thereof.
- If the retained hardware blocks guide pin placement or completely interferes with drilling the new tunnel, or if there is excessive tunnel widening that would prevent adequate fixation, the hardware should be removed and bone void filler should be used (multiple options; see earlier).
  Use of allograft bone dowels (Fig. 55.14).[3,4]
- First, débride the previous tunnel.
- Insert the Beath pin into the center of the tunnel (confirm fluoroscopically).
- Sequential reaming of the tunnel is performed.
  - Start with an 8-mm diameter reamer, and continue until a satisfactory tunnel is created for the allograft bone dowel, with fresh bone margins.
- Select correct size of dowel, and insert arthroscopically (Fig. 55.15).
- Use an over-the-top guide to insert the guide pin in an acceptable position.
- Drill the tunnel over the guide pin.

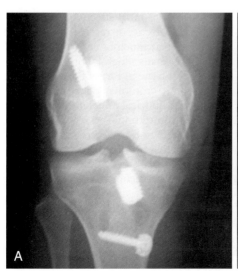
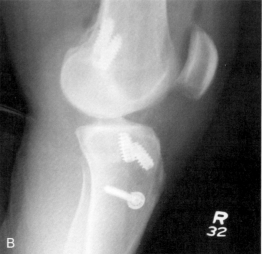

FIG 55.13 Postoperative anterior cruciate ligament (ACL) revision (A) anteroposterior (AP) and (B) lateral x-rays showing divergently placed femoral and tibial tunnels.

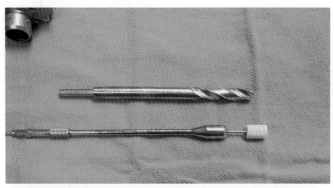

FIG 55.14 Allograft bone dowel and instrumentation for insertion.

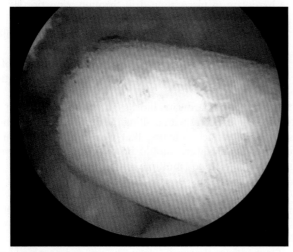

FIG 55.15 Intraoperative photo of dowel being inserted arthroscopically.

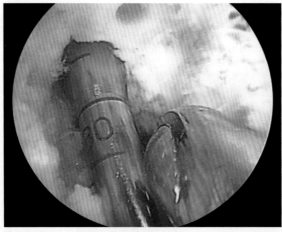

FIG 55.16 New tunnel being drilled adjacent to old tunnel. Note that the allograft bone is partially overdrilled.

- Allograft bone dowel provides sufficient support to allow redrilling of the new tunnels immediately adjacent to the old tunnels (Fig. 55.16).
  Alternatively, replace metal interference screw with bioabsorbable screw of same size.

- Drill the tunnel in standard fashion.
- Insert an ACL graft through the tunnels.
- Use dual fixation (see Fig. 55.10).
  Carry out accelerated rehabilitation protocol postoperatively.

Two-Stage Technique

First Stage. Plan skin incisions carefully to avoid skin sloughing and infection.
- Use previous incision when possible.
  Perform examination under anesthesia.
- Assess medial collateral ligament (MCL) and posteromedial and posterolateral corners.
  Perform diagnostic arthroscopy.
- Address meniscal and chondral lesions.
  Send cultures and biopsy tissue (if infection is suspected).
  Remove hardware (if necessary).
- Universal screw removal sets (see Fig. 55.6) should be available.
- Use adequate soft tissue débridement for proper seating of screw and proper angle of screwdriver to avoid stripping.
  - Metal cross pins (Mitek Slingshot, DePuy Mitek, Raynham, Massachusetts; see Fig. 55.2) may be especially challenging. The bone grows into the hex head, so there is usually a need to overdrill and pull out as a plug, leaving a larger defect than anticipated.
- Bioabsorbable screws may soften or fragment on removal.
  - May still be present several years after implantation, depending on the type of polymer
  Remove previous tendon graft.
- Autograft or allograft should be débrided completely.
- Prosthetic graft should be removed en bloc.[30]
  - Create synthetic fiber particles that incite inflammatory response.
  - May cause more synovitis and scarring.[32]
  Perform revision notchplasty, as needed.
- Notch overgrowth and osteophyte formation are common after primary procedure.
- Resect bone from roof and lateral wall of notch similar to primary procedure.
  Bone graft tunnel
- Identify previous tunnels.
- Débride sclerotic walls of tunnel.
  - A reamer is most effective (Fig. 55.17).
  - A drill, curette, or rasp may also be used.
  - Preserve as much bone as possible.
- Autograft versus allograft bone is patient and cost dependent.
  - Harvest bone in form of dowel grafts from the iliac crest.
  - Allograft croutons (dried morsellized bone) or freeze-dried cylindrical bone graft
- Pack graft into tunnel.
  - On the femoral side, use a bone tamp or screwdriver to ensure that graft is well packed (Fig. 55.18).
  - On the tibial side, be careful not to breach the joint.
  Confirm arthroscopically that the graft is not within the joint.

Interim. Repeat imaging (x-ray or CT scan) 12 to 16 weeks later to assess healing of the bone graft (Fig. 55.19).

Second Stage. Examination under anesthesia and diagnostic arthroscopy
- Assess previous tunnel sites that were bone-grafted during the first stage.

Graft harvest
- Choice of graft is dependent on its availability and individualized to the patient.

Revision ACL technique is similar to the primary procedure.
- Drill tunnels anatomically.
  - Landmarks may be less distinct; consider intraoperative imaging.
- Consider dual fixation.

Carry out accelerated rehabilitation protocol postoperatively.

CASE EXAMPLES

Case 1

(See video on website.)

A 23-year-old female soccer player with a history of a left knee ACL reconstruction with a hamstring allograft 5 years ago presented complaining of left knee pain and instability after a noncontact injury 1 week prior to presentation. She had an uneventful postoperative course, participated in aggressive rehabilitation, and returned to full activity without difficulty until the most recent injury. Her physical examination revealed a trace effusion, a 3+ Lachman test with no endpoint, and a 3+ pivot shift test. Her x-rays (Fig. 55.20) and MRI scans (Fig. 55.21) confirmed a complete tear of the ACL graft and showed adequate tibial and femoral tunnel location with a metal cross pin fixation device on the femur. The patient was consented for a two-stage revision ACL reconstruction because of the expected challenges in removing the metal cross pin device and potential for creating a large transverse bone defect after removal.

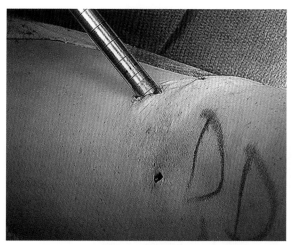

FIG 55.17 Débriding sclerotic bone of old tibial tunnel with reamer.

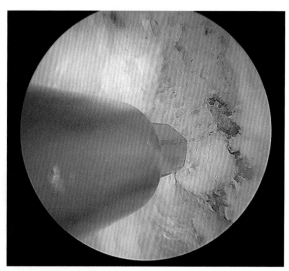

FIG 55.18 Packing allograft cancellous bone chips in femoral tunnel with screwdriver.

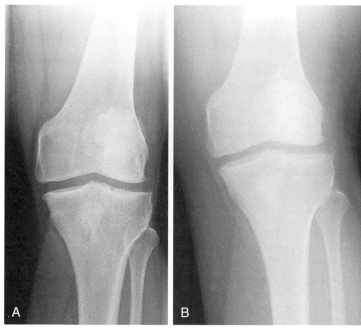

FIG 55.19 (A) Anteroposterior (AP) x-ray at 6 weeks postoperatively showing bone graft in tunnels. (B) AP x-ray at 16 weeks postoperatively showing consolidated and healed bone graft.

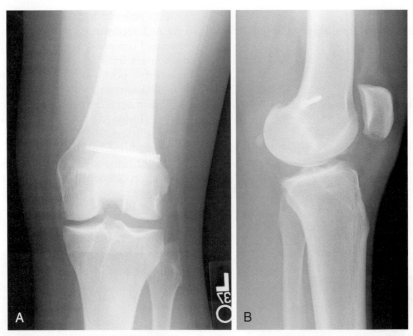

FIG 55.20 (A) Anteroposterior (AP) and (B) lateral x-rays showing metal cross pin fixation in the femur.

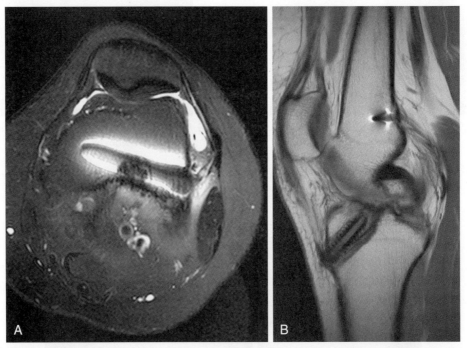

FIG 55.21 (A) Axial and (B) saggital MRI images confirming adequate tunnel location and minimal osteolysis.

During the first procedure, the screw was removed through the previous lateral incision and the resulting defect was packed with cancellous allograft chips. Next, a diagnostic arthroscopy was performed and a small area of chondromalacia was addressed with a shaving chondroplasty. The intercondylar notch was débrided, and the previous tunnel was identified (Fig. 55.22). The tibial and femoral tunnels were reamed to remove sclerotic bone. The articular surface of the tibial tunnel was preserved so that the bone graft did not enter the joint. The femoral and tibial tunnels were then packed tightly with cancellous chips using a bone tamp.

Consolidation of the bone graft was confirmed 4 months postoperatively radiographically (Fig. 55.23). Subsequently, the patient underwent the second-stage procedure. Once again, the notch was débrided, and a revision notchplasty was performed. The lateral wall of the femoral condyle was carefully assessed and there was no evidence of a previous tunnel (Fig. 55.24). The new tibial and femoral tunnels were drilled in standard fashion (Fig. 55.25).

Case 2

(See video on website.)

A 17-year-old male with a history of a right knee ACL reconstruction with a BPTB autograft and a partial lateral meniscectomy 1 year ago presented complaining of right knee pain and swelling after being kicked in his knee playing soccer. He had returned to full activity without difficulty. In the clinic, he was noted to have a positive Lachman test and an effusion. Radiographs demonstrated acceptable but not ideal tunnel positioning, without evidence of significant widening and metal

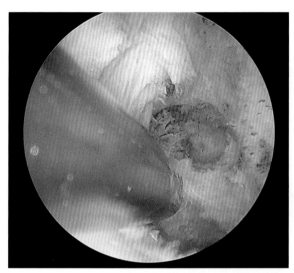

FIG 55.22 Débridement of notch and identification of old femoral tunnel.

interference screws (Fig. 55.26). The femoral tunnel appeared slightly anterior. An MRI was obtained, which confirmed the diagnosis of an ACL tear and further defined tunnel location. Based on the preoperative workup, the surgical plan was to keep the existing hardware in place, attempt to bypass the old tunnels, and drill new tunnels in more anatomic alignment. If the tunnels could not be bypassed, an attempt would be made to drill through a portion of the screw or remove the screw and fill it with bone void filler (bioabsorbable screw or allograft bone dowel).

At surgery, the diagnostic arthroscopy demonstrated a complete tear of his ACL graft. A hamstring tendon autograft (semitendinosus and gracilus [ST and G]) was harvested from the ipsilateral side. The ACL stump on the tibial and femoral surfaces was débrided, and the previous tunnel locations were identified. The femoral tunnel was noted to be slightly vertical and anterior (Fig. 55.27). Next, an attempt was made to drill the tibial tunnel. A guide wire was passed into the tibial tunnel in a satisfactory position; however, the previous metal interference screw blocked the drill (Fig. 55.28). The old interference screw was then removed (Fig. 55.29A), and a matching bioabsorbable interference screw was inserted and used as a bone void filler (see Fig. 55.29B). The tibial tunnel was then drilled partly through the edge of the new bioabsorbable screw. Next, an over-the-top guide was used to insert the femoral guide pin in a more horizontal and posterior location to bypass the previous hardware completely. The femoral tunnel was drilled without interference, and the posterior cortex remained intact (Fig. 55.30). The graft was then passed (Fig. 55.31), and satisfactory fixation was obtained. The patient was discharged home and participated in an accelerated ACL rehabilitation without complications.

Case 3

A 29-year-old man who previously had an ACL reconstruction with an allograft 2 years earlier presented to our clinic

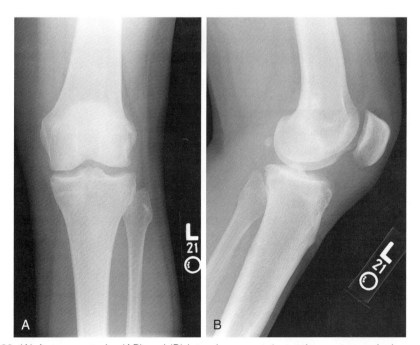

FIG 55.23 (A) Anteroposterior (AP) and (B) lateral x-rays at 4 months postoperatively confirming healing of bone graft in tunnels.

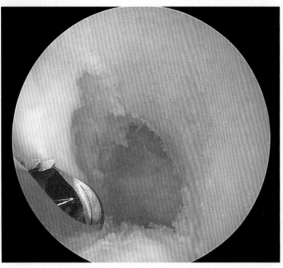

FIG 55.24 Revision notchplasty with no evidence of previous femoral tunnel.

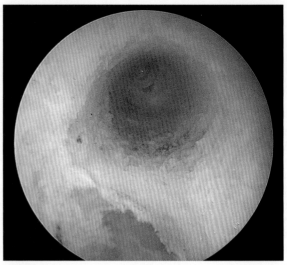

FIG 55.25 New femoral tunnel drilled in anatomic location with intact posterior wall.

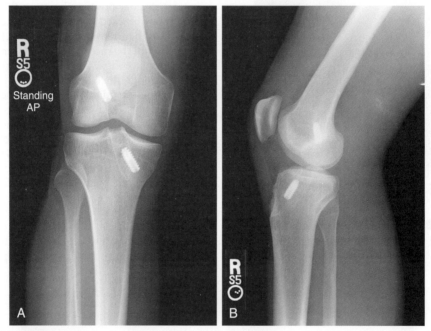

FIG 55.26 (A) Anteroposterior (AP) and (B) lateral x-rays showing acceptable but not ideal tunnel position without significant tunnel widening.

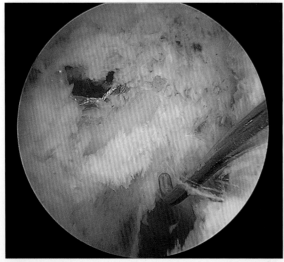

FIG 55.27 Previous tunnel with metal interference screw in a slightly anterior location.

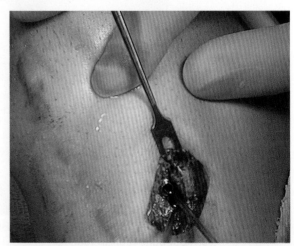

FIG 55.28 Guide wire placed for new tibial tunnel. Metal interference screw blocks drilling of tunnel.

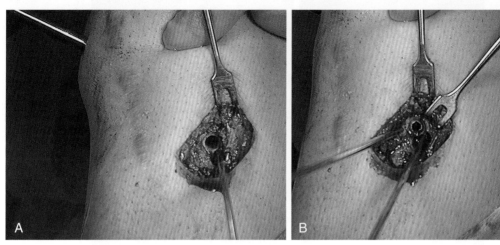

FIG 55.29 (A and B) Metal interference screw removed and replaced by bioabsorbable screw.

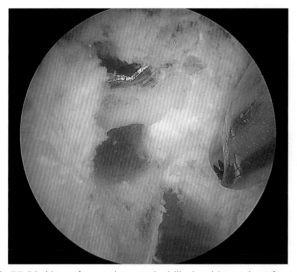

FIG 55.30 New femoral tunnel drilled without interference from previous tunnel.

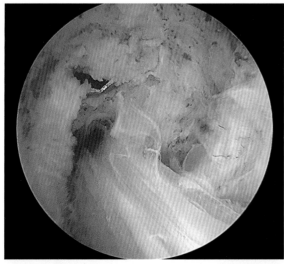

FIG 55.31 Graft inserted and fixed.

complaining of left knee pain and swelling after a twisting injury while playing softball. On examination, he had positive Lachman and pivot shift tests.

Radiographs revealed a metal interference screw in the femur and a screw and washer construct on the tibia. There was significant tunnel osteolysis and a malpositioned femoral tunnel (vertical and anterior; Fig. 55.32). An MRI was subsequently performed, which confirmed the diagnosis of an ACL graft tear (Fig. 55.33A) and again demonstrated significant tunnel osteolysis (see Fig. 55.33B). The patient was consented to undergo a single-stage ACL revision using a hamstring autograft. Although it was thought that this could be performed in one procedure with the use of a cylindric allograft dowel, the patient was informed that if adequate fixation could not be obtained intraoperatively, the surgery might have to be staged.

The patient was subsequently taken to the operating room, and a diagnostic arthroscopy confirmed a complete tear of the ACL graft (Fig. 55.34). The graft was débrided, previous hardware was removed, and the tunnels were débrided with a 12-mm reamer (Fig. 55.35). A 12 × 18 mm cylindrical allograft dowel was then inserted into the prepared femoral tunnel, completely filling the bone void. A guide pin was inserted in the standard fashion, and the tunnel was drilled through a portion of the allograft (Fig. 55.36). The graft was passed into position, and two methods of fixation were used to secure it into position.

OUTCOMES

Currently, no study has directly evaluated the outcomes of one-stage versus two-stage revision ACL reconstructions. However, there have been a few studies that have evaluated one-stage and two-stage revisions versus primary ACL reconstructions. Weiler et al.[35] have evaluated the outcomes of single-stage revision ACL reconstructions versus primary ACL reconstructions with autologous hamstring grafts. In their prospective study, 62 patients met the inclusion criteria and were compared with a matched control group. The postoperative results demonstrated no statistical significance in the objective International Knee Documentation Committee (IKDC) rating between the primary and single-stage revisions. Despite no objective differences, there were differences in the subjective Lysholm scores and functional testing, in which the primary reconstruction group fared considerably better. The authors concluded that factors

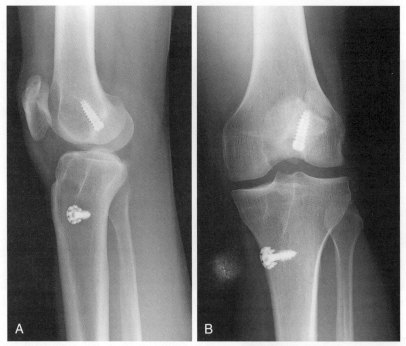

FIG 55.32 (A) Lateral and (B) anteroposterior (AP) x-rays showing a vertical and anterior femoral tunnel and moderate tunnel widening.

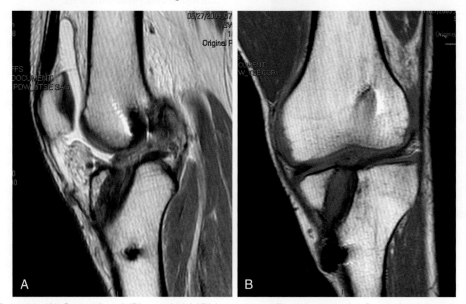

FIG 55.33 (A) Coronal and (B) saggital MRI images confirming tear of ACL graft and moderate tunnel widening.

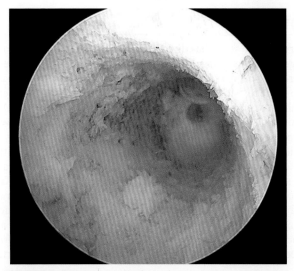

FIG 55.34 Sclerotic wall of old femoral tunnel débrided.

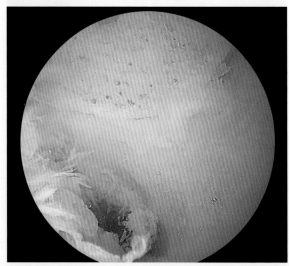

FIG 55.35 Allograft bone dowel inserted in prepared femoral tunnel.

other than objective measures were responsible for the inferior results in the revision group.

Franceschi et al.[10] published outcomes of a group of 30 patients who underwent two-stage revision ACL reconstruction. All patients experienced ACL rerupture following index reconstruction with use of a bone-patellar tendon-bone autograft. Large femoral defects were filled using autograft obtained from the tibial metaphysis. CT scans were performed at the 3-month mark confirming graft integration, at which point a standard single-bundle ACL reconstruction was performed through a transtibial approach. Postoperative IKDC and Lysholm scores were significantly improved as compared with baseline levels, and 20 of the 30 patients returned to the same preoperative sport activity level, leading the authors to conclude that their two-stage approach is a safe and effective procedure for patients with large femoral defects precluding a single-stage procedure.

In another study by Thomas et al.[32] a prospective study comparing the results of a two-stage revision versus a primary ACL reconstruction was performed. They looked at 49 consecutive two-stage revisions and compared the results to that of a matched group that underwent a primary ACL reconstruction. Unlike in the study by Weiler et al.[35] a significant difference between the objective IKDC scores was found in those who underwent primary and two-stage revisions. Overall, the patients who underwent a two-stage ACL revision had a greater degree of passive range of motion deficits, as well as crepitus. The IKDC subjective score was 61.2 in the revision ACL group, whereas it was 72.8 in the primary group. They also found that, although objective scores were often similar, there were statistically significant worse subjective outcomes in patients who underwent a two-stage ACL revision compared with those who underwent a primary ACL reconstruction.

CONCLUSION

As the need for ACL revisions increases, it will be imperative for surgeons to identify the causes of failure of the primary procedure accurately and address them in a systematic fashion (Figs. 55.37 to 55.39). Pitfalls must be recognized and avoided to optimize the success of the revision procedure. The accurate placement of femoral and tibial tunnels should not be compromised by the index tunnel placement.[12] Depending on the type and location of the fixation, the location and size of the existing tunnels, and the quality of the bone, the surgeon must be prepared to use a number of different techniques. Regardless of

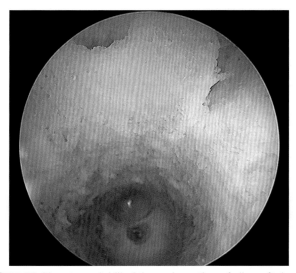

FIG 55.36 New tunnel drilled through portion of allograft dowel.

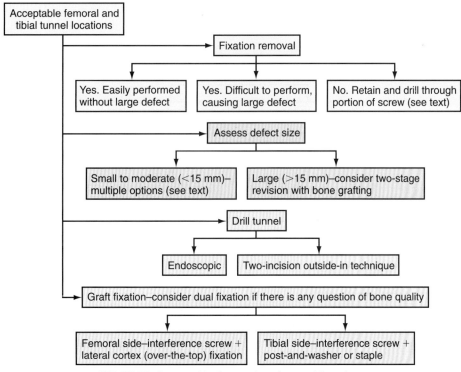

FIG 55.37 Acceptable femoral and tunnel locations.

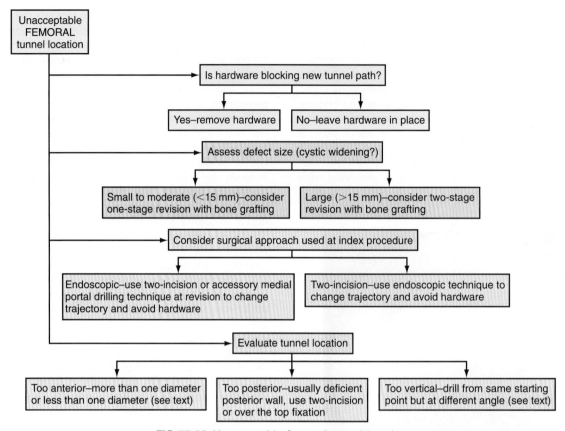

FIG 55.38 Unacceptable femoral tunnel location.

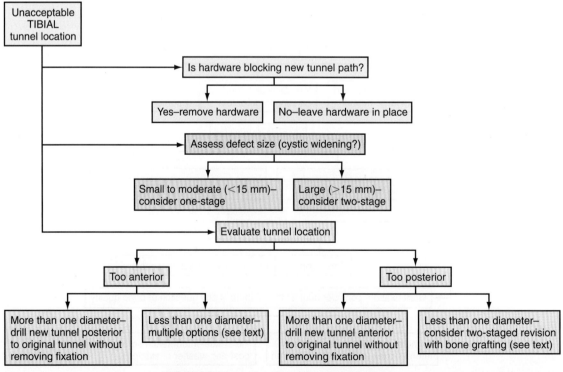

FIG 55.39 Unacceptable tibial tunnel location.

whether a one-stage or two-stage procedure is performed, the goal must be to choose an appropriate graft and fix it in anatomic position in good quality bone, similar to a primary procedure.[32] Both surgical techniques have advantages and disadvantages and should be carefully considered to meet the needs of the individual patient.

KEY REFERENCES

2. Bach BR, Jr: Revision ACL reconstrucion: indication and technique. In Miller MD, Cole BJ, editors: *Textbook of arthroscopy*, Philadelphia, 2004, WB Saunders, pp 675–686.

5. Battaglia TC, Miller MD: Management of bony deficiency in revision anterior cruciate ligament reconstruction using allograft bone dowels: surgical technique. *Arthroscopy* 21:767, 2005.

7. Brown CH, Jr, Carson EW: Revision anterior cruciate ligament surgery. *Clin Sports Med* 18:109–171, 1999.

8. Diamantopoulos AP, Lorbach O, Paessler HH: Anterior cruciate ligament revision reconstruction: results in 107 patients. *Am J Sports Med* 36:851–860, 2008.

12. George MS, Dunn WR, Spindler KP: Current concepts review: revision anterior cruciate ligament reconstruction. *Am J Sports Med* 34:2026–2037, 2006.

15. Harner CD, Giffin JR, Dunteman RC, et al: Evaluation and treatment of recurrent instability after anterior cruciate ligament reconstruction. *J Bone Joint Surg Am* 82:1652–1664, 2000.

20. Lind M, Menhert F, Pedersen AB: The first results from the Danish ACL reconstruction registry: epidemiologic and 2 year follow-up results from 5,818 knee ligament reconstructions. *Knee Surg Sports Traumatol Arthrosc* 17:117–124, 2009.

25. Miller MD: Revision cruciate ligament surgery with retention of femoral interference screws. *Arthroscopy* 14:111–114, 1998.

32. Thomas NP, Kankate R, Wandless F, et al: Revision anterior cruciate ligament reconstruction using a 2-stage technique with bone grafting of the tibial tunnel. *Am J Sports Med* 33:1701–1709, 2005.

35. Weiler A, Schmeling A, Stohr I, et al: Primary versus single-stage revision anterior cruciate ligament reconstruction using autologous hamstring tendon grafts: a prospective matched-group analysis. *Am J Sports Med* 35:1643–1652, 2007.

The references for this chapter can also be found on www.expertconsult.com.

56

Osteotomy and the Cruciate-Deficient Knee

Sebastiano Vasta, Biagio Zampogna, Annunziato Amendola

Estimates report 100,000 new anterior cruciate ligament (ACL) injuries each year in the United States, with an overall incidence of 1/300,000 people.[18] ACL injuries are frequently associated with dysfunction and impairment caused by knee joint instability, loss of proprioception, chondral and meniscal injuries, reduced quadriceps strength, and changes in the biomechanics of knee, with the risk of subsequent posttraumatic arthritis. Risk factors associated with ACL injury and implicated in the development of posttraumatic knee arthritis are meniscal injury, osteochondral pathology, malalignment, high levels of activity, genetic predisposition, obesity, age, and participating in high-level sports activities involving cutting, pivoting, and twisting.[12,32] Long-term follow-up has shown that, although ACL reconstruction helps in restoring knee stability, it has only minimal effect on the development of osteoarthritis (OA)[5,14,50]

CRUCIATE INJURY AND ARTHROSIS

In general, instability of the knee is not well tolerated and eventually posttraumatic arthritis develops. There is a significant amount of literature regarding ACL deficiency and posttraumatic arthritis. Some authors have reported the development of knee OA after ACL injury in 50% of patients on average.[12,31] Others have reported the development of OA in up to 70% of patients with combined ACL and meniscal injuries at 15 to 20 years after injury.[23] Results from a recent meta-analysis demonstrated that after an ACL injury, independent from an associated meniscal injury, there is a greater risk (almost 5 times) to developing grade III or IV radiologic changes compared with the contralateral knees without a history of an ACL injury.[2]

In a systematic review, Øiestad et al.[40] indicated that the most accurate report of knee OA after isolated injury could be as low as 0% to 13% and a prevalence of knee OA in combined ACL and meniscal injuries as high as 21% to 48%. Meniscal resection at the time of ACL reconstruction is a strong risk factor for OA of the medial compartment, with an odds ratio of 3.6.[5]

In the case of ACL deficiency and underlying varus malalignment, with the loss of neuromuscular control, the knee is more likely to go into increased varus and overload the medial compartment. The varus knee with radiographic separation of the lateral tibiofemoral compartment and increased external rotation and hyperextension with an abnormal varus recurvatum position is referred to as a triple varus knee.[9,39] Medial joint pain, instability, and early degenerative joint disease may result in patients with this clinical scenario.

The medial compartment tends to have a posterior medial tibial plateau wear pattern in the triple varus knees (Fig. 56.1).

This is thought to be caused by a chronic anterior subluxation of the tibia with respect to the femur.[8] This pattern is further exacerbated by medial meniscal insufficiency. As the degenerative process progresses and the arthritic changes occur, the knee becomes less unstable. The patient begins to have arthritis-type complaints rather than instability complaints.

It is important to differentiate the cause of the patient's complaints. The surgeon must determine whether he or she is suffering from underlying instability or if the complaints are caused by degenerative joint disease. The surgeon can differentiate between the two by determining which activities cause symptoms. It is important to distinguish whether the patient is complaining of pain with aggressive activities and pivoting types of movement, indicating instability, or of pain with activities of daily living, indicating arthrosis.

Posterior cruciate ligament (PCL)-deficient knees are susceptible to posterior tibial subluxation and posterior instability.[33] Mavrodontidis et al.[37] have discussed two cases of rapid development of posttraumatic arthritis after failed PCL reconstruction. Instability of the knee joint leads to progressive knee arthritis. Much attention is devoted to soft tissue reconstruction, but surgeons may choose to ignore correctable risk factors for reconstruction failure, such as joint malalignment. Frequently, joint malalignment contributes to the ligamentous injury prior to the discussion of reconstruction ever occurring. Geissler and Whipple[19] found a 49% incidence of chondral defects and 36% incidence of meniscal tears in patients with chronic PCL instability. Keller et al.[26] reviewed 40 PCL-deficient patients treated nonoperatively and found that 90% complained of knee pain with activity at 4 years from the time of injury, and only 12% of patients had normal-appearing radiographs. Clancy et al.[11] found that 48% of patients with chronic PCL injuries had moderate-to-severe articular injury to the medial femoral condyle at the time of surgical reconstruction.

Posterior tibial slope and its relationship to instability in cruciate deficiency is also something to consider, particularly when considering osteotomy in these patients. Bonin et al.[8] have described the relationship of pathologic tibial slope and incidence of ACL injury. The greater the slope, the greater the incidence of ACL instability. Giffin et al.,[21,22] Agneskirchner et al.,[1] and Dejour and Bonin[15] have shown that increasing tibial slope alters tibial translation, and this is amplified in the cruciate-deficient knee (Fig. 56.2). Conversely, it has been demonstrated that in the setting of a PCL/posterolateral corner lesion (PLC), increasing posterior tibial slope diminishes static posterior instability, although it has little effect on rotational or dynamic multiplanar instability.[41] Literature shows that soft tissue procedures alone are often unsatisfactory for chronic

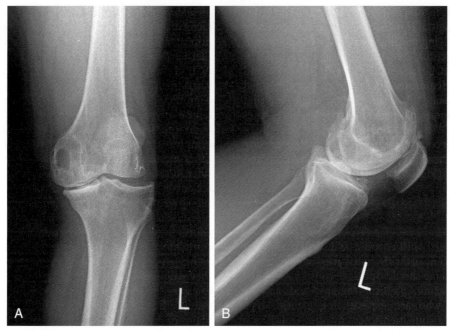

FIG 56.1 Anteroposterior (AP) (A) and lateral (B) views of a 50-year-old male chronic ACL-deficient patient with medial compartment OA, varus alignment, and no previous surgery. Note the medial wear on the AP view and the posterior wear pattern on the lateral view caused by chronic anterior subluxation.

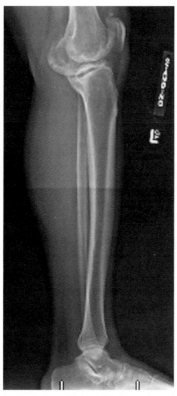

FIG 56.2 Long lateral view of the tibia in a chronic ACL-deficient patient. Note the increased posterior slope and anterior subluxation of the proximal tibia.

posterior instability if alignment is not corrected. In the case of a chronic PCL-deficient knee, with or without a PLC injury, it has been suggested to correct varus deformity and increase tibial slope by means of an opening wedge medial high tibial osteotomy (HTO), reserving soft tissue procedures as a second line of treatment when the patient is still unstable after bony procedure.[38,44]

INDICATIONS FOR OSTEOTOMY

Osteotomies have been used for localized medial and lateral compartment gonarthrosis with varus and valgus malalignment. The principle supporting the use of tibial osteotomy is redistribution of the mechanical force across the joint. Coventry[13] initially described the indications for HTO to include stable knees with no subluxation or thrust, range of motion (ROM) of at least 15 to 100 degrees, localized medial compartment OA, minimal or no patellofemoral symptoms, and age younger than 65 years. Indications for HTOs have since expanded for cases of posterior instability, ACL deficiency, and correcting tibial slope in sagittal instability.[16,39] The senior author's indications for osteotomy in the setting of instability are found in Box 56.1.

In the setting of ACL insufficiency with symptomatic instability and pathologic sagittal tibial slope, one should consider correction of the underlying malalignment issue in addition to ligamentous reconstruction. Previous observations of an increased incidence of ACL tears with increased tibial slope and biomechanical studies demonstrating increased anterior tibial translation with increasing tibial slope have suggested that decreasing the tibial slope would provide a more stable biomechanical environment[15,21,22] (Figs. 56.3 to 56.8). The PCL-deficient knee presents a contrary situation in which decreasing tibial slope causes an increase in posterior tibial translation and symptoms of instability (Fig. 56.9).

TREATMENT OF CRUCIATE DEFICIENCY AND ARTHROSIS

If the patient is diagnosed with chronic ACL deficiency with early medial compartment arthritis and varus malalignment with overload, the physician should optimize conservative care, including unloader bracing, physical therapy, and activity modification. Patients who are experiencing arthritis-type symptoms related to previous meniscectomy, mechanical axis deviation into the medial compartment, and early medial compartment degenerative changes may benefit from an HTO. The painful symptoms from degenerative joint disease secondary to underlying instability and previous injury are termed *pseudoinstability*. In the setting of previously failed soft tissue reconstruction, one must consider malalignment as a contributing factor. A cadaveric study from van de Pol et al.[52] shows that varus malalignment creates higher forces on the ACL or ACL graft, especially for higher varus degrees associated with varus thrust. Therefore the authors suggest addressing the varus alignment with a high tibial valgus osteotomy to prevent a failure of the reconstructed ACL.

In the setting of a younger patient who is experiencing symptoms of instability with underlying malalignment and other meniscal or chondral pathology, the surgeon could consider ACL reconstruction in addition to an osteotomy. Surgeons are currently pushing the limits for ACL reconstruction in older yet active patients with complaints of instability.

To determine whether an ACL reconstruction is indicated in addition to HTO, the physician must consider the patient's complaints at the time of initial presentation. If an older or less active patient is suffering from mechanical overload and pain, they will likely respond to the osteotomy alone. It is important to assess the entire clinical picture and differentiate pseudo-instability from true instability. If the patient continues to complain of instability after HTO, ACL reconstruction can be considered as a secondary procedure. However, ACL reconstruction alone in the face of malalignment is doomed for continuing symptoms of compartment overload and early failure of the ACL surgery.

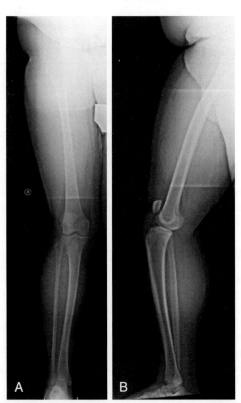

FIG 56.3 X-ray, right long leg AP (A) and lateral (B) view of a 21-year-old male affected by valgus alignment of the right knee with increased anterior tibial slope and tibial translation, in the setting of a congenital ACL absence.

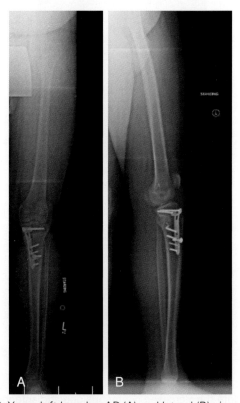

FIG 56.4 X-ray, left long leg AP (A) and lateral (B) view. The left knee was in varus alignment, and it was previously addressed by another surgeon with a medial opening wedge HTO. Notice the iatrogenic increased left tibial slope. This is a complication of opening wedge HTO that the surgeon must avoid, especially in an ACL-deficient knee.

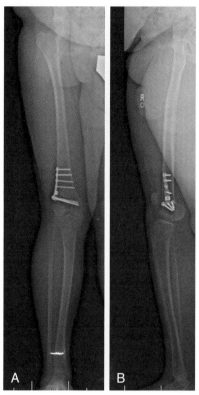

FIG 56.5 The right knee of the patient was addressed by lateral opening wedge distal femur osteotomy. The gap was bonegrafted with bone from a homologous femoral head. X-ray, long leg AP view (A) and long leg lateral view (B) of the right lower limb showing good coronal alignment 6 weeks after lateral distal femur opening wedge osteotomy (DFO), but increased tibial slope (approximately 20 degrees) and anterior translation on the sagittal plane.

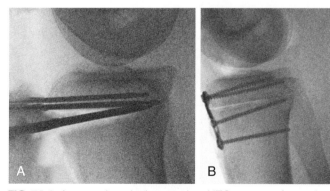

FIG 56.6 An anterior closing wedge HTO was performed to correct malalignment on the sagittal plane. At the same time the ACL was reconstructed to improve knee stability and reduce anterior tibial translation. Intraoperative fluoroscopic view: guide pins and osteotome into the osteotomy wedge (A). Fixation with plate and screw (B).

PREOPERATIVE EVALUATION

Factors considered in the preoperative evaluation and indication for osteotomy include the following: (1) pure valgus or varus malalignment; (2) loss of neuromuscular control associated with ligament injury and loss of proprioceptive feedback

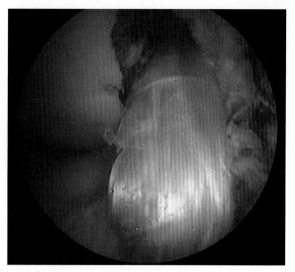

FIG 56.7 Intraoperative scope view after anterior cruciate ligament reconstruction at the same time of anterior closing wedge high tibial osteotomy.

(thrust during stance); (3) abnormal sagittal slope in the setting of ACL or PCL insufficiency; (4) triple varus knee; and (5) unicompartmental degeneration (usually a postmeniscectomy knee).

The preoperative examination should include a detailed history, clinical examination, and imaging studies. Physical examination findings supportive of an osteotomy include joint line tenderness, abnormal gait patterns, with special attention to lateral thrust, and limb alignment in stance. Attention is directed toward instability tests including Lachman, pivot shift, anterior and posterior drawer, reverse pivot shift, and external rotation tests. The examiner should note the double or triple varus knee associated with ACL, PCL, or posterolateral corner deficiency.

Radiographic evaluation begins with assessment of the extent of knee arthrosis and lower extremity alignment with bilateral standard weight-bearing long leg (hip to ankle) anteroposterior (AP) views, standard AP views in full extension, bilateral weight-bearing posteroanterior tunnel views in 30 degrees of flexion, and lateral and Merchant patellar views. Dugdale et al.[17] have described the technique used to calculate the HTO correction. The mechanical axis and weight-bearing axis are determined, and the correction to be made is calculated just lateral to the lateral tibial spine (Fig. 56.10).

Magnetic resonance imaging (MRI) evaluation is helpful for preoperative planning. The astute clinician can determine ACL or PCL insufficiency from the examination, but advanced imaging provides additional information that is often useful in determining soft tissue repair and reconstruction, in addition to the osteotomy, which is determined from plain films and the clinical examination. The senior author uses MRI to evaluate chondral, meniscal, and soft tissue injury, in addition to subtle osseous findings that plain film radiographs are often not sensitive enough to demonstrate.

In active patients who hope to return to a high activity level, we plan the osteotomy so that it will place the weight-bearing line—as measured from the center of the femoral head to the center of the tibiotalar joint—through the center of the knee joint. This is described as just lateral to the tibial spine (or 62%

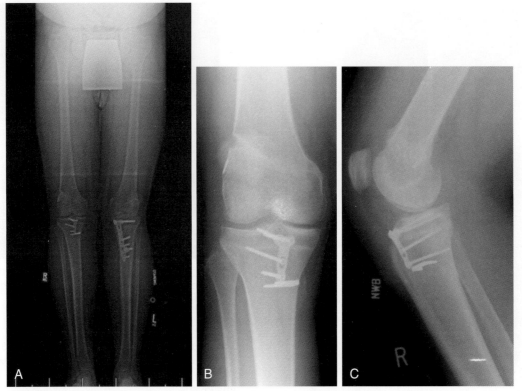

FIG 56.8 X-ray, long leg AP (A), short leg AP (B) and lateral (C) view of the right knee: consolidation of the osteotomy 3 months after anterior closing wedge HTO, ACL reconstruction and DFO plate removal. Notice the improved tibial slope and sagittal alignment.

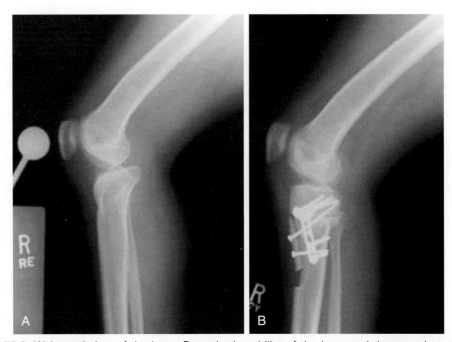

FIG 56.9 (A) Lateral view of the knee. Posterior instability of the knee and decreased posterior tibial slope accentuates posterior subluxation and hyperextension. (B) Same patient treated with proximal tibial osteotomy to increase the slope and prevent hyperextension and posterior instability. Note the improved slope and decreased posterior subluxation. The tibial tubercle osteotomy was performed to move the tubercle proximally to prevent patella baja.

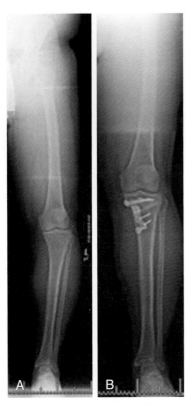

FIG 56.10 (A) Hip to ankle x-ray (the patient is standing with equal weight on both legs) to measure preoperative varus deformity. (B) Postoperative correction of varus deformity with medial opening wedge osteotomy.

of the width of the joint surface referenced from medial joint line). Some authors have recommended overcorrection in the setting of medial compartment arthritis. We do not perform significant overcorrection in younger patients; rather, our goal is to re-create neutral alignment and unload the previously overloaded medial compartment in the varus knee. In the setting of an arthritic knee with ACL or PCL insufficiency, the goal of the osteotomy is to achieve the desired posterior tibial slope in the sagittal plane and thus obtain enhanced stability of the knee (Fig. 56.11).[1,16,21,22,42]

The surgeon must exercise caution in the setting of severe deformity because the accuracy of correction may be more difficult to determine (Fig. 56.12). Patients with osteoporosis present challenges in obtaining suitable fixation and can require prolonged periods for healing. Other considerations must be given to risk factors for failure, including smokers, prolonged dependency of corticosteroids, immunosuppressants, and chronic illness.

SURGICAL PROCEDURE

Authors' Preferred Technique

We prefer the medial opening wedge osteotomy to the lateral closing wedge osteotomy because, in our experience, precise correction is more likely and overcorrection is less likely. Although this approach increases the stability of a malaligned knee, it also avoids osteotomy of the proximal fibula, thereby avoiding potential instability through the tibiofibular joint and posterolateral corner structures and injury to the peroneal

nerve.[10,28,51] The medial opening wedge incision also provides access to the hamstring autograft in the setting of ACL reconstruction. This approach also allows for correction in the coronal and sagittal planes. We use an opening wedge plating system from Arthrex (Naples, Florida). Another advantage of the medial opening wedge tibial osteotomy is that the risk of inadvertently altering the normal tibia slope is decreased. Amendola et al.[4] have shown that by avoiding osteotomy of the proximal fibula, as with a lateral closing wedge technique, the tibial slope will be forced to decrease because of hinging at the proximal tibiofibular joint.

Operative Procedure With Anterior Cruciate Ligament Reconstruction

The patient is administered prophylactic intravenous antibiotics preoperatively. The patient is then positioned supine, and the involved limb is prepared and draped in standard fashion. Arthroscopy using low pressures and frequent compartment checks is performed to evaluate the condition of the articular cartilage and menisci. After the arthroscopy has been completed, the extremity is elevated and exsanguinated, and the tourniquet is used for the remainder of the osteotomy procedure.

The senior author does not perform any articular cartilage resurfacing procedures, such as autologous chondrocyte implantation (ACI) or meniscal transplantation, at the time of this surgery. If they are required, surgery is staged; the osteotomy is performed first, followed by soft tissue reconstruction after the patient has recovered from the osteotomy.

To close the osteotomy wedge anteriorly, a bump is placed underneath the leg to hyperextend the knee. This decreases the tibial slope and thus decreases anterior tibial translation in the ACL-deficient knee.

A vertical incision is made over the pes anserinus insertion halfway between the medial border of the patellar tendon and the posterior margin of the tibia. This is followed by exposure and incision of the sartorial fascia and finally by subperiosteal elevation of the medial collateral ligament (MCL). Blunt retractors are then placed anteriorly to protect the patellar ligament and posteriorly to protect the hamstring tendons and superficial MCL.

Under fluoroscopic control, a guidewire is drilled across the proximal tibia from medial to lateral. The guide is positioned at the level of the superior aspect of the tibial tubercle and oriented obliquely to the end, at least 1 cm below the joint line at the lateral tibial cortex. By aiming approximately 1 cm below the lateral joint line, we can stay proximal to the patellar tendon insertion and still be sufficiently inferior to the articular surface to prevent intra-articular fracture during the cut. The osteotomy maximizes the metaphyseal location and likelihood of healing. If the osteotomy cut is too distal, it becomes extracapsular, thereby reducing the stability of the osteotomy site. The osteotomy is performed with an oscillating saw below the guide pin to prevent superior migration and decrease risk of an intra-articular fracture. The osteotomy is deepened with flexible and rigid osteotomes, using fluoroscopic confirmation.

After the osteotomy has been completed, the medial opening is created with an osteotomy wedge to the predetermined depth. Intraoperative femorotibial alignment is verified by fluoroscopy, and an extramedullary alignment guide is used to ensure that the weight-bearing axis is passing through the center of the knee joint. Sabharwal and Zhao[43] have cautioned that for obese patients or those with substantial malalignment, supine

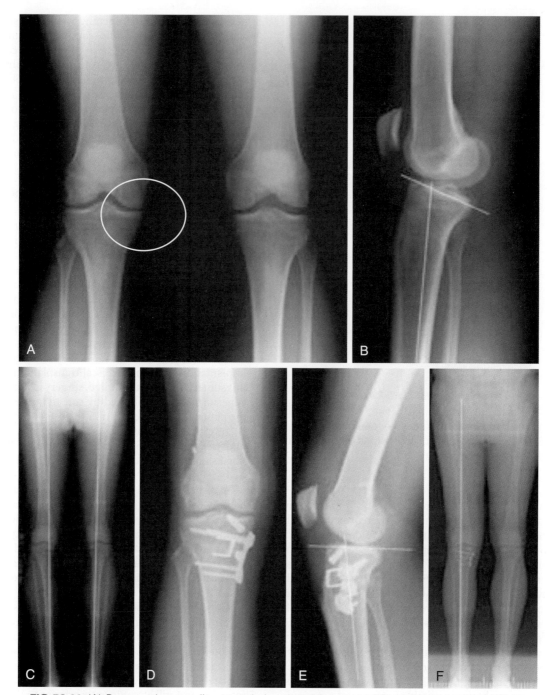

FIG 56.11 (A) Preoperative standing tunnel view in a 30-year-old ACL-deficient patient with no previous surgery. (B) Preoperative lateral view with increased lateral slope, ACL deficiency. (C) Preoperative long leg, hip to ankle radiograph demonstrating medial axis deviation, used for operative planning on the amount of correction. (D) Postoperative AP view with opening wedge osteotomy plus ACL reconstruction using allograft and interference screw fixation on the tibia and EndoButton fixation on the femur. (E) Postoperative lateral view demonstrating decrease in tibial slope to help the ACL deficiency. Often, fixation can be augmented anteriorly to close the wedge and thereby decrease the slope. (F) Postoperative long leg, standing x-ray demonstrating correction of the weight-bearing axis to the lateral tibial spine, avoiding overcorrection.

fluoroscopy alignment measurements without loading of the knee joint does not reflect the axis as accurately as preoperative standing films. In such cases, we think careful scrutinizing of the preoperative weight-bearing films and the intraoperative fluoroscopic images can still lead to favorable results.

The posterior tibial slope is also assessed intraoperatively and can be changed by distracting the osteotomy more anteriorly or posteriorly if the patient has any symptomatic cruciate deficiency or excessive AP translation preoperatively. If the opening is more than 1 cm anteriorly, a tibial tubercle osteotomy

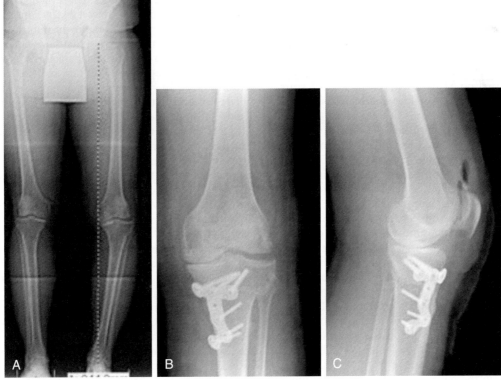

FIG 56.12 (A) Preoperative long-leg standing view from hips to ankles in a chronic anterior cruciate ligament (ACL)-deficient patient with severe deformity. (B) Postoperative anteroposterior view after dome osteotomy, which was performed rather than opening wedge for a large deformity. (C) Postoperative lateral view with decreased slope following a dome osteotomy to help the ACL instability.

is performed to advance the tubercle the same height of the osteotomy. When the desired opening has been achieved, the osteotomy is secured with a plate and bone graft (corticocancellous wedges cut from a femoral head allograft).

The plate is fixed proximally with 6.5-mm cancellous screws and distally with 4.5-mm cortical screws. Placement of fixation is confirmed with fluoroscopic imaging. The tourniquet is released and hemostasis controlled. The wound is closed in layers over a drain placed in the subcutaneous space.

The osteotomy is performed prior to drilling the tunnels for ACL reconstruction to prevent the creation of a possible stress riser through the ACL tunnel. Arthroscopically assisted ACL reconstruction is performed using standard technique with the following considerations. We drill the tibial tunnel anterior and superior to the osteotomy site. A retro drill (Arthrex) technique is useful to avoid the osteotomy site.

A femoral tunnel is drilled in the usual technique. The ACL graft is passed through the tibial tunnel and out the femoral tunnel. The senior author's preference is to use extracortical button fixation. A tibial side interference screw is placed for primary fixation proximal to the osteotomy site. Secondary fixation can be placed below the osteotomy site, if desired. Bone grafting of the osteotomy site is performed at this point (see Fig. 56.6).

POSTOPERATIVE PROTOCOL

Following surgery, the patient is allowed toe-touch weight bearing with ROM performed within a 0- to 90-degree arc for

6 weeks. It is important to begin early postoperative ROM to prevent stiffness in the knee joint. Radiographs are obtained at the 6-week postoperative appointment. If there is evidence of consolidation, the brace is discontinued and full weight bearing is initiated with a strengthening program. At the 10-week postoperative appointment, radiography is repeated. If osseous consolidation has been achieved, sport-specific rehabilitation is initiated.

OUTCOMES

HTO, in addition to ACL, reconstruction in patients with early medial compartment arthrosis has been shown to reduce symptoms and possibly reduce the progression of arthritis.[8] On a series of four patients who underwent ACL reconstruction and concomitant opening wedge HTO, Akamatsu et al.[3] reported, during a second-look arthroscopy at 24 to 64 months from the first surgery, there was no progression of cartilage deterioration in the medial side and progression from grade 1 to grade 2 in the lateral compartment, using the International Cartilage Research Society score. Interestingly, the authors found that in three of the four patients there was a partial tear in the anterolateral regions of the graft, in the point where the graft comes into contact with the lateral wall of the intercondylar notch, requiring notchplasty or renotchplasty. The authors speculated that the morbidity in the anterolateral region of the graft was the result of lateral rotation of the intercondylar notch relative to the tibial plateau, secondary to the changed alignment; therefore intercondylar notchplasty should be performed at the time of the initial operation. ACL tunnel placement should be performed following the osteotomy, as a means of taking this effect into consideration.

More recent studies with larger populations confirm combined procedure of ACL reconstruction with either opening or closing wedge HTO lead to satisfactory outcomes. Zaffagnini et al.[55] in 2013 reported on 34 patients aged 40.1 ± 8.1 years underwent ACL reconstruction with simultaneous lateral closing wedge HTO. Signs of severe medial OA (grade D, International Knee Documentation Committee [IKDC] radiographic score) occurred in 22% of patients at final follow-up (mean: 6.5 ± 2.7 years); nevertheless, all the outcome scores (IKDC, Tegner Activity Level, EuroQol five dimensions questionnaire (EQ-D5), visual analogue scale (VAS) for pain, KT-1000 arthrometer) were improved compared with the preoperative level. Trojani et al.[49] reported their experience on 29 patients with a mean age of 43 (range: 25 to 56) years who underwent medial opening wedge HTO and ACL reconstruction. At a mean 6-year follow-up, 23 patients returned to sports activities (45% in competitive sports); 28 were free of instability and 21 free of pain. An interesting study from Marriott et al.[34] reported on the change in gait biomechanics after concomitant HTO and ACL reconstruction, comparing the operated limbs to the nonoperated ones. After 5 years from surgery, patients showed substantial changes during walking. The authors found a substantial decrease in the knee adduction moment in the surgical limb and a slight increase in the nonsurgical limb, together with a decrease in the knee flexion moment for both the surgical and nonsurgical limbs. Because the external knee adduction moment is considered an index for the mediolateral load distribution across the knee,[25,27] and the knee flexion moment represents net flexor-extensor muscle contraction,[45] results from the study are consistent with a load shift towards the lateral compartment without increasing the total load.

The older patient with ACL deficiency who is suffering from symptoms consistent with advanced arthritis rather than instability would benefit most from joint realignment and unloading of the diseased medial compartment. Lattermann and Jakob[29] have shown that many patients older than 40 years do well with osteotomy alone and do not require later ACL reconstruction. In patients with ACL deficiency who would be indicated for an HTO alone, it is important to consider reduction of the tibial slope to reduce the tendency of the tibia to translate anterior to the femur, as is expected with chronic ACL insufficiency.

There is some discussion as to whether the young patient who is experiencing ACL-related instability, in addition to medial compartment degeneration and malalignment, should undergo a one-step or staged ACL reconstruction with HTO. We prefer to perform one definitive procedure with modern techniques and minimal morbidity. If the surgeon feels inclined to perform a two-stage reconstruction, the senior author recommends performing the HTO first because this is likely to improve symptoms of the degenerative medial compartment, in addition to improving symptoms of instability. Performing an ACL reconstruction alone will lead to inferior results, with a propensity to failure and progression of arthritic symptoms.

COMPLICATIONS

Complications associated with HTO include nonunion, fracture, hardware failure, symptomatic hardware, infection, peroneal nerve palsy, and compartment syndrome. A recent systematic review[30] on studies reporting on simultaneous HTO and ACL reconstruction shows a 24.3% complication rate. The most common were deep venous thrombosis (7.7%), stiffness (6.1%), and hematoma (2.8%). Matthews et al.[36] and Hernigou et al.[24] have noted intra-articular fractures to occur in 11% of cases in medial opening HTO and in 10% to 20% in lateral closing HTO. To avoid this complication, we stay inferior to a guide pin during the osteotomy. The guide pin is aimed 1 cm below the joint line on the lateral side to help to reduce the risk of intra-articular fracture. In the setting of an intra-articular fracture, the priority becomes congruity of the tibial plateau with stable fixation. Nonunion is a more common complication in opening wedge techniques, with risks reported from 0.7% to 4.4%.[6,47,48] Bone autograft and allograft, bone substitutes, and growth factors have been used to fill the void in opening HTO and decrease nonunion. We routinely use a femoral head allograft.

Recent research supports use of a locking plate design to enhance fixation and allow earlier weight bearing to help to decrease risk of nonunion.[53,54] The Contour Lock System (Arthrex) offers polyaxial locked fixation and less often is symptomatic than larger traditional locking plates. In our experience the Arthrex plate usually does not require a second surgery for hardware removal and has not been associated with hardware failure or nonunion. Infection risk with open reduction and internal fixation (ORIF) has been reported to be 4%.[7] The senior author has not encountered the complication of compartment syndrome; the exact incidence of compartment syndrome in HTO is unknown.[24] Nonetheless, concomitant arthroscopic procedures should increase concern and suspicion for compartment syndrome during HTO.[35] When arthroscopy is necessary, we use lower pressures and perform frequent compartment checks during the operation. Reports of the incidence of peroneal nerve palsy associated with closing wedge HTO range from 2% to 16%.[20,46]

KEY REFERENCES

1. Agneskirchner JD, Hurschler C, Stukenborg-Colsman C, et al: Effect of high tibial flexion osteotomy on cartilage pressure and joint kinematics: a biomechanical study in human cadaveric knees. Winner of the AGA-DonJoy Award 2004. *Arch Orthop Trauma Surg* 124:575–584, 2004.
2. Ajuied A, Wong F, Smith C, et al: Anterior cruciate ligament injury and radiologic progression of knee osteoarthritis: a systematic review and meta-analysis. *Am J Sports Med* 42(9):2242–2252, 2014.
4. Amendola A, Rorabeck CH, Bourne RB, et al: Total knee arthroplasty following high tibial osteotomy for osteoarthritis. *J Arthroplasty* 4(Suppl):S11–S17, 1989.
8. Bonin N, Ait Si Selmi T, Donell ST, et al: Anterior cruciate reconstruction combined with valgus upper tibial osteotomy: 12 years follow-up. *Knee* 11:431–437, 2004.
9. Brinkman JM, Lobenhoffer P, Agneskirchner JD, et al: Osteotomies around the knee: patient selection, stability of fixation and bone healing in high tibial osteotomies. *J Bone Joint Surg Br* 90:1548–1557, 2008.
12. Clatworthy M, Amendola A: The anterior cruciate ligament and arthritis. *Clin Sports Med* 18:173–198, 1999.
14. Daniel DM, Stone ML, Dobson BE, et al: Fate of the ACL-injured patient. A prospective outcome study. *Am J Sports Med* 22:632–644, 1994.
17. Dugdale TW, Noyes FR, Styer D: Preoperative planning for high tibial osteotomy. The effect of lateral tibiofemoral separation and tibiofemoral length. *Clin Orthop* 274:248–264, 1992.
22. Giffin JR, Vogrin TM, Zantop T, et al: Effects of increasing tibial slope on the biomechanics of the knee. *Am J Sports Med* 32:376–382, 2004.

24. Hernigou P, Medevielle D, Debeyre J, et al: Proximal tibial osteotomy for osteoarthritis with varus deformity. A ten- to thirteen-year follow-up study. *J Bone Joint Surg Am* 69:332–354, 1987.

28. LaPrade RF, Engebretsen L, Johansen S, et al: The effect of a proximal tibial medial opening wedge osteotomy on posterolateral knee instability: a biomechanical study. *Am J Sports Med* 36:956–960, 2008.

29. Lattermann C, Jakob RP: High tibial osteotomy alone or combined with ligament reconstruction in anterior cruciate ligament–deficient knees. *Knee Surg Sports Traumatol Arthrosc* 4:32–38, 1996.

30. Li Y, Zhang H, Zhang J, et al: Clinical outcome of simultaneous high tibial osteotomy and anterior cruciate ligament reconstruction for medial compartment osteoarthritis in young patients with anterior cruciate ligament-deficient knees: a systematic review. *Arthroscopy* 31(3):507–519, 2015.

33. MacDonald P, Miniaci A, Fowler P, et al: A biomechanical analysis of joint contact forces in the posterior cruciate deficient knee. *Knee Surg Sports Traumatol Arthrosc* 3:252–255, 1996.

41. Petrigliano FA, Suero EM, Voos JE, et al: The effect of proximal tibial slope on dynamic stability testing of the posterior cruciate ligament- and posterolateral corner-deficient knee. *Am J Sports Med* 40(6):1322–1328, 2012.

42. Phisitkul P, Wolf BR, Amendola A: Role of high tibial and distal femoral osteotomies in the treatment of lateral-posterolateral and medial instabilities of the knee. *Sports Med Arthrosc* 14:96–104, 2006.

52. van de Pol GJ, Arnold MP, Verdonschot N, et al: Varus alignment leads to increased forces in the anterior cruciate ligament. *Am J Sports Med* 37(3):481–487, 2009.

The references for this chapter can also be found on www.expertconsult.com.

57

Rehabilitation of the Surgically Reconstructed and Nonsurgical Anterior Cruciate Ligament

Thomas L. Sanders, Jonathan T. Finnoff, Diane L. Dahm

INTRODUCTION

The anterior cruciate ligament (ACL) serves multiple roles within the knee. The ACL is the primary restraint to anterior tibial translation relative to the femur. It also assists in varus and valgus knee stability, provides proprioceptive feedback, guides the "screw-home" mechanism that occurs during knee extension, and prevents knee hyperextension.[48] Consequently, ACL injuries may result in significant functional deficits. Recurrent episodes of joint instability have been associated with meniscal injury and damage to the articular cartilage. Furthermore, ACL injuries, whether treated surgically or nonsurgically, predispose to the development of knee osteoarthritis.[29,89] Whether a patient chooses surgical or nonsurgical management, rehabilitation is an integral part of the treatment program. Rehabilitation techniques have evolved substantially over the past 25 years. The goals of both a nonoperative and postoperative ACL rehabilitation program include return of neuromuscular control, strength, power, and functional symmetry.[81] This chapter will discuss current recommendations for nonoperative and postoperative rehabilitation of ACL injuries.

NONOPERATIVE REHABILITATION OF ANTERIOR CRUCIATE LIGAMENT INJURIES

Traditionally, nonoperative management of ACL injuries has been offered primarily to those participating in International Knee Documentation Committee (IKDC) level III or IV activities (Table 57.1).[68] Several studies have reported poor outcomes and limited success in returning to IKDC level I and II sports with nonoperative treatment of ACL injuries.* Furthermore, a number of studies have demonstrated that the incidence of medial meniscal tears increases over time in ACL-deficient knees, potentially predisposing patients to early-onset knee osteoarthritis.† A study by Levy and Meier[73] found the incidence of meniscal tears in chronically ACL-deficient patients to be 40% at 1 year, 60% at 5 years, and 80% by 10 years post injury. Indeed, the ACL has been referred to as "the guardian of the meniscus."[99] Ultimately, the goal of treatment following ACL injury is to provide the patient with the best functional outcome and to minimize the risk of future injury and/or development of knee osteoarthritis.

Nonoperative treatment is an appropriate option for individuals with an isolated ACL injury who lead a sedentary lifestyle, do not experience instability during activities of daily living (ADL), and have no concomitant injury requiring surgical intervention. However, in patients who participate in IKDC level I or II activities, correctly identifying individuals who can dynamically stabilize their knee (copers) is imperative to meet the goals of optimizing functional outcome and minimizing the risk of future knee injuries and knee osteoarthritis. There is evidence that individuals who meet specific post-ACL injury screening criteria and successfully complete a rehabilitation program involving both perturbation and sport-specific functional training can return to cutting, pivoting, and jumping types of sports 63% to 79% of the time without subsequent episodes of instability, injury, or reduced functional status.[32,40,62,63]

Dynamic knee stability can be defined as the ability to stabilize the knee during the rapidly changing loads created by activity[63] and is dependent upon neuromuscular control when static restraints (ie, the ACL) are absent. Also impacting the ability to regain dynamic knee stability are the proprioceptive deficits that occur in the knee following an ACL injury.‡ Correction of proprioceptive deficits has become a focus of modern nonoperative and postoperative rehabilitation programs following ACL injury.§ This is achieved through controlled stimulation of joint mechanoreceptors and muscle spindles using proprioceptive and balance exercises to increase their sensitivity and improve the ability of muscles to respond to destabilizing forces.[26]

There are a number of stabilization strategies that are used by individuals who sustain an ACL injury. Patients who experience episodes of instability and achieve poor functional outcomes (non-copers) following ACL injury attempt to stabilize their knees through excessive co-contraction of thigh musculature, reduced knee flexion during the load acceptance phase of gait, and a greater posterior tibial displacement when compared with copers and uninjured controls.[21,22,106,107] By restricting knee flexion during load acceptance, non-copers maintain a relatively extended position of the knee, which may predispose to future subluxation episodes.[58] Non-copers also preferentially recruit their quadriceps during unilateral stance postural perturbations, which may further destabilize the ACL-deficient knee.[31]

---

*References 2, 3, 8, 34, 36, 52, 70, and 118.
†References 19, 24, 25, 38, 93, 127, and 137.

‡References 9, 10, 13, 59, 84, and 129.
§References 20, 26, 81, 84, 108, and 128.

TABLE 57.1	International Knee Documentation Committee Activity Levels[53]	
Level	Sports Activity	Occupational Activity
I	Jumping, cutting pivoting	Comparable to level I sports
II	Lateral movements but less pivoting than level I sports	Heavy manual labor on uneven surfaces
III	Linear activities with no jumping or pivoting	Light manual work
IV	Sedentary activities	Activities of daily living

BOX 57.1   Nonoperative Anterior Cruciate Ligament Rehabilitation Summary

Prescreening Examination Phase

Decrease pain and effusion
Re-establish range of motion
Normalize gait pattern
Maintain cardiovascular fitness
Strengthen the trunk, hip girdle, and thigh musculature

Post-Screening Examination Phase

Restore full dynamic stability
Prepare for return to sports

Thus non-copers stabilize the knee through abnormal muscular recruitment patterns and by limiting knee movement, whereas copers attempt to normalize knee movement and recruitment patterns.

Based upon the earlier work of Eastlack et al.,[32] Fitzgerald et al.[40] developed a screening examination by which potential copers and non-copers could be distinguished. This screening examination has been used successfully by other investigators.[63,64] According to the criteria used by Fitzgerald et al.,[40] patients were not considered candidates for the screening examination and were referred to an orthopedic surgeon for ACL reconstruction surgery if they had any of the following: a fracture, repairable meniscal tear, multiligament knee injury, or a full-thickness articular cartilage lesion. In addition, patients could not have experienced more than one instability episode since sustaining the ACL injury. Prior to the screening test, patients participated in a rehabilitation program to resolve their knee effusion, restore full knee range of motion, strengthen their quadriceps muscle to 70% or greater of the isometric strength of their contralateral extremity, and improve their weight-bearing status to the point where they could hop on the injured leg without pain. Patients who did not meet these criteria after 1 month of rehabilitation were not considered candidates for the screening examination and were referred for ACL reconstruction surgery. The screening examination included a timed 6-m single-leg test, global rating of knee function, and Knee Outcome Survey—Activities of Daily Living. Potential copers were identified by hop test scores ≥80% of their contralateral limb, global rating of knee function of ≥60%, and a Knee Outcome Survey—Activities of Daily Living score of ≥80%. Patients who met these criteria were enrolled in a physical therapy program that involved exercises for strength, endurance, agility, balance, and proprioception. A sport-specific functional progression was also included in the physical therapy program. Approximately two-thirds of individuals identified as copers were able to return to IKDC level I or II sports without subsequent episodes of instability, injury, or reduced functional status after completing the physical therapy program.[32,40,62,63]

Using the screening test of Fitzgerald et al.,[40] Hurd et al.[63,64] were able to identify several additional characteristics that assist in differentiating ACL deficient copers from non-copers. A timed single-leg hop test demonstrating less than 10% difference between the injured and uninjured sides was the greatest predictor of a high level of self-assessed global function post injury. In addition, non-copers were more likely to be female, to have sustained an ACL injury via a non-contact mechanism, and to have less quadriceps strength than copers. Furthermore, non-copers participated in fewer hours of IKDC level I and II sports preinjury.

For patients with isolated ACL injuries who have not experienced a post-injury subluxation episode and who only participate in IKDC level III or IV activities, we suggest a trial of nonoperative management. We recommend ACL reconstructive surgery in the following individuals: patients who participate in IKDC level I or II activities, or who have experienced at least one subluxation episode after injury, have sustained a multiligament knee injury, or have a concomitant repairable meniscal and/or significant chondral injury. If a patient who participates in IKDC level I or II activities sustains an isolated ACL injury and requests a trial of nonoperative treatment, we recommend performing the screening examination outlined by Fitzgerald et al.[40] If the patient does not pass the screening examination, we recommend ACL reconstructive surgery. If the screening examination is passed, the patient is enrolled in a nonoperative ACL injury rehabilitation program. The following is a description of this nonoperative ACL injury rehabilitation program (Box 57.1).

Prescreening Examination Rehabilitation Phase

The goals of the prescreening examination rehabilitation phase are to reduce the patient's pain and effusion; re-establish full knee range of motion; normalize the gait pattern; maintain cardiovascular fitness; and strengthen the trunk, hip girdle, and thigh musculature. The patient is given crutches, and weight bearing is gradually progressed as pain, knee range of motion, and ability to dynamically stabilize the knee improves. Crutches are discontinued when the patient is able to ambulate without a limp or pain.

Pain can be reduced through local physical modalities, such as cryotherapy and electrical stimulation, and the judicious use of analgesic medications.[128] Resolution of any knee effusion facilitates knee range of motion, improves the patient's ability to ambulate, and reduces reflex quadriceps inhibition.[30,66,122] Active contraction of the calf musculature with active ankle range of motion exercises also facilitates edema reduction and may prevent complications of venous stasis. Knee range of motion exercises include heel slides, active knee range of motion, active assisted knee flexion with the arms or uninvolved leg, stationary bicycle assisted knee flexion, towel stretches, overpressure knee extension with 2.5 to 10 pounds of weight, prone hangs, and passive knee extension while propping the heel up on a towel.

Isometric quadriceps strengthening exercises can be initiated immediately following the injury and include quadriceps setting and straight leg raises. If the patient is unable to actively contract his or her quadriceps either because of reflex inhibition from a large knee joint effusion or significant pain, high-intensity neuromuscular electrical stimulation can be applied to the quadriceps musculature to facilitate muscle contraction.[120] Closed kinetic chain (CKC) exercises can also be safely used during the prescreening phase of rehabilitation and produce minimal anterior tibial displacement forces across the knee.[14,54,91,92,133] CKC exercises promote normal muscle activation patterns and joint stability through muscular co-contraction, provide proprioceptive input through joint compressive forces and mechanoreceptor stimulation, mimic normal functional movements, and assist in strengthening the quadriceps muscles, as well as ACL antagonist muscles (eg, gastrocnemius and hamstrings).[48] Open kinetic chain (OKC) exercises for the quadriceps can also be used during the prescreening examination phase of rehabilitation but should be limited to the range of motion within 90 to 45 degrees of knee flexion because of the increased anterior displacement of the tibia at lower knee flexion angles.[14,15,48,87,92] OKC hamstring exercises can be performed through the entire knee range of motion.

Proprioceptive exercises begin in this phase of rehabilitation and can be accomplished with a combination of CKC exercises, such as weight shifts, and joint-repositioning exercises.[128] A compressive sleeve used for edema control may also improve knee proprioception and should be worn during rehabilitation exercises.[72] Mini-squats can be progressed to occur on an unstable surface, such as a foam pad, based upon the patient's functional improvements. Functional activities, such as three way lunges, step ups, and cone step-over drills, can also be incorporated into the rehabilitation program. As the patient's ability to bear full weight and sense of knee stability improves, progression to single-leg balance exercises while standing on a stable surface can be attempted. Initially, single-leg balance exercises can be performed between parallel bars so that the subject can use their arms for support if needed. Eventually, the patient can begin moving the non-stance leg in adduction-abduction and flexion-extension directions, and the upper extremities in flexion, extension, abduction, adduction, and diagonal patterns with or without weight, while maintaining knee stability.[128] The amount of extremity excursion, rate of movement, and amount of resistance can be manipulated to alter the level of challenge posed by the exercise. The patient can eventually progress to standing on an unstable surface, such as a foam pad (Fig. 57.1).

To complete the screening examination, the patient must be able to perform various single-leg jumping tasks. Therefore this phase of rehabilitation should prepare the patient for single-leg jumping. Jumping should initially be performed with two legs in a submaximal vertical direction and only involve a single jump. Correct landing mechanics should be emphasized, which include avoidance of excessive lower extremity coronal and transverse plane motions; good balance; and adequate ankle, knee, and hip flexion for shock absorption. When the patient displays good technique during a submaximal double-leg vertical jump, he or she can progress to a maximal double-leg vertical jump. Next, a single forward double-leg jump can be introduced, in which the patient lands softly, with proper technique, and holds the knee in a flexed position for 5 to 10 seconds after landing. This can progress to a double-leg triple jump. When forward jumping can be performed successfully, backward and side-to-side double-leg jumping can be introduced. Eventually double-leg jumping while rotating clockwise or counterclockwise can be performed. Single-leg jumps should be introduced

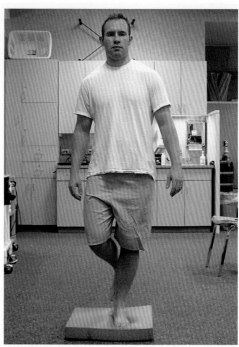

FIG 57.1 Single-leg balance exercises on a foam pad.

after the double-leg jump progression has been successfully completed, but single-leg jumps should not progress beyond the forward direction until the screening examination has been completed.

Finally, during the prescreening examination rehabilitation phase, the patient should maintain cardiovascular fitness through low-impact aerobic conditioning progressing from a stationary bike to an elliptical machine. Running should not occur during this phase. The patient should also incorporate trunk and hip girdle strengthening exercises. In particular, the hip extensors, external rotators, abductors, and flexors should be strengthened to provide concentric (hip extensors, external rotators, and abductors) and eccentric (hip flexors) control of femoral adduction and internal rotation motions, which have been implicated as potential contributing factors to ACL injuries.[57]

While participating in the rehabilitation program, the patient should be monitored for an increase in pain, increased knee effusion, or sensation of knee instability during or following activity. If any of these signs or symptoms should occur, the patient should be instructed to rest, ice, compress, and elevate the lower extremity until they resolve, at which time the rehabilitation program should be reinitiated at a lower level and with a slower rate of progression. If the patient experiences a subluxation episode, he or she should be encouraged to discontinue the nonoperative rehabilitation program and meet with a surgeon for consideration of ACL reconstructive surgery.

Post-Screening Examination Rehabilitation Phase

After the patient has passed the screening examination, they will enter the second phase of the rehabilitation program. The goal of the post-screening examination phase is to restore full dynamic stability to their knee and prepare the patient for a return to sports. The patient's primary sport should be identified and the program tailored accordingly.

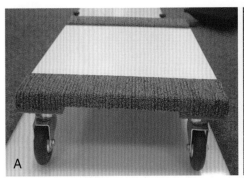
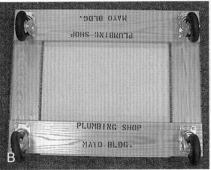
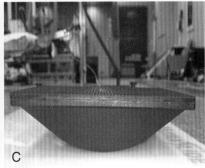

FIG 57.2 Top (A) and bottom (B) views of a roller board. The roller board casters rotate freely, allowing multiple planes of movement during perturbation training. Side view of a tilt board (C).

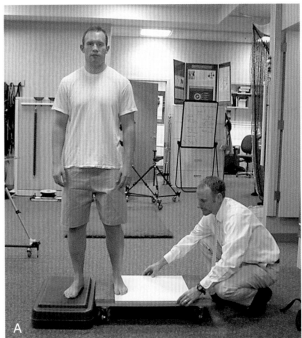
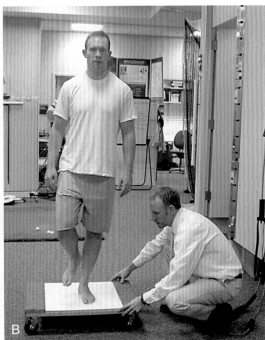

FIG 57.3 During the initial phase of perturbation training, the roller board is placed next to a stable platform so that the patient can place one foot on the roller board and the other foot on the stable platform while a perturbation force is applied to the roller board (A). A walker or parallel bars can be used initially for safety (not shown). Eventually, the patient is advanced to balancing on a single leg on the roller board while perturbation forces are applied to the roller board (B).

A key component to this phase of the patient's rehabilitation program is the addition of perturbation training. Perturbation training has been shown to improve the functional outcomes in ACL-deficient patients when compared with rehabilitation without perturbation training.[41] Perturbation training may be performed on a roller board or a tilt board (Fig. 57.2) and should occur 2 to 3 times per week. The speed, direction, and amplitude of perturbations should be varied by the therapist and applied in a random order as the patient becomes more proficient with the exercises. When the patient is able to perform all perturbation exercises in a single limb position on the tilt board and roller board with minimal disturbance in their balance, sports-specific and functional tasks should be added to the program, with the goal of producing compensatory responses to sports specific and functional activities (Figs. 57.3 and 57.4). By performing perturbation training during sports-specific and functional tasks, improved carryover to athletic or

functional situations may occur, thereby minimizing the chance of a subluxation episode or recurrent knee injury when patients resume activity.[41]

The patient should continue strengthening exercises focusing on the quadriceps, hamstring, gastrocnemius-soleus complex, hip girdle, and trunk. The principles of progressive resistance exercises and periodization are applied during this phase of rehabilitation. A periodized resistance training program may be divided into three phases.[125] The first phase is the hypertrophy/endurance phase, which involves low-to-moderate weight (50% to 75% of the patient's one repetition maximum) and moderate-to-high repetitions (10 to 20) and sets (three to six). The goals of the hypertrophy/endurance phase are to develop good technique during resistance exercises, increase lean body mass, and provide a base of strength in preparation for the later phases of resistance training. During the second, or basic strength, phase of resistance training, muscle strength is

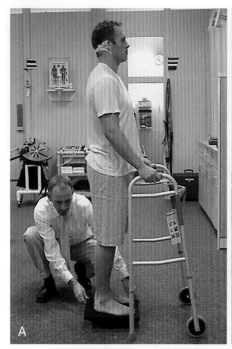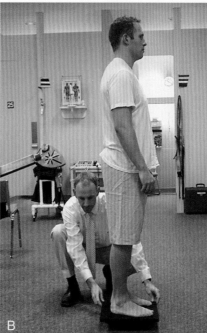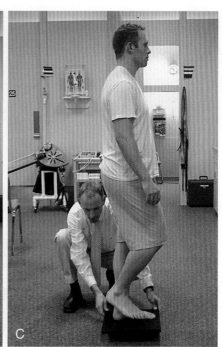

FIG 57.4 The patient begins perturbation training by standing with both feet on the tilt board while a perturbation force is applied to the tilt board (A). Parallel bars or a walker can be used initially for patient safety. The patient is progressed to double-leg perturbation exercises on the tilt board without parallel bars or a walker (B) and finally to single-leg perturbation exercises on the tilt board (C).

increased by progressively increasing the intensity (weight = 80% to 90% of one repetition maximum) and decreasing the volume (three to five sets of four to eight repetitions). Emphasis should be placed upon technique, slow movement, and strengthening the muscles required for the patient's particular sport. The final resistance training phase, the strength/power phase, involves sports-specific exercises performed at or near competition level, at a high intensity (85% to 95% of one repetition maximum) and low volume (three to five sets of two to five repetitions). Throughout the periodized resistance training program, the patient's one repetition maximum for their primary exercises should be determined every 2 to 4 weeks and the amount of resistance applied during their exercises adjusted accordingly.

A combination of CKC and OKC exercises can be used during this phase, with an emphasis on functional movement patterns and strengthening muscles involved in the patient's primary sport. OKC quadriceps strengthening exercises should continue to be limited to knee flexion angles between 45 and 90 degrees for the first 4 weeks after the injury to minimize anterior tibial displacement forces but can be performed through the entire knee range of motion after this time. Other strengthening exercises may include leg curls, squats, calf raises, three way lunges, lunges with trunk rotation, front and lateral step-ups, front step-downs, four-way hip resistance exercises (ie, hip adduction, abduction, extension, and flexion), and hip external rotation resistance exercises. Trunk stability exercises may include prone, supine, and side-lying stability ball bridges, bird-dog exercises, stability ball straight and oblique crunches, and stability ball partial crunch with medicine ball trunk rotations. Single-leg and/or single-arm bridges can add difficulty to the trunk exercise. As the patient's program progresses, the exercises should become more sports specific, not only strengthening the muscles that will be required for their sport, but also improving the neuromuscular movement patterns required for participation in their sport.

Plyometric training should begin in this phase of the rehabilitation program. The therapist should continually reinforce appropriate landing technique, which includes landing softly on the toes with the knees slightly flexed, and absorbing the ground reaction forces associated with landing through adequate hip, knee, and ankle flexion. Plyometric exercises should include double-leg and single-leg tasks.

If the patient participates in running sports, running should be introduced during this phase of the rehabilitation program. The running program should begin on a treadmill at a slow speed on a level surface. A running analysis should be performed to detect gross abnormalities in running gait, including asymmetries in stride length, stance time, and lower extremity joint angles during the load acceptance phase of gait. After the patient's running gait has been normalized and no gross asymmetries are present, the speed and incline of the treadmill workouts can gradually be increased, and the patient may transition, if desired, to running off the treadmill. The patient should begin running on a level surface and hills can be introduced when the patient can run 20 to 30 minutes on a level surface without symptoms. Finally, the patient can begin performing sprint drills. After successfully performing sprint drills, patients can begin drills that involve deceleration and direction change. Finally, sports-specific drills should be incorporated into the patient's rehabilitation program in preparation for a return to sports. Sport-specific training should simulate the functional movement patterns of the patient's sport while incorporating peripheral afferent stimulation (eg, proprioceptive challenges) to facilitate neuromuscular re-education and train dynamic knee stability during functional, sports-specific tasks. For sports that involve running, cutting, and jumping, such as football or soccer, sports-specific drills may include cone drills, side-shuffling, carioca, sudden starts and stops, cutting drills, jumping drills, and ball handling drills. For skating sports, sport-specific drills may include sudden starts and stops, direction changes, figure-of-eights, forward-backward skating, among others.

After the athlete has successfully performed the previously described rehabilitation program, he or she may return to unrestricted sports with use of a functional derotational brace as needed. If the patient has pain, recurrent effusions, or a sensation of knee instability despite completing the rehabilitation program or experiences a subluxation episode during the rehabilitation program, he or she is referred to a surgeon for consideration of ACL reconstructive surgery.

REHABILITATION AFTER ANTERIOR CRUCIATE LIGAMENT RECONSTRUCTIVE SURGERY

Surgical Considerations

Graft healing following ACL reconstruction is a complex biologic process that is influenced by multiple surgical and postoperative variables.[33] These variables include graft type, graft position, graft tensioning and fixation, and individual patient factors. In general, the graft healing process following ACL reconstruction occurs in several phases. An initial inflammatory response occurs almost immediately.[71] Graft revascularization occurs over the next several months and originates primarily from the infrapatellar fat pad, posterior synovial tissue, and endosteal vessels within the femoral and tibial tunnels.[6,33] Over the ensuing months to years, remodeling or "ligamentization" of the intra-articular portion of the graft occurs, which is characterized by cellular repopulation, collagen remodeling, and ligament maturation.[6,80]

In general, options for graft type in ACL reconstruction include bone-patellar tendon-bone autograft, quadruple hamstring autograft, quadriceps tendon bone autograft, bone patellar tendon bone allograft, Achilles tendon bone allograft, and tibialis anterior allograft. The rates and characteristics of the healing process among these grafts differ, and the specifics of these differences are not well understood. Several animal models have shown slower bone tunnel incorporation with soft tissue autograft and allograft compared with bone-patellar tendon-bone autograft.[33,104] Although complete incorporation at the bone-tunnel interface has been shown to occur at 6 to 8 weeks with the use of patellar tendon autograft,[94] the incorporation of soft tissue graft has been shown to be considerably longer at 12 weeks.[46,104] Although allograft tissue appears to heal in a similar manner to autograft tissue, this occurs at a much slower rate.[49] In addition, compared with autograft tissue, allografts lose more of their time zero strength during remodeling. ACL reconstruction with allograft tissue has not been definitively shown to have inferior functional outcomes[49,57] although a large multicenter study demonstrated a four-fold higher failure rate of ACL reconstruction when allograft tissue was used.[69] Nonetheless, these differences should be taken into account when designing a rehabilitation protocol. Two prospective randomized trials have shown that an accelerated rehabilitation program produces no differences in

knee laxity, range of motion, or functional outcomes in patients reconstructed with bone-patellar tendon-bone autograft or hamstring autograft.[17,23] Despite the trials evaluating autograft tissue, insufficient evidence exists regarding the safety of an accelerated rehabilitation program for patients undergoing ACL reconstruction with allograft tissue.

Secure mechanical fixation is required in the early postoperative period to achieve reliable graft incorporation. A host of different fixation devices are available, including metallic and bioabsorbable interference screws for both femoral and tibial fixation, various suspensory and transfixion devices for femoral fixation, and various combinations of aperture and augmentation devices for tibial fixation. A large number of studies have examined differences in the biomechanical properties between various fixation devices at time zero; however, few studies have explored differences in biologic incorporation of grafts relative to individual fixation methods.[33] Graft fixation is influenced by various physical properties, including graft material, bone density, fixation device, and fixation site.[51] Although the majority of fixation techniques have been demonstrated to perform well in clinical studies, it is important that the surgeon is familiar with the biomechanical properties of the individual system being used because the rehabilitation program may need to be adjusted accordingly.

Anatomic tunnel placement has been emphasized to achieve physiologic graft loading, promote bone-graft healing, and restore knee stability.[33,37] In particular, a more anatomic femoral graft placement has been shown to offer significant biomechanical advantages.[33,136] With respect to graft tension, both excessively low tension and excessively high tension have been postulated to reduce the biomechanical properties of the graft.[33] Further study is required to determine the optimal tension that should be applied relative to each graft type and fixation method. Delayed graft healing and tunnel enlargement have been postulated to occur secondary to excessive graft-tunnel motion.[33,60] Motion between the graft and bone tunnel has been correlated with both the type of fixation used and the postoperative rehabilitation program.[33] Although early knee range of motion and weight bearing are considered to be beneficial, an early aggressive rehabilitation protocol may increase graft-tunnel motion, thus impacting graft incorporation and tunnel enlargement. This phenomenon may be more likely to occur in the setting of nonanatomic femoral tunnel placement.[33] Although a study suggested that tunnel enlargement may not affect clinical outcome,[126] further study is required to determine the effects of aggressive rehabilitation on successful graft incorporation after ACL reconstruction.

Timing of Surgery and General Rehabilitation Considerations

Prior to undergoing surgery, the patient should demonstrate minimal knee effusion, and full symmetric extension to minimize the risk of postoperative arthrofibrosis.[85,117] The patient is allowed sufficient time to psychologically cope with the injury and prepare for both the surgery and rehabilitation process, which require significant commitment from the patient to optimize surgical outcome.[113] Shelbourne and Klotz[113] reported that regaining symmetric knee range of motion after surgery is a critical factor related to patient satisfaction. Thus achieving full knee range of motion should be a primary focus of the early postoperative rehabilitation program.

Cryotherapy

Several studies have demonstrated that cryotherapy reduces pain, edema, and inflammation in the postoperative setting.[96,110] In an experimental knee swelling model, cryotherapy was found to be effective in reducing arthrogenic muscle inhibition induced by swelling.[100] In a meta-analysis following ACL reconstruction, it was found that cryotherapy had a statistically significant benefit in postoperative pain control.[98] The study highlighted that cryotherapy is inexpensive, easy to use, and rarely associated with adverse events and has a high level of patient satisfaction.

Range of Motion and Weight Bearing

Immediate postoperative motion has been shown to reduce complications associated with joint immobilization, including detrimental effects to knee ligaments, cartilage, bone, and musculature.[16] Five prospective, randomized controlled trials have demonstrated the benefits of immediate joint mobilization compared with delayed knee motion following ACL reconstruction.[50,56,90,97,105] These studies report improved ACL graft healing and capsular mobility, as well as decreased postoperative pain, scar formation, and adverse articular cartilage changes.

To date, there have been six prospective, randomized controlled trials investigating the use of continuous passive motion (CPM) machines after ACL reconstruction.** Four of the studies did not demonstrate a significant benefit when CPM was added to the postoperative rehabilitation regimen.[101,105] However, a study by Yates et al.[134] reported decreased hemarthrosis, narcotic use, and swelling in patients who received CPM 16 hours per day for the first 3 postoperative days, followed by 6 hours per day for 11 days, when compared with patients who did not receive CPM. In addition, McCarthy et al.[78] demonstrated decreased narcotic pain medication use in patients who received CPM for the first 3 postoperative days when compared with patients who did not receive CPM. Therefore it appears CPM may have a limited role in the early reduction of pain and edema following ACL reconstructive surgery.

There appears to be no benefit to delaying weight bearing after ACL reconstruction.[123] In a randomized trial comparing immediate weight bearing versus delayed weight bearing for 2 weeks, Tyler et al.[123] found a decreased incidence of anterior knee pain in the weight-bearing group. This was thought to be secondary to earlier recruitment of the vastus medialis muscle in the weight-bearing group.

Bracing

The use of a rehabilitation brace during the early postoperative phase of ACL reconstruction appears to reduce effusion, wound drainage, rate of hemarthrosis, and pain but does not appear to affect the long-term clinical outcome.[16,76,119] Wright et al. published a systematic review of 11 studies that showed no increase in adverse effects without the use of a postoperative rehabilitative brace. Specifically there was no evidence found for increased pain, decreased range of motion, or increased knee laxity in patients who were not treated with a rehabilitation brace following surgery.[130] Furthermore, functional derotational braces after ACL reconstructive surgery do not appear to affect long-term functional outcomes and should therefore be reserved for special circumstances.[79,103]

Electrical Stimulation

Several studies have demonstrated that the use of neuromuscular electrical stimulation of the quadriceps during the volitional exercises results in more quadriceps strength and a better gait pattern when compared with volitional exercises alone.[120,121] Fitzgerald et al. evaluated neuromuscular electrical stimulation in a prospective randomized study of 48 patients who underwent ACL reconstruction. The electrical stimulation group was found to demonstrate improved quadriceps strength at 12 weeks after surgery. Activities of daily living scores and the time to begin agility training were improved in the electrical stimulation group versus controls.[42] Based on these studies, neuromuscular electrical stimulation appears to have a beneficial effect; however, for it to be successful, it must be applied in the early postoperative setting and at a high intensity. This requires that the treatment be administered by a physical therapist in a supervised setting. Insufficient data exist regarding the beneficial effect of home-based electrical stimulation units.[131]

Supervised versus Home-Based Rehabilitation

There have been several randomized controlled trials comparing the efficacy of predominantly home-based rehabilitation programs that require intermittent supervision by a physical therapist, to supervised clinic-based rehabilitation programs following ACL reconstructive surgery.[11,39,109] None of the studies demonstrated a higher level of subjective and/or objective outcome measures between the two rehabilitation conditions. These findings suggest that intermittent supervision by a physical therapist to monitor the patient's progress and direct their home-based rehabilitation program may be as effective as a supervised, clinic-based rehabilitation program.

Proprioceptive Training

Multiple studies have demonstrated proprioceptive deficits in knees following ACL injury, regardless of whether the injury is treated with or without surgery.[9,10,13,84,129] It has been suggested that exercises designed to stimulate joint mechanoreceptors and muscle spindles (ie, proprioceptive and balance exercises) may increase their sensitivity, thereby improving the muscles ability to stabilize the joint in response to destabilizing joint forces.[67] Thus multiple prospective, randomized controlled studies have been performed to evaluate the effectiveness of proprioceptive and balance exercises in rehabilitation after ACL reconstruction.†† All of the studies but one[27] demonstrated better subjective and/or objective outcome measures following post-ACL reconstructive surgery rehabilitation with proprioceptive and balance exercises rather than standard post-ACL reconstructive surgery rehabilitation without proprioceptive and balance exercises. Therefore it appears that the addition of proprioceptive and balance exercises to post-ACL reconstructive surgery rehabilitation programs provides a positive benefit to patients.

Closed Kinetic Chain versus Open Kinetic Chain Exercises

A study comparing CKC and open kinetic chair protocols after ACL reconstruction reported significantly better improvements in knee flexion and Lysholm knee scores with a CKC program.[124] However, the addition of OKC exercises to rehabilitation after ACL reconstruction may provide additional quadriceps strength

---

**References 35, 77, 78, 101, 105, and 134.

††References 1, 12, 27, 74, 102, and 135.

when compared with CKC exercises alone[83] and does not appear to be detrimental as long as the OKC exercises are limited to 40 to 90 degrees of knee flexion.[18,61,86,87] For patients treated with a bone-patellar tendon-bone graft, it appears that OKC exercises between 0 and 40 degrees of knee flexion can be safely introduced 4 weeks postoperatively,[17] although the exact timing of introducing these exercises when using other graft materials, such as the four-strand hamstring graft, has not been well established.[132] Furthermore, it has been suggested that early use of OKC quadriceps exercises after hamstring ACL reconstruction may result in significantly increased anterior knee laxity in comparison with both late start and early and late start after bone-patellar tendon-bone ACL reconstruction.[55]

Accelerated Rehabilitation

Finally, there have been limited studies determining the optimal duration of the post-ACL reconstruction rehabilitation program. Shelbourne et al. reported that early postoperative weight bearing and early return to sports was safe and effective.[111,112,114] This form of rehabilitation has frequently been referred to as "accelerated rehabilitation." Two prospective, randomized controlled trials have confirmed that accelerated rehabilitation protocols produce similar results in a shorter duration of time when compared with traditional (ie, delayed) rehabilitation programs.[17,65] One study also suggested that 2.5 hours of rehabilitation performed three to five times per week produced better knee joint position sense and higher Lysholm scores and returned people to work earlier than a rehabilitation program that involved 30 minutes of rehabilitation performed two to three times per week.[43] Further research is required to determine the optimal duration and intensity required for an accelerated rehabilitation program after ACL reconstruction, particularly in the setting of hamstring and allograft reconstruction.[33,44]

Based on the current evidence and considering the goals of returning patients safely and expeditiously to their preinjury level of function, we propose the following postoperative rehabilitation program (Box 57.2).

Preoperative Rehabilitation

The rehabilitation program for patients who undergo ACL reconstructive surgery begins at the initial visit prior to the surgery. A study reported the benefits of a progressive preoperative and postoperative rehabilitation program by demonstrating better Knee Injury and Osteoarthritis Outcome Scores (KOOSs) and quality of life scores preoperatively and for 2 years postoperatively when compared with patients treated with standard protocols.[47] The indications for ACL reconstructive surgery, the risks and benefits of the surgery, the postoperative rehabilitation process and expected return-to-sports date are discussed with the patient during the initial physician appointment. In addition, patients can also benefit from meeting with a sports psychologist and physical therapist. The sports psychologist suggests coping strategies, teaches the patient relaxation and pain management techniques that assist them in the rehabilitation process, and discusses ways to enhance their performance during rehabilitation and return to sports. The physical therapist instructs the patient on the appropriate use of crutches, which the patient will use until he or she is able to ambulate without a limp and has regained adequate dynamic stability of the knee. The patient is instructed on edema control measures, including compression, which is achieved through the use of a

---

BOX 57.2 Postoperative Rehabilitation Summary

Week 1
Pain control
Decrease swelling and edema
Improve quadriceps activation
Achieve full passive knee extension

Weeks 2-4
Maintain full passive knee extension
Improve knee flexion
Re-establish patellar mobility
Resolve effusion
Strengthen thigh and hip girdle and trunk musculature
Improve aerobic fitness—non/low impact
Improve joint proprioception

Weeks 5-12
Maintain full active and passive knee extension
Achieve normal patellar mobility
Re-establish full knee flexion
Advance thigh, hip girdle, and trunk strengthening
Introduce more advanced proprioceptive and functional exercises
Improve aerobic fitness—low/medium impact

Weeks 13-24
Re-establish symmetric lower extremity strength
Introduce plyometrics
Progress to higher-impact aerobic conditioning as tolerated
Enhance proprioception and neuromuscular control
Begin a functional progression of sports-specific drills

---

compressive sleeve, elevation, ankle pumps, and cryotherapy. Cryo-compression devices are occasionally used to assist with resolution of the effusion. The patient is taught knee range-of-motion exercises, including wall heel slides, heel props, and towel stretches. A stationary bicycle can be used to assist with obtaining symmetric knee range of motion. Strengthening exercises during the preoperative phase begin with quadriceps sets and straight leg raises and progress to CKC exercises, such as mini squats, lunges, and step-ups. OKC knee extension exercises can be performed within the knee flexion ranges of 45 and 90 degrees, whereas knee flexion exercises can be performed throughout the entire knee range of motion. Neuromuscular electrical stimulation can be used to facilitate quadriceps contraction if the patient is unable to adequately contract the quadriceps volitionally. The patient should also perform trunk stability exercises (eg, prone, side lying, and supine bridges) and hip girdle strengthening exercises (eg, hip flexion, abduction, extension, adduction, and external rotation against resistance). The patient should be educated on appropriate forms of low-impact aerobic conditioning exercises, such as a stationary bicycle, elliptical machine, or rowing machine, which can be performed to maintain cardiovascular fitness. The therapist also assists the patient in establishing a normal gait pattern.

Postoperative Week 1 Rehabilitation

During the first week, our emphasis is on pain control, decreasing swelling and edema, and improving quadriceps activation. Knee range-of-motion exercises include heel slides, active knee range of motion, active assisted knee flexion using the upper extremities or the uninvolved leg, stationary bicycle assisted knee flexion, towel stretches, sustained overpressure knee extension, prone hangs, and passive knee extension while propping the heel up on a towel. Full knee extension should be achieved within 5 days after surgery.

Cryotherapy is used regularly. A compressive wrap or sleeve is applied to the knee and the knee is elevated in full extension whenever the patient is not performing rehabilitation exercises. Cryo-compression devices may be used to reduce swelling and active ankle range-of-motion exercises help to reduce postoperative edema and venostasis. The patient is provided with a knee immobilizing brace, which is used only until the patient has regained the ability to activate the quadriceps to prevent risk of falls because of quadriceps inhibition. This is typically used for up to 1 week following surgery as a safety precaution. A proper crutch gait is reviewed with the patient, and the patient is allowed to bear weight as tolerated.

Strengthening exercises begin immediately following surgery. Early strengthening exercises should include multiangle isometric thigh-strengthening exercises (between 60 and 90 degrees of knee flexion), quadriceps sets with the knee in full extension, three direction straight leg raises (ie, hip flexion, abduction, and extension), weight shifts, and mini squats. Early quadriceps neuromuscular electrical stimulation is frequently used during volitional exercises to enhance quadriceps muscle recruitment and strengthening. Standing hamstring curls without resistance may begin within the first few days but should be performed with the patient using parallel bars for stability.

In addition to strengthening exercises, the patient should also participate in proprioceptive training, trunk strengthening and stability exercises, and aerobic conditioning exercises. Early proprioceptive training can include knee-repositioning exercises, weight shifts, and CKC exercises, such as mini squats. Aerobic conditioning can be maintained initially by using an upper extremity ergometer. Early trunk stability exercises can include abdominal muscle isometrics, straight and oblique abdominal crunches on a stable surface, and light weight and low-speed medicine ball trunk rotations while sitting on a stable surface.

One potential complication following ACL reconstructive surgery is patellar hypomobility, which can lead to pain, decreased range of motion, and inability to adequately recruit the quadriceps muscle.[128] Therefore the patient should be instructed on performance of mediolateral and superior-inferior patellar mobilization exercises. If the patient's ACL was reconstructed using a bone-patellar tendon-bone autograft, particular attention should be paid to superior-inferior patellar mobilization exercises to prevent excessive infrapatellar scaring, often referred to as infrapatellar contracture syndrome.[95]

Postoperative Weeks 2 to 4 Rehabilitation

By the beginning of the second postoperative week, the patient should have achieved full weight bearing and full passive knee extension, at least 90 degrees of knee flexion, satisfactory patellar mobility, and quadriceps control, and any knee effusion should be nearly resolved. The goals of this rehabilitation phase are to maintain full passive knee extension, improve knee flexion, re-establish normal patellar mobility, resolve any remaining knee effusion, strengthen the thigh, hip girdle, and trunk musculature, and improve aerobic fitness and knee joint proprioception. The patient may discontinue crutches whenever he or she is able to ambulate painlessly without a limp (typically by postoperative day 10 to 14).

Edema control measures, including cryotherapy, elevation, and compression, should continue until the knee effusion has fully resolved. The patient should continue to work on regaining full passive knee range of motion during this rehabilitation phase, with the goal of achieving full knee flexion by 4 weeks postoperatively.[60]

In addition to the strengthening exercises for the hip girdle and thigh musculature that were initiated in the first postoperative week, multiple exercises can be gradually incorporated into the strengthening program during this rehabilitation phase. The patient may begin the following CKC exercises as tolerated: leg press, squats from 0 to 50 degrees of knee flexion, three-way lunges, front and lateral step-ups, or forward and lateral cone step-overs. OKC quadriceps-strengthening exercises between 40 and 90 degrees of knee flexion can begin. Quadriceps contraction during both CKC and OKC exercises can be facilitated with neuromuscular electrical stimulation. OKC hamstring curls with resistance may also be introduced during this phase of rehabilitation unless the patient's ACL was reconstructed with a hamstring graft, in which case hamstring resistance exercises are delayed until 6 weeks post-ACL reconstructive surgery to avoid irritation of the graft harvest site.[128]

Early proprioceptive exercises should be emphasized during this rehabilitation phase. These should include the proprioceptive exercises performed during the first week after surgery (ie, CKC strengthening exercises, weight shifts, and joint repositioning exercises). The compressive sleeve used for edema control may also improve knee proprioception and should be worn during rehabilitation exercises.[72] Mini squats can be progressed to occur on an unstable surface, such as a foam pad, based upon the patient's functional improvements. When able, the patient should begin single-leg balance exercises on a stable surface between parallel bars so that he or she can use arms for support if needed. The proprioceptive challenge can be increased by moving the nonstance limbs while standing on one leg.[128] The amount of extremity excursion, rate of movement, and amount of weight can be manipulated to alter the level of challenge posed by the exercise. The patient can eventually be progressed to standing on an unstable surface, such as a foam pad (see Fig. 57.1).

As the patient's knee range of motion improves, the aerobic conditioning program can switch from an upper extremity ergometer to a stationary bicycle, which has the advantage of promoting knee range of motion and lower extremity strengthening while developing cardiovascular fitness. Furthermore, when the patient's incision site has completely healed, the patient can be allowed to begin aerobic conditioning in the pool with such activities as pool walking. Hip girdle–strengthening exercises can be advanced to include standing four-way hip (ie, abduction, adduction, extension, flexion) isotonic strengthening exercises performed on a stable surface. Trunk strengthening and stability exercises should be incorporated into the routine, including medicine ball trunk rotations performed at different speeds and at different trunk inclination angles while sitting on a stability ball. Double-leg prone, supine, and side bridges on a stable surface can be added during this phase of rehabilitation and progressed to single-leg bridges as tolerated. The patient can also begin straight and side abdominal crunches and back extension exercises while on a stable surface. Gait training should focus on restoration of normal speed and rhythm, as well as an avoidance of walking with a flexed knee gait.

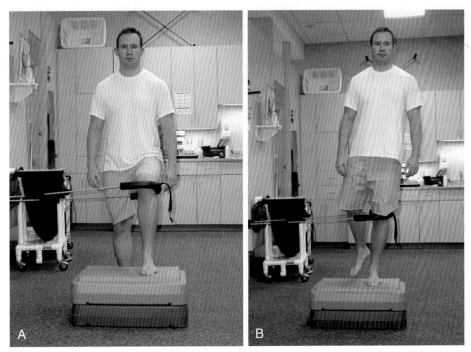

FIG 57.5 (A and B) This figure depicts a patient performing a step-up exercise while a medially directed force is placed upon the patient's left knee using resistance tubing.

Postoperative Weeks 5 to 12 Rehabilitation

By the beginning of postoperative week 5, the patient should have achieved near full knee flexion and have minimal or no knee effusion. The patient's quadriceps strength should be at least 60% of the contralateral side if isometric and/or isotonic strength testing is performed at this time. The goals of this rehabilitation phase are to maintain full passive knee extension and normal patellar mobility, regain symmetric knee flexion, continue to advanced thigh-, hip girdle–, and trunk-strengthening exercises, introduce more advanced proprioceptive and functional exercises, and improve aerobic fitness.

The patient should continue the knee flexion and extension range-of-motion exercises and patellar mobility exercises previously described. The patient's strengthening exercise program should continue using isometric, and CKC and OKC isotonic exercises, but the principles of progressive resistance exercises and periodization, as described in the nonoperative ACL injury rehabilitation program, can now be emphasized. During this rehabilitation phase, the patient is in the hypertrophy/endurance phase of a periodized strength training program, which involves low-to-moderate weight and moderate-to-high repetitions, with an emphasis on developing good technique during resistance exercises, increasing lean body mass, and providing a base of strength in preparation for the later phases of resistance training. Isometric exercises can include multiangle quadriceps strengthening from 0 to 90 degrees of knee flexion. Isotonic exercises for the hip girdle and thigh can include four-way (abduction, adduction, flexion, and extension) standing hip exercises, front and side step-ups, three-way lunges, squats, and hamstring curls. A functional CKC hip external rotator–strengthening exercise involves step-ups while the therapist exerts a medially directed force on the patient's knee with resistance tubing (Fig. 57.5). For patients treated with a bone-patellar tendon-bone autograft, OKC knee extension exercises between 0 and 40 degrees of knee flexion are typically

introduced 6 to 8 weeks after surgery. In contrast, patients who have undergone ACL reconstruction using a hamstring autograft or allograft typically do not perform OKC knee extension exercises in this range of knee flexion until approximately 12 weeks after surgery.[7,55]

Single-leg CKC and OKC exercises should be added to the patient's resistance training program during this rehabilitation phase to improve strength, balance, and coordination. When able, the patient should begin performing single-leg squats focusing on correct technique, including avoidance of contralateral hip drop (ie, Trendelenburg), and either adduction or internal rotation of the femur, which commonly presents as "dynamic knee valgus" or "corkscrewing." As previously discussed, this abnormal movement pattern may lead to traumatic and atraumatic knee injuries and should be corrected. Initially, single-leg squats can be performed to between 20 and 30 degrees of knee flexion. As the patient's ability to perform this exercise improves, the knee should be flexed to 60 degrees. Weight and speed can gradually be added to the single-leg squat exercises as tolerated.

Proprioceptive training, which appears to be one of the keys to successful ACL rehabilitation, should continue to progress during this rehabilitation phase. In addition to the previously mentioned CKC exercises on stable surfaces, these exercises can also be performed on unstable surfaces, such as foam or air pads. The previously described single-leg squatting exercises also rely on proprioceptive feedback and assist in establishing normal neuromuscular patterns required for a variety of activities. Additional proprioceptive exercises can include single-leg balance on an unstable surface with or without extremity movements. The patient can be given a medicine ball or weights that they can hold while they perform functional movements while standing on one leg. A ball can also be thrown to the patient while he or she is standing on one leg, to increase the challenge and sports specificity of this proprioceptive exercise.

Finally, the patient should continue trunk strength, stability exercises, and aerobic conditioning. The patient should continue to use the exercises introduced in the previous rehabilitation phase with the addition of one- and two-legged prone, side-lying, and supine bridges on an unstable surface; forward and side crunches on an unstable surface; back extensions on an unstable surface; and four-way hip strengthening exercises while standing on an unstable surface. Aerobic conditioning may continue on the stationary bicycle, but the patient can progress to using an elliptical machine if he or she plans to return to activities that involve running. In addition, a slide board can be used for patients who would like to return to activities that involve skating. We do not typically encourage our athletes to begin running or plyometric activities during this rehabilitation phase, regardless of the type of graft used to reconstruct the ACL.

Postoperative Weeks 13 to 24 Rehabilitation

By 12 weeks after surgery, the patient should have achieved full knee range of motion, resolution of their knee effusion, and isokinetic and/or isometric quadriceps strength of at least 75% of their uninjured limb, if strength testing is performed at this time. The goals of this phase of rehabilitation are to establish symmetric lower extremity strength, introduce plyometrics, enhance proprioception and neuromuscular control, and complete a functional progression of sports-specific drills prior to releasing the patient to sports. All of the previously described exercises should continue during this phase of rehabilitation, with the following additions. The patient should begin the second or basic strength phase of their periodized resistance training program, which increases the weight and decreases the volume of their resistance exercises. Proper technique, slow controlled movements, and strengthening of the muscles required for their particular sport should be emphasized. Toward the end of this rehabilitation phase, the patient should transition into the strength/power phase of their periodized strength training program, which involves the performance of high-intensity, low-volume, sports-specific exercises at or near competition pace. Exercises include leg extensions, leg press, squats, and deadlifts.

Perturbation training should be incorporated into the proprioceptive exercise regimen of this rehabilitation phase and should follow the same roller board and tilt board progression as described in the nonoperative ACL injury post-screening examination rehabilitation program. After completing the standard perturbation training progression, sports-specific perturbation training exercises can be added, which may include swinging a bat, club, or stick, or catching a ball or hitting a puck while standing on a roller board or tilt board.

The patient should complete the plyometric double-leg jumping progression and progress to the single-leg jumping progression. After finishing the single-leg jumping progression, sports-specific plyometric drills should be incorporated into the patient's rehabilitation program, such as catching a weighted or unweighted ball thrown by the physical therapist to the patient while performing a jumping drill or performing a continuous jumping drill that incorporates unforeseen direction and leg changes as directed by the physical therapist (ie, double-leg straight, right single-leg forward, left single-leg 180 degrees left rotation).

The patient should begin running or skating at the beginning of this rehabilitation phase and may follow the same functional progression outlined in the nonoperative ACL injury post-screening rehabilitation program. Sports-specific agility drills, as described in the nonoperative ACL injury post-screening examination rehabilitation program, should be introduced after they have completed their running or skating functional progression. Particular attention should be paid to proper technique and neuromuscular control during deceleration, cutting, and jumping activities to prevent future knee injury.

Return to Sports Criteria

After successful completion of the rehabilitation program, the patient is prepared to begin reintegration into his or her respective sport. Objective tests include single-leg hop for distance, single-leg hop for height, single-leg triple hop for distance, single-leg triple cross-over hop for distance, and 6-m single-leg hop test for speed. In addition, the patient's technique during single-leg squat and double-leg jumping are evaluated, as well as the patient's concentric quadriceps and hamstring isokinetic strength testing at 60 degrees/s and 180 degrees/s. To clear a patient to resume practice activities, the performance on the single-leg hop test of the injured knee should be at least 90% of the uninjured leg. In addition, the patient should exhibit satisfactory neuromuscular control and correct movement patterns during single-leg squat to 60 degrees of knee flexion and double-leg jumping. Isokinetic strength in the ACL reconstructed knee should be at least 80% of the uninjured leg. Athletes who attain symmetry with respect to sports performance in both limbs prior to sports reintegration after ACL reconstruction may significantly reduce their potential for recurrent ACL injury.[5,81]

Several recent studies have identified predictors for readiness to return to sport after ACL reconstruction. Muller reported that single-leg hop for distance and the ACL-Return to Sport after Injury Scale (RSI) were the strongest predictors of a successful return to sport 6 months after ACL reconstruction.[88] Similarly, Logerstedt et al.[75] reported that lower IKDC scores were predictive of failing functional testing but that normal IKDC scores were not predictive of passing functional tests. They concluded that functional sport testing is the best criteria when determining readiness to return to sport.[75] Finally, several studies have reported that psychologic readiness to return to sport is a strong predictive factor for returning to preinjury levels of activity and that rehabilitation protocols should also focus on improving patient confidence.[4,28]

Rehabilitation Variations Based Upon Concomitant Procedures

ACL injuries frequently are associated with injuries to other ligaments, the menisci, or articular cartilage. Treatment of these injuries, whether surgical or nonsurgical, frequently leads to changes in the rehabilitation program. Commonly associated injuries and their effect upon the rehabilitation process will be discussed in the following section.

The incidence of medial collateral ligament (MCL) injuries associated with acute ACL injuries is approximately 13%.[128] If the MCL injury is treated nonoperatively, ACL reconstruction may be delayed to allow for MCL healing, reduction of the patient's effusion, and re-establishment of knee range of motion.[115] If an MCL repair or reconstruction is also performed at the time of ACL reconstruction, a postoperative brace to prevent valgus stress is typically used for the first 6 weeks postoperatively. Patients with combined ACL/MCL injuries frequently have more pain, effusion, and difficulty achieving full passive knee range of motion after ACL reconstructive surgery.[128] Therefore the physical therapist should pay close attention to effusion control and regaining knee range of motion with an emphasis on achieving full passive knee extension.

Combined ACL/posterior cruciate ligament (PCL) injuries appear to have improved short- and long-term functional outcomes with ligament reconstructive surgery versus nonoperative treatment.[82] The primary differences between the standard ACL reconstruction program and the combined ACL/PCL reconstruction rehabilitation program are a slower progression in weight bearing, resumption of knee flexion, and introduction of strengthening exercises.[128] In general, these patients undergo protected weight bearing for a total of 6 weeks. A gradual progressive knee range of motion program is emphasized, with early establishment of full knee extension, and 90 degrees of flexion by the beginning of postoperative week 7. A PCL brace can be used during the first 8 to 12 weeks after surgery to reduce posterior tibial sagging. CKC exercises and bicycling can begin during postoperative weeks 8 to 12. OKC quadriceps exercises (between 0 and 45 degrees of knee flexion) also begin during this period. Aerobic conditioning with low-impact activities, such as walking and use of an elliptical trainer, may begin at 3 to 4 months postoperatively, and light jogging may begin at 5 to 6 months postoperatively. OKC resisted knee flexion should not occur until at least 6 months postoperatively. More aggressive agility drills should be delayed until 6 to 9 months postoperatively. Return to sports and heavy labor occurs thereafter, after sufficient range of motion, strength, and proprioceptive skills have returned.

Sixty four percent to 77% of ACL injuries are accompanied by traumatic meniscal tears.[116,128] If a partial meniscectomy is performed, the post-ACL reconstructive surgery rehabilitation program will remain essentially unchanged, although it may take longer to introduce running and jumping activities. However, if the meniscal injury is treated with surgical repair, the patient will use crutches with partial weight bearing to be performed with a brace locked in extension for the first 3 to 4 weeks postoperatively. During this time, patients are allowed to perform non–weight-bearing range-of-motion exercises as tolerated, with limits of flexion anywhere from 90 to 120 degrees depending on the complexity of the repair. Rehabilitation then progresses similar to that of the previously mentioned post-ACL reconstructive surgery rehabilitation program. However, the patient is instructed to avoid knee flexion and weight bearing for at least 4 to 6 months after surgery, again, depending on the complexity of the repair.

If the patient requires surgical microfracture treatment of an articular cartilage lesion sustained at the time of the ACL injury, activities that increase articular cartilage shear stress should be delayed.[128] Although passive range-of-motion exercises should be encouraged because of the nutritional benefits of joint movement on articular cartilage, the postoperative weight-bearing progression should be postponed considerably.[128] The actual postoperative weight-bearing status depends on the location of the chondral lesion within the knee.[45] Lesions of the patella and trochlea may bear weight as tolerated in a hinged brace with a 30-degree flexion stop. Alternatively, if the area of microfracture is in the medial or lateral compartment, the patient is kept strictly touch-down weight bearing for 6 weeks. A CPM machine is used for 6 to 8 hours per day during the first 6 weeks postoperatively. After 6 weeks the patients begin gradually progressive weight bearing and progresses to full weight bearing by 12 weeks or as tolerated. Return to sports that require cutting, pivoting, or jumping are restricted for 4 to 6 months postoperatively.

SUMMARY

An optimal rehabilitation program is essential for a fully functional return to sports and other activities in patients who have suffered an ACL tear regardless of surgical management. It is essential that patients progress through the varying stages of the ACL rehabilitation protocol and that patients are able to demonstrate adequate return of neuromuscular control, strength, power, lower extremity symmetry, and proficiency in their sport or activity prior to return. For the postoperative patient, it is critical that the surgeon have an understanding of the biomechanical and biologic properties of the specific ACL graft and fixation construct used and the potential implications for the rehabilitation process. Finally, various aspects of these protocols can be modified based on the individual patient's goals, resources, and response to treatment.

KEY REFERENCES

8. Barrack R, Bruckner JD, Kneisl J, et al: The outcome of nonoperatively treated complete tears of the anterior cruciate ligament in active young adults. *Clin Orthop* 259:192–199, 1990.

17. Beynnon B, Uh BS, Johnson RJ, et al: Rehablitation after anterior cruciate ligament reconstruction: a prospective, randomized, double-blind comparison of programs administered over 2 different time intervals. *Am J Sports Med* 33:347–359, 2005.

57. Hewett T, Lindenfeld TN, Riccobene JV, et al: The effect of neuromuscular training on the incidence of knee injury in female athletes: a prospective study. *Am J Sports Med* 27(6):699–706, 1999.

88. Muller U, Krüger-Franke M, Schmidt M, et al: Predictive parameters for return to pre-injury level of sport 6 months following anterior cruciate ligament reconstruction surgery. *Knee Surg Sports Traumatol Arthrosc* 23(12):3623–3631, 2015.

114. Shelbourne K, Nitz P: Acclerated rehabilitation after ACL reconstruction. *Am J Sports Med* 18:292–299, 1990.

The references for this chapter can also be found on www.expertconsult.com.

58

Knee Bracing for Athletic Injuries

Geoffrey S. Van Thiel, Amer Rasheed, Bernard R. Bach, Jr.

Knee injuries represent the most common problem encountered in sports medicine. As sports participation continues to increase, so does the likelihood of sustaining a debilitating knee impairment. Prevention, treatment, and rehabilitation of these injuries are important to both the athlete and the treating physician. Surgery is often a viable option; however, most of these injuries are treated conservatively with rest, therapy, and use of a knee brace.

The use of braces in sports medicine has long been surrounded by debate. Does the benefit of a brace justify the potential discomfort and cost? This question must be evaluated in the context of brace use and the desired purpose. Different braces serve different functions. The American Academy of Orthopaedic Surgeons (AAOS) has defined three categories of knee braces, as follows[31]:
1. Rehabilitative braces—allow protected range of motion after knee surgery
2. Functional braces—provide stability to an unstable knee and improve function
3. Prophylactic braces—prevent injury to a normal knee

In addition to the three proposed categories, unloader and patellofemoral braces have become popular in contemporary orthopedics. Unloader (knee osteoarthritis [OA]) braces are designed to improve function in patients with unicompartmental arthritis and supplement other conservative management. This chapter evaluates the current literature available for braces in each of these categories and clarifies their purpose, function, and usefulness.

REHABILITATIVE BRACES

Rehabilitative braces are designed to protect a reconstructed/repaired ligament and allow early motion. However, the effectiveness of attaining both of these purposes and the clinical need for them have been called into question by the contemporary literature. These braces can be off-the-shelf types with thigh and calf enclosures, hinges, hinge-brace arms, and straps that encircle the brace components (Fig. 58.1). The hinges can be unlocked to allow restricted range of motion, and the braces are typically long to improve the lever arm and stability. Custom braces are available at an added cost. Rehabilitation braces are most prevalent in anterior cruciate ligament (ACL) reconstruction and postoperative protocols.

Bracing After Anterior Cruciate Ligament Reconstruction

There are two main reasons to use a knee brace after ACL reconstruction: (1) to protect the repair and (2) to avoid loss of extension. Various authors and surgeons have different opinions and protocols regarding brace use; some are based on experience, and some are based on the literature. This was clearly illustrated in a survey conducted by Marx and colleagues[63] of 397 AAOS members with regard to ACL surgery. When surgeons were asked whether they prescribed a brace to patients postoperatively for 6 weeks, 40% responded "no," and 60% responded "yes." When asked if they recommended braces postoperatively for sports participation, 38% responded "no," and 62% responded "yes." Despite the disparity in clinical opinion, there have been many prospective randomized clinical trials that evaluated the effect of a postoperative rehabilitation brace as well as a multitude of systematic reviews (Table 58.1).

Harilainen and associates[42,43] performed a randomized controlled trial with a brace and a no-brace group. The brace group used a rehabilitation brace for 12 weeks postoperatively with a gradual increase in weight bearing, and the no-brace group was allowed immediate range of motion with the use of crutches for 2 weeks. The 1-, 2-, and 5-year follow-up examinations revealed no differences in Tegner activity level, Lysholm knee score, laxity, or isokinetic thigh muscle strength.

Brandsson and coworkers[17] also performed a prospective randomized clinical trial on the usefulness of postoperative rehabilitation braces in 50 patients. ACL reconstruction was completed with a bone–patellar tendon–bone (BPTB) autograft, and patients were randomly assigned to undergo rehabilitation for 3 weeks with or without a brace. Patients were followed for 2 years; at the early follow-up visits, rehabilitation with a brace resulted in fewer problems with swelling, a lower prevalence of hemarthrosis and wound drainage, and less pain throughout the early recovery period compared with rehabilitation without a brace. The 2-year follow-up revealed no differences between groups with regard to Tegner activity level, International Knee Documentation Committee (IKDC) rating, one-legged hop and isokinetic strength, or KT-1000 arthrometer measurement of knee laxity.

Moller and colleagues[72] performed a randomized prospective clinical trial in which they randomly assigned 62 patients to 6 weeks of rehabilitation with or without a brace followed by a specific program for up to 6 months. In the early follow-up period, the brace group had slightly higher Tegner activity level scores. At the 2-year follow-up, there were no differences in Lysholm scores, visual analog scale (VAS) scores, range of motion, isokinetic strength, or laxity. The authors concluded that a postoperative knee brace provided no additional benefit. Risberg and associates[91] compared a no-brace population with a brace population in a prospective randomized study that included the use of a postoperative rehabilitative knee brace for

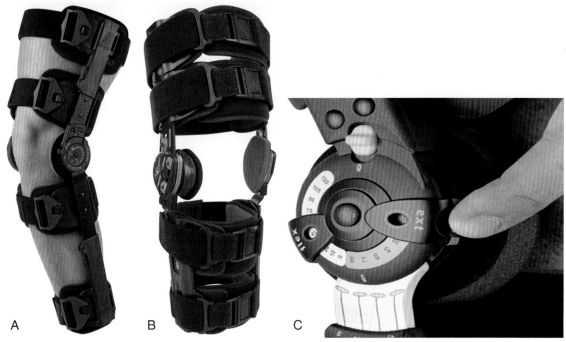

FIG 58.1 Anterior cruciate ligament (ACL) rehabilitation braces. (A) Breg T-Scope; postoperative ACL brace. (B) Donjoy TROM adjuster; postoperative brace. (C) Össur Innovator DLX; dial for the postoperative brace.

2 weeks and then a functional brace for an additional 10 weeks. There were no differences between the groups except at the 3-month point. Despite greater thigh atrophy, the brace group showed an improved Cincinnati Knee Rating System score. Otherwise, KT-1000 laxity, Cincinnati Knee Rating System score, goniometry-measured range-of-motion testing, computed tomography, thigh atrophy measurement, Cybex testing, functional knee tests, and VAS scores all were equal at 6 weeks, 3 months, 6 months, 1 year, and 2 years. Before the 3-month time period, 24% of subjects in the brace group discontinued use.

Mayr and associates[65] also conducted a randomized prospective clinical trial looking at the effects of rehabilitative bracing on 64 patients after ACL reconstruction. All 64 patients followed a defined rehabilitation program for 6 weeks after surgery. In addition to participating in the rehabilitation program, 32 patients were assigned to the brace group and wore a knee brace during the 6 weeks. At 4 years, 52 of the original patients could be examined, and the authors found no significant difference in these patients between the brace and nonbrace groups with regard to 2000 IKDC Subjective Knee Evaluation Form subjective and objective results as well as KT-1000 arthrometer measurement of anteroposterior laxity. VAS pain scores were significantly lower in the nonbrace group under sports activity or heavy physical work. The authors concluded that use of a knee brace after ACL reconstruction showed no advantage over treatment without a brace at 4-year follow-up.

McDevitt and coworkers[67] performed a complete analysis of brace use after ACL reconstruction . In their prospective study, the authors randomly assigned 100 patients over three institutions to brace wear for 1 year after ACL reconstruction or no brace. All patients had a BPTB autograft and were held in extension for 3 weeks postoperatively. In the 95 patients available at 2-year follow-up, no significant differences were found between the brace and nonbrace groups in knee stability, functional testing with the single-leg hop test, IKDC scores, Lysholm scores, knee range of motion, or isokinetic strength testing. Reinjuries occurred in two subjects with braces and three subjects without braces.

The referenced studies are, for the most part, high-quality prospective randomized clinical trials that showed no quantifiable long-term benefit to brace wear after ACL reconstruction with regard to activity level, subjective outcome, or knee laxity. However, some surgeons believe that a brace in the immediate postoperative period can provide the patient additional comfort. Hiemstra and colleagues[45] looked at patients who wore braces for the first 2 days, with a follow-up of 14 days. They found that wearing a brace did not provide any additional pain relief in the acute period above and beyond that for patients who were not immobilized.

Mayr and associates[64] investigated the viability of a soft fluid-filled brace as an alternative to the common hard brace in a randomized clinical trial comprising 72 patients. For 6 weeks after ACL reconstruction, 36 patients wore a hard brace, and 37 patients wore a soft water-filled brace. From 5 days to 12 weeks postoperatively, the soft brace group had significantly less effusion. From 5 days to 12 months, patients in the hard brace group presented with more extension deficit. However, there was no difference between the two groups with regard to complete range of motion, laxity, or thigh atrophy at any follow-up examination. Between 6 weeks and 12 months, the soft brace group had higher IKDC subjective ratings, and at 6 and 12 months, the soft brace group had higher Tegner activity scores and Lysholm knee scores. The results led the authors to conclude that the water-filled soft brace is a safe alternative to and has several advantages over the classic hard brace.

Brace wear has also been proposed as a way to reduce any potential flexion contracture. Petsche and Hutchinson[83]

TABLE 58.1 Summary of Literature: Bracing After Anterior Cruciate Ligament Reconstruction

Study (Year)	Type	No. Patients	Groups	Graft	Follow-Up	Results
Harilainen and Sandelin (2006)[42]	RCT	60	Brace, 12 weeks; no brace, crutches, 2 weeks	BPTB	1, 2, 5 y	No difference: Tegner, Lysholm scores, laxity, muscle strength
Brandsson et al (2001)[17]	RCT	50	Brace, 3 weeks; no brace	BPTB	2 y	Early: brace had less swelling, drainage, pain 2 y: no differences in Tegner, IKDC scores, strength, laxity
Moller et al (2001)[72]	RCT	62	Brace, 6 weeks; no brace	BPTB	2 y	No differences in Lysholm, VAS scores, range of motion, strength, laxity
Risberg et al (1999)[91]	RCT	60	Rehabilitation brace, 2 weeks; functional brace, 10 weeks; no brace	Various	2 y	No differences in laxity, range of motion, strength, functional tests, pain
Mayr et al (2014)[65]	RCT	64	Brace, 6 weeks; no brace	BPTB	4 y	No difference in IKDC 2000 subjective and objective results and KT-1000 Significant difference VAS scores: lower score nonbrace group under sports activity or heavy physical work
McDevitt et al (2004)[67]	RCT	95	Functional brace, 1 y; no brace	BPTB	2 y	No differences in stability, functional testing, IKDC, Lysholm scores, range of motion, strength
Hiemstra et al (2009)[45]	RCT	88	Brace—knee immobilizer, 2 weeks; no brace	Hamstring	2 weeks	No differences in VAS score, pain medication, range of motion
Mayr et al (2010)[64]	RCT	73	Hard brace, 6 weeks; water-filled soft brace, 6 weeks	Hamstring	1 y	Soft brace superior to hard brace regarding effusion, swelling, and patient-measured medium-term outcome
Melegati et al (2003)[68]	Clinical trial	36	Brace locked in extension, 1 week; brace not locked in extension	BPTB	8 weeks, 4 months	Significant differences at 8 weeks: extension greater in extension lock group No differences in KT-1000
Mikkelsen et al (2003)[69]	RCT	44	Brace set at −5 degrees for 3 months; brace set at 0 degree for 3 months	BPTB	3 months	Significant differences in 0-degree group; loss of full extension No differences in flexion, laxity, pain

BPTB, Bone–patellar tendon–bone; *IKDC,* International Knee Documentation Committee; *RCT,* randomized controlled trial; *VAS,* visual analogue scale.

identified loss of knee extension as the biggest problem after ACL reconstruction. Potential causes include surgical technique, graft placement, and postoperative contracture. Melegati and coworkers[68] evaluated the effect of bracing BPTB ACL reconstructions in extension for the first week. In this study, 36 subjects were allocated to an extension bracing group or a brace group with 0 to 90 degrees of motion for the first week. All patients were then allowed unrestricted motion after the first week. The authors found a significant difference in the two groups at the 4- and 8-week postoperative points; the extension bracing group had extension closer to that of the normal knee.

Mikkelsen and coworkers[69] evaluated the concept that the 0-degree setting on a brace does not represent true anatomic 0 degree and that this discrepancy affects postoperative knee extension in patients who have undergone ACL reconstruction. Five subjects were placed in postoperative dressings and extension braces. Radiographs were taken to determine alignment. With the brace set at 0 degree, no subject had an anatomically straight leg (mean, +2.8 degrees) compared with the −5-degree (mean, −2.5 degrees) and −10-degree (mean, −4.1 degrees) settings. Then, in a prospective study of knees after ACL reconstruction, the authors compared the differences between a hyperextension brace (−5 degrees) and an extension brace (0

degree) postoperatively. No significant differences were found between the groups in terms of knee flexion, sagittal knee laxity, or postoperative pain. However, only 2 of 22 patients in the hyperextension brace group had an extension loss more than 2 degrees, whereas 12 of 22 patients in the extension brace group had a loss more than 2 degrees.

In summary, knee bracing in the postoperative period continue to be used by many practicing surgeons for various reasons. However, the evidence that a brace confers additional stability, improves range of motion, protects the graft, reduces pain, or improves subjective outcomes is limited. At long-term follow-up, most prospective randomized clinical trials have shown no difference between subjects with braces and subjects without braces. In contrast, if the brace is used to maintain extension, there is a moderate amount of literature that supports bracing in the acute postoperative period to prevent flexion contractures.

PROPHYLACTIC KNEE BRACES

Many athletes at all levels of competition have experienced significant knee injuries. Prevention and use of prophylactic knee braces have received considerable attention over the last 50 years. This is perhaps most evident in football, in which there is a high percentage of knee injuries; 20% of professional football players never return from ACL reconstruction, and athletes who do return often do not reach their preinjury level of play.[20] Anderson and colleagues[4] were the first to report a prophylactic brace that was predominantly used to protect the medial collateral ligament (MCL) of professional football players; they also speculated that the brace provided increased anterior and posterior stability. They noted that there was no adverse impact on performance for the athletes with braces. No controlled studies were done at that time; however, use of braces in professional and collegiate football players rapidly increased. In this section, we review studies regarding the benefits and drawbacks of prophylactic knee braces (Fig. 58.2 and Table 58.2).

The reports by Anderson and associates[4] led to a significant increase in brace use and studies to evaluate their efficacy in the early and mid-1980s. These early studies failed to demonstrate an appreciable benefit to brace wear, and some studies documented increased injuries and performance impairments. In 1985, the AAOS stated that "Efforts need to be made to eliminate the unsubstantiated claims of currently available prophylactic braces and to curtail the inevitable misuse, unnecessary costs, and medical legal problems."[31] The American Orthopaedic Society of Sports Medicine and the *Journal of Bone and Joint Surgery* took a similar position.[24] The American Academy of Pediatrics went a step further and recommended that prophylactic lateral knee braces not be considered standard equipment for football players because of lack of efficacy and the potential for causing harm.[62]

Two basic types of prophylactic knee braces are designed to prevent or reduce the severity of knee injuries. One type includes lateral bars with a single axis, dual axis, or polycentric hinges. The second type uses a plastic shell that encircles the thigh and calf and has polycentric hinges. The effect on performance and degree of protection provided must be evaluated on an individual basis. There have been a few large studies regarding brace usefulness and functional effects (see later discussion).

Advantages and Disadvantages

No Benefit of Prophylactic Bracing. Teitz and coworkers[115] used the members of Division I in the National Collegiate Athletic Association as its study population. They reviewed statistics from 71 colleges in 1984 and 61 colleges in 1985; 6307 players in 1984 and 5445 players in 1985 were analyzed. The player's position; incidence of injury; type, mechanism, and severity of injury; playing surface; level of skill; and prior knee injury were considered contributing factors. The results showed that players in 1984 and 1985 who wore braces had a significantly higher injury rate than players who did not wear braces. Four different types of prophylactic knee braces were worn, and no attempt was made to differentiate between them with data analysis. The severity of injuries did not differ between the two groups. Player position, playing surface, mechanism of injury, or type of brace did not affect the rates of injury. Injuries were more common during contact and at every skill level in players who used braces. The incidence of ACL injury was similar in both groups, but players who wore braces had more meniscal injuries. The severity of injury was assessed by measuring playing time lost and the need for surgery. Surgical rates were similar for both groups. Although the average playing time lost was less for players who used braces, the increased incidence of injury produced an overall time loss that was greater in players using braces. The authors concluded that prophylactic bracing would not prevent injuries and might actually be harmful.

Hewson and colleagues[44] also performed a study of football players with and without brace wear over an 8-year period

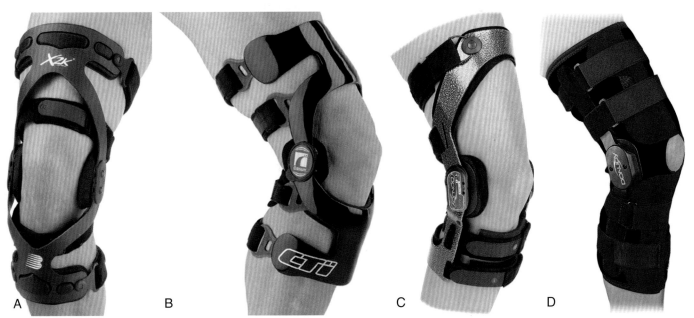

FIG 58.2 Prophylactic and functional knee braces. (A) Breg X2K High Performance; indicated for anterior cruciate ligament (ACL), posterior cruciate ligament (PCL), medial collateral ligament (MCL), and lateral collateral ligament (LCL) instabilities. (B) Össur CTi Custom; custom-made brace; indicated for ACL, MCL, LCL, PCL, rotary, and combined instabilities. (C) DonJoy AirArmor; moderate to severe ACL, PCL, MCL, and LCL instabilities. (D) DonJoy Playmaker; neoprene with hinges, for mild to moderate ligament instabilities.

TABLE 58.2	Summary of Literature: Prophylactic Knee Bracing				
Study (Year)	**Type**	**Subjects**	**Groups**	**Follow-Up**	**Results and Comments**
Teitz et al (1987)[115]	Retrospective case	11,752 players	Brace; no brace	1 season	Players who wore braces had higher injury rates and more meniscal injuries; no controls and 4 braces used; college football players
Hewson et al (1986)[44]	Case control	57,484 exposures	Anderson Knee Stabler; brace; no brace	8 y	No differences in injury rates or severity of injury; college football players
Rovere et al (1987)[95]	Case control	742 player seasons	Anderson Knee Stabler; brace; no brace	1 season	No differences in injury rate; cramping and financial expenditure larger in brace group; college football players
Grace et al (1988)[39]	Prospective clinical trial	580	Single-hinged brace (247); double-hinged brace (83); no brace (250)	2 y	High school football players; significantly greater injury rate in single hinge; significantly greater foot and ankle injuries in brace group
Sitler et al (1990)[102]	RCT	1396 players	Double-hinged brace; biaxial brace; no brace	2 y	Football—military cadets; shoe-, compliance-, and brace-controlled; significantly greater injury rate in nonbrace group
Sanders et al (2011)[96]	Prospective clinical trial	2115	Brace; no brace	1 y	Nonbrace group had significantly higher overall injury rate as well as injury rate for ACL and MCL; no significant difference in rates of any other type of injury
Albright et al (1994)[2,3]	Prospective clinical trial	987	Brace; no brace		Analyzed injury patterns for college football MCL; trend toward decreased injury rates with brace wear, especially for linemen and linebackers

ACL, Anterior cruciate ligament; *MCL*, medial collateral ligament; *RCT*, randomized controlled trial.

(1977–1985). The nonbrace period was reviewed from 1977 to 1981. Following this period, the Anderson Knee Stabler (Omni Life Science, Vista, CA) was mandatory for all practices and games for players at greatest risk, including linemen, linebackers, and tight ends. In the mandatory brace group, 28,191 exposures occurred, and 29,293 exposures occurred in the nonbrace group. Information was analyzed by type of injury, severity of injury, player's position, days lost from practice or games, and rate of knee injury/season per 100 players at risk. Results showed that the number of knee injuries was similar for the brace and nonbrace groups, and the type and severity of injury were similar in all categories. Rovere and associates[95] also performed a 2-year study that included all players on the Wake Forest football team using the Anderson Knee Stabler prophylactically during practice and games. A 2-year nonbrace group control period was evaluated and compared with a subsequent brace group. The time and mechanism of injury, diagnosis, and treatment were noted. Brace use did not significantly alter the relative frequency of injuries by player or position; also, brace wear was associated with cramping and added financial expenditures.

Grace and coworkers[39] evaluated 580 high school football players over a 2-year period; 250 athletes without braces were matched according to size, weight, and position with 247 athletes wearing single-hinged braces and 83 athletes wearing double-hinged braces. The athletes who wore the prophylactic single-hinged braces had a significantly higher knee injury rate ($P < .001$), and the athletes wearing double-hinged braces had a greater number of injuries (no statistical significance). Foot and ankle injuries occurred three times more frequently in the athletes wearing braces ($P < .01$). Different playing surfaces were used, and no documentation of prophylactic ankle taping

was noted. The study results not only questioned the efficacy of prophylactic knee braces but also called attention to the potential adverse effects on adjacent joints.

Potential Benefit of Prophylactic Bracing. The previous studies suggested no benefit and potential detrimental effects of prophylactic bracing. However, some well-designed studies have purported a benefit for specific football positions. Initially, Garrick and Requa[35] conducted a review of available studies and noted two studies that suggested a benefit of prophylactic braces, one by Schriner[99] and one by Taft and associates.[112] However, these studies were presented at conferences and were never published. Furthermore, there were significant methodologic concerns with the study designs. Garrick and Requa[35] were unable to reach a conclusion with regard to brace use secondary to the lack of well-designed clinical trials.

In 1990, Sitler and colleagues[102] reported the results of a prospective, well-controlled research study on the effectiveness of a single, upright biaxial brace in a 2-year study of 1396 United States Military Academy cadets playing intramural tackle football as their mandatory competitive sport. The military population afforded control of the athletic shoe, athlete exposure, brace assignment and compliance, playing surface, and knee injury history. The study was completed over 2 years; at the beginning of each year, the subject was assigned to a brace or nonbrace group. The brace selected was the DonJoy Protective Knee Guard (DonJoy Braces, Coconut Creek, FL) a double-hinged, single, upright, off-the-shelf brace applied to the leg with a brace-constrained, no-slip strap and neoprene thigh and calf straps. Individuals with ACL deficiencies, reconstructions, or repairs were excluded from the study. Knee injuries were defined as injuries that were severe enough to cause a missed practice or game. Nonsurgical evaluation was confirmed by at least two of three orthopedic surgeons, and the injury was classified accordingly. There were 71 injuries, and the overall knee injury rate was 2.46/1000 athlete exposures. The nonbrace group had a significantly higher rate of injury than the brace group (3.40/1000 vs 1.50/1000 athlete exposures). There was also a trend noted toward decreased severity of injury in the brace group. This was a well-designed study with significant control, and the authors concluded that in this study population there is a benefit to prophylactic brace use.

In a more recent study, Sanders and coworkers[96] studied injuries and the use of prophylactic bracing in off-road motorcyclists. The authors obtained data on 2115 motorcycle riders during a 1-year period through an Internet-based survey. The orthoses used in the study included custom-made and commercially available knee braces. Participants reported 39,611 total hours of riding, and 57 riders had at least one riding-related knee injury that fit the inclusion criteria. Only knee injuries that were evaluated by a physician were included in the study. The most common injuries involved the ACL (43%), menisci (20%), and MCL (15%). The overall injury rate was found to be significantly higher in the nonbrace group versus the brace group (3.675 vs 1.587 per 1000 riding h). In addition, rates of ACL and MCL injury were significantly higher in the nonbrace group versus the brace group (1.518 vs 0.701 per 1000 rider h and 0.799 vs 0.111 per 1000 rider h, respectively). No significant difference was found in the rates of any other type of injury.

Another well-done study was completed by the Big Ten Sports Medicine Committee. These investigators conducted a 3-year prospective, multiinstitutional analysis of MCL sprains in college football players.[2,3] In this study, 987 previously uninjured participants were classified according to their frequency of wearing preventive knee braces. These subjects were then studied, and the brace use patterns from 100 injuries were analyzed. The investigators evaluated the following factors:
- Patterns of MCL sprains that occurred in knees without braces
- Daily brace wear records of the study group
- Importance of the relationship between injury patterns in knees without braces and brace wear tendencies in study group participants

Confirmation that a reportable MCL sprain had occurred was the combined responsibility of the team athletic trainer and the team physician; confirmation was based on clinical determination and examination. The total number of injuries was recorded. With regard to brace use, 50.7% of the 55,722 knee exposures were with braces. The pattern of where, when, and how often an individual participant chose to wear a brace most closely paralleled the patterns of his peers playing the same position and their string. The line players tended to wear braces almost 75% of the time in both games and practices. The linebackers and tight ends wore braces 50% of the time in practices and 40% of the time during games. Finally, players in the skill positions wore braces only 26% of the time in practices and 10% of the time during games. The effectiveness of preventive braces was examined by comparing only the injury rates for players with and without braces who were in the same position groups playing during the same sessions. For players in practice, all position groups displayed lower injury rates with brace use. During games, the same trend held true for the linemen and linebacker–tight end group but not for the skill position players.

Although none of these numbers were statistically significant, a consistent trend in favor of the braces did emerge. For players in the two position groups (linemen and linebackers–tight ends) who were at greatest risk of such injury, the injury rates were lower for players wearing braces. The protective tendency of the braces to reduce risk of injury was greatest in the linebacker–tight end positions. However, this group did not wear braces as often as expected because they were allegedly torn between protecting their knees and keeping up with the speed of their competition.

Performance Impairments With Bracing

There does appear to be a potential role for prophylactic brace use in specific situations with specific athletes. However, this preventive benefit must be weighed against any potential performance impairments that the brace could cause. These impairments may be a direct effect of increased intramuscular pressures, muscle performance, knee joint kinematics, and associated energy costs. The following studies must be reviewed in the context of the time during which they were conducted. Many braces in use at the present time have improved on the initial concepts and shortcomings of the braces historically used and reported in the studies reviewed here.

Styf and associates[109] studied the intramuscular pressures associated with functional braces. The intramuscular pressures of eight healthy athletes were recorded at rest and during and after exercise in the supine, sitting, and standing positions. Three braces were used in this study; a catheter was connected to an electromagnetic transducer, and intramuscular pressures were measured by an infusion technique. Pressures at rest increased significantly in all positions in study participants with braces. Muscle relaxation pressure during exercise also increased significantly. Muscle relaxation pressures decreased to pre–brace wear levels after removal of the brace or the distal straps. The results of this study suggested that external compression from a knee brace on leg muscles may induce premature muscle fatigue by reducing perfusion of the working muscle. More recently, Lundin and Styf[60] demonstrated that there is a direct correlation between thigh and tibial strap tensions and intramuscular values. There is also an inverse relationship with local blood perfusion.

Houston and Goemans[48] evaluated the performance of knees with and without braces. Seven athletes with knee instability underwent four tests. Maximal torque output was measured during knee extension. Isometric torque was measured at a knee angle of 90 degrees at increasing velocities (30 degrees/s, 90 degrees/s, 180 degrees/s, and 300 degrees/s). Maximal unloaded angular velocity was measured during leg extension. Vertical velocity and power were determined using a short stair run. In addition, blood lactate concentration was measured 1 minute after a 15-minute ride on a bicycle ergometer. Maximal torque during isokinetic knee extension without braces was found to be significantly higher, and the differences between study participants with and without braces increased as velocity increased. Maximal unloaded knee extension velocity was 20% faster for individuals without braces during the stair run. In addition to reporting impaired performance for study participants with braces, an increased energy expenditure was observed; the blood lactate level increased 41% for participants with braces.

This finding of increased energy expenditure was supported by Zetterlund and associates,[123] who showed increased energy cost during treadmill running at a slow rate in 10 players.

Oxygen consumption and heart rate significantly increased in athletes with braces. Energy consumption is not the only adverse effect reported with brace wear. In the context of proprioception, Osternig and Robertson[80] noted significant changes in joint position sense and electromyographic activity in six healthy volunteers when a brace was worn compared with when it was not worn. However, these claims were not supported in a more recent study by Bottoni and coworkers,[15] who found that knee supports do not influence knee proprioception in healthy active subjects.

Sforzo and colleagues[100] showed that wearing a dual-hinged brace did not affect the performance of 25 male football players, although brace wear did inhibit 10 women's collegiate lacrosse team members. The testing protocol involved the use of a Cybex II lower extremity isokinetic dynamometer to measure peak quadriceps torque, rise time, and time to fatigue. A Monark cycle ergometer (HealthCare International, Langley, WA) fitted with a Lafayette impulse counter (Lafayette Instrument Company, Lafayette, IN) was then used to perform a 30-second maximal effort Wingate test of anaerobic power. Serum lactate accumulation was determined as the difference between postexercise and resting lactate levels. Although the overall performance score was significantly different, the differences were not significant for any one of the parameters.

Veldhuizen and associates[118] did not support the theory that brace wear affects performance. There was no significant difference between healthy study participants with and without braces performing testing for isokinetic muscle strength, a 60-m dash, a vertical jump height test, and treadmill running. Knutzen and coworkers[52-54] studied the knee joint kinematics of six subjects wearing braces who ran a 12- to 13-km/h pace. Knee stability and function were studied during maximum knee flexion in the swing phase, maximum knee flexion during the support phase, maximum external tibial rotation, and maximum internal tibial rotation. It was concluded in this and other reports that rotation and abduction-adduction decrease for individuals wearing braces but do not affect performance.[114]

In a series of studies, Mortaza and colleagues[73,74] also opposed the idea that bracing weakens the knee. The authors had the participants perform a multitude of tests with a knee brace, neoprene sleeve, knee sleeve with four bilateral metal supports, or no brace. One study tested 31 healthy male athletes and showed no statistically significant difference between the four conditions in jump height, crossover hop distance, peak torque-to-body ratio, and average power.[74] Another study tested six healthy male subjects and six subjects with ACL deficiency and found no statistically significant difference between the conditions in vertical-jump, hop, torque-time curve frequency content, peak torque, and average power.[73] In addition, the authors saw some benefits to the brace/sleeves in subjects with ACL deficiency with regard to extension peak torque and power-generating capacity, which could be helpful in reducing bilateral asymmetry.

Baltaci and associates[9] compared the effect of five different knee braces on performance in 24 healthy subjects. They found that the hinged "H" buttress for support of the knee brace (DJO Global, Vista, CA) was more effective than others in balance tests, and the Drytex economy hinged knee brace (DJO Global) was more effective than others in proprioceptive and maximal force tests. Greene and coworkers[40] demonstrated the effects of bracing on speed and agility as well as the tendency of the brace to migrate in 30 college football players. Players in full gear ran

a 40-yard dash and performed a four-cone agility drill either wearing braces on both knees or wearing no brace, serving as matched controls. Brace migration and subjective measures were recorded after each trial. In the 40-yard dash, times did not significantly differ when using the AirArmor 1 (AirArmor Sports, Scottsdale, AZ) and OMNI (OMNI Life Science, East Taunton, MA) braces compared with no-brace control times. Times with other braces were significantly slower, with the Breg (Breg, Vista, CA) having the slowest time, followed by DonJoy, McDavid (McDavid USA, Woodridge, IL), and AirArmor. The AirArmor 1 and McDavid braces showed significantly less superior-inferior migration in the 40-yard dash than the other braces. These findings indicate that specific braces have differential effects on the athlete and that fit is an important factor to prevent migration.

Marchini and colleagues[61] evaluated proprioception, comfort, and muscle force control in conventional and new-generation knee and ankle orthoses. In their randomized controlled trial of 16 healthy subjects, they found that new-generation orthoses produced better dynamic control of submaximal forces and better kinesthesia in the knee joint. The new-generation orthoses were also rated higher in subjective comfort and preference scores. However, there was no difference between the two orthoses in static balance and perceived joint stability.

Rishiraj and associates[92,94] looked at accommodation to brace use and how it might affect performance in 27 healthy male subjects over 6 days. The participants went through five testing sessions without a brace (day 1–3) and five testing sessions using a custom functional knee brace (day 4–6). Each subject participated in two testing sessions per day. The sessions included the repeated high-intensity shuttle and Léger beep/multistage tests as well as tests for acceleration, agility, speed, and lower extremity power. The authors found that performance was initially hindered with the use of a brace; however, after 14 hours of brace use, there was no difference in performance or fatigue between subjects with and without braces.

In summary, use of prophylactic knee braces remains controversial. These braces have not consistently been shown to prevent or reduce the severity of injuries to the ACL or menisci. Several studies have shown a trend toward a reduced incidence of serious MCL injuries, but other studies have shown no change in the incidence of these injuries. Evidence suggests that brace use for specific positions and athletes is beneficial (e.g., for football linemen). However, this recommendation must be weighed against the fact that other studies have shown decreased performance and increased muscle fatigue in subjects wearing a brace. Many of the studies reviewed used older braces that are no longer on the market, and the possibility that newer braces have improved on previous shortcomings is acknowledged. Further brace and sport-specific studies need to be completed before any definitive conclusions can be drawn.

FUNCTIONAL KNEE BRACES

Functional knee braces (see Fig. 58.2) have shown limited clinical usefulness in various studies, although many studies reported improved subjective knee stability with brace use (Table 58.3). Although scientific evidence supporting the clinical efficacy of functional knee braces is limited, they continue to have widespread use. In 1995, a survey of practice patterns for use of functional braces revealed that most sports medicine orthopedic surgeons surveyed prescribed braces for patients with ACL

TABLE 58.3   Summary of Clinical Studies: Functional Knee Bracing

Study (Year)	Type	Subjects	Groups	Follow-Up	Results/Information
McDevitt et al (2004)[67]	RCT	95	Functional brace, 1 y; no brace	2 y	No differences in stability, functional testing, IKDC and Lysholm scores, range of motion, strength
Risberg et al (1999)[91]	RCT	60	Postoperative rehabilitation brace, 2 weeks; functional brace, 10 weeks; no brace	2 y	No differences in laxity, range of motion, strength, functional tests, pain, patient satisfaction
Birmingham et al (2008)[14]	RCT	150	Brace at 6 weeks after ACL reconstruction; neoprene sleeve at 6 weeks postoperative	2 y	No differences in questionnaire, KT-1000, Tegner score
Sterett et al (2006)[106]	Prospective clinical trial	820	Brace—post–ACL reconstruction; no brace	1 season	Skiers: brace group significantly fewer knee injuries
Swirtun et al (2005)[111]	RCT	42	Brace for ACL deficiency; no brace	6 months	Management of acute ACL tears; no differences in functional knee scores; significantly lower subjective instability in brace group

ACL, Anterior cruciate ligament; *IKDC,* International Knee Documentation Committee; *RCT,* randomized controlled trial.

deficiency and ACL reconstruction.[26] Only 1% reported never prescribing braces for patients with ACL deficiency, and 7% reported never prescribing braces for patients with ACL reconstruction. In a follow-up study in 2003, 13% of physicians reported never prescribing braces for patients with ACL reconstruction, whereas only 3% never prescribed braces for patients with ACL deficiency.[25] Half of the respondents reported prescribing braces less frequently than 5 years ago.

The theory behind functional bracing is that normal gait patterns at a low cadence rate generally do not pose any difficulty to these patients, but instability and risk of further injury are possible if above-normal cadence or sudden deceleration movements are encountered. Instability is primarily caused by knee subluxation and tibial rotation during the terminal aspect of knee extension. The contributing factor for such instability seems to be the increased angular velocity of the knee during fast cadence rates when anatomic deficiencies allow increased impact energy at extension, resulting in anterior displacement and rotation of the tibia relative to the femur.[31] Functional braces attempt to control these abnormal moments.

McDevitt and associates[67] conducted a prospective randomized clinical trial comparing rehabilitation using functional bracing for 1 year with rehabilitation without bracing after ACL reconstruction in 95 patients. Both groups were treated for the first 3 weeks after surgery with a rehabilitation brace locked in extension. Then the knee was mobilized gradually from 3 to 6 weeks in the functional brace group, with the rehabilitation brace used intermittently. The patient was then fitted for a functional brace at 6 weeks and allowed full range of motion. The brace was worn full time for the following 6 months and thereafter during all rigorous activities until 1 year after surgery. In the nonbrace group, bracing was discontinued after 3 weeks. At the 2-year follow-up examination, there were no differences between the groups with regard to anterior-posterior knee laxity, one-legged hop distance, IKDC and Lysholm scores, range of motion, and isokinetic strength. Two subjects in the brace group and three subjects in the nonbrace group sustained reinjuries to their ACL graft. It was concluded that there are no significant differences between the brace and nonbrace treatment groups.

In a second prospective randomized clinical trial, Risberg and coworkers[91] compared rehabilitation with functional bracing with rehabilitation without bracing after ACL reconstruction in 60 patients. The brace group was protected by a rehabilitation brace for 2 weeks, and a functional brace was used almost full time for the following 10 weeks. Thereafter, the functional brace was used as needed for sports. The nonbrace group had no brace at any time postoperatively. The authors found no evidence that bracing had an effect on knee joint laxity, range of motion, strength, functional knee tests, patient satisfaction, or pain at final 2-year follow-up. Birmingham and colleagues[14] also performed a randomized prospective study of a brace versus a neoprene sleeve for functional use after ACL reconstruction. In this study, 150 patients were given a brace or a neoprene sleeve at 6 weeks postoperatively and then followed for 2 years. There were no significant differences in any objective scores or adverse events.

Sterett and associates[106] prospectively evaluated skiers who had ACL reconstruction and used or did not use a functional brace; 257 subjects used a functional knee brace, and 563 did not use a brace. Despite the fact that the skiers with braces had a significantly higher percentage of grade II Lachman tests, there was a significantly decreased rate of subsequent knee injuries: 8.9 injuries/100 knees per ski season in the nonbrace group and 4.0 injuries/100 knees per ski season in the brace group.

Swirtun and coworkers[111] prospectively evaluated functional knee braces in the nonoperative management of acute (<5 weeks) ACL tears. In this study, 95 patients were randomly assigned to a brace group for 12 weeks or to a no-brace group; 42 patients completed the study. There were no differences in functional knee scores at 6-month follow-up; however, the brace group had significantly lower subjective instability ratings.

Studies of the Lenox Hill brace (Lenox Hill Brace Shop, New York, NY) by Colville and colleagues[22] showed that the absolute laxity of the deficient knee is unchanged by the brace, but that the relative resistance to displacement is increased. Branch and associates[16] evaluated the contribution of functional bracing to muscle-firing amplitude, duration, and timing, which may result in improved dynamic stability. Ten subjects with ACL deficiency and five normal control subjects were evaluated using foot switches and dynamic electromyography. Bracing did not alter the relative electromyography activity and did not change firing patterns compared with no brace wear. All muscles showed a similar reduction in activity, suggesting that functional braces do not have a proprioceptive influence.

In more recent literature examining the mechanism of how functional braces might act, Stanley and colleagues[105] found that although knee extension braces did not consistently reduce posterior ground reaction forces, they did consistently increase knee flexion angle, which should help reduce ACL loading. Rishiraj and coworkers[93] similarly compared peak ground reaction forces in patients with and without functional knee braces. Their study showed that functional brace use can significantly lower peak vertical ground reaction forces in patients. The authors stated that this may help prevent traumatic forces from reaching the ACL until neuromuscular restraints are activated to protect the knee joint ligaments. Butler and associates[19] looked at motion asymmetry in patients wearing functional knee braces during rehabilitation after ACL reconstruction surgery. The authors performed a motion analysis on 23 subjects during a stop-jump activity both with and without knee braces on the surgical side. They found that functional knee braces may improve symmetry of lower knee mechanics, which could help prevent second ACL tears.

Cook and coworkers[23] performed a dynamic analysis of functional knee braces for athletes with ACL deficiency. Foot switch, high-speed photography, and force plate data were recorded with and without the custom-fitted CTi braces (Össur, Foothill Ranch, CA). Cutting angle, approach time to cut, and time on the force plate showed no significant differences during brace wear. Athletes who did not achieve 80% of the isokinetic quadriceps torque of the normal limb generated significantly more forces during cutting maneuvers while wearing their braces. Athletes also reported better subjective results while snow skiing and waterskiing compared with playing basketball and racket sports. They noted subjectively fewer subluxation episodes and better performance with the brace. Improvements were even more significant in the patients with quadriceps deficiency, suggesting that athletes who do not achieve complete rehabilitation may obtain increased benefit from functional knee bracing.

Rink and colleagues[90] compared the CTi, OTI (DJ Orthopedics, Vista, CA), and TS7 (Omni Scientific, Springfield, UT) knee braces in 14 patients with ACL deficiency as shown on arthroscopy. The subjects evaluated the braces and underwent testing with physical examination, KT-1000 arthrometry, and timed running events. All braces reduced subjective symptoms of knee instability, and a reduction in anterior tibial displacement was seen with all braces at low loads. However, this reduction decreased as forces increased. A timed figure-eight running event did not show any functional advantage, and five subluxation events occurred in four subjects while wearing a brace.

Strutzenberger and associates[107] looked at the effect of two different brace designs in 28 patients with ACL deficiency. The authors evaluated the sleeve brace design and shell brace design by testing subjects wearing a SofTec Genu brace (Bauerfeind Inc., Zeulenroda-Triebes, Germany) and 4Titude Donjoy brace (ORMED GmbH, Freiburg, Germany), respectively. Subjects participated in a series of tests using one of the two braces. The results showed that although both designs had similar effects on functional achievements, such as reduction of knee joint laxity, the sleeve brace design showed a higher effect size and increased rate of force development at the counter-movement-jump. The authors hypothesized that this may be partly because sleeve braces also address proprioceptive mechanisms. The authors further suggested that it may be favorable to incorporate proprioceptive elements in future functional brace designs.

Mishra and colleagues[71] evaluated four functional knee braces and their effect on anterior knee laxity. All braces reduced giving-way episodes and the grade of pivot shift testing. Brace use decreased anterior displacement on KT-1000 measurements at 89-N, high-load passive anterior displacement and with quadriceps contraction active displacement. There was no significant effect on functional test results. Patients with the most functional limitations had the most improvement, whereas patients minimally affected had diminished performance.

Several studies have evaluated metabolic costs of knee brace wear. Highgenboten and coworkers[46] studied four braces in 14 normal subjects performing horizontal treadmill running. The braces caused increases in oxygen consumption, heart rate, and ventilation of 3% to 8% compared with running without the brace. Subjective exertion also was increased 9% to 13%. The authors concluded that the braces caused a consistent increase in metabolic cost, which was related to their weight. These results are consistent with past research on prophylactic braces showing increased energy costs and intramuscular pressures.[48,108,109,123]

In summary, definitive studies supporting or refuting functional brace use have not been done. The treating physician must make educated, patient-specific recommendations. In a patient after ACL reconstruction, there does not appear to be a clear benefit (objective or subjective) to brace use. However, in the setting of ACL deficiency or instability, there is a subjective and biomechanical advantage to brace use. Although this benefit has not translated into a significant functional improvement, brace use should still be considered in this patient subset. Further studies are needed to clarify the usefulness and benefit of functional knee bracing.

BIOMECHANICAL FINDINGS

Clinical studies may provide the highest usefulness and practice application; however, it is notoriously difficult to control all extraneous variables. Thus, biomechanical corollaries provide important information and can direct good clinical research and decision making. The studies reviewed here provide a solid foundation for future clinical research.

Beynnon and colleagues[12] critically evaluated nine subjects with ACL deficiency to determine the effect of functional bracing on knees with chronic ACL deficiency in non–weight bearing and weight bearing and the transition between the two states. They used the Vermont Knee Laxity Device (DJ Orthopedics) and recorded tibial translation relative to the femur in simulated conditions. Bracing resulted in a significant reduction of anterior translation values to a level within normal limits in the non–weight-bearing and weight-bearing states. However, as the knees transitioned from non–weight bearing to weight bearing, the brace group had translation 3.5 times greater than the normal knees. The authors concluded that this is why patients gain partial control of their pathologic laxity but may continue to experience subluxation episodes during activity. Hinterwimmer and associates[47] also showed a decrease in tension in the collateral ligaments in an ACL-deficient cadaveric model with brace use.

Jalali and associates[49] used electromyographic analysis to study functional knee bracing in 10 subjects with ACL deficiency during lunge exercise. The authors found no difference in quadriceps and hamstring activity. They did find that the mean amplitude of the medial gastrocnemius was significantly lower throughout the whole lunge cycle movement and that the lateral gastrocnemius had a significantly lower mean amplitude during the isometric phase of lunge cycle movement. Similarly, Theoret and Lamontagne[116] used electromyographic and three-dimensional kinematic data to evaluate functional bracing in 11 patients with ACL deficiency during running. Few differences were found in the kinematic analysis, and no significant differences were reported in the electromyographic findings; however, based on the data, it was concluded that bracing a knee with ACL deficiency during running has the effect of placing the injured limb in a safer kinematic position, particularly in preparation for and during weight bearing. Bracing also has the effect of increasing the efficiency of the stride by increasing stride length.

Beck and colleagues[11] tested seven functional knee braces on three knees with ACL deficiency with KT-1000 and Stryker knee laxity testers. They found that the hinge, post, and shell types of braces performed consistently better in controlling anterior tibial displacement at low loads. The effectiveness of the functional knee braces in controlling anterior tibial displacement decreased as forces increased. Liu and associates[58] evaluated 10 functional knee braces on a knee model and found that the bilateral hinge–shell models provided the greatest resistance to anterior displacement, whereas the unilateral hinge–shell models provided the least resistance. None of these braces were capable of controlling displacement at high loads. Baker and coworkers[8] evaluated commercially available athletic braces for their effect on abduction forces applied to a cadaveric knee with no instability and with medial instability. Under computer control, abduction forces were applied while simultaneous data were obtained from an electrogoniometer and transducers applied to the ACL and superficial MCL at 0 degree, 15 degrees, and 30 degrees of flexion. Results showed a reduction in abduction angle using functional braces, whereas prophylactic braces showed little or no protective effect.

Pierrat and coworkers[84] studied how well knee braces can replace the mechanical role of the ACL. The authors tested three commercial hinged braces and one knee sleeve using a GNRB arthrometer (GeNouRoB, Laval, France). The testing was done on both pathologic and healthy joints in 16 patients with documented ACL injuries. The results suggested that the braces tested could replace the mechanical role of the ACL only at low anterior tibial displacements.

Beynnon and colleagues[13] used strain transducers applied to the ACL to test scientifically the protective effect of bracing in vivo when different loads were applied to the knee. They found a protective effect of bracing when low anterior shear loads were applied to the knee. However, these low loads were lower than loads during activities of daily living. Along the same lines, Hangalur and coworkers[41] evaluated the effect of knee braces on ACL strain during dynamic activities using a musculoskeletal model, a dynamic knee stimulator on a cadaveric knee, and the Optotrak Certus motion capture system (Northern Digital, Waterloo, Ontario, Canada) on a human subject. They found a significantly lower peak strain in the ACL with the brace (7%)

compared with no brace (20%). The authors concluded that the knee brace could decrease strain in the ACL during dynamic activities in high-risk subjects. They attributed the reduction to altered muscle firing.

Giotis and associates[36-38] studied the effect of knee bracing on tibial rotation in patients with ACL deficiency during high-demand athletic activities. The participants performed two high-demand activities that involved pivoting after either descending from a stair or landing from a platform. The activities were performed wearing a knee brace, knee sleeve, or no brace, and kinematic data were collected during the activities using an eight-camera optoelectronic system (Vicon, Oxford, United Kingdom). The results revealed that brace use can decrease excess tibial rotation in patients with ACL deficiency during high-demand activities, but the brace fails to fully restore normative values.

Cawley and colleagues[21] performed a biomechanical comparison of eight commonly used rehabilitative knee braces using a mechanical limb. Most of the braces significantly reduced translations and rotations compared with the limb with no brace under static test conditions. Factors believed to be important in brace design included overall brace stiffness; the use of nonelastic straps, which adapt to leg contour better; and hinge design, including the presence or absence of joint line contact.

In a biomechanical study using fresh-frozen cadaveric knees, Paulos and coworkers[81,82] measured ligament tension and joint displacement at static nondestructive valgus forces and at low-rated destructive forces. After control knees with no brace were examined, two different laterally applied preventive braces, the McDavid Knee Guard and the Anderson Knee Stabler, were applied to knees. The effects of lateral bracing were analyzed according to valgus force, joint line opening, and ligament tension. Valgus applied forces, with or without braces, consistently produced MCL disruption at ligament tension surprisingly higher than the ACL and higher than or equal to the posterior cruciate ligament. In the first part of the study, no significant protection could be documented with the two preventive braces used. Also, four potentially adverse effects were noted—MCL preloading, center axis shift, premature joint line contact, and brace slippage. In the second part of the study, brace-induced MCL preload in vivo was negated by joint compressive forces. The authors concluded that most prophylactic knee braces presently available are biomechanically inadequate. They noted that before prophylactic knee braces can be categorically recommended, more biomechanical and clinical studies should be initiated.

In 1991, Paulos and colleagues[81] also evaluated the effects of six different prophylactic knee braces on ACL ligament strain under valgus loads using a mechanical surrogate limb. Brace hinge contact with the lateral joint line of the knee reduced the effectiveness. These results should be confirmed clinically, and there is a definite need for improved designs.

Patellofemoral Braces

Patellofemoral pain is a common clinical problem encountered by sports medicine physicians. A retrospective chart review by Taunton and associates[113] found that patellofemoral pain is the primary complaint in patients presenting to a sports medicine clinic. Anterior knee pain has a predilection toward the young female athletes, and patients often present with a history of nontraumatic peripatellar or retropatellar knee pain of gradual onset. The pain is usually worse after exercise activity or after prolonged inactivity, particularly when sitting with the knee in a flexed position. It can be aggravated with ascending and descending stairs. These symptoms are often attributed to the patella and are manifestations of a lateral subluxation force. This can be evident radiographically as a lateral tilt or on examination with lateral laxity. Regardless, initial treatment consists of activity modifications, nonsteroidal antiinflammatory drugs, and physical therapy. The role of bracing in these patients has yet to be clearly delineated (Fig. 58.3). Solinsky and colleagues,[103] surveying 1307 sports medicine professionals, concluded that little overall consensus exists among specialties in the criteria used for prescribing a brace for patellofemoral pain syndrome.

The primary goal of bracing is to centralize the patella within the trochlear groove, improving alignment and tracking. Several studies have demonstrated decreases in pain with brace wear; however, the mechanism whereby braces reduce symptoms has not been elucidated. Although it is assumed that bracing improves patellar kinematics, imaging studies have reported that bracing has little or no effect on patellar alignment or tracking. Apart from changing patellar kinematics, it has been suggested that bracing may have a subtle effect on patellofemoral joint mechanics. For example, the compressive force applied to the patellofemoral joint as a result of bracing could seat the patella more firmly within the trochlear groove, increasing contact area.

In a randomized prospective study, Lun and coworkers[59] evaluated 186 knees with patellofemoral pain in four distinct treatment groups at 3, 6, and 12 weeks of follow-up. The treatment groups included patellofemoral brace only, home exercise, home exercise with patellofemoral brace, and home exercise with knee sleeve. All groups showed reduction in pain and an improvement in function, but there were no differences between the treatment groups. Swart and associates[110] found similar

evidence in their systematic review, which included seven randomized controlled trials and one clinical controlled trial. They concluded that there is no additional benefit to brace wear in terms of pain reduction or functional improvement compared with exercise therapy alone for patients with patellofemoral pain syndrome. These findings were further supported by Miller and colleagues[70] in their study of 59 military cadets during basic training. Subjects presented with anterior knee pain were randomly assigned to therapy only, therapy plus brace type A (Palumbo "Dynamic Patellar Brace," DynOrthotics, Vienna, VA), and therapy plus brace type B (Cho-Pat Knee Strap, Cho-Pat Inc, Hainesport, NJ). At the completion of basic training (6 to 8 weeks), there were no differences between the groups with regard to pain.

Warden and associates[120] performed a systematic review of studies that evaluated patellar bracing and taping. The results of 10 moderate-quality studies demonstrated that, on a 100-mm scale, medially directed patellar tape reduces chronic knee pain by 16 mm compared with no tape. This effect was not dependent on the time course of tape application; pain reductions were observed immediately after tape application and after repeated applications over the short term (3 to 12 weeks), with reductions in pain of 17 mm and 14 mm, respectively. Similarly, the reduction in pain with tape use was independent of diagnosis; medially directed tape reduced pain associated with anterior knee pain by 15 mm and with knee OA by 20 mm. In contrast to the evidence for the benefits of patellar tape, there was disputable evidence for the benefits of a patellar brace. Braces reduced anterior knee pain by 15 mm on a 100-mm scale compared with no brace. This outcome was attributable to the immediate effects in one study,[85] with no differences being found in two studies on the short-term effects of medially directed bracing.[59,70]

Other options exist for treating patellofemoral pain. One option is to use an infrapatellar strap. The evidence is limited,

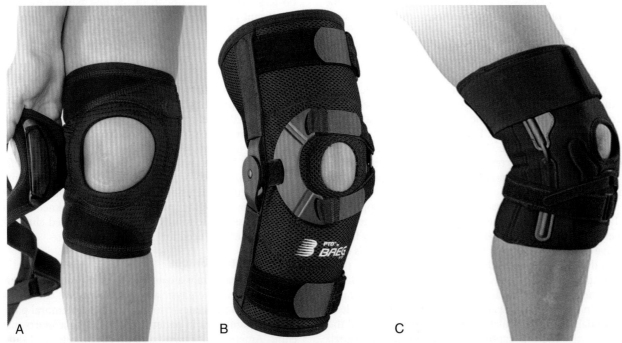

FIG 58.3 Patellofemoral braces. (A) DonJoy Tru-Pull Lite. (B) Breg PTO. (C) Össur patella-stabilizing brace.

but Villar[119] studied the infrapatellar strap in military recruits. The brace was effective in only 24% of recruits in the short term and in 22% at 1 year. Despite these suboptimal results, the strap seems to help some individuals and to have relatively few drawbacks. Another option is the application of Kinesio Tape. Akbas and coworkers[1] compared the use of Kinesio Taping with exercise alone at 3 and 6 weeks of follow-up. In their randomized controlled trial, 31 women with patellofemoral pain syndrome were assigned to either exercise therapy only or exercise therapy with Kinesio Taping at 4-day intervals. Significant improvement in function, soft tissue flexibility, and pain were seen in both groups, although no significant change in patellar shift was seen in either group. However, the authors did see an additional benefit in the Kinesio Tape group of quicker improvement in hamstring muscle flexibility.

The question of whether patellofemoral braces improve knee kinematics has also been evaluated from a biomechanical standpoint. Draper and colleagues[30] used magnetic resonance imaging (MRI) to evaluate patellar mechanics with and without a patellofemoral brace and sleeve. They found an improvement in lateral translation and patellar tilt with the patellofemoral brace. Powers and associates[85] evaluated patellar mechanics and contact pressures in 15 subjects with both MRI and gait analysis for walking and fast walking. They found a significant decrease in peak patellofemoral contact pressures and an increase in patellofemoral contact area in the brace group, with an average 56% decrease in pain perception, suggesting that a possible cause for clinically decreased pain with bracing may be the result of increased contact area between the patella and trochlea. However, in a corollary study, Powers and associates[86] found no significant decrease in peak patellar contact pressure between a brace and nonbrace state for stair climbing. There was an increase in patellar contact area, but the corresponding increase in extensor moment negated any decrease in overall peak contact pressure.

Previously, Shellock and coworkers[101] studied 21 patellofemoral joints with a brace in place. There was restraint to lateral displacement of the patella in 16 knees. They concluded that four of the five other knees did not have a change because these subjects had patella alta. Muhle and colleagues[77] also used MRI data to evaluate the usefulness of a brace in altering patellar kinematics. They studied 24 knees and found no significant improvement in patellar tilt angle, bisect offset, or lateral patellar displacement before or after wearing the patellar brace.

Wilson and associates[121] further addressed the question of the mechanism of action of patellofemoral braces. The authors studied nine cadaveric knees in simulated free speed walking conditions. Each knee was tested with no brace, a knee sleeve, two unique patellar stabilization sleeves, and a wrap-style patellar stabilization brace. All conditions with a brace showed a significant increase in patellofemoral contact area. The knee sleeve and both patellar stabilization sleeves significantly increased patellofemoral contact area compared with the patellar stabilization brace. However, the patellar stabilization brace was the only condition that saw a significant decrease in peak contact pressure. The authors suggested that this was due to the fact that the brace transferred the location of highest pressure to an area with greater articular cartilage thickness.

In conclusion, clinical efficacy has not been reliably shown for bracing for patellofemoral pain. However, despite the dearth of functional evidence, according to Arroll and associates,[7] patients continue to have subjective improvement. A moderate amount of evidence exists showing that taping may provide short-term relief. Regardless, patellar bracing cannot be recommended or denied at this point. More controlled studies must be completed with defined patient populations. The clinical data are inconclusive, but there are biomechanical data that may suggest improvement in knee kinematics.

Unloader Braces

As patients remain active longer into their lives and physiologic age becomes more important than chronologic age, unicompartmental arthritis can pose a significant treatment paradox. Excellent pain relief can be achieved with operative techniques, but the risk of postoperative limitations is significant. A brace that relieves pain can be an attractive option for patients with mild to moderate disease (Fig. 58.4). The question then becomes whether braces work for these patients.

Once a patient begins having medial unicompartmental disease, the adduction moment of the knee can change. Various compensatory mechanisms are then put into play, including redistribution of condylar loads, contraction of antagonist muscle groups, increased tension in the lateral convex soft tissues and cruciate ligaments, increased body sway in the lateral direction, decreased stride length, and decreased inversion moment at the ankle accomplished by out-toeing. When the degeneration overcomes these protective mechanisms, the load becomes excessive, and the result is medial knee pain.

The AAOS has published a consensus statement with an inconclusive strength of recommendation, which does not recommend for or against the use of valgus unloading braces. The AAOS did not evaluate the use of varus unloading braces owing to lack of appropriate studies.[122] In addition, the Osteoarthritis Research Society International has given use of biomechanical interventions for OA, which includes bracing, a recommendation of appropriate, while citing the quality of evidence as fair.[66] These recommendations are largely based on the result of one systematic review[87] and three randomized clinical trials[18,51,117] in the valgus-directing brace group and zero clinical trials in the varus-directing brace group. Kirkley and coworkers[51] were the first to evaluate brace treatment in varus gonarthrosis with a randomized controlled trial. In their study, 119 patients with varus gonarthrosis were randomly assigned to a control group of medical treatment alone, a combined group of medical treatment and a neoprene sleeve, and a combined group of medical treatment and an unloader brace. At the 6-month evaluation, there was a significant improvement in the quality of life and function of the neoprene sleeve group and the unloader brace group. The unloader brace group had significant improvement over the neoprene sleeve group with regard to pain after a 6-minute walking test and a 30-second stair-climbing test. The combination of an unloader brace and medical treatment was the best treatment regimen for varus gonarthrosis.

Brouwer and colleagues[18] completed a multicenter randomized controlled trial comparing brace treatment with standard conservative management. In this study, 117 patients were enrolled and allocated to a brace with conservative treatment arm (60 patients) or conservative management alone arm (57 patients). Follow-up examinations were done at 3-, 6-, and 12-month intervals with VAS, Hospital for Special Surgery, and walking distance scores recorded. The only significant improvement was noted in walking distance, with VAS and Hospital for Special Surgery scores trending toward a decrease in the brace

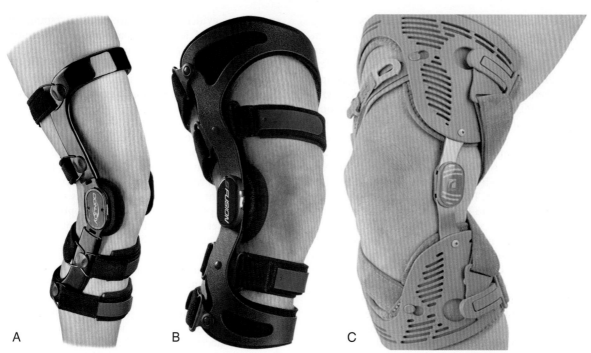

FIG 58.4 Osteoarthritis and unloader braces. (A) DonJoy OA Defiance. (B) Breg Fusion OA. (C) Össur Unloader One; custom knee brace.

group. In the brace group, 25 patients discontinued treatment, and 14 patients in the nonbrace group discontinued treatment. Of the patients who stopped brace treatment, 13 switched to conservative management only and cited "no effect" as the reason. This study led the authors to conclude that brace treatment has a small effect on unicompartmental arthritis, but it also suggests that some patients will not maintain this treatment regimen for an extended period.

The previous studies suggest a benefit of valgus-unloading braces for a varus knee. The question of whether the unloading brace or a control orthosis (neutral knee brace, neoprene knee sleeve, or shoe insert) provides variable levels of pain relief and function improvement was evaluated in a meta-analysis by Moyer and associates.[76] The meta-analysis included six studies with data from 445 patients. When the valgus brace group was compared with the group that did not use an orthosis, there was a moderate statistically significant difference favoring the valgus brace group in both pain and function. However, when the valgus brace group was compared with the group that used a control orthosis, this difference was reduced to a small statistically significant difference favoring the valgus brace group in just pain. Along these same lines, Draganich and coworkers[29] compared the use of an off-the-shelf valgus-directing brace with a custom valgus-directing brace in patients with medial compartment disease; 10 patients participated in a crossover study and served as their own controls. It was concluded that the custom brace is more effective than the off-the-shelf brace in improving the results for pain, stiffness, and function and in reducing the varus angle of alignment of the knee and the peak external adduction moments around the knee during gait and stair stepping.

Nonetheless, the effectiveness of valgus-unloading braces and the cause of pain relief remain controversial. The leading theory—that these valgus-producing braces unload the medial compartment of a varus malaligned knee—has been challenged by some authors. Ramsey and associates[88] suggested that bracing reduces pain and improves function by stabilizing the knee and decreasing antagonistic muscle cocontraction. In their study, 16 subjects were evaluated with no brace and a custom unloader brace in neutral and in 4 degrees of valgus. Pain and function were improved in the brace group but were not significantly different between the neutral and 4 degrees of valgus brace groups. The study suggested that there may be another mechanism for patient improvement in the brace group besides unloading. Moyer and colleagues[75] went further with this idea in their systematic review and meta-analysis including 30 studies with 478 participants. The studies they reviewed suggested that valgus braces can decrease direct and indirect measures of knee compressive forces, decrease quadriceps-gastrocnemius and quadriceps-hamstring cocontraction ratios, and increase medial joint space during gait. The authors concluded that braces can affect knee joint loads through a combination of mechanisms.

To address the question of the effectiveness of unloader braces, Feehan and coworkers[34] conducted a systematic review. The review included 15 studies with a total of 567 participants. The authors stated that all the reviewed studies showed pain reduction in patients, with 73% of the studies showing a statistically significant reduction in pain. Overall, the authors stated that their review indicated strong evidence that pain is relieved with the use of an unloader knee brace. The authors mentioned that eight studies[10,18,33,51,57,89,98,117] in their review looked at the effect of braces on function, and all eight showed significant increases in function for subjects. More recently, Duivenvoorden and associates[32] published a systematic review to address the effectiveness of braces and orthoses in general. The portion of the review that addressed unloader braces included two articles[18,51] that were included in the review by Feehan and coworkers[34] and two[78,97] that were not. The authors stated that evidence was inconclusive in addressing the benefits of bracing for pain, function, stiffness, and quality of life for patients with medial compartment OA of the knee.

One of the biggest problems with unloader braces is that they have a low compliance rate. In a survey administered by Squyer and colleagues[104] to patients fitted for unloader braces, only 25% of the 89 respondents were still using braces regularly after 2 years. The respondents cited brace discomfort, skin irritation, lack of symptom relief, and poor fit as reasons for stopping brace use. A possible solution to increase brace use is to create a more comfortable brace. Della Croce and coworkers,[27] Arazpour and associates,[5,6] and Laroche and colleagues[56] have made progress on this front in their studies looking at the effectiveness of less cumbersome unloading braces. A more immediate solution may be to replace the unloader brace with an option with which patients are more likely to comply. Jones and coworkers[50] conducted a randomized crossover trial comparing valgus knee braces and lateral wedged insoles; 28 participants were exposed to both lateral wedged insoles and valgus knee braces in a random order with a 2-week washout period in between. Although the authors noted that there were no differences in clinical outcomes between the two treatments, insoles demonstrated a greater level of acceptance by patients. Van Raaij and colleagues[117] also performed a study comparing insoles and braces; 91 patients were randomly assigned to either a lateral wedged insole group (45 patients) or a valgus knee brace group (46 patients). The participants were evaluated at baseline and at 6 months. The researchers found no difference between the two groups in VAS pain scores or Western Ontario and McMaster Universities Osteoarthritis Index function scores at 6 months. The authors' analysis also showed that the knee varus malalignment was not reduced in either group. Furthermore, they found a significant difference in compliance between the insole group (71%) and the brace group (45%) and the amount of time each group used its intervention during the week (57.8 h in the insole group and 38.8 h in the brace group). The authors concluded that laterally wedged insoles may be a viable alternative to valgus knee bracing for medial compartment OA of the knee.

Lamberg and coworkers[55] studied 15 patients with medial compartment arthritis. The subjects were assessed at baseline, fitted with a valgus brace, and assessed again at 2 and 8 weeks. Significant decreases of 36% and 34% were found for knee adduction impulse and 26% for second peak adduction moment at weeks 2 and 8, respectively. Similarly, Lindenfeld and colleagues[57] assessed 11 patients with confined medial arthritis using an automated gait analysis to study the adductor moment of a valgus-producing brace. The 11 patients were custom-fitted with a valgus-producing brace and compared with 11 healthy control subjects. The mean adduction moment with the use of the brace decreased 10%, approaching the normal control subjects. The VAS pain score decreased 48%, and the Cincinnati Knee Rating System score increased 79%. This study showed that pain, function, and biomechanics of the knee are improved with the use of an appropriately fitted unloader brace.

Dennis and coworkers[28] and Nadaud and associates[79] published results of a three-dimensional imaging study of the effect of valgus unloading braces and found a small benefit to these braces with the most significant improvement at heel-strike and the smallest effect at midstance. The authors also noted that obese patients experienced less benefit both clinically and radiographically. They also found a wide variability among different manufacturers.

In conclusion, as with the other brace categories, additional randomized controlled trials need to be completed before solid conclusions can be made regarding unloader braces. However, some current studies do suggest a benefit from clinical and biomechanical standpoints. The cause of this pain relief remains under debate. Given the mild adverse effects of bracing (cost and inconvenience), it can be considered for nonobese active patients with mild to moderate unicompartmental arthritis. However, with the low rate of compliance of brace use, it may be important to consider alternative interventions for patients, such as lateral wedged insoles.

SUMMARY

Knee bracing for the prevention and treatment of athletic injuries is prevalent and controversial. With a relatively small downside, bracing gives physicians a tool that can potentially avoid more extensive treatment protocols associated with greater risks. However, the literature fails to support some of these regimens fully. Given the increased complexity and improvements in current knee braces, further studies are needed to define the role of each specific brace for specific patient subsets.

In the post–ACL reconstruction period, the evidence that a brace confers additional stability, improves range of motion, protects the graft, reduces pain, or improves subjective outcomes is limited. However, there are data that support brace use to maintain extension and prevent flexion contractures. Prophylactic knee braces have not consistently been shown to prevent or reduce the severity of injuries to the ACL, MCL, or menisci in the general population. However, evidence suggests that brace use for specific athletic positions and athletes is beneficial (e.g., for a football lineman).

Studies that definitively support or refute functional brace use have not been done. The treating physician must make educated, patient-specific recommendations. In patients with ACL deficiency or instability, there is a subjective and biomechanical advantage to brace use. Although this benefit has not translated into a significant functional improvement, brace use should still be considered for this patient subset.

Bracing for patellofemoral pain has not reliably shown clinical or functional efficacy; nevertheless, some patients continue to experience subjective improvements. Biomechanically, an increased patellar contact area has been described in the laboratory, but more clinical studies are needed to determine the potential patient benefit.

Lastly, limited studies have shown unloader braces to have a biomechanical and clinical advantage. However, the cost of the brace must be weighed against the potential improvements in pain and function. These braces have been shown to be more effective in nonobese active patients with mild disease. In addition, alternative interventions for patients, such as lateral wedged insoles, may need to be considered because of the low rate of compliance associated with unloader braces. Overall, prescribing patterns for knee braces should follow explicit guidelines, with a distinct goal for treatment of each patient.

KEY REFERENCES

18. Brouwer RW, et al: Brace treatment for osteoarthritis of the knee: a prospective randomized multi-centre trial. *Osteoarthritis Cartilage* 14:777–783, 2006.

45. Hiemstra LA, et al: Knee immobilization for pain control after a hamstring tendon anterior cruciate ligament reconstruction: a randomized clinical trial. *Am J Sports Med* 37:56–64, 2009.

65. Mayr HO, et al: Brace or no-brace after ACL graft? Four-year results of a prospective clinical trial. *Knee Surg Sports Traumatol Arthrosc* 22:1156–1162, 2014.

67. McDevitt ER, et al: Functional bracing after anterior cruciate ligament reconstruction: a prospective, randomized, multicenter study. *Am J Sports Med* 32:1887–1892, 2004.

72. Moller E, et al: Bracing versus nonbracing in rehabilitation after anterior cruciate ligament reconstruction: a randomized prospective study with 2-year follow-up. *Knee Surg Sports Traumatol Arthrosc* 9:102–108, 2001.

75. Moyer RF, et al: Biomechanical effects of valgus knee bracing: a systematic review and meta-analysis. *Osteoarthritis Cartilage* 23:178–188, 2015.

92. Rishiraj N, et al: Effect of functional knee brace use on acceleration, agility, leg power and speed performance in healthy athletes. *Br J Sports Med* 45:1230–1237, 2011.

106. Sterett WI, et al: Effect of functional bracing on knee injury in skiers with anterior cruciate ligament reconstruction: a prospective cohort study. *Am J Sports Med* 34:1581–1585, 2006.

The references for this chapter can also be found on www.expertconsult.com.

59

Decision Making and Surgical Treatment of Posterior Cruciate Ligament Ruptures

Frank R. Noyes, Sue D. Barber-Westin

INTRODUCTION

The proper management of complete ruptures to the posterior cruciate ligament (PCL) and other ligaments of the knee involves a series of decisions based on knowledge of the diagnosis, reconstruction options and techniques, and rehabilitation concepts.[95,97] The clinician must be able to diagnose and treat a spectrum of knee injuries, from an isolated PCL rupture to a combined injury involving other knee ligaments (Table 59.1). PCL injuries are classified as either low velocity, such as those that occur from contact with another player in sports, or high velocity, such as a dashboard injury in a motor vehicle accident. The mechanism of PCL rupture in athletes is usually a fall on the flexed knee with a plantar-flexed foot or hyperflexion of the knee.[115,137] High-velocity injuries frequently involve dislocations with multiple ligament ruptures that require immediate medical attention. Traffic-related injuries appear to produce greater posterior tibial displacement values on stress radiography than sports-related injuries.[116]

This chapter will review the current knowledge of the function of the PCL—both alone and in concert with other ligament systems—that form the basis for the diagnosis of abnormal translations and rotations that result in different types of knee subluxations requiring surgical restoration (Table 59.2). Legitimate controversy exists regarding the treatment of complete PCL ruptures because of limitations of natural history studies and lack of Level 1 randomized controlled trials of sufficient numbers of patients to form conclusions. However, there are a number of clinical studies that will be summarized that form the basis for treatment of these ligament injuries.

The steps to diagnose and treat associated problems in knees with PCL ruptures must be systematically accomplished. These include varus malalignment, deficiency of the posterolateral structures (PLS), abnormal gait mechanics including knee hyperextension, and severe muscle atrophy. The detection and treatment of these problems is critical because failure to correct associated conditions may result in an undesirable outcome. Many of these problems are found in patients with chronic knee instabilities who may also have lost one or both menisci and demonstrate advanced articular cartilage damage. In these knees, the goal is to restore knee function for daily activities. Surgical advances in treating acute PCL ruptures hopefully will prevent the chronically unstable knees and resultant arthritis that often present in younger athletes.

This chapter will also review advances from our Center in PCL graft selection and surgical techniques designed to reduce the morbidity of surgical procedures. There are different surgical approaches available for acute knee injuries, dislocated knees with multiple ligament ruptures, chronic knee injuries, and revision surgery. Important decisions must be made regarding the placement of single- and two-strand graft constructs. In addition, differences exist in the postoperative rehabilitation program depending on the surgical procedure(s) performed.[99] A detailed analysis and surgical treatment of other knee disorders that accompany PCL ruptures has been previously published; this chapter represents a synopsis of this work.[93,97,99]

POSTERIOR CRUCIATE LIGAMENT ANATOMY

The PCL arises from a depression posterior to the intra-articular upper surface of the tibia and courses anteromedially behind the anterior cruciate ligament (ACL) to the lateral surface of the medial femoral condyle (Fig. 59.1).[125] The PCL has an average length of 38 mm and width of 13 mm; its cross-sectional area varies and increases from tibial to femoral insertions.[39] The PCL is approximately 50% larger than the ACL at its femoral origin and 20% larger at its tibial insertion. The anterior meniscofemoral ligament (aMFL) (ligament of Humphrey) courses anterior to the PCL, and the posterior meniscofemoral ligament (pMFL) (ligament of Wrisberg) runs obliquely behind the PCL. At least one meniscofemoral ligament is present in 91% of knees, and both ligaments may be found in 50% of knees in young individuals (Table 59.3).[38,78]

Free nerve endings and mechanoreceptors that are believed to have a proprioceptive function in the knee have been identified in the femoral and tibial attachment sites and on the surface of the PCL.[52,114]

The traditional division of the PCL into separate anterolateral and posteromedial bundles (PMBs) oversimplifies PCL fiber function. The PCL is a complex anatomical structure composed of a continuum of fibers of different lengths and attachment characteristics. The length-tension behaviors of the fibers that resist posterior tibial translation (with knee flexion) are controlled primarily by femoral attachment regions.[36,72,113,118] The distal fibers lengthen with increasing knee flexion, and the proximal fibers shorten with knee flexion.[78,113]

Variation exists between knees in the shape of the PCL femoral attachment, from the common elliptical shape to a more rounded and thicker shape (Fig. 59.2).[78] Different measurement systems have been proposed to describe the femoral attachment site. The most common method uses a clock reference position, with measurement lines perpendicular to the

TABLE 59.1 Spectrum of Posterior Cruciate Ligament Injuries

Posterior cruciate ligament rupture, isolated
A. Partial
B. Complete
    1. Bone avulsion
    2. Ligament insertion "peel-off"
    3. Ligament substance
Posterior cruciate ligament rupture combined with other knee joint abnormality
A. Lateral, posterolateral structures
B. Medial, posteromedial structures
C. Anterior cruciate ligament
D. Meniscus tears, partial or complex, medial or lateral
E. Joint arthrosis, articular cartilage damage[a]
    1. Medial tibiofemoral
    2. Lateral tibiofemoral
    3. Patellofemoral
F. Extensor mechanism malalignment, subluxation
Posterior cruciate ligament rupture combined with other system abnormality
A. Lower limb malalignment
B. Neuromuscular system
C. Peripheral vascular system
D. Cutaneous, skin

[a]Classified according to system described in Noyes FR, Stabler CL: A system for grading articular cartilage lesions at arthroscopy. *Am J Sports Med* 17:505–513, 1989.

TABLE 59.2 Clinical Effects of Posterior Tibial Subluxation of the Posterior Cruciate Ligament-Deficient Knee

- PCL forces up to 50% body weight occur during level walking.
- Higher PCL forces occur during stair-climbing, ascending stairs, descending stairs.
- Posterior tibial subluxation occurs in PCL-deficient knees during activities of daily living in high knee flexion positions, but not at low flexion positions in which smaller posterior shear forces are present.
- High PCL forces occur during single-leg lunge between 60 and 120 degrees of flexion.
- Quadriceps neutral angle may vary from 60 to 90 degrees between knees, not objective measurement diagnosis of posterior tibial subluxation.
- PCL-deficient patients frequently note an anterior shifting of the tibia, as the tibia moves forward from its subluxated position, when they attempt to stand from a seated position.
- Significantly increased contact pressures in medial tibiofemoral and patellofemoral compartments occur in PCL-deficient knees.

PCL, Posterior cruciate ligament.
From Noyes FR, Barber-Westin SD: Function of the posterior cruciate ligament and posterolateral ligament structures. In Noyes FR, Barber-Westin SD (eds): *Noyes' knee disorders: surgery, rehabilitation, clinical outcomes,* ed 2, Philadelphia, 2017, Elsevier, pp 406-446.

TABLE 59.3 Meniscofemoral Ligaments

- Most knees have at least one MFL.
- One-third of knees have both MFLs.
- There is insufficient data to support a functional role of these structures.
- Identify aMFL and pMFL (when present) to determine true PCL anatomic footprint for graft placement.
- In some knees with isolated PCL ruptures, secondary ligament restraints (including the MFL structures) resist posterior tibial subluxation, particularly at low knee flexion angles.
- 90 degrees knee flexion, neutral tibial rotation is the best position to test for maximum posterior translation.
- Amount of posterior translation determined by secondary restraints will vary depending on physiologic laxity.

aMFL, Anterior meniscofemoral ligament; *MFL,* meniscofemoral ligament; *PCL,* posterior cruciate ligament; *pMFL,* posterior meniscofemoral ligament.
From Noyes FR, Barber-Westin SD: Function of the posterior cruciate ligament and posterolateral ligament structures. In Noyes FR, Barber-Westin SD (eds): *Noyes' knee disorders: surgery, rehabilitation, clinical outcomes,* ed 2, Philadelphia, 2017, Elsevier, pp 527-577.

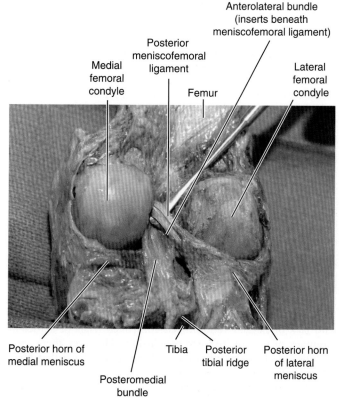

FIG 59.1 The PCL Femoral and Tibial Attachments Note the prominent posterior meniscofemoral ligament and broad posterior tibial attachment. (From Noyes FR, Barber-Westin SD: Posterior cruciate ligament: diagnosis, operative techniques, and clinical outcomes. In Noyes FR [ed.]: *Noyes' knee disorders: surgery, rehabilitation, clinical outcomes,* Philadelphia, 2017, Elsevier, pp 447-526.)

articular cartilage edge and other lines parallel to the femoral shaft. The clock method is a general guide and not highly accurate; therefore, the entire PCL footprint and relationships to other structures should be viewed.

In general, the PCL attachment extends from high in the notch (11:30 to 5 o'clock on a right knee) along the medial femoral condyle notch. The anterior portion of the PCL attachment follows the articular cartilage within 2 to 3 mm of its edge and gradually recedes deeper within the notch until, at the 5 o'clock position, the posterior third is 5 mm from the articular margin. Therefore, the distal boundary of the PCL femoral attachment is furthest away from the cartilage margin posteriorly.

The distal and proximal measurements for the PCL femoral attachment are shown in Table 59.4, and measurements vary from one study to another depending on the method selected. The proximal edge of the PCL is usually straight or partially

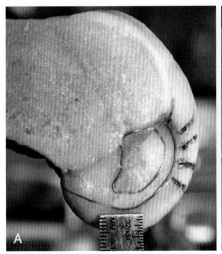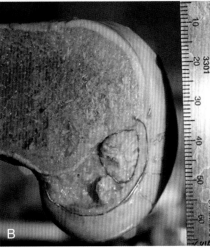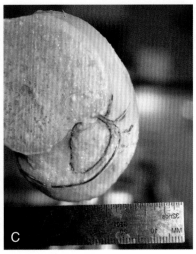

FIG 59.2 Composite of the shapes of different PCL insertion sites as seen on lateral views. Variability is noted between specimens from an oval to an elliptical PCL footprint configuration. Note the differences in anterior to posterior and proximal to distal dimensions in the PCL footprint. The most common shape of the PCL footprint is elliptical. (A) Fibers insert proximally to the intercondylar roof. The PCL footprint is smaller in its anteroposterior dimension. (B) Prominent posterior meniscofemoral ligaments. (C) More oval PCL attachment, with greater proximal to distal width. (From Mejia EA, Noyes FR, Grood ES: Posterior cruciate ligament femoral insertion site characteristics. Importance for reconstructive procedures. *Am J Sports Med* 30(5):643–651, 2002.)

TABLE 59.4   Posterior Cruciate Ligament Femoral Attachment Measurements Made With the Femoral Condyle Articular Cartilage Clock System

Measurement	Distal (mm)	Proximal (mm)	Thickness (mm)
Perpendicular to the Cartilage			
12 o'clock	2.54 ± 1.0	12.92 ± 2.8	10.38 ± 2.8
1 o'clock	2.38 ± 0.7	14.33 ± 2.2	11.96 ± 2.0
2 o'clock	2.38 ± 0.5	14.79 ± 1.8	12.42 ± 1.7
3 o'clock	2.54 ± 0.5	14.83 ± 2.0	12.50 ± 1.7
4 o'clock	2.71 ± 0.7	13.92 ± 2.4	11.21 ± 2.2
Parallel to the Femoral Shaft			
12 o'clock	2.54 ± 1.0	12.75 ± 2.8	10.25 ± 2.8
1 o'clock	2.38 ± 0.7	13.75 ± 2.8	11.38 ± 2.8
2 o'clock	2.46 ± 0.7	14.63 ± 2.0	12.17 ± 1.9
3 o'clock	2.63 ± 0.8	13.42 ± 2.2	10.83 ± 2.2
4 o'clock	3.78 ± 1.0	11.06 ± 2.6	7.39 ± 2.9

From Mejia EA, Noyes FR, Grood ES: Posterior cruciate ligament femoral insertion site characteristics. Importance for reconstructive procedures. *Am J Sports Med* 30(5):643–651, 2002.

oval, with the attachment tapered in width along its posterior portion (Figs. 59.3 and 59.4).

A clear understanding of the anatomy of the native PCL is critical in determining which portion of the ligament will be reconstructed. The terms *high, low, shallow,* and *deep* are only general descriptors. Because there may be confusion regarding femoral graft tunnel placement during PCL reconstruction, the PCL femoral attachment is described using the rule of thirds (Fig. 59.5A and B) to define the proximal-middle-distal thirds (deep to shallow in the femoral notch), and anterior-middle-posterior

thirds (high to low), with a small posterior oblique portion in the sagittal plane.[78,81] This provides a grid for the identification of the tunnel locations for the graft strands and is preferred by the senior author (see Fig. 59.5C).

Vascular Anatomy and Variations

The PCL is covered with a well-vascularized synovial sleeve that contributes to its blood supply. The distal portion also receives some vascular supply from capsular vessels originating from the inferior and middle genicular arteries and the popliteal artery.

Detailed knowledge of posteromedial knee anatomy, especially the vascular structures, is required to avoid complications when using a posteromedial approach for a tibial inlay PCL reconstruction. The popliteal artery originates at the adductor hiatus and passes through the popliteal fossa. Before passing deep to the fibrous arch over the soleus muscle, it divides into the anterior and posterior tibial arteries at the distal aspect of the popliteus muscle.

At the level of the knee joint, four major arteries are distributed: the medial and lateral sural arteries, a cutaneous branch that travels with the small saphenous vein to supply superficial tissues, and the middle genicular artery. The medial and lateral inferior genicular arteries are present just distal to the knee joint.

Two branches deserve particular attention. The medial inferior genicular artery arises from the medial aspect of the distal portion of the popliteal artery and runs medially, deep to the medial head of the gastrocnemius, and approximately 2 to 3 mm from the superior surface of the popliteus muscle. It continues around the medial aspect of the proximal tibia, deep to the superficial medial collateral ligament (SMCL). The middle genicular artery arises at the level of the femoral condyles proximal to the joint line and passes anteriorly to pierce the oblique popliteal ligament and posterior joint capsule and supply the cruciate ligaments.

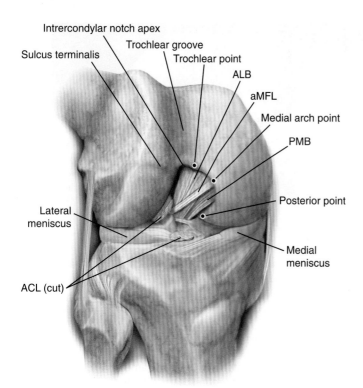

FIG 59.3 Illustration of the anterior view of a right knee flexed to 90 degrees with the PCL intact, demonstrating the characteristic morphology of the cartilage margin of the femoral intercondylar notch. The illustration also shows the trochlear, medial arch, and posterior points as well as the intercondylar notch apex and trochlear groove. *ACL,* Anterior cruciate ligament; *ALB,* anterolateral bundle; *aMFL,* anterior meniscofemoral ligament; *PMB,* posteromedial bundle. (Modified and with permission from Anderson CJ, Ziegler CG, Wijdicks CA, et al: Arthroscopically pertinent anatomy of the anterolateral and posteromedial bundles of the posterior cruciate ligament. *J Bone Joint Surg Am* 94:1936–1945, 2012.)

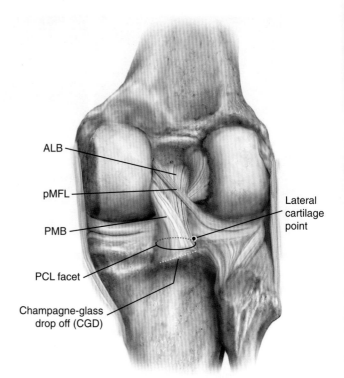

FIG 59.4 Illustration of the posterior aspect of a right knee with the PCL intact, demonstrating the fiber orientation. *ALB,* Anterolateral bundle; *PCL,* posterior cruciate ligament; *PMB,* posteromedial bundle; *pMFL,* posterior meniscofemoral ligament. (Modified and with permission from Anderson CJ, Ziegler CG, Wijdicks CA, et al: Arthroscopically pertinent anatomy of the anterolateral and posteromedial bundles of the posterior cruciate ligament. *J Bone Joint Surg Am* 94:1936–1945, 2012.)

This "normal" vascular pattern has been reported to occur in approximately 88% of knees.[18,77] In approximately 5% to 7%, the popliteal artery will divide at least 2 cm or more proximal to the distal border of the popliteus muscle.[77] In slightly less than half of these knees, with a high division of the popliteal artery, the anterior tibial artery passes anterior, not posterior, to the popliteus muscle belly. A number of variations of the anterior tibial artery were described by Mauro et al.[77] Therefore, with a tibial inlay approach, the dissection is always performed proximal to the popliteus muscle using a meticulous technique because the anterior tibial artery is at risk for transection in approximately 3% to 4% of knees.

An unusual variation in the vascular pattern involves the popliteal artery passing medial and then beneath the medial head of the gastrocnemius. Various subtypes of this abnormal pattern have been described. An abnormal vascular pattern may manifest clinically as the popliteal artery entrapment syndrome, which is characterized by vascular claudication symptoms. Arterial insufficiency occurs most commonly with entrapment of the artery deep to the medial gastrocnemius muscle but may also occur when the artery is entrapped deep to the popliteus muscle (persistence of ventral component of artery), or entrapped deep to an abnormal accessory head of the gastrocnemius. A history of pain in the lower extremity with activity, but none at rest (particularly in a young patient), should alert the surgeon to the possibility that an abnormal vascular pattern may exist. Further evaluation with magnetic resonance vascular imaging may be warranted.

POSTERIOR CRUCIATE LIGAMENT FIBER FUNCTION

The femoral attachment location of a PCL graft strongly influences graft tension and the ability of the reconstruction to restore posterior stability.[2,24,113,118] Investigations by Grood et al.[34] and Sidles et al.[123] have demonstrated that the femoral attachment location, and not the tibial attachment location, determines the graft tibiofemoral separation distance with knee flexion–extension.

On the femur, the proximal-distal location of a graft has a greater effect on the attachment separation distance than the anterior-posterior location (Figs. 59.6 and 59.7), which forms the basis for the rule of thirds. In an investigation at our laboratory,[113] the changes in tibiofemoral length for seven peripheral attachment sites at the proximal and distal origins located around the circumference of the PCL femoral attachment were studied. The data showed that proximal PCL fibers lengthen with knee extension and distal fibers lengthen with knee flexion (Fig. 59.8). In Fig. 59.9, the flexion angles in which the fiber length elongations were the least (within 5% of the maximum

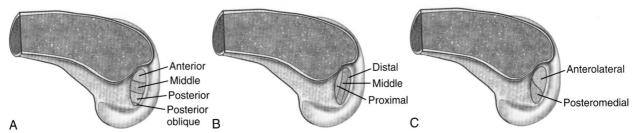

FIG 59.5 (A) Rule of thirds. The PCL footprint is divided into anterior, middle, and posterior thirds. The anterior third extends past the midline (11:30 o'clock, right knee) and the posterior region extends to 5 o'clock. The smaller posterior oblique portion of the PCL footprint is also represented. The PCL footprint is elliptical in most knees, but variations exist. (B) Rule of thirds. The PCL footprint is further divided into the distal, middle, and proximal thirds. This allows for more exact referencing of graft strand placement during PCL reconstruction. The PCL fibers in the distal two-thirds lengthen with knee flexion whereas the proximal fibers shorten. The reverse occurs with knee extension. (C) Typical division of anterolateral and posteromedial bundles provides an incorrect description of PCL fiber length change because it describes anterior PCL fibers that lengthen (AL) and posterior fibers (PL) that shorten with knee flexion. (From Noyes FR, Barber-Westin SD: Posterior cruciate ligament: diagnosis, operative techniques, and clinical outcomes. In Noyes FR [ed.]: *Noyes' knee disorders: surgery, rehabilitation, clinical outcomes*, Philadelphia, 2017, Elsevier, pp 447-526.)

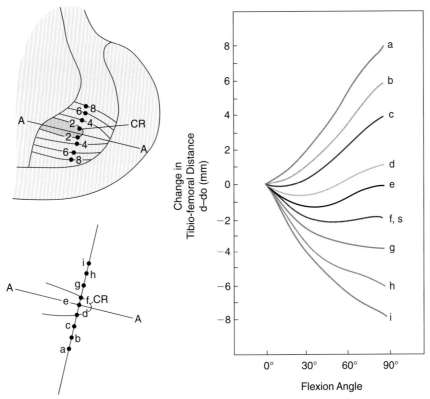

FIG 59.6 Contour map for a typical knee. The number on each contour line indicates the magnitude of the maximum length change. Line A-A represents the most isometric line and runs almost in the AP direction. Point CR indicates the intersection of the best-fit flexion axis with the lateral surface of the medial femoral condyle. Note that line A-A passes near point CR. The curves at the *right* show the changes in the tibiofemoral separation distances that occurred for selected femoral attachments. Attachments proximal to the isometric line were shorter at 90 degrees than at full extension. Attachments distal to the line were longer at 90 degrees. Attachments along line A-A had a length at 90 degrees that was almost identical to its length at 0 degree. (From Grood ES, Hefzy MS, Lindenfeld TN: Factors affecting the region of most isometric femoral attachments. Part I: the posterior cruciate ligament. *Am J Sports Med* 17(2):197–207, 1989.)

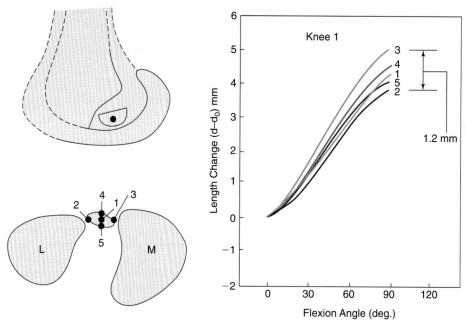

FIG 59.7 *Left,* The curves show the average tibiofemoral separation distance versus knee flexion for three femoral attachment sites located along the most isometric line. *Right,* The bar chart shows the average and the standard deviation of the difference between the maximum and minimum tibiofemoral separation distance for each of the three femoral attachment sites. (From Grood ES, Hefzy MS, Lindenfeld TN: Factors affecting the region of most isometric femoral attachments. Part I: the posterior cruciate ligament. *Am J Sports Med* 17(2):197–207, 1989.)

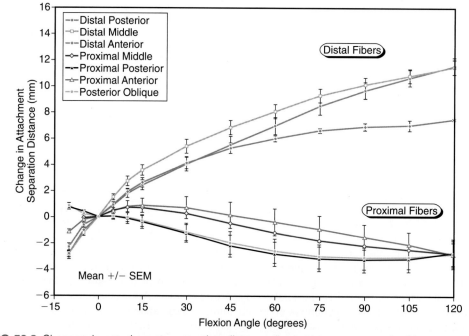

FIG 59.8 Changes in attachment separation distance (in mm) are measured with progressive knee flexion under a 100-N posterior load. Distal fibers lengthen with knee flexion; proximal fibers shorten with knee flexion. (From Saddler SC, Noyes FR, Grood ES, et al: Posterior cruciate ligament anatomy and length-tension behavior of PCL surface fibers. *Am J Knee Surg* 9(4):194–199, 1996.)

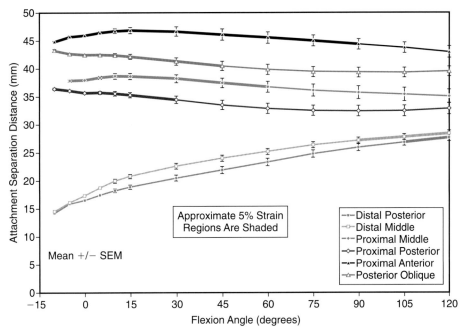

FIG 59.9 The change in attachment separation distance curves have been shifted to begin at the measured absolute length of each fiber. The darker area for each curve represents the 5% strain for each fiber. This, in theory, represents the functional range of knee flexion for each fiber. Note that this model predicts that the proximal-anterior fiber will function over the longest functional range. (From Saddler SC, Noyes FR, Grood ES, et al: Posterior cruciate ligament anatomy and length-tension behavior of PCL surface fibers. *Am J Knee Surg* 9(4):194–199, 1996.)

length and therefore the functional zone) are graphed for each attachment point. The data as a whole show a progressive loading of fibers from distal to proximal within the PCL attachment with increasing knee flexion. There is a smaller effect proceeding from anterior to posterior. These data contradict the description of PCL fiber function that divides the PCL into an anterolateral bundle (which lengthens with knee flexion) and PMB (which shortens with knee flexion).

The surgeon has the option of placing a PCL graft strand into different regions of the PCL femoral attachment site that determine the functional range of the graft with knee flexion and the knee flexion position to tension the graft. In a study from our laboratory,[72] one- and two-strand PCL reconstructions were attached in three different locations within the PCL femoral footprint. A 50-N posterior force was applied to the tibia for the single-strand construct, and a 100-N force was applied to the two-strand PCL reconstruction. The tension in the graft strands was adjusted to restore posterior translation to within ±1 mm of the intact knee. The complex behavior of a two-strand PCL reconstruction is shown in Fig. 59.10, in which the two strands were placed into the more distal locations and tensioned at 90 degrees. Both strands shared the applied load as shown. In contrast, a two-strand construct, in which one strand was placed anterior and the second strand was placed more proximal (deep), resulted in a reciprocal loading relationship between strands (Fig. 59.11). In both situations, posterior translation limits were restored to normal.

Another investigation at our laboratory[118] confirmed that a proximal to distal change in the femoral position of the second strand of a two-strand construct markedly affects strand tension and function. A middle placement of the second strand produced load sharing, which is more ideal in terms of graft

function in the long term in preventing posterior tibial subluxation with increasing knee flexion. These concepts are used to select PCL graft attachment locations and tensioning, described in the operative techniques section. The surgeon should select graft attachment locations that have the least amount of change in tibiofemoral length and tension the graft at the knee flexion position at which the graft length is the longest (and therefore functional). If a graft is tensioned at a knee flexion angle at which the tibiofemoral fiber length is at its shortest, the graft will initially constrain knee flexion or extension and fail as the graft (tibiofemoral distance) lengthens with further knee flexion or extension.

DIAGNOSIS OF POSTERIOR CRUCIATE LIGAMENT FUNCTION AND KNEE JOINT SUBLUXATIONS

Anteroposterior Translation

The normal anterior and posterior translation knee limits are shown in Fig. 59.12A.[36] The increase in these limits when the PCL is cut are shown in Fig. 59.12B, and the further increase in these limits when the PLS are also sectioned are shown in Fig. 59.12C.

The PCL is the primary restraint to posterior tibial translation throughout knee flexion, with the exception of a small increase in posterior translation at full extension when the PLS are cut. The PLS include the popliteus muscle-tendon-ligament (PMTL), popliteofibular ligament (PFL), and posterolateral (PL) capsule. The clinical finding of a knee with increased posterior translation at 30 to 45 degrees of knee flexion, similar to the posterior translation limit at 90 degrees, indicates associated injury to the PLS and the medial structures. In a knee with

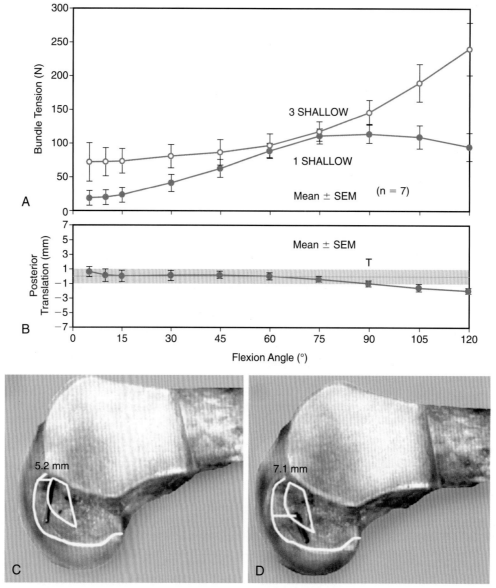

FIG 59.10 The graph shows the strand tension (A) and change in posterior translation from intact (B) for the one shallow and two shallow two-strand reconstruction with a 100-N posterior force. The T indicates the flexion angle where the strands were tensioned. The shaded area for posterior translation represents the translation for the intact knee ±1 mm. The photographs show the (C) one shallow and (D) three shallow femoral tunnel placements. (From Mannor DA, Shearn JT, Grood ES, et al: Two-bundle posterior cruciate ligament reconstruction. An in vitro analysis of graft placement and tension. *Am J Sports Med* 28(6):833–845, 2000.)

a combined deficiency of the PCL and PLS, the abnormal posterior tibial translation is at least four to five times the normal limit throughout knee flexion.

The PLS are some of the most important secondary restraints and have a major effect on lateral tibiofemoral compartment translation. There are marked differences in the amount of posterior tibial translation between isolated and combined PCL injuries. Although the amount of posterior translation may vary among knees,[36] it is generally appreciated clinically that a 10-mm or greater abnormal displacement at 90 degrees flexion indicates some deficiency of the secondary restraints in addition to the PCL. Furthermore, the posterior tibial displacement progressively increases at low flexion angles with injury or

stretching of the secondary ligament restraints. The abnormal forces placed on the patellofemoral and tibiofemoral compartments are expected to increase as greater posterior tibial displacements occur.[124] Clinically, it is advantageous to reconstruct the PCL before the loss of these secondary restraints. Otherwise, the PCL graft is placed under greater forces because the secondary restraints are not able to share a portion of the load in resisting posterior tibial subluxation. In chronic cases, in which the secondary restraints are deficient, we recommend surgical reconstruction of these structures during the PCL reconstruction to allow load sharing and protection of the PCL graft during the healing process. The individual function of each of the PLS has been previously published.[95]

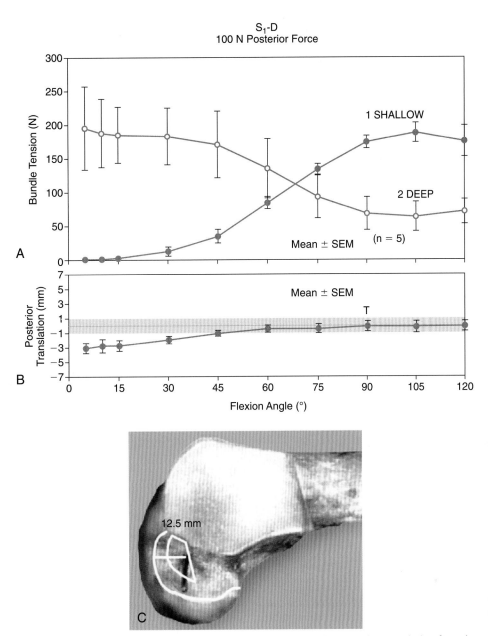

FIG 59.11 The graph shows the strand tension (A) and change in posterior translation from intact (B) for the one shallow and two-deep two-strand reconstruction with a 100-N posterior force. The T indicates the flexion angle where the strands were tensioned. The shaded area for posterior translation represents the translation for the intact knee ±1 mm. (C) Photograph shows the two-deep femoral tunnel placement. (From Mannor DA, Shearn JT, Grood ES, et al: Two-bundle posterior cruciate ligament reconstruction. An in vitro analysis of graft placement and tension. *Am J Sports Med* 28(6):833–845, 2000.)

Varus and Valgus Rotations

Injury to PLS results in increases in lateral joint opening under varus loads and increases in posterior subluxation of the lateral tibial plateau with external tibial rotation. With these ligament injuries, the PCL is placed under higher than normal loading conditions. Figs. 59.13 and 59.14 show the relationship of the primary ligamentous restraints to medial and lateral joint opening and the PCL.[35] Normally, a small force is present in the PCL to both varus and valgus loads.[35,75] With injury to medial or lateral structures, the PCL and ACL may be placed in the role of a primary restraint that is not ideal because their mechanical advantage in the center of the knee joint is not suited to resist medial and lateral joint openings. These biomechanical findings indicate the importance of determining an abnormal medial or lateral joint opening (subluxation) that requires surgical reconstruction. The failure to correct such associated subluxations places the PCL graft reconstruction under high in vivo forces postoperatively and risks graft failure.

Careful examination of the knee preoperatively and under anesthesia is required to determine whether abnormal motions and other ligament injuries are present that require reconstruction at the same time as the PCL. During the arthroscopic

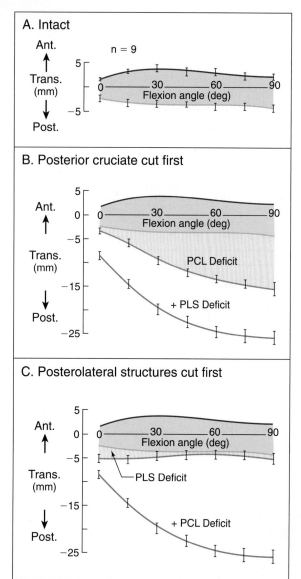

FIG 59.12 The curves show the limits of anterior and posterior translation (*vertical axis*) when a 100-N AP force was applied. (A) Intact knees. The curves show the average limits of motion and the standard deviation for nine knees. The range of total AP translation of the intact knee is shown shaded green in A-C. (B) PCL cut first. The increase in posterior translation after cutting the PCL is shown in the blue shaded area (PCL deficit). The limit of posterior translation, and therefore the amount of increase, is controlled by the remaining intact structures. The unshaded portion (+ PLS deficit) shows the added increase when the posterolateral structures (FCL, capsule, PMTL) were cut after the PCL had first been removed. A concurrent external rotation took place with this cut. (C) Posterolateral structures cut first. There was only a small increase (PLS deficit) in the posterior limit near full extension when the posterolateral structural elements were cut first. A concurrent external rotation was also present. *PCL*, Posterior cruciate ligament; *PLS*, posterolateral structures. (Adapted from Noyes FR, Barber-Westin SD: Function of the posterior cruciate ligament and posterolateral ligament structures. In Noyes FR [ed.]: *Noyes' knee disorders: surgery, rehabilitation, clinical outcomes*, Philadelphia, 2007, Elsevier, pp 406-446.)

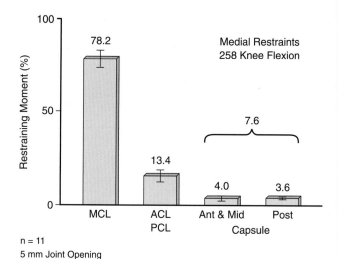

n = 11
5 mm Joint Opening

FIG 59.13 The percent contributions to the medial restraints by the ligaments and capsule at 5 mm of medial joint opening and 25 degrees of flexion. The error bars represent ± one standard error of the mean. *ACL*, Anterior cruciate ligament; *MCL*, medial collateral ligament; *PCL*, posterior cruciate ligament. (Adapted from Noyes FR, Grood ES: The scientific basis for examination and classification of knee ligament injuries. In Noyes FR [ed.]: *Noyes' knee disorders: surgery, rehabilitation, clinical outcomes*, Philadelphia, 2017, Elsevier, pp 83-109.)

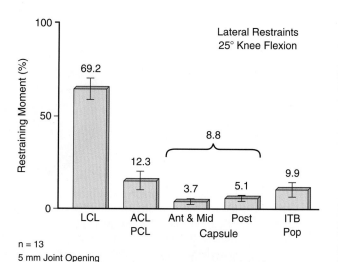

n = 13
5 mm Joint Opening

FIG 59.14 The percent contributions to the lateral restraints by the ligaments and capsule at 5 mm of lateral joint opening and 25 degrees of flexion. The error bars represent ± one standard error of the mean. *ACL*, Anterior cruciate ligament; *ITB*, iliotibial band; *LCL*, lateral collateral ligament; *PCL*, posterior cruciate ligament. (Adapted from Noyes FR, Grood ES: The scientific basis for examination and classification of knee ligament injuries. In Noyes FR [ed.]: *Noyes' knee disorders: surgery, rehabilitation, clinical outcomes*, Philadelphia, 2017, Elsevier, pp 83-109.)

examination, the gap test confirms that excessive medial or lateral joint opening is not present, which would place abnormal loads on a PCL graft (Fig. 59.15). The goal is to restore function of any insufficient ligamentous structure in one surgical setting. Both the ACL and PCL function in combination with the medial and lateral ligamentous structures in a complex system of primary and secondary restraints that establish the limits to rotations and translations that normally occur in the knee joint. Any insufficiency of two ligamentous structures results in a combination of subluxations involving the medial and lateral tibiofemoral compartments.

Tibiofemoral Rotational Subluxations

Injury to the PLS produces an increase in external tibial rotation and a posterior subluxation of the lateral tibial plateau. There are two primary restraints to external tibial rotation: the PLS at low flexion angles and both the PLS and PCL at high flexion angles (Fig. 59.16). Careful examination of knees with suspected injury to these structures may show either a marked increase in external tibial rotation and posterior translation of the lateral tibial plateau, or only a slight increase in these abnormal knee motions.[106] The clinician's first goal is to diagnose all of the possible knee subluxations and define the extent of injury to the PLS. In 1989, we first reported on a modification of existing rotation tests to diagnose tibial rotatory subluxations of the medial and lateral tibiofemoral compartments more accurately (dial or spin rotation test).[105] We then studied the amount of increased posterior subluxation of the medial and lateral tibial plateaus that result from injury to the PCL and PLS.[106] We

found that sectioning of the PLS resulted in a significant mean increase in posterior translation of the lateral tibial plateau of 8.0 mm at 30 degrees of flexion over the intact state ($p < .01$). No significant increase of the lateral tibial plateau occurred at 90 degrees of flexion. There was no significant increase in posterior translation of the medial tibial plateau at either flexion angle. After sectioning both the PCL and PLS, significant increases in posterior translation of both the medial and lateral tibial plateaus occurred at 30 and 90 degrees of flexion ($p < .01$). The increase in posterior translation of the lateral tibial plateau averaged 17.8 and 23.5 mm at 30 and 90 degrees of flexion, respectively, and the increase in posterior translation of the medial tibial plateau averaged 7.6 and 12.3 mm at 30 and 90 degrees, respectively.

From the results of this study, we concluded that the diagnosis of injury to the PLS should be made based on the final position of the lateral tibial plateau and not on the amount of increased external tibial rotation alone. An increase in external tibial rotation can occur with anterior subluxation of the medial tibial plateau, posterior subluxation of the lateral tibial plateau, or a combination of both subluxations. In a prior investigation,[103] we found that clinicians often misdiagnosed injuries to the PLS because of misinterpretation of the increase in external tibial rotation as a posterior subluxation of the lateral tibial plateau, when in fact there was a subluxation of the medial tibial plateau caused by injury to the medial collateral ligament (MCL) alone or in combination with the ACL.

We have recommended that during the rotation tests to determine rotatory subluxations of the tibial plateaus, the

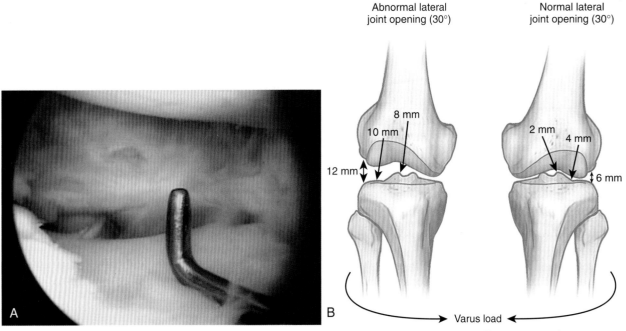

FIG 59.15 (A) Arthroscopic demonstration of the lateral joint opening-gap test. The amount of lateral joint opening is measured with the knee at 25 degrees flexion. (B) Knees with insufficiency of the posterolateral structures will demonstrate 12 mm of joint opening at the periphery of the lateral tibiofemoral compartment, 10 mm of opening at the midportion of the compartment, and 8 mm at the inner most medial edge. (From Noyes FR, Barber-Westin SD: Tibial and femoral osteotomy for varus and valgus knee syndromes: diagnosis, operative techniques, and clinical outcomes. In Noyes FR [ed.]: *Noyes' knee disorders: surgery, rehabilitation, clinical outcomes*, Philadelphia, 2017, Elsevier, pp 773-847.)

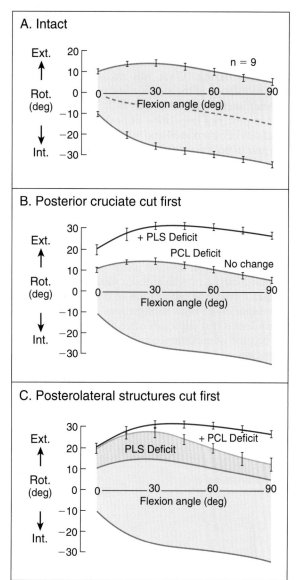

FIG 59.16 The limits of internal and external rotation of the tibia when a 5-N torque was applied. The fully extended position, measured in the intact knee, was used as the zero-rotation reference. (A) Intact knees. The *upper curve* shows the limit of external rotation. The *dashed line* shows the average position of the knee during passive flexion with the tibia hanging freely. The range of tibial rotation in the intact knee is shaded in A-C. (B) Posterior cruciate ligament cut first. No change was found in external tibial rotation. (C) Posterolateral structures (FCL, capsule, PMTL) cut first. Increases in external tibial rotation occurred at low flexion angles. With added PCL sectioning, the increase in external tibial rotation occurred at high flexion angles. *PCL*, Posterior cruciate ligament; *PLS*, posterolateral structures. (Adapted from Noyes FR, Barber-Westin SD: Function of the posterior cruciate ligament and posterolateral ligament structures. In Noyes FR [ed.]: *Noyes' knee disorders: surgery, rehabilitation, clinical outcomes*, Philadelphia, 2017, Elsevier, pp 406-446.)

examiner carefully palpates the position of each tibial plateau to determine qualitatively whether an anterior or posterior subluxation is present. We and others[16,17] have reported that it is not possible to determine the actual millimeters of translation of the medial and lateral tibial plateaus in reference to the femoral condyle. Thus, a qualitative determination of whether the reference tibial plateau is anteriorly or posteriorly subluxated is recommended. The inability to measure tibiofemoral compartment translations precisely, and to quantify the amount of PL subluxation, creates problems when deciding whether surgical correction is warranted. It is important to perform tibial rotation dial tests in a supine position (and not the prone position, as sometimes recommended) so that the medial and lateral tibia plateau positions may be determined.

A classification system of rotatory subluxations was previously described based on two concepts—determining the final position of the medial and lateral tibial plateaus under defined loading conditions (eg, with either internal or external tibial rotation at a defined knee flexion angle) and classifying the position of each plateau.[106] There are three possible positions for each plateau: anterior subluxation, normal position, or posterior subluxation. For each of these positions of the lateral tibial plateau, there are three corresponding positions for the medial tibial plateau (Fig. 59.17).

When a posterior subluxation of the lateral tibial plateau is positively identified by the described tibiofemoral rotation test, the examiner performs additional tests to determine whether ruptures exist in other ligamentous structures. The amount of lateral joint opening at 0 and 20 degrees of knee flexion should be determined (and quantified by stress radiography when possible) to determine the integrity of the fibular collateral ligament (FCL) and other lateral restraints.[36] The presence of a varus recurvatum in both the supine and standing positions must be carefully assessed. The difference in results of these tests between the injured and contralateral normal knee is compared because of inherent physiological looseness that is present in some individuals. The different types of subluxations after PL injuries depends on whether there is a concomitant rupture to the ACL or PCL.

CLINICAL EVALUATION

Physical Examination

A comprehensive examination of the knee joint is required to detect all abnormalities (Fig. 59.18). This includes assessment of the patellofemoral joint and patellar tendon-tibial tubercle alignment (Q angle), which may be increased because of increased external tibial rotation when a PL ligament injury accompanies the PCL rupture. A second factor is patellofemoral and tibiofemoral crepitus, indicative of articular cartilage damage. A third indicator is gait abnormalities (excessive hyperextension or varus thrust) during walking and jogging.[104] Finally, assess for abnormal knee motion limits and subluxations compared with those of the contralateral knee.[105]

Experienced clinicians are aware that patients with chronic deficiency of the PCL and PLS may develop an abnormal gait pattern, which is characterized by excessive knee hyperextension during the stance phase.[104] Subjective complaints of knee instability and giving way during routine daily activities, along with severe quadriceps atrophy, often accompany this gait abnormality. Gait analysis and retraining are required in patients who demonstrate abnormal knee hyperextension patterns

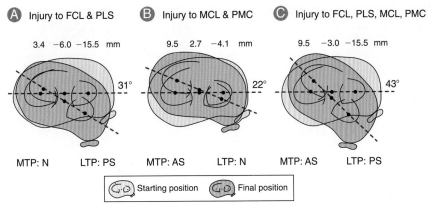

FIG 59.17 Three Types of Tibiofemoral Situations Observed With Increased External Tibial Rotation (A) Abnormal posterior translation of the lateral tibial plateau (at 30 degrees of knee flexion under the loading conditions described in the study). (B) Abnormal anterior translation of the medial tibial plateau under loading conditions of 5 Nm (at 30 degrees of knee flexion). (C) Abnormal posterior translation of the lateral tibial plateau plus abnormal anterior translation of the medial tibial plateau after sectioning both the medial and lateral ligament structures. *AS,* Anterior subluxation; *FCL,* fibular collateral ligament; *LTP,* lateral tibial plateau; *MCL,* medial collateral ligament; *MTP,* medial tibial plateau; *N,* normal position; *PLS,* posterolateral structures (FCL, PMTL); *PMC,* posterior medial capsule; *PS,* posterior subluxation. (From Noyes FR, Stowers SF, Grood ES, et al: Posterior subluxations of the medial and lateral tibiofemoral compartments. An in vitro ligament sectioning study in cadaveric knees. *Am J Sports Med* 21(3):407–414, 1993.)

before proceeding with any ligament reconstruction.[104] The failure to do so may lead to failure of reconstructed ligaments if the abnormal gait pattern is resumed postoperatively. As described in detail elsewhere, several weeks of specific gait adaption training may be required (Fig. 59.19).[104]

Diagnostic Clinical Tests

The medial posterior tibiofemoral step-off on the posterior drawer test is performed at 90 degrees of flexion. The amount of posterior tibial translation will vary among knees with isolated PCL ruptures because of physiological laxity or injury to the secondary PL or medial soft tissue restraints. Posterior tibial translation progressively increases with injury to the secondary restraints.

The exact determination of the extent of a PCL tear (partial vs. complete) can be difficult but is essential from a therapeutic standpoint. The clinical posterior drawer test can be highly subjective, with the forces applied too variable to allow accurate determination of the status of the PCL. Magnetic resonance imaging (MRI) is not always accurate in diagnosing partial PCL tears. Frequently, this test may indicate that the ligament is completely ruptured; however, ligament continuity may still exist, with some portions functioning to limit posterior tibial subluxation to only a few millimeters.

The quantitative measurement of posterior tibial subluxation in knees with PCL ruptures or reconstruction is therefore important.[42] The knee arthrometer is the most frequently used device to measure posterior tibial translation after PCL injury and reconstruction. However, this device underestimates the true amount of posterior translation in PCL-deficient and reconstructed knees, often by several millimeters.[42,73] Stress radiography is the most accurate and reproducible technique currently available.[42,73,116] We recommend that PCL clinical

investigations incorporate stress radiography to provide a more valid measure of posterior tibial translation (Figs. 59.20 and 59.21). Selected tibia and femoral radiographic points are taken on the injured and normal knee, which may include the individual medial and lateral tibiofemoral compartments or a central tibiofemoral point.[46]

The integrity of the ACL is determined by Lachman and pivot shift tests. The result of the pivot shift test is recorded on a scale of 0 to 3, with a grade of 0 indicating no pivot shift; grade 1, a slip or glide; grade 2, a jerk with gross subluxation or clunk; and grade 3, gross subluxation with impingement of the posterior aspect of the lateral side of the tibial plateau against the femoral condyle. Knee arthrometer testing may be done at 20 degrees of flexion (134-N force) to quantify total anteroposterior (AP) displacement.

Medial and lateral ligament insufficiency are determined by varus and valgus stress testing at 0 and 30 degrees of knee flexion. The surgeon estimates the amount of joint opening (in millimeters) between the initial closed contact position of each tibiofemoral compartment, performed in a constrained manner to avoid internal or external tibial rotation, to the maximal opened position. The result is recorded according to the increase in the tibiofemoral compartment of the affected knee compared with that of the opposite normal knee.

The tibiofemoral rotation dial test at 30 and 90 degrees is done to determine whether increases in external tibial rotation exist with posterior subluxation of the lateral tibial plateau as previously described.[105] The presence of a varus recurvatum in both the supine and standing positions is carefully assessed.

Imaging Studies

Radiographs taken during the initial examination include lateral at 30 degrees of knee flexion, weight-bearing posteroanterior

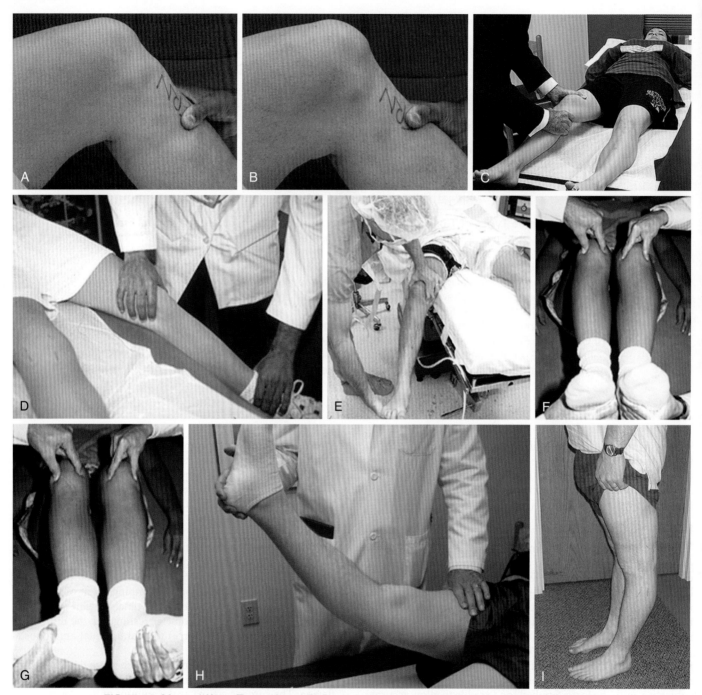

FIG 59.18 Manual Knee Tests (A and B) Posterior drawer test at 90 degrees knee flexion. (C) Lachman test. (D) Valgus manual test for medial joint opening. (E) Varus manual test for lateral joint opening. (F) Dial test at 90 degrees of knee flexion in neutral tibial rotation and maximum external tibial rotation (G). Varus recurvatum in the supine (H) and standing (I) positions. (From Noyes FR, Barber-Westin SD: Tibial and femoral osteotomy for varus and valgus knee syndromes: diagnosis, operative techniques, and clinical outcomes. In Noyes FR [ed.]: *Noyes' knee disorders: surgery, rehabilitation, clinical outcomes*, Philadelphia, 2017, Elsevier, pp 773-847.)

(PA) at 45 degrees of knee flexion, and patellofemoral axial views.

Posterior stress radiographs are done with an 89-N force applied to the proximal tibia (see Figs. 59.20 and 59.21).[42] A lateral radiograph is taken of each knee at 90 degrees of flexion. The limb is placed in neutral rotation with the tibia unconstrained and the quadriceps relaxed. The difference in posterior tibial displacement between the reconstructed knee and the contralateral knee is recorded. More than 8 mm of increase in posterior tibial translation on stress testing indicates a complete PCL rupture.[116]

Medial or lateral stress radiographs may be required of both knees. The patient is seated (20 degrees knee flexion) in neutral tibial rotation with the tibia unconstrained. Approximately 89

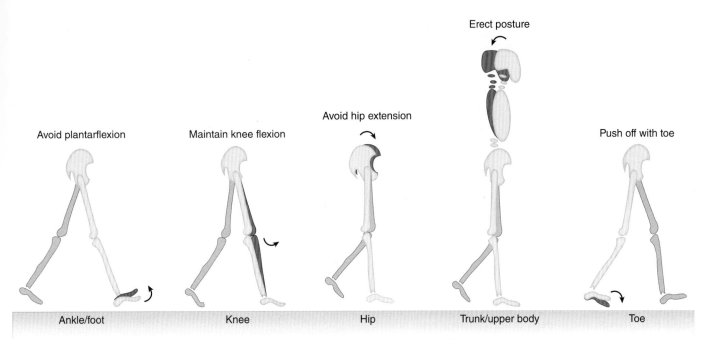

Erect posture

Avoid plantarflexion | Maintain knee flexion | Avoid hip extension | | Push off with toe

Ankle/foot | Knee | Hip | Trunk/upper body | Toe

Look for patellofemoral pain/rotational instabilities with knee flexion   Avoid medial-lateral body sway

FIG 59.19 Graphic representation of gait abnormalities observed in patients before retraining. *Filled gray anatomic structures* represent the correct, retrained positions at the trunk, upper body, hip, knee, foot, ankle, and toes. (From Noyes FR, Dunworth LA, Andriacchi TP, et al: Knee hyperextension gait abnormalities in unstable knees. Recognition and preoperative gait retraining. *Am J Sports Med* 24(1):35–45, 1996.)

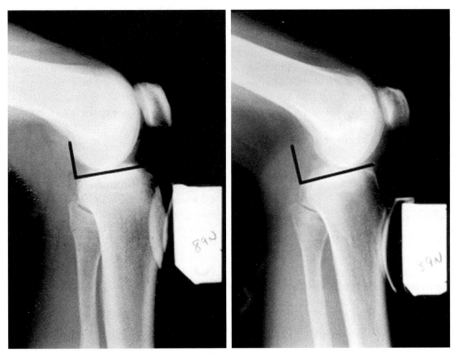

FIG 59.20 Lateral stress radiograph of a PCL-deficient knee demonstrating a 19-mm posterior drop-back (involved–noninvolved knee, 70 degrees knee flexion, 89 N). (From Noyes FR, Barber-Westin SD: Treatment of complex injuries involving the posterior cruciate and posterolateral ligaments of the knee. *Am J Knee Surg* 9:200–214, 1996.)

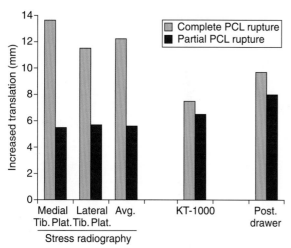

FIG 59.21 The results of lateral stress radiography on 20 patients with PCL deficiency (9 complete ruptures and 11 partial ruptures). The differences in the measurements between complete and partial PCL ruptures for the medial tibial plateau, lateral tibial plateau, and average of both plateaus were statistically significant ($p < .01$). Differences in the KT-1000 and posterior drawer measurements between complete and partial PCL ruptures were not significant. The KT measurements at 70 degrees flexion underestimated the magnitude of posterior tibial subluxation for complete PCL ruptures. *PCL,* Posterior cruciate ligament. (From Hewett TE, Noyes FR, Lee MD: Diagnosis of complete and partial posterior cruciate ligament ruptures. Stress radiography compared with KT-1000 arthrometer and posterior drawer testing. *Am J Sports Med* 25(5):648–655, 1997.)

N of varus or valgus force is applied and comparison made of the millimeters of medial or lateral tibiofemoral compartment opening between knees (in millimeters).

Full standing radiographs of both lower extremities, from the femoral heads to the ankle joints, are done in knees in which varus lower extremity alignment is detected on clinical examination. The mechanical axis and weight-bearing line are measured to determine whether high tibial osteotomy (HTO) is indicated before PCL reconstruction.[20,102] If the varus malalignment is not corrected, there is a risk that either a PCL or ACL graft may fail because of the varus thrusting forces and concurrent increased lateral joint opening producing high graft tension loads.[89]

MANAGEMENT CONSIDERATIONS

Posterior Cruciate Ligament Natural History

The treatment of complete isolated PCL ruptures remains controversial because of the unknown natural history of this injury in regard to long-term symptoms, functional limitations, and risk of joint arthritis. Although some studies (that included large percentages of patients with partial PCL deficiency) reported that patients did well when treated conservatively,[109,120,121] other investigations described noteworthy symptoms and functional limitations after the injury.[5,8] Many knees with complete PCL ruptures develop articular cartilage deterioration over time; this usually occurs on the medial femoral condyle and patellofemoral surfaces because of increased joint

pressures and altered tibiofemoral and patellofemoral kinematics.* Posterior tibial subluxation with activities after PCL rupture has a deleterious effect to the knee, similar to that of a medial meniscectomy[25] because there is loss of medial meniscus function and increased joint contact stress. There is less of a deleterious effect to the lateral tibiofemoral compartment because the lateral meniscus retains load-bearing function. Posterior tibial subluxation with weight-bearing activities results in a loss of normal joint kinematics[31,68,128] and in coupled external tibial rotation with joint loading. Accordingly, a PCL rupture would be expected to have a more deleterious effect in a varus-angulated knee with associated loss of the medial meniscus and, in particular, larger-sized athletes who desire to return to strenuous athletics. All of these factors alone or together result in substantial medial tibiofemoral loads and risk of joint deterioration.

Treatment of Acute Posterior Cruciate Ligament Ruptures

Controversy exists in the treatment of isolated mid-substance complete PCL ruptures, primarily because of the lack of a scientifically proven operative procedure that can restore posterior stability and PCL function predictably. In comparison, surgical procedures to reattach the native PCL in cases of bony avulsion injuries or peel-off injuries directly at the PCL attachment site have more predictable healing rates.[15,33,146] In knees with a PCL rupture directly at the attachment site, there is usually sufficient ligament substance for a direct repair.

In select situations, an augmentation using the semitendinosus tendon may facilitate PCL repair. Augmentation of partial PCL tears is controversial[†] and only indicated in high-grade tears.

The treatment rationale for patients with acute PCL ruptures is shown in Fig. 59.22.[97] The algorithm is divided into three major sections based on the PCL tear (partial, complete, or combined with other ligament ruptures). The 10-mm division is somewhat arbitrary; however, it provides a reasonable guideline for classification of the PCL injury.

The rules for treating partial or acute isolated PCL tears are shown in Table 59.5. These rules are used when the injury is seen within the first 2 weeks; after this time, the program is not instituted. In our experience, 4 weeks of protection to allow initial healing of a complete PCL rupture will frequently restore partial PCL function, with less than 5- to 7-mm of posterior tibial subluxation remaining on examination. The initial PCL healing process involves a low tensile strength, and an additional 4 to 6 weeks of protection is recommended, including avoiding athletics, running, walking on downhill grades, walking down stairs, or other high knee flexion activities that load the PCL. Even in knees with a complete PCL tear and more than 10 mm of increased posterior tibial displacement, healing of the disrupted PCL fibers may still occur, although a residual posterior tibial subluxation of a few millimeters (with a hard endpoint) will remain. The knees in which partial PCL function has been restored should be followed and repeat stress radiographs obtained at 6 months and over the next few years to determine PCL function. These partial PCL tears seldom require reconstruction. A repeat MRI with fast spin-echo cartilage sequences

---

*References 13, 28, 29, 31, 32, 41, 59, 68, 107 and 127-129.
†References 3, 19, 50, 51, 55, 63, 64, 141, 142 and 149.

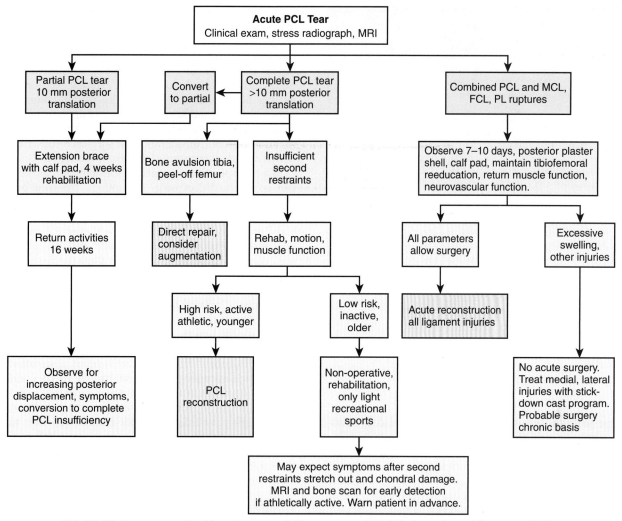

FIG 59.22 Treatment algorithm for acute PCL ruptures. *FCL,* Fibular collateral ligament; *MCL,* medial collateral ligament; *MRI,* magnetic resonance imaging; *PCL,* posterior cruciate ligament; *PL,* posterolateral. (From Noyes FR, Barber-Westin SD: Posterior cruciate ligament: diagnosis, operative techniques, and clinical outcomes. In Noyes FR [ed.]: *Noyes' knee disorders: surgery, rehabilitation, clinical outcomes,* Philadelphia, 2017, Elsevier, pp 447-526.)

helps determine the integrity of the articular cartilage and provides important information for counseling the patient on athletic activities to decrease the risk of future joint arthritis.

In cases of complete isolated midsubstance PCL ruptures (>10 mm of increased posterior tibial displacement) in which the patient is seen late after the injury and the previously discussed program cannot be instituted, one treatment approach in athletes and patients involved in strenuous occupations is PCL graft reconstruction before the secondary restraints stretch out with subsequent reinjuries. We believe that PCL reconstructive procedures have advanced to the point where more predictable results can be expected to restore sufficient PCL function to prevent gross posterior tibial subluxation. Studies have demonstrated, at least in the short term, that most patients with acute PCL ruptures treated with reconstruction are able to return to various levels of sports activities.[67,83] Additional factors to be weighed in the decision to perform early surgery on a complete isolated PCL rupture include athletic goals, body weight, medial meniscus damage, tibiofemoral joint damage, patellofemoral joint damage, and varus malalignment because

these factors add to the effects of the residual posterior subluxation in increasing knee joint loads and subsequent joint deterioration. Sedentary patients with a complete PCL rupture and 10 mm of posterior translation (90 degrees flexion) are not considered surgical candidates; however, they are followed as previously described.

Patients with a PCL disruption and other ligament injuries have an obvious posterior tibial dropback without a firm endpoint on posterior drawer testing (10 mm or more of posterior tibial subluxation). In almost all of these knees, some increase in medial or lateral joint opening or external tibial rotation can be detected, although the findings may be subtle. There may be physiologic laxity of other ligament structures without a true injury that allows for the gross posterior tibial subluxation.

In knees that have associated ruptures of the PLS, acute anatomical repair is planned if possible within 14 days before scarring occurs and the ability to anatomically restore these structures is lost. A similar situation exists for the medial ligament structures; however, these tissues are easier to reconstruct later if surgery cannot be performed during the ideal time

TABLE 59.5   Rules to Treat Partial or Acute Isolated Posterior Cruciate Ligament Tears

1. Immobilize for 4 weeks in a full knee extension brace or bivalved cylinder cast to maintain tibiofemoral reduction. Use quadriceps isometrics, electrical muscle stimulation, leg raises, and 25% weight bearing.
2. Obtain an anteroposterior and lateral radiograph to verify that no posterior tibial or lateral subluxation exists, which can occur in up to 50% of knees.
3. At 2 weeks, the therapist initiates 0 to 90 degrees of motion, maintaining an anterior tibial translation load. The patient must sleep in the brace and is not allowed unsupervised knee motion to prevent posterior tibial subluxation.
4. At 4 weeks, the patient is allowed to perform active quadriceps extension out of the brace, 50% weight-bearing with crutch support, and maintains brace protection. Newer PCL braces that incorporate an anterior tibia loading using a posterior pad and hinge design may be beneficial when ambulation is initiated
5. At 5 to 6 weeks, the patient is weaned from the brace and crutch support, full knee flexion is allowed, and the rehabilitation protocol is followed to protect the healing PCL fibers.

PCL, Posterior cruciate ligament.
From Noyes FR, Barber-Westin SD: Posterior cruciate ligament: diagnosis, operative techniques, and clinical outcomes. In Noyes FR, Barber-Westin SD (eds): *Noyes' knee disorders: surgery, rehabilitation, clinical outcomes*, ed 2, Philadelphia, 2017, Elsevier, pp 447-526.

period for anatomic repair. There may exist a displaced meniscus tear requiring early treatment. As a word of caution, a displaced meniscus should be reduced into the tibiofemoral joint by 3 weeks to prevent meniscus shortening and scarring that compromises a future repair and results in loss of meniscus function. Even in knees that have soft tissue swelling and edema, and in which major ligament reconstruction is contraindicated, a meniscus repair procedure using all-inside techniques can be performed to reduce the meniscus to a normal tibiofemoral position. The mistake is to wait until 6 weeks or later, expecting that the meniscus repair can be performed at that time.

Too frequently, major ligament surgery in dislocated knees performed under acute conditions results in joint arthrofibrosis, compromising the result. Patients should be carefully selected for acute multiligament repairs, realizing that there are proven techniques for reconstruction of the ruptured ligaments that may be performed later under more ideal conditions. When surgery is performed on acute combined PCL and PL ruptures, the procedure includes the use of appropriate grafts to restore lateral stability (for example, FCL graft substitution that allows an early protected range of knee motion program).[97] Most acute knee dislocations should be treated in a staged approach, first by treating the acute injury and then determining whether a ligament reconstruction should be performed within the 10- to 14-day envelope or be delayed. When early surgery is not advisable, the knee is protected for the first 4 weeks to prevent posterior tibial subluxation, as already described for acute isolated PCL ruptures. AP and lateral radiographs are obtained with the knee placed in a posterior plaster shell and a soft bolster positioned beneath the calf to prevent posterior tibial subluxation. The capsular tissues heal in 7 to 10 days to provide enough stability to prevent recurrence of dislocation.

There is a select group of morbidly obese patients who sustain serious knee dislocations with minimal trauma. The lack of protective muscle function and abnormal body weight places excessive tensile loads on ligament reconstructions, and a high rate of failure of a PCL reconstruction and other concurrent ligament repairs in the acute setting is expected. The preferred treatment for these patients is short-term plaster immobilization (and occasionally external fixation) to allow healing of soft tissues, followed by rehabilitation to return muscle function and knee motion. Only in exceptional circumstances would operative repair (acute or chronic) be warranted in these patients. Consideration for surgical reconstruction may be warranted after appropriate weight reduction.

If a nonoperative approach is selected with associated MCL and posteromedial capsular disruptions, the same program is followed, with the lower limb placed in a cylinder cast to allow "stick-down" of the medial soft tissues. Plaster immobilization is required because a soft hinged brace, even if maintained at 0 degree of extension, does not provide sufficient protection to maintain medial joint line closure to allow the disrupted medial tissues to heal. At 7 to 10 days, the cylinder cast is split into an anterior and posterior shell and the therapist assists the patient with range of motion from 0 to 90 degrees in a figure-of-four position, with the hip joint externally rotated to protect the healing medial tissues.

In multiligament knee injuries, a deep venous thrombosis (DVT) program is instituted that involves assessment of risk factors such as family or personal history of DVT and use of estrogen products in women. A lower extremity ultrasound is obtained before surgery. Postoperative care includes initial use of compressive calf devices, ankle pumps, and early mobilization and ambulation to avoid unnecessary bed rest. In the absence of specific risk factors requiring chemical prophylaxis, the senior author routinely uses one aspirin (325 mg) twice daily and pays close attention for signs of a DVT.

Treatment of Chronic Posterior Cruciate Ligament Ruptures

The algorithm for the treatment of chronic PCL ruptures is shown in Fig. 59.23. The symptoms and clinical examination determine the functional limitations, particularly the component of symptoms resulting from medial tibiofemoral or patellofemoral arthritis because these problems are likely to persist after surgical stabilization. Knees with chronic PCL ruptures are arbitrarily divided into three categories—those with varus osseous malalignment (and, rarely, valgus malalignment) in which an osteotomy must be considered, those with an isolated PCL rupture in which reconstruction may or may not be necessary, and those with significant combined ligament injuries that require reconstruction.

Patients who have severe muscle atrophy, loss of knee motion, or hyperextension gait abnormalities require extensive rehabilitation and gait retraining before reconstruction.[104] The amount of joint arthritis must be determined with accuracy. Radiographs (merchant, standing PA at 45 degrees) and MRI articular cartilage fast-spin-echo sequences provide valuable information.

In knees with no or only mild articular cartilage damage, an assessment of the patient's goals and athletic desires may indicate the need to proceed with PCL reconstruction. The indications for surgical reconstruction in these knees are pain and instability with athletics or other activities, swelling, and 10 mm or more of increased posterior tibial translation at 90 degrees flexion.

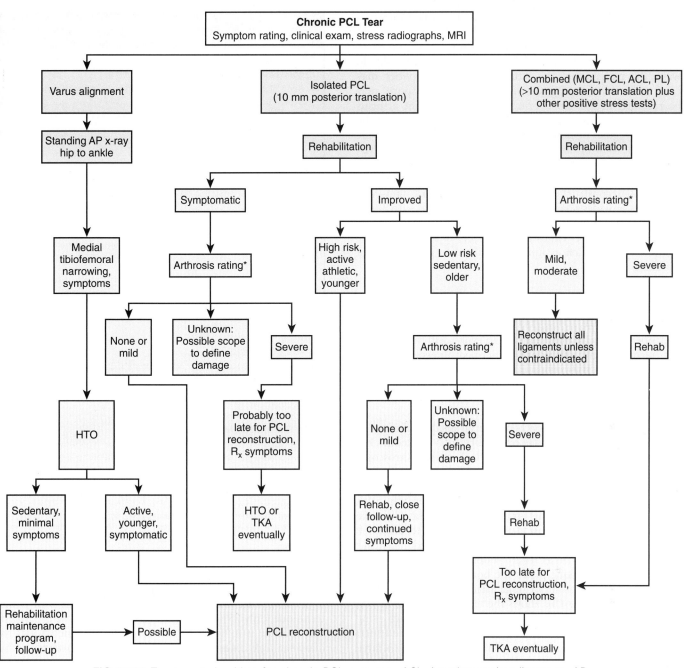

FIG 59.23 Treatment algorithm for chronic PCL ruptures. *ACL,* Anterior cruciate ligament; *AP,* anteroposterior; *FCL,* fibular collateral ligament; *HTO,* high tibial osteotomy; *MCL,* medial collateral ligament; *PCL,* posterior cruciate ligament; *PL,* posterolateral; *TKA,* total knee arthroplasty. (From Noyes FR, Barber-Westin SD: Posterior cruciate ligament: diagnosis, operative techniques, and clinical outcomes. In Noyes FR [ed.]: *Noyes' knee disorders: surgery, rehabilitation, clinical outcomes,* Philadelphia, 2017, Elsevier, pp 447-526.)

Combined ligament ruptures that produce complex instability patterns require careful clinical assessment to detect all of the joint subluxations and ligament deficiencies present. PCL reconstruction is most frequently performed in dislocated knees with gross instability caused by other ligament injuries to the ACL, MCL, or PLS.

The results of PCL reconstruction in knees with chronic ruptures are not as favorable as those that undergo reconstruction for acute injuries. This is because patients present with pain and swelling because of joint deterioration, which often persists, although some benefit may be gained from improved knee stability obtained from the operative procedure.[83] In these knees, areas of exposed bone are frequently encountered in the medial tibiofemoral compartment, along with diffuse cartilage fragmentation in the patellofemoral joint. In these individuals, even mildly strenuous exercises aggravate the joint arthritis symptoms and cannot be performed. The patient's initial experience with rehabilitation, and the inability to perform the required rehabilitation exercises, provides important information regarding the amount of joint arthritis that is present and joint symptoms, which are likely permanent.

If a nonoperative approach is elected, the clinician should warn the patient that the return to athletic activities may carry an uncertain prognosis and that although sports may be resumed in the short term, some form of joint arthritis will eventually ensue. It is therefore important to follow the patient at regular intervals. A bone scan may be used to provide some indication of abnormal blood flow dynamics; however, it is our experience that the onset of pain and swelling usually indicates more advanced joint damage and a poor prognosis after PCL reconstruction. A MRI scan with fast spin-echo sequences provides a baseline for repeated studies at 1- to 2-year intervals. The nonoperative treatment protocol for chronic PCL injuries involves educating the patient to avoid high knee flexion activities such as lunges that increase posterior tibial subluxation.[13,29,31]

OPERATIVE TECHNIQUES: CURRENT CONCEPTS

Surgical Options

PCL operative techniques continue to evolve with many different reconstructive procedures described; however, clinical outcome studies still remain limited to allow precise decision making. The senior author's recommended surgical approaches and relative advantages and disadvantages of each procedure are shown in Table 59.6.

First, the surgical approach of the all-inside technique is recommended. The use of the open tibial inlay procedure has been replaced in recent publications with all-inside arthroscopic techniques. The tibial inlay procedure still has a role in PCL tibial avulsion fractures, in rare revision cases, or when the surgeon prefers a combined tibia inlay approach with arthroscopic femoral tunnel graft placement. The all-inside approach involves the decision regarding where to place the bone portion of the graft when a quadriceps tendon-patellar bone (QT-PB) or Achilles tendon-bone (AT-B) graft is used. Our preferred technique places the bone portion of the PCL graft directly at the posterior tibial attachment, simulating the tibial inlay approach. This allows the technique of one or two femoral tunnels for a single- or two-strand construct using all-inside or outside-in tunnel techniques, as is discussed later.

In our experience, soft tissue grafts placed through a large tibial tunnel have an increased risk of failure because of delayed graft incorporation that may lead to a revision procedure and necessity for staged bone grafting. A sclerotic line often forms in the bone tunnel about the graft periphery, with limited bone ingrowth into the central regions of the graft. From an antidotal standpoint, it has been our experience that an increased success rate of PCL reconstruction occurs when the bone portion of the graft is placed at the tibia, with one or two collagenous graft strands placed at the femoral site. Still, there are many publications that describe the historical technique of placing the bone plug at the femoral site (inside-out or outside-in tunnel) and the collagenous portion through a single tibial tunnel, most frequently using an AT-B allograft. This technique is perhaps the easiest to master and can be used when surgical time is an issue because it is more difficult to pass the bone portion of the graft into the tibial tunnel.

Second, a large-diameter graft is selected that will fill the majority of the anatomic femoral and tibial footprints. At the

---

TABLE 59.6   Recommended Surgical Approaches

All-Inside

Single-Tibial Tunnel Approach
- Bone plug in tunnel at posterior PCL attachment (same as inlay except tunnel)
- Alternative option: Use FlipCutter femoral socket and TightRope plus interference screw
- Avoids posterior dissection, operative time
- Projected results similar to tibial inlay

Two-Tunnel Femoral Approach
- Provides better anatomic positioning along oval PCL attachment
- Advantage graft incorporation over single large-diameter graft
- Outside-in tunnel, graft interference screw with suture post
- Second option: Single femoral tunnel for multiligament reconstruction where time and operative complexity warrant single tunnel

Tibial Inlay
- Reserved for revision knees to bypass misplaced tibial tunnel (staged bone graft may be required)

Graft Selection

Isolated PCL Rupture
- Quadriceps tendon-patellar bone autograft, ipsilateral (rarely contralateral)
- Achilles tendon-bone allograft
- Bone-patellar tendon-bone allograft

PCL Combined Other Ligament Rupture
- Use allograft listed above
- Avoid large-diameter soft tissue allograft through tibial tunnel
- Bone plug placed at posterior tibial tunnel
- No autograft harvest same knee

PCL, Posterior cruciate ligament.
From Noyes FR, Barber-Westin SD: Posterior cruciate ligament: diagnosis, operative techniques, and clinical outcomes. In Noyes FR, Barber-Westin SD (eds): *Noyes' knee disorders: surgery, rehabilitation, clinical outcomes*, ed 2, Philadelphia, 2017, Elsevier, pp 447-526.

---

femoral PCL attachment, a two-tunnel technique is preferred for larger patients; however, in most patients, a single large-diameter tunnel may be used. It is probable that with either technique, only 75% of the femoral attachment site is covered. The mistake is to select a graft construct in which a smaller diameter graft covers less than approximately two-thirds of the footprint.

Third, an autograft or allograft construct is selected with a bone plug at one end for more secure fixation and predictable incorporation, compared with an all soft tissue graft as already discussed. It is important that high strength graft fixation methods be used to withstand the large forces expected postoperatively. For example, the use of a soft tissue interference screw for fixation of a PCL graft, frequently described in publications, still provides lower fixation strength, and a backup procedure with sutures and suture posts is recommended for added graft fixation strength.

Fourth, an autogenous QT-PB graft is used in isolated PCL surgical procedures in athletic patients and patients with high demand activities; our studies show a higher success rate with this graft compared with allografts. This recommendation is in agreement with clinical outcome studies of ACL grafts that report a 4 to 6 times higher failure rate of allografts compared with autografts in high activity demand patients. Allografts are still recommended in sedentary patients and in multiligament knee injuries. In multiligament reconstructions, a QT-PT autograft is not recommended (harvested from the operative knee) because this adds to the morbidity of the operative procedure and subsequent rehabilitation.

Tibial Attachment Techniques: Arthroscopic All-Inside Versus Open Tibial Inlay Approach.

The arthroscopic-assisted placement of the tibial tunnel or socket avoids the added operative time and complexity of the posteromedial tibial inlay approach. The surgeon must have extensive arthroscopic experience to safely perform these procedures to identify the PCL posterior tibial attachment site, avoid penetration into the posterior capsule and subsequent damage to the neurovascular structures, and place the tibial tunnel into the anatomic PCL tibial footprint. Specially designed instruments, drill guides with safety stops for guide pins, and drills are available to lessen the serious risk of inadvertent penetration of instruments posteriorly and damage to neurovascular structures.

The all-inside arthroscopic technique is particularly advantageous in knees with multiple ligament ruptures that require repair and reconstruction. In these knees, high strength grafts are used to reconstruct the PCL and ACL, which are appropriately tensioned and fixed to reduce the tibiofemoral joint to its normal AP position. Medial or lateral operative approaches are used for concurrent medial and PL ligament and soft tissue repairs or reconstructions. A combined ACL/PCL/MCL injury involves an all-arthroscopic approach for the ACL and PCL, followed by a limited medial dissection for repair of the medial tissues and meniscus attachments. A similar operative plan is followed with an ACL/PCL/MCL reconstruction.

Combined ligament injuries, particularly those involving medial ligament and muscle tissues, have a high rate of postoperative motion problems and arthrofibrosis. In these knees, an open posterior tibial inlay procedure and popliteal dissection is purposely avoided by using the all-inside arthroscopic approach.

From a historical standpoint, the open posteromedial tibial inlay technique did have the advantage of placing a tibial inlay graft securely into the posterior PCL tibial attachment site. This approach was often selected when only the PCL required reconstruction. The tibial inlay graft provides ideal graft fixation and early healing. A two-strand autogenous QT-PB graft with two femoral tunnels has been previously described and the clinical outcomes published.[82,88]

One theoretical disadvantage of the all-inside technique is the potential for the collagenous portion of the graft abrading against the angulated posterior tibial tunnel. There are operative techniques designed to diminish this problem. These include creating a more oblique tibial tunnel drilled through the anterolateral tibia and carefully chamfering the tunnel exit. Collagen grafts with a large cross-sectional area and diameter are favored over those with a smaller area and diameter, in which any abrasion compromises graft strength. To decrease soft tissue graft abrasion at the tibial tunnel, the bone portion of the graft may be placed in a tibial tunnel directly adjacent to the tunnel exit or placed in an all-inside tibial socket. The goal is to match the beneficial effect of the tibial inlay procedure to allow prompt osseous healing. Biomechanical studies of PCL reconstructions conducted at our facilities have shown the potential for graft abrasion and failure at the femoral attachment.[119] Operative techniques to protect against graft failure and abrasion are required at both tibial and femoral attachment

sites, and repetitive knee motion in the postoperative period is limited, as will be described.

Posterior Cruciate Ligament Femoral Attachment Technique: Two-Tunnel Versus Single-Tunnel Options.

It is not difficult from a technical standpoint to use two well-placed femoral tunnels within the PCL femoral footprint from outside-in, and this is a recommended technique to master. The outside-in technique, with a limited anteromedial subvastus or muscle-splitting approach, allows graft tensioning, a long femoral tunnel for tendon graft incorporation, and graft fixation with an interference screw and suture post. The posteromedial graft is usually shorter by 15 mm than the anterolateral graft. The outside-in tunnel approach allows accurate tensioning, fixation, and visualization of the graft length change during knee flexion. This allows the surgeon to determine the ideal knee flexion position for graft fixation.

When a single femoral graft is selected, the femoral tunnel may be drilled from inside-out or outside-in. There is an increased obliquity with the inside-out approach; however, in either case, the posterior or deep portion of the tunnel needs to be radicalized and smoothed to decrease graft abrasion effects. A FlipCutter (Arthrex, Naples, Florida) may be selected to create the femoral socket and TightRope (Arthrex) fixation may be used along with a soft tissue interference screw. This avoids a vastus medialis obliquus (VMO) incision, maintains the medial femoral cortex, and is less invasive. This is our preferred technique.

In the alternative technique described, in which the bone portion of the PCL graft is placed at the femoral site, a circular tunnel or a rectangular femoral slot technique may be used. The bone plug is fixed using an inside-out interference screw. The rectangular slot technique places the bone within the PCL femoral footprint and is more ideal than a single large-diameter tunnel, although either technique may be used. We advocate only one tibial tunnel for the collagenous portion of the graft. An exception is in select PCL revision cases with a misplaced femoral tunnel in which the bone portion of the graft is required for adequate femoral graft placement and fixation instead of one or two soft tissue femoral graft tunnels.

A single femoral tunnel drilled from an inside-out anterolateral portal is more difficult because of the narrow intercondylar notch, proximity of the lateral femoral condyle, placement of the tunnel within the PCL footprint, and exact placement required to avoid portions of the graft located outside of the PCL footprint. The outside-in drilling approach or FlipCutter approach for a single large-diameter femoral graft tunnel is often more advantageous and is recommended.[9]

Techniques for fixation of soft tissue grafts at the femoral attachment site using interference screws alone provide a weaker fixation construct[44] and result in lower attachment strength. The outside-in approach allows an interference screw and sutures with a suture post to be used. As an alternative, the use of the Flipcutter and TightRope fixation also allows for an interference screw to be added for graft fixation strength. PCL reconstructions are under high in vivo loads, and it is advantageous to select graft fixation methods that provide for a high tensile strength of the graft construct.

Single-Strand Versus Two-Strand Posterior Cruciate Ligament Graft Constructs.

The advantages and disadvantages of one- and two-strand PCL graft techniques are summarized in Table

TABLE 59.7   Basis for the Selection of One- Versus Two-Strand Posterior Cruciate Ligament Reconstruction

	Single-Strand	Two-Strand
Greater area	−	+
Load-sharing (decreased tensile forces in each graft strand)	−	+
Operative complexity	+	−
Cyclic fatigue	−	+
Clinical results (residual posterior tibial translation)[a]	Unknown	Unknown

+ Denotes relative advantage; − denotes relative disadvantage.
[a]Proven by objective measurements, including stress radiography at 90 degrees of knee flexion. From Noyes FR, Barber-Westin SD: Posterior cruciate ligament: diagnosis, operative techniques, and clinical outcomes. In Noyes FR, Barber-Westin SD (eds): *Noyes' knee disorders: surgery, rehabilitation, clinical outcomes*, ed 2, Philadelphia, 2017, Elsevier, pp 447-526.

59.7. The goal of adding a second strand is to place additional collagenous tissue within the PCL footprint to increase the cross-sectional area of the graft and more closely replicate the native PCL attachment. This theoretical advantage is sometimes referred to as the *mass action effect* of adding additional collagen within the PCL footprint. The improved stability and clinical success of a two-strand graft construct compared with a single-strand graft has not been proven from a clinical standpoint.[59] There are clinical studies that show patients who received a single-strand PCL graft reconstruction obtained results similar to those who underwent a two-strand PCL procedure.[22,54,56,67,122]

The incorporation of a second graft strand has the theoretical advantage of providing additional collagen tissue for load sharing that decreases stress in the collagen fibers, increases graft strength, and reduces cyclic fatigue of the graft construct.[119,135] The two graft strands are tensioned at surgery to share loads, thus decrease the loads compared with those of a single PCL graft construct. This has been shown in the majority (but not all[74]) biomechanical studies that have compared single- with two-strand graft constructs. Studies report that the two graft strands placed in the distal two-thirds of the PCL femoral footprint will function to resist posterior tibial translation with increasing knee flexion. Alternatively, when two graft strands are placed in the proximal and distal (deep and shallow) portion of the PCL footprint, graft loading occurs in a reciprocal manner and the graft strands are under higher loads, which is less ideal.

A justification to add a second PCL graft strand is the observation in clinical studies of a residual posterior tibial subluxation at high knee flexion after single-strand PCL reconstructions.[59,83] Current PCL surgical procedures do not uniformly produce functional restoration of normal joint kinematics and stability postoperatively. This problem is discussed in detail in the "Clinical Studies" section of this chapter. The concern is that a residual posterior tibial displacement changes tibiofemoral contact positions (more anterior on the tibia), with altered and high cartilage pressures and decrease in function of the medial meniscus.[70,110] Increases in patellofemoral contact pressures have also been reported.[28]

There are many different types of two-strand PCL graft constructs reported in the literature. One type consists of two separate grafts placed into two separate femoral and tibial tunnels, or two separate femoral tunnels with both graft strands placed in one tibial tunnel. For purposes of differential load sharing between two graft strands with knee flexion, it is assumed that two separate femoral attachments and a single tibial attachment avoid the necessity and operative complexity of two tibial tunnels.

When an AT-B allograft is selected, it is important that the graft be inspected to discard those that have a narrow tendon section just adjacent to the bone attachment. A QT-PB allograft is a more suitable PCL substitute because of the larger cross-sectional area of the tendon; however, this graft has to have sufficient length and is more difficult to obtain from tissue banks. It should be noted that in some patients the (autogenous) quadriceps tendon portion of the graft is not robust enough to produce two graft strands. In these cases, a single graft is used that represents a large-diameter graft.

Multicenter randomized controlled trials of one- and two-strand PCL reconstructions are required in the future to provide a more scientific basis for selection of one type of PCL reconstructive technique over another. For this reason, more than one PCL technique is described, with recommendations made regarding the technical issues to maximize the clinical result. Our preferred PCL graft procedures are provided, along with the justification and rationale for these selections.

In summary, it appears that there are sound theoretical reasons to warrant a two-strand PCL reconstruction when clinically feasible. These conditions include isolated PCL reconstructions when the added time required to perform a two-strand PCL graft does not represent a contraindication in terms of operative time and complexity. In multiligament reconstructions, the primary goal is to repair and reconstruct all ruptured ligaments. Adding a second femoral tunnel and tensioning and securing two graft strands is time consuming for an already complex surgical reconstruction. Therefore, the surgeon should be prepared, based on the operative findings, to modify the preoperative plan when required. In multiligament injured knees, a single-strand PCL graft construct still has the ability to restore functional stability.[74] Given the complex PCL fiber microgeometry, either a single- or two-strand graft construct still represents an imperfect substitution, providing only a check rein effect in controlling joint motions and subluxations.

Graft Selection. The goal of PCL surgery is to select a graft that matches the structural properties of the PCL as closely as possible. The problem is that the PCL is a highly complex ligament composed of fibers of different lengths that are brought into the loading configuration based on the knee flexion and tibial rotation positions. The initial graft mechanical properties are expected to decline after graft implantation and in vivo remodeling. It is thus not possible to match the complex PCL microgeometry with any tendon substitute. The principles for the selection of all-inside grafts are summarized in Table 59.8.

Recommendations for Surgeons on Selecting a Posterior Cruciate Ligament Operative Technique. The operative techniques available to the surgeon require experience and knowledge at an expert arthroscopic level. There is a building level of difficulty in PCL reconstructive techniques, and the literature reflects marked variability among surgeons in surgical options and graft choices. Based on the senior author's experience, a few suggestions are provided for consideration of this selection process.

Starting from the initial level of surgical complexity, a soft tissue graft (without a bone portion) is the easiest to prepare,

TABLE 59.8 All-Inside Posterior Cruciate Ligament Graft Options

Two-Strand Grafts	Single-Strand Grafts
Preferred	**Preferred**
QT-PB autograft	QT-PB autograft
1. Single tibial tunnel: Bone plug at posterior tunnel exit	1. Tibial tunnel: Bone plug at posterior tunnel exit
2. Femur: Two strand, two tunnels or one strand, one tunnel based on graft size	2. Femoral tunnel: One strand FlipCutter femoral socket Tightrope plus interference screw
Alternatives: Femoral Attachment Two Tunnels	**Alternatives**
QT-PB allograft	QT-PB allograft
AT-B allograft	AT-B allograft
Principles	**Principles**
• Allografts have lower success rate, delayed healing.	• Allograft provides acceptable results in multiligament reconstructions, dislocated knees when operative complexity and time warrant single tunnel procedure.
• Bone graft plug provides secure fixation, faster healing, increased graft construct tensile strength compared with all soft-tissue grafts.	• Preference for bone plug at posterior tibial tunnel to avoid large-diameter soft tissue graft through tibia with delayed graft incorporation.
• Rehabilitation, return to activity delayed with allografts.	
• Avoid single small-diameter B-PT-B autograft, second graft is required to achieve native PCL width.	
• Graft selection rules still empiric until randomized controlled clinical trials are performed.	

AT-B, Achilles tendon-bone; *B-PT-B,* bone-patellar tendon-bone; *PCL,* posterior cruciate ligament; *QT-PB,* quadriceps tendon-patellar bone.
From Noyes FR, Barber-Westin SD: Posterior cruciate ligament: diagnosis, operative techniques, and clinical outcomes. In Noyes FR, Barber-Westin SD (eds): *Noyes' knee disorders: surgery, rehabilitation, clinical outcomes,* ed 2, Philadelphia, 2017, Elsevier, pp 447-526.

pass into the knee joint, and fixate in well-placed femoral and tibial tunnels. There are a variety of fixation methods available. The senior author expresses a level of concern with allograft tissue, particularly in an athletic patient, owing to delayed remodeling and the lack of a beneficial graft hypertrophy after implantation that occurs with autografts. In addition, the use of soft tissue interference screws alone provides a relatively low strength attachment fixation.

The next level of complexity is a PCL graft that has bone attached on one end, such as an AT-B allograft. There is the opportunity for ease of passage, with the tendon portion placed in the tibial tunnel and secure fixation accomplished with an interference screw of the bone plug at the femoral tunnel. The tendon is passed first into the knee joint through an enlarged anterior portal, and then into the tibial tunnel. This allows the bone portion of the graft to be passed next into the joint, docked by a leading suture within the femoral tunnel, and fixed with an interference screw. The tendon portion in the tibial tunnel allows double fixation with an interference screw and backup suture post. This is one of the most frequently used PCL procedures and is done with either an AT-B or QT-PB graft.

The placement of the bone portion of an autograft or allograft within the tibial tunnel represents an added level of difficulty because the bone portion is introduced into the knee joint through an enlarged portal and then guided by a leading suture (always at the end of the bone) and nerve hook into the tibial tunnel. This requires the bone plug to be angled close to a right angle to enter into the tibial tunnel entrance. The tibial tunnel is enlarged 2 mm greater than the bone portion of the graft. With experience, the gentle docking technique of the bone plug within the tibial tunnel is successful. After the bone plug is in the tibial tunnel, the tendon portion is brought into the joint and easily passed into the femoral tunnel. This allows the overall graft to be displaced proximal to distal for appropriate graft lengths in the tunnels and final fixation. The senior author believes the fixation of the bone plug within the tibial tunnel is a distinct advantage. The clinical experience at our Center has shown (in revision cases) a relatively poor healing ability of large allografts within a large diameter tibial tunnel. The bone plug is fixed with both an interference screw and backup suture post. Accordingly, this represents the preferred technique recommended in this chapter. In addition, two tibial tunnels are not necessary to achieve successful results and, therefore, one well-placed tibial tunnel is selected in all PCL surgical cases.

The final level of complexity is adding a second femoral tunnel, and the recommendations for the double-graft construct have already been presented. In summary, the primary indication is in larger patients with corresponding larger PCL femoral attachment sites where a single graft replaces two-thirds or less of the femoral attachment area. Future well-designed Level 1 studies of sufficient numbers of patients are necessary to resolve these controversies; however, the recommendations discussed in this chapter appear warranted at this time.

INTRAOPERATIVE EVALUATION

The patient is instructed to use a chlorhexidine scrub of the body with emphasis on the operative limb (toes to groin) 3 days before surgery and the evening before and morning of surgery. Lower extremity hair is removed by clippers, not a shaver. Antibiotic infusion is begun 1 hour prior to surgery. A nonsteroidal antiinflammatory drug (NSAID) is given to the patient with a sip of water upon arising the morning of surgery (which is continued until the fifth postoperative day unless there are specific contraindications to the medicine). The use of an NSAID and a postoperative firm double-cotton, double-Ace compression dressing for 72 hours (cotton, Ace, cotton, Ace-layered dressing) has proven very effective in diminishing soft tissue swelling. In select knees that demonstrate soft tissue swelling before or after surgery, the judicious use of an intravenous corticosteroid for 2 to 3 days may be necessary. This is especially relevant in larger muscular patients in whom postoperative swelling of the entire lower extremity may occur. In complex multiligament surgery, the antibiotic is repeated at 4 hours and continued for 24 hours. A urinary indwelling catheter is not used unless there are specific indications. The patient's urinary output and total fluids are carefully monitored during the procedure and in the recovery room.

The knee skin area is initialized by the surgeon before entering the operating room, with a nurse observing the procedure. The identification process is repeated with all operative personnel with a "time-out" before surgery to verify the patient name and birth date, knee undergoing surgery, procedure, allergies, antibiotic infusion, and special precautions that apply. All personnel provide verbal agreement.

All knee ligament subluxation tests are performed after the induction of anesthesia in both the injured and contralateral limbs. The amount of increased anterior tibial translation, posterior tibial translation, lateral joint opening, medial joint opening, and external tibial rotation is documented. In acute knee injuries, arthroscopic pressure is maintained at a low setting, with adequate outflow at all times to prevent fluid extravasation, which is carefully monitored during the operative procedure. A thorough arthroscopic examination is conducted, documenting articular cartilage surface abnormalities and the condition of the menisci.

The medial and lateral tibiofemoral gap test is done during the arthroscopic examination.[100] The knee is flexed 30 degrees and a varus and valgus load of approximately 89 N applied. A calibrated nerve hook is used to measure the amount of lateral and medial tibiofemoral compartment opening. Twelve millimeters or more of joint opening at the periphery of the compartment indicates the need for a combined lateral or medial ligament reconstructive procedure to protect and unload the PCL reconstruction.

Appropriate arthroscopic procedures are performed as indicated, including meniscus repairs or partial excision, débridement, and articular cartilage procedures.

POSTERIOR CRUCIATE LIGAMENT GRAFT HARVEST OPTIONS

Quadriceps Tendon-Patellar Bone Autograft

A tourniquet is inflated to 275 mm of pressure. This is usually the only time the tourniquet is used in the reconstructive procedure. An incision is made just medial to the superior pole of the patella and extended proximally 5 to 6 cm (Fig. 59.24). The incision allows access to the anteromedial aspect of the medial femoral condyle and VMO for subvastus placement of the femoral tunnels. A cosmetic approach is used, with subcutaneous dissection performed circumferentially about the incision to allow the skin to be mobilized superiorly and inferiorly for the graft harvest. With this technique, no incision is required over the patella.

The graft length and thickness is marked on the tendon, and the proximal musculotendinous junction is avoided because it would weaken the extensor mechanism. The quadriceps tendon appears more narrow proximally, and it is important not to remove more than one-third of the tendon. In rare cases, there is a shortened quadriceps tendon that is not suitable for harvest; the patient is advised preoperatively and provides consent for either an autograft or allograft approach. A suitable quadriceps tendon must be a minimum of 70 mm, not counting the 22 to 24 mm patellar bone plug. The full-thickness quadriceps tendon graft is taken from the central tendon and is 10 to 12 mm in width and thickness, respectively, depending on the overall size of the tendon. A general rule is to take approximately 30% of the tendon in the middle portion, realizing there may be some narrowing of the tendon proximally. The quadriceps tendon consists of three layers—rectus tendon, VMO-vastus lateralis oblique (VLO) combined tendon, and vastus intermedius tendon. A meticulous technique is followed to incise all three layers in a perpendicular fashion with a new blade. There is a tendency not to harvest the deep layer or to allow the blade to

assume an oblique plane rather than a perpendicular plane. A curved instrument is placed behind the three tendon layers at the proximal aspect of the tendon harvest site to protect the underlying joint synovium. If the synovium is entered, it is closed along with the remaining quadriceps tendon closure to maintain joint distension for the arthroscopic procedure.

An Ellis clamp is placed about the three ends of the tendon to maintain tension. Care is taken at the quadriceps tendon attachment to the patella because the tendon attachment is located at the proximal and anterior third of the proximal patella. There is a plane established at this point just behind the quadriceps tendon attachment to preserve the posterior underlying synovial attachment and adjacent soft tissues. These tissues provide a superior buttress for the bone grafting the patella to close the defect and secure the bone graft.

The patella bone block matches the quadriceps width. The bone block length is 22 to 24 mm and has a depth of 8 to 10 mm. A thin powered saw blade is marked with a Steri-Strip to a depth of 10 mm to prevent a deep penetration. The saw is kept perpendicular to the patella anterior surface for all cuts. After the anterior bone cuts are made, the quadriceps tendon is lifted anteriorly at its attachment site. The posterior portion of the bone block is cut in a transverse plane beneath the quadriceps tendon attachment to a depth of 8 to 10 mm. This allows the bone block to be gently removed for graft preparation. The tourniquet is deflated and hemostasis obtained.

The graft is prepared based on whether the one-strand or two-strand technique is selected. The tendon portion must be 11 to 12 mm wide and thick to be able to fashion graft strands that are 7 to 8 mm in diameter. In smaller patients, a single 10 mm quadriceps tendon with a reduced thickness does not provide sufficient tendon for a robust two-strand graft; therefore, a single-strand construct must be selected. The tendon graft strands are sutured in a meticulous manner using Fiber-Loop or FiberWire sutures (Arthrex). The graft diameter is sized for the appropriate tunnel to be drilled. Two FiberWire sutures are passed in the distal end of the patellar bone. A blood-soaked sponge is wrapped around the graft to provide protection, keep the tissues moist, and potentially maintain some cell viability.

The quadriceps tendon and synovium are closed to provide a fluid tight closure, allowing joint distension. The quadriceps tendon defect is loosely closed with nonabsorbable zero sutures. The tendon is closed in a Z-plasty manner, in which portions of the quadriceps tendon layers are brought together to avoid the circumferential tight sutures placed through all three tendon layers. This technique decreases medial-to-lateral tension in the extensor mechanism.

The patella bone defect is later bone grafted in a meticulous manner with bone obtained with a coring reamer during preparation of the femoral graft tunnels. It is important to obtain a bone graft that completely fills the defect because bone shavings from the tunnel preparations are insufficient. Postoperatively, a bone defect that was meticulously grafted heals without a palpable patella defect and decreases the incidence of graft site harvest pain.

Achilles Tendon-Bone Allograft

The preparation of an AT-B allograft is performed in a similar manner to that of QT-PB already described and is the most commonly used single-strand construct. It is necessary to tube or roll the wide proximal fan shaped portion of the tendon. In the optional technique described, the bone plug is placed into

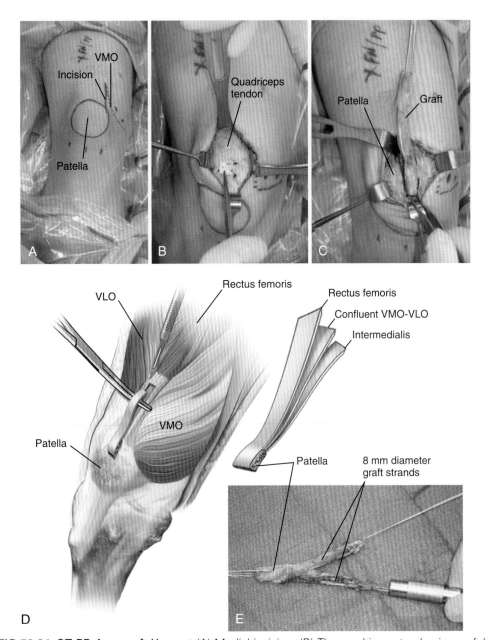

FIG 59.24 QT-PB Autograft Harvest (A) Medial incision. (B) The quadriceps tendon is carefully marked to only remove 30% of its width and not extend to the musculotendinous junction. (C) A central 10- to 11-mm wide full-thickness quadriceps tendon graft is harvested. The defect is later closed to maintain arthroscopic joint distention. (D) Graft harvest. (E) Two-strand 8-mm tendon graft with patellar bone is prepared. *VLO*, Vastus lateralis oblique; *VMO*, vastus medialis obliquus. (From Noyes FR, Barber-Westin SD: Posterior cruciate ligament: diagnosis, operative techniques, and clinical outcomes. In Noyes FR [ed.]: *Noyes' knee disorders: surgery, rehabilitation, clinical outcomes*, Philadelphia, 2017, Elsevier, pp 447-526.)

a rectangular femoral site for all-inside placement, or a 10- to 11-mm diameter graft for a single femoral tunnel is placed using an outside-in technique or FlipCutter technique.

SURGICAL PROCEDURES

Anteromedial Approach and Outside-In Femoral Tunnels

This approach is selected when two femoral tunnels are used and is less traumatic than a muscle-splitting approach, in which the VMO is split for 5 to 6 cm for proper visualization. In addition, this approach allows for good visualization of the graft and suture post fixation. When a single femoral tunnel is selected, a limited muscle-splitting approach is performed or a FlipCutter is used. A vertical skin incision of 3 to 4 cm is made over the anteromedial vastus medialis proximal to the knee joint and just medial to the quadriceps tendon. When an ipsilateral QT-PB is harvested, the same skin incision is used.

The key to the anteromedial approach is to identify the VMO anterior attachment to the medial retinaculum and dissect in this plane, thereby avoiding the muscle and achieving a subvastus elevation of the VMO. Note that no incision is made into the VMO attachment to the patella, and the medial patellofemoral ligament is not incised. Only a limited subvastus exposure is required. The synovium beneath the VMO is protected and not entered. The VMO nerve innervation proximally is not disturbed. A branch of the superior genicular artery that traverses the inferior border of the VMO is protected.

The outside location of the 1 o'clock femoral tunnel entrance is identified with the drill guide. The guide pin is placed 12 mm proximal to the articular cartilage of the medial femoral condyle, at an equal distance medially from the medial trochlear border. The articular cartilage border is carefully palpated. The more distal femoral tunnel decreases graft tunnel angulation at the entrance within the joint. The tunnel should be in line with the obliquity of the PCL graft, but not located too far distally adjacent to the articular cartilage to prevent a breakout of the tunnel into the distal femoral condyle. The location of the 4 o'clock femoral tunnel, to maintain an adequate bone bridge at both the entrance and exit of both tunnels, is also 12 mm from the medial articular cartilage margin and just anterior to the femoral epicondyle.

At the time of graft fixation, the surgeon uses a headlight to view the graft in the tunnels. The graft length is observed as the knee is flexed to determine the knee flexion angle at which the greatest graft length is produced. In addition, the headlight provides adequate visualization for the placement of the interference screw and a graft suture post for added fixation. Routine closure is performed with absorbable sutures used for the VMO retinaculum attachment and subcutaneous tissues.

Posterior Cruciate Ligament All-Inside Technique: One- and Two-Strand Graft Reconstructions

Our graft preference for isolated PCL reconstruction using the all-inside technique is a QT-PB autograft, using a single- or two-strand femoral placement based on the size of the quadriceps tendon as discussed (see Table 59.8). This approach is recommended for athletic patients. The bone plug is placed and fixated in a posterior tibial tunnel directly at the posterior entrance under fluoroscopic control. The goal is to match the results of the tibial inlay procedure, with the bone plug placed directly at the posterior PCL attachment using an oblique tunnel instead of a tibial inlay that requires an open posteromedial approach. In a sedentary patient or multiligament knee injury, an AT-B graft is selected with the bone plug placed in either the femoral or tibial tunnel. However, the senior author advocates a similar approach as already described with the bone portion of the graft placed in the tibial tunnel and soft tissue graft strand in the femur. The operative steps for these techniques are described in the following sections.

Patient Positioning and Setup. An examination under anesthesia is performed to confirm the diagnosis and carefully compare the injured knee to the opposite normal knee. It is important to palpate the medial tibiofemoral step-off at 90 degrees of flexion in both knees. At surgery, the PCL graft will be tensioned in knee flexion and the medial tibiofemoral step-off used as verification that the abnormal posterior translation has been corrected.

The patient is placed supine on the operating table with appropriate padding (Fig. 59.25). The operating table is placed in a 15-degree retroflexed lumbar position to prevent hyperextension of the spine and produce mild flexion of the hip to relieve undue tension on the right and left femoral nerves. The knee portion of the bed is flexed up to 90 degrees. A thigh tourniquet is placed over cast padding. The opposite limb is positioned in a foam leg holder with the hip slightly flexed. A thigh-high compression stocking is placed on the opposite extremity. After appropriate draping, a 4-inch flat padded bolster is placed underneath the operative thigh to protect the

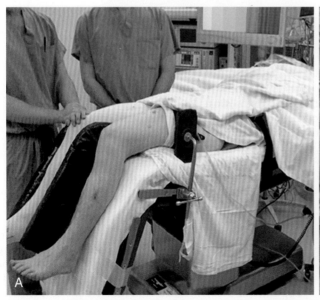
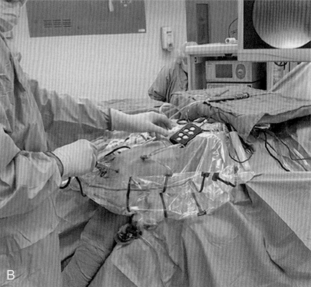

FIG 59.25 (A and B) Patient position with the knee flexed to 70 degrees. Note that the bed is retroflexed to maintain hip flexion. There is no pressure against the posterior popliteal space. The opposite leg is well padded. (From Noyes FR, Barber-Westin SD: Posterior cruciate ligament: diagnosis, operative techniques, and clinical outcomes. In Noyes FR [ed.]: *Noyes' knee disorders: surgery, rehabilitation, clinical outcomes*, Philadelphia, 2017, Elsevier, pp 447-526.)

tissues and allow for knee flexion during the operative procedure. The operative procedure is performed with the knee flexed from 60 to 90 degrees; however, further knee flexion is possible by adjusting the operative table or using an additional thigh bolster. It is important that no undue pressure be placed against the posterior thigh and sciatic nerve during the operative procedure. For this reason, an arthroscopic thigh holder is typically not used. In prolonged surgical cases, a rigid thigh holder may place abnormal pressures on the posterior thigh, which compromises the neurovascular structures. Posterior thigh muscle ischemia and peroneal tibial nerve damage are avoided by ensuring no undue posterior pressures occur.

When a meniscus repair is required, an arthroscopic thigh holder is initially used to allow for adequate joint opening for an inside-out meniscus repair using the patient and limb positioning described. The knee position of the bed is flexed as required. After the meniscus repair is performed, the thigh holder is removed and appropriate posterior thigh padding placed as necessary.

Arthroscopy of the knee begins with a pressure-regulated pump that is adjusted to provide mild joint distention and prevent fluid extravasation. The pump is required to maintain joint distention, particularly during the drilling of the tibial tunnel, so that the fluid expands the posterior capsule out of the operative field. Modern pressure- and volume-regulated pumps allow for a controlled inflow and outflow that maintains a safe pressure. In addition, sufficient fluid inflow is maintained so that a tourniquet is only used selectively, usually during the drilling of the tibia tunnel. Routine arthroscopic anteromedial, anterolateral, and superolateral portals are created. During the PCL reconstruction, a transpatellar central portal is required. Many surgeons recommend a posteromedial portal to débride the PCL tibial fibers and visualize the PCL tibial attachment. The senior author performs a technique in which the posteromedial portal is not required. The use of three anterior portals is advantageous because inadvertent fluid extravasation into the popliteal fossa is avoided, which may limit posterior capsule distention and visualization during drilling of the tibial tunnel.

A standard arthroscopic examination is performed. The gap test is done to assess lateral and medial joint opening at 20 degrees knee flexion with a varus and valgus stress. Any meniscal repairs or partial resections, débridement, or other arthroscopic procedures are performed.

Tibial Tunnel Preparation. The most difficult part of the operative procedure is preparation of the tibial tunnel (located in the distal PCL attachment position) without injuring the popliteal neurovascular structures. To maintain joint distention and allow full visualization, the tourniquet is inflated, a pressure-regulated arthroscopic pump is used, and the femoral tunnels and ipsilateral graft harvest are completed after preparation of the tibial tunnel.

The knee is positioned at 70 degrees of flexion to prevent pressure against the popliteal structures posteriorly, and a proximal thigh pad is used to elevate the thigh. This allows the posterior neurovascular structures to drop away from the posterior aspect of the knee. Matava et al.[76] reported that the mean distance of the PCL from the popliteal artery from 0 to 100 degrees of flexion was 7.6 mm in the axial plane and 7.2 mm in the sagittal plane; however, there may be individual variation between knees. During the operative procedure, the surgeon is constantly aware of the joint pressure, fluid inflow and outflow,

increased thigh tension, and any lack of joint distention. Intermittent palpation of the popliteal and calf region is performed during the operative procedure to detect fluid extravasation by an inadvertent puncture of the posterior capsule.

The preparation of the tibial tunnel is more difficult when the ACL is intact. It is first necessary to identify residual PCL fibers adjacent to the ACL, which are removed with a shaver or basket through the anteromedial portal with the arthroscope in the anterolateral portal. The middle genicular artery enters into the proximal aspect of the PCL and requires electrocoagulation. Some PCL fibers are left on the femoral attachment for later identification and placement of the graft tunnels. The aMFL and pMFL are identified if present. It is usually possible to preserve the pMFL. If these structures impede visualization, they may be removed as long as the lateral meniscus has a confirmed posterior horn attachment to the posterior tibia and is not an anatomic variant, in which the posterior horn is attached by a meniscofemoral attachment.

The 30-degrees arthroscope is next placed into the anteromedial portal and positioned high in the notch adjacent to the PCL femoral attachment. This allows the posterior capsular recess and remaining PCL stump at the tibial attachment to be viewed and instruments to be passed medial to the ACL.

A critical step is the passage of a curved Cobb elevator or commercially available curved Acufex PCL Elevator (Smith and Nephew Endoscopy, Andover, Massachusetts, Fig. 59.26), which has a 90-degree curve and is used to gently free up the capsular space behind the remaining PCL fibers. In some knees, the posterior capsule becomes adherent to the PCL fibers. The PCL Elevator is used to tease the capsule gently off of the PCL fibers and avoid rupture of the posterior capsule. This step requires a gentle approach to push the posterior capsule distally to the level of the distal PCL and capsule attachments, which are at the level of the posterior tibial step-off. Again, this step is emphasized as the key step to prevent damage to the neurovascular structures because the posterior capsular pocket behind the PCL tibial attachment is restored. This allows the PCL Elevator to be placed into this posterior position behind the tibial attachment during the tibial drilling. In some cases, the capsule is so adherent to the remaining PCL ligament fibers that it is not possible to separate the capsule from the PCL fibers. Instead, the plane at the PCL fiber tibial attachment is gently dissected to allow the remaining PCL fibers to displace posteriorly along with the adherent capsule.

If the posterior capsule is violated, a decrease in pump pressure is required and a large anterior fluid outflow portal is established. Close monitoring of any fluid extravasation into the popliteal space and calf is done. It is usually safe to proceed under low-pressure conditions; however, if there is any question of visualization and popliteal space distention, the operative procedure is postponed to allow for capsule healing.

The medial and lateral meniscus posterior tibial attachments adjacent to the PCL tibial fossa are viewed. The shiny white attachment of the medial meniscus is well visualized, and the adjacent lateral meniscus attachment is protected at all times during the preparation of the tibial tunnel. These meniscal attachments are located within a few millimeters of the PCL attachment and may be easily damaged during drilling of the tibial tunnel if it is too proximal or angled to the medial or lateral aspect of the PCL fossa.

The PCL stump is removed with arthroscopic instruments of the surgeon's preference. There are a variety of curved

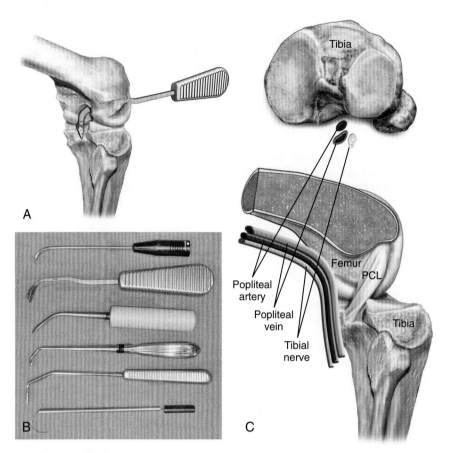

FIG 59.26 (A and B) Tibial preparation. A 30-degrees arthroscope is placed through the anteromedial portal. The arthroscope is placed high in the notch adjacent to the medial condyle to view the posterior region of the joint. Instruments are placed through a central portal, medial to the ACL, carefully protecting the ligament. (A) Acufex PCL Elevator is inserted through the notch to free the posterior capsule carefully and re-create the normal capsular recess behind the PCL because the capsule may be adherent to the ruptured PCL fibers. This step allows the capsule to displace posteriorly with fluid distension, protecting the neurovascular structures. (B) The tibial PCL stump is removed under direct visualization using curved shavers, baskets, Cobb elevators, and radiofrequency instruments. The posterior medial and lateral meniscus attachments are protected at all times. (C) Anatomic illustration shows the close proximity of popliteal neurovascular structures. *PCL,* Posterior cruciate ligament. (From Noyes FR, Barber-Westin SD: Posterior cruciate ligament: diagnosis, operative techniques, and clinical outcomes. In Noyes FR [ed.]: *Noyes' knee disorders: surgery, rehabilitation, clinical outcomes,* Philadelphia, 2017, Elsevier, pp 447-526.)

instruments, including baskets, shavers, and curettes that are helpful. The senior author prefers an electrocoagulation cautery instrument that is manually bent to a 45-degree curve to initially cauterize the PCL fibers at the most proximal portion of the PCL fossa, immediately posterior to the ACL tibial attachment. This initiates a safe plane directly on cortical bone, which is then continued distally to the main PCL attachment. As previously stressed, any remaining PCL fibers that are adherent to the posterior capsule are left alone and displaced posteriorly, exposing the PCL fossa distally to the tibia capsular attachment "champagne glass" step-off. The capsule attachment is not violated to prevent fluid extravasation into the popliteal space. At the conclusion of these steps, the entire posterior PCL tibial fossa (to the level of the posterior capsule attachment) is viewed for identification of the correct placement of the tibial tunnel.

Tibial Tunnel Drilling. A medial skin incision of 3 to 4 cm is made 1 cm medial to the tibial tubercle. The tunnel entrance is medial or lateral to the tibial tubercle (Fig. 59.27). There may be a theoretical advantage for the tunnel to be started just lateral to the tibial tubercle to produce less posterior tunnel graft angulation. However, either tunnel location is acceptable. The senior author usually prefers an entrance medial to the tibial tubercle. When an ACL reconstruction is also performed with a medial tunnel, the PCL graft is placed through a tunnel lateral to the tibial tubercle.

The arthroscope is placed in the anteromedial portal and positioned high in the notch to view the posterior aspect of the tibial PCL attachment to the capsular attachment. In most cases, a 30-degree arthroscope provides an excellent view. On occasion, a 70-degree arthroscope is required. As already discussed, an alternative approach is to place the arthroscope in a

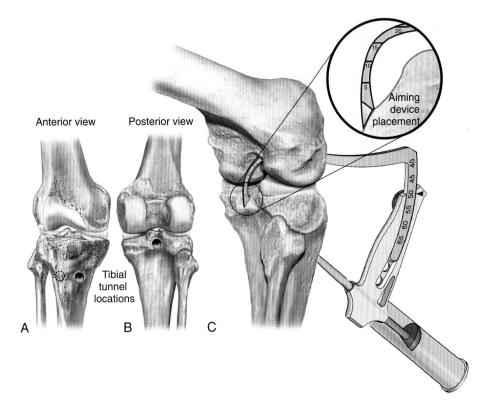

FIG 59.27 Location of Tibial Tunnel (A) Tunnel position may be medial or lateral *(dotted circle)* to the tibial tubercle 3 to 4 cm distal to the joint line. The tunnel position is at a 50-degrees angle or more to decrease the acute angulation at the posterior tibia. (B) Posterior tibial tunnel at distal PCL attachment site. (C) Acufex Director PCL Tibial Aimer is placed through the central portal with the tip of the guide resting on the posterior capsule insertion, with the target 5 mm proximal to the distal aspect of the PCL footprint. This allows sufficient tibial bone proximal to the tunnel to prevent anterior graft migration. (From Noyes FR, Barber-Westin SD: Posterior cruciate ligament: diagnosis, operative techniques, and clinical outcomes. In Noyes FR [ed.]: *Noyes' knee disorders: surgery, rehabilitation, clinical outcomes*, Philadelphia, 2017, Elsevier, pp 447-526.)

posteromedial portal and view the drill guide placed through the anteromedial portal; however, this is seldom required and avoids the potential for posterior fluid extravasation.

The drilling of the tibial tunnel is shown in Fig. 59.28. The drill guide is placed through the central transpatellar tendon portal. The tip of the guide is placed so that the guide pin exits 6 mm proximal to the level of the posterior capsule insertion on the tibia, just before the posterior tibial step-off. This is a critical step because a guide pin placed directly at the distal tibial ridge would allow a large-diameter drill to enter distal to the capsular attachment into the popliteal space. At all times, the drill pin and drill are proximal to the distal capsular attachment of the PCL fossa. Another error is to place the guide pin too proximal in the PCL fossa, which produces a near-vertical PCL graft with limited ability to resist posterior tibial subluxation. The goal is to place the guide pin in the distal central portion of the PCL fossa, 20 to 25 mm from the proximal entrance of the PCL fossa. This leaves 15 mm of the posterior fossa to retain the posterior graft position and prevent a vertical PCL graft. This is a key step of the procedure. The drill guide is angled 50 to 55 degrees to produce an oblique tibial tunnel that will decrease graft angulation effects.

The next step involves use of the drill guide Safety Stop system (Acufex). This is a unique feature of this drill guide system. The guide pin is chucked to a fixed distance with the

safety stop mounted on the drill guide. The safety stop controls the depth of guide pin penetration into the tibia, irrespective of the angle or position of the PCL tibial aimer, and prevents the guide pin from passing beyond the guide tip and damaging neurovascular structures.

The guide pin is drilled into the selected tibial tunnel location. The depth of the guide pin is measured and used during the drilling process to determine the depth of drill penetration. The final position of the guide pin is viewed, and it is again confirmed that the guide pin is distal in the PCL fossa. Fluoroscopic confirmation of the guide pin position is recommended.

The tibial tunnel is drilled to the desired diameter using safety procedures to be described. A commercially available PCL guide pin protector (Acufex) has a wide shape, with a central recess 5 mm from its tip to engage the tibial guide pin before and during the drilling procedure. The tip of the pin is viewed at all times during the drilling process with the arthroscope. The instrument prevents posterior migration of the pin and drill bit. The drilling process involves use of a drill with a drill tip and not a drill twist extending the length of the drill. The drill tip only extends 10 mm with a smooth shank. The drill is advanced in a slow manner. The depth of drill penetration is measured by the calibrated drill and prior drill guide pin measurements. As the drill tip reaches the posterior cortex, there is

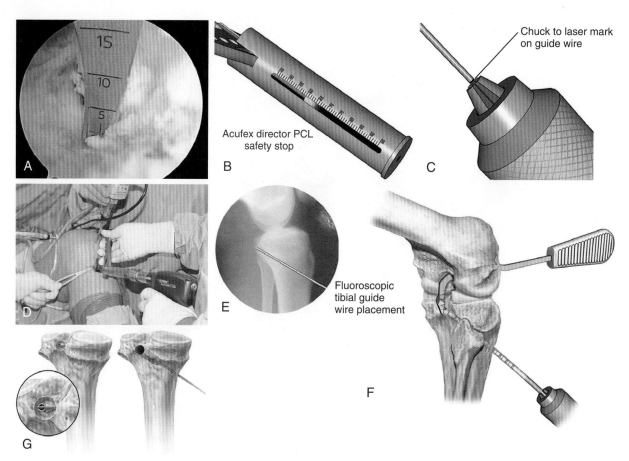

FIG 59.28 Drilling of the Tibial Tunnel (A) Drill guide at distal PCL attachment adjacent to posterior capsule insertion. (B) Acufex guide pin safety stop is attached to the drill guide. (C) The guide wire is chucked on the power drill to the laser mark, which is the maximum length from the safety stop to the drill guide tip. This prevents the guide wire from being advanced beyond the drill guide after passing through the posterior cortex. (D) Placement of guide pin using drill guide system at surgery. (E) Fluoroscopy verifies guide wire placement. (F) Tibial tunnel drilling with PCL Elevator-Wire Catcher to protect posterior neurovascular structures. (G) Alternative technique using a flip-drill to make a posterior tibial socket for the PCL graft bone plug. Four FiberWire sutures (Arthrex, Naples, Florida) placed through the plug are passed to the anterior tibia for graft fixation. *PCL,* Posterior cruciate ligament. (From Noyes FR, Barber-Westin SD: Posterior cruciate ligament: diagnosis, operative techniques, and clinical outcomes. In Noyes FR [ed.]: *Noyes' knee disorders: surgery, rehabilitation, clinical outcomes,* Philadelphia, 2017, Elsevier, pp 447-526.)

a noticeable resistance. At this point, the drill is slowly advanced without sudden penetration. A second option is to remove the power and place a hand chuck over the drill bit to complete the tunnel through the posterior tibial cortex. In younger patients with a thick posterior tibia cortex at the PCL fossa, a two-stage drilling process is used, starting with an 8-mm drill and then progressing to an 11- or 12-mm drill.

When the FlipCutter (Arthrex) technique is selected, a 4-mm drill is initially used to establish the tibial tunnel. The FlipCutter is then advanced under arthroscopic visualization to exit the posterior tibial tunnel. The drill is flipped and held against the posterior tibial cortex, and the tunnel is carefully drilled in a retrograde manner to the desired depth that is determined by the measured length of the FlipCutter. The PCL dilator remains in place posteriorly at all times to displace the posterior capsule away from the drilling procedure sand prevent inadvertent capsule penetration. This technique requires practice and,

importantly, requires an enlarged posterior capsular recess so the drill tip does not engage the capsular tissues when it is first engaged.

To summarize, there are specific safety procedures built into this technique to protect the neurovascular structures. The first procedure involves use of the drill guide system with the Safety Stop and controlled depth of guide pin penetration, with the guide pin placed 5 mm proximal to the distal posterior capsule insertion. The second involves placement of the guide pin protector and slow drill penetration, with direct viewing of the guide pin. The third involves the final drill penetration of the posterior tibial cortex with complete protection posteriorly to prevent inadvertent deep drill penetration.

The proximal edge of the tibial tunnel is carefully chamfered with a rasp to limit graft abrasion effects (Fig. 59.29). Any remaining PCL fibers are removed so that the tibial tunnel entrance does not have soft tissue that would limit graft passage

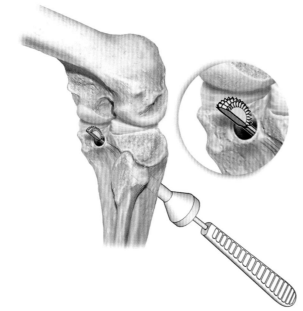

FIG 59.29 Chamfering of the tibial tunnel with a rasp to decrease graft abrasion effects. It is necessary to have 15 mm of bone retained in the posterior tibial fossa above the PCL footprint to prevent the graft from migrating through the tibia. (From Noyes FR, Barber-Westin SD: Posterior cruciate ligament: diagnosis, operative techniques, and clinical outcomes. In Noyes FR [ed.]: *Noyes' knee disorders: surgery, rehabilitation, clinical outcomes*, Philadelphia, 2017, Elsevier, pp 447-526.)

and to ensure the graft will lie flat against PCL tibial fossa. Again, it is necessary to have 15 to 20 mm of the posterior tibial fossa proximal to the tunnel. This maintains the angulation of the PCL graft from the tibial attachment to femoral attachment to prevent a vertical graft and decrease graft tunnel enlargement (windshield-wiper effect). The most common technical mistake is to place the tibial tunnel at the proximal entrance of the PCL fossa, which is proximal to the native PCL tibial attachment.

Posterior Cruciate Ligament Femoral Graft Technique

As described previously, the PCL attachment is elliptical in shape, extending from high in the notch of the distal medial condyle from an approximate 11:30 to 5 o'clock position (right knee). The PCL footprint follows the articular cartilage, with the anterior portion within 2 to 3 mm of its edge, depending on the reference system used.[78] At the 4 o'clock position, the PCL attachment is approximately 4 to 5 mm from the articular cartilage edge.[113] However, if the aMFL is present, the footprint will appear to be 1 to 2 mm from the cartilage edge. There is anatomic variability in the normal proximal-to-distal width of the PCL, and in some knees, a more oval appearance exists because of an increased width of the middle third of the PCL attachment. Because of anatomic variability in the PCL femoral attachment, it is necessary to map out the attachment using remaining PCL fibers to locate the desired graft position within the PCL attachment grid represented by the rule of thirds. The reference system axis used to describe the PCL attachment is distal-to-proximal and anterior-to-posterior, with the knee in full extension. However, the surgeon views the PCL with the knee flexed, and it is also helpful to communicate a graft

position as deep or shallow and high or low in the femoral notch on the medial femoral condyle.

There are two main techniques used for PCL graft femoral placement and fixation. The first technique (our preferred) incorporates two separate femoral tunnels with two separate graft strands. The second technique involves a single femoral tunnel when operative time and complexity of the surgery is a factor, or if the graft size does not allow two separate graft strands to be prepared.

Placement of One or Two Femoral Tunnels and Graft Passage. The technique for femoral placement of two tunnels and graft passage is shown in Fig. 59.30. The PCL footprint is mapped with a calibrated probe and electrocoagulation. The 12, 1, and 4 o'clock position marks on the medial femoral condyle are made. The goal is to create two separate femoral tunnels in the distal two-thirds of the native PCL attachment. This places a graft with an approximate area of 100 mm^2 in cross section, occupying up to 75% or more of the PCL attachment.

If the PCL graft is placed too distal or shallow in the notch, it will be subjected to high tensile forces with knee flexion, resulting in constraining flexion and probable graft failure. If the graft is placed too proximal or deep in the notch, the graft will slacken with knee flexion and allow posterior tibial subluxation. The recommended placement within the PCL footprint is shown in Fig. 59.30, in which the graft replaces the distal two-thirds of the PCL that functions in resisting posterior tibial subluxation with knee flexion.

The PCL guide is used for two separate femoral tunnels to prevent overlap. The anterior tunnel is centered at the 1 o'clock position, 6 to 8 mm deep to the articular cartilage based on the size of the graft and footprint that allows the graft tunnel to come within 1 to 2 mm of the articular cartilage edge. The posterior tunnel is centered at the 4 o'clock position, 8 mm proximal (deep) to the articular cartilage edge. A mark is made at the center position of each tunnel with cautery and then defined with a curette or sharp awl passed from the anterolateral portal. The bone beneath the PCL attachment is dense and requires making a well-defined small entrance hole for the two drill guide pins. Following this technique, the first tunnel is located in the anterior half of the PCL attachment and in the distal two-thirds in the proximal-to-distal direction. The second tunnel is located in the posterior half of the PCL attachment, also in the distal two-thirds. The tunnels are carefully placed in the anterior-to-posterior direction to allow for a 2- to 3-mm bone bridge between tunnels. This placement of the two tunnels ensures that both graft strands will resist posterior tibial translation with knee flexion, sharing the load and not placed too deeply in the notch.

The two femoral tunnels are drilled using the outside-in subvastus technique. The entrance of the 1 o'clock tunnel is 12 mm proximal to the femoral articular cartilage border and medial to the trochlea. The 4 o'clock tunnel entrance is also 12 mm proximal to the articular cartilage border and anterior to the femoral epicondyle. A core reamer is used for the 1 o'clock tunnel to obtain a bone graft for the patellar defect (QT-PB graft, Fig. 59.31). Careful chamfering of the tunnel edges is performed to decrease graft abrasion. A flexible ruler is passed through the tibial and femoral tunnels to measure the intra-articular length of the two graft strands.

The passage of the graft is performed in a stepwise fashion (Fig. 59.32). A 20-gauge wire is passed through the tibial tunnel

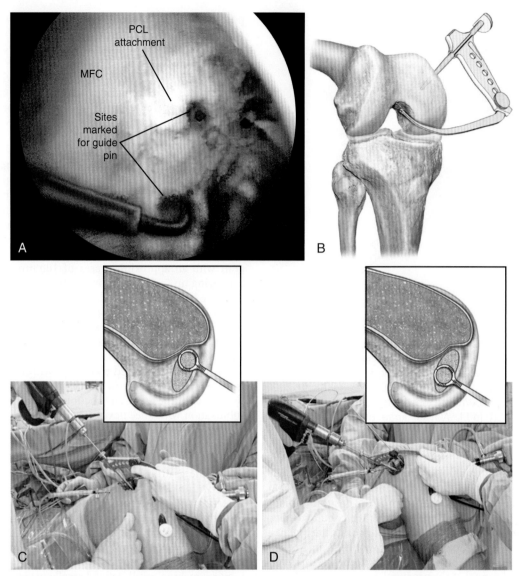

FIG 59.30 Placement of Two Femoral Tunnels (A) Arthroscopic view of two PCL attachment shows 1 and 4 o'clock guide pin marks, 6 and 8 mm from the articular cartilage. (B) PCL guide 15 mm proximal to the outside articular cartilage border. (C) Placement of 1 o'clock tunnel. (D) Placement of 4 o'clock tunnel. *MFC,* Medial femoral condyle; *PCL,* posterior cruciate ligament. (From Noyes FR, Barber-Westin SD: Posterior cruciate ligament: diagnosis, operative techniques, and clinical outcomes. In Noyes FR [ed.]: *Noyes' knee disorders: surgery, rehabilitation, clinical outcomes,* Philadelphia, 2017, Elsevier, pp 447-526.)

and brought out the anterolateral portal, which is enlarged sufficiently to accept the PCL graft. A 22-gauge wire is passed through each of the two femoral tunnels and a grasper or nerve hook is used to bring the two wires out of the same anterolateral portal. The 1 and 4 o'clock wires are marked.

The tibial tunnel bone plug is first passed into the knee joint with the arthroscope placed in the anteromedial portal. A nerve hook facilitates passage adjacent and medial to the ACL and into the tibial tunnel. It is important that all soft tissues have been removed about the tibial tunnel, which is 2 mm larger than the graft to facilitate passage. The nerve hook is used to angle the bone to facilitate the initial entrance into the tibial tunnel. The two femoral graft strands are then passed through the enlarged anterolateral portal spond viewed through the anteromedial portal to have the correct orientation in the 1 and

4 o'clock tunnels. It is preferable to first pass the 4 o'clock and then the 1 o'clock graft.

Fluoroscopy is used to confirm final placement of the bone plug in the tibial tunnel. The graft is marked at the collagenous fiber-bone junction and is viewed arthroscopically to confirm that the bone plug is entirely within the tibial tunnel and placed directly at the posterior tibial tunnel entrance. The sutures are tied over a tibial suture post. An absorbable interference screw (1 mm smaller than the diameter of the tunnel) is used for bone plug fixation at the tibial tunnel, verified by fluoroscopy. The final tensioning of the graft at the femoral side is performed next.

With the selection of one single femoral tunnel, the technique is modified as follows. A FlipCutter is used for the femoral tunnel, the center of which is located at the 2 o'clock position

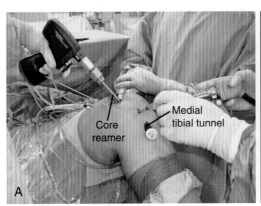
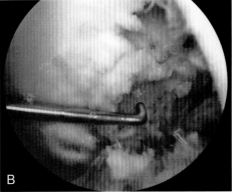

FIG 59.31 (A) Use of core reamer to obtain bone graft for patellar bone defect. (B) Arthroscopic view shows final appearance of two femoral graft tunnels. (From Noyes FR, Barber-Westin SD: Posterior cruciate ligament: diagnosis, operative techniques, and clinical outcomes. In Noyes FR [ed.]: *Noyes' knee disorders: surgery, rehabilitation, clinical outcomes*, Philadelphia, 2017, Elsevier, pp 447-526.)

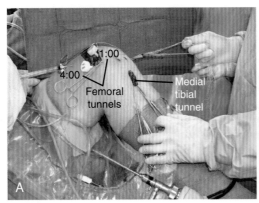
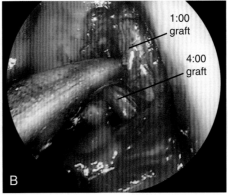

FIG 59.32 (A) Passage of the quadriceps-bone two-strand graft through enlarged anterolateral portal. (B) Final appearance of two-strand graft within femoral tunnels. (From Noyes FR, Barber-Westin SD: Posterior cruciate ligament: diagnosis, operative techniques, and clinical outcomes. In Noyes FR [ed.]: *Noyes' knee disorders: surgery, rehabilitation, clinical outcomes*, Philadelphia, 2017, Elsevier, pp 447-526.)

to span the center two-thirds of the PCL attachment. This is located approximately 8 mm from the articular cartilage edge to produce a graft tunnel that comes to within 1 to 2 mm of the cartilage margin. A TightRope (Arthrex) fixation for the tendon portion of the graft is used, which will be placed in a femoral socket. Three looped FiberWire sutures are passed in a locking stitch at the end of the graft that is tied to the TightRope. The graft passage is the same as already described, with the TightRope sutures passed out the femoral tunnel and the graft tensioned to the correct depth. A bioabsorbable soft tissue interference screw is placed in the femoral socket using the anterolateral portal. This backup fixation is important, particularly in larger size patients given the higher tensile loads that will be placed on the graft.

Graft Tensioning and Fixation. The graft tensioning and fixation steps are the same for all grafts. For grafts with the bone block in the tibial tunnel, initial fixation is performed at the tibia (as described), and final tensioning and fixation are performed at the femoral side (Fig. 59.33). For bone blocks placed at the femoral site, fixation is first performed at the femoral side and final tensioning and fixation performed at the tibial site.

With a single strand femoral graft, the TightRope is tensioned first on the femoral side to seat the graft, the tibial fixation is then performed, and finally the TightRope is tensioned to remove any residual graft laxity.

After the initial fixation of the graft at either the femoral or tibial side, the knee is taken through a full range of motion, with an assistant displacing the tibia forward to correct for the weight of the leg and maintain joint reduction.

The knee flexion position for graft fixation is checked by determining the flexion angle at which the graft strand is the longest (functional zone) to ensure that the graft is not tensioned in its shortest position, which would overconstrain the joint and produce graft failure. A hemostat is placed on each set of graft strand sutures exiting from either the femoral or tibial tunnel(s) and circumferentially wound onto the clamp. The clamp is used to apply a 10-lb (44-N) load to each graft strand. The graft strands are conditioned by taking the knee joint through 0 to 120 degrees of flexion. The knee is placed at 90 degrees flexion and a normal medial tibiofemoral step-off is palpated and confirmed. This is done with the assistant placing approximately 10 lb. (44 N) of pressure against the calf to apply an anterior tibial force (assuming the ACL is intact). The knee

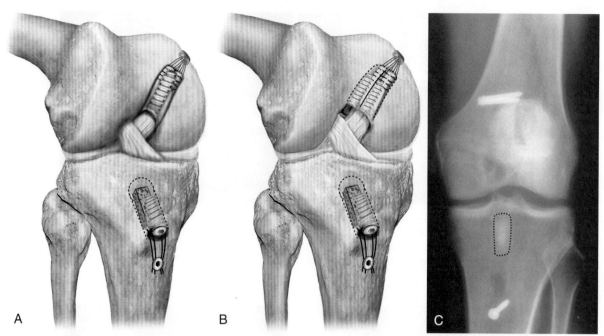

FIG 59.33 PCL graft placement using a single (A) or double-femoral (B) tunnel (see text). (C) Anteroposterior radiographs of a PCL two-strand QT-PB reconstruction using a single tibial tunnel with the bone plug *(dotted)* placed in the posterior tunnel exit with fixation by an absorbable interference screw and suture post. Femoral tendon fixation is with a separate absorbable interference screw in each tunnel and a suture post (staple). (From Noyes FR, Barber-Westin SD: Posterior cruciate ligament: diagnosis, operative techniques, and clinical outcomes. In Noyes FR [ed]: *Noyes' knee disorders: surgery, rehabilitation, clinical outcomes,* Philadelphia, 2017, Elsevier, pp 447-526.)

is again taken through a full range of motion and the change in length of both graft strands noted. With increasing knee flexion, there will be increased tension and a pulling of the sutures and clamp into the tunnel of only 0 to 2 mm as the 90-degree position is reached.

The graft is longest at high knee flexion angles, which is the position selected for graft fixation. In most knees, the 70 degrees flexion angle has the same graft length behavior as 90 degrees, and this position is selected. There are commercially available graft-tensioning devices[23] (as used in ACL reconstructions) that provide measurable length-tension data and may be used for measurement of graft-tensioning loads. The sutures for each graft strand are tied over a femoral or tibial post, maintaining the 44 N of graft load and 44 N of anterior tibial load. These are empiric loading profiles.

The final position of the medial tibiofemoral joint is again verified. An absorbable interference screw is added to the fixation. The arthroscope is again placed and, with a nerve hook, the tension in the PCL graft strand(s) is confirmed. The knee is taken through 0 to 110 degrees flexion.

Although techniques have been described in the literature for the second posterior tunnel to be placed in a deeper, more proximal position, the senior author recommends placing the tunnels in the middle and distal two-thirds of the PCL attachment, as described. This allows both graft strands to share the loading, and therefore tensioning is performed at the 70-degree knee flexion position for both grafts.

It should be noted that if one or both femoral tunnels are too proximal (deep in the notch), the graft strand length decreases with knee flexion, allowing posterior subluxation. In this situation, the final graft fixation was performed at an extended knee position. The proximal graft strand position will function in a reciprocal manner, and the desired load-sharing between graft strands will not be achieved.

Alternatively, if the graft tibiofemoral attachment length is longest at 45 to 60 degrees of knee flexion as the graft is pulled into the tunnel with knee flexion, then the femoral tunnels are too distal (shallow). This is not an acceptable position, and the femoral tunnel is reconfigured, removing 5 mm of the proximal aspect of the tunnel to allow the graft to assume a deeper position. The interference femoral screws are placed distal in the femoral tunnels to secure the grafts in a more proximal (deep) position. With the technique described in the placement of the femoral tunnels, it would be unusual for this graft tunnel adjustment to be performed.

In knees that undergo ACL reconstruction, it is important to determine as accurately as possible the neutral AP position of the medial and lateral tibiofemoral joints (without added internal or external tibial rotation). There is a tendency to displace the tibia into an abnormal anterior position by overtensioning the PCL graft. When the ACL is intact, the graft forces displace the tibial anteriorly, loading the ACL under low loads. When the ACL is insufficient to prevent anterior tibial subluxation, the following steps are performed:

1. Place the knee at full extension with a 10-lb (44-N) force on each graft (or 20 lb for a single graft) and sufficient anterior loading on the calf to overcome gravity weight effects of the leg. This achieves a reduced tibiofemoral joint position when one or both of the medial or FCLs are present.

2. Flex the knee to 90 degrees, maintaining the same approximate graft load and anteriorly directed load on the calf. An anteriorly subluxated tibia at 90 degrees (compared with 0

degrees) will have abnormally increased tibiofemoral attachment site distances, and the graft can be observed to piston into the tibial tunnel. In essence, the graft should be almost similar in its tibial position at both 0 and 90 degrees of flexion.

3. Palpate for a normal tibiofemoral step-off and arthroscopically visualize a normal anterior relationship of the anterior portion of the medial and lateral meniscus in relationship to the respective femoral condyles. If there is any question, a lateral fluoroscopic or radiograph may be obtained intraoperatively. This is especially helpful in large limbs where the neutral AP position is difficult to determine with accuracy.

Placement of a Femoral Single Tunnel: Outside-In Technique. The drill guide is introduced into the anteromedial portal, and the desired femoral tunnel position is located. The arthroscope is placed in the anterolateral portal. The goal is to place the tunnel into the middle two-thirds of the PCL attachment, avoiding too proximal a placement. The entrance of the guide pin is at the 2 o'clock position and approximately 8 mm from the articular cartilage edge. This should produce a tunnel that is 2 mm from the articular cartilage edge. A note of caution is that there is a tendency to place the drill tunnel too proximal (deep in femoral notch) and out of the PCL femoral footprint, producing a graft that only functions at low flexion angles. The ability to determine the native PCL footprint in the patient's knee carefully is important for correct tunnel placement. The preference is for a femoral tunnel of 11 to 12 mm in most knees. If the drill diameter is larger, portions of the graft will be too deep in the notch and outside of the normal PCL footprint.

The entrance position of the guide pin in the outside-in technique is midway between the femoral epicondyle and trochlea, at least 12 mm proximal to the articular cartilage edge. A more proximally placed guide pin would increase the tunnel angulation entering the joint and potentially increase graft abrasion effects.

A small skin incision and VMO muscle-splitting incision is made. A larger incision is not required because the bone block fixation is done with a cancellous screw without an added fixation device. The guide pin is over-reamed or, alternatively, a coring reamer may be used to harvest a bone graft. The tunnel entrance into the knee joint is chamfered to limit graft abrasion effects.

A modification of this technique is used with a FlipCutter placed from outside-in instead of the guide pin and the femoral socket drilled from inside-out. This is an easier technique than placing the femoral tunnel through the anterolateral portal. When a femoral socket is placed with the FlipCutter, the technique involves over-drilling the socket depth so that graft positioning and tensioning are possible.

At the time of graft passage, either an inside-out passage (preferred; enlarged anterolateral portal used for graft passage into the knee) or an outside-in passage (retrograde guide wire from tibial tunnel out through femoral tunnel) is used. The process of graft positioning in the tunnels, graft conditioning, and fixation at the tibial tunnel is the same as described earlier. Femoral graft fixation is easily performed with the TightRope adjustment of tension, and an interference screw is also placed through the anterolateral portal (usually 8 mm diameter, 2 to 3 mm less than the tunnel diameter). With the VMO muscle-splitting approach, the final tension is the same, except it is performed on the femoral side with an interference screw and added suture post. The surgeon uses a headlight and adequate exposure

to advance an interference screw into the anterior aspect of the femoral tunnel for graft fixation. Arthroscopic examination confirms that the screw is not advanced into the knee joint.

There are publications that describe the all-inside drilling of a large single tunnel at the femoral attachment. However, the outside-in approach or inside-out FlipCutter is preferred for the femoral tunnel. From a technical standpoint, the drilling of a large-diameter tunnel through the anterolateral portal is difficult because of the proximity of the lateral condylar articular cartilage and the ACL, and the tendency exists to have a tunnel entrance that is markedly angled distally. In the senior authors' experience, a more precise and less angulated tunnel is obtained with the outside-in or FlipCutter approach.

ALTERNATIVE POSTERIOR CRUCIATE LIGAMENT ALL-INSIDE TECHNIQUES

Femoral Placement of Rectangular (Oval) Tunnel for Bone Plug

An all-inside technique using the QT-PB autograft or allograft or AT-B allograft is described in which the bone plug is placed at the femoral site and the soft tissue graft is placed through a tibial tunnel. This procedure has the advantage of easy passage of the soft tissue graft through the posterior tibial tunnel. This is used in select knees, in which operative time is a factor. In addition, in revision knees, there may be displaced femoral tunnels where the bone plug provides a more stable fixation at the femoral site. As noted, the senior author prefers to reverse the graft with the bone plug at the posterior tibial tunnel.

The patient positioning and initial surgical approach are similar to the all-inside technique described. The posterior PCL stump is removed and PCL tibial attachment is prepared for one tibial tunnel.

The technique for the femoral PCL graft attachment of the bone portion of the graft involves using a rectangular femoral slot or a femoral tunnel. The all-inside technique for the rectangular slot has a theoretical advantage of placing a greater portion of the graft within the PCL femoral footprint, in which approximately 75% of the footprint is occupied by the graft.

The goal is to create a 9- × 13-mm rectangular slot that extends from 1 to 4 o'clock in the distal two-thirds of the PCL footprint. The 12 and 4 o'clock marks are made on the medial femoral condyle. Again, the guide pin mark is 7 to 8 mm from the articular cartilage of the medial femoral condyle for the anterior and posterior tunnels (Fig. 59.34), verified by observing the PCL footprint and the two tunnels in the distal two-thirds of the footprint. A small curette or awl is used to penetrate and define the pilot hole for each tunnel. A 2.4-mm guide pin is placed through the anterolateral portal into the anterior tunnel location, the knee is flexed to 90 degrees, and the guide pin is advanced through the medial femoral condyle, approximately 25 mm deep, based on the patellar bone length.

The second guide pin is placed into the second marked position. The guide pins are over-reamed with an endoscopic drill (Fig. 59.35) to form an oblong tunnel entrance to a depth that corresponds to the graft bone. Care is taken to avoid the lateral femoral condyle articular cartilage as the drill is introduced into the knee joint. The remaining central bone bridge is removed with a curette or burr.

The PCL Dilator (Fig. 59.36) produces an oval 9- × 13-mm shape that is approximately 1 mm larger than the bone portion of the graft. Care is taken to use low forces in dilating the

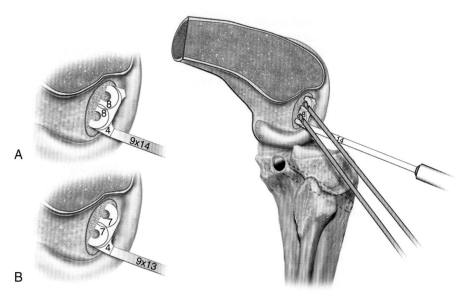

FIG 59.34 (A and B) All-inside femoral tunnel. The PCL femoral template is placed through the anteromedial portal with the arthroscope in the central portal. This defines the position of two overlapping 7- or 8-mm tunnels. The top edge of the template is placed 2 mm from the articular margin, and the bottom edge is 4 mm from the articular margin. This places the center of the anterior tunnel 6 mm from the articular cartilage margin and the center of the posterior tunnel 8 mm from the articular cartilage margin. (From Noyes FR, Barber-Westin SD: Posterior cruciate ligament: diagnosis, operative techniques, and clinical outcomes. In Noyes FR [ed.]: *Noyes' knee disorders: surgery, rehabilitation, clinical outcomes*, Philadelphia, 2017, Elsevier, pp 447-526.)

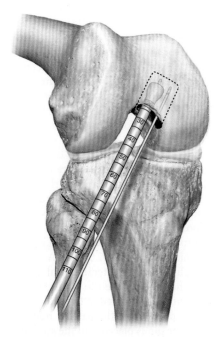

FIG 59.35 The guide pins are placed and then overreamed with an endoscopic drill to a depth of 25 mm, avoiding passage of the drill through the femoral cortex. The central bone bridge is removed with a curette and burr. (From Noyes FR, Barber-Westin SD: Posterior cruciate ligament: diagnosis, operative techniques, and clinical outcomes. In Noyes FR [ed.]: *Noyes' knee disorders: surgery, rehabilitation, clinical outcomes*, Philadelphia, 2017, Elsevier, pp 447-526.)

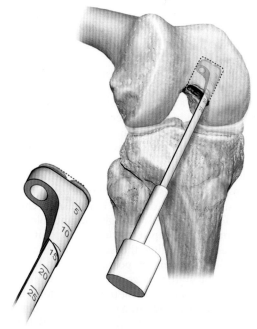

FIG 59.36 The PCL Dilator is used to gently conform the femoral oval footprint to 9 × 13 mm and to an appropriate depth. There is a matching oval opening in the PCL Dilator handle of 9 × 13 mm to size the bone block. (From Noyes FR, Barber-Westin SD: Posterior cruciate ligament: diagnosis, operative techniques, and clinical outcomes. In Noyes FR [ed.]: *Noyes' knee disorders: surgery, rehabilitation, clinical outcomes*, Philadelphia, 2017, Elsevier, pp 447-526.)

TABLE 59.9	Posterior Cruciate Ligament All-Inside Procedures			
Surgical Procedure	**Advantages**	**Disadvantages**	**Options**	
QT-PB two-strand autograft[a]	Autograft, replaces femoral footprint, secure fixation, tensioning two strands, authors' preference athletic patients	Autograft harvest: added time, postoperative pain	Single-strand graft, femoral socket with FlipCutter and TightRope fixation, tibial tunnel entrance lateral to tibial tubercle	
QT-PB, AT-B allograft	All-inside femoral socket, FlipCutter, interference screw, single tibial tunnel, tensioning two strands	Delayed healing allograft	Single strand graft tensioned at tibia, rectangular bone plug, tibial tunnel entrance lateral to tibial tubercle	
QT-PB, AT-B allograft	All-inside femoral socket, TightRope replaces suture post, single tibial and femoral tunnel, bone fixation tibial tunnel	Delayed healing allograft	Tibial socket all-inside fixation using FlipCutter	
QT-PB two-strand autograft tibial inlay	Replaces femoral footprint, secure fixation, tensioning two strands	Open posteromedial approach, time and complexity	Single femoral tunnel, QT-PB, AT-B allografts, replaced by all-inside arthroscopic procedures	

AT-B, Achilles tendon-bone; *B-PT-B*, bone-patellar tendon-bone; *PCL*, posterior cruciate ligament; *QT-PB*, quadriceps tendon-patellar bone; *STG*, semitendinosus-gracilis tendons.
[a]Authors' preference.
From Noyes FR, Barber-Westin SD: Posterior cruciate ligament: diagnosis, operative techniques, and clinical outcomes. In Noyes FR, Barber-Westin SD (eds): *Noyes' knee disorders: surgery, rehabilitation, clinical outcomes*, ed 2, Philadelphia, 2017, Elsevier, pp 447-526.

rectangular slot to avoid fracture of the femoral condyle. In the senior authors' experience, this has not been reported; however, it is worth a cautionary note. The PCL Dilator has a graft sizing slot on the handle for a 9- × 13-mm bone block that is used in preparation of the graft. The distal aspect of the femoral oval opening is chamfered and rasped to create a gentle slope to limit graft abrasion.

The passage of the graft (Fig. 59.37), conditioning, and final fixation are the same as already described. The femoral bone is fixed first with an interference screw, and the tibia portion of the graft is fixed next with a soft tissue interference screw and suture post (see Fig. 59.33). The option exists to use two graft strands that are tensioned separately in the tibial tunnel; however, there is no data to determine if this is required.

Posterior Cruciate Ligament Arthroscopic-Assisted Open Tibial Inlay Technique

The authors have described in detail all of the operative steps required for the open tibial inlay and arthroscopic-assisted femoral tunnel PCL reconstruction.[97] The approach that is recommended is the all-inside technique described previously, in which the bone block is positioned at the posterior tibial tunnel entrance, simulating the tibial inlay approach. The goal is to avoid the added time and potential morbidity of the open posteromedial approach. However, with added experience it should be noted that the open posteromedial approach and tibial inlay procedure remains a suitable technique to use in select cases. The various PCL reconstruction options are summarized in Table 59.9.

POSTERIOR CRUCIATE LIGAMENT AVULSION FRACTURES

Avulsion fractures of the PCL are rare, and treatment options depend on the type and size of the fracture, displacement, comminution, and orientation of the fragment.[33,136] These injuries usually occur at the tibial attachment and may involve a small area at the posterior region of the attachment or a large area that extends anteriorly and outside the PCL attachment. Griffith et al.[33] reported that the entire insertion area was avulsed in all 19 skeletally mature patients in their series of PCL avulsion fractures. The avulsion fracture is usually obvious on routine

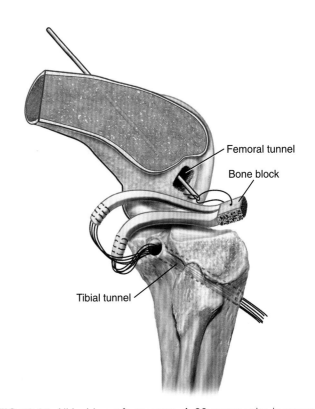

FIG 59.37 All-inside graft passage. A 20-gauge wire is passed through the tibial tunnel and grasped anteriorly through the anterolateral arthrotomy. The tibial portion of the graft is passed through the single tibial tunnel. The pin is then passed through the anterolateral portal into the femoral tunnel. The bone block is passed through the enlarged anterolateral portal and carefully oriented into the correct position with the cancellous bone surface oriented deep in the oval opening. (From Noyes FR, Barber-Westin SD: Posterior cruciate ligament: diagnosis, operative techniques, and clinical outcomes. In Noyes FR [ed.]: *Noyes' knee disorders: surgery, rehabilitation, clinical outcomes*, Philadelphia, 2017, Elsevier, pp 447-526.)

radiographs. Occasionally, a computerized tomography scan or MRI is required to define the extent of the facture pattern in major avulsion fractures extending into the joint.[10,33] Avulsion or peel-off PCL injuries at the femoral site have been reported in the literature but are rare.[30,108]

Patients who have small, partial PCL avulsion fractures, with a negative posterior translation test at 90 degrees knee flexion, are kept in a brace locked in full extension and remain partial weight bearing for 4 weeks to allow healing. The brace is removed for gentle range of motion (avoiding posterior tibial translation) and quadriceps exercises. Overall, the prognosis for healing and PCL function is good to excellent in these cases.[148]

Complete avulsion of the PCL attachment at the tibia and, less frequently, at the femoral attachment (peel-off avulsion) with posterior tibial subluxation is an indication for surgical repair. Authors have reported favorable clinical results with the open reduction and internal fixation of PCL avulsion fractures at the tibial insertion site.[4,45] For example, Inoue et al.[45] reported on 31 patients followed for 2 to 8 years and reported low side-to-side differences (<5 mm, KT-2000) after surgery. Most knees showed a mild residual posterior knee displacement (mean, 3.0 mm). Along with the tibial avulsion, an abnormal MRI signal intensity may be observed within the PCL fibers, indicating partial tearing.

Several authors have described arthroscopic techniques for PCL tibial avulsion fractures.[‡] Gui et al.[37] treated 28 patients using two posteromedial portals and a single tibial tunnel to facilitate suture passage and seating of the bony fragment. The knees were casted for 2 weeks unless a concomitant tibial plateau fracture was present, which necessitated 4 weeks of immobilization. The fractures healed a mean of 2.8 months postoperatively. At 1 year postoperative, 4 of 20 cases followed had arthrofibrosis, two of whom underwent arthroscopic release. The posterior drawer test was negative in all but one knee. International Knee Documentations Committee (IKDC) rating system[40] results were normal in 20 patients and nearly normal in four patients.

Zhao et al.[148] treated 29 patients with PCL tibial avulsion fractures. The PCL and bony fragment were arthroscopically fixed with sutures that were pulled out through Y-shaped bone tunnels and fixed on a titanium button. Immediate knee motion and partial weight bearing were allowed in a brace that was used for the first 4 weeks. Four patients required a manipulation 3 months after surgery for flexion limitations. At follow-up (>2 year postoperatively), all patients except one had a negative posterior drawer test, and all regained full knee motion, except for two patients who had 5 degrees flexion limitations. IKDC results were normal in 28 patients and nearly normal in one patient.

Zhang et al.[146] treated isolated PCL tibial avulsion fractures in 16 patients (with a mean age of 43 years) with a minimally invasive posteromedial approach and suture anchors. The patients all had displaced fractures that exceeded 1 cm and fracture fragments less than 2 cm in diameter. Plaster splints were used for 4 to 6 weeks. At a mean of 18 months postoperatively, all cases showed satisfactory reduction and bony healing, and all but one patient had returned to their former occupation.

Chen et al.[15] treated 36 patients with displaced PCL tibial avulsion fractures (>3 mm of upward displacement of the bony fragment) and posterior knee instability of grade II or higher. Arthroscopic reduction and suture fixation of the bone fragments was accomplished through two tibial tunnels. The knees were immobilized in a brace the first postoperative week, followed by 0 to 60 degrees of motion during weeks 2 to 4 and 120 degrees by week 8. All fractures demonstrated union within 3 months. At a mean of 3 years postoperatively, all but three patients were participating in strenuous or moderate activities, 92% rated their knee function as normal or nearly normal, and three patients (8%) were rated as abnormal as a result of limitations in knee flexion.

The concept of immediate postoperative knee motion is addressed in detail elsewhere.[99] The therapist initiates early and protected knee motion within the first postoperative week, applying an anteriorly directed load to protect the relatively weak suture fixation. The use of a posterior calf pad and careful positioning in the brace is required for the first 4 postoperative weeks until suitable healing has occurred. Knees with suture or pin fixation have relatively low tensile strength repairs and require expert postoperative rehabilitation.

The surgeon should select either an arthroscopic or open technique for tibial avulsion fractures based on experience. In general, it is relatively straightforward to use an arthroscopic approach for cannulated screw fixation for large and medium avulsion fractures. For PCL tibial avulsions with small bony fragments that require a combination of sutures and bone fixation, an open posterior tibial approach is favored by the senior author because it provides good exposure and allows for secure fixation.

A peel-off type of PCL rupture from the femoral attachment has been described as a hyperextension knee injury. This type of PCL rupture directly at the femoral attachment may occur at the fibrocartilaginous junction, with minor associated damage to the bulk of the PCL fibers. The PCL attachment is easily repaired, with sutures passed through small drill holes, avoiding the proximal physeal growth plate. Arthroscopic approaches to PCL femoral soft-tissues avulsions have been described by several authors,[30,108] although clinical data remain scarce. Ross et al.[112] described an arthroscopic approach for repair of acute femoral peel-off tears. Three no. 2 nonabsorbable sutures were passed through the PCL substance, through a femoral tunnel at the PCL footprint, and tied over the medial cortex. Park and Kim[108] reported an arthroscopic technique that used two transfemoral tunnels for the anterior strand and two posterior tunnels for suture repair of the posterior strand. These authors noted that femoral avulsion injuries were exceedingly rare.

The senior authors' preferred technique for femoral peel-off or proximal PCL repairs is to use an arthroscopic-assisted approach in which two to three guide pin tunnels (small-diameter for sutures) are placed at the anterior and posterior aspects of the PCL footprint, distal to the physis, to fan out the PCL fiber attachment. A VMO-sparing approach is used, and respective suture passers are brought into the knee joint. Through a limited medial arthrotomy and under direct visualization using a headlight, multiple nonabsorbable baseball looped sutures are placed at appropriate sites in the PCL fibers to approximate the broad elliptical femoral PCL attachment. The mini-arthrotomy has limited morbidity and allows the surgeon to carefully place multiple sutures into the broad PCL

---

‡References 10, 15, 37, 43, 132 and 148.

fibers. Secure fixation is achieved along with anatomic placement of disrupted PCL fibers.

In PCL injuries that extend away from the femoral attachment and involve the proximal third of the PCL fibers, an augmentation is favored (assuming the growth plate is closed). The postoperative protocol for a direct suture repair should take into account the low repair tensile strength, requiring maximum protection. The knee is maintained in full extension, and the therapist assists in gentle range of knee motion for the first 4 weeks postoperatively. Only toe-touch weight bearing is permitted during this time period. Then the patient may progress to 50% weight bearing with the brace locked at full extension. At 6 weeks postoperative, weight bearing is progressed in the brace. Knee motion is advanced to 0 to 90 degrees. The brace is removed at 8 weeks.

POSTERIOR CRUCIATE LIGAMENT AUGMENTATION APPROACHES AND TECHNIQUES

In select knees, an acute tear of the PCL may occur at the proximal third femoral attachment (and not through the midsubstance). A considerable bulk of the PCL attachment still exists and may be repaired to the femoral attachment, as discussed for the "peel-off" type of tear. In these cases, it is worthwhile to add a graft augmentation to the attachment site, which may be performed in an arthroscopic-assisted manner (assuming the growth plate is closed). An 8-mm femoral tunnel is placed at the desired site where the PCL fibers require a graft augmentation, usually in the more proximal aspect of the femoral attachment.

Sutures are used to repair the more distal fibers to the femoral attachment as already described. The placement of an 8-mm tibial tunnel must be well chosen and not interfere with the PCL attachment site. The tunnel is placed just medial to the tibial PCL attachment, carefully avoiding the medial and lateral meniscal attachments. A lateral tibial tunnel is not used because PCL fibers attach, in part, to the PL meniscus tibial attachment. The authors prefer a three- or four-strand semitendinosus-gracilis (STG) autogenous graft, although an allograft may also be considered.[3,19,51,64,133] Suture fixation to a femoral or tibial post, or absorbable interference tibial and femoral screws in adults, is required.

In skeletally immature knees, Kocher et al.[60] reported the use of a small-diameter graft placed through the distal femoral and proximal epiphysis, avoiding the physeal plate. An augmentation graft has the advantage of maintaining tibiofemoral reduction and preventing posterior tibial subluxation in the early postoperative healing period.

In very select knees with a prior PCL rupture and abnormal posterior tibial subluxation, the remaining PCL fibers may appear healed and intact, although with a residual elongation. Rarely, the senior author has performed a distal advancement of the tibial PCL attachment; this is only considered when the MRI shows a normal signal to the PCL fibers and arthroscopic examination shows also a normal-appearing PCL. The operative approach is similar to a tibial inlay procedure, except the native PCL tibial bone attachment is distally advanced the required amount to restore posterior stability. A proximal advancement (recession) at the femoral insertion is avoided owing to the marked influence of the PCL femoral attachment on PCL fiber function previously described.

POSTOPERATIVE REHABILITATION

The authors' rehabilitation program is summarized in Table 59.10.[99] The protocol consists of a careful incorporation of exercise concepts supported by scientific data and clinical experience. The protocol was developed for a two-strand PCL graft reconstruction (QT-PB, AT-B). The goal is to progress a patient on a rate that takes into account athletic and occupational goals, condition of the articular surfaces and menisci, return of muscle function and lower limb control, and postoperative graft healing. Modifications to the program may be required if articular cartilage deterioration is found during surgery.

The supervised rehabilitation program is supplemented with home exercises that are performed daily. Therapeutic procedures and modalities, and routine examinations, are used as required for successful rehabilitation. Patients are warned to avoid any exercises or activities that place high posterior shear forces on the tibia, such as walking down inclines or squatting for the first 6 postoperative months. In addition, patients are cautioned that an early return to strenuous activities postoperatively carries a risk of a repeat injury or the potential of compounding the original injury.

Passive knee motion from 0 to 90 degrees is begun the first day postoperatively, along with patellar mobilization. Although patients are encouraged to regain full extension as soon as possible, knee flexion is limited to avoid high posterior shear forces. The total number of daily knee motion cycles is limited to 60 (20 cycles, 3 times a day) for the first 4 weeks to lessen abrasion effects on the graft. Knee flexion should reach 120 degrees by 8 weeks and 135 degrees by 10 to 12 weeks.

A long-leg hinged postoperative brace with a posterior calf pad is worn for the first 6 weeks postoperatively, 24 hours a day. A functional PCL brace is indicated when patients return to higher level occupational or sports activities. In patients who undergo a combined PCL-PL procedure, a bivalved cast is used for 4 weeks postoperatively to limit lateral joint opening during ambulation and daily activities. The cast is removed 4 times a day, and active range of knee motion exercises are performed in a seated position. The cast is then carefully reapplied to protect the knee joint during walking activities. After the first 4 postoperative weeks, sufficient healing of the PL ligamentous reconstructive procedure should occur and the patient is placed in a long-leg hinged brace.

Patients are allowed to bear 25% of their body weight during the first 1 to 2 postoperative weeks. Weight bearing is then slowly progressed and crutches are usually discontinued at postoperative week 6. The entire program is described in detail elsewhere.[99]

CLINICAL STUDIES

All of our clinical studies involved a prospective, consecutive patient enrollment, using the validated Cincinnati Knee Rating System for the analysis of function and symptoms. The minimum follow-up of each study described below was 2 years, and the results were evaluated by a senior clinical research associate and not the surgeon.

Posterior Cruciate Ligament Two-Strand Procedures
Quadriceps Tendon-Patellar Bone Autograft, Tibial Inlay.
Nineteen knees with chronic PCL ruptures treated with a

TABLE 59.10　Rehabilitation Protocol After Posterior Cruciate Ligament Reconstruction

	POSTOPERATIVE WEEKS					POSTOPERATIVE MONTHS			
	1-2	3-4	5-6	7-8	9-12	4	5	6	7-12
Hinged long-leg postoperative brace	X	X	X						
Patellar knee sleeve				X	X	X	X		
Functional brace								X	X
Range of Motion Minimum Goals (Degrees)									
0-90	X								
0-110		X							
0-120			X	X					
0-135					X				
Weight Bearing									
25% body weight	X								
50% body weight		X							
Full			X						
Patella mobilization	X	X	X	X					
Modalities									
EMS	X	X	X	X	X				
Pain/edema management (cryotherapy)	X	X	X	X	X	X	X	X	X
Stretching									
Hamstring, gastrocnemius-soleus, iliotibial band, quadriceps	X	X	X	X	X	X	X	X	X
Strengthening									
Quadriceps isometrics, straight leg raises, active knee extension	X	X	X	X	X				
Closed-chain: gait retraining, toe-raises, wall-sits, mini-squats		X	X		X	X	X	X	
Knee flexion hamstring curls						X	X	X	X
Knee extension quads		X	X	X	X	X	X	X	X
Hip abduction–adduction, multi-hip					X	X	X	X	X
Leg press (70-10 degrees)				X	X	X	X	X	X
Balance/Proprioceptive Training									
Weight-shifting, cup-walking, BBS				X	X				
BBS, BAPS, perturbation training, balance board, minitrampoline				X	X	X	X	X	X
Conditioning									
UBC	X	X	X	X	X				
Bike (stationary)		X	X		X	X	X	X	X
Aquatic program						X	X	X	X
Swimming (kicking)						X	X	X	X
Walking					X	X	X	X	X
Stair climbing machine						X	X	X	X
Ski machine						X	X	X	X
Elliptical cross-trainer						X	X	X	X
Running: straight								X	X
Cutting: lateral carioca, figure-eights									X
Plyometric training									X
Full sports									X

BAPS, Biomechanical Ankle Platform System (Camp, Jackson, Michigan); *BBS,* Biodex Balance System (Biodex Medical Systems, Inc, Shirley, New York); *EMS,* electrical muscle stimulation; *UBC,* upper body cycle (Biodex Medical Systems, Inc, Shirley, New York).
From Noyes FR, Barber-Westin SD, Heckmann TP: Rehabilitation of posterior cruciate ligament and posterolateral reconstructive procedures. In Noyes FR, Barber-Westin SD (eds): *Noyes' knee disorders: surgery, rehabilitation, clinical outcomes,* ed 2, Philadelphia, 2017, Elsevier, pp 578-607.

two-strand PCL QT-PB autograft reconstruction (tibial inlay approach) were followed a mean of 2.9 years (range, 2 to 7 years) postoperatively.[88] The PCL reconstructions were performed at a mean of 3.6 years (range, 4 months to 18 years) after the original knee injury. In nine knees, prior PCL procedures had been done elsewhere and failed. Associated procedures included PL procedures in five knees, ACL reconstruction in two knees, MCL STG reconstruction in two knees, and meniscus transplantation[101] in one knee.

The mean increase in posterior tibial translation (compared with the contralateral knee) on stress radiography improved from 11.6 ± 2.9 mm preoperatively to 5.0 ± 2.6 mm at follow-up ($p < .0001$). Preoperatively, all knees were graded C or D (IKDC rating) according to stress radiographic data. At follow-up, 2 knees (10%) were graded A; 12 knees (63%) as B; 3 knees (16%) as C; and 2 knees (10%) as D. All of the associated knee ligament procedures were rated A or B at follow-up. There were no infections, permanent limitations of knee motion, donor site problems, or patellar fractures.

All patients except one rated their knee condition as improved. Before surgery, 11 patients (58%) had pain with daily activities, but only one (5%) had such pain at follow-up. Significant improvements were noted for symptoms and limitations with daily and sports activities. Eleven patients (58%) were participating in low-impact sports at follow-up without problems, and two were participating in more strenuous sports without problems.

The results affirmed the recommendation for early operative treatment for PCL ruptures because by the time surgical reconstruction is necessary for problems with daily activities, the reconstruction may not be effective because of arthritic joint damage. The posterior stability obtained in this study was superior to that previously reported in the our single-strand PCL allograft investigation.[83] Stress radiography revealed that 68% of the knees had no more than 5 mm increase in posterior tibial displacement, compared with 37% of the knees in the allograft population. Still, in acute injury situations, or in dislocated knees that require multiligament reconstructive procedures, allografts may be more suitable.

Quadriceps Tendon-Patellar Bone Autograft, Tibial Tunnel.
Twenty-nine knees that received a two-strand PCL QT-PB autograft reconstruction (all-inside tibial tunnel) were followed a mean of 3.6 years (range, 2 to 7 years) postoperatively.[91] Eighteen patients had the PCL reconstruction for chronic ruptures and 11 for acute injuries. Fifteen knees had an associated ligament reconstruction, including ACL reconstruction in nine knees, MCL repair or reconstruction in six knees, PL procedures in five knees, and meniscus transplantation in one.

The mean increase in posterior tibial translation measured with stress radiography improved from 10.5 ± 2.9 mm preoperatively to 6.5 ± 4.3 mm at follow-up ($p = .06$). Preoperatively, all knees were rated C or D (IKDC) according the stress radiographic data. At follow-up, 3 knees (10%) were rated A; 7 knees (24%) as B; 17 knees (59%) as C; and 2 knees (7%) as D. Eight of the associated ACL reconstructions were rated A or B and one was rated C. All of the MCL and PL procedures were rated as A or B. There were no infections or patellar fractures. Two patients reported residual pain at the patellar donor site.

Ninety-four percent of the patients rated their knee condition as improved. Before surgery, 87% of the patients with chronic PCL ruptures had pain with daily activities compared with 11% at follow-up. Significant improvements were noted for pain, swelling, giving-way, walking, stairs, running, jumping, and twisting/turning ($p < .01$). For all 29 patients, 15 (52%) returned to low-impact sports and 7 (24%) were participating in strenuous sports without problems.

Revision Quadriceps Tendon-Patellar Bone Autograft Reconstruction.
PCL revision reconstructions with a two-strand QT-PB autograft were performed in 15 knees that were followed a mean of 3.7 years (range, 2 to 7 years) postoperatively.[90] A mean of 3.8 years (range, 4 months to 15.6 years) had elapsed between the failed PCL procedures and the revision. Before the PCL revision reconstruction, a staged HTO was required in three knees, and autogenous bone grafting of prior graft tunnels was done in one knee.

The tibial inlay technique was used in nine knees, and the tibial tunnel technique was done in six knees. Six knees had one or more concomitant ligament reconstructive procedures with the PCL revision. Four knees had an ACL allograft reconstruction,[87] one had an MCL autograft reconstruction,[85] and four had a PL reconstruction.

Stress radiograph posterior tibial translation values improved from 11.7 ± 3.0 mm preoperatively to 5.1 ± 2.4 mm at follow-up ($p < .001$). Before the revision, all knees were rated as C or D according to stress radiographic data. At follow-up, one knee was rated A; nine knees as B; four knees as C; and one knee as D. Associated knee ligament reconstructive procedures restored anterior, medial, and PL stability.

Significant improvements occurred in pain, function, and patient perception scores, and 87% believed the overall knee condition was better postoperatively. However, the subjective and functional results were inferior to those reported after primary acute PCL reconstruction. Only 53% returned to light sports without problems.

The QT-PB two-strand revision provided reasonable results in this group of complex knees; however, this is a small series and definitive conclusions cannot be reached. In this study, 13 of 15 knees (87%) had compounding problems of articular cartilage damage, prior meniscectomy, need for associated ligament procedures, or varus malalignment with medial tibiofemoral compartment damage. The results were inferior to those obtainable from primary PCL reconstructions because most patients were in a salvage knee situation.

Causes of Failure of Posterior Cruciate Ligament Reconstructions
A study was conducted to analyze the potential factors that contributed to the failure of PCL operations.[89] Between June 1989 and July 2003, 41 knees in 40 patients were referred to our center for treatment after 52 failed PCL operative procedures. The patients were evaluated a mean of 3.4 years (range, 1 month to 23.7 years) after the failed PCL procedures. There were 24 males and 16 females whose mean age at the initial PCL procedure was 30 years (range, 11 to 51 years). The initial PCL procedures were done for an acute knee injury in 15 knees and for chronic deficiency in 26 knees.

A total of 155 operative procedures had been done in the 41 knees. PCL graft reconstructions had been done in 31 cases, primary repairs in 14, synthetic replacements in 4, and thermoplasties in 3. A single PCL procedure had been done in 32 knees, two procedures in 7 knees, three procedures in 1 knee, and four procedures in 1 knee. Only four knees (10%) had an isolated PCL reconstruction with no associated or further surgery performed.

Reconstruction of other knee ligaments had been done in 27 knees (66%). These involved 21 FCL or PL complex procedures in 14 knees, 19 ACL reconstructions in 16 knees, and 9 MCL procedures in 9 knees.

Medical records, operative notes, radiographs, and MRI scans were reviewed, and a comprehensive knee examination was performed. A single factor that caused the operations to fail was identified in 23 (44%) of the 52 operations, and multiple factors were identified in 29 (56%). The most common probable causes of failure were associated PL deficiency (40%), improper graft tunnel placement (33%), associated varus malalignment (31%), and primary suture repair (25%).

Sixteen of 21 (76%) prior PL procedures had failed, as had 9 of 19 (47%) prior ACL reconstructions. Twenty-nine knees (71%) presented with pain with activities of daily living. Thirty-four knees (83%) had compounding problems of joint arthritis, prior meniscectomy, associated ligament deficiencies, or varus malalignment.

In the patients' rating of their own knee condition, 20 (49%) rated the knee as poor; 12 (29%), as fair; and 9 (22%) as good. Thirty-one (75%) patients had given up sports activities completely and 10 were participating with significant limitations and symptoms. Significant functional limitations were found with walking in 19 (46%) patients and during squatting in 37 (90%) patients.

In 22 knees (54%), a PCL revision reconstruction was performed. In 19 knees (46%), revision was not performed. Eleven of these 19 knees had developed advanced knee joint arthritis with significant loss of joint space on radiographs (with only a few millimeters remaining in tibiofemoral compartments) that contraindicated PCL revision. Eight patients declined further operative treatment.

Failure to restore associated ligament instabilities and incorrect tunnel placement were major factors contributing to surgical failure of PCL operative procedures. The results suggest the need for greater emphasis on the initial reconstruction in graft tunnel placement, correction of associated ligament instabilities, and correction of varus osseous malalignment. Failure of concurrent PL complex reconstructions was frequently encountered, suggesting the need for higher-strength augmentation procedures or anatomic graft replacement. The results of this study were verified in 2012 by Lee et al.,[66] who found, in a cohort of 28 failed PCL-reconstructed knees, that the most common causes of failure were PL deficiency and improper graft tunnel placement. Kim et al.[53] reported that patients with generalized joint laxity (Beighton and Horan criteria) had an increased risk of failure of single-strand PCL reconstruction compared with those without such laxity (9 of 24 patients [37.5%] and 6 of 29 patients [20.7%], respectively).

Results of Posterior Cruciate Ligament Reconstructions From Other Investigators

Inconsistent results have been reported after single-strand isolated PCL reconstructions in restoration of normal posterior tibial displacement and knee function.[§] Generally, improved knee symptoms and activity levels have been reported in most studies, although normal stability was not always restored.[67,130] It is not possible at present to scientifically analyze the effects of various graft materials or surgical techniques on the outcome of isolated single-strand PCL reconstructions. Kim et al.[59] conducted a systematic review of isolated PCL single-strand transtibial reconstruction studies, of which 10 met the inclusion criteria. Autografts were used in 78% of the knees, and allografts were selected in 22%. Stress radiographs were done in only one investigation. The IKDC objective knee evaluation form, completed in six studies, reported 75% of the knees were rated as normal or nearly normal at follow-up. The authors concluded that the procedure improved posterior drawer testing by an average of 1 grade but did not reliably restore normal knee stability.

Few authors have described results of isolated two-strand PCL reconstructions.[14,26,79] Min et al.[79] performed a transtibial two-strand reconstruction with a tibialis anterior allograft in 21 patients who were followed a mean of 4.1 years postoperatively. The graft was passed through two femoral tunnels into one tibial tunnel, which the authors referred to as a single-sling method. At follow-up, a mean KT-2000 90 degrees flexion value of 3.4 ± 0.8 mm (range, 1.6 to 6.3 mm) was reported. Three knees had grade II posterior instability. Overall IKDC grades were normal in 38%, nearly normal in 38%, abnormal in 19%, and severely abnormal in 5%. Chen and Gao[14] performed a two-strand PCL reconstruction in 19 patients in whom a quadruple semitendinosus graft was used to replace the ALB of the PCL and a quadruple gracilis tendon graft was used to reconstruct the PMB. A suture suspension technique was used for fixation. Mean posterior stress radiographs improved from 10.6 ± 2.0 preoperatively to 2.0 ± 1.2 mm postoperatively ($p < .001$). The IKDC subjective score increased from 65.6 ± 5.1 preoperatively to 92.1 ± 3.7 ($p < .001$). One knee had a grade II posterior drawer test.

Comparisons have been made between single- and two-strand PCL procedures, with little to no difference in stability and knee function reported in recent studies.[22,54,56,67,122] The few studies available at the time of writing typically had low evidence levels and were not randomized.[**] One prospective randomized study was conducted by Li et al.,[67] in which fifty patients were randomized to receive either a single-strand or two-strand tibialis anterior allograft. At a mean of 2.4 years postoperatively, the two-strand group had a significantly lower mean amount of posterior translation on KT-1000 testing compared with the single-strand group (2.2 ± 1.3 mm and 4.1 ± 1.3 mm, respectively; $p < .05$). The difference in the mean posterior translation of 1.9 mm has questionable clinical application. The authors did not provide ranges of this test, or the amount of knees with a grade II or III posterior drawer. There was a significantly greater percentage of patients in the two-strand group with overall IKDC knee examination scores of normal/nearly normal compared with the one-strand group (92% and 82%, respectively; $p < .05$). In addition, the mean IKDC subjective knee score was higher in the two-strand group compared with the single-strand group (72 ± 7 and 65 ± 8, respectively; $p < .05$).

Preserving the PCL remnant, in combination with usually a single-strand PCL graft, has been performed by several investigations in an effort to achieve superior results compared with graft reconstructions.[††] A systematic review was recently conducted by Del Buono et al.[19] to determine if significant differences existed between PCL augmentation and PCL reconstruction studies regarding functional and stability results. The review included 24 studies that involved 623 PCL reconstructions and 158 PCL augmentation (remnant preservation) procedures. Overall, equivalent outcomes were found between the two operative techniques for IKDC scores, Lysholm scores, KT-1000 measurements, and stress radiographic measurements. For example, IKDC overall evaluation scores of normal or nearly normal were reported in a mean of 89.8% of patients that underwent PCL augmentation and in 80.1% of those that had PCL reconstruction. Posterior stress radiograph

---

[§]References 1, 7, 12, 41, 47, 61, 67, 69, 71, 80, 117, 131, 138, 139, 144, and 145.

[**]References 22, 44, 54, 56, 122, and 134.
[††]References 3, 21, 50, 51, 55, 63, 64, 141, 142, and 149.

side-to-side differences improved by a mean of 8.6 ± 1.6 mm after PCL augmentation (from 11.1 ± 1.4 mm preoperatively to 2.5 ± 0.4 mm postoperatively) and by a mean of 8.0 ± 5.8 mm after PCL reconstruction (from 11.5 ± 2.2 mm preoperatively to 3.5 ± 1.3 mm postoperatively). The concern was expressed that no long-term data were available and subsequent rates of arthritis remain unknown.

POSTEROLATERAL SURGICAL TECHNIQUE OPTIONS

Fibular Collateral Ligament Anatomic Reconstruction

Perhaps the most common injuries associated with PCL ruptures are PL ligament ruptures. Many investigators have reported clinical outcome data from a variety of PLC reconstructive procedures.[‡‡] We have described in detail the surgical options for correcting lateral and PL ligamentous deficiency, and the reader is referred to these publications which are summarized in this chapter.[92,94,98] Furthermore, the operative approach and surgical techniques for repair of acute PL ligament injuries are detailed elsewhere.[98]

The surgical options are based on the quality and integrity of these tissues determined at the time of surgery and the anatomic structures that are disrupted. Indications for reconstruction of the PLS include abnormal lateral joint opening, increased external tibial rotation, and a varus recurvatum position with hyperextension of the knee.

In cases of acute ligamentous disruptions, primary repair of the FCL is only indicated for bony avulsions that are amendable to internal fixation. Otherwise, graft reconstruction is recommended. We prefer to perform acute PL reconstruction procedures within the first 7 to 14 days of injury. Because PL ruptures are usually accompanied by injuries to one or both cruciates and may represent a knee dislocation, we observe these patients for 5 to 7 days to evaluate the neurovascular structures and skin condition. This short delay also allows appropriate planning of the surgical procedure and, most importantly, the institution of rehabilitation to initiate supervised range of motion and muscle exercises prior to surgery. The specific surgical steps and techniques for acute PL ligament repair and reconstruction are beyond the scope of this chapter and have been published by the authors.[98]

Our preferred technique for FCL reconstruction in either acute or chronic ruptures is an anatomic FCL reconstruction with a B-PT-B allograft or autograft. A second choice is an AT-B allograft with the bone portion fixated into the fibula and tendon fixated at the femoral FCL insertion.

A 10- to 12-cm skin incision is made in a straight line centered over the joint line and 1 cm posterior to the iliotibial band (ITB) attachment at the tibia (Fig. 59.38). The skin flaps are mobilized beneath the subcutaneous tissue and fascia to protect the vascular and neural supply. The peroneal nerve is identified and protected throughout the procedure and usually is not dissected from its anatomic position.

The ITB is incised at the posterior edge and anterior to the biceps tendon. The ITB attachments are excised to the short head of the biceps femoris muscle, and the ITB is gently lifted anteriorly to expose the entire lateral aspect of the lateral

femoral condyle and attachments of the popliteus, FCL, and lateral gastrocnemius muscle tendon attachment.

The interval anterior to the lateral gastrocnemius tendon at the joint line and directly at the top of the fibula is entered, avoiding the inferior geniculate artery. The approach is similar to that described for meniscus repairs.[96] This allows exposure of the PMTL junction, PL capsule, and PFL. A second anterior ITB incision may be required when there is extensive scarring involving all of the PLS. The VLO is lifted gently in an anterior direction, and an S retractor is placed beneath the muscle fibers. A vertical incision approximately 2 cm in length is made into the capsule, just anterior to the popliteus tendon attachment. The joint is entered and the lateral meniscus attachments are inspected and later repaired if torn about the popliteal hiatus.

The normal anatomic attachment sites of the FCL to the lateral femur and anterolateral aspect of the fibular head are identified and a suture is placed between the two attachment sites; the length is measured to determine the required graft size. The bone portion of each end of the graft is 22 to 25 mm in length. The patellar tendon graft must normally be 55 to 60 mm or longer to be suitable for an anatomic FCL reconstruction. Only in select patients is a B-PT-B autograft used, such as a revision situation where autogenous tissue is deemed more ideal. An allograft of the desired size is required, and we ensure that sufficient allograft tissue is available during surgery.

The fibular tunnel is drilled first, using a guide pin to a depth of 25 mm. The drills are gradually increased in diameter to create a final 9-mm tunnel. The femoral tunnel is next placed 5 mm eccentric to the normal FCL attachment to allow the collagenous portion of the graft to occupy the normal FCL anatomic location. Prior to drilling the femoral socket, a suture is attached to the fibular graft position and is also positioned at the desired femoral location to check graft isometry. If an ACL reconstruction is performed, it is necessary to diverge the FCL tunnel in an anterior direction away from the ACL tunnel to maintain integrity of the two tunnels. The edges of the femoral tunnel are smoothed with a rasp to avoid graft abrasion.

Another option is a femoral inlay of the proximal bone portion of the graft, which is only required if there is a 5- to 8-mm discrepancy of graft length that will not allow full coverage of the bone in a femoral tunnel.

The bone portion of the graft is gently tapped into the fibular tunnel so that the bone is entirely seated into the tunnel and level with the proximal fibular head to preserve graft length. The ideal graft fixation is with one or two small-fragment cortical screws placed at the anterolateral bare area to engage the center bone portion of the graft and both fibular cortices (Fig. 59.39). The proximal bone of the graft is advanced into the femoral tunnel. The graft is conditioned by cycling the knee 20 to 30 times. The graft is fixed with a soft tissue interference screw at 30 degrees knee flexion, in neutral tibial rotation, under an approximate 5 lb tensile load (22 N) on the sutures that have been advanced by the Beath needle to the medial aspect of the knee joint. The graft is purposely not overtensioned to avoid overconstraining the lateral tibiofemoral joint.

Popliteus Muscle-Tendon-Ligament Procedures

In acute cases in which partial PMTL function exists and the joint external tibial rotation (PL subluxation) is deemed only moderate (10 degrees increased tibial rotation at 30 degrees of knee flexion), a surgical repair of disrupted tissues is performed. The FCL graft reconstruction protects the PMTL repair and

---

[‡‡]References 6, 11, 27, 48, 49, 57, 58, 62, 64, 65, 111, 126, 140, 143, and 147.

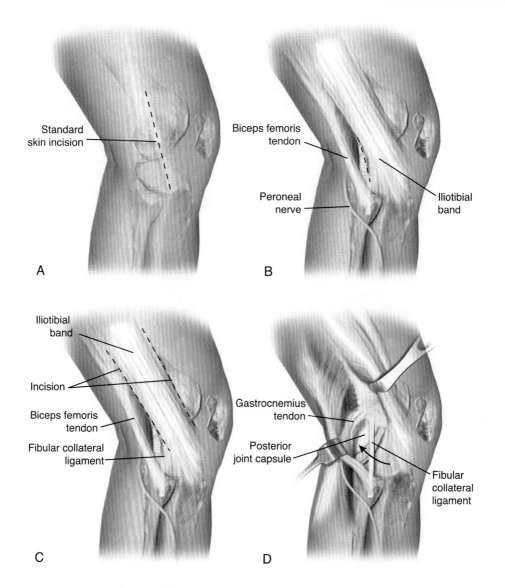

FIG 59.38 Posterolateral Surgical Technique (A) Site for the skin incision. (B) Incision site in the interval between the posterior edge of the iliotibial band (ITB) and the anterior edge of the biceps tendon. (C) In chronic cases with severe scarring, it may be necessary to add an anterior incision and displace the ITB posteriorly during the reconstructive procedure to allow better exposure. (D) With the ITB retracted anteriorly, the interval between the lateral head of the gastrocnemius and the posterolateral aspect of the capsule is opened bluntly, just proximal to the fibular head, without entering the joint capsule proximally. (From Noyes FR, Barber-Westin SD: Posterolateral ligament injuries: diagnosis, operative techniques, and clinical outcomes. In Noyes FR [ed.]: *Noyes' knee disorders: surgery, rehabilitation, clinical outcomes*, Philadelphia, 2017, Elsevier, pp 527-577.)

provides the necessary resistance, in which the popliteus is avulsed at its femoral site, so that a direct repair may be performed. In most cases, the tear is at the distal muscle-tendon junction or fiber attachment.

In chronic cases in which no PMTL function is found, a graft replacement is required (Fig. 59.40). The senior author prefers to use an AT-B allograft. The bone portion of the graft is placed at the anatomic femoral insertion site and the collagenous portion of the graft is passed in the tibial tunnel. An incision is made just beneath Gerdy's tubercle, extending from the bare

area of the anterior fibula to the tibial tubercle, and then 3 cm distally along the anterolateral tibia. A retractor is placed anterior to the lateral gastrocnemius muscle directly behind the posterior tibia to expose the popliteus muscle. The final tibial 8-mm tunnel is at the most lateral aspect of the tibial margin and 15 mm distal to the joint line, passing through the popliteus muscle attachment and just medial to the tibiofibular joint. The total length of the graft is measured from the femoral to tibial tunnels, plus the length for the tibial fixation distal to the anterior tibial tunnel.

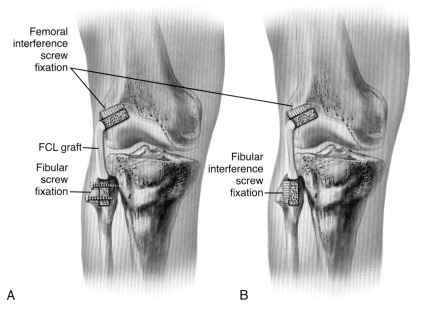

FIG 59.39 Anatomic Substitution of the FCL With a B-PT-B Autograft or Allograft Shows Two Methods for Fibular Graft Fixation (A) (Authors' choice) Two small fragment screws are used to fix the bone into a slot created in the proximal fibula. Interference screw fixation is used at the femoral anatomic site of the FCL. (B) A fibular tunnel is made, the graft seated, and an interference screw is used for fixation. *FCL*, Fibular collateral ligament. (From Noyes FR, Barber-Westin SD: Posterolateral ligament injuries: diagnosis, operative techniques, and clinical outcomes. In Noyes FR [ed.]: *Noyes' knee disorders: surgery, rehabilitation, clinical outcomes*, Philadelphia, 2017, Elsevier, pp 527-577.)

The graft is passed through the femoral tunnel, out the PL capsule and through the tibial tunnel, and fixed at the femoral site by an interference screw. The graft is conditioned by repetitive knee flexion and extension, and fixation is performed with an absorbable interference screw in the tibial tunnel with the leg at 30 degrees of knee flexion, neutral tibial rotation, and approximately 5 pounds (22 N) of tension placed on the graft. A backup suture fixation screw post is used on the anterolateral aspect of the tibia. A final graft assessment is done to determine that it is under adequate tension and resists abnormal external tibial rotation and knee hyperextension. A direct suture of the PMT graft to the FCL graft at the level of the fibular head is done (Fig. 59.40F and G). A plication procedure is performed on the PL capsule at 10 degrees of flexion, avoiding overtension that would limit normal extension (Fig. 59.40H and I).

Femoral-Fibular Reconstruction

Another operative option that we have described for PL instability is a nonanatomic femoral-fibular graft reconstruction.[84] This procedure is recommended for acute knee repairs to provide the stable FCL graft cornerstone about which other soft tissues are repaired. The procedure is advantageous when operative time needs to be considered in dislocated knees and a relatively easy stabilizing procedure can be performed.

The femoral-fibular reconstruction provides a large graft reconstruction of the FCL and a posterior graft arm to augment the PLS (Fig. 59.41). The PL capsule reconstruction is performed by a plication procedure. The popliteus tendon is plicated to the fibular FCL reconstruction to restore the PFL. The procedure is considered a nonanatomic reconstruction because the femoral-fibular graft is placed adjacent but not directly at the FCL femoral and fibular anatomic attachment sites. A modification of this procedure is to place both graft arms into a single femoral socket with interference fixation. These procedures are not recommended for chronic PL ligament ruptures because it is necessary to perform an anatomic reconstruction of both the FCL and popliteus muscle tendon ligament complex, described next.

Another option for FCL reconstruction in acute injuries (already described) is to use an AT-B allograft with the bone portion placed within the fibula in a similar manner described for the B-PT-B graft and fixated with one or two small fragment screws. The tendon is placed into a femoral socket at the FCL femoral insertion and fixed with an interference screw.

Proximal Advancement of the Posterolateral Structures

A third operative approach may be considered in knees in which chronic insufficiency of the PLS results from a minor injury (without a traumatic disruption). In knees with varus osseous malalignment and a varus thrust on ambulation, there is frequently an insufficiency of the PL structures because of chronic interstitial tearing. In these situations, a definitive FCL of normal width and integrity (although lax) may be identified at surgery, and the PMTL attachments are intact although elongated. A graft reconstruction of the FCL and PMTL is not indicated in these knees. Instead, the PL structures are proximally advanced in a more simplified operative procedure that avoids the added complexity and morbidity from major graft reconstructive procedures (Fig. 59.42).[86] The PL structures must be carefully inspected at surgery because this procedure

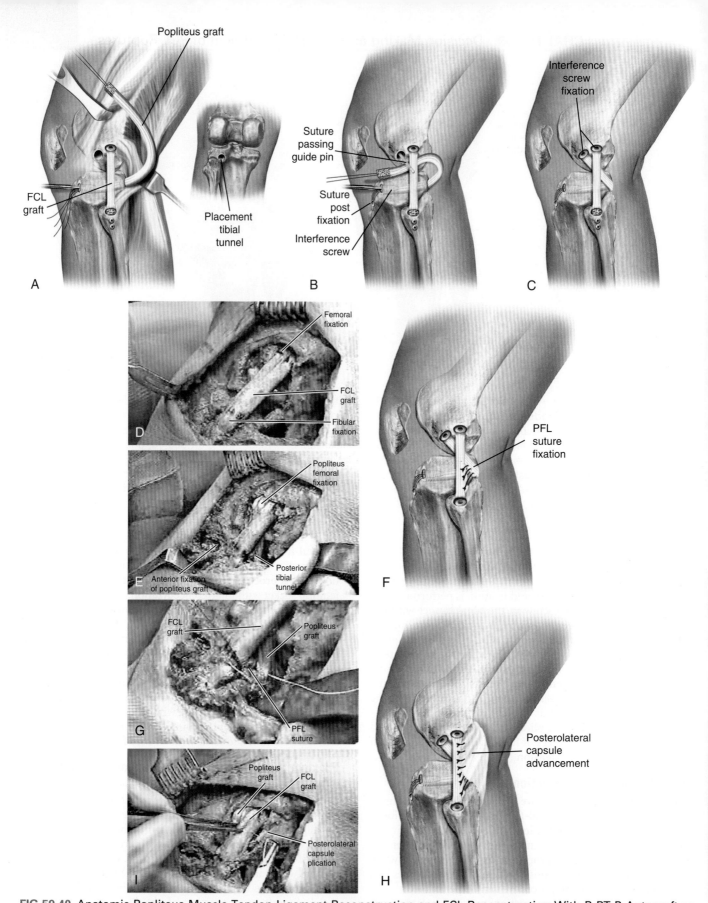

FIG 59.40 Anatomic Popliteus Muscle-Tendon-Ligament Reconstruction and FCL Reconstruction With B-PT-B Autograft or Allograft (A) Location of PL tibial tunnel and graft passage. A soft tissue interference screw and suture post are used for tibial fixation of the popliteus graft. (B) Passage of popliteus graft beneath the FCL B-PT-B graft. (C-E) Final fixation of the popliteus and FCL graft reconstructions. (F and G) Suture of popliteus graft to posterior margin of the FCL graft at the fibular attachment site to restore the PFL. (H and I) Suture plication of the PL capsule to posterior margin of the FCL graft. *FCL,* Fibular collateral ligament; *PFL,* popliteofibular ligament. (From Noyes FR, Barber-Westin SD: Posterolateral ligament injuries: diagnosis, operative techniques, and clinical outcomes. In Noyes FR [ed.]: *Noyes' knee disorders: surgery, rehabilitation, clinical outcomes*, Philadelphia, 2017, Elsevier, pp 527-577.)

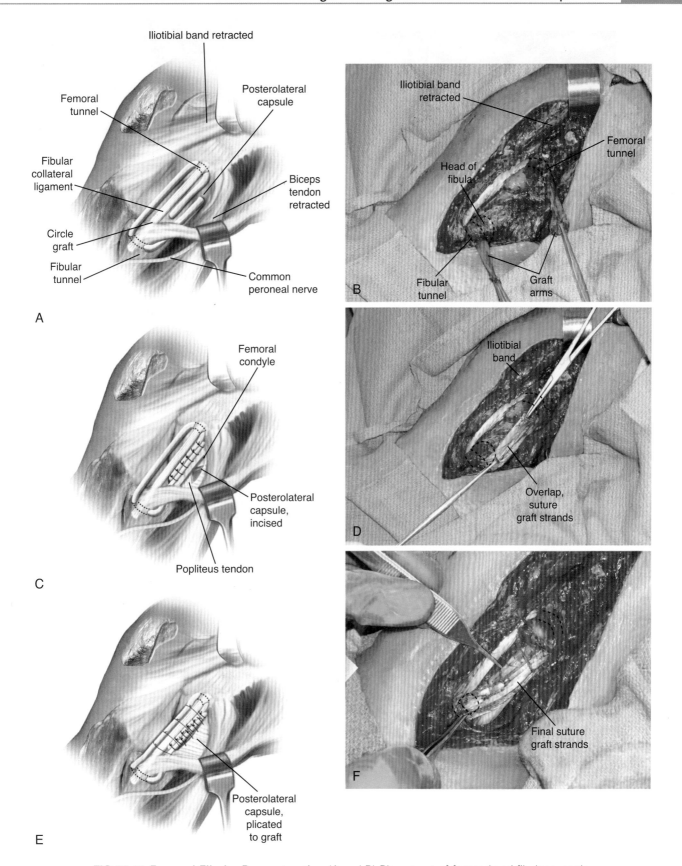

FIG 59.41 Femoral-Fibular Reconstruction (A and B) Placement of femoral and fibular tunnels and FCL graft. (C and D) Suturing and tensioning of graft arms. (E and F) Multiple sutures used through both arms of graft and the slack FCL. Plication of the posterolateral capsule is performed to the graft. (From Noyes FR, Barber-Westin SD: Posterolateral ligament injuries: diagnosis, operative techniques, and clinical outcomes. In Noyes FR [ed.]: *Noyes' knee disorders: surgery, rehabilitation, clinical outcomes*, Philadelphia, 2017, Elsevier, pp 527-577.)

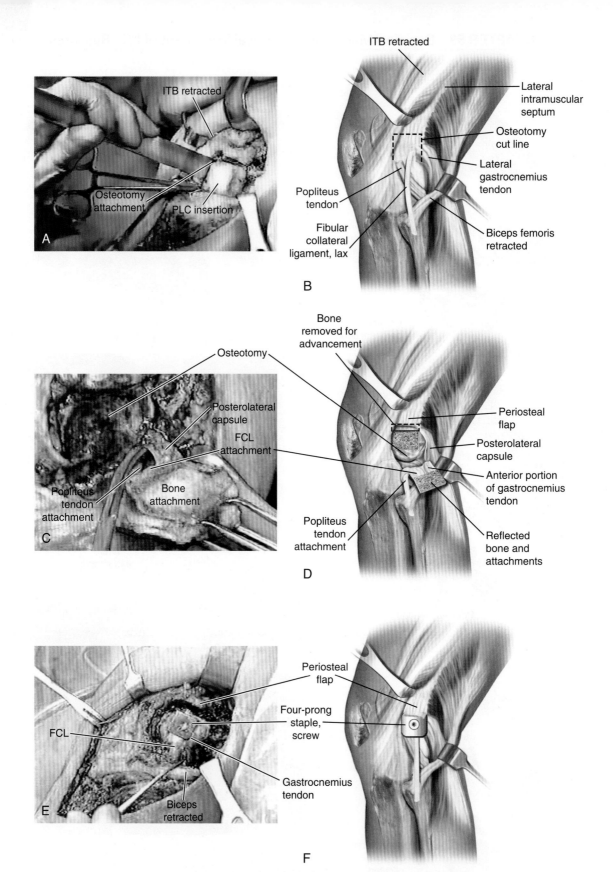

FIG 59.42 Proximal Advancement of Intact but Lax Posterolateral Structures (Top left and right) Posterolateral structures are identified and have a normal appearance, although lax. The line for the osteotomy of the femoral attachment of the FCL, PMT, and anterior portion of the gastrocnemius tendon is shown. (Middle left and right) The osteotomy is 8 mm deep to provide sufficient bone to maintain the attachments of the FCL, popliteus tendon, anterior gastrocnemius tendon, and posterolateral capsule. The posterolateral capsule is incised 15 mm in length. (Bottom left and right) The bone attachment of the posterolateral structures is advanced proximally in line with the FCL, with the knee in neutral tibial rotation and 30 degrees flexion. Reattachment of the bone is achieved with a four-pronged staple and screw. *FCL,* Fibular collateral ligament; *ITB,* iliotibial band. (From Noyes FR, Barber-Westin SD: Posterolateral ligament injuries: diagnosis, operative techniques, and clinical outcomes. In Noyes FR [ed.]: *Noyes' knee disorders: surgery, rehabilitation, clinical outcomes,* Philadelphia, 2017, Elsevier, pp 527-577.)

will fail if there is scar tissue replacement, lack of a normal appearance of the structures (although lax), or if the distal attachments of the PL structures are disrupted. Importantly, the FCL must be at least 5 to 7 mm in width, and the PL structures must be at least 3 to 4 mm thick to be functional when the residual slackness is removed by the advancement procedure. The goal is to advance the FCL in a proximal direction to remove excessive slackness and to use staple fixation at the normal anatomic site.

Posterolateral Capsule Reconstruction for Severe Varus Recurvatum

In patients who demonstrate 15 degrees or more of knee varus recurvatum and hyperextension, severe deficiency exists of the entire posterior capsule and oblique popliteal ligament in addition to possible cruciate, FCL, and PMTL damage (Fig. 59.43). In these severe knee injuries, a PMTL reconstruction and posterior capsule plication will not resist the severe varus recurvatum deformity. A PLC reconstruction is required in addition to a reconstruction of the PMTL and FCL (Fig. 59.44). The operative approach and placement of the tibial tunnel for the capsular reconstruction using an AT-B allograft (8 to 9 mm in diameter) is the same as described for the PMTL reconstruction. The tibial tunnel is enlarged as required for graft passage. The bone portion of the graft is located adjacent to the lateral gastrocnemius tendon origin using either a femoral tunnel or a bone inlay technique. The inlay technique is required when a concurrent ACL reconstruction is performed to avoid a second femoral tunnel. The fixation at the femoral attachment requires a portion of the lateral gastrocnemius tendon insertion (which is

very broad) to be partially incised to expose the site for the AT-B graft fixation. The fixation of the bone inlay is accomplished with two small-fragment cancellous screws and washers (Fig. 59.45). This provides a stable bone-to-bone attachment. If a femoral tunnel is used, a 7-mm interference screw is selected. The graft lies along the PLC, which is plicated, and the graft is passed through the tibial tunnel.

The tendon portion of the graft is fixated at the tibia after graft conditioning similar to that previously described for the PMTL reconstruction. The knee is placed at 10 degrees of flexion with 5 pounds (22 N) graft tension. The knee joint will passively go to 0 degrees. Ultimately, the graft will stretch a few millimeters; the goal is to allow 0 to −2 degrees of hyperextension, which effectively blocks knee hyperextension and varus recurvatum. Frequently, the ACL is ruptured and the two ligaments grafts (ACL and PLC) work in concert to block varus recurvatum. The same is true when a concomitant PCL reconstruction is performed.

POSTEROLATERAL POSTOPERATIVE REHABILITATION

The authors' rehabilitation program is summarized in Table 59.11.[99] The rehabilitation protocol incorporates immediate protected knee motion but stresses maximal protection against undue joint loads to prevent stretching and failure of PL grafts or advancement procedures. Patients are warned to avoid hyperextension and activities that would incur varus loading on the joint. Delays in return of full knee flexion, full weight bearing, initiation of certain strengthening and conditioning

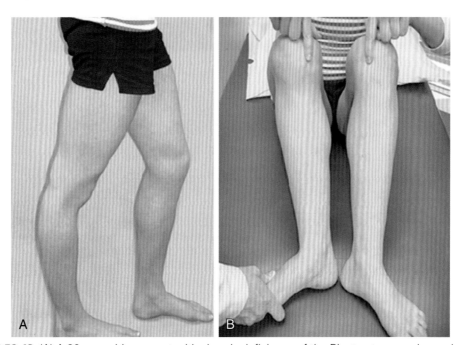

FIG 59.43 (A) A 20-year-old gymnast with chronic deficiency of the PL structures and complaints of recurrent hyperextension injuries with athletic activities. The ACL and PCL were intact, although a prior partial disruption could not be excluded. (B) Dial test at 30 and 90 degrees demonstrates increased tibial rotation of the right knee. (From Noyes FR, Barber-Westin SD: Posterolateral ligament injuries: diagnosis, operative techniques, and clinical outcomes. In Noyes FR [ed.]: *Noyes' knee disorders: surgery, rehabilitation, clinical outcomes*, Philadelphia, 2017, Elsevier, pp 527-577.)

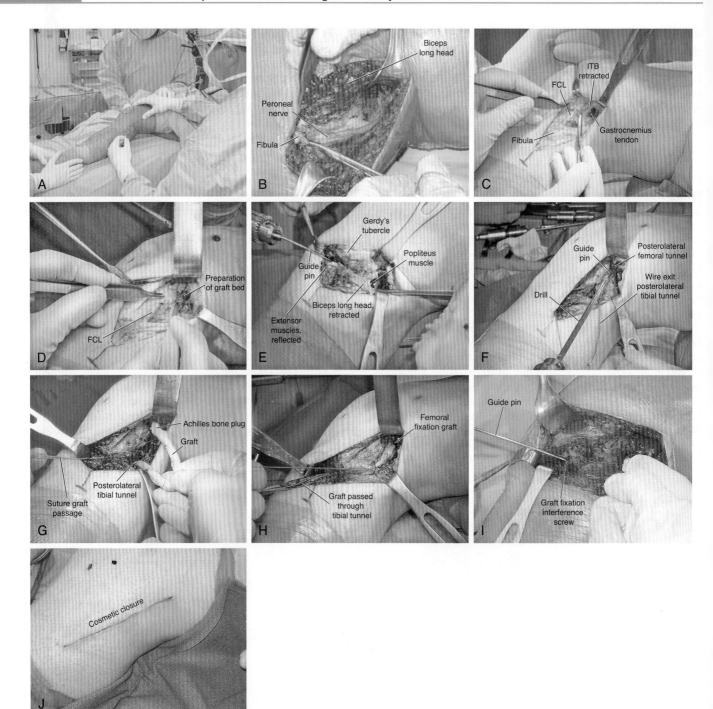

FIG 59.44 PL Capsular Reconstruction for Severe Knee Varus Recurvatum and Hyperextension Using an AT-B Allograft (A) Patient positioning. (B) Identification of the peroneal nerve at fibular neck. (C) Identification of FCL and popliteus muscle-tendon-ligament (PMTL), functionally intact. (D) Exposure of femoral graft site at lateral gastrocnemius tendon attachment. (E) Placement of the tibial drill hole lateral and distal to the joint line. (F) Placement of the femoral drill hole. (G) Placement of the AT-B allograft with bone plug at femoral site. (H) Fixation at the femoral site and graft conditioning with tension of distal graft. (I) Graft fixation at the tibia with interference screw and suture post. (J) Cosmetic closure. *FCL*, Fibular collateral ligament; *ITB*, iliotibial band. (From Noyes FR, Barber-Westin SD: Posterolateral ligament injuries: diagnosis, operative techniques, and clinical outcomes. In Noyes FR [ed.]: *Noyes' knee disorders: surgery, rehabilitation, clinical outcomes*, Philadelphia, 2017, Elsevier, pp 527-577.)

TABLE 59.11 Rehabilitation Protocol After Posterolateral Knee Reconstruction

	POSTOPERATIVE WEEKS					POSTOP MONTHS			
	1-2	3-4	5-6	7-8	9-12	4	5	6	7-12
Brace									
Bivalved cylinder cast	X	X							
Custom medial unloader or hinged soft tissue brace			X	X	X	X	X	X	X
Range of Motion Minimum Goals (Degrees)									
0-90	X	X							
0-110			X						
0-120				X					
0-130					X				
Weight Bearing									
None	X								
Toe-touch-25% body weight		X							
25-50% body weight			X						
Full, cane support				X					
Full					X				
Patella mobilization	X	X	X	X					
Modalities									
EMS	X	X	X	X					
Pain/edema management (cryotherapy)	X	X	X	X	X	X	X	X	X
Stretching									
Hamstring, gastrocnemius-soleus, iliotibial band, quadriceps	X	X	X	X	X	X	X	X	X
Strengthening									
Quad isometrics, straight leg raises	X	X	X	X	X				
Active knee extension	X	X	X	X	X				
Closed-chain: gait-retraining, toe-raises, wall-sits, mini-squats			X	X	X	X	X	X	
Knee flexion hamstring curls (90 degrees)						X	X	X	X
Knee extension quads (90-30 degrees)			X	X	X	X	X	X	X
Hip abduction–adduction, multi-hip					X	X	X	X	X
Leg press (70-10 degrees)					X	X	X	X	X
Balance/Proprioceptive Training									
Weight-shifting, cup-walking, BBS				X	X				
BBS, BAPS, perturbation training, balance board, mini-trampoline						X	X	X	X
Conditioning									
UBC		X	X	X					
Bike (stationary)			X	X	X	X	X	X	X
Aquatic program						X	X	X	X
Swimming (kicking)						X	X	X	X
Walking						X	X	X	X
Stair-climbing machine						X	X	X	X
Ski machine						X	X	X	X
Elliptical cross-trainer						X	X	X	X
Running: straight									X
Cutting: lateral carioca, figure-eights									X
Plyometric training									X
Full sports									X

BAPS, Biomechanical Ankle Platform System (Camp, Jackson, Michigan); *BBS*, Biodex Balance System (Biodex Medical Systems, Inc, Shirley, New York); *EMS*, electrical muscle stimulation; *UBC*, upper body cycle (Biodex Medical Systems, Inc, Shirley, New York).
From Noyes FR, Barber-Westin SD, Heckmann TP: Rehabilitation of posterior cruciate ligament and posterolateral reconstructive procedures. In Noyes FR, Barber-Westin SD (eds): *Noyes' knee disorders: surgery, rehabilitation, clinical outcomes*, ed 2, Philadelphia, 2017, Elsevier, pp 578-607.

exercises, running, and return to full sports activities are incorporated.

The immediate postoperative management is similar to that described for PCL reconstructions. A bivalved cast is used for the first 4 postoperative weeks to provide maximum protection to the knee joint and PLS. The cast is used in this time period because many soft-hinged postoperative braces do not provide sufficient protection against excessive lateral joint opening, which could occur with ambulation and produce a failure of the PL reconstruction. The cast is removed four times per day for passive knee motion exercises, which are performed in a seated position. Patients are cautioned to avoid varus tensioning

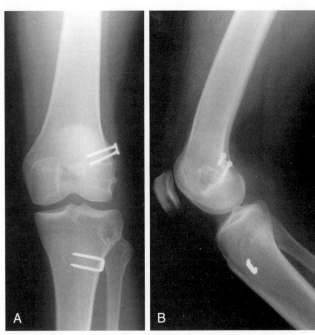

FIG 59.45 AP (A) and lateral (B) radiographs show fixation of PL capsular reconstruction with two 4.0-mm cancellous screws at the femoral site and an absorbable interference tibial screw and suture post. At the femoral site, either a bone inlay or tunnel may be selected. (From Noyes FR, Barber-Westin SD: Posterolateral ligament injuries: diagnosis, operative techniques, and clinical outcomes. In Noyes FR [ed.]: *Noyes' knee disorders: surgery, rehabilitation, clinical outcomes*, Philadelphia, 2017, Elsevier, pp 527-577.)

when performing knee flexion exercises. They are taught (and the assistance of a partner is encouraged) to place a hand on the lateral aspect of the knee and create a 10-pound valgus load to protect the PLS. If associated with a PCL reconstruction, a combined medial-anterior load should be applied to control both varus and posterior loads. At 4 weeks postoperative, a lower extremity, hinged, double-upright brace is applied, locked at 10 degrees of flexion. The brace is removed four times daily for range of motion exercises. At 6 weeks postoperative, the brace is unlocked as knee flexion to 110 degrees is encouraged and partial weight bearing is allowed.

At 7 to 8 weeks, a custom medial unloading brace is applied as weight bearing progresses to full and flexion is advanced to 120 degrees. The brace is also used as patients return to activity to provide protection against knee hyperextension and excessive varus loads.

Patients are not allowed to bear weight for the first 2 postoperative weeks. Then, partial weight bearing (25% of the patient's body weight) is begun at postoperative weeks 3 to 4. There is a slow advancement to full weight bearing by weeks 8 to 10, with the brace unlocked and cane or crutch support, which is used for approximately another 3 to 4 weeks. The patient must have good control of the lower extremity and adequate muscle strength to maintain joint compression and avoid an abnormal lift-off of the lateral tibiofemoral compartment.

Patellar mobilization, flexibility exercises, modality usage, and the strengthening and conditioning programs are all similar to those described in the PCL reconstruction protocol. In select

athletes, a running program is begun at approximately the ninth postoperative month, and plyometric- and sports-specific training programs are initiated at the 12th postoperative month. However, most patients who require multiple ligament reconstructive procedures do not desire to return to high-impact sports, and therefore this advanced conditioning and training is usually not required. Patients who have articular cartilage damage are advised to return to low-impact activities only to protect the knee joint.

KEY REFERENCES

36. Grood ES, Stowers SF, Noyes FR: Limits of movement in the human knee. Effect of sectioning the posterior cruciate ligament and posterolateral structures. *J Bone Joint Surg Am* 70(1):88–97, 1988.

72. Mannor DA, Shearn JT, Grood ES, et al: Two-bundle posterior cruciate ligament reconstruction. An in vitro analysis of graft placement and tension. *Am J Sports Med* 28(6):833–845, 2000.

78. Mejia EA, Noyes FR, Grood ES: Posterior cruciate ligament femoral insertion site characteristics. Importance for reconstructive procedures. *Am J Sports Med* 30(5):643–651, 2002.

88. Noyes FR, Barber-Westin S: Posterior cruciate ligament replacement with a two-strand quadriceps tendon-patellar bone autograft and a tibial inlay technique. *J Bone Joint Surg Am* 87(6):1241–1252, 2005.

89. Noyes FR, Barber-Westin SD: Posterior cruciate ligament revision reconstruction, part 1: causes of surgical failure in 52 consecutive operations. *Am J Sports Med* 33(5):646–654, 2005.

90. Noyes FR, Barber-Westin SD: Posterior cruciate ligament revision reconstruction, part 2: results of revision using a 2-strand quadriceps tendon-patellar bone autograft. *Am J Sports Med* 33(5):655–665, 2005.

92. Noyes FR, Barber-Westin SD: Posterolateral knee reconstruction with an anatomical bone-patellar tendon-bone reconstruction of the fibular collateral ligament. *Am J Sports Med* 35(2):259–273, 2007.

94. Noyes FR, Barber-Westin SD: Long-term assessment of posterolateral ligament femoral-fibular reconstruction in chronic multiligament unstable knees. *Am J Sports Med* 39(3):497–505, 2011.

95. Noyes FR, Barber-Westin SD: Function of the posterior cruciate ligament and posterolateral ligament structures. In Noyes FR, Barber-Westin SD, editors: *Noyes' knee disorders: surgery, rehabilitation, clinical outcomes*, ed 2, Philadelphia, 2017, Elsevier, pp 406–446.

97. Noyes FR, Barber-Westin SD: Posterior cruciate ligament: diagnosis, operative techniques, and clinical outcomes. In Noyes FR, Barber-Westin SD, editors: *Noyes' knee disorders: surgery, rehabilitation, clinical outcomes*, ed 2, Philadelphia, 2017, Elsevier, pp 447–526.

98. Noyes FR, Barber-Westin SD: Posterolateral ligament injuries: diagnosis, operative techniques, and clinical outcomes. In Noyes FR, Barber-Westin SD, editors: *Noyes' knee disorders: surgery, rehabilitation, clinical outcomes*, ed 2, Philadelphia, 2017, Elsevier, pp 527–577.

99. Noyes FR, Barber-Westin SD, Heckmann TP: Rehabilitation of posterior cruciate ligament and posterolateral reconstructive procedures. In Noyes FR, Barber-Westin SD, editors: *Noyes' knee disorders: surgery, rehabilitation, clinical outcomes*, ed 2, Philadelphia, 2017, Elsevier, pp 578–607.

106. Noyes FR, Stowers SF, Grood ES, et al: Posterior subluxations of the medial and lateral tibiofemoral compartments. An in vitro ligament sectioning study in cadaveric knees. *Am J Sports Med* 21(3):407–414, 1993.

118. Shearn JT, Grood ES, Noyes FR, et al: Two-bundle posterior cruciate ligament reconstruction: how bundle tension depends on femoral placement. *J Bone Joint Surg Am* 86-A(6):1262–1270, 2004.

119. Shearn JT, Grood ES, Noyes FR, et al: One- and two-strand posterior cruciate ligament reconstructions: cyclic fatigue testing. *J Orthop Res* 23(4):958–963, 2005.

The references for this chapter can also be found on www.expertconsult.com.

60

Posterior Cruciate Ligament Reconstruction: Posterior Inlay Technique

Adam S. Wilson, Mark D. Miller

The posterior cruciate ligament (PCL) stabilizes the knee against posterior translation of the tibia with respect to the femur and against external rotation of the knee. It is injured at a much lower frequency than the anterior cruciate ligament (ACL). Injuries to the PCL account for 3% to 16% of soft tissue injuries to the knee, and thus PCL injuries have traditionally gained less attention than ACL injuries.[*] If left untreated, isolated PCL injuries can lead to progressive instability and degeneration of the joint.[29,36] Increased interest in PCL reconstruction has been led by improvement in diagnostic techniques and recognition of PCL injuries.[†] Many patients are able to tolerate a PCL-deficient knee, but recent interest and investigation has demonstrated altered biomechanics of the PCL-deficient knee.[29,36] There continues to be considerable debate regarding preferred techniques for operative management of PCL injuries, specifically related to tibia graft fixation. The posterior tibial inlay technique provides a significant advantage in that it avoids the "killer turn"—the major drawback of the transtibial tunnel technique, as it has been shown to be a cause of graft failure.[1] The tibial inlay technique is also believed to provide greater biomechanical resistance to anteroposterior (AP) translation and is less or a risk to neurovascular structures.[3]

The traditional tibial inlay technique has required an open approach to the posterior knee; however, the technique continues to evolve and undergo advances, with some authors more recently advocating for an all-arthroscopic technique.[6,7,20,28,29] The tibial inlay technique has a proven track record and has become a durable method for PCL reconstruction. This chapter describes the traditional tibial inlay technique for PCL reconstruction using a single-bundle autograft.[3]

ANATOMY[‡]

To understand and treat PCL injuries, a familiarity with the anatomy of the PCL is necessary. The PCL is generally 32 mm to 38 mm in length with a cross-sectional area of 11 mm^2 at its midpoint. The PCL originates from the medial femoral condyle, approximately 1 cm proximal to the articular surface. The insertion of the PCL is in a central sulcus on the posterior aspect of the tibia, approximately 1 cm to 1.5 cm distal to the posterior edge of the tibial plateau. The PCL is present within the joint capsule of the knee but is considered extra-articular because it is enclosed within a synovial sheath.

Functionally, the ligament consists of two bundles, the anterolateral (AL) bundle and the posteromedial (PM) bundle. The naming of the bundles is based on the location of the femoral origin to its tibial insertion. The AL bundle is the thicker, stronger bundle and is tight in flexion, and the PM bundle is smaller and tight in knee extension. Although the AL bundle is stronger and provides greater resistance to posterior tibial translation, biomechanical research has verified the importance of the PM bundle and the meniscofemoral ligaments.

The meniscofemoral ligaments (ligaments of Humphrey and Wrisberg) run from the lateral meniscus to the medial femoral condyle and insert anterior (Humphrey) or posterior (Wrisberg) to the PCL. These ligaments may remain intact after a PCL injury and provide some level of knee stability because they can contribute as much as 28% of the resistive forces to posterior tibial translation in ligamentously intact knees.

HISTORY AND PHYSICAL EXAMINATION[§]

The most common mechanism for a PCL injury is an excessive, posteriorly directed force on the tibia with the knee in 90 degrees of flexion. Importantly, foot position at the moment of impact may be predictive of the resultant injury. With the foot in dorsiflexion, a posteriorly directed force can lead to a patellofemoral injury, as opposed to the same force on the tibia with the foot in plantar flexion will likely result in a PCL injury. In contrast to ACL injuries, PCL injuries frequently occur without an immediate subjective feeling of instability or a definitive "pop." Frequently, patients will continue to participate in activities following a PCL injury and present in a delayed fashion because of the late development of pain or subtle instability during activities. They often report an increased difficulty with stairs or inclines, specifically the descent.

Although isolated PCL injuries can, and do, occur, a high suspicion for the potential presence of additional knee pathology must be maintained. Frequently PCL injuries occur in higher energy mechanism as part of a multiligamentous injury. The most common pattern of multiligamentous injuries involves rupture of the ACL, PCL, and posterolateral corner. Physical examination is an important tool in the diagnosis and differentiation of these injuries.

The gold standard examination maneuver for the diagnosis of PCL injury is the posterior drawer test (Fig. 60.1). The

---

[*]References 1-3, 8, 10-12, 24, 25, 31, 34, 36, and 38.
[†]References 11, 12, 24, 25, 29, 34, and 36.
[‡]References 2, 12, 19, 21, 22, and 34-36.

[§]References 3, 11, 13, 21, 24, 25, 27, 34, 37, and 38.

posterior drawer test is 90% sensitive and 99% specific for PCL injury. The posterior drawer test is performed with the knee in 90 degrees of flexion. The examiner must have an understanding of the concept of the starting point to assess PCL and ACL integrity. In the presence of posterior tibial sagging, ACL pseudolaxity can result in a false-positive anterior drawer test and subsequent misdiagnosis of an ACL injury (Fig. 60.2). PCL injuries can be classified by measuring the amount of posterior tibial translation in comparison with the uninjured contralateral knee. PCL injuries are graded I to III, with grade I defined as 5 mm of posterior translation of the tibia, grade II as 6 to 10 mm, and grade III as greater than 10 mm. Placing the thumbs on the anterior joint line to provide tactile feedback of tibial translation is the best way to perform this test. Grade III PCL injuries rarely occur in isolation, thus additional ligamentous injuries must be considered. Injury to the posterolateral corner is frequently associated with grade III PCL laxity.

The dial test should be performed to assess for any posterolateral instability. The dial test should be performed with the patient prone. External rotation asymmetry of more than 15 degrees at 30 and 90 degrees of knee flexion indicates a combined PCL and posterolateral corner injury. Additional physical exam maneuvers that can be used to diagnose posterolateral instability include varus laxity, external rotation recurvatum test, posterolateral and PM drawer tests, and reverse pivot shift.

Other pertinent physical exam maneuvers for diagnosis of a PCL injury include the posterior sag test, Godfrey test, prone drawer test, quadriceps active test, and dynamic pivot shift.

Imaging[23,30]

Initial imaging for a suspected PCL injury should begin with plain x-rays. Standard radiographs can be used to assess for the presence of any bony avulsion or concomitant tibial plateau fracture or fibular head fracture. Plain films can also reveal subtle posterior tibial subluxation. Any of these could hint at additional posterolateral corner injury (Fig. 60.3).

Stress x-rays should then be performed to quantify the extent of the injury. These views should be performed by the physician applying a posteriorly directed force to the proximal tibia, with the knee in 90 degrees of flexion. The authors use the Telos system, which applies 15 decaNewtons of force. The injury is quantified by measuring the amount of posterior translation of the tibial plateau in relation to the femoral condyles. In addition, the authors obtain varus stress x-rays to assess the lateral joint opening because increased opening has been found to correlate with increased likelihood of posterolateral corner injury (Fig. 60.4).

In addition, magnetic resonance imaging (MRI) should be used to confirm a suspected ligamentous injury in the knee. MRI is approximately 100% sensitive for diagnosis of acute PCL

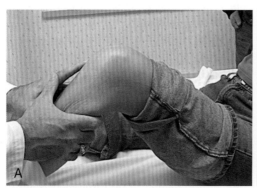
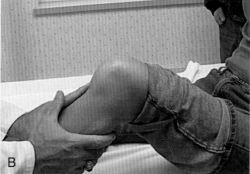

FIG 60.1 Posterior drawer test demonstrating proper starting point (A) with obvious posterior laxity (B) suggestive of PCL pathology.

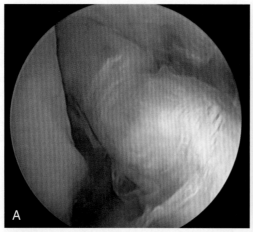
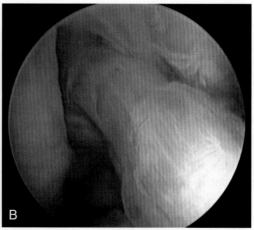

FIG 60.2 (A) Arthroscopic view demonstrating ACL pseudolaxity. (B) ACL tension is subsequently restored following anterior drawer.

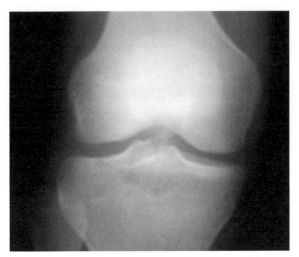

FIG 60.3 Plain film demonstrating PCL avulsion.

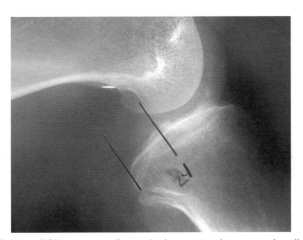

FIG 60.4 PCL stress radiograph demonstrating posterior tibial translation suggestive of PCL injury.

tears. MRI can also aid in assessing for any additional injuries to the structures about the knee. MRI has become critical for preoperative planning. It is important for the surgeon to be aware of any additional injuries prior to the time of surgery for appropriate planning to ensure all injuries are addressed at the time of surgery (Fig. 60.5).

Treatment

Prior to detailed discussion of the posterior tibial inlay technique, it is important to mention initial treatment strategies for PCL injuries. Low-grade, isolated PCL injuries are typically treated nonoperatively, with emphasis placed in reduction of inflammation, regaining full knee motion, and strengthening the quadriceps to counteract the tendency toward posterior tibial subluxation. Patients are allowed to return to activity within 3 to 6 weeks, depending on the severity of the injury and the patient goals.

Operative indications following PCL injury include multiligamentous injuries, symptomatic chronic grade II or III injuries that have failed conservative management, PCL avulsions, and PCL injuries in active patients who are unwilling to alter their activities to comply with conservative treatment options.**

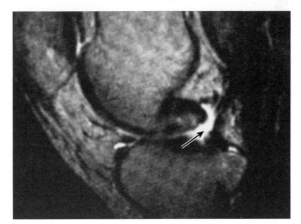

FIG 60.5 PCL tear (black arrow) as seen on MRI.

Posterior tibial avulsion injuries involving the PCL insertion are repaired anatomically with lag screws or suture fixation, whereas midsubstance tears of the PCL require ligamentous reconstruction.[27] Advocates for the tibial inlay technique of PCL reconstruction argue that it reproduces the most anatomic PCL reconstruction while avoiding the "killer turn" associated with tibial tunneling.[1] In addition, patients with tibial osteopenia or prior osteotomies or tibial plateau fractures may require the tibial inlay technique rather than transtibial tunneling to prevent proximal graft migration.

Indications and Contraindications[††]

Indications for operative treatment of PCL injuries using the posterior tibial inlay technique include acute grade III PCL injuries, chronic grade III PCL injuries with symptomatic instability after a trial of nonoperative treatment, PCL injuries with associated bony avulsion injuries or posterolateral corner injuries, and PCL injury as a component of a multiligamentous injury (specifically grade II or higher medial collateral ligament injury or an ACL injury).

Relative indications for posterior tibial inlay reconstruction of the PCL include grade II injuries in a young, active patient with symptomatic instability after attempted nonoperative management.

The primary contraindication to the use of the posterior tibial inlay technique for PCL reconstruction is patients with a prior history of vascular procedures in the operative extremity, such as vascular repair or bypass, because the anatomy becomes distorted and unpredictable, creating an increased risk of complications.

Equipment

Portions of the procedure are performed both using open and arthroscopic techniques; therefore it is important to ensure the surgeon has all equipment available for each portion of the procedure. Many pans and trays do not immediately need to be opened prior to, or at the beginning of, the case but should be easily accessible and readily available.

Prior to the start of the case, a standard knee arthroscopy setup (including both 30- and 70-degrees arthroscopes) should be opened, along with a major orthopedic retractor pan. All

---

** References 3, 13, 24, 25, 27, and 38.

†† References 3, 4, 13, 24, 25, 27, 37, and 38.

necessary equipment for bone-patellar tendon-bone autograft harvest should also be immediately available. The surgeons preferred screws for tibial inlay fixation should be open and available (the authors prefer 4.5-mm cannulated screws with washers, but solid screws can also be used). The authors preferred fixation for the femoral tunnel is an interference screw, but alternative fixation should be available as per surgeon preference. Luque wires should be available for passage of the graft. In addition, PCL guides should be available to assist with femoral tunnel placement. A headlight for the primary surgeon should be available for the posterior approach portion of the procedure. Burrs should be available for creation of the tibial trough. Multiple 3/32 pins should be available to be used for retraction and tunnel placement, as will be further described in the technique portion of the chapter. A Shanz pin with a T-handle (such as from a large external fixator set) should also be present to apply an anterior drawer on the tibia while the PCL graft is being fixed.

TIBIAL INLAY TECHNIQUE IN DETAIL

Examination Under Anesthesia, Patient Positioning, and Diagnostic Arthroscopy

The authors adopted this technique after the initial report by Berg by modifying it and combining it with the posterior approach described by Burks and Shaffer.[3-5,26] This approach has been shown to be effective at restoring the PCL in an anatomic fashion by fixing the graft into a trough at the tibial origin. In addition, the approach has been shown to be safe as the popliteal artery is retracted by the medial head of the gastrocnemius and kept well out of the surgical field.[9,18]

This procedure should be performed under a general anesthetic because this facilitates adequate positioning and examination under anesthesia. The patient should always be examined under anesthesia prior to position and beginning the procedure. This is necessary to confirm PCL injury and ensure there are not any additional, unrecognized ligamentous injuries, including ACL, PM, or posterolateral injuries. Prior to positioning, the contralateral leg should also be examined for comparison. In addition, stress radiographs under anesthesia are frequently performed to document the degree of injury without any patient guarding as you may see in an awake patient.

The patient is then positioned in the lateral decubitus position with the uninjured leg against the bed in extension. It is important to sufficiently pad the uninjured leg and the upper extremities. An axillary roll should be used. The authors use a beanbag or hip positioners to hold the patient in the lateral position. An unsterile tourniquet is placed on the proximal thigh of the operative extremity. After the extremity has been prepped in sterile fashion, the foot and ankle are placed into a bracketed foot holder to aid in positioning for the anterior portions of the procedure (Fig. 60.6).[14]

For patients undergoing acute operative intervention (within 2 weeks of injury), the authors will begin the procedure with an egress incision in the center of any planned corner incision. This is performed to prevent iatrogenic compartment syndrome during the arthroscopic portion of the case. The leg is then abducted and externally rotated and placed in the bracketed foot holder for the arthroscopic, and other anterior portions, of the procedure. Arthroscopy is then performed using standard arthroscopic portals (Fig. 60.7). During diagnostic arthroscopy the joint is visually inspected while addressing any meniscal or

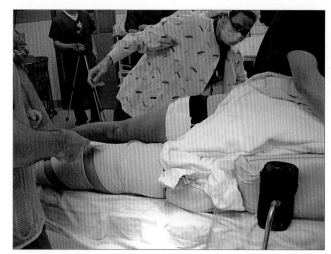

FIG 60.6 The patient is placed in the lateral decubitus position in preparation for PCL reconstruction. The nonoperative extremity is generously padded. A tourniquet is applied to the proximal operative thigh.

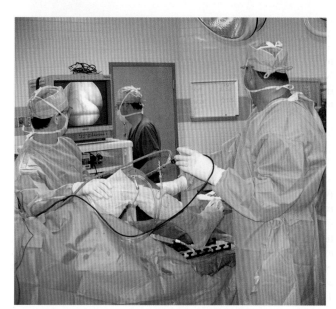

FIG 60.7 Diagnostic arthroscopy and graft harvest are performed with the hip placed in abduction and external rotation while the knee is secured in flexion using a bracketed foot holder. Standard arthroscopic portals are used during diagnostic arthroscopy.

cartilage pathology prior to PCL reconstruction. The presence of a torn PCL is confirmed prior to proceeding to graft harvest (Fig. 60.8). Indicators of PCL injury include hemorrhage and ACL pseudolaxity.[16,17] After confirmation of a PCL injury, the stump is débrided using a combination of biters and a 5.5-mm shaver. Any residual intact fibers of the PCL, as well as intact mensicofemoral ligaments, should be preserved.

Patellar Graft Harvest

The bone-patellar tendon-bone autograft is harvested from the ipsilateral knee, with the operative extremity placed in abduction and external rotation flexed to approximately 90 degrees using the foot holder. A longitudinal incision is made of the

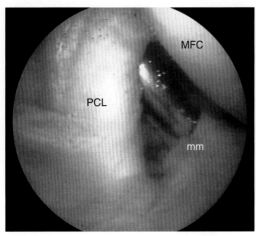 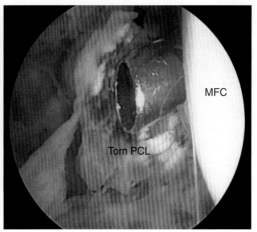

FIG 60.8 Arthroscopic view of an intact PCL *(left)* and a torn PCL with hemorrhage *(right)*. *MFC*, Medial femoral condyle; *PCL*, posterior cruciate ligament.

anterior knee, just medial to the midline of the patellar tendon and beginning at the level of the inferior pole of the patella, and carried approximately 2 cm distal to the tibia tubercle. Full-thickness skin flaps are raised as the dissection is carried down to the paratenon. Using a fresh, sharp blade, a generous 11-mm to 12-mm central one-third of the patellar tendon is defined. Next, an oscillating saw is used to remove bone plugs from the tibial tubercle and patella. The bone plugs are typically 20 mm to 25 mm in length.

Graft Preparation

The bone-patellar tendon-bone autograft is then prepared on the back table by an assistant, while the knee is being prepared for graft incorporation. The authors prefer to use the tibial portion of the graft for the tibial inlay and therefore make it rectangular and 20 to 25 mm in length. The patellar portion of the graft is then contoured into a cylinder with a rounded tip, or "bulleted." The bulleted portion of the graft should be approximately 18 mm in length and fit through a 10- to 12-mm wide femoral tunnel. Two perpendicular drill holes are then placed 5 mm and 10 mm from the tip of the patellar bone plug. Two number 5 sutures are passed through the drill holes to assist in graft passage. In addition, a number 2 Ethibond or Ti-Cron suture may be placed at the junction of the tendon and patellar bone plug to facilitate easier entry into the femoral tunnel. The graft is then placed under tension on a graft board on the back table during the next portions of the procedure (Fig. 60.9).

Femoral Tunnel Placement[16,32,33]

Prior to femoral tunnel placement, the lateral aspect of the medial femoral condyle and any remaining soft tissue in the notch are débrided arthroscopically. A standard PCL guide is introduced into the knee through the anteromedial portal. The PCL guide is then placed approximately 6 to 8 mm from the articular surface of the anteromedial portion of the intercondylar notch. This correlates to the 1:30 clock position in a right knee and 10:30 clock position in a left knee. This position ensures an adequate bone bridge between the articular surface and the femoral tunnel to minimize the risk of avascular necrosis of the medial femoral condyle. Next a 2-cm incision is made along Langer lines over the medial aspect of the knee at the level

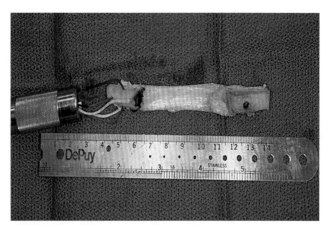

FIG 60.9 Harvested bone-patellar tendon-bone autograft. Predrilled rectangular tibia bone block *(top)* with tapered bone plug and perpendicular sutures for femoral fixation *(bottom)*.

of the medial femoral condyle. Dissection is carried down through the subcutaneous tissue and along the inferior border of the vastus medialis muscle to the level of the condyle. The external portion of the guide is placed on the cortical surface of the condyle. A 3/32 guide pin is then drilled from outside-in. Confirmation that the pin is in the center of the femoral PCL footprint is done arthroscopically (Fig. 60.10). The tunnel is then overdrilled using the appropriately sized cannulated drill. Bone graft from the flutes of the drill bit should be saved for later placement into the patellar harvest site. The edges of the tunnel are then rasped to reduce graft abrasion. A looped, smooth, 18-gauge Luque wire is then placed into the tunnel from outside to inside and arthroscopically positioned in the posterior aspect of the knee. The arthroscopic equipment is then removed from the knee to begin the tibial inlay portion of the case.

Posterior Approach and Tibial Inlay

Next, the authors place the leg in full extension and neutral rotation on a padded Mayo stand (Fig. 60.11). The surgeon sits on an operative stool and uses a headlight for this portion of the procedure. A horizontal incision is then made in the flexion

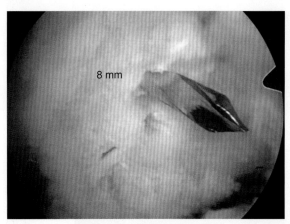

FIG 60.10 Arthroscopic view during femoral guide pin placement. Guide pin entry occurs 8 mm from the articular surface of the medial femoral condyle *(top left)*.

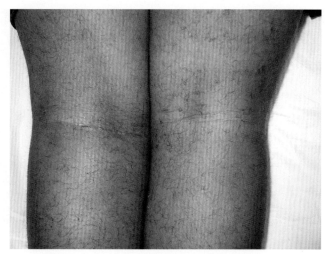

FIG 60.12 Healed surgical scar in the flexion crease of the left knee demonstrating excellent cosmetic results.

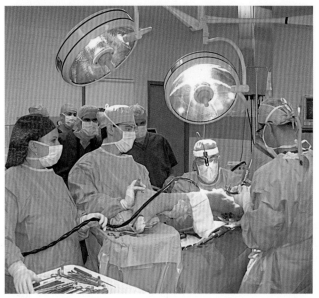

FIG 60.11 The operative extremity is placed in full extension and neutral rotation during the inlay portion of the procedure to facilitate access to the popliteal fossa.

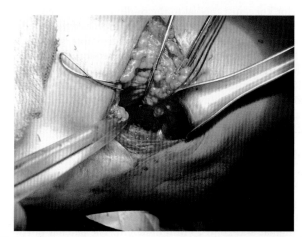

FIG 60.13 Smooth Steinmann pins placed in the posterior tibia allow for static retraction of the medial head of the gastrocnemius, facilitating exposure of the posterior capsule.

crease of the popliteal fossa (Fig. 60.12). A hockey stick incision is then made in the gastrocnemius fascia by incising the fascia perpendicular to the skin incision laterally and curving distally between the medial head of the gastrocnemius and semimembranosus muscles. The medial head of the gastrocnemius is then identified and mobilized by blunt dissection. The medial head of the gastrocnemius should be mobilized sufficiently to retract it laterally past the midline. Slight knee flexion can increase the ability to laterally mobilize the medial head of the gastrocnemius and exposure of the posterior knee capsule. A smooth 3/32 Steinmann pin may then be inserted into the posterior tibia and bent laterally to maintain lateral retraction of the gastrocnemius (Fig. 60.13). Lateral retraction of the medial head of the gastrocnemius provides excellent protection for the neurovascular structures within the popliteal fossa.

The tibial footprint of the PCL is identified by palpating the sulcus between the medial and lateral prominences of the

posterior tibia. The muscle belly of the popliteus is then identified, and a posterior arthrotomy is made along the superior border of the popliteus. A combination of electrocautery and an elevator can be used to clear soft tissue away from the sulcus and expose the posterior cortex of the tibia. A combination of a rongeur, an osteotome, a high-speed burr, and a bone tamp are used to create a trough in the posterior tibia to match the shape and dimensions of the tibial block portion of the graft. The graft is then retrieved from the back table and fit into the tibial trough to assess fit. Care must be taken to ensure that the bone plug of the graft lays flush and snug in trough.

After verifying an adequate fit of the tibial bone plug, the graft is returned to the back table, where two guide pins for the 4.5-mm cannulated screws are placed through the anterior cortex of the tibial bone block. The graft is then brought back to the operative field, where it is secured to the drapes to ensure that the graft cannot be dropped. The Luque wire placed during the preparation of the femoral tunnel is then visualized through the posterior incision and retrieved. Using this Luque wire, the number 5 sutures previously placed through the patellar portion of the graft are used to pull the graft into the joint and into the femoral tunnel. An additional wire may be used to pull the number 2 suture through the anteromedial arthroscopic portal to aid in graft passage. After the graft is pulled into the knee joint, the tibial bone block is secured into the tibia. Provisional fixation is achieved by driving the guide pins through the anterior tibial cortex. After measurement for screw depth, a cannulated drill bit is used to overdrill the pins and two 4.5-mm bicortical screws with flat washers are placed to fix the tibial bone block to the tibia. The guide pins are then removed, leaving the graft well secured to the posterior tibia (Figs. 60.14 and 60.15).

Graft Passage and Fixation

After the tibial bone block has been secured to the tibia, the knee should be cycled through a full range of motion to ensure that the tibial bone block is secure and the graft is free from impingement at the site of the posterior capsulotomy. The leg is then abducted and externally rotated, and the foot is placed back in the bracketed foot holder. The graft is then visualized arthroscopically. The number 5 sutures are passed through the femoral tunnel, and traction on these sutures is used to bring the patellar-bone plug-tendon interface of the graft flush with the articular margin of the femoral tunnel (Fig. 60.16). The number 2 suture, or a right angle clamp, passed through the anteromedial portal may be used to help to toggle the bone plug into position. Failure to properly position the bone plug can result in early graft failure caused by excessive shear stress on the graft. After the graft is correctly positioned, moderate tension is applied to the number 5 sutures and the knee is again cycled through a full range of motion to ensure the graft will

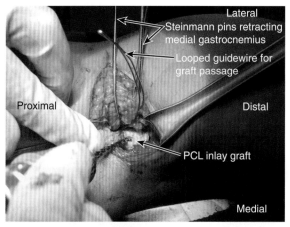

FIG 60.14 Preparing the tibial bone block for definitive fixation. *PCL*, Posterior cruciate ligament.

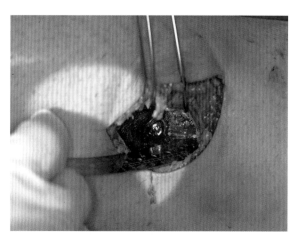

FIG 60.15 Posterior view of the knee following graft passage and tibia bone block fixation.

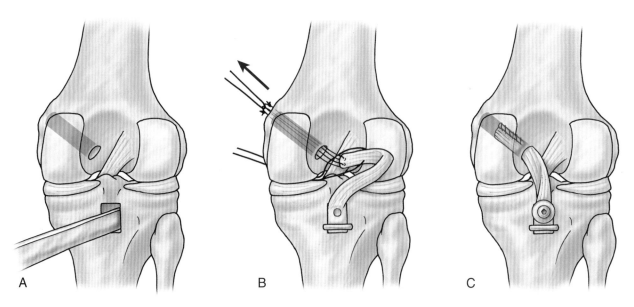

FIG 60.16 **Overview of the Tibial Inlay Technique** (A) The tibia footprint of the PCL is placed in the sulcus between the medial and lateral prominences of the posterior tibia. (B) Prior to fixation, the graft is pulled through the posterior arthrotomy and into the femoral tunnel using the looped wire. (C) After verifying appropriate bone block fitting and graft clearance, the graft is tensioned and definitively secured.

not kink. The bone plug is then secured into the femoral tunnel using a 9 × 20 mm interference screw while an anterior drawer force is applied to the knee in 70 to 90 degrees of flexion. A Shantz pin with a T-handle from the external fixation set can be used for this purpose. Additional fixation can be obtained by tying the number 5 nonabsorbable suture to a plastic button over the cortex at the femoral tunnel entrance. The graft should be visualized arthroscopically to ensure proper fixation. Stability of the PCL should be confirmed by the posterior drawer test.

Closure

Prior to closure, the bone graft set aside from reaming the femoral tunnel is used to pack the defects at the patellar and tibial graft harvest sites. The anterior knee is closed in standard fashion, and a sterile dressing is applied. Posteriorly, the capsule is repaired and a Hemovac drain is placed deep to the medial head of the gastrocnemius to reduce the risk of postoperative hematoma. The tourniquet is deflated prior to the remainder of the posterior closure. The posterior wound is then closed in a standard layered fashion and a sterile dressing is applied. AP and lateral radiographs of the knee are taken following the procedure to ensure appropriate graft and hardware placement (Figs. 60.17 and 60.18). The knee is braced in extension to support the posterior tibia and prevent posterior translation.

Postoperative Rehabilitation Program

Postoperative rehabilitation following PCL reconstruction is often more difficult than rehabilitation following ACL, with full recovery taking up to a year. Rehabilitation is focused on regaining full knee range of motion, reducing pain and edema, and strengthening the quadriceps while preventing posterior tibial translation. Excessive graft stress must be avoided until adequate healing has occurred. Open chain hamstring exercises place excessive posterior force on the tibia and must be avoided for the first 3 months.

The patient is placed into an external hinged knee brace that is locked in full extension for the first 2 weeks (Fig. 60.19). The patient is permitted 50% weight bearing with crutches for the

first 4 to 6 weeks, followed by progression to weight bearing as tolerated. Supervised passive range of motion of the knee from 0 to 90 degrees is started on postoperative day 1. The knee brace is locked at 0 degrees at all other times. This range of motion exercises must be done with the patient in the prone position to avoid early stress on the reconstruction. Quadriceps strengthening using isometric quadriceps training and straight leg raises is initiated as soon as the patient can tolerate the exercises.

After 4 to 6 weeks the hinged knee brace is transitioned to an unlocked position and the patient may begin ambulating and progressing to weight bearing as tolerated, under the direction of a therapist. The brace may be removed after the patient is able to fully weight bear without the use of crutches. At 8 weeks postoperatively, quadriceps strengthening may progress to closed chain terminal knee extension exercises. No hamstring strengthening should be performed prior to 3 months after the reconstruction. Jogging on a treadmill may begin at 10 to 12 weeks postoperatively, but full speed running should be avoided for 4 to 6 months. After 16 weeks the patient may begin plyometrics and sport-specific activities and progress as tolerated. Return to sport, or full activity, is typically 6 to 12 months after PCL reconstruction after the patient has demonstrated adequate return of strength and dynamic control of the limb.

Complications[15]

As with any surgical procedure, infection is a constant concern. There are many steps to this procedure with multiple approaches.

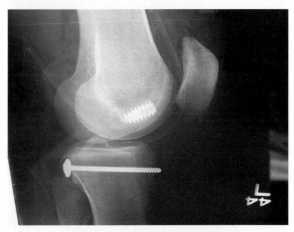

FIG 60.18 Lateral radiograph.

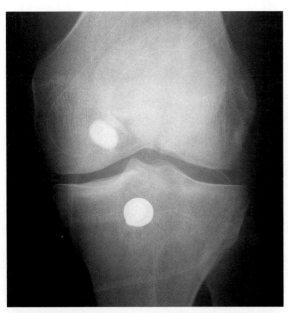

FIG 60.17 Postoperative AP radiograph.

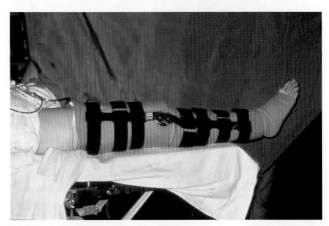

FIG 60.19 Postoperative hinged knee brace with knee locked in extension.

The significant amount of surgeon and staff movement provides many opportunities for breech in sterile technique. Great care must be observed to maintain sterile technique by all staff members. The American Board of Orthopaedic Surgery database from 2003 to 2009 showed that PCL reconstruction has the highest complication rate among arthroscopic procedures; at 20.1%, infection is a common complication.

The most common complication following PCL reconstruction is residual posterior laxity. This is most likely attributed to improper tensioning of the graft during graft placement or graft fixation. Other causes leading to residual laxity include failure to diagnose and treat associated ligamentous injuries and overly aggressive rehabilitation. During the surgical procedure the surgeon must ensure that the graft is properly tensioned and not kinking or impinging on the posterior arthrotomy. During graft fixation the surgeon must ensure that the bone-tendon junction of the graft rests at the articular margin of the femoral tunnel. Failure to do so can result in graft fraying and laxity. PCL reconstruction using the tibial inlay technique has been shown to achieve significantly less residual posterior laxity than the transtibial technique. Double-bundle reconstruction can improve posterior laxity because of more accurate restoration of the anatomic bundles of the PCL but may result in overconstraint of the knee at certain angle of flexion.

The most feared complication during PCL reconstruction is injury to the neurovascular structures in the popliteal fossa (Fig. 60.20). Full understanding of the anatomy of the posterior knee is essential prior to performing the tibial inlay technique. These structures must be protected by fully mobilizing, and properly retracting, the medial head of the gastrocnemius. 3/32 Steinmann pins placed in the posterior tibia provides sufficient, constant retraction and eliminates the risk from repetitive repositioning of retractors. Revision surgeries inherently have an increased risk for neurovascular injury because of scarring and distortion of normal anatomic planes.

Avascular necrosis of the medial femoral condyle has been reported following PCL reconstruction. This is thought to be caused by femoral drilling close to the articular surface and resulting trauma to the subchondral blood supply. Symptoms typically present months to years after reconstruction. Starting the femoral tunnel approximately 10 mm posterior to the articular margin helps to avoid this potential complication.

In addition, early arthrofibrosis can be seen following PCL reconstruction. If an early loss of motion is noted, it may warrant lysis of adhesions and manipulation under anesthesia. Some patients will report anterior knee pain from the graft harvest site. Finally, in patients with multiligamentous injuries, extravasation of fluid during the arthroscopic portion of the case can create an iatrogenic compartment syndrome. The leg should be continually monitored throughout the case. This complication is avoided by making an egress incision at the beginning of the case to allow a path for the arthroscopic fluid to follow without filling the compartments of the leg.

SUMMARY

Indications to perform PCL reconstruction include multiligamentous injuries, symptomatic chronic grade II or grade III injuries that have failed conservative management, PCL avulsions, and PCL injuries in young active patients who do not wish to change activities to comply with conservative management. Chronic, untreated PCL deficiency can lead to increased knee pain and degenerative changes. Following a properly performed PCL reconstruction, patients will have grade I, or better, laxity and rarely complain about functional instability.

The tibial inlay technique more closely replicates the anatomy of the PCL that does transtibial technique. In addition, the tibial inlay technique avoids the "killer turn" thought to be responsible for early failure and residual laxity after transtibial tunneling. All-arthroscopic tibial inlay techniques are continuing to be developed and adapted. Although these procedures are technically challenging, they do not require extensive dissection within the popliteal space, thus eliminating the need for changing patient position during the case. Although all-arthroscopic PCL reconstruction using tibial inlay are being developed, the surgeon must remain vigilant and be very comfortable with the anatomy of the posterior knee. Long-term studies demonstrating potential benefits of double-bundle PCL reconstruction, as well as all-arthroscopic techniques, are not yet available in the literature.

KEY REFERENCES

2. Benedetto KP, Hoffelner T, Osti M: The biomechanical characteristics of arthroscopic tibial inlay techniques for posterior cruciate ligament reconstruction: in vitro comparison of tibia graft tunnel placement. *Int Orthop* 38:2363–2368, 2014.

3. Berg EE: Posterior cruciate ligament tibial inlay reconstruction. *Arthroscopy* 11:69–76, 1995.

10. Curry RPL, Mestriner MB, Kaleka CC, et al: Double-bundle PCL reconstruction using autogenous quadriceps tendon and semitendinous graft: surgical technique with 2-year follow-up clinical results. *Knee* 21:763–768, 2014.

20. Lee DW, Jang HW, Lee YS, et al: Clinical, functional, and morphological evaluations of posterior cruciate ligament reconstruction with remnant preservation: minimum 2-year follow-up. *Am J Sports Med* 42:1822–1831, 2014.

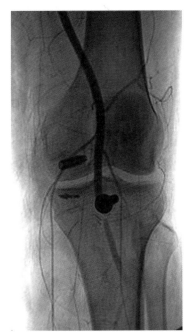

FIG 60.20 Postoperative angiogram demonstrating occlusion of the popliteal artery.

27. Montgomery SR, Johnson JS, McAllister DR, et al: Surgical management of PCL injuries: indications, techniques, and outcomes. *Curr Rev Musculoskelet Med* 6:115–123, 2013.

29. Panchal HB, Sekiya JK: Open tibial inlay versus arthroscopic transtibial posterior cruciate ligament reconstructions. *Arthroscopy* 27(9):1289–1295, 2011.

30. Richter D, Wascher DC, Schenck RC: A novel posteromedial approach for tibial inlay PCL reconstruction in KDIIIM injuries: avoiding prone patient positioning. *Clin Orthop* 472:2680–2690, 2014.

31. Salim R, Fogognolo F, Kfuri M: A new simplified onlay technique for posterior cruciate ligament reconstruction. *J Knee Surg* 27:289–294, 2014.

33. Schoderbek RJ, Golish SR, Rubino LJ, et al: PCL femoral tunnel angles—the graft/femoral tunnel angles in posterior cruciate ligament reconstruction: a cadaveric comparison of three techniques for femoral tunnel placement. *J Knee Surg* 22:106–110, 2009.

36. Voos JE, Mauro CS, Wente T, et al: Posterior cruciate ligament: anatomy, biomechanics, and outcomes. *Am J Sports Med* 40:222–231, 2012.

38. Whiddon DR, Zehms CT, Miller MD, et al: Double compared with single-bundle open inlay posterior cruciate ligament reconstruction in a cadaver model. *J Bone Joint Surg Am* 90:1820–1829, 2008.

The references for this chapter can also be found on www.expertconsult.com.

61

Posterior Cruciate Ligament Reconstruction: Transtibial Double-Bundle Technique

Gregory C. Fanelli

INTRODUCTION

This chapter illustrates the authors' surgical technique of the arthroscopic double-bundle/double femoral tunnel transtibial posterior cruciate ligament (PCL) reconstruction surgical procedure and presents our results of PCL reconstruction using this surgical technique. Because the isolated PCL reconstruction is rarely performed in our practice, this chapter has been written with PCL reconstruction within the context of the multiple ligament injured knee.[10,13]

The incidence of PCL injuries is reported to be from 1% to 40% of acute knee injuries. This range is dependent upon the patient population reported and is approximately 3% in the general population and 38% in reports from regional trauma centers.[1,4,16,26] Our practice, at a regional trauma center, has a 38.3% incidence of PCL tears in acute knee injuries, and 56.5% of these PCL injuries occur in multiple trauma patients; 45.9% are combined anterior cruciate ligament (ACL)/PCL tears, whereas 41.2% are PCL/posterolateral corner tears. Only 3% of acute PCL injuries seen in our trauma center are isolated.

The keys to successful PCL reconstruction are to identify and treat all pathology, use strong graft material, accurately place tunnels in anatomic insertion sites, minimize graft bending, use a mechanical graft tensioning device, use primary and backup graft fixation, and use the appropriate postoperative rehabilitation program. Adherence to these technical points results in successful single- and double-bundle arthroscopic transtibial tunnel PCL reconstruction documented with stress radiography, arthrometer, knee ligament rating scales, and patient satisfaction measurements.*

PCL surgical reconstructions may be unsuccessful because of failure to recognize and treat associated ligament instabilities (posterolateral instability and posteromedial instability), failure to treat varus osseous malalignment, and incorrect tunnel placement.[35-37] This chapter will describe the authors' surgical technique for arthroscopic transtibial tunnel PCL reconstruction and related surgery.

The double-bundle/double femoral tunnel transtibial tunnel (DB/DFT TTT) PCL reconstruction approximates the anatomy of the PCL by reconstructing the anterolateral bundle (ALB) and posteromedial bundle (PMB) of the PCL. This double-bundle reconstruction more closely approximates the broad femoral insertion of the PCL, enhancing the biomechanics of the PCL reconstruction.[34] Although the DB/DFT TTT PCL reconstruction does not perfectly reproduce the normal PCL, the following certain factors lead to success with this surgical technique:

1. Identify and treat all pathology (especially posterolateral instability)
2. Accurate tunnel placement
3. Anatomic graft insertion sites
4. Strong graft material
5. Minimize graft bending
6. Final tensioning at 70 to 90 degrees of knee flexion
7. Graft tensioning
   a. Biomet mechanical tensioning device
8. Primary and backup fixation
9. Appropriate rehabilitation program

SURGICAL INDICATIONS

Our indications for surgical treatment of acute PCL injuries include insertion site avulsions, tibial step-off decreased 10 mm or greater, and PCL tears combined with other structural injuries. Our indications for surgical treatment of chronic PCL injuries are when an isolated PCL tear becomes symptomatic or when progressive functional instability develops.

SURGICAL TIMING

Surgical timing is dependent upon vascular status, reduction stability, skin condition, systemic injuries, open versus closed knee injury, meniscus and articular surface injuries, other orthopedic injuries, and the collateral/capsular ligaments involved. Certain ACL/PCL/medial collateral ligament (MCL) injuries can be treated with brace treatment of the MCL followed by arthroscopic combined ACL/PCL reconstruction in 4 to 6 weeks after healing of the MCL. Other cases may require repair or reconstruction of the medial structures and must be assessed on an individual basis.

Combined ACL/PCL/posterolateral injuries are addressed as early as safely possible. ACL/PCL/posterolateral repair-reconstruction performed between 2 and 3 weeks post injury allows sealing of capsular tissues to permit an arthroscopic approach and still permits primary repair of injured posterolateral structures.

Open multiple ligament knee injuries/dislocations may require staged procedures. The collateral/capsular structures are repaired after thorough irrigation and débridement, and

*References 6-8, 11, 12, 17, 18, 20, 22, 23, 25, and 27-32.

the combined ACL/PCL reconstruction is performed at a later date after wound healing has occurred. Care must be taken in all cases of delayed reconstruction to confirm that the tibio-femoral joint is reduced by serial anteroposterior and lateral radiographs.

The surgical timing guidelines outlined previously should be considered in the context of the individual patient. Many patients with multiple ligament injuries of the knee are severely injured, multiple trauma patients with multisystem injuries. Modifiers to the ideal timing protocols outlined previously include the vascular status of the involved extremity, reduction stability, skin condition, open or closed injury, and other ortho-pedic and systemic injuries. These additional considerations may cause the knee ligament surgery to be performed earlier or later than desired. We have previously reported excellent results with delayed reconstruction in the multiple ligament–injured knee.[10,13]

GRAFT SELECTION

Our preferred graft source for PCL, ACL, posteromedial, and posterolateral reconstruction is allograft tissue. The ALB of the PCL is reconstructed with Achilles tendon allograft, and the PMB of the PCL is reconstructed with tibialis anterior allograft tissue. Posterolateral reconstruction is performed with semiten-dinosus allograft for fibular based reconstructions combined with a posterolateral capsular shift procedure. Fibular head- and tibia-based posterolateral reconstructions are performed with a split Achilles tendon allograft, or semitendinosus allograft for the fibular arm, and a tibialis anterior or semitendinosus allograft for the tibial arm, also combined with a posterolateral capsular shift procedure. ACL reconstruction is performed with Achilles tendon allograft or tibialis anterior allograft. Postero-medial reconstruction is performed with a posteromedial cap-sular shift procedure combined with allograft augmentation as indicated.[8,9,12]

POSTERIOR CRUCIATE LIGAMENT RECONSTRUCTION SURGICAL TECHNIQUE

The patient is positioned on the operating table in the supine position, and the surgical and nonsurgical knees are examined under general or regional anesthesia.[8,10-13] A tourniquet is applied to the operative extremity, and the surgical leg prepared and draped in a sterile fashion. Allograft tissue is prepared prior to beginning the surgical procedure, and autograft tissue is harvested prior to beginning the arthroscopic portion of the procedure. Standard arthroscopic knee portals are used. The joint is thoroughly evaluated arthroscopically, and the PCL evaluated using the three zone arthroscopic technique.[5,26] The PCL tear is identified, and the residual stump of the PCL is débrided.

An extracapsular posteromedial safety incision approxi-mately 1.5 to 2.0 cm long is created. The crural fascia is incised longitudinally, taking precautions to protect the neurovascular structures. The interval is developed between the medial head of the gastrocnemius muscle and the posterior capsule of the knee joint, which is anterior. The surgeon's gloved finger is positioned so that the neurovascular structures are posterior to the finger and the posterior aspect of the joint capsule is anterior to the surgeon's finger. This technique enables the surgeon to monitor surgical instruments, such as the over-the-top PCL

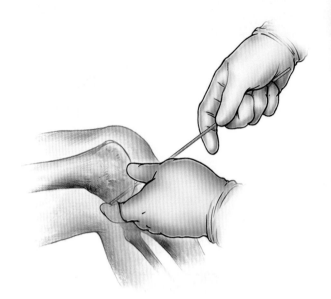

FIG 61.1 The surgeon is able to palpate the posterior aspect of the tibia through the extracapsular extra-articular posteromedial safety incision. This enables the surgeon to accurately position guidewires, create the tibial tunnel, and to protect the neuro-vascular structures. (From Fanelli GC: *Rationale and surgical technique for PCL and multiple knee ligament reconstruction,* ed 3, Warsaw, IN, 2012, Biomet Sports Medicine.)

instruments, and the PCL/ACL drill guide as they are positioned in the posterior aspect of the knee. The surgeon's finger in the posteromedial safety incision also confirms accurate placement of the guidewire prior to tibial tunnel drilling in the mediolat-eral and proximal-distal directions (Fig. 61.1). This is the same anatomic surgical interval that is used in the tibial inlay poste-rior approach.

The curved, over-the-top PCL instruments are used to elevate the posterior knee joint capsule away from the tibial ridge on the posterior aspect of the tibia. This capsular elevation enhances correct drill guide and tibial tunnel placement (Fig. 61.2).

The arm of the Biomet Sports Medicine PCL-ACL Drill Guide (Biomet Sports Medicine, Warsaw, Indiana) is inserted into the knee through the inferior medial patellar portal and positioned in the PCL fossa on the posterior tibia (Fig. 61.3). The bullet portion of the drill guide contacts the anterior medial aspect of the proximal tibia approximately 1 cm below the tibial tubercle, at a point midway between the tibial crest anteriorly and the posterior medial border of the tibia. This drill guide positioning creates a tibial tunnel that is relatively vertically oriented and has its posterior exit point in the inferior and lateral aspect of the PCL tibial anatomic insertion site. This positioning creates an angle of graft orientation such that the graft will turn two very smooth 45-degree angles on the poste-rior aspect of the tibia (Fig. 61.4).

The tip of the guide in the posterior aspect of the tibia is confirmed with the surgeon's finger through the extracapsular posteromedial safety incision. Intraoperative anteroposterior (AP) and lateral x-ray may also be used, as well as arthroscopic visualization to confirm drill guide and guide pin placement. A blunt, spade-tipped guidewire is drilled from anterior to poste-rior and can be visualized with the arthroscope, in addition to

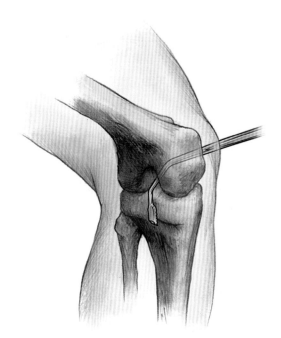

FIG 61.2 Posterior capsular elevation using the Biomet Sports Medicine PCL instruments. (From Fanelli GC: *Rationale and surgical technique for PCL and multiple knee ligament reconstruction,* ed 3, Warsaw, IN, 2012, Biomet Sports Medicine.)

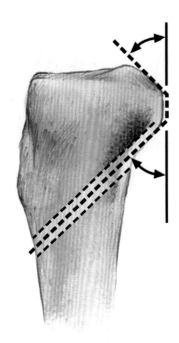

FIG 61.4 Drawing demonstrating the desired turning angles the PCL graft will make after the creation of the tibial tunnel. (From Fanelli GC: *Rationale and surgical technique for PCL and multiple knee ligament reconstruction,* ed 3, Warsaw, IN, 2012, Biomet Sports Medicine.)

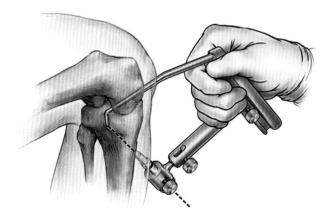

FIG 61.3 Biomet Sports Medicine PCL-ACL drill guide positioned to place guidewire in preparation for creation of the Transtibial PCL tibial tunnel. (From Fanelli GC: *Rationale and surgical technique for PCL and multiple knee ligament reconstruction,* ed 3, Warsaw, IN, 2012, Biomet Sports Medicine.)

being palpated with the finger in the posteromedial safety incision. We consider the finger in the posteromedial safety incision the most important step for accuracy and safety.

The appropriately sized standard cannulated reamer is used to create the tibial tunnel. The closed curved PCL curette may be positioned to capture the tip of the guidewire. The arthroscope, when positioned in the posteromedial portal, may visualize the guidewire being captured by the curette and may help in protecting the neurovascular structures, in addition to the surgeon's finger in the posteromedial safety incision. The reamer is advanced to the posterior cortex of the tibia. The drill chuck is then disengaged from the drill, and completion of the tibial

tunnel reaming is performed by hand. This gives an additional margin of safety for completion of the tibial tunnel. The tunnel edges are chamfered and rasped with the PCL/ACL system rasp.

Double-Bundle Femoral Tunnel Preparation—Outside In

The PCL femoral tunnel may be created from outside in or inside out. Creating the PCL femoral tunnel from outside in, the Biomet PCL/ACL drill guide is positioned to create the femoral tunnel. The arm of the guide is introduced through the inferomedial patellar portal and is positioned such that the guidewire will exit through the center of the stump of the ALB of the PCL (Fig. 61.5A and B). The spade-tipped guidewire is drilled through the guide, and just as it begins to emerge through the center of the stump of the PCL ALB, the drill guide is disengaged. The accuracy of the placement of the wire is confirmed arthroscopically with probing and visualization. Care must be taken to ensure the patellofemoral joint has not been violated by arthroscopically examining the patellofemoral joint prior to drilling and that there is adequate distance between the femoral tunnel and the medial femoral condyle articular surface. The appropriately sized standard cannulated reamer is used to create the femoral tunnel. A curette is used to cap the tip of the guidewire so there is no inadvertent advancement of the guidewire, which may damage the ACL or articular surface. As the reamer is about to penetrate the notch wall, the reamer is disengaged from the drill and the final reaming is completed by hand. This adds an additional margin of safety. The reaming debris is evacuated with a shaver to minimize fat pad inflammatory response with subsequent risk of arthrofibrosis. The tunnel edges are chamfered and rasped.

The Biomet PCL/ACL drill guide is positioned to create the second femoral tunnel. The arm of the guide is introduced

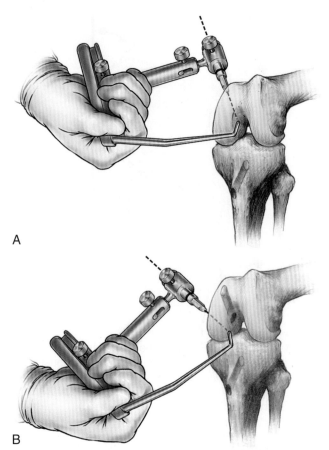

A

B

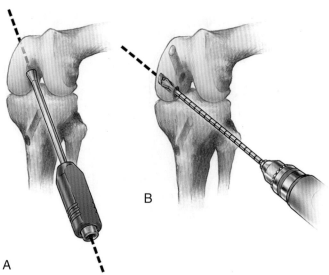

B

A

FIG 61.6 (A) Biomet Sports Medicine double-bundle aimer positioned to drill a guidewire for creation of the PCL PMB femoral tunnel through the low anterolateral patellar portal. (From reference 8, Fanelli GC: *Rationale and surgical technique for PCL and multiple knee ligament reconstruction,* ed 3, Warsaw, IN, 2012, Biomet Sports Medicine). (B) Endoscopic acorn reamer is used to create the PCL PMB through the low anterolateral patellar portal. (From Fanelli GC: *Rationale and surgical technique for PCL and multiple knee ligament reconstruction,* ed 3, Warsaw, IN, 2012, Biomet Sports Medicine.)

FIG 61.5 (A and B) The Biomet Sports Medicine PCL-ACL drill guide is positioned to drill the guidewire from outside in. The guide wire begins at a point half way between the medial femoral epicondyle and the medial femoral condyle trochlea articular margin, approximately 2 to 3 cm proximal to the medial femoral condyle distal articular margin, and exits through the center of the stump of the ALB of the PCL stump. (From Fanelli GC: *Rationale and surgical technique for PCL and multiple knee ligament reconstruction,* ed 3, Warsaw, IN, 2012, Biomet Sports Medicine.)

through the inferior medial patellar portal and is positioned such that the guidewire will exit through the center of the stump of the PMB of the PCL. The blunt spade-tipped guidewire is drilled through the guide, and just as it begins to emerge through the center of the stump of the PCL PMB, the drill guide is disengaged. The accuracy of the placement of the wire is confirmed arthroscopically with probing and visualization. Care must be taken to ensure that there will be an adequate bone bridge (approximately 5 mm) between the two femoral tunnels prior to drilling. This is accomplished using a calibrated probe and direct arthroscopic visualization. The appropriately sized cannulated reamer is used to create the PMB femoral tunnel. Final reaming is completed by hand, and bone debris is removed. The tunnel edges are chamfered and rasped for a smooth transition.

Double-Bundle Femoral Tunnel Preparation—Inside Out

The author's preferred method is to perform a double-bundle PCL reconstruction, making the PCL femoral tunnels from

inside out. The PCL femoral tunnels are made from inside out using the Biomet Sports Medicine double-bundle aimers. Inserting the appropriately sized Biomet Sports Medicine double-bundle aimer through a low anterior lateral patellar arthroscopic portal creates the PCL ALB femoral tunnel. The double-bundle aimer is positioned directly on the footprint of the femoral ALB PCL insertion site. The appropriately sized guidewire is drilled through the aimer, through the bone, and out a small skin incision. Care is taken to ensure there is no compromise of the articular surface. The double-bundle aimer is removed, and an acorn reamer is used to endoscopically drill from inside out the ALB PCL femoral tunnel. The tunnel edges are chamfered and rasped. The reaming debris is evacuated with a shaver. The same process is repeated for the PMB of the PCL. Care must be taken to ensure that there will be an adequate bone bridge (approximately 5 mm) between the two femoral tunnels prior to drilling. This is accomplished using the calibrated probe and direct arthroscopic visualization (Fig. 61.6A and B).

Posterior Cruciate Ligament Graft Passage and Fixation

In preparing for passage of the PCL graft, the Biomet Sports Medicine Magellan suture-passing device is introduced through the tibial tunnel, pulled into the notch region, and retrieved through the femoral tunnel with an arthroscopic grasping tool. The traction sutures of the graft material are attached to the loop of the Magellan suture-passing device, and the PCL graft material is pulled into position.

Fixation of the PCL graft is accomplished with primary and backup fixation on both the femoral and tibial sides. Our most

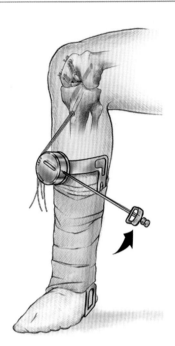

FIG 61.7 Biomet Sports Medicine knee ligament graft-tensioning boot. This mechanical tensioning device uses a ratcheted torque wrench device to assist the surgeon during graft tensioning. (From Fanelli GC: *Rationale and surgical technique for PCL and multiple knee ligament reconstruction,* ed 3, Warsaw, IN, 2012, Biomet Sports Medicine.)

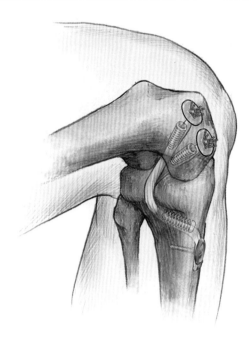

FIG 61.8 Final PCL graft fixation using primary and backup fixation. (From Fanelli GC: *Rationale and surgical technique for PCL and multiple knee ligament reconstruction,* ed 3, Warsaw, IN, 2012, Biomet Sports Medicine.)

commonly used graft source for PCL reconstruction is the Achilles tendon allograft alone for single-bundle reconstructions, and Achilles tendon and tibialis anterior allografts for double-bundle reconstructions. Other graft choices, allograft or autograft, may also be used successfully, as preferred by individual surgeons. Femoral fixation is accomplished with cortical suspensory backup fixation using polyethylene ligament fixation buttons and aperture fixation using Biomet Sports Medicine gentle thread bioabsorbable interference screws. The Biomet Sports Medicine graft tensioning boot is applied to the traction sutures of the graft material on its distal end and tensioned to restore the anatomic tibial step-off. The knee is cycled through several sets of full flexion-extension cycles for graft pretensioning and settling (Fig. 61.7), The PCL graft is tensioned in physiologic knee flexion ranges. Graft fixation is achieved with primary aperture fixation using the Biomet Sports Medicine bioabsorbable interference screw and backup fixation with a ligament fixation button or screw and post or screw and spiked ligament washer assembly (Fig. 61.8).

ANTERIOR CRUCIATE LIGAMENT RECONSTRUCTION

With the knee in approximately 90 degrees of flexion, the ACL tunnels are created using the Biomet PCL/ACL drill guide single incision endoscopic surgical technique. The arm of the Fanelli drill guide enters the knee joint through the inferior medial patellar portal. The bullet of the drill guide contacts the anterior medial proximal tibia externally at a point 1 cm proximal to the tibial tubercle, midway between the posterior medial border of the tibia, and the tibial crest anterior. The guidewire is drilled

through the guide to emerge through the center of the ACL tibial footprint. A standard cannulated reamer is used to create the tibial tunnel. Reaming debris is evacuated, and the tunnel edges are chamfered and rasped.

With the knee in approximately 90 degrees of flexion, an over-the-top femoral aimer is introduced through the tibial tunnel, and used to position a guidewire at the 10 o'clock position (right knee), or 2 o'clock position (left knee) on the medial wall of the lateral femoral condyle. The femoral tunnel is created to approximate the ACL anatomic insertion site, and the offset of the femoral aimer will leave a 1- to 2-mm posterior cortical wall, so interference fixation can be used. The ACL graft is positioned, and fixation is achieved on the femoral side using a Biomet resorbable interference screw and backup fixation with a polyethylene fixation button.

The ACL graft is tensioned on the tibial side using the Biomet graft-tensioning boot. Traction is placed on the ACL graft sutures, and tension is set. The knee is then cycled through full flexion and extension cycles to allow settling of the graft. The process is repeated until there is no further change in the torque setting on the graft tensioner, indicating all laxity is removed from the system. The knee is placed in 20 degrees of flexion, and fixation is achieved on the tibial side of the ACL graft with a resorbable interference screw and back up fixation with Biomet polyethylene ligament fixation button (Fig. 61.9).

Posterolateral Reconstruction Surgical Technique

The free graft, figure-of-eight technique, for posterolateral reconstruction uses semitendinosus autograft or allograft, Achilles tendon allograft, or other soft tissue allograft material. This technique combined with capsular repair and/or posterolateral capsular shift procedures mimics the function of the popliteofibular ligament and lateral collateral ligament, tightens

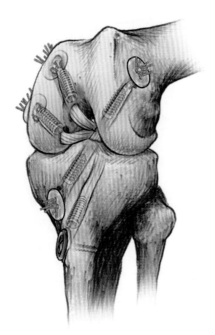

FIG 61.9 ACL reconstruction. (From Fanelli GC: *Rationale and surgical technique for PCL and multiple knee ligament reconstruction,* ed 3, Warsaw, IN, 2012, Biomet Sports Medicine.)

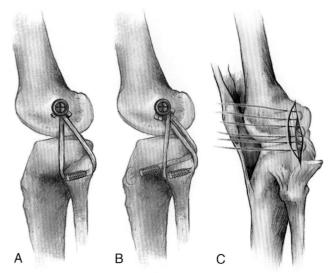

FIG 61.10 (A-C) Posterolateral reconstruction using single- and double-tailed graft. Transfibular head figure-of-eight semitendinosus allograft mimics the force vectors of the fibular collateral ligament and the popliteofibular ligament. Transtibial tibialis anterior allograft mimics the force vectors of the popliteus tendon. Posterolateral capsular shift is also performed. (From Fanelli GC: *Rationale and surgical technique for PCL and multiple knee ligament reconstruction,* ed 3, Warsaw, IN, 2012, Biomet Sports Medicine.)

the posterolateral capsule, and provides a post of strong autogenous tissue to reinforce the posterolateral corner.[†] A curvilinear incision is made in the lateral aspect of the knee extending from the lateral femoral epicondyle to the interval between Gerdy's tubercle and the fibular head. The peroneal nerve is dissected free and protected throughout the procedure. The fibular head is exposed, and a 7-mm tunnel is created in an anterior inferior to posterior superior direction at the area of maximal fibular diameter. The tunnel is created by passing a guide pin followed by a cannulated drill usually 7 mm in diameter. The free tendon graft is then passed through the fibular head tunnel. An incision is made in the iliotibial band in line with the fibers directly overlying the lateral femoral epicondyle. A longitudinal incision is made in the lateral capsule just posterior to the fibular collateral ligament. The graft material is passed deep to the iliotibial band and secured to the lateral femoral epicondylar region with a screw and spiked ligament washer, with the allograft insertion sites corresponding to the anatomic insertion sites of the fibular collateral ligament and the popliteus tendon. The final graft-tensioning position is approximately 30 to 40 degrees of knee flexion. The posterolateral capsule that had been previously incised is then shifted and sewn into the strut of figure-of-eight graft tissue material to eliminate posterolateral capsular redundancy. The anterior and posterior limbs of the figure-of-eight graft material are sewn to each other to reinforce and tighten the construct. The iliotibial band incision is closed.

When there is a disrupted proximal tibiofibular joint or hyperextension external rotation recurvatum deformity, a two-tailed (fibular head, proximal tibia) posterior lateral reconstruction is used.[†] The semitendinosus allograft is passed through the fibular head and secured to the lateral femoral epicondylar

area as described previously. A tibial arm of the reconstruction is passed through a 7-mm drill hole made 2 cm below the joint line through the proximal lateral tibia. This tibial arm of the posterolateral reconstruction follows the course of the popliteus tendon, providing additional support to the posterolateral corner. The procedures described are intended to eliminate posterolateral and varus rotational instability (Fig. 61.10A-C).

Posteromedial and Medial Reconstruction

Posteromedial and medial reconstructions are performed through a medial hockey stick incision (Fig. 61.11A and B). Care is taken to maintain adequate skin bridges between incisions. The superficial MCL is exposed, and a longitudinal incision is made just posterior to the posterior border of the superficial MCL. Care is taken not to damage the medial meniscus during the capsular incision. The interval between the posteromedial capsule and medial meniscus is developed. The posteromedial capsule is shifted anterosuperiorly. The medial meniscus is repaired to the new capsular position, and the shifted capsule is sewn into the MCL. When superficial MCL reconstruction is indicated, this is performed using allograft or autograft tissue. This graft material is attached at the anatomic insertion sites of the superficial MCL on the femur and tibia, using a screw and spiked ligament washer, or suture anchors. The posteromedial capsular advancement is performed and sewn into the newly reconstructed MCL. The final graft-tensioning position is approximately 30 to 40 degrees of knee flexion.[‡]

[†]References 6, 8-10, 12, 13, 23, 25, and 31.

[‡]References 8-10, 12, 13, 24, 25, 29, and 30.

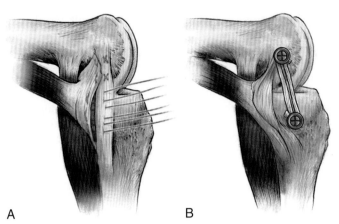

FIG 61.11 (A and B) Posteromedial reconstruction using primary repair, posteromedial capsular shift, and free graft as indicated. (From Fanelli GC: *Rationale and surgical technique for PCL and multiple knee ligament reconstruction,* ed 3, Warsaw, IN, 2012, Biomet Sports Medicine.)

OVERVIEW OF GRAFT TENSIONING AND FIXATION

The PCL reconstruction is commonly performed within the context of the multiple ligament–injured knee. When there are multiple ligaments to be reconstructed, the PCL is reconstructed first, followed by the ACL, followed by the posterolateral complex and medial ligament complex. Tension is placed on the PCL graft distally using the Biomet knee ligament-tensioning device with the knee in full extension, and the tension is set. This reduces the tibiofemoral joint and restores the anatomic tibial step-off. The knee is cycled through a full range of motion to allow pretensioning and settling of the graft. The knee is placed in 70 to 90 degrees of flexion, and fixation is achieved on the tibial side of the PCL graft with a Biomet bioabsorbable interference screw, and bicortical screw and spiked ligament washer. The Biomet knee ligament-tensioning device is applied to the ACL graft and set with the knee in full extension. This reduces the tibiofemoral joint and balances the PCL and ACL reconstructions. The knee is placed in 30 degrees of flexion after cycling, and final fixation is achieved of the ACL graft with a Biomet bioabsorbable interference screw and Biomet polyethylene ligament fixation button for cortical suspensory backup fixation. The knee is placed in 30 to 40 degrees of knee flexion, the tibia slightly internally rotated, slight valgus force applied to the knee, and final tensioning and fixation of the posterolateral corner is achieved. The MCL reconstruction is tensioned with the knee in 30 to 40 degrees of knee flexion with the leg in a supported figure-four position. Full range of motion is confirmed on the operating table.

POSTOPERATIVE REHABILITATION

The knee is maintained in full extension, non–weight bearing for 3 weeks postoperatively in a long leg, hinged knee brace. Progressive range of motion occurs after the third postoperative week. Progressive weight bearing occurs at the beginning of postoperative week 4, progressing at a rate of 20% body weight per week. Progressive closed kinetic chain strength training, proprioceptive training, and continued motion exercises are initiated very

slowly. The long leg range of motion brace is discontinued after the 10th week. Return to sports and heavy labor occurs after the 12th postoperative month when sufficient strength, range of motion, and proprioceptive skills has returned.[2,3,14]

AUTHORS' RESULTS OF POSTERIOR CRUCIATE LIGAMENT RECONSTRUCTION

Fanelli and Edson, in 2004, published the 2- to 10-year (24 to 120 month) results of 41 chronic arthroscopically assisted combined PCL/posterolateral reconstructions evaluated preoperatively and postoperatively using Lysholm, Tegner, and Hospital for Special Surgery (HSS) knee ligament rating scales, KT-1000 arthrometer testing, stress radiography, and physical examination.[18] PCL reconstructions were performed using the arthroscopically assisted single femoral tunnel–single-bundle transtibial tunnel PCL reconstruction technique using fresh frozen Achilles tendon allografts in all 41 cases. In all 41 cases, posterolateral instability reconstruction was performed with combined biceps femoris tendon tenodesis and posterolateral capsular shift procedures. Postoperative physical exam revealed normal posterior drawer/tibial step-off for the overall study group in 29 out of 41 knees (70%). Normal posterior drawer and tibial step-offs were achieved in 91.7% of the knees tensioned with the Biomet Sports Medicine mechanical graft tensioner. Posterolateral stability was restored to normal in 11 out of 41 knees (27%), and tighter than the normal knee in 29 out of 41 knees (71%) evaluated with the external rotation thigh foot angle test. Thirty-degree varus stress testing was normal in 40 out of 41 knees (97%), and grade 1 laxity in 1 out of 41 knees (3%). Postoperative KT-1000 arthrometer mean side-to-side difference measurements were 1.80 mm (PCL screen), 2.11 mm (corrected posterior), and 0.63 mm (corrected anterior). This is a statistically significant improvement from preoperative status for the PCL screen and the corrected posterior measurements ($p = .001$). The postoperative stress radiographic mean side-to-side difference measurement measured at 90 degrees of knee flexion and 32 lb of posterior directed force applied to the proximal tibia using the Telos device was 2.26 mm. This is a statistically significant improvement from preoperative measurements ($p = .001$). Postoperative Lysholm, Tegner, and HSS knee ligament rating scale mean values were 91.7, 4.92, and 88.7, respectively, demonstrating a statistically significant improvement from preoperative status ($p = .001$). The authors concluded that chronic combined PCL/posterolateral instabilities can be successfully treated with arthroscopic PCL reconstruction using fresh frozen Achilles tendon allograft combined with posterolateral corner reconstruction using biceps tendon tenodesis combined with posterolateral capsular shift procedure. Statistically significant improvement is noted ($p = .001$) from the preoperative condition at 2- to 10-year follow-up using objective parameters of knee ligament rating scales, arthrometer testing, stress radiography, and physical examination.

Fanelli et al. in 2005 published the results of allograft multiple ligament knee reconstructions using the Biomet Sports Medicine mechanical graft-tensioning device.[20] The data presents the 2-year follow-up results of 15 arthroscopic assisted ACL/PCL allograft reconstructions using the Biomet Sports Medicine graft-tensioning boot. This study group consists of 11 chronic and 4 acute injuries. These injury patterns included six ACL/PCL/posterolateral corner (PLC) injuries, four ACL/PCL/MCL injuries, and five ACL/PCL/PLC/MCL injuries. All knees had grade III preoperative ACL/PCL laxity and were assessed preoperatively and postoperatively using Lysholm, Tegner, and HSS knee ligament rating scales, KT-1000 arthrometer testing, stress radiography, and physical examination.

Arthroscopically assisted combined ACL/PCL reconstructions were performed using the single incision endoscopic ACL technique, and the single femoral tunnel–single-bundle transtibial tunnel PCL technique. The PCL was reconstructed with allograft Achilles tendon in all 15 knees. The ACL was reconstructed with Achilles tendon allograft in all 15 knees. MCL injuries were treated surgically using primary repair, posteromedial capsular shift, and allograft augmentation when indicated. Posterolateral instability was treated with allograft semitendinosus graft, with or without primary repair, and posterolateral capsular shift procedures as indicated.

Post-reconstruction physical examination results revealed normal posterior drawer/tibial step-off in 13 out of 15 knees (86.6%), normal Lachman test in 13 out of 15 knees (86.6%), and normal pivot shift tests in 14 out of 15 knees (93.3%). Posterolateral stability was restored to normal in all knees with posterolateral instability, when evaluated with the external rotation thigh foot angle test (nine knees equal to the normal knee and two knees tighter than the normal knee). Thirty degrees varus stress testing was restored to normal in all 11 knees with posterolateral lateral instability. Thirty degrees and 0 degrees valgus stress testing was restored to normal in all nine knees with medial side laxity. Postoperative KT-1000 arthrometer testing mean side-to-side difference measurements were 1.6 mm (range: −3 to 7 mm) for the PCL screen, 1.6 mm (range: −4.5 to 9 mm) for the corrected posterior, and 0.5 mm (range: −2.5 to 6 mm) for the corrected anterior measurements, a significant improvement from preoperative status. Postoperative stress radiographic side-to-side difference measurements measured at 90 degrees of knee flexion, and 32 lb of posteriorly directed proximal force using the Telos stress radiography device were 0 to 3 mm in 10 out of 15 knees (66.7%), 4 mm in 4 out of 15 knees (26.7%), and 7 mm in 1 out of 15 knees (6.67%). Postoperative Lysholm, Tegner, and HSS knee ligament rating scale mean values were 86.7 (range: 69 to 95), 4.5 (range: 2 to 7), and 85.3 (range: 65 to 93), respectively, demonstrating a significant improvement from preoperative status.

The authors concluded that the study group demonstrates the efficacy and success of using allograft tissue and a mechanical graft-tensioning device in single-bundle single femoral tunnel arthroscopic PCL reconstruction.

Multiple studies have shown good outcomes with both single-bundle and double-bundle PCL reconstruction.[15,21,34,37] We have published a comparison of the results of arthroscopic transtibial tunnel single-bundle and double-bundle PCL reconstructions using allograft tissue in PCL-based multiple ligament–injured knees.[15]

Ninety consecutive PCL reconstructions were evaluated: 45 single-bundle and 45 double-bundle reconstructions. All PCL reconstructions were performed using the arthroscopically assisted transtibial tunnel PCL reconstruction technique described in this chapter using fresh frozen allograft tissue from the same tissue bank. Achilles tendon allograft was used for the ALB and tibialis anterior allograft for the PMB. The knees were evaluated postoperatively, comparing the single-bundle results to the double-bundle results, with KT-1000 arthrometer testing, three different knee ligament rating scales, and Telos stress radiography.

Postoperative KT-1000 arthrometer mean side-to-side difference measurements were 1.91 mm (PCL screen, 90 degrees), 2.11 mm (corrected posterior, 70 degrees), and 1.11 mm (30 degrees) in the single-bundle group, and 2.46 mm (PCL screen, 90 degrees), 2.94 mm (corrected posterior, 70 degrees), and 0.44 mm (30 degrees) in the double-bundle group ($p = .29, .23,$ and .32, respectively). The postoperative stress radiographic mean side-to-side difference measurement, measured at 90 degrees of knee flexion with 32 lb of posteriorly directed force applied to the proximal tibia using the Telos device, was 2.56 mm in the single-bundle group and 2.36 mm in the double-bundle group ($p = .90$). Postoperative Lysholm, Tegner, and HSS knee ligament rating scale mean values were 90.3, 5.0, and 86.2, respectively, in the single-bundle group and 87.6, 4.6, and 83.3 in the double-bundle group, respectively ($p = .23, .31,$ and .28, respectively). All objective parameters demonstrated no statistically significant difference between the single- and double-bundle PCL reconstructions in both acute ($p = .40$), and chronic ($p = .42$) cases.

We were able to conclude that both the single-bundle and the double-bundle PCL reconstruction surgical techniques using allograft tissue provide successful results in the PCL-based multiple ligament injured knee when evaluated with stress radiography, arthrometer measurements, and knee ligament rating scales.

Our 2- to 18-year postsurgical results in combined PCL, ACL, medial and lateral side knee injuries (global laxity) revealed the following information.[19] Forty combined reconstructions were performed by a single surgeon. Twenty-eight of 40 were available for 2- to 18-year follow-up (70% follow-up rate). The patients were evaluated postoperatively with three different knee ligament rating scales for physical examination and functional capacity (HSS, Lysholm, Tegner). Static stability was assessed postoperatively comparing the normal to the injured knee using the KT-1000 knee ligament arthrometer (PCL screen, corrected posterior, corrected anterior, and 30 degree posterior to anterior translation), and stress radiography at 90 degrees of flexion to assess PCL static stability using the Telos device. All measurements are reported as a side-to-side difference in millimeters comparing the normal to the injured knee. Range of motion, varus and valgus stability, and axial rotation stability of the tibia relative to the femur using the dial test are reported comparing the injured to the normal knee. Incidence of degenerative joint disease and return to preinjury level of function are also reported.

Knee ligament rating scale mean scores were: HSS 79.3 out of 100 (range: 56 to 95), Lysholm 83.8 out of 100 (range: 58 to 100), and Tegner 4 out of 10 (range: 2 to 9). KT-1000 mean side-to-side difference measurements in millimeters were: PCL screen at 90 degrees of knee flexion 2.02 mm (range: 0 to 7 mm), corrected posterior at 70 degrees of knee flexion 2.48 mm (range: 0 to 9 mm), corrected anterior at 70 degrees of knee flexion 0.28 mm (range: −3 to 7 mm), and the 30 degree of knee flexion posterior to anterior translation 1.0 mm (range: −6 to 6 mm). Telos stress radiography at 90 degrees of knee flexion with a posterior displacement force applied to the area of the tibial tubercle mean side-to-side difference measurements in millimeters were 2.35 mm (range: −2 to 8 mm).

Range of motion side-to-side difference mean flexion loss comparing the normal to the injured knee was 14.0 degrees (range: 0 to 38 degrees). There were no flexion contractures. Varus and valgus stability were evaluated on physical examination at hyperextension, 0, and 30 degrees of knee flexion comparing the injured to the normal knee. Symmetrical varus stability was achieved in 93.3% of knees, and symmetrical valgus stability was achieved in 92.6% of knees. The dial test performed at 30 degrees of knee flexion to evaluate axial rotation posterolateral stability comparing the injured to the normal knee was symmetrical in 85.2%, tighter than the normal knee (less external rotation) in 11.1%, and increased laxity (greater external rotation) in 3.7% of knees. Thus posterior lateral axial rotation instability was corrected or overcorrected in 96.3% of knees.

Radiographic posttraumatic degenerative joint disease occurred in 29.6% of injured knees. No degenerative joint disease was found in 70.4% of the injured knees. Postoperatively, patients were able to return to their preinjury level of activity in 59.3% of cases and returned to decreased level of postoperative activity in 40.7% of cases; 93% of patients returned to their preinjury level of activity or one Tegner grade lower level of activity in these severe global laxity knee injuries.

Another study presented the outcomes of knee dislocations with long-term follow-up using the PCL reconstruction surgical technique described in this chapter.[33] This paper presented the outcomes of surgical treatment of knee dislocations with 5- to 22-year follow-up in 44 patients. Knee stability was achieved when evaluated with KT-1000 arthrometer testing (mean: 1.7 mm side-to-side difference), stress radiography (1.9 mm side-to-side difference), physical examination, and knee ligament rating scales. Functional stability was achieved with 92.8% of patients returning to physically demanding work and/or physically demanding recreational activities. In addition, 90.7% of patients lose 0 to 20 degrees of terminal knee flexion; however, this is not a problem with a functionally stable knee. Posttraumatic degenerative joint disease occurs in 22.7% of the knees in this series, with a total knee replacement rate of 6.8%, and the incidence increases as the time from injury increases. This study and the others outlined above demonstrated the long-term effectiveness of the transtibial PCL reconstruction surgical technique.

SUMMARY

Both the single-bundle and double-bundle arthroscopically assisted transtibial PCL reconstruction technique are successful surgical procedures. We have documented results demonstrating statistically significant improvements from preoperative to postoperative status evaluated by physical examination, knee ligament rating scales, arthrometer measurements, and stress radiography. Factors contributing to the success of this surgical technique include identification and treatment of all pathology (especially posterolateral and posteromedial instability), accurate tunnel placement, placement of strong graft material at anatomic graft insertion sites, minimize graft bending, performing final graft tensioning at 70 to 90 degrees of knee flexion using the Biomet Sports Medicine graft tensioning boot, using primary and backup fixation, and the appropriate postoperative rehabilitation program.

KEY REFERENCES

Fanelli GC, editor: *The multiple ligament injured knee. A practical guide to management*, ed 2, New York, 2013, Springer-Verlag.
Fanelli GC, editor: *Posterior cruciate ligament injuries. A practical guide to management*, ed 2, New York, 2015, Springer.

The references for this chapter can also be found on www.expertconsult.com.

62

Posterior Cruciate Ligament Reconstruction: Remnant-Preserving Technique Through the Posteromedial Portal

Sung-Jae Kim, Sung-Hwan Kim

The posterior cruciate ligament (PCL) is the strongest ligament in the knee and provides primary restraint to tibial posterior translation. Although the anatomy and biomechanics of the PCL have been examined in detail, controversy continues regarding the optimal treatment for PCL injuries. If surgical reconstruction is elected, the goals of surgery are to replicate the anatomy and biomechanics of the native PCL. Various surgical options are currently available for PCL reconstruction: transtibial and inlay techniques, single- or double-bundle reconstructions, and one- or two-incision techniques.[32] Surgeons observe preserved continuity of the attenuated PCL in most PCL-insufficient patients.[2,18,23,30,45] In conventional PCL reconstruction the surgeon generally removes the residual stump of the PCL to facilitate visualization and technical performance. Indeed, ligaments around the joints contain mechanoreceptors that are involved in providing the central nervous system with information about joint position and movement.[20] The cruciate ligaments have recently attracted interest and have been studied not only as mechanical and structural stabilizers but also as sensory structures.[11,13,14,20] In addition, it has been suggested that the meniscofemoral ligaments (MFLs) contribute significantly to the cross-sectional area of the PCL complex and act as secondary restraints to tibial posterior translation.[5,34]

Accordingly, it may be of benefit to attempt to preserve the remnant tissue during PCL reconstruction. In this chapter, we describe the scientific rationale, surgical indications, and surgical technique for transtibial PCL reconstruction with remnant preservation.

SCIENTIFIC RATIONALE

Mechanoreceptors in the Posterior Cruciate Ligament

The presence of mechanoreceptors in the cruciate ligaments has led surgeons to suppose that these receptors influence the motor function of the knee joint. Several studies on anterior cruciate ligament (ACL) reconstruction revealed that success of surgery depends not only on the stability of the reconstructed ligament but also on the quality of proprioception.[17,31,37] Unfortunately, in comparison with the ACL, very little research has been carried out exclusively on PCL receptors and proprioception. Franchi et al.[12] found that the PCL possesses a neural network and that mechanoreceptors occupy 1% of the total area of the ligament in histologic study. Afferents from these mechanoreceptors, such as Ruffini endings, Ruffini corpuscles of the Golgi

tendon organlike type, and Pacinian corpuscles, are thought to be involved in the control of proprioception.[8,12,42] Clark and Safran et al.[7,38] reported that proprioception of the affected side was significantly decreased compared with the normal side. In their study, they analyzed the threshold to detection of passive motion (TTDPM) of PCL-injured patients who had not received surgical treatment. Loss of proprioception after ligament injury leads to changes in gait pattern, muscle strength, and timing of muscle activation, which may inhibit protective reflexes and result in degenerative changes.[14]

Mechanoreceptors on the Remnant Fibers

The PCL is known to have better synovial coverage, blood circulation, and healing potential than the ACL.[40,41] Arthroscopic examination of the PCL-insufficient knee usually demonstrates well-maintained continuity of the PCL, even though it might be attenuated.[3,6,19] However, no histologic reports have indicated whether the remnant of the ruptured PCL contains mechanoreceptors. Some studies have revealed the presence of mechanoreceptors even 3 years after ACL injury,[13] and reproducible cortical somatosensory-evoked potentials induced by electrical stimulation were detected in patients with an ACL remnant bridging the femur and tibia or adherent to the PCL.[36] In this respect, the importance of the remnant of the PCL as a proprioceptive organ can be considered similar to that of the ACL. Eguchi et al.[10] documented that proprioceptive function measured by TTDPM during the postoperative follow-up period was maintained over the entire period in patients who underwent PCL reconstruction using remnant-preserving technique. This result was contrary to a previous study by Adachi et al.,[1] which showed that impaired proprioceptive function following surgery did not return to preoperative status until 24 months after surgery in patients who underwent PCL reconstruction without preservation of the remnant.

Functions and Anatomy of the Meniscofemoral Ligaments

The MFLs are composed of the ligament of Humphrey (anterior) and ligament of Wrisberg (posterior), which originate from the posterior horn of the lateral meniscus and insert on the lateral aspect of the medial femoral condyle. The anterior MFL passes anterior to the PCL and attaches adjacent to the femoral condylar articular cartilage, indenting the attachment of the anterolateral fibers of the PCL.[9] The posterior MFL passes posterior to the PCL and attaches proximally, close to the roof of the intercondylar notch.[4] Studies investigating the prevalence of MFLs have shown that 82% to 93% of all knees have at least one MFL, and 26% to 50% possess both.[5,34] The mean strength of the MFLs is approximately 300 N, which is mechanically equivalent to that of the posteromedial bundle of the PCL.[5] Nagasaki et al.[34] reported that the cross-sectional area of MFLs accounted for 17.2% of the area of the PCL proper. Regarding a functional role in knee stability and protection, the slanting arrangement of the MFLs from the posterior horn of the meniscus up to the femoral intercondylar notch can help to withstand a tibial posterior drawer.[15] Amis et al.[4] indicated that the MFLs contributed 28% of the resistance to posterior drawer in the intact knee at 90-degree flexion; this contribution rose to 70% in the PCL-deficient knee. Moran et al.[33] showed that MFLs allowed the posterior horn of the lateral meniscus to be effectively restrained relative to the femur. In some PCL-insufficient knees, where the distal attachment of the MFLs is seen at the relatively mobile lateral meniscus, it is possible for the MFLs to remain intact despite rupture of the PCL.[5] Consequently, preservation of the MFLs may promote stabilization of knees that require PCL reconstruction.

SURGICAL INDICATIONS

Indications for PCL reconstruction are as follows: (1) pain and instability during daily activities of living, with 10 mm or more of increased posterior laxity of the affected knee compared with the intact contralateral knee on posterior stress radiographs or KT-2000 arthrometer (MedMetric Corp., San Diego, California) despite appropriate rehabilitation; and (2) PCL tears combined with other ligament injuries.

SURGICAL TECHNIQUE
Arthroscopic Portals

For more convenient reconstruction of the PCL, three unique portals are used: a high medial parapatellar portal, a far anterolateral portal, and a high posteromedial portal (Fig. 62.1). The high medial parapatellar portal is made first at the highest position on the medial parapatellar line, which is just off the medial edge of the patella tendon and the inferior border of the patella. This portal is more proximal than the conventional anteromedial portal and facilitates access to the attachment area of the PCL through the intercondylar notch, as well as to the posterior capsule, with a 30-degree arthroscope. The far anterolateral portal is made just above the joint line and 5 mm anterior to the lateral femoral condyle. Then, under direct visualization through the high medial parapatellar portal, the high posteromedial portal is made. A spinal needle is inserted through the posteromedial side of the knee as high as possible and just beside the medial gastrocnemius, aiming for the tibial footprint of the PCL. A scalpel is inserted alongside the entry point of the needle and is run parallel with the needle. The back of the scalpel blade should face the femoral condyle to avoid damage to articular cartilage (Fig. 62.2). Through this portal, the tibial attachment of the PCL can be accessed directly while viewing through the intercondylar notch. Furthermore, the high posteromedial portal facilitates excellent visualization of the tibial stump and the posterior capsule as an additional viewing portal.

Tibial Tunnel Preparation

In preparing the tibial footprint of the PCL, the remnant is laterally peeled from the tibial attachment with a narrow osteotome (Fig. 62.3). To create a tibial tunnel, a PCL guide is inserted

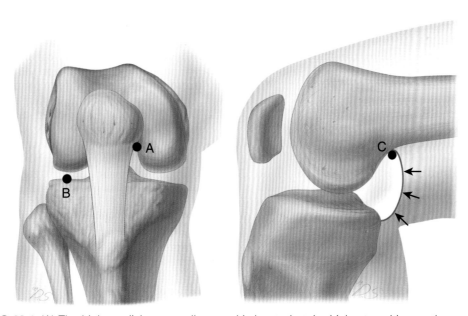

FIG 62.1 (A) The high medial parapatellar portal is located at the highest position on the medial parapatellar line, which is just off the medial edge of the patella tendon and the inferior border of the patella. (B) The far anterolateral portal is made just above the joint line and 5 mm anterior to the lateral femoral condyle. (C) The high posteromedial portal is situated 3 to 5 cm above the joint line and in the superomedial corner of the capsule (*black arrows*).

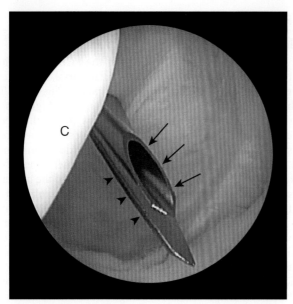

FIG 62.2 Arthroscopic view through the high medial parapatellar portal as the posteromedial portal is created. A scalpel is inserted just beside the entry point of the needle *(black arrows)* and is run parallel with the needle. The back of the scalpel blade *(black arrowheads)* should face the femoral condyle *(C)* to avoid damage to articular cartilage.

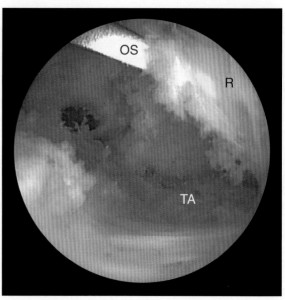

FIG 62.3 Arthroscopic view through the high medial parapatellar portal. The remnant *(R)* is laterally peeled from the tibial attachment *(TA)* with a narrow osteotome *(OS)* through the posteromedial portal.

through the high medial parapatellar portal and is passed through the intercondylar notch while viewing through the high posteromedial portal. The PCL guide is located approximately 1.5 cm below the articular surface and just lateral to the midline on the fossa for the PCL. A 3- to 4-cm longitudinal skin incision is made just lateral to the tibial tuberosity. The tibialis anterior muscle is stripped off and retracted laterally, exposing the starting point of the tibial tunnel 2 cm posterolateral from the anterior tibial crest. Using calibrations on the PCL guide, the distance from the anterolateral cortex of the tibia to the tip of the guide in the fossa for the PCL is accurately measured. The same length as measured on the guide system is marked on the guide pin to prevent past-point drilling (Fig. 62.4). Placement of the guide pin at the ideal site of the PCL footprint is confirmed by visualization through the high posteromedial portal. To enhance visualization during the following procedures, the previously stripped PCL stump and the posterior capsule are pushed back with the arm of the PCL guide. The tibial tunnel is reamed incrementally with a 6- to 11-mm-diameter cannulated reamers. The final tibial tunnel reaming is completed manually to avoid damage to neurovascular structures (Fig. 62.5). Then, chamfering of the upper sharp edge of the aperture is performed using the half-round rasp to reduce abrasion of the graft.

Authors' Tips. In the tibial attachment of the native PCL, the anterolateral fibers are on the anterior (deep) aspect, and the posteromedial fibers are posterior (superficial). Because of this arrangement, when a surgeon performs a single-bundle PCL reconstruction with reproduction of the anterolateral fibers, the graft should be brought up from the tibia underneath (anterior to) the remnant of the PCL.[5] In this respect, lateral peeling of the remnant from the tibial attachment with the osteotome enables not only preservation of the remnant but also

restoration of the anatomic arrangement. In addition, as described earlier, we are in favor of anterolateral tibial tunnel drilling for PCL reconstruction. Concentration of stress from the acutely angled graft at the proximal tibial tunnel margin can cause friction and stretching, followed by failure of the graft during motion against the abrasive edge, in the early postoperative incorporation period. A biomechanical laboratory study showed that the lateral approach for tibial tunnel drilling had the lowest values for maximum shear stress.[28] Moreover, in a cadaveric experiment using pressure films, the lateral tunnel showed a lower reactive force than that of the medial tunnel.[28] A clinical study in our institute supports the superiority of this lateral approach. When cases of anteromedial tibial tunnel and anterolateral tibial tunnel were compared, side-to-side differences in posterior tibial translation were significantly less with the anterolateral tibial tunnel technique (2.87 ± 1.25 mm) than with the anteromedial tibial tunnel technique (3.98 ± 1.27 mm).[21] In addition to decreased stress concentration, technical advantages of the anterolateral tibial tunnel direction include easy inspection of the inside of the tibial tunnel aperture through the posteromedial portal view, making it more convenient to chamfer the abrasive edge (Fig. 62.6), and shorter tibial tunnel length with less surgical damage.

Femoral Socket Preparation

The landmark of the femoral socket is prepared in the center of the footprint of the anterolateral bundle using a blade and osteotome along the fiber direction (Fig. 62.7). This technique minimizes damage to the remnant, including adjacent MFLs. The center of the femoral socket is located 8 mm posterior from the articular junction and at the 10:30 position for the left knee and the 1:30 position for the right knee. A cannulated headed reamer with a plastic sheath is introduced through the far anterolateral portal. The plastic sheath covering the shaft of the reamer prevents damage to the articular surface of the lateral femoral condyle during reaming. To reduce graft socket

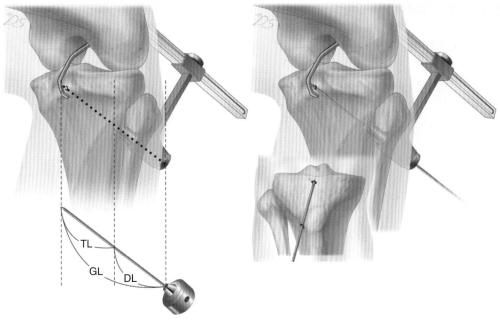

FIG 62.4 (A) The length of the guide pin *(GL)* to prevent past-point drilling is determined as the distance from the anterolateral cortex of the tibia to the tip of the guide tunnel length *(TL)* in the fossa for the posterior cruciate ligament (PCL) plus the length of the device *(DL)*. (B) The ideal site of the PCL footprint is approximately 1.5 cm below the articular surface and just lateral to the midline in the fossa for the PCL. The entry point of the tibial tunnel is 2 cm posterolateral from the anterior tibial crest.

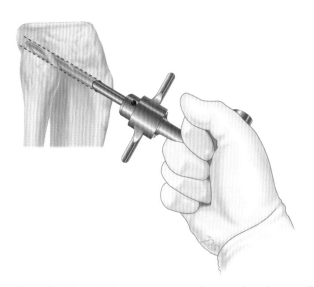

FIG 62.5 The final tibial tunnel reaming is completed manually to avoid damage to neurovascular structures.

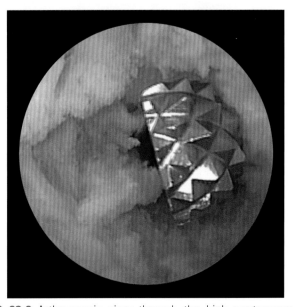

FIG 62.6 Arthroscopic view through the high posteromedial portal. With inspection of the inside of the tibial tunnel aperture, chamfering of the upper sharp edge of the tunnel is performed.

divergence in the femur, the following unique tips are applied: (1) the knee is flexed more than 100 degrees; (2) the proximal tibia is pushed backward as much as possible; and (3) the cannulated headed reamer is introduced through the far anterolateral portal with a plastic sheath, which is pushed posteriorly to contact the lateral femoral condyle (Fig. 62.8). The direction of rotation of the reamer is counterclockwise to allow the socket to be made in the intended location without waggling during reaming and to preserve as much of the PCL remnant as possible. The femoral socket is created to a 35-mm depth, and

chamfering the edge of the femoral socket, especially the posterior half, is important for reducing abrasion.

Authors' Tips. For creation of the femoral tunnel, one-incision (inside-out) and two-incision (outside-in) techniques have been described. We prefer the one-incision technique, which avoids potential injury to the extensor mechanism, especially

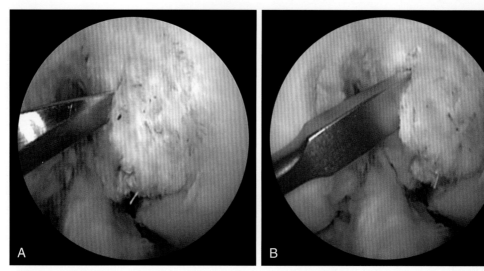

FIG 62.7 Arthroscopic view through the high medial parapatellar portal. The site of the femoral socket is prepared in the center of the footprint of the anterolateral bundle using a blade (A) and an osteotome (B) along the fiber direction.

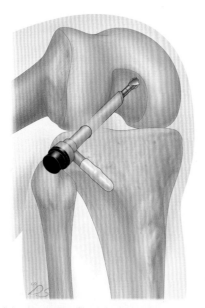

FIG 62.8 With the knee flexed more than 100 degrees and maintaining posterior translation of the proximal tibia, the cannulated headed reamer is introduced through the far anterolateral portal with a plastic sheath to protect the lateral femoral condyle.

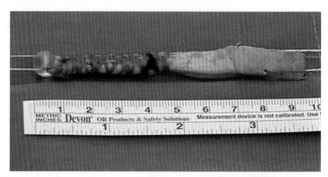

FIG 62.9 The Achilles tendon, of which the tendinous end is to be used for femoral fixation, is threaded in whipstitch fashion for up to 30 mm; then a 9-mm EndoPearl is attached.

the vastus medialis obliquus muscle and the medial patellofemoral ligament.[27] A few authors have alleged that this technique resulted in a greater graft-socket angle, which could lead to attrition of the graft at the edge of the femoral aperture.[16,39] However, this is counteracted by using the three unique tips previously mentioned. A cadaveric three-dimensional model study demonstrated that graft-tunnel angle at the femoral intraarticular aperture using modified inside-out femoral tunneling was significantly increased and maximum contact pressure measured by pressure-sensitive film was also significantly decreased compared with those of tunnel made by conventional inside-out femoral tunneling.[22] A comparison study of one- and two-incision techniques showed no significant postoperative side-to-side differences in posterior translation between the two groups as measured by the KT-1000 or KT-2000 arthrometer (2.38 vs. 2.10 mm; $p = .26$), Lysholm scores (90.6 vs. 90.0; $p = .72$), and Tegner activity level scales (6.5 vs. 6.4; $p = .38$). Moreover, mean Hospital for Special Surgery values were significantly higher in the one-incision group than in the two-incision group (92.6 vs. 87.7; $p = .037$).[27]

Graft Preparation

An Achilles tendon–bone allograft is currently used at our institute because of its high tensile strength, lack of harvest site morbidity, rigid fixation of the osseous end, and short operation time. The bone plug for tibial fixation with the attached Achilles tendon is designed with a width of 11 mm and a length of 25 mm. The Achilles tendon is prepared to be 60 mm in length and 11 mm in width. The end of the Achilles tendon that is to be used for femoral fixation is threaded in whipstitch fashion for up to 30 mm, then a 9-mm EndoPearl (Linvatec, Largo, Florida) is attached to the tip of the tendon to enhance fixation strength (Fig. 62.9).[43]

Graft Passage

The curved portion of plastic tube (intravenous tube) connected to a passing suture is passed through the tibial tunnel and pulled out through a cannula in the far anterolateral portal, using a grasper (Fig. 62.10). A Beath pin is introduced into the femoral socket through the cannula in the far anterolateral portal and then is drilled further through the medial femoral cortex to exit through the skin anteromedially. The passing suture is threaded into the eyelet of the Beath pin, and the pin is pulled out of the medial femoral condyle (Fig. 62.11). The leading suture of the graft is tied to the tibial end of the passing suture and is pulled out of the medial femoral condyle. Then, under arthroscopic guidance, the leading suture is pulled to pass

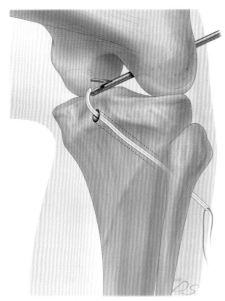

FIG 62.10 A plastic tube (intravenous tube) connected to a passing suture is passed through the tibial tunnel and pulled out using a grasper.

the graft from distal to proximal, and the graft is engaged into the femoral socket.

Graft Fixation

Femoral fixation is achieved with an absorbable interference screw through the far anterolateral portal, with the knee at 100 degrees of flexion. The graft is pretensioned through a range of motion 20 times. This cyclic motion helps to precondition the graft and eliminates creep.[35] The distal bone peg is secured with an absorbable interference screw, with the knee in 70 degrees of flexion while an anteriorly directed force is applied to restore the normal anterior tibial step-off (Fig. 62.12).

ADDITIONAL SURGERY

Most PCL injuries are accompanied by a posterolateral corner injury or a medial injury. PCL reconstruction is performed first, followed by posterolateral or medial reconstruction. We have developed and use the following techniques.[25,26]

For posterolateral corner insufficiency, lateral collateral ligament (LCL) and popliteus tendon (PT) reconstructions are performed with tibialis posterior tendon (TPT) allograft (Fig. 62.13). A cryopreserved TPT allograft longer than 260 mm long is placed in warm saline 30 minutes before surgery for complete thawing. A skin incision is made on the lateral aspect of the knee just anterior to the fibular head and is extended proximally to the lateral femoral epicondyle in an extended position. The interval between the iliotibial tract and the biceps tendon is dissected. The lateral epicondyle of the femur, the fibular head, the posterolateral corner of the tibia, and the lateral head of the gastrocnemius muscle are exposed. Using an ACL guide, the tip is placed on the point 10 mm inferior to the posterior joint line and 5 mm medial to the posterior aspect of the tibiofibular joint, and the anterior portion is placed on Gerdy's tubercle. A guide pin is inserted under fluoroscopic guidance. The tunnel is created with a 7-mm-diameter cannulated reamer. A double-stranded looped wire is inserted into the tibial tunnel in an anterior-to-posterior direction. Then, using the ACL guide, the

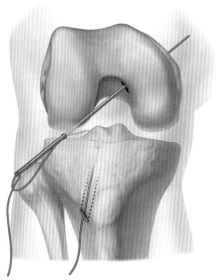

FIG 62.11 The Beath pin is pulled out of the medial femoral condyle with the passing suture.

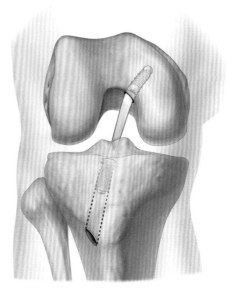

FIG 62.12 Final graft fixation is achieved with absorbable interference screws.

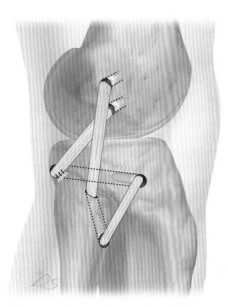

FIG 62.13 For posterolateral corner insufficiency, lateral collateral ligament and popliteus tendon reconstructions are performed with posterior tibialis tendon allograft.

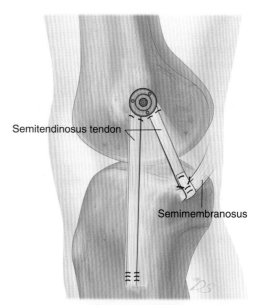

FIG 62.14 For medial instability, medial collateral ligament and posterior oblique ligament reconstructions are performed using the autogenous semitendinosus tendon with preservation of its tibial attachment.

tip is placed at the point just posteromedial to the LCL of the fibular head, and the other end is placed at the anteroinferior aspect of the fibular head 10 mm above the peroneal nerve. The tunnel is at an angle of 70 degrees to the axial plane in an anteroinferior-to-posterosuperior direction. The direction of rotation of the reamer is counterclockwise, avoiding cortical destruction of the fibular head and peroneal nerve injury. A double-stranded looped wire is passed through the fibular tunnel in a posterior-to-anterior direction. To make the leading portion of the graft, the TPT is sutured from the tip with a whipstitch technique. A no. 2 Ethibond suture is whipstitched at the other end of the tendon for approximately 25 mm, and a 7-mm-diameter EndoPearl device is attached to the end. Using the looped wire in the tibial tunnel, the leading suture of the graft is pulled anteriorly through the tibia; then, using the same method, the graft is passed posteriorly through the fibular tunnel. The graft is fixed in the tibial and fibular tunnels using bioabsorbable interference screws through the anterior aperture, respectively.

The lateral femoral epicondyle is then exposed. The position of the patient is changed to lateral decubitus to eliminate the gravitational force of the lower leg in the supine position, and 0.045-inch Kirschner wires are provisionally inserted at tentative isometric points. A PT insertion site is placed at the superior margin of the anterior one-third portion of the popliteal sulcus, which is located approximately 15 mm distal to the femoral epicondyle. An LCL insertion site is placed at the anterosuperior lateral femoral epicondyle. Isometricity is confirmed by migration of less than 2 mm during flexion and extension of the knee. A femoral socket, 40 mm in depth, is created with a 7-mm-diameter cannulated reamer in the anterosuperior direction to the transverse line of the femoral shaft at an angle of 20 degrees for the PT socket and LCL socket, respectively. Using a Beath pin, the graft for the PT, which was passed underneath the LCL, is pulled through the femoral socket and then is fixed at the femur using a bioabsorbable interference screw. The distal popliteal

graft is sutured to the posterosuperior ligamentous tissue of the fibular head to restore the popliteofibular ligament. The other band of graft from the fibular head is managed and fixed using the same method for LCL reconstruction.

For medial instability, medial collateral ligament (MCL) and posterior oblique ligament (POL) reconstructions are performed using the autogenous semitendinosus tendon (ST) with preservation of its tibial attachment (Fig. 62.14). A curvilinear skin incision is made from a point 3 cm proximal to the medial femoral epicondyle to the insertion of the pes anserinus. The fascia is incised along the anterior border of the sartorius muscle, in line with the muscle fibers, and the sartorius and gracilis are retracted medially. After the ST is exposed, the tendon fibers attached to the medial head of the gastrocnemius are carefully dissected to prevent premature cutting of the tendon. The ST is transected at the musculotendinous junction, and then the proximal end of the tendon is whipstitched with a no. 2 Ethibond suture for a 2-cm length. The accessory tibial insertion of the tendon is dissected for the graft to overlap with the anterior bundle of the MCL. A 0.045-inch Kirschner wire is inserted tentatively at the anterior half of the medial femoral epicondyle. After the ST is looped around the wire, isometricity is tested by pulling the suture at the tendon end during flexion and extension of the knee. After the isometric point is confirmed, a 3.2-mm hole is drilled 9 mm (the radius of a washer) proximally. After decortication under the washer, a 6.5-mm-diameter cancellous screw and an 18-mm washer are placed in the drill hole. The ST is looped around the shank of the screw to allow fixation of the tendon at the isometric point on the epicondyle. The screw is tightened with the knee in 30 degrees flexion. After dissection to find the insertion of the direct head of the semimembranosus (SM), the free end of the graft is pulled through the bisected insertion of the direct head to overlap the central arm of the POL. In 30 degrees of knee flexion the end of the graft is fixed by no. 2 Ethibond sutures at the insertion of the direct head of the SM. Additional suture fixation using absorbable sutures is done at the femoral and tibial insertion of the MCL and at the proximal insertion of the POL.

POSTOPERATIVE REHABILITATION

The reconstructed graft is protected by immobilization in extension with a hinge knee brace for 4 weeks with passive range-of-motion exercise allowed three times a day. Isometric quadriceps-strengthening exercise and mobilization of the patella are initiated immediately after surgery. Toe-touch weight bearing is allowed for the first 4 weeks; then patients are allowed to bear their weight and flex their knee as tolerated, with progressive increase in flexion to 90 degrees. At 8 weeks the brace is removed, and closed kinetic chain exercise is started; after 12 weeks, swimming and cycling are permitted. Return to sports involving jumping, pivoting, or side-stepping is permitted after 6 months.

CLINICAL RESULTS

The number of reports on the clinical outcomes of PCL reconstruction using the remnant-preserving technique is a growing trend in recent years. Although most of reports were limited to case series, these reports in which single- or double-bundle PCL reconstruction was performed and accompanied with remnant preservation in various method, have showed good outcomes in postoperative follow-up.[2,18,29,30,44]

As a comparative study, the clinical outcomes of double-bundle PCL reconstruction (DB) and transtibial single-bundle PCL reconstruction with remnant preservation (rSB) were compared by Kim et al.[23] The study subjects consisted of 42 patients who had undergone PCL reconstruction using either technique (rSB group, 33 patients; DB group, 19 patients) combined with anatomic reconstruction of the LCL and PT for posterolateral corner insufficiency. The mean follow-up period was 51.2 months in the rSB group and 44.5 months in the DB group. No significant differences were reported between rSB and DB groups in mean side-to-side differences in posterior laxity as measured with Telos stress radiographs (4.2 vs. 3.9 mm; $p = .628$) and KT-2000 arthrometer (2.9 vs. 1.4 mm; $p = .400$) at latest follow-up. Average Lysholm knee scores were 85.7 in the rSB group and 87.7 in the DB group ($p = .392$). No significant difference was noted between the two groups in IKDC knee score ($p = .969$). Conclusions of this study were that DB combined with posterolateral corner reconstruction did not seem to have advantages over rSB combined with posterolateral corner reconstruction in terms of clinical outcomes or posterior stability. Recently, Kim et al.[24] retrospectively evaluated 53 cases of PCL reconstruction with simultaneous posterolateral corner reconstruction. Of these, 23 cases were performed with a conventional approach without remnant preservation (group C), and 30 cases incorporated a remnant-preserving technique (group R). The mean side-to-side differences in posterior tibial translation, Lysholm knee score, return to activity, and objective IKDC grade were tiny between group C and group R. However, the final Tegner activity scale, near–return to activity, and subjective IKDC score differed significantly between group C (3.5 ± 0.8; 43.5%; 64.5 ± 8.8, respectively) and group R (4.3 ± 1.1; 73.3%; 70.6 ± 7.9; $p = .007, .028, .012$, respectively). Conclusively, techniques combining remnant-preserving transtibial single-bundle PCL reconstruction with posterolateral corner reconstruction were followed by better activity-related outcomes compared with those of approaches without remnant preservation. However, incorporation of remnant preservation does not seem to provide increased posterior stability or result in clinically better outcomes versus techniques without remnant preservation.

CONCLUSIONS

During the past two decades, arthroscopic technology has advanced and the anatomy and biomechanics of the cruciate ligaments have been elucidated. This allows surgeons to preserve the remnants of cruciate ligaments during arthroscopic ligament reconstruction. Although remnant-preserving PCL reconstruction is more demanding than the conventional technique and consensus regarding clinical improvement has not yet been reached, preserving the remnants as much as possible deserves consideration with respect to restoring proprioceptive, sensory, and mechanical functions. Additional investigations are needed to clearly define the benefits of preserving remnants in PCL reconstruction.

ACKNOWLEDGMENTS

The authors thank Dae-Young Lee, MD, for contributions with his view and comments to the manuscript.

KEY REFERENCES

3. Ahn JH, Nha KW, Kim YC, et al: Arthroscopic femoral tensioning and posterior cruciate ligament reconstruction in chronic posterior cruciate ligament injury. *Arthroscopy* 22(3):341, e341–e344, 2006.

4. Amis AA, Bull AM, Gupte CM, et al: Biomechanics of the PCL and related structures: posterolateral, posteromedial and meniscofemoral ligaments. *Knee Surg Sports Traumatol Arthrosc* 11(5):271–281, 2003.

5. Amis AA, Gupte CM, Bull AM, et al: Anatomy of the posterior cruciate ligament and the meniscofemoral ligaments. *Knee Surg Sports Traumatol Arthrosc* 14(3):257–263, 2006.

7. Clark P, MacDonald PB, Sutherland K: Analysis of proprioception in the posterior cruciate ligament-deficient knee. *Knee Surg Sports Traumatol Arthrosc* 4(4):225–227, 1996.

10. Eguchi A, Adachi N, Nakamae A, et al: Proprioceptive function after isolated single-bundle posterior cruciate ligament reconstruction with remnant preservation for chronic posterior cruciate ligament injuries. *Orthop Traumatol Surg Res* 100(3):303–308, 2014.

11. Fontbote CA, Sell TC, Laudner KG, et al: Neuromuscular and biomechanical adaptations of patients with isolated deficiency of the posterior cruciate ligament. *Am J Sports Med* 33(7):982–989, 2005.

13. Georgoulis AD, Pappa L, Moebius U, et al: The presence of proprioceptive mechanoreceptors in the remnants of the ruptured ACL as a possible source of re-innervation of the ACL autograft. *Knee Surg Sports Traumatol Arthrosc* 9(6):364–368, 2001.

14. Grassmayr MJ, Parker DA, Coolican MR, et al: Posterior cruciate ligament deficiency: biomechanical and biological consequences and the outcomes of conservative treatment. A systematic review. *J Sci Med Sport* 11(5):433–443, 2008.

19. Jung YB, Jung HJ, Tae SK, et al: Tensioning of remnant posterior cruciate ligament and reconstruction of anterolateral bundle in chronic posterior cruciate ligament injury. *Arthroscopy* 22(3):329–338, 2006.

20. Katonis P, Papoutsidakis A, Aligizakis A, et al: Mechanoreceptors of the posterior cruciate ligament. *J Int Med Res* 36(3):387–393, 2008.

21. Kim SJ, Chang JH, Kang YH, et al: Clinical comparison of anteromedial versus anterolateral tibial tunnel direction for transtibial posterior cruciate ligament reconstruction: 2 to 8 years' follow-up. *Am J Sports Med* 37(4):693–698, 2009.

22. Kim SJ, Chun YM, Kim SH, et al: Femoral graft-tunnel angles in posterior cruciate ligament reconstruction: analysis with 3-dimensional models and cadaveric experiments. *Yonsei Med J* 54(4):1006–1014, 2013.

23. Kim SJ, Jung M, Moon HK, et al: Anterolateral transtibial posterior cruciate ligament reconstruction combined with anatomical reconstruction of posterolateral corner insufficiency: comparison of single-bundle versus double-bundle posterior cruciate ligament reconstruction over a 2- to 6-year follow-up. *Am J Sports Med* 39(3):481–489, 2011.

24. Kim SJ, Kim SH, Chun YM, et al: Clinical comparison of conventional and remnant-preserving transtibial single-bundle posterior cruciate ligament reconstruction combined with posterolateral corner reconstruction. *Am J Sports Med* 40(3):640–649, 2012.

31. Lee BI, Min KD, Choi HS, et al: Immunohistochemical study of mechanoreceptors in the tibial remnant of the ruptured anterior cruciate ligament in human knees. *Knee Surg Sports Traumatol Arthrosc* 17(9):1095–1101, 2009.

The references for this chapter can also be found on www.expertconsult.com.

63

The Dislocated Knee

Jonathan N. Watson, Verena M. Schreiber, Christopher D. Harner, Volker Musahl

INTRODUCTION

Traumatic knee dislocations (KDs) represent a rare but serious injury to the lower extremity because the damage to multiple soft tissues and stabilizing structures can potentially be limb threatening. Traumatic KDs can be caused by multiple mechanisms. High-energy trauma, as seen in motor vehicle accidents, can result in greater damage to the structures of the knee. Low-velocity KDs generally occur in the setting of sports. Some studies have noted that up to 40% of KDs can happen in overweight patients sustaining low-energy trauma or ultra–low-velocity injuries, such as falling on even ground or slipping while walking.[17,24,54,68,81] The yearly incidence ranges from 1/10,000 to 1/100,000 at various institutions, which accounts for approximately 0.02% to 0.1% of all orthopedic injuries.[7,62] However, this number likely underestimates the true incidence because an unknown percentage of KDs spontaneously reduce and therefore can be missed on initial presentation.[36,76] Dislocations are defined as a complete disruption of the tibiofemoral articulation and result in multiligamentous knee injury. Multiligamentous knee injuries are defined as the rupture of at least two of the four major knee ligament structures (eg, the anterior cruciate ligament [ACL] and posterior cruciate ligament [PCL], posterolateral corner [PLC], and medial collateral ligament [MCL]).[6,34,66,69,80] This is in contrast to subluxations, which are defined as partial disruption of the joint with some tibiofemoral contact remaining.

Dislocations that spontaneously reduce before evaluation can be classified according to the structures that are disrupted. Depending on the mechanism, associated injuries are common and may include injuries to neurovascular structures, in particular the popliteal artery, as well the popliteal vein and tibial and peroneal nerves. In their systematic review, Medina et al. reported an incidence of 18% of associated vascular injuries and 25% of associated nerve injuries.[41] Robertson et al. found common peroneal nerve palsy following KD in 5% to 40%.[64] In addition, the risk of compartment syndrome is increased. Therefore the potential for catastrophic complications is high, and these injuries require timely and accurate diagnosis, stabilization, and treatment.

In the acute setting, treatment goals include prompt reduction and stabilization of the knee joint and, if necessary, revascularization. Initial stabilization should be temporary, and assessment of the patient's neurovascular status should not be delayed. Failure to restore vascularization within 6 to 8 hours increases the risk for amputation and should therefore not be delayed.[18,52,55] Historically most patients were managed nonoperatively; however, more recent literature shows that this results in inferior outcomes in comparison with surgical management.[11,13,34,50,85] In addition, Dedmond and Almekinders[11] showed that surgical management had improved Lysholm scores and range of motion, whereas Levy and Marx[34] found significantly better International Knee Documentation Committee (IKDC) scores, as well as higher return to work and sports rates.

Current treatment approaches include acute, staged repair/reconstruction and chronic reconstruction. There are still controversies in terms of timing of surgery, graft selection, surgical techniques, and rehabilitation.[34] Current literature favors early over staged surgical intervention because better outcomes were seen with early treatment.[20,47]

Because of the severity of these injuries, patients typically require an extensive preoperative workup to identify the specifics of the injury. Meticulous preoperative planning is required to ensure medical stability for surgery. The surgeon must prioritize their evaluation and workup with attention to factors that may predicate early surgical intervention. Initial evaluation that reveals open dislocation, irreducible dislocation, arterial injury, or compartment syndrome requires emergent surgical intervention.

VASCULAR INJURIES

The anatomy of the popliteal artery and vein is critical in understanding the pathophysiology of injury with dislocations. The popliteal artery is the main blood supply to the leg and is the continuation of the superficial femoral artery, which passes through the adductor canal into the popliteal fossa. The artery is tethered proximally at the adductor hiatus and distally by a fibrous arch from the soleus, which increases its susceptibility of injury (Fig. 63.1). The popliteal artery sends off many branches, including the superior medial, superior lateral, inferior medial, inferior lateral, and middle geniculate arteries. Other, less commonly injured structures during dislocation include the medial geniculate, anterior tibial, posterior tibial, superficial femoral, and common femoral arteries.[41]

Two recent reviews noted the incidence of vascular injury after KD, ranging from 3% to 18%.[41,48] These injuries occurred most often in the 20- to 40-year-old age group. Approximately 13% of these injuries required vascular repair in one study, whereas another quoted up to 80%. Vascular injuries associated with KDs represent a surgical emergency, and their care takes precedence over management of the musculoskeletal injuries. Reduction of KDs should be attempted immediately to decrease rates of vascular injury. Delays in care can be disastrous, with one study reporting an increase in amputation rates from 13%

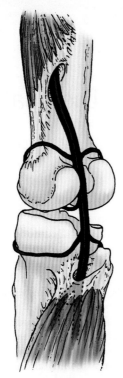

FIG 63.1 Anatomy of the popliteal artery posterior to the knee joint. (From Bloom MH: Traumatic knee dislocation. In Chapman MW (ed): *Operative orthopaedics*, Philadelphia, 1988, JB Lippincott, p 1636. Reprinted with permission of Michael W. Chapman.)

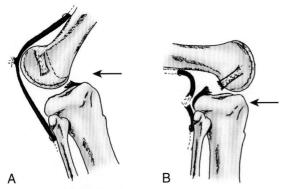

FIG 63.2 Mechanism for popliteal artery injury for anterior (A) and posterior (B) dislocations.

to 86% when revascularization was delayed for longer than 8 hours post injury.[18] Amputation can result from infection or ischemia related to failed repair or secondary to prolonged ischemia or neurovascular deficit. The Lower Extremity Assessment Project (LEAP) cohort had a 20% incidence of amputation in patients with a KD and vascular injury.[52]

There is an equivalent rate of arterial injury regardless of whether the direction of dislocation is anterior or posterior. Theoretically, anterior dislocations can lead to traction injuries and intimal tears, whereas posterior dislocations are thought to have a higher association with arterial transection (Fig. 63.2). In a cadaveric study, Kennedy noted that anterior dislocations were more often associated with intimal injuries because of the vessel stretch over the distal femur.[25] Posterior dislocations

resulted in transection secondary to the thrust of the tibia posteriorly into the vessel. One must be very careful in assessing potential vessel injuries because a KD with spontaneous reduction has the same risk for a vessel injury as does an unreduced KD, so the initial evaluation must always assume that the injury has been a dislocation with potential vascular injury.

A variety of diagnostic studies can aid in diagnosing a vascular injury, including ankle-brachial index (ABI), magnetic resonance angiography (MRA), and arteriography. Physical examination with palpation of the dorsalis pedis and tibialis posterior pulses is the essential first step. Stannard et al. used physical exam to determine the need for angiography.[72] The authors assessed 134 knees with physical examination and found a 7% prevalence of arterial injury. None of the patients with normal examinations developed any vascular complications. There was only one patient with false-positive physical exam findings. Mills et al. examined the accuracy of the ABI in 38 patients with KDs.[43] Patients with an ABI less than 0.9 underwent arteriography and those with an ABI greater than 0.9 underwent serial exams or duplex ultrasonography. All of those who underwent arteriography had a vascular injury requiring surgical repair, and none of the patients with an ABI greater than 0.9 were diagnosed with a vascular injury. Tocci et al. compared MRA to ABI and angiography in evaluating vascular injuries.[75] They prospectively evaluated 16 patients, performing angiography in those with ABI greater than 0.9 and serial physical exams with MRA in those with ABI greater than 0.9. They showed that ABI had 100% sensitivity for vascular injury and argued that MRA could be performed instead of angiography to decrease morbidity. Klineberg et al. argued that use of routine angiography to detect vascular injuries associated with KDs was not necessary.[28] In their study, 57 patients were assessed with physical exam, with an abnormal examination getting arteriography. Forty-eight percent of those who underwent arteriography had a vascular injury. In those with a normal exam, 41% underwent arteriography, with the remaining followed with serial clinical exams. None of these patients had a vascular injury. In addition to arterial injury, venous injury can also result from a KD. It is imperative to obtain an ultrasound to rule out deep venous thrombosis (DVT) prior to any surgical intervention. In conclusion, physical exam and ABI are important initial methods for diagnosis of vascular injuries. When in doubt, it is prudent to obtain computed tomography angiography (CTA) or an arteriogram for diagnosis.[66]

NEUROLOGIC INJURIES

Neurologic injury associated with a KD can be a devastating complication. A systematic review noted the frequency of nerve injury after dislocation to be approximately 25%.[41] Peskun et al. found that elevated body mass index (BMI), fibular head fracture, and vascular injury were the only variables associated with nerve injury, whereas younger age was associated with recovery.[56] The nerves that can be injured during a dislocation include the common peroneal nerve and rarely the tibial nerve. The peroneal nerve is tethered around the fibular head, which puts it at the greatest risk of injury (Fig. 63.3). A thorough neurovascular examination documenting strength and sensation is critical even in cases in which the KD presents spontaneously reduced. The use of electromyography (EMG) is limited in the immediate post-injury period because changes secondary to nerve injury do not appear for 2 to 3 weeks.

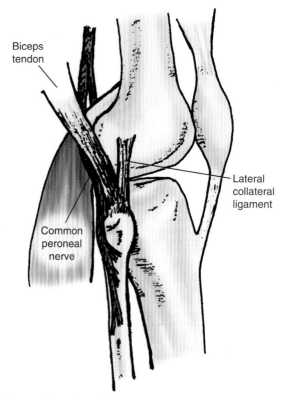

FIG 63.3 Anatomy of peroneal nerve near the knee joint.

Biceps
tendon

Lateral
collateral
ligament

Common
peroneal
nerve

Treatment options for peroneal nerve injury include physical therapy to prevent contractures, bracing with an ankle-foot orthosis (AFO), surgical exploration with neurolysis, primary repair, nerve grafting, and tendon transfers.[23] Surgical exploration with neurolysis has been advocated at time of ligamentous reconstruction if approximately 3 weeks post injury. Complete injuries are also an indication for early surgical exploration. Kim et al. performed neurolysis in 121 patients, half of which in stretch or contusion injuries, with 88% obtaining motor recovery of $\geq$ grade 3. Primary nerve repair or nerve grafting are also options in complete injuries.[27] Molund et al. performed posterior tibial tendon transfers for treatment of peroneal nerve palsy.[44] The authors found a significant improvement in dorsiflexion strength, range of motion, and a mean 6-minute walking test improvement compared with 90% of age-matched controls.

CLASSIFICATION

Two accepted classification systems have been used to describe KDs: descriptive and anatomic. The authors' preference is to use the anatomic classification because this is more accurate in predicting associated injuries and planning for surgical intervention.

Anatomic

The Schenck classification is an anatomic classification based on which ligamentous structure(s) are torn.[61] This system has the advantage that all KDs can be grouped into this classification, and it helps to guide treatment and outcomes. Each KD type is ordered by Roman numeral. A KD-I injury is a cruciate intact injury, including both ACL intact and PCL intact

dislocations. A KD-II is a bicruciate injury with functionally intact collateral ligaments. KD-III is the most common subtype and involves tears of both cruciate ligaments and one of the collateral ligaments. These injuries are subdivided into KD-IIIM and KD-IIIL, which denote medial and lateral injuries, respectively. KD-IV involves complete disruption of both cruciate and both collateral ligaments. KD-V is a knee fracture dislocation, which is a KD in the presence of a major periarticular fracture. Subtypes are also used to denote neurovascular injuries. A subtype C indicates an arterial injury, and subtype N indicates a nerve injury.

EVALUATION

Acute KDs require an expeditious but thorough evaluation consisting of a targeted history and physical examination, paying particular attention to the mechanism of injury and potential associated injuries. Evaluation of patients with multiple ligamentous knee injuries requires a high index of suspicion to exclude the possibility of KD followed by spontaneous reduction. There exist two distinct categories of KD patients: those seen acutely in the emergency room and those seen as an outpatient in the office setting. Patients presenting to an emergency room require adequate resuscitation per Advanced Trauma Life Support (ATLS) protocol followed by careful inspection of the limb, skin integrity, color, vascular assessment, and both visual and tactile joint examination. If the knee is found to be acutely dislocated, it is imperative to perform and document a detailed neurovascular examination without delay in reduction.[40,57,80] If spontaneous reduction occurred, significant swelling and ecchymosis can be suggestive of capsular disruption. In addition, it can be difficult to perform stability tests in the acutely painful joint.

The extremity distal to the involved knee should be examined thoroughly for color, temperature, and capillary refill. Posterior tibial and dorsalis pedis pulses are palpated and compared with the contralateral side. ABI measurements are performed to establish a baseline and for diagnostic purposes. Specific algorithms for diagnosis of vascular injuries are described in a previous section of this chapter.

With regards to the peroneal nerve, sensation in the distribution of both the superficial and deep peroneal nerves should be assessed, and the peroneal nerve motor function graded and documented because common peroneal nerve palsy is found in 5% to 40% of all KDs[64] and most commonly occurs in posterolateral dislocations.[25,70]

Unlike vascular compromise, injury to the common peroneal nerve does not represent a surgical emergency. It is important to keep in mind that injury to this nerve may result in foot drop and gait impairment, in addition to sensory loss. Woodmass et al.[84] performed a systematic review and found that most patients with an incomplete palsy will regain full motor recovery, whereas less than 40% of all patients with a complete palsy will regain the ability to dorsiflex the ankle with an overall poor outcome.

After performing a history and physical examination, radiographs should be obtained to determine the direction of dislocation and assess for concomitant bony injury. Following reduction maneuvers, radiographs should be obtained again to verify the reduction and rule out any additional osseous trauma. If the knee is grossly unstable following reduction and it cannot be maintained in a splint, a joint-spanning external

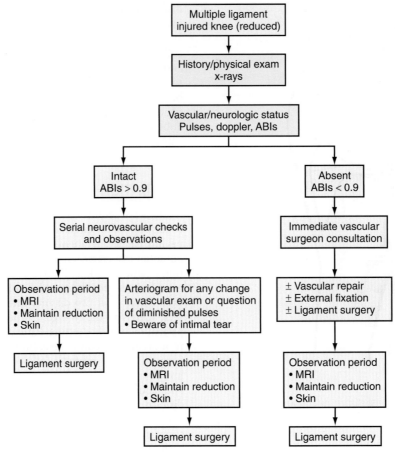

FIG 63.4 Treatment algorithm for the multiligamentous-injured knee. *ABI,* Ankle-brachial index; *MRI,* magnetic resonance imaging.

fixator should be applied. This is also true for open dislocations, as well as dislocations requiring vascular repair. External fixation allows for frequent skin, compartment, and neurovascular checks.[33]

When the patient is medically stable and a complete neurovascular examination has been performed, more attention can be focused on the ligamentous damage to the knee. In the acute setting, it is often difficult to perform a thorough clinical ligamentous examination secondary to the significant pain and edema. However, a knee that has limited motion from 0 to 30 degrees can be assessed for varus-valgus instability, Lachman test, and integrity of the extensor mechanism. The Lachman test is the gold standard for testing the integrity of the ACL. The PCL is tested with the posterior drawer and sag tests, and the collateral ligaments are assessed with varus/valgus stress to the knee joint both in full extension and 30 degrees of flexion. In addition, the PLC should be evaluated with the external rotation dial test at 30 and 90 degrees because misdiagnosis of this entity can lead to poor outcomes after surgery secondary to residual rotatory instability.[22]

Magnetic resonance imaging (MRI) is obtained after the patient has been appropriately medically stabilized and is especially useful in the absence of fracture to assess the extent of damage to the soft tissue structures of the knee because it allows for full ligamentous, meniscal, and osteochondral evaluation and aids in preoperative planning. The actual site of cruciate and collateral ligament injury (ie, avulsion vs. midsubstance rupture) can be defined and be of help in planning reconstruction or primary repair of structures. MRI is also helpful in assessing PLC and popliteal tendon injuries. MRA is also used to identify vascular injuries and has been shown to have both high sensitivity and specificity.[58] At our institution, this study is obtained as standard prior to operative reconstruction because it is extremely useful in planning the surgical approach.

TREATMENT

Surgical Decision Making

After adequate resuscitation and after vascular integrity has been restored or confirmed, a decision in terms of nonoperative versus operative treatment, surgical timing, and operative technique has to be made. Historically, KDs were treated nonoperatively with prolonged immobilization, or "watchful neglect." Nonoperative treatment was mainly described in series published between 1930 and 1984. This kind of treatment was mainly reserved for uncomplicated dislocations; however, studies have shown that nonsurgical treatment results in inferior outcomes compared with surgical management.* Our treatment algorithm is detailed in Figs. 63.4 and 63.5.

There is still no true consensus regarding timing of surgery, repair versus reconstruction, use of autograft or allograft, single

*References 11, 13, 25, 34, 50, 73, 74, and 85.

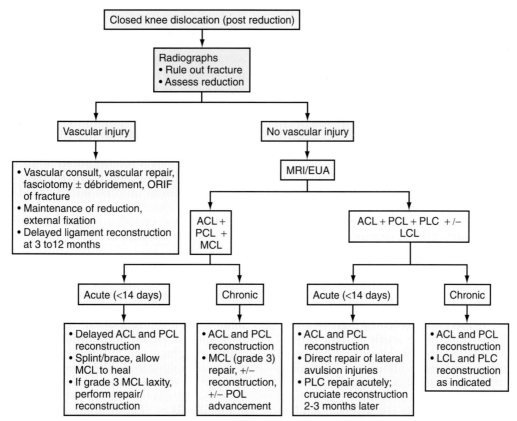

FIG 63.5 Evaluation and management of the dislocated knee. *ACL*, Anterior cruciate ligament; *EUA*, examination under anesthesia; *LCL*, lateral collateral ligament; *MCL*, medial collateral ligament; *MRI*, magnetic resonance imaging; *ORIF*, open reduction internal fixation; *PLC*, posterolateral corner; *POL*, posterior oblique ligament.

versus two stage, and postoperative rehabilitation. In addition, complications related to surgery, such as knee stiffness, wound healing complications, infections, DVT, pulmonary embolism (PE), and the need for reoperation secondary to recurrent instability have to be taken into consideration.[1,5,50]

The following sections will address the indications for acute operative management and the approach to neurovascular injuries that frequently accompany these injuries.

Urgent Surgical Intervention

There are some situations that require immediate surgical intervention. As mentioned previously, any evidence for vascular injury requires immediate consultation and treatment by a vascular surgeon. It has been widely accepted that failure or delay in reperfusion of more than 8 hours can dramatically increase the risk for amputation.[18] In addition, patients with prolonged vascular compromise should undergo fasciotomies at the time of revascularization because they are at significant risk for the development of compartment syndrome. Open dislocations require immediate surgical intervention, with irrigation and débridement (often multiple occasions), intravenous antibiotics, and soft tissue coverage procedures, as needed. These procedures can lead to a delay in ligament repair or reconstruction until the soft tissue envelope has healed.[62]

Irreducible dislocations are a unique case in which urgent surgical intervention is also needed. The most common pattern of an irreducible dislocation is posterolateral, with buttonholing

of the medial femoral condyle through the medial joint capsule with subsequent invagination of the capsule into the joint.[8,78] Multiple other causes of irreducible KD have been described, the majority being case reports including interposition of the vastus medialis,[29,53] muscular buttonholing[26] and interposed menisci.[3]

Operative Management

Although there was no consensus on timing of surgical treatment in the past, more studies currently emphasize early intervention, which is defined as no longer than 3 weeks after the injury. This time period should allow for enough time to decrease the amount of soft tissue swelling and inflammatory response without significant scar tissue formation.[12,33,38,40,60] A study conducted at our institution assessed the outcome of 31 patients, 19 of whom were treated less than 3 weeks after the injury and 12 patients were treated more than 3 weeks after injury. Patients who underwent early surgical intervention had higher knee outcome scores and were less likely to have a positive Lachman test. There was no significant difference in range of motion between the groups.[19] Tzurbakis et al. found that patients who were treated with early surgical intervention (<3 weeks of injury) had normal or near-normal outcomes on the IKDC subjective form.[77] A retrospective study by Richter et al.[60] evaluated 89 traumatic KDs, of which 63 were treated operatively and 26 were treated nonoperatively. The Lysholm and Tegner scores were better in the surgically treated group at longer than 8-year average follow-up. Functional rehabilitation following surgical treatment was the most important prognostic factor. Another study by Rios et al.[63] looked at the results after 26 traumatic dislocations and found that eight of the patients (31%) had a poor result based on the Lysholm scoring system. Five of the eight with poor scores were treated nonoperatively secondary to concomitant visceral or skeletal injuries, making their surgery inadvisable. The other three poor results occurred in patients who underwent primary repair of avulsed lateral collateral ligament (LCL) and posterolateral structures without addressing the cruciate ligaments.

Previously, multiple types of operative stabilization procedures have been proposed for treatment of KDs, achieving generally good results.[1,15,42,71] It has been difficult to establish a consensus regarding these injuries because these studies generally contain few patients with different degrees of knee injury that are approached in different ways. Early reports emphasized primary ligamentous repair of collateral and cruciate ligament injuries. Marshall et al.[39] modified this, in which ligament repair was performed with multiple looped sutures brought out through drill holes in the tibia and femur.[46,71] Meyers and associates recognized the shortcomings of these previous studies and in 1975 published a follow-up article to their original report on 33 patients treated with immobilization (13 patients) or early ligamentous primary repair (20 patients). Outcomes were based on the patients' pain, stability, and ability to perform their previous occupation. The types of injuries in each group were thought to be equivalent and without complications. The patients who underwent early primary repair of all the ligamentous injuries had the best results, as measured by the authors' criteria. Subsequently, other studies have supported this approach.[42] Mook et al.[47] performed a systematic review in which they compared the outcomes of early, delayed, and staged procedures, as well as the subsequent rehabilitation protocols, in 24 retrospective studies involving 396 knees. They found that acute treatment was associated with residual anterior knee instability when compared with chronic treatment. In addition, significantly more patients who were managed acutely were found to have more flexion deficits when compared with those who were managed chronically. Staged treatments yielded the highest percentage of excellent and good subjective outcomes. When compared with chronic treatment, acute and staged treatments were more likely to undergo additional treatments for joint stiffness and concluded that more aggressive rehabilitation may prevent stiffness from occurring. Sisto and Warren[71] reviewed 20 KDs that were treated with early primary repair and showed superior results to those that were treated with immobilization. However, the authors had modest clinical results in both groups, and clinical instability was generally not a problem. Almekinders et al.[1] also showed modest results for these injuries regardless of the treatment method used. Although the operatively treated group seemed to have superior motion and increased objective stability in the anteroposterior plane compared with nonoperatively treated patients, resultant pain, swelling, and degenerative changes by radiographic criteria were similar for both groups.

As surgical techniques advanced for isolated anterior and posterior cruciate intrasubstance ruptures, reconstruction (as opposed to primary ligamentous repair) was considered to produce the best functional results.[51] Shapiro and Freedman[67] reviewed seven patients treated with early allograft stabilization of both cruciates in combination with primary repair of the medial and lateral collateral structures. Results at 4 years were graded as good to excellent in six patients, with arthrofibrosis being the most common postoperative complication encountered (four patients), all of which required manipulation under anesthesia. Similarly, Noyes and Barber-Westin[50] followed 11 patients with combined allograft and autograft reconstruction for bicruciate KDs. At 5-years follow-up, 8 of 11 patients (73%) were asymptomatic with daily activities and 6 of 11 (55%) returned to sporting activities. Frosch et al.[16] performed a meta-analysis of clinical results of anatomic suture repair versus reconstruction of the cruciate ligaments. They showed that nonoperative treatment of combined ACL and PCL ruptures ($n = 27$) leads to poor outcomes in 70% of patients, whereas 40 patients undergoing suture repair of the ACL and PCL showed good to excellent results. There was no statistically significant difference in suture repair versus reconstruction.

In addition, several authors recommend reconstructing the PCL with graft tissue in combination with primary medial or lateral ligament repair. This technique is based on Hughston's experience of addressing the PCL first when both cruciates are injured.[21] This approach delays reconstruction of the ACL for a later time if persistent instability remains a problem. In approaching bicruciate KDs in this manner, the risk of postoperative arthrofibrosis may be lessened.

In terms of graft choice for multiple ligament reconstruction, no graft has been shown to be superior to any other and choice should be made depending on injury pattern, surgeon experience, patient discussion, and graft availability. Ipsilateral autologous hamstrings may be used to reconstruct at least one ligament. Bone-patella tendon-bone ACL reconstruction has the advantage that the hamstrings can be used for another ligament, such as the PCL. Allograft tendons are increasingly used and reduce donor site morbidity but have potential problems with availability and cost. Biomechanical properties may be compromised if allografts are irradiated with 2.5 mrad or greater.[20]

A more recent study by Ibrahim et al.[22] assessed simultaneous reconstruction in 20 patients of the ACL and PCL with gracilis and semitendinosus, respectively, which were both reinforced with the ligament augmentation and reconstruction system (LARS). In addition, the PLC was reconstructed with gracilis and semitendinosus tendon autograft from the contralateral, uninjured knee. At a 44-month follow-up, 80% of patients had good subjective results and functional stability, but according to the IKDC scale only 45% of knees were normal.

Angelini et al.[2] investigated the use of supplementary external fixation in the treatment of chronic multiligament-injured knees. The authors found that its use in comparison with rigid knee bracing in extension can provide the same ligament stability but with improved final range of motion and better Lysholm scores. Seventy-three percent of patients in the external fixation group rated their function as excellent or good, compared with 35% in the brace group ($p < .05$).

Vascular Injuries

Injury to the popliteal artery during KD is caused by stretch of the relatively immobile artery, which then can lead to intimal tears, transection, or complete ruptures. These mechanisms can also injure the popliteal vein. In most cases, surgical treatment is required, and most commonly resection of the damaged portion of the vessel, with reverse saphenous vein interposition grafting, is performed.[4] In addition, endovascular repair with a covered stent has been described, but this technique is applicable only to arteries that are not completely ruptured, and repair can be complicated by fracture or thrombosis of the stent, caused by movement of the tibiofemoral joint.[37,59]

Four-compartment fasciotomies should also be performed in concurrence with vascular repair because the edema that ensues following revascularization can often be associated with development of compartment syndrome.[15] Injury to the popliteal vein, if present, should be addressed. Repair of the ligamentous structures is ill advised at the same time as revascularization because the prolonged surgical time required and manipulation of the knee could potentially jeopardize the arterial repair. Reduction and stabilization of the knee joint is required and placement of an external fixator has been used frequently as a method of initial stabilization as long as excessive manipulation can be avoided.[79] Definitive ligamentous repair often can be performed within the next 10 to 14 days without significant risk to the vascular structures, but this remains controversial.[46]

Neurologic Injuries

Treatment of neurologic injuries, most commonly injury to the common peroneal nerve, remains controversial, with poor results regardless of treatment strategies used. Several studies have shown that less than a third of patients will regain dorsiflexion and that patients with a persistent foot drop have significantly worse outcomes.[49,54,56,63] Woodmass et al.[84] performed a systematic review and found that most patients with an incomplete palsy will regain full function, whereas less than 40% of patients with a complete injury will return to their preinjury full motor status. Krych et al.[30] found similar results in their study of 27 patients with peroneal nerve injury after KD who underwent multiligament knee reconstruction with follow-up of 6.3 years. Overall, 18 patients regained antigravity dorsiflexion (3 patients with complete nerve palsy and 15 with partial nerve palsy) and one patient with complete nerve palsy, and 13 patients with partial nerve palsy regained antigravity extensor hallucis longus strength.

Immediate and delayed treatment of nerve injuries varies, depending on the physician and setting. In the acute setting, nerve repair, neurolysis, and grafting have been associated with poorer results in terms of motor function, and most authors approach these injuries nonoperatively for the first 3 months after injury.[27,31,83] Patients with foot drop should be treated with an AFO and physical therapy (for range of motion) to prevent equinus contracture. If spontaneous resolution does not occur, reconstructive procedures, including nerve grafting, tendon transfers, and permanent bracing, are considered at that time. Results of operative decompression of the peroneal nerve have been reported after an initial period of observation, showing improvement in 97% of the patients studied.[45] Although this study suggests better results with early exploration and decompression, this may be misleading. Only a small subset of the patients included in this study had traumatically induced peroneal nerve injuries, and direct comparisons should not be made with previous reports.

Our approach to these injuries in the acute setting involves the exploration and decompression of the peroneal nerve at the time of the initial operative procedure. Postoperatively the foot is braced in an AFO, and recovery is closely monitored over the ensuing 3 months. If residual deficits are present at this time, tendon transfers are discussed with the patient. In our experience, nerve grafting has been less successful and has not been performed for these injuries.

Rehabilitation

Unlike protocols for isolated cruciate ligament reconstruction, postoperative rehabilitation in the multiligament reconstructed knee should be tailored to the injury pattern. The main goals are to protect the surgical repair, maximize quadriceps function, and restore full passive extension.[9] Hyperextension and open-chain hamstring contractions should be avoided during the first 6 to 8 weeks, and weight bearing can be increased after 6 to 10 weeks, with return to sporting activities at 9 to 12 months at the earliest.

Current Surgical Controversies

Although there has been considerable discussion regarding the most appropriate treatment algorithm for KD, the most recent literature agrees that ligamentous instability should be addressed with surgical treatment. There still remains debate with respect to surgical timing, need to stage the repair/reconstruction, which ligaments to repair/reconstruct, and what types of grafts to use. Staged ligamentous repair/reconstruction, including early PCL reconstruction followed by ACL reconstruction and chronic management of lateral injuries, has been described in multiple studies and is associated with a decreased risk of postoperative arthrofibrosis.[51] Other studies have shown that concomitant reconstruction of the ACL and PCL, with repair or reconstruction of the collaterals or PLC, can be done in the acute setting (<3 weeks) without increasing the risk of late arthrofibrosis.[19,35] Tissue quality, injury severity, and stability dictate the ability to repair the MCL, LCL, and PLC injury. If the repair is deemed inadequate, it is augmented or reconstructed. Our current preference is to acutely repair bony avulsion injuries of the lateral knee and reconstruct ruptures and midsubstance injury patterns. This single-stage procedure eliminates the morbidity of a second surgical procedure. Several studies have shown good results with acute ligament repair or reconstruction. Liow et al.[35] reported on a series of 22 KDs of which eight patients were treated with acute ligament repair/reconstruction (<2 weeks) and 14 were reconstructed at longer than 6 months post injury. They showed that at an average follow-up of 32 months, the mean Lysholm score was 87 in the acute group versus 75 in the delayed group. Similarly the Tegner activity rating was 5 in the acute group versus 4.4 in the delayed group. In addition to the improved results in the acute group, the authors did not see any increased risk of arthrofibrosis.

COMPLICATIONS

In addition to the previously discussed neurovascular injuries, there are several other complications associated with KDs. Some complications include arthrofibrosis, missed fractures, heterotopic ossification (HO), instability, and degenerative joint disease. Whelan et al. found that PCL reconstruction was the only factor associated with HO formation, which occurred in 34%, and that 25% of patients in their series required an additional operation to address knee stiffness.[82] Complications not unique to KDs include DVT, PE, infection, and wound healing complications. Fanelli et al. examined complications associated with multiligamentous knee reconstructions with 10-year follow-up.[14] Approximately 16% of knees had residual instability, 23% developed radiographic evidence of degenerative joint disease, and the mean loss of flexion was 12.5 degrees. Salzler et al. examined the complication rates after knee arthroscopy and found an overall rate of 4.7%, with the highest being from PCL reconstruction (20.1%).[65] The authors' preference for management of arthrofibrosis after multiligament reconstructions is manipulation under anesthesia between 8 and 12 weeks postoperatively if the patient has not obtained 90 degrees of flexion.

AUTHORS' APPROACH

The primary goals in treating KDs include anatomic reduction, restoration of knee motion, and stability. It is important to counsel the patient preoperatively regarding the severity of the injury and the expected outcomes. Associated injuries, patient age, and preoperative level of function influence the final result. From a technical perspective, such variables as surgical timing, operative technique, graft selection, and postoperative rehabilitation are crucial components of the overall treatment plan.

Timing

Delayed and/or staged surgery is acceptable in many cases of multiligament knee injuries. However, the optimal timing for repair of multiligamentous injuries to the knee that include the PLC and certain MCL injuries is within 10 to 14 days from the time of injury. At this time, the soft tissue envelope surrounding the knee has typically had a sufficient time to recover and heal, and the knee's range of motion has been partially restored. Anatomic definition and repair of the collateral ligament structures is often possible at this time. Following reduction and confirmation of vascular integrity, the patient is placed into a long leg, hinged knee brace and is instructed to begin range-of-motion exercises in the brace in conjunction with quadriceps-strengthening exercises until definitive surgical treatment is performed.

In the presence of collateral ligament injuries requiring surgical intervention, operative treatment is delayed up to 3 weeks in the face of vascular or other associated injuries, without compromising the surgeon's ability to perform a primary repair. Beyond 3 weeks, the surgical approach becomes more difficult secondary to scar formation, making anatomic reattachment of the collateral structures much more difficult. Reconstruction of the cruciate ligaments is less affected by surgical delay. In situations in which the severity of injury prohibits acute operative treatment of ligamentous injury, it is best to take a conservative approach, allowing full restoration of motion in a long leg, hinged brace prior to making further decisions regarding surgical management.

In the presence of any vascular injury, orthopedic management is secondary until vascular perfusion has been reestablished. The definitive repair and reconstruction of ligamentous structures is a major undertaking requiring manipulation and dissection of the extremity that potentially could threaten the vascular repair if done simultaneously. Provided that normal perfusion has been reestablished, it is typically considered safe to perform the definitive ligamentous repair and reconstruction 10 to 14 days after revascularization. Because of the potential length of these cases and potential for thrombosis in cases of vascular injury, we no longer use a tourniquet for any of these reconstructions, although a sterile tourniquet is available if needed.

Anesthesia, Positioning, Surface Anatomy, and Examination Under Anesthesia

The choice of anesthesia is made in conjunction with the patient, surgeon, and anesthesiologist. The choice will often depend on patient age, medical comorbidities, and the patient's previous anesthesia history. General anesthesia is our preference. In addition, we recommend that a vascular surgeon be "on call" during the procedure because unexpected vessel injury may occur.

In addition, a thorough neurovascular examination is performed and documented, paying particular attention to the popliteal, dorsalis pedis, and posterior tibial pulses and the function of the tibial and peroneal nerves. Doppler ultrasound is routinely used and vessel location marked for later ease of assessment.

The patient is brought into the operating suite and placed in the supine position on the operating table. Our goal with positioning is to have a full, free range of motion of the knee during the procedure, with the ability to have the knee statically flexed at 80 to 90 degrees without any manual assistance. An example of our surgical positioning is shown in Fig. 63.6.

A skin marker is used to identify surface anatomy and the incisions that will be used. Important osseous landmarks include the patella, tibial tubercle, Gerdy's tubercle, and the fibular head. The peroneal nerve is palpated, and its course is marked superficial to the fibular neck. The medial and lateral joint lines are identified, and the course of the MCL and LCL are marked. The anterolateral (AL) arthroscopy portal is drawn adjacent to the lateral border of the patella, above the joint line and adjusted for patella baja if indicated. The anteromedial

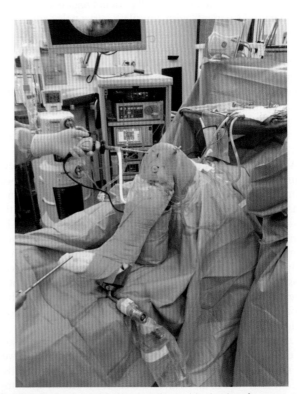

FIG 63.6 Patient positioning supine with the leg free, no tourniquet, and a pneumatic leg holder.

arthroscopy portal is positioned approximately 1 cm medial to the patellar tendon at the same level. A superolateral outflow portal is established proximal to the superior border of the patella and posterior to the quadriceps tendon. A posteromedial (PM) portal, if needed, is made under direct visualization using an outside-in technique and is not marked initially. A longitudinal 3-cm incision approximately 2-cm distal to the joint line and 2-cm medial to the tibial tubercle is drawn on the anteromedial proximal tibia for the ACL and PCL tibial tunnels. In addition, a 2-cm incision is placed medial to the medial trochlear articular surface along the subvastus interval for the PCL femoral tunnel. If there is an MCL injury, the distal incision for the tibial tunnels is traced proximally to the medial epicondyle and extended to the level of the vastus medialis in a curvilinear fashion. The incision for the lateral and posterolateral injuries is a curvilinear 12-cm incision that is drawn midway between Gerdy's tubercle and the fibular head and traced proximally just inferior to the lateral epicondyle while the knee is flexed to 90 degrees. The proximal extent of this incision parallels the plane between the biceps femoris tendon and the iliotibial band. When both collateral ligaments are disrupted, we prefer the above medial and lateral incisions instead of a midline incision, owing to potential complications of skin breakdown over the patella and limited access to the collateral ligaments.

Exam Under Anesthesia. A thorough examination is performed and correlated with the preoperative impression. It is crucial to examine the opposite extremity and use it as a reference. The knee range of motion is documented. The anterior drawer, Lachman test, and pivot shift test assess integrity of the ACL. PCL integrity is assessed by the posterior drawer and posterior sag tests, with associated step-off at 90 degrees of flexion. The MCL is examined with a valgus stress test at both 0 and 30 degrees of knee flexion. The LCL is palpated in the figure-of-four position and tested with a varus stress at both 0 and 30 degrees of knee flexion. The PLC, which consists of the LCL, popliteus, and popliteal-fibular ligament, is tested at 30 degrees and externally rotating the tibia. In addition, applying an external rotation force on the proximal tibia tests the PLC and fibula while the knee is flexed 90 degrees to feel for lateral dropout. A mini C-arm fluoroscope is in the operating suite and draped on the opposite side of the table, whereas a sterile Doppler is used on the surgical field before the initial incision and throughout the case to confirm the presence of the dorsalis pedis and posterior tibial pulses.

Surgical Approach

The two most common combined injury patterns with KDs include the ACL/PCL/MCL or ACL/PCL/PLC ± LCL. Less commonly, the PCL is intact or only partially torn and does not require reconstruction. At our institution, we attempt to augment the PCL if possible. Most commonly, the AL bundle is ruptured, and the meniscofemoral ligament (MFL) and PM bundle are intact. If this injury pattern is identified and present, we preserve the intact portion of the PCL and MFL and reconstruct the torn AL bundle via a single-bundle technique.

Our approach includes repair/reconstruction of all injured collateral structures. The ACL and PCL are most commonly intrasubstance tears and are treated with ligament reconstruction. We perform primary repair of ACL and PCL tibial avulsions, if indicated. The primary repair can be accomplished by passing large nonabsorbable sutures into the bony fragment and through bone tunnels in the tibia or femur. A primary repair of the PCL insertion may be advocated in the case of a "peel off" or a soft tissue avulsion of the PCL at its femoral insertion by a similar technique.

Concerning the MCL, LCL, and PLC, it is our experience that a primary repair is possible if performed acutely within 2 weeks of injury. Chronic injuries are limited by scar formation and soft tissue contractures and often require a ligament reconstruction. The MCL can be repaired directly with intrasubstance sutures or with suture anchors if avulsed off the bone. Repair of the PLC structures and the LCL can be accomplished with direct suture repair or by repair to bone via drill holes versus suture anchors. If direct repair is limited by poor tissue quality, the involved structures are augmented with allograft (preferred), hamstring tendons, biceps femoris, or iliotibial band. Delayed treatment involves reconstruction. In addition, concomitant injuries to the articular cartilage and menisci are operatively addressed at the time of surgery. Arthroscopic assistance is useful but must be used with caution. Extravasation of arthroscopy fluid can lead to compartment syndrome in rare cases, secondary to capsular injury.

Graft Selection

There are many different options available for graft selection in the multiligamentous-injured knee. Graft choice is made depending on the extent of injury, timing of the surgery, and experience of the surgeon. At our institution, we recommend the use of allograft over autograft in multiligamentous reconstruction surgery. The advantages of using allograft tissue include decreased operative time, smaller skin incisions in a knee that has been severely traumatized, and no additional donor site morbidity. We also believe that the use of allograft decreases pain and stiffness postoperatively. However, one must be willing to assume the risks of using allograft tissue, which include an increase in cost, a delay in the incorporation of the graft, and a minimal risk of disease transmission. Autograft tissue may be harvested from the ipsilateral or contralateral extremity and has the advantage of improved graft incorporation and remodeling when compared with allograft tissue.

We prefer the use of bone-patellar tendon-bone allograft for reconstruction of the ACL. The bone-patellar tendon-bone allograft provides adequate biomechanical strength combined with rigid bony fixation at both the femoral and tibial attachment sites.

We use Achilles tendon allograft for reconstruction of the PCL. If a double-bundle technique is indicated (rarely in KDs), an ipsilateral hamstring tendon (semitendinosus) autograft is also harvested. The allograft Achilles tendon is a good choice for PCL reconstruction because of its long length, significant cross-sectional area, and calcaneal bone plug, which provides rigid bony fixation in the femoral tunnel.

The LCL is reconstructed with an Achilles tendon allograft with calcaneal bone plug. The bone plug can be fixed into the LCL insertion at the fibula through a bone tunnel. We do not tubularize the tendon because it is often reinforced to the native LCL tissue. Alternatively, the remaining bone-patellar tendon-bone allograft may be used for the LCL reconstruction.

For the PLC, our graft choice for reconstructing the popliteofibular ligament (PFL) is a tibialis anterior tendon allograft or an ipsilateral hamstring (semitendinosus) autograft. These are prepared using a whipstitch on both ends with heavy nonabsorbable suture.

Intra-Articular Preparation

The arthroscope is introduced through the anterolateral portal, and gravity inflow is used in combination with superolateral outflow. Care must be taken to avoid a compartment syndrome, and the posterior leg and calf region must be palpated intermittently during the procedure. Factors that influence a potential compartment syndrome include an acute reconstruction (<2 weeks from the time of injury) in which the capsular healing was insufficient to maintain joint distention or if the capsule has been breached iatrogenically during the procedure. If extravasation is noted and a potential compartment syndrome is suspected, the arthroscopic technique is abandoned, and the remainder of the procedure is performed with an open technique.

All compartments within the knee are assessed. A PM portal is established to visualize the tibial insertion of the PCL completely. The PM portal is established under direct visualization through the Gilchrist portal. The 70-degree arthroscope is placed into the anterolateral portal and through the intercondylar notch adjacent to the posterior aspect of the medial femoral condyle. An 18-gauge spinal needle is used for placement, anterior to the saphenous nerve and vein, posterior to the MCL, and 1 cm above the joint line.

After completion of the diagnostic arthroscopy, with confirmation of all intra-articular pathology, any concomitant meniscal or cartilaginous injury is addressed. Every effort is made to preserve torn meniscal tissue. Peripheral meniscal tears are repaired via an inside-out technique with zone-specific cannulas and meniscal sutures. Central or irreparable meniscal tears are débrided to a stable rim. Should the meniscus require repair, the sutures are tied down directly onto the capsule at 30 degrees of flexion at the end of the procedure after all grafts have been passed and secured.

The notch and stumps of the torn cruciates are débrided, preserving any remaining intact PCL tissue as previously described. The tibial insertion of the PCL is removed using an arthroscopic shaver, a curette, or both, via the PM portal and gently developing the plane between the PCL and posterior capsule, while looking through the anterolateral portal with the 70-degree arthroscope. Alternatively, the 30-degree arthroscope may be introduced through the PM portal and a PCL curette and rasp used through the anterolateral or anteromedial portals. Every attempt is made to débride the distal most aspect of the tibial PCL insertion because this aids with tibial tunnel guide wire placement later in the procedure.

Cruciate Tunnel Preparation, Graft Passage, and Proximal Fixation

We prefer to address the PCL tibial tunnel initially because of the significant risks that accompany this portion of the procedure. A PCL offset guide is used via the anteromedial portal, placing the tip of the guide at the distal and lateral third of the insertion site of the PCL on the tibia approximately 10 to 15 mm below the joint line. A proximal anteromedial tibial skin incision is made, and the periosteum is sharply dissected from the bone. The starting point of the guide wire is approximately 3 to 4 cm distal to the joint line. The trajectory of the tibial PCL tunnel approximately parallels the angle of the proximal tibiofibular joint. The guide wire is passed in the desired position until it just perforates the far posterior cortex of the tibia at the PCL insertion, under direct arthroscopic visualization. Caution must be taken when passing the guide wire through the

posterior tibial cortex to avoid the neurovascular structures. The PCL insertion often has a soft "cancellous" feel, when the posterior tibial cortex is breached, thus lending to the increased risk when passing the guide wire. Proper guide wire location is then confirmed with a mini C-arm fluoroscopy unit on a true lateral projection of the knee. Occasionally the wire is too proximal on the PCL insertion site and a 3- or 5-mm parallel pin guide is used to obtain ideal guide wire placement. The guide wire for the PCL tibial tunnel is then left in place while attention is directed to the tibial tunnel of the ACL.

The ACL tibial tunnel guide is used via the anteromedial portal, and a guide wire is placed in the center of the ACL footprint adjacent to the anterior horn of the lateral meniscus. The guide wire should rest posterior to Blumensaat line on the full-extension lateral mini C-arm projection to ensure proper placement of the ACL tibial tunnel. The ACL tibial tunnel is proximal and anterior to the PCL tunnel at the proximal medial tibia.

After acceptable placement of the ACL and PCL guide is confirmed, the PCL tunnel is reamed to the predetermined graft diameter. A curette is placed directly on top of the guide wire posteriorly, to prevent protrusion of the wire into the adjacent neurovascular structures. The PCL tunnel is expanded using dilators in 0.5-mm increments to the diameter of the graft. The ACL tibial tunnel is reamed in a similar manner. We prefer at least a 1- to 2-cm bone bridge between the ACL and PCL tibial tunnels anteriorly on the tibia.

Attention is turned to the preparation of the femoral ACL and PCL tunnels. For a single-bundle PCL reconstruction, the insertion of the PCL on the intercondylar notch is identified, and the guide wire is placed from the anterolateral portal to a point approximately 7 to 10 mm from the articular margin within the anterior portion of the PCL femoral footprint at approximately 1 o'clock (right knee) and the knee flexed to 100 degrees. Following reaming over the guide wire, the tunnel is dilated to the size of the graft by 0.5-mm increments. If a double-bundle PCL reconstruction is chosen (in the delayed setting), the anterolateral tunnel is drilled at the 1 o'clock position, approximately 5 to 6 mm off the articular cartilage, and the PM bundle is placed at the 3 to 4 o'clock position, approximately 4 mm off of the articular cartilage. These tunnels are prepared to a depth of 25 to 30 mm.

The ACL femoral tunnel is established with the knee flexed to 120 degrees. The anteromedial portal is used to introduce the guide wire into the desired position on the posterolateral femoral footprint below the lateral intercondylar ridge. The guide wire is placed in the center of the anatomic femoral ACL footprint, approximately 6 mm anterior to the back wall or over-the-top position of the femur. We prefer the medial portal technique to the traditional transtibial technique because of the location of the femoral tunnel is not limited by the position or angulation of the tibial tunnel. If there is any question about femoral tunnel placement, the mini C-arm fluoroscopic machine is used for visualization. A schematic regarding our ACL and PCL tunnel placement is shown in Fig. 63.7.

The Achilles allograft PCL graft is passed first. A long, looped, 18-gauge wire is passed retrograde into the PCL tibial tunnel and retrieved out the anterolateral arthroscopy portal with a pituitary rongeur. The draw suture of the graft is shuttled into the joint with the looped 18-gauge wire via the anterolateral portal and antegrade down the PCL tibial tunnel to exit on the anteromedial tibia. The draw suture securing the calcaneus

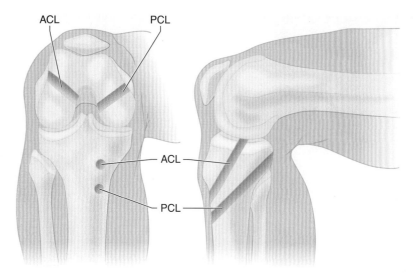

FIG 63.7 ACL and PCL reconstruction tunnel placement *ACL,* Anterior cruciate ligament; *PCL,* posterior cruciate ligament.

portion of the graft is then passed out the anteromedial femur via a Beath pin through the PCL femoral tunnel and out the anteromedial thigh. With arthroscopic assistance, a probe is used to direct the graft in the joint to facilitate passage of the graft.

The ACL graft is passed using the medial portal technique. A Beath pin with a no. 5 suture attached to the eyelet is passed through the femoral tunnel via the medial portal. A pituitary rongeur is passed retrograde through the tibial tunnel, and the no. 5 suture is retrieved. The graft is then passed from the tibial tunnel into the femoral tunnel with arthroscopic assistance.

Femoral fixation of both the PCL and ACL grafts is performed. The fixation at the tibia is performed after the collateral fixation is done. The PCL femoral grafts are fixed with a 4.5-mm Arbeitsgemeinschaft für Osteosynthesefragen (AO) screw and washer, or the grafts are tied and secured over a button. The anteromedial incision is extended proximally and distally adjacent to the exiting Beath pins. The vastus medialis obliquus is split in line with its fibers, or a small subvastus approach is used to gain access to the graft sutures and the bone. Alternatively, an interference screw may be used for the femoral fixation of the calcaneal bone plug for single-bundle reconstructions. For the ACL femoral fixation, a metal interference screw secures the femoral bone plug via the medial portal technique. Other types of fixation are feasible and depend on the type of graft and comfort level of the surgeon.

Cruciate and Medial Sided Injury

If the cruciate ligaments are injured in combination with a medial-sided injury, a standard medial curvilinear incision is made (Figs. 63.8 and 63.9). The PCL femoral tunnel, the ACL and PCL tibial tunnels, medial meniscal repairs, or medial capsular repairs can be addressed through this incision. Peripheral meniscal tears can be repaired by standard meniscal repair techniques, and any capsular disruptions can be repaired with suture anchors. During the approach, the infrapatellar branch of the saphenous nerve should be identified approximately 1 cm above the joint line and protected throughout the procedure.

The MCL should be repaired or reconstructed only for grade 3 injuries that open up with valgus stress testing in the extended

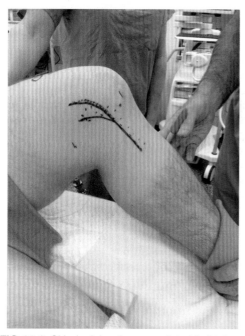

FIG 63.8 Skin incision for a medial-sided injury.

knee. In the acute setting (<3 weeks) the MCL can be repaired at the time of cruciate reconstruction. MCL avulsions off of the tibial or femoral insertions are reattached to bone via suture post and spiked washer or suture anchors, and intrasubstance tears are repaired primarily with no. 2 braided nonabsorbable sutures using a modified Kessler stitch configuration. In the chronic setting a reconstruction may be required to augment the repair, described by Coobs et al.[10] The surgeon must beware of a possible posterior horn medial meniscus root tear associated with combined PCL and MCL injuries.

The posterior oblique ligament (POL), which is confluent with the posterior edge of the superficial MCL, is reinforced by the semimembranosus and is critical to medial knee stability. The plane between the posterior edge of the MCL and the POL is incised longitudinally, and the two flaps are elevated. The

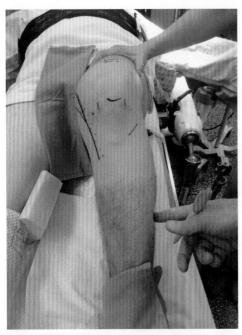

FIG 63.9 Skin incision for a medial-sided injury.

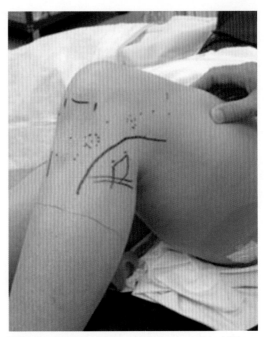

FIG 63.10 Skin incision for a lateral-sided injury.

medial meniscus attachments to the POL must be released to the PM corner of the knee. The peripheral border of the medial meniscus is rasped to prepare the tissue for eventual repair back to the POL. The medial meniscus is repaired to the anteriorly advanced POL with full-thickness outside-in no. 0 cottony Dacron sutures through the meniscus. The POL is advanced anteriorly and imbricated to the MCL in a pants-over-vest fashion using no. 2 cottony Dacron sutures. If needed, the repair can be augmented with a soft tissue graft at the anatomic origin and insertion of the MCL in double-bundle fashion. The graft is looped over a staple placed in the medial epicondyle. The short limb is passed posteriorly to the tibial insertion of the POL, 2 cm distal to the joint line, and the long limb is passed to the tibial insertion of the superficial medial collateral ligament (sMCL), 5 cm distal to the joint line. The graft is fixed on the tibia using interference screws and reinforced to the native MCL in a side-to-side fashion.

Cruciate- and Lateral-Sided Injury

Following femoral fixation of the cruciate ligament reconstructions, a standard lateral "hockey stick" incision is made (Fig. 63.10). The plane between the posterior edge of the iliotibial band and the biceps femoris is incised longitudinally. The peroneal nerve is identified proximally as it travels posterior to the biceps femoris and distally as it travels along the fibular neck and into the anterior tibialis muscle belly (Fig. 63.11). A formal neurolysis generally is not performed unless there is evidence of compromise of the nerve at the time of surgery. The insertion of the iliotibial band at Gerdy's tubercle is partially released to increase visibility of the LCL and popliteus insertions.

If reparable lateral meniscal tears or lateral capsular avulsions are visualized during the diagnostic arthroscopy, a longitudinal capsular incision is made just posterior to the LCL and the lateral inferior geniculate artery is coagulated if encountered. The meniscus is repaired using standard meniscal repair techniques depending on the type and location of the tear.

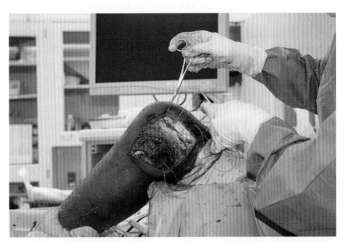

FIG 63.11 Lateral dissection, showing borders of iliotibial band and identification of peroneal nerve, protected with red vessel loop.

Capsular avulsions are repaired with suture anchors. The LCL and PFL are identified. If tissue quality allows, avulsions of the biceps, iliotibial band insertion, LCL, and/or popliteus are repaired directly with no. 2 braided nonabsorbable sutures. If interstitial injury has occurred to these structures or the injury is chronic, reconstruction is usually necessary.

Our preferred method for posterolateral reconstruction is similar to LaPrade et al.[32] The tendinous portion of the Achilles allograft is secured to the femoral LCL insertion by means of drill holes or suture anchors. The native LCL is imbricated to the tendinous portion of the allograft using a whipstitch technique. The injured LCL is then dissected free from its distal insertion on the fibular head, and a tunnel is drilled along the longitudinal axis of the fibula. The allograft calcaneal bone plug is tensioned and secured in the tunnel using a metal interference screw. Alternatively, the calcaneal bone plug can be fixed initially into the fibular tunnel and the tendinous portion recessed into the lateral femoral epicondyle via a small bone tunnel and tied over a post or button on the medial femur.

The goal of reconstruction of the popliteus complex is to re-create its static component, the PFL. We prefer a tibialis anterior allograft or hamstring allograft/autograft. The lateral epicondyle of the femur is exposed, and the popliteus tendon is dissected of its anatomic insertion. A whipstitch is placed in the popliteus tendon with a no. 2 braided nonabsorbable suture. Verification of the correct placement of the whipstitch is confirmed if the whole popliteus complex becomes taut when tension is placed on the suture. A 6-mm femoral tunnel is drilled at the popliteus insertion, 18 mm away from the LCL to a depth of 25 to 30 mm, and the tunnel is expanded to 7 mm in diameter with serial dilators. The posterior border of the fibula at the insertion of the PFL is exposed by incising horizontally just below the biceps insertion proximal to the peroneal nerve. The anterior border of the fibula also is exposed, and a guide wire is passed by hand (with it loaded on a chuck) from anterior to posterior across the fibular head in an attempt to match the oblique angle of the fibular head. The PFL tunnel rests more medial and closer to the proximal tibiofibular joint than the previously drilled LCL tunnel. The fibular head tunnel for the PFL graft is obliquely drilled over the guide wire with a 6-mm drill by hand and dilated to a diameter of 7 mm. The graft is passed from posterior to anterior through the tunnel with a suture passer, but is not fixed to the fibula until the graft is tensioned properly. The graft is passed underneath and medial to the LCL and into the previously drilled femoral tunnel. A beath pin is used to dock the graft into the femoral tunnel as it is pulled through to the medial side. Both the graft and the native popliteus tendon that was previously subperiosteally dissected are pulled into the tunnel together. Approximately 25 mm of the allograft and 10 mm of the popliteus tendon should be paralleled into the tunnel. The sutures from the graft and popliteus tendon are tied over an AO screw with washer or a button on the anteromedial distal femur. The reconstructed tendon is fixed to the fibula with either a bioabsorbable interference screw or over a button at the end of the case.

Cruciate-, Medial-, and Lateral-Sided Injuries

The combination of cruciate-, medial-, and lateral-sided injuries is potentially the most unstable of injuries and is approached through medial and lateral "hockey stick" incisions as described earlier. Cruciate reconstruction is performed first, as described above, followed by medial and lateral repairs or reconstructions. Proximal fixation is performed first, followed by tensioning and distal fixation in a similar sequence.

Tensioning and Distal Fixation

After all grafts are successfully passed and fixed on the femoral side, the final tensioning and distal fixation of the grafts is performed. In a stepwise fashion, we prefer to tension and fix the PCL, ACL, lateral structures, and medial structures. For the PCL the knee is brought to 90 degrees of flexion, and a bolster is placed under the tibia to support its weight against gravity. The medial step-off is reduced with an anterior drawer so that the anterior edge of the medial tibial plateau rests approximately 10 mm anterior to the medial femoral condyle. The graft is fixed to the tibia with a bioabsorbable interference screw or an AO screw and soft tissue washer. The ACL graft is tensioned and

fixed close to full extension with co-axial tension on the draw sutures and axial compression. We prefer a metal interference screw for the bone-patellar tendon-bone allograft fixation on the tibia. The PLC of the knee is reduced with an internal rotation force to the tibia relative to the fixed femur, and the LCL and PFL are tensioned at 30 degrees of flexion. The LCL is fixed with a metal interference screw into the fibular head. The PFL is fixed with a bioabsorbable interference screw in the fibula, and the remaining graft is reapproximated to itself or over the insertion of the biceps in a figure-of-eight pattern with a no. 2 braided absorbable suture. Alternatively, the PFL graft is fixed to the fibula with sutures tied over a button. The MCL is fixed at 30 degrees of knee flexion, and the POL is fixed with the knee near full extension. This method prevents overconstraining the knee during the repair/reconstruction. After all grafts are fixed, the knee should have a tension-free range of motion from 0 to 90 degrees.

Postoperative Regimen

In the early postoperative period, the main goals are to protect the healing structures, maximize quadriceps recovery, and restore full passive extension. We place the limb locked in full extension for the first 4 weeks with a hinged knee brace. Exercises immediately after surgery include passive knee extension to neutral and isometric quadriceps sets with the knee in full extension. At 2 weeks postoperatively, physical therapy begins with passive flexion limited to 90 degrees and should prevent posterior tibial subluxation by applying an anterior force to the proximal tibia (can be performed prone). For the first 6 weeks, active flexion is avoided to prevent posterior tibial translation, which results from hamstring contraction. At 6 weeks, passive and active assisted range-of-motion and stretching exercises are begun to increase knee flexion. The brace is discontinued after 6 weeks. Depending on the combination of injury and the degree of instability, as determined by the examination under anesthesia, a reasonable goal for range of motion is 0 to 120 degrees of flexion.

Quadriceps exercises are progressed to limited-arc, open-chain, knee-extension exercises only from 60 to 75 degrees of knee flexion as tolerated after 4 weeks. These exercises are performed to prevent excessive stress on the reconstructed grafts. Open-chain hamstring exercises are avoided for 12 weeks to prevent posterior tibial translation and excessive stress on the PCL graft. Crutch weight bearing is progressed from partial to weight bearing as tolerated over the first 4 weeks, unless a lateral repair/reconstruction was performed. In this case, we maintain partial weight bearing until the patient has regained good quadriceps control, at which time the brace may be unlocked for controlled gait training. Running is permitted at 6 months if 80% of quadriceps strength has been achieved. Patients may return to sedentary work in 2 to 3 weeks, heavy labor in 6 to 9 months, and sports in 9 to 12 months.

CONCLUSION

KDs are rare but serious injuries that require prompt evaluation and treatment to prevent major complications and poor results. The sequence of events include closed reduction, neurovascular evaluation (including serial physical examination), and ABI measurements with the selective use of arteriography and vascular repair where required. This is followed by evaluation and treatment of soft tissue injuries.

Treatment should involve acute reconstruction of the cruciate ligaments combined with reconstruction or repair of the collateral structures and selective use of preoperative and postoperative joint-spanning external fixation. Primary open reconstruction rather than repair is advised for injuries of the lateral collateral ligament and PLC, whereas repair is usually sufficient for acute treatment of MCL injuries. Collateral ligament repair/reconstruction can be done staged or with concomitant ACL/PCL. Although a more recent study reported similar outcomes of ACL/PCL repair and reconstruction, arthroscopic reconstruction of these structures is still considered the gold standard. This approach has improved knee function with regard to stability and improved mobility of patients with KDs. Long-term outcome for these severe injuries depends on neurovascular status and functional ligament reconstruction. Further research is necessary to define the appropriate timing and optimal types of reconstructions.

KEY REFERENCES

5. Born TR, Engasser WM, King AH, et al: Low frequency of symptomatic venous thromboembolism after multiligamentous knee reconstruction with thromboprophylaxis. *Clin Orthop* 472(9):2705–2711, 2014.

7. Bui KL, Ilaslan H, Parker RD, et al: Knee dislocations: a magnetic resonance imaging study correlated with clinical and operative findings. *Skeletal Radiol* 37(7):653–661, 2008.

9. Chhabra A, Cha PS, Rihn JA, et al: Surgical management of knee dislocations. Surgical technique. *J Bone Joint Surg Am* 87(Suppl 1 Pt 1):1–21, 2005.

11. Dedmond BT, Almekinders LC: Operative versus nonoperative treatment of knee dislocations: a meta-analysis. *Am J Knee Surg* 14(1):33–38, 2001.

12. Fanelli GC: Multiple ligament-injured (dislocated) knee. *Sports Med Arthrosc* 19(2):81, 2011.

15. Frassica FJ, Sim FH, Staeheli JW, et al: Dislocation of the knee. *Clin Orthop* 263:200–205, 1991.

16. Frosch KH, Preiss A, Heider S, et al: Primary ligament sutures as a treatment option of knee dislocations: a meta-analysis. *Knee Surg Sports Traumatol Arthrosc* 21(7):1502–1509, 2013.

28. Klineberg EO, Crites BM, Flinn WR, et al: The role of arteriography in assessing popliteal artery injury in knee dislocations. *J Trauma* 56(4):786–790, 2004.

42. Meyers MH, Moore TM, Harvey JP Jr: Traumatic dislocation of the knee joint. *J Bone Joint Surg Am* 57(3):430–433, 1975.

54. Peltola EK, Lindahl J, Hietaranta H, et al: Knee dislocation in overweight patients. *AJR Am J Roentgenol* 192(1):101–106, 2009.

57. Peskun CJ, Levy BA, Fanelli GC, et al: Diagnosis and management of knee dislocations. *Phys Sportsmed* 38(4):101–111, 2010.

58. Potter HG, Weinstein M, Allen AA, et al: Magnetic resonance imaging of the multiple-ligament injured knee. *J Orthop Trauma* 16(5):330–339, 2002.

79. Varnell RM, Coldwell DM, Sangeorzan BJ, et al: Arterial injury complicating knee disruption. Third place winner: Conrad Jobst award. *Am Surg* 55(12):699–704, 1989.

80. Wascher DC, Dvirnak PC, DeCoster TA: Knee dislocation: initial assessment and implications for treatment. *J Orthop Trauma* 11(7):525–529, 1997.

81. Werner BC, Gwathmey FW Jr, Higgins ST, et al: Ultra-low velocity knee dislocations: patient characteristics, complications, and outcomes. *Am J Sports Med* 42(2):358–363, 2014.

The references for this chapter can also be found on www.expertconsult.com.

64

Dislocation of the Proximal Tibiofibular Joint

Amit Nathani, John A. Grant

INTRODUCTION

Injuries to the proximal tibiofibular joint (PTFJ) are rare, but subsequent instability can be debilitating in the symptomatic patient. There is a paucity of literature regarding these injuries, making diagnosis and management challenging for the treating clinician. Although these injuries are most commonly seen in athletes such as wrestlers, mixed-martial arts fighters, skiers, gymnasts, snowboarders, soccer players, football and rugby players, and parachute jumpers, who participate in sports that require forceful twisting of the flexed knee, they can also occur idiopathically or in the context of high-energy trauma.[28,36,38,49,60] A thorough understanding of the anatomy and biomechanics of the PTFJ as well as the clinical presentation and evaluation of the patient with a suspected injury is crucial to avoid misdiagnosis and choose an appropriate treatment plan.

ANATOMY

The anatomy of the PTFJ is complex and variable, and its clinical significance is still debated. The PTFJ is a hyaline-cartilage-lined diarthrodial articulation between the posterior and inferior aspect of the lateral tibial condyle and the anterior and medial surface of the fibular head. The opposing flat and oval articular facets lack intrinsic stability,[9] and are held together by a strong and thick anterior capsular ligament and weaker posterior capsular ligament (Fig. 64.1).[10,17,36,37,41] The anterior capsule is composed of three broad ligamentous bands that pass obliquely superior and attach to the anterior aspect of the lateral tibial condyle, whereas the posterior capsular ligament is composed of two distinct bands that run in a parallel fashion to attach to the posterior tibial condyle.[10,17,36,37,41]

The PTFJ is in close proximity to and supported by the posterolateral structures of the knee (lateral collateral ligament [LCL], arcuate ligament, fabellofibular ligament, and popliteus muscle) (see Fig. 64.1).[48,58] Posteriorly, the joint is reinforced by the popliteus tendon and superiorly by the biceps femoris insertion and LCL.[9,13,36,38] The biceps femoris tendon primarily attaches to the styloid process and upper surface of the head of the fibula, which stabilizes normal anterior motion of the fibular head with knee flexion. Its deep layer extends anteromedially above the PTFJ anterior capsular ligament to insert into Gerdy's tubercle and further reinforce the joint.[31] The LCL attaches just anterior to the styloid process on the fibular head and supports the PTFJ in a similar manner. At 0 to 30 degrees of knee flexion, the LCL is tight and pulls the proximal fibula posteriorly. With further passive knee flexion, the proximal fibula moves anteriorly as both the LCL and biceps femoris

relax.[2,37] This motion places patients at higher risk for PTFJ injuries during capsular laxity with the knee in a flexed position. The physiologic anterior-posterior movement of the PTFJ is more pronounced in children and decreases with age.[37] The chief function of the PTFJ is to dissipate forces on the lower leg, such as torsional stress on the ankle, lateral tibial bending moments, and tensile weight bearing.[39]

Given the intimate relationship of the PTFJ with the posterolateral structures of the knee, it is not surprising that a recent study showed an overall 9% incidence (12 of 129 knees) of PTFJ instability in the setting of a multiligament-injured knee. Furthermore, restoration of PTFJ stability in patients undergoing fibular-based lateral-sided knee reconstruction resulted in satisfactory patient-reported outcomes (Lysholm and International Knee Documentation Committee [IKDC] scores) and low complication rates.[21] The common peroneal nerve is another crucial structure that wraps around the neck of the fibula, just distal to the fibular head, and is susceptible to injury with posterior dislocations of the PTFJ.[10,40]

Several cadaveric studies have shown the PTFJ is highly variable. Earlier studies suggested that it communicates with the knee joint through the subpopliteal recess in 10% to 12% of adults (Fig. 64.2A and B).[11,47] More recent studies by Puffer et al. demonstrated this communication was present in all 22 patients they examined.[44,45] The inclination of the PTFJ typically has an obliquity of 10 to 30 degrees, but this has been reported to vary anywhere between 0 and 70 degrees across specimens.[37-39,47] This obliquity has implications in overall joint stability because more horizontal-oriented joints demonstrate increased stability (Fig. 64.3). Barnett and Napier showed greater fibular external rotation and thus greater ankle dorsiflexion in more horizontally inclined PTFJs.[4] In addition to rotational stress dissipation, the function of the PTFJ has been suggested to dissipate both axial loads of up to one-sixth of body weight and tensile forces resulting from lateral bending moments.[25,37,38]

CLASSIFICATION

Anatomic Variation

Several classification schemes have been proposed for the PTFJ based on both anatomic variation and instability patterns. The first classification system relates to the obliquity of the PTFJ and is based on Ogden's landmark study in 1974, which first described the PTFJ as either an oblique or horizontal variant based on an arbitrary angle of 20 degrees in the horizontal plane.[37] The horizontal variant, by definition, is less than 20 degrees of inclination (Fig. 64.4A). This configuration allows for increased rotational motion at the PTFJ and thus increased

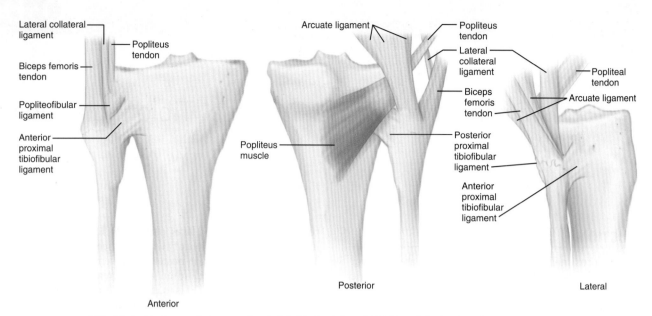

FIG 64.1 Anatomy of the proximal tibiofibular joint. (Whiddon DR, Parker TA, Kuhn JE, Sekiya JK: Disorders of the proximal tibiofibular joint. In Scott NW [ed]: Surgery of the knee, ed 4, Philadelphia, 2006, Elsevier, pp 797–803.)

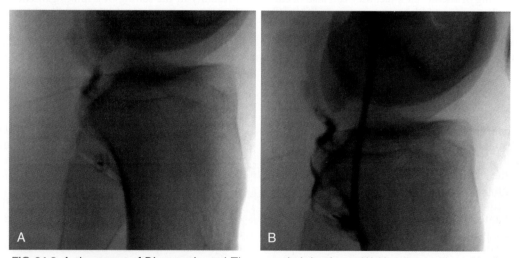

FIG 64.2 Arthrogram of Diagnostic and Therapeutic Injections. (A) Needle positioned in the proximal tibiofibular joint (PTFJ). (B) Radiographic dye is used to verify that the needle is in the correct position. Note the communication of the PTFJ with the knee joint.

ankle dorsiflexion, and is more stable than its oblique counterpart. In the horizontal variant, the fibular head is seated in a groove behind a prominent lateral tibial ridge, which imparts increased stability. Furthermore, horizontal variants have an average surface area of 26 mm² compared to an average of 17 mm² in oblique variants.[38] Ogden found the oblique variant in 70% of PTFJ injuries and suggested that the increased constraint in rotational mobility in this group increased torsional loads during forced ankle dorsiflexion, thus increasing the probability of fibular dislocation (see Fig. 64.4B).

Instability Patterns

Fibular head instability has also been classified by Ogden. In his series of 43 patients he reported four types of instability: 10 had subluxation, 29 had anterolateral dislocation, 3 had

posteromedial dislocation, and 1 experienced a superior dislocation.[38]

Type I injuries are not true dislocations, but rather excessive and symptomatic anteroposterior motion. Patients typically present prior to skeletal maturity and do not report a history of inciting trauma.[38,39,47,50] Type I PTFJ injuries can be associated with generalized ligamentous laxity and are often a self-limiting condition.[38,39]

Type II injuries (Fig. 64.5A) are the most common type of PTFJ instability, accounting for up to 85% of PTFJ injuries.[14,33] The mechanism of anterolateral dislocation is produced from a sudden internal rotation and plantar flexion of the foot combined with external rotation of the leg and flexion of the knee.[12,24] The violent rotatory movement translates the fibular head laterally to the edge of the bony buttress of the lateral tibial

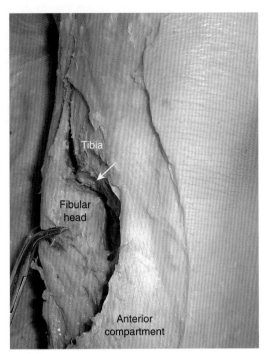

FIG 64.3 Horizontal orientation (<20 degrees) of the proximal tibiofibular joint (*white arrow*).

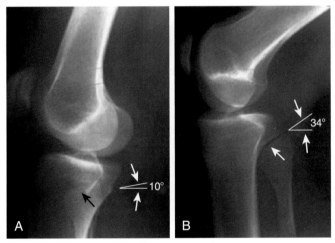

FIG 64.4 Lateral radiographs show the anatomic variations in the joint described by Ogden. An increased slope of the articulation causes instability in the joint by minimizing the surface area of the joint. (A) Horizontal orientation (<20 degrees). (B) Oblique orientation (>20 degrees) is more likely to develop instability. (2003 American Academy of Orthopaedic Surgeons: Reprinted from the Sekiya JK, Kuhn JE: Instability of the proximal tibiofibular joint. *J Am Acad Orthop Surg* 11[2], 120–128, 2003, Fig. 45.2, with permission.)

metaphysis. Knee flexion relaxes the LCL and biceps femoris, producing an environment with less bony and ligamentous restraint.[18] Reflex contracture of the extensor halluces longus, extensor digitorum longus, and peroneus caused by forced ankle inversion and plantar flexion forces the laterally displaced fibula anteriorly. Disruption of both the anterior and posterior ligamentous restraints, and often the LCL, are associated with type II injuries.[38,47]

Type III injuries (see Fig. 64.5B) are posteromedial dislocations and often occur as a result of direct trauma or severe

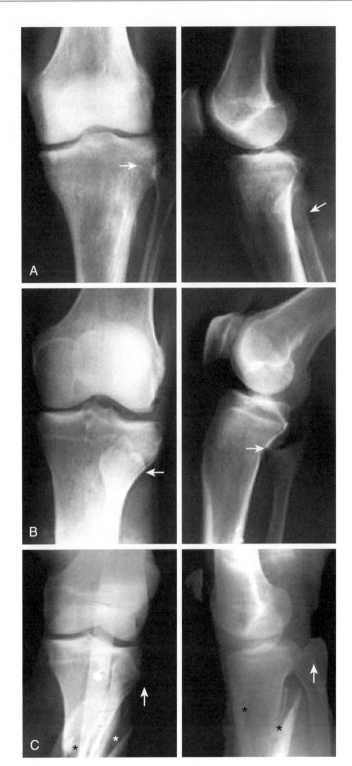

FIG 64.5 (A) Anteroposterior and lateral radiographs of an anterolateral dislocation of the proximal tibiofibular joint (PTFJ). (B) Posteromedial dislocation of the PTFJ. (C) Superior dislocation. Note the tibia fracture (*asterisks*) associated with this high-energy injury. *Arrows* indicate the direction of dislocation. (2003 American Academy of Orthopaedic Surgeons. Reprinted from the Sekiya JK, Kuhn JE: Instability of the proximal tibiofibular joint. *J Am Acad Orthop Surg* 11[2], 120–128, 2003, with permission.)

torsional injuries.[19] With capsular and ligamentous tearing, contraction of the biceps femoris displaces the fibular head posteriorly and medially along the tibial metaphysis.[29] These injuries can be particularly devastating because they have been most commonly associated with peroneal nerve injuries.[10]

Type IV injuries (see Fig. 64.5C) are superior dislocations and the least common. Superior migration of the fibula is associated with high-energy ankle injuries and disruption of the of the tibiofibular interosseus membrane. Commonly associated injuries include lateral malleolar and tibial fractures.[38]

CLINICAL EVALUATION

Clinical Presentation

PTFJ dislocations are rare injuries and often missed if there is not a high degree of clinical suspicion. Early diagnosis is crucial to prevent the potential long-term morbidity and complexity of treatment associated with chronic injuries. In the acute setting, PTFJ injuries should be considered in any patient reporting the sudden onset of lateral-sided knee pain, especially following a torsional event on a flexed knee. This includes multiligamentous knee injuries because any repair or reconstruction of the posterolateral corner (PLC) may fail if the PTFJ is left unstable.[42,43] Recurrence or chronic dislocation of the PTFJ is more difficult to diagnose, and symptoms often resemble numerous other knee pathologies. Identifying these injuries is primarily based on patient history and clinical examination, although radiographs and advanced imaging help confirm the diagnosis.

Patients with type I injuries, or subluxation, typically present in the absence of trauma or inciting event and describe lateral-sided knee discomfort over the fibular head.[38,39] In the absence of injury, there is usually no effusion or asymmetric prominence of the fibular head to suggest frank dislocation. Patients are typically preadolescent females and often report a history of generalized ligamentous laxity or hypermobility disorder, such as Ehlers-Danlos syndrome.[38,39,50] In this clinical situation, the problem is frequently bilateral and the magnitude of symptoms tends to gradually decrease with skeletal maturity.[38-40,50,52,54] Although uncommon, subluxation of the PTFJ has been reported in patients with rheumatoid arthritis, osteochondromas, runners, patients with below-knee-amputations, and those with septic joint infections or osteomyelitis.[3,29,38,39,47]

Patients who present with acute dislocations of the PTFJ typically describe a torsional or traumatic event. In type II injuries the fibula is dislocated anterolaterally and usually associated with a fall onto a flexed knee during sports activities, in which patients often report an audible "pop." Pain is localized to the lateral side of the knee and associated with a prominent fibular head.[14,36] This pain can be felt along the distal biceps femoris tendon, which may be palpated as a tense cord attaching to the anterolaterally dislocated fibular head. Weight bearing is typically avoided because of discomfort. Knee extension and ankle dorsiflexion and eversion exacerbate pain and can reproduce locking and popping phenomena, while ankle plantarflexion and inversion may give partial relief.[39,66] Although more common with posteromedial dislocations, transient peroneal nerve palsies have been reported with type II PTFJ injuries.[60] In these clinical situations, pain may radiate to the dorsal and lateral aspects of the foot.

Type III injuries, or posteromedial dislocations of the head of the fibula, result from direct trauma. Previously reported cases describe patients being struck by a car bumper or sustaining a posteriorly directed force during horseback riding when impacting a gatepost.[38,39] Ogden, Lyle, and Levy have all reported peroneal nerve palsies following posteromedial dislocations.[26,29,38] In the small series of cases reported, these symptoms typically resolve spontaneously.[10]

Type IV injuries involve a superior dislocation of the entire fibula and are associated with disruption of the tibiofibular interosseus membrane. These injuries typically involve high-energy mechanisms. Type IV injuries have been associated with fractures of the tibial plateau, tibial shaft, ipsilateral femoral head or shaft, distal femoral epiphysis, fractures of the ankle, and knee dislocations.[15,38] Shelbourne et al. reported a case of peroneal nerve injury associated with a superior dislocation; thus the examiner must always perform a careful neurovascular examination and avoid a missed diagnosis secondary to severe distracting injuries.[53]

Although not part of Ogden's classification scheme, six cases of inferior dislocation of the PTFJ have been reported in the literature. The injuries were all associated with high-energy trauma, tibial shaft fractures, and injury to the peroneal and tibial nerves. All reported cases had poor outcomes with four of the five cases resulting in either above-knee or below-knee amputations.[16,35] An additional case was reported that caused both a common peroneal injury and injury to the popliteal artery.[64]

Recurrence or chronic dislocation is more difficult to diagnose because symptomatology can mimic a variety of knee pathologies. Most commonly, patients may report lateral knee pain associated with "giving-way" episodes and mechanical clicking or popping.[51,59] These symptoms are exacerbated by activities that require cutting or twisting motion in sports activities, or by climbing stairs.[54] The nature and location of symptoms mimics more common pathologies, and thus the diagnosis is often missed. The differential diagnosis includes lateral meniscal tears, LCL injuries, posterolateral rotatory instability, biceps femoris tendinitis, iliotibial band syndrome, and intra-articular loose bodies within the popliteus tendon sheath, among many other potential causes.[50]

Physical Exam

Examination of the PTFJ should be included as a routine part of any knee examination, but particularly if the patient's history or location of pain suggests possible acute, subacute, or chronic injury to the lateral side of the knee. The complete examination should include gross observation, palpation, and both active and passive range-of-motion testing of the knee and ankle, special tests for the PTFJ, a full knee ligamentous exam including the integrity of the LCL and PLC and a thorough neurovascular exam, especially for the peroneal nerve distribution.

In patients with suspected atraumatic subluxation (type I injuries), the only complaint may be lateral sided knee pain. Because most patients tend to be young and the injuries often associated with states of hypermobility, the Beighton criteria can be used to assess generalized ligamentous laxity.[5] If Ehlers-Danlos or another disorder is suspected, signs and symptoms for each should be screened for or referred for specialist evaluation. An effusion is typically absent. Tenderness to palpation of the fibular head or with proximal fibular translation may reproduce the patient's discomfort. The optimal technique to assess translation of the PTFJ in both atraumatic subluxation and chronic injuries is by holding the patient's knee in 90 degrees of flexion to relax the LCL and biceps femoris muscle. The proximal fibula is grasped between the thumb and index finger and passively translated anteriorly and posteriorly. The patient should be questioned regarding reproduction of pain, feeling of giving way or instability, and apprehension.[54] A side-to-side comparison should be completed for the all tests. This is especially important in adolescent patients before skeletal maturity, in whom increased baseline laxity may be present. Another provocative maneuver is the Radulescu sign, which attempts to sublux the fibula anteriorly by internally rotating the leg with the patient in the prone position, thigh supported, and the knee in 90 degrees of flexion.[3]

In the acute setting and when associated with high-energy trauma, injuries to the PTFJ are often missed, and when they occur in isolation, a high degree of clinical suspicion is required because a knee effusion is rarely present. Particularly with the more common anterolateral dislocations, there may be a visible prominence of the fibular head, especially when compared to the contralateral side. The fibular head may be tender to palpation as well as its associated structures. The biceps femoris tendon may feel cord-like and taught because of stretching.[38] Extension of the knee as well as ankle dorsiflexion and eversion may exacerbate pain, while knee flexion and ankle plantarflexion and inversion may partially relieve discomfort. Examination of the ankle is also important because complete injuries to the interosseous membrane, proximal, and distal tibiofibular joints have been reported, even in the absence of fracture.[8] In high-energy mechanisms, posteromedial and superior dislocations are more commonly seen in association with other bony, ligamentous, and neurovascular injuries. It is important to always assess the status of the peroneal nerve, distal perfusion, and vascular status if knee dislocation is suspected, and integrity of the ankle syndesmosis. If the PTFJ is unstable in knee extension, injury to the LCL and PLC should be suspected.[9]

Imaging

Plain radiographs and advanced imaging can aid in diagnosis of PTFJ injuries. True anteroposterior and lateral images of the knee should be obtained in all cases. The diagnosis of instability is difficult even with good radiographs. Contralateral imaging can be helpful to identify subtle differences when there is a high clinical suspicion but apparently negative radiographs on the affected side.[34] On the anteroposterior view, increased lateral displacement of the fibular head and widening of the interosseus space are clues to possible PTFJ injury.[60] On the true-lateral view, Resnick described a line that follows the contour of the lateral tibial spine distally along the posterior aspect of the tibia (Fig. 64.6).[47] This line defines the most posteromedial aspect of the lateral tibial condyle. In normal knees, this line crosses through the midpoint of the fibular head. In posteromedial dislocations, all or most of the fibular head lies posterior to this line, and in anterolateral dislocations, all or most of the fibular head lies anterior to this line. The role of oblique radiographs with internal rotation of the knee is controversial.[47,65] Internal rotation of 30 to 90 degrees can place the joint in profile for evaluation of joint space widening.[47,65] In select cases, radiographs of adjacent joints should be included if there is concern for proximal injury, tibial or fibular shaft fracture, syndesmotic injury, or ankle fracture. Comparison stress radiographs of the ankles can be obtained to evaluate the talocrural angle and medial clear space in both injured and noninjured ankles to

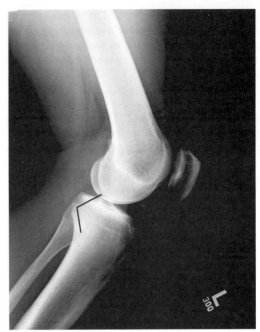

FIG 64.6 Resnick's line (*solid line*) depicted on the lateral radiograph of a normal knee is used to identify instability of the proximal tibiofibular joint. Resnick's line should intersect near the midpoint of the fibular head and defines the posterior border of the tibia. (Whiddon DR, Parker TA, Kuhn JE, Sekiya JK: Disorders of the proximal tibiofibular joint. In Scott NW [ed]: *Surgery of the knee,* ed 4, Philadelphia, 2006, Elsevier, pp 797–803.)

evaluate the integrity of the syndesmosis.[27] Computed tomography is indicated whenever there is uncertainty of PTFJ dislocation, and axial imaging is diagnostic.[23,67] The role of magnetic resonance imaging (MRI) is limited but may demonstrate pericapsular edema. Ultrasound can have both diagnostic and therapeutic uses. Intra-articular injections of local anesthetic can be used to help confirm the PTFJ as the source of lateral-sided knee pain in the elective setting and can be used to assist with reduction maneuvers in the acute setting. Ultrasound is beneficial over blind injections based on bony landmarks because it is 100% accurate compared to blind injections (accuracy = 58%). Inaccurate injections tended to be superficial and inferior.[55]

TREATMENT

Atraumatic Subluxation

Nonsurgical management is the mainstay of treatment for symptomatic atraumatic subluxation of the PTFJ. For patients with substantial pain, a period of rest and immobilization in a cylinder cast for 2 to 3 weeks is typically successful in reducing symptoms, followed by activity modification with avoidance of knee hyperflexion.[39] A trial of formal physical therapy for lower extremity gastrocnemius and hamstring strengthening with gradual return to activities can provide some benefit.[50,54] Bracing or supportive bandages placed just distal to the fibular head can decrease symptoms of instability; however, this can lead to a peroneal nerve palsy if placed too tightly.[18,60]

Atraumatic subluxation of the PTFJ in those with generalized ligamentous laxity tends to be a self-limiting problem with a gradual decrease in symptoms as patients approach skeletal maturity. Surgical intervention is rarely indicated in patients with subluxation of the PTFJ.

Acute Dislocation

If acute dislocation of the PTFJ is confirmed, prompt treatment is mandatory to prevent long-term morbidity. Options for treatment include closed reduction without postreduction immobilization, closed reduction with postreduction immobilization, and open reduction with temporary internal fixation.

Attempted closed reduction in the emergency department or operating theater is advocated in all four types of acute PTFJ dislocation, although types III and IV are typically more difficult.[12] Reduction may be assisted by intra-articular injection of local anesthetic or by an ultrasound-guided regional anesthetic block of the common peroneal nerve.[7,22] The reduction maneuver is performed with the knee flexed to approximately 100 degrees to relax the LCL and the biceps femoris. With direct pressure over the fibular head, the ankle is externally rotated and dorsiflexed.[1] An audible or palpable clunk confirms adequate reduction. Failed closed reduction may occur if the fibular head is perched on the lateral tibial ridge by the LCL. If this maneuver fails to reduce the joint, the patient should be asked to contract their hamstrings muscles at 90 degrees of knee flexion while the physician holds the patient's heel with one hand and performs the proximal fibular reduction with the other.[7] This uses the active contraction of the biceps femoris muscle to help reduce the joint.

After reduction, the knee exam described previously should be repeated paying close attention to the integrity of the knee ligamentous structures, particularly the LCL. Immobilization following successful closed reduction is controversial. Some authors advocate for an elastic bandage and immediate mobilization with full weight bearing if the postreduction exam is considered stable and knee range of motion is pain-free.[24] Others advocate for a period of immobilization in an above-knee cast or splint for 3 to 4 weeks followed by an elastic bandage and progressive weight bearing until 6 weeks postinjury.[63] Results of closed reduction were poor in Ogden's series because 57% of patients with acute PTFJ dislocations later required surgery for persistent symptoms.[38]

Open reduction of PTFJ dislocations is indicated if closed reduction is unsuccessful for anterolateral, posteromedial, and superior dislocations. It can also be considered if there is persistent instability following closed reduction. Several techniques have been described including temporary internal fixation with Kirschner wires, bioabsorbable pins, or cancellous screws.[41,46,61] Despite varying techniques, each author advocates for primary repair of the capsule and injured ligaments at the time of open reduction and temporizing internal fixation. Immobilization is recommended postoperatively for a total of 6 weeks, in which the patient is non-weight-bearing. Temporary fixation is removed between 6 and 12 weeks with the initiation of bracing and gradual weight bearing. Surgical intervention for PTFJ dislocations is also indicated in superior dislocations, which usually have an associated tibia or ankle fracture, and in cases of injury to the posterolateral structures. Controversy exists regarding acute repair versus reconstruction of the PLC in these cases.[49] Stannard et al. reported that the outcomes following primary repair of the PLC structures were significantly worse compared to PLC reconstruction in cases of knee dislocation.[56]

Chronic Instability

Late presentations, malreductions, and unrecognized dislocations of the PTFJ can be a source of significant morbidity. Persistent instability and pain from degeneration of the articular cartilage of the joint can create significant symptoms. In the case of chronic dislocations, closed reduction is no longer a treatment option. Conservative therapy consists of physical therapy and bracing as discussed previously, with goals to improve rotational stability and avoid knee hyperflexion. In cases of recalcitrant pain or instability, surgical intervention can be considered. Many procedures have been described, but there is a relative lack of literature regarding long-term outcomes given the small sample sizes and relative rarity of the condition. Surgical treatment options include temporary fixation of the PTFJ (Kirschner wire or screw fixation), soft tissue ligamentous reconstruction, arthrodesis of the PTFJ, or fibular head resection.

Temporary open fixation of the fibular head using a single cancellous screw with subsequent removal in 6 weeks to 6 months has shown good results.[6,32,62] The procedure is done in combination with a common peroneal nerve release. Van den Bekeron and colleagues have demonstrated excellent results in a series of eight patients with screw fixation. Postoperatively patients were not immobilized and were allowed immediate full weight bearing. All eight had good symptom alleviation at last follow-up.[61] Other authors have been less aggressive using fixation with a single transarticular 1.6 mm Kirschner wire after open reduction of the joint. The wire was cut subcutaneously and the patient treated in a cast brace at 30 degrees flexion and non-weight-bearing for 4 weeks. The brace was unlocked and progressive weight bearing as tolerated was allowed at 4 weeks. The wire and brace were removed at 8 weeks with return to sports (soccer) at 3 months.[6]

Several soft tissue procedures to reconstruct the PTFJ have been described for patients with recurrent instability. These small series all show promising short-term results.[9,43,67] However, they are technically demanding and require a significant amount of soft tissue dissection. There is a risk of injury to the peroneal nerve (Fig. 64.7), and postoperative non–weight-bearing immobilization for a minimum of 4 to 6 weeks is required. Gradual return to full weight bearing is followed by a focus on knee and ankle range of motion. Progressive strengthening then ensues. Strengthening should not be started too early in the recovery phase because early activation of the leg muscles in a patient with an anterolateral dislocation may increase instability and symptoms.

Laprade et al. have described their technique for reconstruction of the posterior proximal tibiofibular ligament and a modification of this procedure for use in patients with open physes.[20,69] After dissection of the fibular head with neurolysis and protection of the common peroneal nerve, an anterior to posterior tunnel is drilled in the fibular head.[69] Dissection is carried anteriorly to identify the flat spot slightly distal and medial to Gerdy's tubercle. Dissection is carried posterior to the fibular head and under the lateral head of the gastroc and popliteus muscle. An anterior to posterior guide pin is then drilled (a tibial anterior cruciate ligamnet [ACL] guide can be used to help with the trajectory) from anterior to posterior through the tibia while maintaining adequate posterior retraction. The tunnel should exit approximately 1 cm medial to the posterior fibular head tunnel. After reaming the tunnel, shuttling sutures are used to shuttle the graft, first anterior to posterior through the fibula and then posterior to anterior through the tibia. LaPrade's technique used a 6-mm semitendinosis autograft fixed in the fibula and tibia with interference screws.[20] The modification for open physes used fluoroscopy to confirm the location of the physes with fibular and tibial tunnels placed more distally to avoid injury to the proximal physes.[69] There has also been a single report of using a double cortical button and suture construct to repair the PTFJ in a patient with open physes.[57]

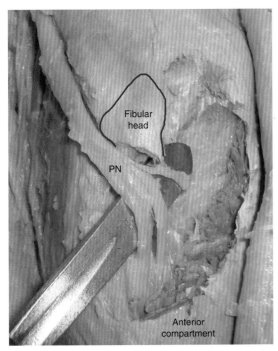

FIG 64.7 Common peroneal nerve and bifurcation in close proximity to fibular head and proximal tibiofibular joint. Particularly in an injury situation, protection of the nerve and its branches during surgery is paramount. *PN,* Peroneal nerve.

An alternate technique using an autogenous gracilis graft has been used by Maffulli et al. in eight patients.[30] The gracilis is harvested with an open-ended tendon stripper through a small medial incision. Through a separate lateral incision, two convergent tunnels are drilled from the fibular head to the medial tibial incision. One tunnel is anterior superior and the other is more inferior and posterior in the fibular head. The gracilis is passed from medial to lateral and then back from the fibular head to the medial opening, where it is fixed with an interference screw. Average follow-up was 44 months with significant improvements in modified Cincinnati and Kujala scores.[30]

Giachino described his technique in a series of two patients, with both returning to their previous level of activity and resolution of instability. His technique harvests half of the ipsilateral biceps femoris tendon still attached distally to the fibular head and a 10-cm rolled strip of deep fascia of the anterolateral compartment of the leg still attached proximally to the fibular head. Both limbs are wrapped around the head of the reduced fibula and tunneled through a tibial drill hole from posterior to anterior and secured anteriorly to the fascia.[17] White described a similar technique in two patients that used a strip of biceps femoris tendon without augmentation.[68] Shapiro and colleagues harvested a 20 × 2-cm strip of the iliotibial band left connected to its insertion into Gerdy's tubercle. The band was first tunneled through a tibial drill hole from anterior to posterior just proximal to Gerdy's tubercle and subsequently passed through the posterior capsule and arcuate complex and through the fibular head from posterior to anterior at the fibular head-neck junction just deep to the LCL. It is then tightened and sutured in place.[51]

In patients who have developed degenerative changes of the PTFJ and report primary complaint of pain, arthrodesis can be considered.[15] PTFJ arthrodesis prevents physiologic rotation of the fibula with ankle motion. The overconstraint caused by PTFJ arthrodesis can lead to ankle pain and instability.[39] Therefore, this technique has been largely abandoned in children and athletes.[49] When performed, 1.5 cm of fibular resection is recommended at the junction of the proximal- and middle-thirds of the fibular shaft to prevent overconstraining the fibula and to protect the arthrodesis site (Fig. 64.8).[3,39] As with soft tissue reconstruction procedures, identification and protection of the

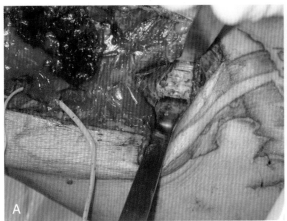
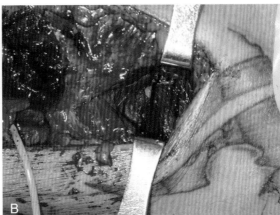
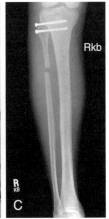

FIG 64.8 Surgical Dissection During Proximal Tibiofibular Joint Stabilization. (A and B) Before and after osteotomy. (C) Anteroposterior radiograph depicting resection of the middle third of the fibula following arthrodesis.

peroneal nerve is important to avoid injury (see Fig. 64.7). Following resection, the articular surfaces are prepared and provisionally compressed with a clamp (Fig. 64.9). The joint is then held reduced with cancellous lag screws (Fig. 64.10). Patients are immobilized for 5 weeks, and full weight bearing is allowed at 8 weeks postoperatively.[54]

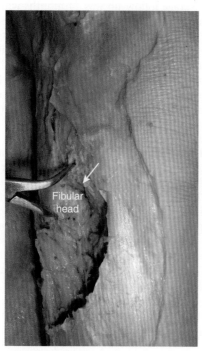

FIG 64.9 Proximal tibiofibular joint surfaces are denuded of articular cartilage and provisionally compressed in preparation for arthrodesis screws.

Lastly, fibular head and neck resection can be considered as a salvage procedure in cases of chronic peroneal nerve palsy resulting from chronic fibular head dislocation.[38] Peroneal tenolysis is performed and the fibular head and neck are excised, while the fibular styloid is preserved and the attached LCL is secured to the underlying tibia. Although care is taken to preserve the posterolateral structures of the knee, posterolateral rotatory instability is a reported complication and this procedure is contraindicated in athletes.[50] The procedure is also avoided in patients with open physes because of the risk of damage to the growth plate and subsequent growth disturbance or arrest.[17]

CONCLUSION

PTFJ dislocations are rare injuries. A significant portion of these injures are missed at initial evaluation. Despite the low incidence, both acute and chronic PTFJ injuries can result in significant short- and long-term morbidity if mistreated. Clinicians should be aware of these injuries to optimize early treatment and functional outcomes. Specific mechanisms should heighten clinical suspicion of PTFJ disruption, and a thorough knee clinical exam should always include the PTFJ. Knowledge of the anatomy of PTFJ and its relationship with the entire lower extremity is paramount for identifying these injuries.

Atraumatic subluxation can usually be treated conservatively, whereas acute dislocations require urgent closed or open reduction. Chronic injuries are more difficult to treat, and a number of soft tissue reconstructive procedures to address recurrent instability have been described in small series with promising short-term results. Temporary screw fixation has recently been proposed with excellent short-term results without a period of immobilization. Salvage operations such as arthrodesis and fibular head resection are considered for pain relief in the setting of end-stage degenerative changes or chronic dislocation of the PTFJ.

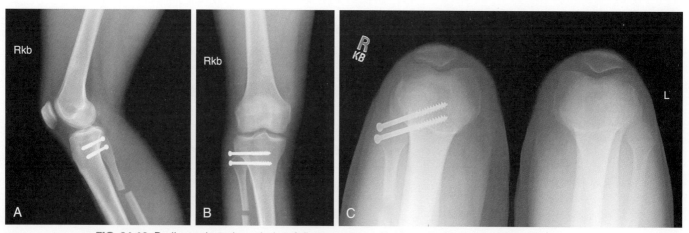

FIG 64.10 Radiographs taken during follow-up show fixation of the proximal tibiofibular joint using cancellous lag screws. (A) Lateral. (B) Anteroposterior. (C) Merchant views.

KEY REFERENCES

3. Baciu CC, Tudor A, Olaru I: Recurrent luxation of the superior tibio-fibular joint in the adult. *Acta Orthop Scand* 45:772–777, 1974.

14. Falkenberg P, Nygaard H: Isolated anterior dislocation of the proximal tibiofibular joint. *J Bone Joint Surg Br* 65:310–311, 1983.

20. Horst PK, LaPrade RF: Anatomic reconstruction of chronic symptomatic anterolateral proximal tibiofibular joint instability. *Knee Surg Sports Traumatol Arthrosc* 18:1452–1455, 2010.

30. Maffulli N, Spiezia F, Oliva F, et al: Gracilis autograft for recurrent posttraumatic instability of the superior tibiofibular joint. *Am J Sports Med* 38:2294–2298, 2010.

36. Ogden JA: Dislocation of the proximal fibula. *Radiology* 105:547–549, 1972.

37. Ogden JA: The anatomy and function of the proximal tibiofibular joint. *Clin Orthop* 101:186–191, 1974.

38. Ogden JA: Subluxation and dislocation of the proximal tibiofibular joint. *J Bone Joint Surg Am* 56:145–154, 1974.

39. Ogden JA: Subluxation of the proximal tibiofibular joint. *Clin Orthop* 101:192–197, 1974.

47. Resnick D, Newell JD, Guerra J Jr, et al: Proximal tibiofibular joint: anatomic-pathologic-radiographic correlation. *AJR Am J Roentgenol* 131:133–138, 1978.

48. Seebacher JR, Inglis AE, Marshall JL, et al: The structure of the posterolateral aspect of the knee. *J Bone Joint Surg Am* 64:536–541, 1982.

49. Sekiya JK, Kuhn JE: Instability of the proximal tibiofibular joint. *J Am Acad Orthop Surg* 11:120–128, 2003.

51. Shapiro GS, Fanton GS, Dillingham MF: Reconstruction for recurrent dislocation of the proximal tibiofibular joint. A new technique. *Orthop Rev* 22:1229–1232, 1993.

56. Stannard JP, Brown SL, Farris RC, et al: The posterolateral corner of the knee: repair versus reconstruction. *Am J Sports Med* 33:881–888, 2005.

58. Terry GC, LaPrade RF: The posterolateral aspect of the knee. Anatomy and surgical approach. *Am J Sports Med* 24:732–739, 1996.

60. Turco VJ, Spinella AJ: Anterolateral dislocation of the head of the fibula in sports. *Am J Sports Med* 13:209–215, 1985.

The references for this chapter can also be found on www.expertconsult.com.

Sports Medicine: Patellar and Extensor Mechanism Disorders

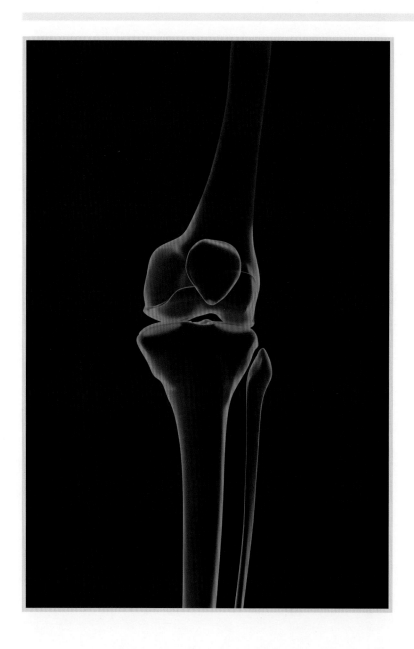

65

Disorders of the Patellofemoral Joint

David DeJour, Paulo R.F. Saggin, Vinícius Canello Kuhn

BASIC ANATOMY AND BIOMECHANICS

The patella is the biggest sesamoid bone in the human body, linking the powerful quadriceps muscle to the patellar tendon. The patella is the connection element in the extensor mechanism, receiving the convergent quadriceps' fibers in its superior pole and transferring its forces to the patellar tendon originated from its inferior pole.

Only the superior two-thirds of the patella have an articular surface. The distal pole is extra-articular and houses the patellar tendon's proximal insertion. Its anterior surface is roughly rounded and convex. On its posterior and articular sides, the patella is similarly convex, divided by a longitudinal median ridge. This ridge divides the patella in medial and lateral facets, but overall seven facets are described. A transverse ridge may also exist. In the most medial zone, there is a secondary ridge, delineating the odd facet. Patellar shape, however, is not constant. Three different types of patella were originally defined morphologically by Wiberg[216] and additional variant types were described later (Fig. 65.1).

The posterior (articular) surface of the patella is covered with the thickest cartilage in the human body. There is a slight difference in the surface geometry of the articular cartilage and the corresponding subchondral bone, which means that the articular apex may not correspond to the osseous apex of the retropatellar surface.[195]

A rich arterial plexus supplies the patella. A complex vascular anastomotic ring lying in the thin layer of loose connective tissue that covers the dense fibrous rectus expansions surrounds the patella. Six main arteries compound this ring: the supreme genicular artery, the medial and lateral superior and inferior genicular arteries, and the anterior tibial recurrent artery. Both of the superior genicular arteries (medial and lateral) run toward each other and anastomose with the supreme genicular artery. The inferior genicular arteries (medial and lateral) divide into three branches: the ascending parapatellar branches, which anastomose with the descending branches from the superior genicular arteries; the oblique prepatellar arteries, which run centripetally in front of the patella with other rami from the vascular ring; and the transverse infrapatellar arteries, which anastomose behind the *ligamentum patellae* and give origin to the polar vessels (Fig. 65.2). Two intraosseous systems were described by Scapinelli[180] that originate from this ring: the midpatellar vessels, which enter the vascular foramina situated in the anterior surface of the patella; and a second system, which arises from the polar vessels, from the anastomosis behind the patellar ligament. Later, Björkstrom and Goldie[22] demonstrated that arteries penetrate the quadriceps tendon and from the synovial tissue into the base of the patella. Arteries have also been demonstrated to penetrate from the synovial tissue on the retinacula through both the medial and lateral patellar borders. Some of the arteries penetrating the medial, superior, and lateral borders of the patella have their origin in deeply situated peripatellar arteries, not arising from the superficial arterial circle.

Opposed to the patella is the femoral sulcus (femoral trochlea), situated in the distal and anterior part of the femur, similarly covered by hyaline cartilage. Normal trochleae are formed by a medial and a lateral facet that project anteriorly, separated by the trochlear groove (TG). The lateral facet is bigger, more prominent, and extends more proximally than the medial facet. Distally, in the transition from the trochlea to the femoral condyles, a groove can be observed in each side. The medial condylar TG is discrete, and at times almost imperceptible, while the lateral is more marked (also designated as the *sulcus terminalis*). If the deepest points of the trochlea are taken into account, then the natural TG is most often aligned so that it deviates distally and laterally in relation to the femoral shaft axis.[5,190] The TG ends in the notch, and this can roughly serve as a reference for establishing the trochlear surgical limits: "v-shaped," the apex distal in the notch, and limited by both the medial and the lateral grooves. Proximal to the trochlear cartilage is the anterior surface of the femur, called the *supratrochlear fossa*, covered by adipose tissue and synovium that prevent patellar contact with the cortical femoral bone.

The quadriceps muscle has four parts: *rectus femoris, vastus medialis, vastus lateralis,* and *vastus intermedius.* These muscles converge to a trilaminar tendon 5 to 8 cm superior to the patella. Fibrous expansions arise from the *vastus lateralis* and *medialis,* blending with the lateral and medial retinacula, respectively. The most inferior part of the *vastus medialis* is also known as the *vastus medialis obliquus* (VMO) and inserts in the patella with mean angulation of 47 ± 5 degrees from the femoral axis in the coronal plane.[81] Similarly, a *vastus lateralis obliquus* (VLO) can be described, but with a more vertical (35 ± 4 degrees) orientation.

The patellar tendon arises from the inferior pole of the patella. It derives primarily from the central fibers of the rectus femoris that extend distally over the anterior surface of the patella. Its average length is 4.6 cm (3.5 to 5.5 cm) and its width varies between 24 and 33 mm.[170] It inserts distally in the tibial tubercle (TT), which is usually lateralized in relation to the long axis of the tibia, thus the distal orientation of the patellar tendon is oblique and lateralized (valgus). A small portion continues past the tubercle to blend with the fascial expansions of the iliotibial tract over the anterior surface of the tibia.[7] The

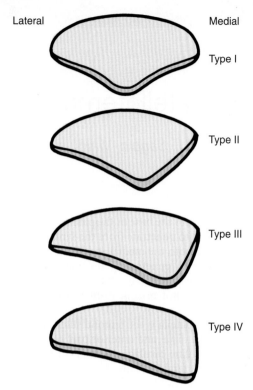

Lateral   Medial

Type I

Type II

Type III

Type IV

FIG 65.1 The types of patella according to the Wiberg classification are illustrated here as seen in axial views.

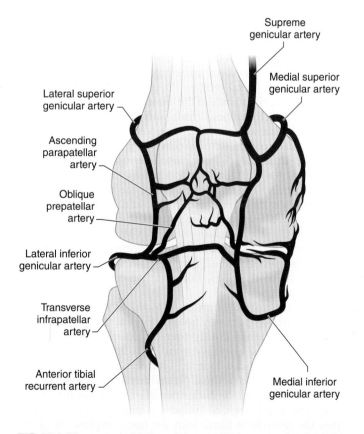

Supreme
genicular artery

Medial superior
genicular artery

Lateral superior
genicular artery

Ascending
parapatellar
artery

Oblique
prepatellar
artery

Lateral inferior
genicular artery

Transverse
infrapatellar
artery

Anterior tibial
recurrent artery

Medial inferior
genicular artery

FIG 65.2 The vascularization of the patella (see text for details).

posterior part of the patellar tendon is separated from the synovial membrane of the joint by the infrapatellar fat pad, and from the tibia, more distally, by a bursa.

On the medial aspect of the knee, the retinacular expansion of the *vastus medialis* merges with the crural fascia. The medial patellofemoral ligament (MPFL) is situated in the second of the three layers described by Warren and Marshal[212] along with the superficial medial collateral ligament, below the deep fascia and superficial to the joint capsule. The MPFL runs transversely from the patella to the femur. Its femoral insertion is proximal and posterior to the medial epicondyle, and distal and anterior to the adductor tubercle. The patellar attachment is wider than the femoral one, extending from the proximal and medial corner of the patella over approximately half of its length.[6] The mean length of the MPFL is 53 to 55 mm, and its width varies between studies, ranging from 3 to 30 mm, widening at its attachments.[6,45,170,205] As it approximates the patella, it is overlaid by the distal part of the VMO, and some of its fibers merge into the deep aspect of the muscle. Other bands, with secondary functions, have also been described linking the patella to the tibia and medial meniscus. One of these bands is the medial patellomeniscal ligament (MPML), which connects the inferior border of the medial patellar edge to the anterior horn of the medial meniscus.[7]

On the lateral side, some controversy exists about the nomenclature and location of the composing anatomic structures. Generally, the lateral aspect can be divided in the superficial oblique retinaculum and deep transverse retinaculum. The superficial oblique retinaculum originates from the iliotibial band (ITB) and interdigitates with the longitudinal fibers of the *vastus lateralis*. Deep to this structure are a separate distinct transverse band to the patella, an epicondylopatellar band and a patellotibial band.[85] The deep transverse retinaculum is the most substantial structure, consisting of the deeper transverse fibers of the ITB, which are dense and anchor the lateral edge of the patella and the tendon of VLO to the ITB. These can be called *ITB–patella fibers* and constitute an intermediate layer.[147] In fact, they are not a distinctly separate layer, but adhere to the deep aspect of the ITB. These transverse fibers lack a direct connection to the femur. The deeper capsular structures that link the patella to the lateral femoral epicondyle and the lateral meniscus are less substantial. Merican and Amis[147] did not find an extracapsular band linking the patella to the lateral epicondyle, and it is probable that the descriptions of the epicondylopatellar band and the lateral patellofemoral (PF) ligament represent the same structure, a capsular thickening linking the osseous elements. The patellotibial band is formed by longitudinal fibers of the quadriceps aponeurosis that descend distally along the lateral border of the patella and the patellar tendon, and attach to the lateral tibial condyle.

PF biomechanics can be understood as a complex interplay of factors that allow the quadriceps to perform its primary functions: knee extension and deceleration, especially during gait. To allow proper function, one must assume that the quadriceps is located in the TG and no instability is present. Continuity of the extensor mechanism should be mandatory to allow proper force transmission, and no pain should be present that would otherwise inhibit the quadriceps function.

The patella increases the moment arm of the extensor mechanism. It concentrates the tension of the converging quadriceps fibers and transmits it to the patellar tendon. In complete extension, a coronal resultant is produced, and no sagittal forces are expected (this is not completely true, as the retinacula exerts some posterior displacement forces in the patella when the knee is in extension). As the knee flexes, however, a posteriorly directed force vector becomes clear, and this raises the PF joint reaction force. The greater the degree of flexion, the greater the resultant force vector (Fig. 65.3).[106]

This posteriorly directed resultant vector is also important to patellar stability in the coronal plane. The trochlear lateral facet is deeper near the TG and becomes more prominent (higher) as it extends laterally. The patellar shape follows this principle: the crest is posterior and the lateral facet more anterior. Thus, the lateral part of the PF joint is not in the coronal plane, but oblique in relation to it, with its more medial part posterior to its more lateral part. As a result of this, when the quadriceps contracts, the resultant posteriorly directed force vector tends to bring the mobile part of the articulation (the patella) medially.[5]

The several quadriceps insertions and their different angles of action should be noted in the coronal plane. The VMO and VLO act in an oblique manner in the longitudinal direction, so malfunctioning of one (VMO) or hyperfunctioning of the other (VLO) can cause coronal displacement, and to a greater extent, instability. If the force-producing capacity of each muscle head is in proportion to its cross-sectional area, the

VMO could contribute to 10% of total quadriceps tension, and if completely relaxed, it can cause tension to swing laterally to approximately 6 degrees (Fig. 65.4).[81]

The difference between the quadriceps insertion angle and the patellar tendon insertion angle is another cause of a laterally directed force vector (valgus orientation of the extensor mechanism). This difference can be measured during the physical examination by tracing two lines that intersect each other in the center of the patella: one is traced from the patella to the anterior iliac spine, representing the quadriceps tension; the other is traced from the patella to the TT, and represents the patellar tendon reaction force. This is called the *Q angle*, and in normal subjects it is expected not to exceed 15 or 20 degrees. Women have the greatest values.

Lower extremity torsions (specifically, femoral internal torsion or tibial external torsion) accentuate the valgus resultant over the patella as they shift the TG medially and the extensor mechanism laterally.

Soft tissue restraints also play a fundamental role in the coronal plane force balance. In complete extension, normal patellae are not engaged in the TG. This engagement starts at approximately 20 degrees of flexion, when the distal and lateral parts of the patella touch the upper and proximal parts of the trochlea. As the patella is not engaged before this point, only soft tissue stabilizers act to ensure its coronal location. On the lateral side, because the retinaculum is directly linked to the ITB, tension to the ITB causes the patella to track in a more lateral position.[125] On the medial side, the MPFL contributes

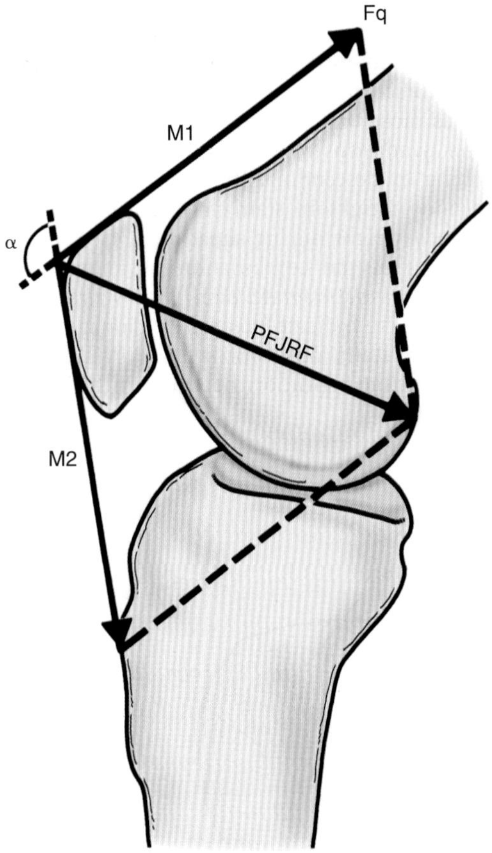

FIG 65.3 The PF joint reaction force becomes higher as the knee flexion angle increases. In complete extension, M1 and M2 are in opposite directions, but in the same plane; the resultant PFJRF is almost zero. As flexion increases, M1 and M2 converge, and the vector PFJRF increases. *PFJRF,* Patellofemoral joint reaction force.

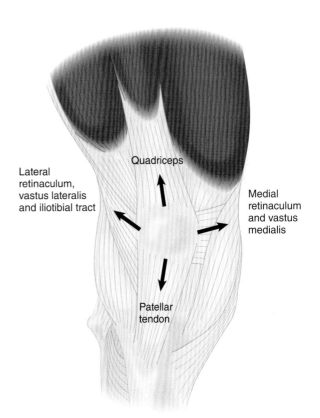

FIG 65.4 Anatomic view showing the valgus alignment of the extensor mechanism and the contributions of the medial retinaculum, vastus medialis, lateral retinaculum, vastus lateralis, and iliotibial tract.

50% to 60% of the restraint to patellar lateral displacement at 0 to 20 degrees of flexion, with a mean failure load of 208 N.[6,151] Although not the cause of lateral dislocation, one cannot assume lateral dislocation without MPFL insufficiency or rupture (Fig. 65.5).

Relative movement occurs between the patella and the trochlea in the longitudinal plane during flexion-extension. In initial PF contact, as a result of the articular surface orientation, a medial patellar shift is produced before the patella engages and follows the TG. As the flexion angle of the knee is increased, the contact area of the patella progresses proximally, while the trochlear contact area progresses distally. From extension to 90 degrees of flexion, the patella holds the quadriceps tendon away from the femur, but in further degrees of flexion, an extensive

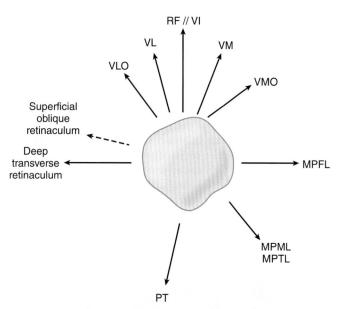

FIG 65.5 Diagram demonstrating the several forces acting on the patella in the coronal plane. *MPFL,* Medial patellofemoral ligament; *MPML,* medial patellomeniscal ligament; *VLO,* vastus lateralis obliquus; *VMO,* vastus medialis obliquus.

area of contact between the tendon and the trochlea is formed. Between 90 and 135 degrees of flexion, the patella rotates and the ridge that separates the medial and odd facets engages the femoral condyle. At 135 degrees, separate lateral and medial (limited to the odd facet) contact areas are formed (Fig. 65.6).[89,90]

Clinical Evaluation

Symptoms. When collecting the clinical history, the physician should have in mind that PF disorders can be some of the most difficult pathologies of the knee to manage. Some patients have visited numerous clinicians with variable degrees of success with treatment. Therefore, it is essential to listen carefully and give the patient enough time to talk about their symptoms, anguish, and expectations.

There are three main complaints in PF disorders: pain, instability (or feeling of instability), and locking (or catching), which will be explained below. It is also important to investigate common associated conditions, such as low back pain, hip catching, ankle pain or sprains, and, of course, symptoms in the opposite knee. A positive family history can suggest some constitutional causes and influence prognosis.[163] Time from the onset of symptoms must be determined. Frequency of symptoms and number of episodes (such as dislocations) have to be scrutinized.

Pain. Pain is usually anterior, diffuse, and not well localized. It may be referred to the medial or the lateral retinaculum. Sometimes the pain is referred below the patella, as a bar. Posterior knee pain, although less common, may also be possible, especially if an intra-articular effusion is present. Usually, the pain is worse during or after activities that overload the joint, such as those that demand jumping, running, squatting, or vigorous quadriceps contraction. It can be evoked during stair climbing or descending. PF joint reaction force reaches 3.3 times body weight in stair climbing or descending, and 7.6 times body weight during squatting.[120,171] Stefanik et al.[197] demonstrated that the combination of anterior knee pain (AKP) and at least moderate pain with stairs had the best specificity (97%) to indicate isolated PF damage, and that isolated pain with stairs does not specifically differentiate the structurally damaged location between PF and tibiofemoral

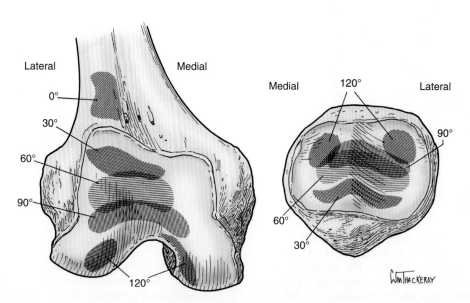

FIG 65.6 Illustration demonstrating the PF joint contact areas according to the knee flexion angle.

(TF) joints. Prolonged sitting with the knees flexed is a classic situation that produces or increases PF pain; this is commonly known as the *movie sign* (or *theater sign*). Although classic, this sign is not specific.

Instability. The symptom of instability better describes the subjective feeling of an unstable knee. It may be objective, as found in patellar dislocation, when it is a mechanical phenomenon whereby the patella completely loses contact with the trochlea. The first episode generally occurs during high-energy activity and is followed by an effusion, hemarthrosis, or sometimes even hematoma caused by capsule rupture and subcutaneous blood diffusion. Objective instability may also occur during subluxations, when these features are absent. Instability may also be subjective, caused by quadriceps inhibition (reflex) as the result of pain and fear, without loss of contact of the articulating surfaces. It occurs generally with low-energy activities that demand quadriceps effort, such as walking, ascending or descending stairs, and rising from a squat. Careful analysis of the clinical history and the patient's description of the episode is useful in differentiating the mechanisms of instability. Objective instability is easy to diagnose when the patella is still dislocated, when a medical report indicates that a physician relocated it, or when imaging has been taken and demonstrates the dislocation or objective signs of it.

Locking (or catching). Locking and catching are the third most frequent complaints and must be differentiated from those produced by meniscal tears. The main difference from meniscal locking is that the knee is not able to flex or extend, but in a bucket-handle tear, the knee is able to flex. Sometimes, locking in extension can be produced by a reflex mechanism of quadriceps and hamstring contracture because of pain to avoid contact of the opposed cartilage surfaces. Locking episodes are usually momentary, but in some cases can last for longer periods and can be extremely painful. Catching may be produced by cartilage lesions or by irregularities in the opposed patellar or trochlear surfaces as they glide over each other.

Physical Examination. Physical examination starts by inspecting how the patient rises from the chair and walks into the physician's office. This information is interesting because the patient is acting naturally. In the office, the evaluation starts with the patient standing. Asymmetry at the level of the shoulders or pelvis is noted when the patient is standing and sitting. The patellae should face forward. If femoral anteversion is present, they will face inward. Coronal and rotational alignments are observed. Genu valgus, tibial torsion, and limb discrepancy are also noticed at this time. The overall extensor mechanism alignment is checked and the Q-angle can be estimated. Subtalar eversion, which would produce compensatory internal tibial rotation, is best identified while standing behind the patient.

The same observations performed when the patient is standing should be done when he/she is walking. Rotational deformities are especially exacerbated during gait. Muscle hypotrophy can be noted and any limp will become evident.

The spine and the pelvis (and therefore the sacroiliac articulation) must be assessed thoroughly. Stiffness of this "system" avoids adequate stretching of the quadriceps (remember the *rectus femoris* originates from the pelvis). Irreducible lordosis is an indicator of anterior pelvic tilt and its commonly associated features (weak abdominals, weak glutes and hamstrings, and tight hip flexors). Anterior pelvic tilt may cause femoral internal rotation (and relative lateralization of the patella) because of

changes in acetabular orientation. The inspection begins when the patient was seated in front of the physician (thoracic abnormal kyphosis may already be apparent) and continues when the patient is asked to stand up (pelvic anterior tilt and lumbar hyperlordosis can be evaluated from the side of the patient). A simple test may be performed asking the patient to stand with the back against the wall. The patient must be able to touch the wall with the heels, the back of the knees, the buttocks, the back (lumbar region), and the shoulders. Inability to do so and stand flat against the wall reflects stiffness and muscular imbalance.

With the patient supine and the hips and knees extended, the Q-angle measurement can be done effectively. Care should be taken because a laterally displaced patella will cause underestimation of its value. Knee flexion can correct this by bringing the patella into the center of the TG, but no agreement has been reached on the best *Q angle* measurement method (flexion or extension), nor even on its applicability.[194] Normal individuals, in general, will not present with values greater than 20 degrees.

Asking the patient to contract both quadriceps will allow comparison of the contraction pattern and the muscular mass. The VMO bulk should also be noted at this time. Active and passive movements of flexion and extension of the knee will allow patellar tracking assessment. The J-sign, seen when the patella shifts abruptly medially and then down in the TG as flexion progresses, similar to an inverted J, is sometimes found, and indicates patellar lateral displacement in extension. Palpation and specific tests are then performed (Fig. 65.7).

Palpation. Palpation should start in the less painful areas. The patella, patellar tendon, quadriceps tendon, and lateral and medial retinacula should be investigated for tenderness. The patellar facets may even be palpated and inspected for tenderness, but it should be noted that some structures (retinacula) are interposed, and this can confuse the interpretation

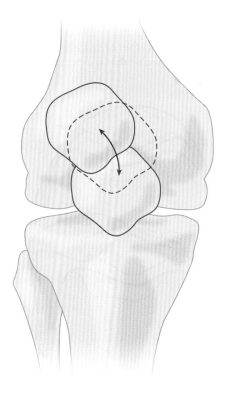

FIG 65.7 The "J-sign."

of the pain source. The distal-to-proximal position of the patella can be assessed by observation and palpation.

Anterior palpation should be done during the arc of movement in the search for pain and crepitus. Schiphof et al.[181] showed, with magnetic resonance imaging (MRI) analysis, that crepitus is an important clinical finding that indicates PF lesions, but not lesions in the TF joint. Crepitus is more important when accompanied by pain and recurrent effusion, because it can be found sometimes even in normal knees. The degree of flexion at the time crepitus or symptoms are produced should be noted.

Patellar compression test. The knee is positioned in full extension. The examiner uses two hands to posteriorly compress the patella against the TG. While compressed, the patella is moved superiorly and inferiorly. The test is positive if it produces pain, suggesting articular cartilage injury. This test is frequently painful and the clinician must be aware that it is not specific to cartilage damage.

Glide test. Patellar medial and lateral glide should be tested at full extension and at 30 degrees of flexion. For this purpose, the examiner can divide the patella into four vertical quadrants. Displacement of less than one quadrant or more than three is considered abnormal (Fig. 65.8). The main value of this test is to indicate the competency of the MPFL.

Tilt test. The lateral and medial margins of the patella should be in the same horizontal plane, and it should be possible to elevate its transverse axis beyond the horizontal plane. Significant tilt in the physical examination correlates with MRI[94] or computed tomography (CT) scan tilt measures greater than 10 degrees. The main value of this test is to indicate tightness or laxity of the lateral retinaculum.

Smillie test,[193] apprehension test, or Fairbank test.[80] This test may be performed with the knee extended or at 30 degrees of flexion. The examiner grasps the patella with his fingers and applies a laterally directed force, trying to dislocate the patella while holding the tibia with the other hand. This laterally directed force applied over the patella causes apprehension in the patient as he/she feels that the patella is about to dislocate. It is also called the *apprehension test* because it is the patient's

positive reaction that determines if the test is positive. For adequate examination, the quadriceps should be relaxed. The test should be performed bilaterally and comparison with the opposite side may help. It is not useful in acute dislocations because pain and fear will be present even before physical examination is undertaken. In chronic cases, it specifically reflects the insufficiency of the patellar restraints (notably the MPFL) (Fig. 65.9).

A new variation of the apprehension test has been described, called the *moving apprehension test*. It is divided into two steps. In both steps, the knee is flexed from 0 to 90 degrees. During the first step, a laterally directed force is used over the patella. During the second step, a medially directed force is applied. The test is considered positive when the patient feels apprehension during the first step, but not throughout the second. Ahmad et al. showed that the moving apprehension test has a sensitivity of 100% and a specificity of 88.4% when compared to the ability to dislocate the patella under anesthesia.[2]

Muscle stiffness. Hamstrings are tested with the patient supine and the opposite leg extended and flat in the table. The hip is flexed to 90 degrees and the knee is then extended as far as possible. The popliteal angle is observed and compared with the opposite side. The quadriceps is tested with the patient prone, and in most patients the heels should touch the buttocks. The ITB is tested with the Ober test: with the patient in the lateral decubitus position (the side to be tested is up), the hip is extended and abducted, and the knee is extended. From this position, the thigh is released and is allowed to adduct. Most patients will be able to touch the examination table with the medial aspect of the knee.

IMAGING

X-ray Analysis

X-ray analysis is the first step in the investigation of the knee. Combined with the history and physical examination, it will

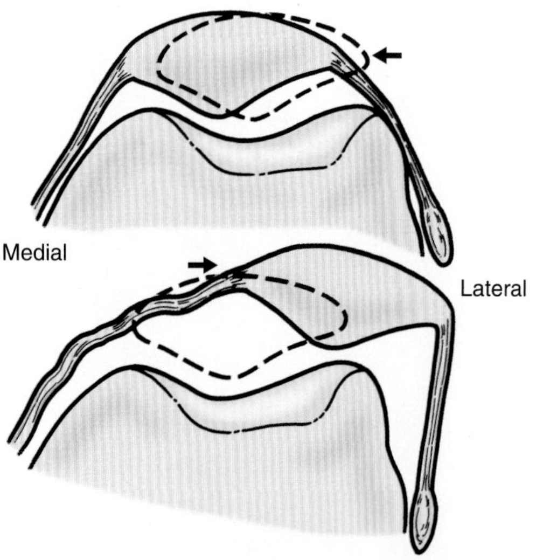

FIG 65.8 Clinical evaluation of the mediolateral displacement of the patella. It should be tested at 0 and 30 degrees of knee flexion and recorded in millimeters or quadrants.

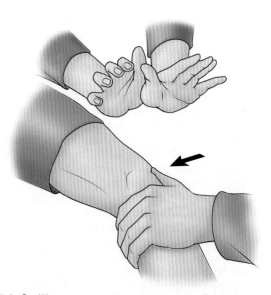

FIG 65.9 Smillie test, apprehension test, or Fairbank test. The physician laterally displaces the patella and the patient shows apprehension and fear of dislocation. Test positivity is determined by the patient's reaction and not the physician's ability to dislocate or subluxate the patella.

guide subsequent imaging procedures, and at times it will even make them unnecessary. The basic protocol is almost uniform in the various situations, chronic or urgent. Basic standard x-rays are described in the following paragraphs.

Anteroposterior View. The anteroposterior (AP) view must be obtained in monopodal stance if the patient is able to do so. In younger patients (less than 50 years old), it should be performed in 15 to 20 degrees of flexion; in older patients and in those who have antecedents of trauma or surgery around the knee, it should be performed in 30 or 45 degrees of knee flexion (Schuss or Rosenberg). The AP analysis is not very helpful for PF problems. It will allow the evaluation of bone quality, alignment assessment, and assessment of femorotibial-associated pathology. Major patellar displacement can already be observed in this view (Fig. 65.10), along with malformations such as bipartite patella or fractures. Loose bodies in the lateral gutter may be found, representing patellar or lateral condyle fractures that occurred during patellar dislocation.

In the AP view we can observe a bipartite or a multipartite patella. These conditions are the result of incomplete fusion of an ossification center and are described to have a frequency between 0.005% and 1.66%.[25,199] The accessory fragments are commonly located close to the superolateral border. The edges of the fragment are smooth, which allows the differentiation from fractures. Bipartite or multipartite patellae are often bilateral.

Lateral View. This is the most interesting view of the knee. The reliability of its interpretation depends on the technical quality of the image. It is essential to achieve perfect superimposition

of both the posterior femoral condyles. The image is obtained in monopodal weight bearing with the knee flexed between 15 and 20 degrees. Some authors propose taking the lateral view in full extension, but its accuracy in determining patellar height is controversial because different degrees of quadriceps contraction could modify the patellar height. Moreover, if the patient exhibits knee hyperextension, this could yield a false-positive *patella alta* with consequent false information about patellar engagement. Nevertheless, the location of the patella in relation to the trochlea provides interesting data.

Lateral x-ray analysis has to be systematic and should follow the guidelines provided in the following sections.

Trochlea. In normal knees, the Blumensaat line is continued anteriorly by the TG line, which should stay posterior to the projection of the femoral condyles (facets). The crossing sign characterizes trochlear dysplasia (TD) on the sagittal view. The crossing point represents the exact location where the deepest point of the trochlear sulcus reaches the same height as the femoral condyles, meaning that the trochlea becomes flat in this location (Fig. 65.11).[62,138] The crossing sign has been found in 96% of the population with antecedents of true patellar dislocation and in only 3% of healthy controls.[63]

Not only the shape, but also the position of the trochlear sulcus line is abnormal in relation to the anterior femoral

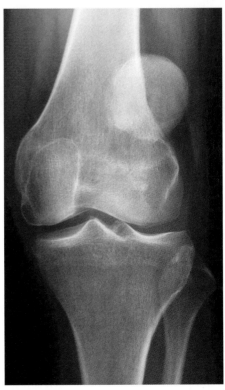

FIG 65.10 In rare cases, patellar tilt and subluxation are so pronounced that they can be seen even in AP views. In this case, note the high and tilted patella.

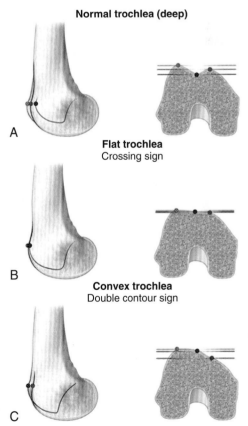

Normal trochlea (deep)

A

Flat trochlea
Crossing sign

B

Convex trochlea
Double contour sign

C

FIG 65.11 In a normal trochlea, the TG is posterior to the facets (A). In flat trochlea, the facets and the TG are in the same plane. In the lateral view, this is demonstrated by the crossing sign (B). When the trochlea is convex, the "groove" does not exist and the lateral part of the trochlea rests in front of the medial facet, what can be demonstrated in the lateral view as the double-contour sign (C).

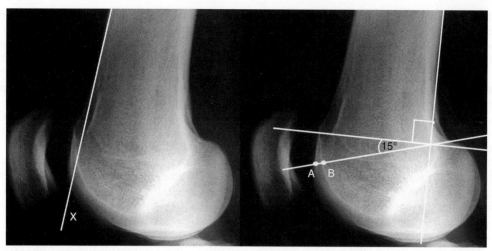

FIG 65.12 TG position and trochlear depth in relation to the anterior femoral cortex. A line (X) is drawn tangential to the anterior femoral cortex along its most distal 10 cm, extending below the articular surface. The trochlear sulcus is anterior to this line *(left figure)*. The trochlear depth is the distance A-B (measured in millimeters) along a line subtended 15 degrees from the perpendicular to the tangent of the posterior femoral cortex *(right figure)*.

cortex. In a study performed by Dejour et al.,[63] in normal knees the trochlear sulcus line was at a mean distance of 0.8 mm posterior to a line projected from the anterior femoral cortex (line X), while in knees with dysplastic trochleae, its mean position was 3.2 mm forward of the same line, increasing the contact force between the patella and the trochlea (anti-Maquet effect). Another sign was the depth of the trochlea measured from the contours of the condylar crests to the floor of the sulcus through a line subtended 15 degrees from another line perpendicular to the femoral shaft and tangential to the posterior cortex (Fig. 65.12).

The first published classification of TD (Henri Dejour) divided dysplasia into three grades, according to the level of the crossing sign. The classification in three grades has some limitations, as it has been corroborated by the work of Remy et al.[172] Remy et al. showed that interobserver reproducibility of trochlear analysis was low, especially for type II dysplasia. This led to a new study performed in 1996 by Dejour (Dejour, D.) and Le Coultre, which analyzed 177 cases of patellar instability and included radiographs along with preoperative and postoperative CT scans. Based on this analysis, a new and more precise classification with four grades of TD was defined.[58,60] Two new signs were added to the crossing sign. The first is the supratrochlear spur, which represents the prominence of the trochlea and plays a role similar to a "ramp" when the patella engages the trochlea. The second sign is the double contour, which is the radiographic line that ends below the crossing sign and represents the subchondral condensation of the hypoplastic medial facet on the lateral view. In 2002, the Lillois group conducted a new interobserver study[173] and concluded that "this new classification system is more reproducible than the former three-type system proposed. The crossing sign and the supratrochlear spur are the most reproducible signs" (Fig. 65.13).

This classification system (Figs. 65.14 and 65.15) is based mainly in the lateral view, but to increase the specificity, it must be combined with slice imaging (like CT axial views or MRI), which may assist in the differentiation between types. Four types, based on the three dysplastic signs described, are included:

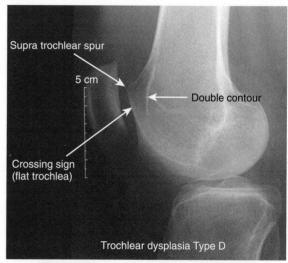

FIG 65.13 Adequate analysis of TD requires a true profile, with perfect superimposition of the posterior femoral condyles. The three signs of TD: 1. the crossing sign; 2. the supra-trochlear spur; 3. the double-contour ending below the crossing sign.

- Type A: The crossing sign is the only one of the three signs present. On axial views, the trochlea is shallower than normal ones (abnormal sulcus angle).
- Type B: The crossing sign and the supratrochlear spur are present. On axial views (slice imaging) the trochlea is flat.
- Type C: The crossing sign and the double contour sign are present, but there is no spur. On axial views (slice imaging) the medial facet is hypoplastic.
- Type D: Combines the three signs: crossing sign, supratrochlear spur, and double contour. On axial views (slice imaging) there is a cliff pattern (square link between lateral and medial facet).

Patella. The shape of the patella on lateral views is correlated with tilt and with its global morphology. In normal patellae,

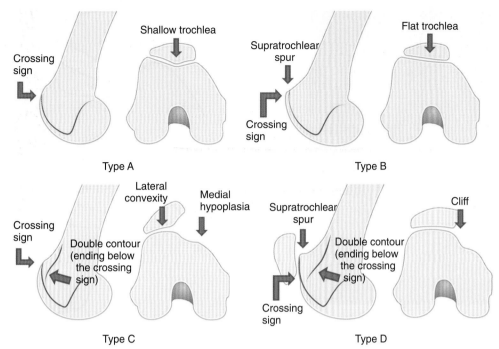

FIG 65.14 TD classification according to D. Dejour: *Type A*, presence of the crossing sign in lateral true view. The trochlea is shallower than normal, but still symmetric and concave. *Type B*, crossing sign and trochlear spur. The trochlea is flat or convex in axial images. *Type C*, presence of the crossing sign and the double-contour sign, representing the densification of the subchondral bone of the medial hypoplastic facet. In axial CT scan views, the lateral facet is convex. *Type D*, combines all the mentioned signs—crossing sign, supratrochlear spur, and double-contour sign going below the crossing sign. In axial CT scan views, there is a cliff pattern.

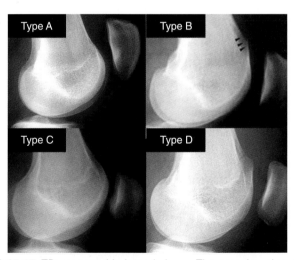

FIG 65.15 TD assessed in lateral views. The crossing sign, the supratrochlear spur, and the double-contour sign should all be assessed to classify the TD.

with no tilt, the most posterior part visible in the lateral view should be the median longitudinal ridge. The lateral facet projection is located slightly anterior. In tilted patellae, these relations are lost, and the overall AP size of the patella looks larger (Fig. 65.16).

Tilt categorization has been described by Maldague and Malghem.[138] Three positions are described: normal position, in which the lateral facet is anterior to the crest; mild tilt, in which

the two lines (lateral facet and crest) are on the same level; and severe tilt, which shows the lateral facet behind the crest (Fig. 65.17).

Grelsamer et al.[93] performed a study to evaluate the sagittal shape of the patella. Three types of patella were described based on the ratio between the length of the patella and the length of the articular surface. Most patellae exhibit a ratio between 1.2 and 1.5, and are classified as type I. Type II has the appearance of a long nose, and exhibits ratios above 1.5. Those with a ratio below 1.2 (short-nosed) are classified as type III (Fig. 65.18).

Patellar height. Patella *alta* or *infera* are essentially diagnosed on the lateral views, which are the key to the measurement of patellar height. Several methods of measurement (and diagnosis) using the tibia as reference have been described. The three main ratios are:

- Caton-Deschamps[39,40] is the ratio between the distance from the lower edge of the patellar articular surface to the antero-superior angle of the tibia (AT) outline, and the length of the articular surface of the patella (AP). A ratio (AT/AP) of 0.6 and smaller determines patella infera, and a ratio greater than 1.2 indicates patella alta (Fig. 65.19).
- Insall-Salvati[111] is the ratio between the length of the patellar tendon (LT) and the longest sagittal diameter of the patella (LP). Insall determined that this ratio (LT/LP) is normally 1. A ratio smaller than 0.8 indicates a patella infera and greater than 1.2, patella alta (Fig. 65.20).
- Blackburne-Peel[23] is the ratio between the length of the perpendicular line drawn from the tangent to the tibial plateau to the inferior pole of the articular surface of the

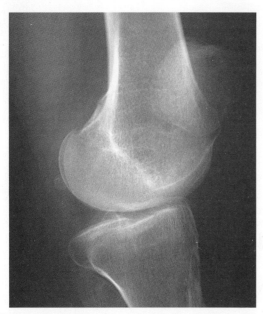

FIG 65.16 Lateral view of severe patellar tilt and subluxation. Note that the projection is a perfect lateral view (perfect posterior condyles superimposition). The patella, however, is not in front of the femur, but lateral to it, and the patellar AP diameter is increased. Additionally, severe TD can be noticed.

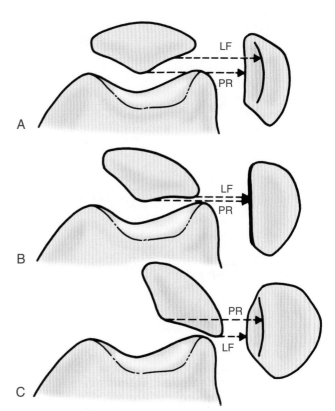

FIG 65.17 Tilt evaluation in lateral views as described by Maldague and Malghem. In the normal position, the lateral facet is in front of the crest. When mild tilt is present, the lateral facet and the crest are on the same level. When severe tilt occurs, the lateral facet is behind the crest.

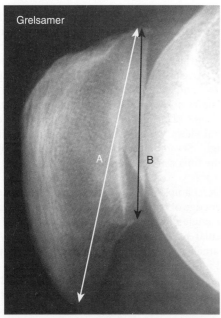

FIG 65.18 Patellar shape in lateral views according to Grelsamer. The ratio (*A/B*) between the length of the patella (*A*) and the length of its articular surface (*B*) is calculated. Most patellae exhibit ratios between 1.2 and 1.5.

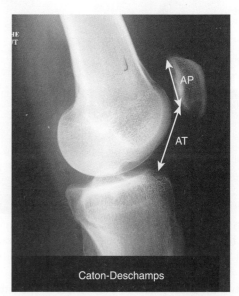

FIG 65.19 The Caton-Deschamps index (AT/AP) is the ratio between the distance from the lower edge of the patellar articular surface to the AT outline, and the length of the AP. *AP,* Articular surface of the patella; *AT,* anterosuperior angle of the tibia.

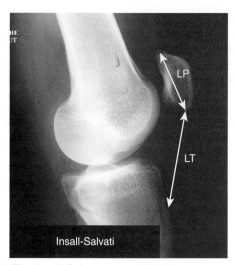

FIG 65.20 The Insall-Salvati index (LT/LP) is the ratio between the LT and the LP. *LP,* Longest sagittal diameter of the patella; *LT,* length of the patellar tendon.

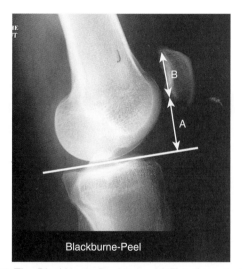

FIG 65.21 The Blackburne-Peel index (*A/B*) is the ratio between the length of the perpendicular line drawn from the tangent to the tibial plateau to the inferior pole of the articular surface of the patella (*A*) and the length of the articular surface of the patella (*B*).

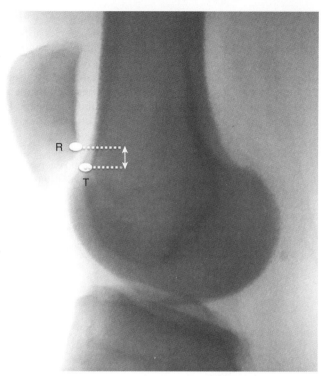

FIG 65.22 Patellar height measurement according to Bernageau. Patella alta is defined if *R* is more than 6 mm above *T*.

patella (*A*) and the length of the articular surface of the patella (*B*). The normal ratio (*A/B*) was defined as 0.8. In patella infera, it is smaller than 0.5, and in patella alta it is greater than 1.0 (Fig. 65.21).

Several factors must be considered when deciding which which index to use. Blackburne-Peel needs good superimposition of medial and lateral tibial plateaus. Insall-Salvati is not a good choice in the presence of Osgood-Schlatter disease or sequelae of it. Finally, the Caton-Deschamps method seems the easiest to use, especially for surgical planning.

Another method to measure patellar height uses the femoral trochlea as reference. Bernageau et al.[17] described this method on lateral x-rays with the knee in extension and the quadriceps contracted. If the inferior edge of the articular surface of the patella (*R*) is more than 6 mm above the superior limit of the trochlea (*T*), there is patella alta, and if *R* is more than 6 mm beneath *T*, patella infera is present (Fig. 65.22).

Other indexes have also been described using the distal femur as reference. Most of them are influenced by the variation of the knee flexion angle and are not widely used clinically. Chareancholvanich et al.[41] described a new method that does not change between 0 and 60 degrees of knee flexion. It is calculated as the ratio between the distance from the posterior angle of the intercondylar roof to the TT, and the distance from the midpoint of the patellar articular facet to the TT. The normal value is 1 (±0.1) (Fig. 65.23).

Axial View. The axial view has been described at different angles of knee flexion and different positions of the x-ray cassette. Our common approach is to perform 30-degree axial views as described by Ficat, who also described axial views at 60 and 90 degrees (Fig. 65.24). Radiographs are obtained with the knee flexed over the edge of the table, the beam directed proximally, and a perpendicular cassette in place. Images beyond 45 degrees of flexion are less informative as they show the lower part of the trochlea and the patella as fully engaged, at times correcting tracking abnormalities (Fig. 65.25). Thus, these high-flexion angle images are dispensable.[52] Lower flexion angles, although capable of more accurately showing the maltracking signs, are technically demanding, and at times impossible. With adequately performed images, the relation between the femoral trochlea (at 30 degrees, the lateral facet should appear with two-thirds total trochlear width [TW]) (Fig. 65.26) and the patella (with the lateral facet also composing two-thirds) can be effectively assessed. Tilt, congruence, and cartilage thickness can also be appreciated.

The classic methods that were proposed in the past and originated the described approach are discussed later.

Merchant View.[146] The Merchant view is obtained with the patient in the supine position, the knees in 45 degrees of flexion over the edge of the table, and the lower limbs resting on an angled platform. The x-ray beam is angled toward the feet, 30 degrees from the horizontal, and the film cassette is positioned 30 cm below the knees. The x-ray beam strikes the cassette at a 90-degree angle, imaging both knees simultaneously. Two angles are measured on this view: the sulcus angle and the congruence angle.

- Sulcus angle (Fig. 65.27) (defined by Brattström[28]): This is the angle formed by two lines drawn from the deepest point of the TG to the highest point on the medial and lateral femoral condyles. This measurement reveals the shape of the groove; the greater the sulcus angle, the flatter is the trochlea. The average sulcus angle on the merchant view measures 138 degrees (standard deviation [SD] ± 6) and is equal in males and females. Values in excess of 150 degrees are considered abnormal.

- Congruence angle (Fig. 65.28): This angle is measured by bisecting the sulcus angle to construct a reference line, and then projecting a second line from the apex of the sulcus angle to the lower point of the subchondral articular surface of the patella (apex). If the line drawn from the patellar apex is lateral to the reference line, then the angle is positive; if the patellar apex is medial to this line, a negative value is assigned; measurement of the normal congruence angle averages −6 degrees (SD ± 11 degrees; abnormal if greater than +16 degrees).

Laurin View.[128,129] This image is obtained with the patient sitting and the knee flexed 20 degrees. The x-ray cassette is held approximately 12 cm proximal to the patellae and is pushed against the anterior thighs. The x-ray beam is directed

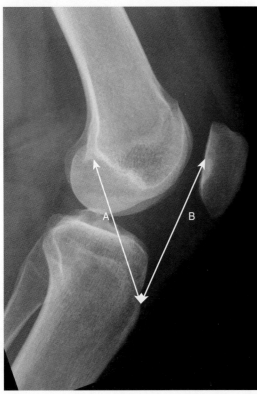

FIG 65.23 New method to measure patellar height. It is determined by the ratio between the distance from the posterior angle of the intercondylar roof to the TT (*A*), and the distance from the midpoint of the patellar articular facet to the TT (*B*). The normal value is 1 (±0.1).

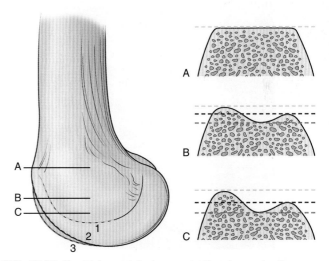

FIG 65.25 Sagittal model demonstrating how, in the same patient, different images can fail to show the abnormal trochlear shape. Proximally (A), the trochlea is flat, while it deepens distally (B and C). For this reason, it is important to have a full CT scan acquisition of the trochlea. Axial views performed with angles superior to 30 degrees could miss the proximal TD.

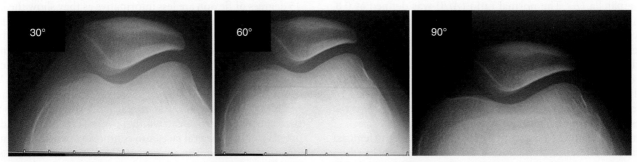

FIG 65.24 Axial views performed at 30, 60, and 90 degrees of knee flexion. Note how the trochlear shape changes as flexion increases and the medial facet seems bigger. There is no need to routinely perform 60 and 90 degrees flexion x-rays in common PF disorders.

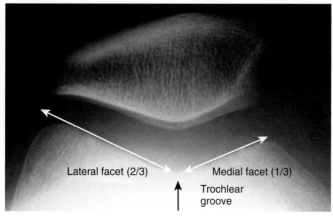

FIG 65.26 Axial view of the PF articulation at 30 degrees of knee flexion. The medial facet appears smaller and corresponds to 1/3 of the TW, while the lateral facet corresponds to 2/3 of the TW. The patella is centered and its long axis is horizontal, meaning that no tilt is present.

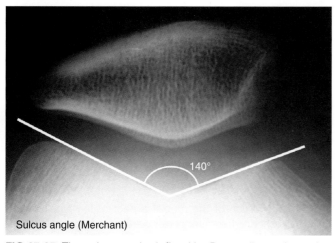

Sulcus angle (Merchant)

FIG 65.27 The sulcus angle defined by Brattström and popularized by Merchant is the angle formed by the two lines drawn from the deepest point of the TG to the highest point on the medial and lateral femoral condyles.

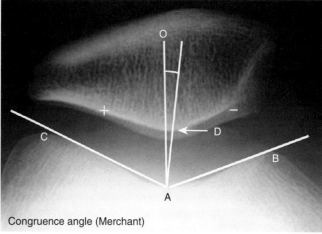

Congruence angle (Merchant)

FIG 65.28 The congruence angle is measured by bisecting the sulcus angle to construct a reference line and then projecting a second line from the apex of the sulcus angle to the lower point of the subchondral articular surface of the patella (apex). If the line drawn from the patella apex is lateral to the reference line, then the angle is positive; if it is medial to this line, a negative value is assigned.

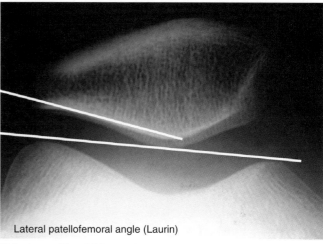

Lateral patellofemoral angle (Laurin)

FIG 65.29 The LPFA is formed by one line connecting the superior points of the medial and lateral trochlear facets and a second line tangent to the lateral facet of the patella. *LPFA,* Lateral patellofemoral angle.

cephalically and 20 degrees superiorly from the horizontal. Two measurements are made on this view: the lateral patellofemoral angle (LPFA) and the PF index.
- LPFA (Fig. 65.29): This angle is formed between one line connecting the superior points of the medial and lateral trochlear facets and a second line that is tangent to the lateral facet of the patella. It measures tilt and subluxation; it should open laterally in normal knees (97% open laterally and 3% are parallel; no LPFA opening medially was found in normal knees in Laurin's study).
- PF index (Fig. 65.30): This index is the ratio (M/L) between the thickness of the medial joint space (M) and the thickness of the lateral joint space (L). It should be 1.6 or less (Fig. 65.31).

Malghem and Maldague Lateral Rotation View (30 Degrees Lateral Rotation).[139]
This view is obtained in 30 degrees of knee flexion while one examiner pulls the forefoot laterally. The cassette is held over the patient's thighs, and the x-ray beam is

directed cranially. Patellar position (centered or subluxated) is defined according to Merchant's congruence angle. In the authors' series, the 30-degree lateral rotation (LR) view was superior to standard 45-degree axial views to detect patellar subluxation. In 27 knees operated on for patellar instability, 45-degree routine views depicted subluxation in only seven cases, while 30-degree LR views demonstrated it in all cases. Additionally, when both views showed signs of instability, the degree of subluxation was greater in the 30-degree LR view.

In acute or chronic patellofemoral instability (PFI), medial patellar avulsions (Figs. 65.32 and 65.33) can be demonstrated and should not be confused with bipartite patella. Haas et al.[98] retrospectively studied the presence of a linear or curvilinear osteochondral fragment arising from a fractured patella or lateral femoral condyle visualized in radiographic studies of patients with acute knee trauma and effusion. The history of patellar dislocation was confirmed with history and MRI. The fragment, called the *sliver sign*, was found in 15% of the axial radiographic views, and is a specific sign for the diagnosis of patellar dislocation. This sign can help in cases when the history of dislocation is unclear. It is important, however, not to misinterpret the fragment in other views with tibial spine avulsions.

Other important data provided by axial views include patellar shape and joint line thickness. Patellar shape is evaluated according to the Wiberg classification (Fig. 65.34). In osteoarthritis (OA), joint space thickness is diminished. Axial views allow assessment of which side of the articulation is affected, provide information on the size of osteophytes, and permit joint line narrowing quantification. Iwano et al.[113] proposed the following simple staging system of lateral patellofemoral osteoarthritis (PFOA) (Fig. 65.35):

- Stage I, mild OA: joint space measures at least 3 mm.
- Stage II, moderate OA: joint space measures less than 3 mm, with no bony contact.
- Stage III, severe OA: bony contact in less than one-quarter of the joint surface.
- Stage IV, very severe OA: joint surfaces entirely touch each other.

Computed Tomography

Many parameters observed in CT images are similar to those observed in axial views. The contribution of CT in this aspect, however, is the ability to produce such images in complete extension. This is particularly helpful when PF tilt or subluxation are considered, because flexion of the knee causes the patella to engage the trochlear sulcus, correcting (or at least reducing) these abnormalities (Fig. 65.36).[109,184] CT also provides a constant reference for the performance of several

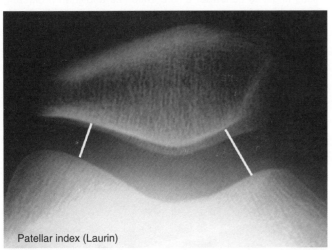

Patellar index (Laurin)

FIG 65.30 The PF index is the ratio (*M/L*) between the thickness of the medial joint space (*M*) and lateral joint space (*L*).

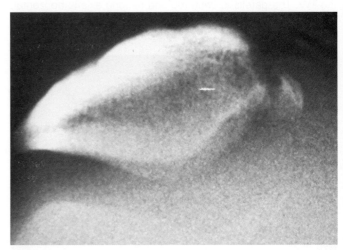

FIG 65.32 Avulsion of the medial aspect of the patella. Note the small osseous fragment corresponding to the patellar insertion of the MPFL and retinaculum. In addition, a large effusion can be seen. *MPFL,* Medial patellofemoral ligament.

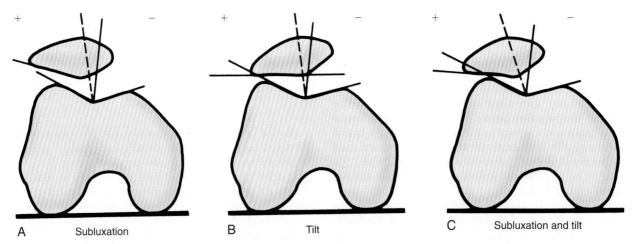

A   Subluxation   B   Tilt   C   Subluxation and tilt

FIG 65.31 Radiologic Differentiation Between Tilt and Subluxation. (A) Subluxation can be detected using the congruence angle (the normal range is demonstrated in the figure). (B) The congruence angle is within the normal range, but tilt is noted as the patellar transverse axis is lifted off from the horizontal. Another possible method of assessment could be the LPFA (in CT scans, the posterior femoral condyles could be used as reference). (C) Both tilt and subluxation are present. *CT,* Computed tomography; *LPFA,* lateral patellofemoral angle.

alignment measures—the posterior femoral condyles—otherwise not visualized in axial views.

CT plays an important role in the evaluation of anatomic abnormalities. Trochlear shape evaluation is essentially improved by its axial (Fig. 65.37) and sagittal views. Tri-dimensional reconstructions are also performed after image acquisition, and a precise judgment can be obtained.

Another important contribution of CT is the superimposition of images, allowing assessment of torsional deformities such as femoral anteversion and external tibial torsion (using the posterior condyles as a reference). By superimposing images, additionally, one can assess the tibial tubercle–trochlear groove (TT-TG) distance and patellar tilt (referenced to the posterior condyles, which is more reliable than the trochlea, which may vary in dysplasia).

As patellar tilt is dependent on the degree of the knee flexion (even in normal knees) and quadriceps contraction, the analysis of tilt and subluxation with variable conditions adds important information to the understanding of patellar tracking and to the determination of any abnormalities. Delgado-Martins[64] compared extension CT images and axial radiographs at 30, 60,

and 90 degrees of flexion in normal knees and found that in complete extension, with the quadriceps relaxed, only 13% of the patellae were centered in the trochlea (the median crest corresponded exactly with the intercondylar groove), while this rate increased to 29% at 30 degrees, 63% at 60 degrees, and 96% at 90 degrees of flexion. Schutzer et al.[183] found, in healthy subjects, a mild degree of lateral shifting and tilting from 0 to 5 degrees of flexion, and a central or medialized patella at 10 degrees of flexion. The study of Martinez et al.[142] did not corroborate these findings—19 of 20 patients had the patella well centered in the TG in complete extension with the quadriceps relaxed.

Dejour et al.[63] analyzed CT images of 143 knees post symptomatic patellar instability surgery and 27 controls, determined methods of measurement, and defined their normal and pathologic values in patellar instability. This protocol is known as *Lyon's protocol*.

The Protocol (Lyon's Protocol)

Image acquisition. The patient is imaged in the supine position, while lying on a rigid table with the knee in full extension and the patella positioned strictly anterior ("looking to the roof"), which usually places the feet in 15 degrees of external rotation. The feet are then fixed to the table with straps.

Image acquisition is performed for hip, ankle, and knee, the last with and without quadriceps contraction.

The following specific axial sections should be acquired for measurement:

- Section through both femoral necks at the top of the trochanteric fossa.
- Section through the center of the patella, through its larger transverse axis.
- Section through the proximal trochlea (where the intercondylar notch looks like a Roman arch, and a slight condensation of the trochlear lateral facet subchondral bone can be observed).
- Section through the proximal tibial epiphysis, just beneath the articular surface.
- Section through the proximal part of the tibial tuberosity.
- Section near the ankle joint, at the base of the malleoli.

Tibial Tubercle–Trochlear Groove Distance.
The TT-TG distance was described first by Goutallier and Bernageau[92] in 1978 on x-ray axial views at 30 degrees of knee flexion. The TT-TG distance is a direct measure of the extensor mechanism valgus

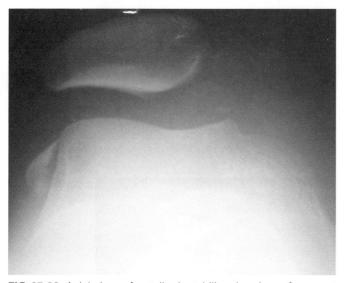

FIG 65.33 Axial view of patellar instability showing a fragment of the lateral femoral condyle fractured during the acute dislocation. The TD can also be seen. *TD*, Trochlear dysplasia.

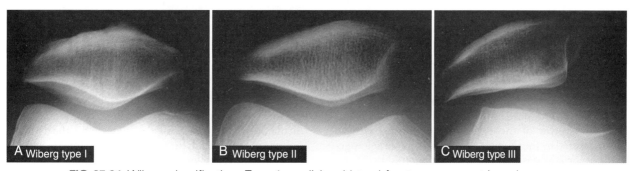

A Wiberg type I   B Wiberg type II   C Wiberg type III

FIG 65.34 Wiberg classification: *Type 1*, medial and lateral facets are symmetric and concave (A). *Type 2*, the lateral facet is bigger than the medial, accounting roughly for 2/3 of the PW (B). *Type 3*, there is a predominant lateral facet, while the medial facet is smaller than in type 2 and assumes a convex shape (C). *PW*, Patellar width.

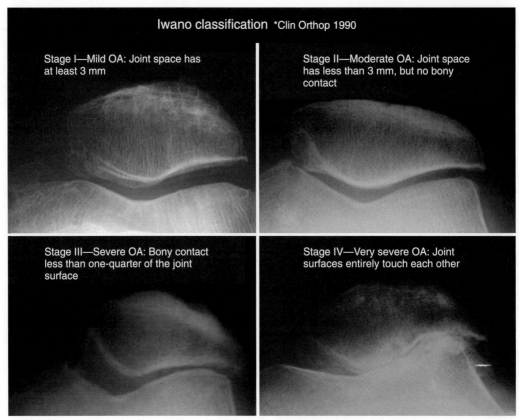

FIG 65.35 Iwano's OA classification system, based on axial x-rays: Stage I is mild OA; the joint space is at least 3 mm. Stage II is moderate OA; the joint space is less than 3 mm, but no bony contact can be seen. Stage III is severe OA; there is patellar-trochlear bony contact in less than one-quarter of the joint surface. Stage IV is very severe OA; the joint surfaces entirely touch each other. *OA, Osteoarthritis.*

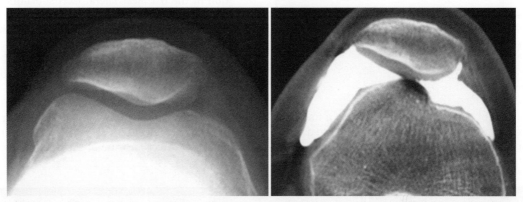

FIG 65.36 X-ray axial view and arthro-CT of the same patient. Note how the TD and the patellar tilt that are hidden on the x-ray can be clearly identified in the arthro-CT preformed in complete extension. *TD, Trochlear dysplasia.*

alignment, but it incorporates information about the forces acting on the patella produced by femoral and tibial torsion. This resulting valgus vector of the extensor mechanism has been classically measured by the Q-angle, with considerable heterogeneity of the reported measurement methods and results. Moreover, lateral displacement of the patella underestimates this angle. This bias is not present in CT measurements.

The TT-TG distance is calculated from a CT scan protocol that superimposes two previously described cuts: one through the bottom of the TG (proximal trochlea) and another through the most proximal part of the TT. Both cuts should be perpendicular to the long axis of the bones, and the two reference points are projected in the bicondylar line (line traced tangential to both posterior femoral condyles). The distance between their projections is the TT-TG value, expressed in millimeters. The average normal value in full extension is 12 mm, and 56% of knees with at least one episode of patellar dislocation presented with values in excess of 20 mm in Dejour et al.'s study.[63]

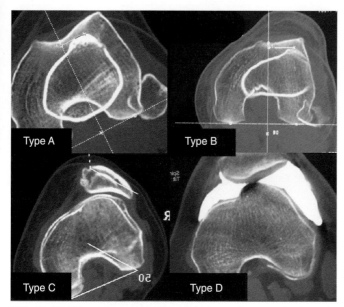

FIG 65.37 TD assessed in CT axial views: In type A, there is mild flattening, but the groove is still present. In type B the trochlea is flat, with no groove (if proximal cuts were performed, they would show the spur). In type C, the trochlea is convex (the patellar tilt is high). In type D, there is a cliff pattern (abrupt transition from lateral to medial facet). *CT,* Computed tomography; *TD,* trochlear dysplasia.

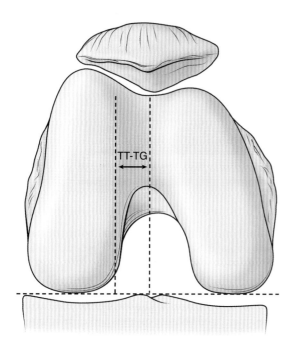

FIG 65.38 TT-TG measurement. *TT-TG,* Tibial tubercle–trochlear groove.

Thus, 20 mm is considered the uppermost limit (Figs. 65.38 and 65.39).

Patellar Tilt. Patellar tilt is measured on CT views with and without quadriceps contraction. Its method of measurement is different from the one used with x-ray axial views. Two lines are drawn: one tangent to the posterior femoral condyles and

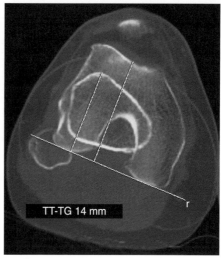

FIG 65.39 TT-TG Distance. Two CT scan cuts are superimposed: one through the superior part of the trochlea and the other through the proximal patellar tendon tibial insertion. The deepest point of the TG and the TT are projected on the posterior condylar line. The distance between them is the TT-TG value in millimeters. *TT-TG,* Tibial tubercle–trochlear groove.

another through the transverse axis of the patella (alternatively, one cut through the Roman arch level and another through the patellar longer transverse axis can be superimposed). The angle between the two lines is the patellar tilt (Fig. 65.40). Eighty-three percent of patients with PFI, with at least one episode of dislocation, presented values above 20 degrees in Dejour's original series. If instead of using only the relaxed quadriceps measure, a mean is calculated between the measures obtained when relaxed and in contraction, sensitivity and specificity are improved if the threshold value remains the same—90% of patients with at least one previous patellar dislocation have values above 20 mm while only 3% of controls have such values in a subsequent series (Fig. 65.41).[63]

Femoral Anteversion. Two cuts are superimposed. The trochlear reference cut with the posterior condylar tangent line is used again. In the femoral neck section, a line is traced joining the center of the femoral head with the center of the femoral neck. This line and the posterior condylar line form the femoral anteversion angle (Fig. 65.42).[153,219]

In Dejour et al.'s study,[63] the femoral anteversion mean value was 10.8 ± 8.7 degrees in controls and 15.6 ± 9 degrees in patients with at least one patellar dislocation. Some overlapping of values was noted in both groups, and no statistical threshold could be set.

External Tibial Torsion. The proximal (beneath the articular surface) and the distal (ankle) tibial cuts are superimposed. One line is drawn tangent to the posterior aspect of the plateau, and another through the bimalleolar axis. The angle between these lines is measured.[114,115,220] In Dejour's study, the mean tibial external rotation was 33 degrees in the patellar instability group and 35 degrees in the control group. Too much variation was present, and no particular significance could be demonstrated (Fig. 65.43).

Table 65.1 summarizes the CT scan protocol proposed by Dejour (Dejour, H.) et al. (Lyon's protocol).

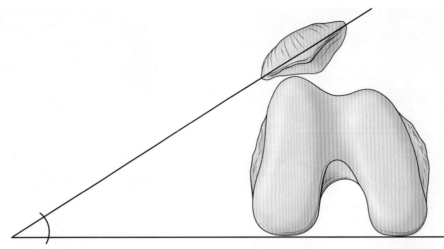

FIG 65.40 The patellar tilt measurement in CT scans (in extension) is performed by drawing two lines: one tangent to the posterior femoral condyles and another through the patellar transverse axis. The angle between these lines is the patellar tilt angle. *CT*, Computed tomography.

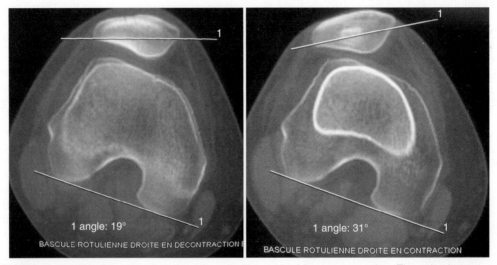

1 angle: 19°
BASCULE ROTULIENNE DROITE EN DECONTRACTION

1 angle: 31°
BASCULE ROTULIENNE DROITE EN CONTRACTION

FIG 65.41 Patellar tilt measurement with and without quadriceps contraction. The value increases from 19 degrees (within the normal range) to 31 degrees (abnormal) after the patient effectively contracts his quadriceps.

Finally, CT may help in the evaluation of joint cartilage thickness. Ordinary CT scans do not provide much information about cartilage status unless advanced OA is established. However, cartilage can be successfully analyzed if intra-articular contrast is injected (Fig. 65.44). Double-contrast methods use room air and positive contrast material. The use of arthro-CT allows identification of several types of chondral lesions: fissures, fibrillation, ulcers, and erosion. Overall cartilage thickness can also be assessed. Ihara[108] showed that for PF cartilage, when arthro-CT findings were compared with arthroscopy or arthrotomy, CT diagnosis was accurate in 68 of 70 knees (97.1%). Arthro-CT is also useful for diagnosis of plica syndromes and for detection of loose bodies.

Magnetic Resonance Imaging

Compared with CT scans, MRI provides superior anatomic and pathologic definition of soft tissues and articular cartilage. Conventional arthrography or arthro-CT allows visualization of surface anatomy but does not allow delineation of subchondral bone. In MRI, subchondral bone edema is a clue to cartilage damage. Similar to CT, MRI produces axial images in full extension, but with thinner slices.

Some of the measurements applied to x-ray or CT scanning can be applied to MRI when instability or maltracking is evaluated. Of great importance, MRI allows bony and cartilaginous shape assessment, and because osseous and cartilaginous shapes do not match exactly,[195] the true articulating surfaces can be revealed. In fact, if the measures used for CT scanning are considered in MRI, a significant difference using the subchondral bone as reference will be noted from those measures using the cartilaginous shape (Fig. 65.45).[152]

Because of the extensive information available using MRI to evaluate PF disorders, it is essential to have a systematic approach to this exam. Several instability factors have also been extensively studied and are described in detail next.

Cartilage and Soft Tissue. On sagittal views, the entire extent of trochlear and patellar surfaces can be evaluated. The thickest

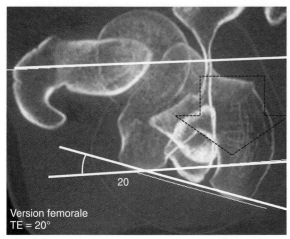

FIG 65.42 Femoral Anteversion Measurement The trochlear reference cut provides the posterior condyle line. In a proximal cut, through the femoral neck, a line is drawn joining the center of the femoral head and the center of the femoral neck. These cuts are superimposed and the angle between the lines is calculated. *TE,* Trochlear entrance.

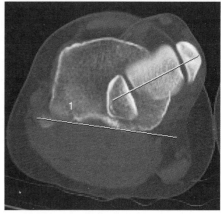

FIG 65.43 Tibial Torsion Measurement Two cuts are superimposed: one through the proximal tibia, beneath the articular surface, and another through the ankle joint, at the base of the malleoli. The angle between the line tangent to the posterior plateau and the bimalleolar axis is the tibial torsion value, in degrees.

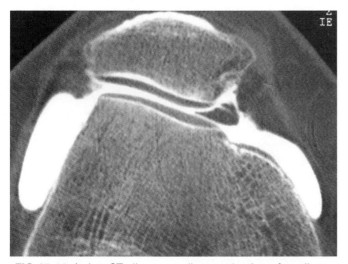

FIG 65.44 Arthro-CT allows excellent evaluation of cartilage.

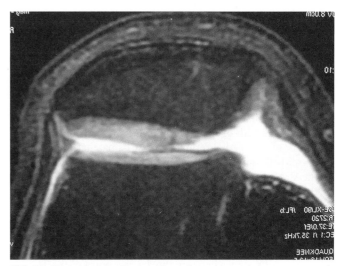

FIG 65.45 In dysplastic trochlea, the mismatch between cartilaginous and bony anatomy is less important. A flat or convex trochlea will be covered by similar flat or convex cartilage.

TABLE 65.1	**The Lyon's Protocol**			
Measure	**How to Measure (Computed Tomography)**	**Patients With at Least One Episode of Patellar Dislocation (Mean ± SD)**	**Controls (Mean ± SD)**	**OBS**
Femoral anteversion	Angle between center of femoral head/neck and posterior condyles	15.6 ± 9.0	10.8 ± 8.7	
TT-TG	Distance between trochlear groove and tibial tuberosity in 2 overlapped cuts	19.8 ± 1.6	12.7 ± 3.4	Pathologic threshold = 20 mm
External patellar tilt	Angle formed by the transverse axis of the patella and posterior femoral condyles	28.8 ± 10.5 Average increase of 6 with quadriceps contraction	10 ± 5.8 Average increase of 1.5 with quadriceps contraction	Pathologic threshold without quadriceps contraction = 20
External tibial torsion	Angle formed by the tangent to the posterior aspect of the plateau and the bimalleolar axis	33	35	Too much variation, no particular significance found

part of the patella corresponds to the median ridge; medial and lateral to it are the patellar facets. The distal quadriceps and the entire patellar tendon are visualized with their anterior insertions on the patella. Tendon signal alterations should be examined for tendinopathy and partial tears. Hoffa's infrapatellar fat pad lies posterior to the patellar tendon. The infrapatellar plica is identified in midline sagittal sections as a band linking the intercondylar notch to Hoffa's fat pad. In the presence of joint fluid, the suprapatellar bursa is seen proximal to the superior pole of the patella and a suprapatellar plica may be identified in its superior aspect.

On axial images, PF osseous and cartilaginous relationships become evident. Trochlear cartilage can be assessed, but overlapping Hoffa's fat pad and adjacent synovium may produce false-positive fissuring. The medial plica is best visualized in the presence of joint fluid, extending from the medial capsule toward the medial patellar facet. Patellar and quadriceps tendons are visualized in their axial plane; intrasubstance signal intensity abnormalities can be observed.[175]

Intravenous gadolinium enhances areas of pannus in inflammatory arthritis; intra-articular contrast or distention with saline improves the identification of plicae.

Patellar dislocation may not be suspected before MRI examination in up to 50% of cases.[127] MRI is particularly helpful in the recognition of acute dislocations recognition and evaluation of associated lesions. Positive findings include the following[66,78,122,210]:

- Lateral femoral condyle contusion and/or osteochondral lesion.
- Injury of the MPFL at its femoral origin (Fig. 65.46).
- Medial patellar facet contusion and/or osteochondral lesion, sometimes with osteochondral fragment avulsion.
- Injury of the medial retinaculum at its patellar attachments or midsubstance (Fig. 65.47); tearing of the distal belly of the VMO.
- Patellar tilt and subluxation.
- Joint effusion.

Trochlear Shape. On magnetic resonance (MR) transverse images 3 cm above the joint line, trochlear depth may be measured: the AP distance between the deepest point of the TG and the line paralleling the posterior outlines of the femoral condyles is subtracted from the mean of the maximal AP distance of the medial and lateral condyles from the same posterior line. In Pfirrmann's study,[167] dysplastic knees showed a mean of

−0.6 mm (range −6.5 to −2.7 mm) while controls showed a mean of 5.2 mm (range 2.4 to 10.5 mm). If a threshold is set at 3 mm, specificity of 100% and sensitivity of 96% could be expected. In the same study, facet asymmetry (medial facet/lateral facet) below 40% provided similar specificity and sensitivity to dysplasia diagnosis (Fig. 65.48).

Carrillon et al.[38] investigated the lateral trochlear inclination (LTI) angle calculated by means of a line tangential to the subchondral bone of the posterior aspect of the two femoral condyles crossed with a line tangential to the subchondral bone of the lateral trochlear facet. A significant difference between healthy and patellar instability patients was recorded. The mean value in patellar instability patients was 6.17 degrees; in the

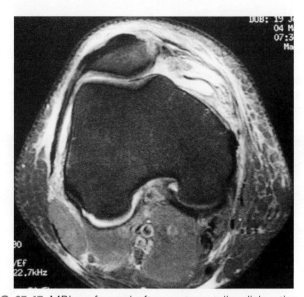

FIG 65.47 MRI performed after acute patellar dislocation. In addition to the medial retinaculum and MPFL disruption, edema in the lateral femoral condyle and medial patellar osteochondral lesion can be clearly visualized to set the diagnosis.

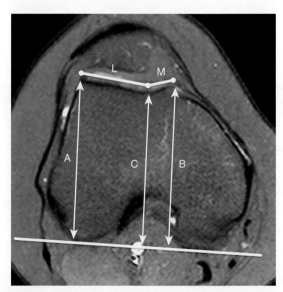

FIG 65.48 Trochlear depth on MR axial images ((A + B)/2 − C). Facet asymmetry in percentage (M/L × 100). MR, Magnetic resonance.

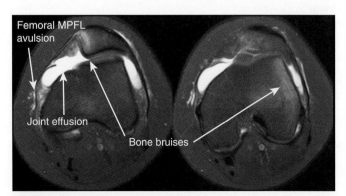

FIG 65.46 Several findings indicating acute dislocation of the patella. MPFL, Medial patellofemoral ligament.

control group, it was 16.9 degrees. When 11 degrees was chosen as the threshold value for LTI, results were excellent in discriminating between the two groups, with sensitivity of 93%, specificity of 87%, and accuracy of 90% (Fig. 65.49).

Biedert et al.[20] proposed the lateral condyle index, which identifies the length of the lateral trochlear cartilage. This index

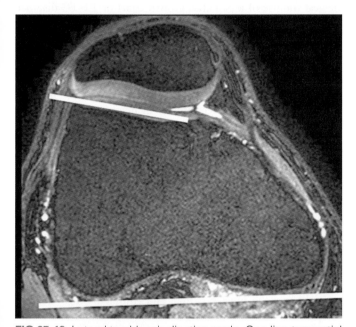

FIG 65.49 Lateral trochlear inclination angle. One line tangential to the subchondral bone of the posterior aspect of the two femoral condyles is crossed with a line tangential to the subchondral bone of the lateral trochlear facet.

is measured on sagittal MRI views, with the knee extended and the foot 15 degrees externally rotated. First, in the slice that images the entire length of the anterior cruciate ligament (ACL), the femoral shaft axis is determined (drawing two circles and connecting the center of them). Next, the most lateral image that still shows cartilage of the lateral condyle is used. The distance of the most anterior and the most posterior parts with cartilage are measured on lines tangent to the cartilage and parallel to the axis line. The lateral condyle index is the ratio between the anterior and posterior distances described as a percentage (Fig. 65.50). Twenty-eight knees in 23 patients with patellar subluxation and 46 controls were analyzed. Their mean index values were 86 ± 9% and 93 ± 7%, respectively. The authors concluded that a lateral condyle index of 90% or less had a sensitivity of 79% and a specificity of 37% for a lateral cartilaginous condyle that is too short. With this find, the authors suggested a new form of trochlea dysplasia (a trochlea that is too short), as another potential contributor to patellar instability.

Lippacher et al.[131] analyzed intraobserver and interobserver agreement of radiographic and MRI-based Dejour (Dejour, D.) classification for TD. They concluded that the four-grade analysis showed fair intraobserver and interobserver agreement, whereas a two-grade analysis (type A, low grade, vs. types B, C, and D combined, representing high-grade dysplasia) showed good to excellent agreement. They also concluded that the best overall agreement was found for the two-grade analysis on MRI scans, and that lateral radiographs tended to underestimate the severity of dysplasia compared with axial MRI views.

Tibial Tubercle–Trochlear Groove Distance. Several authors have investigated TT-TG distance on MRI. Schoettle et al.[182] evaluated the reliability of the TT-TG distance on MRI

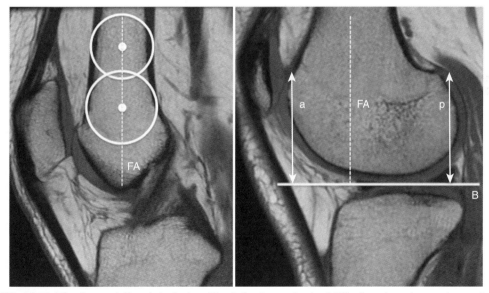

FIG 65.50 The Lateral Condyle Index The left picture is the MRI slice that shows the entire length of the ACL. The FA is determined by the center of the two circles, one proximal and the other distal. The next step *(right picture)* uses the most lateral MRI image that still shows the cartilage of the lateral condyle. A perpendicular line (B) to the axial line is drawn, tangent to the distal femoral cartilage. The distance of the most anterior (a) and the most posterior (p) parts of the cartilage to this line are measured. The lateral condyle index is calculated as a ratio between the anterior and posterior distances, multiplied by 100, and described as a percentage. *FA,* Femoral shaft axis.

compared with CT scan in 12 knees with PFI or AKP. The mean TT-TG distance referenced on bony landmarks was 14.4 ± 5.4 mm on CT scan, and 13.9 ± 4.5 mm on MRI. The mean TT-TG distance referenced on cartilaginous landmarks was 15.3 ± 4.1 mm on CT scan, and 13.5 ± 4.6 mm on MRI. They conclude that TT-TG distance can be determined reliably on MRI using cartilage or bony landmarks, and that additional CT scans are not necessary.

Pandit et al.[164] evaluated MRI exams of patients with clinically and arthroscopically normal PF joints. Using cartilage landmarks and the midpoint of the distal insertion of the patellar tendon at the tibial tuberosity, they showed that MRI is a reliable method for accessing the TT-TG distance, with a mean normal value of 10 ± 1 mm, with no difference between the sexes. This value was inferior to the 12.7 mm determined by Dejour H. on CT scans.

Thakkar et al.[202] also compared measurements between CT and MRI in 32 patients without PF disorders. The mean values of the TT-TG distance for CT and MRI were 15.3 ± 3 mm and 14.7 ± 2.8 mm, respectively. They achieved the same conclusion that TT-TG distance can be calculated on MRI, and duplicate CT scans are not necessary. They also concluded that the trochlear angle and the trochlear depth can be determined reliably on MRI. Similarly, Skelley et al.[192] showed that MRI has high intra- and interobserver reliability when measuring TT-TG distance in populations with and without patellar instability. Their mean TT-TG value in knees with instability was 18.2 mm, lower than previous CT values, but still within the statistical range.

Camp et al.[35] analyzed 59 knees with patellar instability and compared the TT-TG distance between CT and MRI. They found that both methods have an excellent inter-rater reliability, but their values are different, and the same cutoff values should not be used for the two exams. In their results, MRI values were always lower, with a mean difference of 2.3 mm from the entire cohort and 3.8 mm in patients with TT-TG distance greater than 20 mm. In the same way, Anley et al.[8] found a mean difference of 4.16 mm between CT and MRI, with lower values for MRI. They support the idea that the TT-TG measures from these two exams are not interchangeable. Ho et al.[103] also concluded that the TT-TG distances measured on the two exams might not be considered equivalent. They found lower values in MRI compared with CT, with a mean of 2.8 mm. The authors attributed this discordance to differences in imaging protocol techniques, including patient positioning.

In conclusion, the reliability of measuring TT-TG distance on MRI has been tested in several studies that proved it is a reliable method. Generally, MRI values are less than CT values. Two studies,[68,69] however, demonstrated that as TD increases, inter- and intra-observer correlation for the measurements of TT-TG distance decrease, because of the difficulty in defining the TG in these cases. Thus, caution should be exercised before deciding to perform a TT osteotomy based on MRI TT-TG distance.

Other questions have been raised concerning individual variables that can affect the measurement of the TT-TG distance, including the age of the patient, weight, height, and distal femoral size.

Dornacher et al.[68] analyzed the MRIs of 60 patients with a history of patellar dislocation and TD and 60 patients without PF problems. They looked for correlations between TT-TG distance, body height, and femur width, but found no difference. Using MRI, Balcarek et al.[13] investigated the relationship between TT-TG distance, age, femur width, in a population of young athletes, with and without patellar instability. Their results did not show differences among different ages or femur widths. They suggest this population must be evaluated like adults. In contrast, Dickens et al.[65] showed, in a young population, that the TT-TG distance increases with age. These authors suggest the use of a pediatric growth chart of TT-TG distance relative to chronological age.

Pennock et al.[165] studied the variations in TT-TG distance by MRI according to patient age, height, weight, body mass index (BMI), and femur width; 45 patients with patellar instability and 180 without instability were analyzed. In their results, TT-TG distance increased as a function of height in both groups; each additional centimeter in height correlated to an increase in TT-TG distance of 0.12 mm. With these results, they concluded that the normalization of TT-TG distance by height makes more logical sense.

To achieve better measurements of the TT-TG distance according to the knee size, Hingelbaum et al.[101] created a new method using MRI called the *TT-TG index*. It consists of the ratio between the TT-TG distance and the trochlear entrance–tibial tubercle (TE-TT) distance (distance between the chondral proximal TE and the TT (Fig. 65.51). The TT-TG distance is measured using the method described by Schoettle et al.[182] The TE-TT is measured as follows: the deepest point of the cartilaginous TE in the axial view is localized and transferred to the sagittal view; the most proximal and complete attachment of the patellar tendon into the TT is determined and also transferred to the sagittal sequences; the proximal-to-distal distance between these two transferred points can then be measured (Fig. 65.52).

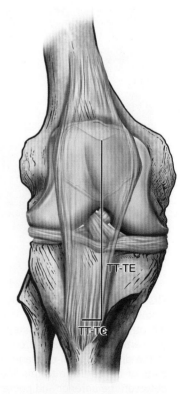

FIG 65.51 TT-TG Index.

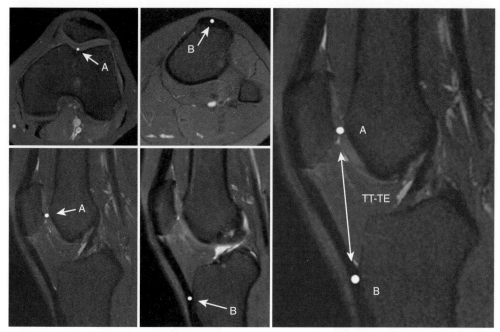

FIG 65.52 TT-TG Index The TT-TG distance is measured using the method described by Schoettle et al. To measure the TT-TE, the deepest point of the cartilaginous TE in the axial view is found (1), and transferred to the sagittal view (2). Then, the height of the most proximal, complete attachment of the patellar tendon to the TT is found (3), and also transferred to the sagittal sequences (4). Now, the proximal–distal distance between these two transferred points can be measured, which is the TT-TE (5). The index is the ratio TT-TG/TT-TE. *TT-TE*, Tibial tubercle–trochlear entrance.

This new index was tested in patellar instability and in a control group. The authors found high intra- and inter-observer reliability for both groups. The control group presented a mean TT-TG index of 0.12 ± 0.05. Using the TT-TG distance threshold of 20 mm proposed by Dejour et al.[63] it was established that a TT-TG index higher than 0.23 is pathological, with a 95% confidence interval. Their results showed that of the 51 patients in the instability group, only 6 had a TT-TG distance greater than 20 mm, but 20 patients had a TT-TG index of more than 0.23. Based on the new index, more medial transfer osteotomies of the TT should have been indicated, compared with evaluating only the TT-TG distance. This finding shows that the knee size can change the surgical indications. The authors further concluded that this new index is a reliable approach to TT-TG evaluation, particularly when it is between 15 and 20 mm, or when the patient has a very small or a very large joint.

In line with this tendency of individualizing the TT-TG distance, Camp et al.[34] compared patients with one single patellar dislocation and patients with multiple (more than two) dislocations. They found that the ratios between TT-TG and trochlear width (TT-TG/TW) and TT-TG and patellar width (TT-TG/PW) are more predictive of recurrent dislocations than the TT-TG alone.

Another point of view was introduced by Seitlinger et al.[185] They advocate that not every patient with elevated TT-TG distance presents lateralization of the TT. To overcome this limitation, they proposed to measure the tibial tubercle–posterior cruciate ligament (TT-PCL) distance, defined as the mediolateral distance between the TT midpoint and the medial border of the PCL, measured parallel to the dorsal aspect of the proximal tibia. Comparing patients with two or more patellar

dislocations and controls with no history of dislocation, they found different values between the groups (mean 21.9 and 18.4 mm, respectively).

Patellar Height. Miller et al.[148] analyzed patellar height on sagittal MRI of the knee. They applied the Insall-Salvati method to 46 knees and compared MRI with radiographs. Good to excellent correlation between values was found, and the investigators concluded that patellar height could be assessed reliably on sagittal MRI using the patellar tendon-to-patella ratio. On sagittal MRI, patella alta is suggested at values greater than 1.3.

Neyret et al.[154] used radiography and MRI to measure patellar tendon length in 42 knees with a history of patellar dislocation and 51 control knees. On MRI, the mean length was 44 mm in controls and 52 mm in the dislocation group. The distance between the tibial plateau and the point of tendon insertion was also measured and was found to be 28 and 29 mm in the control and dislocation groups, respectively. The investigators concluded that patella alta is caused by a long patellar tendon rather than by a low insertion into the tibia. Additionally, they did not find significant differences between x-ray and MRI tendon length measurements (Fig. 65.53).

Biedert and Albrecht[19] described the patellotrochlear index on sagittal cuts of MRI, performed with the knees in extension, the foot 15 degrees externally rotated, and the quadriceps consciously relaxed. The length of the articular cartilage of the patella (baseline patella [BLp]) is measured first. The second measure is the length from the most superior aspect of the trochlea to the most inferior part of the trochlea facing the patellar articular cartilage (baseline trochlea [BLt]). The ratio BLt/BLp is calculated as a percentage; values above 50% indicate

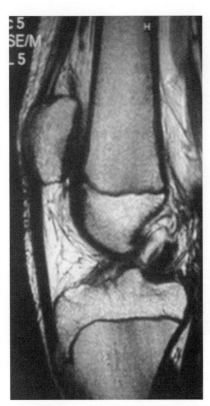

FIG 65.53 Sagittal MRI showing excessive length of the patellar tendon and consequent patella alta. The tibial insertion remains in its usual location. *MRI,* Magnetic resonance imaging.

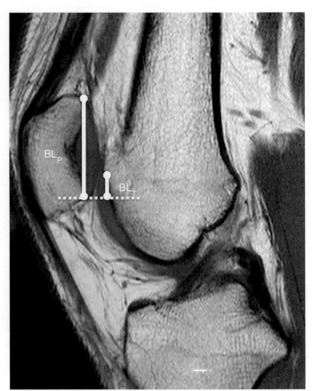

FIG 65.54 Patellar height measurement according to Biedert and Albrecht. The ratio BLt/BLp is calculated as a percentage. Patella alta is indicated if the ratio is less than 12.5%. *BLp,* Baseline patella; *BLt,* baseline trochlea.

patella baja, whereas values below 12.5% indicate patella alta. This index is not always measurable because it uses a single MRI slice, thus it cannot be measured in cases of a dislocated patella (Fig. 65.54).

Dejour (Dejour, D.) et al.[57] introduced a new index that emphasizes the importance of the relationship between the patellar and trochlear articular cartilages, called the *sagittal patellofemoral engagement (SPE) index.* Standard MRI is performed with the knee close to full extension. Because the position of the patella in the axial plane in patients with patellar dislocation is inconsistent, two distinctive sagittal cuts are selected to allow all cases to be measurable. The first cut is the sagittal MRI section where the patella shows the longest articular cartilage. On this image, a patellar length (PL) line is drawn, measuring the entire length of the patellar articular cartilage. The second cut is the sagittal section where the trochlear cartilage extends more proximally. On this section, the PL line that was copied is inserted. A second line is then drawn, the trochlear length (TL) line, parallel to the PL, extending from the most proximal trochlear cartilage to the distal end of the PL. The SPE is the ratio between the TL and the PL (Fig. 65.55).

Analyzing the results of one group with objective patellar dislocation (OPD) and another group without OPD, the authors showed 95% probability that patients with patellar dislocation and an SPE index less than 0.45 had patella alta and insufficient functional SPE. The authors also showed a 95% probability that a patient with patellar dislocation and an SPE index of more than 0.45 did not have patella alta and had adequate functional SPE. The SPE index did not correlate with the Caton-Deschamps index. Based on this fact, the authors concluded that even if a

patient has a normal patellar height, he/she can have an insufficient PF engagement, and the need to distalize the patella must be considered. On the other hand, a patient with patella alta can have a normal PF engagement and patellar distalization can be unnecessary. This index does not exclude the necessity of measuring patellar height with the established methods, but it is an additional tool to evaluate the patellar position.

Patellar Tilt (and Subluxation). Grelsamer et al.[94] described results using an MRI tilt angle similar to that proposed by Dejour et al.[63]; they also used the lines connecting the medial and lateral borders of the patella and the posterior femoral condyles as references. Thirty patients with tilt and 51 patients without tilt were evaluated. Patients with significant tilt on physical examination could be expected to have an MRI tilt angle of 10 degrees or greater, whereas an angle of less than 10 degrees was associated with absence of significant tilt on physical examination.

Guilbert et al.[96] introduced a new method to assess patellar instability, the axial engagement index (AEI) of the patella. This index measures patellar lateral displacement and evaluates the severity of instability. Like the SPE, it can be measured in every case, because it uses two different MRI slices. The first slice is the axial view, where the most lateral point of the lateral border of the trochlea is identified. A line (T) is drawn from this point perpendicular to another line drawn tangent to the posterior condyles. The two lines are copied to the second selected MRI image, the axial view, where the patella presents the widest diameter. In this slice, another line (P) is drawn perpendicular to the posterior condylar line, but from the most medial point

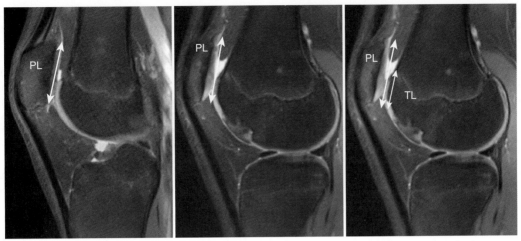

FIG 65.55 The SPE: The left image represents the MRI slice where the patella shows the longest articular cartilage. On this image, a PL line is drawn, measuring the entire length of the patellar articular cartilage. The second cut is the sagittal section where the femoral trochlear cartilage extends more proximally. On this slice, the PL line that was copied is inserted (middle image). In the right image, a second line is drawn parallel to the PL, which starts from the most proximal articular trochlear cartilage and finishes at the distal end of the PL, providing the TL line. The SPE is the ratio TL/PL. *PL*, Patellar length; *TL*, trochlear length.

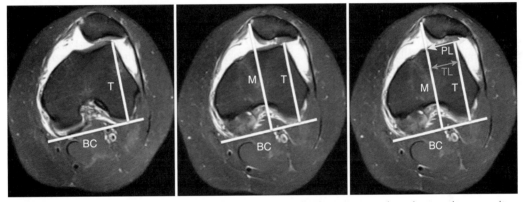

FIG 65.56 AEI: This index measures patellar lateral displacement and evaluates the severity of instability. The index is the ratio LT/LP, where LT represents the length of the surface of the joint engaged in the trochlea, and LP the width of the patellar surface. *PL*, Patellar length; *TL*, trochlear length.

of the patellar cartilage. The two distances are measured from line P to line T (LT) and from line P to the most lateral cartilaginous point of the patella (LP). The index is the ratio LT/LP, where LT represents the length of the surface of the joint engaged in the trochlea, and LP the width of the patellar surface. In the authors' study, the mean AEI of the 135 patients with objective patellar instability (OPI) was 0.83 ± 0.16, which was statistically different from the controls. The normal values were close to 1 in the controls, indicating complete transversal engagement of the patella (Fig. 65.56).

Dynamic MR imaging of the PF joint has been described to evaluate tracking during early flexion.[188,189] Axial images are acquired sequentially with increments of flexion. These images can be analyzed individually or as a cine-loop display, thus facilitating interpretation and recognition of abnormal tracking.[29] In normal tracking, the ridge of the patella is situated over the center of the trochlea (the groove), and this relation is maintained through increments of knee flexion, as the patella moves distally in the vertical plane. Quantitative assessments have also been described,[124] but despite all the studies produced, no consensus on measurement protocols and abnormal values exist. At the moment, dynamic MRI remains a promising procedure, but without a well-defined clinical application.

Patellofemoral Instability. PF dislocations annual incidence varies between 7/100.00011 and 43/100.000155 in different studies. It is more common among young females, 10 to 17 years old.

PF stability is of great importance for proper functioning of the extensor mechanism of the knee. The PF articulation, however, has a low degree of congruency, which is established by the balance of bony architecture and soft tissue restraints. Anatomic aberrations are not unusual, and as a result of mechanical imbalance, instability may occur.

The clinical presentation of instability includes a spectrum of manifestations. On this basis, it is important to differentiate patients who only have symptoms from those who have subluxation and/or dislocation. Dislocation is defined as the total loss of contact between the two articular surfaces, while subluxation refers to partial loss of contact.

According to Dejour (Dejour, H.),[61] there are three major groups in which patients with PF pathology associated with instability may be classified:
- OPI or OPD: This group includes patients who have had at least one dislocation of the patella. These patients will always present at least one anatomic abnormality; otherwise they would not have had the dislocation (rare cases of pure traumatic dislocations are excluded).
- Potential patellar instability (PPI) or potential patellar dislocation (PPD): These patients typically complain of knee pain and present anatomic abnormalities, but they do not present previous patellar dislocations. Maltracking and subluxation are usually found in the affected knee and commonly in the opposite side.
- Painful patellar syndrome (PPS): Patients who complain of knee pain but have no objective anatomic abnormalities and no history of subluxation. Many of these patients actually do not belong to the instability spectrum.

Factors in Patellar Instability

The four major anatomic factors leading to instability were described by Henri Dejour et al. in 1994[63]:

Trochlear Dysplasia. The abnormal shape of the trochlea leads to the loss of the osseous guide to patellar tracking (Fig. 65.57). TD is the single factor most associated with patellar instability, and is present in up to 96% of patients with OPI.[63] Instead of being concave, the trochlea is flat or convex. The normal trochlear constraint to lateral patellar displacement is lost and, as a consequence, dislocations can occur.

TD seems to be an inherited disorder. The asymmetrical orientation of the human trochlea seems to have been acquired during hominid evolution and bipedal locomotion. Comparative anatomy provides interesting information about the origin of TD. In apes, the femoral shaft is vertical (no obliquity), the TG is wide and symmetrical, and the patella is flat. In contrast,

humans have asymmetrical TGs where the lateral facet is higher and more prominent. This seems to be a response to the laterally directed forces acting on the patella that are created by the femoral shaft obliquity acquired with the process of walking.[100,200,201] Additionally, several authors[87,88,116,211] have demonstrated that fetal anatomy resembles that of adults, with an asymmetrical groove and facets. Because this asymmetrical trochlear shape is found in the fetus (where walking is irrelevant), it seems reasonable to assume that TD is an inherited condition and infer that TD is primitive.

Excessive TT-TG Distance. The coronal valgus alignment of the extensor apparatus and the forces produced by femoral internal and tibial external torsion produce lateral forces acting on the patella; this vector can be demonstrated by the tibial tuberosity–trochlear groove (TT-TG) distance.

Patellar Tilt. Patellar tilt and subluxation refer to an abnormal position of the patella in relation to the TG. Tilt was formerly believed to be one of the leading factors in the genesis of instability, caused by VMO insufficiency. Actually, it seems to be the result of a complex interplay of factors, including trochlear and patellar shape and congruence, insufficiency of medial restraints and lateral retinacular tightness. Whether a cause or consequence of instability, tilt must be considered in the diagnosis and in determining adequate treatment of instability.

Patella Alta. In normal knees, patellar engagement with the trochlea occurs at around 20 degrees of knee flexion. Patella alta refers to an abnormally high riding patella that engages the osseous restraint to dislocation (the TG) later in flexion, increasing the patellar "free" arc of movement and facilitating dislocation (Fig. 65.58).

Minor or secondary instability factors described include excessive femoral anteversion, excessive tibial external rotation, *genu recurvatum*, and *genu valgus*. Many of these factors

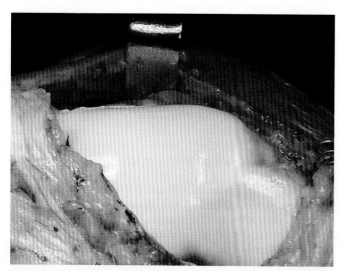

FIG 65.57 TD. Note that there is no sulcus and no distinct facets. The trochlea is flat (type B). *TD,* Trochlear dysplasia.

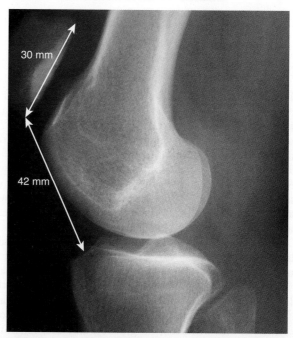

FIG 65.58 Patella alta. The Caton-Deschamps index is 1.4.

are already considered in TT-TG distance evaluation, which resumes the valgus and torsional alignment of the extensor mechanism.

Another important factor that must be considered is the MPFL disruption and the consequent medial restraint insufficiency. Despite the possible anatomic abnormalities and the consequent overall intrinsic instability that may be present between the trochlea and the patella, dislocations cannot occur if the MPFL is competent.

Natural History

The rate of subsequent dislocations after the first episode varies from 15% to 44% following conservative management, and this rate is increased in those that have had more than one episode.[44,83,99] In a natural history study, Fithian et al.[83] demonstrated that only 17% of first-time dislocators suffered a second dislocation within the next 2 to 5 years. In contrast, patients who presented with recurrent patellar instability were much more likely to sustain subsequent dislocations than patients who had only one dislocation. The risk of an additional dislocation within 2 to 5 years was around 50% in patients with a history of prior patellar instability (and therefore, at the moment of the study, suffering at least the second episode).

Complaints of pain and subjective instability are common following the initial episode, and frequently disabling. MacNab et al.[135] described a 33% rate of symptoms following first-time patellar dislocation, although the rate of redislocations was only 15%. Hawkins et al.[99] noted that at least 30% to 50% of all patients having sustained a primary patellar dislocation will continue to have symptoms of instability and/or AKP.

Clinical Evaluation

When evaluating the patient, adequate interviewing will promptly show the most frequent symptoms: instability and pain. Subjective instability is usually reflex, while objective instability may arise from abnormal tracking and subluxation. True dislocations must be recognized; usually the gross anatomy disruption followed by significant swelling makes diagnosis easier, at least after the first episode. Quantification of the patient's previous dislocations is of major importance and will guide treatment.

The imaging protocols (described in earlier sections) are particularly rich in findings, allow the identification of major and minor anatomic abnormalities, and help establish the treatment plan.

First Dislocation Management. The ideal approach to a first-time dislocation should not only avoid subsequent dislocations, but also prevent persistent symptoms, while allowing full recovery to sports as promptly as possible.

The classic treatment is conservative, consisting of immobilization followed by rehabilitation. Initial immobilization must permit the healing of the soft tissues (that provide the medial restraint), but longer periods of immobilization can cause stiffness; therefore, the ideal period should achieve a compromise between healing (stability) and mobility. This ideal period is not clear, nor is the method of immobilization, but accepted regimens include immobilization with a cast, splint, or brace for periods ranging from 2 to 6 weeks.[207]

Arthrocentesis to evacuate the hemarthrosis in the emergency setting is certainly a good option because it diminishes the pressure in the joint and allows the medial structures to heal with adequate tension because the patella is in its proper position.

After immobilization, and once swelling and pain have subsided, range of motion (ROM) restoration should be achieved. Quadriceps strengthening is another goal of the conservative management strategy. Good quadriceps strength seems to alleviate symptoms, but whether it prevents further dislocations is unclear.

The most important contraindication to conservative treatment in the acute setting is the presence of a dislocated osteochondral fracture, which should be fixated. Some authors propose acute repair when there is substantial disruption of the medial structures or in cases of a laterally subluxated patella in the presence of a normally aligned opposite knee (which would indicate important medial disruption because the affected knee is expected to have a similar alignment before the dislocation).[196]

Surgical management of the first dislocation has grown in popularity in recent years. Surgical strategies are diverse, but most commonly include acute repair of the torn MPFL and retinacula or primary reconstruction. Several studies have addressed the possibility of superior results following immediate surgery after the primary dislocation, and although some studies suggest a lower redislocation rate in the surgical group, several meta-analyses have failed to prove the superiority of the surgical strategy over conservative management. A lower redislocation rate seen in some studies[21,33,191] is not confirmed across different series,[43,163] and even if present, it may be counterbalanced by inferior functional outcomes and higher rates of OA.[42,79,174]

Chronic/Recurrent Dislocations Management. Surgical treatment is usually indicated in chronic dislocators, once the risks are considered. Surgery's main objective is prevention of recurrent dislocations; results for pain are less predictable. Substantial controversy exists on the choice of the procedure to be used. From a logical standpoint, the procedure (or the procedures) adopted should correct the observed root abnormalities. It is probable that a combination of procedures rather than any single procedure would correct each of the abnormalities to achieve stability. To remedy patellar instability, the surgeon will need to combine soft tissue and bony procedures to address all the involved factors, and correct each individually (Figs. 65.59 and 65.60).[9]

Soft tissue procedures. The most commonly used soft tissue procedures are lateral retinacular release, proximal VMO realignment, and MPFL reconstruction. Lateral retinacular release may be performed open or arthroscopically, to address lateral retinacular tightness. Variable amounts of release may be performed as it is extended proximally until the VL insertion or distally along the patellar tendon. The results are poor if other procedures are not associated.[208] The absence of lateral tightness (assessed mainly on physical examination through the patellar glide) contraindicates the release, and caution should be exercised when distal realignments are performed simultaneously as the risk of iatrogenic medial dislocation is increased.[82]

VMO advancement is another possible method, and is usually referred to as proximal realignment. The VMO insertion may be advanced in line with its fibers or a medial placation may be performed as part of the procedures described by Hughston[105] or Elmslie and Trillat.[204] Another option is the complete overlap of the medial structures described by Insall.[110]

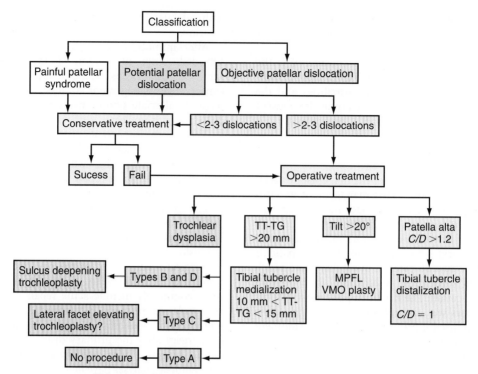

FIG 65.59 Algorithm for treatment of patellar instability.

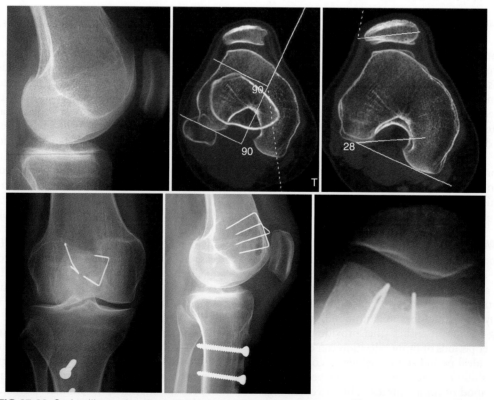

FIG 65.60 Series illustrating the individual instability factor treatment. The patient presented with high-grade TD (type D), increased TT-TG (23 mm), and increased patellar tilt (28). He was treated with sulcus deepening trochleoplasty, TT medial transfer, and MPFL reconstruction. Postoperative images show the correction of the abnormalities and adequate patellar position. The patient did not experience any further dislocations.

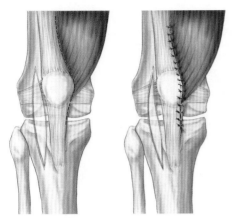

FIG 65.61 Medial advancement of the VMO and medial retinaculum. Lateral release is also demonstrated. These procedures can be performed alone or as part of more complex procedures.

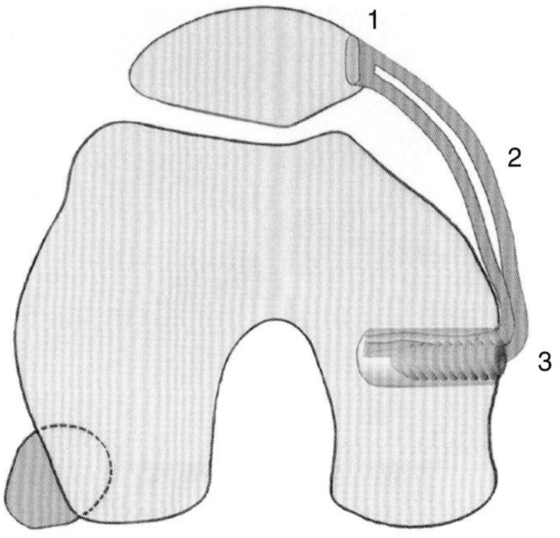

FIG 65.62 Schematic representation of MPFL reconstruction. A doubled-gracilis tendon is passed in a loop through the patella and fixed with an absorbable interference screw into the femur.

Proximal realignments are commonly performed in conjunction with lateral release and distal realignments (TT transfers). Alone, proximal realignments most probably address patellar tilt and exert some medial traction on the patella (Fig. 65.61). The VMO advancement or plasty has been progressively replaced by the MPFL procedure.

The MPFL, in conjunction with the VMO and the medial retinaculum, opposes lateral patellar displacement. Although not the primary cause of instability, MPFL reconstruction is an effective procedure to prevent redislocations and may alone avoid lateral patellar dislocation. Its rupture in previous abnormal but stable knees predisposes the patient to subsequent dislocations, corroborating its effectiveness despite the presence of the classic instability factors. Several techniques have been proposed,* with different grafts and fixation methods, but the overall principle remains the same: provide a checkrein to oppose lateral patellar displacement, especially in early flexion. Some degree of tilt correction may be achieved, but the principle of reconstruction is to avoid providing an element that exerts constant medial traction on the patella. If the reconstructed ligament is constantly tense and must exert permanent traction to avoid lateral displacement, it is probable that it will fail in the long term. In these cases, the classic factors causing instability must be addressed and the ligament must be unloaded. Isolated MPFL reconstruction is an excellent alternative in patients with mild instability and no major abnormalities (Fig. 65.62).

Tibial tubercle transfers. This procedure involves displacing the insertion of the patellar tendon, with the purpose of realigning the extensor mechanism and/or correcting patellar height. Medial TT transfers have been classically indicated in patients with extensor mechanism "malalignment." The goal of medial TT transfer is to reduce the abnormal TT-TG (above 20 mm) to values between 10 and 15 mm. Goutallier[42] stressed that the shape of the trochlea must also be taken into account in the correction of the TT-TG distance: the deeper the trochlea, the greater the risk of overmedialization, which would result in patellar impingement on the medial facet of the trochlea, and pain (Figs. 65.63 and 65.64). If the patella is high, the tubercle

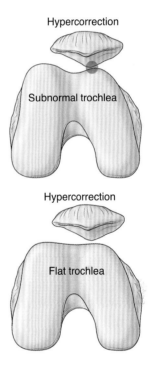

FIG 65.63 Hypermedialization is more likely to cause impingement in normal or subnormal trochleae. In flat or convex trochlea, the absence of the medial facet's prominence causes hypermedialization to be more tolerable. The amount of medialization has to take into account the trochlear shape.

should be distalized by the amount needed to correct the indexes to normal values.

In the earlier descriptions of TT transfers, a lateral incision was used. Following the advances in PF surgery, and in knee arthroplasty in particular, an anteromedial incision is now the preferred approach. This allows the association of medial soft tissue procedures like MPFL reconstruction without an additional incision.

Regardless of the type of transfer that is undertaken, complete exposure of the TT must be obtained. The proximal limit

*See references 18, 36, 43, 46, 53, 130.

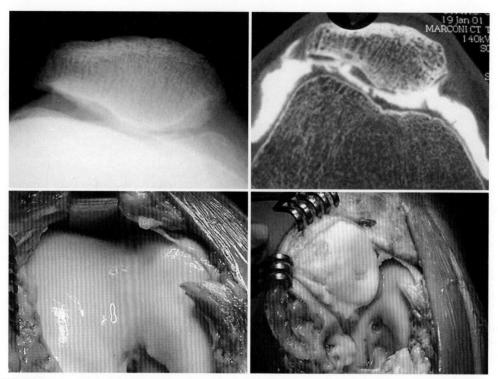

FIG 65.64 An example of hypermedialization with medial impingement. Note that the cartilage damage predominates in the medial patellar aspect. The patient was submitted to lateral TT transfer.

of the insertion of the patellar tendon is identified, and the outline of the osteotomy is traced with a scalpel in the periosteum. An oscillating saw or an osteotome is used to fashion a 6-cm-long bone block. To decrease the risk of nonunion, the cut must be made sufficiently deep in cancellous bone.

Medial tibial tubercle transfer. The TT is fully detached on three sides only, leaving a distal bony hinge. The pilot hole for the screw is made prior to the osteotomy, with a 3.2-mm drill bit, and overdrilled with a 4.5-mm drill bit, to allow lagging. The bone bed to receive the block is prepared medially. The block must be trimmed to ensure that it can be medialized with sufficient ease, and that it will not sit above the surface of the tibia. The proximal portion of the tubercle is pried off, using an osteotome, and medialized as planned, while the distal portion of the osteotomy is broken, but the periosteum is maintained intact. Fixation is achieved with a single screw. A hole is drilled in the opposite cortex with a 3.2-mm drill bit, and the tubercle is attached with a 4.5-mm screw (Figs. 65.65 and 65.66).

Distal tibial tubercle transfer. In this procedure the TT is detached completely, requiring fixation with two screws. The screw sites are prepared 2 cm apart prior to the actual osteotomy. The osteotomy block length should be increased by the amount of distal displacement planned. The proximal portion of the TT is pried off and grasped with bone-holding forceps while the distal portion is cut to the required length. The distal portion is tapered and trimmed to fit flush into its bone bed. It must not stand above the surface of its bone bed because any prominence would interfere with kneeling. The block is held in its distalized position, and fixation is started with the lower screw. The screws are inserted perpendicular to the tibia, to prevent the tubercle moving back up the tibia during lagging, with loss

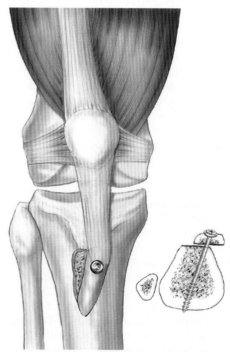

FIG 65.65 **Medial TT Transfer** A distal bone-periosteum hinge is left, and one screw is used to fixate the osteotomy.

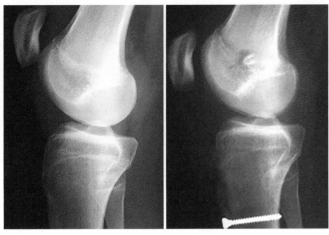

FIG 65.66 Pre- and Postoperative Lateral Views of Patella Alta After the distal TT transfer, the patellar height is corrected (1.5 preoperatively to 1 postoperatively). Associated MPFL reconstruction was also performed, but note that the MPFL femoral insertion is too anterior and high.

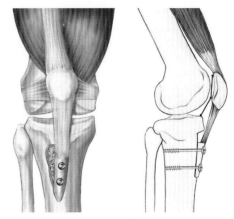

FIG 65.67 Medial and Distal TT Transfer Two screws are used. This procedure is used to correct increased TT-TG distance and patella alta. Caution should be taken not to overmedialize the tubercle, because the distalization procedure alone induces automatic medialization. Screws must be perpendicular to the tibial shaft to allow good compression.

of correction. Bicortical fixation is required for proper lagging of the TT.

Tibial tubercle distal transfer induces coupled medialization of 3 to 4 mm as a function of the tibial torsion. This phenomenon should be included in the calculations of the desired correction as it could contribute to "overmedialization."[187] Additional medialization may be provided after the first screw is inserted but not tightened. Once the desired amount of medialization has been obtained, the second screw is inserted (Fig. 65.67).

Patellar tendon tenodesis. Described by Neyret,[154] this is an adjuvant procedure to distal TT transfer surgeries. It is indicated when the patellar tendon length is greater than 52 mm, an excessively long tendon. This measurement can be obtained on radiographic examination, but it is far more reliable when MRI is used. After TT osteotomy for distalization, two anchors with sutures are fixed at both sides of the patellar tendon, about 29 mm distal to the tibial plateau, at the level of normal tendon insertion. The sutures are tied, attaching the patellar tendon to the underlying bone and reducing the patellar tendon length.

Postoperative care is common to all TT osteotomies. The patient wears a straight-leg splint, and is allowed to walk with full weight bearing. ROM exercises are started on the first postoperative day; to avoid excessive stress on the fixation of the TT, flexion is limited to 100 degrees. After 45 days, the splint is removed and full flexion is allowed. Return to sports is permitted 6 months postoperatively.

Trochleoplasties. Trochleoplasty is indicated to correct severely dysplastic trochlea. Lateral-facet elevating trochleoplasty is indicated in patients with flat or shallow trochlea, without trochlear prominence. Care must be taken to ensure that the procedure does not result in greater trochlear prominence, which might give rise to impingement in flexion. This procedure is certainly efficient to achieve stability but can lead to further PF arthritis as it increases the compression forces. Sulcus-deepening trochleoplasty is more anatomic and is indicated in severe dysplasia (D. Dejour types B or D), when the trochlea spur is prominent and the patella impinges on the trochlea. The best indication occurs when abnormal patellar

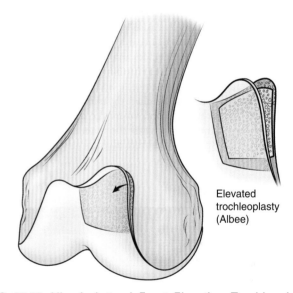

Elevated trochleoplasty (Albee)

FIG 65.68 Albee's Lateral Facet Elevating Trochleoplasty After the lateral facet osteotomy, a bone wedge is interposed, thus elevating the trochlear lateral facet and restraining patellar lateral displacement.

tracking with a J-sign is found in patients with previous dislocations. The deepening trochleoplasty decreases the TT-TG distance because it repositions the TG, and this must be considered when adding distal realignment procedures.[161]

Lateral-facet elevating trochleoplasty. Described in 1915 by Albee,[3] this procedure consists of an osteotomy of the lateral condyle producing a hinge near the intercondylar groove. The osteotome enters the condyle 5 mm away from the cartilage to preserve adequate thickness and prevent necrosis of the trochlea. The lateral condyle is then pried open to create a 5-mm gap, and a wedge of corticocancellous bone (iliac crest or local bone graft) or of bone substitute is inserted. Fixation, if needed, is achieved with transosseous sutures. In this way, the lateral facet is elevated sufficiently to block any further tendency of the patella to dislocate (Fig. 65.68).

Sulcus-deepening trochleoplasty. This procedure was first described by Bilton Polar in 1890 in a small article, described later by Masse in 1978,[143] and was subsequently modified and formalized by H. Dejour.[62,55] It is designed to abolish the prominence of the trochlear sulcus and to establish a groove of correct depth. After surgical exposure, the new trochlea is planned. Cancellous bone is removed from under the trochlea. Two osteochondral flaps, corresponding to the lateral and medial facets, are created and fixed to re-create the trochlear shape with a deeper central groove and higher facets diverging from it (Figs. 65.69 and 65.70).

Bereiter's trochleoplasty.[16] It is somehow similar to the sulcus deepening trochleoplasty, but with a thinner and malleable osteochondral flap. After bone is removed from under the trochlea and the bone bed is prepared, the osteochondral flap is fixed to it with vicryl stripes.

In postoperative care, immediate weight bearing is permitted after trochleoplasty. No limitation is placed on the ROM. Knee movement is encouraged to restore the nutrition of the cartilage and to allow further molding of the trochlea by the patella.

Patellar osteotomy. Morscher[150] described an anterior closing-wedge osteotomy, fixed with transosseous sutures, designed to restore the two facets of the patella. The procedure is technically demanding because the patella is a small and poorly vascularized structure with a high proportion of cortical bone. It is also difficult to decide how much space each facet should occupy, and where exactly the ridge must be placed. There is a major risk of necrosis and nonunion. Patellar osteotomy is indicated in patellar dysplasia such as Wiberg type III and "Jaegerhut" patella, when the articular surface is flat. In such cases, the reshaping of the patella is an adjunct to trochleoplasty. Despite its theoretical indication, it is rarely

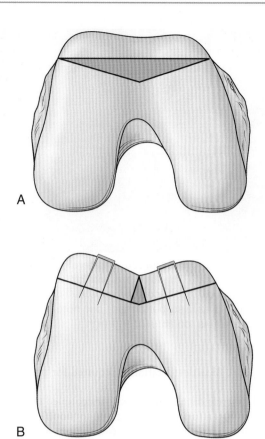

FIG 65.69 Sulcus Deepening Trochleoplasty Schematic Model (A) Cancellous bone from the trochlear undersurface is removed to allow modeling *(gray zone)*. (B) The bone-cartilage flap is then modeled and fixation is performed.

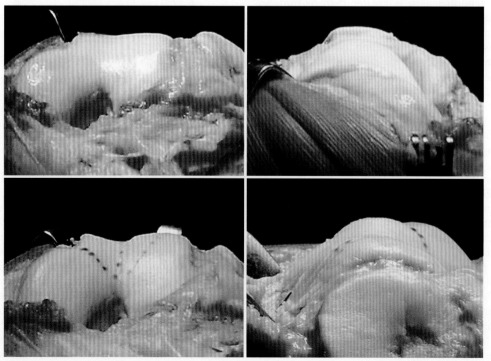

FIG 65.70 Trochlear shape before *(up)* and after *(down)* sulcus deepening trochleoplasty. The trochlear sulcus is restored and more "anatomic" shape is achieved.

recommended because of the numerous complications and remains an unpopular procedure.

Femoral and tibial osteotomies. In a small number of cases, patellar instability is the consequence of lower limb malalignment in excessive valgus or in torsion.

Valgus deformity increases the Q angle and enhances the dislocating pull on the patella. A valgus angulation should be considered abnormal if it is very pronounced (>10 degrees). The problem usually arises from the femur, but full-length radiographs must be examined for precise localization of the deformity. This pattern may be corrected by a lateral opening-wedge or a medial closing-wedge osteotomy performed at the distal femur.

Excessive femoral anteversion or external tibial rotation are most likely the torsional deformities. Surgery should be considered in carefully selected cases, bearing in mind that osteotomy is a major procedure. Femoral derotation osteotomy is best performed at the intertrochanteric level, while the preferred site for tibial derotation osteotomy is proximal to the TT.

PATELLOFEMORAL INSTABILITY AND OSTEOARTHRITIS

Patellar dislocations are associated with a high prevalence of chondral injury. Damage to the patellar articular cartilage has been reported in up to 95%[160] of first-time dislocations and 96% of recurrent dislocations.[158] Although the prevalence of chondral injuries is very high in acute dislocations, only a small number correspond to more severe osteochondral injuries. The most frequent lesions are cracks of the cartilage without full-thickness damage. Femoral-sided lesions are less common, with reported prevalence ranging from 5% to 32%.[133]

Chondral damage may result from an acute traumatic event and/or from altered joint loading caused by preexisting anatomic abnormalities.[133] In fact, the same anatomic factors associated with patellar instability are associated with PF cartilage damage and OA.[107,118,133,157] Ultimately, the sum of the chronic abnormal loading because of anatomic abnormalities and the acute damage during the dislocation(s) determine the prognosis of the articulation.

The multitude of procedures proposed to treat instability has not solved the problem of progressive degeneration. It is true from a logical standpoint that improving the mechanical environment of the articulation and avoiding prejudicial abnormal loading must prevent (or at least reduce) the progression of degeneration, but clinical observations failed to prove this logic. In fact, some series have even demonstrated the opposite—worse osteoarthritic prognosis following surgical management.[10,47,136] A possible explanation is that the stabilizing procedures used would achieve stability by non-anatomic means, therefore not appropriately correcting the underlying anatomic abnormalities nor avoiding the deleterious mechanical stresses imposed on the cartilage.

In contrast, some studies have shown minimal progression of degenerative changes following patellar dislocation treated with soft tissue procedures[47] or MPFL reconstruction,[123,159] in line with the theory that avoiding recurrent dislocation without the aggravation of biomechanical overload could achieve the best results in terms of OA progression. Because adequately designed randomized studies comparing diverse procedures in different groups of patients and at different follow-up intervals have not been performed, the osteoarthritic evolution following

dislocations remains unclear. Instability and recurrent dislocations are still indications for surgery. Prevention of OA is debatable, at least, and the indication for surgery considering OA progression in cases of severe malalignment or several recurrences of dislocation is based ultimately on the belief of the surgeon that it will improve the biomechanical environment in the long term.

PATELLOFEMORAL PAIN SYNDROME/ANTERIOR KNEE PAIN

The term *patellofemoral pain syndrome* (PFPS) encompasses pain in the anterior aspect of the knee (also called anatomic) that arrives from the PF articulation and is because of a multitude of factors, but frequently without a clearly defined cause. The sporting and general population's true epidemiology is not known.[217] In military personnel, the annual incidence in men is 3.8% and in women is 6.5%, with a prevalence of 12% and 15%, respectively.[27] AKP is common among adolescents, with a high point prevalence between 12 and 17 years.[169]

There is considerable overlap of the terms used to describe PF pathology, and some patients considered as AKP sufferers in some series may be classified as chondropathy/chondromalacia sufferers by different authors. The variable relationship between abnormality and pain creates most of the controversy regarding AKP diagnosis. PF chondral pathology (chondromalacia or chondropathy) and malalignment may cause pain, but there are many asymptomatic individuals who have these conditions. On the other hand, individuals with apparently normal knees may complain of pain. From this perspective, it becomes clear that some individuals may suffer from pain that in fact does not originate from the evident abnormalities the orthopedic surgeon may diagnose on a first evaluation.[54,72,74,77] This is especially important because effective treatment must address the true causes of pain, and not the confounding findings.

Pain may arise from several mechanisms. The soft tissues around the knee are common sources of pain and histologic studies have demonstrated abnormalities that could possibly create pain. This is particularly true considering the lateral retinaculum, where fibrosis, demyelination, and tissular neuromas have been found.[86,178] Other soft tissue potential sources of pain are the medial retinaculum, the infrapatellar fat pad, and the synovium.

Cartilage damage alone cannot cause pain because cartilage is aneural. Chondral pathology, however, may contribute to pain. Despite the evidence showing that advanced chondral damage may exist in asymptomatic individuals, the lack of cartilage and its protective effect over bone favors overload on the subchondral bone, which is richly innervated and thus a possible cause of pain. Also, synovitis may arise from the cartilage debris.

The PF articulation (as any other articulation) may be subjected to a variable range of load while keeping its homeostasis. Particularly in high-demand activities, excessive loading of the joint may alone be responsible for homeostasis loss, generating inflammation and nociceptive output (pain). These overuse/overload injuries are common when increasing frequency or intensity of sports. Most of the time the history is clear, and so the overuse diagnosis is straightforward. Other times, however, the abuses are not elicited and the diagnosis becomes cloudy.

Skeletal anatomy and muscular balance determine patellar tracking and joint mechanics. From this standpoint, it becomes clear that the interplay of many factors can potentially lead to abnormal loading of the PF joint even in the absence of evident overuse. Sometimes there is clear maltracking causing overload, but most of the time, anatomic and functional characteristics that contribute to overload are minimal, do not reach a pathological threshold to be diagnosed on clinical examination and imaging evaluation, and cannot even be considered significantly different from the averages in the general population. This is particularly true when we consider the wide range of anatomic patterns that are considered normal in anatomy and become even more complicated when we add to this formula the multitude of muscular imbalance possibilities. Based on this logic, it is understandable that fully extending the knee against tight hamstrings, ITB, or gastrocnemius muscles can increase the PF joint reaction force and precipitate pain.[4] Similarly, tight quadriceps may lead to the same consequences in deep flexion.

Recently, the dynamic valgus theory has gained popularity. It advocates that subtle maltracking of the patella in some patients with AKP may not be part of a structural fault but rather a dynamic or functional malalignment.[166] Potential risk factors involved in the genesis of dynamic valgus include hip weakness (abductors and external rotators), ITB tightness, excessive quadriceps (Q) angle, abnormal VMO/*vastus lateralis* reflex timing, and rear-foot eversion (causing compensatory tibial and femoral internal rotation). Quadriceps dysfunction through weakness, selective VMO weakness, or altered activation pattern of the VMO relative to the *vastus lateralis* has been associated with AKP development.[213]

Proximal musculature (core musculature) imbalance and weakness have also been associated with AKP. Hip weakness and adduction and greater femoral internal rotation have been shown in AKP patients.[26,214] These conditions could theoretically lead to overload of the lateral PF joint, because they produce relative medialization of the trochlear sulcus under the patella (Fig. 65.71). Despite the proven association, the causative role of hip weakness in AKP is still a topic of debate, and hip weakness may in fact be a consequence rather than a cause of knee pain.[168]

Obvious anatomic (and consequent tracking) aberrations may be classified as structural abnormalities, and may contribute to the overload of the PF joint. Torsional abnormalities and elevated TT-TG distance increase the lateralizing vector acting on the patella during flexion, increasing the PF reaction force on the lateral facet and allowing symptomatic overload to manifest. Simultaneously, insufficient load of the medial facet may generate loss of homeostasis and equally provoke pain.

TD is another potential contributor to the genesis of AKP. Keser et al.[121] demonstrated considerably higher prevalence of TD in AKP patients compared to controls (16.5% vs. 2.7%). In their study, TD was assessed with the LTI angle on MR. The prominent position of the trochlear sulcus in relation to the anterior femoral cortex increases the contact force between the patella and the trochlea (anti-Maquet effect) possibly contributing to overload and pain generation (Fig. 65.72).

Pain can be understood as the unpleasant sensory and emotional sensation associated with actual or potential tissue damage.[209] From a different perspective, emotional aspects can predispose the patient to pain in the absence of tissue damage. In fact, psychological distress (anxiety and depression) is intimately correlated with chronic musculoskeletal pain. Furthermore, pain and disability are only moderately correlated,

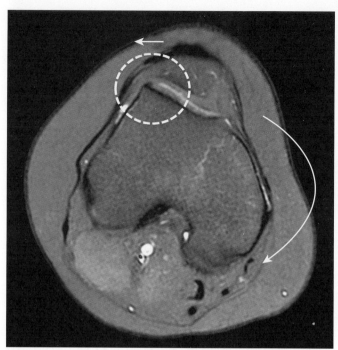

FIG 65.71 The relative displacement of the patella occurs in some circumstances because of internal rotation of the femur. In fact, the trochlea is medialized under the patella. Note how the relative lateralization of the patella can increase PFJRF on the lateral compartment of the PF joint.

suggesting that pain cannot account for all the disability present in some patients, and somehow explain anomalous responses of exaggerated pain in the absence of corresponding tissue damage. Following this same logic, maladaptive responses to pain like catastrophization (the belief that pain will worsen and nothing can be done to avoid it) and kinesiophobia (the belief that movement will aggravate or cause a new injury) worsen the problem in the case of long-lasting pain, aggravating disability and lowering pain experience threshold, creating a vicious circle.[67,177]

History and Clinical Examination

In AKP, pain is usually anterior, not well localized, and diffuse. It is usually aggravated by activities that increase the compressive forces over the PF joint (like squatting, ascending or descending stairs, prolonged sitting with the knees flexed) or cause repetitive loading (like running). Complaints of instability may occur because of quadriceps inhibition (reflex) as a result of pain, but without loss of contact of the articulating surfaces.

Adequate examination must search for different causes of pain and potential contributors to pain generation. Tenderness over the medial and lateral retinacula is frequent. As structural abnormalities are absent most of the time, physical examination is not noteworthy.

Abnormalities that increase the valgus vector acting on the patella, like increased Q angle and malalignment (increased femoral anteversion and increased external tibial torsion), may be evident in the static inspection and may become worse when the patient is asked to walk (dynamic inspection). Tightness of the posterior and anterior muscular chains must be assessed. The feet must be evaluated from behind the patient. Crepitation

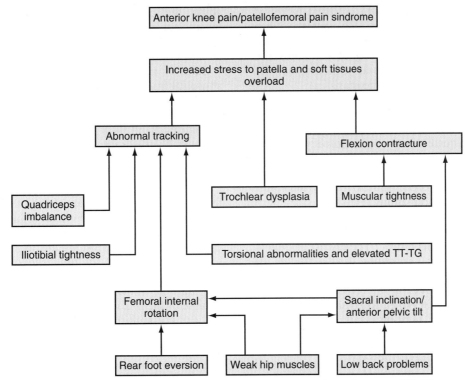

FIG 65.72 Proposed mechanisms of AKP generation. (Adapted from: Petersen W, Ellermann A, Gösele-Koppenburg A, et al: PFPS. *Knee Surg Sports Traumatol Arthrosc* 22:2264–2274, 2014.)

usually correlates with chondral pathology and effusion must be an alert signal for associated intra-articular pathology.

The functional "malalignment" or dynamic valgus can be visualized clinically with one-legged squats (Fig. 65.73). Crossley et al.[50] demonstrated that a valgus collapse of the knee joint during one-legged squat indicates weakness of the hip abductors.

Hip abduction and knee extension strength can be evaluated manually, but imprecision is a concern. Isokinetic devices are not widely available in the clinical setting. To overcome this limitation, handheld isometric dynamometry has been advocated,[137] and although no clinical standards have been defined yet, it may be useful to verify treatment progression, and it may develop a promising value in clinical practice.[186]

Imaging

Because pain is subjective, routine imaging modalities are useful only for identifying the associated structural abnormalities and quantifying them. TD, increased TA-GT distance, patella alta, tilt, and other abnormal tracking measurements may be present. OPI (previous dislocations) must be ruled out.

Despite the multitude of possible associated features, imaging is frequently normal. Several authors have shown that x-rays are not useful for AKP diagnosis, and the alignment parameters used for instability are within normal values in many AKP patients. MRI findings are also not useful in differentiating AKP patients from a control group.[134] Thus, imaging is complementary to the physical examination, but cannot predict the onset of pain or quantify the contribution of the evidenced abnormality to the final pain status.

Bone scans may provide some functional information. Scintigraphy can demonstrate metabolic changes not visualized

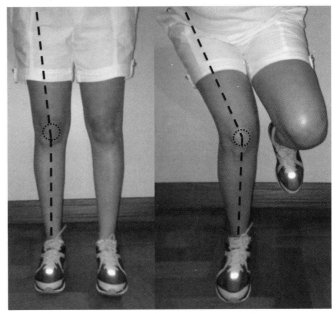

FIG 65.73 Apparently well-aligned limbs can demonstrate dynamic valgus when the patient is asked to perform a single-leg squat.

in other imaging modalities, but its contribution to treatment or diagnosis remains to be established. Dye and Boll[75] noted that about one-half of patients with PF pain demonstrated increased patellar uptake in technetium 99m–methylene diphosphonate scintigraphy, compared with only 4% of the control subjects. The increased osseous metabolic activity of the patella, detected by the bone scan, was biopsy proven to represent increased remodeling activity of bone compared with controls. When these patients underwent follow-up imaging, it was noted that many who experienced resolution of painful symptoms also demonstrated resolution of the bone scan to normal activity, representing restoration of osseous homeostasis.[76]

Treatment Strategy

Conservative treatment is always the first line. In the short term, a period of rest and adequate pain control are usually sufficient to alleviate symptoms. Pharmacologic treatment is aimed at reducing pain. With this purpose, nonsteroidal antiinflammatory drugs and weak analgesics can be used. Ice may contribute to pain reduction during exacerbations.

The importance of rest (or activity decrease) in the initial phase cannot be overemphasized, because it reduces load and allows homeostasis to be reestablished.[73] The absence of evident tissue damage on the imaging evaluation usually hinders the physician from prescribing sports suspension, delaying complete recovery and in some cases, worsening the symptoms. Pain must not be withstood, but rather avoided. The common strategy of "no pain, no gain" must be abandoned.

Flexibility training or muscular tightness improvement should always be part of a successful PFPS treatment strategy. Stretching exercises can be started in the initial phase and must be maintained during the late rehabilitation phases. Stretching exercises aim to loosen potentially tight anatomic structures that could predispose the patient to PFPS. Patients must be informed that flexibility is a lifetime goal.

After the pain subsides, physical therapy becomes the mainstay of treatment. Quadriceps and hip strengthening are the most important goals, and appropriate exercises can be prescribed almost universally to patients, provided they do not cause further pain.

The best way to achieve quadriceps strengthening is still a subject of controversy. Both open and closed kinetic chain exercises can apparently be used with success, but from a logical standpoint, these exercises must be performed in a way that does not impose excessive load on the PF joint. To this end, closed kinetic chain exercises must be performed from knee extension to 45 degrees of flexion, while open kinetic chain exercises must be performed from 90 to 45 degrees of flexion.[145,214,218] Exercises must be performed without pain, and the patient must remain pain-free in the following hours (many times pain arises after exercise cessation because of a cytokine flare). Preferential activation of the VMO during quadriceps strengthening is of particular importance to treatment, but its feasibility remains a topic of debate.

Hip strengthening is targeted preferentially to abductors and external rotators, but the addition of hip flexors and extensors must be considered. Most of the data concerning strengthening of the proximal musculature are still experimental and inconclusive, but it leads us in an important direction. Roughly, it can be proposed that strengthening can restore more normal kinematics, and avoid non-physiologic loading resulting from abnormal kinematics because of insufficient musculature. Although more conclusive data are missing, the prescription of strengthening exercises must not neglect the hip musculature.

Van der Hejiden et al.[206] recently reviewed the available literature regarding exercise for PFPS and found very low-quality but consistent evidence that exercise therapy may result in clinically important reduction in pain, improvement in functional ability, and enhanced long-term recovery. However, there is insufficient evidence to determine the best form of exercise therapy and it is unknown whether this result would apply to all people with PFPS.

Knee or patella orthotics or taping may act in correcting abnormal tracking or unloading compromised areas. Interestingly, these modalities may also provide alternative afferent stimuli, *compete* with the nociceptive information, and thus alleviate pain and allow an exercise program to be developed or initiated. Their efficacy is still controversial, but despite the lack of consensus, adverse events from their use are improbable and short-term usage remains an option for pain control.[14,32]

Foot orthoses are another commonly suggested option for AKP. The evidence supporting its use is controversial, and potential mild adverse effects around the ankle and foot are a concern.[104] The current trend is to avoid indiscriminate use of orthoses, and target specific individuals based on measures of pronation of the feet, who could benefit from this intervention.[15,126]

Failure of initial conservative management is common because of the lack of validated standardized treatment protocols and the multitude of possible approaches. The physician should be aware of the used exercise regimens before the efficacy of treatment is questioned. Patient adherence is another crucial factor in treatment success.[217] Periodic evaluations are therefore essential before complete pain relief is achieved. Persistence is an indispensable quality to the team assisting the patient, and several trials of conservative management are the rule before a failure can be defined.

Surgery decisions for patients complaining exclusively of pain are exceptions and must be made for correctable (treatable at least) structural abnormalities that cause pain with a reasonable amount of probability. Surgical procedures used for AKP are usually TT transfers in patients with evidence of malalignment and cartilage procedures for those who suffer from chondral pathology. In the absence of clear indications, surgery may even aggravate the symptoms.

Prognosis

Pediatric and adult populations seem to represent distinct groups regarding the cause of pain. Overuse and mechanical causes are more probable in pediatric individuals, while adults most commonly present with a diagnosis of OA, with obviously poorer results.

The common belief that AKP is a self-limited and benign condition cannot hold true in several circumstances. Several authors demonstrated high prevalence of persistent symptoms after variable intervals, despite a decrease in pain intensity. Overall, most patients are able to continue sports, but complete remission of pain is improbable in most patients.[24,119,156,179]

Regarding AKP evolution to PFOA, the available evidence is weak, but there seems to be an increased risk of OA development in young patients suffering from AKP.[203] As some of the anatomic variations associated with patellar instability and PFOA are also present in some patients with AKP,[107,118,133,157] it seems logical to expect increased risk of OA progression in this subgroup. Similarly, in patients with evidence of chondral damage, progression is expected. Conclusive evidence to confirm these assumptions is still missing.[217]

If the possibility of progression from pain to OA is considered, then the approach to these patients should include education about management of their joint load and realistic expectations about cure. Decisions related to sports practice and professional activities should consider that higher joint loads are a risk factor for OA when the joint is abnormal, but because weight gain and lower limb weakness should be avoided, exercises should not be abandoned.[48]

PATELLOFEMORAL OSTEOARTHRITIS

Because arthritis affecting the PF joint is less studied than tibiofemoral osteoarthritis (TFOA), various questions about this form of OA remain unanswered. Recently, many studies have been conducted on this particular kind of arthritis, and some of the findings contrast with the old knowledge about this pathology.

PFOA is usually bilateral and predominates in the female sex. It can be observed as an isolated form in which only the PF joint is affected, or combined with TFOA. It is important to note that this joint cannot be overlooked in PFOA. It has been demonstrated that the levels of pain and functional limitation are similar in patients with moderate or severe arthritis in any of these three forms of arthritis: isolated PFOA, isolated TFOA, and combined.[71]

The old belief that PF articulation was less frequently affected than the other compartments of the knee seems not to hold true. Recent studies demonstrate a high prevalence of OA in this joint. Duncan et al.[70] examined radiographs of 777 patients aged 50 years old and over presenting with knee pain. They found 40% prevalence of combined arthritis, 24% of isolated PF joint arthritis, and 4% of isolated TF arthritis. Similarly, Stefanik et al.[198] used MRI to determine the compartmental prevalence of knee joint structural damage in 970 patients older than 50 years from a population-based cohort. The prevalence was different depending on the definition of structural damage that was used. Isolated PF joint damage was found in 15% to 20% of knees, while isolated TF joint damage was found in 8% to 17%. The PF joint was always more affected, except when a definition that included only bone marrow lesions was used. In patients with knee pain, PF damage was at least as common as TF damage. Hinman et al.[102] examined 224 patients older than 40 years, complaining of anterior or retropatellar knee pain. Using radiographs, 30% displayed no evidence of OA, 44% presented mixed OA, 25% presented the isolated PF form, and in only 1% the TF joint was affected alone. From the total, 69% of patients displayed PFOA and 45% TFOA. From these data, the obvious conclusion is that the PF compartment may be the predominant compartment affected in OA.

Considerable controversy exists on the location of wear and on the several causes for PFOA. Extensor mechanism malalignment is one possible protagonist. This theory is based on the valgus quadriceps angle and its lateral resultant force. Because of these assumptions, the common belief is that valgus knees are more associated with PF arthritis, especially on the lateral facet. Therefore, this location has been classically considered to be the most affected, while the medial facet OA is basically associated with varus knees or iatrogenic hypermedialization. In line with this, Cauhe et al.[31] showed that the lateral facet was the most affected and that it had more risk of OA progression than the medial facet. Additionally, varus-valgus alignment influenced the likelihood of PFOA progression in a compartment-specific manner—valgus knees were associated with lateral PFOA progression and varus knees with medial PFOA progression.

The available literature, however, provokes controversy. Gross et al.[95] analyzed three large OA studies to determinate the most prevalent location of PFOA and its relation to knee alignment. In all studies, the medial facet was more affected than the lateral one. Even among knees with valgus malalignment, the prevalence of lateral PF cartilage damage equaled or surpassed that of medial PF damage only when the analysis was restricted to severe OA. Hinman et al.[102] also supported the idea that the medial facet is more commonly affected than previously believed. In patients with PFOA, they found that 63% had both facets affected, 22% had exclusively the lateral facet, and in 15% the medial side was affected alone. Two studies that analyzed PF wear in cadaveric knees also demonstrated high prevalence of medial facet wear.[91,112] The high prevalence of arthritis on the medial patellar facet suggests that although the lateral forces influence the incidence of OA in the PF articulation, other causative mechanisms exist and must be studied.

Other possible PFOA causes are hypermobile kneecap, excessive lateral hyperpressure syndrome (ELHPS), patella alta and patella infera, sequela of articular fractures, and rheumatic diseases. ACL surgery has also been associated with PFOA progression. There are events that occur during ACL injury and after reconstruction that may have specific implications for the PF joint. Such events include concomitant damage to articular cartilage and meniscus, inflammation, biomechanical changes, and quadriceps strength deficits, which may contribute to a greater risk of developing PFOA after ACL reconstruction regardless of the graft used.[51]

In 2003, the senior author (D. Dejour) organized a symposium[56,97] in the French Orthopedic Society (SOFCOT) to understand isolated PF arthritis. A total of 367 cases of isolated PF arthritis from several centers in France were reviewed. Similar to arthritis of the TF compartment, OA of the PF joint was found predominantly in females (72%). Most patients (51%) demonstrated symptoms in the opposite knee. The average age at the time of the first symptoms was 46 years. Radiologic progression was slow; an average delay of 18 years to pass from Iwano stage I to stage IV was observed. Twenty-nine percent of patients were obese and 38% overweight. Activities that load the PF joint were mainly altered. The ability to use stairs was problematic for 65% of patients; 15% did not use stairs. Limitations on flat ground were equally important; 80% of patients reported that they could not walk for more than 1 km. In this symposium, four main causes were identified:

- Primary arthritis (49%): patients with no orthopedic antecedent, and especially no history of dislocation.
- Post PFI (33%): patients with history of OPD (at least one dislocation).
- Posttraumatic (9%): patient with history of PF fractures.
- Chondrocalcinosis and rheumatoid disease (9%).

TD was found as a major factor in this series. Seventy-eight percent of patients demonstrated TD with the crossing sign. Higher-grade dysplasia was more frequent in the population with objective instability (66%) than for those with primary arthritis (38%). The absence of dislocations, however, does not exclude potential instability and maltracking as contributing factors in the primary arthritis group. Confirming this finding, Jungmann et al.[117] also demonstrated high association between TD and more severe PF joint degeneration. Other interesting findings from the symposium were the rates of patients who progressed to TF arthritis: 41% in the primary cases and 32% in the post-instability group.

Diagnosis

Lateral radiographic views may already allow the diagnosis of PF arthritis and TD, but skyline views are the most informative ones. Remodeling of subchondral bone, joint space narrowing, and osteophytes are the classic findings (Fig. 65.74). Malalignment is also a feature to be evaluated; axial x-rays may show subluxation and tilt. The Iwano[113] classification based on skyline views can be used. CT allows more precise alignment assessment, and arthro-CT is useful in assessing the cartilage. Finally, MRI shows the cartilage damage in detail, even in initial stages, as it may show bone marrow lesions.

Treatment

Because the PF joint is less studied than the TF joint, few studies focusing on treatments specifically to this joint are available. The principles of treatment management are similar to OA affecting other articulations.

There are no guidelines focused specifically on the treatment of PFOA, but because the guidelines of knee osteoarthritis (KOA) include patients with OA in all the compartments of the knee, some of the classic options can be used. Similarly, some of the procedures adopted for PF pain are used and aimed at decreasing PF reaction forces. It must be considered, however, that the incidence of arthritis on the medial facet of the joint is higher than previously believed; if this is the case, treatment options that decrease the lateral forces applied to the PF joint will not be universally effective and may even worsen the medial overload.

The patient must be evaluated in a global context; treatment decisions cannot consider only the radiographic severity. The characteristics of pain, the limitations imposed in the patient's daily life, the expectations about the problem and the treatment, and the patient's objectives for the future (high-performance sport vs. low-demand routine activities) are far more important to evaluate than the radiographic severity of OA.

Conservative treatment is the first option in PF arthritis. Patient education is essential. Patient awareness of the origin of the problem, prognosis, and treatment options is crucial to successful treatment. The management follows a staged approach, starting with non-pharmacologic interventions, most of which have to be incorporated into the patient's lifestyle. Pharmacologic treatment can be recommended depending on the severity of the symptoms, after failure of the non-pharmacologic treatment alone or during pain crisis. Finally, failure of conservative interventions may lead to surgical treatment.

The recommendations of non-pharmacologic treatment for KOA are weight management, land-based or water-based exercises (both for strength), active ROM, and aerobic activity.[144] These treatments can all be applied to the PF joint; regarding the PF joint, strength must focus on quadriceps and hip musculature. Stretching exercises can be included. Tapping and bracing may be used as well, but with unconfirmed evidence. No consensus exists concerning whether these interventions are better performed with or without a physiotherapist. A clinical trial compared one group treated with exercises, education, manual therapy, and taping, and another group that received an OA educational program that focused on the PF joint. After 3 months, the first group presented superior results for patient-perceived improvement and pain, but no difference in activities of daily living was observed between groups. After 9 months, the positive effects were not maintained, and the results between groups were equivalent.[49] The inferior results of patients without assistance after 3 months could be caused by poor adherence to the treatment program. As there is no consensus, the physician should fell the patient motivation to a self-management program, or the need for physiotherapist assistance.

The pharmacological recommendations for KOA are mainly nonsteroidal anti-inflammatory drugs and tramadol. Care must be taken in patients with comorbidities; the use should be

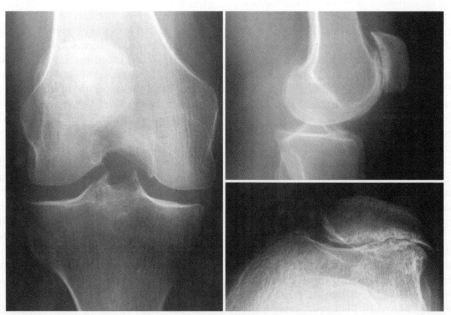

FIG 65.74 Isolated PF Arthritis The anteroposterior view is useful to assess tibio-femoral involvement. The diagnosis can already be made in the lateral view, but the axial view is the most informative.

restricted to short periods.[30,144] Divergences exist between the available KOA guidelines concerning the use of acetaminophen and intra-articular corticosteroids, which are recommended by one set of guidelines (2014 Osteoarthritis Research Society International [OARSI]),[144] but not by the other (2013 American Academy of Orthopedic Surgeons [AAOS]).[30] No study has tested these interventions for PFOA specifically. There is no strong evidence supporting the use of intra-articular hyaluronic acid on KOA[30,144]; thus, its use cannot be supported in PFOA either.

When surgical treatment is planned, two main factors must be assessed: dysplasia (trochlea or patella) and malalignment. Nonprosthetic treatment is best suited for PF arthritis without dysplasia and malalignment, because the anatomic distortion is minimal, which favors postoperative tracking with consequent improved results. In patients without dysplasia but with malalignment, realignment procedures are helpful and may alleviate symptoms. In those who present TD, prosthetic replacement seems to be the most logical procedure, followed by realignment procedures as needed (Fig. 65.75).

Lateral Retinacular Release and Vertical Lateral Patellectomy (Facetectomy).
Lateral release has been proposed as a method of treatment, but its indications and results are unclear. It is helpful in decreasing the PF joint reaction forces, especially in the presence of a tight retinaculum. It seems more appropriate to perform the release in patients with patellar tilt but no subluxation.[1,82,176] It has been demonstrated as effective in pain relief, although inferior to realignment procedures, and only for the short term.[208]

Vertical lateral patellectomy may be an option combined with lateral release and resection of lateral osteophytes. Only part of the degenerated lateral patellar facet (no more than 1.5 cm) can be resected (Fig. 65.76). Wetzels and Bellemans[215] demonstrated that lateral patellectomy for isolated PFOA can produce satisfactory results in half of patients 10 years after surgery. Their survival rates, measured by reoperation rates, were 85% after 5 years, 67.2% at 10 years, and 46.7% at 20 years. The same procedure was studied by López-Franco et al.[132]: after 10 years of surgery, up to 66% of patients did not need a total knee replacement. Montserrat et al.[149] performed partial lateral facetectomy plus Insall's procedure to treat isolated PF arthritis. After 13 years of follow-up, their survival rates (patients that did not need total knee arthroplasty [TKA]) were 59.3%. Factors that increased the risk of failure were the presence of preoperative medial TF pain, flexum of the knee, and incipient TFOA. They found that higher anatomic and total Knee Society Knee Scoring System (KSS) scores, absence of knee effusion, higher

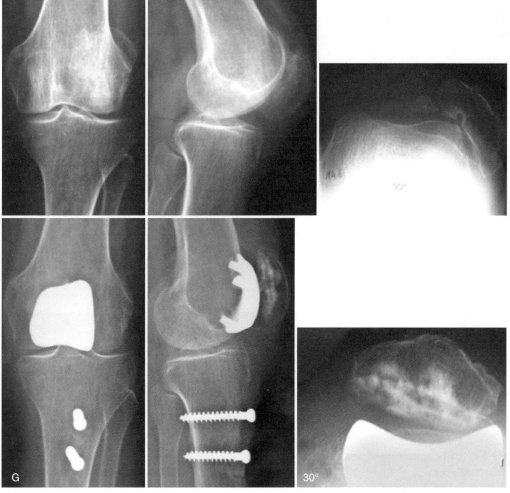

FIG 65.75 **Clinical Case** Severe PFOA in a patient with TD and malalignment (elevated TT-TG). Tibial tubercle osteotomy was added to a PFA, achieving excellent tracking.

Caton-Deschamps index values, and lateral position of the patella contributed to success of this procedure. Lateral retinacular release and partial lateral facetectomy seem to be less-invasive alternatives to treat PF arthritis, and do not preclude subsequent surgeries.

Tibial Tubercle Osteotomies. The rationale for anterior TT transfer derives from biomechanical studies showing that this procedure reduces PF stress levels. This technique was first described by Maquet.[140,141] It consists of an anterior transfer of the tibial tuberosity. The procedure is in part similar to a medial transfer; however, an iliac crest graft is inserted between the tubercle and the tibia. A modification with the same principle has been proposed by Fulkerson,[84] involving anteromedialization of the TT but without the use of a graft; an oblique osteotomy is performed and fixed with screws. It unloads the lateral and inferior parts of the patella; thus, forms of arthritis confined to these locations are best suited for the procedure. Anteromedialization, which is different from the procedure proposed by Maquet, may correct malalignment, which should be taken into account when choosing the procedure.

Atkinson et al.[12] treated 50 knees presenting PF arthritis with TT advancement osteotomy using bone allograft. In their series, 77% of patients had good or excellent results at a mean follow-up of 81 months. Carofino and Fulkerson[37] analyzed a cohort of

19 patients over 50 years old who were submitted to Fulkerson's osteotomy with an average follow-up of 77 months; 63% had good or excellent results, and only 5% had poor results. They suggest that the anteromedialization osteotomy is a good procedure for older active patients who do not have compromised bone healing, like smokers or obese individuals.

Prosthetic Replacement. The presence of PF dysplasia makes procedures like TT transfers or lateral facetectomy hazardous. Dysplasia will not be modified and the imbalance of the PF joint will persist. In this situation, partial or total arthroplasty are more interesting because they permit the substitution of the dysplastic component. In this way, trochlear prominence and orientation are corrected, and congruence between trochlea and patella is established. The TT-TG distance can be diminished, performing a slight lateralization of the femoral component without any procedures on the TT. Concerning the correction of the patella, it is necessary to conserve a satisfactory thickness, if possible, with a minimum of 13 to 14 mm. Slightly undersized patellar components will allow mediolateral- and distal-to-proximal positioning, aiding in the alignment correction.

Prosthetic replacement may be complete (TKA) or partial (patellofemoral arthroplasty [PFA]). TKA is an option in older patients with degenerative changes that are confined to the PF compartment, but is debatable in young patients in the same situation (Fig. 65.77). PFA seems more suited to them. Partial arthroplasty preserves bone stock and does not sacrifice a good TF articulation. PFA is indicated in isolated arthritis of this joint after failure of the conservative treatment, in patients presenting important symptoms and limitations in daily activities, and after failure of previous surgical procedures. As partial arthroplasty produces less surgical trauma, it can also be considered in older patients (Fig. 65.78).

The most common cause of failure in the second generation of PF implants is progression of TF arthritis.[162] Associated TF disease should be ruled out, and failure to identify other causes of pain is a great cause of failure. Revision of an adequately performed PFA to a TKA is possible with no great technical challenges. Newer implants are compatible with TKA implants, at times eliminating the need for patellar exchange.

Patella Baja. Patella baja (or infera) is the opposite of patella alta (using latine roots). It represents the inferior (distal) position of the patella in relation to the trochlea. Its real importance is in the biomechanical abnormality caused by the abnormal

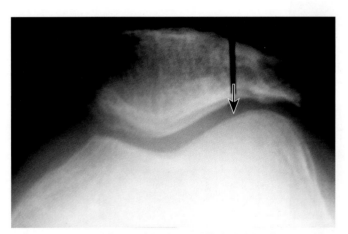

FIG 65.76 Axial View of Isolated PF Arthritis. Preoperative planning of vertical lateral facetectomy. A 15-mm bone removal is necessary. The lateral retinaculum is not always released.

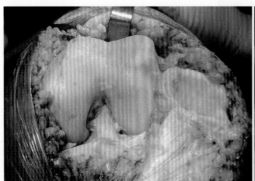
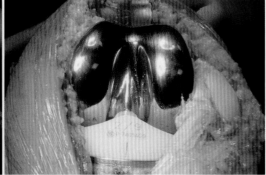

FIG 65.77 Advanced PF arthritis with no TD (evolution to global arthritis is higher than in PF dysplasia) treated with TKA. No particular technical tricks are needed.

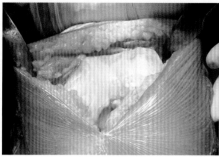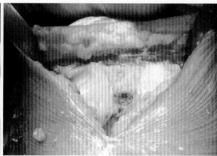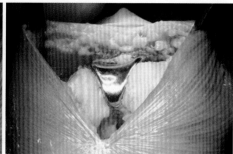

FIG 65.78 Isolated PF arthritis with a flat trochlea. The positioning of the PF arthroplasty is based on the preop CT scan planning to correct PF dysplasia and malalignment.

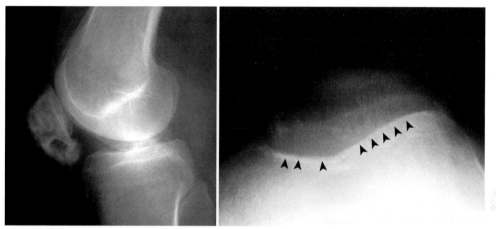

FIG 65.79 Patella Baja On the lateral view, the distance from the lower edge of the articular surface of the patella to the anterosuperior angle of the tibia outline is almost zero. On the axial view, the "sunset pattern" is shown, as the articular space cannot be seen.

situation of the patella, with increased PF stresses. In almost all cases, patella baja is acquired, either post-traumatically or iatrogenically (postoperative, especially TT transfers). Insufficiency of the quadriceps is another possible cause. Rarely, patella baja may have an inflammatory origin.

This condition is frequently symptomatic. Knee stiffness and AKP are the usual complaints. PF arthritis may be associated. The diagnosis is confirmed in lateral views. On adequate 30-degree axial views, the patella has an unmistakable pattern: it appears superimposed on the TG, and the joint space cannot be seen. Compared with the 30-degree "sunrise" view of the healthy side, the affected knee will show a "sunset" pattern (Fig. 65.79).

Conservative (symptomatic) treatment may be tried, but it is unlikely that the patellar height will change after this diagnosis is established. Thus, the mainstay of treatment is operative. The technique will differ according to the cause. When the origin of the problem is in the TT, a proximal transfer will correct it. When the origin is in the quadriceps tendon, and especially when the patellar tendon is retracted, the procedure of choice is patellar tendon lengthening. The postoperative goal is to reach a Caton-Deschamps index near 1.

Proximal Transfer of the Tibial Tubercle[40]. After an anteromedial approach, dissection of the patellar tendon and section of the peripatellar retinacula are performed. Arthrotomy, allowing arthrolysis of the knee and verification of the intra-articular

space (this may also be done under arthroscopy) is then carried out. The TT is detached with a hammered chisel and transferred upward according to the preoperative planning. It is then fixed with two screws. The distal screw maintains the height of the patella, while the second and more proximal screw is inserted after correction of the mediolateral position of the patellar tendon, depending on the TT-TG measurement performed preoperatively. The medial retinaculum is then closed, but the lateral is left open. Postoperative care includes a splint or cast in 45 degrees of flexion. The patient is non-weight bearing for three weeks. Removal of the splint is allowed for ROM exercises. The goal of these exercises is to preserve knee mobility and good tension of the patellar tendon.

Treatment by Lengthening of the Patellar Tendon.[59] An anteromedial approach from the superior part of the patellar tendon to the medial edge of the TT is performed, followed by extensive dissection of the medial and lateral aspects of the patellar tendon. Arthrotomy allows evaluation of the status of the patellar cartilage, and fibrous adhesions of the suprapatellar pouch are then cut. Patellar tendon lengthening is then carried out dividing it longitudinally through its central part over its whole length (Z-plasty). The lateral part remains anchored to the tibia, and the medial part remains anchored on the medial aspect of the patella. The patella should rise naturally while the tendon's stumps slide over each other. Tendon edges are sutured and reinforced by an absorbable polydioxanone suture (PDS) band

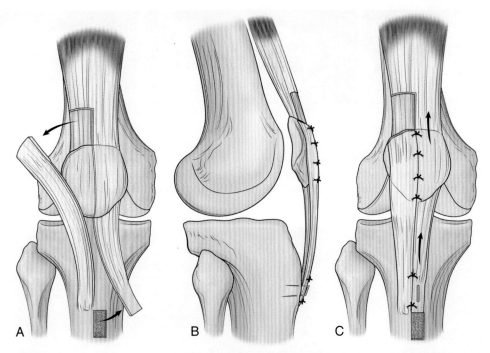

FIG 65.80 Patellar Tendon Lengthening The three steps include Z-plasty of the patellar tendon, perioperative x-ray evaluation of patellar height, and fixation with stitches protected with a metallic wire for 6 months.

or a semitendinosus tendon. The lateral retinaculum is left completely open and the medial retinaculum is closed. Immobilization of the knee in the postoperative period is accomplished in a cast or a posterior plaster splint at more than 40 degrees flexion, but ROM exercises are initiated as pain subsides. After 45 days, knee flexion can be progressed beyond 90 degrees and the splint removed (Fig. 65.80).

KEY REFERENCES

9. Arendt EA, Dejour D: Patella instability: building bridges across the ocean a historic review. *Knee Surg Sports Traumatol Arthrosc* 21:279–293, 2013.

15. Barton CJ, Lack S, Hemmings S, et al: The "Best Practice Guide to Conservative Management of Patellofemoral Pain": incorporating level 1 evidence with expert clinical reasoning. *Br J Sports Med* 49:923–934, 2015.

42. Cheng B, Wu X, Ge H: Operative versus conservative treatment for patellar dislocation: a meta-analysis of 7 randomized controlled trials. *Diagn Pathol* 9:60, 2014.

55. Dejour DH: The patellofemoral joint and its historical roots: the Lyon School of Knee Surgery. *Knee Surg Sports Traumatol Arthrosc* 21:1482–1494, 2013.

57. Dejour D, Ferrua P, Ntagiopoulos PJ, et al: The introduction of a new MRI index to evaluate sagittal patellofemoral engagement. *Orthop Traumatol Surg Res* 99:S391–S398, 2013.

63. Dejour H, Walch G, Nove-Josserand L, et al: Factors of patellar instability: an anatomic radiographic study. *Knee Surg Sports Traumatol Arthrosc* 2:19–26, 1994.

79. Erickson BJ, Mascarenhas R, Sayegh ET: Does operative treatment of first-time patellar dislocations lead to increased patellofemoral stability? A systematic review of overlapping meta-analyses. *Arthroscopy* 31:1207–1215, 2015.

96. Guilbert S, Chassaing V, Radier C, et al: Axial MRI index of patellar engagement: a new method to assess patellar instability. *Orthop Traumatol Surg Res* 99:S399–S405, 2013.

101. Hingelbaum S, Best R, Huth J, et al: The TT-TG index: a new knee size adjusted measure method to determine the TT-TG distance. *Knee Surg Sports Traumatol Arthrosc* 22:2388–2395, 2014.

126. Lack S, Barton C, Vicenzino B, et al: Outcome predictors for conservative patellofemoral pain management: a systematic review and meta-analysis. *Sports Med* 44:1703–1716, 2014.

131. Lippacher S, Dejour D, Elsharkawi M, et al: Observer agreement on the Dejour trochlear dysplasia classification: a comparison of true lateral radiographs and axial magnetic resonance images. *Am J Sports Med* 40:837–843, 2012.

161. Ntagiopoulos PG, Dejour D: Current concepts on trochleoplasty procedures for the surgical treatment of trochlear dysplasia. *Knee Surg Sports Traumatol Arthrosc* 22:2531–2539, 2014.

174. Saccomanno MF, Sircana G, Fodale M, et al: Surgical versus conservative treatment of primary patellar dislocation. A systematic review and meta-analysis. *Int Orthop* 2015. doi: 10.1007/s00264-01502856-x.

175. Saggin PRF, Saggin JI, Dejour D: Imaging in patellofemoral instability: an abnormality-based approach. *Sports Med Arthrosc* 20:145–151, 2012.

185. Seitlinger G, Scheurecker G, Högler R, et al: Tibial tubercle–posterior cruciate ligament distance: a new measurement to define the position of the tibial tubercle in patients with patellar dislocation. *Am J Sports Med* 40:1119–1125, 2012.

The references for this chapter can also be found on www.expertconsult.com.

66

Distal Realignment of the Patellofemoral Joint: Indications, Effects, Results, and Recommendations

Jeffrey T. Spang, William R. Post, John P. Fulkerson

Effective surgical treatment of patellofemoral pain and/or instability depends on an accurate diagnosis, understanding of the pathophysiology of the condition, and knowledge of the effects of a given surgical treatment on the mechanics and biology of patellofemoral function. Anterior knee pain, often caused by a patellofemoral disorder, is a common disabling complaint in young adults, predominantly women. Fortunately, nonoperative treatment, including quadriceps strengthening, stretching, core stability training, McConnell taping, and bracing, is usually effective.* However, when conservative treatment fails, and a specific treatable cause of anterior knee pain can be identified after careful physical, radiographic, and in some cases, arthroscopic examination, successful surgical treatment of patellofemoral disorders is likely. Similarly, in the event of recurrent patellar instability, when anatomic variables are correctly defined, a logical choice can be made for successful treatment. The purpose of this chapter is to define the situations in which tibial tubercle transfer is indicated for anterior knee pain and/or patellar instability and to present appropriate techniques for safe and reproducible treatment.

PATHOPHYSIOLOGY OF PATELLOFEMORAL PAIN AND INSTABILITY: IMPLICATIONS FOR TREATMENT

Patients with patellofemoral pain problems typically have various degrees of articular pain, soft tissue pain from overuse or chronic stretch, and mechanical instability from malalignment or dysplasia of the joint. Quadriceps weakness almost always accompanies anterior knee pain and may be a cause or result of knee pain. Restoration of quadriceps strength and flexibility is critical to improving load acceptance. A primary function of the quadriceps is to absorb energy during gait.[146] If the quadriceps is relatively weak and stiff, it can neither generate the desired force concentrically nor absorb the necessary energy eccentrically. In knees with a deficiency of muscular energy absorption as a result of eccentric quadriceps weakness, this energy must be absorbed elsewhere in the extensor mechanism, which may result in painful overload of patellar subchondral bone or excessive stretch of peripatellar soft tissues. Should the peripatellar soft tissues be less compliant and flexible than normal, such loads may be poorly tolerated. When the problem

is viewed as a deficiency in energy absorption, one can imagine that nonoperative management must focus on improving strength and flexibility throughout the lower extremities. The rehabilitation regimen must not overload the system. The concept of staying within the "envelope of function" during patellofemoral rehabilitation is especially critical to success.[32,33] Rehabilitation efforts that attempt to increase strength and function by working the knee as hard as possible are destined to fail in patients with patellofemoral disorders. The prime example is the effect of isokinetic exercise on patients with anterior knee pain. Because isokinetic equipment is designed to produce resistance proportional to the force applied, the joint is forced to work at its upper limits. Already overloaded tissue tolerates this situation poorly. Instead, flexibility, strengthening, judicious use of anti-inflammatory medication, and patience should be emphasized to allow overloaded tissues to heal.

Surgery is not necessary in every anterior knee pain patient with objective radiographic patellofemoral malalignment with or without arthrosis. Only if a dedicated effort at nonoperative management of these patients fails *and* if malalignment is objectively present, surgery to realign the extensor mechanism and/or decrease patellofemoral joint reaction force may be appropriate. Although our discussion is limited to patellofemoral problems, it is important to remember that anterior knee pain does not necessarily come from patellofemoral disease.[118] Other causes of pain to be considered before surgery on the patellofemoral joint itself is planned include symptomatic chondromalacia patellae, patellofemoral arthrosis, plica or fat pad syndrome, iliotibial band friction syndrome, vastus lateralis tendinitis, quadriceps or patellar tendinitis, retinacular strain,[51,120] referred pain, and chronic effusion from mechanical (meniscal and/or instability) or inflammatory problems. In addition, one must remember to examine the patient for posterior cruciate ligament (PCL) deficiency, a condition sometimes associated with anterior knee pain.[134,144] Anterior cruciate ligament (ACL) deficiency has been reported to produce anterior knee pain in 20% to 27% of patients with chronic tears.[11,14] ACL reconstruction, particularly performed with the use of a bone–patellar tendon–bone autograft, is well known to activate anterior knee pain in some cases.

Postoperative neuromas or reflex sympathetic dystrophy may further complicate the initial diagnosis. Referred, neoplastic, and nonorganic causes of knee pain must also be excluded.[143] Most diagnoses can be made on the basis of the history and physical examination and require only confirmation by radiographic and arthroscopic examination. Patients

---

*See references 1, 45, 54, 72, 95, 108.

with patellofemoral problems, including recurrent dislocation, malalignment causing subluxation and/or tilt, osteoarthrosis, traumatic chondromalacia, and postpatellectomy pain, at times are candidates for surgery. It is imperative for the clinician to understand the pathophysiology of each diagnosis and whether the goal of surgery should be realignment, soft tissue débridement, and/or relief of pressure.

A rational approach to patellofemoral disorders requires the understanding that various problems are evidenced by different combinations of articular pain, soft tissue pain, and lateral instability of the joint. The search for the correct diagnosis therefore requires a search for the cause of the pain and/or instability. Of course, painful stimuli can only originate from tissues that contain pain receptors. Anatomic sources of pain in the patellofemoral joint include retinacular tissue, synovium, and subchondral bone (articular cartilage is devoid of nerve tissue).[35] In knees with patellofemoral degenerative disease, afferent pain-transmitting substance P–containing fibers were isolated in the retinaculum, fat pad, periosteum, and subchondral plate of the patella, thus suggesting that anterior knee pain may have multiple origins.[147] Conversely, a deficiency of such fibers has been seen in the case of congenital insensitivity to pain.[27]

In contrast, causes of patellar instability are less limited and may include both dynamic and static components. Dynamic (muscular) contributions to lateral instability may result from an increased Q angle or from an unbalanced quadriceps contraction (relative weakness of the vastus medialis obliquus [VMO], delayed VMO firing pattern, or relative hypertrophy of the vastus lateralis muscle). Anteversion of the femoral neck, poor muscular control of external rotation at the hip, pathologic tibial torsion, hindfoot pronation, contracture of the retinaculum and/or patellofemoral ligaments, and dysplasia of the patella or trochlea are examples of influences that may increase lateral patellar instability. While performing the history and physical examination on a patient who is suspected to be a surgical candidate, the physician must keep in mind the question of pain versus instability.

Careful examination is indispensable for proper diagnosis of patellofemoral disorders. The diagnosis of patellofemoral pain is dependent on the physician's ability to reproduce the patient's complaints by physical examination. The search for specific clues, such as an underlying malalignment pattern, abnormally tight soft tissue structures, generalized ligamentous laxity, and patterns of tenderness, is critical to understanding the pathophysiology of each individual.

Observation

Examine the patient while standing and ambulating for evidence of an increased Q angle, torsional deformities of the femur or tibia, knee varus/valgus, pronation of the hindfoot, leg length discrepancy, ankle deformity, scars, and other factors that may affect patellar alignment. Have the patient perform a single-leg knee bend as you watch from the front to see whether the knee rolls inward, thus suggesting weakness of external rotation at the hip. Quadriceps atrophy should also be noted, although we believe that apparent "isolated" VMO atrophy is not a true finding, but rather a superficial reflection of generalized quadriceps atrophy, as suggested by Lieb and Perry.[80,81]

The Q angle is classically measured in extension from the anterior superior iliac spine to the midpoint of the patella and onward to the tibial tuberosity (Fig. 66.1). An increased Q angle

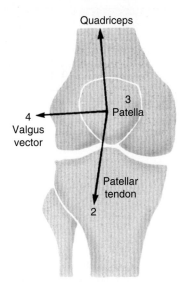

FIG 66.1 The Q Angle Lateralization of the proximal part of the quadriceps, or the tibial tuberosity will increase the resultant valgus vector. (From Fulkerson JP: *Disorders of the patellofemoral joint*, Baltimore, 1990, Williams & Wilkins, p 36.)

should be considered to potentially increase the lateral vector of quadriceps force, possibly causing at least a theoretical tendency toward lateral patellar translation (subluxation). Although the Q angle has always been part of the traditional evaluation of the patellofemoral joint, careful review of the available literature reveals that Q angle measurements are not well standardized. Measurements of the Q angle are made while the patient is supine and standing. We favor the standing measurement because it includes physiologic loading. Unfortunately, the Q angle has not been proved to correlate with the incidence of pain or the results of treatment.[106] Normal populations have been measured, and the results are summarized in Table 66.1. Although the importance of understanding the lateral extensor moment and its potential effects on patellar alignment is undeniable, the role of Q angle measurement is less clear.

At 90 degrees of flexion, the tuberosity is normally directly inferior to the patella. Examining the patient in a seated position allows good visualization of the femur/patella/tuberosity relationship.[78] Observation of these relationships allows the clinician to estimate the degree of valgus in the knee, as well as the position of the tibial tuberosity, which may be laterally displaced out of proportion to the tibiofemoral valgus. Lateral displacement of the tibial tubercle is more common in patients with patellofemoral pain and arthrosis and can be detected by physical examination and documented with advanced imaging which will be more fully discussed in the imaging section. The Q angle, as measured clinically, does not directly correlate with patellofemoral pain, and although it is related to patellofemoral mechanics, it is only one of the many factors that influence patellar balance. However, once nonoperative management maximizes dynamic factors, static alignment, including tubercle position relative to the trochlear groove, should be considered. Patellar tracking must be considered as well. Normally, the patella lies superior and lateral to the trochlea on the supratrochlear fat pad in full extension. One may recognize patella alta on examination by the abnormally proximal position of the patella, but it is more accurately diagnosed radiographically.

TABLE 66.1 Normal Population Q Angle Review

SUPINE			STANDING		
Author	Q Angle, Degrees	No. Knees/Age (Years)	Author	Q Angle, Degrees	No. Knees/Age (Years)
Insall et al.[a]	14	50/not specified	Woodland[b]	F 17.0 ± .072	57/20.0
				M 13.6 ± .072	69/22.3
Aglietti et al.[c]	F 17 ± 3	75/23	Fairbank et al.[d]	F 23 ± 1.2	150/14.8 ± 0.1
	M 14 ± 3	75/23		M 20 ± 1.2	160/14.6 ± 0.1
Hsu et al.[e]	F 18.8 ± 4.7	60/not specified	Horton and Hall[f]	F 15.8 ± 4.5	
	M 15.6 ± 3.5	60/not specified		M 11.2 ± 3.0	
Woodland and Francis[b]	F 15.8 ± .072	57/20.0			
	M 12.7 ± .072	69/22.3			

[a]Insall J, Falvo KA, Wise DW: Chondromalacia patellae: a prospective study. *J Bone Joint Surg Am* 58:1, 1976.
[b]Woodland LH, Francis RS: Parameters and comparisons of the quadriceps angle of college-aged men and women in the supine and standing positions. *Am J Sports Med* 20:208, 1992.
[c]Aglietti P, Insall JN, Cerulli G: Patellar pain and incongruence. *Clin Orthop Relat Res* 122:217, 1983.
[d]Fairbank JCT, Pynsent PB, van Poortvliet JA, et al: Mechanical factors in the incidence of knee pain in adolescents and young adults. *J Bone Joint Surg* 66:685, 1984.
[e]Hsu RWW, Himeno S, Coventry MB, et al: Normal axial alignment of the lower extremity and load-bearing distribution at the knee. *Clin Orthop Relat Res* 255:215, 1990.
[f]Horton MG, Hall TL: Quadriceps femoris muscle angle: normal values and relationships with gender and selected skeletal measures. *Phys Ther* 69:897, 1989.
F, Female; *M*, male.
From Fulkerson JP: *Disorders of the patellofemoral joint*, Baltimore, 1997, Williams & Wilkins.

The patella enters the trochlea smoothly from its superolateral position at 10 degrees of flexion and, with increasing flexion, is centered and drawn into the trochlea. If during early flexion the patella tracks laterally and then suddenly shifts medially into the trochlea with active or passive flexion, the J sign is positive.[9] In a review of 210 asymptomatic adults, Johnson et al.[70] found no subject with a positive J sign. Also, it should be kept in mind that the reverse J sign, in which the patella of a patient with medial patella subluxation slides in a medial-to-lateral direction on knee flexion, is clearly an abnormal pattern, but is often very subtle. As with all tests of tracking, flexibility, and alignment, comparison with the other side is important.

Provocative Tests

Strong compression of the patella resulting in pain and crepitus during flexion and extension of the knee is helpful in determining whether the patient's pain syndrome has a significant patellofemoral component. If the patient remains relaxed, the examiner can stabilize the knee in multiple angles of knee flexion while applying a substantial force on the patella. This allows direct patellofemoral joint compression and avoids stretching the peripatellar soft tissues or muscle firing.[107] Another method of provocative testing is isometric contraction of the quadriceps at different angles of flexion.[87] Isometric contractions, which should be sustained for 10 seconds, provide the advantage of avoiding direct palpation in patients who are particularly apprehensive. If one or both of these methods reproduce the patient's complaint, it is likely that the pain has a patellofemoral origin. These techniques of examination do not, however, distinguish between soft tissue and articular sources of pain because soft tissue stretch and articular compression are noted when the knee is moved or the quadriceps fires during these examinations.

In an attempt to confirm whether a patient has medial patella subluxation, hold the patella slightly medial with one finger and the knee in extension, then abruptly flex the knee. If this maneuver reproduces the symptoms, the patient may have a problem with medial subluxation, most commonly in the clinical setting of previous lateral release, medial retinacular reconstruction, or overaggressive tibial tubercle transfer.[44,119]

Palpation

The subcutaneous position of the patellofemoral joint makes it uniquely available for careful examination. Palpation of the patellofemoral joint has two goals: (1) to differentiate between soft tissue and bony pain, and (2) to precisely localize the soft tissue or articular area that reproduces the patient's complaint. Firm compression of the patella directly into the trochlea while the knee is held in various angles of flexion, combined with the knowledge that articulation starts distal on the patella and moves proximally with increasing flexion, can provide information to localize the articular disease. This can be accomplished by direct compression (with care taken to avoid compressing adjacent soft tissue structures). Meaningful specific palpation of medial or lateral patellar facets seems anatomically unlikely, given the interposition of innervated synovium and retinacular tissue. The degree of crepitus is more significant when absent or asymmetrical with the contralateral knee. When evaluating the presence or absence of crepitus, remember that Johnson et al. found that 94% of asymptomatic women have crepitus.[70] It is more important to note whether articular compression reproduces the patient's pain. Also, noting the character of the crepitus is helpful. Harsh, sustained grinding is different from the faint click that is common on flexion and extension of a normal knee.

Soft tissue palpation should systematically include the retinacular structures, the insertions of the quadriceps tendons into the superior pole of the patella, and the patellar tendon. Structures are generally best palpated in a position that places them on stretch and allows gentle palpation to achieve relative isolation from the underlying structures. This strategy allows discovery of specific points prone to overuse-type injury. We have previously described in detail a thorough anatomically and functionally oriented soft tissue examination, and the reader is encouraged to practice and master these techniques.[43,45,47,108,106] Points of intersection between structures, such as the junction of the medial patellar tendon, the inferior pole of the patella, and the medial retinaculum, seem particularly prone to tenderness, perhaps because of the stress concentration at locations where two or more different structures under load meet. These locations are frequently tender in patients with excessive lateral patellar tilt. A cautious search for such locations will often uncover the origin of a patient's soft tissue pain.

Such differentiation between soft tissue and articular pain helps in surgical planning. Stress-relieving anteriorization should be considered in patients with predominantly articular-based complaints and normal alignment. In contrast, coronal (medial/lateral) realignment may be adequate in cases of malalignment in which the articular surface has not degenerated. With severe articular degeneration, the patella may not tolerate even the relatively lower loads present after completion of a procedure that corrects alignment.

Stability Testing

Just as examination for ACL deficiency includes evaluation of the static stability of a joint in several planes, examination of the patellofemoral joint is not complete without evaluation of static constraints in both the sagittal (tilt) and coronal (medial/lateral) planes. Evaluation of patellar tilt and medial-to-lateral restraints provides important information.

The passive patellar tilt test is performed with the knee in full extension. While the patella is held in the center of the trochlea, the examiner attempts to correct the patellar tilt to neutral or beyond, if possible (Fig. 66.2). We agree with Kolowich et al.[74] that tilt should normally correct at least to neutral, although normal patellae often tilt up to 10 degrees or more past neutral. It is also possible to gain an impression of the nature of the resilience of the lateral retinaculum. Some patients seem to have a springy endpoint, whereas others have a very stiff and unyielding restraint. Comparison with the opposite knee often reveals relatively limited correction of lateral patellar tilt on the symptomatic side. Because the iliotibial band fibers contribute to the lateral retinacular tissue, poor iliotibial band flexibility frequently accompanies abnormal lateral tilt.

Medial and lateral patellar glide testing has been well described by Hughston et al and by Kolowich et al.[65,74] It is similar to the passive hypermobility testing described by Hughston.[65] We believe that these tests should be performed with the patella in neutral tilt if possible to allow consistent comparison of the medial/lateral restraints. As described, medial patellar glide is tested with medially directed pressure on the patella and the knee in 20 to 30 degrees of flexion to

effectively engage the patella in the trochlea (Fig. 66.3). This test is also effective with the knee in extension and lesser degrees of flexion. Near full extension, the ligamentous and muscular restraints may be more isolated because of less bony constraint before engagement of the patella in the trochlea. Through testing of lateral glide with the knee in extension, it is possible to palpate an endpoint to lateral translation similar to that palpable with the Lachman test. Absence of such an endpoint, together with increased translation, is highly suggestive of medial patellofemoral ligament (MPFL) deficiency. Any abnormal tightness found in the retinaculum at these lesser angles of flexion can affect the direction of patellar entry into the trochlea. Medial patellar glide is judged abnormal if medial translation is seen in less than one quadrant, as described by Kolowich et al.[74] Laterally directed pressure on the neutral patella that results in displacement of three quadrants or more is consistent with an abnormally lax medial restraint. Ligamentous laxity itself, as might be measured by quadrant displacement, should not be confused with actual subluxation and, if found, should generate caution if a realignment procedure is contemplated. Evidence of systemic ligamentous laxity should be sought in such patients before any conclusions are drawn regarding specific isolated incompetence of peripatellar restraints or malalignment. In hypermobile patients, dynamic muscular control of patellar position is even more critical. Emphasis should be placed on active muscular control and on being patient. Involuntary quadriceps contraction during positive lateral glide testing or the classic apprehension reaction to the perception of imminent dislocation is strong evidence of clinically relevant patellar instability.

Several tests have been developed to assist in the diagnosis of medial patellar instability, a condition that almost always occurs as a complication of patellar realignment. In patients with symptomatic medial patellar instability, one can displace the patella medially and then passively flex the knee, and the symptoms will be reproduced as the patella moves laterally from the subluxated position into the trochlea.[106] Although the patella is moving laterally, it is moving from a subluxated position into the trochlea, essentially a "reverse apprehension" test. Another helpful test in the setting of potential medial instability

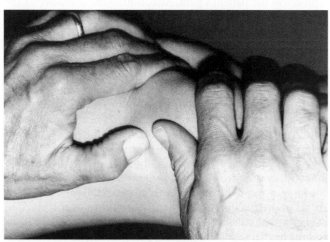

FIG 66.2 Physical examination for patellar tilt. Tilt should correct to neutral. (From Scott WN: The knee, vol 1, St Louis, 1994, Mosby-Year Book, p 445.)

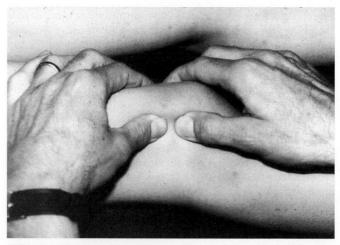

FIG 66.3 Physical examination for patellar glide. Medially directed force is applied to the lateral aspect of the patella. (From Scott WN: The knee, vol 1, St. Louis, 1994, Mosby-Year Book, p 445.)

is the gravity subluxation test.[99] This test requires that the patient be placed in the lateral decubitus position. The patella is then manually displaced medially. Because of previous operative transection of the vastus lateralis, the patient cannot actively reduce the patella into the trochlea. Although provocative testing for medial patellar instability is not routinely necessary, these tests should be regularly included in the evaluation of patients after failed patellofemoral realignment.

Flexibility

Systematic evaluation of the quadriceps, hamstring, iliotibial band, and gastrocnemius/soleus muscle groups is important because each can contribute to anterior knee pain. Quadriceps tightness is often associated with patellar tendinitis and "failed" postoperative patellar pain patients. Quadriceps tightness is best tested with the patient prone, thereby stabilizing the pelvis. Hamstring contracture may result in abnormally increased knee flexion during the stance phase and, therefore, increased patellofemoral joint reaction force. Iliotibial band tightness has a more direct effect through its insertion into the lateral retinaculum and, consequently, abnormally increases posterolateral pull with increasing flexion. Increased hindfoot pronation is a result of gastrocnemius and/or soleus contracture in some patients. This causes the subtalar joint to compensate for the relative lack of tibiotalar dorsiflexion with increased hindfoot pronation. Increased subtalar pronation results in increased internal rotation of the tibia and femur and contributes to patellofemoral malalignment. When diminished flexibility is detected, nonoperative management must include stretching.

Radiologic Evaluation. Once a complete history and physical examination have been performed, radiologic studies are frequently indicated to confirm and document the clinical impression. The patellofemoral joint is a complex articulation and advancements in imaging have made acquiring radiographs and advanced imaging (computed tomography [CT] scans and magnetic resonance imaging [MRI]) a necessity in preoperative planning.[135] Standing anteroposterior and lateral x-ray films are important to search for associated conditions and patella alta. A normal ratio of patellar ligament length to patellar length of less than 1.2 has been described by Insall and Salvati. Blackburne and Peel[10] described the ratio of the articular length of the

patella to the height of the lower pole of the patellar articular cartilage above the tibial articular surface (normal, <1.0). These ratios can be used to quantify patella alta if desired. In cases in which patella alta is prominently abnormal, distal transfer of the tuberosity should be part of the surgical plan.

Axial tangential views of the patellofemoral joint, such as those described by Merchant et al.[89] and Laurin et al.,[77] may be used as screening tests for malalignment, but can be difficult to interpret because of image overlap (unless the image is precisely tangential to the joint). The congruence angle of Merchant and Mercer and the lateral patellofemoral angle of Laurin and Dussault are estimations of lateral subluxation and tilt, respectively. The symmetry of subchondral sclerosis of the patellar facets should also be evaluated for signs of localized sclerosis (indicating unbalanced stress). These authors and their colleagues recognized the importance of imaging the patella early in flexion in the less constrained proximal femoral sulcus. Kujala et al.[76] emphasized imaging of the patellofemoral joint in early flexion. They found greater MRI differences in tilt and lateral subluxation in views with less than 30 degrees of flexion in a group of patients with recurrent patellar dislocations than in a normal control group. CT scans, first suggested by Delgado-Martins[26] in 1979, offer a significant advantage by providing imaging of earlier degrees of flexion with absolutely no image overlap.[93]

When distal realignment including tibial tuberosity transfer is considered, we believe it is wise to measure the position of the tuberosity relative to the trochlea. The most acceptable method for this consists of CT measurement of the tibial tuberosity–trochlear groove (TT-TG) distance (Fig. 66.4). Dejour and associates first described this measurement, and upon comparing normal patients with those with patellar instability, found that the threshold for normal was 20 mm.[25] This measurement is done by measuring the lateral distance of the tibial tuberosity from the most posterior point in the femoral sulcus, along a line parallel to the axis of the posterior femoral condyles. When the TT-TG distance is 20 mm or greater, available data suggest that such a measurement is abnormal on MRI or CT scan. Medialization of the tuberosity should then be considered. The amount of medialization needed can also be estimated from this measurement, and the most often targeted goal for postoperative TT-TG distance is

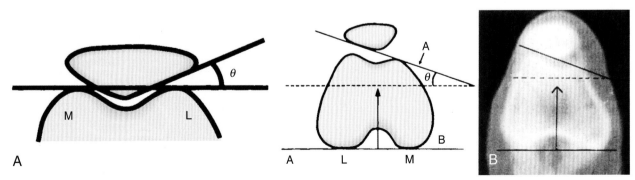

FIG 66.4 TT-TG distance. Axial image through the tibial tuberosity superimposed on a cut through the femoral trochlea at the level where the intercondylar notch appears to be a "Roman arch." TT-TG equals the lateral distance of the tibial tuberosity from the most posterior point in the femoral sulcus, along a line parallel to the axis of the posterior femoral condyles. Normal TT-TG distance should measure less than 20 mm. (Image courtesy of Dr. Rick Cautilli, Philadelphia, Pennsylvania.)

approximately 10 mm. Measurement of the TT-TG distance is helpful in confirming that tuberosity medialization is appropriate in a clinical situation that otherwise warrants medial or anteromedial transfer. It is very important when evaluating measurement of the TT-TG distance to be certain that whoever measures this does so reproducibly and ideally that would be the treating surgeon.

Further work on CT technique, evaluation, and classification of patellofemoral disorders has been done by Schutzer and associates.[123,124] Several significant advantages of CT evaluation are now clear. Use of the posterior femoral condyles as a reference plane for measurement of the patellar tilt angle has proved significantly more consistent than use of the anterior intercondylar line, as reported by Laurin and Dussault. This increases the precision with which tilt can be measured and it eliminates the variable of femoral rotation[49] (Fig. 66.5). Measurement of the congruence angle is also enhanced by the nature of the CT scan "slice" because it ensures that the trochlear and patellar images being measured are, in fact, at the same level and are not artifacts of image overlap (Fig. 66.6). Patterns of patellofemoral malalignment on CT images are usually classified into three types. Type I is lateral subluxation, type II combines lateral subluxation and lateral tilt, and type III includes lateral tilt without subluxation (Fig. 66.7). Type IV has been defined as radiographically normal alignment.[50] This classification has been very helpful in confirming the clinical impression of specific patellar malalignment patterns (tilt and/or subluxation).

Bone scans or single-photon emission computed tomography (SPECT) scans (combination of CT and bone scan) can provide crucial information for understanding the pathophysiology of anterior knee pain patients. Because the uptake of radionuclide is a measure of the bone biology/overload and homeostasis, it adds an important factor in understanding patellofemoral complaints. When considering realignment procedures designed to unload pathologically overloaded tissue, the judicious use of nuclear medicine studies often clarifies the tissue that needs to be unloaded. Static malalignment on imaging studies does not prove overload. It simply proves static abnormality of alignment, which in itself is certainly not a surgical indication.[30,34]

MRI has been helpful in understanding TT-TG distance and how the soft tissues and articular cartilage can be better defined in this relationship. As MRI has become more prevalent, multiple studies have been undertaken to determine the benefits and drawbacks of applying the original CT-based methods of calculating TT-TG distance to MRI imaging. Authors have found that CT and MRI TT-TG measurements may differ in patient groups, making it important to evaluate each study separately and in concert.[17,64] MRI has been used to establish growth-based norms in a pediatric population, allowing better understanding of TT-TG measures in younger patients.[29] Others have emphasized that TT-TG distance may change with patient age and height, and that normalizing MRI-based TT-TG distance to patient height may control for size variations while still noting that elevated TT-TG values were associated with patellar instability in children and adolescents.[103] Skelley et al. reported that surgeons and musculoskeletal radiologists had high intra- and interobserver reliability when measuring the TT-TG distance and the trochlear dysplasia index (TDI) on MRI.[130] MRI has also allowed clinicians to better examine the trochlea by

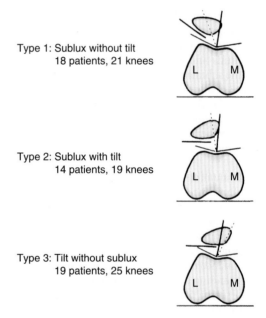

Type 1: Sublux without tilt
18 patients, 21 knees

Type 2: Sublux with tilt
14 patients, 19 knees

Type 3: Tilt without sublux
19 patients, 25 knees

FIG 66.6 Congruence angle as measured on a midtransverse patellar CT scan. (From Scott WN: The knee, vol 1, St Louis, 1994, Mosby-Year Book, p 446.)

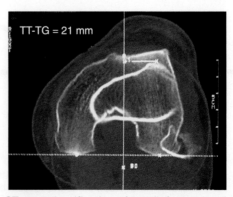

FIG 66.5 (A) Patellar tilt angle of Laurin measured from an axial radiograph. (B) Patellar tilt angle measured from a transverse midpatellar CT scan. (From Fulkerson JP: Disorders of the patellofemoral joint, Baltimore, 1990, Williams & Wilkins, pp 50, 60.)

FIG 66.7 CT scan classification of patellofemoral malalignment. (From Schutzer SF, Ramsby GR: Computed tomographic classification of patellofemoral pain patients. Orthop Clin North Am 17:235, 1986.)

evaluating the bone and cartilage as a unit, thus improving accuracy and understanding of trochlear dysplasia, which is one of the major factors noted in MRI imaging of the patellar dislocation patient cohort along with increased TT-TG distance and patella alta.[131] In an effort to further capitalize on the advantages of MRI imaging (presence of non-bone tissues and multiple viewing planes when compared with CT), authors have proposed modifications in the classic TT-TG measurement to try to improve its predictive value. Consideration of the TT-TG and a TT-TG that incorporated trochlear width (TT-TG/TW) led to a ratio that may be more predictive of recurrent patellar instability.[16] In addition, authors have proposed using a TT-PCL ratio to account for individual patient variability in size while creating a measure independent of trochlear dysplasia.[2] The TT-TG ratio still represents the cornerstone of patellar preoperative planning, even as it is refined and updated for modern imaging techniques. Despite the emphasis in the literature on measurement of these anatomic factors, it must be remembered that any such measurements are only one part of the puzzle in deciding what treatment is most appropriate in a given patient.

Nonoperative Management. Most patients with patellofemoral disorders improve without surgery.[104,110] Dye has provided excellent reviews and a theoretical model that he calls the *envelope of load acceptance model* to enhance understanding of the mechanisms and reasons for improvement of patients with patellofemoral pain by rest and activity modification.[33] Initial management of patellofemoral disorders should include the goals of normal flexibility and balanced quadriceps strength. One should remember to include the entire extremity in rehabilitation, especially hip strengthening. This program should be directed by specific physical examination findings. Discussion of specific techniques exceeds the scope of this chapter. In addition to reassurance, strengthening, stretching, core stability training, taping techniques, anti-pronation orthotics, and patellar braces may be very beneficial in selected patients. Weight loss in obese patients is imperative in controlling patellofemoral pain. It is sometimes surprising how well patients, even those with severe radiographic findings, do without surgery.[109] Therefore, before surgery, it is always important to confirm that a comprehensive nonoperative treatment program has been followed.

A RATIONAL APPROACH TO DISTAL REALIGNMENT

Realignment operations, including distal realignments, should be considered only when objective anatomic malalignment has been diagnosed and nonoperative treatment has failed. Patients with malalignment may have pain and/or symptomatic patellar instability. It is very important to differentiate whether the goal of surgery is simply realignment with improvement in the balance of forces across the patellofemoral joint, or whether discrete episodes of patellar instability have occurred preoperatively. If dislocations have occurred, one must consider whether stabilization of the patella might be needed by MPFL imbrication or reconstruction, along with correction of underlying malalignment, if objective malalignment can be proven. The decision to add imbrication or reconstruction must be made carefully and only after consideration of whether this would unwisely increase load on medial facet chondral lesions.

Rational realignment and unloading patellar and trochlear lesions can help restore bony homeostasis even in the presence of articular damage.

For patients who have severe symptomatic articular degeneration in a normally aligned patellofemoral joint, surgical choices include anteriorization, patellectomy, and patellofemoral arthroplasty. Patellofemoral resurfacing and patellectomy are rarely necessary unless no adequate articular cartilage remains. None of these operations restores the knee to "normal," and nonoperative management is often indicated. Frequently, multiple localized foci of soft tissue inflammation and overload and pain from articular degeneration are noted in such patients with severe arthrosis after blunt trauma. Patient and persistent treatment directed at the soft tissues (eg, stretching, strengthening, activity modification) can often produce satisfactory improvement without surgery. Distal realignment is *not* indicated in such patients, even as a "last resort."

Distal Realignment Procedures
Theory
Medialization. Distal realignment of the patellofemoral joint by medial transposition of the patellar tendon insertion decreases the laterally directed moment that causes patellar subluxation upon quadriceps contraction. Ideal candidates for distal realignment have laterally displaced tibial tubercles. Lateral release or lateral lengthening often accompanies the various methods of medialization and is important when required to relieve any lateral tether that is present. In patients with patellar instability, lateral lengthening may be preferable to release considering that the lateral retinaculum contributes 10% of the resistance to lateral patellar translation in laboratory testing.[28] Additionally, the medial patellofemoral complex can be reconstructed or repaired leading to improved medial soft-tissue tethering of the patella. MPFL reconstruction, when attempted as a stand-alone graft, might potentially create abnormally increased medial patellar facet pressure by attempting to counteract forceful, laterally directed pull on the patella using a posteromedially directed tether on the extensor mechanism. Complications arising from excessive medial tension within the patellofemoral joint can be severe.[101,140] The concept that we wish to put forth here is that the extensor mechanism should be balanced first, before incompetent medial structures such as the MPFL are reconstructed. Amis et al. suggested that MPFL ligament reconstruction may be sufficient in patients with limited TT-TG distances (balanced extensor mechanism), but that in patients with more excessive TT-TG distances (>15+ mm) tibial tubercle transfer may be indicated.[132] This concept does not, however, mean that treatment of medial tissue incompetence should be excluded. Careful consideration of underlying patient anatomy including trochlear dysplasia, TT-TG distance, patella alta, and medial tissue incompetence may lead the physician to apply MPFL reconstruction or medial imbrication and tibial tubercle transfer in the same setting with generally good results.[92,138] It is important to understand, however, when considering medial tuberosity transfer in the setting of patellar instability, that there are not, to our knowledge, any studies comparing MPFL reconstruction alone to MPFL reconstruction and distal transfer.

An alternative medial graft technique has recently been put forth by Edgar and Fulkerson in which a soft tissue graft is secured on the extensor mechanism side by weaving it through the distal and medial quadriceps mechanism, thus avoiding a

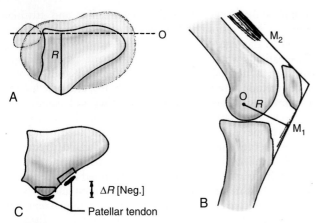

FIG 66.8 (A) Note the lateral position of the tubercle with respect to the tibial plateau and the posteromedial slope of the anteromedial tibial cortex. Distance R illustrates the lever arm of the quadriceps. (B) Lateral view illustrating the quadriceps lever R. (C) Posterior displacement of the tibial tubercle as a result of medial transposition of the tibial tubercle (classic Hauser procedure). The decreased mechanical advantage of the quadriceps mechanism in this situation results in the need to generate greater quadriceps muscle force to accomplish the same work, and this leads to increased patellofemoral joint reaction force. (From Fulkerson JP: Disorders of the patellofemoral joint, Baltimore, 1990, Williams & Wilkins, p 144.)

bone tunnel in the patella, which may facilitate graft passage and eliminate the possibility of patella fracture after tunnel drilling.[48]

Distalization

Distal transfer of the tuberosity when pathologic patella alta is present helps the patella to enter the trochlea earlier in flexion and can be very helpful in some patients with patellar instability.

Anteriorization/Posteriorization

The biomechanics of posterior displacement of the tibial tuberosity dictates an increase in joint reaction force to accomplish the same work, and this should be avoided (Fig. 66.8). Anteriorization will decrease the patellofemoral joint forces and can be used alone or in concert with medialization. A careful understanding of native patellofemoral anatomy and biomechanics can help clinicians understand the effects of various tibial tubercle transfers.[127]

Clinical Data. Distal medialization procedures may be divided into two categories: (1) those involving soft tissue only and (2) those involving transfer of the tibial tuberosity. Skeletal immaturity in a patient being considered for distal realignment mandates selection of a procedure that does not violate the proximal tibial physis or the apophysis of the tibial tubercle—a mistake that could cause complications such as genu recurvatum or continued distal migration of the tibial tuberosity with growth.[†]

[†]See references 22, 23, 40, 58, 62, 83.

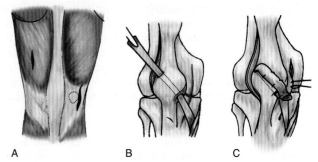

FIG 66.9 Galeazzi semitendinosus tenodesis, an option for soft tissue distal realignment in the skeletally immature patient. (From Baker RH, Carroll N: The semitendinosus tenodesis for recurrent dislocation of the patella. J Bone Joint Surg Br 54:103, 1972.)

Soft Tissue Medialization or Medial Reconstruction. Historically, options for distal realignment in a skeletally immature patient have included (1) the Roux-Goldthwait procedure, in which the lateral half of the patellar tendon is detached distally, passed behind the medial half of the tendon, and sutured to the pes anserinus insertion, and (2) the Galeazzi semitendinosus tenodesis. Each procedure would normally be done with a lateral release. Reports of the Roux-Goldthwait procedure vary from good success rates in two series[19,41] to a high failure rate in another.[12] Another more recent study found a higher rate of patellofemoral osteoarthrosis when the Roux-Goldthwait procedure was compared with MPFL reconstruction.[128] The mechanics of this operation, however, creates the risk of inducing undesirable lateral patellar tilt and this procedure is no longer recommended. The Galeazzi tenodesis procedure uses the distally attached semitendinosus tendon to pull the patella distally and medially (Fig. 66.9). Baker et al.[4] achieved 81% good and excellent results with only 4% recurrent dislocations when using this technique.

Mini-proximal imbrication with MPFL and VMO advancement through a 2-inch incision can be very helpful in many patients and is preferable to alternative procedures when it can restore normal patellar tracking. MPFL reconstruction procedures that involve attaching a graft to the region of the medial femoral epicondyle are contraindicated in skeletally immature patients because of the risk of physeal damage. Immediate range of motion is imperative.

MPFL reconstruction by the technique of Deie et al.[24] using a distally attached semitendinosus graft transferred to the medial proximal patella through a soft tissue attachment in the posterior part of the proximal medial cruciate ligament (MCL) provides good soft tissue stabilization in skeletally immature patients. Others have presented successful medial reconstruction techniques that are appropriate for patients who have open growth plates.[97] We have rarely found that skeletally immature patients require management with distal realignment and recommend other management until skeletal maturity.

Tuberosity Transfers. The Hauser procedure, as described in 1938, includes medial and distal transplantation of the tibial tuberosity.[60] Several authors have noted only 67% to 74% rates of good to excellent pain relief and functional improvement after Hauser procedures for diagnoses of chondromalacia resulting from malalignment,[66] recurrent patellar dislocation,[19] and acute and recurrent dislocations.[40] Recurrent dislocation has occurred at similarly steady rates of 17% to 20%.[23,40,71] Generalized ligamentous laxity has been strongly associated with poor results and recurrent dislocation.[23] Furthermore, in some series, a distressingly high percentage of patients (68% to 71%) have had evidence of progression to osteoarthrosis at average follow-up of 7.3 years, 16 years,[57] and 18 years.[71] Unfortunately, because of the anatomy of the proximal end of the tibia, this procedure has resulted in posterior tuberosity displacement (see Fig. 66.8). The high incidence of articular degeneration is consistent with biomechanical theory, which predicts increased stress with distal and posterior transfer of the tuberosity. Posteromedial transfer of the tibial tubercle is rarely, if ever, justified.

Dougherty et al.[31] and Grana and O'Donoghue[55] reported modifications of the Hauser procedure in which a slot-block method of fixation of the tibial tuberosity was used for lateral patellar instability. Both had 83% successful results, although Grana and O'Donoghue experienced a 26% rate of significant complications and labeled this procedure technically demanding. Dougherty and Wirth noted worse results in patients with more severe chondromalacia, although specific criteria were not cited. Again, this type of surgery is rarely appropriate and is primarily of historical interest.

Cox[20,21] successfully accomplished distal realignment by medial displacement of the tuberosity while avoiding any posterior displacement with the Roux-Elmslie-Trillat procedure (Fig. 66.10). This technique classically combines lateral release, medial capsular reefing, and medial displacement of the bony insertion of the patellar tendon with distal displacement titrated according to the degree of patella alta measured preoperatively. Excellent and good results were achieved in 77% of 116 patients, with only a 7% recurrence rate. Factors associated with poor outcomes included failure to adequately correct the Q angle or the patella alta, concomitant ACL deficiency, and preexisting patellar degeneration. Using the same procedure, Brown et al.[13] found that adequate postoperative correction of the Q angle to 10 degrees or less correlated well with good to excellent results. Shelbourne et al.[126] found that postoperative alignment (as measured radiographically by the congruence angle) correlated with the presence of recurrent instability. In their series, 26% (9/34) of patients with preoperative instability had postoperative subluxation. Although postoperative improvement in the congruence angle was the same for patients with stable patellae, these patients had higher preoperative and postoperative congruence angles. Durable results from tibial tubercle transfer have been reproducible with 10-year minimum follow-up in a number of reports.[18,23,69] No progression of osteoarthrosis was noted, and theoretically one would expect it to be less than with the Hauser procedure, which classically includes posterior tubercle displacement. The Elmslie-Trillat procedure may be combined with arthroscopic lateral release and medial retinacular surgery to obtain results consistent with those described previously.[6] In reviewing series of patients treated by distal realignment, one notes that the procedure is often modified in potentially important ways. Tomatsu et al.[139] compared two groups of similar patients treated with Elmslie-Trillat procedures, but with omission of medial capsulorrhaphy in one group. Results were identical in both groups and were very similar to those reported by previous authors. The series of Shelbourne et al.[126] also omitted medial capsulorrhaphy. Rantanen and Paananen[115] reported on 35 knees treated by medial transfer of the tibial tubercle; they omitted the lateral release in 14 patients. Their results were, again, practically identical to those reported by Cox. Rillmann et al.[116] reported yet another modification in which only the medial third of the patellar tendon was transferred and lateral release was included in only 2 of 39 patients. Again, similar outcomes occurred with no redislocations and an 11% rate of postoperative subluxation. Some authors specifically measure patella alta and routinely include distal transfer of the tubercle.[13,20,21,115] Others specifically omit consideration of distal transfer to correct patella alta.[116,126,139] Although the data currently do not allow for definitive guidelines regarding specific operative procedures, we believe that factors such as systemic hypermobility, skeletal alignment, and articular surface condition should be considered when the best procedure to correct instability in any given patient is selected. Patients with severe radiographic malalignment may require medial imbrication, but based on previous studies, it is apparent that many patients do not require medial capsular imbrication.

Anteriorization

Theory. Anterior elevation of the tibial tuberosity, as proposed by Bandi[5] and Maquet, enhances the efficiency of the quadriceps by increasing the lever arm while decreasing the patellofemoral joint reaction force. As illustrated in Fig. 66.11, increasing the angle between the vector of quadriceps pull and the patellar tendon decreases the joint reaction force. The goal is to reduce articular stress by reducing the force and increasing the area of joint contact, thus further decreasing articular stress. Maquet's calculations of patellofemoral compressive force predict approximately a 50% reduction during the stance phase after a 2-cm elevation.

Laboratory data. This hypothesis is generally confirmed by a progressive reduction in patellofemoral compressive force as cadaver tibial tubercles are advanced. Ferguson et al.'s comparison[38] of six locations on the articular surface of the patella after 1.2-, 2.5-, and 3.7-cm anterior elevation demonstrated significant relief of stress. Overall stress relief with 1.2-cm advancement at 45 degrees of flexion was 57%. Further elevation to 2.5

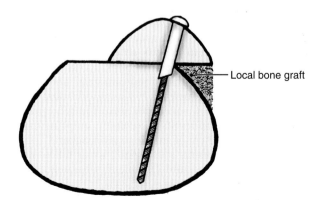

Local bone graft

FIG 66.10 Roux-Elmslie-Trillat procedure. Note that this medialization of the tibial tubercle results in no posterior displacement of the tuberosity. (From Cox JS: Evaluation of the Roux-Elmslie-Trillat procedure for knee extensor realignment. Am J Sports Med 10:303, 1982.)

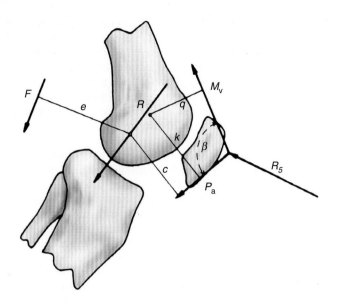

FIG 66.11 Anteriorization of the tibial tubercle decreases the angle β, thereby resulting in decreased patellofemoral joint reaction force. It also tips up the distal patella, thereby unloading distal patellar chondral lesions. (From Maquet P: Mechanics and osteoarthritis of the patellofemoral joint. Clin Orthop Relat Res 144:70, 1979.)

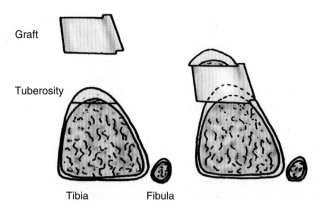

FIG 66.12 Maquet Technique A notched iliac crest graft is used to produce anterior and medial displacement of the tibial tuberosity. This procedure is rarely indicated. (From Maquet P: Advancement of the tibial tuberosity. Clin Orthop Relat Res 115:225, 1976.)

and 3.7 cm resulted in additional progressive decreases in average stress of only 30% and 9%, respectively. In a review of these data, Radin[112] noted, however, that the absolute value of total contact stress after 1.2-cm elevation was more than twice that measured after an elevation of 2.5 cm. Ferguson and Brown's study used averaged values obtained from retropatellar sensors and assumed them to be equivalent to the overall average because their model did not permit measurement of contact areas. They concluded that most contact stress was relieved with the first 1.2 cm of tendon elevation, and that additional decreases were believed to represent decreasing returns in exchange for increasing risk of skin complications. In a similar study using retropatellar piezoelectric transducers, Ferrandez et al.[39] confirmed close to a 50% decrease in pressure in the first 1 cm and a more gradual decline with further tubercle elevation.

Lewallen et al.[79] used pressure-sensitive film to measure the joint contact force and area after 1.2-cm and 2.5-cm tubercle elevations in eight knees with variable degrees of chondromalacia (Outerbridge grades I to IV). They found significant decreases in joint contact force of 29% and 23% after 1.2-cm elevation at 60 and 90 degrees of flexion, respectively. Contrary to the findings of Ferguson et al.'s study,[38] elevation to 2.5 cm resulted in significant additional 60%, 53%, and 55% decreases in force in comparison with "preoperative" values at 30, 60, and 90 degrees. The patellar contact area was observed to shift proximally and laterally with progressive elevation. With regard to the suggestion that anteriorization shifts the load proximally, this may occur secondary to the slight distal transfer that occurs as the shingle is rotated forward (and distally).[100] Logically, this effect is increased with shorter shingle length, which produces relatively more distal transfer for the same anteriorization as would a longer shingle. Overall, these findings substantiate the concept of further relief of joint reaction force with increasing

elevation, even if these particular models do not specifically support or refute Maquet's contention that contact area is increased.

Clinical experience. Maquet[85] reported on 37 patients with patellar arthrosis and chondromalacia an average of 4.7 years after 2- to 3-cm advancement of the tuberosity; 36 knees were stable with relief of pain and range of motion that approximated preoperative motion. His recommendations included medialization of the tubercle when the patella was subluxated, and osteoarthritis was limited to the lateral facet. Medialization was accomplished by notching the graft. Early postoperative motion was possible because of the stable geometry of the iliac graft (Fig. 66.12). Radin's[111] 36 patients had successful results from a modified Maquet procedure, including elevation of at least 2 cm, lateral release, and medialization of approximately 1 cm (as necessary to correct subluxation) in 94% with posttraumatic osteoarthrosis, in 88% with chronic patellar subluxation and osteoarthrosis, and in 66% with postpatellectomy pain. Mendes et al.,[88] in their series of 27 patients with primarily patellofemoral osteoarthritis, achieved 76% subjective satisfactory results at 5.5 years after a 2.5-cm elevation. Heatley et al.[61] reported 65% excellent and good results in 29 patients.

Engebretsen et al.'s results[37] correlated with the pattern of articular degeneration; the best postoperative results were seen in patients with lateral facet degeneration. No improvement was noted in 18 of 20 patients with medial facet involvement. At long-term follow-up of 8 to 15 years, anteriorization was found to be durable; Jenny et al.[68] reported a 62% success rate. Silvello et al.[129] treated patients with "chondromalacia" and patellofemoral arthritis with somewhat less anteriorization (1.2 to 1.5 cm) than the classic Maquet procedure and achieved only 53% good and excellent results. Conversely, emphasizing the importance of at least 2 cm of anteriorization, Schmid[122] found 80% good/very good results at a mean 16-year follow-up. In articles that reported posttraumatic patients separately, successful results were achieved in at least 84%.[30,112] If a localized articular lesion has been identified, care should be taken that the anteriorization will effectively unload the lesion. Heatley et al. presented a modified anteriorization in which anteriorization is typically 1 to 1.5 cm. They presented excellent results in a patient cohort treated for arthroscopically proven chondomalacia.[67] Similarly, Atkinson et al. presented an anteriorization technique using allograft behind a tibial tubercle osteotomy for the treatment of primary patellofemoral arthritis with good results shown.[3] When the use of anteriorization is considered for treatment of anterior knee pain, we believe it is important to recognize that the severity and the pattern of articular degeneration are critical. Distal lateral lesions are probably best suited for relief with this procedure; however, many successes have been reported in the literature with other lesions. Nonetheless, patients and surgeons must realize that this is generally a salvage procedure, and function is rarely truly normal after the procedure. Patients must also understand that the tubercle appears prominent after surgery and is usually uncomfortable when kneeling. It is wise preoperatively to show patients photographs of knees after anteriorization to avoid cosmetic dissatisfaction postoperatively.

Anteromedialization. Although anteriorization procedures have at times included medialization to control subluxation or recurrent dislocation, several procedures that routinely combine some degree of anteromedialization have been designed for patients with malalignment. Laboratory evaluation of this concept in a cadaver model with increased lateral facet overload induced by alteration of the proximal vector of the quadriceps showed excellent reduction of lateral facet pressure.[47] This study reported a 30% reduction in lateral facet pressure with anteriorization of 8.8 mm and medialization of 8.4 mm, and 65% relief after additional anteromedialization to 14.8/8.4 mm. By 20 to 30 degrees of knee flexion, reduction and equalization of medial and lateral facet pressure were noted, with greater reduction in the more anteriorized group. When compared with previous studies of tubercle anteriorization, a similar slight proximal shift in contact area occurred, although no significant undesirable decrease in area was observed, as occurred with some previous laboratory evaluations of anterior tubercle transfer.[79,94] Other more recent biomechanical studies have confirmed that anteromedialization profoundly alters the biomechanical environment of the patellofemoral joint. In a sophisticated biomechanical study, Cole and colleagues performed a complex evaluation of the patellofemoral joint using electroresistive sensors and determined that anteromedial tibial tubercle osteotomy decreased the total contact pressure of the patellofemoral joint while unloading the lateral trochlea and shifting contact pressures medially.[7] Similarly, Saranathan et al. used force sensors placed within the patellofemoral joint to evaluate the effects of anteromedialization. They found that medial joint pressures increased slightly while substantially reducing the pressure applied to the lateral patellar and trochlear cartilage.[121]

Clinical experience. Anteromedialization of the tibial tuberosity via an oblique osteotomy was introduced by John Fulkerson in 1983 (Fig. 66.13). This procedure allows variable anterior and medial displacement of the tubercle with rigid fixation and early motion, while maintaining a broad cancellous surface for primary bone healing.[42] The results of this procedure on 30 knees with patellofemoral pain, moderate articular degeneration, and clinical malalignment indicate good or excellent subjective results in 93%.[47] Objectively, 89% good or excellent results were documented, and 12 patients monitored for longer than 5 years showed no deterioration with time. Mean anteriorization was 10.6 mm. Even 75% of eight patients with advanced deterioration (Outerbridge grades III to IV) had good results, although excellent results were not achieved in this

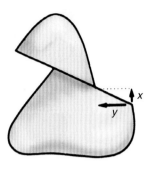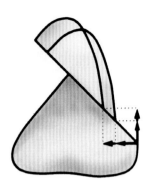

FIG 66.13 An oblique osteotomy allows anterior and medial displacement of the tibial tuberosity without a bone graft. A steeper osteotomy plane will produce increased anteriorization, along with medialization. (From Fulkerson JP: Anteromedialization of the tibial tuberosity for patellofemoral malalignment. Clin Orthop Relat Res 177:176, 1983.)

group. Morshuis et al.[91] described a series of 25 similar osteotomies and reported 84% good and excellent short-term results. Anteriorization was less than 10 mm, and the best results were achieved in patients with mild articular degeneration. Bellemans et al.[8] found consistent clinical improvement and correction of preoperative radiographic pathologic tilt and subluxation in 29 patients after anteromedialization by Fulkerson's technique. One noteworthy procedural modification was the omission of lateral release in 14 patients with CT-documented normal tilt angles preoperatively.

Pidoriano et al.[105] studied the correlation between the pattern of articular degeneration and the result of anteromedialization and confirmed the theoretical and laboratory findings that distal and lateral lesions should respond best to anteromedialization. Distal lesions and lateral facet lesions, of varying severity, correlated with 87% good to excellent functional results (Fig. 66.14). Conversely, medial facet lesions had just 55% good to excellent functional results. Eight percent of patients with diffuse or proximal patellar lesions did poorly. Patients with severe central trochlear lesions also did poorly. It is interesting to note that the location of the articular lesion correlated much better with the result than did the absolute degree of articular degeneration, as described by the Outerbridge classification, despite the fact that 28 of 36 patients in the series had grade III or IV articular cartilage degeneration. As predicted by patellofemoral mechanics, the location of the lesion is critical in selecting patients for anteromedialization.

In a later review, Buuck and Fulkerson established effective long-term success of the anteromedial tibial tubercle transfer procedure in a 4- to 12-year follow-up study.[15] Other techniques of anteromedialization have also been studied. Combined rotation and elevation of the tibial tuberosity with lateral release was reported in 1986 by Miller and LaRochelle.[90] This technique, which uses a wedge-shaped graft rotated medially and fixed with a cortical lag screw, raises the tuberosity 9 to 11 mm and is probably less stable than the technique described by Fulkerson. Casts were maintained for 4 to 5 weeks postoperatively. Indications for surgery were refractory patellofemoral pain with normal or increased Q angles. Fifty-five percent of patients had a positive apprehension sign. Pain was decreased in 86% of 38 patients postoperatively, and no patient had residual patellar

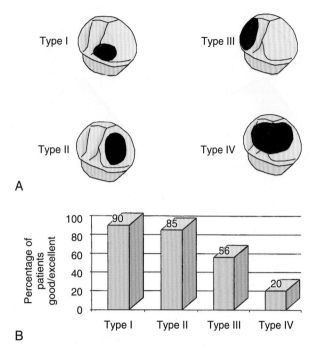

A

B

FIG 66.14 (A) Classification of the location of patellar chondral lesions. (B) Correlation of good/excellent results after antero-medialization with location of the chondral lesion. (From Pidoriano AJ, Weinstein RN: Correlation of patellar articular lesions with results from anteromedial tibial tubercle transfer. Am J Sports Med 25:533, 1997.)

instability. Another potential problem with this method could be proximal shingle fracture caused by lack of support under the most proximal tip of the shingle.[111] Noll et al.[98] reported a 1.25-cm elevation with transposition of the tubercle straight medially onto a tapered bony bed with fixation by a cancellous screw, thereby avoiding the need for bone grafting. Three weeks of cast immobilization followed. Patients had a variety of diagnoses, primarily patellofemoral pain with an increased Q angle, but no patellar instability. Good to excellent relief was attained in 12 of 14 patients.

In an alternative patient population, tibial tubercle transfer and anteromedialization proved to be reliable treatments for recurrent patellar instability with pre-disposing lateralization of the patella. In patients with a high TT-TG distance, large Q angle, and recurrent patella dislocations, many authors have reported excellent clinical results. A research group directed by Wymenga et al. reported excellent results at both 2-year and 10-year follow-up for patients who had tibial tubercle transfer for recurrent patellar instability.[73,136] Porteous et al. reported 79% good or excellent results four years after tibial tubercle transfer and 63% good or excellent results 10 years after the index surgical procedure.[96] In the high-intensity athletic population with patellar instability, Bradley and colleagues reported only one recurrence of instability in a patient cohort of 41 athletes who underwent anteromedialization.[137]

In summary, although these series of distal realignment procedures differ in specific details, the results are generally very good. If the clinician exhausts nonoperative treatment, documents preoperative malalignment sand instability, reserves anteromedialization for patients with distal and lateral facet

lesions, and avoids technical pitfalls, patient satisfaction is very high.

Complications of Distal Realignment. Upon review of the combined findings of six separate reports, potentially disastrous skin necrosis over the tibial tubercle was noted in 8.8% of 182 reported cases treated by a Maquet procedure with advancement of more than 2 cm.[63,85,88,111] In contrast, skin necrosis, to our knowledge, has not been reported with lesser advancements and has not been reported or seen by the authors after antero-medial tibial tubercle transfer. Other serious complications, including acute or stress fractures of the bony shingle, deep venous thrombosis, arthrofibrosis, and compartment syndrome, are less common but can occur. Acute fracture of the proximal end of the tibia was reported in 6 of 234 patients who were encouraged to initiate immediate full weight bearing after anteromedialization; accordingly, patients should be gradually advanced to full weight bearing after about 6 weeks, with some radiographic evidence of consolidation of the tibial shingle.[133] In addition, clinicians who reported proximal tibial fractures recommended tapering the osteotomy and leaving the distal portion intact if possible. Creating a step cut for the distal tubercle was associated with an increase in fractures at the proximal tibia.[36,82] Compartment syndrome occurred in 12 cases after the Hauser procedure,[145] but this procedure is no longer recommended. Emphasis has been placed on strict technique to avoid many of these complications, and indeed, several series have documented a decreased rate of complications as their experience with this procedure increased.[111,114] Radin and Labosky wrote an important article on methods used to minimize complications associated with the Maquet procedure; clinicians planning this procedure would be well advised to study it.[113] A comprehensive review noted that the risk of serious complications was 3% with more modern tibial tubercle transfer techniques. The authors noted that osteotomies requiring a complete detachment of the tuberosity had a higher rate of complications.[102] Special care should be taken in patients with multiple scars from previous surgery. Avoidance of complications entails careful handling of skin edges, techniques to minimize skin tension, postoperative use of suction drains, and early motion whenever possible. Before proceeding with tibial tubercle transfers, clinicians should not only review techniques in detail, but also "complication avoidance" reviews, which provide a wealth of hard-earned knowledge.[46,59]

Fulkerson's Technique of Anteromedialization. After arthroscopic confirmation of the preoperative diagnosis and examination of the medial and lateral joint compartments for associated disease, a straight incision, slightly lateral of midline, is made just lateral to the patellar tendon and tibial crest to a point approximately 5 cm distal to the tibial tuberosity (Fig. 66.15A). It is desirable to make this incision in such a way that a later midline or paramidline incision is possible if arthroplasty or further surgery becomes necessary. Lateral retinacular release or lengthening of the lateral patellofemoral ligaments (patello-tibial and epicondylopatellar bands), synovium, and vastus lateralis obliquus is almost always performed (either arthroscopic or open).[56] Proximally, the main tendon of the vastus lateralis is protected. Care is taken distally to avoid injury to the lateral meniscus, which is at the inferior extent of the release. If the release is adequate, 90 degrees of patellar eversion should be possible to allow direct examination and palpation of articular

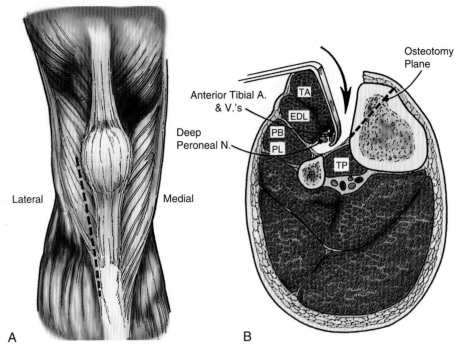

Lateral   Medial

A   B

FIG 66.15 (A) The *dotted line* indicates the suggested skin incision. (The surgeon must consider previous surgical scars and must modify the incision to prevent skin complications.) (B) Plane of dissection. Note the potentially vulnerable position of the neurovascular bundle. During tibial drilling and osteotomy, these structures must be protected. (From Scott WN: The knee, vol 1, St Louis, 1994, Mosby-Year Book, p 458.)

surfaces. Careful observation of the pattern and degree of articular changes and correlation with the patient's symptoms and preoperative evaluation are important in deciding the need for lateral release versus anteromedialization if the patient has an isolated tilt, or in deciding the degree of anteriorization appropriate for those undergoing anteromedial transfer.

Next, the musculature of the anterior compartment is sharply released from the tibial crest and is elevated atraumatically in a posterior direction to expose the posterolateral corner of the proximal end of the tibia. The anterior tibial artery and the peroneal nerve are at this level (Fig. 66.15B) and must be protected. The medial and lateral borders of the patellar tendon are then defined, with particular care taken to delineate the entire insertion into the tibial tuberosity (Fig. 66.16). Next, a longitudinal incision is made just medial to the tibial crest along the planned osteotomy (closer to the crest for a steeper osteotomy). The osteotomy plane is also tapered anteriorly at its distal extent to create a proximally based pie shape on the medial surface of the tibial narrowing down to a 2- to 3-mm apex 5 to 7 cm distal to the tuberosity (see Fig. 66.16). The periosteum is carefully elevated from the line of the planned osteotomy. Although exquisite care is taken to have the posterolateral aspect of the tibia under direct vision at all times, a series of 4.0-mm drill bits may be placed parallel with use of the Hoffmann drill guide or a similar device in a plane from the anteromedial toward the posterolateral aspect of the tibia. Each drill bit should be carefully observed as it penetrates the lateral cortex to avoid injury to the anterior tibial vessels and peroneal nerve. Maintaining bicortical drill bits in the most superior and inferior positions along the drill guide helps place the remaining parallel drill holes accurately, but these bits must be checked frequently to prevent inadvertent and potentially dangerous advancement. A lateral osteotomy must then be made from the superior posterior drill hole to an anterior point proximal to the patellar tendon insertion to prevent propagation of the osteotomy into the proximal end of the tibia (Fig. 66.17). The cortical bone anterior and proximal to the tibial tuberosity is cut next with a half-inch osteotome, while care is taken to avoid injury to the tendon (Fig. 66.18). Alternatively, the Tracker AMZ Guide (DePuy Mitek, Raynham, Massachusetts) may be used to design this osteotomy and make the cut. Arthrex (Naples, Florida) also makes a special guide for this procedure.

The main osteotomy is completed with an osteotome or a saw, while the superior and inferior drill bits are used as guides to the desired plane (Fig. 66.19). A perfectly flat osteotomy plane is critical to the ultimate apposition of the broad flat cancellous surfaces and the stability of fixation. Once the osteotomy is complete, the bone pedicle is hinged distally and is pushed up the inclined plane. Patellar tracking is then observed, and the optimal amount of medialization is maintained while two countersunk 3.2-mm AO bicortical screws are placed (Fig. 66.20). Special care is exercised when drilling through the posterior cortex. Anteriorization of 12 to 15 mm is routine without a bone graft, although locally available bone (proximal lateral tibial metaphysis) can be used to neutralize the medialization and add anteriorization in selected rare cases. If pure medialization is desired, the osteotomy is simply modified to eliminate the anterior-to-posterior obliquity. The tourniquet is released and meticulous hemostasis ensured before placement of a suction drain and closure of the subcutaneous and skin layers.

Postoperative care. A cooling device is placed over light bandages in the operating room to apply continuous

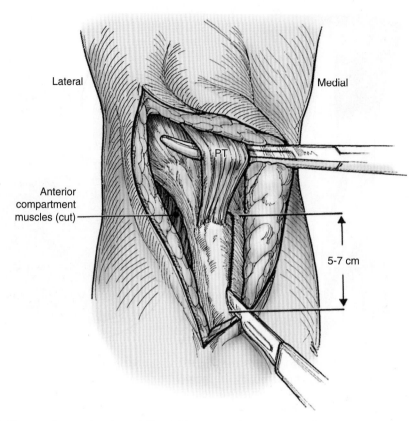

FIG 66.16 The patellar tendon is mobilized. The osteotomy plane is planned. (From Scott WN: The knee, vol 1, St Louis, 1994, Mosby-Year Book, p 459.)

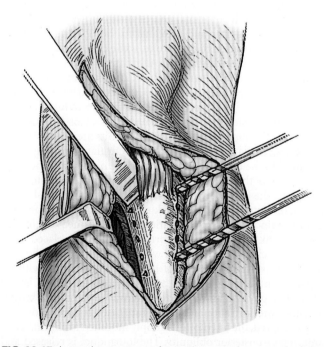

FIG 66.17 Lateral osteotomy frees the superior aspect of the tibial tubercle shingle and prevents propagation of the osteotomy into the proximal end of the tibia. (From Scott WN: The knee, vol 1, St Louis, 1994, Mosby-Year Book, p 460.)

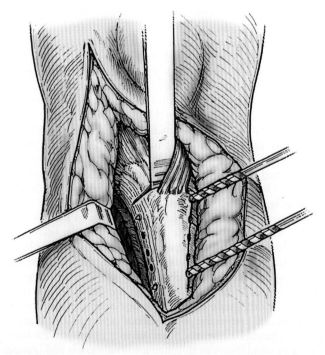

FIG 66.18 Completion of the superior aspect of the osteotomy. (From Scott WN: The knee, vol 1, St Louis, 1994, Mosby-Year Book, p 460.)

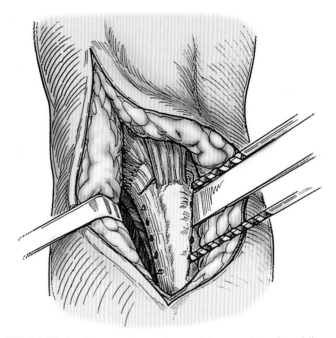

FIG 66.19 A wide osteotome is used to complete the oblique osteotomy along the plane defined by the drill bits previously placed with the parallel drill guide. Care should be taken to make sure that the osteotomy plane is completely flat to ensure good bony apposition. (From Scott WN: The knee, vol 1, St Louis, 1994, Mosby-Year Book, p 460.)

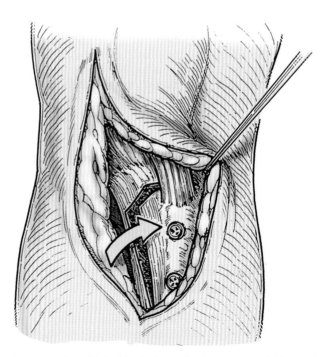

FIG 66.20 The tibial shingle is pushed anteromedially up the inclined plane and is rigidly fixed with two bicortical large-fragment AO cortical lag screws. (From Scott WN: The knee, vol 1, St Louis, 1994, Mosby-Year Book, p 460.)

cryotherapy and gentle compression. Drains, if used, are usually removed in the recovery room or within approximately 24 hours when the drainage diminishes. Quadriceps-setting exercises are encouraged on the day of surgery, and with the assumption of secure fixation of the shingle, early active and gentle passive motion is begun the next day. Touch-down weight bearing is allowed with crutches and a knee immobilizer. At 6 weeks, quadriceps strength is improving, bony union has generally occurred, and crutches can be discontinued, usually with the help of a physical therapist, when the patient can perform a single-leg knee bend without support on the operated side. Full recovery for activities of daily living is generally achieved between 3 and 4 months, but running and vigorous activity should be delayed until 6 to 8 months from the time of surgery to maximize bony recovery. Comprehensive reviews and rehabilitation plans are available.[117]

OUR RECOMMENDED TREATMENT APPROACH

Patellofemoral Malalignment

Patients with patellofemoral pain who have failed nonoperative management may have various degrees of articular pain, soft tissue pain, and instability. Preoperative history and physical examination findings, supplemented by radiographs, and when necessary, advanced imaging (CT, bone scan, SPECT scan, MRI), are used to assess the degree of articular degeneration and the degree of tilt and subluxation. An appropriate procedure can then be selected to address all components of the problem.

Tilt. Recognized on physical examination and confirmed by x-ray film or more reliably by MRI, tilt, when isolated (no lateral subluxation or significant articular degeneration), can result in disabling soft tissue pain. A tight contracted lateral retinaculum draws the patella into increasing lateral tilt with knee flexion as a result of progressive posterior displacement of the iliotibial band (to which a strong portion of the retinaculum is anchored). Soft tissue pain can result from neuromatous degeneration in the lateral retinaculum under these conditions, or from tension overload in the medial tissues. Excessive pressure on the articular surface of the lateral facet is possible and may conceivably result in progressive degeneration if not corrected in a symptomatic patient. Patients with pure tilt probably represent a subgroup of those labeled as having "chondromalacia" without subluxation in many series. Nonoperative management includes quadriceps strengthening, stretching of the tight lateral retinaculum and iliotibial band, McConnell taping, and bracing, and may be supplemented by nonsteroidal anti-inflammatory medication. With proper and thorough nonoperative treatment, lateral release is not often necessary. In the unusual situation where pain persists and is focal to the lateral retinaculum, lateral release is our procedure of choice in this situation when surgery is necessary and has resulted in 92% excellent or good results in patients with CT-documented tilt and mild cartilage degeneration (Outerbridge grade II chondromalacia or less).[125] CT evaluation of tilt in patients with preoperative tilt and no lateral facet collapse showed consistent improvement to within the normal range 3 to 4 months after lateral release.[49] Medial imbrication has not been necessary to achieve this correction. MRI imaging can provide detailed information about the status of the articular cartilage on both the lateral trochlea and the lateral patellar facet. When lateral patellar tilt is present with significant lateral facet arthrosis, anteromedialization with lateral release is a more dependable procedure than lateral release alone.

Lateral Translation (Subluxation) and Tilt Without Severe Chondral Damage. Patients whose knees fall into this category based on the history, physical examination findings, and radiographic studies respond less consistently to lateral release alone after failure of conservative care. Coronal malalignment related to the quadriceps vector and tibial tubercle position is not consistently improved by lateral release, as noted by unchanged postoperative Q angles[75] and by unchanged CT scans.[49] Medialization of the tibial tubercle helps decrease the Q angle, thus reducing the laterally directed component of the extensor force, which has been shown to contribute significantly to patellar subluxation. Thus, straight medialization of the tibial tubercle in conjunction with lateral release should be the appropriate procedure in the absence of significant articular damage. We have not found imbrication of the VMO to be routinely necessary.[139] This may be a clinical reflection of the findings of Mariani and Caruso,[86] who found electromyographic evidence of improved VMO function after lateral release and distal realignment.

When chronic lateral translation of the patella is seen radiographically, we do not believe MPFL reconstruction or medial imbrication alone should be used to pull the patella back into the trochlea. Such attempts at realignment by increasing medial soft tissue tension can produce increased medial facet pressure and increased patellofemoral pain. In cases of radiographically clear lateral translation on patellar axial films and/or CT and MRI scans, distal realignment is usually needed. In select patients with a discrete history of ongoing recurrent traumatic instability episodes, a procedure that includes restoration of medial ligament integrity is combined with distal realignment.

Lateral Translation (Subluxation) and Tilt With More Severe Chondral Damage or Arthrosis. In this situation, one must consider adding pressure relief to the procedure by including anteriorization to the lateral release and tuberosity medialization. In making this decision, one should recall the characteristic proximal and medial load transfer of anteromedialization in cadaver models and should not transfer increased loads onto damaged proximal articular surfaces. One must also remember that progressive elevation of the tubercle brings increasing relief of force but also increases the risk for complications. Anteriorization of up to 17 mm may be attained by using Fulkerson's technique of anteromedialization without the addition of an iliac graft. Advantages of the oblique osteotomy as described by Fulkerson over other techniques with similar goals include a broad flat surface for cancellous healing, rigid internal fixation allowing immediate motion, early functional recovery, and avoidance of skin complications.

In recent years the development of new invasive treatments for articular cartilage lesions has led to renewed interest in unloading the lateral portion of the patellofemoral joint because this is an area that commonly suffers articular cartilage damage. Anteromedialization has proven to be an invaluable adjunct when paired with autologous chondrocyte implantation (ACI).[53] Gallo and Feeley noted that tibial tubercle osteotomy was an important and successful adjunct for ACI and

allograft procedures in the femoral trochlea.[52] For all current articular cartilage restoration procedures (microfracture, ACI, osteochondral autograft, and osteochondral allograft transfer) tibial tubercle transfer is an invaluable method for appropriately offloading areas of cartilage concern, thereby allowing an increased chance of success. Trinh et al. noted, in a comprehensive review, that outcomes were improved if ACI was paired with tubercle osteotomy.[141] Yanke et al. had similar reports about the value of an unloading osteotomy.[148]

Lateral Translation (Subluxation). Without articular changes greater than Outerbridge grades I to II and in the absence of tilt, medialization is the primary goal. As noted earlier, a medial procedure is recommended to avoid pulling the patella into the trochlea. Patients with static lateral translation without tilt often seem to have some degree of systemic hypermobility. In such cases, careful evaluation by CT or MRI scan for evidence of skeletal dysplasia (excessive hip anteversion, trochlear dysplasia, lateralization of the tuberosity, external tibial torsion) is very important. Soft tissue tightening or lateral release in such cases, which include hypermobility, must be done cautiously to avoid iatrogenic medial instability. Most often in such cases, we would not include lateral release, but if the lateral retinaculum was tight intraoperatively, lateral lengthening would be preferred over release.

When necessary in a *skeletally mature* individual with severe subluxation, our preferred method is a Trillat-type procedure with medial rotation of a flat osteotomy, rigid fixation, and concomitant lateral release supplemented by MPFL advancement. Avoidance of posterior transposition of the tubercle is imperative to avoid increasing patellofemoral joint contact forces and the resultant high risk for osteoarthrosis.

Patella Alta With or Without Patellar Instability. Fortunately, distal transfer of the tuberosity occurs with any distally based rotation of a shingle, whether the rotation is straight medial, anterior, or somewhere in between. With a longer tibial shingle, less distal displacement occurs. Thus, the degree of patella alta that is present can be a consideration in selecting the length of the tibial shingle. In patients with severe patella alta in the setting of patellar instability, one may want to be certain that the tubercle osteotomy allows adequate distal transfer for correction. Patella alta is not to be overlooked when considering tibial tubercle osteotomy for the treatment of patellar instability. A review of patients who had recurrent instability after an anteromedialization procedure noted postoperative patellar instability correlated with uncorrected preoperative patella alta.[142] A review of five studies of patients with patella alta and patella instability noted that tibial tubercle transfer, when it included distalization, could normalize patellar height ratios while preventing recurrent dislocations.[84]

Medial Patellofemoral Ligament Reconstruction Without Tibial Tubercle Transfer

Suffice it to say for the purposes of this chapter that isolated MPFL reconstruction by imbrication, advancement, or tendon graft reconstruction should be reserved for patients who have an otherwise balanced extensor mechanism. MPFL reconstruction should not be used to displace the structural tracking vector of the extensor mechanism, because this is likely to seriously alter articular pressures and increase the likelihood of failure.

SUMMARY

Most patients with patellofemoral disorders do not require surgery. Careful attention to the basics of restoring strength and flexibility and of correcting instigating factors in the patient's history is often all it takes to treat these problems successfully. When surgery is necessary, meticulous history and physical examination are invaluable. Diagnoses of malalignment should be documented radiographically before surgical realignment. The clinician should be patient during rehabilitation of deconditioned patients after patellofemoral surgery. As long as the clinician is careful to precisely define the indications for patellofemoral surgery, accurately perform the surgery, and patiently rehabilitate the patient, successful results are probable in most cases.

KEY REFERENCES

7. Beck PR, Thomas AL, Farr J, et al: Trochlear contact pressures after anteromedialization of the tibial tubercle. *Am J Sports Med* 33:1710–1715, 2005.

15. Buuck D, Fulkerson J: Anteromedialization of the tibial tubercle: a 4-12 year follow-up. *Oper Tech Sports Med* 8:131, 2000.

33. Dye SF: The pathophysiology of patellofemoral pain: a tissue homeostasis perspective. *Clin Orthop Relat Res* 436:100–110, 2005.

35. Dye SF, Vaupel GL, Dye CC: Conscious neurosensory mapping of the internal structures of the human knee without intraarticular anesthesia. *Am J Sports Med* 26:773–777, 1998.

37. Engebretsen L, Svenningsen S, Benum P: Advancement of the tibial tuberosity for patellar pain: a 5-year follow-up. *Acta Orthop Scand* 60:20–22, 1989.

45. Fulkerson JP: Diagnosis and treatment of patients with patellofemoral pain. *Am J Sports Med* 30:447–456, 2002.

47. Fulkerson JP, Becker GJ, Meaney JA, et al: Anteromedial tibial tubercle transfer without bone graft. *Am J Sports Med* 18:490–496, discussion 496–497, 1990.

25. Dejour H, Walch G, Nove-Josserand L, et al: Factors of patellar instability: an anatomic radiographic study. *Knee Surg Sports Traumatol Arthrosc* 2:19–26, 1994.

49. Fulkerson JP, Schutzer SF, Ramsby GR, et al: Computerized tomography of the patellofemoral joint before and after lateral release or realignment. *Arthroscopy* 3:19–24, 1987.

106. Post W: History and physical examination of patients with patellofemoral disorders. In Fulkerson J, editor: *Disorders of the patellofemoral joint*, Baltimore, 1997, Williams & Wilkins.

108. Post WR: Anterior knee pain: diagnosis and treatment. *J Am Acad Orthop Surg* 13:534–543, 2005.

127. Sherman SL, Plackis AC, Nuelle CW: Patellofemoral anatomy and biomechanics. *Clin Sports Med* 33:389–401, 2014.

The references for this chapter can also be found on www.expertconsult.com.

67

Surgery of the Patellofemoral Joint: Proximal Realignment

Andrew B. Old, Andre M. Jakoi, W. Norman Scott, Giles R. Scuderi, Gabriel Levi

INTRODUCTION

Disorders of the patellofemoral joint are numerous and of great importance because they seriously limit patients' function in generally young and active patients.[59,61,101] Successful treatment of these conditions is highly dependent on an accurate diagnosis and determination of the correct pathology.[65] Within the spectrum of disorders of the patellofemoral joint, one of the more common is patellar instability. Instability is the topic of multiple studies and reviews,[31,76,100,109] a commentary on not only how common it is but also on the continued debate of how best to diagnose and treat it. Instability can present with a variety of symptoms that mimic other pathology of the knee, such as pain, mechanical "clicking," feelings that the knee is unstable or "gives out," weakness, and limited range of motion. We begin with a review of the presentation and pathophysiology of patellofemoral disorders, including patellofemoral instability. We then review physical examination of the patellofemoral joint, imaging modalities and the surgical technique of proximal realignment.[93] The techniques of patellofemoral arthroplasty, trochleoplasty, and distal patellar realignment (including medial patellofemoral ligament [MPFL] reconstruction) are beyond the scope of this chapter and are discussed elsewhere in the text.

Pathophysiology of Patellar Instability

The stability of the patellofemoral joint is dependent on many factors. Specifically, it depends on the congruence of the femoral trochlea and patella, as well as both static and dynamic stabilizers. Bony and cartilaginous constraint is determined by the shape of the trochlea and patella, which can be extremely variable. For example, a hypoplastic lateral condyle or a shallow trochlea can predispose to acute patellar dislocation after trauma or can lead to chronic subluxation and dislocation. Yamada et al.[141] used magnetic resonance (MR)-derived computer models to map out the three-dimensional morphology of the femoral trochlea in recurrent dislocators versus controls. They looked at 12 knees of recurrent dislocators and compared them with 10 controls. The models were able to analyze the shape of the articular surface, convexity of the surface, and proximal and mediolateral distribution of articular cartilage. They found a mean convexity of 24.9 degrees for instability patients and 11.9 degrees for controls ($p < 0.001$). The mean height of the articular cartilage was 91.3 degrees for the patients and 83.3 degrees for the control group ($p = 0.03$). This showed

that patients with recurrent patella dislocations have differences in the shape and distribution of cartilage when compared with normal, asymptomatic people.

In addition to bony and cartilaginous constraints are the static ligamentous constraints. The MPFL has been shown to be the primary static stabilizer for lateral translation of the patella.[32,42,43,113] Baldwin et al.[13] showed the MPFL to be present in all 50 of their fresh frozen specimens. It was a discrete structure that has two origins on the femur, the sulcus between the medial epicondyle and the adductor tubercle, and the superficial medial collateral ligament. The ligament inserts along the ventral edge of the patella.

Finally, and perhaps most importantly, is the quadriceps mechanism. The coordinated contraction of the quadriceps mechanism centralizes the patella in the trochlea throughout range of motion (Fig. 67.1). Among the quadriceps musculature it is the vastus medialis obliquus (VMO) that is the primary dynamic stabilizer of the patellofemoral joint (Fig. 67.2). Dysfunction of the VMO, whether by trauma or by atrophy, may lead to patellar instability. The sum of these factors defines the ultimate stability of the joint. If any single factor or multiple factors are deficient or dysplastic, the remaining structures must compensate. The ability of these factors to collectively stabilize the joint determines the degree of joint stability. In the remainder of this chapter we will describe how the history, physical findings, and radiographic studies are used to determine the relative contribution of each of these factors to the instability of the patellofemoral joint.

Presentation of Patellofemoral Disorders

Patellofemoral disorders and especially instability may present with a variety of symptoms. The history is important in determining the cause of the instability. A patient with instability will often but not always present with a history of trauma. A valgus and external rotational injury is commonly the culprit. First-time dislocators may describe a traumatic event in which the patella dislocates laterally and then self-reduces or is reduced by the patient. Other first-time dislocators feel "their knee pop out of place." Patients often seek treatment in the emergency department (ED) and commonly describe a twisting movement of the knee, combined with a palpable snap as the knee gives way. The patient may report a brief period in which the patella remains dislocated on the lateral aspect of the knee. Often, simple extension of the knee allows the patella to reduce. These events are usually followed by rapid swelling of the knee, which

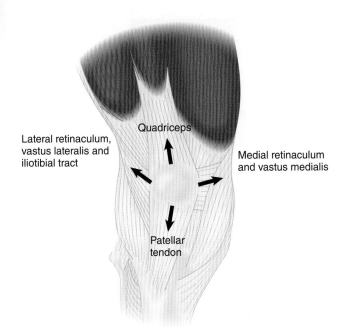

FIG 67.1 The patella is anchored and stabilized to the knee by four structures in a cruciform fashion: the patellar tendon inferiorly, quadriceps tendon superiorly, and retinacula medially and laterally.

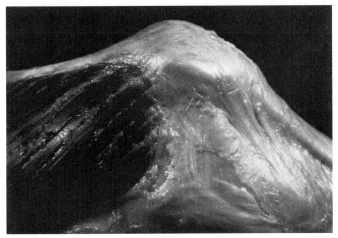

FIG 67.2 The VMO becomes tendinous just a few millimeters proximal to the patella. Because of the oblique direction of its fibers, it is best suited to resist lateral displacement of the patella. The patellotibial ligament is visible as a distinct structure medial to the patellar tendon.

may be the only finding on physical examination because it is rare for the patella to remain dislocated on arrival to the ED.

If the patient has observed abnormal lateral displacement of the patella, the diagnosis is straight forward; otherwise, it can be difficult.[137] The physician is faced with a swollen and tender knee and a nonspecific history of giving way.[135] Aspiration of the joint demonstrates hemarthrosis, and fat droplets may be present if an associated osteochondral fracture has occurred, both of which may be nonspecific findings for patellofemoral dislocation. Careful inquiry into the mechanism of injury often

reveals that the patient was changing direction ("cutting") with the foot planted and the femur internally rotating with respect to the tibia. By definition this increases the quadriceps (Q) angle and directs the pull of the quadriceps laterally. This mechanism has also been described in baseball pitchers.[53] More rarely a direct blow to the medial side of the knee may cause patellar dislocation in a knee with underlying malalignment.

It is rare for a knee to sustain a patella dislocation in the absence of malalignment or dysplasia.[94] In addition, disruption of medial soft tissue restraints, such as the MPFL, is now thought to be almost obligatory.[43,112,113] Concomitant osteochondral injury is common and has a predictable pattern on the medial facet of the patella and the lateral femoral condyle[32,42,108] (Fig. 67.3).

Conlan et al.[32] performed an anatomic study that helped to define the contribution of medial soft tissue structures to lateral restraint of the patella. A lateral displacing force was placed on the patella, and medial structures were sectioned. It was determined that the MPFL is responsible for 53% of static restraint against lateral translation of the patella. In a similar study Hautamaa et al.[57] reported consistent results. After isolating a section of the MPFL, they noted that the force required to displace the patella laterally was reduced by 50%.

Panagiotopoulos et al.[108] confirmed the findings of Conlan et al.[32] and Hautamaa et al.[57] in their cadaveric study. They also found that the MPFL contributes at least 50% of the static medial stability of the patella. Panagiotopoulos emphasized the importance of what he described as "meshing" of the MPFL to the undersurface of the VMO. The MPFL femoral attachment is just anterior to the medial epicondyle, and distally its fibers blend with the undersurface of the VMO as it reaches the superior medial pole of the patella. On account of this meshing, they suggest that the MPFL is pulled taut (shortens) by the contracting VMO, thus pulling the patella medially into the sulcus and working in concert with the dynamic restraint of the VMO in centralizing and stabilizing the patella.[57,108] It is now broadly accepted that the VMO is the primary dynamic restraint and the MPFL is the primary static restraint to lateral displacement of the patella.

Recurrent dislocators often feel catching, locking, or instability. However, many patients with patellar instability do not describe instability on presentation, and for this reason it should be considered in all patients with patellofemoral discomfort and mechanical knee pain. Similar to acute episodes of instability, chronic dislocations or subluxations almost always occur in the setting of dysplasia or misalignment or both. The combined contribution of increased Q angle, valgus alignment of the knee, increased femoral anteversion, and tibial external rotation leads to a lateral force vector on the patella. This results in chronic patellar subluxation and dislocation. The VMO is unable to function at its optimal angle and produces a temporary dynamic destabilizing effect on the patellofemoral joint.

Pain

Patients with patellar complaints typically have an aching pain situated behind the patella, often on the medial side of the joint, and sometimes located posteriorly in the popliteal fossa. The pain is aggravated by activities that require a strong quadriceps contraction, such as squatting, stair climbing, skiing, or riding a bike uphill. Descending stairs requires a strong eccentric quadriceps contraction to proceed to the next step smoothly.

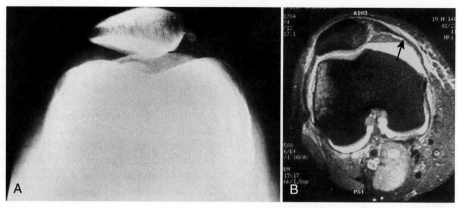

FIG 67.3 Lateral Patellar Dislocation (A) A tangential view of the patella demonstrates an osseous fragment at the medial margin of the patella, consistent with previous lateral patellar dislocation. (B) An axial, fat-suppressed, magnetic resonance image shows a partial tear of the medial patellar retinaculum manifested as increased signal on either side of it *(arrow)*. Signal is increased in the medial aspect of the patella and at the lateral margin of the lateral femoral condyle, indicative of bone contusions, and a large joint effusion is apparent. This constellation of findings is characteristic of a recent lateral patellar dislocation.

This is often more painful than ascending stairs, which requires a concentric quadriceps contraction. Prolonged periods with the knee flexed are usually painful (the movie sign). The reason for this phenomenon is not completely understood but may involve increased tension in the soft tissues or increased compression on the articular surfaces.

Pain may be bilateral, and the onset of symptoms is usually gradual and unrelated to any significant traumatic episode. However, a bout of strenuous activity or a minor injury may seem at times to have initiated the complaint, although questioning generally demonstrates that such events merely served to worsen a preexisting disorder. Bilaterality and insidious onset are most characteristic of patellar pain.

The location of the pain is nonspecific to patellofemoral instability and can therefore mimic other knee pathology; the most common site is the anteromedial side of the knee, which is the same location as pain from a meniscal disorder—this has contributed to inappropriate surgical intervention. Less frequently the patient may experience posterolateral pain, and when local tenderness is noted in this region the diagnosis of bicipital or popliteal tendinitis may be entertained. Popliteal pain is a frequent symptom of patellofemoral arthritis; when an associated popliteal cyst is present, it might be assumed that the cyst is causing the pain, whereas both are secondary to patellar arthritis.

Instability

Instability is the second major symptom of patellar dysfunction. Instability sometimes represents an episode of dislocation or subluxation that can be reproduced upon examination (objective instability), but episodes occasionally occur in patients in whom it is impossible, even under anesthesia, to displace the patella passively from the femoral sulcus (subjective instability). For this reason the boundaries between subjective instability, subluxation, and dislocation should not be too fine because other patients with passively dislocatable patellae will not complain of clinical instability. Instability of patellar origin may mimic the buckling caused by meniscal injury or ligamentous insufficiency, but most often it is a different sensation. Although

instability may occur with pivoting or twisting movements, such as when cutting in sports, the patient is usually aware that it is the kneecap that has slipped. Otherwise, when the patient does not recognize the nature of the buckling, the event is described in such terms as the knee having "collapsed" or "gone forward." There is not the sensation of the joint "coming apart" or of "one bone sliding on the other," which is typical of ligament insufficiency. Episodes of patellar instability may or may not be followed by pain and swelling lasting for a few days to several weeks.

Locking

A grating sensation, particularly when the patellofemoral joint is loaded as in stair climbing or arising from a chair, is a fairly common complaint and sometimes may be audible. It is usually an incidental finding and is rarely of great importance clinically. Momentary "catching" may also be experienced, and interruption of smooth patellar gliding may precipitate buckling or giving way. Actual locking of the knee sometimes happens, and it is curious that patellar locking is not always transient but may give the impression of a true mechanical block. In the case of patellar dislocation, it is not uncommon for a patient to present with an inability to extend the knee.

Swelling

Many patients with patellofemoral disease complain of swelling. This is sometimes a subjective sensation because, on examination, an effusion is not found and circumferential measurement of the joint does not show an increase when compared with the opposite side. Synovitis with distention by synovial fluid or blood occurs after an episode of patellar subluxation and sometimes with chondromalacia or arthritis. Patients with acute patellar dislocations often present with a large hemarthrosis and may require an aspiration prior to physical examination to optimize one's diagnostic abilities. Cartilaginous or osteocartilaginous loose bodies may be generated from the articular surfaces and may contribute to giving way and transient locking, although the patient is usually aware of a free body within the joint that may also be directly felt in the suprapatellar pouch.

In this scenario the aspirate of the joint typically contains fat droplets resulting from disruption of the subchondral bone.

Physical Examination

Thorough examination of the knee, with a focus on the patellofemoral joint, is essential to diagnosing patellofemoral instability or any associated patellofemoral or intra-articular pathology that often accompanies patellofemoral instability. During the physical examination the patient should be examined sequentially while standing, walking, sitting, supine, and prone.

The examination begins with the patient standing with the feet together. Genu varum or valgum can be observed readily, as can rotatory malalignment, such as in-facing or "squinting" of the patellae in patients with an increased Q angle and hip anteversion (Fig. 67.4). Quadriceps tone and development can be appreciated in the standing position or during a half squat. Hypoplasia of the VMO should be noted. The vastus medialis normally inserts on the upper third or half of the medial border of the patella. In knees with patellofemoral dysplasia the muscle belly may end a few centimeters short of the superior patellar margin. The presence of quadriceps atrophy implies decreased dynamic muscle control on the patella.

The position of the foot also deserves attention. Eversion at the subtalar joint is accompanied by compensatory internal tibial torsion, which increases the Q angle and consequently the stress on the patellofemoral joint. The subtalar joint is a single-axis joint that acts like a hinge connecting the talus to the calcaneus. The axis of the subtalar joint deviates an average of 23 degrees medially and anteriorly to the long axis of the foot and

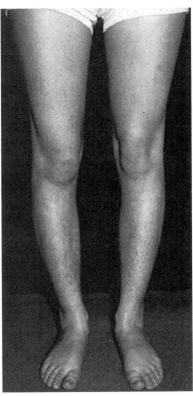

FIG 67.4 Squinting of the Patellae Caused by Rotational Malalignment of the Limb This phenomenon is accompanied by an increase in the Q angle.

41 degrees inferiorly and posteriorly in relation to the horizontal plane. Therefore internal rotation of the leg causes eversion of the heel and depression of the medial side of the foot. External rotation of the leg produces the opposite effect.[29] Subtalar joint eversion may be primary or secondary, as in knees with varus alignment or tibia vara, wherein compensatory subtalar joint eversion is required to produce a plantigrade foot. This phenomenon is probably more important in long-distance runners.[73] Eversion of the heel (heel valgus) is readily appreciated by looking at the patient in the standing position from the back side. Abduction of the forefoot is evaluated in the standing position by palpation of the talar head on the anterior aspect of the ankle. The neutral position is defined when the head of the talus can be equally palpated on the medial and lateral sides. During weight bearing, a normal foot is in mild pronation, and additional pronation should still be possible.[24]

Gait is observed, and if possible the patient is asked to squat and hold the halfway position briefly because pain in this position is usually patellar in origin (half-squat test). Whenever possible, stair climbing and descending should be observed because this activity also provokes patellar symptoms.

With the patient seated on the examining table, the position of the patella is first checked. It normally sinks between the femoral condyles with the knee at 90 degrees of flexion. If patella alta is present, its anterior surface points to the ceiling, with the knee in the same 90-degree position. Active extension is observed, and the presence of patellar crepitus and painful catching, as well as abnormal patellar tracking, is recorded.

Ficat and Hungerford[45] stress the importance of observing the entrance and exit of the patella into and out of the sulcus between 10 and 30 degrees of flexion. They describe four common abnormalities in patellar tracking. Normal patellar tracking is present when the patella glides smoothly into the sulcus, and only minimal lateral displacement may be appreciated in the final extension when the patella exits the trochlear groove. We define more marked lateral displacement as lateralization, whereas greater degrees of pathologic tracking are defined as subluxation or dislocation. This finding is also called the J sign because the path resembles an upside-down J (see video on the website). Furthermore, evaluation of the tilt of the patella should be attempted. In normal knees the medial border of the patella should be at the same level as the lateral border, with a minor lateral tilt in full extension. It should be noted that most abnormalities in patellar tracking involve lateral displacement and lateral tilt of the patella in extension, which reduces in flexion. Therefore we find it useful to roughly estimate patellar subluxation and tilt during the physical examination (Fig. 67.5) and to verify this later with radiographic axial views or computed tomography (CT). Other abnormalities in patellar tracking, including medial dislocation or subluxation of the patella in flexion (after over-release of the lateral structures and excessive medial displacement of the tibial tuberosity) or lateral dislocation in flexion (as in habitual or permanent dislocation), may be encountered more rarely.

Wilson et al.[139] analyzed patella tracking in subjects with patellofemoral symptoms, while squatting, compared with a control group. Using an optoelectronic motion capture system, they found that patients with patellofemoral pain showed lateral spin (distal pole of the patella rotating laterally) compared with medial patella spin in nonsymptomatic patients. They also showed that, as the knee was flexed, the patella tracked significantly more lateral in subjects with patellofemoral pain, and

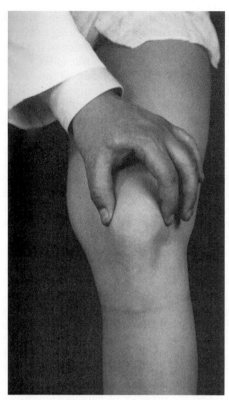

FIG 67.5 Clinical Evaluation of Patellar Tracking The patient is sitting on a firm examining table with the knee flexed at 90 degrees. The examiner places his hand on the knee so that the medial and lateral borders of the patella are palpated with the index finger and thumb. The patient is asked to actively extend the knee. An effort is made to detect the presence of lateral subluxation (displacement) or lateral tilt (lateral border of the patella lower than the medial border) during tracking.

unlike the healthy control group, remained laterally displaced instead of tracking to the medial side as the knee reached 90 degrees. Interestingly they did not find any difference between the two groups with respect to patella tilt. This finding is perhaps subtle but may be appreciated on physical exam.

Patellar crepitation is appreciated during active extension and is recorded as absent, mild, moderate, or severe. It should be evaluated in the sitting position and is enhanced by the application of manual resistance on the lower part of the leg. Because crepitation beyond 90 degrees of flexion cannot be evaluated in the sitting position, it is better assessed during a full squat.

Hughston and Walsh[62] described a lateral position of the patella in the flexed knee for which they coined the term *frog-eye* patella. This seems to be associated with patella alta, which can be suspected clinically when the fat pad is unusually prominent. Indeed the fat pad may, on inspection, be mistaken for the patella because it occupies the femoral sulcus with the knee in extension while the patella is situated in the supracondylar pouch.

With the patient supine on the examining table, tenderness around the patella is evaluated systematically. Tenderness, erythema, and swelling in the prepatellar area may be indicative of prepatellar bursitis. Evaluation of tenderness around the patella includes assessment of the medial and lateral retinacula, quadriceps, and patellar tendons, including their insertions. Point tenderness over the medial facet of the patella, as well as the

MPFL insertion onto the femur on the medial femoral condyle, may point to patella instability. Joint line tenderness should also be evaluated. Tenderness is usually evoked easily in the setting of an acute dislocation and may be most prominent with palpation of the medial retinaculum and medial femoral epicondyle. Ahmad et al.[6] advocated for a modified apprehension test, known as the moving patella apprehension test (MPAT), secondary to concerns that the original test is not sensitive enough. Savallay et al. reported that only 39% of patients had a positive apprehension test.[112] The MPAT is performed in two phases. In phase one the knee is taken from full extension with a laterally directed force on the patella. Pain or subjective apprehension causing the patient to fire their quadriceps to prevent the knee from flexing is considered positive. The second part of the test brings the leg back into full extension, but this time with the examiner's index finger pushing a medially directed force on the patella. If the patient has relief of the pain or sense of instability, then the second part of the test is deemed positive. Both parts of the test must be positive for the MPAT to be considered positive. When compared with a test under anesthesia, Ahmad reported a sensitivity of 100% and a specificity of 88.4%. The positive predicitve value (PPV) was 89.2%, and the negative predictive value (NPV) was 100%.

Testing for ligamentous stability is rendered more difficult by muscle contracture, but with some patience, one should be able to confirm the presence of an intact anterior cruciate ligament with a gentle Lachman test.

The differential diagnosis while examining the knee should include anterior cruciate ligament injury or rupture of the quadriceps or patellar tendon. The latter diagnosis can be excluded by asking the patient to perform a straight-leg raise. If the patient is unable to do this exercise and a defect that is proximal or distal to the patella is appreciated, the diagnosis is confirmed.

Quadriceps Angle. The Q angle is measured by drawing an imaginary line connecting the center of the patella and the anterior superior iliac spine to produce a surface marking that approximates the line of pull of the quadriceps tendon (Fig. 67.6). A second line drawn from the center of the patella to the center of the tibial tubercle indicates the direction of the patellar tendon. The intersection of these two imaginary lines forms the Q angle. Because this measurement is affected by rotation of the hip, an effort is made to note the position of the medial border of the patient's foot during walking and to reproduce this position during measurement.

Active pronation or supination of the foot should be avoided because, as mentioned earlier, these movements are associated with internal and external rotation of the leg, respectively,[106] and consequently increase and decrease the Q angle.

Aglietti et al. measured the Q angle in 150 normal subjects and found it to be 15 degrees (range: 6 to 27 degrees; standard deviation [SD]: 3 degrees) (Table 67.1).[3] It was lower in men (14 degrees; SD: 3 degrees) than in women (17 degrees; SD: 3 degrees), and the difference was significant ($p = 0.001$). Only 11 subjects, all women, had Q angles greater than 20 degrees (7%). Therefore it seems that a Q angle greater than 20 degrees may reasonably be considered abnormal. The Q angle was also measured in a group of pathologic knees, including 53 patients with patellar pain and 37 with recurrent subluxation or dislocation. In the knees with patellar pain the Q angle was significantly increased to 20 degrees; this was true for both men and women.

In contrast, the Q angle was not significantly different from normal in knees with recurrent subluxation or dislocation (average: 15 degrees), and the same applied to both men and women. In patients with patellar subluxation or dislocation, the Q angle is usually underestimated for at least two reasons: first, the patella is displaced laterally in extension; second, the quadriceps tendon frequently lies more lateral than predicted when the superior iliac spine is used as the surface marking (Fig. 67.7).

To overcome the problem of lateral patellar displacement and consequent underestimation of the Q angle, Fithian et al.[46] measured the Q angle with the knee in 30 degrees of flexion. They simultaneously applied a posteriorly directed force so that the patella symmetrically contacted the trochlea. With this method the Q angle was 12 degrees in control subjects (11.2 degrees in men and 13.4 degrees in women). A significantly higher value was found in a group of knees with patellar dislocation (average: 19.2 degrees). The contralateral knee of patients

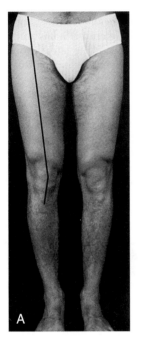
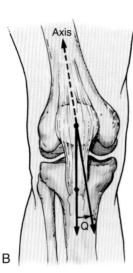

FIG 67.6 The quadriceps angle is measured by drawing two lines from the center of the patella. The first line is drawn up to the anterior superior iliac spine and represents the line of pull of the quadriceps muscle. The second line is drawn down to the tibial tubercle and indicates the line of the patellar tendon.

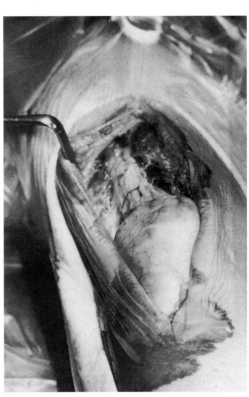

FIG 67.7 The quadriceps tendon often lies more laterally than the surface marking of the Q angle predicts.

TABLE 67.1	**Measurement of Quadriceps Angle and Radiographic Measurements of Patellar Height and Patellofemoral Congruence**					
			CONGRUENCE		**Sulcus Angle,**	
	No. of Subjects	Q Angle, Degree	T/P Ratio[a]	A/B Ratio[b]	Degrees	Angle Degrees
Normal knees[c]	150	15 (3)	1.04 (0.11)	0.95 (0.13)	137 (6)	−8 (6)
Males	75	14	1.01	0.97	137	−6
Females	75	17 ($p < .001$)	1.06 ($p < .05$)	0.94 (NS)	137 (NS)	10 ($p < .001$)
Patella subluxation	37	15 (NS)	1.23 ($p < .001$)	1.08 ($p < .001$)	147 ($p < .001$)	16 ($p < .001$)
Males	16	13 (NS)	1.23 ($p < .001$)	1.07 (NS)	149 ($p < .001$)	15 ($p < .001$)
Females	21	16 (NS)	1.22 ($p < .005$)	1.08 ($p < .001$)	146 ($p < .001$)	17 ($p < .001$)
Patellar pain	53	20 ($p < .001$)	1.08 ($p < .01$)	1.91 (NS)	139 ($p < .01$)	−2 ($p < .001$)
Males	18	20 ($p < .001$)	1.11 ($p < .001$)	0.93 (NS)	140 ($p < .005$)	−1 ($p < .005$)
Females	35	19 ($p < .001$)	1.07 (NS)	0.90 (NS)	139 (NS)	−2 ($p < .001$)

The values of statistical significance reported in normal knees refer to the difference between males and females. The values reported in the pathologic groups (patellar pain and patellar subluxation) refer to the difference from normal knees.
NS, Not significant.
Data from Aglietti P, Insall JN, Cerulli G: Patellar pain and incongruence. I. Measurements of incongruence. *Clin Orthop Relat Res* 176:217, 1983.
[a]T/P ratio: tendon-patella ratio of Insall and Salvati[59] (see text).
[b]A/B ratio: Blackburne and Peel[38] ratio (see text).
[c]Numbers in parentheses indicate standard deviation.

with patellar dislocation also showed an increased value of the Q angle (average: 18.4 degrees).

It is debated whether the Q angle is better measured in the supine or the standing position. Woodland and Francis[140] measured the Q angle in the supine and standing positions in a large number of normal men[91] and women.[89] Average values in the supine position were 12.7 degrees for men and 15.8 degrees for women. Changing to the standing position increased the Q angle 0.9 degree in men and 1.2 in women. The difference was statistically significant but probably is less significant clinically. It is relevant to note that the values determined by Woodland and Francis[140] are close to those detected by Aglietti et al.[3]

It has been suggested that the Q angle should be measured at 30 degrees of knee flexion and with maximum external tibial rotation[127] because this position would give a more reliable measurement of the maximal valgus vector imposed on the patella. However, the difficulty involved in achieving standardized knee flexion and hip rotation makes the reproducibility of this measurement less reliable. We recommend measurement of the tubercle-sulcus angle (TSA), as described by Kolowich et al.[77] The TSA is measured with the knee at 90 degrees of flexion (Fig. 67.8). This allows the patella to engage in the sulcus and highlights any rotational abnormalities. It is defined as the angle formed by a line perpendicular to the transepicondylar axis and a line from the tibial tubercle to the center of the patella. The normal value for the TSA is 0 degrees, and values greater than 10 degrees are considered pathologic. However, consistent identification of the transepicondylar line is not easy, especially in obese patients.

In the supine position and with the knee in extension, the patient is asked to contract the quadriceps, and upward movement of the patella is noted (lateral pull test). In a normal knee the patella is pulled predominantly upward, with an associated minor lateral displacement. The lateral pull test result is considered abnormal if lateral displacement is excessive.[77]

Patellar mobility should be evaluated with the knee in full extension and at 30 degrees of flexion. With the knee in extension the patella is out of the trochlear groove and may be easily displaced medially and laterally. Gross hypermobility, as seen in patients with patella alta and a dysplastic extensor apparatus, is easily detected in this position. With the knee flexed 20 to 30 degrees, the patella is normally drawn into the trochlear groove and stabilized. Excessive displacement in the lateral direction indicates laxity of the medial retinaculum, or vice versa. In contrast, reduced medial mobility indicates the presence of a tight lateral retinaculum. Kolowich et al.[77] suggested that patellar mobility is best evaluated by dividing the patella into longitudinal quadrants (Fig. 67.9). With the knee at 20 to 30 degrees of flexion, mobility in the medial or lateral direction should not exceed two quadrants. A medial glide of one quadrant or less suggests a tight lateral retinaculum, which may also be investigated by trying to lift the lateral border of the patella with the knee in extension (passive patellar tilt) (Fig. 67.10). If the transverse axis of the patella cannot be elevated beyond the horizontal plane, a tight lateral retinaculum is demonstrated.[77]

Medial and lateral displacement of the patella has been measured with a displacement transducer[46] or axial radiographs.[132] Fithian et al.[46] used a displacement sensor to record motion in the coronal plane with the knees bent at 30 degrees. Forces of 2.5 and 5 lb were applied with a handheld force applicator with a load cell. Under a 5-lb force, medial patellar displacement averaged 9.2 ± 3.5 mm and lateral displacement was 7.7 ± 2.6 mm in a group of 188 normal knees. In a group of 22 patients with symptomatic lateral patellar dislocation, medial displacement at 5 lb was 8.3 ± 4.5 mm and lateral displacement was 11.5 ± 4.7 mm. Using the lateral minus medial displacement index, control knees had an average value of -2.1 ± 2.8 mm. Symptomatic knees had a lateral minus medial

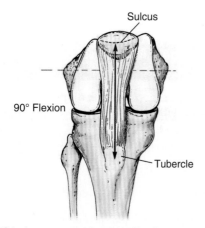

FIG 67.8 TSA is measured with the knee at 90 degrees of flexion. The patella is engaged in the sulcus. The angle is formed by a line perpendicular to the transepicondylar axis and a line form the tibal tubercle to the center of the patella. Normal TSA is 0 degrees and abnormal is greater than 10 degrees. (From Scuderi GR: *The patella*, New York, 1995, Springer-Verlag.)

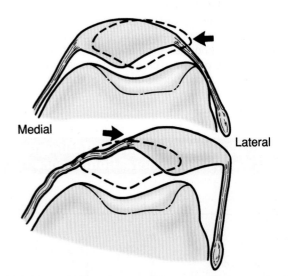

FIG 67.9 The mobility of the patella is best evaluated with the knee flexed to 20 to 30 degrees to engage the patella into the femoral sulcus. Displacement of the patella in the medial or lateral direction is best recorded in quadrants. Displacement in the medial direction of one quadrant or less indicates a tight lateral retinaculum. Displacement in the lateral direction over two quadrants indicates weakened medial stabilizers. (From Kolowich PA, Paulos LE, Rosenberg TD, Farnsworth S: Lateral release of the patella: indications and contraindications. *Am J Sports Med* 18:359, 1990.)

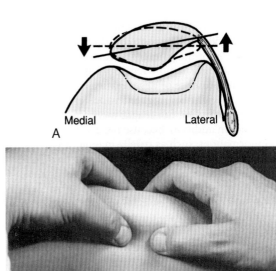

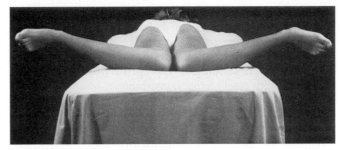

FIG 67.11 Excessive internal rotation of the hips in a patient with recurrent patellar dislocation. Increased femoral neck anteversion is usually present in these cases.

FIG 67.10 (A and B) Passive Patellar Tilt Test In a normal knee in full extension it is possible to lift the transverse axis of the patella beyond the horizontal. An inability to perform this maneuver indicates a tight lateral retinaculum. (From Kolowich PA, Paulos LE, Rosenberg TD, Farnsworth S: Lateral release of the patella: indications and contraindications. *Am J Sports Med* 18:359, 1990.)

displacement of 3.2 ± 3.4 mm. The difference was statistically significant. In summary, total mediolateral displacement of the patella in normal knees under a 5-lb force was close to 17 mm in normal knees and almost 20 mm in knees with patellar instability. The lateral minus medial displacement was useful for differentiating between normal and unstable patellae. Medial displacement was larger than lateral displacement in 81% of control subjects. In unstable patellae, lateral displacement was larger than medial displacement. Asymptomatic knees in patients with unilateral patellar dislocation could not be used as controls because they showed abnormal patellar mobility, similar to symptomatic knees. The authors offered the concept of balance between medial and lateral structures. A normal knee should have greater medial than lateral displacement. If lateral displacement exceeds medial displacement, the restraining structures are unbalanced.

Teitge et al.[132] evaluated medial and lateral patellar mobility with an axial radiograph at 30 to 40 degrees of flexion and a spring-loaded scale to apply a 16-lb force (7.3 kg). In a group of 20 asymptomatic knees, medial displacement averaged 11.1 ± 3.6 mm and lateral displacement was 11.6 ± 8.1 mm. These values are higher than those reported in the study by Fithian et al.,[46] but the displacing force was also greater (16 lb versus 5 lb). In a group of knees with lateral instability, medial displacement was comparable (11.6 mm on average), whereas lateral displacement was highly increased to 21.9 mm on average.

Torsional abnormalities of the femur and tibia have been described as a possible factor leading to patellar pain or instability. The pattern would involve increased femoral neck anteversion so that the trochlear groove faces inward, the Q angle is increased, and the patellae are squinting. Compensatory external tibial torsion is required to produce a foot aligned in the sagittal plane.

Turner and Smillie[134] measured tibial torsion with a tropometer in 836 patients. They found an average lateral tibial torsion of 19 degrees in control knees, which was increased to 24.5 degrees in knees with patellofemoral instability, and to 24 degrees in those with chondromalacia. Because increased tibial rotation was also noted in Osgood-Schlatter disease, this finding does not seem to be specific for patellofemoral joint disorders.

The amount of femoral neck anteversion has often been indirectly estimated by measuring the proportion of internal to external rotation of the hips in extension (Fig. 67.11), which would be its major determinant.[10,129,130] Carson et al.[24] suggested that if internal rotation of the hip in extension exceeds external rotation by more than 30 degrees, femoral neck anteversion is increased. Insall et al.[69] suggested that increased femoral neck anteversion may be present in knees with patellofemoral malalignment. Hvid and Andersen[63] measured the Q angle and internal rotation of the hip in 29 patients with patellofemoral complaints. They found that both the Q angle and internal hip rotation were higher in women than in men. A significant correlation between the Q angle and hip rotation was noted, thus suggesting that the Q angle is in fact increased because of excessive femoral neck anteversion. However, other authors[44] have failed to identify any significant differences in Q angle, genu valgum, and anteversion of the femoral neck between normal adolescents and adolescents or adults with anterior knee pain. They concluded that because those affected by knee pain are also those most interested in sports activities, the probable cause is chronic overloading rather than faulty mechanics.

Dejour et al.[38] reported CT measurements of femoral anteversion and tibial torsion in normal controls and in knees with instability of the patella. They found that femoral neck anteversion was increased in knees with patellofemoral instability (15.6 degrees) as compared with controls (10.8 degrees). Tibial torsion was a less important factor. It was 33 degrees in the control group and 35 degrees in the knees with patellar instability.

In light of the data reported in the literature and our own clinical experience, we think that torsional abnormalities of the lower limb, including femoral neck anteversion and, less significantly, external tibial torsion, may contribute to and play a role in patellofemoral disorders by increasing lateral pull on the patella. However, because these deformities are often less marked and remote from the knee, their importance is minor from therapeutic and surgical points of view.

The ultimate goal, in addition to an accurate diagnosis, is to identify any malalignment, mediolateral restraint imbalance, and patellofemoral articular disease. The history and physical examination, in combination with the correct imaging studies, are essential in developing an appropriate treatment plan for the patient with patellofemoral instability.

Summary of Physical Examination for Patellofemoral Instability

Alignment of the limb is examined in standing and supine positions. Special attention is paid to the Q angle, varus and valgus alignment, and rotation of the limb. Increased Q angle, excessive femoral anteversion, genu valgum, pronation of the foot, and external tibial rotation all lead to excessive lateral force on the patella.

The TSA is measured with the knee at 90 degrees of flexion. The patella is engaged in the sulcus. The angle is formed by a line perpendicular to the transepicondylar axis and a line from the tibial tubercle to the center of the patella. The normal TSA is 0 degrees, and an abnormal TSA measures greater than 10 degrees (see Fig. 67.8).[119]

Atrophy of the quadriceps muscle, especially the VMO, is noted.

Tightness and laxity of the medial and lateral soft tissue restraints are assessed. With the knee flexed to 20 to 30 degrees the patella is displaced medially and laterally. Medial displacement of less than one quarter of the patella, or 5 mm, indicates a tight lateral retinaculum. Lateral displacement of more than three quadrants indicates medial soft tissue incompetence (see Figs. 67.9 and 67.10). Inability to tilt the patella past horizontal is indicative of a tight lateral retinaculum.[77]

A patella apprehension test is performed with the relaxed patient lying supine and the knee flexed to about 20 degrees. The examiner attempts to gently displace the patella laterally. Patients with instability will feel uncomfortable and apprehensive and will inadvertently contract the quadriceps muscle to attempt to stabilize the patella.

Patellar tracking is assessed throughout a range of motion. A J sign,[45] in which the patella is tracking in an inverted J pattern, represents the patella that is tracking centrally and then shifts laterally as the knee is extended (see video on the website). At 90 degrees the patella should be centered between the femoral condyles in a normal patellofemoral joint.

Crepitus in the patellofemoral joint should be noted throughout range of motion. Pain is noted with patellofemoral compression. Tenderness to palpation should be noted with direct palpation of the medial/lateral facets, medial/lateral retinacula, and medial and lateral femoral condyles.

Ligamentous examination of the entire knee, as well as provocative tests for meniscal injury, should be performed.

Radiographic Studies in the Diagnosis and Treatment of Patellofemoral Instability

Standard radiographic evaluation, including anteroposterior, lateral, and axial views, should be obtained in each patient with patellofemoral disorders to assess the height and congruence of the patella and to exclude other bone disorders. CT has been used widely to study the patellofemoral joint because it provides substantially more detail about the bony anatomy. Magnetic resonance imaging (MRI) has also been used to investigate the patellofemoral relationship in extension and early flexion, as well as to detect cartilage lesions and ligamentous injuries.

Radiography

Anteroposterior View. The anteroposterior view does not allow visualization of the patellofemoral joint; however, it does provide valuable information regarding overall alignment of the limb and the presence of degenerative changes in the tibiofemoral joint. Weight-bearing anteroposterior views of the knees, as well as standing full-length mechanical axis views, are recommended. In addition, because the outline of the patella is visible, abnormalities, such as patella magna or parva, bipartite patellae, and fractures, can be seen. Marked lateral subluxation of the patella can also be detected in the anteroposterior view.

Lateral View. The lateral view is taken with the knee in at least 30 degrees of flexion to place the patellar tendon under tension and to demonstrate the functional relationship between the patella and the femur. Excessive rotation should be avoided because it may obscure some of the bony landmarks, such as the tibial tubercle, and may make interpretation difficult. The patella is not visualized on the lateral view in rare cases of congenital absence and when it is completely displaced laterally, as in habitual dislocation. In children younger than 5 years the ossific nucleus has not yet appeared, and thus the patella is nonvisible.

Patellar position is related to the length of the patellar tendon. Patella alta, in particular, is associated with patellar instability, dislocation, and abnormalities of the trochlear groove. Several methods of measurement have been described, including those reported by Blumensaat,[21] Insall and Salvati,[70] Blackburne and Peel,[20] Caton et al.,[26] Rünow,[111] and Grelsamer and Meadows.[51]

Blumensaat line. Blumensaat[21] states that on a lateral radiograph with the knee flexed 30 degrees, the lower pole of the patella should be on a line projected anteriorly from the intercondylar notch (Blumensaat line). It is difficult to obtain routine radiographs with the knee flexed exactly the required number of degrees; this limits the usefulness of the method. The Blumensaat method is also inaccurate. Of 44 radiographs of the knee that were flexed exactly 30 degrees, in no case did the lower pole of the patella lie on Blumensaat line; rather the patella was positioned above this line (Fig. 67.12).

Insall-Salvati method. Insall and Salvati[70] sought a method that would fit the following requirements: (1) simple and practical, as well as accurate; (2) applicable to the range of knee positions used during routine radiography, which in the lateral view is usually 20 to 70 degrees of flexion; and (3) independent of the size of the joint and the degree of magnification of the radiograph. Because the ligamentum patella is not elastic, its length determines the position of the patella, provided that the point of insertion into the tibial tubercle is constant.

Insall and Salvati[70] describe an expression for normal patellar height in terms of the length of the patellar tendon. Measurements were made on 114 knees in which the diagnosis of a torn meniscus had been clearly established by clinical history and examination, by positive arthrographic results, and by the finding of a meniscal tear at arthrotomy. Any case in which the slightest doubt existed was excluded, and it was assumed that the joints examined were structurally normal before a traumatic episode produced a torn meniscus. All patients were adults, and none showed radiologic evidence of osteoarthritis. The following measurements were taken (see Fig. 67.12):

1. T (length of tendon): The length of the patellar tendon was measured on its deep or posterior surface from its origin on

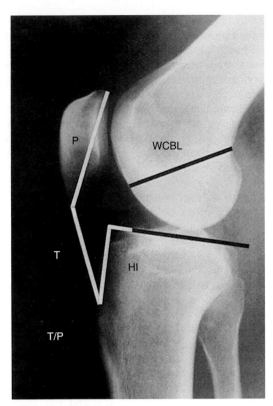

FIG 67.12 Insall-Salvati Measurements to Determine the Height of the Patella *HI,* Height of insertion, or perpendicular distance between the joint line and the insertion of the patellar tendon; *P,* greatest diagonal length of the patella; *T,* length of the tendon measured on its deep posterior surface; *WCBL,* width of the femoral condyles at Blumensaat line. (From Insall JN, Salvati E: Patella position in the normal knee joint. *Radiology* 101:101, 1971.)

the lower pole of the patella to its insertion into the tibial tubercle. The point of insertion is usually represented on the radiograph by a clearly defined notch.

2. P (length of patella): The greatest diagonal length of the patella was measured.

3. WCBL (width of the femoral condyles at Blumensaat line): Both condyles were measured at the level of Blumensaat line, and an average value was obtained. This measurement determined whether great variation in patellar size was present. Patellar size was considered to be acceptably constant.

4. HI (height of insertion): The perpendicular distance from the level of the tibial plateau surface to the point of insertion of the patellar tendon was measured to determine whether a constant relationship could be seen between the level of the tibial tubercle and the tibial plateau. Great variation in tendon insertion would have invalidated the measurements, but the insertion appeared to be acceptably constant. Therefore this measurement may be disregarded in clinical evaluation.

The length of the patellar tendon (T) was found to be approximately equal to patellar length (P), and this was expressed as a ratio (because of variations in the size of individual knee joints and their projection on radiographs). The average value of the T:P ratio was 1.02, with a mean SD

of 0.13. It was concluded that in a normal knee the length of the patellar tendon should not differ from that of the patella by more than 20%.

Measurements were repeated on bilateral knee radiographs in 50 asymptomatic volunteers by Jacobsen and Bertheussen,[72] who confirmed a similar degree of accuracy. Aglietti et al. also measured patellar height according to the Insall-Salvati method in a group of 150 normal knees[3] (see Table 67.1). The T:P ratio was found to be 1.04 on average (range: 0.8 to 1.38; SD: 0.11). The patella was significantly higher in women (1.06) than in men (1.01). In the same group of knees the distance from the plateau level to the tibial tuberosity and the diagonal length of the patella varied only with gender, with larger values in men than in women. In 53 knees with patellar pain the patella was slightly but significantly higher than in normal knees, with an average T:P ratio of 1.08 (range: 0.88 to 1.29; SD: 0.09). In a group of 37 knees with recurrent subluxation the average T:P ratio was clearly increased to an average of 1.23 (range: 0.78 to 1.60; SD: 0.18). In conclusion, according to the Insall-Salvati method, an index greater than 1.2 indicates patella alta, whereas an index below 0.8 indicates a low patella.

Blackburne-Peel ratio. Blackburne and Peel[20] criticized the T:P ratio on the basis of the following two observations:

1. The radiographic marking on the tibial tubercle may be indistinct or even unrecognizable when the tibial tuberosity has been affected by Osgood-Schlatter disease.

2. The nonarticular portion of the lower pole of the patella varies considerably in size; it is instead the position of the articular surface that is of greatest clinical significance.

To overcome these difficulties, the authors suggested a ratio between the perpendicular distance from the lowest articular margin of the patella to the tibial plateau (A) and the length of the articular surface of the patella (B), as measured on a lateral view of the knee in at least 30 degrees of flexion (Fig. 67.13). The A:B ratio in 171 normal knees was 0.80 (SD: 0.14). No difference between genders was noted.

Aglietti et al. measured the A:B ratio in a group of 150 normal knees[3] and found a slightly higher value than the original authors did: an A:B ratio of 0.95 on average (range: 0.65 to 1.38; SD: 0.13), with an insignificant difference between men and women (see Table 67.1). In a group of patients with anterior knee pain the A:B ratio was 0.91, an insignificant difference from the ratio in control knees. On the other hand, the A:B ratio was significantly increased in knees with recurrent subluxation (average: 1.08; range: 0.76 to 1.89; SD: 0.19).

Modified Insall-Salvati ratio. Grelsamer and Meadows[51] observed that the Insall-Salvati index does not account for the shape of the patella. They found that patients with patella alta and a long distal nose may have a falsely normal Insall-Salvati index. The presence of patella alta in these patients can be easily verified by indices that use the patellar articular surface and the upper part of the tibia as landmarks (the Blackburne and Peel or Caton ratio). The variable relationship between the length of the patella and length of the articular surface as expressed by the morphology index[52] has been presented in the section on anatomy (Fig. 67.14).

To overcome the problem of variable morphology of the patella, the Insall-Salvati ratio was modified. It was suggested that the ratio of the distance between the inferior articular facet of the patella and the tibial tuberosity and the length of the articular surface be used (Fig. 67.15). In other words, this method uses the same distal reference point as the Insall-Salvati

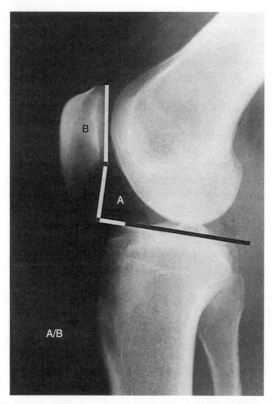

FIG 67.13 Blackburne and Peel Method of Measuring Patellar Height Height is expressed as the ratio between *A* and *B*. (From Blackburne JS, Peel TE: A new method of measuring patella height. *J Bone Joint Surg Br* 59:241, 1977.)

method (the tibial tuberosity) and the same proximal reference point as the Caton method. In a group of 100 control knees the modified Insall-Salvati ratio was 1.5 on average (range: 1.2 to 2.1). Ninety-seven percent of control knees had a ratio less than 2.0. Therefore for practical purposes a ratio of 2 or more can be used as an index of patella alta.

Lyon School. The Lyon School[26] criticized the previously existing methods of measuring the height of the patella. Members of this group found it difficult to define the insertion of the patellar tendon into the tibial tuberosity in knees with previous transposition of the tuberosity. They further observed that the use of a tangent to the tibial plateaus in the Blackburne and Peel method[20] may be a source of significant error. Perfect superimposition of the tibial plateaus is necessary to draw the line. The posterior slope of the tibial plateaus is not constant and may vary 15 degrees or more in subjects who have undergone anterior tibial epiphysiodesis. To overcome these difficulties, they tried to develop an easy method that could be used on lateral radiographs in flexion between 10 and 80 degrees and that was not influenced by radiographic magnification, by previous transposition of the tibial tuberosity, or by fractures of the tip of the patella. In this method a ratio is calculated using the distance between the inferior point of the articular surface of the patella and the anterosuperior edge of the tibia, as the numerator (AT), and the length of the articular surface of the patella as the denominator (AP) (Fig. 67.16). The AT:AP ratio was calculated in 141 normal subjects and was found to be 0.960^7 in 80 men and 0.990^6 in 61 women. Based on these findings the authors considered the patella to be infera with a ratio of 0.6 or less and alta if 1.3 or more.

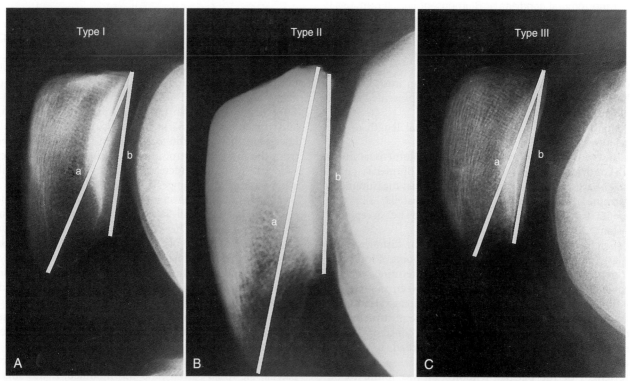

FIG 67.14 Different Shapes of the Patella in the Sagittal Plane According to Grelsamer et al.[52] Patellar shape is described by the morphology ratio (ie, the ratio of patellar length to length of the articular surface). (A) A normal type I patella has a morphology ratio between 1.2 and 1.5. (B) Type II patella, with a morphology ratio greater than 1.5 (ie, with a long inferior pole) (Cyrano appearance). (C) Type III patella with a morphology ratio below 1.2 (ie, with a short inferior pole).

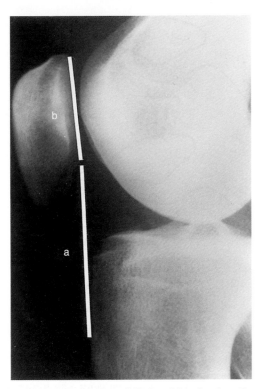

FIG 67.15 The Modified Insall-Salvati Method as Described by Grelsamer and Meadows[51] The distance between the lowest point of the articular surface of the patella and the tibial tuberosity (distance *a*) is divided by the length of the articular facet (distance *b*). A value of 2 or more indicates patella alta.

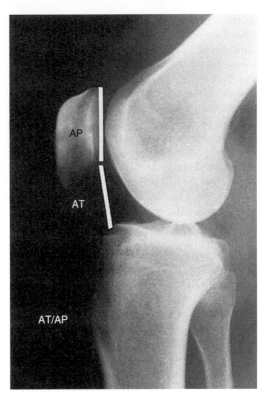

FIG 67.16 Caton Method to Measure the Height of the Patella Height is expressed as the ratio between the distance *(AT)* from the lowest point of the articular facet to the most prominent part of the tibial plateau and the length *(AP)* of the articular facet of the patella. See text for discussion of the ratio AT:AP. (From Caton G, Deschamps G, Chambat P, et al: Les routules basses: à propos de 128 observations. *Rev Chir Orthop* 68:317, 1982.)

Norman index. Norman et al.[104] observed that the Insall-Salvati method does not describe the relationship between the patella and the femoral sulcus and that proximal or distal transposition of the tibial tuberosity may be performed without affecting the T:P ratio. To overcome these difficulties, Norman et al. described a method wherein a lateral radiograph is obtained with the knee in full extension (hyperextension) and in quadriceps contraction to straighten the patellar tendon. The film–focus distance should be kept constant (1 m) and the cassette placed in contact with the lateral aspect of the knee. Various parameters were measured in this radiograph, including the length of the tendon, patella, and articular facet and the vertical position of the patella (ie, the distance from the lowest point of the articular facet to the joint line). These measurements were related to the height of the patient, and it was found that the vertical position of the patella was constant without gender-related differences (Fig. 67.17). The Norman index, defined as the ratio between the vertical position of the patella (in millimeters) and body length (in centimeters), is 0.21 in a normal knee (SD: 0.02). In patients with recurrent dislocation without associated generalized laxity, the index is 0.23 on average; in patients with associated generalized laxity, it is 0.25.

Conclusions and authors' recommendations. Various methods of measuring the height of the patella have been described. Despite some literature[14] supporting the use of the Caton-Deschamps or Blackburne-Peel due to reported increased interobserver reliability, in our opinion, the Insall-Salvati T:P ratio remains a reliable and reproducible method. It does not

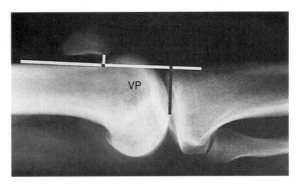

FIG 67.17 Norman Method to Measure the Height of the Patella A lateral radiograph is obtained with perfect superimposition of the femoral condyles, the knee hyperextended, and the quadriceps contracted to straighten the patellar tendon. A line is drawn tangential to the distal third of the anterior femoral cortex. Two perpendicular lines are then drawn that pass through the femorotibial contact point and through the inferior point of the articular facet. The distance between the two perpendicular lines, defined as the vertical position *(VP)* of the patella, is related to the height of the patient in centimeters. The Norman index is expressed as follows: vertical position of the patella (mm)/body height (cm). In a normal knee its average value is 0.21. (From Norman O, Egund N, Ekelund L, Rünow A: The vertical position of the patella. *Acta Orthop Scand* 54:908, 1983.)

require perfect alignment of the knee in the lateral view and does not need correction for magnification. Values greater than 1.2 are diagnostic of patella alta. The method may not be applicable in knees with previous Osgood-Schlatter disease, and the method is not suitable for evaluating patellar position after distal transfer of the tibial tuberosity. In this setting one may use the Blackburne and Peel or the Caton method; these methods measure the height of the patella in relation to the tibial plateau and joint line. The main drawback of the Blackburne and Peel method is that it requires a lateral view with superimposition of the femoral condyles to accurately identify the joint line. An image amplifier is required to consistently obtain this degree of accuracy. The same problem is encountered with the Norman technique, which has the additional difficulty of requiring an effective quadriceps contraction. Furthermore, the film–focus distance (1 m) must be kept constant, and the patient's height must be known. In the presence of abnormal patellar morphology with a long or short distal pole, the modified Insall-Salvati method should be used.

Evaluating for patellofemoral dysplasia. Attention has been drawn to evaluation of the anatomy of the trochlea and subluxation of the patella as seen on the lateral view. Maldague and Malghem[87] first described the radiographic appearance of the patella and trochlea femoralis on lateral views of normal knees and knees with patellar instability. It is necessary to obtain lateral views with satisfactory superimposition of the posterior and distal femoral condyles, which requires the use of an image amplifier. In the lateral view of a normal knee the posterior aspect of the patella is represented by two lines: the most posterior one is the patellar ridge, the other is the lateral facet (Figs. 67.18 and 67.19). In knees with mild lateral tilt of the patella, the two lines superimpose. When the patella is more markedly tilted, the lateral facet overhangs the patellar ridge line posteriorly, and the anteroposterior diameter of the patella is greatly increased. The normal trochlea is composed of three lines: the two anterior lines are projections of the top of the medial and lateral facets of the trochlea; the posterior line, in continuation with the intercondylar roof line, represents the deepest point of the sulcus (Fig. 67.20). The distance between the two anterior lines and the posterior line represents the depth of the sulcus. Maldague and Malghem observed that its depth is normally greater than 1 cm as it is measured 1 cm distal to the upper part of the trochlea. In knees with patellar instability the depth of the trochlea is reduced throughout the length of the sulcus (totally deficient sulcus) or only in its upper part (focally deficient sulcus). The authors emphasized the importance of the lateral view in patients with clinically suspected patellar instability and axial views showing negative results. Because axial views are often obtained in more than 30 degrees of flexion, a lateral view taken at 15 degrees of flexion allows exploration of the patellofemoral congruence at a degree of flexion that cannot be visualized with conventional axial views.

These concepts have been carried a step farther by the Lyon School.[38] Members of this group examined the lateral views of 143 knees with recurrent or acute dislocation of the patella and compared these with the radiographs of 190 control knees. They studied two quantitative measurements—trochlear bump and trochlear depth—and one qualitative sign—the crossing sign.

On a lateral view with superimposition of the femoral condyles, a line is drawn tangent to the last 10 cm of the anterior cortex of the femur. The line of the femoral sulcus may end in

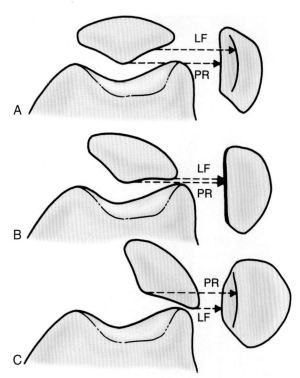

FIG 67.18 Patellar shape on lateral view with the knee flexed 10 to 15 degrees and good superimposition of the femoral condyles. (A) In a normal knee, the posterior profile of the patella is represented by two lines: the most posterior one is the patellar ridge (PR); the anterior one is the lateral facet (LF). (B) If the patella is slightly tilted laterally, the two lines superimpose. (C) If the patella is severely tilted, the LF overhangs the ridge line posteriorly, and the anteroposterior diameter of the patella is increased. (Modified from Maldague B, Malghem J: Apport du cliché de profil du genou dans le dépistage des instabilites rotuliennes: Rapport préliminaire. Rev Chir Orthop 71[Suppl 2]:5, 1985.)

front of (positive value), over, or behind (negative value) the line of the anterior cortex. The distance between the anterior cortex line and the sulcus (saille or bump) is measured in millimeters (Fig. 67.21). The bump of the sulcus line in relation to the anterior femoral cortex was found to be highly useful in differentiating between knees with instability (average: 3.2 mm) and normal knees (average: −0.8 mm). A pathologic threshold value for measurement of trochlear bump was identified: 3 mm. Sixty-six percent of knees with patellar instability had anterior trochlear translation of 3 mm or more as compared with only 6.5% of control knees.

The depth of the trochlea was measured as the distance between the floor of the trochlea and the most anterior condylar contour line. First, a line tangent to the posterior cortex of the femur was drawn. A second line was drawn perpendicular to the posterior femoral cortex line and tangent to the posterior aspect of the femoral condyles. A third line was finally drawn that subtended an angle of 15 degrees to the second line and passed through the intersection of the first and second lines. Trochlear depth was measured along this third line (Fig. 67.22). Trochlear depth was 7.8 mm in the control group and 2.3 mm in knees with patellar instability. A trochlear depth of 4 mm or

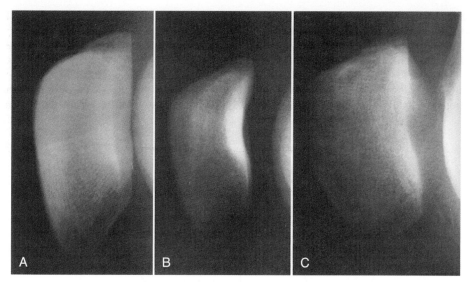

FIG 67.19 Lateral Views (A) The patella in a normal knee. (B) A knee with a mildly tilted patella. (C) A knee with a markedly tilted patella.

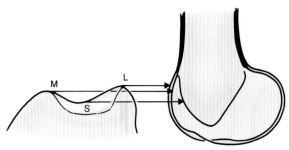

FIG 67.20 Morphology of the trochlea in a lateral radiograph with superimposition of the femoral condyles. The two anterior lines are the projection of the medial *(M)* and lateral *(L)* facets of the trochlea. The posterior line is in continuation with the intercondylar roof line and corresponds to the deepest part of the sulcus *(S)*. (Modified from Maldague B, Malghem J: Apport du cliché de profil du genou dans le dépistage des instabilites rotuliennes: rapport préliminaire. *Rev Chir Orthop* 71[Suppl 2]:5, 1985.)

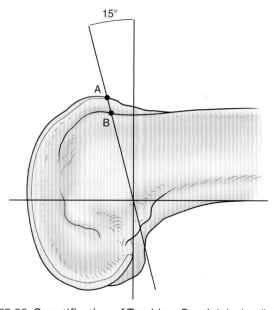

FIG 67.22 Quantification of Trochlear Depth It is the distance *A-B* measured in millimeters along a line subtended 15 degrees from the perpendicular to the posterior femoral cortex line and crossing a line tangential to the posterior femoral condyles and perpendicular to the posterior cortex line.

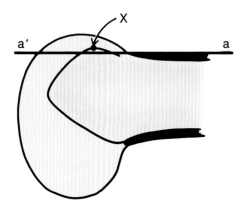

FIG 67.21 Quantification of the Trochlear Bump A line (ac-a) is drawn tangential to the last 10 cm of the anterior femoral cortex. The line of the sulcus at its most anterior point *X* may pass in front of (positive value) or behind (negative value) the tangent line. The bump is measured as the distance between the femoral cortex line and the sulcus line in millimeters.

less was considered pathologic. This value was found in 85% of knees with patellar instability and in only 3% of controls.

Dysplasia of the trochlea can be divided into three types according to the point at which the sulcus line crosses the lines of the condyles (the croisement, or crossing, sign) The crossing sign is a simple qualitative criterion defined as the crossing between the floor line and the lateral condylar line. At that level the trochlea is considered flat (Figs. 67.23 and 67.24)[39]:

Type I dysplasia: This form is the mildest. The lines of the condyles are symmetrical, and they are crossed at the same point in the proximal part of the trochlea by the floor line. Only the very proximal part of the trochlea is flat.

Type II dysplasia: The lines of the condyles are not superimposed; the line of the sulcus crosses the medial condyle line first, and the lateral one crosses at a higher level. Separate crossing of the medial and lateral condyle lines is characteristic of this type.

Type III dysplasia: This form is the most severe. The condyle lines are superimposed, but they are crossed low on the trochlea by the sulcus line. Most of the trochlea is therefore flat.

Two types of normal trochlea were identified:

Type A (50%): The sulcus line is posterior to the condyle lines throughout its length (see Fig. 67.23).

Type B (50%): The sulcus line joins the line of the medial condyle but only in the highest part of the trochlea.

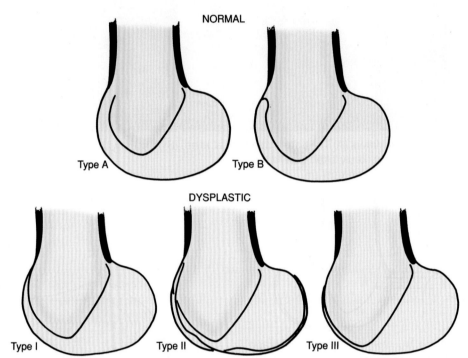

FIG 67.23 The Croisement (Crossing Sign) In normal knees the sulcus line may be posterior to the condyle lines throughout its length *(type A)* or may join the medial condyle line only in the upper part of the trochlea *(type B)*. Therefore there is no crossing between the sulcus line and the condyle line in normal knees. The presence of the crossing sign indicates dysplasia of the femoral trochlea. See text for further discussion. (From Dejour H, Walch G, Neyret P, Adeleine P: La dysplasie de la trochlee femorale. *Rev Chir Orthop* 76:45, 1990.)

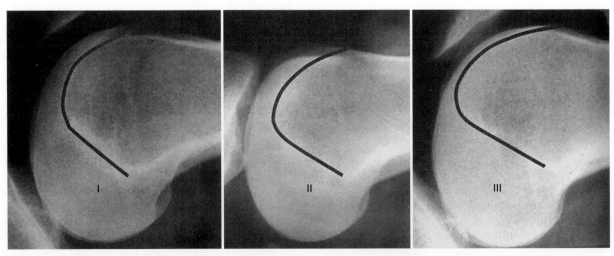

FIG 67.24 Trochlear dysplasia, types I, II, and III. See text for explanation. (From Dejour H, Walch G, Neyret P, Adeleine P: La dysplasie de la trochlee femorale. *Rev Chir Orthop* 76:45, 1990.)

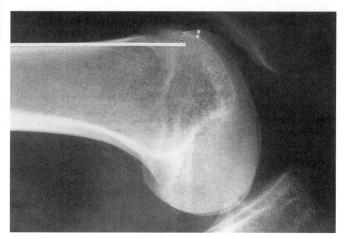

FIG 67.25 Lateral Radiograph of a Knee With Recurrent Patellar Instability. The sulcus line is anterior to the femoral cortex line (bump of +4 mm), the sulcus depth is only 3 mm, and a crossing sign is present between the sulcus and condyle lines (type I dysplasia).

Dysplasia of the femoral sulcus, as evidenced by the crossing sign, was present in the majority of knees with patellar instability (96%) (Fig. 67.25); the same was true in only 3% of control knees. In light of this study the authors concluded that in trochlear dysplasia, the trochlea is flat in a zone of variable length and has a shallow groove more distally. According to the authors trochlear dysplasia is better evaluated on a lateral radiograph than on CT. Such dysplasia is best recognized with the crossing sign, a qualitative factor that was present in 96% of knees with patellar instability. Two other quantitative measurements, trochlear bump (positive when ≥3 mm) and trochlear depth (positive when ≤4 mm), were both positive in 85% of cases.

The Lyon School[131] has modified this classification and has introduced new radiographic signs. The supratrochlear spur is located in the proximal aspect of the lateral trochlea in an attempt to keep the patella in the groove. The double-shape sign has been described as a vertical line of sclerosis that is the projection of the medial trochlea. Based on these new signs, trochlear dysplasia has been described as follows:

Grade A: crossing sign (symmetrical but less deep trochlea).
Grade B: crossing sign and trochlear spur (flat or convex trochlea).
Grade C: crossing and double-shape signs (asymmetrical trochlea, laterally convex, and medially hypoplastic).
Grade D: crossing and double-shape signs, trochlear spur (asymmetrical trochlea with rapid mediolateral change).

It is suggested that treatment of instability of the patella should be based on recognized anatomic abnormalities. Re-creation of a sulcus of normal depth is theoretically desirable to improve the stability of the patella. Van Haver et al.[136] investigated the effects of trochlear dysplasia on the biomechanics of the patellofemoral joint. Using three-dimensional printing, they replaced the native trochlear in four cadaveric knees with dysplastic trochlears and then subjected them to squat simulation, open chain extension, and a patella stability test. They measured the contact area, pressure, kinematics, and stability of the patella and compared the dysplastic models to the native trochlear. They found increased lateral patella tilt,

lateral translation and internal rotation in the dysplastic trochleas when compared with native control trochleas. Grade D trochleas showed the greatest PF contact areas and largest degree of maltracking.

Restoring the PF joint congruency and normal trochlear depth may be achieved by elevating the lateral femoral condyle[7] or by depressing the central part of the trochlea.[92] Elevation of the lateral condyle is a logical approach if the saille of the sulcus is normal; it is contraindicated in knees with a positive saille. Deepening of the sulcus (trochleoplasty) seems to be more logical because it re-creates normal anatomy. However, the procedure is technically more demanding and involves violation of the articular cartilage.

Axial views. An axial view of the patellofemoral joint adds considerably to our knowledge when performed in a correctly standardized manner. Unfortunately, all too often this portion of the examination is omitted or is performed haphazardly. Various techniques are available.

In the method attributed to Settegast[121] the patient lies prone with the knees acutely flexed. The x-ray plate is placed beneath the knees with the tube directed above so that the beam is at a right angle. This is an easy examination for the technician to perform. Unfortunately, it is also uninformative because, if the angle of flexion is poorly controlled, the image of the patella is often distorted and the patella lies on the femoral condyles rather than in the sulcus, which is the most important and functional position.

Ficat and Hungerford[45] described a technique in which the patient's knees were flexed over the end of the x-ray table. The tube is placed at the patient's feet, and the cassette is held proximally against the anterior of the thigh. In this position the tube is perpendicular to the beam. Flexion views can be obtained at 30, 60, and 90 degrees. This technique is widely used in Europe but seems less popular in the United States, probably because of technical difficulties involved in obtaining good views.

Merchant et al.[96] described a technique whereby the patient is positioned supine with the knees flexed 45 degrees over the end of the table. The knees are elevated slightly to keep the femurs horizontal and parallel with the table surface. The x-ray tube is kept proximally over the patient's head and is then angled down 30 degrees from horizontal. The film cassette is placed approximately 30 cm below the knees, resting on the shins and perpendicular to the x-ray beam (Fig. 67.26). The legs are strapped together at about calf level to control rotation, and both knees are exposed simultaneously. It is important for the quadriceps muscle to be relaxed. The position of 45 degrees of knee flexion has been selected as the position of least flexion with which satisfactory results could be obtained.

Two angles are measured on the Merchant view: the sulcus and congruence angles (Fig. 67.27). The congruence angle measures the relationship of the patella to the intercondylar sulcus. For this measurement the sulcus angle is bisected to establish a zero reference line. A second line is then projected from the apex of the sulcus angle to the lowest point on the articular ridge of the patella. The angle measured between these two lines is the congruence angle. If the apex of the patellar articular ridge is lateral to the zero line, the congruence angle is designated positive. If it is medial, the congruence angle is negative. In a group of 100 normal knees, 50 males and 50 females, Merchant et al.[96] measured an average sulcus angle of 138 degrees (SD: 6 degrees) and an average congruence angle

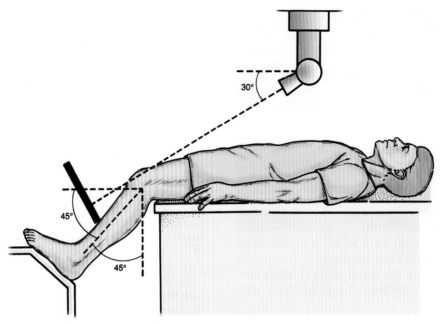

FIG 67.26 Merchant Technique to Obtain Axial Views of the Patella The patient is supine with the knees flexed 45 degrees over the edge of the table and resting on a support. The cassette rests on the shins about 30 cm below the knees. It is struck at a right angle by the x-ray beam, which is angled 30 degrees down from the horizontal. (From Merchant AC, Mercer RL, Jacobsen RH, et al: Roentgenographic analysis of patello-femoral congruence. *J Bone Joint Surg Am* 56:1391, 1974.)

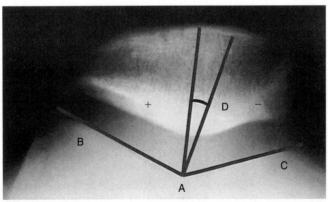

FIG 67.27 Measurement of the Sulcus Angle and the Congruence Angle on a Merchant View The sulcus angle *(BAC)* is bisected by the reference line. A second line *(AD)* is drawn from the sulcus to the PR. If the apex of the PR is lateral to the reference line, the value of the angle is positive; if it is medial the value of the angle is negative. (From Merchant AC, Mercer RL, Jacobsen RH, et al: Roentgenographic analysis of patello-femoral congruence. *J Bone Joint Surg Am* 56:1391, 1974.)

of −6 degrees (SD: 11 degrees). Based on these data it was suggested that any sulcus angle greater than 150 degrees and any congruence angle greater than 16 degrees is abnormal at the 95th percentile. In a group of patients with recurrent patellar dislocation (number not specified), the average congruence angle was +23 degrees, which is well beyond the 95th percentile of normal subjects.

Aglietti et al. repeated the measurements proposed by Merchant and associates in normal and pathologic knees.[3] In a group of 150 normal knees the average sulcus angle was 137 degrees (SD: 6 degrees), with no differences noted between males and females. This is very close to the results of Merchant and associates. On the other hand, Aglietti et al. measured an average congruence angle of −8 degrees (SD: 6 degrees), thus suggesting a lower upper limit in normal knees (+4 degrees) than that proposed by Merchant (+16). In 53 knees with anterior knee pain the sulcus angle was similar to that of controls (average: 139; SD: 4 degrees), and the congruence angle was slightly increased (average: −2; SD: 9 degrees). In 37 knees with recurrent dislocation, both the sulcus angle (average: 147 degrees; SD: 7 degrees) and the congruence angle (average: −16; SD: 13 degrees) were clearly increased over those of controls (Fig. 67.28).

Laurin et al.[83,84] described a similar method in which the x-ray tube is positioned distally between the feet, and the cassette is held proximally against the anterior of the thighs (Fig. 67.29). The following details should be observed:

• The patient should be seated with the feet at the very edge of the table. The x-ray beam is directed parallel to the anterior border of the tibia and the longitudinal axis of the patella. The x-ray beam is thus parallel to the specific proximal segment of the patellofemoral joint that must be visualized.

• The knees must be in a position of 20 degrees of knee flexion, and the quadriceps must be relaxed. A special adjustable support under the knees is recommended to maintain the position.

• The x-ray plate is held by the patient such that it is at 90 degrees to the long axis of the tibia and x-ray beam; it must not be laid flat against the thighs, nor should it be at 90 degrees to the tabletop. The patient must forcibly press the lower edge of the plate against the thighs. Otherwise, especially in muscular or obese patients, only the patella appears at the bottom of the x-ray film, and the femoral trochlea is not included. Under such circumstances, the radiographs must be repeated and the technique modified by pushing on the x-ray plate more forcibly or by holding the x-ray plate more proximal on the thighs. The knees must not be flexed more than 20 degrees.

In a correctly obtained Laurin view the patellofemoral compartment is clearly visualized. The lateral prominence of

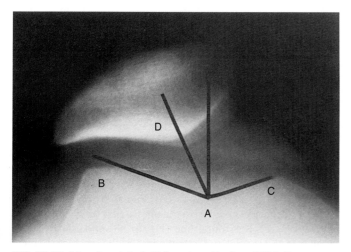

FIG 67.28 Merchant Axial View in a Patient With Recurrent Dislocation of the Patella Both the sulcus angle *(BAC)* and the congruence angle *(CAD)* were clearly increased over normal values.

the trochlea has a rounded contour, whereas the medial prominence is sharp. The lateral patellofemoral angle (Fig. 67.30) can be measured by drawing a line tangent to the top of the medial and lateral femoral condyles and a second line tangent to the lateral facet of the patella.[84] The lateral facet of the patella was chosen as a reference because, given the wide variations in patellar morphology described by Wiberg[138] and Baumgartl,[15] it retains a relatively constant shape. In a group of 100 normal knees the lateral patellofemoral angle was open laterally in the great majority (97%), whereas the lines were parallel in only 3%. In 30 knees with patellar subluxation the lines were parallel in 60% and were open medially in 40% (Fig. 67.31). The lateral patellofemoral angle was of no assistance in the evaluation of knees with patellar pain because it was normal (open laterally) in 90%, and the lines were parallel in the remainder. In an effort to individuate a radiographic measurement diagnostic of chondromalacia, Laurin et al.[83] proposed the patellofemoral index (Fig. 67.32). The basic abnormality underlying patellar subluxation and patellar pain is the same, but it is less severe in the second condition. The lateral patellofemoral angle therefore is not altered, whereas the patellofemoral index may show a "mini-tilt" of the patella. The patellofemoral index is the ratio of the thickness of the medial to the lateral patellofemoral interspace. In normal knees the medial interspace was equal or slightly wider than the lateral, and the patellofemoral index was 1.6 or less. In contrast, the patellofemoral index was higher than 1.6 in 97% of knees with patellar pain. An increased patellofemoral index with widening of the medial interspace indicates a mini-tilt of the patella.

Malghem and Maldague[88] suggested that axial views should be obtained at 30 degrees of flexion and external tibial rotation. This method takes advantage of the lateral pull of the patellar tendon to detect subluxability of the patella. Lateral rotation is produced manually by external rotation of the forefoot.

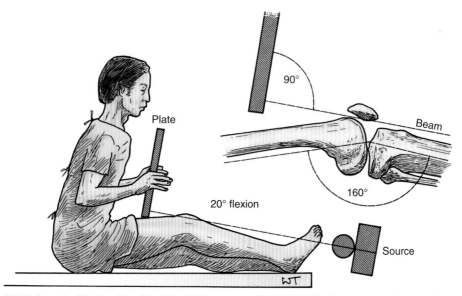

FIG 67.29 Laurin Method to Obtain Axial Views of the Patella The patient is seated on the examining table with the feet near the edge. The x-ray beam is parallel to the anterior border of the tibia, and the knees are flexed 20 degrees. The cassette is held by the patient against the thighs and at 90 degrees to the beam. See text for further discussion. (From Laurin CA, Levesque HP, Dussault R, et al: The abnormal lateral patellofemoral angle: a diagnostic roentgenographic sign of recurrent patellar subluxation. *J Bone Joint Surg Am* 60:55, 1978.)

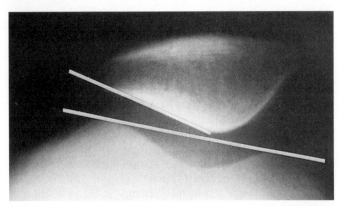

FIG 67.30 Measurement of the Lateral Patellofemoral Angle on a Laurin View The lateral patellofemoral angle (LPFA) is measured by drawing a line tangential to the top of the medial and lateral condyle and a second line tangential to the lateral patellar facet. It is open laterally in normal knees.

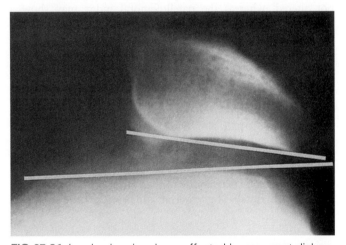

FIG 67.31 Laurin view in a knee affected by recurrent dislocation of the patella. The lateral patellofemoral angle is open medially.

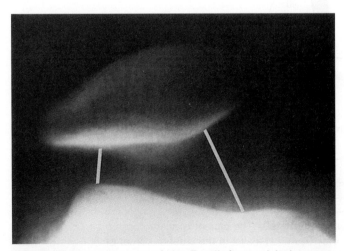

FIG 67.32 Measurement of the Patellofemoral Index on a Laurin View The ratio of the medial interspace to the lateral interspace is up to 1.6 in normal knees. In this case the measurement is clearly pathologic.

Counterpressure on the lateral side of the thigh is necessary to keep the knee within the beam axis. The examination is performed sequentially for both knees. The tube is positioned between the feet of the patient, and the cassette rests against the thighs. In 27 knees that underwent surgery for patellar instability, the congruence angle was measured according to the method of Merchant et al.,[96] and a value greater than 16 degrees was considered evidence of subluxation. Subluxation was evident in 26% of cases by the 45-degree axial view and in 100% by the 30-degree lateral rotation view. Of these 27 knees 13 had a centered patella in the 45-degree axial view and showed subluxation in the 30-degree lateral rotation view. In these knees a 30-degree axial view without external rotation was added. This modification yielded a result (average congruence angle: +10.3 degrees) that was intermediate between the 45-degree (average congruence angle: +1.5 degrees) and the 30-degree (average congruence angle: +26.7 degrees) views with external rotation.

Toft[133] suggested that axial radiographs of the patella in the weight-bearing position can detect narrowing of the patellofemoral joint line.

An alternative method used to measure tilt of the patella was described by Grelsamer et al.[50] They elected to use a line connecting the two edges of the patella (the corner-to-corner line) instead of the more usual line tangent to the subchondral bone of the lateral facet, as recommended by Laurin et al.[84] They reasoned that the corner-to-corner line is independent of patellar morphology, it is easy to draw, and it corresponds more closely to clinical evaluation of the tilt. Patellar tilt was evaluated in relation to a horizontal line (Fig. 67.33) and not to a line tangent to the medial and lateral edges of the trochlea. Using a horizontal line as a reference has a drawback because it requires consistent rotational control of the leg and alignment of the cassette parallel to the ground. Rotational alignment of the leg was judged from the foot, which had to point directly upward. The purpose of using a horizontal line is to be independent of the morphology of the anterior trochlea, which is highly

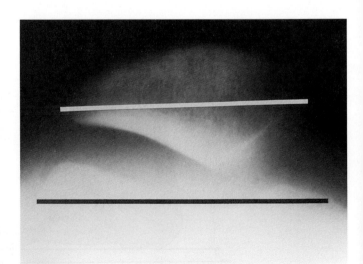

FIG 67.33 Tilt of the Patella Evaluated According to Grelsamer et al.[50] The tilt is the angle joining the edges of the patella and a line drawn parallel to the floor. The axial view is obtained with the knee flexed 30 degrees and with careful control of rotation of the leg with the foot pointing directly upward and the lower border of the film parallel to the ground.

variable and may induce underestimation or overestimation of a tilt.

A second alternative is to use a line tangent to the posterior condyles, but this requires a CT scan. Axial views were obtained at 30 degrees of flexion via a Merchant technique. In a group of 100 knees with patellar malalignment the average tilt angle was 12 ± 6 degrees, and 85% of cases had a tilt greater than 5 degrees. In a control group of 100 knees the average tilt angle was 2 ± 1 degree ($p < 0.01$), and 92% of cases had a tilt of 5 degrees or less. Patellar tilt greater than 5 degrees is therefore 85% sensitive, 92% specific, and 89% accurate in the diagnosis of patellofemoral malalignment. This method of measuring patellar tilt may thus be advantageous if a dedicated radiologist is available to accurately position the patient and the cassette.

In conclusion, standard anteroposterior and lateral radiographs with a Merchant axial view can reasonably be accepted as a first step in the diagnosis of patellofemoral disorders. A lateral view with perfect superimposition of the femoral condyles is necessary to evaluate the morphology of the trochlea for any evidence of dysplasia (flat trochlea). According to Aglietti et al. (see Table 67.1)[3] a normal knee has on average a Q angle of 15 degrees, an Insall-Salvati T:P ratio of 1.04, a Blackburne and Peel A:B ratio of 0.95, a sulcus angle of 137 degrees, and a congruence angle of −8 degrees. Slightly but statistically significantly higher values for the Q angle and the T:P ratio have been found in females. For clinical purposes we consider the following values to be pathologic: a Q angle greater than 20 degrees, a T:P ratio greater than 1.2 and certainly greater than 1.3, an A:B ratio greater than 1.2, a sulcus angle greater than 150 degrees, and a congruence angle greater than +4 degrees. Knees with patellar pain showed a clearly increased Q angle (average: 20 degrees), with minor and clinically insignificant differences in the T:P ratio, A:B ratio, and sulcus angle, as well as minor lateralization of the patella (average congruence angle: −2 degrees). Knees with recurrent subluxation or dislocation of the patella showed a high-riding patella with an average T:P ratio of 1.23 and an average A:B ratio of 1.08, a more open femoral sulcus (average sulcus angle: 147 degrees), and gross lateral displacement of the patella (average congruence angle: +16 degrees) (Fig. 67.34). In view of clear anatomic abnormalities in knees with recurrent dislocation of the patella,

these simple radiographic measurements are diagnostic in most cases. Conversely, patients with anterior knee pain frequently have normal height of the patella and normal-appearing axial views at 45 degrees. In these cases it is worthwhile to request an axial view at 20 degrees[84] or a CT scan of the patellofemoral joint to detect minor abnormalities in the first 30 degrees of flexion.

Computed Tomography

The use of CT has made it possible to investigate patellofemoral relationships in the arc between full extension and 45 degrees of flexion. Traditional axial views can be obtained in 20 degrees of flexion according to the method of Laurin et al.,[84] but the technique is not easy. Obese or muscular patients render the examination more difficult, and a skilled technician is required to obtain consistent results. Furthermore, the use of CT avoids image overlapping and distortion. For these reasons, CT has gained increasing popularity in the evaluation of patellofemoral disorders.

Delgado-Martins[40] first used CT to evaluate the patellofemoral joints of 12 normal subjects with the knee in extension and compared these images with traditional axial views at 30, 60, and 90 degrees. The patella was considered to be centered when the median crest fit exactly in the intercondylar groove. The author reported that the patella was centered in the groove in 96% of cases at 90 degrees, 63% at 60 degrees, 29% at 30 degrees, 13% in full extension with the quadriceps relaxed, and 4% in full extension with the quadriceps contracted. Although the images reported by Delgado-Martins suggest that some of these patients may suffer from subluxation of the patella, it is well emphasized that evaluation in the first degrees of flexion is far more informative than at 60 or 90 degrees.

Martinez et al.[91] made the same observation; they used CT to evaluate 10 normal volunteers and 5 patients with recurrent subluxation. Images were obtained at 0, 20, and 45 degrees of flexion with a special device used to position the knee.[90] The authors measured the sulcus angle and used a line tangent to the posterior condyles as a reference to evaluate patellar tilt angle, height of the lateral condyle, and centralization of the patella. In extension 95% of normal patellae were centralized with the quadriceps relaxed, but this percentage decreased to

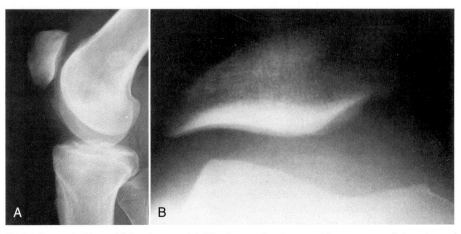

FIG 67.34 Lateral (A) and Merchant axial (B) views of a knee with recurrent dislocation of the patella. Clear anatomic abnormalities, including a high-riding patella, a flat sulcus, and a positive congruence angle, are evident.

85% with quadriceps contraction. Centralization of the patella was maintained in most control subjects at 20 and 45 degrees of knee flexion. The patellar tilt angle was positive (open laterally) in all normal knees in extension (average: 11 degrees) and did not change with flexion. The sulcus angle was 143 degrees in extension and decreased with flexion. In the five knees with subluxation, the patella was clearly displaced laterally in extension but tended to reduce in flexion. The patellar tilt angle was negative (open medially) in extension but tended to reverse to a positive value (decreased patellar tilt) with flexion. The height of the lateral femoral condyle was decreased and the sulcus angle increased when compared with these values in controls. Martinez and colleagues concluded that axial or CT images at 20 and 45 degrees of flexion can falsely indicate a normal patellofemoral joint.

Sasaki and Yagi[114] used CT to investigate the patellofemoral joint with the knee in extension. They studied 24 knees with patellar subluxation and 24 controls. Lines tangent to the medial and lateral prominences of the trochlea and the transverse axis of the patella were used to measure tilt of the patella. Lateral shift of the patella was measured in relation to the most prominent aspect of the lateral femoral condyle. The results were compared with conventional axial views at 30 degrees of flexion. Mean patellar tilt angles in normal knees with the quadriceps relaxed and contracted were 15 degrees and 14 degrees, respectively. The same values in knees with patellar subluxation were 31 degrees and 40 degrees, respectively. The lateral shift of the patella measured in relation to the transverse diameter was 14% with the quadriceps relaxed and 28% with muscle contraction in the normal knees. These values increased to 31% and 59%, respectively, in knees with subluxation. Values of patellar tilt and shift were significantly higher in patients with subluxation than in controls, and the differences were more evident with the quadriceps contracted. Values of patellar tilt and shift in the knees with subluxation were higher on CT images in full extension than on axial views at 30 degrees. Among the 46 knees that underwent extensor mechanism realignment (proximal or distal), the values of patellar tilt and shift returned to nearly normal on postoperative CT scans. The 35 knees with satisfactory postoperative results showed greater improvement in patellar shift (14%) when compared with the five knees with unsatisfactory results (4.3%).

Fulkerson et al. have further progressed in CT evaluation of the patellofemoral joint by obtaining images at various degrees of flexion between 0 and 30 degrees and by emphasizing the importance of accurate and standardized scanning. They recommend the use of midtransverse patellar sections and a line tangent to the posterior condyles as reference for the measurements.[47,117,118] Care should be taken to position the patient in the gantry so that normal standing alignment is reproduced and to obtain the cuts through the same point of the patella. Fulkerson et al. used the Merchant method to measure the sulcus and congruence angles,[96] tilt of the lateral patellar facet with respect to a line tangent to the posterior condyles (patellar tilt angle), and height of the lateral condyle from the deepest point of the sulcus.[117] These authors reported the measurement of 10 normal knees and 54 symptomatic knees, including 49 suffering from patellar pain and 5 from patellar dislocation. Evaluation of the congruence angle in the normal knees revealed that the patellae were slightly lateralized in extension (average congruence angle: +2.5 degrees); however, by 10 degrees of flexion, all were centered or slightly medial. Therefore a patella can be

considered subluxated if the congruence angle remains positive beyond 10 degrees of flexion. The patellar tilt angle of control knees was always positive (open laterally) in the first 30 degrees of flexion. None of the normal knees had a patellar tilt angle of less than 8 degrees in the first 30 degrees of flexion. Therefore a patella was considered tilted if it showed a tilt of less than 8 degrees in any position between 0 and 30 degrees of flexion.

It should be remarked that both the congruence angle and the patellar tilt angle are necessary to describe an abnormal position of the patella. An abnormal congruence angle indicates lateral displacement of the patella (or lateral subluxation), whereas an abnormal patellar tilt angle indicates that the patella is tilted. These changes may occur independently. Based on measurements in normal knees, it was established that a normal patella should be centered by 10 degrees of flexion (congruence angle, 0 degrees or less) and that the patellar tilt angle should be open laterally at least 8 degrees in the arc of motion between 0 and 30 degrees.

According to these criteria, three categories of abnormal patellar position were defined: subluxated, tilted, and tilted and subluxated (Fig. 67.35). Knees with subluxation showed a high congruence angle (average: +23 degrees) in extension, which progressively reduced (average: +8 degrees) at 30 degrees of flexion. Knees with subluxation could be further divided into those with an associated tilt and those without. The first group had a patellar tilt near 0 degrees throughout the range of motion, which is significantly different from controls. A third group included knees with an isolated patellar tilt. In these cases the patellar tilt angle was slightly decreased in extension (10 degrees versus 18 degrees in controls) and was decreased further with flexion at 30 degrees (when it was 2 degrees versus 16 degrees in controls).

The use of CT is recommended in patients with persistent knee symptoms and normal-appearing axial radiographic views at 30 and 45 degrees. Results from different centers seem to confirm that a normal patella is slightly displaced laterally in full extension (with a positive congruence angle) but that it reduces early in flexion by 10 or 15 degrees of flexion. The patellar tilt angle, measured as the angle between the lateral patellar facet and either the tangent to the posterior condyles[47] or the tangent to the medial and lateral trochlear facets,[64] should be open laterally throughout the same arc of motion in normal knees. Knees affected by patellar subluxation or dislocation show excessive lateral displacement and lateral patellar tilt, which are more evident in extension but tend to reduce in flexion.

In 1978 Goutallier and Bernageau[49] described the method of radiologic measurement (with 30-degree axial views) of the distance between the apex of the tibial tuberosity and the deepest point of the trochlear groove. The tibial tuberosity–sulcus femoralis (TT-SF) distance, also termed the tibial tubercle–trochlear groove (TT-TG) distance, gives a measure of the valgus vector that is imposed on the extensor mechanism at a given degree of flexion. Because the tibial tuberosity lies lateral to the sulcus femoralis, the greater the TT-SF distance, the higher the valgus vector. The TT-SF distance gives a true measure of the Q angle because it is independent of the position of the patella. It is well known that the clinical Q angle in extension may be normal in knees with recurrent subluxation or dislocation. This is due to the lateral displacement of the patella, which leads to an underestimate of the true Q angle. Goutallier and Bernageau[49] reported that the average value in a

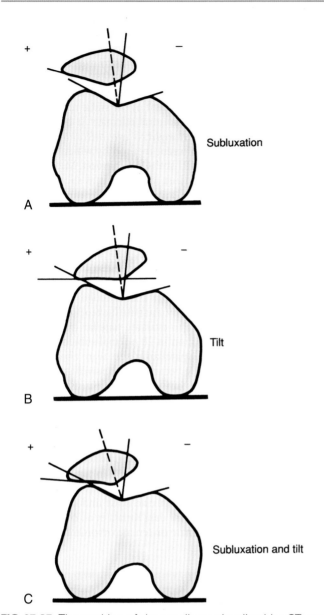

FIG 67.35 The position of the patella as visualized by CT may present the following abnormalities: (A) Subluxation with a positive congruence angle persisting beyond 10 degrees of flexion. (B) Tilt with a lateral patellofemoral angle less than 8 degrees in the first 30 degrees of flexion. (C) Subluxation and tilt when both abnormalities are present.

group of 16 normal knees was 13 mm (range: 7 to 17 mm). This distance was increased in most knees with patellofemoral osteoarthritis or recurrent subluxation of the patella. The introduction of CT offered the possibility of measuring the TT-SF distance in full extension by obtaining a first cut through the proximal part of the femoral sulcus and a second cut through the tibial tuberosity. Both should be perpendicular to the long axis of the bones. Dejour et al.[38] later reported that the average TT-SF distance in normal knees in extension is 12.7 mm, whereas in knees with patellar instability it is 19.8 mm. When 20 mm was used as the borderline value, the distance was greater than this value in 3% of control knees; the same was true in 56% of knees with patellar instability. The reproducibility of the measurement was fair, within 4 mm.

Anley et al.[11] analyzed imaging from 141 knees in patients with patellofemoral disorders. They reviewed both MRI and CT scans of the same knee and found the TT-SF to be statistically different when measured by MRI (13.56 ± 6.07 mm) versus CT (17.72 ± 5.15 mm). The intraclass correlation coefficient (ICC) was only fair (0.54 and 0.48) and, from this, implied that the established values for TT-SF based on CT should not be applied to MRI.

Aglietti used axial views according to Merchant et al.[96] and Laurin et al.[84] and CT in 20 and 30 degrees of flexion to evaluate patellofemoral congruence in a group of 86 knees.[4] Aglietti et al. included 20 controls, 25 knees with patellar instability, and 41 knees with patellar pain. In the patellar instability group the height of the patella was significantly increased in comparison with controls when both the Insall-Salvati and Blackburne and Peel methods were used, whereas the group with patellar pain did not significantly differ from controls. In the Merchant view the sulcus angle and the congruence angle of the patellar pain group were not significantly different from controls, whereas both values were significantly increased in the instability group. In the Laurin view the lateral patellofemoral angle and the patellofemoral index were significantly increased in the instability group but not in the pain group. In the CT scan at 30 degrees, values of the sulcus angle, congruence angle, patellar tilt angle, and sulcus depth were significantly different in the instability group, with a shallower sulcus, a subluxated and tilted patella, and reduced height of the lateral femoral condyle. The patellar pain group showed a significant difference (at the lowest level) from the control group in only congruence angle and sulcus depth. The average TT-SF distance was 8.7 mm in controls, 10.2 mm in the pain group, and 14.7 mm in the instability group. The difference between controls and the instability group was significant. Measurements of these parameters on scans with the knee at 20 degrees of flexion did not significantly differ from those at 30 degrees.

We continue to use CT in the evaluation of knees with patellofemoral disorders and have expanded its use to include four degrees of flexion: 0, 15, 30, and 45 degrees. At each angle of flexion, two cuts are made: through the tibia and through the patellofemoral joint. The tibial cut is made through the tibial tuberosity and at 90 degrees to the tibial axis (Fig. 67.36). The femoral cut is oriented to pass through the middle of the patella and the posterior femoral condyles. Because the apex of the patella is a nonarticular surface, a cut passing through the middle of the patellar height actually passes through the lower third of the articular surface. This is the part that contacts the femoral trochlea in the first 30 degrees of flexion. The femoral cut should pass posteriorly through the most posterior aspect of the femoral condyles, so that a reference line tangent to the condyles can be reliably identified. On the femoral cut we measure the sulcus and congruence angles,[96] the patellar tilt angle,[117] and the sulcus depth.[117] Furthermore, by superimposing the femoral and tibial cuts, the TT-SF distance can be measured (Fig. 67.37). Examples of CT at 0, 15, 30, and 45 degrees of flexion in a knee with recurrent dislocation and patellar pain are given in Figs. 67.38 to 67.40, respectively.

Use of CT imaging for exploration of the patellofemoral relationship has led to a better understanding of the dynamics of this joint in normal and pathologic knees, and its usefulness for scientific purposes is widely accepted.[54,102] However, in knees with recurrent episodes of patellar dislocation the degree of anatomic abnormality is such that it is promptly appreciated on a traditional axial view. If distal realignment is being considered, knowledge of the TT-SF distance may allow more anatomic reconstruction of the joint and thus avoid overcorrection of the transposition itself in knees with a normal TT-SF distance. The usefulness of CT images is probably greatest in knees with patellofemoral disturbances and normal-appearing axial views if some abnormality can be disclosed in a more extended position.

Magnetic Resonance Imaging. MRI is now an established diagnostic modality for the knee.[71,99,128] It has been reported to be an accurate diagnostic tool for meniscal and cruciate

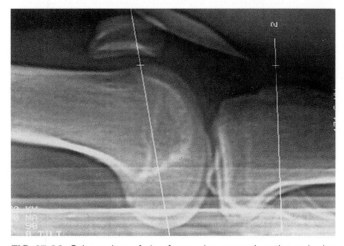

FIG 67.36 Orientation of the femoral cut passing through the middle of the patella, which corresponds to the lower third of the articular surface, and through the posterior aspect of the femoral condyles. Orientation of the tibial cut through the tibial tuberosity and at 90 degrees to the tibial axis.

ligament lesions. Because both osseous and soft tissue structures are visualized, it may be used to assess patellar tracking in the 0- to 30-degree arc of motion, as well as to evaluate lesions in patellar cartilage and the trochlea groove. MRI is also a valuable tool for detecting loose bodies in the knee after patellar dislocation, as well as accurate assessment of the static restraints, such as the MPFL, and any subchondral edema.[12] It has also been used to measure the patella height.

Biedert[13] proposed a different method by which to evaluate patellar height based on MRI scans in extension. Measurements are taken in the central or just lateral sagittal slice, where the articular cartilage is thicker. Patellar articular cartilage is projected on trochlear cartilage, and the height of its projection is calculated. The ratio between trochlear articular cartilage height and patellar articular cartilage height is deemed the patellar index. Normal values are 12.5% to 50%. An index less than 12.5% signifies patella alta, whereas an index higher than 50% indicates patella baja. The main advantage of this method is that it takes into consideration only the articular cartilage very precisely and is not affected by the patellar tendon.

Kujala et al.[79] used MRI to evaluate patellar tracking in the 0- to 30-degree arc of motion in 20 normal subjects (10 males and 10 females). Axial midpatellar images were obtained. They found that the sulcus angle became progressively sharper from full extension to 30 degrees of flexion and decreased 13 degrees on average. The lateral patellofemoral angle[84] increased an average of 6 ± 5 degrees during flexion, and lateral patellar displacement[83] decreased an average of 4 ± 3 mm with flexion. The congruence angle[96] shifted 31 degrees (±13 degrees) medially during flexion. In extension the congruence angle was positive (open laterally) in all knees except in one male. At 30 degrees of flexion the congruence angle was negative (open medially) in all knees except in one male and one female, in whom it was zero. Citing these data Kujala et al. concluded that a normal knee (whether male or female) should be congruent

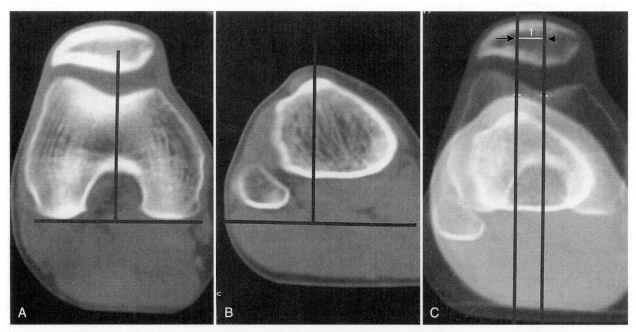

FIG 67.37 (A–C) Measurement of the (TT-SF) distance. By superimposing the femoral and tibial cuts, the distance between the deepest point of the sulcus and the tibial tuberosity can be measured. Values greater than 20 mm with the knee in extension are considered pathologic.

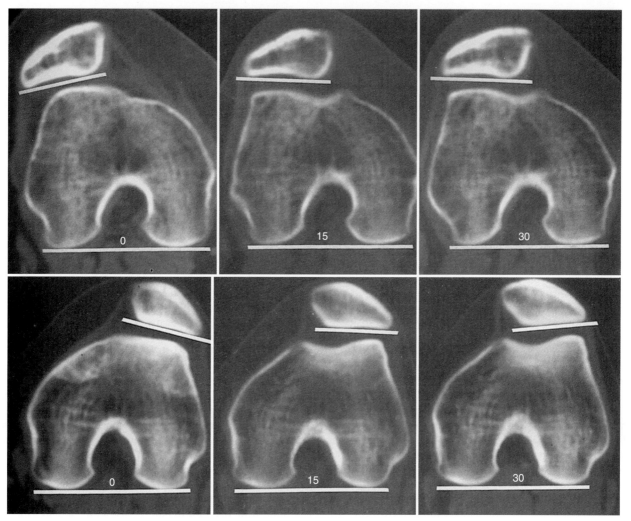

FIG 67.38 CT images at 0, 15, and 30 degrees of flexion in two knees affected by recurrent dislocation of the patella. Proceeding from extension to flexion, the congruence angle, the sulcus angle, and the PT angle are reduced, mainly between 0 and 15 degrees of flexion.

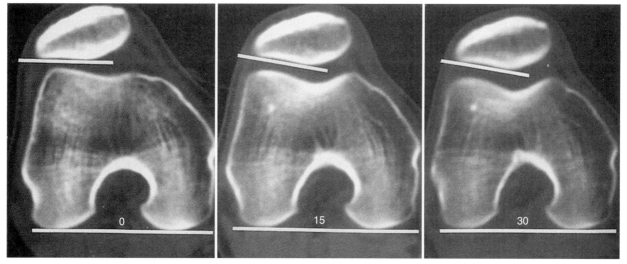

FIG 67.39 CT images of a knee affected by patellar pain. The patella is tilted laterally in extension, but almost normal congruence is restored by 15 degrees of flexion.

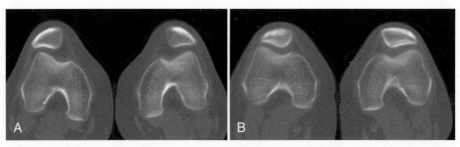

FIG 67.40 (A) CT of patella at 30 degrees demonstrates that the patellae are subluxated laterally. (B) CT of patella at 40 degrees demonstrates that the same patellae are tracking centrally in the sulcus.

(congruence angle: 0 degrees or negative) by 30 degrees of flexion (but not necessarily in a lesser degree of flexion). Females were found to have significantly more laterally displaced patellae at 10 and 20 degrees of flexion, but the other differences were not significant.

Kujala et al.[80] compared the measurements obtained from normal knees and knees affected by recurrent patellar dislocation. For this study 10 women with normal knees and 11 women with recurrent subluxation were selected. Midpatellar sagittal and axial images were used to measure patellar length, patellar tendon length, Insall-Salvati ratio (T:P), sulcus angle, congruence angle, lateral patellofemoral angle, lateral patellar displacement, and depth of the femoral sulcus. Knees with recurrent patellar dislocation showed higher values for sulcus angle, lateral patellar displacement, and congruence angle, and lower values for the lateral patellofemoral angle, which indicates that dislocating patellae were more lateralized and were tilted laterally. The differences were more evident in extension and were gradually reduced when proceeding toward flexion. Statistical analysis showed that the two groups were most clearly differentiated by the sulcus angle at 10 degrees and by the lateral patellofemoral angle at 0 degrees. Kujala et al. concluded that in patients with recurrent dislocation, tilt and lateralization of the patella are more evident in early flexion. All control patellae were congruent at 30 degrees, but the same was true for most (77%) of the dislocating patellae. Therefore differences between normal and dislocating patellae are most evident at the beginning of flexion (0 to 10 degrees).

MRI has been used to investigate knees with acute patellar dislocation.[112] This has led to a better understanding of the pathoanatomy of this condition. A series of 23 knees were examined with x-ray and MRI, followed by arthroscopy (19 knees) and open exploration of medial soft tissues (16 knees). Clinically 83% of the knees exhibited moderate-to-large effusion, and 70% had tenderness over the posteromedial soft tissues and the adductor tubercle (Bassett sign). Radiographs revealed osteochondral fracture of the patella in 21% of cases and fracture of the lateral femoral condyle in 5%. MRI showed moderate-to-large effusion in all knees. A tear of the femoral insertion of the medial patellofemoral ligament (at the adductor tubercle) was present in 87% (20 knees). Two knees had a significant sprain of the medial patellofemoral ligament without detachment. One knee had a detachment of the medial retinaculum from the margin of the patella. Variable amounts of retraction of the VMO and increased signal were present in 78%. Bony injuries were noted in 87% of lateral femoral condyles near the sulcus terminalis and in 30% of patellae medially.

Balcarek et al.[12] used MRI to identify the injury pattern to the MPFL status post acute lateral patellar dislocation, considering trochlear dysplasia, patella alta, and TT-TG distance. They compared a study group of 73 knees following acute patellar dislocation with an age- and gender-matched control group. Inclusion criteria were joint effusion, contusion (edema) on the lateral femoral condyle or medial patellar facet, and osteochondral fragments and injuries to the medial soft tissue stabilizers, including the MCL, MPFL, VMO, and medial retinaculum. Injury to the MPFL was found in 98.6% of their study group. In accordance with prior studies the MPFL was injured most commonly from the femoral insertion (36 of 73), midsubstance in 10 of 72, and at the patella insertion in 10 of 73. The average patella height index was found to be significantly increased in the study group, as was the number of dysplastic trochleas and the TT-TG distance, when compared with the control group.

It appears that detachment of the medial patellofemoral ligament from its insertion into the adductor tubercle is the most frequent lesion in acute dislocation of the patella. This is consistent with the biomechanical work of Conlan et al.,[32] who showed that the medial patellofemoral ligament was the primary restraint to lateral patellar dislocation and provided 53% of the total restraining force, followed by the patellomeniscal ligament, which contributed 22%. Detachment of the VMO from the adductor tubercle was also evident from MRI and surgical findings.

A predictable pattern of soft tissue injury and bony contusions can be seen in MRI studies of patients with prior dislocation of the patella. Soft tissue findings include joint effusion, disruption of the MPFL, injury to the medial retinaculum, and disruption of the VMO attachment. The typical osteochondral pattern of injury occurs when the medial facet of the patella impacts the lateral femoral condyle. This results in osteochondral fracture or contusion of the medial patellar facet and the lateral femoral condyle. Elias et al.[42,43] compared MRI of 81 knees with previous lateral patellar dislocation versus 100 knees with no history of dislocation. In knees with prior lateral dislocation, investigators found contusions on the lateral femoral condyle in 80% and on the medial patella in 61%. They concluded that the specific finding of a concave impaction deformity in the inferomedial aspect of the patella has 44% sensitivity but 100% specificity for lateral patellar dislocation. Furthermore, they found injury to the MPFL in only 49% of patellae in which the MPFL was visualized and edema surrounding the VMO attachment in only 45% of knees with lateral patellar dislocation. The authors stated that perhaps transverse images, as were used in this study, are not optimal for imaging these oblique structures and that transverse oblique images may be of higher yield for detecting injury to these structures. This may account for their low rate of medial soft tissue injury compared with other studies.[32,112] It is important to note that the MPFL cannot always be visualized on MRI studies,[113] and in this study it was visualized in only 87% of patients with dislocation and 80% of control subjects. The authors suggest that increased edema surrounding this structure after patellar dislocation may lead to higher rates of visualization in patients with prior dislocation compared with controls.

Sanders et al.[113] compared MRI findings in 14 knees with known dislocation versus surgical findings in these same knees. MPFL injury was detected in all 14 knees on MRI, and this was confirmed at the time of surgical exploration. MRI detected complete disruption of the MPFL in 57% and wavy or partial disruption in 43%. At the time of surgery the MPFL was found to be completely disrupted in 50% of cases and partially disrupted in the other 50%. The authors concluded that the MPFL was injured in 100% of cases, and that MRI was 85% sensitive and 70% accurate in diagnosing MPFL injury. They also compared VMO findings in these 14 knees versus 100 control MR images of knees that had no clinical or radiographic evidence of dislocation. The VMO was found to be elevated off the medial femoral condyle in 85% of injured knees, and edema was noted within the VMO tendon and muscle in 93% of all dislocators. No evidence of edema in the VMO was found in any of the 100 control knees. Furthermore, a significant difference was noted between the extent of elevation of the VMO in dislocators and in the 100 control knees. Average elevation of the VMO in dislocators was 1.7 cm compared with 0.18 cm in control knees.

MRI is frequently used to investigate patellar cartilage. Yulish et al.[143] compared the results of 23 MRI examinations with findings at arthroscopy: 3 patients were asymptomatic volunteers and 20 had patellar symptoms. Normal patellar cartilage appears uniformly smooth on axial and sagittal MRI views, with a signal intensity that is intermediate between that of cortical and cancellous bone. MRI alterations in patellar cartilage were classified as follows:

Stage 1: Areas of swelling with decreased signal intensity.

Stage 2: Irregularity of the articular surface with focal thinning.

Stage 3: Absence of cartilage with exposure of subchondral bone or synovial fluid extending through the ulcer to subchondral bone.

MRI correctly predicted arthroscopic findings in 20 of 22 knees (91%). It missed a knee with softening of the patella and diagnosed a chondral fracture that was not confirmed by arthroscopy. The presence of joint fluid visible on T2-weighted images was useful in detecting the presence of cartilage ulcers, through which fluid leaked to subchondral bone.

An experimental study has compared the accuracy of CT-arthrography and MRI in detecting patellar cartilage lesions. Drill holes ranging from 0.8 to 5 mm in diameter and from 1 to 2 mm in depth were produced in cadaver knees. Double-contrast CT-arthrography easily detected 3- and 5-mm holes, but 50% of 1.5- and 2-mm lesions were missed. The 0.8-mm holes were not recognized at all. On the contrary, MRI detected the smallest 0.8-mm lesions because they were precisely delineated by intra-articular fluid, which appears bright on T2-weighted images.

In a clinical study 54 knees were examined by MRI, and evidence of a cartilage lesion was found in 44 cases. However, at arthroscopy the corresponding lesion was found in only 34 knees (77%), whereas no chondral lesion or softening was noted in the remaining 10 knees. When compared with arthroscopy, MRI had 81.5% accuracy, 100% sensitivity, and 50% specificity. As far as staging of the lesion, it was correctly predicted by MRI in 76% of cases, overrated in 5.8%, and underrated in 17.6%. Using these data, Handelberg et al.[56] proposed an MRI classification of chondral lesions. It is recognized that MRI yields a discrete incidence of false-positive results, possibly because of detection of early lesions in deep layers of cartilage that are not visualized at arthroscopy. They are evident as linear, dark areas in the gray signal of cartilage. Additional studies are needed to confirm whether these findings represent early lesions or a variation of normal anatomy.

Stage I lesions, described as softening at arthroscopy, are usually visible as round areas of low signal intensity on "proton density" and T2-weighted images.

Stage II lesions correspond to fissures that appear as zones of low signal surrounding the high signal of fluid leaking into the cleft.

Stage III lesions correspond to superficial or deep defects that appear as bright images because of the synovial fluid that fills them.

Stage IV lesions involve thinning and irregularity of cartilage, as found in degenerative arthritis.

MRI is most useful in predicting the location and extent of articular cartilage disease, which is an important factor in determination of which surgical intervention is appropriate. A distal realignment can be added to a proximal realignment in an attempt to unload the affected area of cartilage; however, a lesion in the proximal pole does not lend itself well to unloading because the zone of contact becomes more and more proximal as the knee flexes. Furthermore, MRI can be used to identify patellar congruence, patellar tilt, patellar morphology, trochlear morphology, and soft tissue injury, such as MPFL and VMO injury. Osteochondral fractures of the medial facet of the patella and the lateral femoral condyle are commonly detected by MRI. Use of MRI in the treatment of patellar instability is increasing and may become the one image modality of choice, as quality of the images improves, allowing bony anatomy traditionally imaged with CT to be more clearly visualized, without ionizing radiation. More recent analysis does suggest that MRI could be used to assess all of the measurements associated with patellofemoral instability. Charles et al.[27] analyzed 40 patients with recurrent patella instability and compared their measurements to 81 controls. Measurements of patellar tilt, trochlear morphologic characteristics, TT-SF, patellar height (Insall-Salvati and Caton-Deschamps ratios), and trochlear shape were found to be statistically different from the controls. Further studies are required to fully establish the pathologic cut-offs for these measurements using MRI instead of radiographs and CT.

Our approach to imaging of patellofemoral instability begins with standing anteroposterior and lateral views, as well as a Merchant view of the patella. We evaluate the knee joint for coronal and rotational alignment. Attention is paid to identifying patella alta and any trochlear or patellar dysplasia that would predispose to patellar instability. On the axial view of the patellofemoral joint, we pay particular attention to the congruence and sulcus angles. The lateral patellofemoral angle is assessed for evidence of lateral patellar tilt. CT scan may be used to better evaluate rotational abnormalities and the anatomy of the patellofemoral joint. MRI is used when cartilage injury or loose body is suspected and to rule out other soft tissue and ligamentous injuries.

Classification of Patellar Subluxation and Dislocation

Patellar subluxation and patellar dislocation can be grouped together as patellar instability. The difference is one of degree and not of nature. Subluxation is an alteration in the normal tracking of the patella but with the patella still within the femoral sulcus. Dislocation means that the patella has been completely displaced out of the sulcus. Therefore, unless the patient has noted the patella lying on the lateral aspect of the knee, it appears that it may be impossible to know whether the patella was subluxated or dislocated during the single episode of instability. Furthermore, the patella may show lateralized tracking without episodes of instability (chronic subluxation of the patella).

Many classifications of patellofemoral disorders are known, all of which include several types of patellofemoral instability. These classification systems include the presence or absence of trauma, malalignment, and articular cartilage damage (Boxes 67.1 and 67.2). When classifying patellofemoral instability, we believe that it is important to consider three main factors: chronicity, presence or absence of malalignment, and the condition of the articular cartilage.[37] In doing so we can define patellar instability as acute (generally traumatic) or recurrent (chronic). This classification system helps to guide treatment tailored to the individual patient, as seen in Table 67.2.

Treatments

Nonoperative Treatment. Conservative treatment should be attempted in knees with acute and recurrent patellar instability. It is based on strengthening of the quadriceps and VMO and stretching of the tight lateral structures, as previously described. The frequency of the episodes of instability may be reduced so that surgery is no longer necessary. If disabling symptoms persist, surgical treatment is indicated. Because of the high rate of recurrence and dissatisfaction, many are advocates for early surgical intervention.[22] Unfortunately, the results in the literature are mixed, and it is still unclear whether nonoperative treatment or early surgical intervention will lead to better long-term outcomes and more satisfied patients. A review

---

BOX 67.1   Insall's Classification of Patellofemoral Disorders

Presence of Cartilage Damage

Chondromalacia
Osteoarthritis
Osteochondral fractures
Osteochondritis dissecans

Variable Cartilage Damage

Malalignment syndromes
Synovial plicae

Usually Normal Cartilage

Peripatellar causes: bursitis, tendinitis
Overuse syndromes
Reflex sympathetic dystrophy
Patellar abnormalities

Data from Insall JN: Disorders of the patella. In Insall JN (ed): *Surgery of the knee*, New York, 1984, Churchill Livingstone, p 191.

BOX 67.2   Merchant's Classification of Patellofemoral Disorder

I. Trauma (conditions caused by trauma in an otherwise normal knee)

A. Acute trauma

1. Contusion
2. Fracture
   a. Patella
   b. Femoral trochlea
   c. Proximal tibial epiphysis (tubercle)
3. Dislocation (rare in a normal knee)
4. Rupture
   a. Quadriceps tendon
   b. Patellar tendon

B. Repetitive trauma (overuse syndromes)

1. Patellar tendinitis ("jumper's knee")
2. Quadriceps tendinitis
3. Peripatellar tendinitis (eg, anterior knee pain in an adolescent as a result of hamstring contracture)
4. Prepatellar bursitis ("housemaid's knee")
5. Apophysitis
   a. Osgood-Schlatter disease
   b. Sinding-Larsen-Johansson disease

C. Late effects of trauma

1. Post-traumatic chondromalacia patellae
2. Post-traumatic patellofemoral arthritis
3. Anterior fat pad syndrome (post-traumatic fibrosis)
4. Reflex sympathetic dystrophy of the patella
5. Patellar osseous dystrophy
6. Acquired patella infera
7. Acquired quadriceps fibrosis

II. Patellofemoral dysplasia

A. Lateral patellar compression syndrome

1. Secondary chondromalacia patellae
2. Secondary patellofemoral arthritis

B. Chronic subluxation of the patella

1. Secondary chondromalacia patellae
2. Secondary patellofemoral arthritis

C. Recurrent dislocation of the patella

1. Associated fractures
   a. Osteochondral (intra-articular)
   b. Avulsion (extra-articular)
2. Secondary chondromalacia patellae
3. Secondary patellofemoral arthritis

D. Chronic dislocation of the patella

1. Congenital
2. Acquired

III. Idiopathic chondromalacia patellae
IV. Osteochondritis dissecans
A. Patella
B. Femoral trochlea

V. Synovial plicae (anatomic variant made symptomatic by acute or repetitive trauma)
A. Medial patellar ("shelf")
B. Suprapatellar
C. Lateral patellar

From Merchant AC: Classification of patellofemoral disorders. *Arthroscopy* 4:235, 1988.[95]

of the literature by Smith et al.[126] suggested that there were not enough quality studies devoid of bias to make a clear statement of operative versus nonoperative treatment; however, it is possible that a population of patients would benefit from early intervention.

Several authors have attempted to define the prognosis after conservative treatment of acute patellar dislocation (Table 67.3). Cofield and Bryan[30] reported a discouraging experience in which 52% of their 50 cases were rated as failures. In light of their experience they recommend selective immediate repair in patients with anatomic variants that would contribute to recurrence in high-level athletes and in knees with displaced intra-articular fractures. Larsen and Lauridsen[81] reviewed 79 acute patellar dislocations. A relevant primary trauma was reported in 41 cases (52%), whereas in 38 (48%), the trauma had been minor or absent. Patella alta and increased passive patellar mobility were more frequent in patients with atraumatic dislocations. Dislocation was more frequently atraumatic in females (57%) than in males (32%). Younger patients had a higher incidence of predisposing factors, which were present in 84% of patients younger than 14 years, in 69% between 15 and 19 years, and in 41% between 20 and 29 years. In agreement with this finding, redislocation was more likely in younger patients (<20 years of age).

Mäenpää and Lehto[86] reviewed a series of 100 acute patellar dislocations with long-term follow-up (average: 13 years; range: 6 to 26 years). Patients were treated initially with a cast (60 knees), a splint (17 knees), or a bandage (23 knees), according to the physician's preference. At follow-up, 13% had restricted extension, 21% had restricted flexion, 61% had retropatellar crepitation, and the apprehension test yielded positive results in 52%. Redislocation had occurred in 44% of knees. The redislocation rate per follow-up year was 0.29 in the patellar

TABLE 67.2 Classification of Patellofemoral Diagnosis and Suggested Surgical Treatment

Diagnosis	Surgical Treatment
Lateral patellar compression syndrome	Lateral release
Patellar subluxation	Lateral release
	Proximal realignment
	Proximal and distal realignment
Acute patellar dislocation	Repair medial retinaculum and lateral release
	Proximal realignment
Recurrent patellar dislocation	Proximal realignment
	Proximal and distal realignment
Malalignment with severe chondromalacia	Fulkerson anteromedialization
	Maquet osteotomy
	Patellectomy

With kind permission of Springer Science+Business Media.
From Scuderi GR: *The patella*, New York, 1995, Springer-Verlag, p 223 (see Table 11.1).

TABLE 67.3 Prognosis After Conservative Treatment of Acute Patellar Dislocation

Author	Year	No. of Knees	Treatment	AVERAGE Follow-Up, Mo	Redislocation, (%)	Remarks
Cofield and Bryan[30]	1977	50	Conservative	44	High redislocation rate	52% of knees were considered unsatisfactory; 27% required further surgery
McManus et al.[94]	1979	26	Cast for 6 weeks	31	19	Dislocations in children; 42% complained of instability without dislocation; 38% were asymptomatic
Larsen and Lauridsen[81]	1982	79	Cast or bandage	71	NA	Unable to define factors that may predispose to redislocation except age younger than 20 years
Hawkins et al.[58]	1986	20	Arthroscopy (9), cast (11)	40	15	All patients who experienced redislocation had obvious lower limb malalignment; some degree of pain was present in 75% of cases
Cash and Hughston[25]	1988	74	Cast	96	36	Recurrence rate is higher in presence of signs of patellofemoral dysplasia of the opposite knee (43%) than when these are absent (20%); higher redislocation rate in younger patients
Garth et al.[48]	1996	39	Functional padded sleeve	46	20	One third of cases remain unsatisfactory according to subjective and objective criteria
Mäenpää and Lehto[86]	1997	100	Cast (60), splint (17), bandage (23)	156	44	44% redislocation, 19% patellofemoral pain or subluxation; only 37% without complaints

NA, Not available.

bandage group, 0.12 in the cast group, and 0.08 in the splint group. Beyond the 44% incidence of recurrent dislocation, a 19% incidence of patellofemoral pain or subluxation was reported. Only 37% of patients had no complaints at the time of follow-up. This series suggests that application of a splint may be preferable to both cast and bandage. However, the duration of immobilization was different in each of the three groups. Therefore redislocation rates are influenced by both type and length of immobilization. Furthermore, immobilization was found to result in a high rate of stiffness in this series.

Garth et al.[48] reported the results of 39 knees with acute patellar dislocation that were treated functionally. Treatment included immediate straight-leg raising exercises followed by the application of a laterally padded knee sleeve and immediate mobilization. Average follow-up was 46 months (range: 24 to 71 months). Six patients (15%) experienced recurrent instability. Good or excellent results were achieved in 67% of knees subjectively and in 69% objectively. This means that results after functional treatment of acute patellar dislocation were not satisfactory in approximately a third of the knees. These results are similar to those achieved with cast immobilization. However, functional treatment avoids the deleterious effects of immobilization and decreases the convalescence time.

A prospective nonrandomized study compared 40 patients with acute first-time patellar dislocation who were treated with nonoperative or acute operative repair of injured medial structures.[123] The nonoperative group was immobilized from 0 to 30 for 3 weeks, then from 0 to 90 until week 6, at which point full range of motion was permitted and a guided muscle-strengthening program was initiated. The surgical group was treated with surgical stabilization at an average of 7 days after injury. Fourteen patients were treated with reefing of the medial soft tissues, and four patients were treated with the Roux-Goldthwait procedure, in which the lateral aspect of the patellar tendon was sutured to the medial aspect of the tibia. The surgical group had no redislocations and only two (12%) painful subluxations at a 7-year follow-up. The nonoperative group had six (29%) redislocations and four painful subluxations. Thus the nonoperative group had 10 (48%) patients with symptomatic instability.

Bitar et al.[19] performed a randomized controlled trial of nonoperative versus MPFL reconstruction using patellar tendon graft. Forty-two knees were randomly assigned to one of the two groups with a minimum of 2 years of follow-up. The surgical group reported fewer (0% versus 35%) recurrences and higher Kujala[78] scores (71.43% good or excellent versus 25%) when compared with the nonoperative group.

A high rate of recurrent instability is clearly seen with nonoperative treatment; however, most of the authors would agree that a trial of nonoperative treatment should be attempted. Further studies are required to elucidate which factors contribute to successful nonoperative management. A summary of the studies that have looked at nonoperative treatment of acute patellar dislocation is provided in Table 67.3.

Operative Treatment
Lateral Release and Proximal Realignment
Lateral retinacular release. Although the results of isolated lateral retinacular release (LRR) for patellar instability have been notoriously poor, this procedure was popular for many years and has now mostly falling out of favor. Ostermeier et al.[107] performed an in vitro study on eight fresh frozen cadaver

specimens, investigating the effects of lateral release on contact pressures of the patellofemoral joint. They found that contact pressures within the joint did not change significantly; however, the central contact point moved more medial between 60 and 120 degrees of flexion, thus unloading the lateral facet of the patella. The authors were therefore guarded on its use for patella instability but thought it may help for anterior knee pain.

Results in knees affected by recurrent patellar subluxation and dislocation are reported in Table 67.4. The reported percentage of satisfactory results varies between 30% and 100%. However, rating systems used were not uniformly stringent. We think that any patient with persistent symptoms of instability cannot be included among satisfactory results. Dandy and Griffiths[36] report on 41 knees that underwent lateral release for recurrent dislocation. The average follow-up was 4 years. Ninety percent of knees were classified as satisfactory according to the rating system of Crosby and Insall.[33] However, only 44% of the patellae were stable, 24% were occasionally insecure, and 32% underwent at least one redislocation.

Using an average follow-up of 8 years, Dandy and Desai[35] reviewed 33 knees in which the previous follow-up had been 4 years.[36] The percentage of satisfactory results decreased from 90% at 4 years to 72% at 8 years. Thirty-two percent of the patellae had dislocated at least once before the 4-year follow-up. Twenty-one percent (seven knees) continued to dislocate and underwent tibial tubercle transposition. Subluxation in extension and generalized ligamentous laxity correlated with an increased failure rate. The authors concluded that with these conditions, lateral release does not correct recurrent dislocation.

Aglietti et al. reported that their experience with LRR for recurrent dislocation of the patella was not completely satisfactory either. They reviewed 21 knees.[2] The group included 12 females and 9 males whose age averaged 21 years (range: 12 to 48 years). The operation was performed with the arthroscopic technique described by Metcalf[97] in 18 cases and with an open technique in 3 knees; 20 patients (95%) were reviewed, with an average follow-up of 66 months (range: 22 to 101 months). Most patients (90%) had no pain or swelling at follow-up, but one knee (5%) showed instability during sports activity and six knees (29%) during daily living activities. Therefore only 66% of results could be considered satisfactory. On the axial view at 45 degrees of flexion[96] the congruence angle was 19 degrees preoperatively and decreased to 3 degrees at follow-up, but it was still abnormal in 37% of cases. When satisfactory and unsatisfactory results were compared to identify predictive factors, investigators found that the prognosis was worse in females ($p = 0.05$) and in knees with more than five preoperative dislocations ($p = 0.05$). The persistence of lateral patellar tracking at follow-up was evaluated clinically ($p = 0.02$), and a deficit on the one-leg hop test for a distance greater than 15% ($p = 0.05$) correlated with an unsatisfactory result. No correlation was found between the results and generalized joint laxity, passive patellar tilt, congruence angle at follow-up, patellar height, and degree of chondromalacia.

Lattermann et al.[82] performed a review of the literature on lateral release. They found no level I evidence and only level V evidence in the literature. After review of these retrospective studies they concluded that isolated lateral release had little or no place in the treatment of patellar instability. They recommend the use of isolated lateral release in cases of lateral patellar compression syndrome with a clearly tight lateral retinaculum.

TABLE 67.4   Results of Lateral Retinacular Release for Recurrent Patellar Subluxation and Dislocation

Author	Year	No. of Knees	Follow-Up, Mo	Type of Release	AVERAGE % Satisfactory Result	Remarks
Metcalf[97]	1982	14	48	Arthroscopic	100	No redislocations
Chen and Ramanathan[26a]	1984	39	72	Closed	86	Includes 15 acute dislocations, 9 recurrent subluxations, and 15 recurrent dislocations, with similar success rates in the 3 groups
Simpson and Barrett[124]	1984	32	15	Arthroscopic	86	Worse results with age <30 years, incomplete release, quadriceps weakness, and generalized laxity
Ogilvie-Harris and Jackson[105]	1984	46	60	Arthroscopic	44	Results correlate closely with degree of chondromalacia: 100% satisfactory with grade I chondromalacia but only 25% with grade III
Schonholtz et al.[115]	1987	15	48	Closed	67	Better results than in pain syndromes
Betz et al.[17]	1987	31	48	Closed	74	Knees with subluxation had a higher recurrence rate (64%) than those with dislocation (14%); one patient experienced medial subluxation
Sherman et al.[122]	1987	45	28	Arthroscopic	75	One recurrence among 15 dislocations (6%); poor results more frequent in dislocators (39%) than in subluxers (15%)
Christensen et al.[28]	1988	30	54	Open	30	Deterioration of satisfactory results from the 1-year (73%) to the 4-year (30%) follow-up
Dandy and Griffiths[36]	1989	41	48	Arthroscopic	90	44% of patellae were stable; 24% were occasionally insecure, and 32% had had at least one redislocation; worse results in hyperlaxity and knees with dislocation in flexion
Aglietti et al.[5]	1989	20	66	Arthroscopic	65	35% experienced recurrent instability; worse results in females and knees with more than five preoperative dislocations
Dandy and Desai[35]	1994	33	96	Arthroscopic	72	

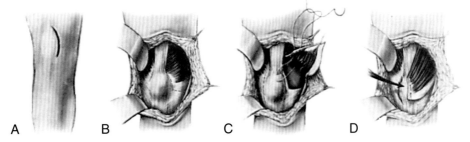

FIG 67.41 Technique of Quadricepsplasty Described by Madigan (A) Medial longitudinal incision. (B) Interrupted line indicating capsular incision to mobilize VMO. (C) Interrupted line indicating lateral retinacular relaxing incision. (D) Insertion of VMO is transferred laterally and distally. (From Madigan R, Wissinger HA, Donaldson WF: Preliminary experience with a method of quadricepsplasty in recurrent subluxation of the patella. *J Bone Joint Surg Am* 57:602, 1975.)

Lateral release is still indicated in proximal and distal realignment surgery.

Richetti et al.[110] performed a similar literature search comparing LRR versus LRR with medial soft tissue realignment (MR). They were only able to find level 3 and 4 evidence studies, and 14 studies met their inclusion criteria, which included 247 knees with LRR and 220 with LRR and MR. There were 56 patients with recurrent instability in the LRR group and only 14 in the LRR and MR group. The frequency-weighted mean success with respect to instability in the LRR studies was 77.3% compared with 93.6% in the LRR with MR studies.

In light of the high rates of failure and recurrent instability noted with lateral release alone, we have moved away from using this technique alone for the treatment of instability. We reserve the use of isolated lateral release for those patients with evidence of tight lateral retinaculum and with no evidence of malalignment and/or instability.

Insall's proximal realignment. The proximal realignment procedure was described by Insall et al. in 1976[69] and again in 1979.[68] This was a modification of the quadricepsplasty procedure described by Madigan et al. in 1975[85] (Fig. 67.41). Insall originally described the "tube" realignment (Fig. 67.42), which

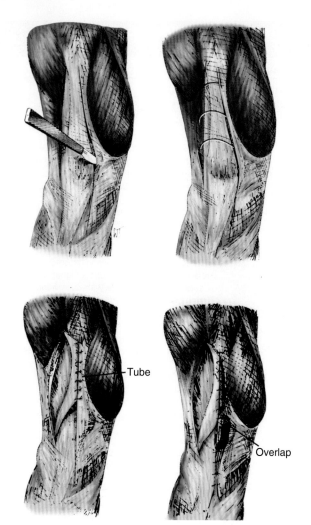

FIG 67.42 Proximal "tube" realignment as described by Insall (From Insall J, Bullough PG, Burstein AH: Proximal "tube" realignment of the patella for chondromalacia patellae. *Clin Orthop Relat Res* 144:63, 1979.)

he did not perform for very long before he modified it to the proximal realignment procedure that is now referred to as the Insall proximal realignment (Fig. 67.43). The procedure, as Insall stated, "... should not be considered merely a lateral retinacular release combined with a medial capsular reefing: it is in fact a quadricepsplasty in which the vastus lateralis is divided and the vastus medialis is advanced so that the line of pull of the quadriceps tendon is moved in a medial direction, thereby reducing the quadriceps angle ..."[68,69] The procedure as Insall described it is indeed an extensive lateral retinacular release combined with lateralization of the insertion of the vastus medialis muscle.[68,69] Specifically it improves the medial pull of the VMO, making it a more effective dynamic centralizing and stabilizing force on the patella. The method can be applied for both patellar pain and patellar dislocation syndromes.

The operation (see Figs. 67.43 and 67.44) is performed under tourniquet control after exsanguination of the limb by elevation or with an Esmarch bandage. A midline skin incision is made over the patella and the extensor mechanism (see video on the website). The incision should be sufficiently extensive that the components of the quadriceps muscle are clearly visible (Figs.

67.45 and 67.46). We have modified our technique by creating a smaller skin incision; however, adequate visualization should not be compromised for a smaller incision (see video on the website). Skin flaps should be raised deep to the fascia to make the skin flaps as thick as possible. Both the vastus medialis and vastus lateralis must be exposed, as well as the proximal extent of the quadriceps tendon and the insertion of the fibers from the rectus femoris. The arthrotomy is performed by making an incision beginning proximally at the apex of the quadriceps tendon and placed within the tendon close to the border of the vastus medialis. The incision is continued distally to the patella and is extended across the medial border of this bone, then distally medial to the patellar tendon. The incision described therefore is almost straight (see Fig. 67.43). The fibers of the quadriceps expansion medial to the incision are dissected from the bone with a scalpel (see video on the website).

Because of vertical ridges on the anterior surface of the patella, the incision can be difficult and should be performed with care to preserve the expansion intact without lacerations. This is necessary to obtain secure closure when the quadriceps repair is completed. The fibers of the expansion can be separated easily from the bone if the dissection proceeds from above and below alternately, thus forming a "V" and leaving the thinnest central part until last. When the procedure is performed in this manner, the central portion separates from the bone easily and can be fully preserved. After the medial border of the patella is reached, the synovial lining is incised. Proceeding distally, the fat pad is divided in the line of the capsular incision until the patella can be everted for inspection of the joint. Partial excision of the fat pad may be performed to avoid bulging of the fat pad through the lateral release.

After the medial arthrotomy is completed, the lateral release must be performed to adequately realign the extensor mechanism (Fig. 67.47). A second capsular incision is made on the lateral side, beginning proximally in the muscle fibers of the vastus lateralis and extending distally to the tibial tubercle (see video on the website). It is desirable but not essential to maintain the integrity of the synovium. Sometimes this is not possible because of tight fibrous bands in the substance of the synovium itself. A number of substantial vessels cross to the patella in the lateral retinaculum. At the level of the superior pole of the patella are two or three branches of the superior lateral geniculate vessels, which are large and bleed profusely if not ligated or coagulated. The branches of the inferior lateral geniculate vessels are smaller vessels that run beneath the retinaculum more distally at the lower pole of the patella; they are generally one or two in number. These vessels should also be identified and ligated or coagulated. Alternatively, an attempt can be made to preserve them.

The interior of the knee is thoroughly explored, and selective débridement is performed when necessary. In the malalignment syndrome, regardless of the extent of the patellar lesion, the femoral sulcus is usually normal. The exception is occasional evidence of an osteochondral fracture at the lateral border of the femoral sulcus caused by patellar dislocation (Fig. 67.48).

At this stage of the operation, the tourniquet should be released to enable coagulation of any bleeding points not previously identified. The knee should be flexed and slowly brought into extension while the bleeding vessels are systematically cauterized. Deflating the tourniquet ensures that the tourniquet does not alter the mechanics of the quadriceps muscle during realignment. The quadriceps must then be reconstructed in

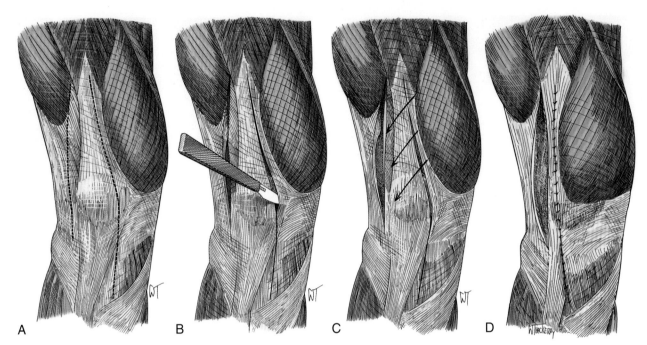

FIG 67.43 Insall's Proximal Realignment (A) After exposure of the quadriceps mechanism, two incisions are made. The first enters the knee joint by a capsular incision placed at the margin of the vastus medialis over the medial quarter of the patella and medial to the patellar tendon. The second is a lateral release extending into the fibers of the vastus lateralis. (B) To preserve continuity of the medial flap, the quadriceps expansion crossing the patella must be carefully preserved and separated by sharp dissection. (C) Realignment is effected by advancing the medial flap containing the vastus medialis laterally and distally in the line of the fibers of the oblique portion of the vastus medialis. (D) After suturing, the incision lies in a straight line across the front of the patella, and the lateral release should open widely.

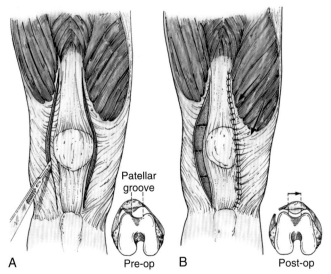

FIG 67.44 Proximal Realignment (A) The medial parapatellar arthrotomy and lateral release. (B) The medial flap is advanced laterally. (With kind permission of Springer Science+Business Media. From Scuderi GR: *The patella*, New York, 1995, Springer-Verlag, p 231.)

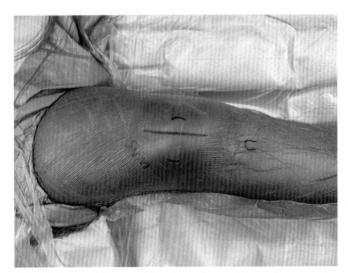

FIG 67.45 A midline incision is performed from the superior pole of the patella to about the level of the joint line. This incision may be extended to obtain adequate exposure.

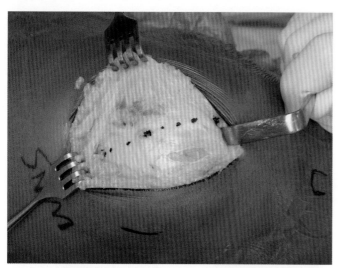

FIG 67.46 Thick skin flaps are made deep to the fascia over the extensor mechanism. A mobile window is created to keep the incision as small as possible so the procedure can be performed safely.

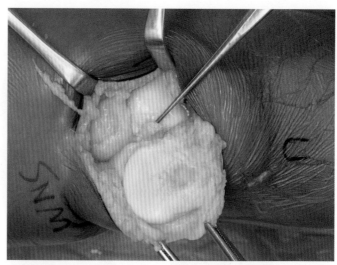

FIG 67.48 A common pattern of osteochondral injury seen on the medial facet of the patella and the lateral border of the femoral sulcus is caused by patellar dislocation.

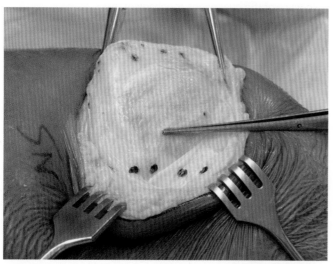

FIG 67.47 A capsular incision is made on the lateral side, beginning proximally in the muscle fibers of the vastus lateralis and extending distally to the tibial tubercle.

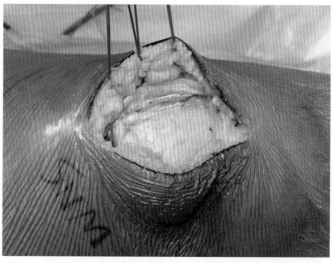

FIG 67.49 Two to three sutures are placed along the medial arthrotomy at the upper and lower poles of the patella. These sutures determine the extent of realignment of medial tissues. Proper patellar tracking is verified before the remaining sutures are placed.

such a way that the subsequent line of pull will be in a more medial direction. This is the purpose of the operative procedure, and by altering the direction of quadriceps action, patellar congruence is restored and patellar instability prevented. Two critical sutures are placed: first at the proximal pole, then at the distal pole of the patella (see video on the website). The first suture is placed on an angle so that the most distal part of the vastus medialis is brought laterally and distally to overlap the upper pole of the patella and the adjoining quadriceps tendon (Fig. 67.49). Before the overlap is executed, the synovium should be removed from the deep surface of the medial flap, which includes the vastus medialis, the medial part of the quadriceps expansion, and distally the medial capsule of the knee. The amount of overlap that should be achieved depends on the preoperative laxity of the tissues. The suture is passed in a mattress fashion through the prepatellar tissue and the medial

flap, then back through the flap and the prepatellar tissue. The point of penetration of the prepatellar tissue determines the amount of transposition of the medial flap over the patella (Fig. 67.50).

The amount of overlap is usually 10 to 15 mm, but if necessary it may be advanced as far as the lateral border of the patella. A second suture is inserted at the lower pole of the patella in the same fashion described previously. This suture will bring the medial flap across as tight as necessary, and often the tightness is determined by however much the soft tissue allows. The suture material may be absorbable or nonabsorbable, according to the surgeon's preference. The two initial sutures determine the remainder of the closure, and after they are placed, the knee should flex to 90 degrees without breakage of the sutures. The

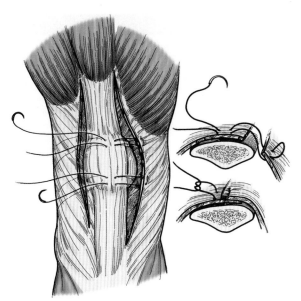

FIG 67.50 Suture of the medial arthrotomy after transposition of the tibial tuberosity in a combined proximal and distal realignment. Two critical stitches are placed at the upper and lower poles of the patella with nonabsorbable no. 5 Ethibond sutures. The suture is passed through the prepatellar tissues, the medial flap, and back through the flap and prepatellar tissues. The point of penetration through the prepatellar tissues determines the amount of overlap of the medial flap over the patella.

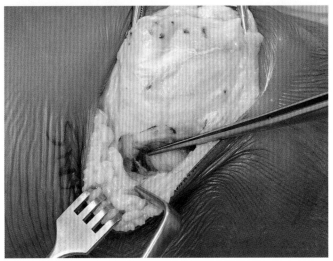

FIG 67.51 The lateral release should extend proximally into the muscle fibers of the vastus lateralis.

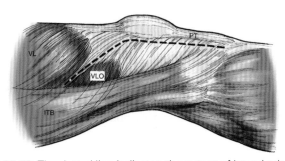

FIG 67.52 The dotted line indicates the extent of lateral release recommended. Note that it extends proximally between the vastus lateralis *(VL)* and the vastus lateralis obliquus *(VLO)*. *PT,* Patellar tendon. (From Scott WN: *The knee,* vol 1, St Louis, 1994, Mosby-Year Book, p 451.)

tension in these sutures is adjusted until the tracking of the patella is acceptable (see video on the website). The remaining closure is completed distally by suturing the flap as it lies and proximally, with decreasing overlap of the vastus medialis over the quadriceps tendon. According to Insall it is not possible to overtighten the medial structures; however, it appears that overtightening may lead to iatrogenic medial subluxation and a poor result.

Occasionally in patients with recurrent dislocation and an extreme lateral position of the patella, the medial flap is so stretched that overlapping to the lateral patellar border is still insufficient to hold the patella in the center of the femoral sulcus. In these circumstances the medial flap, including the vastus medialis, should be everted and the free border rolled back on itself. A series of sutures are inserted, so that a tuck is made in the muscle. The reefed vastus medialis and the quadriceps expansion are sutured anterior to the patella and the quadriceps tendon. The tuck must be sufficient to keep the patella centralized. The resulting bulk of the muscle and capsule lying anterior to the patella may appear aesthetically unpleasant, but the tissue atrophies rapidly, so that within a few weeks the enlargement disappears.

Two features of the repair should be emphasized. First, the lateral incision into the vastus lateralis must extend proximally almost as far as the medial incision. The most common error is reluctance to make an adequate division of the vastus lateralis; unless this is performed, proximal rearrangement of the quadriceps is not possible (Figs. 67.51 and 67.52). It might be expected that extensive division of the muscle would cause quadriceps weakness, but in practice this has not been observed. Insall emphasized that this was instrumental to the success of

the procedure. In practice the lateral release should extend as far proximal as necessary to centralize the patella.

Second, the more distal part of the closure must be snug but not excessively tight. In practice it is almost impossible to overdo the overlapping in this area because it is prevented by soft tissue tension and the anatomy of the femoral sulcus. Excessive tightness is revealed through observation of the behavior of the patella when the knee is flexed.

After routine closure of the subcutaneous tissue and skin, a compression dressing is applied. We no longer routinely close over a hemovac drain.

We are currently using an accelerated rehabilitation protocol. Full weight bearing as tolerated is permitted immediately postoperatively. The patient is discharged on the day of surgery. Continuous passive movement (CPM) is started the night of surgery at the patient's home. Physical therapy is started on postoperative day 1, with a focus on quadriceps strengthening and range of motion. We encourage full active and passive range-of-motion exercises.

Results of Insall Proximal Realignment Procedure

Results of Insall's technique have been reported by different centers (Table 67.5). Insall[66] reviewed 75 realignments performed between 1969 and 1979 for patellar pain and instability.

TABLE 67.5		Results of Proximal Realignment With Insall's Technique				
				AVERAGE		
Author	Year	No. of Knees	Diagnosis	Follow-Up, Mo	% Satisfactory Result	Remarks
Insall et al.[67]	1983	75	Pain and subluxation	48	91	Better results when the patella is centered in the sulcus after the operation; no correlation with the severity of chondromalacia
Scuderi et al.[120]	1988	60	Subluxation and dislocation	42	81	Only one redislocation (1.7%); females and older patients had inferior results; better results with patellar centralization
Abraham et al.[1]	1989	35	Pain and dislocation	76	62	Less satisfactory results in knees with patellofemoral pain (53%) than in knees with recurrent dislocation (78%)
Aglietti et al.[5]	1989	11	Dislocation	102	91	Only one case was unsatisfactory because of insufficient quadriceps rehabilitation

Ten operations were bilateral. The procedures were performed in 40 female and 25 male patients, and the average patient age was 20 years (range: 13 to 32 years). Patients were selected for surgery very carefully. All had dysplasia of the extensor mechanism and serious complaints of pain or instability for a long time, ranging from 1 to 5 years. All had undergone lengthy conservative treatment. Symptoms were always severe enough to interfere with everyday activity, not only with sports. Absence from school was a frequent problem in younger patients.

Of 75 knees, 36 had an increased quadriceps angle (at least 20 degrees), 21 had a high-riding patella (average T:P ratio: 1.19), and 18 had both conditions (quadriceps angle: >20 degrees; average T:P ratio: 1.23); a preoperative Merchant view had been obtained in 20 knees, and findings for the sulcus and congruence angles were in accord with measurements reported by Aglietti et al.[3] Thus the 10 knees with an increased quadriceps angle had an average sulcus angle of 138 degrees and an average congruence angle of 0 degrees. The six knees with a high-riding patella had a sulcus angle averaging 161 degrees and a congruence angle that averaged 25 degrees. The four knees with both variants had an average sulcus angle of 143 degrees and a congruence angle of 19 degrees. The 75 knees were divided according to primary symptoms into 40 knees with patellar pain (32 with an increased quadriceps angle, 3 with a high-riding patella, and 5 with both), 29 knees with subluxation (18 with a high-riding patella, 4 with an increased quadriceps angle, and 7 with both), and 6 knees with both pain and subluxation (all with an increased quadriceps angle and a high-riding patella).

The findings at surgery for patellar surface lesions were normal or grade I in 76%, grade II in 12%, grade III in 4%, and grade IV in 8% of cases. Pain was moderate to severe in 32 of 57 grade I lesions (56%), in 7 of 9 grade II lesions (78%), in no grade III lesions, and in 4 of 6 grade IV lesions (67%). At surgery, 14 patellae were shaved and 7 were shaved and drilled.

The grading system was similar to that described by Bentley.[16] At follow-up ranging from 2 to 10 years with an average of 4 years, the results were as follows: excellent in 37%, good in 54%, fair in 5%, and poor in 4%. Excellent and good results were obtained in 93% of stage I cartilage lesions, 100% of stage II lesions, 33% of stage III lesions, and 83% of stage IV lesions.

Of 21 knees in which the patella was shaved or drilled, 86% had satisfactory results. Postoperatively only 14 patients could not participate in sports.

In 57 knees a postoperative Merchant view was obtained. Among 52 satisfactory knees the average congruence angle was −11 degrees; 35 knees had a negative angle, 5 measured 0 degrees, and 12 had a positive congruence angle. Five knees were rated fair or poor, and in these knees the average congruence angle was 0 degrees. (Two knees had a positive congruence angle, 2 measured 0 degrees, and 1 had a negative angle.) One must naturally not put too much store in radiographic measurements of any kind, and some inconsistencies are to be expected. However, these findings suggested a trend, in that clinical improvement correlated with correct alignment, whereas no such correlation existed with the severity of chondromalacia or with its treatment by patellar shaving.

The complications of proximal realignment were relatively few and minor. They included superficial phlebitis, hematoma, delayed wound healing, and culture-negative drainage. Five knees (7%) required manipulation under anesthesia to allow better range of motion. One subsequent patellectomy was performed because of persistent patellar pain.

Scuderi et al.[120] reported the results of a group of 60 knees with patellar subluxation (34 knees) or dislocation (26 knees) that were treated by Insall's proximal realignment. In this study 20 knees had undergone previous surgery (33%), including proximal and distal realignment, lateral retinacular release, anterior cruciate ligament surgery, meniscectomy, and removal of loose bodies. Postoperatively a cast was applied for 1 month. The follow-up period was 3.5 years (range: 2 to 9 years). Results were excellent in 30%, good in 52%, fair in 10%, and poor in 8%. Results were significantly better in males and in younger patients. No patients younger than 20 years had an unsatisfactory result. The preoperative diagnosis (subluxation or dislocation), the length of follow-up, and the severity of chondromalacia did not correlate with the result. Knees with a satisfactory result showed a greater change in the congruence angle (medial displacement of the patella) than did those with an unsatisfactory grading. The complications were as follows: seven patients (12%) needed postoperative manipulation to increase range of motion, one patient experienced a single episode of recurrent dislocation, three patients underwent arthroscopy for recurrent patellofemoral pain, and one patient underwent bilateral patellectomy for degenerative joint disease. Although the overall results did not correlate with the severity of chondromalacia, it is noteworthy that all patients who needed a reoperation had severe, degenerative osteoarthritis.

Abraham et al.[1] reported the results of Insall's proximal realignment in 15 knees with patellofemoral pain and 9 knees with recurrent dislocation, with an average follow-up period of 6.3 years. Satisfactory results in the group of knees with patellofemoral pain decreased from 87% at 2 years to 53% at 5 years. It should be noted that a quarter of these patients had severe grade IV chondromalacia at the time of the operation: none of these knees obtained a satisfactory result. Better results were achieved in knees with recurrent patellar dislocation: 92% were satisfactory at 2 years, and 78% remained so at 5 years. Two knees required additional surgery for recurrence of dislocation. An anatomic study in cadaver knees was undertaken to define the innervation of the patella. It was noted that branches of the femoral and lateral femoral cutaneous nerves innervated the patella. All these branches are cut by the skin and subcutaneous incisions and by the medial capsulotomy plus lateral release. In light of these findings, Abraham et al. suggested that pain relief may be attributed in part to denervation. No radiographic data were presented to describe the relationship between clinical results and restoration of congruence.

Aglietti et al.[2] reported the results of proximal realignment in 11 knees affected by recurrent patellar dislocation that were reviewed with a long average follow-up of 102 months. Only one case was considered unsatisfactory because of poor quadriceps rehabilitation. No recurrences of dislocation were reported. Eight of these patients (73%) were interested in sports preoperatively, and all returned to their desired sport, including soccer (2), running (3), and aerobics (3). Analysis of Merchant axial views revealed that preoperatively, the average congruence angle was +16 degrees, with 80% of knees considered abnormal. At follow-up only one knee was still abnormal (9%), and the average congruence angle was reduced to −8 degrees. No signs of degenerative arthritis were seen during the long period of follow-up.

More recent studies have reported less success with the Insall technique. Efe[41] evaluated 45 patients status after proximal realignment with a mean follow-up of 49 months. Using the Kujala and Tegner scores, they documented a mean Kujala score of 85 postoperatively ("good") but that 36% scored in the "fair" or "poor" category. They reported a higher redislocation rate of 22% when compared to previous studies and stated 27% were subjectively dissatisfied. Schuttler et al.[116] retrospectively reviewed 42 patients that had undergone proximal realignment using the described Insall technique, a mean 52 months following their surgery. Using plain radiographs and MRI, they documented osteoarthritic changes in the patellofemoral joint. They concluded that Insall's proximal realignment technique led to a significant progression of patellofemoral osteoarthritis. They also noted that recurrent patellar stability had no correlation with osteoarthritis development but that trochlear dysplasia did. The authors did highlight some of the limitations of the study, specifically the lack of a control group and limited preoperative MRI data. However, it is not hard to believe that a nonanatomic procedure may lead to the possibility of abnormal biomechanics of the joint and therefore advanced degenerative changes.

There is a paucity of new literature on isolated proximal realignment procedures. Most of the current literature reports results of proximal and distal combined procedures or of medial patellofemoral ligament reconstruction. Because no new comparative studies have been performed, it is difficult to compare these newer techniques with the results of proximal realignment alone. Therefore we conclude that proximal realignment remains a good surgical intervention for patients with patellar instability. It appears to improve the congruence of the patellofemoral joint by redirecting the pull of the quadriceps mechanism. Some evidence suggests that the procedure is more successful when performed for instability as opposed to advanced articular degeneration. In the face of severe deformity with large Q angles or rotational abnormalities, this procedure may be combined with a distal bony procedure to improve patellofemoral mechanics.

Arthroscopically Assisted Proximal Soft Tissue Plication Procedures

Arthroscopically assisted procedures have been described in the literature. Basically they include lateral retinacular release and plication of the medial capsule. Plication is achieved percutaneously or through short skin incisions with the use of spinal needles, straight or curved, which are used to deliver sutures into the joint and are then extracted and tied over the capsule.

These procedures are not simply less invasive forms of the same proximal realignment procedure that Insall described in 1976.[69] The procedures do not realign or advance the VMO. By including plication of the medial capsule and remaining soft tissue without advancement of the VMO, these procedures functionally shorten the medial restraints on the patella. In theory, these techniques may shorten the MPFL, which is the primary restraint to lateral displacement of the patella.[32] Distal extension of the plication to the tibial tuberosity (through a short incision) may give additional support by shortening the patellomeniscal and patellotibial ligaments.

We favor traditional proximal realignment over the arthroscopic approach. Our concern is that exact tensioning of medial structures and secure repair may be more difficult to achieve by arthroscopic than by more traditional open techniques. Results from small series of arthroscopically assisted repairs are encouraging.[8,23,55,103,125] However, we think that larger series with longer follow-up are needed.

Ali et al.[9] published medium-term results of 7-year follow-up in 36 patients treated with their technique of arthroscopic medial plication and lateral release. The results are promising, with excellent outcomes in 50%, good results in 28%, and poor results in only four knees (11%). Investigators reported two (5%) cases of recurrent instability that improved with reoperation. Overall, 89% of patients were satisfied with the operation, and only three (8%) patients were disappointed at follow-up. Of note, the authors reported no radiographic measurements on these patients because it is their belief that the best assessment of patellar instability is arthroscopic visualization of the patellofemoral joint.

Halbrecht[55] described a technique of all-inside arthroscopic medial plication and arthroscopic lateral release performed on 45 knees with recurrent patellar instability. His technique involves percutaneous passage of sutures and arthroscopic knot tying within the joint to reef the medial soft tissues. Halbrecht reported that at 2-year follow-up 93% of patients experienced significant improvement. Significant improvement was observed in all radiographic measures, such as congruence angle and lateral patellofemoral angle. In this series no complications, such as dislocation or recurrent instability, were reported.

Conclusion and Summary of Chapter

Treatment of patellofemoral instability with proximal realignment dates back to at least 1975, with Madigan's description of the quadricepsplasty.[85] Insall then described the proximal realignment procedure, which consisted of lateral and distal translation of the vastus medialis, as well as an obligatory lateral retinacular release.[68,69] The combination of translation of the vastus medialis and lateral retinacular release is what is now referred to as the Insall proximal realignment procedure. This technique can be combined with distal realignment procedures when the malalignment is severe. We have seen very good results with this technique over the years, although similar to many other treatments for patellar instability, this technique is not perfect, and some recurrence of symptoms is seen.

In recent years many attempts have been made to modify the original technique. Most of these modifications involve arthroscopic assistance or smaller incisions. It is important to remember that all of the described arthroscopic techniques to date omit a very important aspect of the procedure (ie, transposition of the medial tissue). For this reason we do not advocate the use of these arthroscopic techniques. We have modified our technique by performing the procedure through a much smaller incision than was originally described. However, we must emphasize that adequate exposure should not be compromised for a smaller incision. We have also maintained the two main tenets of this procedure: redirecting the pull of the vastus medialis and performing an adequate lateral retinacular release.

An accurate diagnosis is paramount in the treatment of patellofemoral instability. The combination of a thorough physical examination and multiple imaging studies is essential for determining the cause of the instability. Patellofemoral anatomy, as well as angular and rotational malalignment, may contribute to the instability. Only after all of these factors have been identified can the appropriate treatment be provided. The sum of these factors ultimately produces an abnormal, laterally directed force on the patella, and treatment must be directed at restoring patellofemoral congruency by re-establishing a centralizing force vector on the patella. The proximal realignment procedure, as described by Insall, restores patellofemoral congruency and centralizing force by combining lateral translation of the vastus medialis insertion on the patella with extensive lateral release.

ACKNOWLEDGMENTS

The authors thank Paolo Aglietti, Francesco Giron, and Pierluigi Cuomo for their work on the previous edition of this chapter. These were Edition 4 authors.

KEY REFERENCES

1. Abraham E, Washington E, Huang TL: Insall proximal realignment for disorders of the patella. *Clin Orthop Relat Res* 248:61, 1989.
2. Aglietti P, Buzzi R, De Biase P, et al: Surgical treatment of recurrent dislocation of the patella. *Clin Orthop Relat Res* 308:8, 1994.
3. Aglietti P, Insall JN, Cerulli G: Patellar pain and incongruence. I: Measurements of incongruence. *Clin Orthop Relat Res* 176:217, 1983.
32. Conlan T, Garth WP, Lemons JE: Evaluations of the medial soft-tissue restraints of the extensor mechanism of the knee. *J Bone Joint Surg Am* 75:682, 1993.
33. Crosby BE, Insall JN: Recurrent dislocation of the patella: relation of treatment to osteoarthritis. *J Bone Joint Surg Am* 58:9, 1976.
43. Elias DA, White LM, Fithian DC: Acute lateral patellar dislocation at MR imaging: injury patterns of medial patellar soft-tissue restraints and osteochondral injuries of the inferomedial patella. *Radiology* 225:736, 2002.
57. Hautamaa PV, Fithian DC, Kaufman KR, et al: Medial soft tissue restraints in lateral patellar instability and repair. *Clin Orthop Relat Res* 349:174, 1998.
67. Insall JN, Aglietti P, Tria AJ: Patellar pain and incongruence. II: Clinical application. *Clin Orthop Relat Res* 176:225, 1983.
68. Insall JN, Bullough PG, Burstein AH: Proximal "tube" realignment of the patella for chondromalacia patellae. *Clin Orthop Relat Res* 144:63, 1979.
69. Insall JN, Falvo KA, Wise DW: Chondromalacia patellae: a prospective study. *J Bone Joint Surg Am* 58:1, 1976.
85. Madigan R, Wissinger HA, Donaldson WF: Preliminary experience with a method of quadricepsplasty in recurrent subluxation of the patella. *J Bone Joint Surg Am* 57:600, 1975.
108. Panagiotopoulos E, Strzelczyk P, Herrmann M, et al: Cadaveric study on static medial patellar stabilizers: dynamizing role of the vastus medialis obliquus on medial patellofemoral ligament. *Knee Surg Sports Traumatol Arthrosc* 14:7, 2006.
113. Sanders TG, Morrison WB, Singleton BA, et al: Medial patellofemoral ligament injury following acute transient dislocation of the patella: MR findings with surgical correlation in 14 patients. *J Comput Assist Tomogr* 25:957, 2001.
120. Scuderi G, Cuomo F, Scott NW: Lateral release and proximal realignment for patellar subluxation and dislocation: a long-term follow-up. *J Bone Joint Surg Am* 70:856, 1988.

The references for this chapter can also be found on www.expertconsult.com.

68

Repair and Reconstruction of the Medial Patellofemoral Ligament for Treatment of Lateral Patellar Dislocations: Surgical Techniques and Clinical Results

M. Tyrrell Burrus, Marc A. Tompkins, Betina B. Hinckel, David R. Diduch, Elizabeth A. Arendt

LATERAL PATELLA DISLOCATIONS: SURGICAL INDICATIONS

Medial patella soft tissue constraints consist of the medial patellofemoral ligament (MPFL), the medial patellotibial ligament (MPTL), and the medial patellomeniscal ligament (MPML). The MPFL is the primary soft tissue restraint to lateral patellar displacement in early flexion,[13] when most noncontact lateral patellar dislocations occur. As the knee progresses into deeper flexion, patellofemoral bony congruence provides the major restraint to lateral patellar displacement.[24] Surgical treatment to stabilize the patella against lateral dislocation is most often accomplished by restoring the medial patellar check rein afforded by the MPFL. Thus, the goal of MPFL repair or reconstruction is to restore the loss of this medial patellar soft tissue stabilizer that has been rendered incompetent by injury or is chronically lax as seen with recurrent lateral patellar dislocations.

Surgical intervention should be aimed at treating specific injuries, including the torn MPFL, and correcting any additional relevant risk factors for patellar instability. Isolated MPFL reconstruction is indicated when the bony morphology is deemed sufficient, and a soft tissue medial restraint in isolation will stabilize the patella against lateral translation. In situations in which there is trochlear dysplasia and/or patella alta, the MPFL may play a greater role as a biomechanical restraint compared to when the trochlear groove and patellar height are within normal limits. A seminal work established the thresholds of anatomic (imaging) factors associated with recurrent lateral patella dislocations, that is, patella alta greater than 1.2 as measured by Caton-to-Deschamps ratio, trochlear dysplasia as viewed in the true lateral radiograph, patellar tilt on slice imaging greater than 20 degrees, and a quadriceps vector greater than 20 mm as measured by tibial tubercle–trochlear groove (TT-TG) distance.[18] The authors further successfully treated lateral patellar instability by surgically "correcting" all anatomic risk factors greater than the threshold measurements. With the addition of MPFL reconstruction to the surgical armamentarium, the threshold of these measurements has changed, that is, when is a bony procedure necessary? There are no evidence-based guidelines available for the clinician from current published outcomes.[79] Published literature to date has reported on isolated MPFL reconstructions with primarily homogeneous

populations, selecting patients with favorable surgical outcomes whose anatomic risk factors are within normal threshold measurements.[79] Most recent studies have focused on MPFL reconstruction as opposed to repair, as the preferred technique for chronically lax medial patella tissue associated with lateral patellar dislocations.

An ideal candidate for an isolated MPFL repair or reconstruction has the following profile with regard to anatomic risk factors:

- Trochlear morphology; normal or type A dysplasia.[17,75]
- Tibial tubercle–trochlear sulcus angle of 0 to 5 degrees valgus or a tibial tubercle–trochlear groove distance less than 20 mm with the knee at 0 degrees of flexion.
- Absence of "excessive" patella alta as measured by a Caton-Deschamps index if less than 1.2 or Insall-Salvati index of less than 1.3 as measured by lateral radiographs; or on magnetic resonance (MR) imaging (MRI) and engagement factor of less than 12%.[6]
- Patellar tilt less than 20 degrees when measured on an axial slice image, using the posterior femoral condyles as a reference line, or minimal tilt but no lateral tightness on physical examination with the patella reduced.

ANATOMY OF THE MEDIAL SIDE OF THE KNEE: SURGICAL IMPLICATIONS

Knowledge of the medial side knee anatomy is necessary for proper surgical execution of MPFL reconstruction techniques. The capsuloligamentous structures on the medial aspect of the knee have been described in three layers.[81] Layer 2 is where the MPFL and superficial medial collateral ligament (MCL) are located.

The MPFL runs transversely from the medial patellar border to the femur. Although some of the femoral insertion fibers fan out and have a broad attachment, the most consistent attachment site is the saddle between the epicondyle and the adductor tubercle. LaPrade et al. noted this location to be 1.9 mm anterior and 3.8 mm distal to the adductor tubercle.[43] The patellar attachment of the MPFL is wider than the femoral attachment and approximates the upper third of the medial border of the patella, typically at the location where the perimeter of the patella becomes more vertical. As a percentage of the longitudinal length of the patella, Nomura et al.[56] reported that the

MPFL insertion is 27% ± 10% from the proximal extent of the patella. These anatomic measurements were cadaveric measurements made in non-dysplastic knees.

The MPTL is in a more superficial plane than the MPFL and is an oblique condensation of the medial patellar retinaculum. It attaches to the tibia approximately 1.5 cm below the joint line, close to the insertion of the medial collateral ligament, although individual components of the medial retinaculum are more difficult to assess distally.[81] The MPTL is uniquely positioned to help resist superior and superolateral translation of the patella because of the oblique orientation of its fibers. However, the role of the MPTL in resisting lateral patellar displacement is debated, ranging from being an important secondary stabilizer[37] to being functionally unimportant.[13]

MEDIAL PATELLOFEMORAL LIGAMENT REPAIR

Primary Repair of the Medial Patellofemoral Ligament

Imbrication of the medial retinaculum has long been a component of surgical procedures for lateral patellar dislocations. However, with the increasing focus on MPFL reconstruction, there has also been greater scrutiny of the results of primary and secondary repair of the ligament. Multiple studies have shown inferior results with repair compared to reconstruction. In a prospective trial of 80 patients randomized to either conservative treatment or MPFL repair, Christiansen et al. demonstrated no significant difference in redislocation rates (20% vs. 17%) or Kujala scores at 2-year follow up.[12] This result was echoed by Palmu et al. in the pediatric population after acute injuries.[58] Arendt et al. noted a 46% redislocation rate after MPFL repair for recurrent patellar dislocation events.[3] In a level 1 study, Nikku et al.[52] reported the 7-year results of a variety of medial repair procedures in primary patellar dislocations compared with nonoperative treatment. The outcomes were similar between the two groups both in regard to patients' self-assessed outcomes and patellar redislocation rates. Furthermore, there are many variations in the techniques of MPFL repair, making it difficult to accurately compare studies. On the other hand, there are studies that support medial repair. A recent level 1 study[68] compared nonoperative treatment versus open medial repair in younger, predominantly male patients. Preoperative MRI in the operatively treated group helped define the location of the MPFL lesion. Fourteen of 18 operatively treated subjects had a medial reefing at the injury site and 4 had a Roux-Goldthwait procedure. The surgical decision was based on surgeon preference. At 7-year follow-up there were no redislocations in the operative group compared with further dislocations in 6 of 21 patients in the nonoperative group. However, there were no subjective differences between the two groups. A level 2 study[10] also reported improved outcomes for acute patellar dislocations treated surgically. Preoperative MRI was again used to determine the location of MPFL injury. Lesions close to the patella were repaired arthroscopically with an outside-to-inside technique, whereas femoral avulsion injuries were repaired with suture anchors in the epicondyle. At an average of 40-months follow-up, there were no redislocations in the 17 patients in the operative group compared with 8 of 16 redislocations in the nonoperative group.

A variety of arthroscopic techniques of medial soft tissue repair have been developed over recent years.[20,29,34,36] There are numerous studies both supporting and discouraging arthroscopic repair techniques for patellar instability,[2,20,34,36,67] but the results are confounded by various combinations of open and arthroscopic techniques. In one such prospective but nonrandomized study, the results of initial arthroscopic medial repair of the MPFL were compared with those of nonoperative management.[65] At a median 7-year follow-up, initial arthroscopic repair was not associated with a reduced incidence of redislocation. Further detailed outcome studies are needed to clarify the role of arthroscopic repair and to endorse any particular arthroscopic procedure over another.

The indications for repair of the MPFL in primary (first time) lateral patellar dislocations are debated. A clearly defined isolated ligamentous avulsion from the patella or the femur may represent an indication for repair, although they are rare. Repair of an isolated lesion at or near the patella or femoral MPFL attachment is favored by some, especially if open surgery is already planned to address an osteochondral lesion of the patella or trochlear groove. The indications for imbrication of midsubstance ruptures of the ligament are more controversial. Surgical techniques will continue to develop, as will the relative merits of MPFL repair versus MPFL reconstruction versus management as more outcome data becomes available. When approaching MPFL repair, there are certain surgical principles to which the orthopedic surgeon should adhere:

1. Evaluate each patient for anatomic risk factors. Measurements above established thresholds place more stress on this repair tissue.
2. A single location of MPFL injury must be identified (eg, femoral/patellar) and the repair should be focused on this site.
3. Based on the available literature, open repair techniques outperform current arthroscopic techniques. Proper tensioning of the MPFL is critical. Intraoperatively, the knee should easily flex beyond 90 degrees after repair. Overtightening of the MPFL should be avoided.
4. Suture repairs should be stout and anchors used to further strengthen the repair. In a biomechanical evaluation, MPFL repairs using suture anchors plus sutures failed at 142 N, whereas suture repair alone failed at 37 N.[48]

In the authors' practices, repair of the MPFL is rarely and only performed for peel-off lesions of the patella or femur because of the ability to achieve more consistent results and minimal complications with reconstruction. Simply put, a more reliable result can be achieved with a reconstruction using a graft.

Primary repair is rarely indicated in our practices.

Medial Patellofemoral Ligament Repair Technique

Diagnostic arthroscopy is first performed to address any associated intra-articular pathology. Occasionally, the point of disruption to the MPFL can be visualized arthroscopically. If a distal realignment procedure is to be performed, it should be done prior to the repair of the MPFL to allow for proper tensioning. The following repair technique is offered as one option for surgical management.

Most commonly, the MPFL is torn from its femoral origin. For primary repair, a longitudinal incision is made in the deep fascia and periosteum just proximal to the medial epicondyle. In the initial dissection, the MPFL may be more readily palpated than seen. By holding tension on the tissue with forceps, the patella is translated laterally, and the MPFL is identified as the tissue that resists translation (Fig. 68.1). The insertion site should be identified fluoroscopically. (See description for

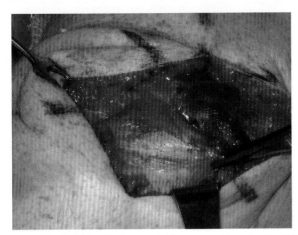

FIG 68.1 Medial Patellofemoral Ligament Repair The MPFL has been localized deep and distal to the vastus medialis obliquus. Traction is applied to the patella to determine the point of ligament disruption. (From Redziniak DE, Diduch DR, Mihalko WM, et al: Patellar instability. *J Bone Joint Surg Am* 91:2264, 2009.)

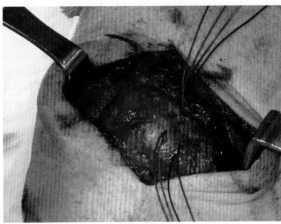

FIG 68.3 Medial Patellofemoral Ligament Repair Horizontal mattress sutures are placed through the MPFL origin and tied at 30 to 40 degrees of knee flexion. (From Redziniak DE, Diduch DR, Mihalko WM, et al: Patellar instability. *J Bone Joint Surg Am* 91:2264, 2009.)

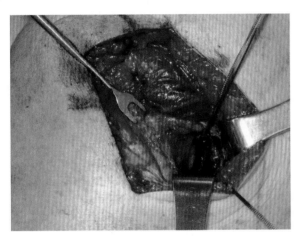

FIG 68.2 Medial Patellofemoral Ligament Repair A longitudinal incision in the deep fascia and periosteum permits exposure of the MPFL origin for the placement of two suture anchors in the femur. (From Redziniak DE, Diduch DR, Mihalko WM, et al: Patellar instability. *J Bone Joint Surg Am* 91:2264, 2009.)

identifying Schottle's point during reconstruction later.) Two suture anchors are then placed into the femur at the attachment site of the MPFL, and mattress sutures are used to repair the ligament with the knee in 30 to 40 degrees of flexion (Figs. 68.2 and 68.3).

If the MPFL is torn off the patella, traction on the medial end of the ligament will not restore patellar stability. In these cases, the MPFL is repaired back to the patella with the use of nonabsorbable sutures placed through drill holes or suture anchors in the patella, in a manner similar to reconstruction techniques[29,36] (discussed later in the chapter). After the sutures are tied, patellar tracking is again assessed and a firm end point to lateral patellar displacement should be appreciated. The investing fascia is repaired prior to skin closure.

If a repair is performed, it is imperative that the surgeon ensure that there is no secondary site of tearing or attenuation because a repair with residual laxity in the ligament will not

result in patellar stability. In general, MPFL repair is not the recommended technique because of concerns of residual laxity.

Rehabilitation After Medial Patellofemoral Ligament Repair

There is presently no evidence to support any specific postoperative rehabilitation regimen after MPFL repair. The published series rarely include a description of postoperative management. Those studies that report their rehabilitation regimen describe a period of restricted range of motion using a hinged brace from 2 to 6 weeks. Weight-bearing status also varies considerably in the published series, ranging from minimal to full weight bearing.

Increasing the range of motion and weight bearing should be based on the surgeon's confidence in the quality of the repair tissue and repair fixation, coupled with an appropriate progression to full strength and agility before a full return to sports. Most authors advocate introducing more demanding rehabilitation tasks from the 10- to 12-week mark, with unrestricted activities commencing from 4 months onward.

MEDIAL PATELLOFEMORAL LIGAMENT RECONSTRUCTION

Basic Principles

Documenting an increase in passive lateral patellar translation beyond the confines of the trochlear groove is a necessary first step because it implies laxity of the MPFL. This is most often established by physical examination with the knee at 20 to 30 degrees flexion, but stress radiographs can also be used.[76] If the diagnosis is in question, an examination under anesthesia can be used to document laxity without guarding or apprehension confounding the findings. Arthroscopy is used to identify and address articular cartilage lesions. However, because distention of the joint during arthroscopy usually results in lateral tilt and translation of the patella, one should not attempt to assess lateral patellar tilt and translation based on arthroscopic appearance alone.

Numerous techniques for MPFL reconstruction have been described. All reconstruction techniques aim to re-create a functional MPFL. Various autologous grafts, such as the semi-tendinosus (ST), gracilis (G), quadriceps, and semimembranosus tendons, as well as the medial retinacular tissues, have been used. The use of allograft tendon and synthetic grafts has also been described. Regardless of the technique used, the surgical principles are the same and should be followed to produce an effective reconstruction that does not impair normal knee function.

The selection of graft type will in part dictate the site and method of fixation of the reconstruction. Free tendon grafts are the most frequently used, usually the G or ST tendons. Alternatively, tendon grafts may be left attached at one end—for example, ST or G tendons left attached to the tibia, a strip of quadriceps tendon left attached to the patella, or a strip of adductor magnus tendon left attached to the femur.

When selecting a graft type, consideration should be given to the biomechanical properties of the native MPFL. The ideal tissue for the graft would have similar stiffness and strength compared to the native MPFL. All current grafts have both strength and stiffness that are significantly greater than those of the native MPFL. Accordingly, it seems preferable to use a graft with stiffness that is closest to the native ligament. For this reason, the G tendon may be preferable to the stiffer ST tendon.[26]

The incisions used will also in part depend on the tendon being harvested and whether any concomitant procedures, such as a tibial tubercle osteotomy, are being performed. Regardless, for the placement of the graft, access to the medial aspect of the patella and the region between the adductor tubercle and medial femoral epicondyle is required. This can be accomplished with a single incision or two separate smaller incisions. The orientation of the incision(s) can be longitudinal, oblique, or transverse. Oblique and transverse incisions may be associated with less sensory disturbance from injury to the prepatellar and infrapatellar branches of the saphenous nerve and may leave a more cosmetically acceptable scar. Longitudinal incisions are, however, more versatile for potential future surgical procedures.

The graft can be fixed to the patella with bone anchors, interference screws, or one or two bone tunnels. If two fixation points are chosen, one is at the superomedial corner of the patella, and the other is at or just distal to the junction of the upper and middle thirds of the medial border of the patella. Nomura et al. noted the MPFL inserted on the medial patella at 27 ± 10% from the upper end of the patella measured longitudinally.[56] LaPrade et al. quantified the midpoint of the MPFL patella attachment as being located at 41.4% of the length from the proximal tip of the patella compared to the total patella length.[43] Thus, it is important to keep the distal insertion site above the midline of the cartilaginous portion of the patella. Stephen et al. noted that the patellar attachment, although important to accurately localize, does not affect graft behavior as much as femoral attachment.[74] A recent study at our institution demonstrated no difference in clinical outcome or recurrent patellar instability when two suture anchors or two short, oblique bone tunnels were used.[42] If bone tunnels are used, they should be just large enough to allow passage of the graft. If two tunnels are used, the graft can be passed through one and into the other to create a sling (Fig. 68.4). Some authors believe that to reduce the risk of fracture, it is important not to breach the anterior cortex of the patella, whereas some techniques

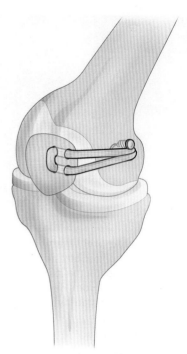

FIG 68.4 MPFL reconstruction using a G tendon that is looped through two tunnels in the medial half of the patella. The tunnels exit in the midline of the patella, avoiding tunnels that pass across the full width of the bone. The femoral fixation at the adductor tubercle is by means of an interference screw. (Courtesy M. Lind.)

deliberately have the tunnel exit the bone anteriorly rather than laterally. Transverse tunnels that traverse the entire width of the patella should be avoided because of the large stress riser and potential fracture risk this creates. Whichever fixation method is chosen, the reconstructed ligament should be placed in the second layer of the medial knee soft tissue structures. It should lie deep to the distal end of the vastus medialis oblique anteriorly, deep to the deep fascia more medially, and superficial to the capsule of the joint.

The femoral attachment site can be referenced from the medial femoral epicondyle, 10 mm proximal and 2 mm posterior; or from the adductor tubercle, 4 mm distal and 2 mm anterior. The femoral insertion point, termed Schöttle's point, can also be identified with fluoroscopic imaging of a true lateral view of the knee (Fig. 68.5).[64] The authors recommend using this technique based on radiographic landmarks to help reproduce the normal anatomy with near isometric graft motion. However, a critical aspect of MPFL reconstruction is to reproduce the normal tightening of the ligament in extension and relaxation in flexion. The ligament functions as a check rein in early flexion (0 to 30 degrees) and is therefore under the greatest tension in this range of knee flexion. Excessive tension in deeper flexion can lead to painful restriction of flexion and articular cartilage overload in the medial half of the patellofemoral compartment.

The ideal tension at the time of fixation of the graft is unknown, but, using a cadaver model, Stephen et al. demonstrated that only 2 N (roughly one-half pound) of graft tension appears to accurately restore contact pressure and patellar tracking.[73] In addition to femoral malpositioning, an overtensioned graft is another common surgical error. Surgical

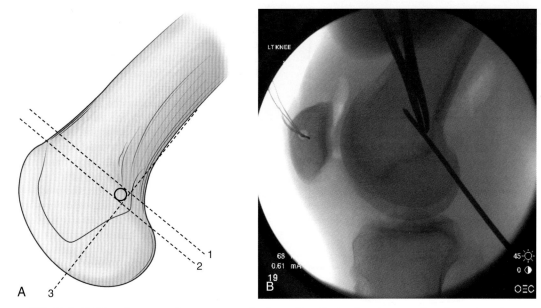

FIG 68.5 (A) Two lines are drawn perpendicular to line 3, the first intersecting the point where the margin of the medial condyle meets the posterior cortex *(line 1)* and the second intersecting the most posterior point of Blumensaat line *(line 2)*. A line is drawn extending distally from the posterior femoral cortex *(line 3)*. A circle of 5-mm diameter is drawn contacting the line drawn from the posterior cortex. The MPFL femoral insertion should fall within this circle. (B) A fluoroscopic intraoperative image of a knee marking the insertion point of a K-wire entering the femur, identifying the position of the femoral tunnel for the MPFL reconstruction. (Courtesy E. Arendt.)

attention to these details is paramount for a successful surgical outcome.

The literature contains varying recommendations for the degree of knee flexion at the time of graft fixation, with the knee flexion ranging from 0 to 90 degrees. However, an unpublished cadaveric study concluded that 30 to 45 degrees of knee flexion is likely the safest option.[8] Because the patella engages the trochlear groove at around 30 degrees of knee flexion, this provides an estimate of where the patella should lie on the femur. This study demonstrated that any mistakes in the femoral tunnel location are magnified as the graft is fixed in increasing amounts of knee flexion. For example, if the femoral location is too distal and the femur is fixed in 90 degrees of knee flexion, the graft will be too tight in knee extension and may cause the patella to medially subluxate. This effect is magnified as the amount of knee flexion increases (Fig. 68.6). The patella should not be pulled medially by the reconstructed ligament, but lateral translation beyond the lateral margin of the trochlea should be prevented.

As with the patella, there are many options for graft fixation to the femur. These include suture anchor fixation and direct soft tissue fixation by looping the graft around the adductor magnus tendon or by looping it around the proximal MCL. Fixing the end(s) of the graft directly into a drilled tunnel offers the advantages of tendon-to-bone healing and precise tunnel placement using fluoroscopy. If a bone tunnel is created, interference screw fixation is commonly used. This can be augmented or even replaced by securing the whip-stitched ends of the tendon to the lateral side of the femur, usually by means of a fixation post or ligament button. Cycling of the knee through flexion and extension prior to fixation may help reduce subsequent creep in the construct.

Troubleshooting

A useful method of assessing the length-tension behavior of the planned femoral attachment site is to insert a Beath pin or Kirschner wire (K-wire) into the planned site. The ends of the graft itself or the ends of temporary sutures or wires attached to the patella are wrapped around the pin. The knee is then cycled through flexion and extension and the movement of the graft relative to the pin is assessed to ensure that the distance between the patellar and femoral attachment sites of the graft decreases or does not change with increasing knee flexion.

Although Schottle's point is likely the ideal landmark to use for locating the correct femoral insertion point, there is variability in the distal femur that may necessitate adjustments to this location. With or without fluoroscopy, testing one's intraoperative fixation points is a necessary step for a successful surgical outcome.

Because of the posterior location of the MPFL insertion on the femoral cortex, placing the guidewire too posterior is not a likely scenario. Being too proximal, distal, or anterior are much more likely, and thus knowing how grafts behave at these locations is important for intra-operative decision making. A recent cadaveric study showed that an anterior femoral location is mostly isometric up to around 30 degrees of knee flexion and then behaves like a proximal femoral location as the knee continues to flex.[8]

A proximal femoral location results in increasing tension in the graft during knee flexion because more graft length would be needed to maintain the same tension because of the cam shape of the distal femur (Fig. 68.7). This surgical malposition can lead to significant postoperative symptoms including stiffness, knee pain, and patellofemoral chondrosis. While flexing the knee prior to graft fixation, if the graft becomes too tight in

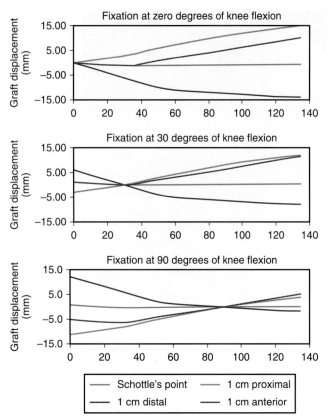

FIG 68.6 Graphic depictions of graft length changes during knee range of motion based on femoral location and amount of knee flexion during fixation. Notice that as the knee flexion during fixation increases, there is increasing length variability during lower degrees of knee flexion. For this reason, we recommend graft fixation in low degrees of knee flexion (30 to 45 degrees).

knee flexion, then likely the femoral position needs to be more distal. "High and tight" is a way to remember that if your location is too high (proximal) the graft will become too tight. Similarly, if the graft becomes too loose in flexion, then the femoral location is too distal (Fig. 68.8). "Low (distal) and loose" is one way to remember this relationship.[9]

Tips for a Successful Medial Patellofemoral Ligament Reconstruction

- Keep the patellar insertion above the proximal half of the cartilaginous patella surface.
- Be anatomic in the femoral insertion location. Using fluoroscopy and Schottle's point is our preferred method.
- After placing a K-wire at this location, take the knee through a range of motion to test graft kinematics. If the graft becomes too tight or loose during testing, the femoral location needs adjustment. Remember "high and tight" and "low and loose."
- Secure the graft in 30 to 45 degrees of knee flexion.
- Do not pull hard on the graft during fixation. Only 2 N (0.5 pounds) of tension is recommended.

Procedures

Double-Strand Gracilis Autograft. This technique uses two transverse tunnels in the patella through which a G tendon autograft is passed to create a double-stranded MPFL

reconstruction (see Fig. 68.4). The two strands of tendon are inserted into a tunnel in the femur in the region of the adductor tubercle and fixed with an interference screw. This technique secures the graft to the patella first and makes adjustments in the length-tension relationship by adjusting the location of the femoral fixation point.

The G tendon is harvested in a standard fashion through a 2- to 3-cm incision over the pes anserine. The ends of the G tendon are secured with an absorbable no. 1 whipstitch. Two incisions, 2 cm in length, are made over the medial border of the patella at the junction of the upper and middle thirds of the bone and over the adductor tubercle.

Via the more anterior incision, the medial border and anterior aspect of the patella are exposed. This involves retracting the distal end of the vastus medialis muscle proximally and sharply dissecting into the attachment of the native MPFL. Alternatively, a single longitudinal incision is made along the medial border of the patella from the superior pole to the pes insertion to allow access to the G insertion and patella and femoral MPFL attachment points.

Two oblique tunnels, 3.2 mm in diameter, depending on the size of the graft, are then drilled through the patella. The start points for the two tunnels are located on the medial border of the patella, one at the superomedial corner and the other at the junction of the upper and middle thirds of the medial border. It is important to start both tunnels in the deeper half of the medial patellar border, but care should be taken not to violate the articular surface. Both tunnels exit anteriorly short of the midline of the patella, angled as obliquely as possible to still maintain an adequate bone bridge. Slight divergence of the tunnels anteriorly may reduce the risk of fracture of the intervening patellar segment. A variation of this technique is to drill the patellar tunnels to exit on the lateral side of the bone (Fig. 68.9). This requires an additional exposure of the lateral aspect of the patella and greatly increases fracture risk.[11]

The adductor tubercle of the medial femoral condyle is then identified through the more medial incision. The G tendon is passed through the patellar bone tunnels using a suture-passing loop. The tendon is first passed through one tunnel from medial to lateral and then back through the other tunnel from lateral to medial. This results in two free tendon ends on the medial side of the patella (Fig. 68.10). Using a hemostat or similar clamp to create a soft tissue tunnel, these tendon ends are then passed to the deep fascia to the adductor tubercle, exiting through the more medially placed incision (Fig. 68.11). The path of the most anterior portion of the graft is through the anterior aspect of the vastus medialis aponeurosis.

A Beath pin is used to find the best point at which to place the femoral tunnel. Graft isometry is tested and adjusted as described previously. Aim the Beath pin transversely or slightly proximally to avoid the intercondylar notch. A 7-mm drill is then passed over the wire to a depth that will comfortably accommodate the free tendon ends. After overdrilling the tunnel, the whip-stitched sutures from the two tendon ends are threaded through the eye in the Beath needle, which is advanced through the far cortex and used to pull the tendon ends into the bone tunnel. A working length of 23 to 25 cm of G graft will allow adequate graft within the femoral tunnel for fixation without risking abutting the far femoral cortex, which would affect graft tensioning.

With traction applied to the whipstitches exiting the lateral femoral cortex, the knee is cycled through a range of motion to

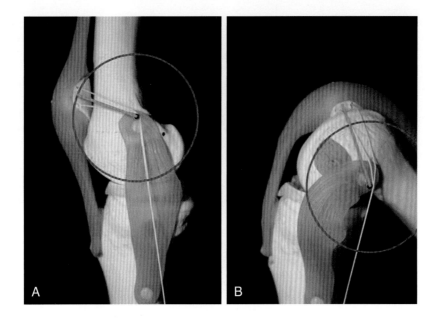

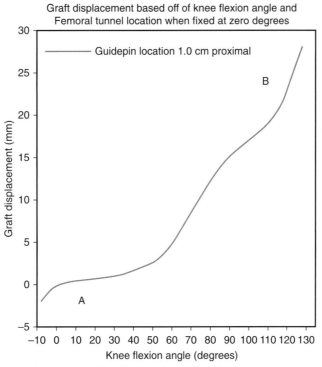

Graft displacement based off of knee flexion angle and Femoral tunnel location when fixed at zero degrees

— Guidepin location 1.0 cm proximal

FIG 68.7 Sawbones and corresponding graphic depiction of how a poorly placed proximal MPFL femoral attachment creates too much tension in the graft during knee flexion; a longer graft would be required to maintain the same amount of tension. The red circle matches the radius of the graft at full extension. The blue line represents the distance from the femoral insertion to the patellar insertion. In other words, if the blue line ends outside the red circle, then the graft would be too tight. Thus, "high and tight." (From Burrus MT, Werner BC, Conte EJ, et al: Location, location, location: troubleshooting the femoral MPFL attachment. *Orthop J Sports Med* 3(1), 2015.)

fully seat the ends in the tunnel and to reduce subsequent creep of the construct. With the knee in 20 to 30 degrees flexion, enough traction is applied to the whipstitches to allow the patella to be centered within the trochlear groove (2 N or 0.5 pounds). The graft is then fixed with an interference screw 7 mm in diameter, depending on the bone quality (see Fig.

68.4). Typically, a 7-mm absorbable interference screw in a 7-mm diameter tunnel with a two-tailed G graft provides excellent fixation. It is important to bury the head of the screw subcortically to avoid local irritation of the soft tissues.

There are variations of this technique that avoid drilling through the anterior patellar cortex but use essentially the

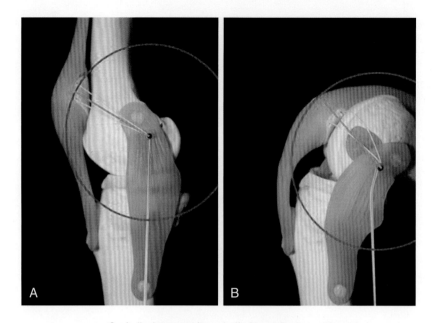

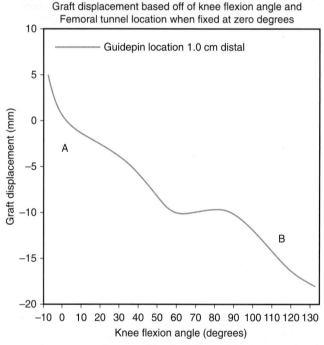

Graft displacement based off of knee flexion angle and Femoral tunnel location when fixed at zero degrees

— Guidepin location 1.0 cm distal

FIG 68.8 Sawbones and corresponding graphic depiction of how a poorly placed distal MPFL femoral attachment creates too much laxity in the graft during knee flexion; a shorter graft would be required to maintain the same amount of tension. The red circle matches the radius of the graft at full extension. The blue line represents the distance from the femoral insertion to the patellar insertion. In other words, if the blue line ends inside the red circle, then the graft would be too loose. Thus, "low and loose." (From Burrus MT, Werner BC, Conte EJ, et al: Location, location, location: troubleshooting the femoral MPFL attachment. *Orthop J Sports Med* 3(1), 2015.)

same attachment points of the graft. One is to use suture anchor fixation of a free tissue graft on the medial aspect of the patella and an interference screw in the medial femoral condyle (Fig. 68.12).[25] The same technique has been modified to use small-diameter tenodesis screws in the patella instead of anchors.[63]

A similar technique is to use a G graft and secure it first on the femur with a bone anchor and then to pass the free ends through two 2.5-mm very oblique (deep to superficial) tunnels in the medial border of the patella. As they exit the anterior aperture of the patellar tunnels, the tendon ends are folded back on themselves and secured with a suture technique.[28,77] If all bone tunnels are to be avoided, the patellar tunnels can be replaced with suture anchors and the medial cortex of the patella can be roughened with a rongeur to encourage the tendon-bone healing response.

Combined Medial Patellar Tibial Ligament Reconstruction. Both the MPTL and MPML originate in the distal pole of the patella and cross distal and medial to insert on the anteromedial aspect of the tibial and medial meniscus, respectively, with some variations in their distal attachment among the study descriptions.[13,19,59,80] The MPTL is more superficial (in the first and second layers), has a length of 35 to 45 mm, a width of 4 to 6 mm, originates medially at the inferior pole of the patella, and inserts 10 to 20 mm distal to the joint line and 15 to 20 mm medial to the patellar tendon, forming an angle of 20 to 25 degrees in relation to the patellar tendon. The MPML is deeper, in layer 3, and has a length of 20 to 25 mm, width of 3 to 5 mm, originates at the inferior pole of the patella, and inserts in the anterior horn and coronary ligament of the medial meniscus, forming an angle of 15 to 30 degrees in relation to the patellar tendon.

Biomechanically, the contributions of the MPTL and MPML as a unit against lateral translation have shown to increase from 26% in extension, to 46% at 90 degrees of flexion. Additionally, the MPTL and MPML at 90 degrees of flexion are responsible for 72% of patellar tilt and 92% of patellar rotation.[60] Near full extension, the MPTL is important to prevent lateral subluxation.[21]

Based on anatomy and biomechanical studies, the MPTL and MPML are more important in two moments during knee range of motion: terminal extension, when it directly counteracts quadriceps contraction,[21,31] and deeper flexion, when it tightens and its contribution to lateral translation restraint

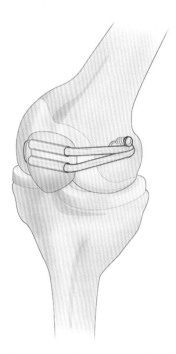

FIG 68.9 MPFL reconstruction using a free G tendon that is passed through two transverse tunnels in the proximal part of the patella. The femoral fixation at the adductor tubercle is by means of an interference screw. (From Christiansen SE, Jacobsen BW, Lund B, et al: Reconstruction of the medial patellofemoral ligament with gracilis tendon autograft in transverse patellar drill holes. *Arthroscopy* 24:82, 2008.)

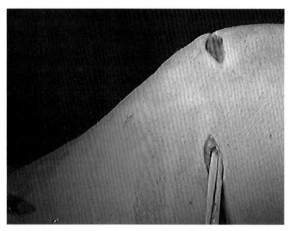

FIG 68.11 Photograph of the medial aspect of the right knee during MPFL reconstruction using a free G tendon graft that is looped through two tunnels in the patella. The free ends of the graft have been passed medially deep to the deep fascia to exit through the more medial wound before being passed into a tunnel in the femur. (Courtesy J. Feller.)

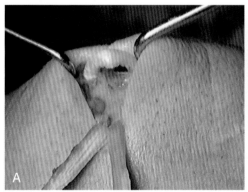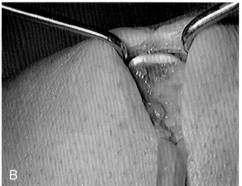

FIG 68.10 (A) Photograph of the anterior incision of the right knee during MPFL reconstruction using a free G tendon graft that is looped through two tunnels in the patella. The free ends of the graft can be seen at the bottom of the picture. (B) Photograph of the anterior incision of the right knee during MPFL reconstruction using a free G tendon graft that is looped through two tunnels in the patella. The loop of tendon has been snugged down onto the anterior aspect of the patella. (Courtesy J. Feller.)

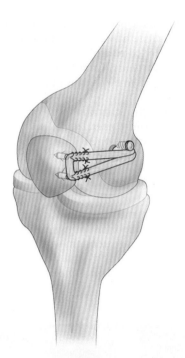

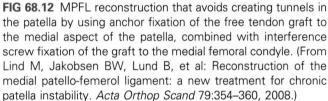

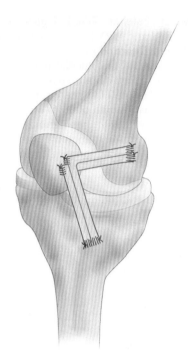

FIG 68.12 MPFL reconstruction that avoids creating tunnels in the patella by using anchor fixation of the free tendon graft to the medial aspect of the patella, combined with interference screw fixation of the graft to the medial femoral condyle. (From Lind M, Jakobsen BW, Lund B, et al: Reconstruction of the medial patello-femerol ligament: a new treatment for chronic patella instability. *Acta Orthop Scand* 79:354–360, 2008.)

FIG 68.13 Technique that combines reconstruction of the MPFL with reconstruction of the MPTL. The semitendinosus (ST) and G tendons are sutured to the medial border of the patella and medial femoral condyle. The distal limb of the tendon grafts is sutured to the proximal medial tibial periosteum to reconstruct the MPTL. (From Lind M, Jakobsen BW, Lund B, et al: Reconstruction of the medial patello-femerol ligament: a new treatment for chronic patella instability. *Acta Orthop Scand* 79:354–360, 2008.)

increases.[60] It also improves kinematics of patellar tilt and rotation throughout range of motion, especially in deep flexion.[60]

Some types of reconstruction of MPTL without the MPFL (isolated or with other associated procedures, eg, lateral release, medial reefing, and transfer of the patellar tendon, such as Roux-Goldthwait) have been described since 1922 by Galeazzi.[30] Good outcomes were reported in many clinical studies,* however, Grannatt et al. found an 82% rate of dislocation and subluxation after the procedure.[33] Combined reconstruction of the MPFL and the MPTL have reported good outcomes[7,15,21,32,69] when performed in patients without risk factors.[7,15,69] There are isolated studies of combined MPFL and MPTL reconstruction combined with correction of large quadriceps vectors with TT medialization,[21] and in children with associated anatomic risk factors,[32] that also report good results. Therefore, although the MPTL reconstruction can be performed safely and has reported good outcomes, the clinical indications are still imprecise.

Based on the reviewed literature and on the authors' experience, possible indications for this procedure are as follows:
- Extension subluxation (defined by patellar lateral translation during quadriceps contraction with the knee passively positioned in extension): to contribute with MPFL to restraint lateral translation, specially opposing the proximal and lateral quadriceps muscle pull.[31]
- Flexion instability (habitual dislocation and lateral glide during flexion): to contribute, in higher levels, to lateral translation restraint, as it tightens with flexion.[41,46,60]

- Children with risk factor (trochlear dysplasia, large quadriceps vector and patella alta): to add additional support during extension and flexion when there is the risk of complications when doing bony procedures with open physes.[32,41,50,57]
- Knee hyperextension associated to generalized laxity: to add additional support to functional patella alta during hyperextension, and functional large quadriceps vector because of increased knee rotation between femur and tibia that would result in overcorrection with TT osteotomy.[40,41]

The isolated reconstruction of the MPTL was described with the ST or the G[30,33] or the medial portion of the patellar tendon.[46,61,83] The techniques described for the combined reconstruction of the MPFL and MPTL use the ST or G, maintaining its tibial insertion,[7,21,32,69] or as free grafts,[15] using the same graft for both the MPFL and the MPTL; or the reconstruction of the MPFL with the quadriceps tendon and the MPTL with the patellar tendon.[38] Another possibility is the use of allograft (typically G allograft) with the fixation on the anatomic landmarks.

One technique combining reconstruction of the MPFL and the MPTL is detailed. Either the ST or G tendon alone or both tendons are harvested but left attached distally. The graft is then passed to the medial border of the patella, where it is passed through a bone tunnel or sutured to periosteum before being passed in layer 2 to the standard attachment point on the femur. Here it can be fixed by any of the methods already described. A variation is to use a free graft and to suture the distal end to the tibial periosteum approximately 1.5 cm distal to the joint line (Fig. 68.13).[15,51] The disadvantage of this technique is that

*See references 4, 5, 30, 35, 44, 61, 83.

one must tension two arms of the same graft in an attempt to duplicate both the MPFL and MPTL. Little is known about the length-tension characteristics of the MPTL. Other techniques have MPTL and MPFL as separate grafts with their own fixation points.

In conclusion, the MPTL and MPML are secondary in lateral patellar restraint in extension, where the MPFL plays a major role. The role of the MPTL and MPML are important to prevent superior-lateral subluxation in extension and are fundamental to stability in flexion. The reconstruction of the MPTL in isolation or associated with other procedures, including the MPFL reconstruction, has good clinical outcomes but further studies are needed to determine the best indications for the procedure.

Single-Strand Middle Third Quadriceps Tendon Autograft. An alternative graft is the central portion of the quadriceps tendon.[70] A 5-cm midline incision is made over the distal quadriceps tendon and another 2-cm vertical incision is made over the medial femoral condyle. A 10- to 11-cm-long and 10-mm-wide graft is harvested. Only half the thickness of the tendon needs to be harvested and the defect can be repaired with absorbable sutures. The distal end of the graft is left attached to the patella. The released tendon is reflected 90 degrees toward the medial condyle (folded upside down) and is passed subcutaneously to the MPFL attachment site on the medial femoral condyle (Fig. 68.14). It can be fixed by any of the techniques already described. The disadvantage of this technique is that one cannot always predict the length of the tendon that can be harvested, which may compromise the femoral fixation point. Typically, a longer anterior incision is required to harvest the distal quadriceps

tendon than with other techniques. Sutures can be placed at the corners of the graft where it crosses the medial patellar border to help re-create the patellar attachment points of the MPFL. This technique can work well when the physes are open with significant growth remaining, as the graft does not require any drill holes other than for anchor placement at Schottle's point on the femur, distal to the physis.

Single-Strand Adductor Magnus Split Tendon Transfer. This technique uses an adductor magnus tendon autograft left attached to the femur.[66] A 3- to 4-cm skin incision is made between the adductor tubercle and proximal half of the patella. The adductor magnus tendon is exposed and split at the junction of its middle and posterior thirds. The split is continued proximally with a tendon harvester to a length of 12 to 14 cm, where the anterior two thirds are released. The free end of the graft is passed through a soft tissue tunnel created in layer 2, deep to the distal part of vastus medialis and superficial to the joint capsule. The graft is then fixed with two suture anchors to the superomedial aspect of the patella, with the knee in 30 degrees flexion (Fig. 68.15). The disadvantage of this technique is also that one cannot always predict the length of the tendon that can to be harvested, which may compromise the ultimate patellar fixation.

Adductor Sling Technique. A 2- to 3-cm incision is made along the medial border of the patella. A K-wire is passed transversely through the patella from medial to lateral, starting at the junction of the upper and middle thirds of the patella and exiting at the lateral border of the patella, passing through a small stab incision in the skin. This K-wire is over-drilled with a 4.0- or 4.5-mm cannulated reamer to a depth of 10 to 15 mm, 10 mm

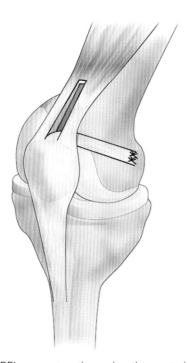

FIG 68.14 MPFL reconstruction using the central portion of the quadriceps tendon. The tendon is released proximally and the patellar insertion left intact. The tendon flap is passed subcutaneously to the medial femoral condyle. (From Lind M, Jakobsen BW, Lund B, et al: Reconstruction of the medial patello-femerol ligament: a new treatment for chronic patella instability. *Acta Orthop Scand* 79:354–360, 2008.)

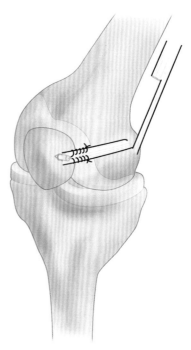

FIG 68.15 MPFL reconstruction using the anterior two-thirds of the adductor tendon. The tendon is released proximally and the femoral insertion left intact. The tendon flap is passed subcutaneously to the proximal patellar edge. (Courtesy M. Lind.)

for a small patella (<35 mm in width) and 15 mm for most patellae.

A looped passer is used to pass a single-strand G graft through the patella from medial to lateral using the ends of a whipstitch in the graft. The graft is secured on the lateral side using the two ends of the whipstitch. One limb of the stitch is passed through the lateral retinaculum with a free needle. It is then tied to the other limb. On the medial side of the patella, a cuff of medial retinaculum is sutured to the graft as it exits the medial border.

The adductor magnus tendon is approached through a separate 3-cm-long incision that extends proximally from a point slightly superior and posterior to the medial femoral epicondyle. The adductor magnus tendon is identified; it can often be palpated before it can be seen. Dissection of the distal tendon insertion includes freeing all interdigitations of the tendon down to its insertion to allow the graft subsequently to lie as distal as possible, approaching the MPFL's anatomic insertion.

The free end of the graft is passed medially from the patella, deep to the deep fascia. It is then passed distal to the adductor tubercle and reflected proximally around and deep to the distal adductor magnus tendon. From here, the free end of the graft is passed anteriorly, again deep to the deep fascia, to reach the midpoint of the medial aspect of the patella. The knee is flexed to 30 to 40 degrees, locating the patella in the trochlear groove. The graft is tensioned just enough to eliminate redundancy in the graft. Where the two arms of the graft pass over one another, just anterior to the adductor insertion, a single stitch is used to secure them to each other. Finally, the free end of the graft is sutured to the periosteum over the middle third of the medial border of the patella (Fig. 68.16).

Medial Collateral Ligament Sling Technique. This technique uses an ST autograft tendon to reconstruct the MPFL (Fig. 68.17).[16] The tendon is harvested and the tibial attachment at the pes anserine is retained. The proximal end of the tendon is transferred to the femoral insertion of the medial collateral ligament.

A 2-cm incision is made over the medial femoral epicondyle and a short longitudinal split is made in the posterior third of the proximal end of the medial collateral ligament. This split subsequently acts as a pulley through which the free end of the ST graft is passed. The free end of the graft is then passed to the anteromedial aspect of the patella. The transferred tendon is sutured to the anterior surface of the patella with the knee flexed to 30 degrees. The criticism of this technique is that it places the femoral insertion of the MPFL lower than its anatomic location. In addition, the more vertical arm does not anatomically duplicate the MPTL.

REHABILITATION AFTER MEDIAL PATELLOFEMORAL LIGAMENT REPAIR RECONSTRUCTION

As with MPFL repair, there is at present no evidence that supports any specific postoperative rehabilitation regimen after MPFL reconstruction.[27] Most of the published series have described a period of restricted range of motion using a knee immobilizer or a hinged brace for 2 to 6 weeks. Typically, the

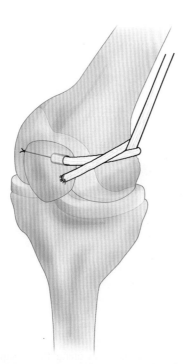

FIG 68.16 MPFL reconstruction using the free ST and G tendons looped around the adductor magnus femoral insertion and fixed to the patella via a short tunnel proximally and a direct suturing to the middle third of the patella. (Courtesy M. Lind.)

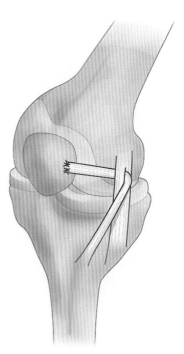

FIG 68.17 MPFL reconstruction using the ST tendon and soft tissue fixation. The tendon insertion is retained and the proximal end of the tendon is transferred to the femoral insertion of the MCL. The graft is passed through a split in the proximal MCL and then sutured to the medial aspect of the patella. (From Lind M, Jakobsen BW, Lund B, et al: Reconstruction of the medial patello-femoral ligament: a new treatment for chronic patella instability. *Acta Orthop Scand* 79:354–360, 2008.)

range of motion is limited to 0 to 60 degrees, although the rationale for this is not entirely clear, given that the reconstruction should be under maximum tension in early knee flexion. Weight-bearing status also varies considerably in the published series, ranging from minimal to full weight bearing. If a graft has been positioned and fixed appropriately, it should be able to withstand full range of motion, with rehabilitation limitations based more on patient comfort and ambulation safety. For isolated MPFL reconstructions, we typically use a hinged knee brace from 0 to 70 degrees of flexion for weeks 0 to 2, increasing to 0 to 90 degrees from weeks 2 to 4, then discontinue the brace. Partial, 50% weight bearing is used the first 2 weeks then advanced as tolerated. Physical therapy works with the patient out of the brace to advance the range of motion as tolerated throughout the recovery.

Using interference screw femoral fixation of a G tendon graft that has been looped through two patellar bone tunnels, we have not experienced problems with a less restrictive regimen, in which a full range of motion and full weight bearing are allowed within the limits of comfort. However, if direct soft tissue fixation is used, some limitation of range of motion and reduced weight bearing may be appropriate until sufficient healing can be expected to have taken place.

With regard to a return to sports activities, it is suggested that closed kinetic chain quadriceps strengthening be introduced from between 3 and 6 weeks and controlled open kinetic strengthening from 3 months.[47] This is followed by a return to noncontact sports, with a resumption of contact sports being considered from 4 to 6 months, depending on individual strength, agility, and confidence.

SKELETALLY IMMATURE PATIENTS

In the skeletally immature, it is preferable not to create bone tunnels or dissect the periosteum in the region of the distal femoral physeal plate. This may require a modification of the femoral fixation method used. Some of the techniques described are suitable for patients with open growth plates. These include the adductor magnus tendon transfer, adductor sling technique, and MCL sling technique. The combined MPFL and MPTL reconstruction can also be safely used, provided that appropriate fixation is used at the femoral and tibial attachment. The central quadriceps tendon graft turned down from above can also be fixed to the medial femur using suture anchors, thereby avoiding larger or deeper drill holes that put the physis at risk.[50a] It is important to remember that the medial femoral anatomic origin of the MPFL is distal to the physis. Because of the curved shape of the distal femoral physis, this can be confusing on a lateral fluoroscopic view and appear to be proximal. Viewing from the AP direction after selecting Schottle's point on the lateral can confirm the true location distal to the physis.

COMPLICATIONS

As with all surgical procedures, there are nonspecific complications such as infection and hematoma formation, as well as complications such as the morbidity of harvesting a tendon autograft and sensory disturbances related to the location of incisions. In particular, the prepatellar and infrapatellar branches of the saphenous nerve can be damaged, with resultant alteration of sensation over the anterior aspect of the knee and proximal leg.[49,62] Another issue relating to the incisions is the potential for widened and unsightly scars on the medial aspect of the knee.[15]

Complications related specifically to the reconstructive procedure include recurrent lateral patellar dislocation, pain and stiffness, and patellar fracture. The rate of redislocation can be affected not only by the surgical technique, but also by the presence of predisposing factors such as patellar alta, trochlear dysplasia, and lateralization of the tibial tubercle as well as the overall alignment of the lower limb. Properly addressing any additional anatomic aberrations will reduce the risk of subsequent patellar dislocations.

Pain and stiffness can have a number of causes. They may be transient and simply the result of surgical intervention on the highly innervated medial aspect of the knee.[1,49] Painful restricted range of motion (ROM) in the immediate postoperative period may lead to adhesion formation and a persistent loss of flexion,[15,77] which may occasionally require manipulation under anesthesia to restore a satisfactory ROM.[12,62] Prominence of fixation hardware on the medial aspect of the medial femoral condyle may also cause local irritation and potentially restrict motion.[14,53,71,72] Even in the absence of prominent hardware, a tunnel in the medial femoral condyle can be a source of ongoing pain. Pain and stiffness may also relate to underlying damage to the articular surfaces of the patellofemoral compartment. As noted, all injuries to the knee need to be addressed, not just the deficient MPFL.

From a surgical point of view, an important cause of postoperative pain and/or stiffness is inappropriate positioning of the graft.[25,78] A graft that is positioned so that it is tighter in flexion than extension can cause anteromedial pain and a restriction of flexion as well as an increase in the force on the articular surface of the medial half of the patellofemoral compartment as the knee moves into greater flexion.[22] Overtensioning the graft will exacerbate these problems.

Patellar fracture is uncommon but usually relates to the use of bone tunnels for graft attachment.[77] Excessively large tunnels may increase the risk of fracture.[45] Some authors believe that penetration of the anterior cortex of the bone may also increase the risk.[12] When a transverse tunnel is used, a displaced transverse fracture of the patella may occur, which is a disabling complication. For those techniques using tunnels that breach the anterior cortex, the fracture is typically an oblique or vertical fracture of the medial border of the patella.

CONCOMITANT SURGICAL PROCEDURES

In the presence of predisposing factors such as trochlear dysplasia, patella alta, an increased TT-TG distance, and tight lateral retinaculum, additional procedures may be necessary to help stabilize the patella. Despite various published protocols, at present there is no evidence to indicate when a supplementary procedure should be performed in conjunction with an MPFL reconstruction. It should, however, be kept in mind that a successful MPFL reconstruction effectively restores the stabilizing anatomy of the individual to the predislocation state. The decision to use one or more concomitant procedures needs to be based on the perceived risk of further challenges to patellar stability in a given individual. In the case of a tight lateral retinaculum, this may need to be addressed with a concomitant lateral retinacular release or lengthening. Patella alta may be addressed with tibial tubercle distalization or patellar tendon shortening. An increased TT-TG distance may be addressed with an anteromedialization osteotomy. Trochlear dysplasia may be addressed with a trochleoplasty. As noted previously, when to perform these additional procedures concomitantly with an MPFL reconstruction is not yet clear.

CLINICAL RESULTS

Reconstruction of the MPFL is a relatively new surgical solution for recurrent lateral patellar dislocation. There have been no level 1 or level 2 studies that report the outcome of this type of surgery. The evidence for clinical outcome results after MPFL reconstruction is, therefore, based on level III and IV studies involving less than 100 patients, except in one study.[39] Two studies reach greater than 10-year follow-up,[55,67] but the remainder involve less than 5-year follow-up. Moreover, studies involving patients undergoing isolated MPFL reconstruction have been inconsistent in their evaluation and reporting of preoperative variables including demographics, history, examination findings, and imaging findings, making comparison among studies difficult. The studies have also included a variety of clinical outcome tools and follow-up examination parameters, again making comparison among studies difficult. The published studies are summarized in Tables 68.1 and 68.2.

In general, MPFL reconstruction results in very good patellar stability, with no redislocations in many studies and an overall redislocation rate below 10%. The incidence of further episodes of patellar subluxation, as opposed to dislocation, has been inconsistently reported and no conclusions can be drawn about this entity. This situation is also, in part, the result of the lack of consistency in terminology and clinical assessment of patellar subluxation.

Success rates based on clinical scores have generally been good, with increases in Kujala scores from as low as 50, often to greater than 90 postoperatively. Lysholm, Fulkerson, and International Knee Documentation Committee (IKDC) scores have generally followed the same pattern. Tegner activity scale scores generally improve by a couple points, suggesting that many patients return to recreational sports. Although a variety of operative techniques and graft choices have been evaluated, graft type and surgical technique do not seem to have influenced the clinical results. When reported, several studies have, however, demonstrated clinical outcomes that are worse in patients with patellofemoral articular cartilage lesions at the time of surgery.

It is again important to point out here that most of the studies evaluating patients following isolated MPFL reconstruction have used exclusion criteria to carefully select patients.[79] Generally, the patients included in these studies have had few risk factors for further dislocation, and are therefore more likely to do well following MPFL reconstruction. It is not yet clear how best to apply MPFL reconstruction and what concomitant procedures should be done when there are risk factors present such as patella alta, trochlear dysplasia, or an increased TT-TG distance.

CONCLUSIONS

In general terms, there are three surgical approaches to the restoration of function of the MPFL:
1. Acute repair. At this time, the literature yields a mixed picture of results. Using redislocation rate as an end point, the literature does not support acute MPFL repair as a best practice option. However, in the setting of a surgical intervention to

TABLE 68.1	**Duration of Follow-Up by Study**			
Study	Patients (Knees) Recruited	Patients (Knees) With Follow-Up	Average Length of Follow-Up	Range
Ahmad	21	20	2.6 years	2.0-3.3 years
Bitar	21	21	3.2 years	2.0-4.0 years
Christiansen	44	44	1.8 years	1.0-2.7 years
Deie	29 (31)	29 (31)	3.2 years	2.0-5.0 years
Drez	19	15	2.6 years	2.0-3.6 years
Ebied	21 (25) 16 (17) minus tibial tuberosity	21 (25)[a]	2.8 years	Minimum 2.0 years
Gomes	24	24	4.4 years	2.5-5.9 years
Goyal	39	32	3.2 years	1.0-5.7 years
Hinterwimmer	19	19	1.3 years	Minimum 1.0 year
Howells	201 (219) 188 (206) minus tibial tuberosity	193 (211)[a]	1.3 years	0.5-3.5 years
Kang	90	82	2.0 years	2.0 years
Kita	71	24 (25)	1.1 years	0.5-2.2 years
Kohn	15	15	2.0 years	2.0 years
Ma	32	32	3.3 years	2.0-4.6 years
Matthews	21 (25)	21 (25)	2.6 years	0.3-7.3 years
Nelitz	22	21	2.8 years	2.0-3.6 years
Nomura 2006	12	12	4.2 years	3.1-5.6 years
Nomura 2007	Not stated (39)	22 (24)	11.9 years	8.5-17.2 years
Panni	48 (51)	45 (48)	2.8 years	2.0-4.5 years
Ronga	28	28	3.1 years	2.5-4 years
Sillanpaa	18	15	10.1 years	8.0-13.0 years
Steiner	36	34	5.5 years	2.0-10.8 years
Wagner	50	50	Not stated	1.0-2.0 years
Witonski	19	10	Not stated	Minimum 2.0 years

[a]Total group reported on at follow-up.

TABLE 68.2 Subjective Outcome Tools and Recurrence Rate by Study		
Study	Redislocation/ Subluxation	Patient-Reported Outcome Measure
Ahmad	0	Kujala, Tegner, Lysholm, IKDC
Bitar	0	Kujala
Christiansen	1 dislocation/3 subluxation	Kujala, Tegner
Deie	0 (1 re-do 3 years out for medial instability, resolved)	Kujala
Drez	1 dislocation/1 subluxation	Kujala, Tegner, Fulkerson
Ebied	Not reported	IKDC, Insall
Gomes	Not reported/1 subluxation	Kujala
Goyal	0	Kujala
Hinterwimmer	0	Kujala, Tegner, Insall
Howells	0	Kujala, Tegner, Fulkerson, IKDC
Kang	0	Kujala, Tegner, Lysholm
Kita	0	Kujala
Kohn	0	Kujala, Tegner, IKDC
Ma	Not reported	Kujala, Tegner
Matthews	0	Kujala, Tegner
Nelitz	0	Kujala
Nomura 2006	0	Kujala
Nomura 2007	1 dislocation/not reported	Kujala
Panni	0	Kujala, Lysholm, Fulkerson
Ronga	3 dislocation/not reported	Kujala, IKDC
Sillanpaa	1 dislocation/2 subluxation	Kujala, Tegner
Steiner	0	Kujala, Tegner, Lysholm
Wagner	1 dislocation	Kujala
Witonski	0	Kujala

stabilize an osteochondral fracture of the patella or trochlea, MRI localization of the site of an MPFL tear that may be amenable to repair seems prudent. A decision regarding repair can then be made at the time of surgery.

2. Delayed tightening or imbrication of the MPFL (for chronic laxity). This is not recommended as a best practice option at this time.

3. Reconstruction of MPFL with graft. This has been shown to produce the most consistent results. There is currently no consensus regarding which surgical technique provides the best clinical results. Graft and technique choice also do not seem to influence the clinical results, as long as key surgical principles are followed.

KEY REFERENCES

3. Arendt EA, Moeller A, Agel J: Clinical outcomes of medial patellofemoral ligament repair in recurrent (chronic) lateral patella dislocations. *Knee Surg Sports Traumatol Arthrosc* 19(11):1909–1914, 2011.

13. Conlan T, Garth WP, Jr, Lemons JE: Evaluation of the medial soft-tissue restraints of the extensor mechanism of the knee. *J Bone Joint Surg Am* 75(5):682–693, 1993.

22. Elias JJ, Cosgarea AJ: Technical errors during medial patellofemoral ligament reconstruction could overload medial patellofemoral cartilage: a computational analysis. *Am J Sports Med* 34(9):1478–1485, 2006.

25. Farr J, Schepsis AA: Reconstruction of the medial patellofemoral ligament for recurrent patellar instability. *J Knee Surg* 19(4):307–316, 2006.

26. Feller JA, Amis AA, Andrish JT, et al: Surgical biomechanics of the patellofemoral joint. *Arthroscopy* 23(5):542–553, 2007.

37. Hautamaa PV, Fithian DC, Kaufman KR, et al: Medial soft tissue restraints in lateral patellar instability and repair. *Clin Orthop Relat Res* 349:174–182, 1998.

45. Lind M, Jakobsen BW, Lund B, et al: Reconstruction of the medial patellofemoral ligament for treatment of patellar instability. *Acta Orthop* 79(3):354–360, 2008.

Monson J, Arendt EA: Rehabilitative protocols for select patellofemoral procedures and nonoperative management schemes. *Sports Med Arthrosc Rev* 20:136, 2012.

Nelitz M, Dornacher D, Dreyhaupt J, et al: The relation of the distal femoral physis and the medial patellofemoral ligament. *Knee Surg Sports Traumatol Arthrosc* 19:2067, 2011.

48. Mountney J, Senavongse W, Amis AA, et al: Tensile strength of the medial patellofemoral ligament before and after repair or reconstruction. *J Bone Joint Surg Br* 87(1):36–40, 2005.

63. Schottle PB, Fucentese SF, Romero J: Clinical and radiological outcome of medial patellofemoral ligament reconstruction with a semitendinosus autograft for patella instability. *Knee Surg Sports Traumatol Arthrosc* 13(7):516–521, 2005.

65. Sillanpaa PJ, Maenpaa HM, Mattila VM, et al: Arthroscopic surgery for primary traumatic patellar dislocation: a prospective, nonrandomized study comparing patients treated with and without acute arthroscopic stabilization with a median 7-year follow-up. *Am J Sports Med* 36(12):2301–2309, 2008.

72. Steiner TM, Torga-Spak R, Teitge RA: Medial patellofemoral ligament reconstruction in patients with lateral patellar instability and trochlear dysplasia. *Am J Sports Med* 34(8):1254–1261, 2006.

81. Warren LF, Marshall JL: The supporting structures and layers on the medial side of the knee: an anatomical analysis. *J Bone Joint Surgery Am* 61(1):56–62, 1979.

79. Tompkins MA, Arendt EA: Patellar instability factors in isolated medial patellofemoral ligament reconstructions. What does the literature tell us? A systematic review. *Am J Sports Med* 43(9):2318–2327, 2015.

The references for this chapter can also be found on www.expertconsult.com.

69

Sulcus-Deepening Trochleoplasty

David DeJour, Paulo R.F. Saggin, Vinícius Canello Kuhn

NORMAL AND PATHOLOGIC ANATOMY

A normal trochlea is located in the anterior aspect of the distal femur. It is composed of two facets divided by a longitudinal groove, the trochlear sulcus. The lateral facet is the largest; it extends more proximally than the medial one and is more protuberant (higher) in the anteroposterior aspect. Proximally the trochlea extends until the junction of the articular cartilage with the femoral anterior cortex, which is covered by adipose tissue and synovium. Distally it is limited by the condylotrochlear grooves, one in each division of the facets with the correspondent femoral condyle. The trochlear sulcus extends distally until the notch deviating slight laterally from the femoral axis.[31]

Dysplastic trochleae are shallow, flat, or even convex. It is easier to consider and define their abnormality in terms of function or deviation from the normal pattern. Radiologic features are also easier to define and measure than those observed during surgical procedures. However, it is common sense that the surgical mark of these trochleae is their abnormal shape. A bump in the superolateral aspect is common (Fig. 69.1).

Radiographic lateral projections of normal trochleae, obtained with perfect superimposition of both femoral condyles, will typically show the contour of the facets and, posterior to them, the line representing the deepest points (floor) of the sulcus.[23,24] In this projection, the lateral facet is distinguished from the medial one by its more visible condylotrochlear groove and because of the greater opacity to the rays of the lateral condyle, which is more perpendicular than the medial one to the x-ray beam. The line representing the bottom of the groove is continuous with the intercondylar notch line (Blumensaat line), extending anteriorly and proximally. It may end posteriorly to the condyle line (type A) or join the medial condyle line in the superior part of the trochlea (type B).[15]

On lateral projections, trochlear dysplasia is defined by the crossing sign: the radiographic line of the trochlear sulcus crosses (or reaches) the projection of the femoral condyles. The crossing point represents the exact location where the floor of the trochlear sulcus reaches the same elevation of the femoral condyles, meaning that the trochlea becomes flat in this exact location. The position of the floor of the trochlear sulcus is abnormal in relation to the anterior femoral cortex. In normal knees it is usually 0.8 mm posterior to a line tangent to the anterior femoral cortex; in knees with dysplastic trochlea its mean position is 3.2 mm anterior to this same line[16] (Fig. 69.2).

Two other features are typical of dysplastic trochleae in lateral views: the supratrochlear spur and the double-contour sign. The supratrochlear spur is a protuberance in the superolateral aspect of the trochlea. The double contour represents the medial hypoplastic facet, seen posterior to the lateral one in this projection. To be considered pathologic, the double contour must be observed below or distal to the crossing sign. Based on these signs, trochlear dysplasia may be classified into the following four types[13,14,35]:

- Type A: Presence of crossing sign in the true lateral view. The trochlea is shallower than normal but still symmetrical and concave.
- Type B: Crossing sign and trochlear spur. The trochlea is flat or convex in slice images.
- Type C: Presence of crossing sign and the double-contour sign on the lateral view. There is no spur. In slice images the lateral facet is convex and the medial hypoplastic.
- Type D: Combines all the mentioned signs—crossing sign, supratrochlear spur, and double-contour sign. In the slice images there is clear asymmetry of the facet's height, also referred as a cliff pattern. (Fig. 69.3)

Axial views obtained with 45 degrees of knee flexion (Merchant view) allow the measurement of the sulcus angle. From the deepest point of the bottom of the groove, two lines are drawn, connecting it with the most superior point of each facet. The mean normal value defined by the Merchant view was 138 degrees (standard deviation [SD] ± 6); angles superior to 150 degrees are considered abnormal. Alternatively, 30-degree flexion axial views will provide those measurements with better trochlear shape assessment.[10] Dysplastic trochleae will show higher angles, some of which cannot even be measured because there is no sulcus. In addition, the subjective impression of the trochlear shape is important and should be performed in no more than 45 degrees of knee flexion. Greater flexion angles show the lower part of the trochlea, which is more normal. Any other signs of patellar instability, such as those evidenced in other projections and with other methods, serve as clues to the dysplasia diagnosis because 96% of patients with a patellar dislocation will present with it.[16]

The computed tomography (CT) scan improves the visualization on the axial plane. Three-dimensional reconstruction can be obtained for global shape assessment. Magnetic resonance imaging (MRI) is another modality in which dysplasia is well documented. The cartilaginous shape of the sulcus can be evaluated; this is particularly interesting because the cartilaginous anatomy does not follow exactly the underlying bony anatomy.[33] However, in higher-grade dysplastic trochleae, bony and cartilaginous anatomies usually match (flat or convex bone will be covered by flat or convex cartilage). MRI axial images help to better evaluate trochlear dysplasia while allowing differentiation of low- from high-grade dysplasia with better

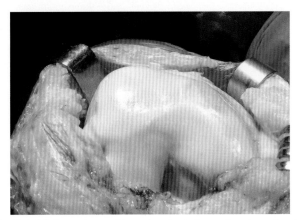

FIG 69.1 High-grade trochlear dysplasia (*anterior view* of a right knee). There is no sulcus, and in the lateral aspect *(right)* a big bump can be observed.

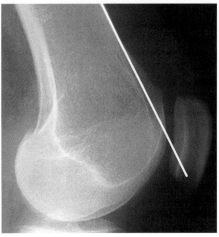

FIG 69.2 The trochlear bump is calculated as the amount of trochlea which is in front of a line parallel to the anterior femoral cortex. Alternatively the sulcus floor position can also be calculated from this line.

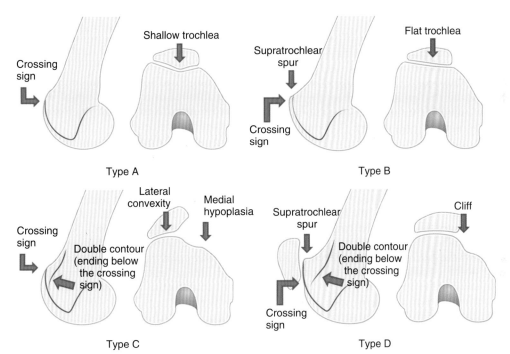

FIG 69.3 Trochlear dysplasia according to D. Dejour. Trochlear dysplasia type A: presence of crossing sign in the lateral view. The trochlea is shallower than normal, but still symmetrical and concave. Trochlear dysplasia type B: crossing sign and trochlear spur. The trochlea is flat in axial images. There is prominence of all the trochlea. Trochlear dysplasia type C: there is the presence of crossing sign and the double-contour sign on lateral view. There is no prominence and in axial views the lateral facet is convex and the medial hypoplastic. Trochlear dysplasia type D: crossing sign, supratrochlear spur, and double-contour sign. In axial view, there is clear asymmetry of the height of the facets, also referred as a cliff pattern.

inter-observer agreement than lateral radiographs.[21] Another interesting feature of dysplastic trochleae is demonstrated by condylar and sulcus height measurements from the posterior condyles in axial views: the lateral facet seems to have a normal height, whereas the groove and medial facet are protuberant.[6]

FUNCTION AND BIOMECHANICS

Trochlear function must be well known to understand the principles of modifying its shape. The lateral facet of the trochlea is oriented obliquely in both the sagittal and coronal planes.

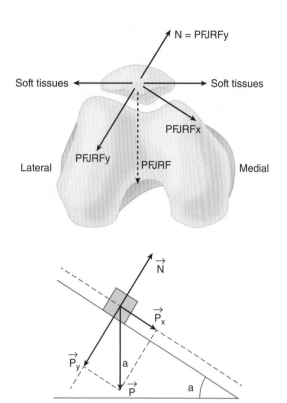

FIG 69.4 Diagram illustrating the several forces acting on the patella in the axial plane. The lateral part of the patellofemoral (PF) joint is inclined medially. The patellofemoral joint reaction force (PFJRF) (*P*) may me decomposed in two vectors: P_y, which is canceled by the reaction force (*N*); and P_x, which pulls the patella medially.

It deviates anteriorly and laterally from the bottom of the groove. The articulating opposed lateral patellar surface follows this orientation. The patella rests in front of the femoral cortex in total extension but engages the trochlea in early flexion. A posteriorly directed force, the patellofemoral reaction force, pushes the patella against the trochlea and, as a result of the obliquity of the two opposed articulating surfaces in relation to the coronal plane, a medializing vector of force is created, directing patellar tracking.[2] From this brief biomechanical explanation, one conclusion is obvious: the trochlea guides patellar tracking (Fig. 69.4).

Not only patellar subluxation or lateral displacement is dependent on trochlear shape but also patellar tilt. There is a high statistical correlation between patellar tilt and the type of trochlear dysplasia.[34] Incongruence between the two opposing surfaces has a major role in tilt generation. The higher the degree of dysplasia, the higher the patellar tilt.

Another feature not included in trochlear function but derived from the same principle is that the patellofemoral reaction force depends on the trochlear prominence. The bigger the trochlear prominence, the greater the reaction force. Inversely, by diminishing the protrusion, the reaction force is also expected to be diminished (Fig. 69.5).

INDICATIONS

Trochleoplasty indications are precise—recurrent patellar dislocations with concomitant high-grade trochlear dysplasia,

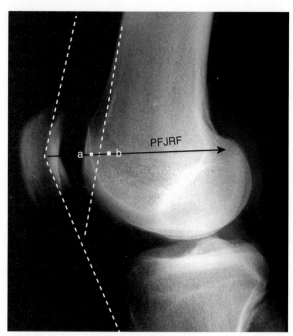

FIG 69.5 Note how the patellofemoral joint reaction force is diminished when the position of the floor of the trochlear sulcus is moved posteriorly (from "a" to "b").

often associated with abnormal patellar tracking, in the absence of established osteoarthritis, which would otherwise indicate a patellofemoral arthroplasty. Open growth plates are a contraindication to trochleoplasty.

The type of dysplasia should be observed when determining the procedure because not all procedures fit all deformities. Types B and D are the most suitable to deepening trochleoplasty because they present prominence. Lateral facet–elevating trochleoplasty is proposed by some authors and, although no consensus of indication exists, type C dysplasia would be the best candidate for this procedure.

In our opinion type A dysplasia does not need to be surgically addressed. It is also not considered severe trochlear dysplasia. Major instability or maltracking, if present, should be attributed to other anatomic abnormalities (eg, tibial tubercle–trochlear groove [TT-TG] distance, patellar tilt, patella alta).

The degree of instability should also be taken into account when surgery is proposed. Trochleoplasty, like any other surgical procedure, is liable to failure. This should be known when discussing the procedure with the patient with mild symptoms and when conservative treatment has not yet been proposed.

As important as a precise indication, the evaluation and correction of associated abnormalities have to be accomplished. No procedure will be successful if there are other important issues neglected. The TT-TG distance should be assessed preoperatively. Its correction is not always necessary because the trochleoplasty procedure lateralizes the trochlear groove, diminishing the TT-TG distance between 5 and 10 mm.[27,29] The sulcus-deepening trochleoplasty is only one of several specific procedures for addressing each of the main factors in patellar instability.

PROCEDURES AND OPTIONS

Three main techniques are described.

Lateral Facet–Elevating Trochleoplasty

Albee pioneered this procedure in 1915.[1] It consists of an oblique osteotomy under the lateral facet, where a corticocancellous bone wedge is interposed, with the apex medial and the base lateral. The osteotomy advances to the base of the trochlear groove but does not disrupt it, producing a hinge in its medial aspect. The result is that it elevates the more lateral aspect of the trochlear lateral facet and increases its obliquity, thus increasing the containment force acting on the patella. At least 5 mm of subchondral bone should be maintained to avoid trochlear necrosis (Fig. 69.6).

The procedure is effective for patellar containment, but it increases the patellofemoral reaction force when it increases the trochlear protuberance. Pain and arthritis may result from this. Nowadays, this procedure is rarely indicated, but it might be used in cases when trochlear dysplasia is a consequence of reduced height of the lateral facet or in cases of short trochlea.[20]

Sulcus-Deepening Trochleoplasty

This procedure was first described by Bilton Polar in 1890, then by Masse in 1978[25]; it was modified and standardized by Dejour et al. in 1987.[11,15] The main goal is to decrease the prominence

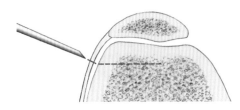
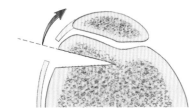

FIG 69.6 Albee's lateral facet–elevating trochleoplasty. The osteotomy is performed under the lateral facet. The medial osteochondral hinge is preserved intact and subsequent grafting under the flap will increase the lateral facet height.

of the trochlea and to create a new groove with normal depth and orientation. This procedure is technically more demanding than the lateral facet–elevating trochleoplasty, but it is more anatomic and acts on the essential cause of the problem. It has the advantage of treating the cause of the dislocation because it corrects the abnormal patterns underlying the different grades of trochlear dysplasia.[3]

The procedure can be performed under regional anesthesia and sedation. The patient is positioned supine. The entire extremity is prepared and draped. The incision is performed with the extremity flexed to 90 degrees; a straight midline skin incision is performed from the superior patellar margin to the tibiofemoral articulation. The extremity is then positioned in extension, and a medial full-thickness skin flap is developed. The arthrotomy is performed through a midvastus-adapted approach: medial retinaculum sharp dissection starting over the 1- to 2-cm medial border of the patella and blunt dissection of *vastus medialis obliquus* (VMO) fibers starting distally at the superomedial pole of the patella, extending approximately 4 cm into the muscle belly (Fig. 69.7).

The patella is briefly everted for inspection of chondral injuries and proper treatment (flap resection, microfracture, autologous chondrocyte implantation) if needed, and then retracted laterally. The trochlea is exposed, and the peritrochlear synovium and periosteum are incised along their osteochondral junction and reflected from the field using a periosteal elevator. The anterior femoral cortex should be visible to determine the amount of deepening that should be undertaken (Fig. 69.8). Changing the knee's degree of flexion allows improved view of the complete operative field and avoids extending the incision.

After the trochlea is fully exposed, the new one is planned and drawn with a sterile pen. The native trochlear groove is marked. Two additional divergent lines starting at the notch and going proximally through the condylotrochlear grooves *(sulcus terminalis)*, representing the lateral and medial facet limits, are also traced. They should not enter the tibiofemoral articulation. Finally, the new trochlear groove is marked in a more lateral position according to the preoperative TT-TG value. The superior limit is the osteochondral edge and the inferior is the intercondylar notch (Fig. 69.9).

The next step is accessing the undersurface of the femoral trochlea. For this purpose a thin strip of cortical bone is removed around the trochlea. The width of the strip is equal to the prominence of the trochlea from the anterior femoral cortex

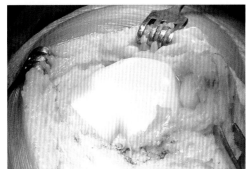
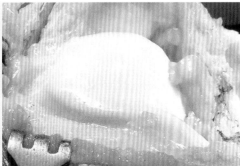

FIG 69.7 Trochlear dysplasia. Anterior *(left)* and lateral *(right)* view during surgical exposure showing the absence of the sulcus and the prominence of the trochlea in relation to the anterior femoral cortex.

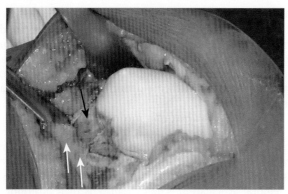

FIG 69.8 Surgical exposure. The periosteum is incised along the osteochondral edge and reflected away from the trochlear margin *(white arrows)*. The anterior femoral cortex should be visible to guide the bone resection *(black arrow)*.

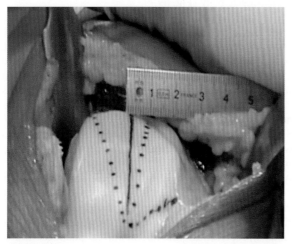

FIG 69.9 After the surgical exposure the new trochlea is drawn. From the intercondylar notch, the native trochlear groove and two divergent lines, representing the lateral and medial facet limits, are marked *(dashed lines)*. The new trochlear groove is marked in a more lateral position according to the preoperative TT-TG value *(continuous line)*.

(ie, the bump formed). A sharp osteotome is used and gently tapped. A rongeur is used next to remove the bone (Fig. 69.10).

Subsequently, cancellous bone must be removed from the undersurface of the trochlea. A first drill is used to make initial holes under the cartilage. It has a guide that is fixed on the cartilage, anteriorly to the notch. The maximum proximity between the tips of the drill and the guide is 5 mm, preventing violation of the cartilage surface (Fig. 69.11). After this, another drill with a depth guide set at 5 mm is used to ensure uniform thickness of the osteochondral flap, maintaining an adequate amount of bone attached to the cartilage (Fig. 69.12). The guide also avoids injuring the cartilage or getting too close to it, which could result in thermal injury. The shell produced must be sufficiently compliant to allow molding without being fractured. Cancellous bone removal is extended until reaching the notch. More bone is removed from the central portion, where the new trochlear groove will rest (Fig. 69.13).

Light pressure should be able to mold the flap to the underlying cancellous bone bed in the distal femur (Fig. 69.14). The groove and sometimes the lateral facet external margin should be cut to allow further molding, which is achieved by gently tapping a bone tamp over a scalpel (Fig. 69.15). If the correction obtained is satisfactory, the new trochlea is fixated: one absorbable anchor is applied near the notch (vertex) (Fig. 69.16); one absorbable no. 2 suture (doubled) spans each facet from the anchor in the notch to another anchor applied in the supratrochlear fossa, proximal to the end of the cartilage. The system used precludes knots; the sutures are tensioned and fixated as the proximal anchors are inserted. Pressure is applied posteriorly while the sutures are being tensioned, ensuring that the prominence is removed and that the facets are flush with the anterior femoral cortex (Fig. 69.17). Patellar tracking is tested. Periosteum and synovial tissue are sutured to the osteochondral edge.

We routinely associate a soft tissue procedure to trochleoplasty, such as a medial patellofemoral ligament (MPFL) reconstruction, which is our procedure of choice.

Deepening trochleoplasty plays a triple role in cases of trochlear dysplasia: it creates a new trochlear shape with a central groove and oblique facets; it reduces the patellofemoral joint reaction force by decreasing the trochlear prominence; and it performs a proximal realignment, reducing the TT-TG distance. It is recommended for patients with types B and D dysplasia, in which the prominence of the trochlea is important.

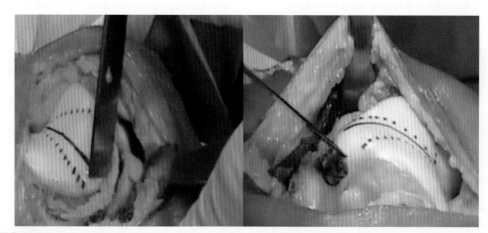

FIG 69.10 A sharp osteotome is used to remove a thin strip of cortical bone around the trochlea to access its undersurface.

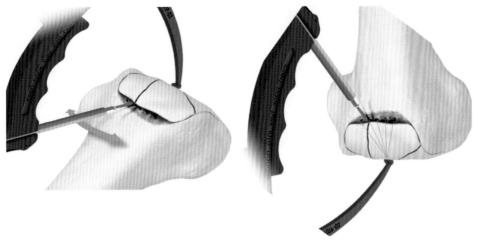

FIG 69.11 Drill with guide to initiate removing the cancellous bone under the cartilage of the trochlea. It is fixed anteriorly to the notch and prevents injuring the cartilage.

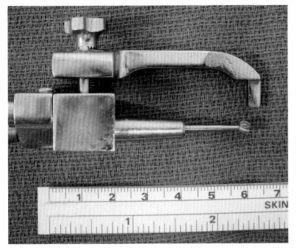

FIG 69.12 Drill with depth guide used to remove the cancellous bone from the trochlear under surface.

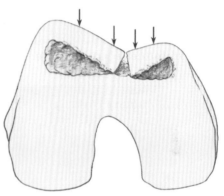

FIG 69.14 After the cancellous bone has been removed, the osteochondral flaps can lie over the new bone bed and the sulcus shape can be corrected.

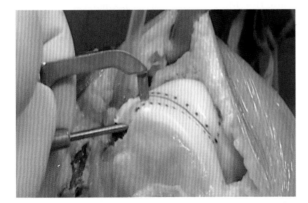

FIG 69.13 The guide avoids injuring the cartilage or getting too close to it. More bone is removed from the central portion.

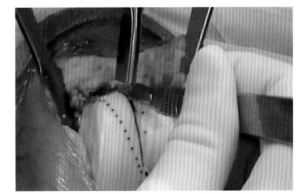

FIG 69.15 To allow further modeling to the underlying bone bed, the osteochondral flaps may be cut in the sulcus and facets lines.

This procedure is not adequate for type C patients, in whom there is no trochlear prominence (Fig. 69.18).

Bereiter Trochleoplasty

This technique was described by Bereiter and Gautier in 1994.[5] In this method a lateral parapatellar approach is performed, the trochlea exposed, and the synovium dissected away from it. Then a thin osteochondral flake with 2 mm of subchondral bone is elevated from the trochlea, extending till the intercondylar notch. The distal femoral subchondral bone is deepened and refashioned with osteotomes and a high-speed burr. Next the osteochondral flap is seated in the refashioned bed and fixated with 3-mm-wide Vicryl bands, passing through the center of the groove and exiting in the lateral femoral condyle. The periosteum is reattached to the edge of the cartilage, and the wound is closed.

Based on Bereiter trochleoplasty, Blønd and Schöttle[9] described in 2010 the deepening trochleoplasty performed under arthroscopy. In 2015 the first author has published an

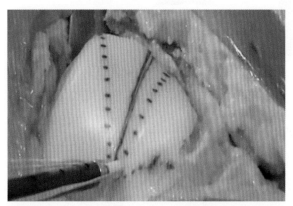

FIG 69.16 The first absorbable anchor is applied near the notch.

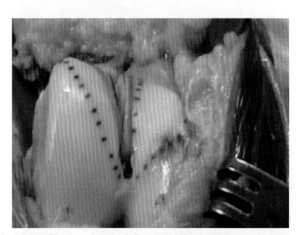

FIG 69.17 Final aspect of fixation. Two other anchors were applied proximal to each facet, while posteriorly pressure and tension to the sutures were maintained.

optimized description of this technique.[7] Using suprapatellar portals, a thin osteochondral trochlear flap is elevated, and the cancellous bone behind it is undermined using a shaver. The flap is then fixated with anchors and absorbable sutures. The arthroscopic trochleoplasty can be an option when open surgery is not required by any associated procedures.

POSTOPERATIVE CARE

The main principles guiding rehabilitation have to respect the associated procedures, and rehabilitation must also apply to them. Trochleoplasty does not need weight protection or range of motion limitation. Movement may in fact improve cartilage healing and further molding of the trochlea; continuous passive movement (CPM) is usually used during the first days. Partial weight bearing is allowed with an extension brace and aided by crutches in the first 15 days, when they can be discontinued if possible. The brace must be removed during the exercises.

During the first 6 weeks patients are encouraged to perform exercises for range of motion, as tolerated, including isometric quadriceps and hamstring strengthening. Range of motion is gradually recovered, avoiding forced or painful postures. Quadriceps strengthening with weights on the feet or tibial tubercle is discouraged.

After 45 days the protocol also includes closed-chain and weight-bearing proprioception exercises. Cycling is usually possible, with weak resistance initially. Active ascension of the patella can be performed seated, with the leg stretched and the knee unlocked, by static and isometric quadriceps contractions. Quadriceps strengthening with weights on the feet or tibial tubercle is still discouraged. The anterior and posterior muscular chains are stretched. Weight-bearing proprioception exercises are started when full extension is complete, first in bipodal stance and later in monopodal stance when there is no pain.

After 12 weeks, running can be initiated on a straight line. Closed kinetic chain muscular reinforcement between 0 and 60 degrees with minor loads but long series are allowed. Stretching of the anterior and posterior muscular chains is continued. The patient is encouraged to proceed with the rehabilitation on his or her own. After 6 months, sports on a recreational or competitive level can be resumed.

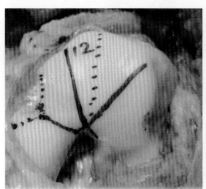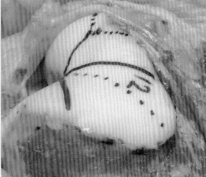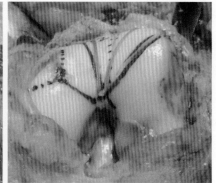

FIG 69.18 High-grade trochlear dysplasia after exposure and planning, with the new trochlea drawn 12 mm lateral to the native trochlea *(left figure)*. A thin strip of cortical bone around the trochlea is removed to access its undersurface *(middle figure)*. After fixation with absorbable sutures the new trochlea is flush with the anterior femoral cortex and does not show the prominence presented before *(right figure)*.

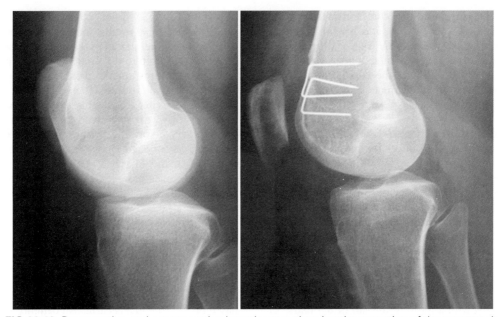

FIG 69.19 Preoperative and postoperative lateral x-rays showing the resection of the supratrochlear bump and trochlear prominence correction. In addition, patellar tilt is clearly improved. Fixation was made by staples.

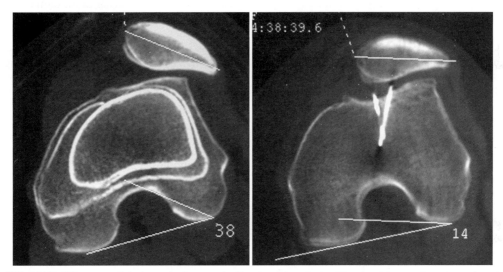

FIG 69.20 CT scan axial views before and after trochleoplasty. The trochlear sulcus is restored and patellar tilt is corrected. Patellar subluxation is also improved. Fixation was made by staples.

Six weeks postoperatively radiographs, including anteroposterior view, lateral view, and axial view in 30 degrees of flexion, are taken (Fig. 69.19). After 6 months a CT scan is obtained to document the obtained correction (Fig. 69.20).

RESULTS

Several series analyzing the results of trochleoplasty are found in the literature. Most of them have short-term or midterm follow-up. They are not homogeneous concerning type of trochleoplasty, inclusion criteria, outcomes, associated procedures, and the presence or absence of previous surgery, obscuring comparative analysis. Studies comparing different techniques or comparing trochleoplasty with other procedures are also missing. Nevertheless, the studies generally demonstrate good results, with improvements in clinical scores and radiographic

parameters. Most of the patients do not sustain a redislocation after the procedure and are satisfied, whereas only few still complain of instability or positive apprehension sign. The best results are demonstrated in patients with objective patellar instability, high-grade trochlear dysplasia (type B and D), and when all risk factors for instability are treated concomitantly.

A systematic review compared the results of trochleoplasty versus nontrochleoplasty procedures in patients treated for patellofemoral instability with the presence of high-grade trochlear dysplasia. Improvement was observed in all patients, regardless of the realization of trochleoplasty or not. However, the trochleoplasty group showed superior results in redislocation rates and degenerative patellofemoral osteoarthritis progression, although with inferior outcomes in range of motion.[32]

Verdonk et al.[37] reported 13 procedures (deepening trochleoplasty), with a mean follow-up of 18 months. Patients were assessed using the Larsen-Lauridsen score considering pain, stiffness, osteopatellar crepitus, flexion, and loss of function. Seven patients scored poorly, three fairly well, and three well. However, on a subjective scoring system six patients rated the result as very good, four as good, and one as satisfactory. Only two patients found the result inadequate and would never undergo the procedure again. Thus, 77% were satisfied with the procedure.

Donell et al.[17] described 15 patients (17 knees) submitted to deepening trochleoplasty, with a mean follow-up of 3 years. Trochleoplasty was indicated if there was a boss larger than 6 mm, and associated procedures were performed as required. Of the 17 knees, 9 had undergone previous surgery for patellar instability. The boss height was reduced postoperatively from an average of 7.5 to 0.7 mm. Tracking became normal in 11 knees and 6 had a slight J sign. Seven knees had mild residual apprehension. Seven patients were very satisfied, six were satisfied, and two were disappointed. The Kujala score improved from an average of 48 to 75 out of 100.

Von Knoch et al.[38] studied 45 knees that had underwent Bereiter trochleoplasty, with a mean follow-up of 8.3 years; 15 had undergone previous surgery. None of them had recurrence of dislocation after the trochleoplasty. Thirty-five knees had pain preoperatively. Postoperatively pain became worse in 15 (33.4%), remained unchanged in 4 (8.8%), and improved in 22 (49%). Four knees that had no pain preoperatively (8.8%) continued to have no pain. Of 33 knees available for radiologic assessment postoperatively, all but 2 knees (93.9%) achieved radiographic correction of trochlear dysplasia. Degenerative changes of the patellofemoral joint developed in 30% (10) of the knees.

Schottle and colleagues[29] reported 19 knees that underwent trochleoplasty (Bereiter) in 16 patients, with a mean follow-up of 3 years. None of the patients sustained a redislocation. Sixteen of 19 knees improved subjectively. The mean Kujala score improved from 56 points preoperatively to 80 points in the latest visit. In 12 knees the pain level became reduced, whereas there was increased pain in 2 knees postoperatively. Four patients reported persistent apprehension while the examiner attempted to lateralize the patella in the extended leg.

Utting et al.[36] analyzed 40 patients (59 knees) with patellofemoral instability secondary to trochlear dysplasia that were submitted to Bereiter trochleoplasty. Only 42 knees were followed for more than 12 months, with a mean follow-up of 24 months. At the time of surgery, from the 59 knees operated, 27 (46%) needed associated procedures. The patients were analyzed in 5 clinical scores: Oxford Knee Score (OKS), Western Ontario and McMaster Universities (WOMAC), International Knee Documentation Comitee (IKDC), Kujala, and Lysholm. All patients that were followed for more than 12 months had improvements in these scores. One patient sustained a traumatic dislocation after a fall, with posterior successful conservative treatment. No other patients presented recurrent patellofemoral dislocations.

Zaki and Rae[39] reported a consecutive series of 25 patients (27 knees) with patellar instability associated with trochlear dysplasia and the presence of a femoral boss, with a mean follow-up of 54 months. They were submitted to a modified trochleoplasty, similar to Bereiter technique, but the trochlea fixation was achieved with four to five anchor sutures that passed through fine drill holes in the articular cartilage. Twenty knees (74%) presented previous surgery. Associated procedures were performed as needed. No redislocations were observed.

According to the Lysholm score 19 knees (70%) had good-to-excellent functional results, and 8 knees (30%) had poor results. The radiographic analysis showed a decrease of the femoral boss height from 6 to 0.4 mm. Nine of the patients (33%) had residual symptoms, such as pain, swelling, and crepitus.

Fucentese et al.[19] studied the results of 38 patients (44 knees) in whom a Bereiter trochleoplasty was performed, with a mean follow-up of 4 years. Thirteen knees had undergone previous knee surgery before the trochleoplasty. According to the classification described by Dejour et al., there were 9 type A, 15 type B, 9 type C, and 11 type D trochlear dysplasia knees. In their results the Kujala score increased from 68 to 90. Pain remained unchanged in 27 knees, decreased in 14, and increased in 3. The results were ranked excellent in 27 knees, good in 10, fair in 2, and poor in 5 knees. This study has showed that the only significant predictor of a better outcome was the type of dysplasia, with better subjective outcome in dysplasia type B and D.

Dejour et al.[12] described 22 patients (24 knees) submitted to the sulcus-deepening trochleoplasty, with a mean follow-up of 66.5 months. Additional procedures were performed as needed, based on the "menu a la carte." All patients presented preoperatively recurrent patellar dislocation, severe trochlear dysplasia (types B and D), and history of previous surgery for the treatment of patellar dislocation. Postoperatively none of the patients sustained recurrent patellar dislocation or complained of instability. The apprehension sign was negative in 75% of the cases, and all patients achieved normal patellar tracking. IKDC score increased from 51.4 to 76.7, and Kujala score increased from 44.8 to 81.7. Radiographically the sulcus angle decreased from 153 to 141 degrees, TT-TG distance decreased from 16 to 12 mm, patellar tilt decreased from 31 to 11 degrees, and no cases of patellofemoral arthritis were observed. In the last follow-up, 95.4% of the patients returned to their previous activities, and all the patients were satisfied with the surgery. No major complications were reported.

Ntagiopoulos et al.[27] analyzed retrospectively 27 patients (31 knees) with recurrent patellar dislocations and the presence of high-grade trochlear dysplasia without any previous surgery, with a mean follow-up of 7 years. All patients underwent sulcus-deepening trochleoplasty combined with other procedures to correct causative factors that were necessary. Their results showed improvement in IKDC and Kujala scores, from 51 to 82 and from 59 to 87, respectively. No recurrence or feeling of instability was observed, and the patellar tracking was normal in all cases. The apprehension sign remained positive in 19.3% of cases. Radiographically the mean sulcus angle decreased from 152 to 141 degrees, the TT-TG distance decreased from 19 to 12 mm, and the patellar tilt decreased from 37 to 15 degrees. No cases of patellofemoral arthritis were detected at the final follow-up, and 93.6% of patients responded that they were satisfied with the surgery.

Nelitz et al.[26] evaluated 23 patients (26 knees) with patellofemoral instability and severe trochlear dysplasia who underwent combined Bereiter trochleoplasty and anatomic reconstruction of the MPFL, with a mean follow-up of 2.5 years. Patients with a TT-TG distance greater than 22 mm were excluded. Thirteen patients had undergone a previous surgery before the index surgery. The results did not show any recurrent dislocation, but one patient still presented apprehension. Kujala score improved from 79 to 96, IKDC score improved from 74 to 90, mean VAS score decreased from 3 to 1, and 95.7% of patients were satisfied or very satisfied with the surgery.

TABLE 69.1   Results From Clinical Studies of Trochleoplasty

Author (Year)	Procedure	N (Knees)	Average Follow-Up (Years)	Results	Conclusion
Verdonk et al.[37] (2005)	Deepening trochleoplasty	13	1.5	• No redislocation • 38.4% stiffness (manipulation) • Larsen-Lauridsen score: 7 poor, 3 fair, 3 well • Subjective: 6 very good, 4 good, 1 satisfactory, 2 inadequate	77% were satisfied with the procedure—good subjective outcome despite poor objective outcomes.
Schottle et al.[29] (2005)	Bereiter trochleoplasty	19	3	• No redislocation • 21% apprehension • Pain: decreased: 63%, increased: 10% • 84% good or excellent results • 26% medial parapatellar tenderness • Kujala score: 56 → 80	Trochleaplasty is an effective and safe procedure, which prevents patellar subluxation or dislocation.
Donell et al.[17] (2006)	Deepening trochleoplasty	17	3	• No redislocation • 41% apprehension sign • 5.8% stiffness (arthrolysis) • 82.3% satisfaction • Kujala score: 48 → 75	Early results have been satisfactory with an acceptable level of complications.
von Knoch et al.[38] (2006)	Bereiter trochleoplasty	45	8.3	• No redislocation • 2.2% apprehension sign • No stiffness • Pain: unchanged: 8.8%, decreased: 33.4%, increased: 49% • 30% PFOA • Final Kujala score: 94.9 • 1 patella baja • 1 tendency of subluxation (distal realignment)	Trochleoplasty is a reasonable treatment for recurrent patellar instability with trochlear dysplasia but may not prevent the development of PFOA.
Utting et al.[36] (2008)	Bereiter trochleoplasty	42	2	• 2.3% redislocation • 2.3% stiffness (manipulation) • Kujala score: 62 → 76 • IKDC score: 54 → 72 • OKS: 26 → 19 • Lysholm score: 57 → 78 • WOMAC score: 23 → 17	Surgery was successfully in patients with symptomatic recurrent patellar instability, with high level of patient satisfaction.
Zaki and Rae[39] (2010)	Modified deepening trochleoplasty	27	4.5	• No redislocation • Functional results: 70% good to excellent / 30% fair • No stiffness	This modified technique of trochleoplasty for recurrent patellar instability showed results for instability, but patients may have residual pain.
Fucentese et al.[19] (2011)	Bereiter trochleoplasty	44	4	• 2.27% redislocation • 4.5% residual instability (needed surgery) • 25% apprehension sign • 3 arthroscopic débridement due pain • Pain: unchanged: 61.3%, decreased: 31.9%, increased: 6.8% • Kujala score: 68 → 90 • 84% ranked good or excellent • 36% deterioration of lateral trochlear cartilage	This surgery is best indicated for young patients with severe dysplasia (types B and D) and without highest sports activities or heavy labor.
Thaunat et al.[35] (2011)	Recession wedge trochleoplasty	19	2.8	• 10.5% redislocation • 94.1% satisfaction • 5.8% stiffness (arthrolysis) • 35% PFOA • Final Kujala score: 80 • Final IKDC score: 67 • Final KOOS score: 70	The procedure should be considered in cases of painful instability with a major dysplastic trochlea or in failed cases.
Faruqui et al.[18] (2012)	Deepening trochleoplasty	6	5.7	• No redislocation • 100% satisfaction • 66% residual pain • Sulcus angles: 149° → 128°	Trochleoplasty can reliably improve stability in patients with severe trochlear dysplasia.

Continued

TABLE 69.1   Results From Clinical Studies of Trochleoplasty—cont'd

Author (Year)	Procedure	N (Knees)	Average Follow-Up (Years)	Results	Conclusion
Dejour et al.[12] (2013)	Deepening trochleoplasty	24	5.5	• No redislocation • 25% apprehension sign • No stiffness • 100% satisfaction • No PFOA • Kujala score: 44.8 → 81.7 • IKDC score: 51.4 → 76.7 • Sulcus angle: 153° → 141° • Tilt: 31° → 11° • TT-TG: 16.6 mm → 12.6 mm	In patients with previous failed surgery for patellar instability, with recurrent dislocations, trochleoplasty is an important option when the trochlear dysplasia was neglected. Midterm follow-up showed good stability and patient satisfaction.
Ntagiopoulos et al.[27] (2013)	Deepening trochleoplasty	31	7	• No redislocation • 19.3% apprehension sign • No stiffness • 93.6% satisfaction • No PFOA • Kujala score: 59 → 87 • IKDC score: 51.2 → 22.9 • Sulcus angle: 152° → 141° • Tilt: 37° → 15° • TT-TG: 19 mm → 12 mm	Trochleoplasty showed satisfactory stability and knee scores, with good to excellent patient satisfaction and no major complications in selected patients with recurrent dislocations and high-grade trochlear dysplasia.
Nelitz et al.[26] (2013)	Bereiter trochleoplasty	26	2.5	• No redislocation • 3.8% apprehension sign • No stiffness • 95% very satisfied or satisfied • 5% partially satisfied • Kujala score: 79 → 96 • IKDC score: 74 → 90 • Pain VAS: 3 → 1 • Tegner score: 5.5 → 5 (not statistically) • ARS score: 6.5 → 6 (not statistically)	Combined trochleoplasty and anatomic MPFLR improved knee function and had good patient satisfaction in young patients with severe trochlea dysplasia and instability.
Banke et al.[4] (2014)	Bereiter trochleoplasty	18	2.5	• No redislocation • No apprehension sign • 94% satisfaction • 11% stiffness (arthrolysis) • No PFOA • 1 painful medial subluxation (reassessed MPFLR) • Kujala score: 51.1 → 87.9 • Tegner score: 2 → 6 • IKDC score: 49.5 → 80.2 • Pain VAS: 5.6 → 2.5 • Sulcus angle: 154° → 143.3° • Tilt: 24.2 mm → 15.8 mm • TT-TG: 16.2 mm → 10.7 mm	The combination of trochleoplasty and MPFLR serves as a successfully procedure to patellar instability in revision cases and also in primary cases.
Blond and Haugegaard[6] (2014)	Arthroscopic deepening trochleoplasty	37	3	• No redislocation • No apprehension sign • No stiffness • 5 patients needed new surgery (2 TTM and 3 lateral releases) • Kujala score: 64 → 95 • Tegner score: 4 → 6 • Improvement in 5 KOOS scores	Arthroscopic deepening trochleoplasty in combination with MPFLR is a safe and reproducible procedure in recurrent patellar instability, but sometimes other associated procedures are necessary.
Rouanet et al.[28] (2015)	Deepening trochleoplasty (Masse)	34	15.3	• No redislocation • 11% apprehension sign • 23% early stiffness (<90° flexion) • 20% failure (need for surgery due PFOA or pain) • Kujala score: 55 → 76 • IKS score: 127.3 → 152.4 • Lille score: 53.3 → 61.5 • 65% Iwano ≥ 2 / 50% Iwano 4	Trochleoplasty is a reliable procedure to objective patellofemoral instability, in the presence of trochleae dysplasia grade B and D. It does not prevent the development of PFOA.

ARS, Activity rating scale; *IKDC*, International Knee Documentation Committee; *IKS*, International Knee Society Score; *KOOS*, Knee Injury and Osteoarthritis Outcomes Score; *MPFLR*, medial patellofemoral ligament reconstruction; *OKS*, Oxford Knee Score; *PFOA*, patellofemoral osteoarthritis.; *TTM*, tibial tubercle medicalization; *TT-TG*, tibial tubercle–trochlear groove distance; *VAS*, visual analogue scale.

Banke et al.[4] reported 17 patients (18 knees) with recurrent patellar instability, presence of apprehension sign, and trochlear dysplasia types B, C, and D, which were submitted to Bereiter trochleoplasty associated with MPFL reconstruction, with a mean follow-up of 30.5 months. Postoperatively there was no case of patellar dislocation, and no patient presented apprehension sign. Results showed significant reduction in pain, with a VAS score decrease from 5.6 to 2.5. All scores tested improved. Tegner score increased from 2 to 6, Kujala score from 51.1 to 87.9, and IKDC score from 49.5 to 80.2. In the radiographic analysis, sulcus angle decreased from 154 to 143.3 degrees, TT-TG distance was reduced from 16.2 to 10.7 mm, and the patellar tilt decreased from 24.2 to 15.8 mm. Only one patient was not satisfied with the procedure.

Blønd and Haugegaard[8] reported the results for the arthroscopic trochleoplasty. Thirty-one patients (37 knees) with recurrent patellar instability, trochlear dysplasia grade B or D, and a positive apprehension test were analyzed, with a mean follow-up of 29 months. Sixteen of these knees had previously undergone surgery for patellar instability, with unsatisfactory results. In their results no redislocations or positive apprehension signs were observed. Five patients needed further surgery during the follow-up. Two of them, who presented the highest TT-TG distances (28 and 40 mm), had a tibial tubercle medialization performed with success. The other three presented anterior pain with knee flexion, caused by a tight lateral retinaculum. Lateral releases were then made with good response. All scores assessed showed improvements. Kujala score increased from 64 to 95, Tegner score increased from 4 to 6, and all KOOS scores were better postoperatively.

Rouanet et al.[28] presented the longest follow-up series after sulcus-deepening trochleoplasty, with a mean of 15.3 years. Thirty-four patients who presented objective (dislocation) or subjective (apprehension without dislocation) patellofemoral instability, associated with trochlear dysplasia, and displayed at most stage 1 patellofemoral osteoarthritis according to Iwano's classification, were submitted to the trochleoplasty described by Masse.[25] Thirteen patients had been previously submitted to surgery, 7 of them because of patellar instability. Insall procedure was associated in all patients, and other risk factors of instability were treated during the same procedure. Their results demonstrated no recurrent dislocation. All the functional scores analyzed improved, with better results in patients operated for severe dysplasia (grades B and D) and that presented objective instability. Despite these improvements, 20% (7 patients) were considered failures. Six underwent revision arthroplasty because of patellofemoral osteoarthritis, and one underwent a tibial tubercle transfer because of pain and because the knee frequently gave out at 3 years. Of patients whose knees did not fail, 81% were satisfied or very satisfied. The apprehension test was negative in 89% of cases, and 37% reported occasional instability. At the final follow-up, 65% were classified as having patellofemoral osteoarthritis (Table 69.1).

COMPLICATIONS

Patients submitted to trochleoplasty are at risk of the same complications inherent to any surgical procedure (eg, infection, deep venous thrombosis). Specific complications include trochlear necrosis, cartilage damage, incongruence with the patella, and hypocorrection or hypercorrection. Schottle and coworkers[30] performed biopsies in three patients after trochleoplasty,

showing cartilage cell viability and flap healing, and concluded that the risk of cartilage damage is low.

Incongruence with the patella is another concern. Studies with longer follow-ups are needed before any assumptions can be made about its consequences. In addition, osteoarthritis development is multifactorial. Patients with patellofemoral instability are prone to develop osteoarthritis, and those patients operated on for patellofemoral instability seem even more prone to degeneration than those treated conservatively.[22]

Recurrence of instability is very rare after such procedures and is more likely to result from missed associated abnormalities. The results for pain are not consistent; although it seems to improve, some patients may even complain of worsening.

In a systematic review performed by Song et al.[32] of the 329 patients that had undergone trochleoplasty procedures, 13.4% (44) had complications. Of these, 6.8% (3) were related to a redislocated patella, 27.3% (12) to a deficit of range of motion, and 65.9% (29) to increased patellofemoral pain level. Among 142 patients that were evaluated for patellofemoral osteoarthritis according to Iwano's classification, 7.9% (13) were reported to present at least Iwano grade 2, at a mean follow-up of 69.9 months.

The longest series of patients presented by Rouanet et al.[28] showed the highest rates of patellofemoral osteoarthritis at the final follow-up (mean of 15.3 years). Sixty-five percent of patients were classified as having patellofemoral osteoarthritis of at least grade 2, according to Iwano (described in this study as joint space narrowing thickness greater than 3 mm, different from the original description in which grade 2 is defined as a thickness less than 3 mm), and 50% had Iwano grade 4 (described in this study as bone surfaces in contact). An important factor that could have increased the osteoarthritis (OA) rate is that the trochleoplasty was made according to the procedure described by Masse,[25] in which the groove is depressed by hammering the cartilaginous trochlea, potentially damaging the chondrocytes.

CONCLUSION

Sulcus-deepening trochleoplasty is a demanding procedure that is indicated for a few cases of patellofemoral dislocation. It has the advantage of treating its essential cause, but trochleoplasty indications are selective. It should not be performed in cases of pain, arthritis, or open growth plates. As with any surgical procedure, it carries a risk of complications.

KEY REFERENCES

3. Arendt EA, Dejour D: Patella instability: building bridges across the ocean a historic review. *Knee Surg Sports Traumatol Arthrosc* 21:279–293, 2013.

5. Bereiter H, Gautier E: Die trochleaplastik als chirurgische Therapie der rezidivierenden Patellaluxation bei Trochleadysplasie des Femurs. *Arthroskopie* 7:281–286, 1994.

7. Blønd L: Arthroscopic Deepening Trochleoplasty: The Technique. *Op Tech Sports Med* 23:136–142, 2015.

11. Dejour DH: The patellofemoral joint and its historical roots: the Lyon School of Knee Surgery. *Knee Surg Sports Traumatol Arthrosc* 21:1482–1494, 2013.

12. Dejour D, Byn P, Ntagiopoulos PG: The Lyon's sulcus-deepening trochleoplasty in previous unsuccessful patellofemoral surgery. *Int Orthop* 37:433–439, 2013.

13. Dejour D, Le Coultre B: Osteotomies in patello-femoral instabilities. *Sports Med Arthrosc* 15:39–46, 2007.

14. Dejour D, Saggin P: The sulcus deepening trochleoplasty-the Lyon's procedure. *Int Orthop* 34:311–316, 2010.

16. Dejour H, Walch G, Nove-Josserand L, et al: Factors of patellar instability: an anatomic radiographic study. *Knee Surg Sports Traumatol Arthrosc* 2:19–26, 1994.

19. Fucentese SF, Zingg PO, Schmitt J, et al: Classification of trochlear dysplasia as predictor of clinical outcome after trochleoplasty. *Knee Surg Sports Traumatol Arthrosc* 19:1655–1661, 2011.

20. Hinckel BB, Arendt EA, Ntagiopoulos PG, et al: Trochleoplasty: historical overview and Dejour technique. *Op Tech Sports Med* 23:114–122, 2015.

21. Lippacher S, Dejour D, Elsharkawi M, et al: Observer agreement on the Dejour trochlear dysplasia classification: a comparison of true lateral radiographs and axial magnetic resonance images. *Am J Sports Med* 40:837–843, 2012.

27. Ntagiopoulos PG, Byn P, Dejour D: Midterm results of comprehensive surgical reconstruction including sulcus-deepening trochleoplasty in recurrent patellar dislocations with high-grade trochlear dysplasia. *Am J Sports Med* 41:998–1004, 2013.

30. Schöttle PB, Schell H, Duda G, et al: Cartilage viability after trochleoplasty. *Knee Surg Sports Traumatol Arthrosc* 15:161–167, 2007.

32. Song G-Y, Hong L, Zhang H, et al: Trochleoplasty versus nontrochleoplasty procedures in treating patellar instability caused by severe trochlear dysplasia. *Arthroscopy* 30:523–532, 2014.

The references for this chapter can also be found on www.expertconsult.com.

70

Quadriceps and Patellar Tendon Disruption*

Jourdan M. Cancienne, F. Winston Gwathmey, Jr., David R. Diduch

ANATOMY

Musculature

The extensor mechanism of the knee consists of the quadriceps musculature, quadriceps tendon, patella, and patellar tendon. The quadriceps musculature is composed of the rectus femoris, vastus medialis, vastus lateralis, and vastus intermedius, which coalesce in a trilaminar fashion to form the quadriceps tendon. The direct head of the rectus femoris takes origin from the anterior inferior iliac spine and the indirect head from the anterior hip capsule. These muscle heads unite distally and form the rectus femoris muscle, the most superficial component of the quadriceps musculature. The muscle bodies narrow to a tendon approximately 3 to 5 cm superior to the patella. The fibers of the quadriceps tendon continue over the anterior surface of the patella and into the patellar tendon. The vastus medialis is divided into two groups: the vastus medialis obliquus and the vastus medialis longus. The muscle fibers of the vastus medialis continue toward the superomedial border of the patella and become tendinous a few millimeters before their insertion. The muscle fibers of the vastus lateralis terminate more proximally than those of the vastus medialis and become tendinous approximately 3 cm from the superolateral border of the patella. The vastus intermedius lies deep to the other three muscles, and its tendinous fibers insert directly into the superior border of the patella and blend medially and laterally with the vastus medialis and vastus lateralis. Aponeurotic fibers from the vastus lateralis and vastus medialis contribute to the lateral and medial retinaculum.

The patellar tendon is primarily derived from the central fibers of the rectus femoris, which extend over the anterior surface of the patella and form a flat tendinous structure that inserts into the tibial tubercle. It continues past the tubercle and blends with the iliotibial band on the anterolateral surface of the tibia. Proximally the tendon width is approximately that of the adjacent patella, with the tendon thickness in the sagittal plane averaging 4 mm and not exceeding 7 mm.[41] The tendon both thickens and narrows distally, with an average thickness of 5 to 6 mm at its insertion at the tibial tubercle.[93] The average length of the patellar tendon is 4.6 cm (range: 3.5 to 5.5 cm).[130]

Biomechanics

Functionally the extensor mechanism transmits forces from the quadriceps to the proximal tibia, with the patella acting as a fulcrum to increase the lever moment arm of the quadriceps. Huberti et al. first described the extensor mechanism force ratio concept that describes forces across the quadriceps and patellar tendon at varying degrees of flexion.[59] The greatest forces in the patellar tendon are found at 60 degrees of knee flexion. At flexion angles less than 45 degrees the patellar tendon to quadriceps tendon force ratio is greater than 1.0, giving the quadriceps tendon a mechanical advantage. The opposite is true at flexion angles greater than 45 degrees, and the patellar tendon has the greater mechanical advantage. This helps to explain the clinical correlate of most extensor mechanism injuries occurring when the knee is in flexion, undergoing eccentric contraction.[52,163]

Vascular Supply

The quadriceps tendon is normally vascularized by three contributions, termed *arcades*.[160] The medial arcade supplies the medial tendon. This arcade is located at the musculotendinous junction and is formed from the anastomosis of the muscular branches of the middle and inferior arteries of the vastus medialis divisions of the femoral artery, the descending genicular artery branch of the superficial artery, and the superior medial genicular artery division of the popliteal artery.[160] The lateral arcade supplies the lateral side of the tendon. The long descending branch of the lateral circumflex femoral artery and divisions of the superior lateral genicular artery create this arcade. This arcade also contributes to the formation of the proximal peripatellar vascular ring and vascular supply of the superior pole of the patella. The peripatellar vascular ring or peripatellar arcade is found deep to the vastus intermedius and capsule and is formed from the deep branches of the superior genicular arteries, in addition to the lateral and medial arcades. This arcade supplies the distal 1 cm of the quadriceps tendon. The overall pattern of blood supply to the tendon has been described as a triangle, with more vascularity at the boundaries and a less vascular center.

The patellar tendon receives its blood supply primarily from the infrapatellar fat pad and retinacular structures.[7] The infrapatellar fat pad supplies the posterior aspect of the tendon and receives its supply from the inferior medial and lateral genicular arteries, whereas the retinaculum supplies the anterior portion of the tendon and receives its supply from branches of the recurrent tibial and inferior medial genicular arteries.[7] The proximal and distal attachments of the tendon are relatively

*This chapter was modified from Seidenstein AD, Farrell CM, Scuderi GR, Easley ME: Quadriceps and patellar tendon disruptions. In Insall JN, Scott WN (eds): Surgery of the knee, ed 5, New York, 2012, Churchill Livingstone, pp 697–708.

avascular and are primarily composed of fibrocartilage, thus making these the most common sites of rupture.[138,139]

CAUSES OF QUADRICEPS TENDON DISRUPTION

Mechanism and Causes

The structural and biomechanical properties of the extensor mechanism allow it to sustain loads up to 17.5 times body weight without rupture.[21,163] Tendon deformation within the extensor mechanism displays the viscoelastic properties of creep and stress relaxation, and sudden and eccentric contractions of the quadriceps can exceed the phase of plastic deformity and lead to an incomplete or complete rupture.[141] Furthermore, experimental studies have shown that a normal quadriceps tendon will not rupture when a longitudinal stress is applied and that the normal quadriceps tendon may be able to tolerate up to 30 kg/mm of longitudinal stress before failing. A sudden and eccentric contraction of the quadriceps musculature is the usual mechanism of injury leading to failure of the quadriceps tendon. A recent meta-analysis examined 319 patients who had acute quadriceps tendon ruptures and reported the most common injury mechanisms to be simple falls (61.5%), fall from stairs (23.4%), sport (6%), and agricultural penetrating direct trauma (2.3%).[30] The low-energy pattern of injury reported in the large majority of cases suggests that rupture will occur in an area of weakened tendon. Age-related changes of tendon tissue display fatty and myxoid degeneration, tendon sclerosis, a decrease in the quantity, and change in type and cross-links of collagen fibers predisposing to rupture.[131]

In addition to the age-related changes of tendon tissue, several pathologic conditions have been shown to affect the extensor mechanism, including renal disease, diabetes mellitus, hyperparathyroidism, rheumatoid arthritis, systemic lupus erythematosus, gout, osteomalacia, infection, obesity, steroid use,[86,99] and other metabolic diseases. These metabolic diseases cause microscopic damage to the vascular supply to the tendons or alter the architecture of the tendon. Diabetes has been shown to cause arteriosclerotic changes in the tendon vessels, whereas chronic synovitis causes fibrinoid reactions within the tendon. Long periods of hemodialysis and uremia associated with renal disease affects the maturation of collagen and causes quadriceps muscle atrophy that significantly weakens the tendon.[146,147] Advancing age and hyperparathyroidism can both cause dystrophic calcifications and subperiosteal bone resorption, weakening the osseotendinous junction between the quadriceps tendon and patella.[120,147] Although quadriceps tendon rupture tends to occur in older patients or those with systemic disease or degenerative changes, literature has suggested that there may also be a genetic link implicated in bilateral quadriceps tendon rupture with the *COL5A1* gene.[51] This variant, known to be associated with Achilles tendon and anterior cruciate ligament (ACL) ruptures, encodes the protein for type V collagen, and a decrease in this collagen is thought to weaken tendon strength.

The most common site of spontaneous rupture of the quadriceps tendon occurs within 1 to 2 cm of the patella and corresponds to the most hypovascular region of the tendon.[160] Age has also been reported to be associated with site of rupture. Rasul et al. suggested that patients older than 40 years of age have more frequent tendon ruptures in the tendon-bone junction, whereas patients younger than 40 years have tears in the mid-tendinous area.[125] Numerous cases of bilateral quadriceps tendon rupture have been reported. Although most ruptures

occur in patients with predisposing conditions, such as obesity, systemic illness, * and use of anabolic steroids, several reports have noted bilateral tendon rupture in healthy patients without predisposing factors.† In a retrospective review of bilateral and unilateral quadriceps tendon rupture, Konrath et al.[73] noted a significant correlation between bilateral simultaneous rupture and systemic disease.

Other conditions that may alter the local properties of the extensor mechanism include total knee arthroplasty (TKA)[88] and lateral retinacular release.[10,38,144] Local steroid injection has similarly been implicated as a cause of tendon rupture. Finally, rupture of the quadriceps tendon has also been reported after patellar dislocation.[107]

Diagnosis

Disruption of the extensor mechanism is a significant disabling injury and should be diagnosed early.[123,142] Patients usually have an acute onset of knee pain, swelling, and loss of function after a stumble or fall. Although rare, acute compartment syndrome of the thigh secondary to a quadriceps rupture has also been reported.[77] The physical examination generally reveals a palpable defect in the quadriceps tendon with a low-lying patella. When asked to perform a straight-leg raise, the patient may be unable to do so or will demonstrate an extensor lag. However, some degree of active extensor function may be preserved if either the medial or lateral retinaculum or the iliotibial band remains intact.[149] In addition, partial ruptures seen in a younger, more athletic demographic may represent a diagnostic challenge because a degree of extensor function may be preserved.[78]

Imaging of Extensor Mechanism Disruption

Although extensor mechanism disruptions are typically diagnosed from the history and physical examination, imaging studies often prove useful in confirming the diagnosis of quadriceps and patellar tendon tears or differentiating complete from incomplete tears.[122] Initial imaging work up of suspected extensor mechanism disruption should start with orthogonal plain radiographs of the affected knee. The lateral view should be used to determine the Insall-Salvati ratio to identify patella alta, which suggests patellar tendon disruption, or patella baja (Fig. 70.1), which suggests quadriceps tendon disruption. Other radiographic clues to injury include disruption of the quadriceps tendon shadow with quadriceps tendon rupture and disruption of the patellar tendon shadow or the infrapatellar fat pad contour with patellar tendon rupture.[28,65,70,106] Despite relatively obvious findings on physical examination and standard radiographs, missed diagnosis of extensor mechanism rupture still occurs with reported rates of 10% to 50%.[126] Several diagnostic imaging modalities may be used in addition to standard radiographs to confirm the diagnosis, including arthrography, ultrasound, and magnetic resonance imaging (MRI). Before the advent of MRI, arthrography was widely used. In the presence of an extensor mechanism tendon rupture, extravasation of radiopaque dye into the defect occurs.[4] However, arthrography has been largely replaced by noninvasive methods, such as ultrasound and, more commonly, MRI. High-resolution ultrasonography‡ may reveal a hypoechogenicity across the entire

---

*References 2, 23, 29, 54, 56, 104, 110, 137, 148, and 154.
†References 5, 23, 35, 55, 67, 79, 128, 148, 151, and 154.
‡References 5, 12, 13, 30, 42, and 51.

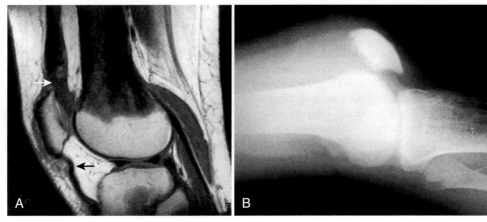

FIG 70.1 (A) MRI scan of a torn quadriceps tendon *(white arrow)*. Note the laxity of the patellar tendon *(black arrow)*. (B) Radiograph showing the low position of the patella associated with quadriceps tendon rupture. This patient has chronic renal failure and hyperparathyroidism. (From Scott WN (ed): *The knee,* vol 1, St. Louis, 1994, Mosby-Year Book, p 470.)

thickness of the tendon with an acute rupture or tendon thickening and alteration of the normal echo signal with chronic tears. Advantages of ultrasonography include collection of images in real time without exposure to ionizing radiation and relatively limited expense. However, operation of the ultrasound equipment plus interpretation of the images require the skills of a highly trained and experienced technician and radiologist. Hence, the reliability is highly operator-dependent. In a retrospective study of 66 patients Perfitt et al. reported a sensitivity of 100%, specificity of 67%, and positive predictive value of 0.88, with the use of ultrasound for diagnosing quadriceps tendon ruptures.[117] In the same study four patients out of the initial study group of 47 were inaccurately diagnosed, either clinically or by ultrasound, leading to surgical exploration of an intact quadriceps tendon. This reinforced the group's recommendation for improved preoperative diagnosis by MRI. MRI is regarded as the imaging study of choice when the diagnosis cannot be established from the clinical and radiographic examination alone.[10,38,143,150,153] In addition, MRI may be useful to identify other intra-articular pathology within the knee.[161] Perfitt et al. noted the sensitivity, specificity, and positive predictive value of MRI in diagnosing quadriceps tendon ruptures to be 100% in their study.[117] The group concluded that patients with a suspected extensor mechanism disruptions on exam undergo ultrasound, and those with positive findings undergo MRI to eliminate false-positive diagnoses.

QUADRICEPS TENDON RUPTURE

Quadriceps tendon rupture is a relatively uncommon injury, with an incidence of approximately 1.37/100,000 patients per year, and predominantly affects middle-aged males.[32] In the literature the quadriceps tendon has been subdivided into three zones. Zone 1 is located between 0 and 1 cm, zone 2 between 1 and 2 cm, and zone 3 more than 2 cm from the superior pole of the patella. Ciriello et al. performed a systematic review of the literature and reported on 319 acute quadriceps tendon ruptures in adults. Using this subdivision 35.6% ruptures occurred in zone 1, 41.4% in zone 2, and 12.1% in zone 3.[30] These ruptures usually occur at the osteotendinous junction or through an area of degenerative tendon. The rupture originates in the tendon of the rectus femoris, often extending into the

vastus intermedius tendon or transversely into the medial and lateral retinacula. Quadriceps tendon rupture may be complete or incomplete. Nonoperative management of quadriceps tendon ruptures is reserved for incomplete tears with an intact extensor mechanism function. The literature has recommended long leg cast immobilization with the knee in extension for at least 6 weeks with aggressive elevation and management of the associated knee effusion. The cast is then replaced by a movable splint until full active extension without pain can be demonstrated.[60,82,136] We recommend surgical treatment for all complete or near-complete tears, with nonoperative treatment reserved only for incomplete tears with intact extensor mechanism function. A hinged knee brace can be used instead of a cast, allowing for progressive range of motion with therapist supervision as healing progresses.

Overview of Surgical Management

Operative management of quadriceps tendon rupture is indicated for incomplete tears with functional extensor mechanism deficits and for all complete tears.[60,82] Acute repair is advocated to avoid tendon retraction and achieve a tension-free construct.[60,135,149] Although Konrath et al.[73] found no detrimental effect of delay in repair, others have shown a delay in surgical repair to be the single most important factor predictive of a poor outcome. Rougraff et al.[135] suggested that a delay of 1 week compromises the outcome of quadriceps tendon repair, with significantly worse functional results and lower satisfaction scores. These findings were supported by Siwek and Rao[149] and Scuderi,[141] who observed worse results with a delay in surgical repair of 2 weeks and 3 days, respectively. In a study of 29 quadriceps tendon repairs, Wenzl et al.[155] demonstrated a significantly higher probability of a successful outcome with repairs performed within 2 weeks from the time of injury. Levy et al.[84] also noted the best results in patients managed acutely with a Dacron graft.

Numerous techniques have been described in the literature for repair of acute and chronic rupture of the quadriceps tendon.[§] Over the years the repair techniques have progressed from simple suture with catgut or silk to wire-reinforced repairs,

---

§References 70, 79, 84, 112, 132, and 149.

suture anchors, autografts xenografts, allografts, and the use of synthetic material.[48,100] McLaughlin[96] and McLaughlin and Francis[97] have even recommended a two-stage procedure with traction for better approximation of the tendon. All techniques largely adhere to the same basic principles of tendon repair. A midline longitudinal incision is used with dissection carried to the level of the quadriceps tendon and retinaculum. It is important to carry dissection laterally and medially enough with full-thickness flaps to assess the full extent of retinacular tears.[82] After the tendon is identified and the extent of the tear localized, the edges are sharply débrided and irrigated of hematoma to fresh edges. At this point, repair options depend on tear location and tendon mobility.

Procedures

Acute Midsubstance Disruption. With an acute midsubstance rupture with adequate proximal and distal tendon, direct primary end-to-end repair may be performed with multiple, interrupted, high-strength no. 2 or no. 5 nonabsorbable sutures. The sutures may also be placed in a running, locked fashion using a Krackow or equivalent technique in both the proximal and distal ends of the tendon.[90] In both techniques the suture ends are tied with the knee in full extension, and the retinaculum is then repaired with multiple interrupted no. 0 absorbable sutures. After the repair is complete, careful assessment of patellar rotation and tracking should be performed. The knee is then extended and the repair may be protected with a cerclage wire or nonabsorbable suture. The wound is closed in layers and the leg placed in a cylinder cast for 6 weeks. When the cast is removed, a control dial, hinged-knee orthosis (Fig. 70.2) is used so that flexion can be gradually increased. The brace is discontinued when more than 90 degrees of flexion has been achieved and quadriceps strength is sufficient to support the limb.

Another widely used option for repairing acute rupture of the quadriceps tendon is the Scuderi technique[60,64,141,145] (Fig. 70.3). Using a midline longitudinal incision, the tendon rupture is exposed and the tendon edges are débrided until solid tendinous material is achieved. The knee is extended, and the tendon edges are pulled with clamps, overlapped, and repaired with interrupted absorbable suture. A triangular flap 2.4 to 3.2 mm thick, 7.5 cm long on each side, and 5.0 cm at the base is fabricated from the anterior surface of the proximal part of the tendon. The base of the flap is left attached approximately 5.0 cm proximal to the rupture. The flap is folded distally over the rupture and sutured in place. A Bunnell pullout wire may be placed along the medial and lateral side of the quadriceps tendon, patella, and patellar tendon. The wound is closed in layers and the leg placed in a cylinder cast or hinged knee brace, with the knee locked in the extended position. Postoperatively the cylinder cast is maintained for 6 weeks and at 3 weeks the pull-out wires are removed. When the cast is removed, a control dial hinged-knee orthosis is used so that flexion can be gradually increased. It is also recommended that the patient undergo physiotherapy including a quadriceps-strengthening program.

Acute Osteotendinous Disruption. When the rupture occurs at the osteotendinous junction, which is the most common location, direct end-to-end repair is not possible, and the use of transosseous sutures represents the gold standard repair (Fig. 70.4).[60] The MRI and repair technique are illustrated in Fig. 70.5. A straight midline incision will expose the quadriceps tendon rupture (see Fig. 70.4C). The hematoma is evacuated

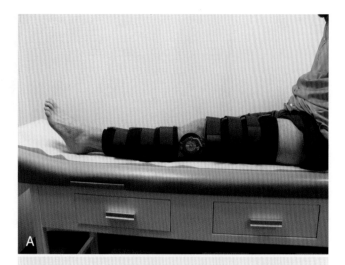

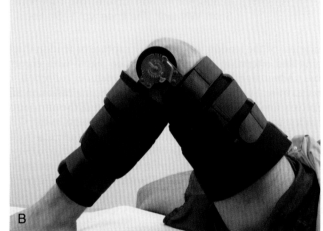

FIG 70.2 A control dial, hinged-knee orthosis with a drop lock to keep the knee in extension (A) during early ambulation and allow flexion when exercising (B). (Courtesy Breg, Vista, California.)

(see Fig. 70.4D), the proximal end of the rectus femoris and vastus intermedius tendon is cut fresh to normal tendon, and the superior pole of the patella is débrided of residual tendon (see Fig. 70.4E). A no. 5 nonabsorbable suture is secured with an interlocking stitch along the lateral portion of the tendon.[74] A second no. 5 nonabsorbable suture is placed in similar fashion along the medial portion of the tendon (see Fig. 70.4F). A transverse trough is then made in the superior pole of the patella with a high-speed bur (see Fig. 70.4G). To avoid patellar tilt, the trough should be placed as posterior as possible in the patella. Next, three marks are made with a methylene blue pen, approximately 1.0 to 1.5 cm apart in the trough (see Fig. 70.4H). A Beath pin is used to drill through the medial mark, exiting at the inferior pole of the patella (see Fig. 70.4I). An ACL drill guide may be used to facilitate precise placement of the drill holes.[111] The medial free end of suture is next placed through the eyelet of the Beath pin, and the pin is pulled distally (see Fig. 70.4I). The Beath pin is then used to drill and pass the sutures in the central and lateral transosseous patellar tunnels (see Fig. 70.4J). The proximal end of the tendon is pulled into the trough, and the sutures are held provisionally with a hemostat. The knee is then flexed so that patellar tracking and rotation can be assessed. The repair is completed by tying the no. 5

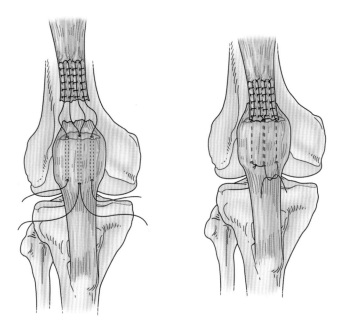

FIG 70.3 Scuderi technique for repairing acute tears of the quadriceps tendon. (Redrawn from Scuderi GR: Extensor mechanism injuries: treatment. In Scott WN (ed): *Ligament and extension mechanism injuries of the knee,* St. Louis, 1991, Mosby-Year Book, p 190.)

nonabsorbable suture distally with the knee in full extension (see Fig. 70.4K). Because the medial and lateral retinacula act as frontal plane stabilizers and play a complementary load-sharing role with respect to the patellar tendon, they are both repaired with multiple interrupted no. 0 absorbable sutures (see Fig. 70.4L).[119] The repair is then checked to ensure that gapping at the repair site does not occur at 20 to 30 degrees of flexion (see Fig. 70.4M). Augmentation is typically not necessary.[73,89,149] However, if the strength of the repair is in doubt, augmentation may be achieved with wire or Mersilene tape.[96,101] After closure of the subcutaneous layer and skin, a cylinder cast or hinged knee brace is applied with the knee in full extension. Postoperatively the cylinder cast is maintained for 6 weeks and the patient is allowed weight bearing as tolerated with a walker or crutches. After the cast is removed, a control dial, hinged-knee orthosis is used until 90 degrees of flexion is achieved and quadriceps strength returns. Although we prefer immobilization in the immediate postoperative period, some authors advocate early passive and active assisted range of motion of the knee after quadriceps tendon repair.[84,156]

Alternatively, satisfactory results have also been obtained with suture anchors in lieu of transosseous sutures.[132] Initially described in the early 2000s, this technique uses two to three anchors in the superior pole of the patella following preparation of a patellar trough.[20,91,132] The heavy, nonabsorbable free suture ends are then tied in a modified Mason-Allen, Kessler, Krackow, or Bunnell interlocking technique proximally into the tendon.[20] Using suture anchors in lieu of transosseous sutures has been backed by biomechanical comparison studies that have shown decreased gap formation during cyclic loading and higher ultimate failure loads than transosseous suture repairs.[85,118] Furthermore, proponents of the suture anchor technique point to several potential advantages over the use of transosseous bone tunnels. Dissection of the distal pole of the patella can be avoided

with suture anchors, and potential trauma to the patella tendon can be avoided. Furthermore, knots within the patellar tendon, which oftentimes are palpable and can cause discomfort for patients while kneeling, can be avoided. Secondarily, decreased exposure may lead to shorter operative times, decreased wound healing complications, and blood loss. However, the main disadvantage of using suture anchors as compared with the transosseous technique is the increased cost associated with the use of anchors versus sutures alone.

Chronic (Neglected) Disruption. Neglected or chronic rupture of the quadriceps tendon presents a difficult reconstruction in the form of having enough tendon length and excursion to perform a tension-free repair, and the results after repair of such tears are less satisfactory than after treatment of acute tears.[135] A longitudinal midline incision is the preferred approach, and the exposure may reveal a large gap between the tendon edges. Next, elevation and release of the quadriceps muscle group from the femur is performed, and mobilization is attempted. When the tendon edges can be apposed, the ends are débrided and repaired with the Scuderi technique, as described earlier. However, when there is contraction of the tendon and apposition cannot be obtained, a Codivilla tendon-lengthening and repair procedure is recommended (Fig. 70.6). An inverted V is cut through the full thickness of the proximal part of the quadriceps tendon, with the lower margin of the V ending approximately 1.3 cm proximal to the rupture. The tendon ends are apposed and repaired with multiple no. 0 nonabsorbable sutures. The medial and lateral retinacula are also repaired at this time with multiple interrupted no. 0 absorbable sutures. The flap is brought distally and sutured in place. The open upper portion of the V is closed with interrupted no. 0 absorbable sutures. The reconstruction should be protected with a pull-out cerclage wire. Postoperative treatment is similar to that after the Scuderi procedure.

In rare, often revision settings, when tendon length cannot be achieved using the Codivilla technique, hamstring autograft in combination with prolene mesh reinforcement has been recently described in case reports.[94,129]

Results of Surgical Management of Quadriceps Tendon Rupture

Results of repair and/or reconstruction of acute midsubstance and osteotendinous quadriceps tendon disruptions are generally favorable.[73,84,123,125,135] Negrin et al. conducted a retrospective review of 93 patients who underwent acute quadriceps tendon repair with transosseous nonabsorbable sutures in a Krackow technique and retinacular repair with absorbable Vicryl suture.[109] After a mean follow-up of 10.3 years, Knee Society (KS) knee scores averaged 93.1, KS function scores 89.7, Oxford Knee Scores (OKSs) 14.6, and Western Ontario and McMaster Universities (WOMAC) scores 95.7. The group concluded that functional restitution and resumption of activities of daily living could be achieved in most cases following repair, especially if performed within 5 days of injury. Boudissa et al. reported on 68 patients who underwent acute quadriceps tendon repair[11]; 91% of the cohort underwent repair with a transosseous technique, with end-to-end repair in the remaining 9% at an average of 2.7 days from injury. The 50 knees that were available for an average follow-up of 76 months averaged a Lysholm score of 93.7; 98% had good or very good subjective results, and 97% of working patients returned to their preinjury

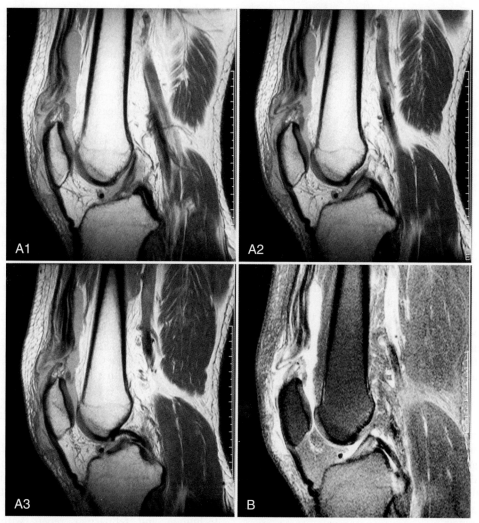

FIG 70.4 Technique for Repair of a Quadriceps Tendon Tear (A and B) Sagittal MRI scans demonstrating a quadriceps tendon tear at the osteotendinous junction.

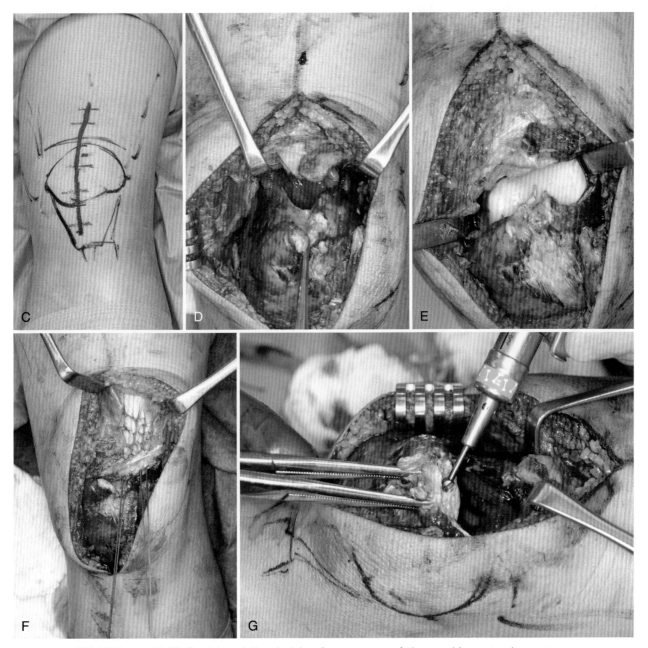

FIG 70.4, cont'd (C) Straight midline incision for exposure of the quadriceps tendon rupture. (D) Hematoma is evacuated and the free tendon ends exposed. (E) The proximal rectus femoris and vastus intermedius tendon edges are débrided to healthy tendon, and the superior pole of the patella is débrided of residual tendon. (F) Two no. 5 nonabsorbable sutures are placed along the medial and lateral borders of the quadriceps tendon in an interlocking fashion. (G) A bur is used to create a transverse trough in the superior pole of the patella near the chondral surface.

Continued

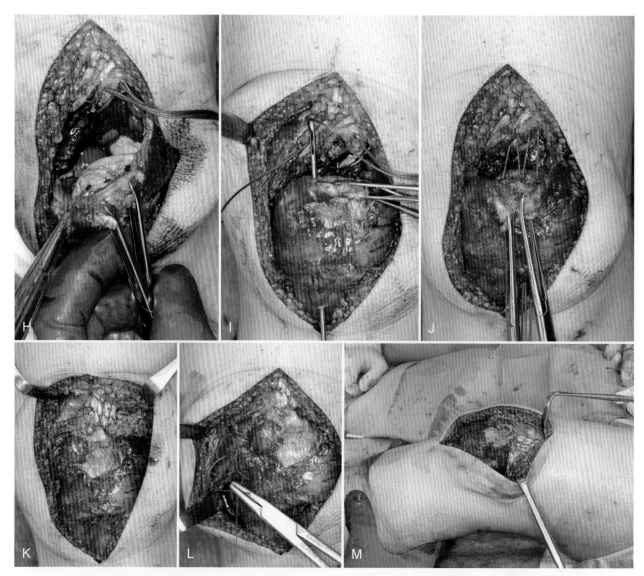

FIG 70.4, cont'd (H) A methylene blue pen is used to mark the site for transosseous drill holes to be placed 1.0 to 1.5 cm apart in the trough. (I) A Beath pin is used here to drill and pass the suture through the medial tunnel. (J) The step is repeated for the central and lateral tunnels so that the central two suture ends are passed through one central tunnel. (K) The sutures are tied with the knee in full extension. (L) The medial and lateral retinacula are closed. (M) The repair is checked to ensure that no gapping at the repair site occurs with 20 to 30 degrees of flexion.

occupations. Furthermore, at final follow-up the average active flexion was 133 degrees. The group concluded that good results could be expected following quadriceps tendon repair if the injury is diagnosed and treated quickly. West et al. reported on a case series of 50 total patients with acute extensor mechanism disruptions, 20 of which were quadriceps tendon ruptures at the osteotendinous insertion.[156] The group used the transosseous suture technique and augmented this with "relaxing suture" tied at 30 degrees of flexion to take tension off the repair in flexion. The group was able to achieve 120 degrees of flexion and brace-free ambulation at a mean of 7.2 weeks and 7.7 weeks, respectively, and by 6 months all patients reached their preinjury level of activity. At a mean follow-up at 4 years there were no postoperative complications and Lysholm scores averaged 92 points. Puranik et al. used three distinct repair techniques in 21 patients with acute quadriceps tendon ruptures. Ten repairs were performed with the transosseous suture technique, nine end-to-end repairs using a Bunnell interlocking suture technique, and three repairs with wire augmentation following end-to-end repair.[121] Patients were graded using the 25-point outcome score described by Rougraff et al.[135] Patients who underwent transosseous repair had the highest outcome scores, followed by the end-to-end repair and finally the wire augmentation group. Finally, Wenzl et al. reported on 30 quadriceps tendon rupture repairs with simple sutures for midsubstance tears and transosseous repair with wire augmentation for osteotendinous injuries[155]; 91% of patients were able to return to their primary occupation following repair, and the overall mean Lysholm score was 92.5. The group reported no significant difference in the functional outcome based on repair technique,

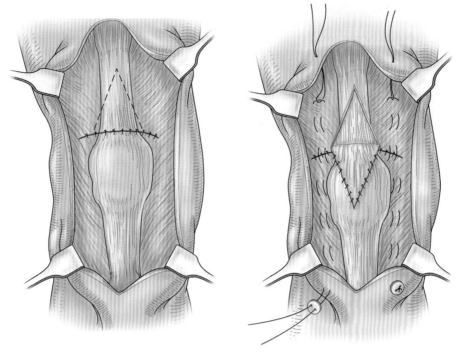

FIG 70.5 Acute repair of the quadriceps tendon into a bony trough. (Redrawn from Scott WN (ed): *The knee*, vol 1, St. Louis, 1994, Mosby-Year Book, p 472.)

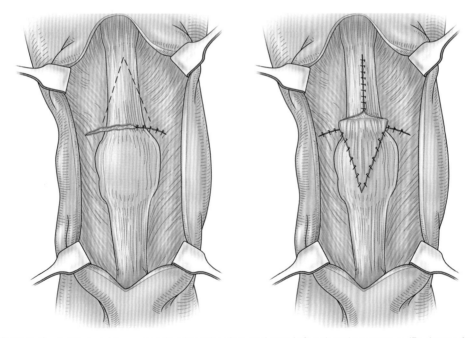

FIG 70.6 Codivilla quadriceps tendon lengthening and repair for chronic ruptures. (Redrawn from Scott WN (ed): *The knee,* vol 1, St. Louis, 1994, Mosby-Year Book, p 473.)

but did report significantly decreased functional outcome based on timing of repair.

Literature on bilateral quadriceps tendon repair is limited. Chang et al. reported on a series of five patients who underwent acute repair of bilateral quadriceps tendon ruptures using transosseous sutures with a minimum 1-year follow-up.[26] Patients were age-matched to a control group with unilateral injuries with similar medical history. The group reported no

statistical significant between the two groups with regard to range of motion, International Knee Documentation Committee (IKDC) score, and return to activity and concluded that patients with early surgical repair of bilateral, simultaneous extensor mechanism ruptures can exhibit adequate recovery with return to high level of function.

Partial tears of the quadriceps tendon are typically treated conservatively with a brief period of immobilization followed by progressive range of motion and strengthening.[60] However, if the patient remains symptomatic, excision of scar tissue and closure of tendon has been shown to be effective.[122]

Complications include rerupture and wound compromise. In the largest series of 93 repairs, Negrin reported an 8% rerupture rate in addition to an 8% wound-healing complication rate.[109] In a series of 53 repairs Rougraff et al.[135] observed two reruptures; in a series of 51 patients by Konrath et al.[73] one rerupture was noted. No large series of surgical repair of chronic or neglected quadriceps tendon rupture is available; however, a number of case reports have suggested favorable results with several different reconstruction methods.

PATELLAR TENDON RUPTURE

Mechanism and Causes of Patellar Tendon Disruption

Rupture of the patellar tendon is a relatively infrequent injury and is estimated to be six times less common than rupture of the quadriceps tendon. Unlike quadriceps tendon rupture, it typically occurs in active patients younger than 40 years.[69,93,136,149] Known risk factors for patellar tendon rupture include systemic inflammatory diseases, such as lupus and rheumatoid arthritis, chronic metabolic disorders, anabolic steroid abuse, local steroid injections and most commonly progressive patellar tendinopathy and microtrauma.** Patellar tendon rupture caused by indirect trauma has been shown to be the result of chronic tendon degeneration secondary to repetitive microtrauma. Several studies have evaluated biopsy specimens of spontaneously ruptured patellar tendons and compared them to intact tendons from age-matched controls and reported up to 97% of the pathologic findings were degenerative tendon changes on histologic analysis.[66,69] Rarely, patella tendon rupture occurs following ACL reconstruction using the central third of the patellar tendon for bone-patellar tendon-bone (BPTB) autograft; however, the reported incidence is less than 0.1%.[81] Finally, patellar tendon ruptures can also occur with high-energy trauma and have been reported with tibiofemoral dislocations.[113,158]

With increasing amounts of knee flexion, the patellofemoral contact area shifts proximally, affording the patellar tendon a mechanical advantage during active extension. Moreover, biomechanical studies have shown that the greatest forces in the patellar tendon occur with the knee at approximately 60 degrees of flexion.[59] Thus most ruptures tend to occur with the knee in a flexed position.

Most of these ruptures occur at the inferior pole of the patella but may also take place in the midsubstance of the tendon or rarely at the insertion of the tubercle.[33,92] This is because of a much higher tensile load that is concentrated at the insertion sites of the patellar tendon than in the midsubstance portion of the tendon.[159] Disruptions through the substance of the patellar tendon can also occur spontaneously but are more often caused by trauma or laceration.

Diagnosis

The history is often helpful and consistent in diagnosing patellar tendon rupture. Patients typically present following a sustained forceful quadriceps contraction with the knee in a flexed position with the inability to weight bear and a tense

hemarthrosis. Physical examination reveals a high-riding patella with tenderness, ecchymosis, and a palpable defect in the tendon. If the rupture extends completely through the tendon and retinaculum, there will be complete loss of active extension. However, similar to quadriceps tendon rupture, if the rupture involves only the tendon and the retinaculum remains largely intact, some active extension will remain. Other intra-articular injuries, such as cruciate ligament tears and meniscal pathology, must be ruled out, given similar mechanisms of injury.

Imaging

Imaging modalities for corroborating a diagnosis of patellar tendon rupture have been discussed previously. In brief, radiographs will reveal patella alta and may demonstrate an avulsion injury from the inferior pole of the patella. A retrospective study on 38 acute patella tendon ruptures reported that 90% of radiographs demonstrated patella alta and 37% had an identifiable avulsion injury.[134] Ultrasound can also be a useful imaging modality, with MRI remaining the most sensitive and specific way of diagnosing a patellar tendon rupture. MRI can also help to identify the exact tear location and rule out other associated intra-articular pathology, especially in cases of high-energy trauma.[95]

Overview of Surgical Management

Partial ruptures of the patellar tendon with intact extensor mechanism function can be treated nonoperatively. The *author* recommends a short period of immobilization in full extension for 2 weeks, followed by progressive range of motion with active flexion and assisted passive extension for 4 weeks and initiation of strengthening after 6 weeks.

Surgical intervention is indicated for incomplete ruptures with functional deficits and for all complete patellar tendon ruptures, irrespective of age or functional level. The surgical technique chosen depends predominantly on the length of time between injury and surgery and the quality of viable tissue available for repair. Surgical repair should be performed as soon after the injury as possible to have the best chance of achieving a tension-free tendon apposition. This also prevents chronic, proximal migration of the patella, alongside degeneration and scarring of the tissue quality that will ultimately preclude primary repair.

The approach typically consists of a straight midline incision, with small full-thickness medial and lateral subcutaneous skin flaps developed to assess the retinaculum. The paratenon overlying the patellar tendon is identified and carefully incised longitudinally. The paratenon is elevated medially and laterally and preserved for subsequent repair at the time of closure. Hematoma within the disrupted tendon is evacuated, the tear location is then assessed, and repair technique is chosen.

Procedures

Acute Disruption. Complete patellar tendon rupture requires surgical intervention to restore extensor mechanism function. Similar to quadriceps tendon rupture, repair technique largely depends on tear location and chronicity. In situations in which rupture of the patellar tendon occurs at the osteotendinous junction, transosseous repair is the technique of choice.[36] The free tendon is freshened, and a horizontal trough is then made along the posterior half of the inferior pole of the patella near the articular cartilage surface (Fig. 70.7). One study by Lu et al. demonstrated in a rabbit model that greater healing occurred

---

**References 12, 27, 31, 61, 66, 75, 99, 103, and 133.

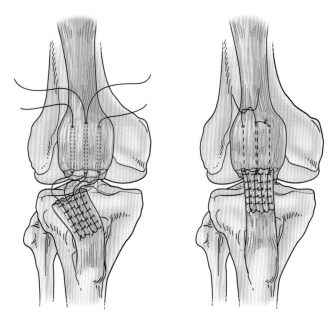

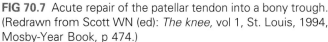

FIG 70.7 Acute repair of the patellar tendon into a bony trough. (Redrawn from Scott WN (ed): *The knee,* vol 1, St. Louis, 1994, Mosby-Year Book, p 474.)

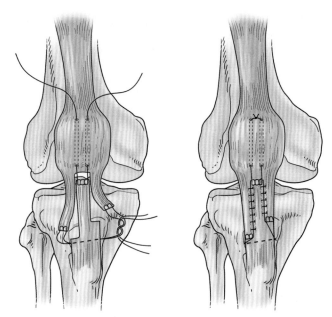

FIG 70.8 Acute repair of intrasubstance tears of the patellar tendon. (Redrawn from Scott WN (ed): *The knee,* vol 1, St. Louis, 1994, Mosby-Year Book, p 475.)

at the cartilage-tendon interface than the bone tendon interface.[87] These results might support the idea of creating the trough closer to the articular cartilage for facilitating earlier biologic repair. Two to three no. 5 nonabsorbable sutures are then placed along the medial and lateral halves of the distal patellar tendon with an interlocking (Krackow) stitch such that the four (or six) free ends of suture exit the proximal portion of the tendon.[74] The number of sutures is based on the width of the patient's patella to accommodate drill holes. Using a Beath pin, a longitudinal drill hole is placed centrally in the patella at the base of the trough, exiting at the superior pole of the patella. An ACL drill guide may be used to place the patellar drill holes more precisely.[111]

The two central free ends of suture are then placed through the eyelet of the beath pin, and the pin is pulled proximally. The Beath pin is used to drill and pass the sutures on the medial and lateral sides of the patella approximately 1.0 to 1.5 cm apart. The sutures are pulled taut, and the free end of the patellar tendon should be seated within the trough. The sutures are held provisionally with a hemostat to assess patellar tracking and rotation. It is important to ensure that the repair has not produced patella baja. At 45 degrees of flexion, the inferior pole of the patella should be above the roof of the intercondylar notch. A mosquito clamp is used to pass one of the central sutures medially and the other laterally so that the suture knots may be placed over bone rather than the quadriceps tendon. The medial and lateral retinacula are repaired with no. 0 absorbable sutures. In most cases we prefer to tie the sutures with the knee in full extension. Optional reinforcement can be performed to augment the repair with Mersilene tape or heavy nonabsorbable suture placed circumferentially around the repair through drill holes in the patella and the anterior cortex of the proximal end of the tibia. The knee is then flexed to 90 degrees of flexion to confirm construct stability.

Alternatively, as with quadriceps tendon ruptures the patellar tendon may be repaired with suture anchors rather than with this transosseous technique.[57] Capiola and Re described their

technique of using three suture anchors that incorporate a six-stranded Krackow technique.[24] The sutures are placed along the medial and lateral halves of the patellar tendon with an interlocking technique (Bunnell or Krackow-Bunnell) following placement of the anchors at the inferior pole of the patella.[19,50] Advantages of suture anchors for repair of patellar tendon ruptures are the avoidance of iatrogenic patellar cartilage or quadriceps injury seen with the transosseous technique.[24] Ho and Lee also proposed that intraosseous wires that pull the free tendon edges through the tunnels carry the theoretical risk of shortening already débrided tendon, resulting in patella baja.[57] In addition, a major concern of the transosseous technique has been loosening through the bone tunnels, which has been shown to occur in some studies in as few as 25 cyclic loads, leading to eventual cutout of the sutures through the tunnels.[14] In a cadaveric biomechanical study by Ettinger et al. 30 patellar tendons underwent tenotomy followed by repair with suture anchors or transpatellar suture tunnels.[43] Compared with transosseous sutures, tendon repair with suture anchors yielded significantly less gap formation during cyclic loading and had significantly higher ultimate failure loads. However, these findings have not been borne out in the literature. In a retrospective review Bushnell et al. reported a 21% failure rate with suture anchors in 14 patients with patellar tendon ruptures.[19] Prospective randomized clinical trials are required to further delineate any superiority between the two techniques. With each repair technique the wound is then closed in layers, and a cylinder cast or hinged brace with the knee in extension is applied and maintained for 6 weeks. The patient may ambulate with full weight bearing, as tolerated, with crutches. When the cast is removed, the control dial, hinged-knee orthosis allowing progressive flexion of the knee is used. When the patient has achieved more than 90 degrees of flexion and sufficient quadriceps strength to support the limb, the orthosis is discontinued.

Acute ruptures that occur within the midsubstance of the patellar tendon can be repaired with running interlocking sutures of no. 2 nonabsorbable suture material (Fig. 70.8). The distally based tendon is reinforced through longitudinal drill holes in the patella, whereas the proximally based tendon is repaired through a horizontal drill hole in the tibial tubercle. Each flap is repaired side to side with interrupted no. 0 absorbable sutures. The medial and lateral retinacula are also repaired with no. 0 absorbable sutures at this time. The postoperative course is similar to that described earlier.

Augmentation. If secure repair of the patellar tendon cannot be achieved with either of the repairs described earlier, augmentation with the semitendinosus or gracilis tendon is recommended (Fig. 70.9).[68,80] The insertion sites of the semitendinosus and gracilis are identified through the original midline incision. While preserving the distal insertion, a tendon stripper is used to divide the tendon proximally. If only the semitendinosus is used for augmentation, it should be passed through an oblique drill hole at the tibial tubercle in a medial to lateral direction. The graft is pulled superiorly, passing laterally to medially through a transverse drill hole in the inferior aspect of the patella, and then sutured to the origin of the semitendinosus with no. 0 nonabsorbable sutures. This technique creates a box around the patellar tendon. The corners of the graft are sutured with nonabsorbable sutures to prevent slippage. If the semitendinosus tendon is thin and further augmentation is needed, the gracilis tendon can also be used. The insertion of the gracilis tendon is maintained distally, and the tendon is passed in a medial to lateral direction through a second horizontal drill hole in the patella; it then circles the patellar tendon and returns in a lateral to medial direction through the oblique tibial drill hole.

The postoperative course is similar to that described earlier, with 6 weeks of immobilization in a cylinder cast. We prefer a postoperative course of immobilization in a cylinder cast before initiation of a physical therapy program. However, Larson and Simonian[80] suggested that immediate mobilization with initial passive and active assisted exercises after reconstruction of the patellar tendon with semitendinosus augmentation may be beneficial. Bhargava et al.[9] have reported on 11 patients treated with primary repair protected by a cerclage wire and early mobilization, and all did well. However, patients with a history of systemic collagen vascular disorders or previous steroid injection were excluded. Levy et al.[84] also recommended immediate postoperative mobilization after reconstruction with a Dacron graft. Marder and Timmerman[92] used early mobilization in athletes younger than 40 years after primary repair without augmentation.

Fulkerson and Langeland's technique, in which the central quadriceps tendon is harvested with a patellar bone graft for ACL reconstruction, has also been applied to repair or reconstruct patellar tendon disruptions.[49] Williams et al. reported success with this technique in three cases of patellar tendon compromise—one acute, one chronic, and one with patella infera.[157] The patellar bone graft is inset into the tibial tubercle, and the quadriceps tendon graft is secured with sutures passed through the patella in a distal to proximal direction. In a case report Edwards et al. used this technique to reconstruct an acute patellar tendon disruption associated with bony compromise of the tibial tubercle.[40]

Reinforcement of Repair. Historically, McLaughlin[96] and McLaughlin and Francis[97] recommended that repair of the patellar tendon be reinforced with the use of stainless steel wire anchored to a bolt placed in the tibial tubercle. Hsu et al.[58] reported a technique of primary repair reinforced with a

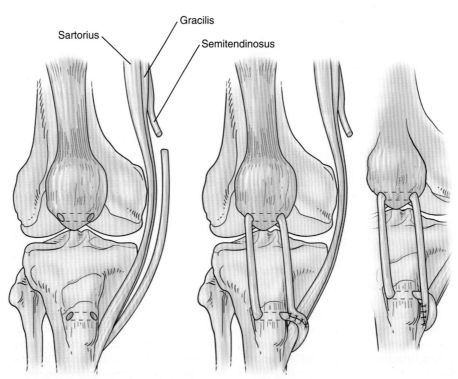

FIG 70.9 Augmentation of a patellar tendon repair with the semitendinosus tendon. (Redrawn from Scuderi GR: Extensor mechanism injuries: treatment. In Scott WN (ed): *Ligament and extension mechanism injuries of the knee*, St. Louis, 1991, Mosby-Year Book, p 191.)

neutralization wire. Siwek and Rao also recommended that all immediate repairs of the patellar tendon be reinforced by external devices.[149] Several reports have described reinforcing the repair with various augmentation grafts, including autografts, allografts[39,68] (fascia lata, semitendinosus, gracilis), and synthetic grafts (Mersilene,[100] Dacron,[46,47,84] carbon fiber,[44] and a poly-p-dioxanone cord[72]). In a study by Ravalin et al. 12 fresh-frozen cadaveric specimens were used to compare standard repair with transosseous sutures without augmentation, with repair using a no. 5 Ethibond suture and with augmentation using 2.0-mm Dall-Miles cable.[127] Gap formation at the repair site was assessed after cycling the knees in a custom knee jig; it was greatest in the repairs without augmentation and least in the group augmented with the cable. However, clinical reports have demonstrated satisfactory results of acute patellar tendon disruption repaired without augmentation. In a series of 15 consecutive patients Marder and Timmerman published excellent results with primary repair of acute patellar tendon disruption treated by suture repair alone.[92]

Chronic (Neglected) Disruption.   Chronic rupture of the patellar tendon poses a particular problem, especially if there is retraction of the quadriceps tendon with proximal migration of the patella. Previously a two-stage reconstruction with preoperative traction through a transverse Steinmann pin placed in the patella was described. More recent techniques describe one-stage techniques using hamstring tendons to reconstruct the extensor mechanism. Mobilization of the patella and quadriceps tendon can be achieved by clearing the medial and lateral gutters into the suprapatellar pouch and subperiosteally elevating the vastus intermedius from the anterior aspect of the femur.[3] A lateral retinacular release is also performed. If necessary, a medial retinacular release can be performed, but this may increase the risk for avascular necrosis of the patella.[142,143] Several techniques have been described for reconstruction of chronic tears of the patellar tendon, including direct repair with augmentation using cerclage wires, autograft, allograft, and synthetic grafts. Direct repair may be performed with transosseous sutures or the more recently described suture anchors.[18,19] Regardless of the technique performed, it is important that care be taken to maintain normal patellar tracking, rotation, and height. Preoperative planning should include a lateral radiograph of the contralateral knee to determine patellar height. Intraoperatively, the inferior pole of the patella should be above the roof of the intercondylar notch at 45 degrees of flexion. The knee should be able to achieve 90 degrees of flexion and, when in full extension, the patellar tendon should be lax, approximately 1.0 to 1.5 cm.

Reconstruction of chronic patellar tendon rupture is performed through a longitudinal midline incision. The paratenon is incised longitudinally to expose the patellar tendon. If sufficient tendon is available, the ends are cut fresh and sutured, as described earlier for the acute repair, but augmentation with a semitendinosus and/or gracilis autograft is typically recommended. A bone tenaculum can be used to pull the patella distally, and the semitendinosus and gracilis are sutured under tension. Casey and Tietjens[25] have reported on their series of four patients with neglected patellar tendon rupture repaired primarily and augmented with three 1.5-mm cerclage wires in a figure-of-eight pattern from the quadriceps tendon to the tibial tubercle. All underwent a supervised therapy program and immediate mobilization in a brace. Average range of motion

was 112 degrees, and no extensor lag was reported. All patients had the hardware removed between 3 and 13 months postoperatively. More recently, Adbou reported on his prospective analysis of 17 chronic patellar tendon ruptures that underwent reconstruction with hamstring autograft and reinforced with stainless steel wire.[1] Twelve patients were able to return to their previous activities, 16 had loss of less than 5 degrees of extension compared with the healthy, contralateral side, and the mean Lysholm score at final follow-up was 85.

When there is a deficiency of remaining tendon or the remaining tendon is attenuated and scarred, a Z-shortening of the patellar tendon and a Z-lengthening of the quadriceps tendon can be performed (Fig. 70.10). This technique requires intraoperative radiographs to determine appropriate patellar height and position because of the increased tendency for patella infra with this reconstruction. After the proper position of the patella has been determined, the Z-plasty is reinforced with multiple interrupted no. 0 nonabsorbable sutures. This reconstruction requires augmentation with the semitendinosus and gracilis tendons, which are harvested as two free tendons and sutured end to end. The hamstring tendons pass through a transverse drill hole in the midportion of the patella and then through a transverse hole in the tibial tubercle in a figure-of-eight fashion. The semitendinosus and gracilis grafts are secured to the patellar tendon with absorbable suture. Alternatively, the quadriceps tendon–patellar bone graft technique described earlier may be applied.[50,157] The postoperative course is similar to that described previously. Some authors have suggested that a judicious program of immediate postoperative mobilization is possible when the repair is augmented with the semitendinosus tendon or a Dacron graft.[80,84]

Allografts[34,85,99] have been used for reconstruction of neglected patellar tendon rupture (Fig. 70.11).[45,63,98] The Achilles tendon with a corticocancellous calcaneal bone block is a convenient allograft. The tibial tubercle is prepared with an

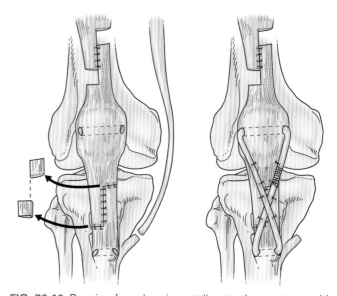

FIG 70.10 Repair of a chronic patellar tendon rupture with a Z-shortening of the patellar tendon and a Z-lengthening of the quadriceps tendon plus augmentation with the semitendinosus and gracilis tendons sutured end to end. (Redrawn from Scott WN (ed): *The knee,* vol 1, St. Louis, 1994, Mosby-Year Book, p 476.)

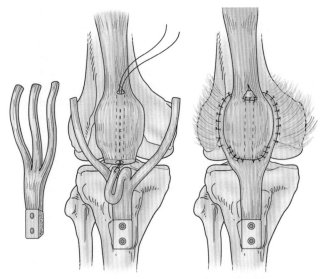

FIG 70.11 Allograft reconstruction for neglected patellar tendon rupture. (Redrawn from Scott WN (ed): *The knee,* vol 1, St. Louis, 1994, Mosby-Year Book, p 476.)

oscillating saw or bur to create a trough measuring 2.5 to 3.0 cm long, 1.5 to 2.0 cm wide, and 1.5 cm deep. The bone block is contoured and press-fit into the trough. It is then secured with two 4.0-mm cancellous screws. The Achilles tendon graft is divided into thirds. The central third, which should measure 8 to 9 mm in width, is pulled through a slit in the residual patellar tendon. The graft is then passed through a longitudinal 8- to 9-mm-wide drill hole in the patella. This drill hole enters the inferior pole of the patella and exits at the superior border proximally, 3 mm posterior to the central portion of the quadriceps tendon. The tendon is then pulled through a vertical slit in the quadriceps tendon. The tendon is sutured at the inferior pole of the patella and at the quadriceps tendon with multiple interrupted no. 0 nonabsorbable sutures. Patellar height should be determined at this time. The knee should flex to 90 degrees and, at 45 degrees of flexion, the inferior pole of the patella should be superior to the roof of the intercondylar notch. After the patellar position has been determined to be correct, the medial and lateral flaps are sutured to the medial and lateral retinacula with multiple no. 0 nonabsorbable sutures. If the paratenon is present, it should be closed over the graft with 2-0 absorbable sutures.

The wound is closed in layers, and a cylinder cast is applied. The cast is worn for 5 weeks, and then a control dial, hinged-knee orthosis is worn until 90 degrees of flexion has been achieved and quadriceps strength is sufficient to support the limb during ambulation. Wascher and Summa described a technique in which an Achilles tendon allograft is used to reconstruct a ruptured extensor mechanism after patellectomy that had failed two previous attempts at primary repair.[153] Bermúdez et al. described a similar technique in which an Achilles tendon allograft was used to reconstruct a ruptured extensor mechanism in a 20-year-old woman 6 months status post-partial patellectomy.[8] Park et al. described reconstructing the extensor mechanism of a patient with a large patella and patellar tendon defect with an extended medial gastrocnemius flap, including a tendinous portion of the Achilles, while simultaneously using a saphenous neurocutaneous flap for additional soft tissue coverage.[114]

Results of Surgical Repair of Patellar Tendon Disruption

As for quadriceps tendons, the results of patellar tendon repair are favorable, regardless of the location of the rupture or the method of repair.[††] Again, delayed repairs have worse outcomes than repairs performed in the acute setting. When the patellar tendon is repaired in the acute setting, range of motion approaching that of the contralateral knee is typically regained and in athletic individuals premorbid activity levels and strength can be expected. A meta-analysis examined 354 acute repairs with eight different operative techniques.[53] The most popular acute repair technique was a primary repair augmented with cerclage wire, Dall-Miles cable, or nonabsorbable sutures in 43% of patients. This was followed by primary repair alone in 31% of patients, and primary repair augmented with tape in 8% of patients. Although reported scoring systems varied, preventing adequate comparison and evaluation, Lysholm scores for primary repair, primary repair with cerclage wire, Dall-Miles cable, or nonabsorbable sutures, and primary repair with autograft augmentation were 94, 95, and 95, respectively. Primary repair augmented with cerclage wire, Dall-Miles cable or nonabsorbable sutures reported the best mean range of motion, from 0 to 129 degrees, followed by primary repair alone with mean range of motion of 11 to 102. Repairing acute ruptures with an allogeneic graft augmented with cerclage wire had the highest rate of failures and complications at 50%, while primary repair augmented with either cerclage wire, Dall-Miles cable, or nonabsorbable sutures had both the lowest failure rate (2%) and complication rate (2%). Combined, the primary repair methods in this study reported 3% failure rate versus a combined 8% failure rate of all other methods. The group concluded that primary repair augmented with cerclage wire, Dall-Miles cable, or nonabsorbable sutures is the method of choice in acute repairs. In the same study 149 chronic repairs were performed using eight different operative techniques. The most popular chronic repair technique was an autogenous graft of gracilis, gastrocnemius, quadriceps, patellar, or semitendinosus tendons in 23% of patients. Autogenous grafts had no failures and a complication rate of 6%, suggesting that autogenous repair is the method of choice in the chronic setting. No large series of neglected patellar tendon ruptures managed with patellar ligament reconstruction have been published. Complications include rerupture, wound problems, and patellofemoral symptoms. Rerupture is generally related to return to rigorous activity before completion of proper physical therapy. Wound complications are more common than with quadriceps tendon disruption because of the thinner skin at the tibial tubercle; therefore it is recommended that the skin incision be made adjacent to but not directly over the tubercle. Patellofemoral symptoms have been managed with lateral release.[73] Obtaining an intraoperative radiograph at completion of the patellar tendon repair is prudent to ensure that patella baja has not been created.

Quadriceps and Patellar Tendon Disruption Associated With Total Knee Arthroplasty

Complications involving the extensor mechanism of the knee following TKA have a reported prevalence of 1% to 12%.[115]

---

††References 53, 58, 76, 80, 93, and 149.

Although the disruption typically occurs in the postoperative setting there are several intraoperative, postoperative, and patient-related factors that affect the overall risk of quadriceps or patellar tendon complications. Depending on the surgical approach and soft-tissue dissection, the blood supply to the entire extensor mechanism may be compromised or completely disrupted.[105,116] The medial parapatellar arthrotomy is the most common surgical approach used to perform TKA and can disrupt the descending genicular and superior and inferior medial genicular arteries that supply the extensor mechanism, as discussed previously. Furthermore, excision of the lateral meniscus and infrapatellar fat pad can disrupt the inferior lateral genicular artery and recurrent branch of the anterior tibial artery, disrupting the blood supply to the patella.[105] Pawar et al. reported that the prevalence of transient patellar hypovascularity was 3.95 times higher in patients who required a lateral release intraoperatively.[116] Another known risk factor for increased risk of extensor mechanism dysfunction following TKA is over-resection of the patella during patellar resurfacing, which increases the risk of iatrogenic damage to the quadriceps and patellar tendons. Finally, as in quadriceps and patellar tendon ruptures in the native knee, systemic disorders, such as obesity, inflammatory arthritis, diabetes mellitus, and hyperthyroidism, in addition to chronic corticosteroid use and multiple corticosteroid injections, increase in the risk of quadriceps and patellar tendon rupture.[88]

Tears of the quadriceps tendon after TKA are rare, with a reported incidence ranging from 0.1% to 1.1%.[37,88] Although a traumatic event may result in a quadriceps tendon tear, the contribution of other factors, such as systemic disease, local injury, and factors related to the TKA technique, such as excessive reaction of the patella and a prior quadriceps snip or V-Y turndown, may predispose an individual and contribute to the rupture.[88,115] With only a few series in the literature these factors may only be speculated on but play an important role; they may include rheumatoid and other inflammatory arthritides, diabetes mellitus, chronic renal failure, hyperthyroidism, and systemic and local steroid use.

Furthermore, Dobbs et al. conducted a review of 24 patients with postoperative quadriceps ruptures of more than 23,000 TKAs and reported that only 9 sustained the rupture as a result of a substantial traumatic mechanism.[37] Physical exam and diagnostic work-up is similar to that in the native knee. As in the case of the native knee, incomplete tears of the quadriceps tendon with intact extensor mechanism function in patients with a TKA generally do well with nonoperative treatment. In the same series from Dobbs et al., seven partial quadriceps tendon ruptures were treated nonoperatively, all with a satisfactory outcome.[37] One of these seven ruptures was diagnosed 1 year after partial rupture and had no further treatment. This patient had a persistent extensor lag of 10 degrees and a palpable defect in the quadriceps tendon. Sixteen patients with a partial quadriceps tendon rupture underwent primary repair. These patients had a high complication rate (5 of 16), and four ultimately had an unsatisfactory result. This suggests that early diagnosis is imperative and nonoperative management, consisting of immobilization of the knee in extension for 4 to 6 weeks with weight bearing as tolerated, can yield good results for partial quadriceps tendon tears.

In contrast to the native knee the results of repair of complete quadriceps tendon tears in patients with a TKA are less predictable with reported rerupture rates of 33% to 36% and overall rates of complications of 33% to 100%.[37,88,162] In the series of Dobbs et al. 11 patients were identified with a complete quadriceps tendon tear.[37] Ten underwent primary repair and only four had a satisfactory result. Complications included four reruptures, two infections, and one patient with symptomatic recurvatum and instability. Similarly, Lynch et al. reported unsatisfactory results with direct suture repair for three quadriceps tendon ruptures, with one sustaining a rerupture and the other two demonstrating limited knee flexion and significant extensor lag.[88] Because of the discouraging results of operative treatment by direct suture repair, augmentation with autogenous graft material, such as semitendinosus tendon, or graft material, such as Marlex mesh, should be considered. Augmentation options described in the literature include semitendinosus or gracilis autograft, synthetic graft, and Achilles tendon or complete extensor mechanism allografts. Achilles tendon allograft reconstruction and synthetic mesh augmentation will be discussed at the end of this section.

Rupture of the patellar tendon after TKA is a rare but devastating complication, with a reported prevalence ranging from 0.17% to 2.5%.[88,102,115,124] Ruptures may occur intraoperatively, in the immediate postoperative period, or at some time after the postoperative period. Intraoperative ruptures typically occur during exposure while trying to evert the patella in a stiff knee with patella baja and occur at the tibial tubercle insertion.[105] Patients with multiple operated knees are at a significant risk, because of soft tissue scarring, stiffness, and devascularization of tissues. Previous distal alignment procedures, excessive patellar resection, and hinged implants have all been implicated as potential contributors to patellar tendon rupture after TKA.[42,101] The most common injury mechanism is a fall on a hyperflexed knee; however, atraumatic rupture can also occur during manipulation of a stiff knee. It may also occur as a delayed complication after chronic attrition from repetitive contact or impingement against the polyethylene tibial insert or an anteriorly overhanging tibial tray. The presentation and work-up is similar to that of patellar tendon ruptures in the native knee.

Prevention is of paramount importance. Awareness of this potential problem should be raised preoperatively in patients with a stiff or multiple operated knee. Intraoperatively, if difficulty with exposure is encountered, several techniques may aid in safely performing a TKA. Posteromedial dissection from the tibia may help to allow external rotation of the tibia, which can markedly relieve tension on the patellar tendon. Incising the lateral patellofemoral ligament in primary TKA and excision of scar tissue in the lateral gutter and beneath the patellar tendon in revision TKA can often allow the extensor mechanism to sublux laterally more easily. A quadriceps snip should be performed if there is still significant tension. Finally, if none of these measures adequately decrease tension on the patellar tendon, a tibial tubercle osteotomy or quadriceps turndown may be required to expose the knee safely.[115]

Treatment options depend on the acuity and location of the injury, the quality of remaining tissue, and the demands of the patient. Bracing may be indicated in patients with low functional demands, poor surgical candidates, and with partial tendon tears.

Patellar tendon avulsions that occur intraoperatively or in the immediate postoperative period and have an intact periosteal sleeve may be reattached with staples, transosseous sutures,[1] or suture anchors.[115,124,140] However, even in the acute setting

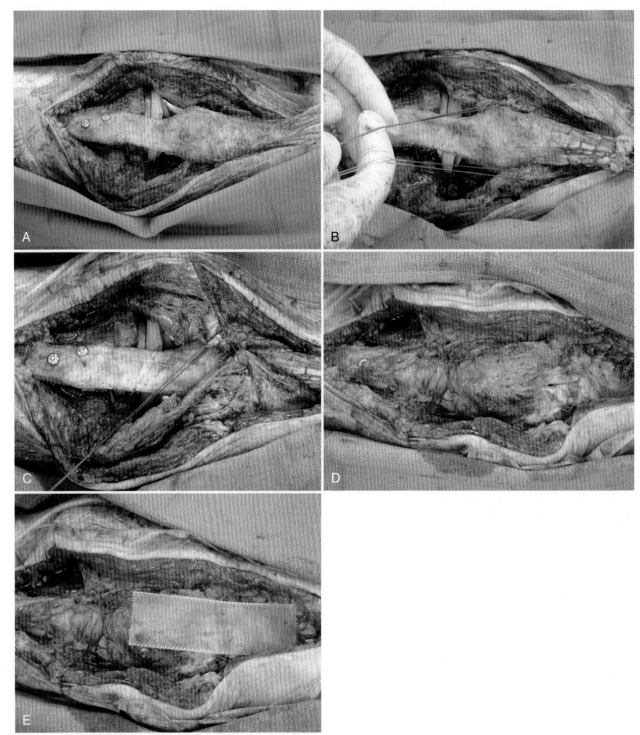

FIG 70.12 Extensor Mechanism Allograft Reconstruction for Patellar Tendon Disruption in a Total Knee Arthroplasty (A) An allograft tibial tubercle is fixed to host bone through an interference fit of the allograft-host junction and the use of two 4.5-mm bicortical screws. The allograft quadriceps tendon is secured proximally with two no. 5 nonabsorbable sutures in the Krackow method, with the knee in full extension. The length of the allograft is adjusted to ensure that the allograft patella lies in the trochlear groove. (B) Two sutures are then placed in the host retinacular tissue. (C and D) The residual host extensor tissue is then sewn over the allograft reconstruction in a pants-over-vest method. (E) Marlex mesh is used to reinforce the repair. (Adapted from Scuderi GR, Easley ME: Quadriceps and patellar tendon disruptions. In Insall JN, Scott WN (eds): *Surgery of the knee,* vol 1, New York, 2001, Churchill Livingstone, pp 1074–1086.)

and in the presence of poor tissue quality, augmentation is recommended to avoid complications, such as rerupture.[13,115,140] Ruptures late in the postoperative course or in the chronic setting are much more difficult to treat, and augmentation should always be used to supplement the repair. Options for reconstruction are numerous and include primary repair augmented with semitendinosus tendon autograft, Achilles tendon allograft, and quadriceps tendon–patella–patellar tendon–tibial tubercle allograft.[16,34,83,124] Browne and Hanssen describe a surgical technique using a knitted, monofilament polypropylene graft to reconstruct the patellar tendon and encourage ingrowth of the host tissue to the graft.[13] They reported on 13 patients, nine of which had an extensory lag of less than 10 degrees with preserved knee flexion, and significant increases in mean KS scores for pain and function.

Cadambi and Engh described a technique for primary repair augmented with an autogenous semitendinosus tendon.[22] In this procedure the semitendinosus tendon is harvested at the musculotendinous junction, with the distal insertion left intact. The tendon is routed medially through a drill hole in the distal pole of the patella and then sutured to itself at its distal insertion. The knee was immobilized for 6 weeks, and patients were permitted to bear weight as tolerated. In their series of seven patients the average extensor lag was 10 degrees, with an average flexion of 79 degrees. The authors concluded that the use of autogenous semitendinosus tendon augmentation of primary patellar tendon repairs could restore sufficient quadriceps strength and motion.

Achilles tendon allograft has also been used to reconstruct chronic patellar tendon rupture after TKA. Crossett et al. reviewed their experience with fresh-frozen Achilles tendon allograft with an attached calcaneal bone graft in nine knees.[34] The calcaneal bone block is cut to match a defect created in the tibia and the bone block is impacted with an interference fit. The bone block is secured with a screw or wires. The allograft tendon is then sewn to the underlying extensor mechanism with nonabsorbable suture while the knee is in full extension. Postoperatively the knees were immobilized in extension for 4 weeks and then progressive flexion was allowed. The average extensor lag improved from 44 degrees preoperatively to 3 degrees postoperatively and, although two grafts had failed, both were repaired successfully.

Emerson et al. were the first to describe an allograft reconstruction using the quadriceps tendon, a patella with a cemented prosthesis, the patellar tendon, and the tibial tubercle.[42] In their description the allograft tubercle is fixed to the host tibia with screws or wire and the patella is placed on the anterior flange of the femoral component. The allograft quadriceps tendon is then sutured to the host tendon with nonabsorbable sutures while the extensor mechanism construct is placed under slight tension. There was a high complication rate, with one-third of patients demonstrating an extensor lag of 20 to 40 degrees. Leopold et al. reconstructed seven extensor mechanisms with Emerson's technique and rated all seven as failures based on persistent extensor lag of more than 30 degrees.[83]

Nazarian and Booth have studied a larger series of 36 patients with chronic extensor mechanism disruption and used a modification of Emerson's technique.[108] In their technique the distal extensor allograft was tensioned with the knee in full extension. The average extensor lag was 13 degrees; 23 achieved full active extension that equaled passive extension. However, eight knees required a repeat allograft reconstruction. This modification

seems to provide improved active knee extension, a finding supported by Burnett et al., who evaluated 20 extensor mechanism allografts: group I consisted of seven knees reconstructed with the allograft slightly tensioned and group II consisted of 13 knees with the allograft tightly tensioned in full extension.[15] The average postoperative extensor lag was 59 degrees in group I and 4.3 degrees in group 2. All seven knees reconstructed with the graft slightly tensioned were clinical failures, whereas all 13 reconstructed with the allograft tightly tensioned in full extension were clinical successes.

Other techniques described include a medial gastrocnemius flap,[17] the use of synthetic ligament augmentation,[6] and patellotibial fusion.[71] Itälä et al. conducted a canine study reattaching distal patellar tendons to porous tantalum washers and suggested that tendon healing into a prosthetic material can be achieved with sufficient soft tissue ingrowth and mechanical strength to withstand physiologic loading.[62] In a study by Sundar et al. the patella tendons of six ewes were reattached to a hydroxyapatite-coated titanium implant (attached to the proximal tibia), using a four-ply Vicryl mesh and then augmented the construct with demineralized bone matrix (DBM), cancellous autograft, and iliac crest autologous bone marrow.[152] The study results demonstrated good functional outcomes at 6 weeks and a direct-type enthesis at 12 weeks.

The technique for extensor mechanism allograft that we prefer (Fig. 70.12) is similar to that described by Nazarian and Booth.[108] A long midline incision is used to provide wide exposure and preserve as much of the residual extensor mechanism tissue as possible. The host tibia is exposed by subperiosteal dissection. Full passive extension of the knee is achieved. The allograft tibial tubercle is then prepared with a microsagittal saw to fashion a bone block approximately 3 cm long, 1.5 cm wide, and 1 cm deep and an oblique dovetail proximal cut.[22] The host tibia is then prepared to create a lock and key fit. The allograft tibia is secured with screws or wires. Two nonabsorbable no. 5 sutures are then secured to the allograft quadriceps tendon with a locking Krackow stitch. The residual extensor mechanism tendon is sewn over the extensor mechanism allograft construct in a pants-over-vest technique. As emphasized by Nazarian and Booth[108] and Burnett et al.[15,16] the graft is tensioned with the knee in full extension. Marlex mesh is used to reinforce the repair. This is just one method to reconstruct the extensor mechanism in TKA. A more comprehensive review of this problem is found elsewhere in this text.

KEY REFERENCES

30. Ciriello V, Gudipati S, Tosounidis T, et al: Clinical outcomes after repair of quadriceps tendon rupture: a systematic review. *Injury* 43(11):1931–1938, 2012. doi: 10.1016/j.injury.2012.08.044.

36. DeBerardino TM, Owens BD: Repair of acute and chronic patell tendon tears. In Wiesel S, editor: *Operative techniques in orthopaedic surgery*, Philadelphia, 2011, Lippincott Williams & Wilkins, pp 402–406.

37. Dobbs RE, Hanssen AD, Lewallen DG, et al: Quadriceps tendon rupture after total knee arthroplasty. Prevalence, complications, and outcomes. *J Bone Joint Surg Am* 87(1):37–45, 2005. doi:87/1/37 (pii).

57. Ho HM, Lee WK: Traumatic bilateral concurrent patellar tendon rupture: an alterative fixation method. *Knee Surg Sports Traumatol Arthrosc* 11(2):105–111, 2003. doi: 10.1007/s00167-002-0332-9.

60. Ilan DI, Tejwani N, Keschner M, et al: Quadriceps tendon rupture. *J Am Acad Orthop Surg* 11(3):192–200, 2003.

64. Kamali M: Bilateral traumatic rupture of the infrapatellar tendon. *Clin Orthop Relat Res* 142(142):131–134, 1979.

82. Lee D, Stinner D, Mir H: Quadriceps and patellar tendon ruptures. *J Knee Surg* 26(5):301–308, 2013. doi: 10.1055/s-0033-1353989.

90. Malik K: Repair of acute and chronic quadriceps tendon ruptures. In Wiesel S, editor: *Operative techniques in orthopaedic surgery*, Philadelphia, 2011, Lippincott Williams & Wilkins, pp 407–412.

93. Matava MJ: Patellar tendon ruptures. *J Am Acad Orthop Surg* 4(6):287–296, 1996.

105. Nam D, Abdel MP, Cross MB, et al: The management of extensor mechanism complications in total knee arthroplasty. AAOS exhibit selection. *J Bone Joint Surg Am* 96(6):e47, 2014. doi: 10.2106/JBJS.M.00949.

115. Parker DA, Dunbar MJ, Rorabeck CH: Extensor mechanism failure associated with total knee arthroplasty: prevention and management. *J Am Acad Orthop Surg* 11(4):238–247, 2003.

128. Razzano CD, Wilde AH, Phalen GS: Bilateral rupture of the infrapatellar tendon in rheumatoid arthritis. *Clin Orthop Relat Res* 91(91):158–161, 1973.

133. Rose PS, Frassica FJ: Atraumatic bilateral patellar tendon rupture. A case report and review of the literature. *J Bone Joint Surg Am* 83-A(9):1382–1386, 2001.

136. Saragaglia D, Pison A, Rubens-Duval B: Acute and old ruptures of the extensor apparatus of the knee in adults (excluding knee replacement). *Orthop Traumatol Surg Res* 99(Suppl 1):S67–S76, 2013. doi: 10.1016/j.otsr.2012.12.002.

149. Siwek CW, Rao JP: Ruptures of the extensor mechanism of the knee joint. *J Bone Joint Surg Am* 63(6):932–937, 1981.

160. Yepes H, Tang M, Morris SF, et al: Relationship between hypovascular zones and patterns of ruptures of the quadriceps tendon. *J Bone Joint Surg Am* 90(10):2135–2141, 2008. doi: 10.2106/JBJS.G.01200.

The references for this chapter can also be found on www.expertconsult.com.

Knee Arthritis

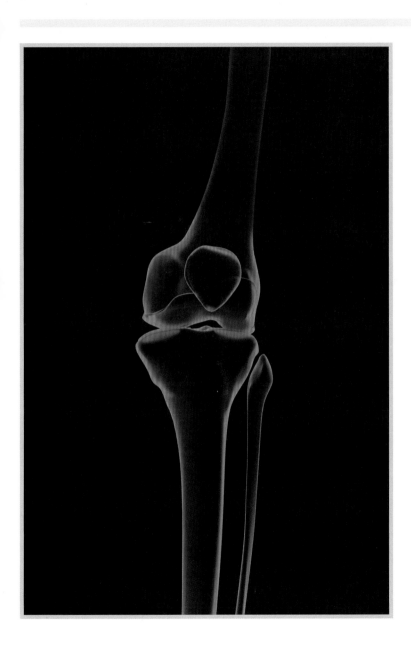

71

Gout and Other Crystalline Arthropathies

Aryeh M. Abeles, Michael H. Pillinger

CRYSTALLINE ARTHROPATHIES

Although there are a number of crystal-related arthropathies, the most common are gout and pseudogout, caused by urate and calcium pyrophosphate crystals, respectively. In this chapter we will focus on gout, with a brief discussion of calcium pyrophosphate and other crystalline diseases.

Gout

Gout, first described in antiquity, is the most common inflammatory arthritis.[15] Nonetheless, gout remains underdiagnosed and inadequately managed in the clinic.

Gout is the end result of sodium urate crystal deposition in joints and soft tissues, as a consequence of chronic hyperuricemia. Uric acid is generated via the metabolism of purines (ie, adenine and guanine). Breakdown of guanine and adenine converges at an intermediate purine product, xanthine, which is then converted to uric acid by the action of xanthine oxidase. In most mammals the enzyme uricase then breaks uric acid down to allantoin, a highly soluble, easily excreted molecule. However, humans and other primates developed inactivating mutations in the uricase gene approximately 15 million years ago.[12] As a result primates have higher serum urate levels than other mammals.[22] Serum urate levels are also determined by the kidney, which excretes about two-thirds of the daily urate load. Accordingly, any failure of renal urate excretion, whether innate or acquired, may result in hyperuricemia.[20]

Uric acid (typically in its deprotonated form of urate) is soluble in serum at 37°C, up to a concentration of approximately 6.8 mg/dL, above which deposition of urate crystals can occur. Peripheral joints are typically the sites of urate deposition because of the effects of temperature on crystal solubility; at lower temperatures (peripheral joints are several degrees cooler than core body temperature), urate crystals are less soluble in serum and precipitate out of solution into joints and soft tissues. Other factors promoting crystal formation in joints, including pH and differences in synovial fluid protein composition, may also play a role. Although serum uric acid concentrations greater than 6.8 to 7.0 mg/dL predispose to developing gout, only a minority of patients with elevated uric acid levels actually develop gouty arthritis, and the diagnosis of gout should never be made solely on the basis of hyperuricemia. However, the higher the serum uric acid level the more likely a given patient will ultimately develop gouty arthropathy.

Most patients suffering their first gouty attack are men between 30 and 60 years. Male sex hormones may contribute to rising serum urate levels (ie, by reducing renal urate excretion), and therefore gout in males is typically delayed at least until several years after puberty. Conversely, estrogen is uricosuric (ie, promotes renal urate excretion), so women rarely develop hyperuricemia or gout before menopause.[8] Aside from androgens and estrogen, other factors influencing serum uric acid concentration include diet and, as noted earlier, renal function. Not surprisingly, a diet rich in purines increases the risk of gout. Purine-rich foods include oily fish (eg, sardines, herring, mackerel), shellfish, beer, and organ meats, such as sweetbread and liver. Although many of these foods are also high in protein, protein consumption per se does not increase serum urate levels and may actually stimulate renal urate excretion. Alcohol consumption increases metabolic urate production, and some alcoholic beverages (eg, beer, spirits) are simultaneously high in purines. Often, patients with gout present with an acute arthritic attack shortly after ingestion of a large purine load (eg, heavy beer consumption, shrimp), which leads to a sudden and precipitous rise in serum uric acid levels.[4] Excessive consumption of fructose (a common food additive as high-fructose corn syrup) also contributes to hyperuricemia by driving metabolic urate production.[5] Urate clearance declines with kidney function, so that patients with impaired renal function have hyperuricemia and a higher incidence of gout.[13] Some medications block urate excretion, such as thiazide diuretics used for hypertension. Because a number of these secondary risk factors for hyperuricemia have epidemiologically increased, the prevalence of gout has risen in the United States by as much as fourfold in the past few decades.[24]

Acute Gout: Presentation and Evaluation. As a rule, gout attacks occur acutely and, although gout attacks can occur at any time of day, patients most typically are awakened by the onset of symptoms. Patients describe severe localized pain in combination with marked tenderness, as well as swelling and redness. The peak of an attack generally occurs within hours of onset, and the attack can last from days (in the case of early gout) to weeks or even months (in established gout). First-ever attacks of gout most typically occur in the first metatarsophalangeal (MTP) joint, although there are many exceptions to this rule, particularly among female sufferers. Diagnostic clues in the history include recent dietary indiscretions (see earlier) or systemic insults, such as surgery, physical trauma (which may liberate crystals from preestablished deposits), infection, or any other problem leading to systemic acidosis; because it is very common for patients with a crystalline arthropathy to have a disease flare-up with these precipitants, gout flare-ups appear to occur at an increased frequency among hospitalized patients.

Importantly, acute drops in serum urate can also precipitate gout, through a process of releasing already-deposited crystals from periarticular aggregates.

On examination the acutely involved joint(s) is generally warm, red, swollen, and markedly tender. Loss of motion because of pain and swelling is the norm. Signs of systemic inflammation may be present, including fever and tachycardia. Joint effusions are usually noted with knee involvement and, if the diagnosis has not already been definitively made, fluid should be withdrawn not only to relieve pain but also for cell count (to assess degree and type of inflammation), crystal identification, and Gram stain and culture. Definitive diagnosis is achieved by the identification of urate crystals under a polarizing microscope (Table 71.1). Urate crystals are negatively birefringent, such that the needle-shaped crystals appear yellow when viewed parallel to the optical axis of the polarizer and blue when perpendicular (Fig. 71.1). Extracellular urate crystals confirm that the patient has gout but may persist in the joint long after prior attacks; consequently, only intracellular crystals in neutrophils unequivocally confirm that the patient is in the midst of an acute attack (ie, that the crystals are activating neutrophils).

TABLE 71.1 Common Crystal-Associated Arthropathies

Parameter	Gout	Pseudogout
Crystal	Sodium urate	Calcium pyrophosphate
Radiograph	Early: Soft tissue swelling Later: Radiolucent erosions around edge of articular cartilage	Fine, radiopaque, linear deposits in the menisci and articular cartilage
Frequency of occurrence in knee	Common	Very common; increases with age, degenerative joint disease
Laboratory studies	Elevated serum uric acid	None
Crystal shape	Needle shape	Rhomboid
Crystal character with compensated polarized light	Parallel, yellow; perpendicular, blue (negatively birefringent)	Parallel, blue; perpendicular, yellow (positively birefringent)

Adapted from Vigorita VJ: The synovium. In Vigorita VJ, Ghelman B, editors: *Orthopaedic pathology*, Philadelphia, 1999, Lippincott Williams & Wilkins, p 596.

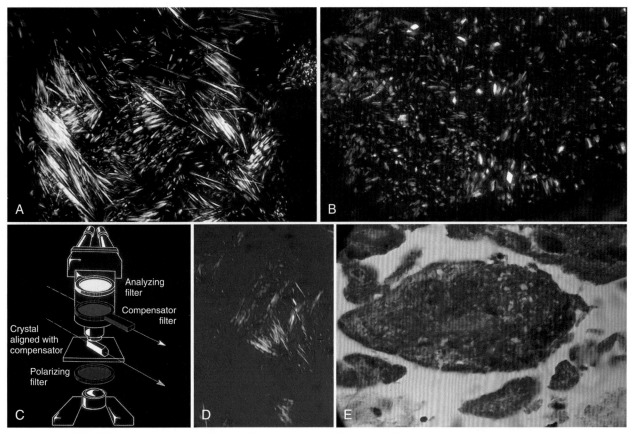

FIG 71.1 Gout Versus Calcium Pyrophosphate Crystals (A) On polarized light microscopy, sodium urate crystals appear needle shaped and brilliantly refractive. (B) Calcium pyrophosphate crystals are less refractile, and crystals are rhomboid in shape. (C) On polarized light microscopy with a red compensator filter, gout (urate) crystals (D) appear yellow when oriented parallel to the axis of compensation and blue when perpendicular (negatively birefringent). (E) Conversely, CPPD crystals appear blue when parallel to the axis of compensation and yellow when perpendicular (positively birefringent). (From Vigorita VJ: The synovium. In Vigorita VJ: *Orthopedic pathology*, Philadelphia, 1999, Lippincott Williams & Wilkins, pp 516–576.)

In addition to synovial fluid analysis, laboratory evaluation should also include assessment of inflammatory markers (eg, erythrocyte sedimentation rate, C-reactive protein [CRP]), renal function (to identify possible and perhaps remediable risk factors for hyperuricemia), and serum uric acid concentration. However, checking the serum uric acid concentration is not as straightforward as it might seem. Because serum uric acid concentration can actually drop during an acute gouty attack, serum urate measured during that period may sometimes be normal or even low, leading the clinician to incorrectly rule out gouty arthritis. Serum urate should therefore be rechecked 2 or 3 weeks until after an attack has subsided, to assess the true baseline level. Plain radiographs are not particularly useful for gout diagnosis early in the course of disease but may be invaluable for ruling out alternative diagnoses. More advanced imaging modalities might be considered in cases in which the diagnosis is unclear (eg, visualizing the double-contour sign on ultrasound may be diagnostic[17]).

Chronic Gout. Patients whose gout has persisted for many years, typically with excessive hyperuricemia and multiple episodic acute attacks annually, may proceed to a more chronic phase characterized not only by continued episodic attacks but also by a persistent, smoldering inflammatory arthritis in the affected joints. In addition, such individuals may go on to develop tophi (Latin for porous stones)—the deposition of crystal aggregates, often large and surrounded by a corona of inflammatory cells. These tophi are most visible in soft tissue areas, such as the olecranon bursa, but may be present in almost any tissue (Fig. 71.2). In the bone and cartilage they may invade and contribute to joint destruction. On plain x-ray, patients with chronic tophaceous gout may have typical erosive changes, particularly of the feet and hands (see Table 71.1). These distinctive erosive changes appear as punched-out lesions, with overhanging edges of bony cortex, and are diagnostic.

Diagnosing Gout. Diagnosing gout can be straightforward, but a few caveats deserve mention. Although an acute gouty attack involving the first MTP joint is typically enough to merit its own name, podagra, acute gouty arthritis can present in a multitude of ways. Even initial attacks can instead occur in the ankles, knees, olecranon bursae, hands, or soft tissue of the feet—almost anywhere—and can be monoarticular or polyarticular. Polyarticular gout attacks become more common as the disease progresses. As noted earlier, women rarely develop the disease until several years after menopause and less typically experience podagra. In contrast to men, women may more commonly experience initial and/or subsequent attacks in the upper extremities and in particular in small joints affected by osteoarthritis, possibly because urate crystals have a predilection to deposit in previously damaged joints.[6] Older women with gout not uncommonly develop tophaceous deposits in osteoarthritic nodes in their distal and proximal interphalangeal (DIP and PIP, respectively) joints, and an examiner should look for chalky white subcutaneous deposits in these joints (as well as the finger pads) in this patient population.

Because some patients with gout do not present to a physician until late in the disease course or have been misdiagnosed with another condition, patients should always be examined for subcutaneous tophi, even on the first visit. Common areas for examination include the olecranon processes, Achilles tendons, and the interphalangeal joints in the fingers and toes.

Because active gouty arthritis can occur concurrently with septic arthritis, appropriate diagnostic and therapeutic measures are necessary if the clinical picture is compatible with infectious arthritis, even in a patient with an established diagnosis of gouty arthropathy.

Treating Gout. In treating gout, one must consider three separate aspects of addressing the disease: (1) treating acute gouty attacks, (2) prophylaxis of future attacks, and (3) addressing the underlying cause of gout (ie, treating the hyperuricemia).

Treating acute gouty arthropathy. A patient presenting with an acute gouty attack can be treated in a number of ways, all of which are directed at reducing inflammation. These include short courses of (1) a nonsteroidal anti-inflammatory drug (NSAID), (2) colchicine, or (3) systemic oral or intramuscular glucocorticoid.[11]

NSAIDs are anti-inflammatory and have the added benefit of providing analgesia. However, they have multiple potential side effects that may preclude their use in a large swath of the gout population, who commonly have multiple comorbidities.[9] Contraindications to NSAIDs include concomitant warfarin therapy, renal insufficiency, congestive heart failure, and a

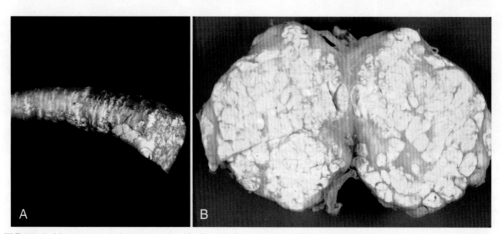

FIG 71.2 Urate crystals seen grossly involving the Achilles tendon (A) and synovium (B) The chalk white deposits have a pastelike consistency. (From Vigorita VJ: The synovium. In Vigorita VJ: *Orthopedic pathology,* Philadelphia, 1999, Lippincott Williams & Wilkins, pp 516–576.)

history of upper gastrointestinal (GI) bleeding. Relative contraindications include age older than 65 years, history of lower GI bleed, chronic liver disease, hypertension, aspirin use, and coronary artery disease. Short courses of NSAIDs in healthy younger patients without comorbidities tend to be well tolerated and should be administered at the highest approved dose. Although indomethacin is the historically preferred NSAID for treating gout, its superiority to other NSAIDs has been repeatedly questioned, whereas its relatively high potential for side effects (eg, GI bleeding, nephrotoxicity, hepatotoxicity, central nervous system [CNS] symptoms) is well established. Consideration should therefore be given to using other NSAIDs with fewer toxicities, selected according to the individual profile of the patient.

Colchicine, derived from the autumn crocus, was previously the drug of choice for acute attacks. The use of one or two doses may abort an attack in patients sensing very early symptoms. Based on safety and efficacy studies the approved colchicine dose for most patients with acute gout is 1.2 mg orally (PO) initially, followed by 0.6 mg PO 1 hour later.[21] However, colchicine is not the ideal choice for abrogating an established gout attack, and the American College of Rheumatology recommends colchicine for acute gout only within the first 36 hours after onset.[11] The US Food and Drug Administration (FDA) banned IV colchicine in 2008 because of its narrow therapeutic range and potential for severe toxicity (eg, severe bone marrow suppression, sloughing of the GI lining, death).

Glucocorticoids can rapidly and effectively resolve acute gout attacks and may be administered as a short course of an oral agent (eg, prednisone at 0.5 mg/kg for several days or a Medrol dose pack) or as a single intramuscular methylprednisolone acetate (Depo-Medrol) injection, often followed by a brief course of low dose of daily prednisone. Polyarticular or well-established attacks may require higher dosing or prolonged treatment, generally 3 weeks or less, depending on the severity of the attack and the underlying disease. Systemic glucocorticoids may be a good option for patients with chronic kidney disease but should generally be avoided in diabetics. Patients with monoarticular gout may be most easily and effectively managed with a single intra-articular steroid injection, which concentrates the medication in the joint and may help to avoid systemic side effects. However, intra-articular steroid injections should be given only after drainage of joint fluid and confirmation that the joint is not infected. Intra-articular injection may not be appropriate for patients with a polyarticular presentation, soft tissue involvement, involvement of joints not amenable to injection (eg, DIP joint), in those who decline an intra-articular injection, or when technical expertise is lacking.

When the previously mentioned treatments are contraindicated or prove inadequate, newer but more expensive therapeutic approaches may be tried. Anti-interleukin (IL)-1 therapy with anakinra or canakinumab has proven effective.[14,18] Adrenocorticotropic hormone (ACTH) intramuscular injections (Acthar gel) both promote adrenal glucocorticoid production and act to block inflammation by engaging melanocortin stimulating hormone 3 receptors and may be particularly useful in hospitalized patients who cannot take oral therapy.

Urate lowering: addressing the root of the problem. After the acute attack has been properly treated, most gout patients should be considered for urate-lowering therapy. Urate lowering not only reduces or abrogates the risk of attacks but also prevents future urate tissue damage and may help to reduce the comorbidities associated with gout, including renal and cardiovascular disease. Patients with two or more gout attacks annually or with one attack in the setting of tophi, kidney stones, or any chronic kidney disease should all be considered for urate lowering.[10] There are currently three pharmacologic approaches for lowering the serum urate level: blocking urate production by inhibiting the urate-producing enzyme xanthine oxidase (allopurinol and febuxostat); increasing renal urate excretion (probenecid and other agents); and metabolism of urate to soluble allonatoin (pegloticase). In almost all cases monotherapy with a xanthine oxidase inhibitor should be used first.[10]

Allopurinol is a purine analogue that lowers urate levels by inhibiting xanthine oxidase, thus blocking the conversion of hypoxanthine to xanthine and of xanthine to uric acid. Allopurinol use is convenient for both physicians and patients. It is most commonly used once or (at higher doses) twice daily and is effective for both underexcreters and overproducers. Dosing of allopurinol should be titrated to achieve a target serum urate level, usually defined as less than 6.0 mg/dL in patients without tophi and less than 5.0 mg/dL in patients with tophi. Dosing should begin at 100 mg daily (50 mg for patients with stage 4 to 5 kidney disease) but may go as high as 800 mg daily for some resistant patients (including those with kidney disease). Primary care physicians may wish to consider referral to a rheumatologist if such high doses are needed. During allopurinol titration, we recommend checking urate levels frequently (every 2 to 4 weeks) and adjusting the allopurinol dose by 100 mg after each assessment. Although generally well tolerated, allopurinol nonetheless carries a less than 1% risk of causing a hypersensitivity syndrome characterized by a morbilliform rash, fever, eosinophilia, and more rarely bone marrow and renal failure (formerly known as allopurinol hypersensitivity syndrome, it now falls under a more general term, DRESS syndrome, for drug rash with eosinophilia and systemic symptoms).[2] Risk factors for allopurinol hypersensitivity include chronic kidney disease and diuretic use (particularly in combination). If allopurinol is not discontinued in patients with hypersensitivity, the syndrome may carry as high as a 50% mortality risk. Physicians should therefore warn patients about the symptoms of hypersensitivity when initiating allopurinol therapy; should a rash or other symptoms occur, the patient must discontinue the drug at once and seek medical advice. Asian and African-American patients should be tested for the presence of HLA B*5801, which conveys a markedly increased risk for allopurinol hypersensitivity.

Febuxostat, a xanthine oxidase inhibitor that is not a purine analogue, received FDA approval for treating gout in 2009. Two daily dosage forms are available, 40 and 80 mg. In head-to-head trials with allopurinol, 40 mg of febuxostat was as effective, and 80 mg was more effective at urate lowering than allopurinol 300 mg daily.[1] Although there have been reports of febuxostat hypersensitivity, it appears to occur much less commonly than for allopurinol. Importantly, febuxostat use rarely if ever results in cross-reactivity with allopurinol hypersensitivity,[3] and febuxostat therefore represents a treatment option for individuals who cannot tolerate allopurinol.

Probenecid inhibits the urate transporter-1 (URAT1) in the proximal renal tubule, resulting in decreased urate resorption. Although safe and effective in the right setting, the drug is uncommonly used for first line therapy because it requires intact renal function (estimated glomerular filtration rate [eGFR] greater than 50 mL/min), twice-daily dosing, and adequate hydration (and possibly urine alkalinization) to prevent formation of renal urate stones. Moreover, probenecid is of limited effectiveness in individuals whose hyperuricemia is caused by urate overproduction (as opposed to renal tubular defects leading to uric acid underexcretion), so prior to initiating probenecid, a 24-hour urine collection should be performed to confirm uric acid underexcretion. If the 24-hour uric acid excretion is greater than 800 mg, probenecid will likely be ineffective and should be avoided. Lesinurad, a highly potent URAT-1 inhibitor intended for use in conjunction with a xanthine oxidase inhibitor and can work even in the presence of kidney disease, was recently approved by the FDA. In patients with a partial response to a xanthine oxidase inhibitor, the addition of probenecid (or losartan or fenofibrate, which also promote uric acid excretion) may also provide additional benefit.

The third and newest way of treating gout is by intravenous infusion of pegloticase, a recombinant pegylated uricase. Pegloticase directly converts uric acid into allantoin and brings serum uric acid down to almost 0 mg/dL shortly after the first infusion. However, approximately 60% of patients develop resistance to the drug within 1 month, because of antipegloticase antibody formation.[19] In addition, pegloticase is expensive, requires infusions every 2 weeks, and causes a high rate of "mobilization flares" (see later). For these reasons it should be reserved for patients with severe and/or refractory gout (usually but not always patients with tophaceous disease) after failure or intolerance of other appropriate agents.

Prophylaxis of attacks. One consequence of lowering the serum urate level is a transient period of increased risk for gouty attacks, thought to result from the liberation of proinflammatory urate crystals during the dissolution of urate deposits. Accordingly, any urate-lowering drug should be co-administered with colchicine or another anti-inflammatory prophylactic agent. Barring any contraindications, colchicine or other anti-inflammatory drug should be continued for at least 6 to 12 months after the target serum urate is achieved.[23]

Although colchicine is not always the favored drug for managing acute gout, it remains the anti-inflammatory treatment of choice for the prevention of gouty attacks. The standard dose of colchicine for prophylaxis is 0.6 mg once or twice daily. Although once-daily dosing is usually sufficient, twice-daily dosing may be required (although GI side effects—principally diarrhea—may occur with the higher dose). Colchicine dosing must be renally adjusted and for patients with an eGFR of 30 to 50 mL/min the dose should be 0.6 mg daily. Patients with an eGFR between 10 and 30 mL/min should receive alternate-day dosing, and those with an eGFR lower than 10 mL/min should not receive colchicine. Those who are intolerant of colchicine or who experience recurrent gouty attacks despite its use may be considered for prophylaxis with a daily low-dose NSAID (eg, naproxen 250 mg bid) or low-dose prednisone, although these strategies are less well studied.

Pseudogout

The clinical presentation of pseudogout, also known as calcium pyrophosphate dehydrate (CPPD) deposition disease, is similar to acute gout; attacks are highly inflammatory (although often less inflammatory than gout), occur acutely, and may be mono-articular or polyarticular.[7] In contrast to gout, attacks most commonly occur in the knee, followed by the wrist. The results of laboratory studies are often similar to those seen in gout and/or joint infection, with elevated erythrocyte sedimentation rate, CRP level, and peripheral blood white cell count. In contrast to gout, which is a systemic disease characterized by elevated serum urate levels, pseudogout is almost invariably a local disease that results from local production of calcium pyrophosphate in a joint with abnormally functioning cartilage (eg, pseudogout is not uncommonly seen in joints affected by osteoarthritis). X-rays of an affected joint often demonstrate chondrocalcinosis, the hallmark of CPPD deposition, appearing as a thin white line running parallel to and just beneath the surface of the cartilage (Fig. 71.3). However, calcium pyrophosphate crystals may appear and pseudogout attacks may occur in the absence of radiographic chondrocalcinosis. Conversely, radiographic chondrocalcinosis may be incidentally observed in asymptomatic patients.

As with gout, definitive diagnosis of pseudogout is made via crystal identification under polarizing microscopy (see Fig. 71.1). In contrast to uric acid, calcium pyrophosphate crystals are positively birefringent and most typically rhomboid-shaped (see Table 71.1). Pyrophosphate crystals are smaller, paler, and more difficult to appreciate than urate crystals and are therefore easily missed. Cell counts from joint fluid are inflammatory, although often less inflammatory than in gout, with neutrophil

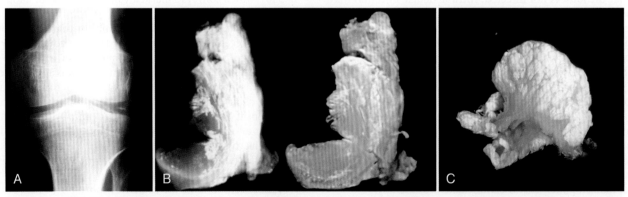

FIG 71.3 Calcium Pyrophosphate Deposition (A) Specimen x-ray film indicating linear calcium deposition in the cartilage. (B) Specimen x-ray film and gross anatomy of dissected meniscus with calcium pyrophosphate deposition. (C) Synovial involvement. (From Vigorita VJ: The synovium. In Vigorita VJ: *Orthopedic pathology*, Philadelphia, 1999, Lippincott Williams & Wilkins, pp 516–576.)

predominance. As in gout the presence of intracellular crystals unequivocally confirms that an inflammatory attack is crystal driven. Also as in gout, pseudogout and infection may occasionally coexist, so vigilance is warranted.

The therapy for acute pseudogout is similar to that for acute gout.[16] NSAIDs and intramuscular, oral, or intra-articular glucocorticoids are effective. Colchicine, 1.2 mg followed by 0.6 mg 1 hour later, may also be tried. Long-term management of calcium pyrophosphate deposition can be difficult because no known therapies regulate the deposition of the calcium pyrophosphate crystals. Low-dose colchicine may be used prophylactically in patients who experience frequent attacks, and NSAIDs may also afford prophylaxis in patients with coexistent osteoarthritis. A small number of patients with pseudogout may have underlying metabolic conditions that promote CPPD deposition (eg, hypomagnesemia, hypothyroidism, hyperparathyroidism, hemochromatosis). These should be addressed, although it is unclear that such treatment ameliorates the risk of ongoing crystal arthritis.

Other Crystal Deposition Diseases

A number of other crystal diseases may occur more rarely and more sporadically than gout or pseudogout. The most common of these is basic calcium phosphate (BCP) deposition. The calcium crystals in BCP disease may take several chemical forms; perhaps most common is the deposition of hydroxyapatite.[7] BCP deposition is seen most typically in older individuals; women may be more commonly affected. Characteristically, BCP disease presents as an acute periarthritis or peritendinitis; x-rays of the affected region may reveal calcium deposition within the tendons or capsular structures. BCP disease can also affect the joint itself. Shoulder involvement (Milwaukee shoulder) is perhaps the most common presentation. Aspiration of the joint characteristically reveals a neutrophilic infiltrate; because the crystals are not birefringent, they are not seen on polarizing microscopy but can be visualized after staining with alizarin red S (a calcium stain) or when viewed under electron microscopy. The condition may resolve spontaneously, persist, or in some cases result in a severe destructive arthropathy. Treatment includes rest and anti-inflammatory agents, including oral or intra-articular steroid injections.

Calcium oxalate crystals may produce arthritis in patients with renal disease, particularly those on dialysis or with familial forms of early onset renal failure. Attacks tend to be acute and resemble those of gout or pseudogout. Examination of joint fluid under polarizing microscopy reveals bipyramid-shaped birefringent crystals. Given the potential toxicities of NSAIDs and colchicine in patients with renal failure, these attacks may be best managed with low-dose oral steroids; some experts express concern about using intra-articular injections because of the risk of infection.

In patients with chronic arthritis, particularly those with long-standing rheumatoid or osteoarthritis, cholesterol crystals may be identified in joints or more typically in the olecranon bursa. These birefringent platelike crystals appear to have limited inflammatory potential and do not require therapy beyond appropriate management of the underlying condition.

KEY REFERENCES

1. Becker MA, Schumacher HR, Jr, Wortmann RL, et al: Febuxostat compared with allopurinol in patients with hyperuricemia and gout. *N Engl J Med* 353:2450–2461, 2005.

4. Choi HK, Curhan G: Gout: epidemiology and lifestyle choices. *Curr Opin Rheumatol* 17:341–345, 2005.

9. Keenan RT, O'Brien WR, Lee KH, et al: Prevalence of contraindications and prescription of pharmacologic therapies for gout. *Am J Med* 124:155–163, 2011.

10. Khanna D, Fitzgerald JD, Khanna PP, et al: 2012 American College of Rheumatology guidelines for management of gout. Part 1: systematic nonpharmacologic and pharmacologic therapeutic approaches to hyperuricemia. *Arthritis Care Res (Hoboken)* 64:1431–1446, 2012.

11. Khanna D, Khanna PP, Fitzgerald JD, et al: 2012 American College of Rheumatology guidelines for management of gout. Part 2: therapy and antiinflammatory prophylaxis of acute gouty arthritis. *Arthritis Care Res (Hoboken)* 64:1447–1461, 2012.

13. Krishnan E: Reduced glomerular function and prevalence of gout: NHANES 2009-10. *PLoS ONE* 7:e50046, 2012.

17. Sivera F, Andrés M, Falzon L, et al: Diagnostic value of clinical, laboratory, and imaging findings in patients with a clinical suspicion of gout: a systematic literature review. *J Rheumatol Suppl* 92:3–8, 2014.

21. Terkeltaub RA, Furst DE, Bennett K, et al: High versus low dosing of oral colchicine for early acute gout flare: twenty-four-hour outcome of the first multicenter, randomized, double-blind, placebo-controlled, parallel-group, dose-comparison colchicine study. *Arthritis Rheum* 62:1060–1068, 2010.

23. Wortmann RL, Macdonald PA, Hunt B, et al: Effect of prophylaxis on gout flares after the initiation of urate-lowering therapy: analysis of data from three phase III trials. *Clin Ther* 32:2386–2397, 2010.

24. Zhu Y, Pandya BJ, Choi HK: Prevalence of gout and hyperuricemia in the US general population: the National Health and Nutrition Examination Survey 2007–2008. *Arthritis Rheum* 63:3136–3141, 2011.

The references for this chapter can also be found on www.expertconsult.com.

72

Knee Osteoarthritis

Pamela B. Rosenthal

INTRODUCTION

Osteoarthritis (OA) is the leading cause of musculoskeletal disability worldwide. The incidence and prevalence of OA increase with aging. For several decades OA has been recognized as a major public health concern. In 1996 the estimate was that 9.6% of men and 18% of women ≥60 years of age suffered from symptomatic OA worldwide.[53] Although OA is more prevalent in the developed than the developing regions of the world,[7,62] in 2004 OA made the World Health Organization's top 10 causes of years lost to disability for both low- and middle-income countries, as well as high-income countries.[60] In the United States estimates include that 85% of the population ≥75 years old are afflicted.[20] OA of the knee represents an important subset of the overall OA burden and is the leading cause of functional disability. A European study estimated that the prevalence of radiographic knee OA is 13% for women and 8% for men between the ages of 45 and 49, rising to 55% and 22%, respectively, for persons 80 years of age and older.[58] These data were corroborated by a groundbreaking study in Johnston County, NC, which concluded that the lifetime risk of symptomatic knee OA was 44.7%.[36] In the United States in 2004 the hospital and associated costs of total knee replacement was estimated to be $14.3 billion dollars, representing costs associated with approximately 450,000 surgeries.[52] The number of total knee replacements has climbed since. The Centers for Disease Control and Prevention (CDC) estimates that there were 719,000 total knee replacements in 2010.[22]

OA presents with a complaint of pain and swelling resulting in decreased joint mobility. Traditionally, diagnostic criteria include characteristic radiologic changes inclusive of joint space narrowing and associated bone changes. The diarthrodial joint is a complex organ composed of a variety of tissue and cell types, all of which are modified in the setting of active OA.

Hominid knees have evolved in response to the constraints and requirements of a bipedal gait. Our earlier hominid ancestors were arboreal. Obligate hominid bipedalism evolved approximately 4 million years ago, with resultant skeletal changes to accommodate the increased demands of weight bearing across two rather than four limbs. The vertebral column assumed its characteristic curve, and the pelvis evolved a dorsal projection, resulting in the placement of our center of mass above our hips and allows for the translation of force through our knees and feet.[59] There are many intriguing theories as to the evolutionary selection pressures that resulted in this transformative stance and gait, including the secondary benefits of an upright head and the advantages of liberated upper extremities, but intriguingly the elongated lower limb and upright posture allows for an energetically more efficient gait than a quadruped gait.[48] Although OA is a general cost of a vertebral skeleton, the vulnerability of our lower lumbar spine, hips, and knee to OA processes maybe a consequence of the unique mechanical forces associated with a bipedal gait.

The knee is the largest joint in the body. The knee is routinely subjected to forces that are three to five times body weight during normal gait. The added weight bearing and stability requirements of the human knee resulted in expanded femoral and tibial condyles relative to the knees of other vertebrates. In addition, the human patellar is notable for its large size and concomitant role in knee stabilization. In addition, the menisci of human knees are much larger than that of other vertebrates.[23]

Lessons From Epidemiology and the Role of Joint Stress

OA is conceived of as a process that is initiated and perpetuated by mechanical stress. Normal healthy joints are defined by their near frictionless excursion and physiologic loading, as maintained and limited by constraints on the joints' range of motion. Increased mechanical stress resulting from traumatic ligamentous and cartilage injuries, as well as the increased mechanical forces associated with obesity, are prominent risk factors for the development of knee OA. In addition, there is an evolving interest in the role of gait variance as an OA risk factor, yet OA is a tissue-based process. The mechanical forces that result in OA are translated into biochemical and cellular perturbation that manifest as and are a consequence of focal loading defects.

As with all disease, OA is a consequence of the interplay between host and environmental factors. Lifestyle and lifecycle events influence the natural history of OA. OA is described as primary (idiopathic) or secondary and localized or generalized. OA that is associated with trauma, congenital defects, inflammatory arthritis, neuropathic, or metabolic disease is conceived of as secondary.[45] Knee OA can present in isolation or associated with polyarticular OA, especially OA of the hands.[24]

Aging, female sex, and underlying predisposing risk genes are invariant risk factors associated with increase incidence of knee OA. By contrast, obesity and trauma are life experience variables that correlate with knee OA incidence and progression. In all cases knee OA can be conceived as resulting from excessive joint loading resulting from perturbations of joint biomechanics that initiates a microinflammatory process, which in turn results in a loss of joint homeostasis.

Explanations for the increased incidence and prevalence of OA with aging include factors attributable to events earlier in life and special circumstances of aging. For example, radiographic knee OA may present in old age, but the events that initiated the

OA may have occurred years earlier. The natural history of OA is such that it likely takes years to manifest as radiographic damage. Even after OA is established radiographically, detectable cartilage volume loss by x-ray may be as little as less than 2% per year.[26] Muscle strength, reaction time, and proprioception are all factors implicated in joint stability and health and are all impaired with aging. As a consequence, aging is characterized by an increased inclination to injury. The risk of OA in aging is magnified by a decreased capacity for cellular repair. These two characteristics of the aging process alone may contribute to increased risk of knee OA incidence and progression,[45] although microscopic changes of aging are also likely to play a role.

The predilection of women's joints to OA is less well understood. In the Framingham cohort, women developed symptomatic radiographic OA at a rate of 1% per year as compared with 0.7% per year for men. At baseline, the women in this cohort had a mean age of 71. Estrogens are presumed to be protective, and in the postmenopausal state their relative deficiency may correlate with accelerated cartilage loss. However, there is no clear consensus with respect to the role of estrogen biology as pertains to the risk of incidence or progression of OA. The reported increased risk may instead correlate with other genetic and phenotypic variables. A Dutch study reported the protective effect of an allelic variation of one of the bone morphogenic proteins, growth differentiation factor 5 (GDF5), on the incidence of hand and knee OA in women, but intriguingly not in men, suggesting that as of yet unidentified biochemical variables may influence the observed OA gender dimorphism.[54,57] Equally, well-documented differences between men and women, such as longer life expectancy, more relative adiposity, less muscle mass, increased ligamentous laxity, decreased joint stability, and increased propensity to obesity in women may influence the increased risk of OA in women.

Furthermore, the experience of knee pain from OA may also be a sexually dimorphic trait. Women are known to have a greater propensity to central pain sensitization. Reports suggest that women with knee OA pain also have increased central pain sensitization. The relationship of increased central pain sensitivity to the pathogenesis of OA is uncertain.[4,16]

The obesity epidemic has wide-ranging implications for public health. An earlier analysis reported that if current obesity trends continue the deleterious effects of weight gain on life expectancy will shortly outweigh the positive impact on life expectancy of decreased rates of smoking.[50] Obesity rates vary by ethnicity, geography, age, and socioeconomic status in the United States. Non-Hispanic black individuals have the highest age-adjusted rates of obesity (47.8%), followed by Hispanic (42.5%), non-Hispanic white (32.6%), and non-Hispanic Asian (10.8%) populations. The highest obesity rates continue to be among middle-aged adults (40 to 59 years old) at 39.5%, followed closely by a prevalence rate of 35.4% among adults over 65 years old. Young adults have an obesity prevalence rate 30.3%, followed by a childhood obesity prevalence of 17%. Over the past decade these rates have stabilized, yet there is ongoing concern that by 2030 the overall population rate of obesity could be as high as 42% and extreme obesity (body mass index [BMI] >40) as high as 11%.[14,37]

Obesity has a profound impact on joint health. The incidence of knee OA across all population studies is highly correlated with BMI. The initial observations of the Framingham Study correlating knee OA with obesity continue to be substantiated.[11] The Johnston County, NC, cohort study concluded that lifetime

risk of knee OA for obese (BMI ≥30) persons is 60.5% versus 46.9% for the overweight (BMI 25 to <30) and 30.2% for those with a BMI less than 25.[36] There is likely an influence of childhood obesity on lifetime OA risk. Several studies have demonstrated a correlation between increased BMI early in life and the development of subsequent knee OA.[15] However, the Johnston Country cohort found that obesity at the baseline and follow-up visits more strongly correlates with lifetime OA risk than BMI at 18 years of age. Equally, although obesity is clearly and strongly correlated with risk for OA, several studies have suggested that obesity does not necessarily correlate with OA progression. In a study of 60 obese and 81 nonobese women followed by x-ray over 12 months, the obese women demonstrated greater initial radiographic OA severity, whereas their joint space widths did not diminish.[31] Another study found a correlation between radiographic progression and obesity for patients with a neutral or valgus alignment but not a varus alignment, lending further insight into the complexity of the relationship between obesity and knee OA progression.[9] Furthermore, the biomechanics of fat distribution likely influences knee joint loads. Messier et al. reported that thigh fat, despite its smaller volume, had the same impact on knee joint forces as larger-volume abdominal fat in older adults.[34]

Obesity in combination with cardiovascular risk factors may enrich a patient's risk for knee OA. In an intriguing analysis Sowers et al. evaluated 482 women (mean age of 47) with knee films and evaluated patients for evidence of diabetes mellitus and/or dyslipidemia and hypertension, with the result that the obese patients with cardiometabolic clustering had a knee OA prevalence of 23.2% versus the obese women without the cardiometabolic clustering who had a knee OA prevalence of 12.8%. In addition, the women with the cardiometabolic syndrome reported more knee pain than the women without the cardiometabolic syndrome. These data point to the influence of metabolic factors on joint health.[49] It was reported in data from the Framingham Heart Study that symptomatic hand OA but not radiographic hand OA without pain was associated with increased coronary heart disease events.[21] Conversely, it is well understood that knee pain from knee OA limits activity, which in turn contributes to risk of metabolic syndrome, suggesting that the relationship between OA and metabolic syndrome may at times be bidirectional.[33]

The medial and lateral compartments of the tibiofemoral knee joint do not load bear equally. In a neutrally aligned knee the medial compartment bears 60% to 70% of the force across the knee in weight-bearing activities. Therefore, not surprising, the medial compartment of the knee is disproportionately afflicted with OA, with medial OA representing up to 75% of the disease burden. Equally patellofemoral OA is also disproportionately medial.[27]

By extension knee malalignment is the single biggest risk factor for OA disease progression. Varus-valgus malalignment correlates with OA progression, in isolation and/or synergy with other risk factors. Varus malalignment increases the predisposition to OA disease progression by upwards of fourfold and valgus malalignment by as much as fivefold in some studies.[44] Intriguingly the data on the role of malalignment as a risk factor for initiation of disease are not as consistent as they are for progression. Traditionally, mechanical knee malalignment is assessed with static limb x-rays. Mechanical axis and dynamic adduction moment are highly correlated. Yet forces across the joint during the dynamic phase of gait may have an even more powerful effect on disease progression than the effect of malalignment measured during a static stance. During normal gait the adduction moment is approximately 3.3% of body weight × height, compared with 4.2% body weight × height in patients with medial knee OA.[42] The degree of joint space loss has been shown to correlate with the degree of adduction moment. Persons with more adduction moment lost joint space faster.[35]

Static knee alignment is determined by a variety of biomechanical factors. Tibiofemoral congruence, integrity of the anterior cruciate ligament and meniscal integrity, and supporting muscular strength all influence joint alignment.[27] Torn anterior cruciate ligament (ACL) and damaged and extruding menisci have long been known to be associated with the progression of knee OA. Standard of care for debilitating knee pain used to include total meniscectomy, until the insight that surgical meniscal resection correlated with accelerated OA. Menisci tear both as a consequence of trauma (a very common athletic injury) and secondary to degenerative change. The advent of magnetic resonance imaging (MRI) scanning as an OA investigational tool allowed for the prospective examination of 121 case and 294 control knees over a 30-month period as part of the Observational Multicenter Osteoarthritis Study. The age of the patients ranged from 50 to 79 years, and all were selected to be at high risk for OA because they were overweight, had persistent knee pain, or had a history of knee trauma. The patients were followed in two cohorts, one with incident OA and the other as controls. Meniscal damage at baseline was more frequent in the knees with progressive joint space loss, as a marker of cartilage degeneration, than in the radiologically stable knees (54% versus 18%; $p < 0.001$). Intriguingly there was a dose effect of meniscal damage, with more severe baseline meniscal disease correlating with increased progressive radiologic OA. Not surprisingly the 30-month MRIs captured new meniscal tears in both the OA and non-OA cohort, although more in the OA than non-OA group. Taken together these data demonstrate the pivotal role that meniscal integrity plays in knee health but also raises compelling questions about the pathoetiologic role of meniscal deformities. Do they initiate or propagate OA? No doubt their role is complex; meniscal injuries at once result in and signifying the biomechanical derangement and modification of associated joint structures.[9]

Lessons From Radiology

Adapting to changing load is a requirement of a healthy joint. Each tissue and cell type contributes. OA results when the capacity to adapt is exceeded, resulting in structure modifications that result in characteristic tissue change. Insights provided by MRI studies of knee OA have expanded our understanding of the pathophysiology. Historically, OA was thought of as a primary condition of articular hyaline cartilage. It is currently appreciated that all joint tissues are concurrently involved (cartilage, synovium, and bone together) and that tissue inflammation and inflammatory pathways play a prominent role in OA pathophysiology. Enthesitis, synovitis, and bone marrow lesions, as well as cartilage loss, are all lesions of evolving interest in OA. In particular there is evolving evidence that synovitis and bone marrow lesions correlate both with joint pain and OA initiation and progression.[41]

Bone is the defining characteristic of skeletal anatomy. Bone is at once brittle and resilient. It is characterized by its ability to respond to mechanical stress with upregulation of

bone formation with osteoblast activation and resorption with osteoclast activation, allowing for the dynamic response of the skeleton to environmental forces. This homeostatic remodeling process is perturbed in OA, resulting in characteristic subchondral sclerosis and subchondral plate thickening. In several studies these changes have preceded cartilage volume loss.[6]

The subchondral bone is the interface between the overlying articular cartilage and underlying cortical and trabecular bone. Although the volume of trabecular bone may also increase in OA, paradoxically, perhaps in response to altered mineralization kinetics, the stiffness of this new bone may actually decrease.[17]

Bone marrow lesions first came to the attention of investigators more than 20 years ago and were originally described as bone marrow edema.[61] Almost a decade ago the correlation between bone marrow lesions and OA progression and pain was first identified.[13] More recently 70% of patients with bone marrow lesions were found to have pseudocysts on histopathologic examination of surgical specimens.[51] These lesions corresponded to the areas of most severe damage in the overlying cartilage and likely correlate with areas of focal bone necrosis.

Bone marrow lesions are of interest not only because of their pathophysiologic significance but also because they correlate with knee pain. In a 2001 study Felson et al. showed that 37% of patients with documented x-ray OA and knee pain had bone marrow lesions versus only 2% of patients with x-ray OA but without knee pain ($p < 0.001$).[12]

Osteophytes are a pathognomonic radiologic finding of OA. They are also known to precede joint space narrowing and cartilage degradation. It has been suggested that they may be a compensatory response to ligamentous injury or laxity. Anterior and posterior osteophytes form in response to anterior cruciate ligament (ACL) tears and limit tibiofemoral excursion.[55] As such, although conceived of as pathogenic, they may contribute to joint stability. They form in areas of active joint loading. They form as a result of endochondral ossification. Initially periosteal cells proliferate then differentiate into chondrocytes, which in turn hypertrophy and ossify.[17]

Synovial hypertrophy is a hallmark of advanced OA and on MRI strongly correlates with knee pain. Synovial lining hypertrophy correlates topographically with areas of underlying cartilage denudation and bone damage. Several prospective MRI studies of OA cohorts have concluded that a decrease in synovitis on MRI correlates with a decrease in pain score. Not surprisingly synovitis is often correlated with joint effusions and joint capsular swelling. The size of a joint effusion itself correlates with the degree of knee pain. The synovium is an extremely bioactive tissue. In addition to the role of synovial-like fibroblasts in the production of synovial fluid, it is also home to various monocytes and macrophages, which when activated assume an inflammatory phenotype. The relevance of inflammation to OA has taken on new importance as the role of synovium in OA has become better appreciated with the advent of newer radiologic techniques.[41]

Lessons From Cell Biology and Genetics

OA is a heterogeneous disorder. Age, trauma, obesity, and gender are all independent risk factors for knee OA. Although they share the common pathway of the disruption of biomechanical joint integrity, the mechanism by which aberrant loading is translated into a biochemical event is less well understood. On a macromolecular level OA cartilage demonstrates fibrillation, fissuring, neovascularization, areas of focal necrosis, and other hallmarks of stress. On a molecular level OA is characterized by the disruption of the extracellular cartilaginous matrix associated with the upregulation of matrix metalloproteinases (MMPs) and proinflammatory and counter-regulatory signaling molecules.

Chondrocytes live in an avascular environment. Presumably the avascular setting is an adaptive constraint to the biomechanical demand placed on cartilage. No doubt the regular shear forces experienced by joints and their shock-buffering cartilage would result in routine vessel shear. Consequently, chondrocytes have a low metabolic rate, yet are responsible for the production of the extremely elaborate and long-lived extracellular matrix. The dominant molecule of the extracellular matrix is type II collagen. The stability of this molecule is marked by its exceptional half-life of 100 years, making it among the few macromolecules that journey with us from cradle to grave.[46] The chondrocyte is also the source of cartilage remodeling and repair. Chondrocytes use the cellular machinery of autophagy to maintain cellular function and homeostasis. When the demands of repair outpace the chondrocytes reparative capacity and autophagy is lost, OA ensues. Impaired chondrocyte mitochondrial function is implicated in loss of autophagy and impaired bioenergetics in OA.[18]

Chondrocytes have the capacity to respond to mechanical stress via integrin and related surface receptors. Many of these receptors also engage type II collagen fragments and glycoprotein fragments. After being activated these receptors can lead to production of MMPs, as well as chemokines and cytokines. MMP-13 is of particular interest in the degradative processes that characterize degradation of type II collagen in OA. The chondrocytes located closer to the cartilage surface assume a more activated catabolic phenotype and deeper in the matrix, closer to the bone margin, assume a more regenerative phenotype, synthesizing more extracellular matrix proteins. In OA the catabolic outpaces the regenerative/anabolic phenotype. The type II collagen fragments themselves feedback to activate the production of more metalloproteinases. Binding of type II collagen fragments bind to the discoidin domain receptor-2 (DDR-2) and upregulate MMP-13.[19]

Collagen provides tensile strength to the cartilage matrix. The matrix proteoglycans and glycoproteins help to stabilize the collagen matrix and contribute to cartilage's biomechanical properties. For example, aggrecan's hydroscopic properties contribute to the compressive strength of cartilage. In addition to collagen degradation by MMPs, the collagen associated glycoproteins and proteoglycans are actively degraded in OA. The increased expression of aggracanase, a specific aggracan proteinase, is a hallmark of OA.[29] Not only are there increased levels of glycoprotein breakdown proteins found in the OA joint tissues themselves, but they are also found in increased levels in the peripheral circulation. Members of the Cartilage oligomeric matrix protein (COMP) family, notably thrombospondin 5, circulate in high levels in OA serum and is associated with both radiographic progression and increased OA associated joint pain.[38] Structurally compromised extracellular matrix perpetuates the OA cycle, in part through the binding of constituent breakdown products to cell surface receptors.

Historically, OA was not considered an inflammatory arthritis because of the dearth of neutrophilic infiltrate and the absence of systemic inflammatory biomarkers. In particular the leukocyte count in osteoarthritic effusions is by definition noninflammatory because it is less than $2000/mm^3$.

Nonetheless, the central role of synovial inflammation is now appreciated as a central driver of the osteoarthritic phenotype, and the term *microinflammatory* is sometimes now applied to describe the OA joint environment. The classic proinflammatory cytokines, better known for their role in erosive inflammatory arthritis, such as rheumatoid arthritis, are also present in OA joint in low but above baseline concentrations. They include tumor necrosis factor (TNF), interleukin (IL)-1β, IL-6, and IL-17. Counter-regulatory cytokines, such as IL-4, Il-10, IL-13, and IL-1Ra, are also present. These cytokines are produced by synovial macrophages. The OA synovial membrane is hypertrophied with an increase in the synovial lining cells and an increase in infiltrating monocytes, including macrophages in the sublining. The chronology and topology of OA synovial hypertrophy and activity evolve in response to biochemical and mechanical signals over the long course of osteoarthritic joint decline. Although the synovial OA phenotype is thought to be initiated by cartilage tissue breakdown products that result from mechanical stress, nonetheless the role of synovitis as an early marker of OA is increasingly appreciated.[43] Work from the OA initiative documents that Hoffa synovitis and effusion synovitis by MRI both predate the presence of plain radiographic knee OA by as much as 2 years.[40]

The role of complement activation in OA is not well appreciated. However, recent work demonstrates that the extracellular matrix proteins fibromodulin, osteoadherin, and lumican can activate the classic complement pathway and that biglycan and decorin can act as counter-regulatory elements and can inhibit complement activation.[47] Activation of the late complement components membrane attack complex likely contributes to OA pathway propagation.

Nitric oxide (NO), traditionally thought of as a proinflammatory mediator, also acts in a counter-regulatory fashion, limiting catabolism. Functional effects of NO may act along a gradient in part contingent on the topographical location of the chondrocyte in the matrix. NO can inhibit the synthesis of proteoglycans and collagens, as well as accelerate their degeneration through the upregulation of MMPs. NO stimulates proinflammatory cytokines and their upstream activating enzymes, such as Interleukin-1 (IL-1) converting enzyme. NO also induces Prostaglandin E2 (PGE2) and Cyclooxygenase-2 (COX-2) synthesis through the activation of nuclear factor kappa-light-chain-enhancer of activated B cells (NFκB). NO can also induce apoptosis. However, NO is part of a complex system of reactive species, including superoxide and its reactive product with NO, peroxynitrite. Peroxynitrite and NO themselves demonstrate discrete functions. Of interest NO in tendons has been demonstrated to increase collagen synthesis, although there may be a dose-dependent response, with moderate amounts of NO yielding increased collagen synthesis, but higher doses resulting in a net collagen loss.[8] Importantly NO and other reactive oxygen species (ROS) are important mediators of pain. Peroxynitrite in particular is known to induce hyperalgesia through the COX-prostaglandin E2 pathway. Taken together these data point to the complex role of NO and its associated ROS in OA.[1]

The Wnt signaling pathway is the central signaling pathway controlling bone morphogenesis. Mechanical loading results in the Wnt signaling through frizzled receptors (LRP5), which leads to the activation of the nuclear transcription factor β-catenin, which results in the increased production of osteoprotegerin (OPG), bone morphogenic proteins (BMPs), osteocalcin, and insulin-like growth factor (IGF). Wnt stimulated osteoblasts are apoptosis resistant. In addition, OPG binds RANK-L, which results in the downregulation of osteoclast activation. Another protein in this system is sclerostin (SOST), which is an inhibitor of Wnt signaling. SOST provides another link between mechanical stimuli and cellular response. Under mechanical loading conditions SOST expression is diminished, hence favoring osteoblast activity.[39] It is presumed that this system plays a role in the pathophysiology of OA. However, the evidence supporting this contention is largely genetic. Frizzled-related proteins, such as sFRP3 and FRZB, are direct antagonists of Wnt, which can lead to osteoblast apoptosis. Polymorphisms in these genes are of interest with respect to contributing to OA risk.[19] Polymorphisms in the FRZB genes have been identified that inhibit MMP induction in mouse chondrocytes by attenuating the activation of the Wnt signaling pathway.[2]

OA is polygenetic. The effect size of any one gene in the contribution to the propensity to OA is small, yet OA runs in families, and twin studies have suggested that genetic factors may contribute as much as 70% of the OA risk. To date, as many as 95 different genes have been proposed to contribute to this risk. Polymorphisms in extracellular matrix component molecules, such as type II and IX collagens and aggrecan, have been proposed, as have polymorphisms in signaling molecules, such as estrogen receptors and the IL-1 gene cluster.[5,19] Insight into the contribution of genes to OA risk is just beginning. More data are awaited from large population Genome-Wide Association Scans.[32] However, a pattern is emerging that confirms what is known epidemiologically, namely that OA at different anatomic sights represents variations on the OA pathway theme. For example, polymorphisms in the *GDF5* gene, a member of the transforming growth factor superfamily, implicated in regulating proteoglycans synthesis, are more strongly correlated with a risk for knee OA than at any other site.[10] As previously mentioned another polymorphism in this gene may reduce the OA risk for women.[54]

Therapy

OA of the knee is a debilitating and complex medical problem. Research into its epidemiology and associated pathophysiology is rapidly advancing with the implicit goal that the research insights will lead to better therapies. Ideally, strategies will be found that can both blunt progressive joint damage and promote healing. Although there are many pipeline compounds based on the biologic insights discussed previously, disease-modifying compounds remain elusive to date. Instead, the 2012 American College of Rheumatology (ACR) recommendations for the treatment of OA are significant for reliance on traditional analgesics and non-pharmacologic interventions. For knee OA the strong recommendations include land-based aerobic and resistance exercise, as well as aquatic exercise and weight loss in the setting of overweight and obese patients. Conditional recommendations include a variety of strategies to improve joint angulation, including medially wedged insoles for valgus knee and medially directed patellar taping, as well as subtalar strapped lateral insoles for varus knees. In addition, self-management program participation, psychosocial intervention, manual therapy in combination with supervised exercise programs, walking aids, and tai chi are all also conditionally recommended. With respect to pharmacologic recommendations, if the patient has no cardiovascular, gastrointestinal, or renal contraindication, topical and/or oral NSAIDs are

conditionally recommended, as are acetaminophen, tramadol, or intra-articular corticosteroids.[25]

Next-generation targeted pain relief is an important goal, with compounds actively under study. That said, the role of pain as potentially joint protective was demonstrated in a clinical trial involving a targeted antinerve growth factor antibody, tanezumab, which controlled knee OA pain but also resulted in excess nontarget joint failures.[30] Although the mechanism of the nontarget joint failures is not fully understood, these compounds continue on clinical hold.[3] Although the promise of targeted OA and pain therapies has yet to realized, there are many innovative strategies in development, stem cell therapy to promote cartilage healing perhaps most intriguing among them.[28]

Conclusion

OA is common to all vertebrates, and we share with all vertebrates this problem as a condition of aging. The biology of aging is itself complex. Senescence and its associated biology are thought to be independent of evolutionary selection pressure. Selective forces are meant to act on maximizing reproductive fitness. Whatever happens to an individual after their peak reproductive period is merely a consequence of the biologic trade-offs and optimizations selected for the benefit of propagating one's genes into the next generation. Historically, the human life span was considerably less than now, approximately 35 years versus our current 78.74 years in the United States in 2012. It is not a coincidence that the prevalence of OA starts to emerge just past the limit of our historical life span, around 40 to 45 years of age. However, as we have seen, the risk factors for OA are diverse and not just aging alone.

Age-related changes in the joint may predispose to the vulnerability to OA, even if the more discrete risk factor might be trauma and/or even obesity. In other words, the effect of aging and abnormal joint loading are likely synergistic. It may be that some of the age-related cartilage changes sensitize the joint to mechanical stimuli. Cartilage may lose its resiliency as a consequence of the aging-related breakdown of aggregan and an age-related increase in type II cartilage cross-links. Aging is also associated with accumulation of glycation end products in articular cartilage, which results in the increased stiffness of the extracellular matrix. The natural history of chondrocytes may itself switch to an aging phenotype, resulting in modification of the signaling pathway thresholds.[56] Human knees may be especially vulnerable to OA as a consequence of our unique bipedal gait.

Regardless of the causality of OA, it needs to be treated. The pain and disability associated with knee arthritis results in substantive disability. The OA research community will continue to investigate causality in an effort to improve therapy and patient outcome.

KEY REFERENCES

7. Cross M, et al: The global burden of hip and knee osteoarthritis: estimates from the Global Burden of Disease 2010 study. *Ann Rheum Dis* 73:1323–1330, 2014.
11. Felson DT, et al: Obesity and knee osteoarthritis. The Framingham Study. *Ann Intern Med* 109(1):18–24, 1988.
12. Felson DT, et al: The association of bone marrow lesions with pain in knee osteoarthritis. *Ann Intern Med* 134(7):541–549, 2001.
13. Felson DT, et al: Bone marrow edema and its relation to progression of knee osteoarthritis. *Ann Intern Med* 139(5 Pt 1):330–336, 2003.

18. Goldring M, Berenbaum F: Emerging targets in osteoarthritis therapy. *Curr Opin Pharmacol* 22:51–63, 2015.

19. Goldring MB, Goldring SR: Osteoarthritis. *J Cell Physiol* 213(3):626–634, 2007.

25. Hochberg M, et al: American College of Rheumatology 2012 recommendations for the use of nonpharmacologic and pharmacologic therapies in osteoarthritis of the hand, hip, and knee. *Arthritis Care Res* 64:465–474, 2012.

26. Hunter DJ, et al: Cartilage markers and their association with cartilage loss on magnetic resonance imaging in knee osteoarthritis: the Boston Osteoarthritis Knee Study. *Arthritis Res Ther* 9(5):R108, 2007.

28. Jiang Y, Tuan R: Origin and function of cartilage stem/progenitor cells in osteoarthritis. *Nat Rev Rheumatol* 11:206–212, 2015.

40. Roemer F, et al: What comes first? Multitissue involvement leading to radiographic osteoarthritis: magnetic resonance imaging–based trajectory analysis over four years in the osteoarthritis initiative. *Arthritis Rheumatol* 67:2085–2096, 2015.

43. Sellam J, Berenbaum F: The role of synovitis in pathophysiology and clinical symptoms of osteoarthritis. *Nat Rev Rheumatol* 6:625–635, 2010.

48. Sockol MD, Raichlen DA, Pontzer H: Chimpanzee locomotor energetics and the origin of human bipedalism. *Proc Natl Acad Sci USA* 104(30):12265–12269, 2007.

58. van Saase JL, et al: Epidemiology of osteoarthritis: Zoetermeer survey. Comparison of radiological osteoarthritis in a Dutch population with that in 10 other populations. *Ann Rheum Dis* 48(4):271–280, 1989.

59. Whitcome KK, Shapiro LJ, Lieberman DE: Fetal load and the evolution of lumbar lordosis in bipedal hominins. *Nature* 450(7172):1075–1078, 2007.

The references for this chapter can also be found on www.expertconsult.com.

73

Overview of Psoriatic Arthritis

Gary E. Solomon

Psoriatic arthritis (PsA) is a chronic inflammatory disorder with clinical features that overlap with those of rheumatoid arthritis (RA). There are, however, important differences in pathophysiology and clinical course, which has implications for the medical and surgical management of patients with this disorder. This chapter will review the epidemiology, genetics, pathophysiology, and immunopathogenesis of PsA in an effort to provide the orthopedist treating a patient with this disorder a firm understanding of unique treatment issues.

GENERAL CONSIDERATIONS

PsA is defined as arthritis, spondylitis, or dactylitis occurring in association with the skin disease psoriasis (PsO). The recent Classification Criteria for Psoriatic Arthritis (CASPAR) criteria for PsA (Box 73.1) dramatically explain the spectrum of this disorder by allowing the inclusion of patients who do not currently have PsO, but have a past history of PsO or a family history of PsO.[10] The criteria also recognize the importance of changes in the nails, as well as changes in the skin.

Epidemiology

The National Psoriasis Foundation has estimated that PsO affects 1% to 3% of the population.[4,5] Estimates of the prevalence of PsA in patients with PsO are 15% to 39%, with the higher estimates being based on patient series in which patients have actually been examined. As a consequence, PsA is likely a more common disorder than RA.

Unlike RA, which affects women more frequently than men, the incidence of PsA is equal between men and women, and the disorder may present at any age. PsO usually precedes the appearance of PsA, but in up to 15%, arthritis may precede PsO, making the diagnosis more difficult. In patients in whom the skin disease occurs first, the mean delay until the onset of PsA is 10 years.

Although there is no linear correlation between severity of skin disease and severity of arthritis, patients with more severe PsO are more likely to develop arthritis. Patients with psoriatic nail changes often have distal interphalangeal joint (DIP) arthritis.

Patterns of Arthritis

Moll and Wright have described five patterns of PsA, which are listed in Box 73.2.[6] Any given patient may present with a combination of arthritis, spondylitis, dactylitis, and enthesitis (insertional tendinitis).

The arthritis itself tends to preferentially involve large joints, is lower extremity predominant, and is often asymmetrical (Fig. 73.1). It frequently involves the foot and ankle and may involve the axial skeleton. The arthritis is often palindromic, unlike the additive pattern seen in RA. Spine involvement often begins in the cervical spine rather than the lumbar spine, which serves to distinguish it from ankylosing spondylitis. Insertional tendinitis is a prominent feature that may dominate the clinical presentation. The net effect of the disease is to cause stiffening rather than gnarling and the end result may be ankylosis of the spine or arthrofibrosis of the knee. Each of these criteria serve to distinguish it from RA (Table 73.1).

Radiographic Features

PsA may be distinguished from RA by its radiographic findings. These are summarized in Table 73.2. The earliest lesion of PsA is bone marrow edema, best demonstrated on T2 images. Fig. 73.2 contrasts the magnetic resonance imaging (MRI) appearance of PsA with that of RA. As expected, the inflammation in PsA centers on the enthesis rather than the synovium as seen in RA.

Unique radiographic features of PsA include osteolysis (Fig. 73.3) and pencil in cup deformities, as well as asymmetrical sacroiliitis (Fig. 73.4).

Immunogenetics

RA is associated with class II major histocompatibility complex (MHC) loci, most notably human leukocyte antigen (HLA)-DR4. PsA is associated with class I MHC loci, most notably HLA-Cw6. Other associations for PsA include B13, B38, B39, B41, and HLA-B27 with psoriatic spondylitis and all forms of PsA associated with human immunodeficiency virus (HIV).

Because of the strong MHC associations, PsA tends to run in families—unlike RA, which usually is sporadic. Families that have members with PsA often also have members with PsO, inflammatory bowel disease, uveitis, and aphthous stomatitis.

Immunopathogenesis and Synovial Histology

PsA likely involves the interplay between genetic predisposition (most notably in the form of HLA) and environmental events, including infection and physical trauma. Up to half of all cases of PsO follow streptococcal infections, and other bacterial infections may also precipitate the first appearance of PsO or PsA. The Koebner phenomenon refers to PsO occurring at sites of skin trauma, including surgical incision sites, burns, and abrasions. A similar musculoskeletal Koebner phenomenon may result in response to skeletal trauma such as sports impact or accidents and may explain the acute appearance of PsA following significant trauma.[11] It may also explain the prominent foot and ankle involvement, as well as the frequency of common sports injuries, such as rotator cuff tendinitis and epicondylitis, which often recur in the absence of significant risk factors (Table 73.3).

Although psoriatic synovium is indistinguishable under light microscopy from rheumatoid synovium, there are ultrastructural and immunohistochemical differences between the two conditions. Compared with RA, there is more vascularity, lymphocyte rather than neutrophil predominance, and less lining cell hyperplasic. There is also a CD163+ macrophage

infiltrate. The cytokine profile is Thy-1 predominant, with elevated levels of both tumor necrosis factor-alpha (TNF-α) and interleukin-1 (IL-1). More recently, it has been appreciated that IL-12/23, IL-22, and IL-17 play a key role in PsA and may be responsible for some of the unique clinical features of this disease.[2] Another important and unique feature of PsA is the

---

BOX 73.1 CASPAR Criteria for Psoriatic Arthritis

Established inflammatory articular disease (joint, spine, or entheseal) with three or more of the following:
1. PsO
   • Current: Psoriatic skin or scalp disease present today as judged by a physician
   • History: History of PsO that may be obtained from patient, family physician, dermatologist, or rheumatologist
   • Family history: History of PsO in a first- or second-degree relative according to patient report
2. PsO: Typical psoriatic nail dystrophy including onycholysis, pitting, and hyperkeratosis observed on current physical examination
3. Negative test for RF: By any method except latex but preferably by ELISA or nephelometry, according to the local laboratory reference range
4. Dactylitis
   • Current: Swelling of an entire digit
   • History: History of dactylitis recorded by a rheumatologist
5. Radiologic evidence of juxta-articular new bone formation: Ill-defined ossification near joint margins (but excluding osteophyte formation) on plain radiographs of hand or foot

ELISA, Enzyme-linked immunosorbent assay; *PsO*, psoriasis; *RF*, rheumatoid factor.
From Taylor WJ, Gladman D, Helliwwell P, et al: Classification criteria for psoriatic arthritis; development of new criteria from a large international study. *Arthritis Rheum* 54(8):2665–2673, 2006.

TABLE 73.1 Contrasting Clinical Features of Rheumatoid Arthritis and Psoriatic Arthritis

Rheumatoid Arthritis	Psoriatic Arthritis
Female predominance	No gender predominance
Peak onset at 45-55 years	Variable age of onset
Sporadic	Familial occurrence
Symmetrical	Asymmetrical
Upper extremity	Lower extremity
Small joint	Large joint
Polyarticular	Oligoarticular
No axial disease	Axial disease
Synovitis	Enthesitis

TABLE 73.2 Radiographic Differences Between Rheumatoid Arthritis and Psoriatic Arthritis

Rheumatoid Arthritis	Psoriatic Arthritis
Periarticular osteoporosis	Periarticular osteosclerosis
Small marginal erosions	Atypical, large erosions
No periostitis	Periostitis
MCP, PIP changes; no DIP changes	DIP common
Bone resorption	Proliferative changes
Spine changes limited to C1-2	Sacroiliitis, spondylitis

DIP, Distal interphalangeal joint; *MCP*, metacarpal-phalangeal; *PIP*, proximal interphalangeal.

BOX 73.2 Moll and Wright Classification of Psoriatic Arthritis[a]

• Symmetrical polyarticular pattern—RA-like (small joints of hands, metacarpophalangeal joint, proximal interphalangeal joint [sparing DIP], symmetrical)
• Asymmetrical oligoarticular pattern—Four joints or less
• DIP-predominant pattern—Nail and distal involvement predominate
• Spondylitis predominant pattern—Progressive low back pain, morning stiffness, sacroiliac and axial joint involvement
• Arthritis mutilans—Destructive form of arthritis, telescoping, joint lysis, typically in phalanges and metacarpals

DIP, Distal interphalangeal joint; *RA*, rheumatoid arthritis.
[a]These subtypes are not fixed and patients can change over time to different patterns.

TABLE 73.3 Enthesitis by Anatomic Site

Site	Features
Shoulder	Rotator cuff tendinitis
Elbow	Medial and lateral epicondylitis
Wrist	De Quervain tendinitis, flexor carpi ulnaris tendinitis
Hand	Trigger fingers
Hip	Trochanteric tendinitis, anterior quadriceps tendinitis
Knee	Pes anserine tendinitis, patellar tendinitis, hamstring tendinitis
Foot and ankle	Achilles tendinitis, plantar fasciitis, anterior and posterior tibial tendinitis, peroneal tendinitis

---

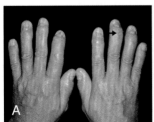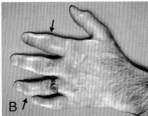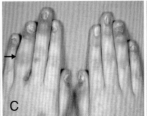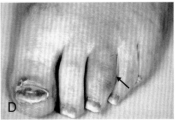

FIG 73.1 Psoriatic Arthritis: Joint Inflammation (A) Distal interphalangeal synovitis. (B) Proximal interphalangeal and distal interphalangeal synovitis. (C) Asymmetrical oligoarthritis. (D) Dactylitis with nail changes.

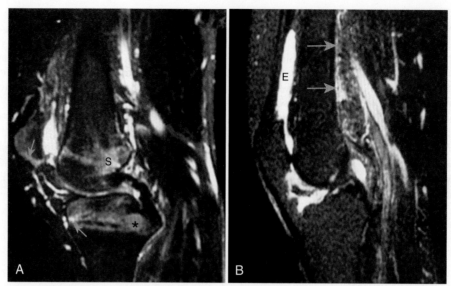

FIG 73.2 Fat-Suppressed Magnetic Resonance Imaging Scan of Psoriatic Arthritis, Enthesitis (A) PsA (*upper arrow,* anterior patella; *lower arrow,* patellar tendon insertion; *S,* superior insertion of the posterior cruciate ligament; *,* inferior insertion of the posterior cruciate ligament). (B) RA (*E,* knee effusion; *arrows,* vessels posterior to the distal femoral diaphysis). (From McGonagle D, Gibbon W, O'Connor P, et al: Characteristic magnetic resonance imaging entheseal changes of knee synovitis in spondylarthropathy. *Arthritis Rheum* 41:694–700, 1998.)

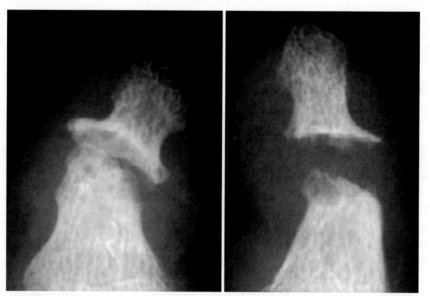

FIG 73.3 Osteolysis *Left,* Pencil cup osteolysis (erosions = 6; joint space narrowing [JSN] = 5). *Right,* Gross osteolysis (erosions = 7; JSN = 5).

presence of. CD8+IL-17+ lymphocytes. The presence of these cells is strongly linked to erosive disease. IL-23 induces enthesitis and new bone formation via activation of resident T cells. IL-22 promotes osteoproliferation, one of the clinical features of PsA.

A unique feature of PsA is large numbers of activated macrophages that differentiate in the presence of TNF-α or receptor activator of nuclear factor κB (RANK) ligand into activated osteoclasts, which serve to digest subchondral bone. Joint destruction in PsA occurs from the outside (proliferative synovitis) and from the inside (activated osteoclasts).[8] Both processes may be interrupted with aggressive treatment with biologic agents directed at TNF-α or other cytokines.

Synovial-Enthesial Complex. In PsA there is a close relationship between synovitis and enthesitis. Inflammation at both sites can be triggered by mechanical trauma, which causes nociceptors to release IL-23 and in turn activates T cells to produce both IL-17 and TNF. This coupling of biomechanical stress to inflammation via cytokine-mediated mechanisms explains the Koebner phenomenon, both in the skin and in the musculoskeletal system.[7]

Intestinal Micorbiota (Biogenome) and the Gut-Joint Axis. Patients with PsA have subclinical mucosal inflammation in the small bowel. They also have a higher incidence of Crohn

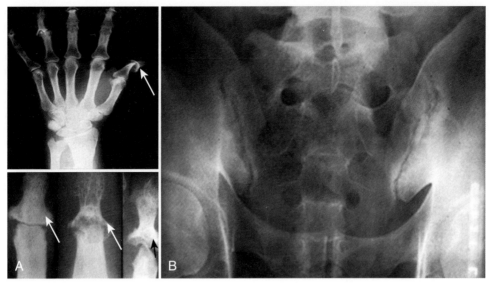

FIG 73.4 Psoriatic Arthritis, Radiologic Features (A) Productive pencil in cup joint erosions. (B) Sacroiliitis.

BOX 73.3 Definition of Metabolic Syndrome

Metabolic syndrome is defined by the presence of at least three of the following five symptoms:
- Increased waist circumference or abdominal obesity
- Hypertension
- Hypertriglyceridemia
- Reduced HDL
- Insulin resistance

Here is some additional information about metabolic syndrome:
- Chronic inflammatory state
- Associated with markedly increased cardiovascular mortality
- Prevalence in the United States = 25% of the population; Australia = 20%; France = 10%

HDL, High-density lipoprotein.
Data from National Cholesterol Education Program (NCEP) Expert Panel on Detection, Evaluation, and Treatment of High Blood Cholesterol in Adults (Adult Treatment Panel III): Third Report of the National Cholesterol Education Program (NCEP) Expert Panel on Detection, Evaluation, and Treatment of High Blood Cholesterol in Adults (Adult Treatment Panel III) final report. *Circulation* 106:3143–3421, 2002; Eckel RH, Grundy SM, Zimmet PZ: The metabolic syndrome. Lancet 365:1415–1428, 2005.

TABLE 73.4 Agents Used to Treat Psoriatic Arthritis

Agent	Half-Life
Topical steroids	NA
Topical tacrolimus and picrolimus	NA
Topical retinoids	NA
Oral retinoids (soriatane [Acitretin])	NA
Methotrexate	Hours
Cyclosporine	Hours
Azathioprine (Imuran) and mercaptopurine (Purinethol)	Hours
Etanercept (Enbrel)	4 days
Adalimumab (Humira)	14 days
Infliximab (Remicade)	8-9.5 days
Golimumab (Simponi)	14 days
Certolizumab (Cimzia)	14 days
Ustekinumab (Stelara)	14.9-45.6 days
Aprmilast (Otezla)	—
Secukinumab (Cosentyx)	—

NA, Not applicable.

disease (CD). Patients with both PsA and CD have a decreased diversity of bacterial species in the bowel as well as a decrease in the level of medium chain fatty acids that are protective against inflammation.

PsO and PsA are both exacerbated by weight gain and improved with weight loss. A gluten free diet may result in clinical improvement, even in patients who do not have actual celiac disease.

Medical Comorbidities

In contrast to RA, patients with PsA tend to be male, heavier, with a higher prevalence of serious medical comorbidities, including diabetes, hypertension, hyperlipidemia, and coronary artery disease. They are far more likely to be smokers and to consume excess alcohol. Many will have full-blown metabolic syndrome (Box 73.3). These medical issues need to be addressed prior to surgical intervention to ensure a good surgical outcome

and minimize the risk of surgical complications. More recently, it has been demonstrated that active PsA confers an augmented risk of coronary artery disease. These risks can be minimized by addressing both the underlying metabolic syndrome and by treating the inflammation with appropriate medication.[9]

Agents Used to Treat Psoriasis and Psoriatic Arthritis

PsA and PsO are treated with a diverse array of medications, including topical therapies, retinoids, nonbiologic disease-modifying antirheumatic drugs (DMARDs), and a growing array of biologic agents directed against specific cytokine pathways that are relevant to the pathogenesis of these disorders. Whereas a review of these agents is beyond the scope of this chapter, it is important to understand the risks associated with each of these agents, their effective half-life, and by extension the appropriate time interval that these drugs should be held before total joint replacement. This is summarized in Table 73.4.

UNIQUE MANAGEMENT ISSUES

Surgical Problems

Psoriasis at Incision Site. PsO at the proposed incision site poses an increased risk of infection because the psoriatic plaque is frequently colonized with bacteria. Every effort should be made to have the proposed incision site clear of psoriatic plaque. When this cannot be accomplished with the use of topical steroids, the patient should be referred to the dermatologist or rheumatologist to address this issue with systemic medications and/or light therapy. Refractory cases can be treated with an excimer laser, which can clear selected areas of the skin for weeks to months.

Heterotopic Ossification. Patients with PsA are at high risk for heterotopic ossification.[1] This can be prevented with the administration of radiation to the joint immediately before surgery or the postoperative administration of nonsteroidal antiinflammatory drugs (NSAIDs) for 6 months after surgery. Indomethacin is the best-studied NSAID for this purpose, but there is no reason to believe that newer NSAIDs will not be similarly efficacious and likely better tolerated.

Axial arthritis. Patients with PsA often have limited mobility in the cervical spine, which may complicate elective intubation. All patients requiring general anesthesia should have a thorough evaluation of the cervical spine, including both range of motion and current radiographs. When warranted, endoscopic intubation should be performed.

Other Issues

Immunosuppressive Therapy. For patients on biologic and nonbiologic immunosuppressive therapy, similar guidelines should be followed as those used for RA. Methotrexate or leflunomide should be discontinued for at least 2 weeks prior to surgery and may be reinstituted 1 to 2 weeks postoperatively, provided that the wound is healing without complication. For patients on biologic therapy, it is reasonable to hold a drug for at least four half-lives. The half-lives of the common agents are listed in Table 73.4. These agents can also be restarted at 1 week if the patient is healing well. Withholding drugs for longer periods of time may result in arthritis flares, which compromise the patient's ability to rehabilitate following total joint replacement. There is no evidence that either methotrexate or anti-TNF-α agents have any impact on wound healing, and there is no need to withhold these agents for long periods.

Thromboembolic Disease. Patients with inflammatory diseases are more prone to thromboembolic disorders than patients without evidence of inflammation. Comorbidities such as obesity or diabetes may further predispose patients to vascular problems. All patients with PsA should be anticoagulated according to current guidelines from the American Academy of Chest Physicians. Acceptable modalities would include coumadin, enoxaparin (Lovenox), and fondaparinux (Arixtra).[3]

Arthrofibrosis. Patients with PsA often develop arthrofibrosis and may achieve a lesser degree of range of motion than patients who have similar surgical procedures for OA and RA. The intensity of physical therapy should be adjusted accordingly, and the orthopedist should pay close attention to postoperative milestones. Modalities such as the use of a Dynasplint or postoperative manipulation under anesthesia may be needed to ensure that a satisfactory range of motion is achieved.

Enthesitis. Patients with PsA may present with postoperative pain that is not the result of failure of the surgical procedure but rather of acute enthesitis of the tendons attaching to the knee. The pes anserine complex is particularly vulnerable, and inflammation at this site can create severe pain that limits postoperative physical therapy. Prompt identification and treatment of this problem is essential.

Postoperative Inflammation of the Operative Site. Koebnerization (discussed previously) of the surgical incision site may mimic wound infection or tape allergy and should be treated promptly to prevent secondary bacterial superinfection. The dermatologist may need to be consulted for diagnosis and treatment of this condition.

KEY REFERENCES

4. Gelfand JM, Gladman DD, Mease PJ, et al: Epidemiology of psoriatic arthritis in the population of the United States. *J Am Acad Dermatol* 53(4):573, 2005.
5. Gladmann DD: Psoriatic arthritis. *Rheum Dis Clin North Am* 24(4):829–844, 1998.
6. Moll J, Wright V: Psoriatic arthritis. *Semin Arthritis Rheum* 3(1):55–78, 1973.
8. Ritchlin CT, Haas-Smith SA, Li P, et al: Mechanisms of TNF-alpha and RANK L mediated osteoclastogenesis and bone resorption in psoriatic arthritis. *J Clin Invest* 111(6):821–831, 2003.

The references for this chapter can also be found on www.expertconsult.com

74

Systemic Allergic Dermatitis in Total Knee Arthroplasty

Gideon P. Smith, Andrew G. Franks, Jr., David E. Cohen

Metal sensitivity in orthopedics was first reported in 1966 by Foussereau and Laugier. Sensitivity to implants containing nickel, stainless steel, cobalt, chromium, and titanium and to the components of the cements used in prostheses has been well documented and remains a consideration in the differential diagnosis of osteolysis and aseptic joint loosening. This chapter focuses on the systemic allergic dermatitis (SAD)–type reactions that may be associated with these events in some patients.

SYSTEMIC ALLERGIC DERMATITIS

SAD or systemic contact dermatitis (SCD) is a type IV or delayed cell-mediated hypersensitivity in the skin.[86] It is caused by systemic exposure to a specific allergen to which the patient has a prior exposure and preexisting sensitization. This systemic re-exposure may come from ongoing contact with an internal substance, either consumed, such as foodstuffs or medications, or implanted, such as prostheses. Although traditionally described following topical exposure, in the case of medications the primary exposure may also be systemic, such as prior exposure to the same drug or a cross-reacting medication.[109] With implants, although it is theoretically possible for the primary exposure to be from a systemic exposure, it is believed that usually these sensitizing exposures occur first in the skin from environmental exposure to components of the implant or a cross-allergen.[38] In such cases the patient may report a prior history of dermatitis occurring in localized areas from contact with external allergens, a syndrome termed allergic contact dermatitis (ACD). Indeed, this is supported by prospective trials looking at patients' contact sensitivity pre- and postimplant, with very similar rates of sensitivity at both stages.[61] SAD is also known by other names including mercury exanthema, internal-external contact-type hypersensitivity, systemically induced ACD, baboon syndrome, paraptic eczema, nonpigmented fixed drug eruption, symmetrical psychotropic and nonpigmented drug eruption, intertriginous drug eruption, drug induced intertrigo, and flexural eruptions,[52] although some of these syndromes may have been erroneously classified as SAD.

In orthopedic patients this syndrome is important because it may lead to cutaneous findings ranging from mild hypersensitivity dermatitis to a chronic and debilitating skin condition but also may be associated with failure of joint prosthesis. The latter remains somewhat controversial but is supported by observations of a high rate of metal sensitivities in patients with prosthetic loosening,[48] the shorter joint life span in patients with positive patch tests,[43] and common finding of hypersensitivity-like reactions on histopathologic testing of the tissue surrounding loosened joints.[123]

Pathophysiology

The pathophysiology of a dermatitis becoming systemic is poorly understood. However, in SAD the initial sensitization is traditionally described as coming from external exposure, and thus the pathomechanism of this stage is identical to that of ACD. On primary exposure to a chemical or contact allergen responsible for SAD or ACD, haptens from these allergens bind to proteins found on the epidermis and this complex is processed by dermal dendritic cells and Langerhans cells.[79] This is termed the afferent stage of sensitization. Subsequently, these antigen-bearing dendritic cells migrate to the lymph nodes where they present haptenated peptides on major histocompatibility complex class I and II molecules. The change in the MHC molecule surface[118] results in the induction of hapten-specific CD8+ and CD4+ T cells, respectively.[15,60] This initial sensitization stage takes approximately 10 to 14 days. However, on re-exposure, the response is much quicker, typically taking between 12 and 48 hours. During this latter, efferent stage, cloned memory Th-1 cells are activated, releasing a cascade of inflammatory cytokines, promoting spongiosis and dermal edema; classic histopathologic features on the skin. In ACD the re-exposure is from direct skin contact, whereas in SAD the hapten must be distributed hematogenously from its site of origin, to the skin site to elicit a cutaneous response. Conversely response at the site of implant may cause inflammation leading to implant complications (see later).

Histopathologic immunophenotyping of cutaneous SAD to systemic nickel reveals both CD4+ and CD8+ T lymphocytes in the epidermis and dermis[39] but decreased CD4+ and CD8+ T-cells, along with decreased CD3+, CD45RO+, and CD19+ T and B cells in peripheral blood.[13] Similarly in the gastrointestinal mucosa of nickel-sensitive patients CD4+, CD45RO+, and CD8+ lymphocytes are increased when orally challenged.[28] Nickel-sensitive patients have also been shown to have a higher fraction of skin-homing CLA+ (cutaneous lymphocyte antigen) CD3+ CD45RO, CD4+ CD45RO, and CD8+ CD45RO T cells when compared with healthy controls but a decrease in blood CLA+ CD8+ CD45RO memory T cells after nickel provocation. This suggests that these cells may have migrated to the skin and is consistent with a delayed cell-mediated hypersensitivity.[57]

Cytokine dysregulation is also consistent with a Th-1–driven delayed-type hypersensitivity. Tumor necrosis factor-alpha (TNF-α), soluble TNF receptor type 1 (sTNF-R1), interleukin-1 (IL-1) receptor antagonist, and neutrophil gelatinase-associated lipocalin (NGAL) have been shown to be upregulated in gold-sensitive patients when challenged.[75] In nickel-sensitive patients similar challenge only provoked increases in sTNF-R1,[76] although other studies using high-dose nickel also noted upregulated IL-2, IL-5,[13] IL-6, and IL-10.[57] In a zinc-sensitive patient both TNF-α and migration inhibitory factor (MIF), which upregulates TNF-α, were found to be increased.[124] In addition, upregulation of IL-1beta, TNF-α, IL-6, and PGE2 have been associated with proinflammatory cytokine-induced bone resorption via activation of osteoclasts and suppression of osteoblasts,[84] providing a theoretical mechanism for the observed aseptic loosening, although more recent studies have also suggested a critical importance for adenosine signaling in this pathway.[69]

Other Types of Reaction to Implants

This type of reaction should be distinguished from other forms of inflammation that may exist at times ranging from during surgery to months or years afterwards. One such reaction is an immunoglobulin (Ig)E-mediated immediate hypersensitivity response, which presents with a variety of clinical signs, including contact urticaria, angioedema, asthma, and anaphylaxis, within minutes of exposure and is most commonly associated in the clinical setting with natural rubber latex allergy. A second type is a granulomatous reaction, which often occurs in response to a foreign body, such as plastic particulate matter from a worn prosthesis or talc from surgical gloves, although the skin and internal organs, such as the lungs, can demonstrate granulomatous inflammation in response to metals.[32,111] This type of reaction is also associated with joint loosening.[8] These reactions may not show clinical significance for weeks to months after particle deposition. The normal healing and repair response also invokes significant stages of inflammation and repair in the weeks to months after surgery. Finally, an autoimmune reaction in which the body produces antibodies against itself is theoretically also possible to trigger with prosthesis placement. A humoral type III immune reaction mediated by circulating antigen-antibody complexes that cause inflammation on tissue deposition has been postulated; it is supported by the identification of antibodies against hapten-albumin complexes in the blood.[85,115]

Epidemiology

More than 3000 environmental chemicals have been identified as causing SAD or ACD. Interpretation of diagnostic patch test findings is critical because assessment and assignment of clinical relevance can be difficult in the setting of suspected orthopedic prosthetic implant hypersensitivity reactions.

Allergenic Substances Used in Orthopedics. There are a variety of designs of knee prosthesis used throughout the world. However, because their components generally do not vary greatly we will review here standard constituents and not specific designs. In orthopedic prostheses the metals used are alloys, or combinations of metals, very rarely pure metals. At times minor metal alloy constituents and trace impurities can be the detected allergens.

Vitallium, a commonly used alloy, is composed of 70% cobalt, 25% to 30% chromium, 6% to 7% molybdenum, with trace amounts of nickel. Austenitic stainless steel, which is also commonly used, occasionally contains up to 35% nickel but generally contains 8.5% to 14% nickel, 17% to 20% chromium, 2% to 3% molybdenum, and less than 1% carbon, nitrogen, manganese, silicon, sulfur, phosphorus, and niobium. Alloys of cobalt-chromium-tungsten-nickel with 9% to 11% nickel and cobalt-chromium-molybdenum with 2% nickel are also sometimes used. Titanium is used in its pure form and can be alloyed with 6% aluminum or 4% vanadium for improved tensile strength.[38]

In addition to the metals in prosthesis, bone cement is sometimes used. The most common bone cement is polymethylmethacrylate (PMMA) based, but this and others may have allergenic additives, the most common of which are gentamicin and benzoyl peroxide.[102] These chemicals are likely less significant than the metal sensitivities given the lower prevalence of these allergies in the general population, their transient presence at the surgical sites, and the lower amounts of these substances in prostheses. The allergenicity of all these standard components is reviewed later.

Genetics of Contact Sensitization. In general, there is no known genetic predilection for the development of contact sensitization to prosthesis components. The potential for increased prevalence of nickel allergy in monozygotic over dizygotic twins might suggest a genetic predisposition, although the magnitude of this risk factor is likely small and further studies are needed.[19,72] Null mutations in filaggrin have been found to be associated with nickel allergy.[82] Filaggrin is a highly phosphorylated, histidine-rich polypeptide important in keratin filament aggregation and formation of the skin barrier.[24] This may be particularly important in nickel-sensitive patients because histidine-rich polypeptides are strong nickel-chelating agents and thus may also cause the accumulation of nickel in the stratum corneum.[103] The failure of definitive epidemiologic study findings noted earlier may therefore partly be explained by the fact that the study showing no correlation included a significant number of patients exposed via ear piercing, thus circumventing the need for a genetic basis for barrier disruption, whereas the earlier study looked primarily at patients with topical clothing-based exposures.

Prevalence of Contact Sensitization. Risk factors for the development of SAD are linked to the risk factors for developing an initial cutaneous sensitization. These will therefore be reviewed to facilitate patient risk stratification for SAD. Because exposure risk is controlled by the environment, prevalence data and risk factors vary by geographic location and therefore need to be assessed based on the patient population. For example, nickel allergy rates are lower in Denmark and Germany than in the United States presumably because nickel content for clothing (buttons, fasteners) and piercings is more stringently regulated in Europe.[73,95,105] The effects of such regulatory practices on prevalence can be seen by the decline in nickel allergies after these nickel content regulations were introduced in these countries.

Metal allergy prevalence is most often presented as percentage of patients with positive patch test reactions. There is potential for selection bias because patients who are patch tested are those already suspected of having ACD. Rarely are data presented for well individuals. Nickel allergy is among the most common contact allergies, with an estimated prevalence based on positive patch testing of 16.7%[65] to 19%[127] in the United States. In Thailand this figure is reported to be as high as 33.8%,[122] whereas in Europe a similar incidence has been reported but with a clear disparity between women (17%) and men (3%).[30,108] This gender discrepancy may be explained by a discrepancy in the rates of ear piercing,[80] with 80% of women and 10% of men estimated to have piercings in this population.[108] However, as noted the prevalence of nickel allergy in Denmark is reported to have dropped to 6.9% ($p = 0.004$) in piercings in women since the introduction in 1990 of more stringent nickel content restrictions.[106] Cobalt and chromium sensitivity are estimated to be approximately 1% to 3%,[73,95,105,108] although chromium sensitivity is believed to be increasing in Denmark,[104] Singapore,[41] and the United States.[78]

When the results of 10 European patch-testing centers were pooled, cobalt sensitivity was seen to have an age-dependent prevalence of 6.2% to 8.8% and chromium of 2.4% to 5.9%. Gold[12,87] and palladium[1] allergies are seen in approximately 10% of dermatitis patients. Patients with gold-containing dental[2] and cardiac[31] implants demonstrated substantially higher rates of positive patch tests of up to 30. In contrast, aluminum sensitivity is rarely reported.[59]

Titanium hypersensitivity is regarded as extremely rare.[64] However, it has been reported in hip replacement[63] and with a static titanium implant, in which dermatitis was observed overlying the site and a positive lymphocyte transformation test (LTT) result was obtained.[100]

Co-reactivity to metals is common, with one study showing nickel reactivity in 79% of cobalt-sensitive patients, 39% of chromium-sensitive patients, and 95% of palladium-sensitive patients.[59] This high rate of co-reactivity between nickel and palladium and the low rate of palladium exposure outside the electronics and chemicals industry has led many to question whether this is simply a cross-reaction to a nickel allergy.[113] In contrast, the high rate of concordance of cobalt and nickel sensitization is believed to be caused by concomitant sensitization rather than cross-sensitization because of the prevalence of cobalt in consumer products and is thus clinically relevant.

Risk Factors

For Nickel Sensitivity. Nickel allergy has been identified in a variety of occupational exposures. These include plating industry workers,[110] retail clerks, hairdressers, domestic cleaners, metal workers and caterers,[97] locksmiths, and carpenters.[66] Nickel dermatitis has also been reported as being caused by clothing, ranging from suspenders[23] to jean buttons and zippers.[17] Other sources include head sets and mobile phones.[107] Jewelry and body piercings are a common cause in women,[14,33] and the number of body piercings has been shown to positively correlate with the risk of nickel allergy.[119] Significant, long-time exposure to metals that release nickel are also likely to be a risk factor. These include white gold, gold plating, German silver, Monel solder, nickel plating, and stainless steel. Finally, some reports have implicated nickel-containing cosmetics and devices, such as eye shadow,[40] mascara,[114] eyeliner pencils,[126] and eyelash curlers.[16]

For Chromium Sensitivity. Occupational exposure to chromium is possible in locksmiths and carpenters[66] and those working with cement,[125] dyeing agents, metal alloys, pottery, colorant, and anti-rust agents in coolants, such as mechanics.[5] Although cement workers have historically been the most important of these, addition of iron sulfate to reduce the amount of water-soluble hexavalent chromium reduced chromium sensitivity from 12.7% in 1989 to 1994 prior to its addition to 3.0% in 1995 to 2007.[104] In contrast, in the same time period chromium sensitivity from consumer exposure to leather has increased from 24.1% to 45.5%.[35,96,104]

For Cobalt Sensitivity. Occupational exposures to cobalt include hard metal workers, painters in the glass and pottery industry,[34,91] locksmiths, carpenters, cashiers, and secretaries.[66] In consumer exposure many of the same risk factors are present as in nickel because chromium has historically often been mixed with nickel. These include jewelry and piercings.[70,80]

SENSITIVITY TO IMPLANTS

Systemic Allergic Dermatitis to Implants

Metal implants have been used for repair of fractures since the 1950s and in joint replacements since 1962 with the first prosthetic hip. All metal implants, even static ones, such as those used to repair fractures or in pacemaker devices, are inevitably in contact with body fluids. Therefore they can corrode and release metal ions, which have the potential to bind proteins and activate T cells[46,74] and macrophages.[22] As noted, T-cell activation can lead to an ACD in the overlying skin in pacemakers[20] and joints[90] or to a more extensive SAD. In contrast, macrophage activation has been associated with device failure.[22]

The degree of allergenicity in stainless steel implants has been shown to be directly related to the sulfur content, which reflects the alloy's ability to liberate nickel ions. High sulfur (0.3%) stainless steel AISI 303 can release up to 1.5 µg/cm^2/week, sufficient to induce dermatitis in nickel-sensitive patients.[50,71] In contrast, stainless steel with less than 0.03% sulfur release only 0.03 µg/cm^2/week and does not result in nickel dermatitis. Despite multiple reports of localized dermatitis over a static implant,[68,88] in a prospective study of 48 subjects receiving static stainless steel orthopedic implants, none developed dermatitis, even the three subjects shown by patch testing prior to implantation to have a nickel allergy.[38] However, restenosis of stainless steel stents, which contain nickel, cobalt, and molybdenum, have been associated with the presence of a nickel allergy,[55,58,92] although this association continues to be debated.[53,98] In contrast, coronary artery stent restenosis is strongly associated with gold allergy in gold-plated stents.[31]

In nonstatic implants, there is an even greater theoretical potential for metal ion exposure because of the mechanical wear inherent in the device's function. Today the most commonly reported SAD associated with an implanted orthopedic joint prosthesis is that following hip replacement. This may be caused by a combination of factors, including that hip replacement is the most common type of implanted joint prosthesis performed, the high load and frictional forces of this joint contributing to high wear and particulate production, and the materials and design used, most especially in early hip prostheses, which were more prone to allergenic particulate production. Early prosthetic hips consisted of metal-on-metal components, resulting in much higher frictional wear, subsequent release of particulate metals and metallic ions, and eventual loosening in up to a quarter of cases.[38]

Subsequent to this, hips with metal femoral but plastic acetabular components were introduced. The former is most commonly austenitic stainless steel, and the latter is composed of high or ultra–high-molecular-weight polyethylene (UHMWPE), ceramic, or carbon fiber. In younger patients porous coated implants are sometimes used that require no cement, but in older and other higher risk patients, PMMA bone cement is used. Because acrylic bone cements are not easily biodegraded, inflammatory reactions to PMMA and other bone cements have been occasionally reported.[44] In addition, additives, such as benzoyl peroxide[112] and gentamicin,[45,67] can be allergenic. In one study 28 of 113 patients with cemented prostheses had a sensitivity to bone cement components[101]; 16.8% were sensitive to gentamicin and 8.0% to benzoyl peroxide, although N,N-dimethyl-p-toluidine and hydroquinone sensitivities were also identified in a minority of patients. With the metal-on-plastic hips many reports exist of patch test-confirmed metal-sensitive patients receiving implants with no development of cutaneous problems or loosening.[7,21] The downside of these metal-on-plastic hips is that, although they release less metal, they do produce greater overall wear, the loss of 0.2 mm/year from the polyethylene surface[117] in comparison to 0.1 to 10 µm/year for the ball and 0.2 to 6 µm/year for the cup in all-metal prosthesis. The polyethylene particles also tend to be larger, inducing greater tissue reaction and thus more osteolysis. For this reason metal-on-metal hips consisting of a cobalt alloy femoral stem and a titanium acetabular cup were reintroduced in the 1980s. Three years after prosthesis insertion, serum levels of titanium were found to be threefold higher and that of chromium fivefold higher,[18,56] leading to the potential for development of SAD long after implantation.

After hip, the knee is the next most common prosthetic joint replacement. Although many of the same concerns that exist for hip replacement could be extended to knee prostheses, the design and biomechanics of the two joints are different. In particular, in knee prostheses the articulation in more commonly metal on plastic leading to decreased metal debris. Despite this, SAD cases have been reported in nickel- and cobalt-sensitive patients even after preoperative patch testing.[9] Localized dermatitis over an artificial knee joint has also been reported, occurring 2 months after the use of a condylar knee joint replacement.[49] This prosthesis contained a $Cu^{2+} Cr^{3+}$ alloy femoral component. The patient did not go on to SAD, and serum levels of copper, nickel, and chromium were normal, but the patient had a positive patch test result to copper sulfate and cobalt chloride but not to nickel. An 80-year-old Japanese patient also developed knee dermatitis after total knee arthroplasty (TKA) with a Co-Cr alloy knee.[83] The patient patch tested positive to Co, Ni, Cr, Mn, Pt, Ir, In, Hg, Sn, and Zn, and the dermatitis was resolved when the prosthesis was replaced with a titanium-ceramic device. In cases such as this it is unclear if the dermatitis developed because of one of the more common metal-allergies, such as nickel or chromium, or a less common metal. However, cases of implant complications caused by the less common metal allergies, such as manganese, have also been documented.[120] As this problem becomes increasingly recognized and increasingly investigated it is possible more cases due to rare sensitivities will continue to be identified, making pre-identification of at-risk patients at the least challenging and in many cases unrealistic.

In one case series 30 patients were observed to develop localized dermatitis around the knee 1 to 3 months after joint revision with a total condylar knee prosthesis (DePuy Orthopaedics, Warsaw, Indiana).[116] This prosthesis contains a femoral component consisting of a cobalt chrome alloy made up of 27% to 30% chromium, 5% to 7% molybdenum, 0.7% nickel, 59% to 64% cobalt, and 4% other elements. The tibial component was a titanium alloy containing 5.5% to 6.5% aluminum, 3.5% to 4.5% vanadium, and 88% to 91% titanium. Of the 30 original patients 15 consented to patch testing. Testing was performed to nickel sulfate (5% in pet), cobalt chloride (1% pet), and potassium dichromate (0.5% pet). At day 3 of testing, 7 of 15 patients showed a positive metal sensitivity: 4 to nickel, 2 to chromium, and 1 to cobalt.

In a different case series four German female patients were reported to have persistent dermatitis after a Co-Cr alloy TKA.[29] Each patient underwent an LTT to Ni, Cr, Co, Mo, Mn, and Ti and patch testing to a standard series containing Ni, Cr, and Co, an expanded metal series, including Mn, Mo, V, and Ti, and a bone cement series, composed of 2-hydroxyethyl methacrylate, PMMA, copper sulfate pentahydrate, benzoyl peroxide, gentamicin sulfate, hydroquinone and N,N-dimethyl-p-toluidine. The first patient in the series had a positive nickel sensitivity. The second patient was sensitive to both cobalt and nickel, and in the third patient patch testing was positive to cobalt and the LTT showed elevated sensitivity to both nickel and cobalt. The final patient was sensitive to nickel and cobalt but was also sensitive to ethylene glycol dimethacrylate, 2-hydroxyethylmethacrylate, and 2-hydroxypropylmethacrylate. Resolution of all symptoms in all patients, including joint effusion and dermatitis, was achieved after switching to a titanium-plated prosthesis and in the case of the final patient removal of residual cement at the time of titanium prosthesis implantation.

In a prospective study of 92 patients undergoing TKA between 2000 and 2002 preoperative modified lymphocyte stimulation tests (mLSTs) to Ni, Co, Cr, and Fe were performed.[81] Of these, 26% showed positive sensitivity to at least one of these metals. Five of the patients with preoperative metal sensitivity went on to develop implant-related dermatitis, although the only association reaching statistical significance was with Cr ($p < 0.05$). Two of the metal-sensitive patients had TKA revision, with resolution of the dermatitis.

In a different study 94 subjects were recruited, 20 prior to TKA, 27 with a well-functioning TKA, and 47 with loosening of the joint after revision.[42] Patch testing for 5% nickel sulfate, 1% cobalt chloride, 2% chromium trichloride, 0.5% potassium dichromate, 2% ferric chloride, 2% molybdenum chloride, 1% niobium chloride, 2% titanium dioxide, 5% PMMA, 2% butyl methacrylate, 2% triethylene glycol dimethacrylate, 2% ethylene glycol dimethacrylate, 2% N,N-dimethyl-p-toluidine, 5% hydroxylethylmethacrylate, 2% benzoyl peroxide, and 1% hydroquinone monobenzyl ether was performed. In preimplant patients a positive patch test result was seen in 20% of patients. In postimplant patients positive patch tests were shown to be higher in both groups tested after TKA, with a slight increase in patch test positives in patients with TKA loosening (59.6%) over those with stable TKA (48.1%). The most important factor identified in this study in predicting joint loosening was a prior history of contact allergy to metals. This single item in the history increased the risk of failure fourfold.

Finally, one case has been reported in which TKA failure was attributed to a preexisting contact sensitivity to PMMA.[51] The patient had previously had a periungual dermatitis believed to be from acrylic nail use, which resolved with the avoidance of acrylic nails and glues. She subsequently underwent TKA with a PMMA-containing bone cement. The patient went on to experience significant early joint loosening and was patch tested to both the bone cement and metals. PMMA was positive but metal patch testing was negative. The patient subsequently underwent joint revision with a cementless prosthesis, with no recurrence of the problem.

Development of a New Hapten Sensitization From Prosthesis Implantation

Although the initial sensitization event is classically described as coming from topical exposure, it is theoretically possible that the initial exposure could be from a systemic event. In this regard a metal orthopedic implant could potentially serve as the sensitizer for a new dermatitis in a patient, although the degree of risk is unknown. In retrospective studies of 112 patients after metal-on-metal hip replacement, one was found to have a new nickel allergy and two a new cobalt allergy.[25] In another series of 85 patients post hip replacement, two nickel, five cobalt, and one chromate nickel allergy were documented after surgery.[121] In addition, three nickel and one new (patch testing performed before and after surgery) cobalt allergy were documented in 66 hip surgeries.[27] Of 1400 patients receiving joint replacement and 200 internal fixations, only 2 of 13 with a persistent eczematous dermatitis patch tested positive to a metal.[62]

However, to assess this rigorously, patch testing has to be prospectively examined and needs to be performed before and after prosthesis implantation. Ironically, in one study in which 69 patients were patch tested before and after prosthesis implantation, five subjects who initially tested positive to nickel, chromium, or cobalt tested negative post surgery.[89] This may reflect the sensitivity of the test or induction of immunologic tolerance after prosthesis insertion, although another study of 85 patients did show induction of sensitivity to cobalt (four patients), and in individual patients, PMMA, nickel, cobalt, and chromium post implantation.[121] Because studies are equivocal, with some supporting a low rate of induction of tolerance and some supporting a low rate of induction of sensitivity, this is probably not of high clinical concern.

WORK-UP PRIOR TO IMPLANTATION

History and Physical Examination

There are no established guidelines of care that outline preoperative work-ups for the detection or prevention of prosthesis hypersensitivity. SAD from knee prostheses appears rare, screening may be considered only for highly suspect patients prior to prosthesis implantation or after surgery when dysfunction is detected and other common causes are excluded. As noted, the most significant historical factor is a known clinical sensitivity or prior positive patch test to metals. Patients may not be specifically aware of contact sensitivities, and the physical examination could assess for unexplained dermatitis, especially if located in proximity to a likely contactant, such as a nickel-containing jeans stud or button. In such a case the patient should be referred to a dermatologist for full evaluation. Other important factors are history and number of piercings, occupational exposures—including metal workers, retail clerks, hairdressers, domestic cleaners, caterers, locksmiths, and carpenters, and those exposed to cements, dyeing agents, metal alloys, pottery, colorants, and antirust agents in coolants (eg, mechanics, painters in the glass or pottery industry). In addition, although atopic dermatitis has variably been described as both a risk and protective factor for the development of contact dermatitis, contact dermatitis can sometimes be incorrectly diagnosed as atopic dermatitis or another skin rash. Thus any patient with an ongoing or history of recurrent rash should be evaluated by a dermatologist.

Serology

Although several blood tests exist and are purported to diagnose allergen sensitivity, these are not standardly performed in the work-up of or screening for ACD. In the LTT, radioactive H^3-labeled thymidine is placed in vitro, with lymphocytes from the patient as a marker. Proliferation of lymphocytes causes uptake of the radioactive thymidine into cellular DNA upon division. This can then be quantified via liquid scintillation after 3 to 6 days of incubation with the suspected allergen. Although showing good sensitivity, even in patch test negative patients,[99] the test is prohibitively expensive for routine use and requires very specialized laboratory facilities, limiting its clinical usefulness. Further studies are needed to clinically correlate the laboratory findings and clinical outcomes.

The lymphokine MIF test is another in vitro test for allergen sensitivity.[47] First, lymphocytes are isolated from a sample of the patient's blood. These are then mixed with solutions of the allergens to be tested, such as nickel, chromium, cobalt, or titanium ions. The function of MIF is to prevent lymphocytes from leaving an area where foreign antigens are present. If lymphocytes react to the suspected allergen, they therefore remain in proximity to it, and the MIF test is read as positive. If there is no sensitivity, the lymphocytes are seen to migrate away, giving a negative MIF test. This test also suffers from the same limitations of cost, availability noted previously for the LTT, and lack of clinical correlation and therefore has limited clinical usefulness.

Patch Testing

Patch testing is seen as the gold standard for the evaluation of ACD. However, the usefulness of the test is affected by a number of factors. The testing must be performed by someone experienced in appropriate patient selection, selection of allergens, patch application, appropriate reading of the skin reactions to patches, and interpretation of the clinical relevance of the results.[77]

Patch testing consists of the application of nonirritating concentrations of allergens suspected of causing ACD in the particular patient. The skin must be intact and noninflamed prior to application. The upper back is the most common site chosen because it provides a large surface area for the application of series of patches. The patches should remain on for approximately 2 days; during this period the patient is unable to bathe her or his back because this would risk washing away allergens, moving patches, or erasing marks identifying patches. The first read is performed on removal of the patches at 48 hours. Different scales exist for this initial read but generally include no reaction, weak reaction (eg, mild macular erythema), positive reaction (eg, edema with erythema), strong reaction (eg, bullae), and irritant. The locations of the patches are marked on the skin with tape or surgical marker. To differentiate between allergic and irritant reactions, a second read is performed at day 4 or 5. Very strong positive patch test results may cause negative allergen sites to appear mildly positive; thus repeat isolated testing of the weaker positive may be required in this case. Because the patch test relies on the patient being able to mount an immune response to the applied patches, the patient cannot have ongoing treatments or engage in activities that would interfere with this testing, such as treatment with systemic steroids or other immunosuppressive drugs and activities, such as tanning.

In the United States the most common patch testing performed is the thin-layer rapid-use epicutaneous (TRUE) test, which consists of 28 common skin sensitizers and one negative control. Unfortunately, of the substances relevant to prosthesis, this contains only nickel sulfate and cobalt dichloride. Therefore the examiner will ideally use a nonstandard test patch series, sometimes individually prepared in aluminum (Finn) or foam chambers mounted on hypoallergenic paper tape.[10] This often requires referral to a dermatologist specializing in contact dermatology. A variety of patch test series have been suggested for the work-up[93]; however, when clinical concern is particularly high, such as in a patient with known metal allergies, specific allergens may be included in otherwise established series. In SAD the use of patch testing is less conclusive than in ACD, in part because the epicutaneous application of metal salts is likely biologically distinct from exposure to metal ions within the joint. Use of subcutaneous metal implants prior to prosthesis implantation has been attempted but has its own dissimilarities to the long-term joint environment.[9] Because contact sensitivity is more prevalent than post-prosthesis SAD, patch testing may overpredict sensitivities. Finally, metal allergens likely to be the most significant allergens in prostheses can be difficult to reproduce. Consequently, patch testing was not designed for detection of systemic allergic phenomena from implanted devices, and the magnitude of the correlation of test findings to clinical orthopedic activity remains unknown. Despite this, patch testing should theoretically be able to provide some level of reassurance when a negative result is obtained requiring, like SAD, prior cutaneous sensitization. It also allows for rapid screening of a large number of potential allergens. Indeed, in a questionnaire study of 119 individuals attending the European and American Contact Dermatitis meetings in 2012 patch testing was the top choice for evaluation.[94] Few participants made use of lymphocyte transformation or intradermal tests. However, 38% of respondents recommended foregoing all testing and using instead a titanium implant for decreased risk. Despite this questionnaire study, a study of 72 patients undergoing implant did suggest improved rates of outcomes with preimplant patch screening.[4] Thus where screening is deemed appropriate by the clinician, patch testing remains the best and certainly most cost-effective screening tool for determining sensitivity to prosthesis components.

POST KNEE ARTHROPLASTY

Clinical Cutaneous Signs of Sensitivity

Clinical features of patients with hypersensitivity to their prosthetic implant are variable but often reflect the standard symptoms of prosthetic failure, including loosening, pain, and instability. Local inflammatory reactions are possible, such as warmth and erythema, and skin dermatitis may be localized or, more commonly, generalized. The exact appearance of SAD lesions will vary, depending on the stage of the disease. During the early acute phase, like other dermatitides, lesions are often edematous and/or erythematous and may produce papular or vesicular lesions. If vesicles rupture, oozing ensues and patients may develop secondary bacterial infection. In the chronic stage, scaling, lichenification, and excoriations predominate. Because clinical signs of hypersensitivity can mimic those of infection, careful consideration of the most pressing issue should be evaluated.

Work-Up After Implantation

If after implantation a rash fitting the clinical characteristics of SAD should occur, especially if the patient had risk factors, postimplantation patch testing may be performed. This is important because no curative medical atherapy exists; if the artificial joint is the cause, prosthetic revision might be

considered prior to joint failure. Patch testing may also be considered in a patient subsequently presenting with symptoms of joint loosening who has risk factors for sensitivity, to allow adequate selection of the replacement prosthesis. In either case x-rays of the joint should be obtained.[3,11] Signs that may be attributable to loosening from hypersensitivity include radiolucencies around the implant, screw migration, or change in implant position. In hypersensitivity-induced osteolysis, cystic changes may also be seen. Magnetic resonance imaging (MRI) and computed tomography (CT) scans have not proven additionally helpful in the assessment, and bone scans, although sometimes positive, are nonspecific. Although serum levels of different suspected allergens may be determined, standard levels above which an allergic event is likely have not been established because sensitivity depends on the individual patient, making clinically significant interpretation impossible.[37] In addition, a high serum level does not imply sensitization and cannot be determined to provide evidence of future sensitization. This may be seen in the lack of prognostic significance of elevated serum metal levels.[26]

The list of medications causing SAD is long. It includes many common medications, including antibiotics, antihistamines, and heart medications, which the patient may not think are related to the exanthema. The list of such agents has recently been updated,[109] but new medications are continually being identified; the list should be reviewed on an ongoing basis when clinical suspicion is high—for example, because of the timing of the exanthema in relation to the administration of new medications. Medications should always be excluded because this does not affect the prognosis of the joint and elimination of the drug is curative. Therefore SAD is best assessed by an experienced dermatologist who can evaluate all its potential causes.

CONCLUSIONS

In conclusion, SAD after knee arthroplasty is a rare but important condition. Consequences include chronic systemic dermatitis and joint prosthesis failure secondary to the hypersensitivity reaction and chronic inflammation. In patients with an identified risk of SAD, or SAD itself, alternative knee prosthesis components may be considered, depending on the quality and severity of the cutaneous eruption. These include prostheses with ceramic rather than metal components, use of nonallergenic metallic implants, such as titanium or Zn-Nb alloys, or a prosthesis with a suitable coating to mask the allergenic components.[6] At a 5-year follow-up no patients receiving oxidized zirconium femoral prosthesis showed SAD[54]; SAD is therefore a syndrome of which generalists and specialists dealing with these patients, such as orthopedists, dermatologists, and rheumatologists, should be well aware. Despite awareness, even with the greatest clinical care, some patients may still develop SAD. This is evidenced by studies showing that patient's history does not always reveal existing metal sensitivities and that metal sensitivities may arise after implantation.[36] Determining causation of hypersensitivity still remains an exercise in conjecture.

KEY REFERENCES

11. Berquist TH: Imaging of joint replacement procedures. *Radiol Clin North Am* 44:419–437, 2006.
26. Dahlstrand H, Stark A, Anissian L, et al: Elevated serum concentrations of cobalt, chromium, nickel, and manganese after metal-on-metal

alloarthroplasty of the hip: a prospective randomized study. *J Arthroplasty* 24:837–845, 2009.

29. Dietrich KA, Mazoochian F, Summer B, et al: Intolerance reactions to knee arthroplasty in patients with nickel/cobalt allergy and disappearance of symptoms after revision surgery with titanium-based endoprostheses. *J Dtsch Dermatol Ges* 7:410–413, 2009.

38. Gawkrodger DJ: Metal sensitivities and orthopaedic implants revisited: the potential for metal allergy with the new metal-on-metal joint prostheses. *Br J Dermatol* 148:1089–1093, 2003.

42. Granchi D, Cenni E, Tigani D, et al: Sensitivity to implant materials in patients with total knee arthroplasties. *Biomaterials* 29:1494–1500, 2008.

48. Hallab N, Merritt K, Jacobs JJ: Metal sensitivity in patients with orthopaedic implants. *J Bone Joint Surg Am* 83:428–436, 2001.

50. Haudrechy P, Foussereau J, Mantout B, et al: Nickel release from nickel-plated metals and stainless steels. *Contact Dermatitis* 31(4):249–255, 1994.

59. Kranke B, Aberer W: Multiple sensitivities to metals. *Contact Dermatitis* 34:225, 1996.

64. Lalor PA, Revell PA, Gray AB, et al: Sensitivity to titanium. A cause of implant failure? *J Bone Joint Surg Br* 73:25–28, 1991.

74. Merritt K, Rodrigo JJ: Immune response to synthetic materials. Sensitization of patients receiving orthopaedic implants. *Clin Orthop Relat Res* 326:71–79, 1996.

81. Niki Y, Matsumoto H, Otani T, et al: Screening for symptomatic metal sensitivity: a prospective study of 92 patients undergoing total knee arthroplasty. *Biomaterials* 26:1019–1026, 2005.

84. Otto M, Kriegsmann J, Gehrke T, et al: Wear particles: key to aseptic prosthetic loosening? *Pathologe* 27:447–460, 2006.

102. Thomas P, Schuh A, Ring J, et al: [Orthopedic surgical implants and allergies: joint statement by the implant allergy working group (AK 20) of the DGOOC (German Association of Orthopedics and Orthopedic Surgery), DKG (German Contact Dermatitis Research Group) and DGAKI (German Society for Allergology and Clinical Immunology)]. *Orthopade* 37:75–88, 2008.

123. Willert HG, Buchhorn GH, Fayyazi A, et al: Metal-on-metal bearings and hypersensitivity in patients with artificial hip joints. A clinical and histomorphological study. *J Bone Joint Surg Am* 87:28–36, 2005.

The references for this chapter can also be found on www.expertconsult.com.

75

Rheumatoid Arthritis of the Knee: Current Medical Management

Andrew G. Franks, Jr.

There has been substantial transformation in the evaluation and treatment of rheumatoid arthritis (RA) over the past decade. This has been accelerated by expanded understanding of the immune pathways of the disease itself (Fig. 75.1), the rapid development of novel therapeutics, especially the biologics, and the recently developed recommendations for treating both early and established RA "to target," with the therapeutic goal of remission or goals that bring disease activity to the lowest achievable level.[26] Despite classification criteria that have been updated and refined, the diagnosis of RA still requires clinical expertise.[23] For patients with newly diagnosed, early RA, methotrexate (MTX) is widely recommended as the first-line therapy for most patients. In those who do not respond to MTX monotherapy, switching to other disease-modifying antirheumatic drugs (DMARDs) or treatment with an antitumor necrosis factor (TNF) biologic agent is usually the next step. The "treat to target" paradigm in patients not in remission also includes the addition or dose escalation of a nonsteroidal anti-inflammatory drug (NSAID), an intra-articular steroid injection, or low-dose short-course oral steroids.[2]

Steroids, NSAIDs, and nonbiologic DMARDs have been used for many years to treat RA. Because of its safety profile, long-term effectiveness, and low cost, MTX has been the most commonly used DMARD. Other nonbiologic DMARDs used less frequently include sulfasalazine, antimalarials, gold salts, leflunomide, azathioprine, mycophenalate mofeteil, cyclosporine, and minocycline. Despite this large choice of drugs, about one-third of patients will discontinue conventional DMARD therapy because of a lack of efficacy.[18]

Although most of the NSAIDs have had more limited use than in the past because of their cardiovascular risks through cyclooxygenase-2 (COX-2) inhibition[8] or their risk for gastrointestinal intolerance,[12] treatment goals that bring disease activity to the lowest possible level may now include those currently available. In addition, use of low dose corticosteroids has also been advocated by some to reduce symptoms and systemic manifestations of RA; however, they do not appreciably prevent disease progression,[22] MTX and other DMARDs used early and over time can control symptoms and are thought to delay progression of the disease (Fig. 75.2) and remain the most often used agents by rheumatologists throughout the world for the treatment of RA.[17] In fact, recent evidence suggests that MTX, when used concomitantly, actually increases the efficacy of some biologics.[19] Nevertheless, recent advances, such as tumor necrosis factor-alpha (TNF-α) inhibitors, costimulatory T cell blockers, interlukin-1 (IL-1) and IL-6 inhibitors, and

anti-CD20 monoclonal antibodies as well as Janus kinase (JAK) inhibitors, have allowed many patients with RA to experience improvement in symptoms, function, and quality of life to a degree they might not have achieved in the past.[4] Etanercept, infliximab, adalimumab, anakinra, golimumab, certolizumab pegol, rituximab, abatacept, tocilizumab, and the JAK inhibitor tofacitinib are currently US Food and Drug Administration (FDA) approved for the treatment of RA.[10] Thus, therapeutic decision making for this disease has become more complex for clinicians, with many conflicting factors including cost playing increasingly important roles. According to the most objective measures of RA progression, early intervention with conventional DMARDs, especially MTX, is cost effective, whereas that of early intervention with biologics remains unclear.[15] However, more recent data indicate that biologic therapy is associated with increases in workforce participation in patients typically expected to experience progressively deteriorating ability, which could result in significant indirect cost benefits to society.[13] In addition, recent studies suggest that biosimilar biologics may have equal efficacy at reduced cost.[21] The recently released American College of Rheumatology 2015 Guidelines for the Treatment of Rheumatoid Arthritis (Figs. 75.3 and 75.4) distinguish early versus established RA and take into consideration all of the above in an attempt to maximize patient outcomes.[25]

Biomarkers have been important in understanding pathogenesis and developing new therapies, but there is no single biomarker that can be used in diagnosis, prognosis, and monitoring of all patients. Therefore, a multi-biomarker disease activity score (MBDA) has recently been introduced and may prove more useful.[16] The Clinical Disease Activity Index (CDAI), Routine Assessment of Patient Index Data 3 (RAPID3), and other patient and physician-reporting instruments have been in clinical use for some time. However, there appears to be poor correlation between physician global assessment of disease activity and biomarkers such as acute phase reactant results indicating that the physician global pain visual analog scale with joint counts remain important in clinical settings. The Rheumatoid Arthritis Impact of Disease (RAID) score is a patient-derived composite score also in use. Ultrasound has become a useful adjunctive tool in the assessment of RA (Fig. 75.5) and may identify occult active synovitis, allowing more aggressive "treat to target" therapy.[1,6]

In addition to cost, the overall safety profile of the biologics remains a central issue, and a number of side effects have been reported. Reactivation of tuberculosis and other opportunistic infections has occurred after introduction of these agents,

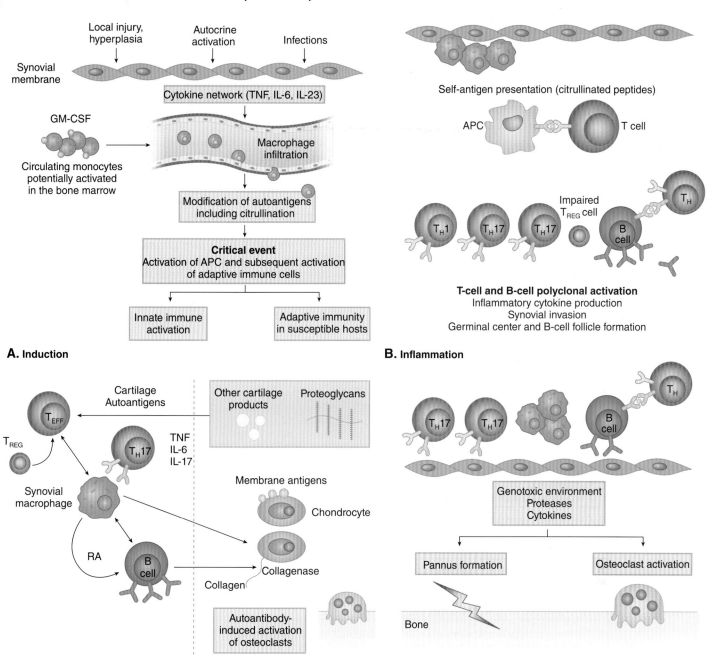

FIG 75.1 Stepwise Development of Arthritis in Rheumatoid Arthritis *APC,* Antigen presenting cells; *GM-CSF,* granulocyte-macrophage colony-stimulating factor; *IL,* interlukin; *RA,* rheumatoid arthritis; *TNF,* tumor necrosis factor. (Burmester GR, Feist E, Dörner T: Emerging cell and cytokine targets in rheumatoid arthritis *Nat Rev Rheumatol* 10:77–88, 2014.)

mandating testing prior to initiation of therapy.[9] Data suggest that anti-TNF therapy may be safe in chronic hepatitis C; however, TNF-α antagonists have resulted in reactivation of chronic hepatitis B if not given concurrently with antiviral therapy, also mandating pretreatment testing.[20] Solid tumors do not appear to be increased with anti-TNF therapy,[20] although variable rates of increased lymphoma risk have been described. Compared with those in the general population, no increase over patients with RA in general has been reported.[3] Use of

TNF-α antagonists in patients with heart failure remains an unsettled issue but probably should be avoided if possible in those with advanced heart disease.[7] The formation of autoantibodies may occur, including antinuclear antibody (ANA) and anti-double-stranded DNA (anti-dsDNA), and these autoantibodies may uncommonly be associated with clinical syndromes.[24] Rare cases of aplastic anemia, pancytopenia, vasculitis, and demyelinating disorders have also been reported. Progressive multifocal leukoencephalopathy (PML), a lethal rare brain

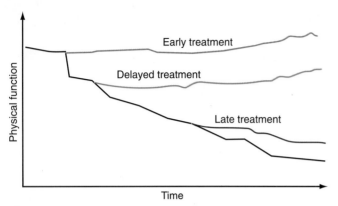

FIG 75.2 Why is early classification of rheumatoid arthritis (RA) needed? Over time, structural damage increases and physical function declines if RA is not treated effectively. Although institution of therapy in late RA can improve function to only a small extent, earlier treatment has the potential to stabilize physical function before permanent disability occurs. (In Aletaha D: Classification of rheumatoid arthritis. In Emery P, ed: *Atlas of rheumatoid arthritis*. London, 2015, Springer Healthcare Ltd.)

disease caused by reactivation of the JC virus, has been rarely described with anti-TNF therapy.[11] Finally, whether adverse events after orthopedic intervention are higher with these agents than with conventional DMARDs remains inconclusive, although recent data suggest that they are equally safe and may not require discontinuation. Previously, it was generally suggested they be discontinued 1 week prior to surgery and reinstituted 1 week thereafter, or depending on the frequency of administration of the agent itself, that surgery be performed at the latter end of the biologic half-life of the drug.[5]

Despite recent advances with biologic therapies, newer small molecules, and combination DMARD strategies, remission rates still remain suboptimal and patients with RA are still missing a considerable number of work days. More sensitive early diagnostic criteria are needed to ensure that appropriate treatment is initiated early to prevent joint damage, but there remains considerable discordance with those currently in place. Patients who develop RA have normal radiographs more than 75% of the time at presentation, whereas magnetic resonance imaging (MRI) can detect changes in most early RA patients whose x-rays are normal.[14] As mentioned earlier, high-resolution ultrasound can detect synovitis and classic erosions in many of

Recommendations for Patients With Symptomatic *Early RA*	Level of evidence (evidence reviewed)
1. Regardless of disease activity level, use a treat-to-target strategy rather than a non-targeted approach (PICO A.1).	Low (17)
2. If the disease activity is low, in patients who have never taken a DMARD: • Use DMARD monotherapy (MTX preferred) over double therapy (PICO A.2). • Use DMARD monotherapy (MTX preferred) over triple therapy (PICO A.3).	Low (18–21) Low (22–25)
3. If the disease activity is moderate or high, in patients who have never taken a DMARD: • Use DMARD monotherapy over double therapy (PICO A.4). • Use DMARD monotherapy over triple therapy (PICO A.5).	Moderate (18,20,21) High (22–25)
4. If disease activity remains moderate or high despite DMARD monotherapy (with or without glucocorticoids), use combination DMARDs *or* a TNFi *or* a non-TNF biologic (all choices with or without MTX, in no particular order of preference), rather than continuing DMARD monotherapy alone (PICO A.7).	Low (26–28)
5. If disease activity remains moderate or high despite DMARDs: • Use a TNFi monotherapy over tofacitinib monotherapy (PICO A.8). • Use a TNFi + MTX over tofacitinib + MTX (PICO A.9).	Low (29) Low (30)
6. If disease activity remains moderate or high despite DMARD (PICO A.6) or biologic therapies (PICO A.12), add low-dose glucocorticoids.	Moderate (31–37) Low (31–37)
7. If disease flares, add short-term glucocorticoids at the lowest possible dose and for the shortest possible duration (PICO A.10, A.11).	Very low (38–43)

FIG 75.3 2015 American College of Rheumatology Guideline for the Treatment of Rheumatoid Arthritis. Guidelines and recommendations developed and/or endorsed by the American College of Rheumatology (ACR) are intended to provide guidance for particular patterns of practice and not to dictate the care of a particular patient. (From Singh JA, Saag KG, Bridges SL Jr, et al: 2015 American College of Rheumatology guideline for the treatment of rheumatoid arthritis. *Arthritis Care Res* 68:1–25, 2016.)

Recommendations for Patients With *Established RA*[1]	Level of evidence (evidence reviewed)
1. Regardless of disease activity level, use a treat-to-target strategy rather than a non-targeted approach (PICO B.1).	Moderate (44–46)
2. If the disease activity is low, in patients who have never taken a DMARD, use DMARD monotherapy (MTX preferred) over a TNFi (PICO B.2).	Low (47,48)
3. If the disease activity is moderate or high in patients who have never taken a DMARD: • *Use DMARD monotherapy (MTX preferred) over tofacitinib (PICO B.3).* • *Use DMARD monotherapy (MTX preferred) over combination DMARD therapy (PICO B.4).*	*High (49)* *Moderate (18,20–25)*
4. If disease activity remains moderate or high despite DMARD monotherapy, use combination traditional DMARDs *or* add a TNFi *or* a non-TNF biologic *or* tofacitinib (all choices with or without MTX, in no particular order of preference), rather than continuing DMARD monotherapy alone (PICO B.5).	Moderate to very low (23,26,29,30,47,48,50–59)
5. If disease activity remains moderate or high despite TNFi therapy in patients who are currently not on DMARDs, add one or two DMARDs to TNFi therapy rather than continuing TNFi therapy alone (PICO B.6).	High (60–65)
6. If disease activity remains moderate or high despite use of a single TNFi: • *Use a non-TNF biologic, with or without MTX, over another TNFi with or without MTX (PICO B.12 and B.14).* • *Use a non-TNF biologic, with or without MTX, over tofacitinib with or without MTX (PICO B.13 and B.15).*	*Low to very low (66–72)* *Very low[4]*
7. If disease activity remains moderate or high despite use of a single non-TNF biologic, use another non-TNF biologic, with or without MTX, over tofacitinib, with or without MTX (PICO B.16 and B.17).	*Very low[4]*
8. If disease activity remains moderate or high despite use of multiple (2+) sequential TNFi therapies, first use a non-TNF biologic, with or without MTX, over another TNFi or tofacitinib (with or without MTX) (PICO B.8, B.9, B.10, B.11).	*Very low (73–75)*
9. If the disease activity still remains moderate or high despite the use of multiple TNFi therapies, use tofacitinib, with or without MTX, over another TNFi, with or without MTX, if use of a non-TNF biologic is not an option (PICO B.23 and B.24).	*Low (29,30)*
10. If disease activity remains moderate or high despite use of at least one TNFi and at least one non-TNF-biologic: • *First use another non-TNF biologic, with or without MTX, over tofacitinib (PICO B.21 and B.22).* • *If disease activity remains moderate or high, use tofacitinib, with or without MTX, over another TNFi (PICO B.19 and B.20).*	*Very low (29,30)* *Very low (29)*
11. If disease activity remains moderate or high despite use of DMARD, TNFi, or non-TNF biologic therapy, add short-term, low dose glucocorticoid therapy (PICO B.26 and B.27).	*High to moderate (33,41,76,77)*
12. If disease flares in patients on DMARD, TNFi, or non-TNF biologic therapy, add short-term glucocorticoids at the lowest possible dose and the shortest possible duration (PICO B.28 and B.29).	*Very low (40–43)*
13. If the patient is in remission: • *Taper DMARD therapy (PICO B.31)[2].* • *Taper TNFi, non-TNF biologic, or tofacitinib (PICO B.33, B.35, B.37) (please also see #15).*	*Low[3] (78)* *Moderate to very low[3] (79,80)*
14. If disease activity is low: • **Continue DMARD therapy (PICO B.30).** • **Continue TNFi, non-TNF biologic or tofacitinib rather than discontinuing respective medication (PICO B.32, B.34 and B.36).**	Moderate (78) High to very low (79,80)
15. If the patient's disease is in remission, *do not* discontinue all RA therapies (PICO B.38).	Very low[4]

FIG 75.4 2015 American College of Rheumatology Guideline for the Treatment of Rheumatoid Arthritis. Guidelines and recommendations developed and/or endorsed by the American College of Rheumatology (ACR) are intended to provide guidance for particular patterns of practice and not to dictate the care of a particular patient. (From Singh JA, Saag KG, Bridges SL Jr, et al: 2015 American College of Rheumatology guideline for the treatment of rheumatoid arthritis. *Arthritis Care Res* 68:1–25, 2016.)

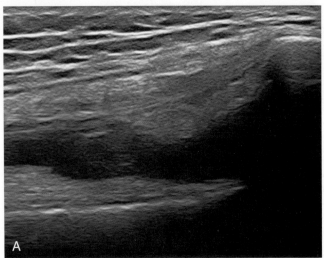
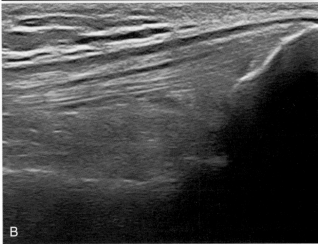

FIG 75.5 Ultrasound of the Knee Joint in an Rheumatoid Arthritis Patient Anterior longitudinal scan at the level of the suprapatellar recess. (A) Synovial hypertrophy and joint effusion are detected at baseline. (B) No evidence of synovitis is present at follow-up. (Iagnocco A, Finucci A, Ceccarelli F, et al: Power Doppler ultrasound monitoring of response to anti-tumour necrosis factor alpha treatment in patients with rheumatoid arthritis. *Rheumatology* 54:1890–1896, 2015. [Advance Access publication 11 June 2015].)

those patients not identified on x-ray as well. Better prognostic markers are also needed to identify patients with the potential for poor outcomes, for whom more aggressive strategies can be applied at the outset. For example, anticyclic citrullinated peptides (anti-CCP) in patients with early RA is a predictor of more active disease.[27] Patient preference is also important and may depend on mode and frequency of administration and, finally but significantly, the risks versus benefits as they continue to unfold. The newly released 2015 guidelines of the American College of Rheumatology (see Figs. 75.3 and 75.4) clearly define the role of the biologics and newer small molecules such as the JAK inhibitors in RA, as well as the role of conventional DMARDs, NSAIDs, steroids, and combinations thereof, as they relate to onset and severity of disease, and to early versus late intervention and prior treatment failures. Continued discussion and controversy will remain as more sensitive diagnostic criteria and their related tools such as ultrasound and newer biomarkers as well as more novel agents are introduced for the treatment of RA worldwide, and it will remain the clinician's task to keep their patients wisely informed.

KEY REFERENCES

1. Aaltonen KJ, Virkki LM, Malmivaara A, et al: Systematic review and meta-analysis of the efficacy and safety of existing TNF blocking agents in treatment of rheumatoid arthritis. *PLoS ONE* 7(1):e30275, 2012.

11. Codreanu C, Damjanov N: Safety of biologics in rheumatoid arthritis: data from randomized controlled trials and registries. *Biologics* 9:1–6, 2015.

26. Smolen JS, Breedveld FC, Burmester GR, et al: Treating rheumatoid arthritis to target: 2014 update of the recommendations of an international task force. *Ann Rheum Dis* 75:3–15, 2016.

The references for this chapter can also be found on www.expertconsult.com.

76

Hemophilia and Pigmented Villonodular Synovitis
Hemophilia and the Knee

Andrew G. Franks, Jr.

The knee is the most frequently affected joint in patients suffering from hemophilia. Hemophilia A and B are inherited X-linked bleeding disorders caused by a deficiency in specific clotting factors. The incidence of hemophilia is rare. About 1 in 10,000 people are born with it. The most common type of hemophilia is Factor VIII deficiency, also called hemophilia A or classic hemophilia. The second most common type is Factor IX deficiency, also called hemophilia B. The clinical hallmark of hemophilia is bleeding into the joints and muscles, which can occur spontaneously in the severe forms of the diseases or secondary to minor trauma. Recurrent hemarthroses produce deposits of hemosiderin and synovitis (Fig. 76.1). In the acute phase, hypertrophy of synovium occurs, causing a higher risk of repeated bleeding. A pannus may form, as in rheumatoid arthritis, with underlying cartilage destruction. With time, synovial fibrosis occurs, resulting in stiffness, pain, and subsequent disabling limited range of motion.[6] Differential diagnosis includes anterior cruciate ligament tear, intra-articular fracture, meniscus tear, capsular tear, and traumatic hemarthroses.

Imaging studies early in the disease reveal soft tissue swelling associated with the hemarthroses. Later stages include widening of epiphyseal regions caused by overgrowth from increased vascularity. Skeletal changes are initially manifested as subchondral sclerosis and cyst formation, with later loss of cartilage and secondary osteophyte formation. Squaring of the patella is seen, possibly resulting from overgrowth[14] (Fig. 76.2). Magnetic resonance imaging demonstrates the extensive synovitis that is commonly present (Fig. 76.3).

The principles adopted for replacement therapy as prophylactic cover for surgery are beyond the scope of this chapter. The development and availability of efficacious clotting factor concentrates over the last four decades has enabled surgeons to safely manage surgery in hemophiliac patients where even "minor" procedures have the potential for life-threatening bleeding complications. Unfortunately, commercial concentrates transmitted infections such as hepatitis and human immunodeficiency virus (HIV), which dramatically changed lives in the hemophiliac community and is still heavily affecting patients and doctors dealing with this disease.[7]

Patients with hemophilia require a specialized team and a hospital capable of supporting intense factor concentrate use and timely laboratory monitoring. A multidisciplinary approach is optimal, and includes the coordination and resources of a hematologist and if possible a comprehensive hemophilia treatment team working closely with the surgeon and anesthesiologist. With planning, teamwork, and careful postoperative follow-up, major and minor procedures can be performed with high rates of success.[27]

Patients are usually admitted 2 to 3 days prior to surgery to undergo all the biochemical and instrumental assessments that are useful for the intervention and general anesthesia. Blood is crossmatched according to the normal surgical blood-ordering policy of the hospital, taking into account that patients at high risk of bleeding may need more units than patients without hemophilia. The coagulation laboratory should be alerted to the potential need for frequent and/or unscheduled assays.[25]

Arthrocentesis is indicated to extract the hematic contents of the joint to reduce pain, improve the general condition, and prevent articular cartilage damage owing to the action of hemosiderin. Arthrocentesis is usually very easy because of capsular distension. The joint should be drained completely and washed if clots are present or there is any suspicion of septic arthritis. It is advisable to perform arthrocentesis in the following situations:

- A bleeding, tense, and painful joint that shows no improvement 24 hours after conservative treatment
- Joint pain that cannot be alleviated
- Evidence of neurovascular compromise of the limb
- Unusual increase in local temperature (septic arthritis)

A relative contraindication is the presence of an inhibitor, and an absolute contraindication is local skin infection. For postprocedure care, a splint and Jones dressing immobilization for 3 to 5 days helps to alleviate symptoms and prevent recurrence. Isometric exercises must be performed with the limb.[23]

PIGMENTED VILLONODULAR SYNOVITIS

Pigmented villonodular synovitis (PVNS) or intra-articular giant cell tumor, is a benign, locally aggressive, and recurrent disease arising from the synovial membrane.[17] The knee is the most commonly affected joint and the tumor usually occurs in patients between the ages of 30 and 40.[28] PVNS is

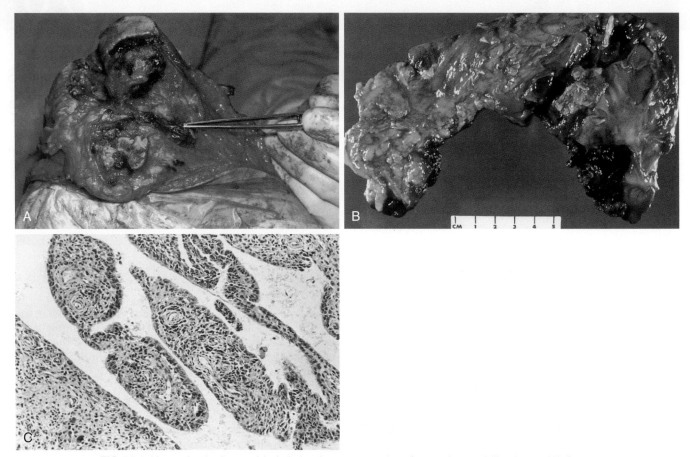

FIG 76.1 Hyperplastic, hemosiderin-laden brown synovium from a hemophiliac knee. (A) Gross appearance on arthrotomy. (B) Surgical specimen. (C) Microscopic specimen. (Fig. 73.2 from previous version.)

rare with an estimated incidence in the United States of 1.8 cases in 1 million people and does not seem to have any gender predisposition.[20]

Although the cause of PVNS remains unclear, it may be associated with chronic inflammatory disease within the joint and may occur after trauma or orthopedic intervention.[29] Recently, it has been suggested that PVNS is a neoplastic process with specific genetic features, but further studies are needed.[8] The typical histopathological finding, locally or diffusely within the joint, is synovial hyperplasia that appears villous, nodular, or villonodular with varying amounts of hemosiderin deposition[1] (Figs. 76.4 and 76.5).

The clinical presentation of PVNS is nonspecific with symptoms of pain and/or swelling being most common, often leading to a delay in diagnosis. Other reported symptoms such as limited range of motion and mechanical "locking" are less common.[16] Serum erythrocyte sedimentation rate (ESR) and C-reactive protein (CRP) may be elevated in some patients. Radiographs are also nonspecific, often just demonstrating an effusion.[1] Ultrasonography has revealed heterogeneously hypoechoic masses in the Hoffa fat pad, hyperemia, and a markedly thickened synovium, but these findings are nonspecific.[4] The most accurate screening method to obtain a diagnosis is magnetic resonance imaging (MRI), which reveals prominent

low signal intensity (seen with T2-weighting) and a "blooming" artifact from the hemosiderin (seen with gradient-echo sequences)[19] (Fig. 76.6A to C).

The goal of treatment of PVNS is to remove as much or all abnormal synovial tissue to relieve pain and lower the risk of joint destruction. Depending on whether involvement is local (LPVNS) or diffuse (DPVNS) the main therapeutic options for PVNS are arthroscopic synovectomy or open synovectomy.[3] Variations abound including arthroscopic partial synovectomy, arthroscopic total synovectomy, open anterior synovectomy, open total synovectomy, combined anterior arthroscopic synovectomy and open posterior synovectomy, and ultimately total knee arthroplasty.[9,15,20,12] Nonsurgical modalities alone or in combination with previous surgery, have also been widely used including external beam radiation and intra-articular radioactive isotopes.[18,13] Recently, anti-tumor necrosis factor (anti-TNF) alpha and Janus kinase (JAK) inhibitors have been tried in small case series.[24,26]

Recurrence rates with the different options and follow-up durations in the literature vary considerably because large randomized controlled trials have not been performed owing to the rarity of the disease.[10,22,5] However, a lower rate of postoperative complications has been reported after arthroscopic surgery techniques.[11,2]

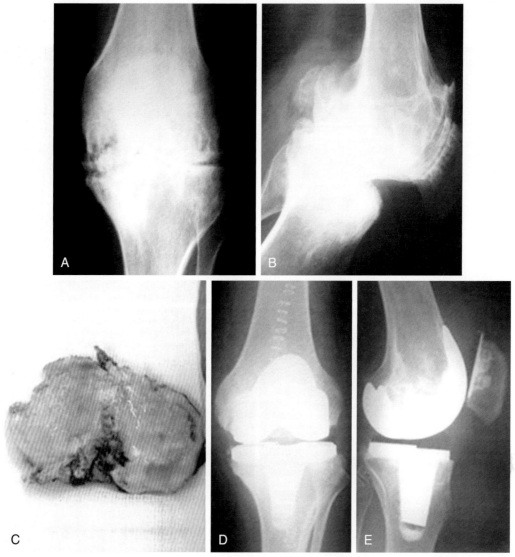

FIG 76.2 Total knee arthroplasty for severe hemophilic arthropathy: (A) Anteroposterior preoperative radiograph. (B) Lateral preoperative view. (C) Intraoperative view of the resected proximal tibia. (D) Postoperative anteroposterior view. (E) Lateral postoperative radiograph. (From Rodriguez-Merchan EC: Management of the hemophilic knee. In Caviglia HA, Solimeno LP, eds: Orthopedic surgery in patients with hemophilia, 2008, Springer-Verlag, Italia, p 146.)

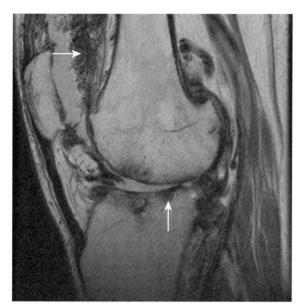

FIG 76.3 Hemophilic arthropathy of the knee seen on a sagittal proton density-weighted magnetic resonance image. Extensive synovitis of very low signal intensity is present in the suprapatellar recess, consistent with hemosiderin from recurrent hemarthroses *(horizontal arrow)*. In addition, full thickness cartilage loss and subchondral cysts are evident in the lateral compartment of the knee *(vertical arrow)*. (From Bleasel JF, ed: Hemophilia and von Willebrand disease. In *Rheumatology*, ed 6, Philadelphia, 2015, Mosby, pp 1615–1622.)

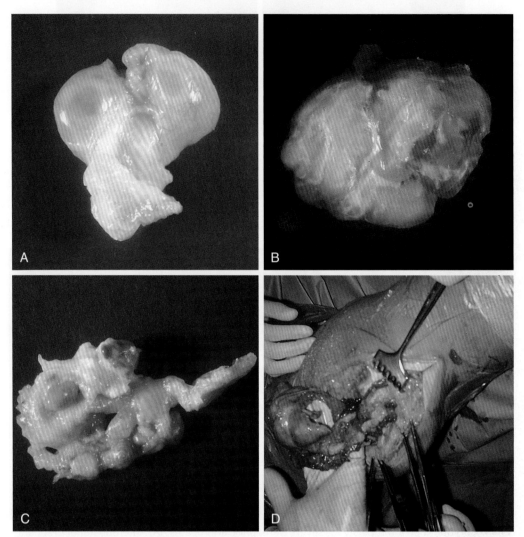

FIG 76.4 Pigmented villonodular synovitis/giant cell tumor of the tendon sheath. (A) Loose body. (B) Localized nodule (gross appearance, cross section). (C) Localized aggregate of multiple nodules. (D) Diffuse type throughout joint. (From Vigorita VJ: The synovium. In Vigorita VJ, Ghelman B, editors. *Orthopaedic pathology.* Philadelphia, 1999, Lippincott Williams & Wilkins.) [This was Fig. 73.9 from the previous edition]

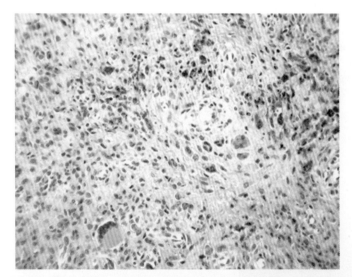

FIG 76.5 Pigmented villonodular synovitis. Photomicrograph (H&E, x20) demonstrates bland polyhedral cells surrounded by collagen. Giant cells and hemosiderin are present. (From Toy PC, Heck RK: Soft tissue tumors. In Canale ST, Beaty, JH, eds: Campbell's operative orthopaedics, ed 3, Philadelphia, 2013, Elsevier, pp 947-978.)

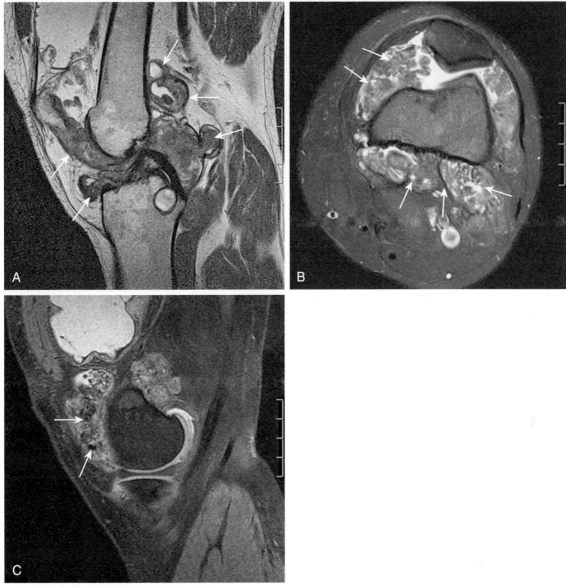

FIG 76.6 A 27-year-old male with pigmented villonodular synovitis of the left knee. Sagittal (A) and axial (B) T2-weighted images show an intra-articular synovial-based mass with predominantly hypointense signal intensity *(arrows)*. Gradient echo sequence sagittal plane image shows susceptibility artifacts *(arrows)* from hemosiderin deposition within this mass that are quite typical of pigmented villonodular synovitis (C). (From Ilaslan H, Barazi H, Sundaram M: Radiologic evaluation of soft tissue tumors. In Goldblum JR, Weiss SW, Folpe AL, eds: Enzinger and Weiss's soft tissue tumors, ed 6, Philadelphia, 2014, Elsevier. pp 25-75.)

The references for this chapter can also be found on www.expertconsult.com.

Human Immunodeficiency Virus Infection and Its Relationship to Knee Disorders

Henry Masur

When evaluating patients with human immunodeficiency virus (HIV) infection for knee surgery, orthopedists should recognize that many HIV-infected patients, especially those with CD4 counts >200 cells/mm^3, are excellent candidates for surgery. Complication rates are not substantially different from HIV-uninfected patients with other comparable comorbidities. HIV infection should have little impact on the decision to perform surgery or the postoperative results.

Patients who are well managed for their HIV infection with durable viral suppression have almost equal life expectancy compared with their non–HIV-infected peers. They are living active lives and are capable of participating in amateur or professional athletics and thus are susceptible to the same traumatic, degenerative, and infectious processes as the HIV-uninfected population.

Orthopedists must recognize that 15% to 30% of HIV-infected individuals in the United States are unaware of their HIV status. Their medical encounter with an orthopedics service is an excellent opportunity to test them for HIV infection because the Centers for Disease Control and Prevention (CDC) encourages that testing be done on an "opt-out" basis (ie, patients should be informed that HIV testing will be performed routinely unless the patient specifically declines).[15,106,126] Counseling prior to testing is not a requirement in most states and institutions (there are some exceptions) unless the patient is found to be HIV-infected, in which case counseling is required.

HIV poses a very small but finite risk for transmission in the operating room or during other procedures involving sharp objects or blood fluid exposure. There has never been a surgeon documented to have acquired HIV in the operating room, and there have been no occupational HIV infections reported in the United States since 2000.[32] Other blood-borne pathogens are much more worthy of attention in terms of likelihood of transmission from patient to health care provider via accidental exposures, such as hepatitis B and C.

EPIDEMIOLOGY OF HUMAN IMMUNODEFICIENCY VIRUS INFECTION

The CDC estimates that there are approximately 1.2 million Americans living with HIV infection. There are approximately 50,000 new cases in the United States each year, and this number of new cases has not changed substantially in 30 years. Approximately one-half are age 15 to 35 years. These demographics point out that in the United States, prevention efforts[25,33] have not been impressively effective (http://www.cdc.gov/hiv/statistics/index.html).[26] They also point out that many cases of undiagnosed HIV infection occur in young individuals who may be cared for in orthopedic practices.

In terms of transmission categories 30,000 new cases in 2013 were caused by male-to-male sexual contacts, 11,000 by high-risk heterosexual contacts, and 3000 to 5000 by injection drug use.

In many urban areas of the United States the rates of HIV infection are astonishingly high. For example, in Washington, DC,[24] 2.7% of the adult population is infected, including 6% of African American males.[65] In many urban areas in the United States 25% to 40% of HIV-infected individuals are estimated to be unaware of their HIV status and up to 50% of HIV-infected adolescents may be unaware of their infection. Some of these patients are not aware that they are participating in high-risk behavior. Others do not recognize the advantages of early diagnosis and treatment. Thus a considerable number of patients consulting orthopedists about musculoskeletal problems are unaware that they are infected.[36,48,85,128]

HIV-infected patients often lead active lives, participating in activities for fitness and recreation, as well as in competitive high school, college, and professional sports. Furthermore, weight training to build lean muscle mass is considered a standard component of treatment and prevention of wasting syndrome and lipodystrophy in HIV-infected individuals. Consequently, these persons experience trauma and degenerative processes just like their uninfected counterparts. These persons will come to orthopedic attention for processes that are clearly related to HIV infection and for syndromes that are related to the same traumatic and aging processes that afflict HIV-uninfected patients.

HUMAN IMMUNODEFICIENCY VIRUS VIROLOGY

Human T-cell lymphotropic virus type I (HTLV-I), HTLV-II, and HTLV-III (HIV-1 and HIV-2) are the four known human retroviruses. HIV-1 is by far the most important retrovirus of humans currently known and has been established as the causative agent of acquired immune deficiency syndrome (AIDS). Retroviruses are a group of RNA viruses that produce reverse transcriptase, an enzyme that converts viral RNA to proviral DNA. This proviral DNA is then integrated into the chromosomal DNA of the host cell.

The hallmark of HIV disease is a profound immunodeficiency resulting primarily from a progressive quantitative and qualitative deficiency of CD4 helper T lymphocytes.[70]

This subset of CD4 helper T cells is defined by the presence of the CD4$^+$ T-lymphocyte molecule on its surface. HIV infection is persistent and associated with an extended period during which the patient has no symptoms and has normal routine laboratory values. Infection stimulates an immune response to HIV that initially appears to hinder viral replication but fails to eradicate the virus.[4,42,64] Without therapy, almost all infected individuals ultimately experience a progressive deterioration in immune function that results in susceptibility to HIV-related complications and opportunistic infections.[20,48,53,70] Contemporary combination antiretroviral therapy reduces circulating virus, augments CD4 counts, reduces HIV-related complications, and prolongs survival.[48] Regardless of CD4 count and antiretroviral therapy, patients have an elevated lifetime risk for tuberculosis, pneumococcal disease, and malignant neoplasms.

TRANSMISSION OF HUMAN IMMUNODEFICIENCY VIRUS

HIV is transmitted between humans by the exchange of body fluids via two principal routes: sexual contact and parenteral inoculation. In the United States vertical transmission from an infected mother to her child is a rare event.[40] Fewer than 200 children are perinatally infected in the United States per year.

Body fluids identified as significant sources of HIV exposure include blood, semen (including pre-ejaculatory fluid), vaginal secretions, breast milk, and any body fluid containing blood.[29,100] Body fluids considered to represent minimal risk for transmission of HIV include feces, nasal secretions, sputum, saliva, sweat, tears, urine, and vomitus, unless contaminated with visible blood. Synovial fluid can be infected by HIV.

The quantity of virus isolated from a body fluid varies by site and stage of HIV infection. Viral burden in blood and other fluids is highest during acute infection before seroconversion.[42,64] However, even when the circulating viremia is quantitatively high, HIV has not been shown to be transmitted by casual contact or by insect vectors, such as mosquitoes.

Sexual Transmission

Throughout the world the predominant mode of HIV transmission is sexual contact. Homosexual contact has accounted for the preponderance of sexual transmission in developed countries. In developing countries most sexual transmission of HIV has been through heterosexual contact. Heterosexual transmission has been increasing in the United States.

Among men having sex with men, transmission of HIV is strongly associated with receptive anal intercourse. Even when intact, the thin, fragile rectal mucosa offers little protection against infection from deposited semen. Moreover, anal intercourse, as well as other sexual practices involving the rectum (such as "fisting" and insertion of objects), traumatizes the rectal mucosa, thereby increasing the likelihood of infection during receptive anal intercourse.

HIV can be transmitted to either partner through vaginal intercourse. There is an estimated 20-fold greater chance of transmission of HIV from a man to a woman than from a woman to a man by this means. This greater risk in women is thought to be due in part to the prolonged exposure to infected seminal fluid by the vaginal, cervical, and endometrial mucosa. Transmission of HIV is also closely associated with genital ulceration.

Although oral sex appears to be a less efficient mode of transmission of HIV, it is a misperception that oral sex is a form of "safe sex." HIV transmission has been reported as resulting solely from receptive fellatio and insertive cunnilingus. The risk appears to be increased by the presence of oral ulcerations and gum bleeding.

Transmission Associated With Intravenous Drug Use

HIV infection in intravenous drug users is highly prevalent throughout the world. Risk factors for HIV infection in intravenous drug users include the frequency of injection, the number of persons with whom needles are shared, anonymous sharing of needles and other paraphernalia, cocaine use, and the use of injection drugs in geographic locations with a high prevalence of HIV infection, such as inner-city areas.[38] This population appears to be functioning as the primary reservoir for the rapid spread of HIV infection into the heterosexual population throughout the world.[3,95]

Although the risk of infection is highest with direct sharing of needles, the sharing of drug paraphernalia, such as syringes, water, "spoons" and "cookers" (used to dissolve drugs in water and to heat drug solutions), and "cottons" (small pieces of cotton or cigarette filters used to filter out particles that could block the needle), can also increase the risk of transmission. An outbreak in rural Indiana was associated in 2015 with shared drug paraphernalia and heroin use. In one small community 153 cases of HIV infection were related to multigenerational drug use among the rural poor, living in an area with poor health care services.[41]

Street sellers of syringes and needles often repackage and sell such equipment as "sterile." Needle or syringe sharing for any use, including skin popping and injecting anabolic steroids, can put persons at risk for HIV and other blood-borne infections, such as hepatitis B and C.

Athletes have transmitted HIV to each other by sharing syringes for injection of illicit drugs designed to enhance performance.

Transmissions by Blood Transfusion and Bone Grafts

Currently, because of current screening programs, blood products almost never transmit HIV infection in the United States (http://www.cdc.gov/mmwr/preview/mmwrhtml/mm5941a3.htm). In this country, all blood products are screened for HIV for antibody and RNA and by donor questionnaire inquiring about high-risk behaviors and past infections. Such screening may fail to detect occasional cases of HIV infection, usually in very recently infected donors. Such transmission occurs only a few times per decade in the United States when blood is appropriately screened. The current risk is estimated to be 1 in 2 million transfused units in the United States.*

HIV transmission by blood transfusion is a substantial risk in many parts of the world. In the developing world, travelers or expatriates are often reassured that the blood they received came from reliable donors or was screened, but often the screening processes are far inferior to those used in this country.[129]

Orthopedists must also be aware that HIV can be transmitted by bone grafts. HIV infection of bone is well documented, although such events in the current era of screening should

---

*References 21, 31, 50, 88, 89, and 129.

be extremely rare, at least in the United States and western Europe.[19,28,103,125] The primary safeguards against potential transmission of HIV by bone allograft are serologic testing of donor patients, as well as carefully questioning regarding high-risk behavior.[88] The freezing step in bone tissue banking probably results in further reduction of the risk of transmission.[19,125]

Transmission Related to Sports

The transmission of infectious agents during sports has become a major interest in the United States, with attention focused on methicillin-resistant *Staphylococcus aureus* (MRSA) and herpes simplex. Close person-to-person contact on the athletic field and in the locker rooms, as well as sharing clothing, combs, razors, and towels, provide ample opportunity for transmission of microorganisms by skin-to-skin contact or skin-to-inanimate object contact.

However, in contrast to MRSA and herpes simplex virus (HSV), no cases of HIV transmission have been documented to date during participation in athletic activities. The risk of transmission during sports participation is estimated to be extremely low, and it would be expected to occur only after blood from an infected individual came into contact with mucous membranes or open skin of an uninfected athlete or trainer. Without visible blood, there appears to be no measurable risk of HIV transmission through sports activities.

Human bites could in theory transmit HIV, but such bites are also very, very low risk. When the health care staff deal with injured players, the risk of HIV transmission is therefore extremely remote, especially if the athletic staff have intact skin and if they use gloves and barriers to prevent blood contact.

In their joint position statement on HIV and other blood-borne pathogens in sports, the American Medical Society for Sports Medicine and the American Academy of Sports Medicine in 1995 recommended that sports medicine practitioners should play a role in the education of infected and uninfected athletes, their families, and the sports community regarding disease transmission and prevention.[132]

This approach to educate athletes about HIV still seems prudent because the advice is relevant to several blood-borne pathogens, especially hepatitis C virus (HCV) and hepatitis B virus (HBV). Athletes should be advised that it is their responsibility to report wounds and injuries in a timely manner. If an athlete is bleeding, sports participation should be interrupted. After the wound stops bleeding and has been antiseptically cleaned and securely bandaged, participation may be resumed. Universal precautions (usually satisfied by the treating providers wearing disposable gloves) and basic principles of hygiene should be observed.

The position statement asserts that sports medicine practitioners should be knowledgeable about management issues involving HIV-infected athletes and should maintain the confidentiality of HIV-infected athletes. Such confidentiality policies clearly mandated that some athletes (those with HIV infection) should not be managed in public forums differently from uninfected athletes.

Occupational Transmission of Human Immunodeficiency Virus From Patient to Provider

As of December 31, 2013, 58 confirmed occupational transmissions of HIV, plus 150 possible transmissions have been reported in the United States since the beginning of the epidemic in 1982. Remarkably, only one confirmed case has been reported since 1999. As noted previously no surgeon has been documented to have acquired HIV from patient contact inside or outside the operating room.

Health care workers who are exposed to a needlestick involving HIV-infected blood at work have a 0.23% risk of becoming infected. Risk of exposure because of splashes with body fluids is thought to be near zero, even if the fluids are overtly bloody. Fluid splashes to intact skin or mucous membranes are considered to be extremely low risk of HIV transmission, whether or not blood is involved.

In the 1980s prominent orthopedic surgeons refused to perform orthopedic procedures on HIV-infected patients because of the risk to staff, and the short life expectancy of the patients. As more information has become available, data-based policies have been established that confirm the concept that the risk of transmission of HIV to operating room staff by any mechanism (needlesticks, mucosal splashes, bone dust or fragments) is not zero but is vanishingly small.[61,62,71,77] Other pathogens, such as hepatitis B and C, pose far greater risks to nonimmune health care providers.[35,90]

Given their prolonged and repeated exposure to potentially large volumes of blood, surgeons' concerns about possible occupational acquisition of HIV infection are understandable. However, studies have documented that inpatient and outpatient nurses, followed by house staff and operating room nurses and technicians, are at greatest risk for occupational sharp instrument injuries,[102] the type of injury most likely to be associated with transmission of HIV infection.

Factors that may influence the risk of HIV transmission during surgery include the skill and training level of the surgeon, the surgical procedure being performed, the volume and duration of blood exposure during the procedure, the number of procedures performed, and conditions under which the procedure is performed (ie, emergency versus elective).[8] Practices undertaken to reduce the risk of exposure to HIV and other blood-borne pathogens include restriction of operating room personnel to essential and experienced staff, double-gloving, use of protective eyewear and appropriate garment shields, and minimization of sharp instrument use.[8,23,97,116]

Although HIV has been demonstrated to remain viable in the cool vapors and aerosols produced by several common surgical power instruments, aerosols have not been documented to cause any transmissions of HIV.[79] Interestingly, no infectious HIV has been detected in aerosols generated by electrocautery or manual wound irrigation syringes.

The risk of becoming infected with HIV after any exposure to body fluid of any type is low. When blood or infected fluids come into contact with intact skin, the risk of transmission is negligible. For mucosal exposure the risk is approximately 0.09%. For needlestick injuries the likelihood of transmission is approximately 0.33%.

Each exposure must be individually evaluated in terms of determining risk. How much circulating virus the source patient had at the time of the event, what type of body fluid or tissue was involved, how deep or extensive was the wound or exposure, and how thoroughly and rapidly the injured area was irrigated are all relevant factors. There is no formula for assessing these factors and estimating the risk for transmission.

Although nurses have fewer exposures per year than surgeons, there are more nurses in the United States than surgeons. Thus nurses have been the most heavily represented among HIV occupational exposures. As a group evaluated for lifetime exposures a higher percent of nurses have had an exposure (37.9%) than physicians who are residents or fellows (11.4%), attending physicians (10.7%), attending surgeons (9.0%), phlebotomists (5.4%), and nonlaboratory technologists (4.7%).

In one notable study a survey performed with 699 surgeons-in-training at 17 medical centers found that the mean number of needlestick injuries by the final year of residency was 7.7 and that 99% of residents had at least one needlestick injury, often with a high-risk patient. Many of these occurred because of haste or fatigue.[58,94]

Orthopedic procedures have generally been shown to have a relatively low percutaneous injury rate when compared with other surgical subspecialty procedures. In one observational study, total knee replacement and open reduction plus internal fixation of the hip were shown to have percutaneous exposure rates of 8% and 7%, respectively. All other orthopedic procedures were shown to have a combined percutaneous exposure rate of 2%.[136] The incidence of skin and mucous membrane contact with blood has been estimated to be 16.7 contacts per 100 orthopedic procedures.[137] To date, there are no confirmed seroconversions among surgeons and no seroconversions because of suture needle exposures.[49,58,90,94]

Universal precautions recommended by the CDC to protect health care workers from contact with potentially infected body fluids emphasize barrier techniques to prevent skin and mucous membrane exposure to blood and other body fluids.[1,27] As noted previously, it is not always obvious who has an HIV infection because a substantial fraction of cases are unrecognized and because so many patients are unwilling to recognize that they are at high risk because of sexual or drug-using behavior. Hospitals are encouraged to test patients universally, allowing patients to "opt out" rather than "opt in." However, many hospitals have not yet adopted this policy. Therefore all patients should be assumed to have blood-borne pathogens, such as HIV or some other known or unknown pathogen.

In 1992 the United States Occupational Safety and Health Administration (OSHA) established mandatory regulations requiring national standards for the prevention of occupational exposure to hepatitis B and HIV, including guidelines for disposal of sharp instruments, such as using designated boxes and not recapping needles. A review of the circumstances of reported exposures suggests that the risk of transmission could have been decreased or prevented if universal precautions and OSHA guidelines had been followed. This observation is supported by an observational study of percutaneous injuries during surgery, in which injuries often occurred when fingers were used instead of instruments to hold tissue or suture needles during suturing or when instruments were being handled by a coworker.[136]

Thus, although health care workers often worry more about HIV than other blood-borne pathogens, more health care workers die each year because of occupationally acquired hepatitis B than HIV. Thus vaccination against blood-borne pathogens should be mandatory for health care workers. There is an effective vaccine against hepatitis B, but unfortunately there is no effective vaccine against HIV or hepatitis C.

HUMAN IMMUNODEFICIENCY VIRUS–INFECTED HEALTH CARE WORKERS: RISK OF TRANSMISSION TO PATIENTS

In the past there was concern that health care workers infected with HIV might transmit HIV to their patients.[55] Few controversies involving HIV infection have generated as much media or public sector commentary as the highly publicized incident of HIV transmission from a Florida dentist to at least six of his patients in 1991.[34,39] Documentation that the dentist was the source of infection was based on the lack of alternative substantive risk factors in several of his patients, all patients undergoing multiple procedures (including extractions) after onset of the dentist's symptomatic disease, and genetic analysis of HIV strains. Although it is evident that the dentist was the source of infection in these patients, the mechanism of transmission remains unclear.

Two reports from Europe have also reported possible transmissions. Lot et al. reported a case of probable transmission of HIV from an orthopedic surgeon to a patient in France.[92] Other reports followed.[14,37,62]

In another investigation, after HIV infection was diagnosed in a surgeon in Israel in 1995, serologic tests were obtained from 983 patients of the infected surgeon. One patient tested positive. That patient, a 67-year-old woman, had no other identifiable risk factors for HIV exposure. She tested negative for HIV before placement of a total hip prosthesis with a bone graft. She subsequently underwent hip aspiration and removal of the prosthesis by the same surgeon. This woman received two units of packed red blood cells after the third procedure. However, the donor of the bone graft and both units of blood tested negative for HIV infection. The patient had no reported sexual exposure to HIV. In addition, the surgeon reported a high frequency of intraoperative injury. Molecular analysis indicated that the viral sequences obtained from the surgeon and patient were closely related.[12] The patient did undergo noninvasive tooth whitening in Indonesia, where HIV infection is prevalent. Thus the mechanism and date of transmission could not be definitively established. It appears as though the most likely source of infection was the surgeon.[62]

Using look-back studies and other data, the CDC estimated the risk of HIV transmission from provider to patient to be 1 in 2.4 million to 24 million cases.[†] Thus the risk of provider-to-patient transmission of HIV during invasive procedures does exist, but this risk is exceedingly small. Since 1995 there have been no well-documented cases of such transmission.

The Infectious Disease Society of America and the Society of Health Care Epidemiology have issued guidelines regarding the management of health care workers who are infected with HIV, HBV, and HCV. These guidelines represent the opinions of professional societies. The CDC has also issued guidelines.[10,86,113]

DIAGNOSIS OF HUMAN IMMUNODEFICIENT VIRUS INFECTION

Testing for HIV infection is accurate, sensitive, and specific in all but a few unusual situations. Antibody tests become positive within 3 to 12 weeks in most cases, and nucleic acid amplification tests become positive within 3 to 4 days of infection acquisition for the common strains of HIV seen in the United States.

All patients should consider undergoing HIV testing even if they do not perceive themselves to be at risk. How often

---

[†]References 11, 14, 35, 37, 46, 92, and 117.

testing should be done depends on the frequency of high-risk behavior.

Virtually every patient who is HIV antibody positive will have detectable, circulating viremia. This should be measured by one of several approved nucleic acid amplification tests.

Informed consent is not necessary in most states with regard to HIV testing. Most states are reducing the barriers to widespread testing by reducing time-consuming counseling for uninfected persons, although such counseling is always useful if staff are available to perform it. However, HIV results can have devastating personal and financial repercussions, and thus confidentiality is important, as is the responsibility to follow-up with positive patients to ensure that they are informed and referred to care and to ensure that the result is reported to the health department.

In the United States high-risk activities include any type of unprotected intercourse, sharing of needles, or receipt of blood or organs from other individuals. This logically leads to regular testing for those with a prior sexually transmitted disease, pregnancy, and exposure to contaminated needles, as soon as their infection is recognized if the individual is willing to take oral therapy reliably.

CLINICAL MANIFESTATIONS OF HUMAN IMMUNODEFICIENT VIRUS INFECTION

The clinical manifestations of HIV infection include (1) an acute syndrome associated with primary infection, (2) a prolonged asymptomatic state, and (3) a period of profound immunosuppression during which clinical manifestations occur.

Natural history studies of HIV infection in individuals not receiving antiretroviral therapy or prophylaxis for *Pneumocystis jiroveci* pneumonia (PCP) indicate that the average time from initial infection to an AIDS-defining diagnosis is approximately 10 years and the time from an AIDS-defining diagnosis to death is approximately 1 year, although significant variation exists.[3,111] In contrast, patients receiving potent antiretroviral combinations and aggressive prophylaxis and treatment of opportunistic infections are living longer.[36,48] Some have been clinically and immunologically stable for two to three decades.

With few exceptions, the level of CD4[+] T-lymphocyte cells in blood decreases gradually and progressively in untreated HIV-infected individuals and is the classic marker for disease progression. The rate of decline in CD4[+] T-lymphocyte cell counts and the absolute viral burden have been shown to correlate with the time to development of clinical manifestations.[104] Patients often remain asymptomatic during this progressive decline. Active viral replication and progressive immunological impairment occur throughout the course of HIV infection in most patients, even during the clinically latent stage.[111] CD4[+] T-lymphocyte cell dysfunction has been demonstrated in patients early in the course of infection, even when the CD4[+] T-lymphocyte cell count is in the low-normal range. Immunological activation by HIV appears to cause this qualitative dysfunction. Most AIDS-defining opportunistic infections and malignancies occur in the advanced stage of disease. Some manifestations, such as tuberculosis, bacterial respiratory infections, and lymphoma, can occur at all stages of HIV infection.

Three basic mechanisms are thought to underlie the production of AIDS-defining complications: depletion and functional impairment of CD4[+] T-lymphocyte cell counts resulting in

susceptibility to opportunistic infections and malignancies; development of immune complex–mediated events, such as glomerulonephritis and thrombocytopenia; and damage to specific organs, such as the heart, brain, peripheral nerves, and lungs, because of direct or indirect retroviral effects. The time-frame in which these events unfold and the precise disease manifestation in an individual are highly variable, impossible to predict, and presumably the result of a complex interaction between viral factors and host defense mechanisms. Viral factors include size of the inoculum, strain-specific virulence, and viral replicative accuracy and efficiency. Host factors that may predispose to disease progression, such as age at the time of infection, route of transmission, sex, ethnicity, and coinfection with other infectious agents, are less defined.

There is growing recognition that HIV viremia is associated with systemic inflammatory responses that can be measured by serum cytokine levels, serum CRP levels and erythematous sedimentation rates (ESRs). As patients live longer and develop AIDS-related opportunistic infections less often, patients are developing chronic liver, kidney, and heart disease, which seem to be accelerated by this systemic inflammatory response.[87,107,119]

Primary Human Immunodeficiency Virus Infection

Orthopedists should recognize that acute myalgias, arthralgias, and even arthritis can be manifestations of primary HIV infection. When individuals acquire HIV infection, 50% to 70% experience an acute clinical syndrome 3 to 6 weeks after the acquisition of infection.[‡]

Clinical manifestations may include generalized symptoms, such as fever, fatigue, malaise, pharyngitis, headache, photophobia, myalgias, anorexia, nausea, vomiting, and diarrhea, as well as neurologic complications, such as meningitis, encephalitis, peripheral neuropathy, and myelopathy. Findings may include a morbilliform rash, mucocutaneous ulcerations, thrush, generalized lymphadenopathy, hepatosplenomegaly, elevated transaminase levels, and leukopenia with atypical lymphocytes. Arthralgias, but not usually arthritis, can be a prominent aspect of primary infection. The severity and constellation of manifestations vary. The illness is self-limited, with resolution of symptoms within days to weeks.

Seroconversion occurs within 3 to 12 weeks after the acquisition of HIV in 99% of exposed persons.[75,84] Viremia can be detected by nucleic acid amplification tests within 4 to 7 days after the acquisition of infection and thus is the best approach to early identification of the infection.

Well-documented cases of seroconversion more than 12 weeks after infection are extremely rare. Thus, although patients are often followed with serology and polymerase chain reaction (PCR) tests for 24 weeks, the likelihood that they are truly infected is remote.

The clinical manifestations of acute HIV syndrome coincide with a rapid rise in the plasma level of viral RNA and p24 antigen, widespread dissemination of virus, and a drop in the CD4[+] T-lymphocyte cell count.[57] The associated immunodeficiency at this stage results from both reduced numbers and functional impairment of CD4[+] T-lymphocyte cells and can be accompanied by opportunistic infections. An immune response subsequently develops and leads to a decrease in the plasma level of viral RNA, an increase in the CD4[+] T-lymphocyte cell

---

[‡]References 43, 47, 56, 59, 84, and 135.

count, and gradual resolution of symptoms. In most patients the CD4$^+$ T-lymphocyte cell count remains mildly depressed for a period before progressively declining to more markedly abnormal levels. There is considerable biologic variability among patients: a few will have fulminant falls in CD4$^+$ counts within the first few years. On the other end of the spectrum, a few will survive with intact immune systems and low viral loads for many years. These latter patients, termed *long-term nonprogressors*, or *elite nonprogressors*, appear able to control their viral infection and to avoid long-term consequences of their infection.[118]

Asymptomatic Infection

The asymptomatic stage of HIV infection is referred to as *clinical latency*. Active viral replication continues during this asymptomatic period. Although viral loads in many patients, particularly those taking potent antiretroviral combinations, may be determined to be below the level of detection in the blood with currently available tests, it has been shown that the virus is still replicating in other reservoirs such as lymphoid tissue.[114]

The rate of disease progression is directly correlated with HIV RNA levels. In most cases a patient with high levels of HIV RNA will progress to symptomatic disease faster than will a patient with low levels of HIV RNA. Although the length of time from initial infection to development of clinical disease varies greatly, the median time is approximately 10 years in the absence of antiretroviral therapy or PCP prophylaxis. Multiple studies have shown that progression to AIDS, the frequency of opportunistic infections, and survival correlate directly with CD4$^+$ T-lymphocyte cell counts.[30,99,115,130]

The term *long-term nonprogressor* refers to the rare individual who has been infected with HIV for 10 or more years and whose CD4$^+$ T-lymphocyte cell counts have remained in the normal range despite lack of antiretroviral therapy. These patients generally have a low level of viremia and some may have such a low level that commercial assays will not detect the virus.[118]

Early Symptomatic Disease, Acquired Immune Deficiency Syndrome, and Opportunistic Infections, and Tumors

All patients with HIV infection have an enhanced likelihood of developing tuberculosis, pneumococcal diseases, and malignant neoplasms. After the CD4$^+$ T-lymphocyte cell count falls below 500 cells/mm^3, most signs and symptoms of clinical illness characteristically begin to develop. Common clinical features of early symptomatic disease include vulvovaginal and oropharyngeal candidiasis (thrush), oral hairy leukoplakia, persistent generalized lymphadenopathy, dermatomal herpes zoster (shingles), recurrent herpes simplex, aphthous ulcers, molluscum contagiosum, condyloma acuminatum, and thrombocytopenia. Individuals may also experience constitutional symptoms, such as persistent fever to 38.5°C or diarrhea lasting more than 1 month. The occurrence of these events in an otherwise asymptomatic individual should prompt consideration of underlying HIV infection.

Opportunistic infections are defined as infections that occur in a specific population with greater frequency or severity than in a normal patient population. Opportunistic infections are generally encountered when the CD4$^+$ T-lymphocyte cell count declines below 200 cells/mm^3. Many of the organisms that cause

opportunistic infections, such as *P. jiroveci*, *Mycobacterium avium* complex (MAC), and cytomegalovirus (CMV), are ubiquitous in nature and do not ordinarily cause disease in the absence of a compromised immune system. Opportunistic infections can also be caused by common bacterial and mycobacterial pathogens. Such infections are the leading cause of morbidity and mortality in HIV-infected individuals who are not receiving drug therapies. With the development of more effective management of HIV and more aggressive treatment and prophylaxis of opportunistic infections, the clinical spectrum of disease caused by opportunistic organisms will continue to change.

The median time from the onset of severe immunosuppression (CD4$^+$ T-lymphocyte cell count <200 cells/mm^3) to an AIDS-defining diagnosis is 12 to 18 months in persons not receiving antiretroviral therapy.[53,81] Studies have shown that in patients receiving monotherapy with zidovudine (AZT) (a monotherapy regimen with modest activity) this timeframe was delayed by 9 to 10 months.[66] For patients adherent to currently recommended regimens, patients can be stable for many years, and perhaps lifelong if they are adherent to their therapy.

The most common opportunistic infections encountered in HIV-infected persons are PCP, pneumococcal pneumonia, mucocutaneous candidiasis, cryptococcosis, toxoplasmosis, CMV retinitis and colitis, dermatomal herpes zoster, tuberculosis, and disseminated MAC. Patients are also predisposed to certain neoplastic processes, including Kaposi sarcoma, lymphoma, cervical and rectal carcinoma, multicentric Castleman disease, and primary effusion cell lymphoma. Some of these occasionally involve bone, such as Kaposi sarcoma and lymphoma.[105]

Neoplastic processes also are overrepresented among HIV-infected patients. Kaposi sarcoma and lymphoma have been considered AIDS-defining diseases. However, other solid tumors appear to be overrepresented because of HIV infection itself or because of overrepresentation of traditional risk factors. For instance, tobacco abuse is very frequent among HIV-infected patients: lung carcinoma is becoming a more and more common complication in this population.

Other tumors that are overrepresented included hepatoma, often related to hepatitis B or C or alcohol abuse; and cervical and rectal carcinoma related to human papillomavirus infection. Thus, when evaluating patients for orthopedic problems, clinicians need to consider primary and metastatic tumors. There is no evidence that primary bone tumors are overrepresented among HIV-infected patients.

HIV-related manifestations that appear to be related to the virus and immune response, can also be prominent clinical features, including cardiomyopathy, encephalopathy, and cytopenias.[6]

TREATMENT OF HUMAN IMMUNODEFICIENCY VIRUS INFECTION

Management of Antiretroviral Drugs

The explosion of information regarding HIV, the increasing number of antiretroviral medications, the development of resistance to these medications, and the long-term survival of many patients with HIV have led to increasing complexity in the treatment of HIV-infected individuals.[85,128]

This complexity has necessitated the formalization of guidelines for the management of antiretroviral agents, management and prophylaxis of opportunistic infections, and management of occupational exposure to HIV and recommendations for postexposure prophylaxis. These guidelines are prepared by a panel of leading experts in the field of HIV care and the US Department of Health and Human Services. They are frequently updated and readily available online (www .aidsinfo.nih.gov).[1,111]

Antiretroviral therapies are medically complex and associated with a significant number of adverse effects and drug interactions, which can complicate both physician management and patient adherence. Although the guidelines recommend that management of HIV-infected individuals be supervised by a physician experienced in HIV care, almost all physicians will participate in the care of HIV-infected individuals at some time and thus should be familiar with the principles set forth by the guidelines. They should be particularly aware that whenever new drugs are prescribed, drug interactions require expert management by an experienced clinician.

SPECIFIC ISSUES RELATED TO PERIOPERATIVE MANAGEMENT OF HUMAN IMMUNODEFICIENCY VIRUS-INFECTED PATIENTS

Perioperative Morbidity and Mortality

There is little convincing evidence that HIV infection has significant impact on surgical morbidity or mortality for patients with suppressed viremia and good performance status. HIV-infected patients with advanced immunosuppression, active opportunistic infections, widespread neoplastic disease, or poor performance status would plausibly have additional risk.[‡]

Preoperative Evaluation of Human Immunodeficiency Virus-Infected Patients

No formal guidelines have been established for the preoperative evaluation of HIV-infected patients. In general, consultation with a clinician experienced in the care of HIV-infected individuals is appropriate.

Patients with HIV infection must be assessed in the context of how advanced their HIV disease is, what morbidities and comorbidities they have, and what drugs they are taking. There is no evidence that routine HIV screening prior to surgery is useful or cost effective in terms of surgical management now that universal precautions are the standard of care for all patients. However, as noted, hospitals should aggressively screen patients for HIV to identify patients and get them into care before they develop a serious complication.

Patients must also be screened for active infections. Patients at all CD4 levels are predisposed to tuberculosis, although admittedly tuberculosis is not common in the United States among US-born individuals.

Patients with advanced HIV infection often have hematologic abnormalities that are an important issue prior to surgery. Thrombocytopenia, anemia, leucopenia, and coagulopathies should all be screened for.

Patients also have endocrinologic issues. Adrenal insufficiency can be seen in patients with advanced disease, and hypothyroidism is also seen on occasion. Testing patients with advanced disease for adrenal function prior to surgery would be prudent in many situations.

Prior to surgery, there must also be careful assessment of current medications by a clinician with HIV expertise. The advice of an expert is needed to determine whether antiretroviral agents should be continued during surgery or discontinued. Most antiretroviral agents are available only as oral agents. Poor absorption of drugs and low serum levels can lead to lifelong drug resistance and the loss of classes of agents for antiretroviral therapy. In some situations discontinuation of antiretroviral drugs is preferable to erratic absorption.

Many antiretroviral agents inhibit or augment hepatic drug metabolism. Thus careful consideration must be given to the effects of antiretroviral agents on narcotic and sedative doses, anticoagulant doses, or other agents used in perioperative management. Although there are excellent websites reviewing such interactions, the advice of an expert is extremely useful. Antiretroviral effects on hepatic metabolism can persist for days after the antiretroviral agents are stopped.

Postoperative Management of Human Immunodeficiency Virus–Infected Patients

Postoperative management of HIV-infected patients should not differ markedly from that of HIV-uninfected patients. As noted previously, drug doses for any agent that is hepatically metabolized must be carefully calculated based on knowledge of that interaction.

HIV-infected patients need to resume their preoperative medications as soon as feasible. This is important not only for antiretroviral agents, but for chemoprophylactic drugs aimed at preventing opportunistic infections as well.

HIV-infected patients should develop the same postoperative infections as other patients. Wound infections and pneumonia are most likely to be caused by the same pathogens as HIV-uninfected patients.

Should patients respond to conventional therapy slowly, opportunistic infections should be considered. If patients are septic or hypotensive, surgeons should be cognizant that adrenal insufficiency is more likely in this population. Again, evaluation of such patients is optimally performed in conjunction with a clinician experienced in managing HIV-infected patients.

MANAGEMENT OF OCCUPATIONAL EXPOSURE TO HUMAN IMMUNODEFICIENCY VIRUS

Many experts suggest that all health care workers consider the pros and cons of postexposure prophylaxis before an occupational exposure occurs so that they may be better prepared to take immediate action and to cope with the anxiety of decision making and the uncertainty of outcome. All known and suspected exposures should be reported, regardless of how small the perceived risk, because the collective data continue to provide much of our understanding regarding transmission risk.[80,86]

Guidelines for the drugs to use in postexposure prophylaxis are updated regularly. An expert should be consulted to determine if there is relevant information about the likely or documented drug susceptibility of the source virus and if there are host factors favoring one drug regimens versus another in terms of toxicities or drug interactions.

- Start postexposure prophylaxis as soon as possible after exposure—if possible, within hours of the exposure and certainly within 72 to 96 hours.

[‡]References 2, 52, 67, 68, 91, 93, 124, 133, and 142.

- Use a highly potent regimen, similar to those recommended for treatment, to which the infecting virus is not likely to be resistant.
- Reassess after 48 to 72 hours to be certain that the facts of the case warrant prophylaxis.
- Reassess after 48 to 72 hours to make certain that the drugs chosen are appropriate given the source of virus.
- Monitor the health care provider carefully for tolerance and adherence; health care providers have a poor record of completing a full 4-week regimen.
- Continue for 4 weeks of therapy.
- Retest the health care worker at 4, 12, and 24 weeks to determine whether HIV infection has occurred, recognizing as noted previously that in the current era occupational transmission of HIV is an exceedingly rare event in the United States.

The drugs recommended for therapy are changing regularly based on new data and new drug availability. Because there are now almost 30 different drugs in six mechanistic categories, the selection of the best regimen should be made by a clinician who has expertise and experience in dealing with HIV infection on a regular basis.

HUMAN IMMUNODEFICIENCY VIRUS INFECTION AND MUSCULOSKELETAL DISEASE

Almost 75% of HIV-infected individuals report musculoskeletal symptoms.[24,82,110,141] Infectious, inflammatory, and neoplastic processes are all represented in the spectrum of rheumatic manifestations of HIV disease. The frequency and type of processes clinically manifested appear to be a function of the patient's level of immunosuppression and primary risk factor for HIV infection. Infectious, neoplastic, and rheumatologic processes are all part of the differential diagnosis.

Musculoskeletal Infections

Septic arthritis, osteomyelitis, pyomyositis, avascular necrosis, and bursitis are the most common orthopedic infectious complications seen in patients with HIV infection.[§] Infection occurs with conventional or atypical bacteria, fungi, or other opportunistic organisms. The diagnosis depends on isolation of the infecting organism from synovial fluid, bone, muscle, or blood.

Mycobacterium tuberculosis has been associated with infectious musculoskeletal disorders in HIV-infected patients, especially among immigrants from countries where tuberculosis is endemic. Classic Pott disease still occurs. Tuberculosis appears to be a very aggressive disease associated with frequent dissemination, multidrug resistance, and high mortality in patients with HIV infection. Consequently, orthopedic surgeons must be aware that pulmonary disease may coexist and must take appropriate respiratory isolation precautions to prevent the spread of infection to other patients and health care workers.

Septic arthritis is usually monoarticular, with the knee[76] and hip[109] most commonly involved. Unusual sites of joint infection, including the sternoclavicular and sacroiliac joints and the intervertebral disks, have been described in intravenous drug users.[82] Infection of the joint occurs via hematogenous spread

---

§References 63, 76, 106, 108, 109, and 140.

or direct extension from an adjacent soft-tissue or bone infection. Polyarticular involvement is generally seen in the setting of disseminated disease.

S. aureus and *Candida albicans* are the most frequently isolated causes of septic arthritis and osteomyelitis.[76,108,109] In addition to a variety of conventional bacterial organisms, several uncommon organisms have been isolated, including fungi, *M. tuberculosis*, and atypical mycobacteria.[120] Clinically, septic arthritis caused by *S. aureus* is manifested similarly in seropositive and seronegative patients. Erythema, effusion, and tenderness are usually noted on examination. Although atypical organisms, such as fungi and mycobacteria, often result in a chronic infectious arthritis in seronegative individuals, an acute or subacute infectious arthritic process may ensue in seropositive patients.[82]

Even though effusion is often present, synovial fluid cultures may be negative despite the presence of organisms on Gram stain, wet mount, or acid-fast bacillus smears.[76] Blood cultures may be helpful in definitively establishing a microbiological diagnosis.[44,98] Synovial biopsies may be necessary to isolate fungi and mycobacteria from joints. Imaging studies, such as serial radiograms and/or radionuclide bone scans, should be performed in patients with septic arthritis to eliminate the possibility of coexistent osteomyelitis.[82] In addition, septic bursitis caused by *S. aureus* has been reported in a number of patients with HIV infection.[140]

Septic arthritis occurs more frequently in patients with intravenous drug use and hemophilia as risk factors.[108,109] The degree of immunosuppression does not appear to be a contributing factor for infection with pathogens commonly introduced via needles. However, infection with opportunistic pathogens tends to occur in patients with more advanced HIV disease and CD4+ T-lymphocyte cell count of less than 100.[140]

The most common causes are *S. aureus* and atypical *Mycobacterium* species.[140] The rate of infection with atypical mycobacteria and *M. tuberculosis* was 676-fold and 35-fold higher, respectively, in HIV-infected patients than in the general population.[74] Generally, fungal osteomyelitis is uncommon, but when it does occur, it is hematogenously spread and thus often develops in more than one bone.[122]

Osteomyelitis is more frequently seen in advanced HIV disease, with a median CD4+ T-lymphocyte cell count of 41 documented in one study.[140]

Bacillary angiomatosis associated with disseminated *Bartonella henselae* has been reported to cause lytic bone lesions.[7,72,139] This clinical syndrome is characterized by subcutaneous nodules and osteolytic lesions that are typically culture negative on biopsy and aspirate samples. Electron microscopy and histopathologic examination of vascular soft tissue may verify the presence of *B. henselae*.

Once primarily seen in tropical climates, pyomyositis appears to be associated with advanced HIV infection in temperate climates. By far the most common organism identified in HIV-infected individuals is *S. aureus*.[45,140] Other organisms reported include *Streptococcus* and *Salmonella* species, *Toxoplasma gondii*, *Cryptococcus neoformans*, MAC, and microsporidia.[82,140]

Noninfectious Inflammatory Conditions of the Joints

As noted earlier, the most common musculoskeletal manifestation seen during the course of HIV infection is arthralgia.[108,121,160] Diffuse arthralgias may be seen in the setting of acute primary infection, as well as at other times during the course of HIV infection. The large joints, such as the knee, shoulder, and elbow, are most commonly involved. Symptoms are usually of moderate intensity and intermittent, but rarely, they can be extremely severe and debilitating. Often the clinical examination is without evidence of inflammatory signs. Simple analgesics are generally adequate for treatment of arthralgia in HIV-infected individuals.

Reiter syndrome is reported as a common rheumatologic syndrome in HIV infection. The signs and symptoms are similar to those of idiopathic Reiter syndrome and consist of asymmetrical oligoarthritis of the large joints (knees, shoulders, and ankles). Inflammation of the Achilles tendon, plantar fascia, and anterior and posterior tibial tendons is common. Patients may have gait disturbances secondary to these enthesopathies combined with multidigit dactylitis of the toes.[82]

The classic triad of arthritis, urethritis, and conjunctivitis is seen in a much smaller proportion of patients. Urethritis has been found in 59% of HIV-infected individuals with Reiter syndrome, conjunctivitis in 47%, keratoderma blennorrhagicum in 25%, and circinate balanitis in 29%.[82]

Organisms that trigger reactive arthritis, such as *Salmonella typhimurium, Shigella flexneri, Campylobacter fetus, Ureaplasma urealyticum*, and *Yersinia* species have been found in less than a third of HIV-infected patients with reactive arthritis. However, an antecedent culture-negative diarrheal illness often precedes the onset of Reiter syndrome and reactive arthritis in HIV-infected patients.[82] In a patient with a Reiter syndrome–like arthritis but lacking the other defining features, it may be more appropriate to classify the patient as having nonspecific reactive arthritis.[54]

Patients with Reiter syndrome are likely to be HLA-B27 seropositive. In contrast, in a cohort of 13 African American patients with Reiter syndrome and HIV infection, no HLA-B27 seropositivity was found. This finding may reflect the low prevalence of HLA-B27 in African American people in general.[82]

HIV-associated arthritis is an oligoarthritis that primarily involves the knees and ankles. It is characterized by brief episodes of debilitating pain. The peak intensity occurs within 1 to 4 weeks and often remits within 6 weeks to 6 months. Intense pain may necessitate the use of narcotics, nonsteroidal anti-inflammatory drugs (NSAIDs), and intra-articular corticosteroids. Arthrocentesis reveals fluid that is noninflammatory. Synovial biopsy reveals a chronic mononuclear infiltrate. The antecedent infections, mucocutaneous lesions, and ophthalmologic and urogenital features commonly seen with Reiter syndrome and psoriatic arthritis are not associated with these patients. Rheumatologic markers (HLA-B27, rheumatoid factor, antinuclear antibodies) and bacterial and viral cultures are also negative in these patients. The pathophysiology is unknown; however, a direct viral infection, immune complex deposition in the joint, and a form of reactive arthritis have been proposed as possible mechanisms.[5,82,112]

Psoriasis and psoriatic arthritis are more frequent in HIV-infected individuals than in the general population.[54] Psoriatic arthritis may precede, occur concomitantly, or follow the clinical onset of AIDS. It is frequently an asymmetrical, polyarticular disease that can be accompanied by enthesopathy and dactylitis. The clinical course is variable, ranging from mild to rapidly progressive and deforming.[45] Psoriatic arthritis may occur alone or in conjunction with psoriatic skin lesions. Various types of psoriatic skin lesions, including vulgaris, guttate, seborrheic,

pustular, and exfoliative erythroderma forms, have been described in both HIV-positive and -negative individuals.

Painful articular syndrome involves the acute onset of painful arthralgias in up to three joints. The physical examination is not suggestive of synovitis. The pain usually resolves within 24 hours, but narcotics may be required because NSAIDs often do not adequately control the pain. This syndrome appears to be unique to HIV-infected patients. Other considerations include infections with parvovirus B19 and hepatitis C.

Some of these syndromes have been associated with the institution of antiretroviral therapy. These "immune reconstitution syndromes" occur within weeks or months after the initiation of antiretroviral therapy. They may represent an enhanced inflammatory response to latent microorganisms or to nonviable antigens. After appropriate diagnostic evaluation to rule out active infection, these syndromes are managed symptomatically with anti-inflammatory agents, sometimes including corticosteroids.

Avascular Necrosis

Avascular necrosis of one or more joints will develop in approximately 4.4% of patients with HIV infection. It has been recognized most often in the hip but has been described in almost every joint. Some patients have unilateral disease; others have bilateral disease involving many different joints.[78,143]

If patients with HIV infection are scanned, silent lesions consistent with avascular necrosis can be found.[69,83] These lesions do not necessarily fit the paradigm that might have been expected from experience with other patient populations, such as those with hemoglobinopathies (eg, sickle cell disease) or those receiving chronic steroid therapy. Their progression to structural collapse and pain may be more subacute than with other populations.

The cause of aseptic necrosis has not been identified. Pathologic examination of the head of the femur has not demonstrated any unusual findings. HIV infection and antiretroviral therapy may each have roles in promoting the lesions. Epidemiologic studies have associated the occurrence of such lesions with vigorous activity, yet such activities may simply cause the ultimate damage after the initial weakening of the substrate that brought the patient to medical attention. These lesions have also been linked to previous corticosteroid use. It is conceivable that HIV-infected patients who receive corticosteroids, especially those who are taking antiretroviral agents that increase the area under the curve for corticosteroids, may be predisposed to avascular necrosis.

Hip replacement has been performed in hundreds of patients with HIV-related avascular necrosis, with good results. Postoperative complications seem to be no different in HIV-infected patients than in HIV-uninfected patients with similar comorbidities. There is no known way to prevent this complication.

Osteoporosis and Fragility Fractures

Bone and calcium disorders are being recognized with greater and greater frequency among HIV-infected patients. HIV-infected patients have multiple risk factors for osteopenia and osteoporosis.[†]

Although some HIV-infected patients have active lifestyles and minimize risk, other HIV-infected patients, especially those

---

†References 9, 13, 16-18, 51, 63, 73, 96, 101, 123, 127, 131, and 134.

with advanced immunosuppression, may have poor nutrition, physical inactivity, long-term tobacco abuse, low testosterone levels, heavy use of alcohol and opiates, and chronic use of drugs that promote bone demineralization.

Antiretroviral therapy naïve patients have a higher incidence of osteopenia than HIV-uninfected patients.[17] In one study 67% of patients had decreased bone mineralization and 15% met the criteria for osteoporosis.[17]

The clinical significance of these bone mineralization losses has not been definitively demonstrated. Some studies have shown increased risk of fragility fractures, but others have not.[96,101,127,138]

As this population ages and as more patients are exposed to preferred antiretroviral drugs, such as tenofovir, that are associated with osteopenia, the clinical relevance of this will become more apparent. Other drugs often used by HIV-infected patients, including foscarnet and pentamidine, can also promote demineralization.

Currently, there is no recommendation for routine screening of HIV-infected patients for osteoporosis, and no consensus recommendations on regimens to reduce bone demineralization in this patient population.[123]

SUMMARY

Virtually all physicians, including orthopedic surgeons, will encounter individuals with HIV infection in their practice of medicine. Orthopedic surgeons need to be familiar with the risk of acquiring HIV from needlesticks, other surgical accidents, and blood transfusions, as well as the principles of risk reduction to ensure the safety of both patients and the entire health care team. Moreover, individuals infected with HIV are living longer, healthier, and more active lives. Consequently, orthopedists need to be aware of the possibility that their patients may have orthopedic complications not only because of HIV but also independent of HIV infection. Thus individuals with HIV infection deserve the same careful diagnostic and therapeutic management as uninfected patients. Finally, almost all practicing physicians will encounter patients who are at risk for acquiring HIV infection or who are infected but have not yet been tested; frank discussion about prevention of transmission and testing, as well as referral to an HIV specialist when indicated, will contribute to the overall health of the individual and efforts to stem the tide of the HIV epidemic and are part of every health care professional's responsibilities.

KEY REFERENCES

1. AIDSinfo. <www.aidsinfo.nih.gov>.
9. Battalora L, Buchacz K, Armon C, et al: Low bone mineral density and risk of incident fracture in HIV-infected adults. *Antivir Ther* 21(1):45–54, 2016.
10. Beekmann SE, Henderson DK: Prevention of human immunodeficiency virus and AIDS: postexposure prophylaxis (including health care workers). *Infect Dis Clin North Am* 28(4):601–613, 2014.
16. Brown TT, Hoy J, Borderi M, et al: Recommendations for evaluation and management of bone disease in HIV. *Clin Infect Dis* 60(8):1242–1251, 2015.
24. Castel AD, Choi S, Dor A, et al: Comparing cost-effectiveness of HIV testing strategies: targeted and routine testing in Washington, DC. *PLoS One* 10(10):e0139605, 2015.
25. Castel AD, Magnus M, Greenberg AE: Update on the epidemiology and prevention of HIV/AIDS in the United States. *Curr Epidemiol Rep* 2(2):110–119, 2015.
26. CDC HIV/AIDS Facts: HIV/AIDS in the United States. <http://www.cdc.gov/hiv/resources/factsheets/us.htm>.
37. Centers for Disease Control and Prevention: Investigation of patients treated by an HIV-infected cardiothoracic surgeon—Israel, 2007. *MMWR Morb Mortal Wkly Rep* 57(53):1413–1415, 2009.
39. Ciesielski C, Marianos D, Ou CY, et al: Transmission of human immunodeficiency virus in a dental practice. *Ann Intern Med* 116(10):798–805, 1992.
41. Conrad C, Bradley HM, Broz D, et al: Community outbreak of HIV infection linked to injection drug use of oxymorphone—Indiana, 2015. *MMWR Morb Mortal Wkly Rep* 64(16):443–444, 2015.
60. Fox C, Walker-Bone K: Evolving spectrum of HIV-associated rheumatic syndromes. *Best Pract Res Clin Rheumatol* 29(2):244–258, 2015.
78. Issa K, Naziri Q, Rasquinha V, et al: Outcomes of cementless primary THA for osteonecrosis in HIV-infected patients. *J Bone Joint Surg Am* 95(20):1845–1850, 2013.
80. Joyce MP, Kuhar D, Brooks JT: Notes from the field: occupationally acquired HIV infection among health care workers—United States, 1985–2013. *MMWR Morb Mortal Wkly Rep* 63(53):1245–1246, 2015.
86. Kuhar DT, Henderson DK, Struble KA, et al: Updated US Public Health Service guidelines for the management of occupational exposures to human immunodeficiency virus and recommendations for postexposure prophylaxis. *Infect Control Hosp Epidemiol* 34(9):875–892, 2013.
143. Whitlock GG, Herbert S, Copas A, et al: Avascular necrosis in HIV patients: a case-control study. *Int J STD AIDS* 24(10):799–803, 2013.

The references for this chapter can also be found on www.expertconsult.com.

Anesthesia for Knee Surgery

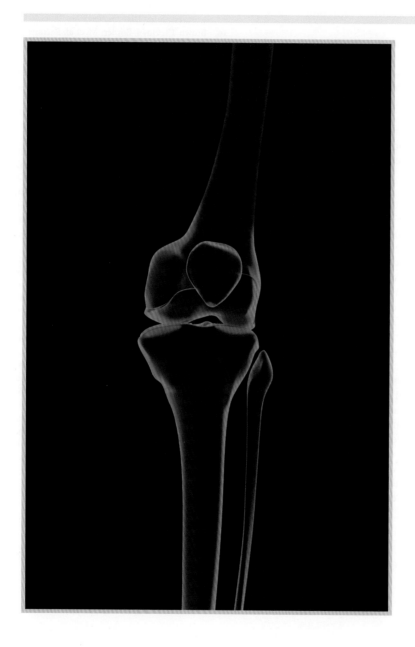

PART I

Preoperative Evaluation

77

Basics, Preoperative Assessment, and Medical Optimization

Milad Nazemzadeh

A thorough preoperative assessment of the orthopedic patient is pivotal to identify and optimize medical comorbidities, quantify risk, formulate an individualized anesthetic plan and reduce postoperative complications. During the preoperative assessment, the patient's preexisting medical problems, allergies, previous anesthetic complications, current medications, and cognitive or physical aspects that would affect their suitability for different anesthetic and postoperative pain management techniques should be addressed.[1] A focused physical examination should be performed, and appropriate lab testing and imaging should be ordered (Table 77.1). Ideally the patient should also undergo a preoperative educational session that describes the surgical procedure, anesthetic and analgesic options, and the postoperative rehabilitation plan.

Overall, patients undergoing major lower extremity orthopedic procedures are considered at intermediate risk (~5%) for cardiac complications perioperatively (Table 77.2). Particularly in the geriatric population, cardiac disease is common and remains the leading cause of postoperative mortality.[1] Assessment of exercise tolerance is often difficult because of the limitations in mobility induced by the underlying orthopedic condition. Therefore in the presence of clinical predictors of preoperative cardiovascular risk (ischemic heart disease, congestive heart failure [CHF], cerebrovascular disease [CVD], diabetes mellitus [DM], and renal insufficiency [serum creatinine >2.0 mg/dL]), patients are advised to undergo a thorough cardiac evaluation, including physical or pharmacologic stress testing (Fig. 77.1). Without these predictors, patients may proceed for surgery without further evaluation.[3] Elective orthopedic procedures should be postponed in patients with a history of recent myocardial infarction (MI), unstable/severe angina, decompensated heart failure, significant arrhythmias or severe valvular disease until these issues are addressed. In patients who have received percutaneous coronary intervention (PCI), surgical interventions should be delayed 14 days after balloon angioplasty, 4 to 6 weeks for bare metal stents, and 1 year for drug-eluting stents.[4] After PCI, most patients are placed on antiplatelet therapies for secondary prevention of cardiovascular disease, and therefore early termination of these agents for nonurgent surgeries increases the risk of perioperative stent thrombosis and its consequences of MI or death. Emergent operations should be performed under continued dual antiplatelet therapy unless the risk of surgical bleeding outweighs the benefit of continuing antiplatelet therapy.[2]

The patient's medications should be reviewed and the patient specifically instructed on which medications are to be continued until the time of surgery. Specifically, antihypertensive medications, such as β-blockers and calcium channel blockers, should NOT be discontinued because of the risk of perioperative cardiac events. It is recommended that angiotensin-converting enzyme inhibitors (ACEIs), angiotensin receptor blockers (ARBs), and diuretics be avoided on the day of surgery to avoid treatment-resistant hypotension. Similarly, patients who require long-term opioid medications should be allowed to maintain their usual dosing regimen. Steroid-dependent patients will require steroid replacement in the perioperative period. Finally, the patient should be queried regarding the use of any medications that affect hemostasis, including nonsteroidal antiinflammatory drugs (NSAIDs), oral anticoagulants, and over-the-counter herbal drugs (Box 77.1).

Patients should be assessed for limitations in mouth opening or neck extension/flexion, Mallampati classification of the airway, interincisor distance, adequacy of thyromental distance, tonsillar size, tongue size, and state of dentition (Box 77.2). The heart and lungs should be auscultated. The site of proposed injection of regional anesthesia should be evaluated for evidence of infection and anatomic abnormalities or limitations. A brief neurologic examination to identify deficits is particularly important in the elderly who commonly have dementia or neurodegenerative diseases. The functional and cognitive status and any neurologic symptoms should be documented.[1] In addition, the patient should be evaluated for any potential positioning difficulties (during block performance or intraoperatively) related to arthritic involvement of other joints or body habitus.

Many patients undergoing orthopedic surgery have chronic inflammatory joint diseases that may impact other organ systems. One particular example is rheumatoid arthritis. Systemic manifestations of this disease include pulmonary, cardiac, and musculoskeletal involvement. Particularly significant to the anesthesiologist is involvement of the cervical spine, temporomandibular joint, and larynx. Rheumatoid involvement of the cervical spine may result in limited neck range of motion, which interferes with airway management. Atlantoaxial instability, with subluxation of the odontoid process, can lead to spinal cord injury during neck extension. Therefore, it has been suggested that these patients receive cervical spine lateral extension and flexion radiographs prior to manipulation.[1] Mouth opening may also be limited secondary to temporomandibular

TABLE 77.1 Framework for Preoperative Diagnostic Testing Based on Patient's Medical History

Preoperative Diagnosis	ECG	Chest Radiograph	Hct/Hb	CBC	Electrolytes	Creatinine	Glucose	Coagulation	LFTs	Drug Levels	Ca
Cardiac Disease											
History of MI	X	—	—	X	±	—	—	—	—	—	—
Chronic stable angina	X	—	—	X	±	—	—	—	—	—	—
CHF	X	±	—	—	—	—	—	—	—	—	—
HTN	X	±	—	—	Xª	X	—	—	—	—	—
Chronic atrial fibrillation	X	—	—	—	—	—	—	—	—	Xᵇ	—
PAD	X	—	—	—	—	—	—	—	—	—	—
Valvular heart disease	X	±	—	—	—	—	—	—	—	—	—
Pulmonary Disease											
COPD	X	±	—	X	—	—	—	—	—	Xᶜ	—
Asthma			(PFTs only if symptomatic; otherwise no tests required)								
Diabetes	X	—	—	—	±	X	X	—	—	—	—
Liver Disease											
Infectious hepatitis	—	—	—	—	—	—	—	X	X	—	—
Alcohol or drug induced hepatitis	—	—	—	—	—	—	—	X	X	—	—
Tumor infiltration	—	—	—	—	—	—	—	X	X	—	—
Renal disease	—	—	X	—	X	X	—	—	—	—	—
Hematologic disorders	—	—	—	X	—	—	—	—	—	—	—
Coagulopathies	—	—	—	X	—	—	—	X	—	—	—
CNS Disorders											
Stroke	X	—	—	X	X	—	X	—	—	X	—
Seizures	X	—	—	X	X	—	X	—	—	X	—
Tumor	X	—	—	X	—	—	—	—	—	—	—
Vascular disorders or aneurysms	X	—	X	—	—	—	—	—	—	—	—
Malignant disease	—	—	—	X	—	—	—	—	—	—	—
Hyperthyroidism	X	—	X	—	X	—	—	—	—	—	X
Hypothyroidism	X	—	X	—	X	—	—	—	—	—	—
Cushing disease	—	—	—	X	X	—	X	—	—	—	—
Addison disease	—	—	—	X	X	—	X	—	—	—	—
Hyperparathyroidism	X	—	X	—	X	—	—	—	—	—	X
Hypoparathyroidism	X	—	—	—	X	—	—	—	—	—	X
Morbid obesity	X	±	—	—	—	—	X	—	—	—	—
Malabsorption or poor nutrition	X	—	—	X	X	X	X	—	—	—	—
Select Drug Therapies											
Digoxin (digitalis)	X	—	—	—	±	—	—	—	—	X	—
Anticoagulants	—	—	X	—	—	—	—	X	—	—	—
Phenytoin (Dilantin)	—	—	—	—	—	—	—	—	—	X	—
Phenobarbital	—	—	—	—	—	—	—	—	—	X	—
Diuretics	—	—	—	—	X	X	—	—	—	—	—
Corticosteroids	—	—	—	X	—	—	X	—	—	—	—
Chemotherapy	—	—	—	X	—	±	—	—	—	—	—
Aspirin or NSAIDs	—	—	—	—	—	—	—	—	—	—	—
Theophylline	—	—	—	—	—	—	—	—	—	X	—

ªIf the patient is taking diuretics.

ᵇIf the patient is taking digoxin.

ᶜIf the patient is taking theophylline.

±; *Ca*, Calcium; *CBC*, complete blood count; *CHF*, congestive heart failure; *CNS*, central nervous system; *COPD*, chronic obstructive pulmonary disease; *ECG*, electrocardiogram; *Hb*, hemoglobin; *Hct*, hematocrit; *HTN*, hypertension; *LFTs*, liver function tests; *MI*, myocardial infarction; *NSAID*, nonsteroidal antiinflammatory drug; *PAD*, peripheral arterial disease; *PFT*, pulmonary function test; *X*, obtain.

From Miller RD: *Miller's anesthesia*, ed 8, Philadelphia, 2015, Elsevier, p 1142.

TABLE 77.2   Stratification of Perioperative Cardiac Risk for Noncardiac Surgical Procedures

Risk Stratification	Estimated Risk of Cardiac Death or Nonfatal MI	Examples of Procedures
Vascular	>5%	Aortic and other major vascular surgery Peripheral vascular surgery
Intermediate	1-5%	Intraperitoneal and intrathoracic surgery Carotid endarterectomy Head and neck surgery Orthopedic surgery Prostate surgery
Low[a]	<1%	Endoscopic procedures Superficial procedure Cataract surgery Breast surgery Ambulatory surgery

[a]These procedures do not require further preoperative cardiac testing unless the patient has an unstable cardiac condition.

MI, Myocardial infarction.

From Miller RD: Miller's anesthesia, ed 8, Philadelphia, 2015, Elsevier, p 1096. From Fleisher LA, Beckman JA, Brown KA, et al: 2009 ACCF/AHA focused update on perioperative beta blockade incorporated into the ACC/AHA 2007 guidelines on perioperative cardiovascular evaluation and care for noncardiac surgery: a report of the American College of Cardiology Foundation/American Heart Association Task Force on Practice Guidelines. *Circulation* 120:e169–e276, 2009.

joint ankylosis, so appropriate equipment should be prepared in advance.[1]

Preoperative risk assessment and optimization is an area of medicine that has gained much interest in recent years. This is particularly true for the geriatric population because they have higher rates of perioperative complications. Preoperative optimization of medical comorbidities is key to the perioperative outcomes of this population. Important general strategies in their preoperative management include rapid optimization for early surgical repair, avoidance of perioperative hypotension, medication adjustment, pain control, delirium prevention, avoidance of polypharmacy and overtesting.[8] Perioperative blood management is essential for the orthopedic patient. Perioperative anemia and allogenic blood transfusion are some of the strongest predictors of adverse clinical outcomes.[5] Therefore it behooves the perioperative anesthesia provider to detect, diagnose, and treat the underlying cause of anemia prior to surgical intervention whenever possible.[7] Indeed, Munoz et al. dispel the misconception that intravenous (IV) iron is hazardous and advocates its use in both elective and nonelective surgical patients with suboptimal Hb, to improve Hb concentrations rapidly and decrease blood transfusions and its related complications. If significant blood loss is expected, implementation of different blood-conserving strategies may be prudent but does not preclude adequate perioperative management of anemia, especially in Jehovah's Witness patients who are known to refuse blood products.[7] Prior to major surgery, the patient's

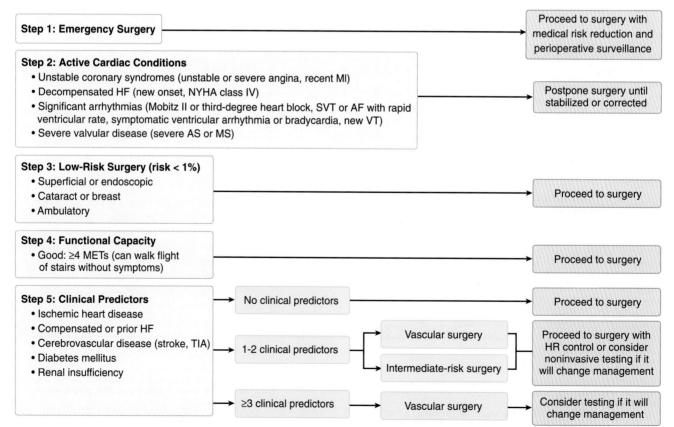

FIG 77.1 Simplified cardiac evaluation for noncardiac surgery. (From Miller RD: *Miller's anesthesia,* ed 8, Philadelphia, 2015, Elsevier, p 1094.)

BOX 77.1 Preoperative Management of Medications

Instruct patients to take these medications with a small sip of water, even if fasting.

1. Antihypertensive medications
   Continue on the day of surgery.
   - Possible exception
   For patients undergoing procedures with major fluid shifts or for patients who have medical conditions in which hypotension is particularly dangerous, it may be prudent to discontinue ACEIs or ARBs before surgery.
2. Cardiac medications (eg, β-blockers, digoxin)
   Continue on the day of surgery.
3. Antidepressants, anxiolytics, and other psychiatric medications
   Continue on the day of surgery.
4. Thyroid medications
   Continue on the day of surgery.
5. Birth control pills
   Continue on the day of surgery.
6. Eye drops
   Continue on the day of surgery.
7. Heartburn or reflux medications
   Continue on the day of surgery.
8. Narcotic medications
   Continue on the day of surgery.
9. Anticonvulsant medications
   Continue on the day of surgery.
10. Asthma medications
    Continue on the day of surgery.
11. Steroids (oral and inhaled)
    Continue on the day of surgery.
12. Statins
    Continue on the day of surgery.
13. Aspirin
    Consider selectively continuing aspirin in patients where the risks of cardiac events are felt to exceed the risk of major bleeding. Examples would be patients high-grade CAD or CVD. If reversal of platelet inhibition is necessary, aspirin must be stopped at least 3 days before surgery. Do not discontinue aspirin in patients who have drug-eluting coronary stents until they have completed 12 months of dual antiplatelet therapy, unless patients, surgeons, and cardiologists have discussed the risks of discontinuation. The same applies to patients with bare metal stents until they have completed 1 month of dual antiplate-

let therapy. In general, aspirin should be continued in any patient with a coronary stent, regardless of the time since stent implantation.
14. Thienopyridines (eg, clopidogrel, ticlopidine)
    Patients having cataract surgery with topical or general anesthesia do not need to stop taking thienopyridines. If reversal of platelet inhibition is necessary, then clopidogrel must be stopped 7 days before surgery (14 days for ticlopidine). Do not discontinue thienopyridines in patients who have drug-eluting stents until they have completed 12 months of dual antiplatelet therapy, unless patients, surgeons, and cardiologists have discussed the risks of discontinuation. The same applies to patients with bare metal stents until they have completed 1 month of dual antiplatelet therapy.
15. Insulin
    For all patients, discontinue all short-acting (eg, regular) insulin on the day of surgery (unless insulin is administered by continuous pump). Patients with type 2 diabetes should take none, or up to one half of their dose of long-acting or combination (eg, 70/30 preparations) insulin, on the day of surgery. Patients with type 1 diabetes should take a small amount (usually one-third) of their usual morning long-acting insulin dose on the day of surgery. Patients with an insulin pump should continue their basal rate only.
16. Topical medications (eg, creams and ointments)
    Discontinue on the day of surgery.
17. Oral hypoglycemic agents
    Discontinue on the day of surgery.
18. Diuretics
    Discontinue on the day of surgery (exception: thiazide diuretics taken for hypertension, which should be continued on the day of surgery).
19. Sildenafil (Viagra) or similar drugs
    Discontinue 24 hours before surgery.
20. COX-2 inhibitors
    Continue on the day of surgery unless the surgeon is concerned about bone healing.
21. NSAIDs
    Discontinue 48 hours before the day of surgery.
22. Warfarin (Coumadin)
    Discontinue 4 days before surgery, except for patients having cataract surgery without a bulbar block.
23. Monoamine oxidase inhibitors
    Continue these medications and adjust the anesthesia plan accordingly.

ACEI, Angiotensin converting enzyme inhibitors; *ARB*, angiotensin receptor blocker; *CAD*, coronary artery disease; *COX-2*, cyclooxygenase-2; *CVD*, cerebrovascular disease; *NSAID*, nonsteroidal antiinflammatory drugs.
From Miller RD: *Miller's anesthesia*, ed 8, Philadelphia, 2015, Elsevier, p 1098.

BOX 77.2 Components of the Airway Examination

Length of the upper incisors
Condition of the teeth
Relationship of the upper (maxillary) incisors to the lower (mandibular) incisors
Ability to advance the lower (mandibular) incisors in front of the upper (maxillary) incisors
Interincisor or intergum (if edentulous) distance
Visibility of the uvula
Presence of heavy facial hair
Compliance of the mandibular space
Thyromental distance
Length of the neck
Thickness or circumference of the neck
Range of motion of the head and neck

From Miller RD: *Miller's anesthesia*, ed 8, Philadelphia, 2015, Elsevier, p 1092.

blood type should be determined and an antibody screen performed. Depending on the patient's preoperative hemoglobin level, presence of antibodies, overall medical condition, and anticipated surgical procedure, several units of blood products may be cross-matched preoperatively. Preoperative autologous blood donation may be an option for selected patients. Other laboratory testing and imaging are conducted, as indicated by the preoperative medical condition. Of note, preoperative screening for methicillin-resistant *Staphylococcus aureus* (MRSA) and urinary tract infection (UTI) are performed by some to decrease joint and surgical site infections.[4]

Prevention of postoperative pulmonary complications is yet another growing body of research. Postoperative pulmonary complications are reported to be as common as cardiac complications in surgical patient and account for a great deal of their morbidity and mortality. The identification of risk factors, including advanced age, obstructive sleep apnea (OSA)/obesity, CHF, ASA ≥2, chronic obstructive pulmonary disease

(COPD), functional dependency, recent respiratory infection, major surgery, prolonged or emergent surgery, and preoperative anemia, is an important task of the perioperative provider.[10] In high-risk patients, anesthesia providers may consider neuraxial blockade over general anesthesia, avoidance of long-acting neuromuscular blockade, use of lower tidal volumes with positive end-expiratory pressure (PEEP), and a restrictive fluid management strategy to reduce the risk of postoperative pulmonary complications.[10] Malnutrition is another well-established risk factor for pulmonary complications and poor surgical outcomes. Patients should be screened by measuring body mass index (BMI), serum albumin, and prealbumin.[9] Severely malnourished patients should at least be assessed by a dietician preoperatively to optimize them for surgery.[9]

The references for this chapter can also be found on www.expertconsult.com.

78

Patients With Stents

Ghislaine M. Isidore

Worldwide, coronary artery disease (CAD) is the most common cause of morbidity and mortality.[21] Yearly, more than 500,000 Americans and 1,000,000 patients worldwide undergo a coronary artery interventional procedure.[29] Management of CAD has evolved from coronary artery bypass grafting (CABG) and percutaneous transluminal coronary angioplasty (PTCA) to percutaneous coronary intervention (PCI) with stents.[17] Management of surgical patients who have undergone PCI with stents and are presenting for noncardiac surgery is a major safety issue confronting clinicians.[34,35,39] The American Heart Association (AHA) and American College of Cardiology (ACC) have coauthored a guideline on preoperative cardiac risk stratification and management of patients with stents undergoing noncardiac procedures.[29,39]

CORONARY ARTERY STENTS AND MANAGEMENT

Bare Metal Stents Versus Drug-Eluting Stents

There are two broad groups of stent devices[29]: (1) balloon expandable and (2) self-expanding. Each system is designed to help decrease stent thrombosis and possible restenosis. Based on the delivery method, they are further subdivided into sheathed stents, or drug-eluting stents (DES), versus bare metal stents (BMS).

A milestone in PCI was reached with the development of BMS in the late 1980s.[23] BMS effectively reduces stenosis when compared to PTCA alone and significantly decreases the rates of major adverse cardiac events (MACE), myocardial infarction (MI), and death. DES, a stent combined with a drug, was devised to respond to a problem associated with BMS: in-stent restenosis (ISR). DES, approved by the US Food and Drug Administration (FDA) in 2002 to 2003, greatly reduced ISR by 50% to 70%.[13,23,32,33]

Antiplatelet Therapy and Coronary Stents

The Role of Aspirin and Clopidogrel. Current guidelines recommend dual platelet inhibition with aspirin (ASA) and clopidogrel to prevent postprocedure adverse events after elective PCI with stent implantation.[2]

Aspirin. Platelets are key mediators in the pathophysiology of thrombosis, making antiplatelet therapy the cornerstone of treatment in patients with acute coronary syndrome (ASA) following PCI, reducing the risk of thrombotic events, improving long-term outcome, and reducing the risk of MACE.[10,14] Most cardiovascular events are not prevented by ASA because it only blocks one of several pathways involved in the platelet activation and aggregation.

ADP receptor antagonist. Ticlodipine (Ticlid), clopidogrel (Plavix), prasugrel (Effient), and ticagrelor (Brilinta) are adenosine diphosphate (ADP) receptor antagonists that are used in conjunction with ASA in patients with acute ACS and/or undergoing PCI.[25] The active metabolite of clopidogrel irreversibly binds to platelet P2Y12 ADP receptors, thereby inhibiting ADP-induced platelet aggregation.

Guidelines currently recommend dual platelet inhibition with ASA and clopidogrel to prevent postprocedure adverse events after elective PCI with stent implantation.[2]

IN-STENT THROMBOSIS AND RESTENOSIS: ASPIRIN AND CLOPIDOGEL RESISTANCE AND THE DIABETIC DILEMMA

Antiplatelet drug response is multifactorial; older age, diabetes mellitus, elevated body mass index (BMI), renal function, and left ventricular ejection fraction are independent risk factors that predict high rates of cardiovascular events.[2,15] Patients with high risk scores have an increased probability and higher rate of major cardiovascular events. Diabetic patients are at a disadvantage for several reasons[2,11,15,18]:

1. Diabetics have a prothrombic state that includes increased platelet reactivity. Many diabetics are relatively resistant to or have insufficient response to several antithrombic agents in addition to higher baseline risk of ACS. Diabetics have less antiplatelet response to both ASA[27] and clopidogrel. A significant reduction (19%) in cardiovascular death, MI, and stroke is observed with prasugrel at 450 days, compared to clopidogrel, except in patients with previous transient ischemic attacks (TIA) or cerebro-vascular accidents (CVA). Bleeding is significantly higher with prasugrel.[16] A high correlation exits between insulin-treated diabetes mellitus patients and the risk of restenosis within 1 year of DES implantation.[41] With regard to the type of stent, there are no differences in outcome using second generation DES.

2. Clopidogrel is an inactive prodrug that is oxidized to its active metabolite via hepatic cytochrome (CY) P450 systems. The allele variant CYP2C19*2 is associated with high levels of ADP-induced platelet aggregation, leading to higher risk of adverse cardiovascular events, including ST. In contrast, recent data have shown that the CYP2C19*17 polymorphism is associated with enhanced response to clopidogrel and increased risk of bleeding.[1,3,17,36] In addition to carriers of CYP2C19*2, diabetes and BMI are major predictors of insufficient response to clopidogrel.[7]

The FDA, recently added a boxed warning to the clopidogrel label, emphasizing the increased risk of adverse cardiovascular events in patients with genetic polymorphism.[9]

The presence of newly formed immature platelets, suggestive of platelets turnover, is key in the antiplatelet effect of ASA and the development of acute coronary thrombosis.[10,24,27] In cases of high platelet turnover, ASA alone may not provide adequate protection.[24] Most cardiovascular events are not prevented by ASA because it only blocks one of several pathways involved in the platelet activation and aggregation. Platelets also contain a variable amount of cyclooxygenase (COX-2).

Experience with coronary stents has elucidated several predictors of stent thrombosis, including residual dissection, underexpansion of the stent, combining/overlapping different stents, and longer total length.[38] Formation of a smooth muscle cell-rich neointima at the site of vascular injury is considered the primary mechanism of restenosis after coronary stent implantation.[31] There is evidence that the inhibition of thrombus formation at early stages after vascular injury can prevent subsequent neointimal formation at later stages. Abnormal vessel wall linings, abnormal blood-flow patterns, and abnormal blood constituents favored late stent thrombosis (LST).[5] Antiplatelet therapies are not effective at reducing restenosis rates. DESs can be considered as the gold standard for the prevention of restenosis.[12,19,31] Switching types of DESs, preferably different generations, has been found to be more effective in managing ISR.[8,19,36]

GUIDELINES

A serious consequence of discontinuing antiplatelet medication is LST (>30 days after stent implantation), leading to MI in the territory of DES.[5,22] The incidence of acute MI is 50%, with a mortality rate of 20%.[7] Administration of dual antiplatelet therapy for 45 days (BMS) and 12 months (DES) can counterbalance the thrombogenicity favored by delayed vessel healing and local inflammation.[30] Risk of perioperative MACE is highest when major nonelective surgery is performed less than 45 days after coronary stent implantation.[7,28,36] The delay allows for neointimal hyperplasia. The process peaks at around the third month and reaches a plateau at between 3 and 6 months after the procedure.[43] Beyond 1 year after implantation, with either BMS or DES, physicians can be assured that the perioperative cardiac risk has reached a plateau.

When evaluating a patient with a coronary stent, considerations should be given to the following factors:

1. Surgery-related factors. The urgency of the procedure and bleeding risks.
2. Lesion- and stent-related factors. Types of stents, the date of implantation, number, location, and length of stents.
3. Current oral antiplatelet agents (OAA). The duration of therapy.[28,35,39]
4. Patient-related factors. Diabetes mellitus, renal insufficiency, low ejection fraction.

The combination of stopping protective OAA, along with hypercoagulable perioperative state and a poorly endothelialized stent, leads to a high risk of acute stent thrombosis. In contrast, the administration of OAA therapy in the perioperative period should be done in a way that considers bleeding associated with the surgery or procedure.[20]

The following guidelines to perioperative management are derived from several consensuses and the 2014 ACC/AHA guideline*:

1. Discussion and coordination of care must involve anesthesiologist, surgeon, primary care physician and cardiologist. It is crucial for the patient to be evaluated by his cardiologist, who will assess surgical risk with regard to patient's functional capacity.
   a. Further testing will depends on those factors. Individualized preoperative cardiac evaluation is emphasized. Preoperative testing should provide information on these cardiac risk factors: left ventricle (LV) dysfunction, myocardial ischemia, and valve abnormalities, all of which are major determinants of postoperative outcome. Asymptomatic patients (following PCI with stents) do not require preoperative stress testing.
   b. According to current guidelines, statins should be continued throughout the perioperative period. In patients not previously treated, ideally, statins therapy should be initiated at least 2 weeks before the intervention. Treatment onset and the optimal choice of beta-blocker dose are closely linked. Bradycardia and hypotension should be avoided. Dose should be slowly titrated, when indicated, and tailored to appropriate and target heart rate and blood pressure. All cardiac medications must be continued unless there is a specific contraindication.
2. Discuss whether surgery can be safely performed in a hospital where a catheterization lab is immediately available.
3. If emergent surgery, proceed under antiplatelet therapy; manage bleeding as needed.
4. If semiurgent surgery:
   a. Implant BMS.
   b. Complete dual antiplatelet therapy as indicated (45 days).
   c. Proceed to surgery.
5. If elective surgery:
   a. Patient with DES:
      i. If less than 12 months from insertion of stent, defer procedure until completion of appropriate course of dual antiplatelet therapy (12 months) and then perform procedure on ASA.
      ii. If patient is still taking clopidogrel after 12 months (because deemed high thrombosis risk by cardiologist):
         1. Discontinue clopidogrel and have surgery on ASA.
         2. If ASA is not recommended for that type of surgery because of a high bleeding risk (intracranial and spine surgery, urologic surgery, surgery of the retina), discontinue ASA preoperatively and restart as soon as possible.
   b. Patient with BMS:
      i. Delay procedure for 45 days (until completion of dual antiplatelet therapy), and then perform procedure on ASA if possible.
      ii. If ASA not recommended, discontinue ASA preoperatively and resume postoperatively as soon as possible.

Both regional and general anesthesia are used to manage patients with stents, but the use of neuraxial techniques is subject to debate.[33,39] A reasonable approach is to avoid continuous neuraxial techniques.

---

*References 5, 23, 28, 35, 39, 20, 46, and 47.

REGIONAL ANESTHESIA

Dual antiplatelet therapy also presents problems for regional anesthesia. Neuroaxial blocks cannot be recommended unless platelet transfusion is given before the procedure and platelet function is within acceptable limits.[18,19] Platelet dysfunction is present for 5 to 7 days after discontinuation of clopidoprel and 10 to 14 days with ticlodipine. With prasugrel, which inhibits platelets more rapidly, more consistently, and to a greater extent than standard and higher doses of clopidogrel, platelet aggregation normalizes in 7 to 9 days after discontinuation of treatment.

The waiting period prior to performing regional anesthesia is 14 days for ticlodipine, 5 to 7 days for clopidogrel, and 7 to 10 days for prasugrel.[15,20,38,39] Regional anesthesia can be performed safely in patients receiving therapy with ASA.

SUMMARY

Patients with a previous PCI may be at higher risk of cardiac events during or after subsequent noncardiac surgery, particularly in cases of unplanned or urgent surgery. Cardiac events, in relation to perioperative stent thrombosis when surgery is performed off dual OAA therapy, approach 25%. The risk of stent thrombosis and perioperative bleeding must be considered. The recommendations are as follows: regarding the perioperative management of dual OAA, following BMS implantation, the patients must wait 45 days before elective noncardiac surgery, whereas those with DES stents must wait 12 months. ASA should be continued perioperatively, except in those cases where the risk is too high. Mortality rates remain high when surgery is performed. The management of OAA therapy in patients who have undergone recent coronary PCI with stents and are scheduled for noncardiac surgery should be discussed by anesthesiologists, surgeons, and cardiologists so that the risk of life-threatening stent thrombosis and bleeding can be fully understood.

KEY REFERENCES

12. Fleischer LA, Fleischmann KE, Auerbach AD, et al: A report of the American College of Cardiology/ American heart association Task Force on Practice Guidelines. 2014 ACC/ AHA Guideline on perioperative cardiovascular evaluation and management of patients undergoing noncardiac surgery: executive summary. *J Am Coll Cardiol* 2014. doi: 10.1016/j.jacc.2014.07.945.

15. Guarracino F, Baldassari R, Priebe HJ: Revised ESC/ESA guidelines on non-cardiac surgery: cardiovascular assessment and management. Implications for preoperative clinical evaluation. *Minerva Anestesiol* 81:226–233, 2015.

The references for this chapter can also be found on www.expertconsult.com.

79

Diabetes Mellitus and the Knee

Jesse Ng

Diabetes mellitus affects 20 million people in the United States,[6] with approximately 26.9% of adults 65 and over suffering from this systemic disease. Evidence has shown that diabetes itself is an independent risk factor for the development of osteoarthritis and is often associated with more severe osteoarthritis.[18] In the United States, approximately 46 million people suffer from arthritis, with the prevalence of arthritis among adults with diabetes estimated to be 48% to 52%.[2,6] And in the population of patients with diabetes and arthritis, the risk factors of obesity and cardiovascular disease are also more prevalent.[2] It has been reported an estimate of anywhere from 8% to as high as 22% of patients undergoing total knee arthroplasty suffer from diabetes mellitus.[11]

TREATMENT OF DIABETES

The management of diabetes can be divided into three subcategories: (1) glycemic control, by way of managing diet, making lifestyle changes, increasing exercise, and implementing an appropriate medication regimen, including oral glucose lowering agents and/or insulin; (2) the treatment of diabetes-associated comorbidities, including dyslipidemia, hypertension, obesity, and coronary artery disease; and (3) the screening for and managing of complications of diabetes (such as retinopathy, cardiovascular disease, nephropathy, and neuropathy). The current recommendation of the American Diabetes Association for adult patients is a hemoglobin A1c goal of less than 7%,[12] and the current recommendation of the American Association of Clinical Endocrinologists for adult patients is a hemoglobin A1c goal of less than 6.5%.[19] The aim of treatment is to achieve a hemoglobin A1c as close to normal as recommended by the guidelines without significant hypoglycemia. Glycemic control, however, must be individualized, as the goals of therapy should include medical, social, and lifestyle factors, including age of the patient, ability of a patient to implement a complex treatment regimen, and presence/severity of diabetic complications.[15]

This section will focus on the common medications used in the management of glucose levels in diabetic patients. Hypoglycemic agents can be divided into two categories, oral glucose lowering agents and insulin, with their derivatives.[15]

The goal of oral glucose lowering agents is to reduce toxicity to the islet cells by glucose and to improve endogenous insulin secretion, requiring some level of functioning pancreatic islet cells to be effective. The mechanisms of action of these medications include (1) the increase of insulin secretion, (2) the reduction of glucose production, (3) the increase in insulin sensitivity,

and (4) the enhancement of glucagon-like peptide-1 (GLP-1) action.[15]

Biguanides

The most commonly prescribed medication found in this category is metformin. This class of drugs decreases glucose levels by reducing hepatic glucose production, as well as improving the use of peripheral glucose. As a result, the benefits include a reduction in plasma glucose and insulin levels, an improvement in a patient's lipid profile, and modest weight loss. Metformin usage can result in diarrhea, anorexia, nausea, and more seriously, lactic acidosis.[15] Given risk of lactic acidosis, especially in the event of compromised renal function, it is recommended that patients stop metformin 24 hours before any procedure.[14] Its use should be avoided in patients with renal insufficiency or glomerular filtration rate (GFR) less than 60 mL/min, any form of acidosis, congestive heart failure, liver disease, or severe hypoxemia, and discontinued in patients who become are seriously ill, nothing by mouth (NPO), or receiving radiographic contrast material.[15]

Insulin Secretagogues

Insulin secretagogues are agents that act on the ATP-sensitive potassium channels, resulting in the stimulation of insulin secretion. One class of insulin secretagogues are the sulfonylureas, which include glimepiride, glipizide, and glyburide. These drugs have a rapid onset of action and should therefore be taken shortly before a meal to avoid hypoglycemia, which is more commonly seen in older adults and with delayed meals, increased physical activity, alcohol intake, and renal insufficiency.[15]

The other insulin secretagogues that are not sulfonylureas are repaglinide and nateglinide. They have the same mechanism of action but have a short half life and are therefore given with or immediately before each meal.[15]

Alpha Glucosidase Inhibitors

Alpha glucosidase inhibitors include acarbose and miglitol. They are administered before each meal and postprandial hyperglycemia is reduced by the delay of glucose absorption. The enzyme that serves to cleave oligosaccharides into simple sugars in the intestinal lumen is inhibited, which therefore slows the absorption of glucose. These agents do not affect the use of glucose or insulin secretion. Side effects include diarrhea, flatulence, abdominal distention, and an increased incidence of hypoglycemia when used with sulfonylureas. Its use should be avoided in patients using bile acid resins and/or antacids, patients with inflammatory bowel disease, gastroparesis, or serum creatinine greater than 2 mg/dL.[15]

Thiazolidinediones

This category includes pioglitazone, rosiglitazone, and troglitazone, but only pioglitazone and rosiglitazone are available on the market, as troglitazone has been withdrawn because of reports of hepatotoxicity and hepatic failure. They decrease glucose levels by reducing insulin resistance via the peroxisome proliferator-activated receptor gamma (PPAR-gamma), which is found at the highest level in adipocytes, as well as promotion of redistribution of fat from central to peripheral locations. Administration of thiazolidinediones is associated with a decrease in circulating insulin levels, suggesting a reduction in insulin resistance. Side effects include weight gain, small reduction in hematocrit, mild increase in plasma volume, peripheral edema, and congestive heart failure. Its use is contraindicated in liver disease or history of congestive heart failure (class III or IV) and avoided in those with diabetic macular degeneration. Liver function should be monitored during this therapy.[15]

Other Agents

Colesevelam can be used for hypoglycemia purposes, but the mechanism of action is unknown. Side effects include constipation, abdominal pain, and nausea. It has been associated with an increase in plasma triglycerides and should therefore be used cautiously in patients with hypertriglyceridemia.[15]

Pramlintide is injected immediately before meals. It functions to slow gastric emptying and suppresses glucagon but does not alter insulin levels. It is associated with a modest reduction in hemoglobin A1c and dampens meal-related glucose increases. Side effects include nausea and vomiting.[15]

Insulin

In patients who partially or completely lack endogenous insulin production, insulin regimens are often added to mimic physiologic insulin secretion for the treatment of hyperglycemia. The regimen includes basal insulin administration as well as insulin replacement at meals. Basal insulin regulates the breakdown of glycogen, gluconeogenesis, lipolysis, and ketogenesis. Insulin replacement at meals should be given based upon carbohydrate intake and serves to promote the normal use and storage of glucose.[15]

Short-acting insulin, such as insulin lispro, insulin aspart, insulin glulisine, and regular insulin, is preferred for prandial coverage. It is rapidly absorbed, has a short onset of action, has short duration of action, and therefore is most useful for action against rising plasma glucose levels following meals.[15]

Long-acting insulin, such as Neutral Protamine Hagedorn (NPH) insulin, insulin glargine, and insulin detemir, are used for basal maintenance of glucose levels. Insulin glargine has a duration of action of approximately 24 hours and has a less pronounced peak of action, resulting in a decreased incidence of nocturnal hypoglycemia. Insulin detemir usually requires twice-daily injections to provide 24-hour coverage. It is important to note that the mixing of long-acting and short-acting insulin formulations may result in altering of the absorption.[15]

Insulin can also be delivered as a continuous subcutaneous infusion, which includes a basal insulin infusion and preprandial boluses delivered by the infusion device based on instructions programmed by the patient following individualized algorithms. Continuous subcutaneous infusions, or "insulin

pumps," should be managed by health professionals with considerable experience with insulin devices. The benefits of insulin pumps include the ability to program multiple infusion rates to accommodate for altered periods of requirements (such as exercise and nocturnal versus daytime requirements), as well as the use of different infusions with meal-related boluses to meet the needs of differing meal compositions. Complications include infection, hyperglycemia when infusion is obstructed, and diabetic ketoacidosis with disconnected pumps.[15]

COMPLICATIONS OF DIABETES

Diabetes not only affects glycemic control but also affects multiple organ systems and must therefore be a consideration for both short-term perioperative outcomes and long-term postoperative outcomes in patients undergoing total knee arthroplasty. Uncontrolled diabetes can result in both acute and chronic complications. There are three life-threatening acute complications of diabetes: hypoglycemia, diabetic ketoacidosis, and hyperosmolar nonketotic coma.

Hypoglycemia

Hypoglycemia is caused by an absolute or relative excess of insulin relative to carbohydrate intake and exercise. Symptoms of hypoglycemia include anxiety, lightheadedness, confusion, convulsions, and coma. The normal response to hypoglycemia is secretion of glucagon and/or epinephrine to increase glucose levels, but this mechanism fails in the diabetic patient (also known as *counterregulatory failure*). Because of the excess catecholamine, patients may also experience nervousness, diaphoresis, and tachycardia during episodes of hypoglycemia. Treatment includes glucose administration either via oral or intravenous route.[14]

On the other hand, diabetic ketoacidosis and hyperosmolar nonketotic coma are caused by an absolute or relative deficiency of insulin, which can lead to volume depletion and acid-base abnormalities, and are both potentially serious complications if diagnosis and treatment are not promptly carried out.[15]

Diabetic Ketoacidosis

Diabetic ketoacidosis is often seen in type 1 diabetics but can also be seen in patients with type 2 diabetes. There is a result of absolute or relative insulin deficiency concomitant with a counter-regulatory hormone excess, including glucagon, catecholamines, cortisol, and growth hormones. When there exists a decreased ratio of insulin to glucagon, the body stimulates gluconeogenesis, glycogenolysis, and ketone body formation as a result of fatty acid release from adipocytes.[15]

Symptoms of diabetic ketoacidosis include nausea and/or vomiting, thirst, polyuria, abdominal pain, shortness of breath, and changes in sensorium. Physical findings include signs of dehydration (tachycardia, hypotension), respiratory distress (tachypnea, Kussmaul breathing, respiratory distress), abdominal tenderness, as well as progressive changes in mental status (lethargy, obtundation, cerebral edema, and coma). The diagnosis of diabetic ketoacidosis includes findings of hyperglycemia, ketosis with positive urine ketones, and metabolic acidosis with an increased anion gap (arterial pH 6.8 to 7.3). There is not always a correlation between level of hyperglycemia and degree of acidosis, as diabetic ketoacidosis can be present in mildly elevated glucose levels but ketonemia is a consistent finding in diabetic ketoacidosis.[14,15]

Other electrolyte abnormalities found in diabetic ketoacidosis include serum bicarbonate less than 10 mmol/L, elevated serum potassium level with a total body potassium deficit, elevated BUN and Cr (signifying intravascular depletion), and decreased serum sodium level with a normal serum sodium level signifying a profound water deficit. Other findings include leukocytosis, hypertriglyceridemia, and hyperlipoproteinemia.[15]

Diabetic ketoacidosis is often precipitated by inadequate insulin administration (such as a malfunction of an insulin delivery system) or an increase in insulin requirements that occurs during a concurrent illness, including infection (pneumonia, urinary tract infections, gastroenteritis, sepsis) and infarction (cerebral, coronary, mesenteric, peripheral); with drug use (cocaine); and during pregnancy.[15]

The differential diagnosis of diabetic ketoacidosis incudes starvation ketosis, alcoholic ketoacidosis (serum bicarbonate >15 mEq/L), or other increased anion gap acidosis.[15]

Treatment of diabetic ketoacidosis includes IV fluid replacement, insulin therapy, and treatment of the precipitating agent or event. There is an approximate fluid deficit of ~3 to 5 L, which should be replaced with normal saline. When hemodynamic stability and adequate urine output are achieved, 0.45% normal saline should be used to reduce the trend toward hyperchloremia. When glucose is less than 200 mg/dL, fluids should be switched to 5% glucose + 0.45% normal saline.[15]

Insulin therapy is started with an initial bolus of IV short-acting insulin of 0.1 units/kg, followed by IV regular insulin of 0.1 units/kg/hour. IV insulin should be continued until the acidosis resolves, where it is then transitioned to long-acting subcutaneous insulin. Short-acting subcutaneous insulin is added when patient resumes oral intake.[15]

Electrolyte abnormalities should also be addressed. As glucose moves intracellularly with insulin therapy, it is followed by potassium. In addition, the patient has a total body potassium deficit that should be repleted once adequate urine output is achieved and normal serum potassium documented. Bicarbonate replacement is usually not necessary. Bicarbonate administration and rapid reversal of acidosis may impair cardiac function, resulting in reduction of tissue oxygenation and promoting hypokalemia.[15]

Ketoacidosis will resolve with insulin therapy as it reduces lipolysis, increases peripheral ketone body use, suppresses hepatic ketone body formation, and promotes bicarbonate regeneration. Acidosis and ketosis resolves more slowly than hyperglycemia. Successful treatment often results in a hyperchloremic acidosis that resolves as the kidneys regenerate bicarbonate and excrete chloride.[15]

Hyperglycemic Hyperosmolar State

The hyperglycemic hyperosmolar state is primarily seen in patients with type 2 diabetes and is secondary to a relative insulin deficiency and inadequate fluid intake. It is usually precipitated by a serious illness, including myocardial infarctions, strokes, sepsis, or pneumonia. The insulin deficiency results in increased hepatic glucose production and impaired glucose use in skeletal muscles. The resulting hyperglycemia leads to an osmotic diuresis and subsequent intravascular volume depletion, exacerbated by inadequate volume replacement. Unlike diabetic ketoacidosis, the hyperglycemic hyperosmolar state presents with an absence of ketosis.[14,15]

The prototypical patient is an elderly patient with type 2 diabetes presenting with symptoms of prolonged polyuria, weight loss, and diminished oral intake, leading to subsequent mental confusion, lethargy, and coma. Because of profound dehydration caused by a hyperglycemia-induced diuresis, physical exam findings will include hypotension, tachycardia, altered mental status, kidney failure, lactic acidosis, intravascular thrombosis, and seizures. In comparison to diabetic ketoacidosis, the following symptoms are generally absent: nausea, vomiting, abdominal pain, and Kussmaul respirations. On laboratory examination, the patient has glucose levels greater than 1000 mg/dL, serum osmolality greater than 350 mOsm/L, prerenal azotemia, and ketonuria, which may be present because of starvation.[14,15]

Similar to treatment of diabetic ketoacidosis, the treatment of the hyperglycemic hyperosmolar state involves IV fluid replacement therapy and insulin treatment. Fluid replacement is with 1 to 3 L of 0.9% normal saline over 2 to 3 hours to stabilize hemodynamic status. Rapid fluid replacement may worsen neurologic function because of a rapid reversal of a hyperosmolar state. If serum sodium is greater than 150 mEq/L, 0.45% saline should be administered. When hemodynamic stability has been achieved, fluid administration should be directed at reversing free water deficit, estimated at approximately 9 to 10 L, using hypotonic fluids, then 5% dextrose in water over the next 1 to 2 days.[15]

Insulin treatment begins with a bolus of 0.1 units/kg, then an infusion of 0.1 units/kg/hour. During therapy, glucose should be added to IV fluids when plasma glucose is 250 to 300 mg/dL. Electrolyte replacement is often necessary, especially for potassium and phosphate.[15]

Chronic Complications

Symptoms of hyperglycemia resolve when glucose is less than 200 mg/dL, but the risk of chronic complications increases as a function of the duration and degree of hyperglycemia. Chronic complications of diabetes mellitus can be divided into microvascular versus macrovascular complications. Microvascular complications include those related to retinopathy, neuropathy, and nephropathy. In contrast, macrovascular complications include coronary heart disease, peripheral arterial disease, and cerebrovascular disease. It is therefore imperative to keep in consideration the multiorgan effects of diabetes mellitus.[15]

Ocular. Retinopathy is the leading cause of blindness between the ages of 20 and 74 and is because of progressive diabetic retinopathy as well as macular edema. The duration and degree of glycemic control are the best predictors of the development of retinopathy.[15]

Nonproliferative disease generally occurs late in the first decade or early in the second decade of the disease process. During this stage, retinal vascular microaneurysms form that result in blot hemorrhages and cotton wool spots. As this progresses, there will be changes in venous vessel size, intraretinal microvascular abnormalities, and thereby more numerous microaneurysms and hemorrhages, with the end result of retinal ischemia. Severe nonproliferative disease has a higher likelihood of progression to proliferative disease.[15]

Proliferative retinopathy has the appearance of neovascularization in response to retinal hypoxemia. Newly formed vessels are visible near the optic nerve and/or macula. These vessels rupture easily, which then leads to vitreous hemorrhage, fibrosis, and possible retinal detachment.[15]

Nerves. Neuropathy is present in approximately 50% of patients with diabetes. The development of neuropathy correlates with the duration of diabetes and glycemic control, with additional risk factors of body mass index (BMI) and smoking. It can present as a polyneuropathy, mononeuropathy, or an autonomic neuropathy. The most common neuropathy seen in diabetic patients is a distal symmetrical polyneuropathy affecting the lower extremities, which may be accompanied by motor weakness. In contrast, mononeuropathy is less common but most commonly affects the third cranial nerve.[15]

In diabetic patients with a concurrent diagnosis of hypertension, there is a 40% to 50% likelihood of coexisting autonomic neuropathy.[14] Diabetes mellitus–related autonomic neuropathy involves multiple systems, including cardiovascular, gastrointestinal, genitourinary, sudomotor, and metabolic.

Cardiovascular effects may potentially alter hemodynamic responses to anesthesia and surgery. Autonomic neuropathy limits the cardiovascular system's ability to compensate for intravascular volume changes, such as via mechanisms of tachycardia and increased peripheral vascular resistance, and therefore may predispose patients to cardiovascular instability following induction and with blood loss, increasing the risk for sudden cardiac death. The risk of cardiovascular instability is increased with concomitant use of ACE inhibitors and angiotensin receptor blockers (ARBs), which are commonly used for treatment of hypertension and renal protection in diabetics.[14] Signs of autonomic neuropathy of the cardiovascular system include resting tachycardia and orthostatic hypotension.[15]

Autonomic neuropathy affecting the gastrointestinal system results in gastroparesis, contributing to a delayed gastric emptying, increasing the risk for aspiration during surgery.[14] Premedication with a nonparticulate antacid (to decrease stomach content acidity in the event of aspiration) and metoclopramide to increase gastric motility can be used.

Genitourinary effects include cystopathy, where the patient has the inability to sense a full bladder and often experiences failure to void completely, urinary hesitance, decreased voiding frequency, incontinence, and therefore recurrent urinary tract infections. Patients should therefore be screened with urinalyses and treated accordingly.

Sudomotor effects of autonomic neuropathy include hyperhidrosis of the upper extremities and anhidrosis of the feet, which increases the risk of dry skin and foot ulcers in the diabetic patient.

Autonomic neuropathy can also affect the diabetic patient's ability to compensate for hypoglycemia. The diabetic patient loses the ability to sense hypoglycemia, which results in a reduction of the normal counter-regulatory mechanism of catecholamine release to stimulate an increase in glucose level. These patients are therefore at risk of severe hypoglycemia during the perioperative period.

Renal. Diabetes mellitus is the leading cause of end stage renal disease in the United States and also the leading cause of morbidity and mortality in type 1 diabetics. Microalbuminuria can be seen when there are changes in the glomerulus, which is an important risk factor for progression to macroalbuminuria. The presence of macroalbuminuria is usually associated with a concomitant decline in GFR, and the pathologic changes at this point are typically irreversible. Hemodialysis in diabetic patients is often associated with more frequent complications including

hypotension secondary to autonomic neuropathy and loss of reflex tachycardia, difficult vascular access, and accelerated progression of retinopathy.[15]

Type IV renal tubular acidosis may also develop in patients with compromised renal function, and it leads to a propensity for hyperkalemia that can be exacerbated by medications such as angiotensin converting enzyme (ACE) inhibitors and angiotension receptor blockers (ARB). These patients are also predisposed to contrast-induced nephrotoxicity.[15]

ACE inhibitors and ARBs are often used in diabetic patients for renal protection. There is evidence that these slow the progression of nephropathy, slow progression to macroalbuminuria, and slow the decline of GFR. Diabetic patients should therefore have their serum potassium and renal function investigated prior to surgery.[15]

Cardiovascular. There is an extremely high prevalence of underlying cardiovascular disease in diabetic patients, as evidenced by the Framingham Heart Study, which revealed a marked increase risk of peripheral arterial disease, congestive heart failure, coronary heart disease, myocardial infarction, and sudden death in diabetic patients. The American Heart Association considers diabetes mellitus to be a coronary heart disease risk equivalent.

A thorough cardiac evaluation should be considered in patients undergoing surgical procedures such as total knee arthroplasty. Evidence of atherosclerotic disease should be investigated, looking for symptoms of chest pain, atypical chest pain, or abnormal resting electrocardiogram (ECG), such as ST segment and T wave abnormalities, suggesting cardiac ischemia.[14,15] Preoperative chest radiographs may show cardiac enlargement, pulmonary vascular congestion, and/or pleural effusions but should be obtained on a clinical basis and not routinely indicated for every patient.[14] Patients can often also present with evidence of peripheral arterial disease or carotid arterial disease.[15]

Skin. Hyperglycemia in diabetic patients leads to glycosylation of tissue proteins that results in limited mobility of joints. Therefore, the temporomandibular joint and cervical spine should be assessed to reduce the likelihood of unanticipated difficult intubations.[14]

Infections. Diabetic patients experience infections with greater frequency and severity. The mechanism is proposed to be because of abnormalities in cell-mediated immunity and phagocyte function that is secondary to hyperglycemia, as well as diminished vascularization. Hyperglycemia secondarily also increases risk of infection by providing a hospitable area for colonization and growth of bacteria. Common infections in this patient population include pneumonia, urinary tract infections, and skin and soft tissue infections.[15]

SURGICAL COMPLICATIONS

Glucose control may difficult to maintain in the perioperative period, and assessment of control should be ascertained through history and/or laboratory testing. Diabetes mellitus has been shown to portend a higher risk of postoperative complications, including myocardial infarction, cerebrovascular accident, urinary tract infection, ileus, deep venous thrombosis, and/or pulmonary embolism, pneumonia, sciatic injury, nonroutine or delayed discharge, higher hospital charges, increased postoperative mortality, worse functional outcomes, and most importantly surgical site infections.[1,8]

Diabetes has been identified as a possible modifiable risk factor for both surgical site infections and periprosthetic joint infections.[4,10] Surgical site infections and prosthetic joint infections are rare but devastating complications[4] and are the most common reason for reoperations, with an incidence of 0.5% to 10%.[9,13] The superficial wound infection rate is reported to be 6% to 12% in the diabetic patient, compared to a 1.7% to 10.5% infection rate in the general population. Periprosthetic joint infections have been quoted to be 0.34% to 5.3% in diabetic patients, compared to 0.5% to 2% in the general population.[7,9]

Periprosthetic joint infections add significant expense to the health care system, as well as a societal burden, so there has been much investigation to determine the most appropriate optimization prior to surgery.[4] Theoretically, a patient with controlled blood glucose levels or controlled diabetes would have improved outcomes. The current American Diabetes Association guidelines recommend the following for adults patients: (1) hemoglobin A1c less than 7%, (2) preprandial capillary plasma glucose level of 90 to 130, and (3) peak postprandial capillary plasma glucose level less than 180 mg/dL.[12] Because of the potential for significant financial and personal burden secondary to complications from total knee arthroplasty, candidates who are at higher risks of complications should be identified using clinically accessible risk markers to decrease these risks.[8]

A retrospective study by Hwang et al. in 2015 evaluated glycemic markers that are used to assess the efficacy of glycemic control and their correlation with postoperative complications.[10] The most commonly used marker for glycemic control is preoperative hemoglobin A1c level, which is a measurement of glycated or glycosylated hemoglobin and is a standard method for assessing long-term glycemic control.[15] It provides an indication of degree of glycemic control over a 3-month period or an average glucose concentration over this 3-month period. This compares to blood glucose level measurements, which will fluctuate with diet and only represent acute glycemic control at the time of measurement.[10] The other markers assessed by Hwang et al. include preoperative fasting blood glucose, preoperative 2-hour postprandial glucose level, and postoperative random glucose level (taken on postoperative days 2, 5, and 14).[10]

This study found positive correlations among the values of the four glycemic markers and their chosen endpoints, which included surgical site infections, both superficial and deep, and wound complications, such as drainage, hemarthrosis, skin necrosis, and dehiscence.[10] The strongest correlation was noted between preoperative hemoglobin A1c levels, and correlations with preoperative glycemic markers were stronger than those between postoperative markers. Based on their study, a hemoglobin A1c level of greater than or equal to 8 and fasting blood glucose of greater than or equal to 200 were identified as markers associated with an increased risk of superficial surgical site infections. No patient in the study developed periprosthetic infections. Similarly, Giori et al. also found an increased risk of postoperative complications, but this was also not significant for periprosthetic infections, associated with an increased hemoglobin A1c values.

However, although there is substantial evidence for an increased incidence in wound infections in diabetic patients,[4,6,11]

the evidence is controversial in regard to the value of the preoperative markers (ie, hemoglobin A1c) that would increase the risk substantially enough to warrant a delay in total knee arthroplasty for optimal control. Because blood glucose fluctuates with diet and measurement therefore only represents acute glycemic control at the time of measurement, hemoglobin A1c has been traditionally used as a marker for perioperative glycemic control, as it represents a degree of glycemic control over a 3-month period.[10] Hemoglobin A1c is a measurement of glycated hemoglobin, but the results can be affected by assay methodology, hemoglobinopathies, anemia, reticulocytosis, and transfusion.[15] However, the data for hemoglobin A1c as a preoperative screen tool are conflicting.

In 2007, the American Diabetes Association recommended a target goal hemoglobin A1c for adult patients to be less than 7%, with a normal range of 4% to 7%.[12] Kremers et al. found higher infections rates in diabetics, with results not significant for periprosthetic joint infections, but their infection rates were not found to be associated with specific hemoglobin A1c values.[11] Similarly, Iorio et al. found a higher incidence of infection with diabetic patients, these findings were also not associated with hemoglobin A1c values.[6,10a]

Chrastil et al. found no difference in terms of infection between well controlled versus poorly controlled diabetics, but found that there was an inability to adequately identify diabetic patients at higher risk for infection using hemoglobin A1c alone. They did find that poor preoperative glucose control, as indicated by preoperative glucose level, increased the risk of periprosthetic joint infection. In addition, they found only a moderate correlation between hemoglobin A1c and preoperative glucose levels.[4] Reategui et al. also studied the effects of hyperglycemia and found that immediate postoperative hyperglycemia correlated with an increased risk of medical and infectious complications.[16]

In contrast, Marchant et al. found a 2.28 times higher incidence of wound infection in uncontrolled diabetic patients.[6,12] Lai et al. also found a higher incidence of infection with suboptimally controlled diabetes.[11a,19] Stryker et al. investigated both blood glucose and hemoglobin A1c levels and found an increased odds ratio for wound complications with blood glucose levels greater than 200 and hemoglobin A1c levels greater than 6.7%.[19] Jamsen et al. also found a direct correlation between hyperglycemia levels and hemoglobin A1c levels in association with infections.[10b,19] Han and Kang also found that poor preoperative glycemic control, as defined by a hemoglobin A1c level of greater than 8%, was associated with a significantly higher risk of postoperative wound infection.[7]

Evidence is therefore conflicting as to what extent the disease itself, perioperative hyperglycemia control, or diabetes management around the time of surgery modify the risk of surgical site infections. The evidence suggests that the presence of diabetes mellitus and hyperglycemia is associated with an increased risk of surgical site infections, but the evidence is inconsistent with respect to the role of diabetes control on the risk of surgical site infections.[11]

In addition, although it is necessary to decrease surgical risks by ensuring patients have appropriately controlled diabetes prior to total knee arthroplasty, this needs to be balanced with surgical access and the potential for surgical benefit. Therefore, there should be some threshold set to identify those patients in which a delay in surgery for medical optimization would be beneficial. If this threshold is set too low, it could delay surgery for more patients without avoiding significantly more complications. However, if this threshold is set too high, this may result in delaying surgery for those who otherwise would not have had any complications.[5,8] It is important to note that many studies have been retrospective and therefore rely on International Classification of Diseases Ninth Revision (ICD-9) codes for diagnoses of uncontrolled versus controlled diabetes, which may be confounding results. Further investigative studies are needed to elucidate appropriate markers and thresholds to consider for risk stratifying diabetic patients prior to total knee arthroplasty.[1]

It is also prudent to consider other risk factors for infections in this patient population. A meta-analysis showed that being male, having a BMI greater than 30, diabetes mellitus, hypertension, rheumatoid arthritis, and steroid therapy are all independent risk factors for infection after primary total knee arthroplasty.[3] Looking specifically at deep infections or periprosthetic joint infections, it was found that male gender, obesity, rheumatoid arthritis, posttraumatic arthritis, and longer operative times were risk factors. Every 15 minute increase in operative time was found to be associated with a 9% increase in deep surgical site infection. A lower proportion of infections were found in patients receiving spinal anesthesia and antibiotic irrigation for infection prophylaxis.[13]

Diabetic patients also experience other nonsurgical complications at a higher rate than nondiabetic patients and controlled diabetic patients, including length of stay, mortality, cerebrovascular accidents, myocardial infarction, urinary tract infections, ileus, thrombophlebitis, pneumonia, postoperative hemorrhage, and increased rates of transfusions.[12] One study showed that patients had a twofold increase in 30-day mortality when comparing those with diabetes to those with normal glucose values on admission.[9] Another study showed that diabetic patients had a 2.71-fold higher risk in developing deep vein thrombosis following total knee arthroplasty. And specifically patients with higher blood glucose levels were more prone to venous thromboembolisms, even when adjusted for age, gender, ethnicity, and BMI.[20]

FUNCTIONAL OUTCOMES

The other outcome measure that can be affected by diabetes is the functional outcome following total knee arthroplasty. Patients with diabetes have been identified to have worse functional outcome compared to their nondiabetic cohorts. Robertson et al. found that diabetic patients had a lower maximal flexion and decreased overall range of motion.[17] Amusat et al. delved deeper and hypothesized that patients with diabetes who identified preoperatively that their diabetes affected their routine activities would have a slower recovery after total knee arthroplasty than those whose routine activities were not affected. There was no statistical difference at 1 month, but at 3 and 6 months, it was found that diabetes that affected routine activities also resulted in poorer function.[2] Singh and Lewallen also found that diabetes increased the odds of moderate to severe daily living limitations in patients undergoing primary total knee arthroplasty by almost twofold. In addition, they found that those with diabetes associated with complications preoperatively had a stronger risk of daily living limitations.[18] The importance of these results is as a predictive marker of recovery after total knee arthroplasty, and they encourage closer monitoring by physiotherapy.[2]

The references for this chapter can also be found on www.expertconsult.com.

80

Rheumatoid Arthritis

Cheng-Ting Lee, Arthur Atchabahian

BACKGROUND

Rheumatoid arthritis (RA) is a chronic, systemic autoimmune disease that is characterized by erosive polyarthropathy, most commonly involving synovium-lined joints in the body. The progressive joint inflammation in RA is a result of the destruction of the synovial membrane by cell-mediated immunity in the body. While the exact mechanism remains unclear, activated CD4+ cells and cytokines such as tumor necrosis factor (TNF)-α and interleukin 1 (IL-1) recruit inflammatory cells such as neutrophils, macrophages, lymphocytes, and plasma cells to the synovial membrane.[7] This chronic inflammation process at the articular junctions stimulates the normal fibroblast-like synoviocytes and chondrocytes to proliferate and become hyperplastic. The altered, dysfunctional synoviocytes and local cells form a layer of metabolically active tissue called *pannus* and also begin to secrete matrix-metalloproteinases (MMPs) instead of producing synovial fluid that normally provides nutrition to the synovium and lubricates the joint.[30] Pannus interfaces with cartilage and bone cause the joint to be swollen, spongy, and warm to touch on physical exam, and ultimately destroys the joints as observed in the progress of RA. Erosions are the key end point of the rheumatoid inflammatory process that treatments aim to prevent, as they represent irreversible damage and disability.

The diagnosis of RA is based on detailed clinical history and thorough physical examination, and confirmed with laboratory tests with specific antibodies and biomarkers. Diagnostic criteria include symptoms lasting more than 6 weeks, the presence of inflammatory arthritis in more than three joints, and the exclusion of other diseases with similar clinical presentations such as systemic lupus erythematosus, acute viral polyarthritis, or other erosive or calcium pyrophosphate deposition diseases.[1] Positive rheumatoid factor and anticyclic citrullinated peptide antibodies tests have a high diagnostic sensitivity, although both can be negative in 50% of the patients with RA.[21] Erythrocyte sedimentation and serum C-reactive protein levels are often used to monitor treatment and as indicators for severity and progress of the disease.

PREOPERATIVE

The preoperative investigation of an RA patient undergoing surgery should focus on the state of the disease, the extent of systemic effects, and drug toxicities. Patients with RA often have multisystem diseases that are crucial to their perioperative management (Fig. 80.1; see Fig. 32.1 in Basics of Anesthesia). Common pulmonary involvement includes pleural effusion, interstitial fibrosis, or pulmonary fibrosis as a side effect of medications such as methotrexate.[17] Costochondral involvement affecting chest wall movement can lead to restrictive lung changes resulting in decreased total lung volume and functional residual capacity.[31] These manifestations contribute to increased ventilation perfusion mismatch, arterial hypoxemia, and inadequate oxygenation. Rheumatoid nodules in the lungs can also be found in the parenchyma and pleural surface, mimicking tumor masses or tuberculosis on chest radiographic films, and causing fluid accumulation in the lungs and shortness of breath.[8] Arterial blood gas and pulmonary function tests should be considered in cases of severe pulmonary involvement in order to gauge the severity of the disease.

Cardiovascular disease is responsible for 50% of the deaths in people with RA.[11,14] Common manifestations include coronary artery disease or arteritis, valvular defects, and accelerated coronary atherosclerosis. While a third of RA patients are found to have pericardial thickening and effusion,[14] aortic regurgitation can be observed in patients who have aortitis with dilation of the aortic root. Because conduction abnormalities are often present, obtaining an electrocardiogram should be part of the routine preoperative evaluation. If severe valvular heart disease and pericarditis are suspected, echocardiography should be conducted to rule out underlying heart failure or cardiomyopathy before surgery.

Rheumatoid vasculitis caused by the deposition of immune complexes in the arteries can develop in various stages of the disease. When the immune complexes are deposited in the vasa nervorum, neuropathy in the form of mononeuritis multiplex often presents as numbness, tingling, and weakness.[19] Affecting all vessels, from small synovial blood vessels to medium and large arteries, RA vasculitis can cause bleeding skin ulcerations, purpura, and visceral ischemia, leading to small bowel ulceration, myocardial infarction, and even cerebral infarction.[23,26,34]

Anemia of chronic disease and thrombocytosis consistent with chronic inflammation are often present in RA patients, the severity of which usually correlates to the state of the disease. Felty's syndrome consisting of arthritis, splenomegaly, and leukopenia can also be observed and is more prevalent in 50-70-year-old Caucasian females.[8] Because erythropoiesis can also be inadequate in patients with RA as a result of damaged kidneys, it is important to consider perioperative transfusion to ensure proper hemoglobin content for optimized oxygen carrying capacity before surgery.

Subclinical renal dysfunction is believed to be present in 40% of the RA patients, essentially because of amyloidosis, small vessel vasculitis, and drug toxicity.[3,9] Subclinical liver function

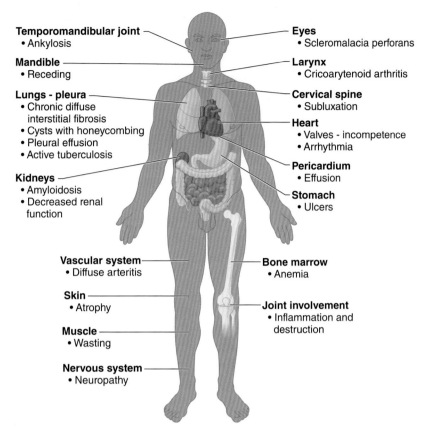

Temporomandibular joint
• Ankylosis

Mandible
• Receding

Lungs - pleura
• Chronic diffuse
  interstitial fibrosis
• Cysts with honeycombing
• Pleural effusion
• Active tuberculosis

Kidneys
• Amyloidosis
• Decreased renal
  function

Eyes
• Scleromalacia perforans

Larynx
• Cricoarytenoid arthritis

Cervical spine
• Subluxation

Heart
• Valves - incompetence
• Arrhythmia

Pericardium
• Effusion

Stomach
• Ulcers

Vascular system
• Diffuse arteritis

Skin
• Atrophy

Muscle
• Wasting

Nervous system
• Neuropathy

Bone marrow
• Anemia

Joint involvement
• Inflammation and
  destruction

FIG 80.1 Systemic manifestations of rheumatoid arthritis (see Fig. 32.1 in Basics of Anesthesia).

test abnormalities are also often present. Because anesthetic drugs are typically eliminated by the kidney or the liver, and can have renal and liver toxicity, it is critical to assess patients' baseline functions to devise the safest anesthesia plan for the surgery.

ANATOMICAL ABNORMALITIES AND DIFFICULT AIRWAYS

Airway management and patient positioning remain the two biggest challenges in the anesthesia plan for RA patients undergoing orthopedic surgery. The most drastic changes in a RA patient are usually found in the osteoarticular system. Prolonged RA can lead to changes in blood supply to the synovium, resulting in decreased sympathetic innervation and sensation defects.[24] These articular changes can compromise patient positioning during surgery, and can limit access for regional anesthetic techniques such as peripheral nerve blocks. Patients with RA can also have frail skin because of either underlying vasculitis or chronic steroid use,[23] leading to a higher risk of tissue ischemia, skin breakdown, and positioning injuries during surgery.

RA patients often suffer from destruction of synovial joints, affecting mainly the small joints, especially the temporomandibular joint and spine joints for anesthesia purposes.[28] The anesthetic plan will depend on the type of surgery and the general condition of the patient. The most common procedures performed on RA patients are hip and knee arthroplasty, while synovectomy is usually the first surgery needed.[22] Hand and foot surgeries are frequently performed for symptom control.

Regional anesthesia has the advantage of better postoperative pain management. Conversely, general anesthesia has the advantage of better control of cardiovascular and respiratory functions, and allows keeping patients in unusual positions without limiting the duration of the procedures because of patient discomfort.

Head and neck involvement in RA patients poses a major challenge for airway management and manipulation. It is estimated that over 80% of the RA patients have cervical spine abnormalities and at least 30% of them experience symptoms of pain from instability in the affected spinal segments.[27,37] Isolated atlantoaxial subluxation (AAS), especially anterior AAS, cranial settling, subaxial subluxation, and a combination of these are among the four most common cervical spine instability in patients with RA[37] (Fig. 80.2; see Fig. 32.2 in Basics of Anesthesia). Extension of the atlantoaxial joint during laryngoscopy or worsening of the subaxial subluxation during transport can exacerbate the underlying deformity and greatly increase the risk of superior migration of the odontoid, myelopathy, spinal cord impingement; pyramidal symptoms such as plantar extension and hyperreflexia; or in extreme situations, sudden death.[29] In fact, it has been recommended that the sniffing position, flexion of the neck, and extension of the head on the neck for direct laryngoscopy be avoided in patients with RA. Instead, the "protrusion position" using a donut-shaped pillow on top of a flat pillow during anesthesia has been found to reduce anterior atlantodental interval and increase posterior atlantodental interval, while optimally increasing the C1-C2 angle, and is recommended as a desirable intubation position for RA patients with AAS.[35]

Radiologic investigations of the cervical spine in anteroposterior, lateral, open-mouth odontoid, and lateral flexion-extension dynamic views are recommended in high-risk patients as part of their preoperative evaluation (Fig. 80.3; see Fig. 32.5 in Basics of Anesthesia). Although magnetic resonance imaging (MRI) in neutral, flexed, and extended positions can provide better assessment of the cervical spine and the surrounding soft tissue, it is not recommended before surgery because of its poor correlation with clinical presentation and lack of impact on

airway manipulation.[37] When general anesthesia and tracheal intubation are necessary for a procedure or when the patient is symptomatic from cervical instability, fiberoptic laryngoscopy is the preferred intubation technique. Patients with confirmed severe cervical instability, a history of difficult intubation, or a high risk for aspiration of gastric contents should be treated as trauma patients with unstable cervical spine and receive awake fiberoptic intubation under sedation.[15,36] This technique decreases the risk of respiratory depression and allows for the assessment of neurological symptoms in case of spinal cord injury. Anesthetized or asleep fiberoptic or videolaryngoscopy intubation can also be used in asymptomatic RA patients deemed at lower risk of difficult mask ventilation. In patients with fused cervical spines presenting with difficult airways, preinduction intubation and the use of videolaryngoscopy can be preferred for maximizing patient safety and comfort. Videolaryngoscopy is a relatively new technique, and its exact indications, as well as the role of the various tools (Glidescope, Airtraq, McGrath, etc.), remain to be defined by further investigations.

Bilateral or unilateral temporomandibular joint (TMJ) arthritis is found in 70% of RA patients and is frequently associated with cervical fixation and a higher prevalence of obstructive sleep apnea (OSA).[17,33] TMJ dysfunction and restricted mouth opening are found to be a result of the articular fibrosis leading to surface ankylosis in both upper and lower jaws as part of the RA process. Joint deformities also lead to acquired retrognathia or micrognathia, which is often seen in juvenile rheumatoid arthritis. These clinical features make appropriate mask ventilation difficult and limit endotracheal intubation with direct laryngoscopy. Fiberoptic laryngoscopy is the recommended intubation method, while the supine patient position is found to increase the risk of obstructed upper airway in patients with TMJ arthritis.[33]

Asymptomatic or symptomatic rheumatoid involvement of the larynx, such as mucosal erythema and limited mobility of vocal cord or arytenoid, is present in 69% of RA patients.[6] Cricoarytenoid arthritis is a rare larynx abnormality found in

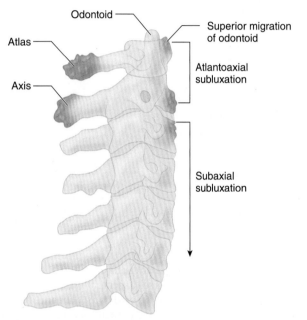

FIG 80.2 Sites of potential involvement of rheumatoid arthritis in the cervical spine (see Fig. 32.2 in Basics of Anesthesia).

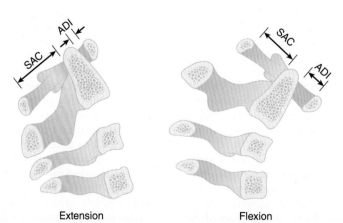

FIG 80.3 Flexion and extension views demonstrating how flexion increases ADI and decreases the SAC. In extension, the ADI is decreased and the SAC is increased (see Fig. 32.5 in Basics of Anesthesia). *ADI,* Atlasdens interval; *SAC,* safe area for the spinal cord.

RA and is associated with narrowed glottis and increased risk of laryngospasm, sometimes observed incidentally with direct laryngoscopy during intubation.[18] It presents as a fixated cricoarytenoid joint on suspension laryngoscopy and clinically as a sensation of a foreign body stuck in the throat or dysphagia. The most important complications of cricoarytenoid arthritis are upper airway obstruction, inspiratory stridor, and postextubation respiratory distress or failure that sometimes leads to emergent tracheostomy. Preoperative fiberoptic laryngoscopy exam is the definitive technique to diagnose cricoarytenoid arthritis, and postoperative vigilance with adequate monitoring is critical in the management of a patient after surgery.

In advanced stages, as the cervical spine collapses and the neck shortens, the trachea will twist in a characteristic manner, further increasing the difficulty of intubation.

REGIONAL ANESTHESIA

When planning for the most appropriate anesthesia for patients with RA undergoing orthopedic surgeries, achieving adequate pain control with the optimization of postoperative quality of life should be taken into consideration. The cost of spinal anesthesia for orthopedic surgery is about half the cost of general anesthesia.[12] Patients who received general anesthesia for orthopedic surgery have also been found to require more analgesic during the postoperative recovery period. Therefore, the use of regional anesthesia as a sole anesthetic or as a combination with other anesthetic plans is important.

PHARMACOLOGICAL MANAGEMENT

Patients with RA undergoing surgery are often concurrently treated with medical regimens for symptom relief and disease modification. Understanding the toxicities and the perioperative management of these drugs is therefore critical to patient safety. Based on recent studies, traditional disease-modifying antirheumatic drugs (DMARDs) such as methotrexate, hydoxychloroquine, azathioprine, and sulfasalazine are safe to be used during the perioperative period, provided renal function is not significantly altered and side effects are monitored.[13,29] Leflunomide should be discontinued 1 week before operation, because of its increased association with postoperative wound complications. Biological agents such as anti-TNF-α should be discontinued at least 2 to 6 weeks, or 3 to 5 times the half life of the drug, before surgery.[13] Cytokines such as TNF-α and interleukins are prominent initiators of the innate immunity, and literature has shown an increase in postoperative skin and soft tissue infection, especially associated with *Staphyloccocus aureus* in patients on TNF-α inhibitors therapy.[4,10] Microorganisms also have the ability to form biofilms at the bone-prosthesis interface, leading to bacterial resistance and implant destruction.[2] Therefore, the management of TNF-α inhibitors in patients with RA undergoing orthopedic surgeries is particularly important and should be discussed with the rheumatologist ahead of time (Table 80.1).

Corticosteroids are reportedly used in 65% of RA patients, usually at a lower dose (<10 mg of prednisone/day) as a bridge therapy for the long-term establishment of a definitive disease-modifying treatment.[5] Higher dosages can also be used to manage other manifestations in RA, such as vasculitis. In addition to the well-recognized higher infection rate and poor wound healing, chronic corticosteroid use is associated with a wide range of complications, including osteoporosis, osteonecrosis, myopathy, and hyperglycemia. Intra-articular corticosteroid injections are sometimes used to provide pain relief of up to 3 months in patients with RA, but repeated injections may result in further cartilage destruction and osteonecrosis. Lastly, patients who have been treated with more than 20 mg/day of prednisone or equivalent for at least 3 weeks are considered to be on chronic steroid treatment and are at risk for adrenal insufficiency. Definitive guidelines for perioperative corticosteroid therapy are lacking, but 50 to 100 mg of hydrocortisone every 8 hours for 24 hours starting the evening before or on the morning of surgery is generally recommended in patients at risk for adrenal insufficiency who are undergoing major surgery.[25] Interestingly, some recent studies have shown no perioperative hypotension with only the usual daily dose of corticosteroids, suggesting that unnecessary higher doses of corticosteroids given perioperatively might expose patients to higher postoperative infection rates.[13]

Nonsteroidal anti-inflammatory drugs (NSAIDs) and cyclooxygenase-2 inhibitors (celecoxib) are effective pain relievers used in RA patients. Together, they can cause disturbance in thromboxane, prostacyclin, and prostaglandin synthesis and interfere with glomerular filtration. Common side effects of NSAIDs include gastrointestinal ulceration, gastric irritation, as well as liver and kidney toxicity. Although celecoxib has been found to reduce the risk of gastrointestinal bleeding by 50% to 60% compared to NSAIDs,[20] it is associated with a higher risk of cardiovascular events when used for prolonged periods and thus is now mostly used for 48 to 72 hours perioperatively for pain relief, as it can be given preoperatively because it does not significantly increase bleeding.[32]

While studies investigating pharmacokinetics in RA patients are lacking, assessing anesthetic drug interactions and potential changes in plasma protein concentration is important. Some drugs can cause a reduction in serum protein levels and an increase in alpha-1-glycoprotein (AAG), which may affect the free fraction of drugs.[38] For example, diazepam has a 98% albumin binding rate, and its effects can be exaggerated in the presence of hypoalbuminemia. On the other hand, drugs such as verapamil, propranolol, and metoclopramide have a high AAG affinity, and RA may lead to a reduction in their therapeutic effects because of a decreased free fraction. This could be an advantage when considering local anesthetics and the possibility of systemic toxicity.

POSTOPERATIVE CARE

Postoperative management of patients with RA should focus on providing effecting analgesia, shortening the immobilization period, and minimizing the risk of respiratory failure more frequently associated with opioid use. Pain management remains a challenge in RA patients. Nerve blocks placed preoperatively are effective for immediate postoperative pain control.[16] The use of opioids should be carefully monitored given that most RA patients are more sensitive to drugs and are more vulnerable to respiratory depression with a baseline of low or restricted lung volumes.[22] Providing adequate postoperative ventilatory support is especially critical in patients with other comorbidities such as obesity, mandibular hypoplasia, obstructive sleep apnea, chronic obstructive pulmonary disease (COPD), or abnormal preoperative lung function tests.

TABLE 80.1   Common Rheumatoid Arthritis Medications and Their Perioperative Management Recommendation[13,29]

Medications	Dosing Interval	Stopping Time Prior to Operation	Important Information/Potential Toxicities
Disease Modifying Anti-Rheumatic Drugs			
Methotrexate	Every week	None	Interstitial lung disease Liver toxicity Monitor renal function
Hydroxychloroquine	Every day	None	Ocular toxicity Monitor renal function
Leflunomide	Every day	1 week	Severe hepatoenteric recirculation Liver toxicity
Azathioprine	Every day	None	Some people are slow acetylators Pancreatitis Monitor renal function
Sulfasalazine	Every day	None	Stevens-Johnson syndrome Monitor renal function
Cyclosporine	Every day	None	Hypertension Monitor renal function
Anakinra	Every day	None	Pneumonia
TNF-α Inhibitors			
Etanercept	Every week	2 weeks	Possible higher infection risk
Adalimumab	Every 2 weeks	3 weeks	Possible higher infection risk
Infliximab	Every 4-8 weeks	6 weeks	Possible higher infection risk
Golimumab	Every month	6 weeks	Possible higher infection risk
Certolizumab	Every 4 weeks	6 weeks	Possible higher infection risk
Rituximab	Every 16-24 weeks	None, can continue	Infection risk has been shown not to be correlated to interval between dose and surgery
Abatacept	Every week for subcutaneous injection; every 4 weeks for intravenous injection	Hold subcutaneous injection for 2 weeks; hold intravenous injection for 4 weeks	Possible higher infection risk
Tocilizumab	Every 1-2 weeks for subcutaneous injection; every 4 weeks for intravenous injection	Hold subcutaneous injection for 3 weeks; hold intravenous injection for 4 weeks	Temperature, C-reactive protein (CRP) or other signs of infection might be masked

Perioperative RA flares also pose a challenge for the recovery of patients, especially after orthopedic surgeries. The most common sign of RA flare is fatigue or inability to carry out activities postoperatively, preventing patients from properly carrying out rehabilitation activities or returning to a better quality of life.[37] These should be managed in collaboration with a rheumatologist.

KEY REFERENCES

4. Bongartz T, Sutton AJ, Sweeting MJ, et al: Anti-TNF antibody therapy in rheumatoid arthritis and the risk of serious infections and malignancies: systematic review and meta-analysis of rare harmful effects in randomized controlled trials. *JAMA* 295:2275–2285, 2006.
5. Caplan L, Wolfe F, Russell AS, et al: Corticosteroid use in rheumatoid arthritis: prevalence, predictors, correlates, and outcomes. *J Rheumatol* 34:696–705, 2007.
11. Galvin EM, O'Donnell D, Leonard IE: Rheumatoid arthritis: a significant but often underestimated risk factor for perioperative cardiac morbidity. *Anesthesiology* 103:910–911, 2005.
13. Goodman S: Rheumatoid arthritis: perioperative management of biologics and DMARDs. *Semin Arthritis Rheum* 44:627–632, 2015.
14. Goodson N: Coronary artery disease and rheumatoid arthritis. *Curr Opin Rheumatol* 14:115–120, 2002.
21. Lindqvist E, Eberhardt K, Bendtzen K, et al: Prognostic laboratory markers of joint damage in rheumatoid arthritis. *Ann Rheum Dis* 64(2):196, 2005.
22. Lisowska B, Rutkowska-Sak L, Maldyk P, et al: Anaesthesiological problems in patients with rheumatoid arthritis undergoing orthopaedic surgeries. *Clin Rheumatol* 27:553–556, 2008.
23. Margo CM, Crowson AN: The spectrum of cutaneous lesions in rheumatoid arthritis: a clinical and pathological study of 43 patients. *J Cutan Pathol* 30(1):1–10, 2003.
29. Samanta R, Shoukrey K, Griffiths R: Rheumatoid arthritis and anaesthesia. *Anaesthesia* 66:1146–1159, 2011.
30. Shingu M, Ngai Y, Isayama T, et al: The effects of cytokines in metalloproteinase inhibitors (TIMP) and collagenase production by human chondrocytes in TIMP production by synovial cells and endothelia cells. *Clin Exp Immunol* 94:145–149, 1993.
31. Skues MA, Welchew EA: Anaesthesia and rheumatoid arthritis. *Anaesthesia* 43:989–997, 1993.
33. Sugahara T, Mori Y, Kawamoto T, et al: Obstructive sleep apnea associated with temporomandibular joint destruction by rheumatoid arthritis: report of case. *J Oral Maxillofac Surg* 52:876, 1994.
35. Tokunaga D, Hase H, Mikami Y, et al: Atlantoaxial subluxation in different intraoperative head positions in patients with rheumatoid arthritis. *Anesthesiology* 104:675–679, 2006.
36. Vieira EM, Goodman S, Tanaka PP: Anesthesia and rheumatoid arthritis. *Rev Bras Anestesiol* 61(3):367–375, 2011.
37. Wasserman BR, Moskovich R, Razi A: Rheumatoid arthritis of the cervical spine clinical considerations. *Bull NYU Hosp Jt Dis* 69(2):136–148, 2011.

The references for this chapter can also be found on www.expertconsult.com.

81

Bilateral Total Knee Replacement: Indications for Sequential and Simultaneous Surgery

Daniel C. Smith, Shawna Dorman, Jonathan M. Vigdorchik, Richard Iorio

Although the health care community continues to prepare for and react to an increasing population seeking surgical treatment of knee arthritis, an additional area of concern involves patients with bilateral knee involvement. Educating surgeons and patients regarding the surgical options for bilateral knee arthritis is important. Twenty percent of patients undergoing unilateral total knee arthroplasty (UTKA) will complain of contralateral knee pain, with up to 10% of UTKA patients seeking contralateral total knee arthroplasty (TKA) within 1 year of surgery.[24,43] Although the rate of patients seeking surgical treatment of both knees at the same time remains low, at approximately 6% of patients with bilateral knee arthritis, the number of simultaneous bilateral total knee arthroplasty (SBTKA) procedures has doubled over the past 20 years.[43]

Total knee arthroplasty of both knees in the same patient may be performed via one of three pathways: (1) separate UTKA, two distinct TKA procedures with the second procedure occurring after at least 1 year; (2) staged BTKA, two UTKA procedures within a year, during either the same or two separate hospitalizations; or (3) simultaneous BTKA, both TKA procedures during the same anesthesia, with either one team performing sequential procedures or two teams operating in parallel. Historically, a 3-month window was commonly used between staged TKA events, as a 90-day interval corresponds to the reset timing of the global period for Centers for Medicare & Medicaid Services (CMS) reimbursement. The 3-month delay between surgeries also allowed prevention of a "second hit" to the patient that could increase risk for venous thromboembolism (VTE), although with the assistance of early mobilization and pharmacologic anticoagulation, the VTE risk does not appear to increase significantly if staged procedures are performed as little as 1 week apart.[7] Despite a lack of definitive evidence concerning the appropriate timeframe between TKAs, current recommendations call for maintaining the 3-month delay.[20]

Further understanding the surgical treatment options in bilateral symptomatic knee arthritis will help surgeons, anesthesiologists, and patients work together to optimize and personalize surgical planning and management. Optimal shared decision making will then result in choosing a safe procedure for the patient that may maximize surgical and rehabilitation efficacy while minimizing economic costs.

PATIENT SELECTION

When determining which approach is best suited for a given patient, one must consider patient selection based on age and comorbidities, preoperative dysfunction and deformity, intraoperative blood management, postoperative rehabilitation and return-to-work goals, and cost to the patient, hospital, and insurer.

Age and Comorbidities

Morbidity and mortality rates in patients undergoing TKA have been shown to increase with age, body mass index (BMI), American Society of Anesthesiologists (ASA) classification level, and operative time.[1] Major morbidity and mortality rates of SBTKA have been reported to be as high as 9.5%, predominantly occurring in older patients and in those with preexisting comorbidities.[21] Common theories explaining the adverse events in these patients following SBTKA revolve around the patient's poor ability to compensate for small vessel insult because of either embolic load entering the vascular system or fluid shifts associated with extensive surgery.[16,23] Identifying those patients particularly at risk for insult via fat emboli should affect surgical planning with regard to tourniquet management. Embolic debris can be released into the circulation within 1 minute of tourniquet deflation, which occurs at an increased incidence and volume with longer tourniquet time.[10,44] An alternative explanation for the increased cardiopulmonary risk associated with bilateral TKA is that tourniquet release may lead to increased pulmonary vascular resistance.[8,26] The pulmonary vascular resistance can remain elevated for as long as a full day following surgery.[4]

Regardless of the physiologic intraoperative cause, increased cardiopulmonary complications of SBTKA have been suggested as the source of higher mortality rates reported in patients undergoing SBTKA as compared to those undergoing staged BTKA, with some authors recommending strict patient selection criteria based solely on cardiopulmonary health.[34] Further supporting this notion is the finding that patients with preexisting cardiovascular disease have higher rates of postoperative myocardial infarction, postoperative intensive care unit (ICU) admission, and increased ICU length of stay after undergoing SBTKA as compared to their matched peers undergoing the procedure without preexisting cardiovascular disease.[30] Obstructive sleep apnea should be considered a condition of interest in the same manner as cardiovascular disease, because of the high association of sleep apnea with right-sided heart disease, congestive heart failure, and pulmonary hypertension.[32]

Age limitations are somewhat controversial, as physiologic age does not necessarily match chronologic age. However, although elderly patients have demonstrated benefits from simultaneous BTKA in prior studies, with no increase in mortality as compared to matched controls undergoing UTKA, they more commonly experienced postoperative complications that, given their limited physiological reserve, could be more problematic.[5,24] Elderly patients undergoing simultaneous BTKA demonstrate an increased risk of urinary tract infection, delirium, and pressure ulcers following the procedure as compared to their peers undergoing UTKA. Additionally, one study linked the risk of myocardial infarction after simultaneous BTKA to patients in their 80s as compared to those in their 70s, with no myocardial infarctions occurring in any patient under 70 years old.[5] Conversely, undergoing SBTKA at a younger age may result in no increase in perioperative cardiovascular-associated morbidity and mortality, while allowing the patient to limit the number of surgical and rehabilitation events.[36]

Additional preoperative conditions to monitor include those that could result in alternative end-organ damage secondary to embolic debris, especially following tourniquet deflation. Metabolic changes, including metabolic acidosis or hyperkalemia, may lead to renal injury or death in patients with preexisting renal disease.[26] Less commonly, rhabdomyolysis has been reported following tourniquet deflation and can also lead to acute renal failure.[29] Perioperative cerebrovascular accident (CVA) occurs in less than 1% of patients but has also been reported to occur in association with extended tourniquet times, prior history of CVAs, or patent cardiac foramina.[25] Although not directly tied to outcomes following staged versus simultaneous BTKA, end-stage or poorly controlled diabetes may also be interpreted as a surrogate for end-stage organ insult susceptibility.[45]

A comprehensive manner of assessing patients for their ability to undergo SBTKA should therefore begin with a history and physical examination to rule out preexisting cardiac, pulmonary, central nervous, or renal conditions that would make SBTKA patients susceptible to further insult following extended anesthesia and tourniquet times. Next, an anesthesiologist should assess the patient to determine the patient's ASA score. As a predictor of the risk for end-organ damage following surgery, the ASA score has proven helpful in understanding which patients have statistically similar outcomes with SBTKA when compared to their peers undergoing UTKA or staged BTKA. A score of ASA 1 or 2 often results in similar outcomes between these groups of patients with regard to perioperative morbidity and mortality.[21,34,40] Additionally, echocardiography can be used to assess for patent foramina or preexisting right-sided heart strain, especially in patients with obstructive sleep apnea.[43]

Uncovering and using these preexisting conditions may help provide an initial means by which to determine which patients should not undergo SBTKA. In those who still qualify after this step, additional areas of concern are addressed to determine the patient's candidacy for SBTKA.

Preoperative Dysfunction and Deformity

Patients with a severe preoperative deformity in both knees warrant strong consideration for SBTKA, as they may not be able to rely on the nonoperative leg for stability and strength while recovering from the first-stage TKA. Such patients, especially those with rheumatoid arthritis, have been shown to have similar clinical outcomes after SBTKA when compared to patients of similar demographics who undergo UTKA for unilateral osteoarthritis, with similar rates of postoperative

morbidity and mortality.[13] Conversely, patients with significant preoperative deformity of both knees—particularly severe varus deformity and/or flexion contracture—who undergo UTKA may have clinically significant limb length discrepancy or poorer functional outcomes after surgery when compared to matched patients undergoing SBTKA, suggesting that those patients may actually benefit more from SBTKA.[42]

Venous Thromboembolism and Hematologic Concerns

Extended surgical and tourniquet times, while increasing the risk of fat embolism and pulmonary hypertension, are also of concern with regard to VTE. Studies comparing VTE risk of SBTKA to staged BTKA and UTKA have demonstrated mixed results, with some reporting higher VTE rates in patients undergoing SBTKA[12,34,47] and others reporting no statistically significant difference in VTE rates.[2,19,27] However, much of the available literature assessing the safety of SBTKA provides a comparison of VTE following SBTKA to that of UTKA, suggesting inherent bias within the reported differences in VTE rates.[2,18] Instead, comparing the VTE rate in SBTKA to that of staged BTKA, in which two separate operative events carry their own VTE risk, SBTKA has demonstrated lower VTE risk, a finding that is further supported by the decreased number of anesthetic events and decreased overall surgical time of SBTKA as compared to the cumulative anesthesia and surgical time of two separate TKA events.[19]

The risk of VTE in SBTKA appears to have improved over time from early studies, with some attributing the relatively low VTE rate to early mobilization, mechanical DVT prophylaxis, and pharmacologic prophylaxis, including aspirin, low molecular weight heparin, and/or warfarin.[27] Additionally, the recent increased use of regional anesthesia has been associated with a lower rate of VTE regardless of the procedure and may further protect against the earlier reported increased risk of VTE in SBTKA patients.[9] However, because of the overall lack of clarity regarding VTE risk, recommendations for SBTKA routinely warn against performing the procedure in patients with prior VTE or with preexisting medical conditions putting them at risk for VTE.[20,43,47]

Another aspect of SBTKA that has improved with current perioperative medical advances is intraoperative blood loss. The routine use of tranexamic acid in recent years has resulted in overall decreased reported blood loss and transfusion requirement in patients undergoing TKA.[46] Similar results have been duplicated in patients receiving tranexamic acid while undergoing SBTKA, with decreased amounts of blood loss and rates of postoperative transfusion as compared with those not receiving tranexamic acid.[2,17] However, patients with coagulopathy (including hepatic disease) or hypercoagulable states were excluded from receiving tranexamic acid in these studies and as such should be considered patients who may warrant further consideration for staged BTKA rather than SBTKA. It should also be noted that (1) much of the literature assessing blood loss and transfusion rates in SBTKA uses strict criteria that often excludes patients with anemia who are already at risk for postoperative allogeneic transfusion, and (2) staged BTKA may also be recommended for these patients. Still, comparisons of total blood loss from SBTKA as compared with the cumulative blood loss from staged BTKA have demonstrated no significant differences in the total intraoperative or intra-articular drain-associated blood loss on a "per knee" basis.[48]

One additional group of patients to note as possible candidates for SBTKA with low baseline hematocrit levels are those with hemophilia. Patients with severe hemophilia tend to be young patients with bilateral knee arthritis and severe deformity, who may require infusion of replacement clotting factors.[37] Because of a combination of the high cost of clotting factors and the patients' otherwise common lack of additional comorbidities, patients with hemophilia who undergo SBTKA have good long-term outcomes with shorter recovery periods and lower infection rates than their peers who undergo staged TKA—and at a lower economic cost to the health care system. However, recovery is difficult because of preexisting contracture and requires significant analgesia and hands-on intervention to prevent recurrence and thus requires careful patient selection for SBTKA.[39]

Postoperative Rehabilitation and Return to Work

Many of the patients who qualify for SBTKA with regard to physiologic safety are considered healthy and are often chronologically (and physiologically) young, as outlined previously. As such, these patients tend to perform well in their postoperative rehabilitation and show long-term functional outcomes similar to their peers undergoing both UTKA and staged BTKA with regard to objective knee scores and patient satisfaction.[32,49] Despite the difficult rehabilitation of both knees at once following SBTKA, the rehabilitation time following SBTKA is not double that following UTKA and is in fact decreased as compared to the overall time required for sequential rehabilitation of each knee following staged BTKA.[28,35]

ECONOMIC COST

Perhaps the most definitive benefit of simultaneous BTKA is the cost savings. Overall cost difference for the surgical episode has been estimated at approximately $28,800 saved by performing simultaneous BTKA rather than staged BTKA.[28] The difference in cost calculated includes savings at all points of the episode. Preoperatively, SBTKA patients undergo half the tests and visits required compared to those undergoing staged BTKA. Intraoperatively, SBTKA requires one preoperative and postoperative room turnover, including one anesthesia episode, one set of anesthetic equipment and medications, as well as decreased cost associated with operating room time and one hospitalization. Postoperatively, earlier return to work in SBTKA patients results in cost savings based on quality of life years gained, while accounting for costs associated with postoperative complications. Additionally, the SBTKA postoperative hospital stay and rehabilitation period, while longer than that of UTKA, does not reach that of combining both episodes of a staged BTKA.[2]

PROCEDURE

Following patient selection based on physiologic health factors, surgeon recommendation, and patient choice to proceed with SBTKA, the procedure is performed with further attention paid to minimizing complications. Although SBTKA requires less surgical time than that accumulated in two TKA surgical events, it still requires more time than UTKA and requires special attention to complications associated with increased surgical and tourniquet time, including increased blood loss, VTE incidence, and death.

One method of decreasing overall surgical time includes performing the operation with two surgical teams working in parallel. However, a prior study has failed to definitively show an improvement in postoperative outcomes in patients undergoing SBTKA with parallel surgical teams as compared to historical controls.[15] Differences in outcomes included a higher rate of cardiovascular complications in at-risk patients undergoing SBTKA as compared to UTKA. There was a similarly low rate of implant malpositioning and long-term component loosening in SBTKA patients as compared to UTKA patients done in separate settings. Postoperative complications were thus attributed not to increased surgical time in SBTKA but rather to the extensive embolic load produced by a combination of tourniquet and cement use, as the rates were unchanged with use of extramedullary femoral alignment rods. A recent study assessing means of decreasing overall surgical time in SBTKA with use of patient-specific instrumentation also failed to demonstrate a significant difference in postoperative complications despite avoiding intramedullary instrumentation. This lends further support to the embolic load associated with tourniquet use and overall surgical trauma as the cause of postoperative complications.[33]

Increased tourniquet time has demonstrated an association with increased cardiopulmonary embolic load and increased pulmonary vascular resistance. In fact, simultaneous bilateral tourniquet use adds to the potential for reperfusion injury and has resulted in cases of cardiac arrest following simultaneous deflation. Additionally, tourniquet use in BTKA has led to more frequent thigh pain at the tourniquet site or nerve injuries in the associated extremity and has been associated with increased rehabilitation time.[14,26] However, although tourniquet use is associated with increased potential postoperative complications, it has been clearly demonstrated to decrease blood loss in total knee arthroplasty,[38] and therefore tourniquet use in SBTKA must still be considered as a reasonable option to optimize the patient's outcome, although care should be taken to limit the duration of tourniquet inflation and avoid simultaneous bilateral tourniquet inflation and deflation.

OUTCOMES

Comparing SBTKA to staged BTKA in young, healthy patients, those undergoing SBTKA tend to have equivalent or better outcomes than those undergoing staged BTKA, especially if assessing staged BTKA against the cumulative results of two UTKAs. Patients undergoing SBTKA have lower total pain medication use, faster overall recovery, and faster return to work than patients undergoing staged BTKA.[22] Periarticular injections, now commonly used during SBTKA, can provide additional perioperative pain control, leading to significantly lower patient pain scores following SBTKA than previously reported.[41] Furthermore, the trauma of multiple surgeries can elicit a central sensitization of pain receptors that can result in increased pain reported following the second procedure of a staged BTKA, resulting in some patients requiring more than double the expected postoperative pain medication overall.[11] Long-term clinical and radiographic outcomes of TKA in these patients are otherwise equivocal.*

With regard to postoperative complications, the major differences between the two bilateral approaches are an increased likelihood of discharge to a rehabilitation facility[49] and a higher

---

*References 6, 15, 18, 32, 36, and 49.

TABLE 81.1 NYULMC Simultaneous Bilateral Total Knee Arthroplasty Exclusion Criteria

1. Age >75 years
2. ASA 3 or 4
3. Ischemic heart disease (positive stress test)
4. Aggressive anticoagulation or clopidogrel
5. Poor ventricular function (LVEF <50%)
6. Oxygen-dependent pulmonary disease
7. Renal insufficiency or end-stage renal disease (Cr >1.6)
8. Steroid dependent asthma or COPD
9. Pulmonary hypertension (PAP >45 mm Hg)
10. Morbidly obese (BMI ≥40)
11. Chronic liver disease (Child class B or worse)
12. Cerebral vascular disease
13. Sleep study proven obstructive sleep apnea without treatment, or STOP/BANG >5
14. Insulin dependent diabetes mellitus (blood glucose >180)
15. History of DVT or PE
16. History of congestive heart failure
17. Hemoglobin concentration <11 g/dL, or Jehovah's Witness

Guidelines

A. Consider echocardiography if there is a question of right-sided heart strain/pulmonary hypertension to assess for dysfunction that would preclude bilateral TKA.

B. Anesthesia will make a determination of inclusion for bilateral, simultaneous TKA at PAT. Anesthesia will identify those that need an echocardiogram at PAT.

C. Consider doing the second TKA of simultaneous bilaterals without tourniquet until the first tourniquet is released.

D. When possible, the second knee of a bilaterally involved patient that does not qualify for same-session bilateral TKA should be done 3 months or more after the first knee to avoid increased risk of VTED.

BMI, Body mass index; *COPD,* chronic obstructive pulmonary disease; *DVT,* deep venous thrombosis; *LVEF,* left ventricular ejection fraction; *NYULMC,* New York University Langone Medical Center; *PAP,* pulmonary artery pressure; *PAT,* preadmission testing; *PE,* pulmonary embolism; *STOP Bang,* scoring system questionnaire for obstructive sleep apnea; *TKA,* total knee arthroplasty; *VTED,* venous thromboembolic disease.

30-day postoperative mortality rate following SBTKA.[6,30,32,34] The latter finding has been largely attributed in prior studies to a lack of exclusion of patients with preoperative cardiovascular risk, as outlined earlier. Current trends toward stricter inclusion criteria for SBTKA have narrowed the difference between simultaneous and staged BTKA with regard to postoperative mortality.[32] Although some debate continues, there is no current definitive evidence that there is an increase in other commonly studied perioperative complications such as VTE, periarticular infection, or readmission risk following SBTKA, when compared to the cumulative results of staged BTKA.[2,3,5,31]

SUMMARY

The choice of simultaneous or staged BTKA is one that the surgeon and patient will make in a combined decision-making process. Patients who are seeking BTKA and are in optimal health can benefit from condensing the surgical and recovery time course, while saving the operating time and minimizing the cost to the health care system as a whole. However, many patients are not fit for extensive surgery or cannot tolerate a more intensive recovery and rehabilitation period (Table 81.1). Certain guidelines can be followed to maximize the patient selection and provide patients a clearer understanding of their options. With a full understanding of the surgical options and the intense but shorter recovery period, the surgeon and patient can then decide which pathway to pursue for treatment of the patient's bilateral knee arthritis.

KEY REFERENCES

2. Bini SA, Khatod M, Inacio MCS, et al: Same-day versus staged bilateral total knee arthroplasty poses no increase in complications in 662 primary procedures. *J Arthroplasty* 29:694–697, 2014.

3. Bolognesi MP, Watters TS, Attarian DE, et al: Simultaneous vs staged bilateral total knee arthroplasty among medicare beneficiaries, 2000–2009. *J Arthroplasty* 28(Suppl 1):87–91, 2013.

5. Bullock DP, Sporer SM, Shirreffs TG: Comparison of simultaneous bilateral with unilateral total knee arthroplasty in terms of perioperative complications. *J Bone Joint Surg Am* 85-A(10):1981–1986, 2003.

20. Memtsoudis SG, Hargett M, Russell LA, et al: Consensus statement from the consensus conference on bilateral total knee arthroplasty group. *Clin Orthop Relat Res* 471:2649–2657, 2013.

34. Restreppo C, Parvizi J, Dietrich T, et al: Safety of simultaneous bilateral total knee arthroplasty. A meta-analysis. *J Bone Joint Surg* 89:1220–1226, 2007.

41. Tsukada S, Wakui M, Hoshino A: Pain control after simultaneous bilateral total knee arthroplasty. *J Bone Joint Surg Am* 97(5):367–373, 2015.

The references for this chapter can also be found on www.expertconsult.com.

PART II

Perioperative Management of Inpatient Procedures

82

Monitoring During Total Knee Arthroplasty

Milica Markovic

Total knee arthroplasty (TKA) is generally considered a safe procedure; however, it can be lengthy and involve significant blood loss and hemodynamic changes. Serious complications, such as cardiac arrest, tachycardia, hypotension, pulmonary embolism, myocardial infarction, and cerebral vascular accidents have been documented perioperatively.[3] Even though the 30-day mortality rate after primary TKA is decreasing, it is still estimated to be 0.18% to 0.28%.[4,9] Therefore, an increased degree of perioperative surveillance is frequently used, both intra- and postoperatively in the recovery room.

Intraoperative tourniquet is frequently used for TKA procedures in order to reduce blood loss and create a bloodless surgical field. On tourniquet deflation, acidotic blood is released into the circulation, and transient systemic metabolic acidosis and increased arterial carbon dioxide have been documented. As acidosis frequently results in hypotension and occasionally even arrhythmias, arterial monitoring is advised in high-risk patients. In addition, even though intraoperative embolic events are uncommon during TKA, they mostly occur following the deflation of the tourniquet. However, they have been detected even while the tourniquet is inflated.[14]

TKA is associated with significant perioperative blood loss, frequently necessitating blood transfusions. As a pneumatic tourniquet is typically used intraoperatively, blood loss mostly occurs because of postoperative drainage and is estimated to be between 0.5 to 1 L, resulting in 1 to 3 g/dL reduction in hemoglobin concentration.[2,8] Patients who require allogenic blood products intraoperatively are more likely to be admitted to the ICU,[1] in part because of complications associated with blood transfusion, ranging from febrile reaction to the more serious transfusion-related acute lung injury.

Acrylic bone cement (methyl methacrylate) is commonly used for joint implantation during TKA. The spectrum of adverse reactions to cement, including systemic hypotension, anaphylactoid reaction, pulmonary hypertension, hypoxemia, and cardiovascular collapse (collectively known as bone cement implantation syndrome) have been well documented.[6] It is difficult to determine the exact incidence of adverse reactions to cement, but it is estimated that 5% of all cemented arthroplasties result in hypotension after femoral stem prosthesis placement.[12] Hypotension can result from a decrease in cardiac output, a reduction in systemic vascular resistance, or a combination of the two. In addition, a sudden decrease in arterial oxygen saturation is frequently observed.

Patients undergoing surgery of any type require standard monitoring, including pulse oximetry, electrocardiography, and blood pressure monitoring. Given the aforementioned complications and hemodynamic alterations, patients undergoing TKA may require a high degree of perioperative surveillance. Invasive hemodynamic monitoring allows for optimizing hemodynamic and fluid management. In high-risk patients such as those with pulmonary hypertension and extensive cardiac disease, or those undergoing revision or bilateral TKA, a higher level of hemodynamic monitoring is necessary[6]:

- Urine output is routinely used for the assessment of patients' intravascular volume status.
- Arterial monitoring allows beat-to-beat measurement of blood pressure and rapid detection of sudden hemodynamic shifts. In addition, arterial monitoring offers an intraoperative point of care measurement of hemoglobin, electrolytes, respiratory, and clotting parameters, and allows customizing blood product and fluid administration. In addition, several devices are clinically available that estimate cardiac output based on arterial pressure waveform analysis.[11] As their validity is becoming established, their use has become more popular in the setting of noncardiac surgery, where arterial line is frequently the only available invasive monitor.
- Even though central venous pressure (CVP) monitoring via a central venous catheter is marginally useful with volume optimization and inotrope administration, it does not detect a rapid fall in cardiac output and stroke volume, nor changes in pulmonary pressures. CVP measurement is a very poor estimate of blood volume, with multiple causes for error.[10]
- Intraoperative pulmonary artery catheters have historically been used to guide fluid management and cardiac output in medically high-risk patients and those patients undergoing one-stage bilateral or revision arthroplasty.[13] However, pulmonary artery catheters are seldom used at present, as improved outcomes have not been demonstrated with their use.[5]
- Transesophageal echocardiography (TEE), or transesophageal Doppler, can also be used to detect the emboli and their effects on cardiac function.[9] TEE is particularly advantageous and is recommended in cases of persistent hemodynamic instability where resuscitative measures are initially unsuccessful.[7] TEE examination is invaluable in detecting emboli, myocardial function, and valvular abnormalities, as well as estimating volume status and cardiac output.

Postoperative abnormalities in heart rate, arterial blood pressure, arterial blood gases, serum electrolytes, and cardiac rhythm disturbances can quickly be recognized and treated when invasive blood pressure monitoring is used in the recovery

Monitor	Indications
Standard Noninvasive Monitors	**Routinely Applied to Monitor**
Pulse oximetry, noninvasive blood pressure, electrocardiogram, capnography, gas/oxygen analyzer, temperature probe, ventilator function monitors	• Circulation (heart rate, blood pressure, electrocardiogram) • Oxygenation (SpO$_2$, inspired oxygen) • Ventilation (end tidal CO$_2$, anesthetic gases) • Temperature
Arterial line	• Beat-to-beat blood pressure monitoring • Rapid detection of hemodynamic shifts • Intraoperative point-of-care measurement of hemoglobin, electrolytes, respiratory, and clotting parameters
Foley catheter	• Measurement of urine output as a measure of intravascular volume and renal perfusion
Central venous pressure line	• Used mostly for administration of inotropes • Poor relationship between central venous pressure and blood volume changes
Pulmonary artery catheter Transesophageal echocardiogram	• Detection of changes in pulmonary arterial pressure, cardiac output, stroke volume • Detect pulmonary emboli • Determine volume status and pulmonary pressures • Determine cardiac output changes • Detect myocardial ischemia/valvular dysfunctions

room. In addition, postoperative hypoxemia is common after TKA because of fat and bone marrow embolism, pulmonary edema, atelectasis, and as a nonspecific reaction to surgical injury, and requires oxygen therapy and diagnostic workup. In addition, blood loss continues postoperatively, and typically 500 to 1000 mL of blood is routinely drained per knee, which can result in hemodynamic compromise following the surgery. Therefore, many centers routinely observe these patients in highly monitored settings for at least 24 hours after surgery.[13]

KEY REFERENCES

1. AbdelSalam H, Restrepo C, Tarity TD, et al: Predictors of intensive care unit admission after total joint arthroplasty. *J Arthroplasty* 27(5):720–725, 2012.

6. Donaldson AJ, Thomson HE, Harper NJ, et al: Bone cement implantation syndrome. *Br J Anaesth* 102(1):12–22, 2009.
7. Jiang FZ, Zhong HM, Hong YC, et al: Use of a tourniquet in total knee arthroplasty: a systematic review and meta-analysis of randomized controlled trials. *J Orthop Sci* 20:110–123, 2015.
12. Memtsoudis SG, Della Valle AG, Besculides MC, et al: Trends in demographics, comorbidity profiles, in-hospital complications and mortality associated with primary knee arthroplasty. *J Arthroplasty* 24:527, 2009.

The references for this chapter can also be found on www.expertconsult.com.

83

Spinal or General Anesthesia?

Chan-Nyein Maung, Milad Nazemzadeh

INTRODUCTION

The anesthetic techniques for knee surgery include general anesthesia (GA) and regional anesthesia. Regional anesthesia includes neuraxial anesthesia (spinal or epidural) and peripheral nerve blocks. The choice of technique depends on numerous factors such as patient preference, contraindications to neuraxial or regional anesthesia based on the patient's medical and surgical history, the anesthesiologist's expertise, the surgeon's particular preference for a specific procedure, the surgical setting (ambulatory vs. hospital admission), tourniquet use, and many others. General and neuraxial anesthesia are used more frequently than peripheral nerve blocks alone for knee surgery. However, peripheral nerve blocks can be combined with general or neuraxial anesthesia, and neuraxial anesthesia can also be combined with general anesthesia. For techniques not involving GA, intravenous (IV) agents can be used to keep patients sedated during the procedure. Finally, the neuraxial technique (if epidural is used) and peripheral nerve blocks (catheter or single shot block) can be used to provide postoperative pain control.[9]

ARTHROSCOPIC KNEE SURGERY

Knee arthroscopy is often performed as an outpatient or ambulatory procedure because it is minimally invasive in nature. It can be used for detecting or treating pathology related to the meniscus and other cartilage, ligaments, tendons, and bones. Although it is minimally invasive, certain procedures such as anterior cruciate ligament (ACL) repair or reconstruction can be very painful for the patient and can present a challenge for the anesthesiologist, especially postoperatively. The patient population for knee arthroscopy can vary from young healthy athletes to elderly patients with multiple comorbidities. For this procedure, the anesthesiologist and surgeon also need to consider the goals of ambulatory surgery, such as efficient operating room use, early ambulation, safe discharge home, and decreased postoperative nausea, vomiting, and pain.

Anesthesia for knee arthroscopy can be accomplished with regional or GA. After induction, GA can be maintained with anesthetic gases, IV agents such as a propofol infusion, or a balanced technique using both IV agents and anesthetic gases. Airway devices such as a supraglottic laryngeal mask airway (LMA) or an endotracheal tube are used with GA. Peripheral nerve blocks alone are usually not used as the main intraoperative anesthetic technique for knee arthroscopy. Blocks such as the adductor canal block are usually combined with GA to provide adjunctive pain control for the postoperative period, especially for more painful procedures such as ACL reconstruction.[13] Neuraxial anesthesia can also be safely performed for outpatient surgery such as knee arthroscopy, with good patient satisfaction as an alternative to GA. However, the spinal technique may prolong recovery room time as compared to the epidural.[35]

A special population to consider for knee arthroscopy are those patients with obstructive sleep apnea. Many of these patients are morbidly obese and are more likely to have lower extremity joint pathology. According to the practice guidelines published by the American Society of Anesthesiologists, neuraxial anesthesia can be considered for peripheral procedures such as knee arthroscopy. If moderate sedation is used in conjunction with neuraxial anesthesia, ventilation should be continuously monitored with capnography to detect airway obstruction. Furthermore, general anesthesia with a secured airway is preferred over deep sedation without a secured airway. More importantly, the anesthetic technique should be discussed in advance with the surgeon and patient. In the setting of apnea at higher doses of sedatives or narcotics, obstructive sleep apnea (OSA) patients can quickly deteriorate without ventilation intraoperatively.[39]

GA reliably provides excellent conditions for unconsciousness, surgical and tourniquet anesthesia, and a faster induction time versus regional anesthesia.[27] However, the incidence of postoperative nausea and vomiting (PONV) is increased after GA, occurring in about 30% of patients. Furthermore, PONV is the main reason for delayed discharge or hospital admission after ambulatory surgery. Prophylaxis is recommended for all at-risk patients, such as females, those who have a history of PONV or motion sickness, and use of opioids.[2,38] Furthermore, the use of opioids intraoperatively is associated with postoperative respiratory depression and urinary retention.[3,25] In addition, anesthetic gases, which are used to maintain anesthesia, have been shown to increase the incidence of PONV when compared to propofol infusions for anesthesia maintenance. However, no differences were shown in postdischarge nausea and vomiting.[23]

Neuraxial anesthesia (spinal, epidural, or combined spinal-epidural) is another option and can be used with IV sedation or GA. This technique provides reliable conditions for the surgery and use of a tourniquet. IV sedation, however, has a shorter time to emergence and orientation, and decreased incidence of PONV compared to GA.[42] Neuraxial anesthesia is associated with a longer time to induction, reduced pain scores, and less need for post-anesthesia care unit (PACU) analgesics.

However, it has not been shown to be associated with decreased PACU time or reduced postoperative nausea despite the need for fewer analgesics such as opioids. In fact, there is an increase in the total ambulatory surgery unit time.[27] If there is a "block room" or a room in the preoperative area, the epidural can be placed prior to entering the operating room, which decreases the overall anesthesia time.

Peripheral nerve blocks can also be used, but are often used in conjunction with GA for postoperative pain control. They are seldom used as the primary anesthetic technique given that surgical anesthesia would require several blocks to target different nerves. Multiple peripheral nerve blocks require more time to accomplish and may not assure total surgical and tourniquet anesthesia if a failed block occurs. Similar to neuraxial anesthesia, the peripheral nerve block technique as the primary anesthetic modality is associated with a longer time to induction, but with reduced pain scores and less need for PACU analgesics. Again, the block can be performed preoperatively to reduce the overall anesthesia time. However, it was not found to be associated with decreased ambulatory surgery unit time.[27] In addition, femoral nerve blocks have been associated with postoperative falls because of quadriceps weakness.[18] The nerve block of the infrapatellar branch of the saphenous nerve has gained increased usefulness in simple knee arthroscopy cases. This is because of a level of analgesia for postoperative pain control similar to a femoral nerve block, but without quadriceps weakness.[17]

Another goal for postoperative pain management in ambulatory surgery, such as knee arthroscopy, involves avoiding large doses of systemic opioids. This goal can be grouped under the umbrella term "multimodal analgesia" and includes intraarticular local anesthetic, systemic nonsteroidal antiinflammatory drugs (NSAIDs), gabapentin, pregabalin, and acetaminophen use. However, the exact role of gabapentin and pregabalin for postoperative pain control after ambulatory surgery has not been well defined.[40]

Finally, another anesthetic method for knee arthroscopy is the use of local anesthetics. Agents such as 2% lidocaine (intermediate-acting) and 0.25% bupivacaine (long-acting) have been used safely for skin infiltration and intra-articular injection.[19,41] A multimodal analgesic regimen with diclofenac administration preoperatively and use of local anesthetics found that 98.5% of the 625 patients tolerated the procedure, and that 95.7% of the patients reported they would undergo the same procedure under the same type of anesthesia. Of note though, the surgery in this study was performed by the same surgeon, and therefore the efficacy may have some limitations.[33] Cost and time effectiveness of performing knee arthroscopy using GA, spinal anesthesia (SA), and local anesthesia (LA) have been also been compared. This study found that there were no differences in surgery time for the three groups. The total hospital stay time was shortest for the local group and longest for the spinal group. However, the time from the start of anesthesia to the start of surgery was longer in the local group. The local group was found to have saved around 1011 Swedish Crowns (or 134.8 USD for December 2003 exchange rate as cited in the article).[14] Postoperative pain was better studied in a prospective observational study in children and adolescents. This cohort received combined LA and IV propofol for outpatient arthroscopic knee surgery; 96.6% of the 147 participants tolerated the procedure well and 71% of the patients required no analgesics during the first two postoperative hours in the recovery room.[29]

KNEE ARTHROPLASTY

Unlike knee arthroscopy, partial and total knee arthroplasties are more invasive procedures. The procedures themselves take longer than knee arthroscopy and require larger incisions. Patients are usually not discharged the same day as they would be for knee arthroscopy. However, discharge can be accomplished as early as 24 hours for partial knee replacement and minimally invasive knee arthroplasty. The surgery might take longer for minimally invasive knee arthroplasty because of the smaller incisions that the surgeon has to work with when compared to the larger incisions in traditional knee arthroplasty.[21]

The anesthetic techniques available for knee arthroplasty (partial, total, or minimally invasive) are GA, neuraxial anesthesia, and peripheral nerve blocks. When choosing an anesthetic technique in this setting, the longer length of surgery and the larger incision size should be considered in addition to the patient's comorbidities, the anesthesiologist's expertise, and the surgeon's preference.

GA provides unconsciousness in addition to surgical and tourniquet anesthesia. Airway protection is also included. The risks of GA include airway trauma (the number one reason for malpractice lawsuit among anesthesiologists),[10] PONV, hypotension because of vasodilating properties of anesthetic agents, increased recovery time in the PACU, postoperative delirium and cognitive dysfunction, and malignant hyperthermia. Other factors such as thromboembolism and cardiovascular events are further discussed in the following text.

Patients that require further consideration are those suffering from joint diseases such as osteoarthritis (OA) and rheumatoid arthritis (RA). Both of these disease processes have major implications for GA. RA patients can be a big challenge for performing anesthesia. IV and radial artery cannulation may be difficult if small joints of hands, wrists, and feet are deformed. Furthermore, RA can involve synovial membranes of the cervical spine and temporomandibular joint (TMJ). Therefore, the airway of these patients can be challenging. If atlantoaxial subluxation is evident radiographically, manual in-line stabilization should be used during tracheal intubation with either video or fiberoptic laryngoscopy. If TMJ involvement limits jaw mobility and range of motion severely, orotracheal intubation might be difficult or even impossible. If GA is used for OA patients, neck manipulation should be minimized during tracheal intubation or LMA placement, because cervical spine disease can also exist in this population.[5,26]

Neuraxial anesthesia can provide surgical and tourniquet anesthesia, but will likely also require IV sedation if it is used as the primary anesthetic modality. Postoperative pain can be controlled with an epidural, whether it is used as the main anesthetic technique or as an adjunct to GA. The risks of neuraxial anesthesia include post-dural puncture headache (more likely with a larger gauge epidural needle in a young female), hypotension from vasodilation secondary to sympathetic inhibition, hematoma formation (greater incidence with epidurals than spinals), paralysis or other neurologic injury such as radiculopathy, transient neurologic syndrome, epidural abscess, lower back pain, meningitis, total SA, intravascular injection, and urinary retention. The contraindications to neuraxial blockade include, but are not limited to, infection at the site of injection, coagulopathy or bleeding disorders, anticoagulation, severe hypovolemia, valvular disorders (severe aortic or mitral stenosis; possible in RA patients although regurgitation is more likely), and preexisting neurological disorders. Prior back surgery at the site of injection is a controversial contraindication.[6]

Lower extremity peripheral nerve blocks are rarely used as the main anesthetic for knee arthroplasty because they would require more than one nerve block to achieve surgical and tourniquet anesthesia, and could increase total anesthesia time. Furthermore, the probability of a failed block is increased given the number of blocks required in this setting. The risks of lower extremity peripheral nerve blocks include, but are not limited to, nerve damage, local anesthetic toxicity from intravascular injection or perivascular absorption resulting in serious events such as seizures and/or cardiovascular collapse, infection, and hemorrhage. Given that patient cooperation is a key factor in performing both neuraxial and peripheral nerve blocks, developmentally delayed patients and those with dementia or movement disorders may not be candidates for regional anesthesia. Also, complications of nerve blocks are increased in patients with preexisting peripheral neuropathy or nerve injury.[7]

The sensory innervation for knee arthroplasty and tourniquet pain are supplied by several nerves: the femoral nerve (anterior thigh, anterior and lateral knee, and medial leg via saphenous nerve), lateral femoral cutaneous (lateral thigh), obturator nerve (portion of mid-medial thigh), and sciatic nerve (posterior thigh and lateral leg). The posterior lumbar plexus or psoas compartment block provides anesthesia to the femoral, lateral femoral cutaneous, and obturator nerves. However, this block has a very high complication rate because of the major structures in its vicinity. The complications include retroperitoneal hematoma, intravascular local anesthetic injection, intrathecal and epidural injections, and renal capsular puncture and hematoma. Complete anesthesia of the knee can be obtained if a proximal sciatic nerve block is added to the psoas compartment block.[8] Femoral nerve or adductor canal blocks are often used for postoperative pain control, usually with a catheter. Recent studies indicate that the adductor canal block provides similar postoperative pain control for total knee arthroplasty and opioid consumption when compared to the femoral nerve block, with the added benefit of less quadriceps weakness.[20,22]

Another option for postoperative pain is intra-articular injection of local anesthetic and opioids. A small, double-blinded, randomized controlled trial with 80 patients compared the efficacy of intra-articular intraoperative injection of morphine, bupivacaine, and betamethasone versus the control group with normal saline. The study found that the intra-articular cocktail injection reduced the need for postoperative opioids and allowed better mobility.[16] A recent study looked at intra-articular analgesia combined with a saphenous nerve block in unilateral total knee arthroplasty patients, compared to a femoral nerve block and epidural anesthesia. It found that although postoperative pain control was similar in both groups, the length of hospital stay was shorter in the intra-articular analgesia and saphenous nerve block group.[11]

Although the previously discussed anesthetic techniques can provide conditions for surgical knee arthroplasty, the perioperative outcomes remain controversial. There have been no large, multicenter, randomized controlled, double-blinded trials to compare the three modes of anesthesia and their outcomes to adequately guide evidence-based practice. Recent studies that retrospectively compared perioperative outcomes of general and neuraxial anesthesia suggest that neuraxial anesthesia is associated with superior outcomes for knee arthroplasty. In one Canadian retrospective study, neuraxial anesthesia for noncardiac surgery identified a small 30-day mortality and benefit of epidural anesthesia, but no significant findings were found for patients undergoing particular procedures.[43] In another study, use of neuraxial anesthesia was associated with lower odds of needing postoperative critical care services in total hip and knee arthroplasty patients.[31] Recently, a major retrospective study of a US national database containing information from 400 acute care hospitals compared perioperative complications after primary hip and knee arthroplasty. Surprisingly, about 75% of these cases were performed under GA alone, and only about 10% under neuraxial anesthesia alone. The authors found that neuraxial anesthesia had superior outcomes in terms of postoperative complications (pulmonary embolism, pneumonia, cerebrovascular events, and acute renal failure), 30-day mortality, length of stay, and cost when compared to GA. No significant differences were found for rate of acute myocardial infarction and other cardiac complications. An interesting finding was that the neuraxial group had a higher average age than the GA group, which is important because advanced age has been shown to be a major predictor of perioperative complications in orthopedic patients. However, this study could not analyze detailed clinical information such as blood loss, intraoperative details, and postdischarge events, such data were not available from the database. Furthermore, complications related to the use of anesthetic techniques such as post-dural puncture headaches, spinal hematoma, and airway trauma during intubation were not included in the study. Finally, because there was no randomization, it is impossible to conclude that there is a causal link between anesthesia technique and outcome.[32]

The use of peripheral nerve blocks has increased significantly in the past decade because of the advent of better technology, mainly ultrasonography. Although neuraxial anesthesia can provide excellent intraoperative anesthesia and prolonged postoperative analgesia, peripheral nerve blocks can target the operative limb, have less effect on motor function, and avoid adverse effects of spinal or epidural techniques. Peripheral nerve blocks can also provide postoperative analgesia via a single-shot or catheter infusion method. However, the block failure rate has been reported to be between 0% and 67%, depending on the particular block, anesthesiologist's experience, and method of nerve block (anatomic, nerve stimulator, and ultrasound techniques).[12] Furthermore, surgical anesthesia for total knee arthroplasty requires several peripheral nerve blocks for both the surgical anesthesia and tourniquet pain.

Similar to the outcome studies of neuraxial anesthesia, there are conflicting results of randomized controlled trials comparing regional to GA and neuraxial anesthesia in total knee arthroplasty. A meta-analysis comparing epidural and peripheral nerve block techniques (including femoral, sciatic, and lumbar plexus blocks; using single shot and catheters) found no significant differences in pain scores, incidence of nausea and vomiting, and consumption of postoperative opioids. This analysis also found that rehabilitation time was similar in both techniques. However, epidurals resulted in a higher incidence of hypotension and urinary retention.[15] In another meta-analysis comparing epidural and patient controlled analgesia (PCA) with femoral nerve block (single shot or catheter, with or without sciatic nerve block), a nerve block resulted in reduced PCA morphine consumption at 24 and 48 hours, pain scores with activity, and nausea and vomiting.[36]

A 2010 landmark review compared epidural and peripheral nerve blocks (RA group) to GA (GA group) in 28 trials. There was no significant difference in mortality between the two groups, which the authors attributed to the safety of modern anesthetic and surgical practices. There was also no significant difference in cardiovascular morbidity, although epidurals were associated with a higher incidence of hypotension than peripheral nerve blocks. Although there was no significant difference in deep venous thromboses (DVTs), the trials in the review that measured DVTs as a specific parameter were inadequately powered. Similar problems were found when comparing differences in blood loss and transfusion requirements. The RA group did have reduced postoperative pain, especially on movement. Although there were no differences in pain scores, patient satisfaction still favored the RA group compared with IV PCA. Furthermore, the RA group had significantly reduced PONV related to opioid use. The length of stay was reduced by 1 day in the RA group and length of rehabilitation stay by up to 13 days.[28] Although this review found pain-related factors to be significant, there is insufficient evidence to conclude if the choice of anesthetic technique had an effect on mortality, cardiovascular morbidity, and DVT and pulmonary embolism (PE) incidence in the setting of routine thromboprophylaxis.

CONSIDERATIONS FOR AN AGING POPULATION

The advanced-age patient population undergoing surgery will continue to increase as medical advances have allowed people with multiple comorbidities to live longer. The number of total hip and knee arthroplasties performed each year in the United States has been increasing and is expected to be greater than 4 million by the year 2030.[24] With advanced age, of particular concern is the role of anesthesia in postoperative cognitive dysfunction (POCD), defined as a range of abnormalities, including postoperative delirium (POD). Although the criteria for POD are stricter than for POCD, they share many overlapping risk factors, which suggest that they share a similar pathogenesis. Of note, POD is different from emergence delirium, a phenomenon attributed to anesthetic agents. In POD, the patient has a lucid post-anesthetic period lasting 1 to 3 days, after which fluctuations in cognition occur. Delirium, in general, has poor short- and long-term outcomes, including increased morbidity, mortality, length of stay, long-term cognitive impairment, and further decline beyond 12 months, all of which

contribute to increased health care costs. The definition of POCD is much broader than it is for POD, and is often dependent on tests to assess cognitive functions such as memory, attention, and executive function.[1,4] The POD mechanism is thought to involve a central cholinergic deficit intra- and postoperatively because of the influence of GA on neuronal processes. Peripheral inflammation from surgery and release of inflammatory substances is also thought to cause neuronal dysfunction. These effects are believed to result in conditions similar to Alzheimer disease, Lewy body dementia, or other central neurodegenerative diseases that manifest as cognitive dynsfunction.[34,37] Today, the debate regarding the role of GA in POCD is ongoing because there have not been any large randomized, double-blinded studies. The studies that exist are smaller studies that may or may not directly compare GA and regional anesthesia. In a meta-analysis of 21 studies, only 5 studies were found suitable for inclusion and were grouped into GA versus non-GA. This study found that the rates of POD are not influenced by the route of anesthesia, an encouraging finding, given POD's short- and long-term consequences. It also found that the incidence of POCD was lower in the non-GA group, but was not statistically significant.[30] More research is needed to elucidate the role of GA in neurodegeneration, because of its mental and health effects on the elderly. There needs to be extensive discussion between the anesthesiologist, surgeon, and the patient and patient's family regarding the route of anesthesia in elderly patients who are at risk for POCD and POD. Unless there are significant contraindications, regional or neuraxial anesthesia with IV sedation might be the best route for these elderly patients.

CONCLUSIONS

There is no one recommended method for performing anesthesia for a patient undergoing knee surgery. The complexity of surgery, patient's history, patient's preference, and the anesthesiologist's expertise need to be considered carefully before choosing a particular technique or combination of techniques. Furthermore, with recent advancements in both technology and medicine, more research is needed to compare the perioperative outcomes of regional and general anesthetic techniques.

The references for this chapter can also be found on www.expertconsult.com.

Revision Total Knee Arthroplasties

Milica Markovic

Given the increased longevity of the population and the burden of osteoarthritis, the rates of both primary and revision total knee arthroplasties (TKA) are on the rise. It is estimated that the overall revision rate for primary arthroplasty of the knee is around 12%,[6] and predictive models estimate the demand for primary TKA to greatly increase in the future.[5] As millions of people are currently living with a TKA and the criteria for primary TKA are widening, the need for revision surgery will be even greater and will potentially represent a large public health burden.[3] In addition, survival rates of TKA revision surgery are estimated to be greater than 80% at 10 years, and therefore re-revision surgery is also expected to be on the rise.[3]

Most studies identify independent patient-related risk factors for perioperative complications and prolonged hospital stay after revision knee arthroplasty (RKA) to be age greater than 75, American Society of Anesthesiologists (ASA) status greater than 2, chronic obstructive pulmonary disease (COPD), and perioperative anemia.[2,7] A low preoperative hematocrit, as the strongest modifiable independent predictor, should be addressed preoperatively, as it may indicate a chronic underlying disease such as cancer or renal failure. Therefore, the patient should be thoroughly evaluated preoperatively. Erythropoietin or preoperative blood restauration strategies may be useful in reducing perioperative transfusion rates, which have been associated with surgical site infections. Urgent surgery is an independent risk factor for perioperative stroke following joint arthroplasty,[8] indicating that perioperative optimizations of medical comorbidities should be achieved whenever possible before the TKA.

It is difficult to analyze the outcome of revisions, as the data are limited and mostly involve small single-center cohorts and multiple variables, such as whether it is a partial or full revision, design of components, and use of cement.[1] However, the outcome of RKA is worse than that of primary procedures. Sepsis and wound infection rates are twice the ones for primary TKA.[7] Revisions for infection have worse outcomes than revisions for aseptic prosthesis failure.[7] Early TKA failure is typically because of infection or instability, whereas later failure involves mostly loosening and mechanical wear.[3] Interestingly, even though the length of stay is shorter after a primary TKA in high-volume hospitals, it is unclear whether hospital volume is predictive of revision after TKR.[9] Revisions performed within 2 years of TKA and those performed in patients of younger age tend to have worse outcomes.[4] The patients are at a significant risk for encountering significant complications (neurovascular

1.8%, thromboembolic 15% to 84%)[10] as well as 12% failure rate from infection (46%), aseptic loosening (19%), and instability (13%).[12]

Revision TKA is a complex and challenging surgery with unpredictable results that requires significant resources. However, component removal is typically less arduous than in revision hip arthroplasty, and the intraoperative time as well as the blood loss are typically only slightly increased compared to a primary surgery, except in cases with major bone loss or when a hinge prosthesis has to be used. Pulmonary embolism of bone debris, fat, clot, air, or cement is more likely when using long-stemmed components, and therefore increased surveillance with invasive monitoring may be necessary for these cases. Even though RKA is associated with increased operating room time, blood loss, and rate of complications, there seems to be no difference in immediate postoperative experience, as the post-anesthesia care unit length of stay and narcotic usage are comparable with those of the primary TKA.[11]

Thirty-day mortality after RKA is estimated to be 0.4% overall[2] and 0.1% for aseptic revisions.[7] High rates of potential life-threatening perioperative complications such as sepsis, cardiac arrest, pulmonary embolism, myocardial infarction, respiratory failure, acute renal failure, and cerebrovascular accident (estimated to be around 1.6%) require that these procedures be performed in centers where critical care units are available.[7] Regional anesthesia is preferred to general, as it is associated with reduced rates of stroke,[8] deep venous thrombosis, pulmonary embolism, pneumonia, bleeding complications, and mortality.[10] In addition, rates of adverse events (both complications and poor surgical results) decrease when these revision procedures are performed in high-volume centers by experienced surgeons.[3] Therefore, it is recommended that these procedures be performed in specialist centers with highly specialized multidisciplinary care providers, including anesthesiologists, intensivists, pain specialists, nurses, and physical therapists.

KEY REFERENCE

3. Hamilton DF, Howie CR, Burnett R, et al: Dealing with the predicted increase in demand for revision total knee arthroplasty. *Bone Joint J* 97-B:723–728, 2015.

The references for this chapter can also be found on www.expertconsult.com.

The Pneumatic Tourniquet

Jean-Pierre Estèbe

INTRODUCTION

The pneumatic tourniquet (PT) is commonly used in knee surgery. It provides a bloodless operative field for better cement implantation, improves surgical visualization of the anatomic structure, and reduces operative time. However, numerous known disadvantages exist.[14] The first recorded use of a tourniquet was by a Roman surgeon in the second century AD. In 1817, French surgeon Jean-Louis Petit described a device for hemostasis, which he named the "tourniquet." Harvey Cushing introduced the PT in 1904 as an adjunct for surgery on extremities. Despite numerous publications concerning use of the PT for total knee surgery (TKA), the interest in its use remains controversial. In a recent meta-analysis comparing outcomes with or without a PT in TKA, minor complications were more common in the PT group.[2] In a more recent meta-analysis, TKA without PT was superior to TKA with PT in terms of thromboembolic events and other related complications.[65] Patient safety has been improved and complications reduced by the development of wide, contoured, and electronically controlled pneumatic cuffs. Despite this, tissue injury by compression under the PT cuff and ischemia-reperfusion (IR) injuries still occur.[13]

MECHANICAL EFFECTS

Limb Exsanguination

Limb exsanguination before tourniquet inflation is usually accomplished by mechanical means. Such devices (Esmarch bandage, Rhys-Davies exsanguinator) increase the risk of disseminating a tumor or infection or dislodging a thrombus from a deep venous thrombosis (DVT). Exsanguination of the limb by elevation alone is a slightly less effective, but safe and easy procedure. It permits better visualization of superficial vessels compared with complete exsanguination, allowing better hemostasis, especially for hand surgery.[5] To achieve maximum exsanguination, it is recommended to elevate the arm at 90 degrees for 5 minutes and elevate the leg at 45 degrees for 5 minutes, without arterial compression, while the limb is being prepped and draped. Recently, a new sterile elastic exsanguination tourniquet was proposed with the aim of improving complete exsanguination.[8] If the PT is effective in occluding the extraosseous blood supply, some intraosseous blood supply is retained, which can make it difficult to obtain a bloodless field.[6]

Pressure Under the Pneumatic Tourniquet

Skin, muscles, nerves, and vessels may be damaged by the mechanical pressure of the tourniquet; sagittal forces cause compression and axial forces cause stretching as a result of uneven distribution of pressure under the cuff (Fig. 85.1).

Instead of using an arbitrary pressure (350 mm Hg for the lower extremity and 250 to 300 mm Hg for the upper extremity), the minimal arterial occlusion pressure (AOP) must be determined before tourniquet application to minimize tissue injury. The AOP depends on the size of the tourniquet used[63] and is determined by Graham's formula: AOP = [(Psys − Pdia)(limb circumference)/3(cuff width)] + Pdia.[17] The tourniquet pressure is set at AOP plus 50 to 75 mm Hg. Using this formula, the PT pressure can be decreased by 20% to 40% in adults[63] and by more than 50% for children,[46] compared to the arbitrary pressure generally used. The tourniquet pressure must be adjusted during surgery relative to blood pressure. Recently a new device was introduced that synchronizes the noninvasive blood pressure with the PT pressure.[23] If the AOP is not determined as explained previously, the tourniquet pressure used can be 75 to 100 mm Hg above systolic arterial pressure.[55] A subsystolic inflation pressure can induce venous congestion (venous tourniquet), which is easily recognized during surgery. Calcified, noncompressible arteries may also cause tourniquet failure.

The Mass of Tissue Under the Pneumatic Tourniquet

The mass of tissue affected by the PT is greater in the lower than the upper limbs (Fig. 85.2, and 85.3). The shape of the PT is critical. A straight tourniquet cannot fit a limb with a conical shape, particularly in obese patients (see Fig. 85.3). A wide cuff is much more effective in the occlusion stage than a narrow cuff and can be painless when pressure is limited to the lowest effective level.[16,35] Despite a possible risk of increased nerve injury, the widest curved cuff appropriate to the size of the extremity should be selected (ie, more than 5 cm for the upper and 9 cm for the lower limb) and must be connected to an integrated cuff inflation system. Conversely, if the width of the PT is increased without decreasing pressure, the combination of these two adverse effects may worsen the outcome.[36]

Tissue Injury

Skin. Wrinkle-free padding beneath the tourniquet is essential to reduce skin damage because of shearing stress.[13] To avoid chemical burns beneath the tourniquet, it must be separated from the operative field by a self-adhesive plastic drape before skin preparation.[10,20] A recent randomized study reported that patients with a cuff pressure of 223 mm Hg or less had a lower rate of wound complications (at discharge and at 2-month follow-up evaluation).[39] There is a correlation between the rate of postoperative wound oozing and the PT time after TKA.[9]

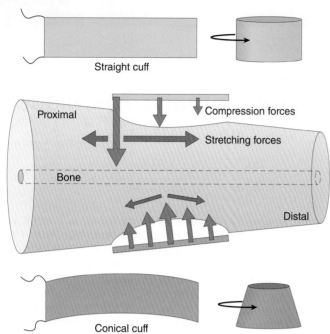

FIG 85.1 Curved tourniquet *(blue)* provides a better distribution of pressure *(purple arrows)* than the straight tourniquet *(green)* and reduces the arterial occlusion pressure. All tissues suffer under the pneumatic tourniquet because of mechanical pressure; sagittal forces are responsible for compression *(purple arrows)*, and axial forces *(red arrows)* are responsible for stretching because of uneven pressure. The intensity of the stretching depends of the level of variation in sagittal pressure.

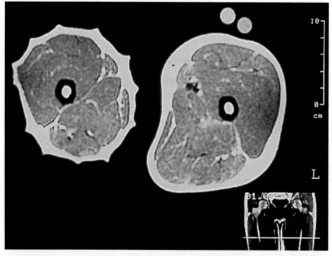

FIG 85.2 Sagittal view of a thigh tourniquet in computed tomography scanning of the left thigh. See the skin pinched under the pneumatic tourniquet set a 350 mmHg. In comparison to the other normal right side, the vascular occlusion is effective.

Because of the high rate of contamination of nonsterile reusable PTs (68%), it could be preferable to use a sterile PT to reduce potential sources of infection.[54] The tourniquet cuff should not be rotated to a new position after it is applied because shearing forces from rotating the cuff may damage underlying tissues.

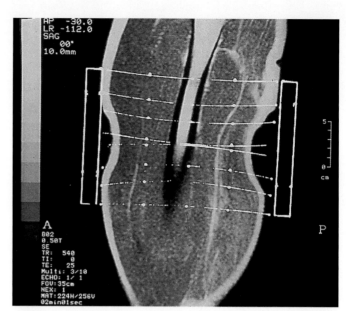

FIG 85.3 Longitudinal view of a thigh tourniquet in computed tomography scanning. The size of the pneumatic tourniquet is too small to apply low occlusion pressure in comparison to the large pneumatic tourniquet.

Muscle. It has been clearly demonstrated in animal and human studies that compression injury owing to the tourniquet results in a more significant loss of muscle functional strength, contractile speed, and fatigability than tourniquet-induced ischemia. Clinically relevant conclusions are difficult to draw from animal studies because small animals have a different muscle fiber composition and vulnerability than humans.[13] A curved cuff designed for animals provides more accurate determination of the magnitude and distribution of tissue pressures caused by tourniquet compression,[42] allowing better interpretation of experimental results.

Nerves. Temporary nerve injuries may be underdiagnosed because of postoperative limb weakness and the rapid recovery of the nerves. Reports of temporary or persistent nerve palsies and functional sequelae are not common in the recent literature, but nerve injuries do occur, especially at higher PT cuff pressures and after prolonged tourniquet inflation.[13,19] Conversely, tourniquet-induced neurologic injuries as a result of shearing forces are not uncommon. Animal models have demonstrated that nerve injury is more pronounced beneath the cuff than distal to it (ie, a combination of ischemia and direct mechanical deformation).[13]

A recent volunteer study showed that directly compressing a nerve causes focal ischemia, inducing localized axonal depolarization, followed by hyperpolarization upon release of the compression.[21] Mechanical deformation is associated with myelin disturbance, demyelination, and Wallerian degeneration. Hyperkalemia also reduces the trans-axonal potassium currents. A short duration (4 to 13 min) of compression is sufficient to impair the transmission of stimuli and cutaneous afferents.[47] The occurrence of electromyography (EMG) abnormalities has been noted during and after tourniquet use, and these abnormalities may persist for up to 6 months afterward.[29]

Tourniquet pain can be explained by ischemia and compression,[14] but it is increased with hyperalgesic phenomena (eg, when a traumatic injury is the primary stimulating factor). Thus, in addition to local mechanisms, sensitization of the central nervous system may also play a part in the tourniquet pain process. Evidence of expansion of the spinal receptive field of nociceptor neurons in response to tourniquet pain has been seen in animal studies.[13]

For the upper limb, the pain tolerance in studies on volunteers is around 20 to 30 minutes.[16,43] In the absence of regional or general anesthesia, the topical application of EMLA cream is effective in providing semicircular subcutaneous anesthesia and reducing tourniquet pain. Morphine added to a lidocaine epidural solution during regional anesthesia significantly delays the onset of tourniquet pain.[13,14]

Vessels. Tourniquet use may also damage the intravascular endothelium. Arterial complications after TKA are rare but the consequences can be disastrous (eg, vascular reconstruction or amputation), particularly in the presence of peripheral arterial disease or ipsilateral prior peripheral arterial reconstruction.[57] Careful monitoring of the vascular status of the limb (ie, distal pulses and capillary refill) is required in the early postoperative period to detect any vascular compromise.[13,14]

ISCHEMIA-REPERFUSION EFFECTS

Duration of Ischemia

The "safe" duration of tourniquet-induced ischemia remains controversial.[13,14] It has been reported that tourniquet application longer than 60 minutes increases the risk of complications after arthroscopy.[48] However, it has also been demonstrated that 3 hours of continuous ischemia will not produce generalized irreversible damage in healthy muscle, although it will result in widespread sublethal injury to cells. The maximum recommended period of tourniquet-induced ischemia is 1 hour.[13,14]

If tourniquet use exceeds one hour, it is common practice to deflate the PT intermittently in an attempt to minimize the ischemic damage. Reperfusion periods can be initiated within 45 to 60 minutes of ischemia (tourniquet downtime technique) and must be longer than 10 minutes to be beneficial. Reperfusion initiated after 2 ischemic hours tends to exacerbate muscle injury. Releasing the PT before wound closure was proposed to reduce the duration of ischemia. On the one hand, a recent meta-analysis confirmed a slight increase in surgical time (around 8 minutes) and blood loss (without significant decrease in hemoglobin) when the PT was released before wound closure. On the other hand, there was a significant decrease in minor and major complications.[64,66] Severe complications such as acute vascular damage can be avoided if the PT is released for hemostasis.

Tourniquet Release, Effects of Reperfusion

Generalities. Tourniquet release is associated with an immediate 10% increase in limb girth, as a result of refilling of the vessels and hyperemia. This causes an increase in intracompartmental pressure in the reperfused limb. Over the first postoperative day, the initial limb girth can increase by as much as 50%.[13,14] Releasing the tourniquet prior to hemostasis and closure reduces inflation time, allowing for a period of reperfusion and swelling before bandage or cast application. This may reduce potential complications associated with an increase in intracompartmental pressure, compared to applying the dressing before tourniquet release. Deflation should be quick to prevent capillary bleeding.[13,14]

IR results in a complex cascade of responses that can lead to muscle degeneration and loss of function. Despite the common use of a tourniquet during limb surgery, it remains difficult to identify manifestations of IR in humans, but animal model studies have shown that tourniquet use might be associated with significant IR injury.[13,14] Signs of primary injury (vasodilation and erythema) have been observed immediately after 1 hour of tourniquet use. Secondary injury presents as a progression of cell injury despite reperfusion, which can lead to a "no-reflow phenomenon" in which blood flow does not return to all areas after a long period of ischemia. Leukocytes play a significant role in this phenomenon, through adhesion to postcapillary venules, microvascular barrier disruption, and edema formation. Described in 1951, the "post-tourniquet syndrome" combines weakness, stiffness, edema, dysesthesia, and pain. These symptoms may be mistakenly attributed to surgical trauma or to lack of patient motivation.[13,14]

Skin. Risk factors for infectious complications include prolonged tourniquet inflation time. The systemic inflammatory response to tourniquet use may be explained by profound and sustained endothelial dysfunction and neutrophil activation.[7] Wound hypoxia during lower limb orthopedic surgery is greater with tourniquet use than without. This may have clinical relevance for wound healing and infection.

Tourniquets (and exsanguinators) can be a potential source of infection.[1,7] Parenteral prophylactic antibiotics must be administered at least 10 to 20 minutes before tourniquet inflation and isolation of the operative site from the systemic circulation. After inflation of the tourniquet, antibiotics may not reach the exsanguinated limb. If the tourniquet has been inflated, regional intravenous injection of an antibiotic is a good alternative. However, antibiotic administration 10 minutes before the PT release seems to be as effective as administration before inflation.[52]

Muscle. Skeletal muscle may be severely affected, even with relatively short periods of ischemia.[13,14] Functional muscle loss seems to be worse if there is hemorrhage before tourniquet application.[59] After anterior cruciate ligament reconstruction, the amount of vastus muscle amyotrophy after tourniquet use is significantly greater than without tourniquet use.[28,37] Similar reduction in quadriceps function was reported after TKA without significant effect on cement interface quality.[34] Cases of rhabdomyolysis with acute renal failure, and compartment syndrome have been reported after tourniquet duration of more than 4 hours, but also with shorter inflation times (45 to 120 min).[30,49] Interestingly, loss of strength, or electromyographic abnormalities, can also be observed in the contralateral limb, suggesting a sensitization of the central nervous system.[13,14]

The mechanism of muscle damage owing to ischemia and subsequent reperfusion is well understood.[40] Complement activation, mast cell degranulation, neutrophil adhesion and infiltration, and microvascular dysfunction all play a role. During ischemia, a cascade of adenosine triphosphate (ATP) depletion, acidosis, and ion imbalance occurs. The production of cytokines, reactive oxygen species (ROS), and rapid calcium influx into the cells, which occurs progressively during reperfusion, is more damaging and causes mitochondrial dysfunction that leads to cellular apoptosis and necrosis. Muscle injury seems to be greater in older patients, probably as a result of greater susceptibility of aged skeletal muscle to IR injury and to local attenuation of insulin-like growth factor-1 gene expression, which reduces regenerative mechanisms.[13,14]

Nerves. Limb dysfunction during ischemia and reperfusion may be largely the result of axonal or neuromuscular junction injury, or both.[13,14] After tourniquet deflation, a warming sensation, quickly turning into an aching sensation of burning is associated with limb reperfusion. During reperfusion the hyperemic flow response in nerves is more prolonged than in muscle. However, the factors that incite the ischemic nerves to spontaneously discharge and cause paresthesia upon reperfusion are not understood.

Postoperative pain control is important for optimal functional recovery from surgery. Pain scores are often similar or lower in orthopedic patients without tourniquet use.[34,58] In a prospective randomized study performed with simultaneous bilateral TKA, a clear decrease in thigh pain was reported in the group with lower PT pressure.[62] Interestingly, the change in systemic pain perception observed after the first knee operation induces greater postoperative pain in the second operated knee after a 1-week interval.[27] To effectively reduce pain, intra-articular injection of local anesthetics must be performed 10 minutes before tourniquet deflation, to allow fixation of local anesthetics before the washout period of tourniquet release, or 30 minutes after PT deflation.[13,14]

Vessels. The risk of DVT is significantly increased with a tourniquet time of more than 60 minutes.[11] Following knee arthroscopy, the incidence of DVT diagnosed using contrast venography is approximately 18% 1 week after surgery. The formation of DVT begins during tourniquet inflation and continues after deflation owing to an increase in circulating markers of thrombosis (plasma D-dimer, tissue plasminogen activator, angiotensin-converting enzyme, antithrombin-III, and protein C).[12,32,33] Inflammation and hemostasis are linked by common activation pathways and feedback regulation. PT use exaggerates these responses, which peak on PT deflation and remain elevated on postoperative days 1 and 2.[24,38,45] Close monitoring of coagulation factors could help detect asymptomatic venous thromboembolism (VTE) after TKA.[60]

In randomized studies, tourniquet use during TKA does not reduce total blood loss.[22,34,53] A meta-analysis of TKA surgery confirms that there is an initial increase in blood loss in groups without PT use, but no significant difference in total perioperative blood loss or transfusion in comparison with PT groups.[51] An increase of local fibrinolysis postoperatively after PT deflation, secondary to the release of anticlotting factors from the surgical site, may explain the increased risk of bleeding into the joint or drains.[31,41] The benefit of surgical hemostasis after tourniquet deflation is still under debate because of the risk of increased blood loss, but prospective studies support intraoperative PT release.[3,44]

SYSTEMIC EFFECTS

General

Just after the deflation of the tourniquet, anesthetic drugs sequestered in the exsanguinated limb are released and may be clinically detected in some cases, eg, when the bispectral index is used.[15,50] This could be clinically important in older adults or debilitated patients.

Cardiovascular

Tourniquet application has significant effects on the cardiovascular system. The mean arterial pressure increases progressively after tourniquet inflation secondary to pain.[13,14] Regional anesthesia is more effective than general anesthesia for moderating the cardiovascular response to tourniquet pain. Preoperative intravenous injection of a small dose of ketamine, dexmedetomidine or clonidine, magnesium sulfate, or dextromethorphan can reduce the increase in systolic arterial pressure associated with tourniquet inflation and have an analgesic effect.

A brief period of hypotension upon PT deflation, secondary to metabolic and lactic acidosis and hyperkalemia, can cause myocardial depression and even cardiac arrest in older adults or debilitated patients after prolonged lower limb surgery.[18] Postoperative hypovolemia may be observed after tourniquet deflation, in part owing to hemorrhage at the surgical site, but mostly to a combination of reactive vasodilation and increased microvascular permeability in the entire reperfused limb during the first hour.[13,14]

Pulmonary

Fatal or near-fatal pulmonary embolism was first reported after use of the Esmarch bandage and/or tourniquet inflation in orthopedic surgery and was subsequently reported after tourniquet deflation.[4] A significant correlation was noted between the occurrence of emboli and the duration of tourniquet application.[13,14] Emboli occur during PT inflation and femur reaming in 27% of patients, and in 100% of patients after tourniquet deflation. Pulmonary embolism occurring during orthopedic surgery can result from a fat embolism owing to invasion of the medullary cavity. Air and cement emboli have also been reported after tourniquet release. The occurrence of emboli in patients undergoing invasive surgery (eg, TKA) is more frequent compared to noninvasive surgery (eg, diagnostic arthroscopy).[13,14] Even in the absence of a patent foramen ovale, cerebral microemboli frequently occur (60%) upon tourniquet release (probably through the opening of recruitable pulmonary vessels).[61]

Acute lung injury can be observed after limb reperfusion, with increased microvascular permeability, sequestration of neutrophils, and generation of oxygen-free radicals. The powerful neutrophil activation causes oxidative stress and has been used in an animal model to develop "tourniquet shock" by applying two tourniquets simultaneously on both lower limbs of an animal.[13,14]

Neurologic

Tourniquet deflation may be accompanied by a dangerous increase in intracranial pressure, mainly owing to a simultaneous increase in CO_2 production and a decrease in systemic blood pressure upon release of the tourniquet; this situation could lead to a severe reduction in cerebral perfusion pressure with potentially disastrous consequences in patients with brain injury.[13,14] When propofol or sevoflurane (but not isoflurane) are used to maintain anesthesia, hyperventilation after tourniquet deflation to prevent or treat hypercapnia can prevent an increase in cerebral perfusion pressure.

TREATMENT OF ISCHEMIA-REPERFUSION INJURY

New treatments have been proposed to help prevent or reduce the effects of IR. Ischemic preconditioning, defined as a brief period of ischemia followed by tissue reperfusion, can be used to decrease the systemic effects of IR after tourniquet use on upper or lower limbs,[56] including attenuation of pulmonary dysfunction.[32] Nitric oxide synthase (NOS) and heme oxygenase (HO) have been implicated in this process. Ischemic preconditioning of limbs also has distant anti-inflammatory effects on remote organs.[13,14,25] Interestingly, pre- and postconditioning can be applied on the contralateral limb with a significant effect on vascular endothelium dysfunction (vasoconstriction and thrombosis). These effects can be partially explained by humoral factors and/or neurologic pathways.[2,14]

Prostaglandins or their analogues do not seem, experimentally, to reduce muscle injury. Antioxidants have a cytoprotective effect that could be attributed to the inhibition of neutrophil adherence activation and scavenging of superoxide radicals. In humans, inhaled nitric oxide (NO) before, during, and after the PT application reduces inflammation in lower limb extremities. HO, which catalyzes the breakdown of heme to iron, biliverdin IXa, and carbon monoxide may also be beneficial because carbon monoxide has a very similar action to NO. Administration of an endothelial xanthine oxidase inhibitor (allopurinol) or a radical scavenger such as vitamin E can decrease oxidative stress and the occurrence of edema in postischemic skeletal muscle.[13,14] Edaravone, another free-radical scavenger, when given during early reperfusion, seems to be effective in reducing nerve injury as a result of oxidative stress. To reduce microvascular reperfusion injury following tourniquet ischemia in striated muscle, buflomedil or flurbiprofen can also be used.

Local hypothermia by cold gel packs reduces metabolic demand by reducing ischemic and anoxic degeneration, but although it could be effective during ischemia, it may aggravate injury after reperfusion.[13,14,26] Phosphodiesterase type 3 inhibitors can be used as inodilators (ie, positive inotropes and arteriovenous dilators) to reduce DVT. A perioperative infusion of milrinone can significantly attenuate platelet activation and monocyte tissue factor expression during a TKA without increasing perioperative blood loss. Regional limb heparinization is not effective in reducing embolic phenomena after PT release.

ECONOMIC IMPACT

The combination of these different mechanical, ischemia-reperfusion, and systemic effects could explain the prolonged hospital length of stay (LOS) and delayed return to work observed in the tourniquet versus nontourniquet groups.[13,14,34] Despite a slight increase in surgical time without PT use, a cost-benefit analysis would have obvious implications for health care management.

CONCLUSION

The variable quality of the articles reviewed makes it difficult to establish an overview of the existing evidence on PT use, but the basic science confirms that there are, at least, transient changes attributable to its use. In practice, the PT is a useful tool for good visualization in extremity surgery but it carries a risk of adverse effects. It is necessary to weigh the advantages and disadvantages before deciding to use a PT. The main indication should not be the hemostatic effect of the tourniquet because elevation, step-by-step hemostasis, and

pharmacologic vasoconstriction may also be used to obtain a bloodless field. Several relative contraindications for use of a tourniquet have been mentioned in the literature, including severe atherosclerotic disease, severe crush injuries, diabetes mellitus, sickle-cell disease, and severe brain injury. Proven or suspected DVT, presence of calcified vessels, rheumatoid arthritis, and other collagen-vascular diseases associated with vasculitis, as well as localized tumors, are also relative contraindications.

To minimize adverse effects, the tourniquet must be used within the framework of strict procedures and protocols, with well-adapted and regularly checked equipment. The location of the PT must be as distal as is surgically possible. The arterial occlusion pressure must be measured, and the PT inflated to an arterial occlusion pressure plus 50 to 75 mm Hg (or 75 to 100 mm Hg greater than systolic blood pressure). Tourniquet duration should ideally be less than 1 hour. Reperfusion periods can be initiated within 45 to 60 minutes of ischemia for longer tourniquet times. To keep the duration of ischemia as short as possible, tourniquet deflation prior to hemostasis and closure is preferable. After deflation, monitoring of the vascular and neurologic status of the limb must be performed regularly, so a temporary bandage or split plaster cast should be used for the first 2 postoperative days to allow space for swelling and to permit evaluation of the limb.

KEY REFERENCES

4. Bharti N, Mahajan S: Massive pulmonary embolism leading to cardiac arrest after deflation following lower limb surgery. *Anaesth Intensive Care* 37:867–868, 2009.

6. Blønd L, Madsen L: Bone narrow perfusion in healthy subjects assessed by scintigraphy after application of a tourniquet. *Acta Orthop Scand* 74:460–464, 2003.

13. Estebe JP: The pneumatic tourniquet. In *Surgical Techniques in Orthopaedics and Traumatology (EFORT)*, Paris, 2002, Ed Elsevier. 55-010-B-20.

14. Estebe JP, Davies J, Richebe P: The pneumatic tourniquet: mechanical, ischaemia-reperfusion and systemic effects. *Eur J Anaesth* 28:404–411, 2011.

15. Estebe JP, Le Corre P, Levron JC, et al: Pilot study on the effect of tourniquet on sufentanil pharmacokinetics. *J Clin Anesth* 14:578–583, 2002.

16. Estebe JP, Le Naoures A, Chemaly L, et al: Tourniquet pain in a volunteer study: effect of changes in cuff width and pressure. *Anaesthesia* 55:21–26, 2000.

30. Lee YG, Park W, Kim SH, et al: A case of rhabdomyolysis with use of a pneumatic tourniquet during arthroscopic knee surgery. *Kor J Int Med* 25:105–109, 2010.

31. Li B, Wen Y, Wu H, et al: The effect of tourniquet use on hidden blood loss in total knee arthroplasty. *Int Orthop* 33:1263–1268, 2009.

37. Nicholas SJ, Tyler TF, McHugh MP, et al: The effect on leg strength of tourniquet use during anterior cruciate ligament reconstruction: a prospective randomized study. *Arthroscopy* 17:603–607, 2001.

60. Watanabe H, Kikkawa I, Madoiwa S, et al: Changes in blood coagulation-fibrinolysis markers by pneumatic tourniquet during total knee joint arthroplasty with venous thromboembolism. *J Arthroplasty* 29:569–573, 2014.

61. Wauke K, Nagashima M, Kato N, et al: Comparative study between thromboembolism and total knee arthroplasty with or without tourniquet in rheumatoid arthritis patients. *Arch Orthop Trauma Surg* 122:442–446, 2002.

62. Worland RL, Arrebondo J, Angles F, et al: Thigh pain following tourniquet application in simultaneous bilateral knee replacement arthroplasty. *J Arthroplasty* 12:848–852, 1997.

64. Zan PF, Yang Y, Fu D, et al: Releasing of tourniquet before wound closure or not in total knee arthroplasty: a meta-analysis of randomized controlled trials. *J Arthroplasty* 30:31–37, 2015.

65. Zhang W, Chen S, Tan Y, et al: The effects of a tourniquet used in total knee arthroplasty: a meta-analysis. *J Orthop Surg Res* 9:13, 2014. doi: 10.1186/1749-799X-9-13.

66. Zhang W, Hu D, Tan Y, et al: Effects of the timing of tourniquet release in cemented total knee arthroplasty: a systematic review and meta-analysis of randomized controlled trials. *J Orthop Surg Res* 9:125, 2014.

The references for this chapter can also be found on www.expertconsult.com.

86

Cement Embolism

Jean-Pierre Estèbe

INTRODUCTION

Bone cement has been successfully used in total knee arthroplasty (TKA) in order to fill the free space between the prosthesis and the bone, and it plays an important role in the elastic zone. Bone cement embolism (BCE) or bone cement implantation syndrome (BCIS), which is because of leakage of cement, is a rare and potentially fatal situation, but the true frequency remains underestimated. The reason for this is that a majority of patients are asymptomatic and complications are probably underreported in the literature. For proximal femur surgery (ie, hemiarthroplasty and cemented total hip arthroplasty), the incidence of BCIS is estimated to be over 20% and the incidence of severe reactions resulting in cardiovascular collapse is 1.7%.[6]

MECHANISMS

Given that the etiology of BCE is poorly understood, several nonmutually exclusive mechanisms have been proposed.

The Monomer-Mediated Model

Bone cement is usually provided as a two-component material composed of small particles of prepolymerized polymethylmethacrylate (PMMA) and liquid monomers of methylmethacrylate (MMA).[2,19] The cement undergoes an exothermic reaction (as high as 86°C) and expands in the space between the prosthesis and bone, trapping air and medullary contents under pressure. The exothermic polymerization of bone cement may induce thermal necrosis of bone.[13] Bone cement acts as a space filler with no intrinsic adhesive properties. As a drug delivery system, various molecules have been successfully mixed with bone cement, such as antibiotics, contrast agents, or additives to increase its bioactivity.[7,8,11] The current process is divided into four stages: mixing, waiting, working, and hardening. One of the local major drawbacks of bone cement in joint replacement is cement fragmentation and foreign body reaction to wear debris, resulting in prosthetic loosening. Some other local effects could be related to the cement, such as local neuropathy, local vascular erosion or occlusion, heterotopic new bone formation, and superficial or deep wound infection. Allergic reactions toward bone cement components are rare.[1]

The Embolic Model

Leakage could be secondary to premature injection of excessively liquid PMMA (circulating MMA monomers could cause vasodilatation) or exaggerated pressure with the aim to improve bone cement interface.[21] Particularly with highly osteoporotic patients, bone embolism could arise during any step of the surgery: intramedullary reaming (just bone and fat), then BCE with cement implantation (cement plus bone and fat), insertion of the prosthesis, or joint reduction. Unfortunately, there is no clear correlation between the amount of emboli and the severity of the clinical symptoms. This may be because of the proportion of fat embolisms being highly variable. In one dog model, it was reported that bilateral femoral intramedullary reaming and bone cement injection induced intraoperative increase of heart rate, central venous pressure, pulmonary capillary wedge pressure, and extravascular lung water, while mean arterial pressure, pH, PaO$_2$, and PaCO$_2$ decreased. At the same time, an increase of TNF-α, IL-1β, and IL-6 was noted.[25] Histologic lung evaluation confirms fat microthrombi in the pulmonary artery, alveolar edema, and hemorrhage.[25]

Paradoxical cerebral embolism, particularly in the case of a patent foramen ovale (ie, right-to-left shunt to the cerebral arterial circulation), has been reported.[12,23] However, in the clinical setting with no neurological abnormalities, an increase of serum protein (S-100B) after cemented TKA has been used as a sensitive marker of cerebral damage.[9]

The Biologic Model

The physiologic consequences of BCE must be considered the result of both a mechanical effect (mechanical occlusion theory) and mediator release (biochemical theory). An inflammatory anaphylactic cascade occurs with the release of cytokines and histamine and the activation of the complement system. This induces pulmonary vascular permeability and increases pulmonary vascular tone, which causes shunting of blood and therefore a decrease in the blood pressure.

DIAGNOSTIC

In most patients, BCIS is nonfatal and is associated with hypoxemia and/or hypotension and occurs at the limb tourniquet (PT) deflation, or around the time of cementation, stem insertion, or reduction of the joint[5] when the PT is not used. Elevated serum gamma-glutamyl-transpeptidase (GGTP) has also been reported. However, in some patients, it causes serious cardiovascular changes, which may produce ventricular tachycardia, other arrhythmias, shock, or cardiac arrest. In the awake patient undergoing regional anesthesia, altered sensorium and dyspnea could be warming signs of bronchospasm. Donaldson et al. recently proposed a severity classification of BCIS: grade 1 is defined as moderate hypoxemia (arterial oxygen saturation <94%) or hypotension (a decrease in systolic arterial pressure [SAP] >20%); grade 2 is severe hypoxemia (arterial oxygen saturation <88%) or hypotension (a decrease in SAP >40%) or unexpected loss of consciousness; grade 3 is defined as cardio-vascular collapse requiring cardiopulmonary resuscitation.[5] Because of poor cardiorespiratory reserve, it is not surprising to find a high risk of cardiac disorders in older patients during the BCIS.[6]

During the perioperative period of TKA, pulmonary embo-lism (PE) could be because of various mixed elements, such as blood clot, fat, bone, and cement. Venous thromboembolism (VTE) with PE is the major life-threatening complication fol-lowing TKA. Symptomatic PE was estimated to be around 0.61% for unilateral and 1.87% for bilateral TKA in a recent study.[22] However, in the postoperative period, we cannot exclude that a PE was built up step by step: fat and bone, then cement, and finally blood clot, as reported after percutaneous vertebroplasty.[15]

BCE is usually diagnosed by imaging technologies (x-ray, computed tomography [CT] scan or CT pulmonary angiogra-phy; magnetic resonance imaging). However, the limited imaging resolution could induce false-negative evidence of BCE. Transthoracic echocardiography can also be a useful tool during surgery.[10]

Few cases have been identified by autopsy. The proportion of cement into emboli remains controversial, as it could be mixed with fat, bone debris, narrow constituents, and platelet and fibrin. Proportions could be evaluated with Fourier-transform infrared spectroscopy.[24] Using intraoperative echo-cardiography to visualize these embolic showers during intramedullary nailing of long bone fractures and during cemented and uncemented arthroplasty, the literature shows that embolic phenomena occurred in essentially 100% of cases.[3] However, in the cemented group, the emboli were most marked (with a 10-fold increase in the number of emboli).[16] It has been shown that the degree of embolism correlates poorly with the extent of hypotension or hypoxemia.[5] Autopsy findings confirm bone marrow elements, fat, and cement not only into the lungs but also into the heart, the brain, and sometimes in the liver and kidneys.[4]

THE TREATMENT

Communication between the surgeon and the anesthesiologist is of utmost importance. A discussion should occur regarding the most appropriate anesthetic and surgical technique based on the comorbidities of the patient. The surgical and anesthesia teams must be extremely vigilant at the time of cementing and/or PT release. Anesthetic risk reduction could include the increase of the inspired oxygen concentration, avoidance of nitrous oxide, and cardiovascular optimization. Surgical mea-sures are proposed with the aim of reducing the incidence of BCE with good hemostasis and venting of the bone medulla. Several methods have been introduced: vacuum drainage, distal venting hole, jet lavage, secondary cementing technique, intra-medullary plugs, and drainage canal in the stem.[14,17,18]

The treatment for symptomatic or central pulmonary cement embolism is surgical embolectomy or percutaneous removal, whereas more conservative management is advocated for smaller or peripherally located emboli. Early detection and supportive care (ie, adequate oxygenation, treatment of coagu-lopathy, anemia, hypovolemia, and cardiovascular dysfunction) are important for improved patient outcome. The use of meth-ylprednisolone remains a topic of discussion. For some patients

at high risk (high body mass index, history of stroke, old age, poor preexisting physical reserve, pulmonary hypertension, and impaired cardiopulmonary function), it is likely better to avoid simultaneous bilateral TKA, and the use of regional anesthesia is recommended.[14] In the presence of asymptomatic peripheral embolism, clinical follow-up and anticoagulation with heparin, followed by vitamin K antagonist (VKA) for 6 months to avoid additional thrombosis, are recommended.

CONCLUSION

The use of cement for TKA remains a topic of discussion. A recent meta-analysis confirms that there is no evidence to support that fixation techniques (ie, with or without cement) alone affect the durability of the TKA.[20] Nevertheless, it remains unclear whether the BCE complication is rare or underdiagnosed.

KEY REFERENCES

3. Christie J, Robinson C, Pell AC, et al: Transcardiac echocardiography during invasive intramedullary procedures. *J Bone Joint Surg Br* 77:450–455, 1995.

4. de Froidmont S, Bonetti LR, Villaverde RV, et al: Postmortem findings in bone cement implantation syndrome-related deaths. *Am J Forensic Med Pathol* 35:206–211, 2014.

5. Donaldson AJ, Thomsom HE, Harper NJ, et al: Bone cement implantation syndrome. *Br J Anaesth* 102:12–22, 2009.

6. Griffiths R, Parker M: Bone cement implantation syndrome and proximal femoral fracture. *Br J Anaesth* 114:6–7, 2015.

9. Kinoshita H, Iranami H, Fujii K, et al: The use of bone cement induces an increase in serum astroglial S-100B protein in patients undergoing total knee arthroplasty. *Anesth Analg* 97:1657–1660, 2003.

10. Lafont ND, Kostucki WM, Marchand PH, et al: Embolism detected by transoesophageal echocardiography during hip arthroplasty. *Can J Anaesth* 41:850–853, 1994.

12. Lee SC, Yoon JY, Nam CH, et al: Cerebral fat embolism syndrome after simultaneous bilateral total knee arthroplasty. A case series. *J Arthroplasty* 27:409–413, 2012.

15. Oh JK, Park HJ, Kim SS, et al: Thread-like bone cement in right-side heart and pulmonary arteries causing diffuse pulmonary embolism as a late complication. *Heart Lung Circ* 24:e104–e107, 2015.

16. Orsini EC, Byrick RJ, Mullen JB, et al: Cardiopulmonary function and pulmonary microemboli during arthroplasty using cemented or non-cemented components. The role of intramedullary pressure. *J Bone Joint Surg Am* 69:822–832, 1987.

19. Vaishya R, Chauhan M, Vaish A: Bone cement. *J Clin Orthop Trauma* 4:157–163, 2013.

20. Wang H, Lou H, Zhang H, et al: Similar survival between uncemented and cemented fixation prostheses in total knee arthroplasty: a meta-analysis and systematic comparative analysis using registers. *Knee Surg Sports Traumatol Arthrosc* 22:3191, 2014.

21. Webb JC, Spencer RF: The role of polymethylmethacrylate bone cement in modern orthopaedic surgery. *J Bone Joint Surg Br* 89:851–857, 2007.

22. Yeager AM, Ruel AV, Westrich GH: Are bilateral total joint arthroplasty patients at a higher risk of developing pulmonary embolism following total hip and knee surgery. *J Arthroplasty* 29:900–902, 2014.

24. Zheng N, Liang M, Zhang HD, et al: Fatal extensive bone cement embolism: histologic findings confirmed by Fourier transform infrared spectroscopy. *Forensic Sci Int* 229:e23–e25, 2013.

25. Zhou F, Qing Song JH, Peng Z, et al: Pulmonary fat embolism and related effects during femoral intramedullary surgery: an experimental study in dogs. *Exp Ther Med* 6:469–474, 2013.

The references for this chapter can also be found on www.expertconsult.com.

87

Tranexamic Acid

Jan Boublik, Arthur Atchabahian

BACKGROUND

Despite the best screening procedures to prevent transmission of infectious agents, a risk remains with any blood transfusion. Another reason for concern is immunologic response and modulation and the fact that allogeneic transfusion by itself leads to negative outcomes and increased morbidity,[12,35] including following knee arthroplasty.[16] In fact, patients who receive red blood cell (RBC) transfusion in the perioperative period have a higher composite morbidity, higher rate of surgical site infection rate, increased chance of mortality, and a longer length of hospital stay.[28]

While optimization of surgical technique and meticulous hemostasis are paramount to reduce bleeding, the use of hemostatic agents has been used more widely in clinical practice. Hemostatic agents can essentially be divided into two major groups: procoagulants such as recombinant factor VII, desmopressin, and fibrinogen; and antifibrinolytics such as serin protease inhibitors (eg, aprotinin) and lysine analogues (eg, aminocaproic acid and tranexamic acid).[38]

Henry et al.[17] found in a Cochrane Review that "antifibrinolytic drugs provide worthwhile reductions in blood loss and the receipt of allogeneic red cell transfusion." While the lysine analogues are slightly less effective than aprotinin in reducing blood loss and blood transfusions, they have a lower risk of death compared with aprotinin, the use of which was abandoned following the BART trial,[10] which found an increased relative risk of death in the aprotinin group, as compared with that in both groups receiving lysine analogues (1.53; 95% CI, 1.06 to 2.22).

TRANEXAMIC ACID (CHEMISTRY, MECHANISM OF ACTION, CLINICAL USE)

The synthetic lysine-analogues tranexamic acid and 1-aminocaproic acid were first described in 1957 by Okamoto[31] (Fig. 87.1).

Tranexamic acid (CYKLOKAPRON, LYSTEDA) is a lysine analogue that reversibly blocks lysine binding sites on plasminogen (and plasmin), thus blocking fibrin binding and degradation (see Figs. 87.1 and 87.2). Aminocaproic acid acts by the same mechanism as tranexamic acid (TXA) but has lower binding affinity to plasminogen. As a result of lower plasmin levels, fibrinolytic activity is diminished, fibrin is not broken down, and thereby bleeding is decreased. The drug has no effect on other blood coagulation parameters such as platelet count, activated partial thromboplastin time, and prothrombin time.[47] TXA has a half-life of 1 to 2 hours, with 100% bioavailability

and wide distribution through intra- and extravascular compartments. Peak levels after intravenous administration occur in the plasma at 30 minutes, in the liver at 60 minutes, and in the heart and muscles at 120 minutes. Hepatic metabolism is minimal, and the medication is primarily eliminated through the urine (65% as unchanged drug, 11% as metabolite); therefore, dose reductions should be considered with renal impairment. As an example, 1 g of TXA achieves plasma levels of more than 1 mg/dL, which achieves therapeutic levels (0.5 to 1.5 mg/dL) for more than 6 hours.

Tranexamic acid can be given intravenously or orally. Another possible route of administration may be topical administration, which has been proven to be efficacious,[21] with a half-life of about 3 hours.

Given the concern that increased systemic thrombotic activity may lead to increased rates of thromboembolism, tranexamic acid was only approved by the US Food and Drug Administration (FDA) to treat menorrhagia in 2009, despite its safe use in other parts of the world for many years. When used for this indication, tranexamic acid usually is given at a dose of 1 g 4 times a day for 4 days.[5b]

While tranexamic acid has been labeled for use in patients with hemophilia or menorrhagia, off-label uses include prevention of surgical blood loss, particularly for orthopedic, gynecological, and cardiac surgery, as well as in the setting of postpartum or posttrauma hemorrhage.

TXA is also used as adjunctive therapy in hemophilia and congenital alpha 2-plasmin inhibitor deficiency,[45] as therapy for bleeding from fibrinolytic therapy, and as prophylaxis for rebleeding from intracranial aneurysms. Treatment success has also been reported in patients with upper aerodigestive tumors,[26] postsurgical gastrointestinal bleeding, postprostatectomy bleeding, and bladder hemorrhage secondary to radiation- and drug-induced cystitis.

Adverse events associated with TXA use have been reported. These include mild to moderate side effects such as nasal stuffiness, hypotension, myopathy, acute gastrointestinal disturbances (nausea, vomiting, and diarrhea, generally dose-related), visual disturbances (blurry vision and changes in color perception, especially with prolonged use), and significant adverse effects such as intravascular thrombosis from inhibition of plasminogen activator, deep venous thrombosis, and pulmonary embolism (Table 87.1). Its use is thus contraindicated in the settings of acquired defective color vision and active intravascular clotting. TXA should be used with caution in the setting of urinary tract bleeding, because ureteral obstruction caused by clotting has been reported.[5a] The favorable risk benefits ratio compounded by the decades-long use for congenital and acquired

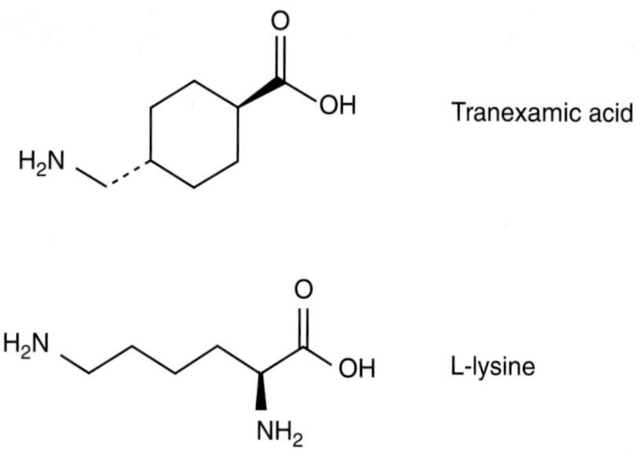

FIG 87.1 Chemical Structure of TXA.

TABLE 87.1	Side and Adverse Effects of Tranexamic Acid
Cardiovascular	Arrhythmia, bradycardia, edema, hypotension, intracranial hypertension, peripheral ischemia, syncope, thrombosis
Central nervous system	Confusion, delirium, dizziness, fatigue, hallucinations, headache, malaise, seizure, stroke
Dermatologic	Rash, pruritus
Gastrointestinal	Abdominal pain, anorexia, cramps, diarrhea, GI irritation, nausea, vomiting
Hematologic	Agranulocytosis, bleeding time increased, leukopenia, thrombocytopenia
Neuromuscular and skeletal	CPK increased, myalgia, myositis, myopathy, rhabdomyolysis (rare), weakness
Respiratory	Dyspnea, nasal congestion, pulmonary embolism
Renal	BUN increased, intrarenal obstruction (glomerular capillary thrombosis), myoglobinuria (rare), renal failure (rare)
Ophthalmic/Otic	Visual disturbances (blurry vision and changes in color perception), vision decreased, watery eyes, tinnitus
Miscellaneous	Allergic reaction, anaphylactoid reaction, anaphylaxis, injection site necrosis, injection site pain, injection site reactions
Rare but important or life threatening	Hepatic lesion, hyperkalemia, myocardial lesion

CPK, Creatine phosphokinase; *BUN*, blood urea nitrogen.

bleeding disorders make tranexamic acid an attractive candidate.[6]

Contraindications to tranexamic acid include a history of or an intrinsic risk for thromboembolic disease (eg, active malignancy). In addition, strong caution is recommended in concurrently prescribing hormonal contraceptives that also increase thromboembolic risk. The drug should not be used in patients with disseminated intravascular coagulation or genitourinary bleeding of the upper tract (eg, kidney and ureters) because of the potential for excessive clotting.[22] TXA is contraindicated in patients with aneurysmal subarachnoid hemorrhage; however, there have been no reported complications associated with intra- or extracranial hemorrhage associated with trauma. TXA should not be given with activated prothrombin complex concentrate or factor IX complex concentrates because these may increase the risk of thrombosis[5a] and possibly be detrimental in patients more than 3 hours after large trauma, given a prothrombotic state.[36] Caution should be exercised in patients with coronary stents[15]; administration of TXA is best be avoided, although strong evidence is lacking.

TRANEXAMIC ACID IN SURGERY

Antifibrinolytic therapy may be particularly useful for patients who are undergoing a repeat operation, for long and complicated procedures, in patients who refuse blood products (such as Jehovah's Witnesses), and in patients who have preexisting coagulopathy or are at high risk for postoperative bleeding because of recent administration of glycoprotein IIb/IIIa inhibitors (eg, abciximab [RheoPro], eptifibatide [Integrilin], or xirofiban [Aggrastat]).[40]

Massicotte et al.[27] observed that TXA was comparable to aprotinin in liver transplantation. Bouet et al.[4] used high-dose TXA (4 g IV) for postpartum hemorrhage after vaginal delivery without any harm or benefit. Song et al.[41] demonstrated in their meta-analysis that TXA reduces perioperative red blood cell transfusions in pediatric craniosynostosis surgery.

Ker et al.[23] performed a systematic review and cumulative meta-analysis on the effect of tranexamic acid on surgical blood loss, thromboembolic events, and mortality. Tranexamic acid reduced the probability of receiving a blood transfusion by a third (risk ratio 0.62, 95%; confidence interval 0.58 to 0.65; $p < 0.001$). The effects of tranexamic acid on myocardial infarction (0.68, 0.43 to 1.09; $p = 0.11$), stroke (1.14, 0.65 to 2.00; $p = 0.65$), deep venous thrombosis (0.86, 0.53 to 1.39; $p = 0.54$), and pulmonary embolism (0.61, 0.25 to 1.47; $p = 0.27$)

were uncertain. Fewer deaths occurred in the tranexamic acid group (0.61, 0.38 to 0.98; $p = 0.04$), although when the analysis was restricted to trials using adequate concealment, there was no statistically significant difference (0.67, 0.33 to 1.34; $p = 0.25$).

TRANEXAMIC ACID IN TRAUMA SURGERY

Emerging therapies in coagulopathy of massive trauma include antifibrinolytic agents. A short review of the coagulopathy of trauma will indicate why it may be an attractive option both in orthopedic trauma and the elective, iatrogenic "trauma" and associated blood loss of elective arthroplasty.

Traditional teaching regarding trauma-related coagulopathy attributed its development to acidosis, hypothermia, and dilution of coagulation factors. Recent data, however, have shown that over one third of injured patients have evidence of coagulopathy at the time of admission. These patients, especially in the first 24 hours after injury, are at a significantly higher risk of mortality. Acute coagulopathy of trauma (ACoT) is a complex problem with multiple mechanisms and not a simple dilutional coagulopathy. Shock and tissue injury are key initiators to the process of ACoT. It is a separate and distinct process from disseminated intravascular coagulation (DIC), with its own specific components of hemostatic failure.

Hypoperfusion causes activation of thrombomodulin (TM) and protein C on the surface of endothelial cells to prevent microthromboembolism. TM binds to thrombin, forming thrombin-TM complexes that limit the availability of thrombin to cleave fibrinogen to fibrin, and induce a hypocoagulable state

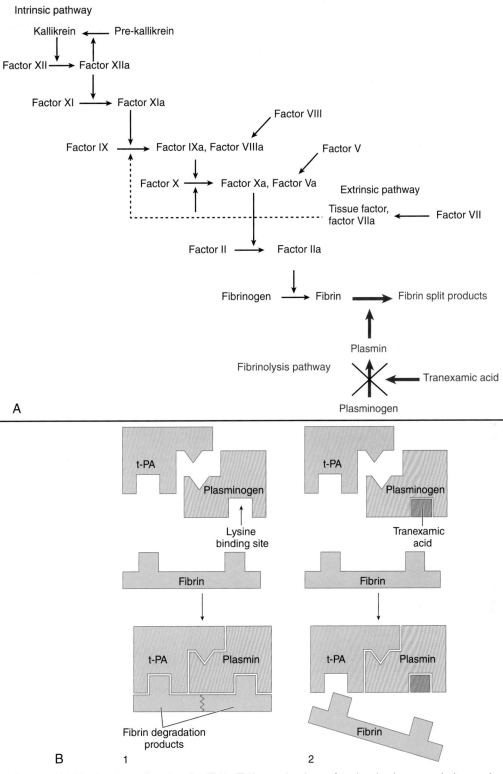

FIG 87.2 (A) Mechanism of action for TXA. TXA mechanism of action in the coagulation pathways. (From Dang PP, Schwarzkopf R: Tranexamic acid and total knee arthroplasty. *Ann Orthop Rheumatol* 1(1):1001, 2013.) (B) Mechanism of competitive inhibition of TXA. (1) Normal activation of the plasminogen and ensuing fibrin degradation. (2) Competitive inhibition of the process in A by TXA. The fibrin binding site on plasminogen is occupied by TXA, preventing fibrinolysis. *FDP,* Fibrin degradation products; *t-PA,* tissue plasminogen activator. (From Santos A-T, Splettstosser JC, Warpechowski P, Gaidzinski MM: Antifibrinolíticos e cirurgia cardíaca com circulação extracorpórea. [Antifibrinolytics and cardiac surgery with cardiopulmonary bypass] *Rev Bras Anestesiol* 57:549–564, 2007 [see Fig. 4].)

through the activation of protein C, which inhibits the extrinsic coagulation pathway by acting on factors V and VIII. However, fibrinolysis is an equally important component as a result of plasmin activity on an existing clot. Activated protein C also inhibits plasminogen activator inhibitor-1 proteins, which increases the tissue plasminogen activator (Fig. 87.3A and B).[5]

The CRASH-2 trial,[36] a randomized control study involving 20,000 trauma patients with or at risk of significant bleeding, found a significantly reduced risk for death from hemorrhage when tranexamic acid therapy (loading dose, 1 g over 10 minutes followed by an infusion of 1 g over 8 hours) was initiated within the first 3 hours following major trauma (Fig. 87.4). Mortality was significantly reduced without an increase in thrombosis or other complications. These results have not only led to the endorsement of tranexamic acid in massive trauma resuscitation guidelines,[43] but also triggered interest and application in other areas of orthopedic surgery such as spine surgery and arthroplasty.

Yuan et al. performed a systematic review regarding the efficacy and safety of antifibrinolytics in spine surgery. They found that antifibrinolytic agents significantly decreased blood loss and the need for transfusion, without an increase of deep venous thrombosis.[50] Another area of concern was that antifibrinolytic agents might decrease the rate of bone fusion. Cuellar et al.[7] found that neither TXA nor aminocaproic acid decreased the rate of fusion compared to saline. A retrospective case control study by Nishihara and Hamada[30] found that the use of TXA did not appear to affect the prevalence of either proximal deep venous thrombosis (DVT) or pulmonary embolism (PE) while increasing the incidence of total DVT on postoperative day 7 compared with the control group; most cases of DVT were isolated distal DVT, with the exception of one patient with proximal DVT in each group. One patient in the control group developed a nonfatal symptomatic PE.

TRANEXAMIC ACID IN TOTAL KNEE ARTHROPLASTY

TXA can have a profound effect on decreasing blood loss in total knee arthroplasty (TKA). One example is the study by Oremus et al.,[32] which found that two doses of TXA 10 mg/kg intravenously (IV) 3 hours apart resulted in a 75.5% decrease for the

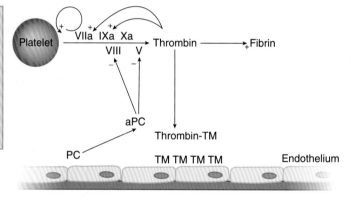

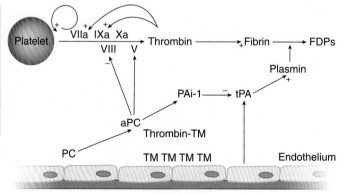

FIG 87.3 Mechanism of Coagulopathy of Trauma and Hyperfibrinolysis. (A) Mechanism of trauma-induced coagulopathy. During periods of tissue hypoperfusion, TM released by the endothelium complexes with thrombin. The thrombin-TM complexes prevent cleavage of fibrinogen to fibrin and also activate PC, reducing further thrombin generation through cofactors V and VIII. (B) Mechanism of hyperfibrinolysis in tissue hypoperfusion. tPA released from the endothelium during hypoperfusion states cleaves plasminogen to initiate fibrinolysis. aPC consumes PAI-1 when present in excess, and reduced PAI-1 leads to increased tPA activity and hyperfibrinolysis. *aPC*, Activated protein C; *FDPs*, fibrin degradation products; *PAI-1* plasminogen activator inhibitor-1; *PC*, protein C; *TM*, thrombomodulin; *tPA*, tissue plasminogen activator. (From Brohi K, Cohen MJ, Davenport RA: Acute coagulopathy of trauma: mechanism, identification and effect. *Curr Opin Crit Care* 13:680–685, 2007 [see Ref. 22].)

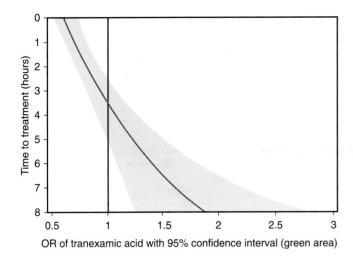

FIG 87.4 Benefits of Tranexamic Acid in Trauma Influence of TXA in preventing death from bleeding. Odds ratios (OR) of TXA with 95% confidence interval *(green area)* on the *x*-axis and time (hours) to treatment on the *y*-axis demonstrate improved survival if TXA therapy is initiated within 3 hours of injury. The area of the curve to the left of OR 1.0 demonstrates the benefits of therapy, while that to the right demonstrates harm from intervention. (From Roberts I, Shakur H, Afolabi A, et al: The importance of early treatment with tranexamic acid in bleeding trauma patients: an exploratory analysis of the CRASH-2 randomised controlled trial. *Lancet* 377:1096, 2011.)

need of transfusion from 85.7% (42/49) to 10.2% of patients, while decreasing the blood loss by an average of 650 mL—320 mL (range, 80 to 930 mL) in the TXA group compared to 970 mL (range, 100 to 2600 mL) in the placebo group ($p < 0.001$).

Hourlier et al.[18] compared the effects of single high dose of TXA (30 mg/kg) compared to a 10 mg/kg loading dose, followed by a continuous infusion of 2 mg/kg per/hour, and observed similar blood loss without any complication in both groups.

Given the adverse effects of tourniquet use, such as local ischemia and postoperative nerve dysfunction, Bidolegui et al.[3] investigated the use of TXA in TKA without tourniquet use, reporting a wide difference, with no transfusions in the treatment group and 32% of transfusion in the control group. The treatment group had higher hematocrit and Hgb level at 24, 48, and 72 hours after surgery (all $p < 0.01$) and lower drain output at 24 hours (363.4 ± 141 vs. 626 ± 260 mL, $p \leq 0.001$).

Poeran et al. performed a retrospective database study with a multivariate regression model use by dose categories (none, ≤1000 mg, 2000 mg, and ≥3000 mg) encompassing 872,614 patients undergoing TKA or THA.[34] TXA administration decreased both the percentage (7.7% vs. 20.2%) as well as the odds for allogeneic or autologous blood transfusions (odds ratio 0.38 [0.35 to 0.42] for ≤1000 mg, 0.38 for ≥2000 mg [0.28 to 0.35]) without significant increase of the risk for thromboembolic complications (odds ratios 0.85 to 1.02), acute renal failure (0.70 to 1.11), and combined complications (0.75 to

0.98) for the respective doses. Huang et al.,[20] in a meta-analysis of 46 trials with 2926 patients undergoing orthopedic surgery, observed that the use of TXA reduced total blood loss by a mean of 408.33 mL (95% confidence interval [CI], −505.69 to −310.77), intraoperative blood loss by a mean of 125.65 mL (95% CI, −182.58 to −68.72), postoperative blood loss by a mean of 214.58 mL (95% CI, −274.63 to −154.52), the number of blood transfusions per patient by 0.78 U (95% CI, −0.19 to −0.37), and the volumes of blood transfusions per patient by 205.33 mL (95% CI, −301.37 to −109.28). TXA led to a significant reduction in transfusion requirements (relative risk, 0.51; 95% CI, 0.46 to 0.56), and no increase in the risk of DVT (relative risk, 1.11; 95% CI, 0.69 to 1.79). Gandhi et al.[11] found a combined weighted mean difference (WMD, referring to the ratio of the differences between the means of the treatment and control groups divided by the standard deviation) of −1.149 for patients undergoing TKA ($p < 0.001$; 95% CI, −1.298, −1.000) (see Fig. 87.3). This indicates that for TKA patients, blood loss was lower in the TXA groups in comparison to the control group at a statistically significant level (Fig. 87.5).

The topical application of TXA has gathered some interest, especially as an alternative to intravenous administration, in order to be able to use it in populations with relative contraindications. Wang et al.[46] performed a meta-analysis investigating topical TXA in total hip arthroplasty and found significant differences in postoperative hemoglobin (Hgb) levels, total blood loss, transfusion requirements, and postoperative drainage volume. Patel et al.[33] compared topical administration of 2 g of TXA versus the IV administration of 10 mg/kg of TXA and showed no significant difference in the primary outcome, perioperative change in Hgb, with a decrease of 3.06 ± 1.02 in the IV group and 3.42 ± 1.07 in the topical group ($p = 0.108$). The study was possibly underpowered with only 89 patients, and may have reached significance in a larger sample.

Another potentially attractive option is the intra-articular application of TXA. Tahmasebi et al.[44] found in a retrospective case control study that intra-articular administration of TXA significantly decreased postoperative blood loss and transfusions. More importantly, Gomez-Barrena et al.[13] compared intra-articular to intravenous application in a randomized controlled trial, and noninferiority was demonstrated for the primary efficacy end point (blood transfusion rate). Noninferiority was also demonstrated for the secondary efficacy end points (visible and invisible blood loss). Soni et al.[42] found no difference in blood loss or Hgb levels when they compared three doses of 10 mg/kg intravenously with 3 g of intra-articular TXA. Lin et al.[25] investigated whether there was a benefit to combining preoperative IV and intraoperative topical administration of TXA in TKA and observed a lower total blood loss in the combined and topical groups (705 mL and 579 mL, respectively) in comparison with the control group (949 mL, $p < 0.001$). There was a significant difference in transfusion rates among groups ($p = 0.009$). The postoperative Hgb decrease and total drain amount were significantly lower in the combined group compared to the other groups.

A meta-analysis by Zhao-Yu et al.[51] showed a significant reduction in total blood loss (mean difference, −344.96 mL; 95% CI, −401.20 to −239.68; $p < 0.01$) and the proportion of patients requiring blood transfusions (risk ratios, 0.28; 95% CI: 0.19 to 0.42; $p < 0.01$) with intra-articular injection of TXA, without significant difference in the incidence of DVT, pulmonary embolism, or other complications among the study groups.

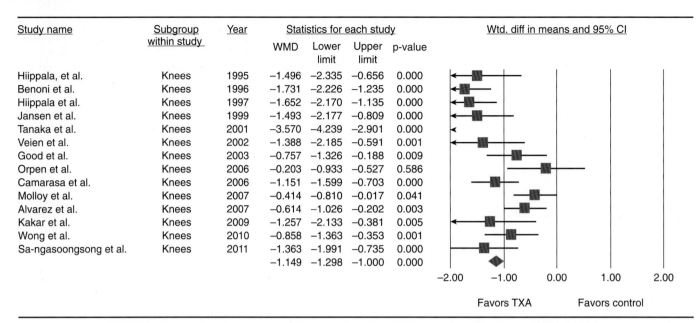

Study name	Subgroup within study	Year	WMD	Lower limit	Upper limit	p-value
Hiippala, et al.	Knees	1995	−1.496	−2.335	−0.656	0.000
Benoni et al.	Knees	1996	−1.731	−2.226	−1.235	0.000
Hiippala et al.	Knees	1997	−1.652	−2.170	−1.135	0.000
Jansen et al.	Knees	1999	−1.493	−2.177	−0.809	0.000
Tanaka et al.	Knees	2001	−3.570	−4.239	−2.901	0.000
Veien et al.	Knees	2002	−1.388	−2.185	−0.591	0.001
Good et al.	Knees	2003	−0.757	−1.326	−0.188	0.009
Orpen et al.	Knees	2006	−0.203	−0.933	−0.527	0.586
Camarasa et al.	Knees	2006	−1.151	−1.599	−0.703	0.000
Molloy et al.	Knees	2007	−0.414	−0.810	−0.017	0.041
Alvarez et al.	Knees	2007	−0.614	−1.026	−0.202	0.003
Kakar et al.	Knees	2009	−1.257	−2.133	−0.381	0.005
Wong et al.	Knees	2010	−0.858	−1.363	−0.353	0.001
Sa-ngasoongsong et al.	Knees	2011	−1.363	−1.991	−0.735	0.000
			−1.149	−1.298	−1.000	0.000

FIG 87.5 Forest plot of a meta-analysis of the benefit of TXA to reduce blood transfusion in TKA. (From Gandhi R, Evans HM, Mahomed SR, Mahomed NN: Tranexamic acid and the reduction of blood loss in total knee and hip arthroplasty: a meta-analysis. *BMC Res Notes* 6:184, 2013.)

Sarzaeem et al.[37] investigated three different methods of TXA administration: intravenous, via the surgical drain, and by irrigation with a solution containing TXA. Intravenous injection of TXA proved to be much more effective in terms of reducing Hgb levels and the need for transfusion, while TXA injection via the drain proved more effective with regard to reducing postoperative drainage.

Aguilera et al.[1] investigated how TXA compared to other hemostatic alternatives such as fibrin glue. In their study, they observed that fibrin glue was no more effective than routine hemostasis in reducing postoperative bleeding and transfusion requirements, while TXA decreased the blood loss by more than 500 mL.

Dahuja et al.[8] looked at role of TXA in reducing postoperative blood loss in TKA and its effect on coagulation profile. While they were unable to demonstrate any effect on the coagulation profile, they found a significant decrease in decline in postoperative Hgb levels with a TXA dose of 15 mg/kg every 8 hours for 24 hours. Longer administration did not result in further reduction in blood loss.

Ultimately, any pharmacological intervention needs to be placed in the context of a comprehensive strategy including preoperative optimization of the Hgb and minimally invasive surgical techniques to minimize blood loss. Moráis et al.[29] described a retrospective analysis of a multimodal blood-loss prevention approach consisting of preoperative Hgb optimization; femoral canal obturation; limited incision and release; peri- and intra-articular use of saline with epinephrine, morphine, tobramycin, betamethasone, and ropivacaine; tourniquet release after skin closure; 24-hour drain under atmospheric pressure; and two doses of intravenous TXA. This strategy resulted in the avoidance of any transfusions, while the matched control group had a transfusion rate of 27.4%.

Duncan et al.[9] found in a large retrospective single-center review with 13,262 elective TKA or THA procedures that neither

the adjusted odds of death (OR = 0.26; 95% CI, 0.04 to 1.80; $p = 0.171$) nor the odds of VTE (OR = 0.98; 95% CI, 0.67 to 1.45; $p = 0.939$) were significantly increased with TXA administration.

DOSING AND TIMING

Benoni et al.[2] found no reduction in postoperative blood loss when TXA was administered at the end of the operation. Whiting et al.,[48] in a retrospective analysis of 2100 primary hip and knee arthroplasty patients, could not identify a preoperative Hgb threshold above which it would no longer be beneficial. Out of the 2100 patients, 1161 (55%) received TXA. Transfusion rates decreased with TXA in all groups; with Hgb > 15, the transfusion rate was 0.5% with TXA and 4.5% without ($p = 0.0086$); with Hgb > 11, the transfusion rate was 4.7% with TXA and 18.7% without ($p < 0.0001$). Patients receiving TXA had a shorter length of stay (LOS) by 0.51 days ($p < 0.0001$), while patients receiving a postoperative transfusion had a longer LOS by 0.69 days ($p < 0.0001$). The authors concluded that TXA should be considered in all arthroplasty patients, independent of their preoperative Hgb level. In a separate study,[49] they also investigated the safety and potential benefits in high-risk patients, defined as presenting at least one of seven risk factors (PE, DVT, myocardial infarction, cerebro-vascular accident, coronary artery bypass graft, coronary artery stent, or prothrombotic condition). They observed no differences in symptomatic thromboembolic events within 30 days of surgery among patients who received TXA and those who did not (2.5% vs. 2.6%, $p = 0.97$). Fewer patients that were treated with TXA received transfusions (11% with vs. 41% without; $p < 0.0001$). In high-risk patients, TXA was not associated with a significant increase in symptomatic thromboembolic events (6.7% with vs. 4.3% without; $p = 0.27$) and was associated with a decrease in transfusion rates (17% with vs. 48% without; $p = 0.001$).

TOWARD A PROTOCOL

Despite the convincing evidence that TXA decreases blood loss without a significant increase of thromboembolic events, morbidity, and mortality, there is no clear consensus on dosing, route, frequency, and duration of the drug. Ker et al.,[24] in their systematic review and meta-analysis of 104 trials, found that TXA reduced blood loss by 34% (pooled ratio 0.66, 95% CI, 0.65 to 0.67; $p < 0.001$). The percentage of reduction in blood loss with TXA differed by type of surgery, timing of TXA administration, and trial quality, but the differences were small. The effect of TXA on blood loss did not vary over the range of doses assessed (5.5 to 300 mg/kg). They concluded that a dose of 1 g of TXA would be sufficient for most adult patients. In the package insert,[19] a dose of 15 mg/kg IV prior to tourniquet release is recommended for TKA and should be repeated every 8 hours for 24 hours for patients without renal disease.

After review of the extensive literature, an initial dose of 1 g or 10 to 20 mg/kg intravenously seems to be the most appropriate dosing in the authors' opinion. It may be beneficial to redose 3 hours after the initial dose and following deflation of the tourniquet; and then every 8 hours for another two doses postoperatively, for a total of four doses. Despite its relative safety, it is prudent to be vigilant about exclusion criteria and relative contraindications to minimize the potential risks with the administration of TXA.

KEY REFERENCES

6. Cap AP, Baer DG, Orman JA, et al: Tranexamic acid for trauma patients: a critical review of the literature. *J Trauma* 71(Suppl 1):S9–S14, 2011.

8. Dahuja A, Dahuja G, Jaswal V, et al: A prospective study on role of tranexamic acid in reducing postoperative blood loss in total knee arthroplasty and its effect on coagulation profile. *J Arthroplasty* 29(4):733–735, 2014.

9. Duncan CM, Gillette BP, Jacob AK, et al: Venous thromboembolism and mortality associated with tranexamic acid use during total hip and knee arthroplasty. *J Arthroplasty* 30(2):272–276, 2015.

11. Gandhi R, Evans HM, Mahomed SR, et al: Tranexamic acid and the reduction of blood loss in total knee and hip arthroplasty: a meta-analysis. *BMC Res Notes* 6:184, 2013. doi: 10.1186/1756-0500-6-184.

13. Gomez-Barrena E, Ortega-Andreu M, Padilla-Eguiluz NG, et al: Topical intra-articular compared with intravenous tranexamic acid to reduce blood loss in primary total knee replacement: a double-blind, randomized, controlled, noninferiority clinical trial. *J Bone Joint Surg Am* 96(23):1937–1944, 2014.

18. Hourlier H, Reina N, Fennema P: Single dose intravenous tranexamic acid as effective as continuous infusion in primary total knee arthroplasty: a randomised clinical trial. *Arch Orthop Trauma Surg* 135(4):465–471, 2015.

21. Ipema HJ, Tanzi MG: Use of topical tranexamic acid or aminocaproic acid to prevent bleeding after major surgical procedures. *Ann Pharmacother* 46(1):97–107, 2012.

24. Ker K, Prieto-Merino D, Roberts I: Systematic review, meta-analysis and meta-regression of the effect of tranexamic acid on surgical blood loss. *Br J Surg* 100(10):1271–1279, 2013.

29. Moráis S, Ortega-Andreu M, Rodríguez-Merchán EC, et al: Blood transfusion after primary total knee arthroplasty can be significantly minimised through a multimodal blood-loss prevention approach. *Int Orthop* 38(2):347–354, 2014.

30. Nishihara S, Hamada M: Does tranexamic acid alter the risk of thromboembolism after total hip arthroplasty in the absence of routine chemical thromboprophylaxis? *Bone Joint J* 97-B(4):458–462, 2015.

34. Poeran J, Rasul R, Suzuki S, et al: Tranexamic acid use and postoperative outcomes in patients undergoing total hip or knee arthroplasty in the United States: retrospective analysis of effectiveness and safety. *BMJ* 349:g4829, 2014.

37. Sarzaeem MM, Razi M, Kazemian G, et al: Comparing efficacy of three methods of tranexamic acid administration in reducing hemoglobin drop following total knee arthroplasty. *J Arthroplasty* 29(8):1521–1524, 2014.

48. Whiting DR, Duncan CM, Sierra RJ, et al: Tranexamic acid benefits total joint arthroplasty patients regardless of preoperative hemoglobin value. *J Arthroplasty* 30(12):2098–2101, 2015.

49. Whiting DR, Gillette BP, Duncan C, et al: Preliminary results suggest tranexamic acid is safe and effective in arthroplasty patients with severe comorbidities. *Clin Orthop Relat Res* 472(1):66–72, 2014.

The references for this chapter can also be found on www.expertconsult.com.

Blood Loss and Fluid Management

Sanford M. Littwin, Alopi Patel

A basic understanding of blood and fluid management is necessary for every surgeon and anesthesiologist taking care of surgical patients. Most perioperative fluid management is coordinated by the anesthesia providers; however, understanding the rationale for varying fluid management strategies depending on the patient's physiologic requirements is key to the continued care of the surgical patient postoperatively. The surgical care team should understand what fluid management and blood therapy might have taken place during the preoperative and intraoperative period. This is especially true when dealing with patients whose physiologic reserves are not normal, based on other disease processes like diabetes, hypertension, chronic renal insufficiency, or who have had marked pathologic changes in the intraoperative period because of blood loss.

BLOOD AND FLUID LOSS

Surgical fluid losses involve blood or body fluids. Blood loss is a difficult but important task for both the surgical and anesthesiology teams to determine and monitor. Two-way communication between surgeons and anesthesiologists regarding blood losses is vital intraoperatively to guide fluid management and transfusions. Common methods for estimating blood loss are visualization of the suction canister volume, surgical sponges, and laparotomy pads. A fully soaked 4 × 4 sponge is estimated to hold 10 mL of blood. A fully soaked "lap pad" holds about 100 to 150 mL of blood.[5] Estimation of the blood in the suction canisters should take into account the surgical irrigation fluid used.

Blood loss can be replaced with crystalloids, colloids, and/or blood transfusions. The decision to transfuse should take into account the risks and benefits of transfusions. The transfusion threshold may vary from patient to patient depending on the clinical scenario and patient history. The key factor to consider is the patient's physiology and preexisting medical conditions. Particular attention must be paid to cardiac reserve and myocardial performance.

Generally, when the hemoglobin concentration drops below 7 g/dL, the cardiac output must increase to maintain normal oxygen delivery. An even higher hemoglobin concentration (eg, 10 g/dL) may be required for a patient with cardiopulmonary disease, especially coronary artery disease.[6] In normal operative settings, anesthesiologists administer crystalloids (eg, lactated Ringer's solution) at approximately 3 to 4 times the volume of blood lost (taking into account the fact that only a portion of the administered crystalloids remains in the intravascular space) or a colloid at a 1:1 ratio, until transfusion risks and benefits have been assessed.[2] When a transfusion is required, blood is most often replaced in a 1:1 ratio of loss to administration with red blood cells (RBCs).

The amount of blood loss needed for the hematocrit to fall below a predetermined threshold (ie, 21% or 30%) is referred to as the "allowable blood loss." This takes into consideration the estimated blood volume for the patient based on their weight. An adult is estimated to have an average blood volume of 70 mL/kg. The following equation is used to calculate the allowable blood loss, where H_i is initial hematocrit and H_f is lowest allowable hematocrit.

$$\text{Allowable blood loss} = [EBV(H_i - H_f)]/H_i$$

Example: An 80-kg man with a preoperative hematocrit of 30% presents for total knee replacement. What is the allowable blood loss for an allowable hematocrit of 21%?[5]

$$\text{Estimated blood volume: } 80\,kg \times 70\,mL/kg = 5600\,mL$$

where H_i is 30% and H_f is 21%.
[5600(30% − 21%)]/30% = 1680 mL allowable blood loss for a minimum hematocrit of 21%.

Of note, clinical guidelines suggest that one unit of RBC (typically about 300 mL with a hematocrit of about 70%) will increase hemoglobin concentration by 1 g/dL and hematocrit by 2% to 3% in average-sized adults.

Fluid Maintenance and Replacement Strategies

Perioperative fluid management includes replacement of preexisting fluid deficits, maintenance requirements, and surgical fluid (ie, body fluids and blood loss).

Preexisting fluid deficits occur from preoperative fasting. The deficit is usually estimated by multiplying the normal maintenance rate, from the common fluid deficit ratio rule (4:2:1 rule), by the duration of the fast. For the first 10 kg of body weight, replace 4 mL/kg/hour; for the next 10 kg, add 2 mL/kg/hour; for each kg above 20 kg, add 1 mL/kg/hour.[20] Usual minimum fasting time is 8 hours. Other preexisting deficits to consider are preoperative bleeding, vomiting, urination, and diarrhea, and occult losses from infected tissue, ascites, and sweating.

Normal maintenance fluid requirements are based on weight, taking into consideration ongoing losses from urine formation, gastrointestinal secretions, sweating, and insensible losses from the skin and lungs. This is also replaced generally by the 4:2:1 rule, which can be applied to both pediatric and adult patients.

BLOOD AND FLUID MANAGEMENT

Volume Assessment

Intravascular volume can be clinically assessed by patient history, physical examination, and laboratory results.

Patient history is useful in the volume assessment of medical conditions such as hypertension, chronic renal insufficiency, and congestive heart failure. Preoperative medical optimization of patients with such systemic illnesses is crucial. These conditions should also be kept in mind when managing intraoperative fluid administration or correcting for fluid deficits.[5,15,16]

Information such as oral intake, vomiting, diarrhea, nasogastric tube losses, blood loss, wound drainage, and hemodialysis are important factors in determining volume status and appropriate resuscitation.

Physical examination markers of hydration or intravascular volume status can be subtle, such as skin turgor, or more pronounced, like the appearance of anasarca. Further signs of decreased intravascular volume include thready peripheral pulses, tachycardia, hypotension, orthostatic changes, and decreased urine output (Table 88.1). Some of these clinical indicators may not be as reliable intraoperatively because of physiologic changes that occur from anesthesia.[5] Of note, pitting edema, whether presacral edema in bedridden patients or pretibial edema in ambulatory surgery patients, are signs of increased extracellular fluid and possibly hypervolemia. Extreme signs of hypervolemia, such as in congestive heart failure, include tachycardia, increased jugular venous pressure, pulmonary crackles, and frothy pulmonary secretions.

Finally, although laboratory evaluation is important, it is perhaps the least accurate under most circumstances. Basic laboratory panels such as a complete blood count or basic chemistry profile change little with moderate volume changes. However, subtle indications of low intravascular volume may be seen such as increased blood urea nitrogen (BUN)-to-creatinine ratio, or a markedly low hemoglobin (Hg) or hematocrit (Hct). Indicators of dehydration include serially increasing hematocrit and hemoglobin, metabolic acidosis (including lactic acidosis), urinary specific gravity greater than 1.010, urinary sodium less than 10 mEq/L, urinary osmolality greater than 450 mOsm/L, hypernatremia, and BUN-to-creatinine ratio greater than 20:1. Radiologic indicators of volume over-load can include increased pulmonary vascular and interstitial markings and diffuse alveolar infiltrates.

Regular comprehensive assessments of intravascular volume status must be made to assure appropriate fluid resuscitation beginning with the preoperative assessment, intraoperative management, and postoperative maintenance.

Intravenous Fluids

Intravenous fluid therapy includes infusion of crystalloids and/or colloids.[2,5,6] Crystalloid solutions are aqueous solutions of ions, which may contain glucose in the form of lactate or dextrose, and redistribute through the extracellular space. Colloids are high-molecular-weight substances that maintain oncotic pressure within the intravascular space. In the ongoing debate regarding the use of crystalloids versus colloids in surgical patients,[5] there is some consensus: crystalloids, when given in sufficient amounts, are just as effective as colloids in replacing intravascular volume; replacing intravascular volume with crystalloids requires three to four times the volume of colloids; severe fluid deficits can be rapidly corrected with colloids; and large amounts of crystalloids (>4 to 5 L) can cause tissue edema.

Crystalloids can be administered in *hypotonic, isotonic,* or *hypertonic solutions. Hypotonic* solutions are used for replacement of water losses in diabetic ketoacidosis. Of note, D5W is considered hypotonic, as the glucose is rapidly consumed and only the water remains. *Hypertonic* solutions (3% saline) can be used for treatment of severe hyponatremia, increased intracranial fibrosis or cystic fibrosis, or rapid volume resuscitation in the trauma setting (as fluid will be pulled out of the extravascular space). *Isotonic* solutions are the mainstay of replacement fluids in the hospital setting, and are used for replacement of both water and electrolyte losses. They are primarily used for maintenance and management of fluid losses perioperatively. Glucose may be added to some solutions, such as lactated Ringer's solution for tonicity and prevention of hypoglycemia. The lactate in lactated Ringer's solution is converted to bicarbonate in the liver, causing lactated Ringer's solution to have a mildly alkalinizing effect. The next commonly used isotonic solution is normal saline, which is 0.9% sodium chloride. Contrary to lactated Ringer's solution, when given in large volumes, normal saline can produce hyperchloremic acidosis.

Colloid solutions differ from crystalloid solutions in their extended intravascular half-life, which is usually between 3 and 6 hours.[1] Although there is still debate regarding colloid use, it is generally accepted that colloids should be used for fluid resuscitation in patients with severe volume deficits (eg, hemorrhagic shock) and for patients with severe hypoalbuminemia or other conditions with protein losses (eg, burns). Some studies also suggest that crystalloids be used intraoperatively for maintenance of fluid requirements and that colloids be used for replacement of blood loss on a milliliter-to-milliliter basis. Colloids are generally derived from human plasma proteins or synthetic glucose polymers.[3] Synthetic colloids, such as hetastarch and dextran, improve intravascular volume, but if given in large volumes, also decrease blood viscosity, leading to coagulopathy.[19] Colloids may increase the risk of renal failure. Dextran has been associated with anaphylactoid and anaphylactic reactions.

Blood Products

Possible administration of blood products during the perioperative period should be anticipated based on patient

TABLE 88.1	Signs of Hypovolemic Shock		
Signs	**5% Loss**	**10% Loss**	**15% Loss**
Mucous membranes	Dry	Very dry	Parched
Mental status	Normal	Lethargic	Obtunded
Orthostatic changes	None	Present	Marked
Urine output	Mild decrease	Decreased	Markedly decreased
Blood pressure	Normal	Mild decrease with respiratory variation	Decreased
Heart rate	Normal or increased	Increased (heart rate > 100)	Marked increase (heart rate > 120)

Butterworth JF, IV, Mackey DC, Wasnick JD: Fluid management & blood component therapy. In Butterworth JF, IV, Mackey DC, Wasnick JD (eds): *Morgan & Mikhail's Clinical Anesthesiology*, 5e, New York, 2013, McGraw-Hill, chapter 51.

comorbidities and type of operation. The surgical team should order appropriate laboratory work prior to the perioperative period based on these factors.

A *type and screen* is ordered to detect the presence of common antibodies associated with nonhemolytic reactions.[12] This test takes approximately 45 minutes and is routinely done when there is a potential need for blood products. A *type and cross* is ordered to confirm the ABO status of the patient and to detect common and uncommon antibodies. This test may take 2 hours and is routinely ordered in patients when there is a high potential for receiving blood products. A type and cross should be ordered prior the perioperative period when there is a high possibility of needing blood products.

RBCs are typically given in the perioperative period to patients who require volume expansion or replacement as well as red cells for oxygen supply.[6-9] Each unit is approximately 300 mL and estimated to increase hemoglobin concentration by 1 g/dL and hematocrit by 2% to 3%. RBCs are frozen for storage and for intraoperative transfusion are warmed to 37°C; transfusion of large amounts of cold blood may lead to profound hypothermia. As with administration of any blood component therapy, RBCs have risks and benefits. Risks include hemolytic reactions, febrile reactions, anaphylaxis, lung injury, graft-versus-host disease, infectious complications, and coagulopathies.

Fresh frozen plasma (FFP) contains plasma proteins including most clotting factors.[5,15] FFP can be administered for clotting factor deficiencies, warfarin reversal, and coagulopathy correction. Each unit of FFP generally increases each clotting factor by 2% to 3%. Once again, risks include infections complications, immune reactions, and exacerbation of coagulopathies.

Cryoprecipitate is another blood component therapy prepared from FFP consisting of fibrinogen, Factor XII, von Willebrand factor, and Factor XIII. It is given for hemophilia, von Willebrand disease, hypofibrinogenemia, disseminated intravascular coagulation (DIC), or massive hemorrhage. It is also costly and thus not a viable means of volume expansion.

Platelet transfusions are given to patients with thrombocytopenia or dysfunctional platelets. They may be given prophylactically or therapeutically. Prophylactic platelet transfusions are indicated in patients requiring major surgery and having a platelet count of less than $50,000 \times 10^9/L$. One unit of platelets is expected to increase the platelet count by 5000 to $10,000 \times 10^9/L$.

SUMMARY

It is important for the perioperative surgical team to be aware of blood loss and fluid management during the perioperative period. Communication between anesthesiology and surgical teams is key for the proper continuation of fluid management. The type of fluids and the need for blood replacement is vital to maintaining smooth hemodynamics in the surgical patient.

KEY REFERENCES

2. Arunachalam L, Macfie J: Colloid versus crystalloid fluid therapy in surgical patients. *Br J Surg* 102(3):145–147, 2014.
5. Butterworth JF, IV, Mackey DC, Wasnick JD: Fluid management & blood component therapy, In Butterworth JF, IV, Mackey DC, Wasnick JD, editors. *Morgan & Mikhail's clinical anesthesiology*, ed 5, New York, 2013, McGraw-Hill, chapter 51.
11. Hiltebrand LB, Kimberger O, Arnberger M, et al: Crystalloids versus colloids for goal-directed fluid therapy in major surgery. *Crit Care* 13:R40, 2009.
15. Liumbruno GM, Bennardello F, Lattanzio A, et al: Recommendations for the transfusion management of patients in the peri-operative period. II. The intra-operative period. *Blood Transfus* 9(2):189–217, 2011.
16. Mythen MG, Swart M, Acheson N, et al: Perioperative fluid management: consensus statement from the enhanced recovery partnership. *Perioper Med* 1:2, 2012.

The references for this chapter can also be found on www.expertconsult.com.

89

Anesthesia for Knee Surgery

Sanford M. Littwin, Neda Sadeghi

Surgery has inherent risk. The decision to proceed with surgery is a balance between the need for the operative procedure and the risks that accompany it. These risks and benefits must be weighed when determining need and timing of operative intervention. As the general population and average life span increase, orthopedic operative procedures are becoming more commonplace. It is interesting to note that compared to a few decades ago, surgical patients have more preoperative comorbidities with a corresponding increase in the incidence of major postoperative complications.[5] After knee surgery specifically, postoperative medical complications can include cardiac complications, hemorrhage or hematoma, infection, thromboembolism, peripheral nerve injury, anesthetic complications, and muscle atrophy. Overall, the incidence of postoperative complications increases with laterality (bilateral more than unilateral), advanced age, body mass index (BMI), American Society of Anesthesiologists (ASA) score, and preexisting pulmonary disease.[13,14]

Optimizing a patient's medical condition before surgery decreases the risk of postoperative medical complications. However, the time frame needed for preoperative optimization is not always practical given the timing of urgent/emergent operations. It is important to bear in mind the preoperative care of a patient when evaluating his or her postoperative status.

Cardiac complications are relatively frequent in the orthopedic population, and the overall incidence is about 0.5% in patients undergoing total knee arthroplasty (TKA).[3] These complications can include myocardial infarction, congestive heart failure, and arrhythmias requiring treatment. The primary pathophysiologic issues underlying cardiac complications are the mismatch between myocardial oxygen supply and demand, problems with the determinants of ventricular performance (preload, afterload, contractility), and cardiac arrhythmias. Thus, it is important to optimize a patient's cardiac status to avoid postoperative cardiac complications.

The overall incidence of a hemorrhage or hematoma in patients undergoing TKA is approximately 0.9% to 2.1% (Huddleston).[3] Hemorrhage/hematoma is defined by continued or increased bleeding at the surgical site that necessitates further medical or surgical intervention. Preoperative medical issues such as coagulopathy and platelet dysfunction can further complicate the bleeding risk. Postoperative hemorrhage/hematoma is a complication that occurs less often after a primary TKA than after a TKA revision and is often this is linked to the length of surgery and the complexity of the surgical revision. The decision to transfuse is multifactorial and is discussed in the prior section.

Acute or early infection is another postop complication that occurs in 0.4% to 0.8% of patients undergoing primary TKA and occurs at a much higher rate in patients undergoing a TKA revision.[8,15] Infection can manifest acutely or can be an indolent process that worsens over time. Signs of infection include fever, an inflamed joint, elevated white blood count (WBC), and elevated synovial WBC. The erythrocyte sedimentation rate/C-reactive protein (ESR/CRP) is always elevated postoperatively and is thus only reliable for late infections. Perioperative precautions such as maintaining sterility and appropriate use of antibiotics help decrease the risk of postoperative infections.

Venous thromboembolism (VTE) can encompass anything from an uncomplicated deep venous thrombosis (DVT) to a life-threatening pulmonary embolism (PE). VTE can occur in up to 84% of patients having a total joint replacement.[7] However, the 3-month incidence of a clinically significant VTE after total knee replacement is 1.79% and the incidence of a fatal PE is 0.15% to 0.41%%.[2,15] The pathophysiology of VTE is because of the triad of causes proposed by Virchow in 1856: stasis, hypercoagulability, and endothelial dysfunction. Encouraging early mobility and proper use of venous thrombus prophylaxis are key factors in preventing VTE.

The overall incidence of permanent peripheral nerve injury is 0.03% to 0.05%, and increases dramatically after TKA to almost 10%.[4] Nerve injury can manifest as paresthesia, numbness, pain, and/or weakness. Peripheral nerve injury can be related to a patient's preexisting deformities or neurologic deficits, underlying disease states (such as rheumatoid arthritis or diabetes), patient positioning, prolonged tourniquet time, type of surgery, tight surgical dressing, and regional anesthesia. Regional anesthesia is commonly blamed for postoperative nerve injury in the postoperative period, but very rarely causes permanent nerve injury. The risk of transient nerve injury is relatively common in the immediate postoperative period, with up to 20% of patients reporting symptoms of nerve injury.[16] These symptoms usually resolve within the first week. By 4 to 6 weeks, the incidence of nerve injury is less than 5% to 8%, and by one year, the incidence of peripheral nerve injury from regional anesthesia is less than 1%.[1,16] Patients who received a peripheral nerve block and were found to have a postoperative peripheral nerve injury were less likely to recover completely.[4] Postoperative nerve complications should be managed in conjunction with the surgeon, anesthesiologist, and pain management consultant. Regional anesthesia is often employed as a technique to minimize or prevent the use of general anesthesia or neuraxial anesthesia. Depending on the patient's preoperative medical problems, avoidance of general anesthesia and even sometimes neuraxial anesthesia may be of great benefit.

Anesthetic complications include sore throat, nausea, fatigue, delirium, and postoperative cognitive dysfunction (POCD). The incidence of delirium after orthopedic procedures ranges from 21% to 63% of patients undergoing knee or hip replacement.[9,18] POCD has been reported in patients undergoing noncardiac surgery at rates of up to 26% after one week and up to 10% after 3 months.[10] The predictors of POCD are advanced age and lower education levels.[11] This unfortunate phenomenon can be extremely unsettling for patients and their families. The best treatment for POCD is still unclear, but most clinicians agree that frequent reorientation, adequate pain control, and early rehabilitation may be helpful measures (Wang). Regional anesthesia, or the avoidance of general anesthesia, might protect against POCD, but this is not currently supported by evidence.[12]

Fatigue and muscle atrophy are particularly frustrating complications because they create a damaging cycle that forms a barrier to physical therapy. The fatigue can be caused by anemia, malnutrition, or drugs (ie, opiates, anxiolytics, and muscle relaxants). Skeletal muscle atrophy is extremely common after orthopedic surgery and is because of the disuse of a muscle group for an extended period of time with subsequent loss of muscle mass. This atrophy begins after a few days of disuse, and the severity is related to the duration of disuse. This muscle breakdown is particularly pronounced in the lower extremities and happens much sooner in the elderly.[6] Early rehabilitation, physical therapy, and adequate nutrition are important in regaining energy and strength in the postoperative period.

Medical complications are part and parcel of any surgical specialty, and present in somewhat unique ways specifically following orthopedic operations such as TKA. Prevention is best achieved by knowledge of the risk factors for the patient undergoing surgery, early intervention should a suspected complication arise, and a high degree of vigilance by both the surgical and anesthesia teams taking care of the patient.

The references for this chapter can also be found on www.expertconsult.com.

90

Specific Considerations for Fractures and Dislocations

Chan-Nyein Maung, Milad Nazemzadeh

INTRODUCTION

Fractures involving the knee can be considered surgical emergencies depending on the acuity and severity of the injury, and the neurovascular structures involved. The anesthetic considerations for fractures are similar to situations involving any major trauma. Although this section solely concentrates on knee fractures, patients with these injuries may also be involved in polytrauma situations, and as such, trauma resuscitative protocols should be followed.

Fractures of the knee are worrisome because of the close proximity of nerves and vessels in and around the joint. The sciatic nerve continues as the popliteal nerve travels in the posterior thigh, eventually branching into the tibial and common peroneal nerves about 6 cm above the popliteal fossa. The tibial nerve continues in the posterior leg, eventually forming numerous branches to innervate the foot. Of interest in fractures, the common peroneal nerve winds around the head and neck of the fibula where it can be injured. The popliteal artery is the deep continuation of the femoral artery where it courses posteriorly in the thigh and through the popliteal fossa, eventually branching out into the anterior and posterior tibial arteries. If a major arterial injury occurs, a patient can present with pallor, cool skin, and decreased pulses in the affected extremity. The patient may also present with an expanding hematoma or massive hemorrhage. The most common knee emergencies include fractures of the distal femur or femoral condyles, tibial plateau, and patella. The head of the fibula can also be fractured, but can usually be treated nonsurgically. However, if the peroneal nerve is injured (ie, the patient develops a footdrop soon after the injury), the fracture must be repaired surgically. Patella fractures are relatively rare and account for 1% of all fractures. Nevertheless, any open, comminuted, or displaced patella fracture requires immediate surgery.[16]

ANESTHETIC CONSIDERATIONS

Knee fractures can present to the orthopedic and anesthesiology teams in a wide variety of situations. The injury can present as an isolated accident, part of a polytrauma scenario, and can also present in elective, urgent, or emergent surgical settings.

Resuscitation: For any trauma patient, the ABCs (airway, breathing, circulation) should be followed. These patients are assessed for resuscitation early by paramedics in the field or by the emergency medicine team in the trauma bay. In a polytrauma situation in which the patient is hemodynamically unstable because of the severity of injuries or requires airway protection, the patient should be emergently intubated with cervical spine precautions. Large-bore IVs (18 g, 16 g, or 14 g) should be placed. If massive resuscitation is anticipated, central and arterial lines should be placed as well. In such a situation, resuscitation should consist of crystalloids, colloids, and blood products.[2]

For many decades, there has been tremendous debate over the use of crystalloids versus colloids for resuscitation. The 2013 multicentered, randomized CRISTAL trial (nonblinded) involving critically ill patients (sepsis, trauma, and hypovolemic shock without trauma or sepsis) concluded that there was no significant difference in 28-day mortality. In addition, the 90-day mortality seemed to be lower in those who received colloids, although this mortality benefit should be interpreted cautiously. The side effects of colloids (especially renal injury) must be considered. Certain shock states cause endothelial leaking with extravasation of protein and other large molecules (including the molecules in colloids), which means that the use of colloids could potentially cause even more hypovolemia and edema because of changes in oncotic pressure.[1,12] Debates aside, in modern trauma situations, the use of fluid resuscitation has decreased because of the shift to early blood product administration. In massive transfusion situations, a balanced transfusion approach involving a 1:1:1 ratio of red blood cells, fresh frozen plasma, and platelets is used to replicate whole blood, but this can result in a pancytopenic solution. However, in practical transfusion situations, red blood cells usually arrive to the operating room first, followed by platelets, plasma, or factors. The anesthesiology and trauma teams must be mindful of the need for early activation of the massive transfusion protocol because this approach can improve survival, reduce total blood product use in the first 24 hours, and decrease the incidence of multiorgan failure.[6]

ANESTHETIC TECHNIQUE

The choice of anesthesia for knee fractures can vary depending on the surgical setting. In a polytrauma situation where surgery is required at multiple sites, general endotracheal anesthesia is the best choice because of its rapid onset, ability to provide airway protection, reliable unconsciousness for any duration, and muscle relaxation. With time constraints and the likelihood of coagulopathy in trauma patients, the performance of an epidural, spinal, or peripheral nerve block may not be feasible because of the gravity of the situation. However, with general anesthesia, the inherent vasodilating properties of the anesthetic agents can make hemodynamic management more challenging, especially if major hemorrhage is involved.[3] If the knee fracture is an isolated injury, neuraxial anesthesia is definitely an option. A spinal block has a quick onset and can provide reliable surgical and tourniquet anesthesia. With bupivacaine, the most common local anesthetic used for spinals, the block can last 1.5 to 2 hours, or even longer if adjuvants are used. An epidural can also be used, although its onset is slightly longer than a spinal. An epidural catheter can be used for redosing if the block appears to be wearing off in longer surgeries, whereas the spinal is usually a single-shot block. An epidural catheter can also be used for postoperative analgesia. Neuraxial anesthesia can cause hypotension, especially with spinals, which may limit its use in situations where vessel damage is involved in the knee fracture. Peripheral nerve blocks are probably best used as adjuvants to general or neuraxial anesthesia. If peripheral nerve blocks are used as the sole anesthetic technique, the number of nerve blocks needed for surgical and tourniquet anesthesia could be too time consuming and may not provide the necessary effects if any one of the blocks fails. The saphenous nerve block ("adductor canal" block) can provide postoperative analgesia without causing quadriceps muscle weakness, which would facilitate early ambulation.[4] Finally, multimodal analgesia, both perioperatively and postoperatively, is encouraged.

COMPARTMENT SYNDROME

Acute compartment syndrome occurs when there is increased pressure within a finite amount of space, compromising neurovascular structures. Tibial and forearm fractures are the most common long bone injuries associated with compartment syndrome, and edema because of muscle injury and hematoma formation are the most common causes.[11] The use of regional anesthesia in surgeries involving fractures is of interest to anesthesiologists and orthopedic surgeons. Neuraxial anesthesia and peripheral nerve blocks have been thought to mask the symptoms of compartment syndrome, but this is a highly controversial issue. Recently, there has been growing evidence that ischemic pain in acute compartment syndrome is not truly affected by regional anesthesia. Kucera and Boezaart presented several case reports where the patient's ischemic pain was apparent despite regional anesthesia for upper and lower extremity orthopedic surgery.[9] Recent evidence also supports the hypothesis that peripheral nerve blocks do not eliminate the pain perception because of ischemia, and that nociceptive activation follows a sympathetic pathway that is not blocked by perineural blockade.[5,15] These symptoms can also be masked by an altered level of consciousness, deep sedation, or large doses of pain medications. Therefore, sedatives, analgesics, and regional anesthesia should be used judiciously. A high index of suspicion coupled with the performance of serial examinations can allow for early detection of this limb-threatening diagnosis.

FAT EMBOLISM SYNDROME

This is an important topic because tibia and distal femur injuries can occur in knee fractures. Fat embolism syndrome usually presents within 72 hours after long-bone or pelvic fractures. Its exact mechanism has not been elucidated, but one hypothesis is that fat globules are released when the fat cells in the fractured bone are disrupted and enter the blood stream. The classic presentation includes dyspnea, confusion, and petechiae. The increased free fatty acid levels cause disruption at the capillary-alveolar membrane, leading to release of vasoactive substances. This can subsequently cause acute respiratory distress syndrome (ARDS). At the level of the brain, the free fatty acids damage the capillaries of the cerebral circulation, leading to agitation, confusion, stupor, or even coma. The fat globules also damage the capillaries in the conjunctiva, skin of the chest, upper extremities, and axillae, forming petechiae in the mentioned areas. Furthermore, coagulation abnormalities (thrombocytopenia, prolonged clotting times) can be present. If a patient is under general anesthesia, a decrease in end tidal CO_2 and arterial PO_2, along with an increase in pulmonary artery pressures can be suggestive of this syndrome. The electrocardiogram may also show ST changes and right-sided heart strain. The best management is prevention, but if a patient develops the syndrome, supportive treatment is indicated. Supportive treatment includes supplemental oxygen therapy, the ARDS protocol such as low lung volume and high positive pressure mechanical ventilation, and possible blood pressure support. Finally, although fat embolism syndrome is uncommon, it can be fatal with a 10% to 20% mortality.[7,10,14]

DEEP VENOUS THROMBOSIS AND THROMBOEMBOLISM

Deep venous thrombosis (DVT) and pulmonary embolism (PE) can occur in patients undergoing pelvic and lower extremity orthopedic surgeries. Risk factors include lower extremity fractures, immobilization for more than 4 days, obesity, age greater than 60 years, a procedure with duration longer than 30 minutes, and tourniquet use. Hip surgery, knee replacement, and major lower extremity surgery after trauma present the greatest risks; DVT rates can reach 80% in these patients if prophylaxis is not used. The mechanism is thought to be because of venous stasis that results in a hypercoagulable state, which is secondary to localized and systemic inflammatory responses from surgery. Prophylaxis is the best method of DVT and PE prevention, as pharmacological agents and routine use of mechanical devices (intermittent pneumatic compression) can decrease the incidence.[8,13] Refer to the "Thromboprophylaxis and Neuraxial Anesthesia" section regarding bleeding risks and neuraxial anesthesia.

The references for this chapter can also be found on www.expertconsult.com.

Note: Page numbers followed by "f" refer to illustrations; page numbers followed by "t" refer to tables; page numbers followed by "b" refer to boxes.

Osteochondral allograft transplantation
  (*Continued*)
  deep venous thrombosis prophylaxis after,
    448
  delayed union after, 452
  description of, 442
  disadvantages of, 453
  exposure technique for, 445–446
  failed cartilage repair after, 462, 465*f*
  graft fragmentation after, 452
  HIV testing, 444
  indications for, 443–444
  infection concerns
    graft transmission, 444
    postoperative, 452
  nonunion after, 452
  osseous component of, 443
  osteochondral lesions treated with, 443
  osteochondritis dissecans lesions treated with,
    409–410
  persistent pain after, 452
  postoperative management, 448–450
  preoperative planning of, 444
  press-fit plug technique for, 446–448,
    446*f*–450*f*
  procurement of, 444
  rehabilitation after, 448–450
  results of, 450–452, 450*f*
  science of, 442–443
  screening of, 444
  shell technique for, 446, 448, 450*f*
  storage of, 444
  surgical techniques for, 444–448, 446*f*–450*f*
  weight-bearing after, 449
Osteochondral autograft plug transfer
  arthroscopic views after, 437*f*
  autologous chondrocyte implantation versus,
    434
  complications of, 432
  contact pressures, 430, 430*f*
  definition of, 427
  description of, 427
  donor site morbidity concerns, 432, 441
  fill pattern, 430–431, 430*f*
  fixation of plugs, 431
  future directions for, 439–440
  harvesting of, 431–432
  indications for, 427–428
  insertion of
    depth for, 431
    description of, 431
    press-fit technique, 431
  juvenile osteochondritis dissecans treated
    with, 1259–1260
  limitations of, 441
  osteochondritis dissecans treated with,
    408–409
  pearls and pitfalls of, 432
  postoperative regimen, 432
  results of
    description of, 432–436, 433*t*–436*t*,
      437*f*–438*f*
    gross morphology and histology, 436,
      437*f*–438*f*
    magnetic resonance imaging evaluations,
      436–439, 439*f*
  summary of, 440–441
  technical considerations for, 428–432
  topographic analysis before, 428–430,
    428*f*–429*f*
Osteochondral autograft transplantation,
  473–474
Osteochondral fractures
  diagnosis of, 116
  impaction, 118*f*
  magnetic resonance imaging staging of,
    403*t*
  stellate fractures and, 121–122

Osteochondral injuries
  classification of, 192*t*
  impaction-related, 193*f*
  lateral patellar dislocation and, 229–231
  magnetic resonance imaging of, 189,
    191*f*–192*f*
  traumatic, 190–191
Osteochondral lesions
  definition of, 192
  hinged, 405
  magnetic resonance imaging of, 12*f*, 116,
    193–194, 194*f*, 445*f*
  radiographic imaging of, 445*f*
  of talus, 194
  traumatic, 193, 193*f*
Osteochondritis dissecans
  adult, 401
  arthroscopic view of, 11*f*
  articular cartilage damaged by, 9
  autologous chondrocyte implantation for,
    409, 409*f*, 413, 414*f*, 417–418, 418*f*, 420*f*,
    474, 1260
  causes of, 1255
  clinical presentation of, 401
  definition of, 193, 401, 1255
  diagnosis of, 1255–1256
  etiology of, 402–403
  failed cartilage repair in patient with, 463*f*
  femoral condylar, 419–420
    illustration of, 410*f*
    osteochondral allograft transplantation for,
      450–451
  fragments
    bone grafting augmentation of, 407
    Guhl's classification of, 404*t*
    surgical management of, 1259
  gender differences, 469
  grading of, 194
  hinged lesions, 405
  idiopathic, 193
  imaging of, 401–402, 402*f*, 1255–1256,
    1257*f*
  incidence of, 1255
  juvenile
    algorithm for, 1258*f*
    arthroscopic drilling for, 472–473, 1259,
      1259*f*
    autologous chondrocyte implantation for,
      1260
    bone scan of, 1256
    cause of, 1255
    clinical presentation of, 1255
    definition of, 469
    description of, 401, 1255
    diagnosis of, 470–471, 470*f*, 1255–1256
    epidemiology of, 469
    gender differences, 469
    historical description of, 469
    immobilization for, 1257–1258
    internal fixation of, 473
    magnetic resonance imaging of, 471, 471*f*,
      1256, 1256*t*–1257*t*
    nonoperative management of, 1257–1258
    osteochondral autograft transfer system
      for, 1259–1260
    pathophysiology of, 469–470
    radiographic imaging of, 470*f*
    summary of, 474
    surgical treatment of, 471–474, 472*f*–473*f*,
      1258–1260, 1259*f*
    trauma as cause of, 469
    treatment of, 471–474, 472*f*–473*f*,
      1257–1260, 1259*f*
  magnetic resonance imaging of, 193–194,
    194*f*, 401, 402*f*, 471*f*, 1256, 1256*t*–1257*t*,
    1257*f*
  natural history of, 402–403
  nonoperative treatment of, 403

Osteochondritis dissecans (*Continued*)
  osteochondral allograft transplantation for,
    450–451
  patellar
    description of, 401
    retrograde fixation of, 405
  physical examination findings, 401, 1255
  prevalence of, 401, 469
  prognosis for, 402–403
  radiographic imaging of, 12*f*, 401, 402*f*, 470*f*,
    1257*f*
  summary of, 1260
  surgical treatment of, 403–404, 408–410
    algorithm for, 404*f*
    antegrade drilling, 405
    arthroscopic reduction, 405–407, 406*f*
    autologous chondrocyte implantation, 409,
      409*f*, 413, 414*f*
    in children, 471–474, 472*f*–473*f*
    drilling, 405, 472–473
    Guhl's classification, 404*t*
    loose body removal, 403–404
    microfracture, 408, 408*f*, 474*f*
    open reduction and internal fixation,
      405–407, 406*f*–407*f*, 473
    osteochondral allograft, 409–410
    osteochondral autograft transplantation,
      408–409
    patient positioning for, 403
    recommendations for, 407–408
    reparative procedures, 405–408, 406*f*–407*f*
    restorative procedures, 408–410
    retrograde drilling, 405
  unstable, 404*f*
Osteochondroma, 264, 265*f*, 2088–2089,
  2089*f*–2090*f*
Osteoclast, 4*f*
Osteocyte, 2
Osteofibrous dysplasia, 2087
Osteoid, 2, 3*f*
Osteoid osteoma, 269–270, 270*f*–271*f*,
  2085–2086, 2086*f*
Osteolysis, 251, 694*f*, 1000*f*, 1872*f*, 1874–1876,
  1937*f*, 1946
  femoral, 106*f*
  tibial, 106*f*
Osteomalacia, 374
Osteomyelitis, 1027
Osteonecrosis
  arthroscopic views of, 12*f*
  definition of, 475
  features of, 13*f*
  medial unicompartmental knee arthroplasty
    for, 1437
  osteochondral fragments in, 9, 13*f*
  patellar fragmentation and sclerosis caused
    by, 249
  in postoperative knee, 478–480
    arthroscopic débridement for, 482
    causes of, 479
    clinical evaluation of, 479
    course of, 479–480
    magnetic resonance imaging of, 479–480
    meniscal tears as cause of, 479
    prevalence of, 478
    radiographic evaluation of, 479
    sites of, 478
    spontaneous osteonecrosis and,
      comparisons between, 479–480, 480*t*
    staging of, 479
  risk factors for, 480*b*
  secondary
    bone scan of, 481*f*
    description of, 480, 480*b*
    risk factors for, 480*b*
    signs and symptoms of, 480
  spontaneous. *See* Spontaneous osteonecrosis
    of the knee